McGraw-Hill Higher Education.

You may know us for our world-class editorial content, instructional development, and design. But … did you know that our engaging, interactive digital platforms and educational services can help instructors meet the learning needs of today's students?

DIGITAL LEARNING PLATFORMS

connect plus+

- Web-based, interactive assignment and assessment platform. Available LMS integration, assignment sharing, and lecture capture help you scale across course formats.
- Engaging student content—tagged and organized by learning outcome and chapter.

BODYANIMAT3D, a component of connect

- Integrated 3D animations help students visualize the most difficult concepts. Pre- and post-assessment questions for every animation.

LearnSmart

- Unique adaptive learning system helps students learn faster, study more efficiently, and retain more knowledge for greater success.

ACTIVSim™

- Realistic patient interactions in a web-based simulation environment based on real photos.
- Unique student debriefing after ever experience—including self-assessment and individualized feedback.

SERVICES FOR EDUCATORS AND INSTITUTIONS

create

- Self-service customization of high-quality textbooks and supplements. Print or e-book, color or black and white.
- Over 45,000 content elements to choose from, including McGraw-Hill textbooks. Add your own content to customize to your course and student needs.
- Account-based project management. Save, share, manage, and create projects with anyone, anytime.

Learning Solutions

- Consultative partnership approach to unique curriculum, print, and technology solutions designed for your specific needs … for a single class or an entire institution.
- Dedicated team of learning specialists focused on your goals and outcomes, including product managers, instructional designers, eLearning specialists, and subject matter experts.

Fifth Edition

MEDICAL ASSISTING

Administrative and Clinical Procedures with Anatomy and Physiology

Kathryn A. Booth, RN-BSN, RMA (AMT), RPT, CPhT, MS
Total Care Programming, Inc.
Palm Coast, Florida

Leesa G. Whicker, BA, CMA (AAMA)
Central Piedmont Community College
Charlotte, North Carolina

Terri D. Wyman, CPC, CMRS
Wing Memorial Hospital
Palmer, Massachusetts

McGraw Hill

Connect
Learn
Succeed™

MEDICAL ASSISTING: ADMINISTRATIVE AND CLINICAL PROCEDURES WITH ANATOMY AND PHYSIOLOGY, FIFTH EDITION

Published by McGraw-Hill, a business unit of The McGraw-Hill Companies, Inc., 1221 Avenue of the Americas, New York, NY, 10020. Copyright © 2014 by The McGraw-Hill Companies, Inc. All rights reserved. Printed in the United States of America. Previous editions © 2011, 2009, and 2005. No part of this publication may be reproduced or distributed in any form or by any means, or stored in a database or retrieval system, without the prior written consent of The McGraw-Hill Companies, Inc., including, but not limited to, in any network or other electronic storage or transmission, or broadcast for distance learning.

Some ancillaries, including electronic and print components, may not be available to customers outside the United States.

This book is printed on acid-free paper.

6 7 8 9 0 DOW/DOW 1 0 9 8 7 6 5

ISBN 978-0-07-340232-1
MHID 0-07-340232-X

Senior Vice President, Products & Markets: *Kurt L. Strand*
Vice President, General Manager, Products & Markets: *Martin J. Lange*
Vice President, Content Production & Technology Services: *Kimberly Meriwether David*
Executive Brand Manager: *Natalie J. Ruffatto*
Director of Development: *Rose Koos*
Managing Development Editor: *Christine Scheid*
Digital Product Analyst: *Katherine Ward*
Associate Marketing Manager: *Jessica Cannavo*
Lead Project Manager: *Susan Trentacosti*
Buyer II: *Debra R. Sylvester*
Senior Designer: *Srdjan Savanovic*

Cover Designer: *Srdjan Savanovic*
Interior Designer: *Maureen McCutcheon*
Cover Image: *bottom 2 hands: © Violin/ww.fotosearch.com; Juggling balls: © Thomas J Peterson, gettyimages.*
Senior Content Licensing Specialist: *Keri Johnson*
Photo Researcher: *Michelle Buhr*
Media Project Manager: *Brent dela Cruz*
Media Project Manager: *Cathy L. Tepper*
Typeface: *10/12 Minion Pro Regular*
Compositor: *MPS Limited*
Printer: *R. R. Donnelley*

All credits appearing on page or at the end of the book are considered to be an extension of the copyright page.

Library of Congress Cataloging-in-Publication Data

Booth, Kathryn A., 1957-
  Medical assisting : administrative and clinical procedures including anatomy and physiology.—
5th ed. / Kathryn A. Booth, Leesa G. Whicker, Terri D. Wyman.
    p.; cm.
  Rev. ed. of: Medical assisting / Kathryn A. Booth . . . [et al.]. 4th ed. c2011.
  Includes index.
  ISBN 978-0-07-340232-1 (alk. paper)—ISBN 0-07-340232-X (alk. paper)
  I. Whicker, Leesa. II. Wyman, Terri D. III. Medical assisting. IV. Title.
  [DNLM: 1. Physician Assistants. 2. Clinical Medicine—methods. 3. Practice Management, Medical. W 21.5]
  610.73'72069—dc23
                                  2012045235

WARNING NOTICE: The clinical procedures, medicines, dosages, and other matters described in this publication are based upon research of current literature and consultation with knowledgeable persons in the field. The procedures and matters described in this text reflect currently accepted clinical practice. However, this information cannot and should not be relied upon as necessarily applicable to a given individual's case. Accordingly, each person must be separately diagnosed to discern the patient's unique circumstances. Likewise, the manufacturer's package insert for current drug product information should be consulted before administering any drug. Publisher disclaims all liability for any inaccuracies, omissions, misuse, or misunderstanding of the information contained in this publication. Publisher cautions that this publication is not intended as a substitute for the professional judgment of trained medical personnel.

The Internet addresses listed in the text were accurate at the time of publication. The inclusion of a website does not indicate an endorsement by the authors or McGraw-Hill, and McGraw-Hill does not guarantee the accuracy of the information presented at these sites.

www.mhhe.com

Brief Contents

UNIT ONE

Medical Assisting as a Career

CHAPTER 1

Introduction to Medical Assisting *1*

CHAPTER 2

Healthcare and the Healthcare Team *12*

CHAPTER 3

Professionalism and Success *28*

CHAPTER 4

Interpersonal Communication *42*

CHAPTER 5

Legal and Ethical Issues *61*

UNIT FOUR

Administrative Practices

CHAPTER 23

The Integumentary System 495

CHAPTER 24

The Skeletal System 509

CHAPTER 25

The Muscular System 525

CHAPTER 26

The Cardiovascular System 540

CHAPTER 27

The Blood 558

CHAPTER 28

The Lymphatic and
Immune Systems 569

UNIT SIX

Clinical Practices

CHAPTER 36

Patient Interview and History 685

CHAPTER 37

Vital Signs and Measurements 706

CHAPTER 38

Assisting with a General Physical Examination 724

CHAPTER 39

Assisting in Reproductive and Urinary Specialties 743

CHAPTER 40

Assisting in Pediatrics *765*

CHAPTER 41

Assisting in Geriatrics *793*

CHAPTER 42

Assisting in Other Medical Specialties *807*

CHAPTER 43

Assisting with Eye and Ear Care *828*

CHAPTER 44

Assisting with Minor Surgery *852*

UNIT SEVEN

Assisting with Diagnostics

CHAPTER 45

Orientation to the Lab 882

CHAPTER 46

Microbiology and Disease 902

CHAPTER 47

Processing and Testing Urine and Stool Specimens 936

CHAPTER 48

Collecting, Processing, and Testing Blood Specimens 962

CHAPTER 49

Electrocardiography and Pulmonary Function Testing 994

CHAPTER 50

Diagnostic Imaging 1021

UNIT EIGHT

Assisting in Therapeutics

CHAPTER 51

Principles of Pharmacology 1041

Procedures

Today's medical assistants juggle many tasks in the medical office. McGraw-Hill is committed to helping prepare students to succeed in the classroom and to be successful in their chosen field. Most textbooks begin with a preface and a long list of features and supplements for both instructors and their students. While keeping with this tried and true format, it is our intention to give you a snapshot of some of the exciting solutions available with the fifth edition of *Medical Assisting: Administrative and Clinical Procedures with Anatomy and Physiology* for your Medical Assisting course. Instructors across the country have told us how much preparation it takes to teach medical assisting—they juggle as much, maybe more, than their students. To help, we have added more detailed information on how to organize and utilize the features in the Information Center of the Online Learning Center (OLC), as well as a breakdown of Learning Outcomes and activities that correspond in the Instructor Resources portion of the OLC at **www.mhhe.com/BoothMA5e**.

The Content—A Note from the Authors

The fifth edition of *Medical Assisting: Administrative and Clinical Procedures with Anatomy and Physiology* has many exciting and noteworthy updates. Along with helpful and important feedback from our users and reviewers, we set out to create a one-of-a-kind, dynamic, practical, realistic, *and* comprehensive set of tools for individuals preparing to become medical assistants.

To begin, the textbook provides students up-to-date information about all aspects of the medical assisting profession, both administrative and clinical and from general to specific. It covers the key concepts, skills, and tasks that medical assistants need to know to become a CMA or RMA. As you enter the book, you will see that it is an interactive experience in learning, rather than merely a reading experience. The book speaks directly to the student, and its chapter introductions, case studies, procedures, chapter summaries, and chapter reviews are written to engage the student's attention and build a sense of excitement about joining the profession of medical assisting.

When you begin the book you will find it is not just about reading the concepts. It is about engaging in a journey by learning as though working at the BWW Associates Clinic. Case studies are based around a set of patients that visit BWW Associates Clinic, and you will get to know these patients as you move through the chapters. The BWW Associates employees include Malik Katahir, CMM, Office Manager; Kaylyn R. Haddix, RMA (AMT) Clinical Assistant; and Miguel A. Perez CMA (AAMA), plus some MA students in training. The practicing

physicians include Paul F. Buckwalter, Alexis N. Whalen, and Elizabeth H. Williams. Most of the patients of BWW Associates you will also work with when using the Medical Assisting ACTIVSim™ 2.0 program.

It is all about consistent, authentic, and correct content and in this fifth edition we have strived to provide all the latest information as of the publishing of the book. Along with tons of minor tweaks and updates, *Medical Assisting*, fifth edition, incorporates the following:

- Expanded coding information, including CPT, HCPCS, ICD-9 and ICD-10 coding.
- Step-by-step instructions for completing CMS 1500, or 1505, claim forms with screen shots.
- A written safety plan to create for the medical office.
- A preparedness plan to implement for pandemic illness.
- New medical terminology practice exercises in all of the anatomy and physiology chapters.
- An exercise to calculate BMI and graph height, weight, and head circumference of infants and children.
- Simplified and enhanced content regarding major pathogens from each group of microorganisms: viruses, bacteria, protozoa, fungi, and multicellular parasites in updated tables.
- American Heart Association's "Chain of Survival" and Guidelines for CPR key components.
- Additional certification exam questions in each chapter, as well as certification exam study tips.
- Dedicated and expanded content in brand new chapters including:
  - Professionalism and Success
  - Electronic Health Records
  - The Blood
  - Assisting in Reproductive and Urinary Specialties
  - Assisting in Pediatrics

- Assisting in Geriatrics
- Assisting with Eye and Ear Care
- Dosage Calculations
- Thirty nine (39) *NEW* procedures

Learning Outcomes and Textbook Organization

If you have seen a previous edition of this book before, one of the first things you will notice is the updated organization of the content. For each of the chapters, we updated the learning outcomes to the latest Bloom's standards and aligned every learning outcome to a level one heading. McGraw-Hill has made it even easier for students and instructors to find, learn, and review critical information.

The chapter organization of the fifth edition was revised to provide a structure that promotes learning based on what a medical assistant does in practice. The chapters build on one another to ensure student understanding of the many tasks they will be expected to perform. The chapters can be easily grouped together to create larger topics or units for the students to learn. For ease of understanding, content can be organized as follows:

- Unit One Medical Assisting as a Career—Chapters 1 to 5
- Unit Two Safety and the Environment—Chapters 6 to 9
- Unit Three Communication—Chapters 10 to 14
- Unit Four Administrative Practices—Chapters 15 to 21
- Unit Five Applied Anatomy and Physiology—Chapters 22 to 35
- Unit Six Clinical Practices—Chapters 36 to 44
- Unit Seven Assisting with Diagnostics—Chapters 45 to 50
- Unit Eight Assisting in Therapeutics—Chapters 51 to 55
- Unit Nine Medical Assisting Practice—Chapters 56 to 58

Content Correlations

Medical Assisting, fifth edition, also provides a correlation structure that will enhance its usefulness to both students and instructors. We have been careful to ensure that the text and supplements provide ample coverage of topics used to construct all of the following:

- CAAHEP (Commission on Accreditation of Allied Health Education Programs) Standards and Guidelines for Medical Assisting Education Programs
- ABHES (Accrediting Bureau of Health Education Schools) Competencies and Curriculum
- AAMA (American Association of Medical Assistants) CMA (Certified Medical Assistant) Occupational Analysis
- AMT (American Medical Technologists) RMA (Registered Medical Assistant) Task List
- AMT CMAS (Certified Medical Assistant Specialist) Competencies and Examination Specifications
- NHA (National Healthcareer Association) Certified Clinical Medical Assistant (CCMA)
- NHA (National Healthcareer Association) Certified Medical Administrative Assistant (CMAAA)
- CMA (AAMA) Certification Examination Content Outline

Correlations to these are included with the instructor materials located on the Online Learning Center at **www.mhhe** .com/BoothMA5e and through Connect® (see later pages for information about Connect®). In addition, CAAHEP requires that all medical assistants be proficient in the 71 entry-level areas of competence when they begin medical assisting work. ABHES requires proficiency in the competences and curriculum content at a minimum. The opening pages of each chapter provide a list of the areas of competence that are covered within the chapter.

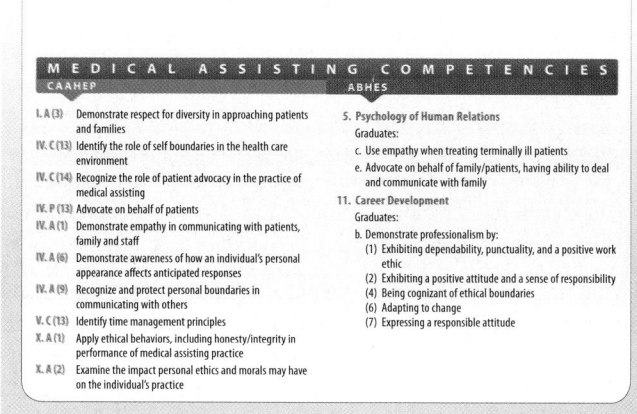

You will also find that each procedure is correlated to the ABHES and CAAHEP competencies within the workbook on the procedure sheets. These sheets can be easily pulled out of the workbook and placed in the student file to document proficiency.

Content Highlights

We have made a consistent effort to discuss patients with special needs:

- **Pregnant women.** Pregnancy has profound effects on every aspect of health, all of which must be taken into account when working with pregnant patients. In the new chapter *Assisting with Reproductive and Urinary Specialties,* we have addressed special concerns for pregnant patients, such as positioning them for an examination, recommending changes in diet, and taking care to avoid harming the fetus with drugs or procedures that would ordinarily pose little or no risk to the patient. There is also a separate procedure for meeting the needs of the pregnant patient during an examination.

- **Elderly patients.** Special care is often required with elderly patients. The body undergoes many changes with age, and patients may have difficulty adjusting to their changing physical needs. The new chapter *Assisting in Geriatrics* deals with the special needs of elderly patients.

- **Children.** The special needs of children are complex, because not only their bodies but also their minds and social situations are very different from those of adults. Dealing with children usually means dealing with their parents as well, and medical assistants must hone their communication skills to meet the needs of both patient and parent when working with children. The new chapter *Assisting with Pediatrics* focuses on children and their special needs.

- **Patients with disabilities.** Many different diseases and disabilities require extra effort or consideration on the part of the medical assistant. Patients in wheelchairs and patients with diabetes, hemophilia, or visual or hearing impairments all require specific accommodations. For example, *The Examination and Treatment Area* chapter addresses the needs of such patients; it includes a section that discusses the Americans With Disabilities Act and the new chapter *Assisting with Eye and Ear Care* includes a procedure for making the examination room safe for patients with visual impairments.

- **Patients from other cultures.** Communicating with patients from other cultures, especially when language barriers are involved, poses a special challenge for the medical assistant. In addition, patients from other cultures may have attitudes about medicine or about social interaction that differ sharply from those of the medical assistants' culture. The *Professionalism and Success* and the *Interpersonal Communication* chapters deal in depth with understanding other cultures including new content for communicating and caring for patients from other cultures.

Because safety is a primary concern for both the patient and the medical assistant, we have emphasized this aspect of medical assisting work. Every clinical procedure includes appropriate icons, discussed in the *Basic Safety and Infection Control* chapter, for safety precautions required by the Occupational Safety and Health Administration (OSHA) guidelines. These icons for the OSHA guidelines appear in order of use within each procedure. The handwashing icon only appears once even though it is always done before and after each procedure. If biohazardous waste is generated during the procedure, the biohazardous waste container icon will appear, and so on.

Chapter Features

Each chapter opens with material that includes the Case Study, the learning outcomes, a list of key terms, the ABHES and CAAHEP medical assisting competencies covered in the chapter, and an introduction. Since the learning outcomes represent each of the level-one headings in the chapter, they serve as the chapter outline. Chapters are organized into topics that move from the general to the specific. Updated color photographs, anatomic and technical drawings, tables, charts, and text features help educate the student about various aspects of medical assisting. The text features include the following:

- **Case Studies** are provided at the beginning of all chapters. They represent situations similar to those that the medical assistant may encounter in daily practice. The case studies include pictures of each of the patients who come to BWW Associates for care. Students will work with these same patients in the ACTIVSim 2.0 program. Students are encouraged to consider the case study as they read each chapter. Case Study Questions in the end-of-chapter review check students' understanding and application of chapter content.

- **Procedures** give step-by-step instructions on how to perform specific administrative or clinical tasks that a medical assistant will be required to perform. The procedures are referenced within the content when discussed. Each of the procedures are found at the end of the chapter. New figures are included with many of the procedures that are taken from the Connect® videos. Again the student can transition between the materials seamlessly.

- **Points on Practice** boxes provide guidelines on keeping the medical office running smoothly and efficiently.
- **Educating the Patient** boxes focus on ways to instruct patients about caring for themselves outside the medical office.
- **Caution: Handle with Care** boxes cover the precautions to be taken in certain situations or when performing certain tasks.
- **Pathophysiology** is featured in each of the chapters on anatomy and physiology. These provide students with details of the most common diseases and disorders of each body system and include information on the causes, common signs and symptoms, treatment, and, where possible, the prevention of each disease.
- **Medical Terminology** practice exercises have been added to all the anatomy and physiology chapters.

Each chapter closes with a summary of the learning outcomes. The summary is followed by an end-of-chapter review with questions related to the case study, as well as 10 multiple-choice exam-style questions.

A list of further readings, including related books and journal articles, is provided for each chapter within the Instructor's Manual and on McGraw-Hill's *Medical Assisting* Online Learning Center. The end-of-chapter questions and activities, as well as the additional online resources, provide supplementary information about the subjects presented in the chapter and allow students to practice specific skills.

The book also includes a glossary and four appendixes for use as reference tools. The glossary lists all the words presented as key terms in each chapter, along with a pronunciation guide and the definition of each term. The appendixes present a list of common medical terminology including prefixes, root words, and suffixes, as well as medical abbreviations and symbols. A brand-new Diseases and Disorders appendix provides a quick reference point for patient conditions that the student may encounter, and the final appendix covers the Electronic Health Record.

Medical Assisting in the Digital World—Supplementary Materials for the Instructor and Student

Knowing the importance of flexibility and digital learning, McGraw Hill has created multiple assets to enhance the learning experience no matter what the class format: traditional, online, or hybrid. This revision is designed to help instructors and students be successful with digital solutions proven to drive student success.

A one-stop spot for presentation, assignment, and assessment solutions available from McGraw-Hill:

McGraw-Hill Connect® Medical Assisting

McGraw-Hill Connect®–Medical Assisting provides online presentation, assignment, and assessment solutions. It connects your students with the tools and resources they'll need to achieve success. With Connect Medical Assisting you can deliver assignments, quizzes, and tests online. A robust set of questions and activities are presented and aligned with the textbook's learning outcomes. As an instructor, you can edit existing questions and author entirely new problems. Track individual student performance—by question, assignment, or in relation to the class overall—with detailed grade reports. Integrate grade reports easily with Learning Management Systems (LMS), such as Blackboard, DesiretoLearn, or eCollege—and much more. **ConnectPlus–Medical Assisting** provides students with all the advantages **of Connect®–Medical Assisting** *plus* 24/7 online access to an eBook. This media-rich version of the book is available through the McGraw-Hill Connect® platform and allows seamless integration of text, media, and assessments. To learn more, visit **www.mcgrawhillconnect.com**.

A single sign-on with Connect® and your Blackboard course:

McGraw-Hill Higher Education and Blackboard

Blackboard®, the web-based course management system, has partnered with McGraw-Hill to better allow students and faculty to use online materials and activities to complement face-to-face teaching. Blackboard features exciting social learning and teaching tools that foster more logical, visually impactful, and active learning opportunities for students. You'll transform your closed-door classroom into communities where students remain connected to their educational experience 24 hours a day.

This partnership allows you and your students access to McGraw-Hill's Connect® and McGraw-Hill Create™ right from within your Blackboard course—all with one single sign-on. Not only do you get single sign-on with Connect and Create, you also get deep integration of McGraw-Hill content and content engines right in Blackboard. Whether you're choosing a book for your course or building Connect assignments, all the tools you need are right where you want them—inside of Blackboard. Gradebooks are now seamless. When a student completes an integrated Connect assignment, the grade for that assignment automatically (and instantly) feeds to your Blackboard grade center.

McGraw-Hill and Blackboard can now offer you easy access to industry leading technology and content, whether your campus hosts it or we do. Be sure to ask your local McGraw-Hill representative for details.

An adaptive learning system to help your students study smarter and learn faster:

McGraw-Hill LearnSmart™

McGraw-Hill LearnSmart™ is available as an integrated feature of McGraw-Hill Connect®—Medical Assisting. It is an adaptive learning system designed to help students learn faster, study more efficiently, and retain more knowledge for greater success. LearnSmart assesses a student's knowledge of course content through a series of adaptive questions. It pinpoints concepts the student does not understand and maps out a personalized study plan for success. This innovative study tool also has features that allow instructors to see exactly what students have accomplished and a built-in assessment tool for graded assignments. **LearnSmart™–Medical Assisting** aids the student in focusing on the information required to successfully pass certification exams and assesses each student's responses to establish a clearly defined learning path that instructors can measure. Visit the following site for a demonstration. **www.mhlearnsmart.com**.

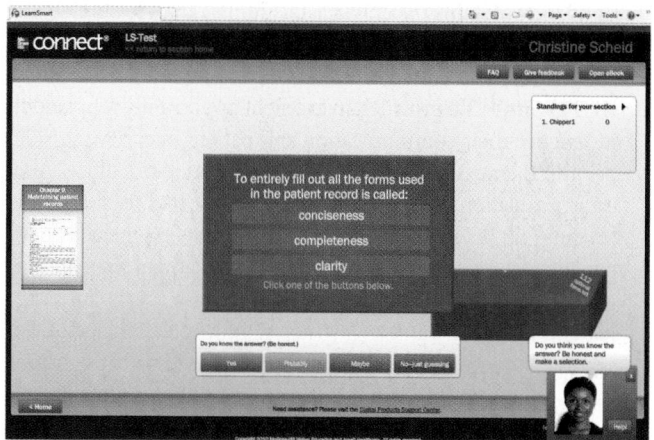

Hands-on emersion activities to help your students apply what they have read in the textbook:

- Ten Electronic Health Record (EHR) live activities are found in the Student Resources on the OLC (**www.mhhe.com/BoothMA5e**):

  - *Building a Patient Face Sheet*
  - *Administering a Patient Instruction*
  - *Recording and Viewing Vitals*
  - *Building an Office Visit Note*
  - *Ordering a Test and Documenting Procedures in an Office Visit*

Students can easily download **Spring Medical Systems, Inc.'s SpringCharts® from the Student Resources on the OLC** and complete these critical EHR tasks to obtain hands-on experience with an ONC-certified electronic health records solution. If you want to include more live EHR exercises, consider *Electronic Health Records*, third edition, by Brian Byron Hamilton (ISBN: 0-07-340214-1).

- In addition to the live activities found on the OLC, **an additional forty-four (44) Electronic Health**

Record (EHR) activities based on SpringCharts® are found in Connect® and provide students with activities that simulate real patient encounters.

- **ACTIVSim™ 2.0 Medical Assisting** Clinical Simulator is made up of two parts: 10 Patient Case Clinical Simulators and 15 Clinical Skills Simulators. The Patient Case Clinical Simulators introduce students to nonacute medical assisting patient case scenarios, procedure simulators and quick e-learning exercises. A large portion of core clinical competencies can be simulated on virtual patients, where the learner can interact with a patient and practice the different tasks that a medical assistant performs in physicians' offices. The focus of **ACTIVSim™ 2.0** is on vital signs and obtaining patient data, including a chart feature, so that the learner can document vital signs and make notes about observations that the medical assistant can brief the doctor about. **ACTIVSim™ 2.0** provides an excellent opportunity for students to practice their communication and patient interviewing skills prior to their externships and working in a doctor's office. After each simulation, the learner receives elaborate feedback (debriefing) on his/her performance. The debriefing includes basic patient assessment issues and recommendations for handling patients who have a particular condition. Instructors can assign patients to students and an instructor gradebook is included. For seamless training, these patients are also used in the textbook case studies. **ACTIVSim™ 2.0** gives extensive, individualized feedback, providing students with a realistic clinical experience. For a demo of **ACTIVSim™ 2.0**, please go to **www.mhhe.com/activsim**, click on Course in the top menu, then on Health Professions in the list provided, where you'll find Medical Assisting.

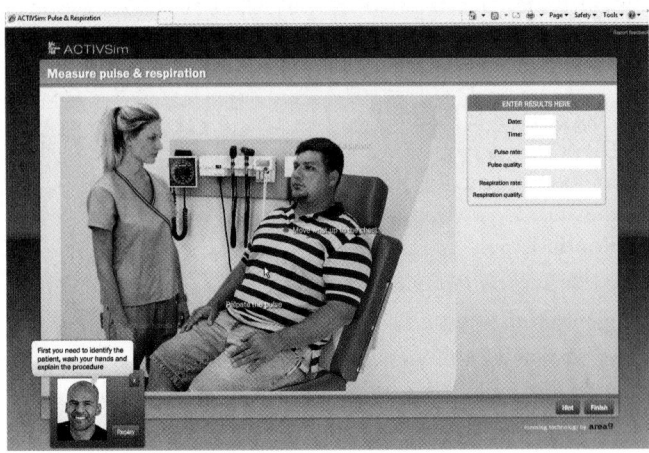

Create™ a textbook organized the way you teach:

McGraw-Hill Create™

With **McGraw-Hill Create™**, you can easily rearrange chapters, combine material from other content sources, and quickly upload content you have written, like your course syllabus or teaching notes. Find the content you need in Create by searching through thousands of leading McGraw-Hill textbooks. Arrange your book to fit your teaching style. Create even allows you to personalize your book's appearance by selecting the cover and adding your name, school, and course information. Order a Create book and you'll receive a complimentary print review copy in 3–5 business days or a complimentary electronic review copy (eComp) via e-mail in minutes. Go to www.mcgrawhill-create.com today and register to experience how McGraw-Hill Create empowers you to teach *your* students *your* way.

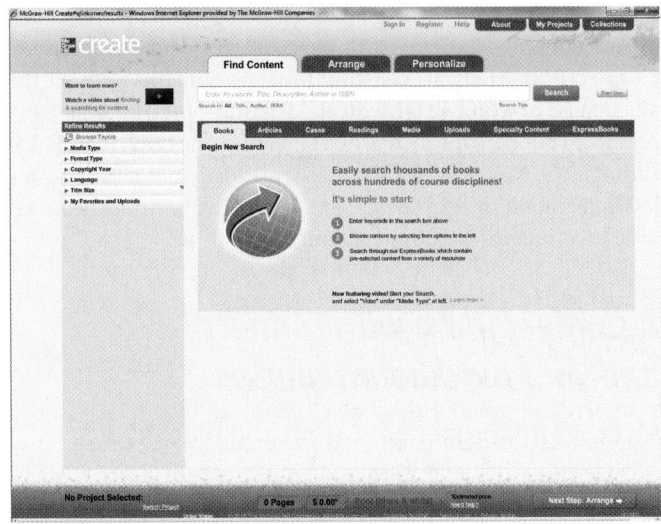

Record and distribute your lectures for multiple viewing:

My Lectures—Tegrity®

McGraw-Hill Tegrity® records and distributes your class lecture with just a click of a button. Students can view anytime/anywhere via computer, iPod, or mobile device. It indexes as it records your PowerPoint® presentations and anything shown on your computer so students can use keywords to find exactly what they want to study. **Tegrity®** is available as an integrated feature of **McGraw-Hill Connect®–Medical Assisting** and as a standalone.

Additional features and activities designed with your students in mind:

- **Fifty (50) BodyAnimat3d Animations,** found in Connect®, including the Cardiac Cycle and Coronary Artery Disease (CAD); Type 1 and Type 2 Diabetes; COPD; Obesity; as well as Medication Distribution, Absorption, and Metabolism; Burns; and Wound Healing.

- **Seventy-five (75) Administrative and Clinical Procedure Videos,** found in Connect®, including Registering a New Patient, Electronically Order and Track Medical Test Results, Manage a Prescription Refill, Interpret a Prescription,

Scheduling Appointments, Completing the CMS 1500 Form, and Locating an ICD-10-CM Code.

All of these assets are available to use with the book and are neatly correlated to enhance the learning experience. The student will notice icons like the above within the chapter as well as the end of each chapter that refer them to interactive learning activities that not only remediate, but that are very visual in nature.

The tried and true: additional supplementary materials for you and your students:

Student Workbook for use with Medical Assisting, 5e—in print and full color (ISBN: 0-07-75258-8)

The Student Workbook provides an opportunity for the student to review and practice the material and skills presented in the textbook. Divided into parts and presented by chapter, the first part provides:

- Vocabulary review exercises, which test knowledge of key terms in the chapter
- Content review exercises, which test the student's knowledge of key concepts in the chapter
- Critical thinking exercises, which test the student's understanding of key concepts in the chapter
- Application exercises, which include figures and practice forms, and test mastery of specific skills
- Case studies, which apply the chapter material to real-life situations or problems

Each section, Clinical and/or Administrative, contains the appropriate procedure checklists, presented in the order in which they are shown in the student textbook. These checklists have been revised for ease of use, and include correlations to the ABHES and CAAHEP competencies mastered with the successful completion of each procedure. Accompanying Work Product Documentation (work/doc) provides blank charting forms for many of the procedure that include a work product or requires documentation to complete. These documentation forms are used when completing many of the application activities as well as procedure competencies. Over 100 procedures as well as multiple application activities in the workbook include correlated work docs.

Pocket Guide for use with Medical Assisting, 5e (ISBN: 0-07-752585-X)

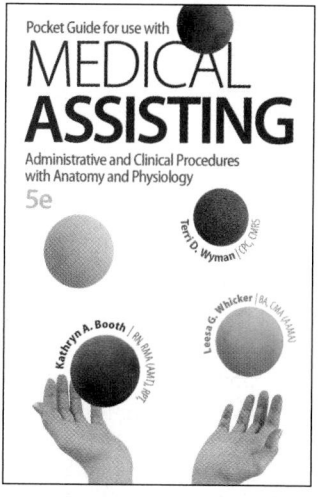

The Pocket Guide is a quick and handy reference to use while working as a medical assistant or during training. It includes critical procedure steps, bulleted lists, and brief information all medical assistants should know. Information is sorted by Administrative, Clinical, Laboratory, and General content.

Online Learning Center (OLC) found at www.mhhe.com/BoothMA5e

Medical Assisting also comes with the instructor resources you've come to expect, and all can be found on the OLC:

- **Instructor's Manual:** An exhaustive resource, containing everything to organize your course, as well as additional tips and exercises; including but not limited to a list of learning outcomes and chapter outline, teaching strategies, and answers for the end-of-chapter material as well as for the Student Workbook. Also included are correlation guides to the many of the accreditation bureaus, including The Accrediting Bureau of Health Education Schools (ABHES) Medical Assisting competencies and curriculum; The Commission on Accreditation of Allied Health Education Programs (CAAHEP) Standards and Guidelines for Medical Assisting Education Programs competencies; American Association of Medical Assistants (AAMA) Occupational Analysis; The Association of Medical Technologists (AMT) Registered Medical Assistant (RMA) Certified Exam Topics; The National Healthcareer Association (NHA) Medical Assisting Duty/ Task List; The Secretary's Commission on Achieving Necessary Skills (SCANS) areas of competence, as well as others.
- **PowerPoint Presentations** have been fully updated to include the latest figures and content. The popular "Test Your Knowledge" slides have been maintained to encourage interaction.
- **A completely revised and enhanced Testbank** with over 5,000 questions, complete with tags for Learning Outcomes; ABHES, CAAHEP, and even some CAHIIM standards (where applicable); and Bloom's and others to organize or modify questions to meet your course needs.

The task of putting together a textbook and all of its supplements both written and digital takes a vast amount of cumulated effort and coordination among multiple individuals and companies. To acknowledge each of them here may take way too long. However, we would like start by acknowledging McGraw-Hill and all of the individuals that are listed on page ii in the front of this book for their continued assistance, encouragement, and support. A special thanks for those who are so close to this edition including Natalie, Chipper, Katie, Edward, Jessica, Sue T., and Srdj. Without McGraw-Hill and its valued employees there would be no need for this acknowledgment to be written.

We would also like to distinguish some individuals that worked tirelessly and directly with us ensuring a completely improved product: Jodie Bernard, for helping us completely update the figures for this edition, changing the face of the book and making it more modern and visually appealing; Lisa Bess Kramer, for helping us make the product one voice, especially her extra effort to keep us all on track as she read each and every chapter; Susan Findley, for taking on the revision of the Power-Point files—this job always takes an extensive amount of time and we appreciate that Susan is willing to take on the task; and Marilee LeBon, for helping us with all of the instructor materials in the Instructor's Manual. Last, but certainly not least, we acknowledge Jody James for picking up the pieces on numerous aspects of the project. Her attention to detail and willingness to help with whatever we needed for this edition has provided us the ability to focus on updating and reorganizing the essential content to make the 5e the best edition ever. We humbly thank each and everyone involved with this *Medical Assisting*, fifth edition.

Contributors and Reviewers

We, along with McGraw-Hill, would like to thank the reviewers and contributors for their assistance in developing content, offering suggestions, and shaping this revision. We appreciate you. Many of the additions, improvements, and changes are due directly to and because of their feedback. We appreciate their insight and commitment to helping us provide information that is relevant and valuable to medical assisting students.

Content Developers and Reviewers for the Fifth Edition:

Connect® Contributors

Elise Clemens
Carrington College
Stephen Clough, Certified Electronic Health Record Specialist
Seacoast Career School–Sanford
Daniele Mbadu, M.A., M.Ed
Vince Ochotoreno, MBA, MAM, BSOE, AAS
Ashford University
Lisa Schaffer, JD, MBA
Newbridge College
Leigh Sullivan, ME BA, NHA
Seacoast Career Schools–Sanford

LearnSmart™ Contributors and Accuracy Checkers

Elisabeth Hoffman, MA Ed, CMA, CPT, ASPT
Baker College
Belinda Beeman, CMA (AAMA), PBT (ASCP), MA Ed
Eastern New Mexico University
Danielle Wilken, MS, MT (ASCP)
Goodwin College

ACTIVSim

Danielle Wilken, MS, MT (ASCP)
Goodwin College

Focus Group Attendees

Kimberly Lehman, BA, CMA (AAMA)
Medtech College
Robin Jones, AA, AAS, BA, CMA, MA, RMA, RT
Pinnacle Career Institute
Kim Hockaday, AS, CMA
Carrington College
Sharon Harris-Pelliccia, AAS, BS, RPA
Mildred Elley
Lorri Christiansen, RN
Centura College Corporate
Danny Pate, AA, BS, RMA
Pima Medical Institute
Terri L. Randolph, BSHA, MBA, HCM
Anthem Education Group
Shauna Phillips
Fortis College
Angela McCray, CMA (AAMA), RMA, NCMA
Brookline College
Michele Crissman, CMA (AAMA), RN, JD
Colorado Technical University
Patti Deitos, BSN, RN, MSN, RN-BC, PWD
Inova Health System Military
Elisabeth Hoffman, CMA (AAMA), CPT
Baker College
Adrian Rios, BA, CPT, MA, RMA, EMT, NCMA
Newbridge College

Page Proof Accuracy Checkers

Ramona Atiles
Career Institute of Health & Technology
Cynthia Bergenstock
Berks Technical Institute
Judy Cornett
Southern Technical College
Lorraine Creadon
Berks Technical Institute
Brian Dickens
Southeastern Institute/Southeastern College
Henry Gomez
ASA College
Mary Koloski
Southern Technical College
Laura Melendez
Southeastern Institute/Southeastern College
Lee Nagy
Southern Technical College
Marion Odom
Illinois School of Health Careers
Jamie Olson
Dorsey Schools–Saginaw
Mia Small
Bryant & Stratton
Gayla Taylor
PCI Health Training Center
Jenny Tiernan
Dorsey Schools–Waterford/Pontiac

Tammy Walsh (McClish)
University of Akron
Petra York
Western Tech College

Testbank Accuracy Checkers
Amy Ensign
Baker College
Carey Mortensen
Southern Careers Institute

Reviewers of the Fifth Edition
Macario Abad, MD
Keiser University–Tallahasee
Diane Alagna, AAS, RMA, RN, AHI, CPT
Branford Hall
Judie Alessi, AHT, CMA (AAMA), GXMO, RMA
Stautzenberger College
Cynthia Allee, MA
Aims Community College
Patrice Allen, CMA (AAMA) AAS
Vance-Granville Community College
Yvonne Alles, MBA, DHA
Davenport University
Jodi Anderson, AA, LVN
Valley Career College
Amy Bacon, CPT-1, CMA, BA
San Joaquin Valley College–Rancho Cucamonga
Junior Basant, RMA, BS, MD
National College–Nashville
Kaye Bathe, CMA (AAMA), BSHA
Tri County Technical College
Jason Belanger, BA, CBCS, CMAA
Loring Job Corps Center
Cynthia Bergenstock, AS
Berks Technical Institute
Norma Bird, BS, CMA (AAMA), M.Ed. State of Idaho
Idaho State University
Cynthia Boles, CMA (AAMA) MT (ASCP)
Bradford School–Pittsburgh
Cheryl Bordwine, BMO, CPI, MS
College Of Mainland
Gerry Brasin, AS, CMA (AAMA), CPC
Premier Education Group
Dan Brewster
Prospect Education–Reno
Carmelita Bronson-Smith, BS, MS, RN, PA
Los Angeles City College
Martina T. Forte Brown, CCMA, CPT, CET
Brookstone College of Business
Mary Ellen Brown, CMA (AAMA), PBT (ASCP)
Lincoln Technical Institute
Candy Bryant, AAS, MA
Carl Sandburg College
Nia Bullock, BS, PhD, RMA
Miller-Motte Technical College
Shirley Buzbee, CMA (AAMA)
Modesto Junior College

Susan Capistrant, BA, BSN, RN
Career College Of Northern Nevada
Cheri Carlson, CMA, RMA, NRMA
Great Lakes Institute of Technology
Lorri Christiansen, AA, RN
Centura College–Virginia Beach
Yicel Cid
Florida Education Institute
Paula Beth Ciolek, CMA (AAMA)
National College–Richmond
Estelle Coffino, BS, CCMA, CPFT, MPA, RRT
College Of Westchester
Sue Coleman
National College–Virginia
Beth Collis
Globe Education Network
Joyce Combs, CMA (AAMA), MS
Bluegrass Community and Technical College
Anne Conway, CCMA-A, ABLE Library-certified
National Career Education
Lorraine Creadon, BSN, MS
Berks Technical Institute
Debbie Cresap, MS, RMA
West Virginia Northern Community College
Michelle Crissman, CMA (AAMA), RN, JD
Colorado Tech University
Joan Crosby, AAS, BS
Remington College–Cleveland
Novella Crowther, AS, CMA, CMAA
Carrington College–New Mexico
Dana Curry, CMA (AAMA)
Carrington College California
Patricia Deitos, BSN, RN, MSN, RN-BC, PWD
Inova Health System Military
Leon Deutsch, BMO, BS, MA, RMA
Keiser University
Pat Devoy, MA, LPN, CMA (AAMA)
Davenport University
Brenda Diaz, MA
Remington College–Nashville
Brian Dickens, MBA, RMA, CHI
Keiser Career College/Southeastern Institute
Jason DiPierro, RMA
Keiser University
Debra Downs, AAS, MBA, LPN
Okefenokee Technical College
Pat Dudek, RMA, RN
McCann School of Business and Tech
Brooke Dunn, CMA
Yti Career Institute–Lancaster
Christine Dzoga, CMA, RMA, RPT, CPCT, CECGT, CPT, AHI
Illinois School of Health Careers
Amy Ensign, CMA (AAMA), RMA (AMT)
Baker College–Clinton Township
Joshua Farquharson, AA, AHI, MA, RMA
San Joaquin Valley College
Pamela Fleming, CMA (AAMA), CPC, MPA, RN
Quinsigamond Community College

Diane Gryglak, BS, CMA (AAMA)
College Of DuPage
Hanaa Guirguis, Bachelor of Medicine and Surgery/Diploma in Maternal Child Health
National Career Education
Sharon Harris-Pelliccia, AAS, BS, RPA
Mildred Elley
Melissa Hilker, BS Psychology, CMA
Blackhawk Technical College
Kimberly Hockaday, AS, CMA
Carrington College–Reno
Elizabeth Hoffman, CMA (AAMA), CPT
Baker College
Melissa Hulsey, CMA (AAMA), MA, RMA
San Joaquin Valley College
Robin Jones, AA, AAS, BA, CMA, MA, RMA, RT
Pinnacle Career Institute–Kansas City
Penny Lee, AAS, CMA, CAHI
Medtech College–Greenwood Campus
Kimberly Leyman, BA, CMA (AAMA)
Medtech College–Fort Wayne
Kathleen Locke
Northwestern College
Angela McCray, CMA (AAMA), RMA, NCMA
Brookline College
Laura Melendez, BS, RMA, RT BMO
Keiser Career College
RobynMoore-Ball, RMA, AHI
Everest College–Bedford Park
Karen Morrow, CPI, CHI
Harris School of Business
Carey Mortensen
Southern Careers Institute–Austin
Marion Odom, RMA, CPCT, CPT, CEKG
Illinois School of Health Careers
Carla Ofhaus, D.C., CST, MBA Healthcare Admin
ATS Institute of Technology
Shelea Oglesby, RMA, RPT, CPhT
San Joaquin Valley College–Fresno
Danny Pate, AA, BS, RMA
Pima Medical Institute
Shauna Phillips
Fortis College
Terri Randolph, BSHA, MBA, HCM
Anthem Education Group, College
David Rice, RMA, BA, AA
Milan Institute
Adrian Rios, BA, CPT, MA, RMA, EMT, NCMA
Newbridge College
Yvette Savala, AA, CMA, CPT
San Joaquin Valley College
Cathy Soto
El Paso Community College–Northwest
Lori Stark, AA, BS, Paramedic, Licensed Radiographic Technologist
Remington College
Jacquelyn Taylor, NCRMA
Sanford Brown College–Dallas

Gayla Taylor, MSM
PCI Health Training Center
Caryn Thomason, RN
Career College of Northern Nevada
Cindy Thompson, RN, RMA
Davenport University–Saginaw
Geraldine Todaro, CMA (AAMA), PBT
(ASCP), MSTE
Stark State College of Tech
Deanne Wilk, RN, CCS, CMS
McCann School of Business and Tech
Kari Williams, AA, BS, DC
Front Range Community College
Mindy Wray, CMA, RMA
ECPI University
Lisa Wright, CMA (AAMA) MT, SH
Bristol Community College
Petra York, AAS, AHI, CCMA, CET, CMA
(AAMA), CMAA, CPT, CPht, NCRMA
Western Technical College

**Previous Edition Content Developers
and Reviewers**

Medical Advisory Board
Gerry A. Brasin, AS, CMA (AAMA), CPC
Premier Education Group
Dr. Marina Klebanov, BDS, MSPH
Mandl College of Allied Health
Tabitha L. Lyons, NCMA, AS
Anthem Education Group
Barry Newman, MD
Lincoln Educational Services
Diane Peavy
Fortis Colleges
Adrienne Predko, M.A. Ed.
MedVance Institute
Dr. Gary Zuckerman
Washington University School of Medicine

Connect® Contributors
Dolly R. Horton, CMA (AAMA), BS, M.Ed.
*Asheville Buncombe Technical Community
College*
Sepanta Jalali, MD
Columbus State
Merideth Sellars, MS
Columbus State Community College
Sherry Stanfield, RN, BSN, MSHPE
Miller-Motte Technical College
Nerissa Tucker, MHA, CPC
Kaplan University School of Health Sciences
Dr. Wendy Vermillion, DVM
Columbus State Community College
Mindy Wray, BS, CMA (AAMA), RMA
ECPI College of Technology
Byron Hamilton, BA, MA
Australian College of Advanced Education

Digital Symposium Attendees
Courtney M. Conrad, MBA, MPH, CMA
Robert Morris University Illinois

Bonnie J. Crist, BS, CMA, AAS, (AAMA)
Harrison College
Patrick J. Debold, Vice President of Academic
Affairs
Concorde Career Colleges, Inc.
Robert Delaney, Chair
Brookline College
Alice Macomber, RN, RMA, AHI, RPT, CPI,
BXO
Keiser University, Port Saint Lucie Campus
Barry Newman, MD
Kathleen Olewinski, MS, RHIA, NHA,
FACHE,
Medical Assisting Program Director,
Bryant & Stratton College—Milwaukee Market
Mickie Roy, LPN, CCMA
Delta College of Arts & Technology
Lisa M. Smith, BS, RMA (AMT), BXMO
Medical Assisting Program & Externship
Coordinator
Keiser University
Michael Weinand
Kaplan Higher Education
Dr. Barbara Worley, DPM, BS, RMA,
Program Manager, Medical Assisting,
King's College
Patti Zint, M.A., N.C.H.I.
Apollo College

Reviewers of the Fourth Edition
Hooshiyar Ahmadi, MD, DC
Remington College
Diana Alagna, RN, RMA (AMT)
Branford Hall Career Institute
Yvonne Beth Alles, MBA
Davenport University
Ramona Atiles, LPN
Allied Health Program Chair
Career Institute of Health and Technology
Vanessa J. Austin, RMA (AMT), CAHI, BS
Clarian Health Sciences Education Center
Dr. Joseph H. Balatbat, MD
Sanford-Brown Institute
Katie Barton, BA, LPN
Savannah River College
Suzanne Bitters, RMA (AMT)-NCPT/
NCICS
Harris Business School
Alecia C. Blake, MD
*Medical Careers Institute at ECPI
College of Technology*
Kathleen Bode, MS
Flint Hills Technical College
Cynthia Boles, CMA (AAMA)
Bradford School
Cindi Brassington, MS, CMA (AAMA)
Quinebaug Valley Community College
Robin K. Choate, LPN, CHI
Pennsylvania Institute of Technology
Stephen M. Coleman, NCMA
Central Florida Institute

Sheronda Cooper, BSD, BSN, MSFN,
RMA (AMT), NRCPT(NAHP), Director of
Medical Assisting
Bradford School of Business
Janet H. Davis, BSN, MS, MBA, PhD
Robert Morris College
Linda Demain, LPN, BS, MS
Wichita Technical Institute
Carol Dew, MAT, CMA-AC (AAMA)
Baker College
James R. Dickerson, AAS
Remington College
Cheryl Lacey Donovan, CMA (AAMA)
Academy of Health Care Professions
Patricia Dudek, RN
McCann School of Business and Technology
Jane W. Dumas, MSN
Remington College
Tamara Epperson Mottler, BA, CMA (AAMA)
Daytona Beach College
Rhonda K. Epps, AS
*National College of Business and
Technology*
Dr. Herbert J. Feitelberg, D.P.M.
King's College
Suzanne S. Fielding, BS
Daytona Beach College
Walter E. Flowers,
Medical Director
Lamson Institute
Martina T. Forte Brown, CCMA (AAMA),
CPT, CET
Brookstone College of Business
Janette Gallegos, RMA (AMT)
ECPI College of Technology
Christine Goldwater, NCMOA, AA,
Campus Director
Ross Medical Education Center
Darlene S. Grayson Harmon, BS
Remington College
Gay Grubbs, MEd
Griffin Technical College
Tiffany Heath, CMA (AAMA)
Porter and Chester Institute
Lisa M. Herrera
Concorde Career College
Claudia N. Hewlett, AS
Remington College
Elizabeth Hoffman, MA Ed., CMA,
(AAMA), CPT (ASPT)
Baker College
Adriane Holliman
Westwood College ATM
Joanna L. Holly, MS, RN, CMA (AAMA)
Midstate College
Deborah Honstad, MA, RHIA
San Juan College
Susan Horn, AAS CMA (AAMA)
Indiana Business College
Janet Hunter, Ph.D.
Northland Pioneer College

Dara A. Indish, CMA (AAMA), EMT
Alpena Community College
Carol Lee Jarrell, MLT, AHI
Brown Mackie College
Shara-Leigh Kauffman, RN
University of Northwestern Ohio
Jody Kirk
Cambria-Rowe Business College
Doris Klein, BA
Concorde Career College
Pam Kowalski, MA
Ross Medical Education Center
Linda E. LaGrange, NCMA
Remington College
Amy L. Lake, RMA (AMT)
Wright Career College
Paul Lucas, CMA (AAMA), CPbt,
PN, AS
Brown Mackie College
Alice Macomber, RN, RMA (AMT)
Keiser University
Gregory Martinez, BS, MS
Wichita Technical Institute
Wilsetta McClain, MBA, ABD
Baker College of Auburn Hills
Diana K. McWilliams
Remington College
Nancy Measell, BS, CMA (AAMA)
Ivy Tech Community College
Maureen Messier, AS, BA
Branford Hall Career Institute
Helen Mills, RN,
MA Instructor
Keiser University
Edward Moreno
STVT
Diane Morlock, BA, CMA (AAMA)
Owens Community College
Roger K. Oatman, DC
Logan Chiropractic College
Thomas O'Brien, AS CCT CST
Central Florida Institute
Londa L. Ogden, RN, BSN
Keiser University E-Campus
Everlee O'Nan, RMA (AMT)
National College
Janet S. Pandzik, BA, CMT, RMA (AMT)
Hallmark College of Technology
June M. Petillo
Capital Community College
Alisa J. Petree, MHSM, MT (ASCP)
McLennan Community College
Robert Plick, BA, BS
Alta/Westwood College
Angela N. Resnick, RMA (AMT)
School of Health Careers
Diane Roche Benson, CMA (AAMA), MSA,
BS
*Wake Technical Community College,
University of Phoenix*
Rebecca Rodenbaugh, CMA (AAMA)
Baker College of Cadillac

Janette Rodriguez, RN
Wood Tobe Coburn
Pratima Sampat-Mar, M. Ed.
Pima Medical Institute
Judy Scire, BS
Stone Academy
Noreen T. Semanski, AS, LPN
McCann School of Business
Lynn G. Slack, BS CMA (AAMA)
Kaplan Career Institute
Robin Snider-Flohr, EdD, RN, CMA (AAMA)
Jefferson Community College
Sherry A. Stanfield, RN, BSN, MSHPE
Miller-Motte Tech College
Judith D. Symons
McCann School of Business
Tricia Taylor
Kaplan College
Catherine A. Teel, AST, RMA (AMT), CMA
(AAMA)
McCann School of Business and Technology
Lynne A. Thomas, BS
Clarita Career College
Cindy Thompson, RN, RMA (AMT),
MA, BS
Davenport University
Carlota Zuniga Tienda, AS
San Joaquin Valley College
Drew D. Totten, CLT, NRCMA
Charter College
Nerissa C. Tucker, BS, MHA
ECPI College of Technology
Marilyn M. Turner, R.N., C.M.A. (AAMA)
Ogeechee Technical College
Sally Vrooman, MA Ed.
Career Quest Learning Centers, Inc.
Judy K. Ward, BS
Ivy Tech Community College
Marsha Lynn Wilson, MA, BS, MS (ABT)
Clarian Health Sciences Education Center
Stacey F. Wilson, BS, MHA
Cabarrus College of Health Sciences
Constance M. Winter, MPH, RN
Bossier Parish Community College
Dr. Barbara Worley
Program Manager, Medical Assisting Program
King's College
Mindy Wray, BS, CMA (AAMA), RMA
(AMT)
ECPI College of Technology
Will L. Wright, BS
Atlanta Medical Academy
Carole A. Zeglin, MS, BS, RMA (AMT)
Westmoreland County Community College
Susan K. Zolvinski, BS, MBA
Brown Mackie College

Reviewers Prior to Fourth Edition

Roxane M. Abbott, MBA
Sarasota County Technical Institute
Dr. Linda G. Alford, Ed.D.
Reid State Technical College

Suzzanne S. Allen
Sanford Brown Institute
Ann L. Aron, Ed.D.
Aims Community College
Emil Asdurian, MD
Bramson ORT College
Rhonda Asher, MT, ASCP, CMA
Pitt Community College
Adelina H. Azfar, DPM
Total Technical Institute
Joseph H. Balatbat, MD, RMA, RPT, CPT
Sanford Brown Institute
Mary Barko, CMA, MA Ed
Ohio Institute of Health Careers
Katie Barton, LPN, BA
Savannah River College
Kelli C. Batten, NCMA, LMT,
Medical Assisting Department Chair
Career Technical College
Nina Beaman, MS, RNC, CMA
Bryant and Stratton College
Kay E. Biggs, BS, CMA
Columbus State Community College
Norma Bird, M.Ed., BS, CMA,
Medical Assisting Program Director/
Master Instructor
Kathleen Bode, RN, MS
Flint Hills Technical College
Natasha Bratton, BSN
Beta Tech
Karen Brown, RN, BC, Ed.D.
Kirtland Community College
Kimberly D. Brown, BSHS, CHES, CMA
Swainsboro Technical College
Nancy A. Browne, MS, BS
Washington High School
Teresa A. Bruno, BA
EduTek College
Marion I. Bucci, BA
*Delaware Technical and Community
College*
Michelle Buchman, BSN, RNC
Springfield College
Michelle L. Carfagna, RMA, ST, BMO, RHE
Brevard Community College
Carmen Carpenter, RN, MS, CMA
South University
Pamela C. Chapman, RN, MSN
*Caldwell Community College and Technical
Institute*
Patricia A. Chappell, MA, BS,
Director, Clinical Laboratory Science
Camden County College
Phyllis Cox, MA Ed, BS, MT(ASCP)
Arkansas Tech University
Stephanie Cox, BS, LPN
York Technical Institute
Christine Cusano, CMA, CPhT
Clark University CCI
Glynna Day, M.Ed,
Dean of Education
Academy of Professional Careers

Anita Denson, BS
National College of Business and Technology

Leon Deutsch, RMA, BA, MA Ed
Keiser College

Walter R. English, MA, MT(AAB)
Akron Institute

Dennis J. Ernst, MT(ASCP)
Center for Phlebotomy Education

C.S. Farabee, MBA, MSISE
High-Tech Institute Inc.

Deborah Fazio, CMAS, RMA
Sanford Brown Institute Cleveland

William C. Fiala, BS, MA
University of Akron

Cathy Flores, BHS
Central Piedmont Community College

Brenda K. Frerichs, MS, MA, BS
Colorado Technical University

Michael Gallucci, PT, MS
Assistant Professor of Practice,
Program in Physical Therapy,
*School of Public Health,
New York Medical College*

Susan C. Gessner, RN, BSN, M Ed
Laurel Business Institute

Bonnie J. Ginman, CMA
Branford Hall Career Institute

Robyn Gohsman, RMA, CMAS
Medical Career Institute

Cheri Goretti, MA, MT(ASCP), CMA
Quinebaug Valley Community College

Marilyn Graham, LPN
Moore Norman Technology Center

Jodee Gratiot, CCA
Rocky Mountain Business Academy

Donna E. Guisado, AA
North-West College

Debra K. Hadfield, BSN, MSN
Baker College of Jackson

Carrie A. Hammond, CMA, LPRT
Utah Career College

Kris A. Hardy, CMA, RHE, CDF
Brevard Community College

Toni R. Hartley, BS
Laurel Business Institute

Brenda K. Hartson, MS, MA, BS
Colorado Technical University

Marsha Perkins Hemby, BA, RN, CMA
Pitt Community College

Linda Henningsen, RN, MS, BSN
Brown Mackie College

Carol Hinricher, MA
*University of Montana College
of Technology*

Elizabeth A. Hoffman, MA Ed., CMA
Baker College of Clinton Township

Gwen C. Hornsey, BS,
Medical Assistant Instructor
Tulsa Technology Center, Lemley Campus

Helen J. Houser, MSHA, RN, RMA
Phoenix College

Melody S. Irvine, CCS-P, CPC, CMBS
Institute of Business and Medical Careers

Kathie Ivester, MPA, CMA(AAMA),
CLS(NCA)
North Georgia Technical College

Josephine Jackyra, CMA
The Technical Institute of Camden County

Deborah Jones, BS, MA
High-Tech Institute

Karl A. Kahley, CHE, BS
Instructor, Medical Assisting
Ogeechee Technical College

Barbara Kalfin Kalish
City College, Palm Beach Community College

Cheri D. Keenan, MA Instructor, EMT-B
Remington College

Barbara E. Kennedy, RN, CPhT
Blair College

Tammy C. Killough, RN, BSN
*Texas Careers Vocational Nursing
Program Director*

Jimmy Kinney, AAS
Virginia College at Huntsville

Karen A. Kittle, CMA, CPT, CHUC
Oakland Community College

Diane M. Klieger, RN, MBA, CMA
Pinellas Technical Education Centers

Mary E. Larsen, CMT, RMA
Academy of Professional Careers

Nancy L. Last, RN
Eagle Gate College

Holly Roth Levine, NCICS, NCRMA, BA,
BSN, RN
Keiser College

Christine Malone, BS
Everett Community College

Janice Manning
Baker College

Loretta Mattio-Hamilton, AS, CMA, RPT,
CCA, NCICS
Herzing College

Gayle Mazzocco, BSN, RN, CMA
Oakland Community College

Patti McCormick, RN, PHD
President, *Institute of Holistic Leadership*

Stephanie R. McGahee, AATH
Augusta Technical College

Heidi M. McLean, CMA, RMA, BS, RPT,
CAHI
Anne Arundel Community College

Tanya Mercer, BS, RN, RMA
Kaplan Higher Education Corporation

Sandra J. Metzger, RN, BSN, MS. Ed
Red Rocks Community College

Joyce A. Minton, BS, CMA, RMA
Wilkes Community College

Grace Moodt, RN, BSN
Wallace Community College

Sherry L. Mulhollen, BS, CMA
Elmira Business Institute

Deborah M. Mullen, CPC, NCMA
Sanford Brown Institute

Michael Murphy, CMA
*Berdan Institute @ The Summit
Medical Group*

Lisa S. Nagle, CMA, BS.Ed
Augusta Technicial College

Peggy Newton, BSN, RN
Galen Health Institute

Brigitte Niedzwiecki, RN, MSN
Chippewa Valley Technical College

Thomas E. O Brien, MBA, BBA, AS, CCT
Central Florida Institute

Linda Oliver, MA
Vista Adult School

Linda L. Oprean, BSN
ACT College

Holly J. Paul, MSN, FNP
Baker College of Jackson

Shirley Perkins, MD, BSE
Everest College

Kristina Perry, BPA
Heritage College

James H. Phillips, BS, CMA, RMA
Central Florida College

Carol Putkamer, RHIA, MS
Alpena Community College

Mary Rahr, MS, RN, CMA-C
Northeast Wisconsin Technical College

David Rice, AA, BA, MA
Career College of Northern Nevada

Dana M. Roessler, RN, BSN
Southeastern Technical College

Cindy Rosburg, MA
Wisconsin Indian Technical College

Deborah D. Rossi, MA, CMA
Community College of Philadelphia

Donna Rust, BA
American Commercial College

Ona Schulz, CMA
Lake Washington Technical College

Amy E. Semenchuk, RN, BSN
Rockford Business College

David Lee Sessoms, Jr., M.Ed., CMA
Miller-Motte Technical College

Susan Shorey, BA, MA
Valley Career College

Lynn G. Slack, BS
*ICM School of Business and Medical
Careers*

Patricia L. Slusher, MT(ASCP), CMA
Ivy Tech State College

Deborah H. Smith, RN, CNOR
Southeastern Technical College

Kristi Sopp, AA
MTI College

Nona K. Stinemetz, Practical Nurse
Vatterott College

Patricia Ann Stoddard, MS, RT(R), MT, CMA
Western Business College

Sylvia Taylor, BS, CMA, CPC-A
Cleveland State Community College

Cynthia H. Thompson, RN, MA
Davenport University

Geiselle Thompson, M. Div.
The Learning Curve Plus NC
Barbara Tietsort, M. Ed.
University of Cincinnati, Raymond Walters
Karen A. Trompke, RN
Virginia College at Pensacola
Marilyn M. Turner, RN, CMA
Ogeechee Technical College
L. Joleen VanBibber, AS
Davis Applied Technology College
Lynette M. Veach, AAS
Columbus State Community College

Antonio C. Wallace, BS
Sanford Brown Institute
Jim Wallace, MHSA
Maric College
Denise Wallen, CPC
Academy of Professional Careers
Mary Jo Whitacre, MSN, RN
Lord Fairfax Community College
Donna R. Williams, LPN, RMA
Tennessee Technology Center
Marsha Lynn Wilson, BS, MS (ABT)
Clarian Health Sciences Education Center

Linda V. Wirt, CMA
Cecil Community College
Dr. MaryAnn Woods, PhD, RN,
Prof. Emeritus
Fresno City College
Bettie Wright, MBA, CMA
Umpqua Community College
Mark D. Young, DMD, BS
*West Kentucky Community and
Technical College*
Cynthia M. Zumbrun, MEd, RHIT, CCS-P
Allegany College of Maryland

Guided Tour

Case Studies
represent situations similar to those that
the medical assistant may encounter in
daily practice.

35
Special Senses

CASE STUDY

PATIENT INFORMATION		
Patient Name	Gender	DOB
Valarie Ramirez	Female	8/4/19XX
Attending	MRN	Allergies
Paul F. Buckwalter, MD	829-78-462	Penicillin

Valarie Ramirez, a 33-year-old female, arrives at the office with something in her eye. While riding her motorcycle yesterday, something flew up under her helmet visor. She has been using Visine® eyedrops, but when

she woke up this morning, her eye felt worse. You notice her right eye is red and swollen. You prepare Valarie for the physician to examine her eye.

Keep Valarie in mind as you study this chapter. There will be questions at the end of the chapter based on the case study. The information in the chapter will help you answer these questions.

🔲ACTIVSim™

CASE STUDY

PATIENT INFORMATION		
Patient Name	Gender	DOB
Mohammad Nassar	M	5/17/20XX
Attending	MRN	Allergies
Elizabeth H. Williams, MD	423-90-687	NKA

Mohammad Nassar is a 15-year-old male who is new to the practice and comes to the office today for his annual physical examination. He has a known past medical history of asthma, which has been relatively stable until recently. He states when he arrives that he has been experiencing an increasing need for his rescue inhaler

in the last several days. His mother has brought him to the appointment, but Mohammad has asked that she remain in the reception area during his appointment. She does give you a list of Mohammad's current asthma medications and the previously completed new patient documents.

Keep Mohammad (and his mother) in mind as you study this chapter. There will be questions at the end of the chapter based on the case study. The information in the chapter will help you answer these questions.

🔲ACTIVSim™

LEARNING OUTCOMES
After completing Chapter 35, you will be able to:
35.1 Describe the anatomy of the nose and the function of each part.
35.2 Describe the anatomy of the tongue and the function of each part.

KEY TERMS

auricle	organ of Corti
cerumen	ossicles
choroid	oval window
cochlea	papillae

LEARNING OUTCOMES
After completing Chapter 17, you will be able to:
17.1 Explain the importance of patient medical records.
17.2 Identify the documents that comprise a patient medical record.
17.3 Compare SOMR, POMR, SOAP, formats.

KEY TERMS

MEDICAL ASSISTING COMPETENCIES

CAAHEP	ABHES
I. C (1) Describe structural organization of the human body	2. Anatomy & Physiology
I. C (2) Identify body systems	Graduates:
I. C (4) List major organs in each body system	b. Identify and apply the knowledge of all body systems; their structure and functions; and their common diseases, symptoms, and etiologies
I. C (5) Describe the normal function of each body system	
I. C (6) Identify common pathology related to each body system	
I. C (7) Analyze pathology as it relates to the interaction of body systems	c. Assist the physician with the regimen of diagnostic and treatment modalities as they relate to each body system
I. C (8) Discuss implications for disease and disability when homeostasis is not maintained	3. Medical Terminology
I. C (9) Describe implications for treatment related to pathology	Graduates:
I. C (10) Compare body structure and function of the human body across the life span	b. Build and dissect medical terms from roots/suffixes to understand the word element combinations that create medical terminology
I. C (12) Describe the relationship between anatomy and physiology of all body systems and medications used for treatment in each	c. Understand the various medical terminology for each specialty
IV. C (11) Define both medical terms and abbreviations related to all body systems	

PROCEDURE 48-3 Performing Capillary Puncture

Procedure Goal: To collect a capillary blood sample using the finger puncture method.

OSHA Guidelines:

Materials: Capillary puncture device (safety lancet or automatic puncture device like an Autolet or Glucolet), antiseptic and cotton balls or antiseptic wipes, sterile gauze squares, sterile adhesive bandages, reagent strips, micropipettes, and smear slides.

Method: Procedure steps.
... the laboratory request form and make sure you ... supplies.

2. Greet the patient, confirm the patient's identity, and introduce yourself.
3. Explain the purpose of the procedure and confirm that the patient has followed the pretest instructions, if indicated.
   RATIONALE: The test may be invalid if the patient did not follow the pretest instructions.
4. Make sure the patient is sitting in the venipuncture chair or is lying down.
5. Wash your hands. Don exam gloves.
6. Examine the patient's hands to determine which finger to use for the procedure. Avoid fingers that are swollen, bruised, scarred, or calloused. Generally, the ring and great (middle) fingers are the best choices. If you notice the patient's hands are cold, you may want to warm them between your own, have the patient put them in a warm basin of water or under warm running water, or wrap them in a warm cloth.
   RATIONALE: Warming the patient's hands improves circulation.
7. Prepare the patient's finger with a gentle "massaging" or rubbing motion toward the fingertip. Keep the patient's

▶ **Introduction**

The special senses are smell, taste, vision, hearing, and equilibrium. They are called special senses because their sensory receptors are located within relatively large sensory organs in the head—the nose, tongue, eyes, and ears. Although the skin is also

receptors. There are also fewer smell receptors in the human nose compared to most animal noses.

Once smell receptors are activated, they send their information to the olfactory nerves. The olfactory nerves send the information along olfactory bulbs and tracts to different areas of the cerebrum. The cerebrum interprets the information as a

Chapter Openers include the CAAHEP and
ABHES competencies covered in the chapter,
a list of learning outcomes, and a list of key
terms.

Procedure boxes Specific administrative
or clinical tasks are illustrated in a step-
by-step format at the end of each chapter.
Over 180 procedures with integrated
photos including, when appropriate, work
documentation forms that are found in
the Student Workbook.

CAUTION: *Handle with Care* boxes
cover precautions to be taken when
performing certain tasks.

CAUTION: HANDLE WITH CARE
Helping Elderly Patients with Depression

Studies published by the National Institutes of Health (NIH) indicate that at least 5% of elderly people attending primary care clinics suffer from depression. For elderly people in nursing homes, that percentage rises to between 15% and 25%. The NIH also indicates that only about 10% of elderly people who need treatment for depression ever receive it. Additionally, the NIH considers depression in people age 65 and older to be a major public health concern. In fact, suicide is more common among the elderly than any other age group. One reason for the low rate of treatment is that many older people—and their families— believe that depression is a normal consequence of growing old. After all, older people may experience many difficult life changes, including enduring the deaths of a spouse and siblings, adjusting to retirement, being alone, dealing with a relocation, suffering economic hardship, and managing a variety of physical ailments. Because of these circumstances, doctors and family may miss the signs of depression.

Recognizing the Symptoms
There is, unfortunately, no specific diagnostic test for depression, so a diagnosis must be made on the basis of symptoms. The symptoms of depression in the elderly are similar to those in other age groups and include the following:

* Decreased ability to enjoy life or to show an interest in activities or people.
* Slow thinking, indecisiveness, or difficulty in concentrating.
* Increased or decreased appetite.
* Increased or decreased time spent sleeping.
* Recurrent feelings of worthlessness.
* Loss of energy and motivation.
* Exaggerated feelings of sadness, hopelessness, or anxiety.
* Recurrent thoughts of death or suicide.

The failure to realize that symptoms like these indicate an illness prevents many older people from seeking help. Yet there is evidence that treatment for depression in the elderly can be highly effective.

Treatment for Depression
Treatment for depression generally combines a course of antidepressant drugs with psychotherapy. Older patients generally

respond to antidepressants more slowly than younger patients, so older patients may not experience relief until more than 6 weeks after starting treatment. For this and other reasons, compliance in taking medications for depression is a problem with the elderly. Many elderly patients do not understand depression and the importance of taking medications as prescribed. They also may be frightened by the idea of taking medication for a mental problem. Psychotherapy aims to help older patients talk through their anxieties, develop coping skills, and improve the quality of their lives. Again, compliance is a problem. Many older adults are unwilling to admit that they have a mental health problem and refuse to follow up on referrals to mental health professionals.

Benefits of Treatment
Elderly patients who follow a course of treatment for depression benefit in several of ways. They gain

* Relief from many of the symptoms associated with depression.
* Relief from some of the pain and suffering associated with physical ailments.
* Improved physical, mental, and social well-being.

Healthcare providers, including you as the medical assistant, can play a significant role in recognizing symptoms of depression in elderly patients and in encouraging them to get the treatment they need.

It is difficult to detect elder abuse. There is no uniform and comprehensive definition of this type of abuse, and bruises from falls and other accidents can be mistaken for abuse. Also, the signs of neglect can be similar to the signs of some chronic medical conditions. There are three basic categories of elder abuse: domestic elder abuse, institutional elder abuse, and self-neglect, or self-abuse. Elders can be abused physically, sexually, or psychologically. Elders may also be neglected, abandoned, or exploited materially or financially. Elders may

even choose to neglect or abuse themselves. More than one type of abuse can occur simultaneously. Elder abuse occurs in all racial, socioeconomic, and religious groups. However, most victims are older women with chronic illness or disabilities. Risk factors or situations that increase the possibility of elder abuse include

* History of alcoholism, drug abuse, or violence in the family.
* History of mental illness in the abuser or victim.

802 CHAPTER 41

Points on Practice boxes

provide guidelines on keeping the medical office running smoothly and efficiently.

Educating the Patient boxes

Patient instruction on self-care outside the medical office is the focus.

Summary and Review

A bulleted summary of the chapter material and an end-of-chapter review close out each chapter. Case study questions and 10 multiple choice questions are found in the textbook. Also media asset icons are included when available for videos, EHR activities, or animations.

Working Efficiently Online

If the medical office where you work is computerized, the system most likely has a modem for sending e-mail and transferring files electronically, as well as accessing various online services and the Internet. If this access is not currently available in the office, it probably will be in the near future, and you may even be asked to help choose the service provider that is most appropriate for your office.

These services, known as *Internet service providers (ISPs)*, allow access to a network of servers that provides a means for healthcare professionals to communicate with one ...

Choosing an Online Ser...

Compare several se...

• Th...

• Use computerized address books. As part of the e-mail system, most services provide an online address book for storing frequently used e-mail addresses. Instead of wasting time searching for an e-mail addres... in a standard card file, you simply click on th... address book and th...
person. You ...

...ne in the
...nt to that
...end the same
...e message
...d copy)

...ddress in
...s of the
...will see
...thus
...ting the

Whenever possible, these guidelines should be recommended to patients of all ages. Good health should be a top priority in life. Although it is best to incorporate healthy behavior before illness develops, remind patients that it is never too late to work toward improving their health.

Protection from Injury

Many accidents happen because people fail to see potential risks and do not develop plans of action. Following safety measures at home, at work, at play, and while traveling can help prevent injury. A discussion of ways to avoid accidents and injury should be part of the educational process. See the Educating the Patient feature Tips for Preventing Injury to help patients avoid injury at home and at work.

Another essential aspect of educating patients about injury prevention is teaching them about the proper use of medications. A prescription includes specific instructions for taking the medication. Emphasize to the patient that these instructions must

be followed exactly. In addition, the patient must not change the dosage or mix medications of any kind without first checking with the physician. Patients who do not adhere to these rules run the risk of potentially dangerous side effects. Tell patients to report to the physician any unusual reactions experienced when taking medications. Patients also must be cautioned to never share their medications with anyone else, no matter how tempting it may be to "help" a family member or friend.

When providing a patient with a new prescription, always ask the patient if he has told the doctor about all the medications he is already taking, including herbs, vitamins, and over-the-counter (OTC) medications. If the patient tells you that he has not, immediately inform the physician before the patient leaves the office. Some medications taken together or with certain foods can interfere with how well the drug works or cause side effects or adverse reactions. The physician needs to know about all drugs as well as herbal preparations and OTC medications that the patient is taking.

Tips for Preventing Injury

To avoid accidents and injury, teach patients to use common sense and follow these guidelines:

At Home

• Install smoke detectors, carbon monoxide detectors, and fire extinguishers.
• Keep all medicines, chemicals, and household cleaning solutions out of the reach of children.
• Purchase products in childproof containers. Lock or attach childproof latches to all cabinets, medicine chests, and drawers that contain poisonous items.
• Keep chemicals in their original containers and store them out of children's reach.
• Install adequate lighting in rooms and hallways.
• Install railings on stairs.
• Use nonskid backing on rugs to help prevent falls, or remove rugs altogether.
• In the bathroom, use nonskid mats or strips that stick to the tub floor.
• Stay with young children when they are in the bathroom.
• Do not rely on bath seats or rings as a safety device for babies and children.
• Set the water temperature on the water heater at 120°F.
• Never use appliances in the bathtub or near a sink filled with water.
• Practice good kitchen safety: Store knives and kitchen tools properly. Unplug small appliances when not in use. Wipe up spills immediately.

• When cooking, take care to turn all handles of pots and pans inward, toward the cooking surface, to avoid spills and burns.
• Shorten long electrical cords and speaker wires, or secure them with electrical tape. Avoid plugging too many electrical appliances into the same outlet.
• Exercise caution when using electrical appliances. Use outlet covers when outlets are not in use.
• To reach high places, use proper equipment, such as stepladders, not chairs.
• Use child safety gates at the top of stairwells.

At Work

• Use appropriate safety equipment and protective gear, as required.
• Lift heavy objects properly: Bend at the knees, not at the waist. As you straighten your legs, bring the object close to your body quickly. That way, strong leg muscles do the lifting, not weaker back muscles.
• Never attempt to move furniture on your own. Request that a member of the office building maintenance staff be engaged to do so.
• Use surge protectors on computer and other electronic equipment to prevent overloading outlets.
• Make sure hallways, entrance areas, work areas, offices, and parking lots are well lit.
• If your job involves desk work, practice proper posture when sitting. Do not sit for long periods of time. Get up and stretch, or walk down the hall and back.

LEARNING OUTCOMES	KEY POINTS
40.1 Relate growth and development to pediatric patient care.	Growth and development occur in stages throughout life, including neonate, infant, toddler, preschooler, elementary school child, middle school child, and adolescent. Each stage of development occurs through physical, cognitive-intellectual, psycho-emotional, and social milestones.
40.2 Identify the role of the medical assistant during pediatric examinations.	The medical assistant must be able to communicate with pediatric patients of all stages, gather and provide educational information to the parent or caregiver, assist with diagnostic and screening procedures, and serve as a liaison between the patient and the physician.
40.3 Discuss pediatric immunizations and the role of the medical assistant.	Immunizations provide patients with protection from infectious diseases. Throughout life, especially during childhood, immunizations are recommended. The medical assistant may schedule appointments, provide education, obtain informed consent, administer the medication, maintain the immunization record, and properly handle and store the immunizations.
40.4 Explain variations of pediatric screening procedures and diagnostic tests.	Screening procedures and diagnostic tests for pediatric patients vary depending upon the age and size of the child. When performing vital signs, body measurements, vision and hearing tests, specimen collection, or administration of immunizations and medications, follow the specific guidelines for the procedure and child.
40.5 Describe common pediatric diseases and disorders and their treatment.	Some childhood diseases include chickenpox, influenza, measles, mumps, rubella, scarlet fever, and tetanus. Other diseases are outlined in Table 40-2.
40.6 Recognize special health concerns of pediatric patients.	The medical assistant should be alert to signs of special health concerns of pediatric patients, including child abuse and neglect; eating disorders; depression, substance abuse, and addiction; violence; suicide; and sexually transmitted infections and birth control.

Now that you have completed this chapter, review the case study at the beginning of the chapter and answer the following questions.

1. Considering Chris Matthews's age, what special aspects of care should you be aware of while caring for him?

2. What information (chief complaint) should you chart regarding Chris?

3. According to his immunization record (see Figure 40-12), what immunizations are missing?

4. What screening and diagnostic tests would you perform or assist the physician in performing?

Introduction to Medical Assisting

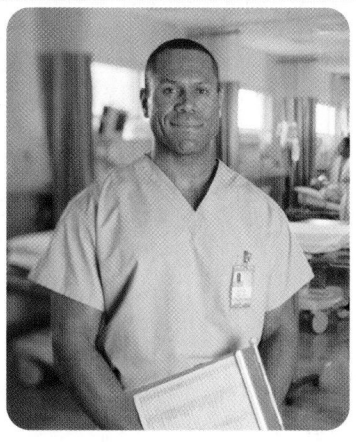

Sandro Peso is a 33-year-old father of four who lost his job at a local factory. He is a medical assistant in-training, and is currently working at BWW Associates. He will be working in the administrative, clinical, and laboratory sections of the office. He wants to decide which area he likes best and where he might like to work when he finishes his training. It will not be long until he graduates and needs to take the test to become credentialed. He is nervous about the exam but really wants to do well to get the best job he can to help support his family.

Keep Mr. Peso in mind as you study this chapter. There will be questions at the end of the chapter based on the case study. The information in the chapter will help you answer these questions.

LEARNING OUTCOMES

After completing Chapter 1, you will be able to:

1.1 Recognize the duties and responsibilities of a medical assistant.

1.2 Distinguish various organizations related to the medical assisting profession.

1.3 Explain the need for and importance of the medical assistant credentials.

1.4 Identify the training needed to become a professional medical assistant.

1.5 Discuss professional development as it relates to medical assisting education.

KEY TERMS

accreditation

Accrediting Bureau of Health Education Schools (ABHES)

American Association of Medical Assistants (AAMA)

American Medical Technologists (AMT)

certification

Certified Medical Assistant (CMA)

Clinical Laboratory Improvement Amendments of 1988 (CLIA '88)

Commission on Accreditation of Allied Health Education Programs (CAAHEP)

continuing education

cross-training

Health Insurance Portability and Accountability Act (HIPAA)

Occupational Safety and Health Administration (OSHA)

professional development

Registered Medical Assistant (RMA)

registration

résumé

IX. C (1) Discuss legal scope of practice for medical assistants

IX. C (5) Discuss licensure and certification as it applies to healthcare providers

IX. P (2) Perform within scope of practice

IX. P (4) Practice within the standard of care for a medical assistant

1. **General Orientation**
   a. Comprehend the current employment outlook for the medical assistant
   c. Understand medical assistant credentialing requirements and the process to obtain the credential; comprehend the importance of credentialing
   d. Have knowledge of the general responsibilities of the medical assistant
   e. Define scope of practice for the medical assistant, and comprehend the conditions for practice within the state that the medical assistant is employed

11. **Career Development**
    Graduates:
    b. Demonstrate professionalism by:
       (9) Conducting work within scope of education, training, and ability

Introduction

Healthcare is changing at a rapid rate. Advanced technology, implementation of cost-effective medicine, and the aging population are all factors that have caused growth in the healthcare services industry. As the healthcare services industry expands, the U.S. Department of Labor projects that medical assisting will be the fastest-growing occupation between 2008 and 2018. The growth in the number of physicians' group practices and other healthcare practices that use support personnel will in turn continue to drive up demand for medical assistants. Medical assisting is the perfect complement to this changing industry.

Medical assistants perform a variety of duties that make them well-qualified to enter a variety of job openings in the healthcare industry. This chapter provides an introduction to the medical assisting profession. It will present a general description of your future duties, credentials, and needed training. Some basic facts about professional associations, organizations, and professional development related to medical assisting are also discussed. All of this will help you to enter your career as a medical assistant.

Responsibilities of the Medical Assistant

LO 1.1

Your specific responsibilities as a medical assistant will probably depend on the location and size of the facility, as well as its medical specialties. Medical assistants work in an administrative, clinical, and/or laboratory capacity. As an administrative medical assistant, you may handle the payroll for the office staff (or supervise a payroll service), obtain equipment and supplies, and serve as the link between the physician and representatives of pharmaceutical and medical supply companies. As a clinical medical assistant, you will be the physician's right arm by maintaining an efficient office, preparing and maintaining medical records, assisting the physician during examinations, and keeping examination rooms in order. Your laboratory duties as a medical assistant may include performing basic laboratory tests and maintenance of laboratory equipment. In small practices, you may handle all duties. In larger practices, you may specialize in a particular duty. As a medical assistant grows in his or her profession, advanced duties may be required. The lists of duties in Table 1-1 are provided to help you better understand what you will be doing when you practice as a medical assistant.

You may also choose to specialize in a specific area of healthcare. For example, podiatric medical assistants make castings of feet, expose and develop X-rays, and assist podiatrists in surgery. Ophthalmic medical assistants help ophthalmologists (doctors who provide eye care) by administering diagnostic tests, measuring and recording vision, testing the functioning of eyes and eye muscles, and performing other duties. A discussion of medical specialties is found in the chapter *Healthcare and the Healthcare Team*. For specific information about medical assistant duties within medical specialty practice, review the following chapters: *Assisting in Reproductive and Urinary Specialties*, *Assisting in Pediatrics*, *Assisting in Geriatrics*, *Assisting in Other Medical Specialties*, and *Assisting with Eye and Ear Care*.

TABLE 1-1   Daily Duties of Medical Assistants

Duty Type	Entry-Level Duties	Advanced Duties
General	• Recognizing and responding effectively to verbal, nonverbal, and written communications. • Explaining treatment procedures to patients. • Providing patient education within scope of practice. • Facilitating treatment for patients from diverse cultural backgrounds and for patients with hearing or vision impairments, or physical or mental disabilities. • Acting as a patient advocate. • Maintaining medical records.	None
Administrative	• Greeting patients. • Handling correspondence. • Scheduling appointments. • Answering telephones. • Creating and maintaining patient medical records. • Handling billing, bookkeeping, and insurance processing. • Performing medical transcription. • Arranging for hospital admissions.	• Developing and conducting public outreach programs to market the physician's professional services. • Negotiating leases of equipment and supply contracts. • Negotiating nonrisk and risk managed care contracts. • Managing business and professional insurance. • Developing and maintaining fee schedules. • Participating in practice analysis. • Coordinating plans for practice enhancement, expansion, consolidation, and closure. • Performing as a HIPAA compliance officer. • Providing personnel supervision and employment practices. • Providing information systems management.
Clinical	• Assisting the doctor during examinations. • Assisting with asepsis and infection control. • Performing diagnostic tests, such as spirometry and ECGs. • Giving injections, where allowed. • Phlebotomy, including venipuncture and capillary puncture. • Disposing of soiled or stained supplies. • Performing first aid and cardiopulmonary resuscitation (CPR). • Preparing patients for examinations. • Preparing and administering medications as directed by the physician, and following state laws for invasive procedures. • Recording vital signs and medical histories. • Removing sutures or changing dressings on wounds. • Sterilizing medical instruments. • Instructing patients about medication and special diets, authorizing drug refills as directed by the physician, and calling pharmacies to order prescriptions. • Assisting with minor surgery. • Teaching patients about special procedures before laboratory tests, surgery, X-rays, or ECGs.	• Initiating an IV and administering IV medications with appropriate training, and as permitted by state law. • Reporting diagnostic study results. • Assisting patients in the completion of advance directives and living wills. • Assisting with clinical trials.
Laboratory	• Performing Clinical Laboratory Improvement Amendments (CLIA)–waived tests, such as a urine pregnancy test, on the premises. • Collecting, preparing, and transmitting laboratory specimens. • Teaching patients to collect specific specimens properly. • Arranging laboratory services. • Meeting safety standards (OSHA guidelines) and fire protection mandates.	• Performing as an OSHA compliance officer. • Performing moderately complex laboratory testing with appropriate training and certification.

▶ Medical Assisting Organizations   LO 1.2

A multitude of organizations guide the profession of medical assisting. These include professional associations such as the American Association of Medical Assistants (AAMA) and the American Medical Technologists (AMT), as well as accrediting and other organizations. As a future medical assistant, knowledge of these organizations will help you make critical decisions about your career.

Professional associations set high standards for quality and performance in a profession. They define the tasks and functions of an occupation, and they provide members with the opportunity to communicate and network with one another. They also present their goals to the profession and to the general public. Becoming a member of a professional association helps you achieve career goals and furthers the profession of medical assisting. Joining as a student is encouraged and some associations even offer discounted rates to students for a specified amount of time after graduation.

American Association of Medical Assistants

The seed of the idea for a national association of medical assistants—later to be called the **American Association of Medical Assistants (AAMA)**—was planted at the 1955 annual state convention of the Kansas Medical Assistants Society. The next year, at an American Medical Association (AMA) meeting, the AAMA was officially created. In 1978, the US Department of Health, Education, and Welfare declared medical assisting as an allied health profession.

AAMA's Purpose The AAMA works to raise standards of medical assisting to a more professional level. It is the only professional association devoted exclusively to the medical assisting profession. Its creator and first president, Maxine Williams, had extensive experience in orchestrating medical assisting projects for the Kansas Medical Assistants Society. She also served as co-chair of the planning committee that formed the AAMA.

AAMA Occupational Analysis In 1996, the AAMA formed a committee whose goal was to revise and update its standards for the **accreditation** of programs that teach medical assisting. The committee's findings were published in 1997 as the "AAMA Role Delineation Study: Occupational Analysis of the Medical Assistant Profession." The study included a new Role Delineation Chart that outlined the areas of competence to be mastered as an entry-level medical assistant. The Role Delineation Chart of the CMA (AAMA) was further updated in 2003 to include additional competencies. In 2009, it was updated again and was renamed the Occupational Analysis of the CMA (AAMA).

The Occupational Analysis provides the basis for medical assisting education and evaluation. Mastery of the areas of competence listed in the Occupational Analysis is required for all students in accredited medical assisting programs. The Occupational Analysis includes three areas of competence: administrative, clinical, and general. Each of these three areas is divided into two or more narrower areas, for a total of 10 specific areas of competence. Within each area, a bulleted list of statements describes the medical assistant's role.

According to the AAMA, the Occupational Analysis may be used to

- Describe the field of medical assisting to other healthcare professionals.
- Identify entry-level areas of competence for medical assistants.
- Help practitioners assess their own current competence in the field.
- Aid in the development of continuing education programs.
- Prepare appropriate types of materials for home study.

Professional Support for CMAs (AAMA) When you become a member of the AAMA, you will have a large support group of active medical assistants. Membership benefits include

- Professional publications, such as *CMA Today*.
- A large variety of educational opportunities, such as chapter-sponsored seminars and workshops about the latest administrative, clinical, and management topics.
- Group insurance.
- Legal information.
- Local, state, and national activities that include professional networking and multiple continuing education opportunities.
- Legislative monitoring to protect your right to practice as a medical assistant.
- Access to the website at www.aama-ntl.org.

American Medical Technologists (AMT)

American Medical Technologists (AMT) is a nonprofit certification agency and professional membership association representing over 45,000 individuals in allied healthcare. Established in 1939, AMT began a program to register medical assistants at accredited schools in the early 1970s. The AMT provides allied health professionals with professional certification services and membership programs to enhance their professional and personal growth. Upon certification, individuals automatically become members of AMT and start to receive benefits. You will read more about the benefits of joining a professional organization later in the chapter. The AMT provides many certifications, including the Registered Medical Assistant RMA (AMT) credential and the Certified Medical Assistant Specialist CMAS (AMT) credential.

Professional Support for RMAs (AMT) The AMT offers many benefits for RMAs (AMT). These include

- Professional publications.
- Membership in the AMT Institute for Education.
- Group insurance programs—liability, health, and life.
- State chapter activities.

- Legal representation in health legislative matters.
- Annual meetings and educational seminars.
- Student membership.
- Access to the website at www.amt1.com.

Other Medical Assisting Organizations

In addition to the AAMA, which provides the CMA credential, and the AMT, which provides the RMA and CMAS credentials, many organizations provide certification testing and medical assisting credentials. Specific information about medical assisting credentials is discussed later in this chapter.

National Healthcareer Association (NHA) This organization was established in 1989 as an information resource and network for today's active healthcare professionals. NHA provides certification and **continuing education** services for healthcare professionals and curriculum development for educational institutions. They offer a variety of certification exams, including Billing and Coding Specialist (CBCS), Medical Administrative Assistant (CMAA), and Clinical Medical Assistant (CCMA). Some of the NHA's programs and services include

- Certification development and implementation.
- Continuing education curriculum development and implementation.
- Program development for unions, hospitals, and schools.
- Educational, career advancement, and networking services for members.
- Registry of certified professionals.

Healthcare educators working in their various fields of study develop the National Healthcare Association certification exams. The NHA is a member of The National Organization of Competency Assurance (NOCA).

National Center for Competency Testing (NCCT) This is an independent agency that certifies the validity of competency and knowledge of the medical profession through examination. Medical assistants and medical office assistants receive the designation of National Certified Medical Assistant (NCMA) and National Certified Medical Office Assistant (NCMOA) after passing the certification examination. The NCCT avoids any allegiance to a specific organization or association.

The National Association for Health Professionals (NAHP) NAHP (www.nahpusa.com) offers multiple credentials for healthcare professionals. The organization, which has been in existence for 30 years, prides itself in making the process of obtaining a credential an accessible, affordable, and obtainable goal for those individuals who wish to show commitment to their chosen profession. Having multiple credentials with one agency makes maintaining continuing education easier for practicing healthcare professionals. The NAHP offers many credentials, including the Medical Assistant, Phlebotomy Technician, EKG Technician, Coding Specialist,

Administrative Health Assistant, Patient Care Technician, Dental Assistant, Pharmacy Technician, and Surgical Technician credentials.

▶ Medical Assistant Credentials LO 1.3

Certification is confirmation by an organization that an individual is qualified to perform a job to professional standards. **Registration** is the granting of a title or license by a board that gives permission to practice in a chosen profession. Once credentialed, you earn the right to wear a pin that is obtained through the credentialing organization (Figure 1-1).

Medical assisting credentials such as certification and registration are not always required to practice as a medical assistant. However, employers today are aggressively recruiting medical assistants who are credentialed in their field. Small physician practices are being consolidated or merged into larger providers of healthcare, such as hospitals, to decrease operating expenses. Human resource directors of these larger organizations place great importance on professional credentials for their employees.

An accredited medical assisting program is competency based; this means that standards are set by an accrediting body for administrative and clinical competencies. Accrediting bodies are discussed later in this chapter. It is the educational institution's duty to ensure that medical assisting students learn all medical assisting competencies and that evidence is clearly documented for each student. Periodic evaluations are performed by the accrediting agencies to ensure the effectiveness of the program.

Competencies and proficiency assessments are parts of the CMA (AAMA) examination. For example, administering medications is a competency required of accredited medical assisting programs and is a component of the CMA (AAMA) examination. The CMA (AAMA) credential and the affiliation with a professional organization demonstrate competence and provide evidence of training. They also lessen the likelihood of a legal challenge to the quality of a medical assistant's work.

FIGURE 1-1 Wearing one of these pins indicates you have obtained a credential in medical assisting. Medical assistants registered by the American Medical Technologists wear the pin on the left. Members of the American Association of Medical Assistants wear the pin on the right.

Basically, there is less chance of malpractice if employees are credentialed through either AAMA or RMA. School accreditation and credentials will be discussed in more detail later in this chapter.

State and Federal Regulations

Certain provisions of the **Occupational Safety and Health Administration (OSHA)** and the **Clinical Laboratory Improvement Amendments of 1988 (CLIA '88)** are making mandatory credentialing for medical assistants a logical step in the hiring process. These two (OSHA and CLIA '88) regulate healthcare but presently do not require that medical assistants be credentialed. However, various components of these statutes and their regulations can be met by demonstrating that medical assistants in a clinical setting are certified. For example, some physician offices perform moderately complex laboratory testing on-site. The medical assistant can perform moderately complex tests if she or he has the appropriate training and skills.

AAMA Credential

The **Certified Medical Assistant (CMA)** credential is awarded by the Certifying Board of the AAMA. The AAMA's certification examination evaluates mastery of medical assisting competencies based on the Occupational Analysis of the CMA (AAMA), which is available at www.aama-ntl.org/resources/library/OA.pdf. The National Board of Medical Examiners (NBME) also provides technical assistance in developing the tests.

CMAs (AAMA) must recertify the CMA (AAMA) credential every 5 years. To be recertified as a CMA (AAMA), 60 contact hours must be accumulated during the 5-year period: 10 in the administrative area, 10 in the clinical area, and 10 in the general area, with 30 additional hours in any of the three categories. In addition, 30 of these contact hours must be from an approved AAMA program. The AAMA also requires you to hold a current CPR card.

The recertification mandate requires you to learn about new medical developments through education courses or participation in an examination. Hundreds of continuing education courses are sponsored by local, state, and national AAMA groups. The AAMA also offers self-study courses through its continuing education department.

As of June 1998, only completing students of medical assisting programs accredited by CAAHEP and ABHES are eligible to take the certification examination. The AAMA offers the Candidate's Guide to the Certification Examination to help applicants prepare for the examination. This guide explains the test format and test-taking strategies. It also includes a sample examination with answers and information about study references. Some schools have also incorporated test preparation reviews into their programs. They do this because the credentialing agencies require a certain percentage of students to pass the program in order for the schools to keep their accreditation.

As of January 2009, the CMA (AAMA) examination is computerized. These computerized tests may be taken any time at a designated testing site in your area. You may search the Internet for an application and test review materials. Once you have successfully passed the CMA (AAMA) examination, you have earned the right to add that credential to your name, such as Miguel A. Perez, CMA (AAMA).

AMT Credentials

The American Medical Technologists (AMT) organization credentials medical assistants as **Registered Medical Assistants (RMA)** or Certified Medical Assistant Specialists (CMAS). Although this section focuses on the RMA credential, you can find more about the CMAS credential on the AMT website at www.amt1.org.

The AMT sets forth both educational and experiential requirements to earn the RMA (AMT) credential. These include

- Graduation from a medical assistant program that is accredited by ABHES or CAAHEP, or is accredited by a regional accrediting commission, by a national accrediting organization approved by the U.S. Department of Education, or by a formal medical services training program of the U.S. Armed Forces.
- Alternatively, employment in the medical assisting profession for a minimum of 5 years, no more than 2 years of which may have been as an instructor in the postsecondary medical assistant program.
- Passing the AMT examination for RMA (AMT) certification.

RMAs (AMT) must accumulate 30 contact hours for continuing education units (CEU) every 3 years if they were certified after 2006. RMAs (AMT) who were certified before this date are expected to keep abreast of all the changes and practices in their field through educational programs, workshops, or seminars. However, there are no specific continuing education requirements. Once a medical assistant has passed the AMT exam, she has earned the right to add RMA (AMT) to her name: Kaylyn R. Haddix, RMA (AMT).

The RMA (AMT) and CMA (AAMA) Examinations

The RMA (AMT) and CMA (AAMA) qualifying examinations are rigorous. Participation in an accredited program will help you learn what you need to know. The examinations cover several distinct areas of knowledge, including

- General medical knowledge, including terminology, anatomy, physiology, behavioral science, medical law, and ethics.
- Administrative knowledge, including medical records management, collections, insurance processing, and the **Health Insurance Portability and Accountability Act (HIPAA)**. HIPAA is a set of government regulations that help ensure continuity and privacy of healthcare, among other things.
- Clinical knowledge, including examination room techniques, medication preparation and administration, pharmacology, and specimen collection.

Each certification examination is based on a specific content outline created by the certifying organization. You should research the Internet to gain additional information regarding any of these certifications. See Procedure 1-1, Obtaining Certification/Registration Information through the Internet.

▶ Training Programs
LO 1.4

With the emergence of formal training programs for medical assistants and the continuous changes in healthcare today, the role of the medical assistant has become dynamic and wide ranging. These changes have raised the expectations for medical assistants. The knowledge base of the modern medical assistant includes

- Administrative and clinical skills.
- Patient insurance product knowledge (specific to the workers' geographic locations).
- Compliance with healthcare-regulating organizations.
- Exceptional customer service.
- Practice management.
- Current patient treatments and education.

The medical assisting profession requires a commitment to self-directed, lifelong learning. Healthcare is changing rapidly because of new technology, new healthcare delivery systems, and new approaches to facilitating cost-efficient, high-quality healthcare. A medical assistant who can adapt to change and is continually learning will be in high demand.

Formal programs in medical assisting are offered in a variety of educational settings, including vocational-technical high schools, postsecondary vocational schools, community and junior colleges, and 4-year colleges and universities. Vocational school programs usually last 9 months to 1 year and award a certificate or diploma. Community and junior college programs are usually 2-year associate's degree programs. Training can be obtained through traditional classroom as well as online settings.

Accreditation

Accreditation is the process by which programs are officially authorized. The U.S. Department of Education recognizes two national entities that accredit medical assisting educational programs:

- **Commission on Accreditation of Allied Health Education Programs (CAAHEP).** CAAHEP works directly with the Medical Assisting Educational Review Board (MAERB) of Medical Assistants Endowments to ensure that all accredited schools provide a competency-based education. CAAHEP accredits medical assisting programs in both public and private postsecondary institutions throughout the United States that prepare individuals for entry into the medical assisting profession.
- **Accrediting Bureau of Health Education Schools (ABHES).** ABHES accredits private postsecondary institutions and programs that prepare individuals for entry into the medical assisting profession.

Accredited programs must cover the following topics:

- Anatomy and physiology
- Medical terminology
- Medical law and ethics
- Psychology
- Oral and written communications
- Laboratory procedures
- Clinical and administrative procedures

High school students may prepare for these courses by studying mathematics, health, biology, keyboarding, office skills, bookkeeping, and information technology. You may obtain current information about accreditation standards for medical assisting programs from the AAMA.

Medical assisting programs must also include a practicum (externship) or work experience. This applied training is for a specified length of time in an ambulatory care setting, such as a physician's office, hospital, or other healthcare facility. Additionally, the AAMA lists its minimum standards for accredited programs. This list of standards ensures that all personnel—administrators and faculty alike—are qualified to perform their jobs. These standards also ensure that financial and physical resources are available at accredited programs.

Graduation from an accredited program helps your career in three ways. First, it shows that you have completed a program that meets nationally accepted standards. Second, it provides recognition of your education by professional peers. Third, it makes you eligible for registration or certification. Students who graduate from an ABHES- or CAAHEP-accredited medical assisting program are eligible to take the CMA (AAMA) or RMA (AMT) immediately.

Work Experience

Your practicum (externship) or work experience is mandatory in accredited schools. The length of your experience will vary, depending on your particular program, so familiarize yourself with the program requirements as soon as possible. Since this is a mandatory part of the program, no matter how good your grades are in class, if the work experience is not completed, you will not graduate from the program.

Your practicum (externship) or work experience is an extension of your classroom learning experience. You will apply skills learned in the classroom in an actual medical office or other healthcare facility. You also earn the right to include this applied training experience on your résumé under job experience, as long as you title it as "Medical Assistant Practicum, Externship, or Work Experience." The *Preparing for the World of Work* chapter will further explain your practical work experience.

▶ Professional Development
LO 1.5

Professional development refers to skills and knowledge attained for both personal development and career advancement. During your training, you should strive to improve your knowledge and skills. This will help you transition into your first job with ease. You can also gain valuable knowledge and skills through volunteering prior to or in addition to work experience obtained as a student.

Once you have entered the world of work as a medical assistant, you will want to continue to develop in your profession. This can be done by gaining more knowledge and skills through additional training, **cross-training,** and/or other forms of continuing education. During your training and practice as a medical assistant, you must know and work within your scope of practice and network to improve yourself professionally.

Volunteer Programs

Volunteering is a rewarding experience. Before you even begin a medical assisting program, you can gain experience in a healthcare profession through volunteer work. As a volunteer, you will get hands-on training and learn what it is like to assist patients who are ill, disabled, or frightened.

You may volunteer as an aide in a hospital, clinic, nursing home, or doctor's office, or as a typist or filing clerk in a medical office or medical record room. Some visiting nurse associations and hospices (home-like medical settings that provide medical care and emotional support to terminally ill patients and their families) also offer volunteer opportunities. These experiences may help you decide if you want to pursue a career as a medical assistant.

The American Red Cross also offers volunteer opportunities for student medical assistants. The Red Cross needs volunteers for its disaster relief programs locally, statewide, nationally, and abroad. As part of a disaster relief team at the site of a hurricane, tornado, storm, flood, earthquake, or fire, volunteers learn first-aid and emergency triage skills. Red Cross volunteers gain valuable work experience that may help them obtain a job.

Because volunteers are not paid, it is usually easy to find work opportunities. Just because you are not paid for volunteer work, however, does not mean the experience is not useful for meeting your career goals.

Include information about any volunteer work on your **résumé**—a computer-generated document that summarizes your employment and educational history. Be sure to note specific duties, responsibilities, and skills you developed during the volunteer experience. Refer to the *Preparing for the World of Work* chapter for examples of résumés.

Continued Training

Continuing education and training are essential to your career as a medical assistant. As discussed earlier, continuing education is mandatory for maintaining your certification or registration. In addition, you may want to become multiskilled. Many hospitals and healthcare practices are embracing the idea of a multiskilled healthcare professional (MSHP). An MSHP is a cross-trained team member who is able to handle many different duties.

Reducing Healthcare Costs As a result of healthcare reform and downsizing (a reduction in the number of staff members) to control the rising cost of healthcare, medical practices are eager to reduce personnel costs by hiring multiskilled health professionals. These individuals, who perform the functions of two or more people, are the most cost-efficient employees.

Expanding Your Career Opportunities Career opportunities are vast if you are self-motivated and willing to learn new skills. If you continue to learn about new administrative techniques and procedures, you will be an important part of the healthcare team.

Following are some examples of positions for medical assistants with additional experience and certifications:

- Medical Office Manager
- Medical Assisting Instructor (with a specified amount of experience and education)
- ECG Technician
- Patient Care Technician
- Medical Biller and Coder

If you are multiskilled, you will have an advantage when job hunting. Employers are eager to hire multiskilled medical assistants and may even create positions for them.

You can gain multiskill training by showing initiative and a willingness to learn every aspect of the medical facility in which you are working. When you begin working in a medical facility, establish goals regarding your career path and discuss them with your immediate supervisor. Indicate to your supervisor that you would like cross-training in every aspect of the medical facility. Begin in the department in which you are currently working and branch out to other departments once you master the skills needed for your current position. This will demonstrate a commitment to your profession and a strong work ethic. Cross-training is a valuable marketing tool to include on your résumé.

Scope of Practice

Professional development includes knowing your scope of practice and working within it. Medical assistants are not "licensed" healthcare professionals and most often work under a licensed healthcare provider, such as a nurse practitioner or physician. Licensed healthcare professionals may delegate certain duties to a medical assistant, providing she or he has had the appropriate training through an accredited medical assisting program or through on-the-job training provided by the medical facility or physician. Questions often arise regarding the kinds of duties a medical assistant can perform. There is no universal answer to these questions. There is no single national definition of a medical assistant's scope of practice. So, the medical assistant must research the state in which he or she works to learn about the scope of practice. In general, a medical assistant may not perform procedures for which he or she was not educated or trained. The AAMA and AMT are good resources to assist you in your research. The AAMA Occupational Analysis is also a helpful reference source that identifies the procedures that medical assistants are educated to perform.

Networking

Networking is building alliances—socially and professionally. It starts long before your job search. By attending professional association meetings, conferences, or other functions, medical assistants generate opportunities for employment and personal and professional growth. Networking, through continuing education conferences throughout your career, keeps the doors open to employment advancement.

PROCEDURE 1-1 Obtaining Certification/Registration Information through the Internet

Procedure Goal: To obtain information from the Internet regarding professional credentialing.

OSHA Guidelines: This procedure does not involve exposure to blood, body fluids, or tissue.

Materials: Computer with Internet access and printer.

Method: Procedure steps.

1. Open your Internet browser and locate a search engine. Search for the credential you would like to pursue; for example, Certified Medical Assistant or Registered Medical Assistant. If you are unsure of the credential you would like to pursue, you may just want to search for "Medical Assisting Credentials."

2. Select the site for the credential you are pursuing. Avoid sponsored links. These links are paid for and typically will not bring you to the site of a credentialing organization.

3. To navigate to the home page:
   - For the CMA (AAMA) credential, enter the site www.aama-ntl.org.

    AMERICAN ASSOCIATION OF MEDICAL ASSISTANTS

   - For the RMA (AMT) or CMAS (AMT) credential, enter the site www.americanmedtech.org.

    AMT American Medical Technologists Certifying Excellence in Allied Health

4. Determine the steps you must take to obtain the selected credential.
   - For CMA (AAMA), go to the drop-down menu "CMA (AAMA) Exam" and select the link "How to Become a CMA (AAMA)" (or "About the Exam" in 2013).
   - For RMA (AMT), look for "Certification," and then "Medical Assistant" for RMA (AMT). Navigate to "Qualifications."

5. Print or write down the qualifications you must obtain. **RATIONALE:** Maintaining a record of needed qualifications will be a reference as you pursue your chosen credential.

6. Once you have met the qualifications, you will need to apply for the examination or certification. Download the application and the application instructions for the RMA (AMT) or the CMAS (AMT) or the candidate application and handbook for the CMA (AAMA).

7. To view or print these instructions, you may need to download Adobe Reader. You can click on a link to download Adobe Reader after you click on the "Apply for Certification" link for AMT or the "Apply for the CMA (AAMA) Exam" (or "Apply for the Exam" in 2013) for AAMA.

8. Before or after you apply for the examination, you will need to prepare for the examination. Select the link "Prepare for the CMA (AAMA) Exam" (or "Study for the Exam" in 2013) on the AAMA site or the "Prepare for Exam" link under the "Medical Assistant" or "Medical Assistant Specialist" drop-down menus on the AMT site.

9. Prepare for the exam by reviewing the content outline, obtaining additional study resources, or taking a practice exam online.

10. Print or save downloaded information in a file folder on your desktop labeled "Credentials" or something that you can recognize. To print, click the printer icon found at the bottom of the Web page or click the printer icon in your browser.

11. Return to the appropriate site if you have additional questions. For the CMA (AAMA) site, you may want to check the "FAQs on CMA (AAMA) Certification" link. On the AMT site for RMA or CMAS, find links for Taking the Exam or FAQs (frequently asked questions).

12. Any questions you have that are not addressed on the sites can be e-mailed to the organizations. For RMA, send an e-mail to the link rma@amt1.com. On the AAMA site for the CMA credential, click the "Contact" link on the top right-hand side of the screen.

SUMMARY OF LEARNING OUTCOMES

LEARNING OUTCOMES	KEY POINTS
1.1 Recognize the duties and responsibilities of a medical assistant.	The duties and responsibilities of a medical assistant include administrative, clinical, and laboratory. Duties range from entry-level to advanced and are listed in Table 1-1.
1.2 Distinguish various organizations related to the medical assisting profession.	Many organizations provide certification and support to the medical assisting profession. The AAMA and AMT are highly recognized professional associations that can help you progress in your medical assisting career.

LEARNING OUTCOMES	KEY POINTS
1.3 **Explain the need for and importance of the medical assistant credentials.**	Certification and registration provide recognition of your education by peers and for advancement in your career. Medical assistants with a credential can expect more and better employment opportunities.
1.4 **Identify the training needed to become a professional medical assistant.**	Professional training for medical assistants includes formal training in a variety of educational settings. Training at a program accredited by CAAHEP or ABHES requires you to obtain work experience while you are still in school.
1.5 **Discuss professional development as it relates to medical assisting education.**	Professional development refers to skills and knowledge attained for both personal development and career advancement. Continuing education, cross-training, and pursuing additional training help you develop within your profession. Medical assistants who network, work within their scope of practice, and are more multiskilled are much more marketable.

CASE STUDY CRITICAL THINKING

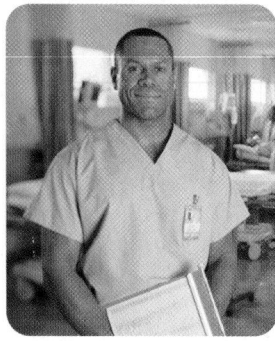

Recall Sandro Peso from the beginning of the chapter. Now that you have completed the chapter, answer the following questions regarding his situation.

1. Describe for Sandro the skills he may perform in each of the three areas (administrative, clinical, and laboratory) of medical assisting at BWW Associates office.

2. Why should Sandro obtain a credential and membership to a professional organization?
3. How can Sandro find out what to expect on his certification test?
4. What suggestions would you give Sandro to assist him in obtaining the best job?

EXAM PREPARATION QUESTIONS

1. (LO 1.3) Two accrediting bodies for medical assisting training programs are
   a. ABHES and OSHA
   b. OSHA and AAMA
   c. ABHES and CAAHEP
   d. CAAHEP and CLIA
   e. CAAHEP and NHA

2. (LO 1.1) Entry-level administrative duties for a medical assistant include
   a. Patient education, drawing blood, and negotiating leases
   b. Taking vital signs and calling in prescriptions
   c. Creating and maintaining patient medical records, and billing and coding
   d. Performing ECGs, infection control, and billing and coding
   e. Checking vital signs and creating and maintaining patient medical records

3. (LO 1.2) The main purpose of the American Association of Medical Assistants (AAMA) is to
   a. Raise the standards of professionalism
   b. Assist with malpractice lawsuits
   c. Provide externships
   d. Support continuing education for CMAs (AAMA) and RMAs (AMT)
   e. Provide accreditation for medical assisting programs

4. (LO 1.2) You want to obtain an RMA credential. Which organization do you need to contact?
   a. NHA
   b. AAMA
   c. CAAHEP
   d. ABHES
   e. AMT

5. (LO 1.5) Which of the following is the best description of networking?
   a. Building alliances that generate opportunities
   b. Practical work experience during training
   c. Official authorization of medical assisting educational programs
   d. Training in every aspect of the medical facility
   e. Using the Internet

6. (LO 1.5) Which of the following is most likely the best reason for you to become multiskilled?
   a. Reduction of healthcare costs
   b. Learning of new skills
   c. Increased employment opportunities
   d. Ability to work two jobs
   e. Reduced wages

7. (LO 1.2) You have become a member of the AAMA. Which of the following is most likely one of your benefits?
   a. Medical transcription
   b. Accreditation
   c. Cross-training
   d. Increased wages
   e. Group insurance

8. (LO 1.1) Which of the following would you be expected to do as an entry-level clinical medical assistant?
   a. Develop public outreach programs
   b. Be a HIPAA compliance officer
   c. Arrange laboratory services
   d. Arrange outpatient diagnostic tests
   e. Sterilize medical instruments

9. (LO 1.3) Which of the following is *least* likely the reason for the increased need to obtain a medical assisting credential?
   a. OSHA regulations
   b. An increase in malpractice
   c. An increase in organizations that require certification
   d. CLIA regulations
   e. An increase in multiskilled employees

10. (LO 1.2) Which of the following does *not* provide a certification examination for the medical assisting profession?
    a. NAHP
    b. AMT
    c. AMA
    d. NCCT
    e. NHA

2 Healthcare and the Healthcare Team

C A S E   S T U D Y

EMPLOYEE INFORMATION

Employee Name	Gender	Date of Hire
Miguel A. Perez	M	6/21/20XX

Position	Credentials	Supervisor
Administrative Assistant	CMA (AAMA)	Malik Katahri, CMM

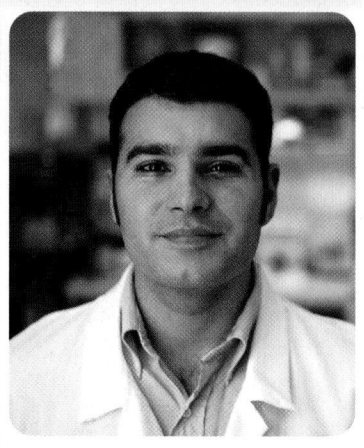

Miguel A. Perez, CMA (AAMA), is the administrative assistant at BWW Associates. He came in early to get caught up on some important duties. He needs to schedule consults for Raja Lautu and Ken Washington, call in a medication refill for Sylvia Gonzales, and verify insurance coverage for Cindy Chen. Just as he is getting started, Kaylyn Haddix, RMA (AMT), calls from one of the exam rooms and tells him to call 911 because a patient has just gone into cardiac arrest. So much for coming in early; looks like it is going to be a busy day.

Keep Miguel in mind as you study this chapter. There will be questions at the end of the chapter based on the case study. The information in the chapter will help you answer these questions.

L E A R N I N G   O U T C O M E S

After completing Chapter 2, you will be able to:

2.1 Discuss healthcare and healthcare trends and their relationship to medical assistant practice.

2.2 Identify medical specialties and specialists certified by the American Board of Medical Specialties (ABMS).

2.3 Recognize the duties of various allied health professionals with whom medical assistants may work.

2.4 Compare specialty careers that a medical assistant may choose for advancement.

2.5 Differentiate professional associations that relate to healthcare and their relationship to the medical assisting profession.

K E Y   T E R M S

anaphylactic shock
autopsy
biopsy
board-certified physician
cardiac rehabilitation
electronic health records (EHR)
meridians

osteopathic manipulative medicine (OMM)
preventive care
primary care physician (PCP)
triage
wellness
whole foods

IV. P (3) Use medical terminology, pronouncing medical terms correctly, to communicate information, patient history, data and observations

IX. C (7) Compare and contrast physician and medical assistant roles in terms of standard of care

IX. P (2) Perform within scope of practice

1. **General Orientation**
   b. Compare and contrast the allied health professions and understand their relation to medical assisting
   d. Have knowledge of the general responsibilities of the medical assistant
   e. Define scope of practice for the medical assistant, and comprehend the conditions for practice within the state that the medical assistant is employed

3. **Medical Terminology**
   Graduates:
   c. Understand the various medical terminology for each specialty

11. **Career Development**
    Graduates:
    b. Demonstrate professionalism by:
       (4) Being cognizant of ethical boundaries
       (9) Conducting work within scope of education, training, and ability

▶ Introduction

Medical assistants are an integral part of a healthcare delivery team. As such, you should recognize healthcare trends and facilities as well as the different physician specialists, allied health professionals, specialty medical assistant careers, and healthcare organizations. Medical assistants work in various roles and must be in contact with multiple other healthcare team members on an ongoing basis. For example, medical assistants are asked to call and process insurance referrals to different specialties and diagnostic departments, or they may need to contact the pharmacy to renew a prescription. A working knowledge of the different specialties and allied health professions demonstrates professionalism and competence, and assists the medical assistant in developing a spirit of cooperation. Recognizing the functions of specialty careers and healthcare associations will help the practicing medical assistant perform his duties, as well as provide for advancement.

▶ Healthcare and Facilities LO 2.1

For as long as human beings have lived on this planet, they have been practicing medicine in some form. Some cultures credited health and illness to the moods of the gods. Others used reason to attempt to explain the causes of disease. Archaeological and anthropological findings tell us that many so-called primitive cultures practiced healing in a variety of ways. Not unlike today, healers in ancient times used natural remedies such as diet, rest, and medications made from herbs and other plants. They even performed surgery. Religion also played an important role in healthcare. Many

cultures combined the use of medications or surgery with religious rites. The evolution of healthcare continues today. Knowledge of current healthcare trends and healthcare practice settings will assist you in determining your future role as a medical assistant.

Healthcare Trends

Consider the following healthcare trends and how they may affect your practice as a medical assistant.

Technology Over the last decade, the advancement of technology has affected all aspects of our life. This holds true in the field of healthcare. Healthcare has always been affected by science and technology. For example, during the 1970s, mobile telephones seemed to be just the imaginings of science fiction. Today, a medical assistant can carry a smartphone in a pocket for easy reference and for professional communication with patients and members of the healthcare team.

Paper charts are becoming a thing of the past. The use of **electronic health records (EHR)** is gaining momentum and should be accomplished by 2014 (Figure 2-1). EHR allows all of a patient's data to be accessible in one location. An electronic chart provides quick access and helps to prevent mistakes with medication and other medical errors. The *Electronic Health Records* chapter will provide details about how to use this essential tool.

Preventive Care and Wellness The terms *preventive care* and *wellness* can bring to mind anything from massage therapy to **whole foods**. Whole foods are those that have little or no processing before they are eaten. The idea of **wellness** includes fitness. The link between exercise, diet, and good health is strong.

FIGURE 2-1 Healthcare employees including medical assistants must be able to use electronic health records.

Screening tests and drugs to prevent disease are common in **preventive care**. A healthy lifestyle goes a long way toward improving your quality of life. Aging baby boomers, physicians, insurance companies, and fitness experts all recognize the value of good health. As a medical assistant, maintaining your own health as well as guiding patients to better health practices is a must.

Aging Population After World War II, the U.S. economy boomed. There were plenty of jobs and people could afford to have large families. This resulted in a phenomenon known as the baby boom, which occurred from 1946 to 1964. Many of these babies are now in retirement age. In 2011, the first boomers began to receive Medicare, our national health insurance for the elderly. Because older adults require more healthcare services, medical assistants will most likely work with these patients.

Ambulatory Care Many procedures, from diagnosis to treatment, are done on an outpatient basis. A patient may walk into a clinic in the morning, have tests or surgery, and go home in the afternoon. Procedures that once required hospitalization now are done in outpatient centers. Outpatient care is also known as ambulatory care. Medical assistants may work in all types of ambulatory care facilities.

Healthcare Facilities

There are numerous types of healthcare facilities where medical assistants may work. These include physicians' offices, clinics, urgent care centers, and hospitals. All four of these types of facilities provide ambulatory care, which is the most common practice area of a medical assistant.

Two other types of healthcare facilities include long-term care and hospice care. Long-term care centers provide care to people who need nursing or other professional healthcare services on a regular basis. These patients may not need round-the-clock nursing services, but it may be unsafe for them to live alone or they may have needs their family cannot meet. Many residents in long-term care facilities are frail or elderly. They also may be handicapped or disabled. Hospice is usually offered only to patients who are thought to have fewer than six months to live. An example of a hospice patient is a person who has terminal cancer (Figure 2-2). Anyone who has a terminal condition is eligible for this type of care.

FIGURE 2-2 Hospice care provides for the needs of patients who are dying including the need for touch.

▶ Medical Specialties LO 2.2

Since the beginning of the 20th century, some physicians have specialized in particular areas of study. According to the American Board of Medical Specialties (ABMS), approximately 24 major medical specialties are now approved in the United States. The primary purpose of the ABMS is to maintain and improve the quality of medical care and to certify doctors in various specialties. This organization helps the member boards develop professional and educational standards for physician specialists.

Within each medical specialty are several subspecialties. For example, cardiology is a major specialty; pediatric cardiology is a subspecialty. As advances in the diagnosis and treatment of diseases and disorders unfold, the demand for specialized care increases and more medical specialties emerge. The education and licensing process for **board-certified physicians** is long—anywhere from 9 to 12 years—and requires multiple board tests. A medical assistant may be the "right arm" to any of the following types of physicians.

Family Practice

Family practitioners (sometimes called general practitioners) are medical doctors (MDs) or doctors of osteopathy (DOs) who are generalists and treat all types of illnesses and ages of patients. The difference between DO and MD is discussed later. Family practitioners are called **primary care physicians (PCPs)** by insurance companies. The term refers to individual doctors who oversee patients' long-term healthcare. Some people, however, have internists or OB/GYNs as their primary care physician.

A family practitioner sends a patient to a specialist when the patient has a specific condition or disease that requires advanced care. For example, a family practitioner refers a patient with a lump in her breast to an oncologist, a specialist who treats tumors, or to a general surgeon. Either of these doctors may order a mammogram or an ultrasound (if these have not already been done). A needle biopsy of the lump is done by the specialist to determine if the lump is malignant.

Working in a general practice, you will encounter patients with many different conditions and illnesses. If you work for a general practitioner, you will often be responsible for arranging patient appointments with specialists. It is therefore important for you to be familiar with the duties of each medical specialist.

Allergy

Allergists diagnose and treat physical reactions to substances such as mold, dust, fur, and pollen from plants or flowers. An individual with allergies is hypersensitive to substances such as drugs, chemicals, or elements in nature. An allergic reaction may be minor, such as a rash; serious, such as asthma; or life-threatening, such as **anaphylactic shock**, which causes swelling of the airways or nasal passages.

Anesthesiology

Anesthesiologists and anesthetists use medications that cause patients to lose sensation or feeling during surgery. These healthcare practitioners administer anesthetics before, during, and sometimes even after surgery. They also educate patients regarding the anesthetic that will be used and its possible postoperative effects. An anesthesiologist is an MD. A certified registered nurse anesthetist (CRNA) is a registered nurse who has completed an additional program of study recognized by the American Association of Nurse Anesthetists.

Bariatrics

Bariatrics is the specialty of medicine that deals with the medical and surgical treatment of obesity. Bariatric surgery may be recommended for extremely obese patients who may suffer impaired health as a result of their weight. Prior to undergoing any type of bariatric surgery, candidates must first undergo counseling and other treatment options for weight management. Therapy before and after bariatric surgery is necessary for successful weight loss and improved health. Several options are available in bariatric surgery, including gastric banding and gastric bypass.

Cardiology

Cardiologists diagnose and treat cardiovascular diseases (diseases of the heart and blood vessels). Cardiologists also read electrocardiograms (ECGs, which are sometimes referred to as EKGs) for hospital cardiology departments. They educate patients about the positive role healthy diet and regular exercise play in preventing and controlling heart disease and recommend cardiovascular rehabilitation when needed (Figure 2-3). **Cardiac rehabilitation** is education, exercise, and therapy for patients who have a cardiovascular disease or disorder, such as patients who have had a heart attack.

FIGURE 2-3 A cardiologist may order a test that monitors the patient's heart while he is exercising.

Dermatology

Dermatologists diagnose and treat diseases of the skin, hair, and nails. Their patients have conditions ranging from warts and acne to skin cancer. Dermatologists treat boils, skin injuries, and infections. They also remove growths such as moles, cysts, and birthmarks; treat scars; and perform hair transplants.

Osteopathy

Osteopathic manipulative medicine (OMM) is a system of hands-on techniques that help relieve pain, restore motion, support the body's natural functions, and influence the body's structure. Osteopathic physicians study OMM in addition to medical courses. Doctors of osteopathy, who hold the title of DO, practice a "whole-person" approach to healthcare. DOs believe that patients are more than just a sum of their body parts, and they treat the patient as a whole person instead of concentrating on specific symptoms. Osteopathic physicians understand how all the body's systems are interconnected and how each one affects the other. They focus special attention on the musculoskeletal system, which reflects and influences the condition of all other body systems.

One key concept that DOs believe is that structure influences function. If a problem exists in one part of the body, it may affect the function in both that area and other areas. DOs focus on the body's ability to heal itself and they actively engage patients in the healing process. By using osteopathic manipulative medicine (OMM) techniques such as muscle energy and counterstrain techniques, DOs can help restore motion to these areas of the body, thus improving function and often restoring health.

Emergency Medicine

Physicians who specialize in emergency medicine work in hospital emergency rooms and outpatient emergency care centers. They diagnose and treat patients with conditions resulting from an unexpected medical crisis or accident. Common emergencies include trauma, such as gunshot wounds or serious injuries from car accidents; other injuries, such as severe cuts; and sudden illness, such as alcohol or food poisoning. Emergency medicine practitioners stabilize their patients so they can then be managed by their PCP or other specialist.

Endocrinology

Endocrinologists diagnose and treat disorders of the endocrine system. This system regulates many body functions by circulating hormones that are secreted by organs and glands throughout the body. An example of a disorder treated by an endocrinologist is hypothyroidism, in which a patient has a lower-than-normal amount of thyroid hormone. This common disorder can cause a variety of symptoms including fatigue, weight gain, dry skin, and constipation.

Gastroenterology

Gastroenterologists diagnose and treat disorders of the gastrointestinal tract. These disorders include problems related to the functioning of the stomach, intestines, and associated organs.

Examples include ulcers, irritable bowel syndrome (IBS), and gastroesophageal reflux disease (GERD).

Gerontology

Gerontologists study the aging process. Geriatrics is the branch of medicine that deals with the diagnosis and treatment of problems and diseases of the older adult. A specialist in geriatrics may also be called a geriatrician. As the population of older adults increases, there is a greater need for physicians who specialize in diagnosing and treating diseases of older patients.

Gynecology

Gynecology is the branch of medicine that is concerned with diseases and conditions of the female genital tract, such as yeast infections, menstrual irregularities, and sexually transmitted infections (STIs). Gynecologists perform routine physical care and examination of the female reproductive system. Many gynecologists are also obstetricians.

Internal Medicine

Internists, or doctors of internal medicine, specialize in diagnosing and treating problems related to the internal organs. The internal medicine subspecialties include cardiology, critical care medicine, diagnostic laboratory immunology, endocrinology and metabolism, gastroenterology, geriatrics, hematology, infectious diseases, medical oncology, nephrology, pulmonary disease, and rheumatology. Internists must be certified as specialists to practice in any of these areas.

Nephrology

Nephrologists study, diagnose, and manage diseases of the kidney. They may work in either a clinic or hospital setting. A medical assistant working with a nephrologist may assist in the operation of a dialysis unit for the treatment of patients with kidney failure, known as end stage renal disease (ESRD). In a rural setting, a medical assistant might help a doctor operate a mobile dialysis unit that can be taken to the patient's home or to a medical practice that does not have this technology.

Neurology

Neurology is the branch of medical science that deals with the nervous system. Neurologists diagnose and treat disorders and diseases of the nervous system, such as strokes. The nervous system is made up of the brain, the spinal cord, and nerves that receive, interpret, and transmit messages throughout the body.

Nuclear Medicine

Nuclear medicine is a fast-growing specialty related to radiology. Nuclear medicine and radiology use radiation to diagnose and treat disease, but radiology beams radiation through the body from an outside source, whereas nuclear medicine introduces a small amount of a radioactive substance into the body and forms an image by detecting radiation as it leaves the body. The radiation that patients are exposed to is comparable to

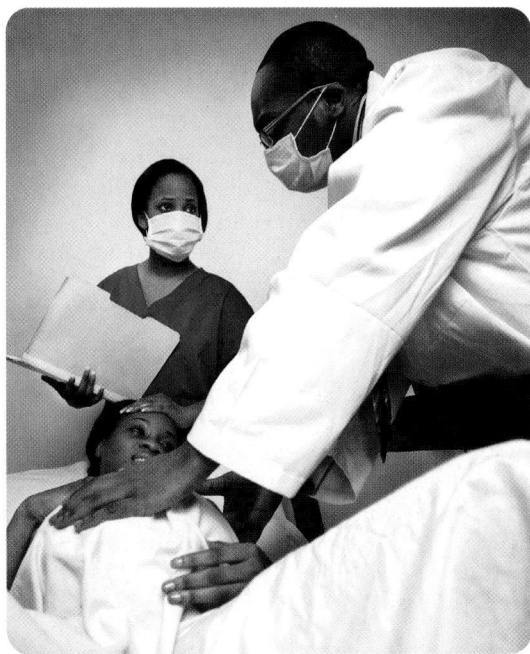

FIGURE 2-4 Obstetricians who are part of a private practice are usually connected with a specific hospital where they help their patients through labor and delivery.

that of a diagnostic X-ray. Radiology reveals interior anatomy, whereas nuclear medicine reveals organ function and structure. Noninvasive, painless nuclear medicine procedures are used to identify heart disease, assess organ function, and diagnose and treat cancer.

Obstetrics

Obstetrics involves the study of pregnancy, labor, delivery, and the period following labor, called postpartum (Figure 2-4). This field is often combined with gynecology. A physician who practices both specialties is referred to as an obstetrician/gynecologist, or OB/GYN.

Oncology

Oncologists determine whether tumors are benign or malignant and treat patients who have cancer. Treatment may involve chemotherapy, which is the administration of drugs to destroy cancer cells. Treatment may also involve radiation therapy, which kills cancer cells through the use of X-rays. Newer therapies include immune therapy, also called immunotherapy, and transplant techniques to urge the body to create healthy tissues to replace those affected by cancer. Oncologists treat both adults and children.

Ophthalmology

An ophthalmologist is an MD who diagnoses and treats diseases and disorders of the eye. This physician specialist examines patients' eyes for poor vision or disease. Other responsibilities include prescribing corrective lenses or medication, performing surgery, and providing follow-up care after surgery. The specialty of ophthalmology includes two other

types of practitioners who are not MDs: optometrists and opticians. An optometrist obtains the credential of OD (optometric doctor) and specializes in diagnosing and treating visual defects with glasses and contacts. An optician is a specialist who works with ophthalmologists and optometrists by filling the prescriptions written by them for glasses and contact lenses.

Orthopedics

Orthopedics is a branch of medicine that specializes in maintaining the function of the musculoskeletal system and its associated structures. An orthopedist diagnoses and treats diseases and disorders of the muscles and bones. Some orthopedists, called sports medicine specialists, concentrate on treating sports-related injuries, either exclusively for professional athletes or for nonprofessionals of all ages.

Otorhinolaryngology

Otorhinolaryngology involves the study of the ear, nose, and throat. An otorhinolaryngologist diagnoses and treats diseases of these body structures. This physician specialist is also referred to as an ear, nose, and throat (ENT) specialist. Otorhinolaryngology is also called otolaryngology, according to the American Academy of Otolaryngology.

Pathology

Pathology is the study of disease. It provides the scientific foundation for all medical practice. The pathologist studies the changes a disease produces in the cells, fluids, tissues, and processes of the entire body. These samples often come from **biopsies** (samplings of cells that could be malignant or cancerous), cultures, and tissue samples. Some pathologists also perform **autopsies**, examinations of the bodies of the deceased, to determine the cause of a patient's death and to advance the clinical practice of medicine.

There are two basic types of pathologists: forensic pathologists and anatomic pathologists. Governments and police departments use forensic pathologists to determine facts about unexplained or violent crimes or deaths. Anatomic pathologists often work at hospitals in a research capacity, and they may read biopsies.

Pediatrics and Adolescent Medicine

Pediatrics is concerned with the development and care of children and adolescents from birth until 18 (in some practices, up to 21) years. A pediatrician diagnoses and treats childhood diseases and teaches parents skills to keep their children healthy.

Physical Medicine

Physical medicine specialists (physiatrists) are physicians who specialize in physical medicine and rehabilitation. They are certified by the American Board of Physical Medicine and Rehabilitation to diagnose and treat diseases and disorders such as sore shoulders and spinal cord injuries. Physiatrists offer an aggressive, nonsurgical approach to pain and injury for both adults and children.

Podiatry

Podiatry is practiced by a licensed doctor of podiatric medicine (DPM). A podiatrist is a podiatry professional devoted to the study and treatment of the foot and ankle. Podiatrists may diagnose, treat, prescribe medication, and perform surgery for disorders of the foot and, in some states, the ankle and leg.

Plastic Surgery

A plastic surgeon performs the reconstruction, correction, or improvement of body structures. Patients may be accident victims or disfigured due to disease or abnormal development. Plastic surgery includes facial reconstruction, facelifts, and skin grafting. Plastic surgery is also used to repair problems such as cleft lip and cleft palate, as well as disfigurement and restrictive scarring due to trauma.

Proctology

Proctology is the branch of medicine that diagnoses and treats disorders of the anus, rectum, and intestines. Proctologists treat conditions such as colitis, hemorrhoids, fistulas, tumors, and ulcers. Proctologists often work closely with urologists.

Radiology

Radiology is the branch of medical science that uses X-rays and radioactive substances to diagnose and treat disease. Radiologists specialize in taking and reading X-rays. X-rays are used mostly for diagnosis; for example, to determine whether bones are broken or whether a patient has pneumonia. Other radioactive substances can be carefully applied to help kill cancer cells and reduce the size of malignant tumors.

Sports Medicine

Sports medicine is an interdisciplinary subspecialty of medicine that deals with the treatment and preventative care of amateur and professional athletes. Sports medicine teams consist of specialty physicians and surgeons, athletic trainers, and physical therapists. Sports medicine involves more than just treating injuries to the musculoskeletal system. Sports medicine can include an array of services, such as prevention and nutritional health.

Surgery

Surgeons use their hands and medical instruments to diagnose and correct deformities and treat external and internal injuries or disease (Figure 2-5). They work with many different specialists to surgically treat a broad range of disorders. General surgeons may, for example, perform operations as diverse as breast lumpectomy and repair of a pacemaker. There are also subspecialties of surgery, such as neurosurgery, vascular surgery, and orthopedic surgery.

Urology

A urologist diagnoses and treats diseases of the kidney, bladder, and urinary system. A urologist's patients include infants, children, and adults of all ages. Urologists also treat male reproductive diseases.

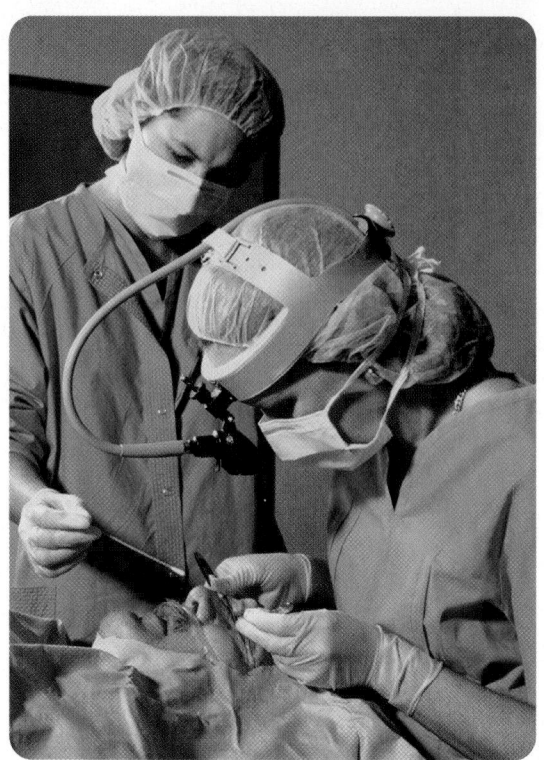

FIGURE 2-5 Most surgeons specialize in a particular type of surgery, such as heart surgery or eye surgery.

▶ Working with Other Healthcare Professionals
LO 2.3

A medical assistant is a member of a healthcare team. Working as a team member is discussed in the chapter *Professionalism and Success*. That healthcare team includes doctors, nurses, specialists, and the patients themselves. Your contact with other members of the team will occur in person, electronically, or by telephone. You should recognize and understand the duties of other allied health professionals in order to be effective in your role as a medical assistant. The following is an introduction to some common allied health professionals.

Acupuncturist

Acupuncturists treat people who have pain or discomfort by inserting thin, hollow needles under the skin. The points used for insertion are selected to balance the flow of qi (pronounced chee), or life energy, in the body. The theory of acupuncture relates to traditional Chinese beliefs about how the body works. Qi is composed of two opposite forces called yin and yang. If the flow of qi is unbalanced, insufficient, or interrupted, then emotional, spiritual, mental, and physical problems will result. The acupuncturist works to balance these two forces in perfect harmony. Although there are variations in types of acupuncture—Chinese, Korean, and Japanese—all practitioners focus on many pulse points along

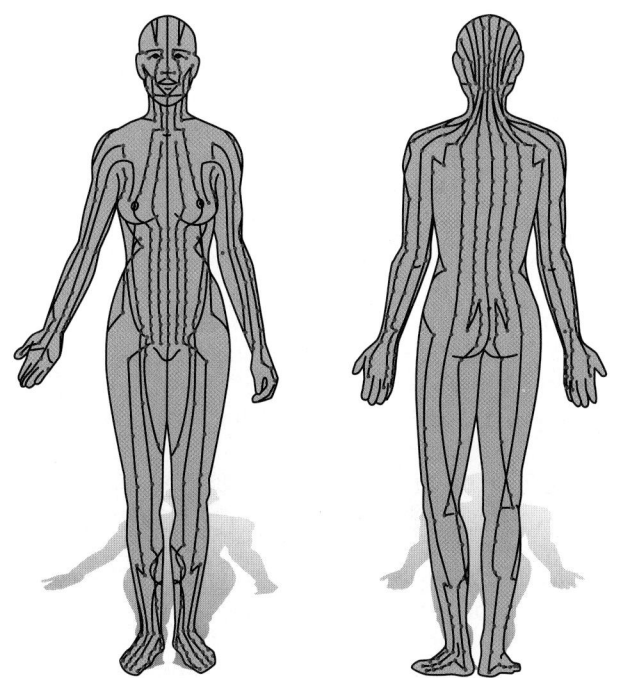

FIGURE 2-6 Meridians are pathways for blood flow in the body that are treated as part of traditional Chinese medicine to restore the body's harmony and wellness.

FIGURE 2-7 Massage uses kneading, pressure, stroking, and human touch to alleviate pain and promote healing through relaxation.

different **meridians**, the channels through which qi flows (Figure 2-6).

Chiropractor

Chiropractors treat people using manual treatments, although they also may employ physical therapy treatments, exercise programs, nutritional advice, and lifestyle modification to help correct problems causing the pain. The manual treatments, called adjustments, realign the vertebrae in the spine and restore the function of spinal nerves. Chiropractors use diagnostic testing such as X-rays, muscle testing, and posture analysis to determine the location of spinal misalignments, also called subluxations. Using their findings, they develop a treatment plan that may require several adjustments per week for several weeks or months.

Electroencephalographic Technologist

Electroencephalography (EEG) is the study and recording of the electrical activity of the brain. It is used to diagnose diseases and irregularities of the brain. The EEG technologist (sometimes called a technician) attaches electrodes to the patient's scalp and connects them to a recording instrument. The machine then provides a written record of the electrical activity of the patient's brain. EEG technologists work in hospital EEG laboratories, clinics, and physicians' offices.

Massage Therapist

Massage is one of the oldest methods of promoting healing. Massage therapists use pressure, kneading, stroking, vibration, and tapping to promote muscle and full-body relaxation, as well as to increase circulation and lymph flow (Figure 2-7). Increasing circulation helps remove blood and waste products from injured tissues and brings fresh blood and nutrients to the areas to speed healing. Massage is used to treat strains, bruises, muscle soreness or tightness, lower back pain, and dislocations. It also can relieve muscle spasms, restore motion and function to a body part, and decrease edema.

Medical Technology

Medical technology is an umbrella term that refers to the development and design of clinical laboratory tests (such as diagnostic tests), procedures, and equipment. Two types of allied health professionals who work in medical technology are the medical laboratory technician and the medical laboratory scientist.

Medical laboratory technicians (CLTs) have 2-year degrees and are responsible for clinical tests performed under the supervision of a physician or medical technologist. They perform tests in the areas of hematology, serology, blood banking, urinalysis, microbiology, and clinical chemistry.

Medical laboratory scientists examine specimens of human body tissues and fluids, analyze blood factors, and culture bacteria to identify disease-causing organisms. They also supervise and train technicians and laboratory aides. Medical laboratory scientists have 4-year degrees and may specialize in areas such as blood banking, microbiology, and chemistry.

Nuclear Medicine Technologist

A nuclear medicine technologist performs tests to oversee quality control, to prepare and administer radioactive drugs, and to operate radiation detection instruments (Figure 2-8). This allied health professional is also responsible for correctly positioning the patient, performing imaging procedures, and preparing the information for use by a physician.

FIGURE 2-8 A nuclear medicine technologist positions the patient, performs imaging procedures, and prepares the information for use by a physician.

Occupational Therapist

An occupational therapist works with patients who have physical injuries or illnesses, psychological or developmental problems, or problems associated with the aging process. This health professional helps patients attain maximum physical and mental health by using educational, vocational, and rehabilitation therapies and activities. The occupational therapist may work in a hospital, clinic, extended-care facility, rehabilitation hospital, or government or community agency.

Pharmacist

Pharmacists are professionals who have studied the science of drugs and who dispense medication and health supplies to the public. Pharmacists know the chemical and physical qualities of drugs and are knowledgeable about the companies that manufacture drugs.

Pharmacists inform the public about the effects of prescription and nonprescription (over-the-counter) medications. Pharmacists are employed in hospitals, clinics, and nursing homes. They also may work for government agencies, pharmaceutical companies, privately owned pharmacies, or chain store pharmacies. Some pharmacists own their own stores. Pharmacists must have 5 to 7 years of education, be registered by the state, and pass a state board examination.

Physical Therapist

A physical therapist (PT) plans and uses physical therapy programs for medically referred patients. The PT helps these patients to restore function, relieve pain, and prevent disability following disease, injury, or loss of body parts. A physical therapist uses various treatment methods, which include therapy with electricity, heat, cold, ultrasound, massage, and exercise. The physical therapist also helps patients accept their disabilities.

Radiologic Technology

A radiographer (X-ray technician) is one of the most common positions for individuals whose education is in radiologic technology. The radiographer assists a radiologist in taking X-ray films, which are used to diagnose broken bones, tumors, ulcers, and disease. A radiographer usually works in the radiology department of a hospital. The X-ray technician may, however, use mobile X-ray equipment in a patient's room or in the operating room.

A radiologic technologist studies the theory and practice of the technical aspects of the use of X-rays and radioactive materials in the diagnosis and treatment of disease. A radiologic technologist may specialize in radiography, radiation therapy, or nuclear medicine.

A radiation therapy technologist assists the radiologist. He may, for example, assist with administering radiation treatments to patients who have cancer. He also may be responsible for maintaining radiation treatment equipment. The technologist shares responsibility with the radiologist for the accuracy of treatment records.

Registered Dietitian

Registered dietitians help patients and their families make healthful food choices. These choices provide balanced, adequate nutrition, particularly when disease or illness makes knowing what to eat to help fight the disease difficult. Dietitians are sometimes confused with nutritionists. A dietician has specialized training to assist ill patients with their nutritional needs; a nutritionist's goal is for those of us who are healthy to maintain a lifestyle of healthful eating. Dietitians may assist food-service directors at healthcare facilities and prepare and serve food to groups. They also may participate in food research and teach nutrition classes. Dietitians work in a variety of healthcare settings and also may teach at colleges and universities.

Respiratory Therapy

A respiratory therapist evaluates, treats, and cares for patients with respiratory problems. The respiratory therapist works under the supervision of a physician and performs therapeutic procedures based on observation of the patient. Using respiratory equipment, the therapist treats patients with asthma, emphysema, pneumonia, and bronchitis. The respiratory therapist plays an active role in newborn, pediatric, and adult intensive care units.

Respiratory therapy technicians work under the supervision of a physician and a respiratory therapist. In addition to performing procedures such as artificial ventilation, they clean, sterilize, and maintain the respiratory equipment and document the patient's therapy in the medical record.

Nursing Aide/Assistant

Nursing aides assist in the direct care of patients under the supervision of the nursing staff. Typical functions include making beds, bathing patients, taking vital signs, serving meals, and transporting patients to and from treatment areas. Certification as a certified nursing assistant (CNA) is available and is required by many healthcare facilities, especially long-term care facilities.

Practical/Vocational Nurse

Licensed practical nurses (LPNs) and licensed vocational nurses (LVNs) are different names for the same type of nurse. Their duties involve taking and recording patient temperatures, blood pressure, pulse, and respiration rates. They also include administering some medications under supervision, dressing wounds, and applying compresses. LPNs and LVNs are not allowed, however, to perform certain other duties, such as some intravenous (IV) procedures or the administration of certain medications. LPNs/LVNs can obtain additional training to become certified in IV therapy.

Practical/vocational nurses assist registered nurses and physicians by observing patients and reporting changes in their conditions. LPNs/LVNs work in hospitals, nursing homes, clinics, and physicians' offices and in industrial medicine. To meet the needs of the growing aging population in this country, employment opportunities for LPNs and LVNs in long-term care settings have increased. LPNs/LVNs must graduate from an accredited school of practical (vocational) nursing (usually a 1-year program). They are also required to take a state board examination for licensure as LPNs/LVNs.

Registered Nurse

A nurse who graduates from a nursing program and passes the state board examination for licensure is considered a registered nurse (RN), indicating formal, legal recognition by the state. The RN is a professional who is responsible for planning, giving, and supervising the bedside nursing care of patients. An RN may work in an administrative capacity, assist in daily operations, oversee programs in hospital or institutional settings, or plan community health services. Registered nurses work in hospitals, nursing homes, public health agencies, physicians' offices, government agencies, and educational settings. They also may work in industry, providing on-site care at manufacturing facilities and other industrial workplaces.

There are three types of nursing education programs that qualify an individual to take a state board examination to become an RN. These include associate degree nurse, diploma graduate, and baccalaureate degree nurse.

Associate Degree Nurse Associate degrees in nursing (ADNs) are offered at many junior colleges and community colleges and at some universities. These programs combine liberal arts education and nursing education. The length of the ADN program is typically 2 years.

Diploma Graduate Nurse Diploma programs are usually 3-year programs designed as cooperative programs between a community college and a participating hospital. The programs combine coursework and clinical experience in the hospital.

Baccalaureate Nurse A baccalaureate degree is awarded by a 4-year college or university program. Graduates of a 4-year nursing program are awarded a bachelor of science in nursing (BSN) degree. The curriculum includes courses in liberal arts, general education, and nursing. Graduates are prepared to function as nurse generalists and in positions that go beyond the role of hospital staff nurses. Some RNs with a BSN will continue their education to earn master's or doctoral degrees.

Nurse Practitioner

A nurse practitioner (NP) is an RN who functions in an expanded nursing role. The NP usually works in an ambulatory patient care setting alongside physicians, but also may work in an independent nurse practitioner practice without physicians. An independent nurse practitioner takes health histories, performs physical exams, conducts screening tests, and educates patients and families about disease prevention.

An NP who works in a physician's practice may perform some duties that a physician would, such as administering physical exams and treating common illnesses and injuries. For example, in an OB/GYN practice, the NP can perform a standard annual gynecologic exam, including taking a Pap smear or a culture to test for a yeast or bacterial infection. The nurse practitioner usually emphasizes preventive healthcare.

The NP must be an RN with at least a master's degree in nursing and must complete 4 to 12 months of an apprenticeship or formal training. With specific formal training, the student may become a pediatric nurse practitioner, an obstetric nurse practitioner (midwife), or a psychiatric nurse practitioner. Clinical medical assistants may work directly with an NP.

Physician Assistant

The physician assistant (PA) practices medicine under the laws of the specific state and the supervision of a physician. PAs provide diagnostic, therapeutic, and preventive healthcare services, as designated by the supervising physician. Physician assistants take medical histories; order laboratory and medical imaging tests; and examine, diagnose, treat, counsel, and follow up with patients. They also perform suturing, casting, and splinting for minor injuries, and some even assist in surgery. PAs also prescribe certain medications. In some cases, managerial duties may be performed, such as purchasing and maintaining equipment and hiring and firing personnel. The physician assistant also may take call duty for the practice and share the responsibility for after-hours call duty with the physician. A medical assistant may work directly with a physician assistant.

Speech/Language Pathologist

A speech/language pathologist treats communication disorders, such as stuttering, and associated disorders, such as hearing impairment. This health professional evaluates, diagnoses, and counsels patients who have these problems. A speech/language pathologist may work in a school, hospital, research setting, or private practice or may teach at a college or university.

▶ Specialty Career Options   LO 2.4

As a medical assistant, you have a multitude of opportunities to specialize by obtaining additional training, education, or certifications. You may determine that you prefer either the administrative or clinical aspect of the work and move forward in your career toward that end. Tables 2-1 and 2-2 highlight some of the careers you may consider.

TABLE 2-1 Administrative Specialty Careers

Career	Duties	Organization(s)
Billing and Insurance Specialist	• Verifies patient insurance coverage. • Processes insurance claims. • Obtains fees for procedures and services performed, from both patients and insurance companies.	American Medical Technologists (AMT), American Medical Billing Association (AMBA)
Certified Medical Reimbursement Specialist (CMRS)	• Facilitates the claims paying process "from patient to payment." • Plays a critical role in the healthcare provider's daily business operations, whether employed by the medical facility or self-employed as a contractor to assist the practice with its accounts receivable processes.	American Medical Billing Association
Compliance Officer	• Reviews and updates the office's policies and procedures manual. • Creates and maintains appropriate coding and billing policies, including audit procedures. • Creates, conducts, and manages compliance education programs for all staff. • Establishes a process for investigating and taking action on all complaints about privacy policies and procedures. • Publicizes the reporting system for all providers, staff, vendors, and business associates. • Analyzes a facility's risk of releasing information incorrectly and sets policies and procedures to avoid these risks.	American Health Information Management Association's Health Care Compliance Association (HCCA), American Academy of Professional Coders (AAPC)
Electronic Claims Professional	• Acts as the link between small-and medium-sized practices and major health insurers such as Medicare. • Contracts with a physician practice or healthcare facility, then enters patient demographic and insurance billing information into the computer billing software and transmits it to the appropriate health insurance provider. • Submits electronic medical (health) insurance claims to an insurance carrier.	Alliance of Claims Assistance Professionals (ACAP), National Association of Claims Assistance Professionals (NACAP)
Medical Biller and Coder, Health Information Coder, or Medical Coder	• Makes sure that all patient charges have been recorded in the billing system. • Enters data such as charges into the patient accounts database. • Prepares claims to send to payers such as insurance agencies. • Prepares bills to send to patients. • Tracks payments due from payers and patients.	American Health Information Management Association (AHIMA), American Academy of Professional Coders (AAPC)
Medical Transcriptionist	• Logs transcriptions of telephone calls or Internet transmissions. • Sorts and distributes transcribed medical reports. • Places the transcribed reports into the appropriate patient accounts in the electronic health records system. • Faxes, e-mails, or uploads transcribed reports to someone other than the originator.	American Association for Medical Transcription
Registered Health Information Technician (RHIT), Medical Record Technician, Medical Chart Specialist	• Manages patient records for a physician, group of physicians, or hospital. • Ensures that all medical information is accurate and complete. • Deals strictly with health information in a hospital and has no patient contact. • Performs additional clerical duties such as answering the telephone in a physician's office. • Checks all patient charts for completeness and accuracy.	American Health Information Management Association

TABLE 2-2   Clinical Specialty Careers

Career	Duties	Organization(s)
Anesthesiologist Assistant	• Provides anesthetic care under an anesthetist's direction. • Gathers patient data and assists in evaluation of patients' physical and mental status. • Records planned surgical procedures, assists with patient monitoring, draws blood samples, performs blood gas analyses, and conducts pulmonary function tests.	American Academy of Anesthesiologist Assistants
Cardiovascular Technologist	• Performs diagnostic examinations and therapeutic interventions of the heart and/or blood vessels at the request or direction of a physician. • Uses various cardiovascular testing techniques to create a foundation of data for patient diagnosis.	Cardiovascular Credentialing International
Dental Assistant	• Performs many administrative and laboratory functions similar to those of a medical assistant. • Serves as chairside assistant, provides instruction in oral hygiene, and prepares and sterilizes instruments.	American Dental Assistant Association
Emergency Medical Technician (EMT)	• Works under the direction of a physician through a radio communication network. • Assesses and manages medical emergencies that occur in private and public locations. • Assesses the urgency and type of condition presented, as well as the immediate medical needs, and initiates the appropriate treatment. This is known as **triage**. • Records, documents, and radios the patient's condition to the physician, describing what has occurred.	National Association of Emergency Medical Technicians
Mental Health Technician (Psychiatric Aide or Counselor)	• Works with emotionally disturbed and mentally challenged patients. • Assists the psychiatric team by observing behavior and providing information to help in the planning of therapy. • Participates in supervising group therapy and counseling sessions.	American Association of Psychiatric Technicians
Occupational Therapist Assistant	• Helps individuals with mental or physical disabilities reach their highest level of functioning through the teaching of fine motor skills, trades (occupations), and the arts. • Prepares materials for activities, maintains tools and equipment, and documents the patient's progress.	American Occupational Therapy Association
Pathologist's Assistant	• May work with forensic pathologists—professionals who study the human body and diseases for legal purposes—in cooperation with government or police investigations. • May prepare frozen sections of dissected body tissue. • May maintain supplies, instruments, and chemicals for the anatomic pathology laboratory. • Performs laboratory work (about 75 percent of the workday) and a variety of administrative duties.	
Pharmacy Technician	• Receives written or electronic prescriptions or telephone requests for prescription refills. • Verifies that the information on the prescription is complete and accurate. • Contacts the insurance company to verify benefits and obtain any patient copay or co-insurance requirements. • Retrieves, counts, pours, weighs, measures, and, if necessary, mixes the medication for the prescription (or script). • Establishes and maintains patient profiles in the pharmacy computer and prepares insurance claim submissions. • Takes inventory of prescription and over-the-counter (OTC) medications. • Assists in equipment maintenance and managing the pharmacy cash register.	National Pharmacy Technician Association and Pharmacy Technician Certification Board
Phlebotomist	• Like a medical assistant, draws blood for diagnostic laboratory testing. • Performs more advanced skills, such as drawing blood under difficult circumstances or in special situations. For example, if a blood sample is needed for an ammonia-level test, it must be drawn and stored in a particular manner only phlebotomists are trained to do.	National Phlebotomy Association (NPA) or American Society of Clinical Pathologists (ASCP)
Physical Therapy Assistant	• Assists with patient treatment by following the patient care program created by the physical therapist and physician. • Performs tests and treatment procedures, assembles or sets up equipment for therapy sessions, and observes and documents patient behavior and progress.	American Physical Therapy Association
Surgical Technician	• Obtains a patient's history and physical data. • Discusses the data with a physician or surgeon to determine what procedures to use to treat the problem. • May assist in performing diagnostic and therapeutic procedures.	National Board of Surgical Technology and Surgical Assisting

▶ Healthcare Professional Associations

Membership in a professional association is important for your professional development and career advancement. As discussed in the *Introduction to Medical Assisting* chapter, being part of organizations such as American Association of Medical Assistants (AAMA) and American Medical Technologist (AMT) enables you to become involved in the issues and activities relevant to your field and presents opportunities for continuing education. It is a good idea to stay informed about other healthcare associations, even those that are open to physicians only, such as the American Medical Association. Also, the physician you work for may ask you to obtain information about a particular group's activities and meetings, and by "staying in the loop," you will have better access to this information. Table 2-3 lists a few organizations that you should be familiar with.

Other organizations and professional associations exist to help regulate healthcare. Some of the most important of these organizations are described here.

American College of Physicians

Founded in 1915, the American College of Physicians (ACP) is the largest medical specialty organization in the world. It is the only society of internists dedicated to providing education and information resources to the entire field of internal medicine and its subspecialties.

American Hospital Association

The American Hospital Association (AHA) is the nation's largest network of institutional healthcare providers. These providers represent every type of hospital: rural and city hospitals, specialty and acute care facilities, free-standing hospitals, academic medical centers, and health systems and networks. The AHA works to support and promote the interests of hospitals and healthcare organizations across the country. Organizations as well as individual professionals may join the AHA. Membership benefits include use of the AHA consultant referral service, accessed, for example, by hospitals that need experts in areas not addressed by in-house personnel. Members also have access to AHA's healthcare information resources, including teleconferencing and AHA database services.

TABLE 2-3   Professional Medical Organizations

Professional Organization	Membership Requirements	Advantages of Membership
American Association of Medical Assistants (AAMA) www.aama-ntl.org	Interested individuals, including medical assisting students and those who practice medical assisting, may join the AAMA.	Offers flexible continuing education programs; publishes *CMA Today*; offers legal counsel, professional recognition, and various member discounts.
American Association of Professional Coders (AAPC) www.aapc.com	Anyone interested in the coding profession. Student memberships are available for those currently in a coding program, as are corporate memberships for groups of six or more employees.	Training, continuing education, multiple certifications for specialties, including compliance, job board, networking, local and state chapter memberships, discounts on coding books, and educational materials.
American Medical Billing Association (AMBA) www.ambanet.net	Interested individuals and those who want to become Certified Medical Reimbursement Specialists (CMRS).	Can prepare for and take the National Medical Billing Certification Exam, also many other services such as online training, insurance, networking, and credit card processing.
Association for Healthcare Documentation Integrity (AHDI) www.ahdionline.org	Interested individuals and those who practice medical transcription may join the AHDI.	Educates and develops medical transcriptionists as medical language specialists; offers advice and support for self-employed medical transcriptionists.
American College of Physicians (ACP) www.acponline.org	Physicians and medical students may join.	Provides education and information resources to the field of internal medicine and its subspecialties.
American Health Information Management Association (AHIMA) www.ahima.org	Members may be students (of approved AHIMA programs only), AHIMA-credentialed members, and noncredentialed members interested in HIM and willing to abide by the association's code of ethics.	Subscription to *Journal of AHIMA*, legislative advocacy, professional development, discounts on services and programs, job postings, members-only website, and automatic enrollment in local and/or state chapter.
American Hospital Association (AHA) www.aha.org	Institutional healthcare providers and other individuals may join.	Provides consultant referral service and access to healthcare information resources.
American Medical Association (AMA) www.ama-assn.org	Physicians and medical students may join.	Provides large information source; publishes *Journal of the American Medical Association (JAMA)*; offers AMA/Net.
American Medical Technologists (AMT) www.americanmedtech.org	Medical assistants, medical technologists, medical laboratory technicians, dental assistants, and phlebotomy technicians may join.	Offers national certification as Registered Medical Assistant (RMA); offers certification to other healthcare professionals, publications, state chapter activities, and continuing education programs.
American Pharmacists Association (APhA) www.pharmacist.com	Pharmaceutical professionals and physicians may join.	Helps members improve skills; active in pharmacy policy development, networking, publishing, research, and public education.
American Society for Clinical Pathology (ASCP) www.ascp.org	Any professional involved in laboratory medicine or pathology may join.	Resource for improving the quality of pathology and laboratory medicine; offers educational programs and materials; certifies technologists and technicians.

TABLE 2-4   2012 Ambulatory Care National Patient Safety Goals

The purpose of the National Patient Safety Goals is to improve patient safety. The goals focus on problems in healthcare safety and how to solve them.

Identify Patients Correctly	Use at least two ways to indentify patients. For example, use the patient's name *and* date of birth. This is done to make sure each patient gets the correct medicine and treatment.
	Make sure that the correct patient gets the correct blood when they get a blood transfusion.
Use Medicines Safely	Before a procedure, label medicines that are not labeled. For example, medicine in syringes, cups and basins. Do this in the area where medicines and supplies are set up.
	Take extra care with patients who take medicine to thin their blood.
	Record and pass along correct information about a patient's medicines. Find out what medicines the patient is taking. Compare those medicines to new medicines given to the patient. Make sure the patient knows which medicines to take when they are at home. Tell the patient it is important to bring their up-to-date list of medicines every time they visit a doctor.
Prevent Infection	Use the hand cleaning guidelines from the Centers for Disease Control and Prevention or the World Health Organization. Set goals for improving hand cleaning. Use the goals to improve hand cleaning.
	Use proven guidelines to prevent infection after surgery.
Prevent Mistakes in Surgery	Make sure that the correct surgery is done on the correct patient and at the correct place on the patient's body.
	Mark the correct place on the patient's body where the surgery is to be done.
	Pause before the surgery to make sure that a mistake is not being made.

*Adapted from The Joint Commission 2012 National Patient Safety Goals from www.jointcommission.org, accessed June 19, 2012.

The Joint Commission

The Joint Commission (TJC) is a U.S.-based nonprofit organization with the goal of maintaining and elevating the standards of healthcare delivery through the evaluation and accreditation of healthcare organizations. TJC employs surveyors who are sent to healthcare organizations to evaluate their operational practices and facilities. Healthcare organizations are highly motivated to do well during a survey because accreditation by TJC is a significant factor in gaining reimbursement from Medicare and managed care organizations. In addition to hospitals, TJC evaluates and accredits ambulatory care, behavioral healthcare, home care, laboratory service, long-term care, and office-based surgery facilities. Starting in 2003, TJC established safety requirements, known as National Patient Safety Goals, to help accredited healthcare organizations address issues of patient safety that can lead to adverse events that can result in lawsuits. The purpose of the goals, found at www.jointcommission.org, is to improve patient safety. The goals focus on problems and how to solve them. Table 2-4 lists the requirements of the National Patient Safety Goals.

Council of Ethical and Judicial Affairs

The Council of Ethical and Judicial Affairs (CEJA) develops ethics policy for the AMA. It is composed of seven practicing physicians, a resident or fellow, and a medical student. The Council prepares reports that analyze and address timely ethical issues that confront physicians and the medical profession. CEJA maintains and updates the AMA Code of Medical Ethics. This code is widely recognized as the most comprehensive ethics guide for physicians who strive to practice ethically.

American Medical Association

The American Medical Association (AMA), founded in 1847, promotes science and the art of medicine and works to improve public health. Its members include physicians from every medical specialty. The AMA is the world's largest publisher of scientific and medical information and publishes 10 monthly medical specialty journals. The AMA also accredits medical programs in the United States and Canada. The AMA provides an online service called AMA/Net for physicians and medical assistants, offering up-to-date information about current medical topics.

SUMMARY OF LEARNING OUTCOMES

LEARNING OUTCOMES	KEY POINTS
2.1 **Discuss healthcare and healthcare trends and their relationship to medical assistant practice.**	Medical assistants typically work in ambulatory care settings using EHR. They can expect to work with many older patients and should practice and assist patients with preventive care.
2.2 **Identify medical specialties and specialists certified by the American Board of Medical Specialties (ABMS).**	The ABMS certifies 24 major medical specialties. Within these specialties are several subspecialties. Medical specialties range from cardiology to oncology. As new medical advances occur, the demand for more specialty areas will emerge.

LEARNING OUTCOMES	KEY POINTS
2.3 **Recognize the duties of various allied health professionals with whom medical assistants may work.**	Medical assistants are members of a healthcare team. The healthcare team includes doctors, nurses, physical therapists, other allied health professionals, and patients. Understanding the duties of other healthcare professionals will assist you as a professional medical assistant. Even if you do not work with some of the team members directly, you may have to contact them through telephone, written, or electronic communication.
2.4 **Compare specialty careers that a medical assistant may choose for advancement.**	A variety of medical specialty careers are available for the practicing administrative or clinical medical assistant. These careers require additional training or education and/or other certifications.
2.5 **Differentiate professional associations that relate to healthcare and their relationship to the medical assisting profession.**	Being a member of a professional association is essential to medical assisting practice. Knowledge of other healthcare and medical organizations allows the practicing medical assistant to function successfully within his profession.

CASE STUDY CRITICAL THINKING

Recall Miguel Perez, the administrative assistant from the beginning of the chapter. Now that you have completed the chapter, answer the following questions about his case.

1. What should Miguel do first and why? What type of healthcare professional will respond to the call?

2. Raja Lautu is going to be evaluated for cancer. What type of physician will Miguel most likely be calling for this consult?

3. Ken Washington will need to have his heart evaluated. What type of physician will most likely be consulted and what type of allied health professional will perform a special test on his heart? What is the name of the test to be performed?

EXAM PREPARATION QUESTIONS

1. (LO 2.2) Medical specialists that deal with the medical and surgical treatment of obesity are
   a. Gastroenterologists
   b. Allergists
   c. Gynecologists
   d. Bariatric surgeons
   e. Neurologists

2. (LO 2.2) The abbreviation for a licensed doctor of podiatric medicine is
   a. DPM
   b. DVM
   c. MD
   d. OD
   e. LDPM

3. (LO 2.5) The Joint Commission (TJC) is a U.S.-based organization that
   a. Offers continuing education for medical assistants
   b. Provides credentialing for physicians
   c. Maintains and elevates the standards of healthcare delivery through credentialing and accreditation
   d. Obtains information for medical groups
   e. Ensures the safety of employees in all facilities

4. (LO 2.4) Which of the following individuals should Miguel contact to verify Cindy Chen's insurance?
   a. Medical administrative assistant
   b. Pharmacy technician
   c. RHIT
   d. Medical billing and insurance specialist
   e. Medical transcriptionist

5. (LO 2.3) Your patient is having treatments based on qi. Which healthcare professional is most likely performing the treatments?
   a. Chiropractor
   b. Doctor of osteopathy
   c. Acupuncturist
   d. Optician
   e. Massage therapist

6. (LO 2.5) Which professional organization develops the National Patient Safety Goals?
   a. ACP
   b. AHA
   c. TJC
   d. AAMA
   e. AMA

7. (LO 2.4) Which professional would *most* likely be working outside of a healthcare facility?
   a. Occupational therapist assistant
   b. Emergency medical technician/paramedic
   c. Anesthetist's assistant
   d. Physical therapy assistant
   e. Surgical technician

8. (LO 2.3) Which healthcare team member can work independently, performing examinations and treating common illnesses?
   a. Associate degree nurse
   b. Radiologic technologist
   c. Physical therapist
   d. Medical records technologist
   e. Nurse practitioner

9. (LO 2.1) Which of the following is a trend in healthcare that has a direct effect on how medical assistants perform their job?
   a. Less hospitalized patients and more long-term-care patients
   b. More hospitalized patients and fewer ambulatory care patients
   c. Lack of preventive healthcare practice and increased patient illness
   d. Increased birth rate and more contact with elderly patients
   e. Increased use of technology and EHR

10. (LO 2.1) What type of healthcare deals with patients who have terminal cancer or less than 6 months to live?
    a. Long-term care
    b. Ambulatory care
    c. Hospital care
    d. Hospice care
    e. Laboratory care

Professionalism and Success

CASE STUDY

EMPLOYEE INFORMATION

Employee Name	Gender	Date of Hire
Kaylyn R. Haddix	F	06/11/XX

Position	Credentials	Supervisor
Clinical Medical Assistant	RMA (AMT)	Malik Katahri, CMM

Kaylyn R. Haddix does well with the "hands-on" skills and gets along fairly well with the other office personnel. However, Kaylyn has a problem with getting to work on time. She seems to show a pattern of poor planning, such as forgetting to set her alarm, losing her car keys, and neglecting to solve her various car problems when they first become apparent (brought on by skipped oil changes, worn tire treads, squeaky brakes, and a rusty muffler). The clinic suffers when Kaylyn is late because she is not ready to see the first patient upon arrival, causing patients to wait and disrupting the routines and schedules of other staff members. Following the third time she was late, Malik, the office manager, noted the problem in Kaylyn's record and informed Kaylyn that chronic tardiness could lead to termination. Although Kaylyn is sometimes afraid to ask questions, her performance is generally above average, so Malik is hoping that Kaylyn will improve.

Keep Kaylyn in mind as you study this chapter. There will be questions at the end of the chapter based on the case study. The information in the chapter will help you answer these questions.

LEARNING OUTCOMES

After completing Chapter 3, you will be able to:

3.1 Recognize the importance of professionalism in the medical assisting practice.

3.2 Explain the professional behaviors that should be exhibited by medical assistants.

3.3 Model strategies for success in medical assisting education and practice.

KEY TERMS

attitude

comprehension

constructive criticism

critical thinking

cultural diversity

empathy

hard skills

integrity

organization

patient advocacy

persistence

prioritizing

problem solving

punctuality

self-confidence

soft skills

teamwork

time management

work ethic

work quality

I. A (3)   Demonstrate respect for diversity in approaching patients and families

IV. C (13)   Identify the role of self boundaries in the health care environment

IV. C (14)   Recognize the role of patient advocacy in the practice of medical assisting

IV. P (13)   Advocate on behalf of patients

IV. A (1)   Demonstrate empathy in communicating with patients, family and staff

IV. A (6)   Demonstrate awareness of how an individual's personal appearance affects anticipated responses

IV. A (9)   Recognize and protect personal boundaries in communicating with others

V. C (13)   Identify time management principles

X. A (1)   Apply ethical behaviors, including honesty/integrity in performance of medical assisting practice

X. A (2)   Examine the impact personal ethics and morals may have on the individual's practice

5. **Psychology of Human Relations**

Graduates:

   c. Use empathy when treating terminally ill patients

   e. Advocate on behalf of family/patients, having ability to deal and communicate with family

11. **Career Development**

Graduates:

   b. Demonstrate professionalism by:

     (1) Exhibiting dependability, punctuality, and a positive work ethic

     (2) Exhibiting a positive attitude and a sense of responsibility

     (4) Being cognizant of ethical boundaries

     (6) Adapting to change

     (7) Expressing a responsible attitude

Introduction

A profession is an occupation or career that is based upon specialized educational training. Professionalism is behavior that exhibits the traits or features that correspond to standards of that profession. Professional standards vary from occupation to occupation, and they also can sometimes vary within the same occupation, depending on the environment. And, of course, these standards go way beyond just personal appearance, although they do include this. Imagine the difference between the professional standards required of a commercial jet pilot who logs thousands of miles despite tough weather conditions and is responsible for the lives of 200-plus passengers at any given time versus those of a hobby pilot who likes to fly his Cessna solo for a few hours on sunny weekends. Will their uniforms or dress code be different? Is punctuality equally important in both cases? Luckily, you will not need to worry too much about airplanes as a medical assistant, but this is just one example of how professional standards may differ in a particular industry.

As discussed in *Introduction to Medical Assisting*, standards for medical assisting education and the profession are developed by professional organizations, such as the American Association of Medical Assistants (AAMA) and the American Medical Technologists (AMT). To be a professional medical assistant, you not only need to know standards of the profession, but you must also be able to exhibit appropriate personal attributes and behaviors.

Success is a favorable or desired outcome. To achieve a favorable or desired outcome from your medical assisting education and in practice, you must follow the standards and exhibit the personal behaviors established by your school and workplace. In this chapter, you will explore the professional behaviors required of a medical assistant in school and in practice, and the attributes and strategies needed for success in your education and career.

Professionalism in Medical Assisting

LO 3.1

The mere fact that you are reading this book means you are embarking on the profession of medical assisting. To understand this profession, you should first understand what a profession consists of. A profession has two areas of competence (abilities):

1. **Hard skills**—specific technical and operational proficiencies.
2. **Soft skills**—personal qualifications or behaviors that enhance an individual's interactions, job performance, and career prospects. These are sometimes called people skills (Figure 3-1).

Hard skills represent the minimum proficiencies necessary to do the job. Some examples of hard skills for medical assisting are

- Scheduling appointments
- Coding for insurance purposes
- Managing medical records
- Interviewing patients
- Taking vital signs
- Assisting a physician with patient examinations

FIGURE 3-1 As a medical assistant, you need to have both technical skills (hard skills) and people skills (soft skills) and maintain a good balance between them.

These are the skills you will learn throughout this program, and the ability to perform them is readily observable. Your hard skills set is the first screen employers use to determine if you are qualified for the position.

Soft skills are less concrete and more difficult to observe and evaluate. These are the characteristics, attributes, or **attitudes** that people develop throughout their lives. Some examples are respect, dependability, and integrity. These personal attributes or qualities, which are sought after and significant for specific jobs, are also professional attributes or behaviors, and they tend to help define an individual's personality. Your professional behaviors together produce what is called a good **work ethic**, which is what employers seek.

A medical assisting credential and the technical skills associated with it are the reasons most graduates are hired. However, the lack of a specific soft skill or poor professional behavior is the reason for most terminations. Weakness in the soft skills is also the major reason that some students do not successfully complete their medical assisting education. So, knowing how to do something is important, but behaving professionally while practicing is essential.

Much of the medical assistant's role involves dealing with other people, whether this is a patient, a patient's family member, a coworker, an insurance agent, a pharmaceutical sales representative, a laboratory staff member, or anyone else with whom you may come in contact in the workplace. Because the majority of professional behaviors and skills are about working with other people, it only makes sense that someone going into a profession that continually deals with people would need these behaviors or skills to do a good job. As a student and in your medical assisting career, you will experience the ongoing assessment of your professional behaviors in the following environments:

- Classroom
- Student work experience
- Hiring process
- Workplace performance evaluation
- Promotion consideration

So, no matter the circumstance, your professionalism contributes to your success and should always be on the top of your list of ongoing self-improvements. For example, what if a medical assistant did not know the proper instructions to give a patient regarding a diagnostic test? She was either too shy (lacked self-confidence) to ask or chose not to ask because of a lack of time or neglect. Consequently, she gave instructions based on what she thought might be appropriate (lacked knowledge). So, it is highly probable that the patient would not be adequately prepared for the test. The results of this poor decision might be

- Difficulty in performing the test on the patient.
- Cancelation of the test, wasting time and resources.
- Repetition of the test, incurring increased costs that may not be reimbursed by insurance.
- Inaccurate test results, leading to incorrect diagnosis and treatment, and a poor patient outcome.
- Potential litigation (lawsuit) against the medical practice.

The issue is not that the medical assistant did not know the correct instructions but that the medical assistant did not use the correct behaviors (communication, cooperation, knowledge, persistence, work quality) to obtain and give the correct instructions. While this scenario seems exaggerated, it has unfortunately occurred. The importance of professional behaviors cannot be overemphasized.

▶ Professional Behaviors   LO 3.2

Certain behaviors distinguish medical assistants who behave professionally from those who just get by, as well as those who do not make it. Professional behaviors contribute to your overall success in life—as a medical assistant and as a human being on this planet. So, let's explore essential medical assisting professional behaviors. As you read each of the following sections, take a moment to consider whether you exhibit this behavior or quality. When you have completed this section, review Procedure 3-1, Self-Evaluation of Professional Behaviors, at the end of the chapter.

Comprehension

Comprehension is the ability to learn, retain, and process information. In order to function as a medical assistant, you must comprehend your role and responsibilities. This means not only to have information but to be able to analyze that information, to know how to use it, and to retain it, no matter how infrequently you might use it. An example of comprehension is learning how to take a blood pressure, including the equipment needed, the steps in the procedure, what results to expect, how to record the results, and when to report a problem.

Persistence

Persistence is continuing in spite of difficulty; being determined and overcoming obstacles. Two other words for persistence are perseverance and tenacity. The slang is "stick-to-itiveness." This attribute ensures that you will finish the job no matter how difficult, boring, annoying, or time-consuming it may be. One example that is not uncommon in the medical office is trying to reach a patient whose contact information is not up-to-date. The issue may be an abnormal laboratory report that requires follow-up or another vital matter. The practitioner must be able to count on you and know that you will follow through and make contact no matter how difficult it may be. The patient's well-being often depends on it.

Self-Confidence

Self-confidence means believing in oneself. It is a trait that puts people at ease. The patient, the physician, and others are more comfortable when they feel that you know what you are doing. The self-assured medical assistant is generally the one that the patient and the physician prefer to work with. However, some people are self-confident to excess, which is not a professional trait. Have you ever felt a test was easy, but when the score came back you did less than great? That is overconfidence. On the other hand, self-confidence is a professional trait that makes you desirable to be around. An overconfident person acts like she knows everything; a self-confident person knows what she knows and what she doesn't know. Display your self-confidence by smiling, making eye contact, and remaining calm no matter what the situation.

Judgment

Judgment is evaluating a situation, reaching an appropriate conclusion, and acting accordingly. It is also referred to as **critical thinking** (Figure 3-2). Critical thinking is defined as purposeful decisions resulting from analysis and evaluation. You will examine the steps of critical thinking in the next section. Applying sound judgment in all situations—even when you are distracted, upset, or annoyed—is necessary as a medical assistant.

Knowledge

Knowledge is understanding gained through study and experience. Medical assisting is a profession that requires

understanding the theory (knowledge) and then applying psychomotor skills or hands-on experience. You will acquire knowledge by learning the principles and then performing the procedures. Students who do not have an understanding of the procedure and only memorize the steps may have difficulty performing when equipment varies or if a procedure is done differently (yet correctly) at the externship site. These students are often unable to function when the procedure does not go as planned. So, it is best to understand the rationale or the "why" for what you are doing. Avoid just memorizing steps.

Organization

Organization is planning and coordinating information and tasks in an orderly manner to efficiently complete the job in a given time frame. This attribute has many aspects, including **time management** and **prioritizing**, which will be discussed in more detail in the next section. Organization is required to know how to prioritize the issues and tasks while addressing them all in an efficient and timely manner. One example is prioritizing your work—deciding which are the most important tasks of the day and which are less important. On a day when everything seems to be "top priority," you must use your professional judgment, knowledge of office policies, and experience with physicians and coworkers to determine what should be completed first, second, third, and so on.

Integrity

Integrity is adhering to the appropriate code of law and ethics and being honest and trustworthy. Ethics is a system of values that determines right or wrong behavior. Integrity involves relatively simple matters, such as not taking pens home from the workplace, to more complex matters, such as always being truthful with patients. It also deals with subjects that are punishable and illegal, such as taking cash, cheating on an exam, or falsifying a time card. Falsifying a time card is clearly dishonest, but knowingly extending breaks or lunches demonstrates a lack of integrity. Knowing that a coworker or a classmate is doing something dishonest is another area of integrity

FIGURE 3-2 Using sound judgment through critical thinking requires (a) identifying a problem, (b) analyzing methods to solve it, and (c) determining an acceptable method to solve it.

FIGURE 3-3 Being dishonest or not reporting something that you observe that is dishonest reduces your integrity and trustworthiness.

(Figure 3-3). If you do not report your facts or suspicion of the act, you could be considered an accomplice and be subject to a penalty. Besides causing harm, once a person is involved in a dishonest act or is seen as lacking integrity, it is very difficult to regain the trust of others. The *Legal and Ethical Issues* chapter provides more details about standards of integrity that involve morals, laws, and ethics.

Growth

Growth is an ongoing effort to learn and improve. Being a professional brings with it an obligation to keep up with new standards, methods, procedures, and technologies in the field. Throughout this text and your medical assisting program, you will learn current practices. However, healthcare practices change frequently. For example, electronic health records (EHR) are replacing paper health records and the standards for cardiopulmonary resuscitation (CPR) change frequently. Growth requires staying informed.

As discussed in the *Introduction to Medical Assisting* chapter, you should join one or more of the medical assisting professional organizations, such as AAMA and AMT. Besides the benefits, you are expected to earn a specific number of continuing education units (CEU) within a specified time frame. These CEU offerings are credits given by the organization for participating in approved professional educational offerings. CEUs help you grow professionally and stay up-to-date with the latest information through taking seminars, reading articles, taking courses, and completing CEU modules, which may be accessed online, on a DVD, or in print.

Teamwork

Teamwork is working with others in the best interest of completing the job. The healthcare team, described in the *Healthcare and the Healthcare Team* chapter, is large and complex. Like any team, its members must work together and cooperate with each other in

order to increase the likelihood of achieving the goal. Also, studies show that in workplaces where staff members cooperate and help each other, job satisfaction and patient (client) satisfaction are high.

In the healthcare practice, the overall goal should be providing good patient care, which is done through cooperation between team members. Everyone in the facility has an important job that depends on someone else. It is important to remember that the patient comes first and everyone is responsible for the care of that patient.

Teamwork also requires coordination, which is the integration of activities. Today's typical patient may have three or more physician specialists, several prescriptions, home healthcare, routine blood work, physical therapy, hospital care, and outpatient procedures. This requires multiple appointments, insurance companies, medical claims, and other processes. These processes require each member of the team to work together for the benefit of the patient. Frequently, coordinating these patient care activities is the role of the medical assistant and requires cooperation and coordination with everyone involved. Team dynamics consist of

- Assisting each other on a daily basis with the duties required.
- Avoiding interpersonal conflict with members of the team.
- Performing extra responsibilities without questioning or complaining.
- Being considerate of all other team members' duties and responsibilities.

Acceptance of Criticism

Acceptance of criticism is the willingness to consider feedback and suggestions to improve; it is taking responsibility for one's actions. In this context, let's focus on **constructive criticism**, which is defined as counseling or advice that is intended to be useful with the goal of improving something. To grow and understand the areas in which you can improve, you must be able to accept feedback or constructive criticism (Figure 3-4). This may come from medical assisting educators, classmates, physicians, other coworkers, or even patients. You will be evaluated throughout your education and workplace experience. Never expect a

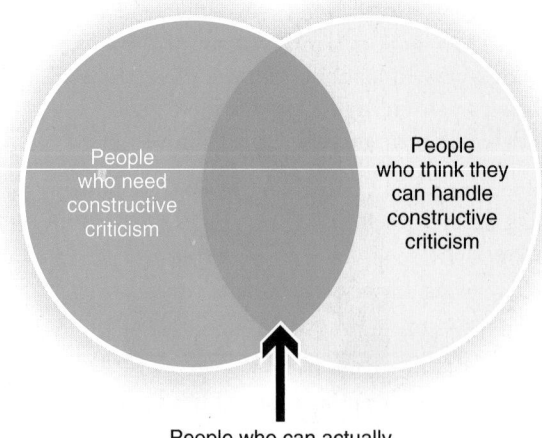

FIGURE 3-4 Accepting constructive criticism to improve your performance is essential to medical assisting practice. Get yourself inside the green zone.

perfect evaluation because no one is perfect and improvements can always be made. Instead, be open to accepting criticism and suggestions and offer your own thoughts on what you may do to improve. Do not be defensive and do not blame others. It is not about what your classmate or coworker does; it is about you.

Relations with Others

Relations with others—the ability to get along with those around you—involves treating everyone with respect and caring even when it is difficult. This sometimes includes **empathy**, feeling and understanding another's experience without having the experience yourself. In the healthcare environment, the medical assistant works with many patients who are experiencing great loss. It may be the loss of health or function or a terminal diagnosis. Or it may be a personal loss, such as the death of a spouse. As in any other workplace, coworkers also experience losses and unfortunate events. Sometimes medical assistants are very kind to patients but do not exhibit the same behaviors with coworkers. With coworkers, they may become involved in gossip and pettiness or display impatience and rudeness.

Caring is showing concern and appropriate attention, while enabling or codependency in this context is doing for others the things that they should be doing for themselves. When you enable, you become part of the disease process. For example, a young medical assistant learned this early in her career when she became attached to a 10-year-old juvenile diabetic patient. Every time the child came into the office, the MA gave her a stuffed animal or cute T-shirt or other gift. The patient started to have more and more problems and the office visits became more frequent. An experienced medical assistant pointed out that the child was being rewarded for not managing her illness. This exemplifies enabling or codependency. Instead of giving a gift (reward) for not managing the disease and becoming ill, the two medical assistants developed a new, more appropriate reward system for the patient if her diabetes was kept under control.

Professional Boundaries Having professional boundaries or limitations means always treating a patient as a client and not becoming involved in issues of his or her private life that do not directly relate to the healthcare. This is often difficult, especially with patients that you see often and particularly enjoy, and with patients you feel you may be able to help in addition to providing care in the medical office. Generally, the guidelines for maintaining professional boundaries are

- Address the patient only by his or her last name unless first asking permission to use his or her first name (children are an exception).
- Avoid offering advice on personal matters.
- Use only tasteful, appropriate humor.
- Avoid becoming excessively friendly.
- Avoid giving or accepting money from a patient.
- Decline meeting a patient outside of the workplace unless you were acquainted prior to taking your position.

Cultural Diversity Have you heard the expression "it takes all kinds"? Professionalism involves understanding people who

FIGURE 3-5 Respect and understanding for everyone is an essential professional behavior for the medical assistant.

are different from you and respecting their right to be different. After all, from their point of view, you are the one who is different! Healthcare facilities serve patients from many countries who speak many languages. The variety of human social structures, belief systems, and strategies for adapting to situations in different parts of the world is referred to as **cultural diversity**. Showing respect to all individuals, regardless of culture or socioeconomic standing, impacts your relations with others (Figure 3-5). Being respectful does not mean that you have to agree with the lifestyles and beliefs of others. It means that you accept the idea that others have every right to be different from you, and, as a medical assistant, you treat them appropriately. The list below gives some ideas that may help you understand and respect diversity.

- Increase your awareness of diversity. Communication with patients and coworkers will help you learn about individual similarities and differences.
- Increase your awareness of your own feelings. Everyone has biases. People tend to stereotype others, and this can lead to discrimination. Examine your own biases. Are they realistic?
- Look at individuals. As you learn about people as individuals, any group stereotypes you may have often begin to break down.

Patient Advocacy As a medical assistant, you may be in a position to speak or act on behalf of the patient or the patient's family. This is called **patient advocacy**. Understanding your scope of practice, as well as being professional in your relations with others and being a good communicator, will help you be an effective advocate for the patient. Be sure you have all the facts before you act, and include your supervisor or licensed practitioner as needed. Table 3-1 provides some examples of possible patient advocacy decisions.

Work Quality

Work quality means striving for excellence in doing the job and having pride in your performance. If you feel you need improvement in an area or would like to learn a new skill, consider taking a course, asking your supervisor or a coworker for help, or spending more time in that area. If you have an idea to improve a work process, make a suggestion. If you see something that is a potential risk, report it. Never say, "It is not my job." If it

TABLE 3-1   Examples of Patient Advocacy

Circumstance	Example	Suggested Action
Concern for the individual's safety.	You suspect an elderly patient is being abused.	Discuss with licensed practitioner; follow legal requirements and office protocols for reporting suspected elder abuse.
A complex situation that requires your level of expertise.	A patient is having difficulty with an insurance claim.	Assist the patient as needed.
A potentially bad situation exists that your knowledge may help to avoid or resolve.	You are aware that a patient will not fill a prescription for an expensive drug because he cannot afford the insurance copay.	Inform the physician, who may prescribe a generic version of the drug, or with the physician's approval, contact the drug company to obtain free or reduced medications, or contact a local pharmacy that provides low-cost medications if available.
Giving extra attention is likely to benefit the patient.	You are reviewing a one-year-old patient's profile and notice that she is probably eligible for a special nutritional program called WIC (Women, Infants, and Children).	Take the time to explain the program to the mother and provide the information for her to enroll.
The patient is capable of advocating for himself or herself.	The patient does not want to tell the physician that he does not understand why he needs a proposed procedure.	Encourage the patient to talk to the physician and assure him it is not unusual for patients to not fully understand the first time information is presented.
Anything that can be considered medical advice or a medical recommendation should be avoided.	The patient is asking your telephone advice regarding his symptoms.	Avoid saying anything that involves a potential diagnosis, such as "that sounds like the flu"; follow the office protocol for scheduling an appointment.
The action interferes with your job duties or presents a potential liability.	A patient asks you to keep an eye on her children during her exam.	Suggest the patient reschedule when she can arrange childcare; if needed, provide a contact number for a facility close to the office.
There are reasonable options.	A patient forgets to fill his monthly prescriptions and is consistently asking for an emergency refill. The office policy is that refills will be processed in three business days. He wants you to call and remind him each month.	Suggest to the patient that many pharmacies provide a monthly automatic refill or a monthly reminder.

is not your job, simply state that you will get the person who can help and then get that person. Getting the job done is the focus. Being flexible is another part of work quality. If a staff member is absent or the schedule changes, the important thing is to get the job done. Again, do not worry about whose job it is as long as you are staying within your scope of practice.

Punctuality and Attendance

Being on time—**punctuality**—and coming to work every day that you are scheduled are essential for maintaining your job. Poor attendance is a frequent reason for termination. You are expected to be at your duty station or in your classroom ready to work at the given time. Whether you are late or absent as a result of poor planning or an emergency, it still means that either your job is not getting done or you created additional work for your teammates. Patient care is impacted when you are not present. Recall Kaylyn in our case study above, who is at risk for termination for frequent tardiness. Do not let this be you.

Professional Appearance

A medical professional always strives to maintain a neat appearance in the workplace, and personal cleanliness is an important part of this. Your appearance is the first impression you make on your patients, coworkers, and the physicians you work with. Medical facilities are considered "conservative" work environments, and your appearance should reflect a conservative style. Listed here are a few professional guidelines to follow in the medical environment:

- Your approved uniform or other clothing worn should be clean, pressed crisply, fit properly, and in good repair.

- Your shoes should be comfortable, white, clean, and in good condition. Open-toed shoes should not be worn in the patient treatment areas to prevent injury or infection to yourself.

- Choose a hairstyle that is flattering and conservative. Hair should be clean and pulled back from your face and off your collar if it is long. Natural colors for hair are the most acceptable colors in a medical environment.

- Your nails should be kept at a short working length, no more than one-fourth of an inch, and of a natural color. Acrylic nails should not be worn, as they pose a risk for infection.

- Body odors, including the odor of smoke, are offensive. Even pleasant odors such as hairspray, perfumes, and lotions may trigger nausea or allergies in some patients and should be avoided.

- Jewelry should be kept to a minimum and in good taste. No more than one ring should be worn. Rings may tear through exam gloves. Ears can be pierced with one hole, and small earrings are appropriate. Avoid dangling earrings, as patients (particularly pediatric patients) can tear these off.

- Visible tattoos, body piercings, and tongue piercings are not acceptable.

Communication

Effective communication involves careful listening, observing, speaking, and writing. Communication even involves good manners—being polite, tactful, and respectful. You must use good communication skills during every patient discussion and in every interaction you have with physicians, other staff members, and other professionals with whom your practice does business.

Communication is giving and receiving accurate information. If a person is a bad communicator, it means that he or she cannot communicate or provide information that is accurate or understandable. Sometimes the patient leaves the office confused because he or she did not understand medical terms that were used and did not communicate that he or she did not understand. Sometimes the student leaves class confused because he or she did not understand the assignment and did not communicate to the instructor that he or she did not understand. In these scenarios, communication was poor from the sender since it was not understood. It was also poor from the receiver since lack of understanding was not communicated back to the sender. Effective communication is a two-way process with a responsibility on both sides. It impacts every aspect of healthcare and is discussed in-depth in the *Interpersonal Communication* chapter.

▶ Strategies for Success   LO 3.3

As you move toward and through your career as a medical assistant, you should be constantly improving your professional behaviors as discussed above. As a medical assistant, you must practice specific strategies to ensure your success. These strategies include critical thinking and problem solving, time management and prioritizing, and stress management. The sections that follow will discuss these strategies, provide examples, and explain how to practice them.

Critical Thinking and Problem Solving

You will develop critical thinking skills over time as you apply your knowledge about and experience with human nature, medicine, and office skills to new situations. Critical thinking skills include quickly evaluating circumstances, solving problems, and taking action. For example, you must use critical thinking skills to assess how to react to emergency situations. If you see a patient suddenly pass out in the physician's waiting room, you must immediately see that the patient receives first aid, notify a physician, and alert the patient's family.

Critical thinking skills are used every day, and critical thinking relies on sound judgment. More specifically, critical thinking involves the ability to

- Analyze situations.
- Determine what aspects of a situation are most important.
- Reach conclusions that go beyond the obvious.

Critical thinking includes both factual problem identification and creative decision-making skills. It is the ability to see the whole picture and to reach reasonable conclusions based on the most important facts.

Problem solving can be broken down into a step-by-step approach (Figure 3-6):

- Identify the problem and define it clearly.
- Identify the potential effects of the problem.
- Clearly identify the objectives to be achieved.

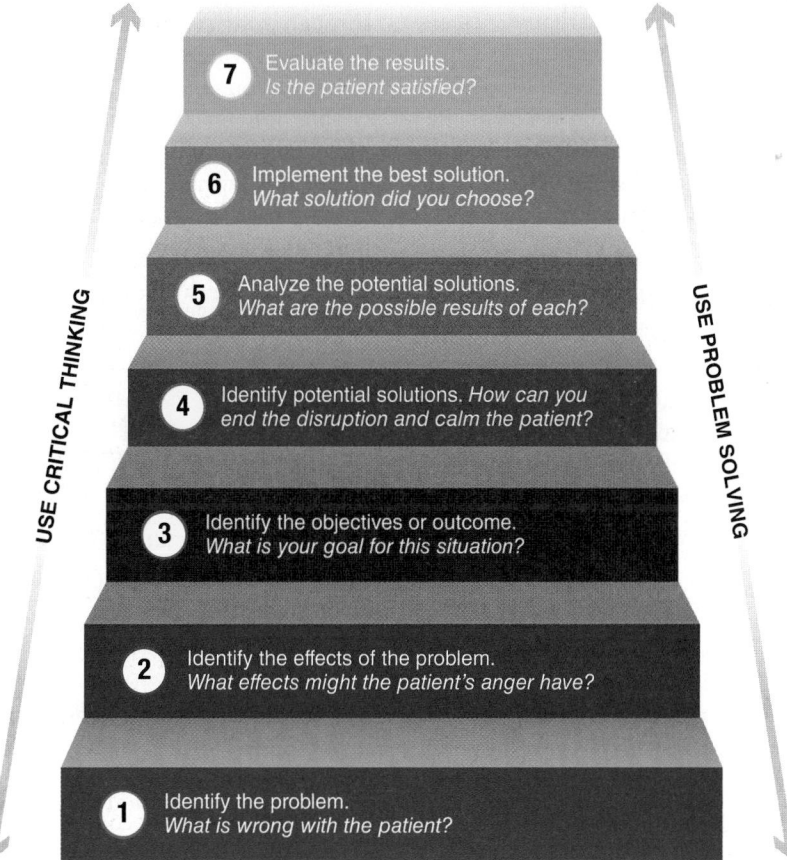

USE CRITICAL THINKING

USE PROBLEM SOLVING

7 Evaluate the results. *Is the patient satisfied?*

6 Implement the best solution. *What solution did you choose?*

5 Analyze the potential solutions. *What are the possible results of each?*

4 Identify potential solutions. *How can you end the disruption and calm the patient?*

3 Identify the objectives or outcome. *What is your goal for this situation?*

2 Identify the effects of the problem. *What effects might the patient's anger have?*

1 Identify the problem. *What is wrong with the patient?*

FIGURE 3-6 Use critical thinking and good judgment when following the steps of the problem-solving process.

- Identify as many potential solutions and strategies as possible.
- Analyze the potential solutions and strategies.
- Implement the strategy that appears to be the best solution.
- Evaluate the results and repeat the steps as needed.

Now, let's use the problem-solving steps to solve a patient problem. A patient approaches your desk and complains loudly that he does not have all day to wait for the doctor to see him. His appointment was at 2:00 and the time is now 2:40. The patient is obviously angry about the delay. What should you do?

Step 1. Identify and define the problem: What is wrong with the patient?

The patient is angry because the physician did not see him promptly at his appointment time.

Step 2. Identify the potential effects of the problem: What effects might the patient's anger have?

The patient is disrupting the office; the practice may lose this client.

Step 3. Identify the objectives to be achieved: What is your goal for this situation?

Your goal is to end the disruption and calm the patient.

Step 4. Identify potential solutions and strategies: What can you do to end the disruption and calm the patient?

This is the step where you may be able to come up with more than one answer. For example, you may want to (a) inform your supervisor that the patient is causing a disruption, (b) ask the physician to talk to the patient, (c) tell the patient there is nothing you can do about it, or (d) explain the situation to the patient quietly and offer to reschedule the appointment. Remember that problem solving is not an exact science. You are attempting to come up with solutions so you can determine the one that will most effectively solve the problem.

Step 5. Analyze the potential solutions and strategies. What are the possible results from each solution?

So let's see. For (a), you discover that the supervisor is busy in a room with another patient, and waiting for her to become available will allow the disruption to continue. For (b), you recall that the physician expects the office staff to take care of this type of incident. For (c), you suspect that telling the patient you cannot do anything will not make him less angry. For (d), you think that talking quietly to the patient and offering to reschedule the appointment might work.

Step 6. Implement the best solution. What solution did you chose?

You explain that an emergency earlier in the day put the physician behind schedule and offer to reschedule the patient's appointment for a more convenient time. Of course, you will need to use your judgment to provide an explanation without violating the confidentiality of the patient who had the emergency earlier.

Step 7. Evaluate the results and repeat the steps as needed. How did it go? Is the patient satisfied and calmer now? If not, try a different strategy.

This step is important because learning from experience counts. If you chose to wait for the supervisor to become available to handle the situation, and the patient stalked out of the office saying he would not be back, you would hopefully do something different if faced with the same circumstance again. In this case, you explained the reason for the delay and offered to reschedule the patient, and he calmed down and decided to wait for the physician to see him.

Time Management and Prioritizing

Personal and professional time management skills are essential for medical assistants. Time management is controlling how you spend your time. People who use time management techniques routinely are the highest achievers in all walks of life, professionally and personally. Using these skills will assist you in functioning exceptionally well in the medical office, even under intense pressure. Even more importantly, you can say goodbye to the often-intense stress of work overload. Setting goals and concentrating on results, not just being busy, is the main focus of time management.

Medical assistant students who are disorganized waste a great deal of time locating assignments and other materials before they get started on their work. Prepare in advance. Make sure you purchase a binder, notebook, or folders for storing your homework assignments, reminders about upcoming tests, your course syllabus, and other pertinent facts, such as your instructor's office hours and contact information and your classmates' information for study sessions. Obtain computer access with an Internet connection at home, through your school, or at the local library. Try practicing the tips provided in the Points on Practice box for Student Organization.

In a busy practice, the medical assistant also must be organized. For example, the phone may be ringing at the same time a patient is trying to schedule a follow-up appointment, while the physician is inquiring about the results of a diagnostic report and a coworker is asking for information about a patient's immunizations. To be an effective medical assistant, you must be able to manage your time and prioritize effectively. Evaluate

POINTS ON PRACTICE
Student Organization

- Make sure you study in a quiet area away from distractions.
- Find a study "buddy" who is just as committed and focused on success as you are.
- Formal classroom courses require at least as much work time outside of class as inside it to prepare.
- Budget your time between school and other responsibilities.
- Set aside study time by creating a study schedule.
- Set daily, weekly, or course-specific goals to accomplish the overall goal of completing your course.

yourself and use the following ideas to improve your ability to manage time and prioritize.

1. Have a plan for your day. Know what needs to be done. Set your daily goals and try to meet them.

2. Take advantage of your own productivity. That is, you may work better at a particular time of day. Choose to do the most difficult tasks when you are working at your best. Remember, everybody has sluggish times, so know when yours are—maybe right after lunch or near the end of the day. Plan your day accordingly.

3. Avoid distractions when you can. Of course, if your job is to answer the phone, then you must do so. But if someone is just chatting or your smartphone is constantly beeping to signal text messages, this probably means you are not accomplishing what needs to be done. Personal phone calls, text messages, tweets, or other communications are not supposed to occur during your working hours. However, business electronic communication is vital. Consider setting specific times during the day to look at business e-mail so you will not have constant interruptions.

4. Evaluate yourself on a daily basis. Consider whether you accomplished your daily goal and come up with a plan to continue or do better the next day.

Stress and Burnout Professionals in the healthcare field, including medical assistants, may experience high levels of stress in their daily work environment. Stress can result from a feeling of being under pressure, or it can be a reaction to anger, frustration, or a change in your routine. Stress can increase your blood pressure, speed up your breathing and heart rate, and cause muscle tension. Stress also can cause you to behave or communicate ineffectively. For example, if you are feeling very pressured at work, you might snap at a coworker or patient, or you might forget to give the physician an important message.

Good or Bad Stress A certain amount of stress is normal. A little bit of stress—the kind that makes you feel excited or challenged by the task at hand—can motivate you to get things done and push you toward a higher level of productivity. For example, your supervisor may ask you to learn a new procedure. Learning something new, although stressful in itself, can be an exciting challenge and a welcome change of pace. Ongoing stress, however, can be overwhelming and affect you physically. For example, it can lower your resistance to colds and increase your risk for developing heart disease, diabetes, high blood pressure, ulcers, allergies, asthma, colitis, and cancer. It also can increase your risk for certain autoimmune diseases, which cause the body's immune system to attack normal tissue.

Some stress at work is inevitable. An important goal is to learn how to manage or reduce stress. Take into account your strengths and limitations, and be realistic about how much you can handle at work and in your life outside work. Pushing yourself a certain amount can be motivating. The Points on Practice box lists the potential causes of stress and ways to reduce stress.

Preventing Burnout Burnout is the end result of prolonged periods of stress without relief. Burnout is an energy-depleting condition that will affect your health and career. Certain personality types are more prone to burnout than others. If you are a highly driven, perfectionist-type person, you will be more susceptible to burnout. Experts often refer to such a person as a characteristic Type A personality. A more relaxed, calm, laid-back individual is considered a Type B person. Type B personalities are less prone to burnout but have the potential to suffer from it, especially if they work in healthcare.

According to some experts on stress, there are five stages of burnout:

1. *The Honeymoon Phase.* During the honeymoon phase, your job is wonderful. You have boundless energy and enthusiasm, and all things seem possible. You love the job and the job loves you. You believe it will satisfy all your needs and desires and solve all your problems. You are delighted with your job, your coworkers, and the organization.

2. *The Awakening Phase.* The awakening stage starts with the realization that your initial expectations were unrealistic. The job is not working out the way you thought it would. It does not satisfy all your needs, your coworkers and the organization are less than perfect, and rewards and recognition are scarce. As disillusionment and disappointment grow, you become confused. Something is wrong, but you cannot quite put your finger on it. Typically, you work harder to make your dreams come true. But working harder does not change anything and you become increasingly tired, bored, and frustrated. You may question your competence and ability, and start losing your self-confidence.

3. *The Brownout Phase.* As brownout begins, your early enthusiasm and energy give way to chronic fatigue and irritability. You become indecisive and your productivity drops. Your work deteriorates. Coworkers and managers may even comment on it. You become increasingly frustrated and angry and project the blame for your difficulties onto others. You are cynical, detached, and openly critical of the organization, superiors, and coworkers. You are beset with depression, anxiety, and physical illness.

4. *The Full-Scale Burnout Phase.* Unless you wake up and interrupt the process or someone intervenes, brownout drifts remorselessly into full-scale burnout. Despair is the dominant feature of this final stage. It usually takes three to four years to get to this phase. You experience an overwhelming sense of failure and a devastating loss of self-esteem and self-confidence. You become depressed and feel lonely and empty. You talk about just quitting and getting away. You are exhausted physically and mentally and prone to physical and mental breakdowns.

5. *The Phoenix Phenomenon.* Just like a phoenix, you can arise from the burnout ashes. But this takes time. First, you need to rest and relax. Do not take work home. If you are like many people, the work will not get done and you will only feel guilty for being lazy. Second, be realistic in your job expectations as well as your aspirations and goals. Third, create balance in your life. Invest more of yourself in family and other personal relationships, social activities, and hobbies. Spread yourself out so that your job does not have such an overpowering influence on your self-esteem and self-confidence.

POINTS ON PRACTICE
Potential Causes of Stress

Sometimes stress can be difficult to measure. Just like varying thresholds for pain, different people can tolerate different amounts of stress. One person's stress may seem a lot worse than another's. For example, who can say that the stress you may be feeling over an upcoming exam is less nerve-wracking than the stress someone else may be feeling about paying off a large credit card balance? Stress can come in many forms from many directions, but here is a list of common potential causes.

- Death of a spouse or family member.
- Divorce or separation.
- Hospitalization (yours or a family member's) due to injury or illness.
- Marriage or reconciliation from a separation.
- Loss of a job or retirement.
- Sexual problems.
- Having a new baby.
- Significant change in your financial status (for better or worse).
- Job change.
- Children leaving or returning home.
- Significant personal success, such as a promotion at work.
- Moving or remodeling your home.
- Problems at work, such as your boss's retiring, that may put your job at risk.
- Substantial debt, such as a mortgage or overspending on credit cards.

Tips for Reducing Stress

Managing your stress levels can benefit your overall well-being, both mentally and physically, at work and at home. The following is a list of helpful, doable tips for lowering stress.

- Maintain a healthy balance in your life among work, family, and leisure activities.
- Exercise regularly.
- Eat balanced, nutritious meals and healthful snacks.
- Avoid foods high in caffeine, salt, sugar, and fat.
- Get enough sleep.
- Allow time for yourself, and plan time to relax.
- Rely on the support that family, friends, and coworkers have to offer. Do not be afraid to share your feelings.
- Try to be realistic about what you can and cannot do. Do not be afraid to admit that you cannot take on another responsibility.
- Try to set realistic goals for yourself. Remember, there are always choices, even when there appear to be none.
- Be organized. Good planning can help you manage your workload.
- Redirect excess energy constructively; clean your closet, work in the garden, volunteer, invite friends for dinner, or exercise.
- Change some of the things you have control over.
- Stay focused. Focus your full energy on one thing at a time and finish one project before starting another.
- Identify sources of conflict and try to resolve them.
- Learn and use relaxation techniques, such as deep breathing, meditation, or imagining yourself in a quiet, peaceful place. Choose what works for you.
- Maintain a healthy sense of humor, as laughter can help relieve stress. Joke with friends after work. See a funny movie.
- Try not to overreact. Ask yourself if a situation is really worth getting upset or worried about.
- Seek help from social or professional support groups, if necessary.

PROCEDURE 3-1 Self-Evaluation of Professional Behaviors

Procedure Goal: To identify necessary professional behaviors and relate them to yourself in order to improve your performance as a medical assistant.

OSHA Guidelines: This procedure does not involve exposure to blood, body fluids, or tissue.

Materials: Self-Evaluation Form (Figure Procedure 3-1).

Method: Procedure steps.

1. Read and review each professional behavior.
2. Rate yourself on each behavior, considering the level at which you exhibit them.
3. Identify at least one measure to improve yourself on each behavior, as needed.
4. Place the completed form in your portfolio and review it on an ongoing basis.
5. Reevaluate your professional behavior prior to your applied training experience (practicum).
6. Compare the two scores and identify any weaknesses.
7. Obtain feedback about your professional behaviors from your instructor, coworkers, classmates, practicum coordinator, or employer.

Behavior	Example(s)	Rate Yourself (5 = Best)					Improvements Needed
		1	2	3	4	5	
Integrity	Consistently honest; able to be trusted with the property of others; can be trusted with confidential information; completes tasks accurately.						
Appearance	Clothing and uniform appropriate for circumstance; neat, clean, and well-kept appearance; good personal hygiene and grooming.						
Teamwork	Places the success of the team above self-interest; does not undermine the team; helps and supports other team members; shows respect to all team members; remains flexible and open to change; communicates with others to help resolve problems.						
Self-confidence	Demonstrates the ability to trust personal judgment; demonstrates an awareness of strengths and limitations; exercises good personal judgment.						
Communication	Speaks clearly; writes legibly; listens actively; adjusts communication strategies to various situations.						
Commitment to diversity	Consistently demonstrates respect for varied cultural backgrounds, ethnicities, religions, sexual orientations, social classes, abilities, political beliefs, and disabilities.						
Punctuality and attendance	Arrives at class and work on the appointed day and time.						
Acceptance of criticism	Listens when constructive criticism is given; does not become defensive with criticism; appreciates constructive criticism and incorporates suggestions into behavior as appropriate.						
Organization	Coordinates more than one task at a time; keeps work area neat and orderly; anticipates future work; works efficiently and systematically.						
Knowledge and comprehension	Learns new things easily; retains new information; associates theory with practice.						

FIGURE Procedure 3-1 Self-evaluation of professional behaviors.

SUMMARY OF LEARNING OUTCOMES

LEARNING OUTCOME	KEY POINTS
3.1 Recognize the importance of professionalism in the medical assisting practice.	Professionalism is behavior that exhibits the traits or features corresponding to the standards of that profession. Standards are developed by professional organizations and, in some states, by governmental entities. The skills are placed in two broad categories: hard skills and soft skills. Hard skills are specific technical and operational proficiencies. Soft skills are personal attributes or behaviors that enhance an individual. Professional behaviors are needed to function at a high level in medical assisting and produce a good work ethic.

LEARNING OUTCOMES	KEY POINTS
3.2 **Explain the professional behaviors that should be exhibited by medical assistants.**	Some essential professional behaviors include comprehension—learning, retaining, and processing information; persistence—continuing in spite of difficulty; self-confidence—believing in oneself; judgment—evaluating and determining an appropriate conclusion; organization—coordinating information and tasks in an orderly manner; integrity—adhering to law and ethics; growth—engaging in ongoing efforts to learn and improve; teamwork—working with others in the best interest of completing the job; acceptance of criticism—willing to consider feedback and suggestions to improve; relations with others—getting along with all people in all circumstances; work quality— striving for excellence in doing the job; punctuality and attendance—showing up on appointed days and times; professional appearance—adhering to the standards and codes of dress; and communication—giving and receiving accurate information.
3.3 **Model strategies for success in medical assisting education and practice.**	Strategies for success as a medical assistant include cultivating your skills, such as critical thinking and problem solving, time management and prioritizing, stress management, and avoidance of burnout. Practicing effective strategies can assist you during your education and employment.

CASE STUDY CRITICAL THINKING

Recall Kaylyn Haddix from the beginning of the chapter. Now that you have completed this chapter, answer the following questions regarding her case.

1. What professional behaviors does Kaylyn need to improve?

2. What strategies for success could Kaylyn use to prevent herself from losing her job?

EXAM PREPARATION QUESTIONS

1. (LO 3.1) The primary reason an employee is hired is usually associated with
a. Hard skills
b. Soft skills
c. References
d. Punctuality
e. Cooperation

2. (LO 3.1) Which of the following is considered a soft skill?
a. Communicating with a patient
b. Measuring the patient's height
c. Taking a telephone message
d. Taking a patient's vital signs
e. Scheduling an appointment

3. (LO 3.2) An indication that a person lacks integrity would be exhibited by
a. Being rude to a coworker
b. Coming into work late
c. Ignoring the dress code
d. Taking money from the cash drawer
e. Gossiping

4. (LO 3.2) A significant part of critical thinking is
a. Memorizing
b. Analyzing
c. Being tenacious
d. Empathizing
e. Criticizing

5. (LO 3.2) Adhering to the dress code and good personal hygiene demonstrates
   a. Persistence
   b. Growth
   c. Respect
   d. Knowledge
   e. Organization

6. (LO 3.2) If a medical assistant is not self-confident, this may lead to the patient feeling
   a. Confident
   b. Neglected
   c. Apprehensive
   d. Ignored
   e. Ill

7. (LO 3.2) An example of enabling or codependency would be
   a. Providing a wheelchair for a patient who is weak
   b. Helping a patient identify a community resource
   c. Scheduling the patient's next appointment
   d. Offering cookies to an obese patient
   e. Calling a taxi for a patient

8. (LO 3.2) Maintaining professional boundaries involves
   a. Showing the patient you care by being personal
   b. Being friendly but not excessively affectionate
   c. Avoiding any touch with the patient
   d. Babysitting for the patient
   e. Buying the patient lunch

9. (LO 3.3) Your coworker likes to talk about her kids and husband, usually right after lunch. What should you do?
   a. Talk with your coworker as much as you can since it is important to have good relationships at work
   b. Talk with your coworker since this is your down time anyway
   c. Consider telling your supervisor that your coworker talks too much and you find it disturbing
   d. Request that your supervisor ask your coworker to not talk to you so much because you cannot get your work done
   e. Realize that the time you speak with your coworker is preventing you from completing your goals, so politely explain this to your coworker

10. (LO 3.3) Once you have considered what the problem is and what effects it will have, what should you do next?
    a. Implement a solution
    b. Identify the problem
    c. Determine multiple solutions
    d. Determine the effects of the solution
    e. Evaluate your solution to determine if it works or worked

4

Interpersonal Communication

LEARNING OUTCOMES

After completing Chapter 4, you will be able to:

4.1 Identify elements and types of communication.

4.2 Relate communication to human behavior and needs.

4.3 Categorize positive and negative communication.

4.4 Model ways to improve listening, interpersonal skills, and assertiveness skills.

4.5 Carry out therapeutic communication skills.

4.6 Use effective communication strategies with patients in special circumstances.

4.7 Carry out positive communication with coworkers and management.

KEY TERMS

active listening

aggressive

assertive

body language

boundaries

closed posture

conflict

customer service

empathy

feedback

hierarchy

homeostasis

hospice

interpersonal skills

open posture

passive listening

personal space

rapport

IV. Concepts of Effective Communications

IV. C (1) Identify styles and types of verbal communication

IV. C (2) Identify nonverbal communication

IV. C (3) Recognize communication barriers

IV. C (4) Identify techniques for overcoming communication barriers

IV. C (5) Recognize the elements of oral communication using a sender-receiver process

IV. C (7) Identify resources and adaptations that are required based on individual needs, i.e., culture and environment, developmental life stage, language, and physical threats to communication

IV. C (15) Discuss the role of assertiveness in effective professional communication

IV. P (1) Use reflection, restatement, and clarification techniques to obtain a patient history

IV. P (11) Respond to nonverbal communication

IV. A (1) Demonstrate empathy in communicating with patients, family, and staff

IV. A (2) Apply active listening skills

IV. A (3) Use appropriate body language and other nonverbal skills in communicating with patients, family, and staff

IV. A (8) Analyze communications in providing appropriate responses/feedback

IV. A (9) Recognize and protect personal boundaries in communicating with others

IV. A (10) Demonstrate respect for individual diversity, incorporating awareness of one's own biases in areas including gender, race, religion, age and economic status

IX. P (2) Perform within scope of practice

5. Psychology of Human Relations

Graduates:

a. Define and understand abnormal behavior patterns

b. Identify and respond appropriately when working/caring for patients with special needs

c. Use empathy with treating terminally ill patients

d. Identify common stages that terminally ill patients go through and list organizations/support groups that can assist patients and family members of patients struggling with terminal illness

e. Advocate on behalf of family/patients, having ability to deal and communicate with family

f. Identify and discuss developmental stages of life

g. Analyze the effect of hereditary, cultural, and environmental influences

8. Medical Office Business Procedures Management

Graduates:

aa. Are attentive, listen, and learn

bb. Are impartial and show empathy when dealing with patients

cc. Communicate on the recipient's level of comprehension

dd. Serve as liaison between physician and others

ee. Communicate on the recipient's level of comprehension

ii. Recognize and respond to verbal and non-verbal communication

kk. Adapt to individualized needs

▶ Introduction

Think about the last time you had a doctor's appointment. How well did the staff and physician communicate with you? Were you greeted pleasantly and invited to take a seat, or did someone thrust a clipboard at you and say, "Fill this out"? If you had a long wait in the reception area or examination room, did someone come in to explain the delay? Did you become frustrated and angry because nobody told you what was happening? The abilities to recognize human behaviors and to communicate effectively are vital to a medical assistant's success. This chapter takes a psychological approach to understanding human behavior and the challenges that influence therapeutic communication in a healthcare setting.

As the key communicator within the healthcare facility, the medical assistant must be able to communicate with each patient with professionalism and diplomacy. This includes patients from different cultures, socioeconomic backgrounds,

educational levels, ages, and lifestyles. The medical assistant sets the tone for the communication circle and must be aware of all the obstacles that can affect human communication. It is important that patients develop a good rapport and feel confident in the care they are receiving from your office. Developing strong communication skills in the medical office is just as important as mastering administrative and clinical tasks.

▶ Elements of Communication   LO 4.1

As you interact with patients and their families, you will be responsible for giving information and ensuring that the patient understands what you, the doctor, and other staff members have communicated. You also will be responsible for receiving information from the patient. For example, patients will describe their symptoms. They also may discuss their feelings or ask questions about a treatment or procedure. The giving and receiving of information forms the communication circle.

FIGURE 4-1 The process of communication involves an exchange of messages through verbal and nonverbal means.

The Communication Circle

The communication circle involves three elements: a message, a source, and a receiver. Messages are usually verbal, written, or nonverbal. (You will explore more about nonverbal messages later in this chapter.) The source sends the message and the receiver receives it. The communication circle is formed as the source sends a message to the receiver and the receiver responds (Figure 4-1).

Consider this example, in which Miguel, BWW's clinical medical assistant, is speaking with Sylvia Gonzales, a patient who is having physical therapy for a back injury. Watch the communication circle at work.

Miguel:	The physical therapist says you're making great progress and that you can start on some simple back exercises at home. I'd like to go over them with you. Then I'll give you a sheet that illustrates the exercises. How does that sound to you?
Sylvia Gonzales:	I'm a little nervous about doing exercises. I still have some pain when I bend over.
Miguel:	I understand. It's important, though, to start using those muscles again. Why don't you show me exactly where it hurts? Then we can go over proper body mechanics, such as bending down to pick something up and getting in and out of chairs, the car, and bed. Then we'll just start with one or two of the exercises and save the rest for next time, when you're feeling more ready.
Sylvia Gonzales:	Okay, I will try, but I only feel up to doing a little bit today.

In this example, the medical assistant (the source) gives a verbal message about back exercises to the patient (the receiver). The patient responds by drawing attention to her pain and uneasiness about certain movements (feedback). The patient's response or feedback is also a message to the medical assistant, who responds in turn. The giving and receiving of information continues within the communication circle until the exchange is finished.

Feedback The patient's response or **feedback** is verbal or nonverbal evidence that the receiver got and understood the message. When you communicate information to a patient or ask a patient a question, always look for feedback. For example, if you calculate a pregnant patient's due date and tell her she's 12 weeks pregnant, look for a response. If she responds, "Oh, good, that means I'm out of danger of having a miscarriage," you may respond by saying that whereas most miscarriages occur in the first 12 weeks, some risk of miscarriage remains throughout the pregnancy. If she responds, "I thought I was 14 weeks pregnant," you would need to clarify how you worked out your calculation and compare it with hers, to uncover any discrepancy. Good communication in the medical office requires patient feedback at every step.

Noise Anything that changes the message in any way or interferes with the communication process can be referred to as noise. Noise refers not only to sounds, such as a siren or jackhammer on the street below the medical office suite, but also to room temperature and other types of physical comfort or discomfort, such as pain, and to emotions, such as fear or sadness. If patients are feeling uncomfortable in a chilly or hot room, upset about their illness, or in great pain, they may not pay close attention to what you are saying. Conversely, if you are feeling upset about a personal problem outside work or if you are unwell or preoccupied with all the things you have on your to-do list, you may not communicate well.

As you deal with each patient, try to screen out or eliminate causes of noise. For example, before you start a conversation with a patient in an examination room, you might ask, "Are you too chilly or too warm? Is the temperature in here comfortable for you?" If there is construction going on outside the building, see if there is a less noisy inner room or office that you might be able to use. If a patient seems nervous or upset, address those feelings before you launch into a factual discussion.

If you are feeling stressed or out of sorts, that feeling constitutes a type of noise. Try to take a "breather" between patients or a break from desk work—walk downstairs, get some fresh air, stretch your legs. Feeling dehydrated or hungry affects your communication efforts, too. Limit your caffeine and sugar intake. Drink plenty of water throughout the day. Eat a good breakfast and lunch and healthful snacks. Leave your personal problems at home.

▶ Human Behavior and Needs   LO 4.2

Medical assistants are exposed to many different personality types in addition to different illnesses. When you understand why a person is behaving in a certain way, you can adjust your communication style to adapt to that person. For example, as highly structured healthcare organizations and technological advances rapidly change the face of healthcare, many patients feel that healthcare is becoming impersonal, and consequently may become difficult. Every time you communicate with patients, you can counteract this perception by playing a humanistic role in the healthcare process. Being humanistic means that you work to help patients feel attended to and respected as individuals, not just as descriptions in a chart. Take care to treat patients as people to help humanize the communication process in the medical office. To humanize and improve communication, you should have an understanding of the developmental stages of the life cycle and Maslow's hierarchy of human needs.

Developmental Stages of the Life Cycle

Understanding the stages of human growth and development will enable you to enhance your communication skills, including patient education, with patients of all age groups, cultures, and religions. Human growth includes physical, psychological, and emotional growth. Many scientists and behaviorists have studied the developmental stages of human life and have developed guidelines to assist healthcare practitioners and staff in applying effective patient communication skills. Figure 4-2 is an example of a lifespan development model created by Erik Erikson (1902–1994).

Maslow's Hierarchy of Human Needs

Abraham Maslow, a well-known human behaviorist, developed a model of human behavior known as the **hierarchy** (classification) of needs (Figure 4-3). This hierarchy states that human beings are motivated by unsatisfied needs and that certain lower needs have to be satisfied before higher needs, such as self-actualization, are met. Maslow felt that people are basically trustworthy, self-protecting, and self-governing and that humans tend toward growth and love. He believed that humans are not violent by nature, but are violent only when their needs are not being met.

Deficiency (Basic) Needs According to Maslow, there are general types of needs—physiological, safety, love/belonging, and esteem—that must be satisfied before a person can act unselfishly. He called these needs deficiency (basic) needs.

Physiological Needs Physiological needs are humans' very basic needs, such as air, water, food, sleep, and sex. When these needs are not satisfied, we may feel sickness, irritation, pain, and discomfort. These feelings motivate us to alleviate them as soon as possible to establish **homeostasis** (that is, a state of balance or equilibrium). Once our basic needs are met and our feelings are alleviated, we may think about other things.

Safety Needs People have the need and desire for establishing stability and consistency. These basic needs are security, shelter, and existing in a safe environment.

Love/Belonging Needs Humans have a desire to belong to groups: clubs, work groups, religious groups, family, and so on. We need to feel loved and accepted by others. Humans are like pack animals—we place great importance in belonging to society.

Esteem Needs Humans like to feel that they are important and valuable to society. There are two types of self-esteem. The first results from competence or mastery of a task, such as completing an educational program. The second is the attention and recognition that come from others.

Self-Actualization Self-actualization is finding self-fulfillment and realizing one's own potential. To reach this level, a person utilizes many tools to maximize potential, such as education, a fulfilling career, and a balanced personal life. Self-actualized people are generally comfortable with who they are and know their strengths and weaknesses.

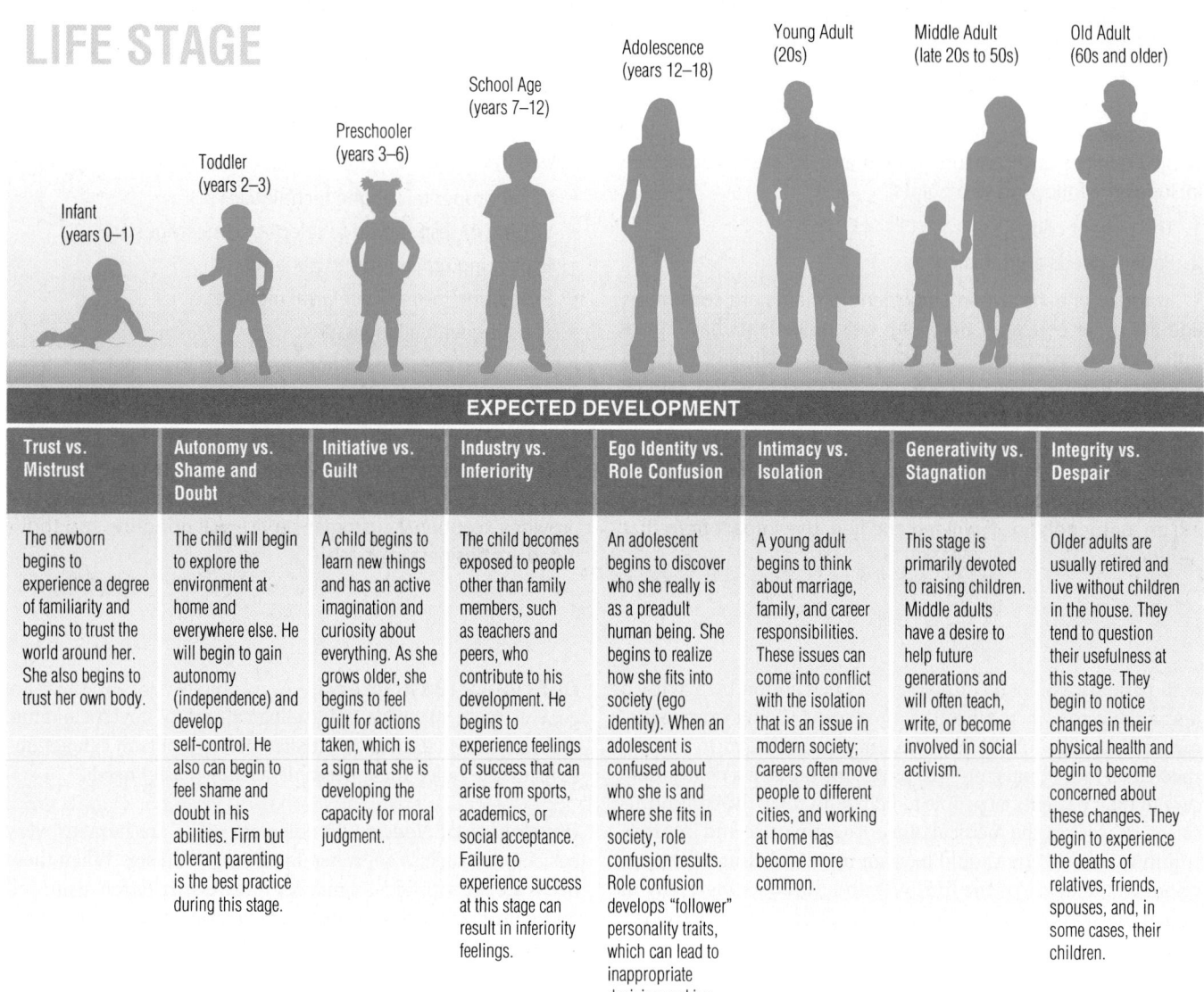

LIFE STAGE

| Infant (years 0–1) | Toddler (years 2–3) | Preschooler (years 3–6) | School Age (years 7–12) | Adolescence (years 12–18) | Young Adult (20s) | Middle Adult (late 20s to 50s) | Old Adult (60s and older) |

EXPECTED DEVELOPMENT

Trust vs. Mistrust	Autonomy vs. Shame and Doubt	Initiative vs. Guilt	Industry vs. Inferiority	Ego Identity vs. Role Confusion	Intimacy vs. Isolation	Generativity vs. Stagnation	Integrity vs. Despair
The newborn begins to experience a degree of familiarity and begins to trust the world around her. She also begins to trust her own body.	The child will begin to explore the environment at home and everywhere else. He will begin to gain autonomy (independence) and develop self-control. He also can begin to feel shame and doubt in his abilities. Firm but tolerant parenting is the best practice during this stage.	A child begins to learn new things and has an active imagination and curiosity about everything. As she grows older, she begins to feel guilt for actions taken, which is a sign that she is developing the capacity for moral judgment.	The child becomes exposed to people other than family members, such as teachers and peers, who contribute to his development. He begins to experience feelings of success that can arise from sports, academics, or social acceptance. Failure to experience success at this stage can result in inferiority feelings.	An adolescent begins to discover who she really is as a preadult human being. She begins to realize how she fits into society (ego identity). When an adolescent is confused about who she is and where she fits in society, role confusion results. Role confusion develops "follower" personality traits, which can lead to inappropriate decision making.	A young adult begins to think about marriage, family, and career responsibilities. These issues can come into conflict with the isolation that is an issue in modern society; careers often move people to different cities, and working at home has become more common.	This stage is primarily devoted to raising children. Middle adults have a desire to help future generations and will often teach, write, or become involved in social activism.	Older adults are usually retired and live without children in the house. They tend to question their usefulness at this stage. They begin to notice changes in their physical health and begin to become concerned about these changes. They begin to experience the deaths of relatives, friends, spouses, and, in some cases, their children.

FIGURE 4-2 Lifespan development.

Considering Patients' Needs When working and communicating with patients, remember this hierarchy of human needs and observe what need a patient is deficient in. For example, if an elderly patient has recently lost her husband, she may feel lonely and deficient in the love need. You may see homeless patients who are deficient in their physiological and safety needs. You may have a young girl as a patient who is overweight and has low self-esteem. On the other hand, you may have a high-level executive as a patient who has reached self-actualization. Each of these scenarios would require a communication style adjustment in order for you to effectively communicate with these patients.

▶ Types of Communication LO 4.3

Each type of communication (verbal, nonverbal, or written) can be positive or negative. An effective communicator is familiar with these different types of communication. This chapter focuses on verbal and nonverbal communication.

Positive Verbal Communication

In the medical office, communication that promotes patient comfort and well-being is essential. Treating patients brusquely or rudely is unacceptable in the healthcare setting. It is your responsibility to set the stage for positive communication.

When information—even bad news—is communicated with some positive aspect, patients are more likely to listen attentively and respond positively themselves. For example, you might explain to a patient who is about to get an injection, "This will sting, but only for a couple of seconds. When we are through, you are free to go." You would not just say, "This is going to hurt."

Other examples of positive communication are

- Being friendly, warm, and attentive ("It's good to see you again, Mrs. Armstrong. I know you're on your lunch hour, so let's get started right away.").
- Verbalizing concern for patients ("Are you comfortable?" "I understand it hurts when I do this; I'll be gentle." "This paperwork won't take long at all.").

FIGURE 4-3 Maslow's hierarchy.

- Encouraging patients to ask questions ("I hope I've explained the procedure well. Do you have any questions, or are there any parts you would like to go over again?").
- Asking patients to repeat your instructions to make sure they understand ("Will you explain to me how you plan to take your medicine?").
- Looking directly at patients when you speak to them.
- Smiling (naturally, not in a forced way).
- Speaking slowly and clearly, being sure to pronounce words correctly.
- Listening carefully.

Negative Verbal Communication

Most people do not purposely try to communicate negatively. Some people, however, may not realize that their communication style has a negative impact on others. Look for and ask for feedback to help you curb negative communication habits. Ask yourself, "Do the physicians and my other coworkers seem glad to speak with me? Are they open and responsive to me?" "Do patients seem at ease with me, or are they very quiet, turned off, or distant?" (Note that some patients may respond this way because of the way they feel, not because of the way you are communicating with them.) Here are some examples of negative communication:

- Mumbling.
- Speaking brusquely or sharply.
- Avoiding eye contact.
- Interrupting patients as they are speaking.
- Rushing through explanations or instructions.
- Treating patients impersonally.
- Making patients feel they are taking up too much of your time or asking too many questions.
- Forgetting common courtesies, such as saying please and thank you.
- Showing boredom.

A good way to avoid negative communication is to open your eyes and ears to others in service-oriented workplace settings.

The next time you buy something at a store, call a company for information over the phone, or eat at a restaurant, take note of the way the staff treat you. Do they answer your questions courteously? Do they give you the information you ask for? Do they make you feel welcome? You expect good customer service and so do your patients as discussed in the Points on Practice: Customer Service box. What specifically makes their communication style positive or negative? Remember, you can always improve your communication skills.

Nonverbal Communication

Verbal communication refers to communication that is spoken. Nonverbal communication is also known as body language. **Body language** includes facial expressions, eye contact, posture, touch, and attention to personal space. In many instances, people's body language conveys their true feelings, even when their words may say otherwise. A patient might say, "I'm OK about that," but if she is sitting with her arms folded tightly across her chest and avoids looking at you, she may not mean what she says.

Facial Expression Your face is the most expressive part of your body. You can often tell whether someone has understood your message simply by his facial expression. For example, when you are explaining a procedure to a patient, look at his expression. Does he seem puzzled? Is his brow wrinkled? Does he look surprised? Facial expressions can give you clues about how to tailor your communication efforts. They also serve as a form of feedback.

Eye Contact Eye contact is an important part of positive communication. Look directly at patients when speaking to them. Looking away or down communicates that you are not interested in the person or that you are avoiding her for some reason. Cultural differences do occur. For example, in some cultures, it is common to avoid eye contact out of respect for someone who is considered a superior. Thus, children may be taught not to look adults in the eye.

Posture The way you hold or move your head, arms, hands, and the rest of your body can project strong nonverbal messages. During communication, posture can usually be described as open or closed.

Open Posture A feeling of receptiveness and friendliness can be conveyed with an **open posture**. In this position, your arms lie comfortably at your sides or in your lap. You face the other person, and you may lean forward in your chair. This demonstrates that you are listening and are interested in what the other person has to say. Open posture is a form of positive communication.

Closed Posture A **closed posture** conveys the opposite—a feeling of not being totally receptive to what is being said. It also can signal that someone is angry or upset. A person in a closed posture may hold his arms rigidly or fold them across his chest. He may lean back in his chair, away from the other person. He may turn away to avoid eye contact. He may even slouch—a kind of closed posture that can convey fatigue or lack of caring. Watch for patients with closed postures that may indicate tension or pain. Avoid closed postures yourself; they have a negative effect on your communication efforts.

Touch Touch is a powerful form of nonverbal communication. A touch on the arm or a hug can be a means of saying hello, sharing condolences, or expressing congratulations. Family background, culture, age, and gender all influence people's perception of touch. Some people may welcome a touch or think nothing of it. Others may view touching as an invasion of their privacy. In general, in the medical setting, a touch on the shoulder, forearm, or back of the hand to express interest or concern is acceptable.

Personal Space When communicating with others, it is important to be aware of the concept of personal space. **Personal space** is an area that surrounds an individual. By not intruding on patients' personal space, you show respect for their feelings of privacy. In most social situations, it is common for people to stand 4 to 12 feet away from each other. For personal conversation, you would typically stand between 1 and 4 feet away from a person. Some patients may feel uncomfortable and become anxious when you stand or sit close to them. Others prefer the reassurance of having people close to them when they speak. Watch patients carefully. If they lean back when you lean forward or if they fold their arms or turn their head away, you may be invading their personal space. If they lean or step toward you, they may be seeking to close up the personal space.

▶ Improving Your Communication Skills

LO 4.4

Sharpening your communication skills should be an ongoing effort and will help you become a more effective communicator. Among the skills involved in daily communication are listening skills, interpersonal skills, and assertiveness skills.

Listening Skills

Listening involves both hearing and interpreting a message. Listening requires you to pay close attention not only to what is being said but also to nonverbal cues, such as those communicated through body language.

Listening can be passive or active. **Passive listening** is simply hearing what someone has to say without the need for a reply. An example is listening to a news program on the radio; the communication is mainly one-way. **Active listening**, on the other hand, involves two-way communication. You are actively involved in the process, offering feedback or asking questions. As seen in Figure 4-4, active listening takes place, for example, when you interview a patient for her medical history. Active listening is an essential skill in the medical office.

FIGURE 4-4 Active listening requires two-way communication and positive body language.

Several ways to improve your listening skills include

- Prepare to listen. Position yourself at the same level (sitting, standing) as the person who is speaking and assume an open posture.
- Relax and listen attentively. Do not simply pretend to listen to what is being said.
- Maintain eye contact and appropriate personal space.
- Think before you respond.
- Provide feedback. Restate the speaker's message in your own words to show that you understand.
- If you do not understand something that was said, ask the person to repeat it.

Interpersonal Skills

When you interact with people, you use **interpersonal skills**. When you make a patient feel at ease by being warm and friendly, you are demonstrating good interpersonal skills. In addition to warmth and friendliness, valuable interpersonal skills include empathy, respect, genuineness, openness, consideration, and sensitivity.

Warmth and Friendliness A friendly but professional approach, a pleasant greeting, and a smile get you off to a good start when communicating with patients. When your approach is sincere, patients will be more relaxed and open.

Empathy The process of identifying with someone else's feelings is **empathy**. When you are empathetic, you are sensitive to the other person's feelings and problems. For example, if a patient is experiencing a migraine headache and you have never had one, you can still let her know you are trying to imagine, or

relate to, her situation. In other words, you can acknowledge the severity of her pain and show support and care.

Respect Showing respect can mean using a title of courtesy such as "Mr." or "Mrs." when communicating with patients. It also can mean acknowledging a patient's wishes or choices without passing judgment.

Genuineness Being genuine in your interactions with patients means that you refrain from "putting on an act" or just going through the motions of your job. Patients like to know that their healthcare providers are real people. In a medical setting, being genuine means caring for each patient on an individual basis, giving patients the full attention they deserve, and showing respect for them. Being genuine in your communication with patients encourages them to place trust in you and in what you say.

Openness Openness means being willing to listen to and consider others' viewpoints and concerns and being receptive to their needs. An open individual is accepting of others and not biased for or against them.

Consideration and Sensitivity You should always try to show consideration toward patients and act in a thoughtful, kind way. You must be sensitive to their individual concerns, fears, and needs.

Assertiveness Skills

As a professional, you need to be assertive—to be firm and to stand by your principles while still showing respect for others. Being assertive means trusting your instincts, feelings, and opinions (not in terms of diagnosing, which only the doctor can do, but in terms of basic communication with patients) and acting on them. For example, when you see that a patient looks uneasy, speak up. You might say, "You look concerned. How can I help you feel more comfortable?" versus asking the patient, "What is the matter with you?" Being assertive is different from being aggressive. When people are **aggressive**, they try to impose their position on others or try to manipulate them. Aggressive people are bossy and can be quarrelsome. They do not appear to take into consideration others' feelings, needs, thoughts, ideas, and opinions before they act or speak. To be **assertive**, you must be open, honest, and direct. Be aware of your body position: an open posture conveys the proper message. When you communicate, speak confidently and use "I" statements such as "I feel . . ." or "I think . . ."

Developing your assertiveness skills increases your sense of self-worth and your confidence as a professional. Being assertive will also help you prevent or resolve conflicts more peacefully and increase your leadership ability. People look up to and respect professionals who are assertive in the workplace. See Table 4-1 for a comparison of nonassertive, assertive, and aggressive behaviors.

TABLE 4-1 A Comparison of Nonassertive, Assertive, Aggressive, and Nonassertive Aggressive Behavior

	Nonassertive Behavior	Assertive Behavior	Aggressive Behavior	Nonassertive Aggressive Behavior (NAG)
Characteristics of the Behavior	Emotionally dishonest, indirect, self-denying; allows others to choose for self; does not achieve desired goal	Emotionally honest, direct, self-enhancing, expressive; chooses for self; may achieve goal	Emotionally honest, direct, self-enhancing at the expense of another; expressive; chooses for others; may achieve goal at expense of others	Emotionally dishonest, indirect, self-denying; chooses for others; may achieve goal at expense of others
Your Feelings	Hurt, anxious, possibly angry later	Confident, self-respecting	Righteous, superior, derogative at the time and possibly guilty later	Defiance, anger, self-denying; sometimes anxious, possibly guilty later
The Other Person's Feelings Toward You	Irritated, pity, lack of respect	Generally respected	Angry, resentful	Angry, resentful, irritated, disgusted
The Other Person's Feelings About Herself/Himself	Guilty or superior	Valued, respected	Hurt, embarrassed, defensive	Hurt, guilty or superior, humiliated

▶ Therapeutic Communication Skills LO 4.5

Therapeutic communication is the ability to communicate with patients in terms that they can understand. At the same time, it helps patients to feel at ease and comfortable with what you are saying. It is also the ability to communicate with other team members in technical terms that are appropriate in a healthcare setting. Therapeutic communication techniques can improve communication with patients. This communication must remain within your scope of practice as discussed in the Scope of Practice Points on Practice box. Therapeutic communication involves the following communication skills:

- *Being silent.* Silence allows the patient time to think without pressure.
- *Accepting.* This skill gives the patient an indication of reception. It shows that you have heard the patient and follow the patient's thought pattern. Some indicators of acceptance include nodding; saying "Yes," "I follow what you said," and other such phrases; and body language.
- *Giving recognition.* Show patients that you are aware of them by stating their name in a greeting or by noticing positive changes. With this skill, you are recognizing the patient as a person or individual.
- *Offering self.* Make yourself available to the needs of the patient.
- *Giving a broad opening.* Allow the patient to take the initiative in introducing the topic. Ask open-ended questions such as "Is there something you'd like to talk about?" or "Where would you like to begin?"
- *Offering general leads.* Give the patient encouragement to continue by making comments such as "Go on" or "And then?"
- *Making observations.* Make your perceptions known to the patient. Say things like "You appear tense today" or "Are you uncomfortable when you . . . ?" By calling patients' attention to what is happening to them, you encourage them to notice it for themselves so that they can describe it to you.
- *Encouraging communication.* Ask patients to verbalize what they perceive. Make statements such as "Tell me when you feel anxious" or "What is happening?" Patients should feel free to describe their perceptions to you, and you must try to see things as they seem to the patients.

- *Mirroring.* Restate what the patient has said to demonstrate that you understand.
- *Reflecting.* Encourage patients to think through and answer their own questions. A reflecting dialogue may go like this:

  Patient: Do you think I should tell the doctor?

  Medical Assistant: Do you think you should?

  By reflecting patients' questions or statements back to them, you are helping patients feel that their opinions about their health are of value.
- *Focusing.* Focusing encourages the patient to stay on the topic.
- *Exploring.* Encourage patients to express themselves in more depth. Try to get as much detail as possible about a patient's complaint but avoid probing and prying if the patient does not wish to discuss it.
- *Clarifying.* Ask patients to explain themselves more clearly if they provide information that is vague or not meaningful.
- *Summarizing.* This skill involves organizing and summing up the important points of the discussion. It gives the patient an awareness of the progress made toward greater understanding.

Ineffective Therapeutic Communication

Often, people think they are communicating thoroughly, but they are not. Here are some roadblocks that can interfere with your communication style:

- *Reassuring.* This type of communication indicates to the patient that there is no need for anxiety or worry. By doing this, you devalue the patient's feelings and give false hope if the outcome is not positive. The communication error here is a lack of understanding and empathy.
- *Giving approval.* This is usually done by overtly approving of a patient's behavior. This may lead the patient to strive for praise rather than progress.
- *Disapproving.* Overtly disapproving of a patient's behavior implies that you have the right to pass judgment on the patient's thoughts and actions. Find an alternate attitude when dealing with patients. Adopting a moralistic attitude may take your attention away from the patient's needs and instead direct it toward your own feelings.

- *Agreeing/disagreeing.* Overtly agreeing or disagreeing with thoughts, perceptions, and ideas of patients is not an effective way to communicate. When you agree with patients, they will have the perception that they are right because you agree with them or because you share the same opinion. Opinions and conclusions should be the patient's, not yours. When disagreeing with patients, you become the opposition to them instead of their caregiver. Never place yourself in an argumentative situation regarding a patient's opinions.

- *Advising.* If you tell the patient what you think should be done, you place yourself outside your scope of practice. You cannot advise patients.

- *Probing.* This means discussing a topic that the patient has no desire to discuss.

- *Defending.* Protecting yourself, the institution, and others from verbal attack is classified as defending. If you become defensive, the patient may feel the need to discontinue communication.

- *Requesting an explanation.* This communication pattern involves asking patients to provide reasons for their behavior. Patients may not know why they behave in a certain manner. "Why" questions may have an intimidating effect on some patients.

- *Minimizing feelings.* Never judge or make light of a patient's discomfort. You need to be able to perceive what is taking place from the patient's point of view, not your own.

- *Making stereotyped comments.* This type of communication involves using meaningless clichés—such as "It's for your own good"—when communicating with patients. These types of comments are given in an automatic, mechanical way as a substitute for a more reasonable and thoughtful explanation.

Defense Mechanisms

When working with patients, it is important to observe their communication behaviors. Patients often develop unconscious defense mechanisms, or coping strategies, to protect themselves from anxiety, guilt, and shame. The following are some common defense mechanisms that a patient may display when communicating with the doctor, medical assistant, or other healthcare team members. These mechanisms may be adaptive (have the ability to change or adjust) or nonadaptive (not have the ability to change or adjust).

- *Compensation*: Overemphasizing a trait to make up for a perceived or actual failing.

- *Denial*: An unconscious attempt to reject unacceptable feelings, needs, thoughts, wishes, or external reality factors.

- *Displacement*: The unconscious transfer of unacceptable thoughts, feelings, or desires from the self to a more acceptable external substitute.

- *Dissociation*: Disconnecting emotional significance from specific ideas or events.

- *Identification*: Mimicking the behavior of another to cope with feelings of inadequacy.

- *Introjection*: Adopting the unacceptable thoughts or feelings of others.

- *Projection*: Projecting onto another person one's own feelings, as if they had originated in the other person.

- *Rationalization*: Justifying unacceptable behavior, thoughts, and feelings into tolerable behaviors.

- *Regression*: Unconsciously returning to more infantile behaviors or thoughts.

- *Repression*: Putting unpleasant thoughts, feelings, or events out of one's mind.

- *Substitution*: Unconsciously replacing an unreachable or unacceptable goal with another, more acceptable one.

▶ Communicating in Special Circumstances   LO 4.6

If you make an effort to develop good interpersonal skills, most patients will not be difficult to communicate with. You will, however, encounter patients in special circumstances that can sometimes inhibit communication, such as when they may be anxious or angry. Patients from different cultures may pose challenges to communication. Others may have some type of impairment or disability that makes communication difficult. Patients with terminal illnesses also may present communication difficulties. Learning about these patients' special needs and polishing your own communication skills will help you become an effective communicator in any number of situations.

The Anxious Patient

It is not uncommon for patients to be anxious in a doctor's office or other healthcare setting. This reaction is commonly known as the "white-coat syndrome." In some cases, the anxiety even raises the patient's blood pressure. There can be many reasons for anxiety. A patient can become anxious because she is ill and does not know what is wrong with her—she may fear the worst. A patient may have recently been diagnosed with an illness that he knows nothing about, which may necessitate a severe lifestyle change. Fear of bad news or fear that some procedure is going to be painful can create anxiety. Regardless of what is causing it, anxiety can interfere with the communication process. For example, because of anxiety, a patient may not listen well or pay attention to what you are saying.

Some patients—particularly children—may be unable to verbalize their feelings of fear and anxiety. Watch for signs of anxiety, which may include a tense appearance, increased blood pressure and rates of breathing and pulse, sweaty palms, reported problems with sleep or appetite, irritability, and agitation. Procedure 4-1, found at the end of this chapter, will help you communicate with anxious patients.

Go to CONNECT to see a video about *Communicating with the Anxious Patient.*

The Angry Patient

In a medical setting, anger may occur for many reasons. Anger may be a mask for fear about an illness or the outcome of surgery. Anger may come from a patient's feeling of being treated unfairly or without compassion, or it may stem from a patient's resentment about being ill or injured. Anger may also be a reaction to frustration, rejection, disappointment, feelings of loss of control or self-esteem, or an invasion of privacy.

As a medical assistant, you will encounter angry patients and will need to help them express their anger constructively, for the sake of their health. At the same time, you must learn not to take expressions of anger personally; you may just be the unlucky target. The goal with angry patients is to help them refocus emotional energy toward solving the problem. Procedure 4-2, found at the end of this chapter, will help you communicate with angry patients.

Patients of Other Cultures

Our beliefs, attitudes, values, use of language, and world views are unique to us, but they are also shaped by our cultural background. Each culture and ethnic group has its own behaviors, traditions, and values. Rather than viewing these differences as communication barriers, strive to understand them (Figure 4-5). For example, many medical facilities are located in heavily populated ethnic locations, and it is important that the medical staff understand the differences among patient cultures. A medical assistant who is employed in a medical facility in which the majority of patients are Latino should learn as much as possible about the specific Latin culture in her area in order to provide good customer service.

It is necessary to understand the difference between stereotyping and generalizing. *Stereotyping* is a negative statement about the specific traits of a group that is applied unfairly to an entire population. A *generalization* is a statement about common trends within a group, but it is understood that further investigation is needed to determine if the trend applies to an individual.

Remember, the beliefs of other cultures are neither superior nor inferior to your own. They are simply different. Never allow yourself to make value judgments or to stereotype a patient, a culture, or an ethnic group. Each patient is an individual in her own right.

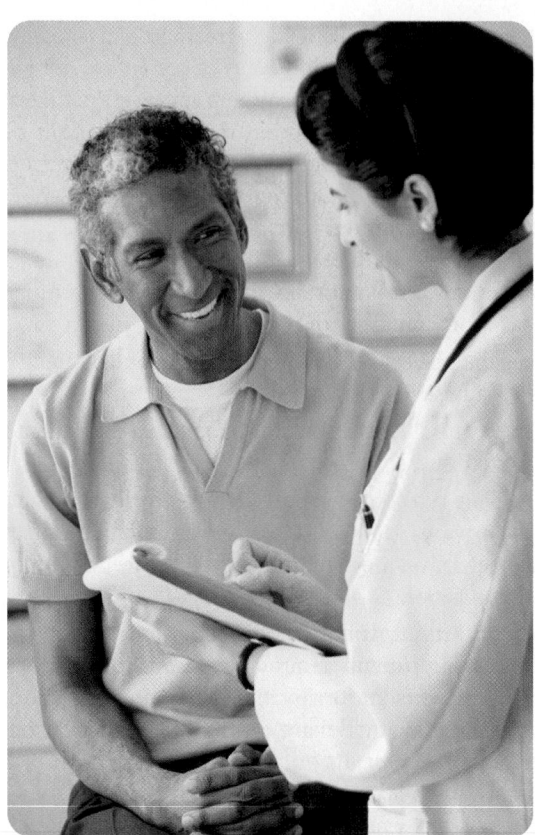

FIGURE 4-5 Knowing how to communicate across cultures is an essential skill of medical assistants.

Cultural Differences Patients' cultural backgrounds have an effect on their attitudes, perceptions, behaviors, and expectations toward health and illness. The following are examples of cultural differences. More information can be found online at the National Institutes of Health website, http://sis.nlm.nih.gov/outreach/multicultural.html.

- Many cultures believe that some illnesses are caused by a change in the "vital energy" or hot and cold forces in the body.
- Certain cultures may differ in the way they perceive and report symptoms. Some may express pain very emotionally because their culture may feel that suppressing pain is harmful. In contrast, people from other cultures may not admit that they are in pain, thinking that acknowledging pain is a sign of weakness.
- Patients of certain ethnic or cultural groups often consult other types of healers before seeing a doctor. They are likely to have different expectations of treatment from each.
- Patients from other cultures may be wary of certain treatments because these treatments are so different from what they are accustomed to. This is especially true of some of the medical procedures and interventions considered to be state-of-the-art, such as laser surgery or diabetes management.
- In some cultures, it may not be appropriate to suggest making a will for dying patients or patients with terminal illnesses; this is the cultural equivalent of wishing death on a patient.

Language Barriers Patients who cannot speak or understand English may have difficulty expressing their needs or feelings effectively. One of the first things you can do is use a family member who is present as an interpreter. However, federal policies require healthcare providers who receive federal funds (i.e., Medicare) to make interpretive services available to their patients with limited English. The interpreter should be a medically trained interpreter, especially for patients having surgery or if a consent form needs to be signed. If your medical office has a large number of non-English speakers, it is a good idea to have forms translated and available for use. Practice Procedure 4-3, Communicating with the Assistance of an Interpreter, at the end of this chapter.

Limited Reading Skills You will find on occasion that some of your patients are functionally illiterate. They may try to hide this by saying, "I didn't bring my glasses with me" or "This is too much to read right now." Be polite, review the information with them, and ask if they have any questions. Send the information home and have them further discuss it with a family member before requesting that they sign forms such as consent forms or forms that need to be signed before having surgery. Several vendors will publish your patient education materials on a specific readability level. It is recommended that patient education brochures not exceed fourth- to eighth-grade reading levels. Visual media can be provided through valid Internet resources that will improve communication as well.

Cultural Competence Your cultural competence relates to your ability to respond to the cultural and language needs of the patients you encounter. Consider the following techniques to improve your communication with patients of various cultures.

- If possible, learn and use a few phrases of greeting and introduction in the patient's native language. This conveys respect and demonstrates your willingness to learn about their culture.
- Use an interpreter whenever needed to assist with communication. Look at the patient, not the interpreter, during communication.
- Be aware of nonverbal communication and respond. For example, look for signs of pain such as a grimace.
- Avoid saying "You must . . ." Instead, teach patients their options and let them decide; for example, "Some people in this situation would . . ."
- Always give the reason or purpose for a treatment or prescription.
- Make sure patients understand by having them explain it themselves.

The Patient Who Is Mentally or Emotionally Disturbed

There may be times when you will need to communicate with patients who are mentally or emotionally disturbed. When dealing with this type of patient, you need to determine what level of communication the patient can understand. Keep these suggestions in mind to improve communication.

- It is important to remain calm if the patient becomes agitated or confused.
- Avoid raising your voice or appearing impatient.
- If you do not understand what the patient said, ask him to repeat what he said.

Terminally Ill Patients

Terminally ill patients are often under extreme stress and can be a challenge to treat. It is important that healthcare professionals respect the rights of terminal patients and treat them with dignity. It is also important that you communicate with the family and offer support and empathy as their loved one accepts her condition. You also should provide information on **hospice**, which is an area of medicine that works with terminally ill patients and their families. Hospice workers often go to the home of the terminally ill patient or work with patients in facilities. Hospice care is usually staffed with RNs and other healthcare providers who have specialized training in issues related to death and dying. They work with the family and patient in the beginning, assisting with medications, comfort care, and emotional support. If the patient dies at home, they may end by making arrangements with the funeral home and coroner.

Elisabeth Kübler-Ross, a world-renowned authority in the areas of death and dying, developed a model that describes the behavior patients will experience on learning their condition. This is called the stages of dying or stages of grief (Figure 4-6). This model is widely used today in work with terminally ill patients.

Patients' Families and Friends

Family members or friends sometimes accompany a patient to the office. These individuals can provide important emotional support to the patient. Always ask patients if they want a family member or friend to accompany them to the examination room, however. Do not just assume their preference. Acknowledge family members and friends, and communicate with them as you do with patients. They should be kept informed of the patient's progress, whenever possible, to avoid unnecessary anxiety on their part. You must always protect patient confidentiality, however. Too often, healthcare workers think that it is acceptable to discuss patient cases in detail with family members, even without the patient's consent.

The Patient with AIDS and the Patient Who Is HIV-Positive

Patients with acquired immunodeficiency syndrome (AIDS) and patients who have the human immunodeficiency virus (HIV), the virus that causes AIDS, may face social stigma or blame themselves. These patients often feel guilty, angry, and depressed.

To communicate effectively with these patients, you need accurate information about the disease and the risks involved. Take the initiative to educate yourself about AIDS and HIV. Patients will have many questions. Part of your role as a good communicator will be to answer as many questions as you can. If a

Kübler-Ross's stages of dying include five stages, which usually—but not always—progress in the following order:

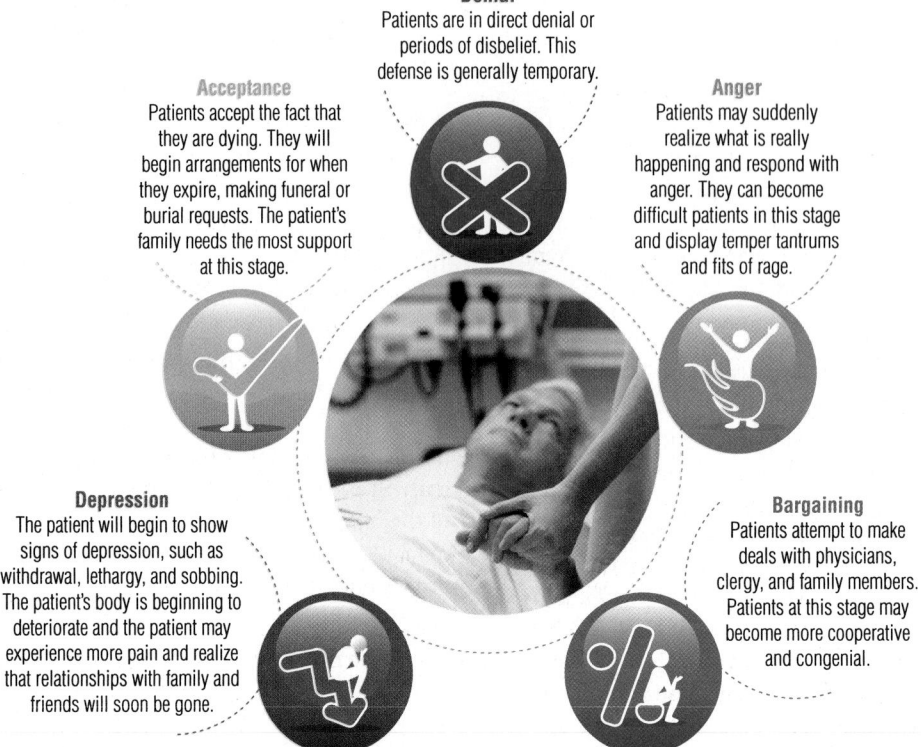

Denial
Patients are in direct denial or periods of disbelief. This defense is generally temporary.

Anger
Patients may suddenly realize what is really happening and respond with anger. They can become difficult patients in this stage and display temper tantrums and fits of rage.

Acceptance
Patients accept the fact that they are dying. They will begin arrangements for when they expire, making funeral or burial requests. The patient's family needs the most support at this stage.

Bargaining
Patients attempt to make deals with physicians, clergy, and family members. Patients at this stage may become more cooperative and congenial.

Depression
The patient will begin to show signs of depression, such as withdrawal, lethargy, and sobbing. The patient's body is beginning to deteriorate and the patient may experience more pain and realize that relationships with family and friends will soon be gone.

Even though these stages have been generalized to dying, many experts have applied them to the grieving process as well. For example, after a stroke, a patient may go through the process of grieving his loss of body function.

FIGURE 4-6 Kübler-Ross's stages of dying.

patient asks a question you cannot answer, tell the physician so he can respond quickly.

Remember, HIV is not transmitted through casual or common physical contact, such as brushing by a person in a crowded hall or shaking hands. It is transferred only through bodily fluids. Patients with AIDS and those who are HIV-positive need to know you are not afraid to be near them, to touch them, or to talk to them. Like any patient whose body is being ravaged by a serious illness, these patients need human contact (verbal and physical) and they need to be treated with dignity.

▶ Communicating with Coworkers LO 4.7

The quality of the communication you have with coworkers greatly influences the development of a positive or negative work climate and a team approach to patient care. In turn, the workplace atmosphere ultimately affects your communication with patients.

Positive Communication with Coworkers

In your interactions with coworkers, use the same skills and qualities that you use to communicate with patients. Have respect and empathy; be caring, thoughtful, and genuine; and use active listening skills. These skills will help you develop **rapport**, which is a harmonious, positive relationship, with your coworkers. Following are some rules for communication in the medical office.

- Use proper channels of communication. For example, if you are having problems getting along with a coworker, try first to work it out with her. Do not go over her head and complain to her supervisor. Your coworker may not have realized the effect of her behavior and may wish to correct it without involving her supervisor. If you go to the supervisor right away, working relationships can become even more strained.

- Have the proper attitude. You can avoid conflict and resolve most problems if you maintain a positive attitude. A friendly approach is much more effective than a hostile approach. Remember, many problems are simply the result of misinformation or lack of communication.

- Plan an appropriate time for communication. If you have something important to discuss, schedule a time to do so. For example, if you want to talk with the office manager about renewing the lease on a piece of office equipment, tell him you would like to discuss that topic and ask him to let you know a time that is convenient.

As an example of good communication with coworkers, consider this exchange between Kaylyn, a clinical medical assistant, and Miguel, her coworker at BWW Associates. Note the way Kaylyn demonstrates assertiveness.

Kaylyn: I know you spent a lot of time choosing the new toys for the reception area. I love the wooden safari animal puzzles.

Miguel: Thanks. I think the children really enjoy themselves now.

Kaylyn: I wanted to mention to you, though, that I'm concerned about the toy tea set with miniature cupcakes and sandwiches. Anything that's smaller than a golf ball is a choking hazard to infants and toddlers.

Miguel: I don't think the little ones pay much attention to the tea set. It's mostly for older kids.

Kaylyn: Yes, but I'm still afraid that a baby could put one of those pieces in his mouth. What if we put up a little shelf in the play area that is low enough for kids 4 years old or more to reach, but high enough to be out of reach of the babies? We could put the tea set on it in a clear plastic box and any other toys with small parts.

Miguel: I see your point. Sounds like a good idea to me.

Kaylyn started with a statement that acknowledged the coworker's situation and feelings. Then she stated her own opinion. When her coworker disagreed, she repeated her concern, describing what might happen if the situation remained unchanged. Then, she made a constructive suggestion for solving the problem without hurting the coworker's feelings. As you interact with coworkers, be sensitive to the timing of your conversations, the manner in which you present your ideas and thoughts, and your coworkers' feelings.

Communicating with Management

Positive or negative communication can affect the quality of your relationships with your supervisor or manager. For example, problems arise when communication about job responsibilities is unclear or when you feel that your supervisor does not trust or respect you, or vice versa. Consider these suggestions when communicating with your direct supervisor:

- Keep your supervisor informed. If the office copier is not working properly, talk to your supervisor about it before a breakdown occurs that will hold everyone up. If several patients express the same types of complaint about the examination rooms, make sure the right people are told. If the doctor asks you to call a patient and you reach the patient, tell the doctor.

- Ask questions. If you are unsure about an administrative task or the meaning of a medical term, for example, do not hesitate to ask your supervisor. It is better to ask a question

before acting than to make a mistake. It is also better to ask than to risk annoying someone because you carried out a task or wrote a term incorrectly. Asking your supervisor or manager a question shows that you respect him or her professionally.

- Minimize interruptions. For example, before launching into a discussion, make sure your supervisor has time to talk. Opening with "Can I interrupt you for a moment, or should I come back?" or "Do you have a minute to talk?" goes a long way toward establishing good communication. It is also better to go to your supervisor when you have several questions to ask rather than to interrupt her repeatedly.

- Show initiative. Any manager or supervisor will greatly appreciate this quality. For example, if you think you can come up with a more efficient way to get the office newsletter written and distributed, write out a plan and show it to your supervisor. He or she is likely to welcome any ideas that improve office efficiency or patient satisfaction.

Dealing with Conflict

Conflict, or friction, in the workplace can result from opposition of opinions or ideas or even from a difference in personalities. Conflict can arise when the lines of communication break down or when a misunderstanding occurs. Conflict also can result from prejudices or preconceived notions about people or from lack of mutual respect or trust between a staff member and management. Whatever the cause, conflict is counterproductive to the efficiency of an office.

Following these suggestions can help prevent conflict in the office and improve communication among coworkers.

- Do not "feed into" other people's negative attitudes. For example, if a coworker is criticizing one of the doctors, change the subject or walk away.

- Try your best at all times to be personable and supportive of coworkers. For example, everyone has bad days. If a coworker is having a bad day, offer to pitch in and help or to run out and get her lunch if she is too busy to go out.

- Refrain from passing judgment or stereotyping others (women are bad at math, men do not know how to communicate, and so on). Coworkers should show respect for one another and try to be tolerant and nonjudgmental.

- Do not gossip. You are there to work. Act professionally at all times.

- Do not jump to conclusions. For example, if you get a memo about a change in your schedule that disturbs you, bring your concern to your supervisor. She may be able to be flexible on certain points. You do not know until you ask.

Setting Boundaries in the Healthcare Environment

As a medical assistant, your professional behavior is extremely important. In many instances, when dealing with patients, physicians, and other staff members, you must set **boundaries**, whether physical or psychological. This will limit undesirable behavior.

If a patient, physician, or staff member is acting inappropriately toward you, you must take immediate action. Do not let the situation "fester." You must act tactfully, assertively, and diplomatically. Let the aggressor know that his actions or language is inappropriate, and that you are not obligated in any way to accept such behavior. If none of the actions assist with stopping the unacceptable behavior, report the behavior to your immediate supervisor so she can assist you in identifying a solution. If the aggressor is your immediate supervisor, follow the office policy and procedure. Make yourself aware of policy and procedures ahead of time by reading the policy and procedure manual, which will be discussed in the *Practice Management* chapter.

PROCEDURE 4-1 Communicating with the Anxious Patient

Procedure Goal: To use communication and interpersonal skills to calm an anxious patient.

OSHA Guidelines: This procedure does not involve exposure to blood, body fluids, or tissue.

Materials: none

Method: Procedure steps.

1. Identify signs of anxiety in the patient.
2. Acknowledge the patient's anxiety. (Ignoring a patient's anxiety often makes it worse.)
   RATIONALE: Good therapeutic communication techniques can help reduce patient anxiety.
3. Identify possible sources of anxiety, such as fear of a procedure or test result, along with supportive resources available to the patient, such as family members and friends.
   RATIONALE: Understanding the source of anxiety in a patient and identifying the supportive resources available can help you communicate with the patient more effectively.
4. Do what you can to alleviate the patient's physical discomfort. For example, find a calm, quiet place for the patient to wait, a comfortable chair, a drink of water, or access to the bathroom.
5. Allow ample personal space for conversation. Note: You would normally allow a 1- to 4-foot distance between yourself and the patient. Adjust this space as necessary.
6. Create a climate of warmth, acceptance, and trust.
   a. Recognize and control your own anxiety. Your air of calm can decrease the patient's anxiety.
   b. Provide reassurance by demonstrating genuine care, respect, and empathy.
   c. Act confidently and dependably, maintaining truthfulness and confidentiality at all times.

7. Using the appropriate communication skills, have the patient describe the experience that is causing anxiety, her thoughts about it, and her feelings. Proceeding in this order allows the patient to describe what is causing the anxiety and to clarify her thoughts and feelings about it.
   a. Maintain an open posture.
   b. Maintain eye contact, if culturally appropriate.
   c. Use active listening skills.
   d. Listen without interrupting.
   RATIONALE: The use of open-ended questioning will result in more information about the patient's feelings of anxiety.
8. Do not belittle the patient's thoughts and feelings. This can cause a breakdown in communication, increase anxiety, and make the patient feel isolated.
9. Be empathic to the patient's concerns.
10. Help the patient recognize and cope with the anxiety.
    a. Provide information to the patient. Patients are often fearful of the unknown.
    b. Suggest coping behaviors, such as deep breathing or other relaxation exercises.
    RATIONALE: Helping them understand their disease or the procedure they are about to undergo will help decrease their anxiety.
11. Notify the doctor of the patient's concerns.
    RATIONALE: The physician must be aware of all aspects of the patient's health, including anxiety, to allow for optimal patient care. Part of your job as a medical assistant is to act as a liaison between the patient and the physician.

PROCEDURE 4-2 Communicating with the Angry Patient

Procedure Goal: To use communication and interpersonal skills to calm an angry patient.

OSHA Guidelines: This procedure does not involve exposure to blood, body fluids, or tissue.

Materials: none

Method: Procedure steps.

1. Recognize anger and its causes. Anger is easy to recognize in most people, but it can be subtle in others. Patients who speak in a tense tone, are stubborn, or appear to ignore your attempts at communication may be angry.

2. Remain calm and continue to demonstrate genuineness and respect. Communicate that you respect and care about the patient's feelings.

3. Focus on the patient's physical and medical needs.

4. Maintain adequate personal space. Place yourself on the same level as the patient. If the patient is standing, encourage him to sit down. Maintain an open posture and eye contact but avoid staring.
   RATIONALE: Open posture and eye contact show the patient you are receptive to listening. Staring at the patient may make the person angrier.

5. Listen attentively and with an open mind to what the patient is saying. Avoid the feeling that you need to defend yourself or to give reasons why the patient should not be angry.
   RATIONALE: Most patients' anger will lessen if they know someone is really listening to them and showing an interest in their emotions and needs.

6. Encourage patients to be specific in describing the cause of their anger, their thoughts about it, and their feelings.

Be empathic and acknowledge the patient's feelings and perceptions. Follow through with any promises you might make concerning correction of a problem, but avoid totally agreeing or disagreeing with the patient. State what you can and cannot do for the patient.

7. Present your point of view calmly and firmly to help the patient better understand the situation. If patients are receptive to your viewpoint, their perspective may change for the better.

8. Avoid a breakdown in communication. Allow the patient to voice anger. Trying to outtalk the patient or overexplain will only annoy and irritate him. If needed, suggest that the patient spend a few moments alone to gather his thoughts or to cool off before continuing any type of communication.

9. If you feel threatened by a patient's anger or if it looks as if the patient's anger may become violent, leave the room and seek assistance from one of the physicians or other members of the office staff.

10. Document any actual threats in the patient's chart.

PROCEDURE 4-3 Communicating with the Assistance of an Interpreter

Procedure Goal: To demonstrate techniques to effectively communicate with a non-English-speaking patient through an interpreter.

OSHA Guidelines: This procedure does not involve exposure to blood, body fluids, or tissue.

Materials: Pen, forms, or computer, and appropriate pictures and other visual aids if available.

Method: Procedure steps.

1. Identify the patient by name and ask if you pronounced the name correctly. Be sure to smile, even if you are feeling slightly awkward or unsure of yourself.
   RATIONALE: A smile is a form of nonverbal communication that will help the patient feel more comfortable.

2. Introduce yourself with your title to the patient and the interpreter.

3. Ask the interpreter to spell his or her full name and provide you with identification, such as his agency's identification or a business card. Retain his business card to file in the patient's medical record. If he or she does not have a business card, obtain contact information, which also will be filed in the patient's medical record.
   RATIONALE: Healthcare facilities are required to provide an interpreter and this information must be documented.

4. Do not take it personally if the patient appears abrupt or even rude; this behavior may be considered appropriate in the patient's culture. For example, in some cultures, male patients may not deal with a female staff member and that should be respected if possible. Ascertain from the interpreter if there is a problem.

5. Inquire of the interpreter if the patient speaks or understands any English and if there are any communication traditions or other customs that you should be aware of. For example, traditional Navajo people consider it rude to have direct eye contact.

6. Provide a quiet comfortable area.

7. Speak directly to the patient and speak slowly if the patient has any understanding of English.
   RATIONALE: Eye contact and other forms of nonverbal communication are important to convey and receive information.

8. If forms are to be completed, instruct the interpreter to translate with appropriate intervals and give opportunities for the patient to ask questions to ensure understanding. For example, if providing general consent for treatment, permission to send information and receive payment directly from the insurance company, and privacy decisions, have one area translated at a time. Instruct the interpreter to ask if there are questions at each portion.

9. If the patient and interpreter are discussing an issue in depth or appear to be leaving you out of the conversation, ask the translator what is being said.

10. Provide the same information, services, and courtesies that you would to a native English speaker. If possible, provide written information in the patient's native language.

11. Document what you would ordinarily document; note on all forms that "translation was done by" and include the name, credential, and agency of the interpreter, as well as the date and time.

LEARNING OUTCOMES	KEY POINTS
4.1 Identify elements and types of communication.	The communication circle involves a message being sent, a source, and a receiver that responds. Feedback is the response to a message and noise is anything that may interfere with or change the message.
4.2 Relate communication to human behavior and needs.	Understanding human behavior and needs, and their correlation with professional relationships, is necessary to practicing as a medical assistant. Understanding the various stages of human life assists you in your communication skills with patients.
4.3 Categorize positive and negative communication.	Communication that promotes comfort and well-being is considered positive communication. Negative communication can be a turnoff. Medical assistants may not be aware of some of the signs of negative communication they display. Lack of eye contact with patients, except in specific cultures, or speaking sharply to a patient is considered negative communication. To assist in avoiding this type of communication, ask yourself, "Does this make me feel good?" or "Do I feel welcome?"
4.4 Model ways to improve listening, interpersonal skills, and assertiveness skills.	Listening and other interpersonal skills can be improved by becoming more involved in the communication process by offering feedback or asking questions of the patient. Understand that assertive medical assistants trust their instincts. They respect their self-worth, while still making the patient feel comfortable and important. Aggressive medical assistants try to impose their positions through manipulation techniques.
4.5 Carry out therapeutic communication skills.	Therapeutic communication is the ability to communicate with patients in terms that they can understand and, at the same time, feel at ease and comfortable in what you are saying. Positive therapeutic skills can enhance communication. Be aware of negative therapeutic skills that can disrupt the communication. Recognize defense mechanisims in patients and note whether the patient is using them to cope or is not able to cope.
4.6 Use effective communication strategies with patients in special circumstances.	Learning about the special needs of patients and polishing your communication skills will help you become an effective communicator. This will assist you with handling diversity in the workplace, with handling anxious and annoyed patients, and in dealing with patients who may have language barriers.
4.7 Carry out positive communication with coworkers and management.	The quality of communication you have with your coworkers and your supervisor greatly influences the development of a positive or negative work climate. Use proper channels of communication. Be open-minded. Keep supervisors informed of office problems as they arise and show initiative in your work habits.

Recall Cindy Chen from the beginning of the chapter. Now that you have completed the chapter, answer the following questions regarding her case.

1. Cindy Chen is nervous. What techniques could you use to improve your communication with her?

2. What should you do regarding Cindy Chen's health status of HIV positive?

3. How would you best answer Ms. Chen's question, "Do you have anything you can give me until I see the doctor?"

1. (LO 4.1) The main elements in the communication circle include
   a. A message (verbal and nonverbal), a source, and a receiver
   b. A message and a receiver
   c. A receiver, a response, a sender, and a source
   d. A source, feedback, and a receiver (verbal and nonverbal)
   e. A message, a receiver, and a response

2. (LO 4.7) Good relationships with coworkers would not include
   a. Professionalism
   b. Stress
   c. Cooperation
   d. Gossip
   e. Integrity

3. (LO 4.3) Which is an example of negative communication?
   a. Speaking sharply to the patient
   b. Listening carefully
   c. Being friendly and warm
   d. Looking directly at the patient
   e. Keeping quiet when appropriate

4. (LO 4.1) Which of the following is an example of positive communication?
   a. Treating patients impersonally
   b. Looking directly at patients when you speak to them
   c. Speaking brusquely or sharply
   d. Showing boredom
   e. Forgetting common courtesies, such as saying please and thank you

5. (LO 4.4) The ability to identify with someone else's feelings is called
   a. Sympathy
   b. Feedback
   c. Empathy
   d. Respect
   e. Assertiveness

6. (LO 4.3) Poor communication could lead to all of the following *except*
   a. Patient satisfaction
   b. Errors in billing
   c. Inefficient care
   d. Malpractice
   e. Anxiety

7. (LO 4.3) Personal space in a healthcare environment is approximately
   a. 7–18 feet
   b. 1–4 feet
   c. 3–6 feet
   d. 4–12 feet
   e. 3–10 feet

8. (LO 4.3) You want to convey an open posture while communicating with a patient. What should you do?
   a. Fold your arms and lean forward while looking into the patient's eyes
   b. Lean back gently while facing the patient
   c. Lean forward in your chair facing the patient
   d. Lean forward and avoid eye contact with the patient
   e. Extend your arms while leaning forward toward the patient

9. (LO 4.6) Your patient has been diagnosed with a terminal illness and makes the following comment: "If you could help me make it to my grandson's graduation next month before I get too sick, that would be perfect." Which of Kübler-Ross's stages of dying is this patient exhibiting?
   a. Denial
   b. Bargaining
   c. Depression
   d. Acceptance
   e. Anger

10. (LO 4.6) Which of the following is a proper technique for demonstrating cultural competence?
    a. Avoid giving the reason or purpose for a treatment or prescription since they will not understand
    b. Do not speak in the patients' native language because it may make them uncomfortable
    c. Look at the interpreter during communication to ensure he or she is making the correct statement
    d. Avoid saying, "You must . . ." Instead, teach patients their options and let them decide; for example, "Some people in this situation would . . ."
    e. Ignore nonverbal communication since it is difficult to interpret

Legal and Ethical Issues

PATIENT INFORMATION

C A S E   S T U D Y

Patient Name	Gender	DOB
Cindy Chen	F	7/15/xx

Attending	MRN	Allergies
Alexis N. Whalen, MD	324-86-542	NKA

Cindy Chen, a 28-year-old female complaining of inability to sleep and nervousness, arrives at the office. She tested positive for HIV in 2005, although she has been asymptomatic on antiviral drugs. Currently, she lives with her aunt and is going to school to become a phlebotomist. As you are preparing to bring Cindy in from the reception area, the externship student, who is new to the office, states that she is afraid to work with you when caring for Cindy because she is afraid she might get AIDS if she works closely with her.

Keep Cindy in mind as you study the chapter. There will be questions at the end of the chapter based on the case study. The information in the chapter will help you answer these questions.

L E A R N I N G   O U T C O M E S

After completing Chapter 5, you will be able to:

5.1 Differentiate between laws and ethics.

5.2 Identify the responsibilities of the patient and physician in a physician-patient contract, including the components for informed consent that must be understood by the patient.

5.3 Describe the four Ds of negligence required to prove malpractice and explain the four Cs of malpractice prevention.

5.4 Relate the term *credentialing* and explain the importance of the FDA and DEA to administrative procedures performed by medical assistants.

5.5 Summarize the purpose of the following federal healthcare regulations: HCQIA, False Claims Act, OSHA, and HIPAA.

5.6 Identify the six principles for preventing improper release of information from the medical office.

5.7 Discuss the importance of ethics in the medical office.

5.8 Explain the differences among the practice management models.

K E Y   T E R M S

abandonment	ethics
assault	expressed contract
battery	felony
bioethics	fraud
breach of contract	implied contract
civil law	law
consent	minors
contract	misdemeanor
criminal law	negligence
durable power of attorney	tort

III. C (4) Identify personal safety precautions as established by the Occupational Safety and Health Administration (OSHA)

IX. C (1) Discuss legal scope of practice for medical assistants

IX. C (4) Summarize the Patient Bill of Rights

IX. C (8) Compare criminal and civil law as it applies to the practicing medical assistant

IX. C (9) Provide an example of tort law as it would apply to a medical assistant

IX. C (10) Explain how the following impact the medical assistant's practice and give examples:
   a. Negligence
   b. Malpractice
   c. Statute of Limitations
   d. Uniform Anatomical Gift Act
   f. Living Will/Advanced directives
   g. Medical durable power of attorney

IX. C (13) Discuss all levels of governmental legislation and regulation as they apply to medical assisting practice, including FDA and DEA regulations

IX. P (1) Respond to issues of confidentiality

IX. P (2) Perform within scope of practice

IX. P (8) Apply local, state and federal legislation and regulations to the practice setting

IX. A (2) Demonstrate awareness of the consequences of not working within the legal scope of practice

IX. A (3) Recognize the importance of local, state and federal legislation and regulations in the practice setting

X. C (1) Differentiate between legal, ethical, and moral issues affecting healthcare

X. C (2) Compare personal, professional and organizational ethics

X. C (3) Discuss the role of cultural, social and ethnic diversity in ethical performance of medical assisting practice

X. C (4) Identify where to report illegal and/or unsafe activities and behaviors that affect health, safety and welfare of others

X. P (1) Report illegal and/or unsafe activities and behaviors that affect health, safety and welfare of others to proper authorities

X. P (2) Develop a plan for separation of personal and professional ethics

X. A (1) Apply ethical behaviors, including honesty/integrity in performance of medical assisting practice

X. A (2) Examine the impact personal ethics and morals may have on the individual's practice

4. Medical Law and Ethics

Graduates:

a. Document accurately

b. Institute federal and state guidelines when releasing medical records or information

c. Follow established policies when initiating or terminating medical treatment

d. Understand the importance of maintaining liability coverage once employed in the industry

e. Perform risk management procedures

f. Comply with federal, state, and local health laws and regulations

11. Career Development

Graduates:

b. Demonstrate professionalism by:
   (3) Maintaining confidentiality at all times
   (4) Being cognizant of ethical boundaries
   (9) Conducting work within scope of education, training, and ability

Introduction

Medical law plays an important role in medical facility procedures and the quality of patient care. Our modern society can be a litigious one, where people are inclined to sue when results or outcomes are not acceptable to them. This is particularly true with healthcare practitioners, healthcare facilities, and manufacturers of medical equipment and products. Patients, their relatives, and others often sue when medical outcomes do not meet expectations. As a result, it is important for all medical professionals to understand medical law, ethics, and the Health Insurance Portability and Accountability Act (HIPAA), which began in 1996 and has expanded since that time.

As a medical assistant, having a basic knowledge of medical law and ethics can help you gain perspective in the following three areas:

1. *The rights, responsibilities, and concerns of healthcare consumers.* Healthcare professionals need to be concerned about how law and ethics impact their respective professions and they also must understand how legal and ethical issues affect patients. As medical technology advances and the use of computers increases, patients know more about their healthcare options and their rights as consumers, and more about the responsibilities of healthcare practitioners to their patients. Patients in the United States have come to expect favorable outcomes from medical treatment, and when these expectations are not met, lawsuits may result.

2. *The legal and ethical issues facing society, patients, and healthcare professionals as the world changes.* Every day new technologies emerge with solutions to biological and medical issues. These solutions often include social issues involving decisions about controversial topics like reproductive rights, fetal stem cell research, and confidentiality with sensitive medical records.

3. *The impact of rising costs on the laws and ethics of healthcare delivery.* Rising costs—of both healthcare insurance and medical treatment in general—can lead to questions concerning access to healthcare services and the allocation of medical treatment. For example, should everyone, regardless of age, race, or lifestyle, have the same access to scarce medical commodities like transplant organs and very expensive medications?

Because medical treatment and decisions surrounding healthcare today have become so increasingly complex, it is important to be knowledgeable about, and aware of, the ethical issues and the laws that govern patient care. As a medical assistant and an important member of the healthcare team, always keep in mind that any health or financial information you obtain regarding a patient (past or present) is protected. It may be shared only with the patient's express permission, except in a few very specific instances that will be discussed in this chapter.

Laws and Ethics
LO 5.1

In order to understand medical law and ethics, it is helpful to know the difference between law and ethics. A **law** is defined as a rule of conduct or action prescribed or formally recognized as binding or enforced by a controlling authority, such as local, state, and federal governments. **Ethics** is a standard of behavior and a concept of right and wrong beyond the legal consideration in any given situation. *Moral values*—formed through the influence of family, culture, and society—serve as a basis for ethical conduct. Ethics will be discussed in further detail later in the chapter.

Classifications of Law

While a crime is any offense committed or omitted in violation of a public law, two types of law pertain to healthcare practitioners: criminal law and civil law.

Criminal Law Criminal law involves crimes against the state. When a state or federal law is violated, the government brings criminal charges against the alleged offender, for example, *Ohio v. John Doe*. Criminal laws prohibit such crimes as murder, arson, rape, and burglary. A criminal act may be classified as a felony or a misdemeanor. A **felony** is a crime punishable by death or by imprisonment in a state or federal prison for more than 1 year. Some examples of a felony include abuse (child, elder, or domestic violence), manslaughter, fraud, attempted murder, and practicing medicine without a license.

Misdemeanors are less serious crimes than felonies and are punishable by fines or imprisonment in a facility other than a federal prison for 1 year or less. Some examples of misdemeanors are thefts under a certain dollar amount, attempted burglary, and disturbing the peace.

Civil Law Civil law involves crimes against the person. Under civil law, a person can sue another person, a business, or the government. Court judgments in civil cases often require the payment of a sum of money to the injured party. Civil law includes a general category of law known as torts. A **tort** is broadly defined as a civil wrong committed against a person or property that causes physical injury or damage to someone's property or that deprives someone of his or her personal liberty and freedom. Torts may be intentional (willful) or unintentional (accidental).

Intentional Torts When one person intentionally harms another, the law allows the injured party to seek a remedy in a civil suit. The injured party can be financially compensated for any harm done by the person guilty of committing the tort. If the conduct is judged to be malicious, punitive damages may also be awarded. Examples of intentional torts include the following:

- **Assault** is the open threat of bodily harm to another, or acting in such a way as to put another in the "reasonable apprehension of bodily harm." In the medical office, if a patient were to feel threatened in any way, assault could be charged.

- **Battery** is an action that causes bodily harm to another. It is broadly defined as any bodily contact made without permission. In healthcare delivery, battery may be charged for any unauthorized touching of a patient, including such actions as suturing a wound, administering an injection, or performing a physical examination.

- *Defamation* is the act of damaging a person's reputation by making public statements that are both false and malicious. The full term for these actions is defamation of character. Defamation can take the form of slander and/or libel. *Slander* is speaking damaging words intended to negatively influence others against an individual in a manner that jeopardizes his or her reputation or means of livelihood. If a patient hears members of the staff speaking about him in an unprofessional manner, or talking about his diagnosis with staff members without a "need to know," it could be considered slanderous. *Libel* is publishing in print damaging words, pictures, or signed statements that will injure the reputation of another.

- False imprisonment is the intentional, unlawful restraint or confinement of one person by another. Preventing a patient from leaving the facility might be seen as false imprisonment.

- **Fraud** consists of deceitful practices in depriving or attempting to deprive another of his or her rights, usually for the gain of another. Healthcare practitioners might be accused of fraud for promising patients "miracle cures" or for accepting fees from patients while using mystical or spiritual powers to heal.

- Invasion of privacy is the interference with a person's right to be left alone. Entering an exam room without knocking can be considered an invasion of privacy. The improper use of or a breach of confidentiality of medical records may be seen as an invasion of privacy.

Unintentional Torts The most common torts within the healthcare delivery system are those committed unintentionally. Unintentional torts are acts that are not intended to cause harm but are committed unreasonably or with a disregard for the consequences. In legal terms, such acts constitute negligence. **Negligence** is charged when a healthcare practitioner fails to exercise ordinary care and the patient is injured. Medical negligence is more commonly known as malpractice, which will be discussed in more detail later in this chapter.

Contracts

A **contract** is a voluntary agreement between two parties in which specific promises are made for a consideration. The elements of a contract are important to healthcare practitioners because healthcare delivery takes place under various types of contracts. To be legally binding, four elements must be present in a contract:

1. *Agreement.* One party makes an offer and another party accepts it. Certain conditions pertain to the offer:
   - It can relate to the present or the future.
   - It must be communicated.
   - It must be made in good faith and not under duress or as a joke.
   - It must be clear enough to be understood by both parties.
   - It must define what both parties will do if the offer is accepted.

   For example, a physician offers a service to the public by obtaining a license to practice medicine and opening a business. Patients accept the physician's offer by scheduling appointments, submitting to physical examinations, and allowing the physician to prescribe or perform medical treatment. The contract is complete when the physician's fee is paid.

2. *Consideration.* Something of value is bargained for as part of the agreement. The physician's consideration is providing service; the patient's consideration is payment of the physician's fee.

3. *Legal subject matter.* Contracts are not valid and enforceable in court unless they are for legal services or purposes. For example, a contract entered into by a patient to pay for the services of a physician in private practice would be *void* (not legally enforceable) if the physician was not licensed to practice medicine. **Breach of contract** may be charged if either party fails to comply with the terms of a legally valid contract.

4. *Contractual capacity.* Parties who enter into the agreement must be capable of fully understanding all its terms and conditions. For example, a mentally incompetent individual or a person under the influence of drugs or alcohol cannot enter into a contract.

Types of Contracts The two main types of contracts are expressed contracts and implied contracts. An **expressed contract** is clearly stated in written or spoken words. A payment contract is an example of an expressed contract. **Implied contracts** are those in which the conduct of the parties, rather than expressed words, indicates acceptance and creates the contract. A patient who rolls up a sleeve and offers an arm for an injection is creating an implied contract.

Legal Elements of a Contract A contract is a legal agreement between two or more people to perform an act in exchange for payment. To be binding, the contract must include these main elements:

- An agreement between two or more competent people to do something legal.
- Names and addresses of the people involved.
- Consideration (whatever is given in exchange, such as money, work, or property).
- Starting and ending dates, as well as the date(s) the contract was signed.
- Signatures of the individuals involved in the contract.

Employment Contract Some medical practices—usually larger practices and hospitals—use employment contracts for their employees. This type of contract could include any or all of the following elements:

- A description of your duties and your employer's duties.
- Plans for handling major changes in job responsibilities.
- Salary, bonuses, and other forms of compensation.
- Benefits, like vacation time, sick days, life insurance, and participation in pension plans.
- Grievance procedures.
- Exceptional situations under which the contract may be terminated by either you or your employer.
- Termination procedures and compensation.
- Special provisions, like job sharing, medical examinations, or liability coverage.

If you are offered an employment contract, study it closely. Consider any local laws that may apply. It is wise to have a lawyer or business adviser review the contract prior to signing it. Figure 5-1 gives an example of a typical MA Applied Training (also known as practicum or work experience) Agreement.

APPLIED TRAINING AGREEMENT

The Medical Assisting student applied training assignments will be created so that experience is obtained in the performance of administrative and clinical skills using applied knowledge. Assignments will encourage the development of professional attitudes for interacting with other professionals in the healthcare environment.

The student MAY NOT receive any compensation for the applied training experience.

SCHOOL RESPONSIBILITIES

1. The school shall obtain an applied training assignment for students taking concurrently one or more academic classes in the medical assisting program.

2. The clinical coordinator at the school shall work with the employer on all phases of the applied training experience.

3. The school will explain as thoroughly as possible to the student all applied training requirements and should any problems or issues arise, will be ready at all times to work with the parties concerned to resolve the issue(s).

4. The clinical coordinator reserves the right to withdraw a student from the applied training program whenever he/she deems it to be in the best interest of the program and the clinical site.

CLINICAL SITE RESPONSIBILITIES

1. The applied training student will be supervised by a clinical supervisor.

2. The clinical supervisor shall rotate the student through the clinical and administrative site areas that were agreed upon.

3. The clinical supervisor shall assist the student in relating the work experience to the student's academic knowledge.

4. The clinical supervisor (or approved representative) will assist the program coordinator by evaluating the student's performance, skills, and attitudes.

STUDENT RESPONSIBILITIES

1. The student will report to the applied training site punctually and at the appointed schedule. The student will, at all times, conduct himself/herself in accordance with the site's rules.If due to illness or emergency, the student is unable to attend the applied training, he/she will notify the clinical supervisor as soon as the absence need is known.

2. The student shall adhere to all medical facility policies and procedures.

3. The student will direct his/her energies to the satisfactory completion of all applied training assignments in a timely and professional manner.

4. The student must adhere to the HIPAA confidentiality guidelines.

STATEMENT OF COOPERATION

I fully understand the responsibilities of all parties involved in the Medical Assisting Applied Training Program and shall make a reasonable effort to do my part to make this a successful learning experience.

Student _____   Date _____

Applied Training Supervisor _____   Date _____

Applied Training Coordinator _____   Date _____

FIGURE 5-1   Example of a Medical Assisting Applied Training (practicum or work experience) Agreement.

The Physician-Patient Contract LO 5.2

A physician has the right, after forming a contract or agreeing to accept a patient under his or her care, to make reasonable limitations (such as expecting the patient to follow through on the agreed-upon treatment plan) on the contractual relationship. The physician is under no legal obligations to treat patients who may wish to exceed those limitations (for example, expecting the physician to accept patient phone calls at home). Under the physician-patient contract, both parties have certain rights and responsibilities.

Physician Rights and Responsibilities

A physician has the right to

- Set up a practice within the boundaries of his or her license to practice medicine.
- Set up an office where he or she chooses and to establish office hours.
- Specialize.
- Decide which services he or she will provide and how those services will be provided.

Within an implied contract, the physician is not expected, or bound, to

- Treat every patient seeking care. A physician is free to use his or her discretion to form contracts within his or her practice, with one exception: if a physician is providing care to patients in a hospital emergency room or free clinic, then the physician must treat every patient who comes for treatment.
- Restore the patient to his or her original state of health.
- Make a correct diagnosis in every case.
- Guarantee the successful result of any treatment or operation. In fact, guarantees of "cures" may constitute fraud on the part of the physician.

Under an implied contract with the patient, the physician does have the responsibility (obligation) to

- Use due care, skill, judgment, and diligence in treating patients, with the same care, skill, judgment, and diligence that peers of the same medical specialty use.
- Stay informed of the best (and current) methods of diagnosis and treatment.
- Perform to the best of his or her ability, whether or not he or she is to receive a fee.
- Furnish complete information and instructions to the patient about diagnoses, options, methods of treatment, and fees for services.

Medical Assistants and Liability All competent adults are liable (legally responsible) for their actions, in both their personal lives and their professional careers. As a medical assistant, it is important to know and understand your scope of practice within the state where you are working. As healthcare providers, medical assistants have general liability in the duties they perform, as well as toward the facility in which they work. By understanding the standard of care and the duty of care, you, as the office medical assistant, can function ethically and legally within the scope of practice for your profession. Medical assistants are held to the "reasonable person standard," which means to carry out your professional and interpersonal relationships without causing harm. This also means that you are held to a higher standard, both inside- and *outside* of the office and both during and *outside* of office hours.

Patient Rights and Responsibilities

Each patient has the right to see the physician of the individual's choosing, although some managed care plans may limit the physician choices to those that are "in-network." Patients also have the right to terminate a physician's services if they wish. Most states have adopted a version of the American Hospital Association's *Patient Care Partnership* (formerly called the Patient's Bill of Rights). The Patient Care Partnership is a list of standards that patients can expect in healthcare. The Joint Commission (TJC) requires hospitals to post a copy of these standards and most managed care organizations also require contracted physicians to post them. Figure 5-2 is an example of a typical patient care partnership list for a medical office. The brochure given to the patient would go into each point in more detail.

Patient Responsibilities Patients are also part of the medical team involved in their treatment. Under an implied contract, patients have the responsibility to

- Follow any instructions given by the physician and cooperate as much as possible.
- Give all relevant information to the physician in order to reach a correct diagnosis. If a patient fails to inform a physician of any medical conditions he or she may have and an incorrect diagnosis is made, the physician is not liable.
- Follow the physician's orders for treatment.
- Pay the fees charged for services provided.

Consent means that the patient has given permission, either expressed or implied, for the physician to examine him or her, to perform tests that aid in reaching a diagnosis, or to treat a known or found medical condition. When the patient makes an appointment to be examined by a physician, the patient has given *implied consent* to the examination and any (simple) diagnostic testing procedures needed for treatment.

Informed consent involves the patient's right to receive all information relative to his or her condition and to make a decision regarding treatment based upon that knowledge. The "doctrine of informed consent" is the legal basis for informed consent (or informed refusal of treatment) and is usually outlined in a state's medical practice acts. Informed consent implies that the patient understands

- Proposed treatment modes.
- Why the treatment is necessary.
- The risks involved in the proposed treatment.
- Available alternative modes of treatment.
- The risks of alternative treatments.
- The risks involved if treatment is refused.

BWW Medical Associates, PC
305 Main Street, Port Snead YZ 12345-9876
Tel: 555-654-3210, Fax: 555-987-6543
Web: BWWAssociates.com

Paul F. Buckwalter, MD
Alexis N. Whalen, MD
Elizabeth H. Williams, MD

Patient Care Partnership
Understanding Expectations, Rights, and Responsibilities

Welcome to our medical practice. As our patient, you have the right to certain expectations, including:

1. High-quality medical care

2. A clean and safe environment for your medical care

3. Informed involvement in your medical care

4. Protection of your privacy

5. Assistance obtaining referrals and appointments with outside providers

6. Help with billing and insurance claim issues

You will receive a brochure outlining the details of these rights for your records. If you have any questions, comments, concerns, or suggestions regarding the information within the brochure or regarding your care with us, please let us know. We are always interested in improving your patient care experience with us.

FIGURE 5-2 Example of a Patient Care Partnership list.

Adult patients who are of sound mind are usually able to give informed consent. Courts have ruled that emancipated minors (those under age 18, not living at home, and self-supporting) understand as a competent adult would and therefore are able to make decisions on their own. Mature minors—although defined differently by each state—are generally minors who, depending on their medical condition, are considered capable of making their own medical decisions and do not require a guardian's consent for certain procedures like contraception, sexually transmitted infection (STI) treatment, and drug or alcohol addictions. Keep in mind, however, that although mature minors may consent to treatment, they may not legally be allowed to enter into a financial contract for payment. The physician or business manager should make decisions regarding payment issues surrounding treatment of mature minors. Figure 5-3 gives state-by-state guidelines defining mature minors and what procedures and treatments they may consent to.

Those patients who cannot give informed consent include the following:

- **Minors** or persons under the age of majority, but excluding married minors.
- The mentally incompetent.
- Those who speak a foreign language—interpreters may be necessary.

Informed consent is a vital part of today's practice of medicine. Physicians are often sued for negligence because of the failure to adequately inform patients of adverse surgical complications, drug reactions, and alternative treatment modes.

Terminating the Physician-Patient Contract

There are times when a physician feels it is necessary to terminate care of a patient. Terminating care is sometimes called withdrawing from a case and must be undertaken very carefully to avoid charges of abandonment. The following are some typical reasons a physician may choose to withdraw from a case:

- The patient refuses to follow the physician's instructions.
- The patient's family members complain incessantly to or about the physician.
- A personality conflict develops between the physician and the patient that cannot be reasonably resolved.
- The patient habitually does not pay for or fails to make satisfactory arrangements to pay for medical services. A physician may stop treatment of such a patient and end the physician-patient relationship only if adequate notice is given to the patient.
- The patient fails to keep scheduled appointments. To protect the physician from charges of abandonment, all missed and canceled appointments should be noted in the patient's chart.

STATE	GENERAL MEDICAL HEALTH[b]	MENTAL HEALTH	SUBSTANCE ABUSE[c]	COMMUNICABLE DISEASES[d]	CONTRACEPTIVES	PRENATAL CARE
Alabama	✓ (3), (8)	✓	✓	✓ (1), (7)		✓
Alaska	✓ (9)			✓	✓	✓
Arizona			✓ (1)	✓	✓	
Arkansas	✓ (15)			✓ (7), (13)	✓	✓ (12), (13)
California		✓ (1), (7)	✓ (1), (7)	✓ (1)	✓	✓ (12)
Colorado		✓ (4), (7)	✓	✓	✓ (11), (19)	
Connecticut		✓	✓	✓		
Delaware	✓ (10)		✓ (1)	✓ (1), (7), (13)	✓ (1), (7)	✓ (1), (7), (12), (13)
District of Columbia		✓	✓	✓	✓	✓
Florida		✓ (2)	✓	✓	✓ (11), (17)	✓ (13)
Georgia			✓ (7)	✓ (7), (13)	✓	✓ (12)
Hawaii			✓ (7)	✓ (3), (7), (14)	✓ (3), (7), (14)	✓ (3), (7), (12), (14)
Idaho	✓		✓	✓ (3)	✓	
Illinois	✓ (11), (13)	✓ (1), (7)	✓ (1), (7)	✓ (1), (7)	✓ (9), (18)	✓ (13), (18)
Indiana			✓	✓		
Iowa			✓	✓ (20)		
Kansas	✓ (13), (21)		✓	✓ (7)	✓ (15)	✓ (13), (22)
Kentucky	✓ (7), (10)	✓ (5), (7)	✓ (7)	✓ (7)	✓ (7)	✓ (7), (12)
Louisiana	✓ (7), (13)		✓ (7)	✓ (7)		
Maine			✓ (7)	✓ (7)	✓ (10), (17)	
Maryland	✓ (7), (10)	✓ (5), (7)	✓ (7)	✓ (7)	✓ (7)	✓ (7)
Massachusetts	✓ (11)	✓ (5)	✓ (1), (23)	✓	✓	✓ (12)
Michigan		✓ (3)	✓ (7)	✓ (7)	✓ (27)	✓ (7)
Minnesota	✓ (7), (10)	✓	✓ (7)	✓ (7)	✓ (7)	✓ (7)
Mississippi			✓ (4), (7)	✓	✓ (10), (19)	✓ (13)
Missouri	✓ (10), (13)		✓ (7), (13)	✓ (7), (13)		✓ (7), (12), (13)
Montana	✓ (7), (11), (13)	✓ (5)	✓ (7), (13)	✓ (7), (13)	✓ (7)	✓ (7), (13)
Nebraska			✓	✓		

FIGURE 5-3 Minors' access to healthcare in the United States.

STATE	GENERAL MEDICAL HEALTH[b]	MENTAL HEALTH	SUBSTANCE ABUSE[c]	COMMUNICABLE DISEASES[d]	CONTRACEPTIVES	PRENATAL CARE
Nevada	✓ (10), (15), (17)		✓	✓		
New Hampshire	✓ (15)		✓ (1)	✓ (3)		
New Jersey	✓ (11)		✓ (7)	✓ (7), (13)		✓ (7), (13)
New Mexico		✓		✓	✓	✓ (24)
New York	✓ (11)	✓ (7)	✓ (7)	✓	✓	✓
North Carolina	✓ (21)	✓	✓	✓	✓	✓ (12)
North Dakota			✓ (3)	✓ (3)		
Ohio		✓ (3)	✓	✓		
Oklahoma	✓ (7), (11)		✓ (7)	✓ (7)	✓ (7), (25)	✓ (7), (12)
Oregon	✓ (4), (7), (13)	✓ (3), (7)	✓ (3), (7)	✓ (13)	✓ (7)	
Pennsylvania	✓ (8)		✓ (7)	✓		✓
Rhode Island			✓	✓		
South Carolina	✓ (5), (26)	✓ (26)	✓ (26)	✓ (26)	✓ (26)	✓ (26)
South Dakota	✓ (21)		✓	✓		
Tennessee		✓ (5)	✓ (7)	✓	✓	✓
Texas		✓	✓ (7)	✓ (7), (13)	✓	✓ (7), (12), (13)
Utah				✓	✓ (7), (16)	✓
Vermont			✓ (1)	✓ (1)		
Virginia	✓ (21)	✓	✓	✓	✓	✓
Washington		✓ (2)	✓ (2)	✓ (3), (13)	✓	✓
West Virginia			✓	✓		
Wisconsin			✓ (1)	✓		
Wyoming				✓	✓	
N =	25	23	46	51	33	31
%	49%	45%	90%	100%	65%	60%

Exclusions and Limitations Key

(1) The minor must be at least 12 years old.
(2) The minor must be at least 13 years old.
(3) The minor must be at least 14 years old.
(4) The minor must be at least 15 years old.
(5) The minor must be at least 16 years old.
(6) The minor must be at least 17 years old.
(7) The heath-care provider may notify parents.

(*Continued*)

(8) The minor must be a high school graduate, married, pregnant, or a parent.

(9) Minor may consent if a parent.

(10) Minor may consent if a parent or if married.

(11) Minor may consent if a parent, married, or pregnant.

(12) Excludes abortive services.

(13) Includes surgical care.

(14) Excludes surgical care.

(15) Minor must be able to understand the nature and consequences of medical or surgical treatment proposed.

(16) Utah Code Ann. § 76-7-325 (LEXIS L. Publg. 2001), "Notice to parent or guardian of minor requesting contraceptive — Definition of contraceptives — Penalty for violation," stating "(1) Any person before providing contraceptives to a minor shall notify, whenever possible, the minor's parents or guardian of the service requested to be provided to such minor. Contraceptives shall be defined as appliances (including but not limited to intrauterine devices), drugs, or medicinal preparations intended or having special utility for prevention of conception. (2) Any person in violation of this section shall be guilty of a class C misdemeanor," was ruled unconstitutional by Planned Parenthood Ass'n v. Matheson, 582 F. Supp. 1001, 1983 U.S. Dist. LEXIS 10330 (D. Utah 1983) with respect to its failure to "provide a procedure whereby a mature minor or a minor who can demonstrate that his or her best interests are contrary to parental notification can obtain contraceptives confidentially." However, the court also noted that it "does not intend to imply by this decision that a law which provided a means for minors to demonstrate maturity or best interests contrary to parental involvement would be constitutional. All that the court has decided is that due to the failure to provide such a process, H.B.343 goes beyond the constitutionally permissible point of regulating the right of minors to make independent decisions concerning whether to bear or to beget children."

(17) If minor is a parent, or provider believes minor will suffer probable health hazard if services withheld.

(18) If minor is a parent, or is referred by a doctor, clergy, or Planned Parenthood clinic.

(19) If minor is a parent, or is referred by a doctor, clergy, family planning clinic, school of higher education, or state agency.

(20) Parental notification required for positive outcome on HIV test.

(21) If parent or guardian is not "immediately available."

(22) If parent is not "available."

(23) Requires diagnosis of two health care providers, and excludes methadone treatment.

(24) Limited to pregnancy testing and diagnosis.

(25) Females can consent if they have ever been pregnant.

(26) Minors of any age when health care provider believes services are necessary; minors at least (16) years old may consent to all health services excluding operations.

(27) Under Mich. Comp. Laws § 400.14b (LEXIS L. Publg. 2001), "Family planning services; notice; referrals; furnishing drugs and appliances," minors may obtain contraceptive services (See Doe v Irwin 441 F.Supp. 1247 (W.D.Mich. 1977), rev'd on other grounds, 615 F.2d 1162 (6th Cir. Mich. 1980), cert denied, 449 U.S. 829 (1980) (the existence, if any, of a fundamental civil right among minors to obtain prescriptive contraceptives does not need to exist to total exclusion of any rights of the minor child's parents) Doe v Irwin 615 F.2d 1162 (6th Cir. Mich. 1980), cert denied, 449 U.S. 829 (1980) (a state-run clinic that distributed contraceptive devices and medication to unemancipated children without the knowledge and the consent of their parents did not infringe parents' constitutional right to care, custody, and nurture of their children).

(a) The age of majority in the 50 states and the District of Columbia is 18, with the exception of Alabama and Nevada, in which it is 19; Pennsylvania, in which it is 21; and Mississippi, in which it is 21, aside from consent for general health care, for which the age of majority is 18.

(b) The Alan Guttmacher Institute did not define the term "general medical health care." However, Minn. Stat. § 144.341 (LEXIS L. Publg. 2001), "Living apart from parents and managing financial affairs, consent for self," provides that "Notwithstanding any other provision of law, any minor who is living separate and apart from parents or legal guardian, whether with or without the consent of a parent or guardian and regardless of the duration of such separate residence, and who is managing personal financial affairs, regardless of the source or extent of the minor's income, may give effective consent to personal medical, dental, mental and other health services, and the consent of no other person is required," while Ala. Code § 22-8-4 (LEXIS L. Publg. 2001), "Minors; consent for self," provides that "Any minor who is 14 years of age or older, or has graduated from high school, or is married, or having been married is divorced or is pregnant may give effective consent to any legally authorized medical, dental, health or mental health services for himself or herself, and the consent of no other person shall be necessary." Thus, this term suggests that statutes indicated provide broad language covering medical, dental, mental, and possibly other, health services.

(c) Statutes typically encompass the broad terms "alcohol" and "drugs."

(d) Includes HIV testing and treatment, with the restriction of testing only in California, New Mexico, and Ohio.

FIGURE 5-3 (*Concluded*).

A physician who terminates care of a patient must do so in a formal, legal manner, following these four steps.

1. Write a letter to the patient, expressing the reason for withdrawing from the case and recommending that the patient seek medical care from another physician as soon as possible. Thirty days is the usual norm allowed for finding another physician. Figure 5-4 shows an example of a letter terminating patient care.

2. Send the letter by certified mail with a return receipt requested. This will provide evidence that the patient received the notification by providing a signature on the return receipt.

3. Place a copy of the letter (and the return receipt, when received) in the patient's medical record.

4. Summarize in the patient record the physician's reason for terminating care and the actions taken to inform the patient.

Just as a physician may choose to end the physician-patient contract, a patient also may choose to end this contract at any time. Often, the ending of the contract on the patient's part is much less formal; he may simply stop coming to appointments. If a patient suddenly stops coming to appointments, as a medical assistant, you should always attempt to reach the patient to ascertain the reason why the patient has stopped coming to the office. If the patient expresses dissatisfaction with the

BWW Medical Associates, PC
305 Main Street, Port Snead YZ 12345-9876
Tel: 555-654-3210, Fax: 555-987-6543
Web: BWWAssociates.com

Paul F. Buckwalter, MD
Alexis N. Whalen, MD
Elizabeth H. Williams, MD

December 12, 20XX

Jack Smallwood
PO Box 3457C
Funton YZ 13254-0987

Dear Mr. Smallwood:

This letter is to inform you of my intent to discontinue providing medical care to you due to habitual and continued noncompliance with your treatment plan. My records indicate that you have missed several appointments and have not complied with ordered testing. In order to allow you sufficient time to establish yourself with another physician, this discontinuation will go into effect 30 days from the date of this letter. My office will be happy to forward your medical records to the physician of your choice.

If you require assistance in locating a new physician, please contact your insurance plan or the Port Snead Medical Society at 1-800-666-9898.

Sincerely,

Paul F. Buckwalter, MD

Paul F. Buckwalter, M.D.

FIGURE 5-4 Sample letter of withdrawal of medical care.

care he has received, inform the physician as soon as possible and document the call in the patient's medical record. You will have a look at patient dissatisfaction and its connection with malpractice claims a little later in this chapter.

Standard of Care

As a medical assistant, you are expected to fulfill the standards of the medical assisting profession by practicing appropriate legal concepts for your profession. According to the AAMA, medical assistants should uphold legal concepts in the following ways:

- Maintain confidentiality.
- Practice within the scope of training and capabilities.
- Prepare and maintain medical records.
- Document accurately.
- Use appropriate guidelines when releasing information.
- Follow legal guidelines and maintain awareness of healthcare legislation and regulations.
- Maintain and dispose of regulated substances in compliance with government guidelines.
- Follow established risk management and safety procedures.
- Meet the requirements for professional credentialing.

Often, state laws dictate what medical assistants may or may not do. For instance, in some states it is illegal for medical assistants to give injections to patients. No states consider it legal for medical assistants to diagnose a condition, prescribe treatment, or allow a patient to believe that the medical assistant is a nurse. In addition to what is stated by law, you and the physician must establish your scope of practice—the procedures that are appropriate for you to perform while working under the physician's supervision. Once that scope of practice is agreed upon, you must continue to stay within that scope of practice unless the scope is updated or changed by mutual agreement. For instance, your scope of practice may change if laws change in your state or if you receive additional training, increasing your skill and/or credential level, which allows an increase in responsibilities for your position.

Closing a Medical Practice

Distressful economic circumstances may cause a medical practice to terminate and close its services to its patients. If this becomes necessary, make sure the medical staff and all physicians do the following:

- Comply with all HIPAA laws for maintaining confidentiality.
- Write letters to all patients, giving them knowledge that your practice will be closing (Figure 5-5).

BWW Medical Associates, PC
305 Main Street, Port Snead YZ 12345-9876
Tel: 555-654-3210, Fax: 555-987-6543
Web: BWWAssociates.com

Paul F. Buckwalter, MD
Alexis N. Whalen, MD
Elizabeth H. Williams, MD

May 23, 20XX

Ms. Gisele Monahan
234 Cutter Lane
Port Snead, YZ 12345-6789

RE: Closing of Medical Practice

Dear Ms. Monahan:

I regret to inform you that our medical practice will be closing on July 30, 20XX. The practice has been purchased by the Vaughn Group, 2345 Williamsburg Court, Port Snead, YZ 12345-6789.

If you wish to use this group of medical practitioners, please sign the enclosed authorization to release medical records form so that your files may be forwarded to them promptly.

Should you choose another physician, please send me a written request with your signature, authorizing the release of your medical records to the physician of your choice. Should we not hear from you prior to the practice closing date, all records will be stored at the Vaughn Group location for retrieval at a future date.

It has been my pleasure to provide your medical care.

Sincerely,

Alexis N. Whalen, MD

Alexis N. Whalen, MD

Enc: Authorization to Release Information

FIGURE 5-5 Sample letter notifying patient of medical practice closure.

- Give patients an option of choosing another physician, or make referrals. If the patient chooses another physician to take over his care, get written consent for his charts to be transferred to that physician properly.
- Keep all files in a secured location for the maximum amount of time files should be saved if contact with patients cannot be made. You will have to choose a vendor that stores files; make sure you choose a reputable vendor.
- Shred files if necessary; again, be sure to choose reputable vendors.
- Stay up-to-date on any HIPAA laws that will affect the practice.

▶ Preventing Malpractice Claims　LO 5.3

Malpractice litigation not only adds to the cost of healthcare, it takes a psychological toll on both patients and healthcare practitioners. Both sides would probably agree that prevention is preferable to litigation. Healthcare practitioners who use reasonable care in preventing professional liability (malpractice) claims are less likely to be faced with defending themselves against these claims.

Risk management is defined as the act or practice of controlling risk. This process includes identifying and tracking risk areas, developing risk improvement plans as part of risk handling, monitoring risks, and performing risk assessments to determine how risks have changed. Proper documentation, patient satisfaction, appropriate behavior, proper medical procedures, and safeguards against exposure assist with decreasing the risk of malpractice lawsuits brought against the medical facility, physicians, and their staff.

Medical Negligence

Malpractice claims are lawsuits by patients against physicians for errors in diagnosis or treatment. Medical *negligence* cases are those in which a person believes that a medical professional did not perform an essential action or performed an improper one, thus harming the patient.

The following are some examples of malpractice:

- *Postoperative complications.* For example, a patient starts to show signs of internal bleeding in the recovery room. The incision is reopened and it is discovered that the surgeon did not complete closure (cauterization) of all the severed capillaries at the operation site.
- *Res ipsa loquitur.* This Latin term means "the thing speaks for itself" and refers to a case in which the doctor's fault is completely obvious; for example, a case in which a surgeon accidentally leaves a surgical instrument inside the patient.

The following are examples of medical negligence:

- *Abandonment.* A healthcare professional who stops care without providing an equally qualified substitute can be charged with **abandonment.** For example, a labor and delivery nurse is helping a woman in labor. The nurse's shift ends, but all the other nurses are busy and her replacement is late for work. Leaving the woman would constitute abandonment.
- *Delayed treatment.* A patient shows symptoms of some illness or disorder, but the doctor decides, for whatever reason, to delay treatment. If the patient later learns of the doctor's decision to wait, the patient may believe he has a negligence case.

The following legal terms are sometimes used to classify medical negligence cases:

- *Malfeasance* refers to an unlawful act or misconduct.
- *Misfeasance* refers to a lawful act that is done incorrectly.
- *Nonfeasance* refers to failure to perform an act that is one's required duty or that is required by law.

The Four Ds of Negligence The American Medical Association (AMA) lists the following "four Ds of negligence":

1. *Duty.* Patients must show that a physician-patient relationship existed in which the physician owed the patient a duty.
2. *Derelict.* Patients must show that the physician failed to comply with the standards of the profession. For example, a gynecologist has routinely taken Pap smears of a patient and then, for whatever reason, does not do so. If the patient then shows evidence of cervical cancer, the physician could be said to have been derelict.

3. *Direct cause.* Patients must show that any damages were a direct cause of a physician's breach of duty. For example, if a patient fell on the sidewalk and damaged her cast, she could not prove that the cast was damaged because it was incorrectly or poorly applied by her physician. It would be clear that the damage to the cast resulted from the fall. If, however, the patient's leg healed incorrectly because of the way the cast had been applied, she might have a case.
4. *Damages.* Patients must prove that they suffered injury.

To go forward with a malpractice suit, a patient must be prepared to prove all four Ds of negligence.

Malpractice and Civil Law Malpractice (medical negligence) lawsuits are part of civil law, coming under the heading of torts. A *tort* is defined as the intentional or unintentional breach of an obligation that causes harm or injury. A *breach of contract* is the failure of one of the parties to adhere to the terms of the contract.

In the case of medical care contracts, which are often implied contracts, either the provider or the patient may breach the contract. The provider may breach the contract by not maintaining patient confidentiality or by not providing adequate medical care (negligence). The patient may breach the contract by not showing up for appointments or by not following the physician's plan of care.

Settling Malpractice Suits Malpractice suits often require a trial in a court of law. Sometimes, however, they are settled through arbitration. *Arbitration* is a process in which the opposing sides choose a person or persons outside the court system, often with special knowledge in the field, to hear and decide the dispute. (Your local or state medical society has information about the policy on arbitration for your state.) If injury, failure to provide reasonable care, or abandonment of the patient is proven to have occurred, the doctor must pay damages (a financial award) to the injured party.

If the physician you work with becomes involved in a lawsuit, you should be familiar with subpoenas. A *subpoena* is a written court order addressed to a specific person, requiring that person's presence in court on a specific date at a specific time. If you were directly involved in the patient case or have knowledge of the events that precipitated the lawsuit, you might be subpoenaed to provide testimony under penalty, known as *subpoena testificandum.* Another important term to know is *subpoena duces tecum*, which is a court order to produce specific, requested documents required at a certain place and time to enter into court records. If you are in charge of patient records at the practice, you will be required to locate, assemble, photocopy, and arrange for delivery of the requested records or be charged with contempt of court if you do not comply.

Law of Agency According to the law of agency, an employee is considered to be acting as a doctor's agent (on the doctor's behalf) while performing professional tasks. The Latin term *respondeat superior*, or "let the master answer," is sometimes used to refer to this relationship. For example, the medical assistant's word is as binding as if it were uttered by the doctor (so you should never promise a patient a cure). With the law of agency, the doctor is responsible, or *liable*, for the negligence of employees. A negligent employee, however, may also be sued directly because individuals are legally responsible for their own actions. So, a patient can sue both the doctor and the involved employee for negligence. The employer, or the employer's insurance company, also can sue the employee. Most likely, in a case of negligence, the doctor would be sued (because you as an employee are acting on the doctor's behalf), and you are usually covered by the doctor's malpractice insurance. Some medical assistants (usually clinical MAs) choose to obtain malpractice insurance. Obtaining personal malpractice insurance is a professional decision that depends on the type of work or facility in which you are employed. The American Association of Medical Assistants (AAMA) offers medical assisting malpractice insurance through various insurance companies at reduced rates.

Courtroom Conduct Most healthcare providers will never have to appear in court, but should you be asked to appear, the following suggestions may prove helpful:

- Attend court proceedings as required. Failure to appear in court could result in charges of contempt of court or in the case being forfeited.
- Do not be late for scheduled hearings.
- Bring required documents to court and present them only when requested to do so.
- Before testifying, refresh your memory concerning all the facts observed about the matter in question, like dates, times, words spoken, and circumstances.
- Speak slowly, clearly, and professionally. Do not use medical terms. Do not lose your temper or attempt to be humorous.
- Answer all questions in a straightforward manner, even if the answers appear to help the opposing side.
- Answer only the question asked, no more and no less.
- Appear well-groomed, and wear clean, conservative clothing.

Professional Liability Coverage Professional liability coverage, also known as malpractice insurance, is specialty coverage to protect the physician and staff against financial losses due to lawsuits filed against them by their clients or others. This coverage protects the physician if she is found to be negligent in her actions, and it protects the physician and her staff members if it is determined that any member is negligent in his or her actions. Professional liability coverage, however, comes at an extremely high cost to the practice. Society in general and patients in particular, have extremely high expectations of physicians and of the medical community. Malpractice lawsuits have become quite commonplace. You have likely seen billboards during a recent commute advertising lawyers who offer assistance for patients who are unhappy with the medical care they have received.

It is no surprise then that malpractice insurance can be one of the most expensive accounts payable for the office. Depending on the type of specialty and the area of the country in which the physician practices, costs for an internist can be as low as $4,000 per year in Minnesota (which has some of the lowest malpractice rates in the country) to a high of $50,000 annually (in 2011) in Florida, which has some of the highest rates in the country. OB/GYNs, who have some of the highest rates of any specialty, can expect to pay anywhere from $15,000 in Minnesota to $80,000–$200,000 per year in Florida for coverage.

Reasons Patients Sue

The following reasons were researched by interviewing families and patients who have sued healthcare practitioners:

1. *Unrealistic expectations.* With modern advancements in medical technology, patients often expect perfection in medical outcomes. They may feel betrayed by the healthcare system when a medical outcome is not what was expected.

2. *Poor rapport and poor communication.* Patients usually do not sue healthcare practitioners that they like and trust. Healthcare providers who do not return telephone calls or are otherwise unavailable to a patient's family members may be perceived as arrogant, cold, or uncaring. When such perceptions exist, patients and family members are more likely to sue if something goes wrong.

3. *Greed and our litigious society.* Financial gain is seldom the reason for medical malpractice, but in some cases it may be an influencing factor. Malpractice attorneys sometimes make it very easy for patients to retain their services, such as contingency arrangements.

4. *Poor quality of care.* Poor quality means that a patient is truly not receiving quality care. Poor quality in "perception" means that the patient believes he or she is not receiving quality care, even if it is not true. Either situation can lead to a malpractice lawsuit.

Statute of Limitations Statutes of limitations are laws that set the deadline or maximum period of time within which a lawsuit or claim may be filed. The most common length of time is 2 years. The deadlines may vary depending on the circumstances and the type of case or claim. The periods of time also vary from state to state and depend on whether the lawsuit or claim is filed in federal or state court. The lawsuit or claim is barred or disqualified if it is not filed before the statutory deadline. Under certain circumstances, a statute of limitations will be extended beyond its deadline. The following are examples for a civil claim for professional malpractice:

- *Medical:* 1 to 4 years from the act or occurrence of injury, or 6 months to 3 years from discovery; certain circumstances will extend the statute, including if the party is a minor, when a foreign object is involved, or in cases of fraud.
- *Legal:* 1 to 3 years from date of discovery, or a maximum of 2 to 5 years from the date of the wrongful act.

Four Cs of Medical Malpractice Prevention

1. *Caring.* As a healthcare professional, caring about your patients and colleagues is your most important asset. Showing patients that you care about them may result in an improvement in their medical condition and, if you are sincere, decreases the likelihood that patients will feel the need to sue if treatment has unsatisfactory results or adverse events occur.

2. *Communication.* If you communicate in a professional manner and clearly ask for confirmation that you have been understood, you will earn respect and trust with your patients and other members of the allied health team.

3. *Competence.* Be competent in your skills and job knowledge by maintaining and updating your knowledge and skills frequently through continuing education.

4. *Charting.* Documentation is proof of competence. Make sure that all current reports and consultations have been reviewed by the physician and are evident in the chart. Chart every conversation or interaction you have with a patient.

How Effective Communication Can Help Prevent Lawsuits Patients who see the medical office as a friendly place are generally less likely to sue. Physicians, medical assistants, and other medical office staff who have pleasant personalities and are competent in their jobs will have less risk of being sued. Medical assistants can help by

- Developing good listening skills and nonverbal communication techniques so that patients feel the time spent with them is not rushed.

- Setting aside a certain time during the day for returning patient phone calls.

- Checking to be sure that all patients or their authorized representatives sign informed consent forms (after all questions and concerns have been addressed) before they undergo medical or surgical procedures.

- Avoiding statements that could be construed as an admission of fault on the part of the physician or other medical staff.

- Using tact, good judgment, and professional ability in handling patients.

- Making every effort to reach an understanding about fees with the patient before treatment so that billing does not become a point of contention.

▶ Administrative Procedures and the Law
LO 5.4

Many of your administrative duties as a medical assistant are related to legal requirements and fall under the heading of risk management. When correct policies and procedures are followed, the risk of lawsuits decreases, but if a lawsuit is brought against the physician, these same policies and procedures will be the physician's best defense. Keep in mind that everything you do and do not do reflects not only on you, but also on the physician and the practice. Always follow office policies and procedures and follow your "best practices" at all times to do your part to avoid lawsuits.

Paperwork for insurance billing, patient consent forms for surgical procedures, and correspondence (like a physician's letter of withdrawal from a case) must be handled correctly to meet legal standards. Documentation of appropriate and accurate entries in a patient's medical record not only provides proof of continuity of care, but it is legally important should the physician ever require the record for a legal case involving the patient. You also may maintain the physician's appointment book—also considered a legal document—especially for tracking missed or canceled appointments. You will explore this aspect of medical assisting in the *Schedule Management* chapter.

In your role as a medical assistant, you also may be responsible for handling certain state reporting requirements. Items that must be reported include births; certain communicable diseases like acquired immunodeficiency syndrome (AIDS) and STIs; drug abuse; suspected child abuse or abuse of the elderly; injuries caused by violence, like knife and gunshot wounds; and deaths. Reports are sent to various state departments, depending on the content of the report. For example, suspected child and elder abuse cases are reported to the state department of social services. Addressing these state requirements is called the physician's public duty.

Phone calls also must be handled with an awareness of legal issues. For example, if the physician asks you to contact a patient by phone and you call the patient at work, you should not identify yourself or the physician by name to someone else without the patient's permission. You can say, for example, "Please tell Mrs. Arnot that her doctor's office is calling." If you do not take this precaution, the physician can be sued for invasion of privacy. You must abide by similar guidelines if you are responsible for making follow-up calls to a patient after a procedure or office visit and when leaving messages on answering machines or on voicemail where someone other than the person you are attempting to reach may pick them up.

Documentation

Patient records are often used as evidence in professional medical liability cases, and improper documentation can contribute to, or cause a case to be lost. Physicians should keep records that clearly show exactly what treatment was performed and when it was done. It is important that physicians be able to demonstrate that nothing was neglected and that the care given fully met the standards demanded by law. One cliché to remember is, "If it is not recorded, then it was not done." (On the same note, if it is recorded, it is assumed that it was done.) Pay attention to spelling in charts and keep a medical dictionary handy if you are not sure of a spelling. Today's healthcare environment requires complete documentation of actions taken and actions not taken. Medical staff members should pay particular attention to the following situations.

Referrals Make sure the patient understands whether you will be making the appointment with the referring physician, whether the specialty physician's staff will be calling to make the appointment with the patient, or whether the patient must call to set up the appointment. Document in the chart that the patient was referred, to whom, and how the appointment is to be made. If the date and time of the appointment are known, document this information also. Follow up with the specialist to verify that the appointment was kept. If a paper referral is necessary, make sure a hard copy is placed in the patient's chart. If the referral is made electronically, note the referral number in the patient's chart. Note whether reports of the consultation were received in your office and document any further care the patient is to receive from the specialty physician.

Missed Appointments At the end of the day, a designated person in the medical office should document the charts of those patients who missed or canceled appointments without rescheduling. Charts should be dated and documented "No Call/No Show" or "Canceled/Not Rescheduled." The appointment book is also considered a legal document; make sure that all missed appointments are documented in the appointment book or within the electronic scheduling system. The treating physician should review these records and note whether follow-up is indicated.

Dismissals To avoid charges of abandonment, the physician must formally withdraw from a case. Be sure that a letter of withdrawal or dismissal has been filed in the patient's records (refer to Figure 5-4). All mailing confirmations should be filed in the record, such as the return receipt from certified mail.

All Other Patient Contact Patient records should include reports of all tests, procedures, and medications prescribed, including prescription refills. Make sure all necessary informed consent papers have been signed and filed in the chart. Make entries into the chart of all telephone conversations with the patient. Correct documentation requires the initials or signature of the person making the notation on the patient's chart as well as the date and time.

Medical Record Correction Errors made when making an entry in a medical record or errors discovered later can be corrected, but corrections must be made in a certain manner so that if the medical records are ever used in a medical malpractice lawsuit, it will not appear that they were falsified. So, when deleting information, never black it out, never use correction fluid to cover it up, and never in any other way erase or obliterate the original wording. Draw a line through the original information so that it is still legible. Write or type in the correct information above or below the original line or in the margin. The *Medical Records and Documentation* chapter describes the proper procedure for correcting paper chart errors and the *Electronic Health Records* chapter discusses the procedure for electronic health records.

Ownership of the Patient Record Patient medical records are considered the property of the owners of the facility where they were created. A physician in a private practice owns his or her charts or records, while records in a hospital or clinic belong to the facility. It is important to remember that although the facility in which the records were created owns the records, the patient owns the information they contain. Upon signing a release, patients may usually obtain access to or copies of their medical records, depending upon state law. Under HIPAA, patients who ask to see or copy their medical records must be accommodated with a few exceptions, such as with mental health records. If the physician decides it may be harmful to the patient to see the contents of the medical record and denies access, the physician is protected under the *doctrine of professional discretion*.

Retention and Storage of the Patient Record As a protection against legal litigation, records should be kept until the applicable statute of limitations period has elapsed, which is

generally 7 years. In some cases, the medical records for minor patients must be kept for a specified length of time after they reach legal age. Some states have enacted statutes for the retention of medical records. Because the federal False Claims Act requires that financial records be kept for 10 years and medical records are often required to back up financial records, many legal experts suggest that medical records also should be kept for a minimum of 10 years. Most physicians retain records indefinitely to provide evidence in medical professional liability suits or for tax purposes. The medical record may provide the patient's medical history for future medical treatment. The chapter on *Managing Medical Records* will go into more detail on this subject.

Credentialing

Credentialing is the term used by various organizations, including insurance carriers, to ensure that healthcare providers are appropriately qualified to provide services and meet all the necessary requirements to do so. The qualifications are determined and approved by unbiased physician peer review groups. Specific criteria vary according to the physician or provider specialty and the provider's scope of practice. Physicians are broken into two types according to medical licensure—MD (medical doctor) or DO (doctor of osteopathy)—and then further broken down according to specialty.

As the office medical assistant, you may be responsible for credentialing any new providers joining the practice. In general, insurance companies require their doctors to hold and maintain the proper credentials. In order for a physician to participate with an insurance carrier like Medicare, he must have the necessary professional credentials and go through the Medicare credentialing process or he will not be allowed to bill Medicare for services provided to Medicare beneficiaries.

Medicare has three forms for credentialing:

1. Form 855B is used to establish or change a practice group number.
2. Form 855I is used to establish or reestablish a physician's individual number.

    In addition to completing this 29-page application, the physician also must provide his or her medical school diploma, individual NPI (national provider identifier), current license number, any board certifications for specialties, work history for at least 5 years, statement of any limitations, history of loss of licensure or felony convictions, history of loss or limitations of privileges or disciplinary actions, and outside verification of information provided.

3. Form 855R is used to link individual provider numbers to group practice numbers.

These forms are not complicated, but they are time-consuming. More information about Medicare's credentialing process may be found on the CMS website at www.cms.gov/manuals/downloads. In addition to the paper-based forms, CMS has established the Internet-based Provider Enrollment Chain and Ownership System (PECOS). This system allows physicians, nonphysician practitioners, and provider and supplier organizations to enroll, make a change in their Medicare enrollment, view their Medicare enrollment information on file with Medicare, or check on the status of a Medicare enrollment application via the Internet. Regardless of the application method used, once the Medicare credential is received, many other insurance plans will follow suit with credentialing or linking so the provider can also bill them for services provided. If a separate credentialing process is required, it is generally much less complicated than that required by Medicare.

The Food and Drug Administration Regulatory Function

The Food and Drug Administration (FDA) requires that drug manufacturers perform clinical tests on new drugs before humans use these drugs. These tests include toxicity tests in laboratory animals, followed by clinical studies (frequently called clinical trials) in controlled groups of volunteers, like the one shown in Figure 5-6. Some volunteers are patients; others are healthy subjects.

Clinical tests are designed to consider the ratio of benefits to the risk of adverse side effects. If the clinical tests prove that the drug is safe and effective, the FDA approves it for marketing. The manufacturer must continue to demonstrate the drug's safety and efficacy (therapeutic value) and must submit reports whenever it discovers unexpected adverse reactions. The FDA can withdraw a drug from the market at any time if evidence suggests that it is no longer safe or effective.

During the clinical trials, the pharmaceutical (drug) company studies all aspects of the pharmacology of the new drug. When the company seeks approval from the FDA, it must document the pharmacodynamics, pharmacokinetics, safety (how many and what kind of adverse effects), and efficacy of the drug. In addition, it must present data regarding the dose—the amount of drug given at one time.

After the FDA approves a drug, it continues its regulatory function to protect patients and consumers. The FDA reviews new-indication proposals (applications from companies for new uses for a drug; for instance, if a side effect of the drug is

FIGURE 5-6 Blood tests provide baseline data on volunteers at the start of clinical drug trials.

weight loss, the company will now propose it also be sold as a weight loss supplement), OTC proposals (applications for OTC status of a prescription drug), and further clinical trial results. If an adverse effect appears many times, for example, the FDA may withdraw the causative drug from the market.

Drug Manufacturing The FDA also regulates drug manufacturing. It ensures that drugs shipped between states have the proper identity, strength, purity, and quality. Each manufacturer must consistently identify each drug by a particular color, form, shape, size, and label. It must produce every dose at the same tested strength, using the exact formula approved by the FDA. The manufacturer also must use high-quality, contaminant-free ingredients.

Nonprescription, or Over-the-Counter, Drugs A nonprescription, or OTC, drug is one that the FDA has approved for use without the supervision of a licensed healthcare practitioner. The consumer must follow the manufacturer's directions to use the drug safely. Some drugs, like aspirin and vitamin supplements, have been OTC drugs for many years. The number of prescription drugs that have been granted OTC status is increasing. Although OTC drugs are safe when used as directed on the package, patient education contributes significantly to their safe use.

Prescription Drugs A prescription drug is one that can be used only by order of a physician and must be dispensed by a licensed healthcare professional, like a pharmacist, physician, podiatrist, or licensed midwife. Some prescription drugs are dispensed as OTC medications at much lower strengths.

Pregnancy Categories Because clinical trials are not typically done on pregnant women, most of the data about the effect of medications on pregnant women is obtained after FDA approval. Some drugs can cause physical defects to the fetus if the mother takes them during pregnancy, especially during the first trimester. To assist physicians who are prescribing medications for pregnant women, the FDA has created drug categories based upon the degree to which available information has ruled out risk to the fetus.

Controlled Substances As stated earlier, a controlled substance is a drug or drug product that is categorized as potentially dangerous and addictive. A greater addictive potential results in more severe limitations on prescribing the drug or substance. Federal laws strictly regulate the use of these controlled drugs. States, municipalities, and institutions must adhere to these laws but may also impose their own regulations.

Comprehensive Drug Abuse Prevention and Control Act

The Comprehensive Drug Abuse Prevention and Control Act, also known as the Controlled Substances Act (CSA) of 1970, is the federal law that created the Drug Enforcement Administration (DEA) and strengthened drug enforcement authority. The CSA designates five schedules, according to degree of potential for a substance to be abused or used for a nontherapeutic effect. Controlled substances and the five schedules will also be discussed in further detail in the *Principles of Pharmacology* chapter.

Doctor Registration Under the CSA, doctors who administer, dispense, or prescribe any controlled substance must register with the DEA and must have a current state license to practice medicine and, if required, a state controlled substance license. They also must comply with all aspects of the CSA. According to the CSA, doctors may issue prescriptions for controlled drugs only in the schedules for which they are registered with the DEA. To register the doctor with the DEA, submit DEA Form 224 (Figure 5-7), called the Application for Registration under Controlled Substances Act of 1970. This form is available online. A fee must accompany the form when sent to the DEA.

Registration must be renewed every three years with DEA Form 224a. The renewal is done by mail or through the Internet via a login process. Doctors who administer or dispense drugs at more than one office must register at each location. Each registration is assigned a unique number, which indicates to suppliers and pharmacies that the doctor is properly authorized. Form 224 can be printed from the U.S. Department of Justice's website. The renewal application (Form 224a) can be completed through registration at this site.

Ordering Drugs That Are Controlled Substances If Schedule II drugs are needed for the practice, they must be ordered by using the U.S. Official Order Forms—Schedules I & II (DEA Form 222), which you can obtain from the DEA through the mail or Internet (Figure 5-8). One copy of the form goes to the DEA for overall surveillance of drug distribution. In most states, this form can be used to obtain Schedule II drugs from the normal drug supplier. When Schedule II drugs are ordered from an out-of-state company, some states require the doctor to send a copy of the purchase agreement (not the DEA Form 222) to the state attorney general's office within 24 hours of placing the order. Schedules III through V drugs require less complicated ordering. They require only the doctor's DEA registration number.

Legal Documents and the Patient

You need to be aware of several legal documents that are typically completed by a patient prior to major surgery or hospitalization, including the advance medical directive, the durable power of attorney, and the uniform donor card. Traditionally, these documents were completed outside the medical office or in the hospital. The current trend, however, is for medical practice personnel, including medical assistants, to assist patients in developing these important documents. Contact your state's Public Health Department website for additional information.

Advance Medical Directive This is a legal document addressed to the patient's family and healthcare providers stating what type of treatment the patient wishes or does not wish to receive if she becomes terminally ill, unconscious, or permanently comatose (sometimes referred to as being in a persistent vegetative state). For example, an advance directive typically states whether a patient wishes to be put on life-sustaining equipment should she become permanently comatose. Some directives contain DNR (do not resuscitate) orders. These orders mean the patient does not wish medical personnel to try to resuscitate her

should the heart stop beating. The directive is signed when the patient is mentally and physically competent to do so. It also must be signed by two witnesses. Advance medical directives are a means of helping families of terminally ill patients deal with the inevitable outcome of the illness. Having these advance directives in place can lower stress levels, as difficult decisions have already been made, and may help limit unnecessary medical costs.

Medical practices can help patients develop an advance medical directive, sometimes in conjunction with organizations that make available preprinted living will forms. The Partnership for Caring (based in Washington, D.C.) is one such organization.

Durable Power of Attorney Patients who have an advance medical directive are asked to name, in the second document, called a **durable power of attorney** (also known as a healthcare proxy), someone who will make decisions regarding medical care on their behalf if they are unable to do so. It is important that the person named in the durable power of attorney knows the patient's wishes ahead of time, so in the event they are required to make medical decisions, they are able to be confident they are carrying out the patient's wishes.

The Uniform Donor Card In 1968, the Uniform Anatomical Gift Act was passed, setting forth guidelines for all states to follow in complying with a person's wish to make a gift of one or more organs (or the whole body) upon death. An anatomical gift is typically designated for medical research, organ transplants, or placement in a tissue bank. The uniform donor card is a legal document that states one's wish to make such a gift. People often carry the uniform donor card in their wallets. Many medical practices offer the service of helping their patients obtain and complete a uniform donor card. In some states, the Department of Motor Vehicles makes the process simple by asking you at the time you renew your driver's license if you would like to be an organ donor, with a card being issued to you at that time and a notation made on the driver's license that you are an organ donor. The patient's family should be aware of his wish to be an organ donor so that the wishes are carried out upon his death.

▶ Federal Legislation Affecting Healthcare
LO 5.5

Congress has passed legislation intended to improve the quality of healthcare in the United States, reduce fraud, and ensure that insurance providers will not discriminate against patients. The most significant healthcare laws passed in recent years are the Health Care Quality Improvement Act of 1986, the False Claims Act, and the Health Insurance Portability and Accountability Act of 1996. In addition, the Occupational Safety and Health Administration regulations are vitally important to the practice of healthcare and the safety of its practitioners, and these, too, are reviewed and often updated by the administration.

Health Care Quality Improvement Act of 1986

The Health Care Quality Improvement Act of 1986 (HCQIA) is a federal statute passed to improve the quality of medical care nationwide. Congress created HCQIA after discovering an increasing occurrence of medical malpractice and a need to improve the quality of medical care. The act requires professional peer review in certain cases, limits damages to professional reviewers, and protects from liability those who provide information to professional review bodies. One of the most important provisions of the HCQIA was the establishment of the National Practitioner Data Bank, designed to improve the quality of medical care nationwide by encouraging effective professional peer review of physicians. Information that must be

---

Form-224

APPLICATION FOR REGISTRATION
Under the Controlled Substances Act

APPROVED OMB NO 1117-0014
FORM DEA-224 (10-06)
Previous editions are obsolete

INSTRUCTIONS **Save time—apply on-line at www.deadiversion.usdoj.gov**

1. To apply by mail complete this application. Keep a copy for your records.
2. Print clearly, using black or blue ink, or use a typewriter.
3. Mail this form to the address provided in Section 7 or use enclosed envelope.
4. Include the correct payment amount. FEE IS NON-REFUNDABLE.
5. If you have any questions call 800-882-9539 prior to submitting your application.

IMPORTANT: DO NOT SEND THIS APPLICATION AND APPLY ON-LINE.

DEA OFFICIAL USE:

Do you have other DEA registration numbers?
☐ NO   ☐ YES

MAIL-TO ADDRESS Please print mailing address changes to the right of the address in this box.

FEE FOR THREE (3) YEARS IS $551
FEE IS NON-REFUNDABLE

SECTION 1 APPLICANT IDENTIFICATION ☐ Individual Registration ☐ Business Registration

Name 1 (Last Name of individual -OR- Business or Facility Name)

Name 2 (First Name and Middle Name of individual -OR- Continuation of business name)

Street Address Line 1 (if applying for fee exemption, this must be address of the fee exempt institution)

Address Line 2

City   State   Zip Code

Business Phone Number   Point of Contact

Business Fax Number   Email Address

DEBT COLLECTION INFORMATION

Mandatory pursuant to Debt Collection Improvements Act

Social Security Number (*if registration is for individual*)

Provide **SSN** or **TIN**.
See additional information note #3 on page 4.

Tax Identification Number (*if registration is for business*)

FOR Practitioner or MLP ONLY:

Professional Degree: *select from list only*

Professional School:

Year of Graduation:

National Provider Identification:

Date of Birth (*MM-DD-YYYY*):

SECTION 2
BUSINESS ACTIVITY

Check one business activity box only

☐ Central Fill Pharmacy
☐ Retail Pharmacy
☐ Nursing Home
☐ Automated Dispensing System

☐ Practitioner (DDS, DMD, DO, DPM, DVM, MD or PHD)
☐ Practitioner Military (DDS, DMD, DO, DPM, DVM, MD or PHD)
☐ Mid-level Practitioner (MLP) (DOM, HMD, MP, ND, NP, OD, PA, or RPH)
☐ Euthanasia Technician

☐ Ambulance Service
☐ Animal Shelter
☐ Hospital/Clinic
☐ Teaching Institution

FOR Automated Dispensing System (ADS) ONLY:

DEA Registration # of Retail Pharmacy for this ADS

An ADS is automatically fee-exempt.
Skip Section 6 and Section 7 on page 2.
You must attach a notarized affidavit.

SECTION 3
DRUG SCHEDULES

Check all that apply

☐ Schedule II Narcotic
☐ Schedule II Non-Narcotic

☐ Schedule III Narcotic
☐ Schedule III Non-Narcotic

☐ Schedule IV
☐ Schedule V

FIGURE 5-7 DEA Form 224 is used to register the physician with the Drug Enforcement Agency. It is usually completed online through the U.S. Department of Justice at www.deadiversion.usdoj.gov.

(Continued).

SECTION 4

STATE LICENSE(S)

Be sure to include both state license numbers if applicable

You MUST be currently authorized to prescribe, distribute, dispense, conduct research, or otherwise handle the controlled substances in the schedules for which you are applying under the laws of the **state** or jurisdiction in which you are operating or propose to operate.

State License Number (required)

What state was this license issued in? _____

Expiration Date (required) ___/___/___ MM - DD - YYYY

State Controlled Substance License Number (if required)

What state was this license issued in? _____

Expiration Date ___/___/___ MM - DD - YYYY

SECTION 5

LIABILITY

IMPORTANT

All questions in this section must be answered.

1. Has the applicant ever been **convicted of a crime** in connection with controlled substance(s) under state or federal law, or is any such action pending?   YES ☐   NO ☐

   Date(s) of incident MM-DD-YYYY: ☐☐–☐☐–☐☐☐☐

2. Has the applicant ever surrendered (for cause) or had a **federal** controlled substance registration revoked, suspended, restricted, or denied, or is any such action pending?   YES ☐   NO ☐

   Date(s) of incident MM-DD-YYYY: ☐☐–☐☐–☐☐☐☐

3. Has the applicant ever surrendered (for cause) or had a **state** professional license or controlled substance registration revoked, suspended, denied, restricted, or placed on probation, or is any such action pending?   YES ☐   NO ☐

   Date(s) of incident MM-DD-YYYY: ☐☐–☐☐–☐☐☐☐

4. If the applicant is a **corporation** (other than a corporation whose stock is owned and traded by the public), association, partnership, or pharmacy, has any officer, partner, stockholder, or proprietor been **convicted of a crime** in connection with controlled substance(s) under state or federal law, or ever surrendered, for cause, or had a **federal** controlled substance registration revoked, suspended, restricted, denied, or ever had a **state** professional license or controlled substance registration revoked, suspended, denied, restricted or placed on probation, or is any such action pending?   YES ☐   NO ☐

   Date(s) of incident MM-DD-YYYY: ☐☐–☐☐–☐☐☐☐   *Note: If question 4 does not apply to you, be sure to mark 'NO'. It will slow down processing of your application if you leave it blank.*

- -

EXPLANATION OF "YES" ANSWERS

Applicants who have answered "YES" to any of the four questions above **must provide a statement to explain each "YES" answer.**

Use this space or attach a separate sheet and return with application

Liability question # _____   Location(s) of incident: _____

Nature of incident: _____

Disposition of incident: _____

SECTION 6   **EXEMPTION FROM APPLICATION FEE**

☐ Check this box if the applicant is a federal, state, or local government official or institution. Does not apply to contractor-operated institutions.

Business or Facility Name of Fee Exempt Institution. **Be sure to enter the address of this exempt institution in Section 1.**

FEE EXEMPT CERTIFIER

Provide the name and phone number of the certifying official

The undersigned hereby certifies that the applicant named hereon is a federal, state or local government official or institution, and is exempt from payment of the application fee.

Signature of certifying official (other than applicant) _____   Date _____

Print or type name and title of certifying official _____   Telephone No. (required for verification) _____

SECTION 7

METHOD OF PAYMENT

Check one form of payment only

☐ Check   Make check payable to: **Drug Enforcement Administration**   See page 4 of instructions for important information.

☐ American Express   ☐ Discover   ☐ Master Card   ☐ Visa

Credit Card Number _____   Expiration Date __–__

Sign if paying by credit card

Signature of Card Holder _____

Printed Name of Card Holder _____

Mail this form with payment to:

U.S. Department of Justice
Drug Enforcement Administration
P.O. Box 28083
Washington, DC 20038-8083

FEE IS NON-REFUNDABLE

SECTION 8

APPLICANTS SIGNATURE

Sign in ink

I certify that the foregoing information furnished on this application is true and correct.

Signature of applicant (sign in ink) _____   Date _____

Print or type name and title of applicant _____

WARNING: Section 843(a)(4)(A) of Title 21, United States Code states that any person who knowingly or intentionally furnishes false or fraudulent information in this application is subject to imprisonment for not more than four years, a fine of not more than $30,000,00 or both.

FIGURE 5-7   (*Concluded*).

reported to the National Practitioner Data Bank includes medical malpractice payments, adverse licensure actions, adverse clinical privilege actions, and adverse professional membership actions. This data bank is a resource to assist state licensing boards, hospitals, and other healthcare entities in investigating qualifications of physicians and other healthcare practitioners.

False Claims Act

The False Claims Act is a federal law that allows individuals to bring civil actions on behalf of the U.S. government for false claims made to the federal government, under a provision of the law call *qui tam* (from Latin, meaning to bring an action for the king and for one's self). The law was enacted because of the rising cost of healthcare,

DEA Form-222
(Oct. 1992)

U.S. OFFICIAL ORDER FORMS - SCHEDULES I & II
Drug Enforcement Administration
SUPPLIER'S Copy 1

See Reverse of PURCHASER'S Copy for Instructions | No order form may be issued for Schedule I and II substances unless a completed application form has been received. (21 CFR 1305.04). | **OMB APPROVAL No. 1117-0010**

To: (Name of Supplier)

Street Address

Address

City | State

Date (MM-DD-YYYY) | Suppliers DEA Registration No.

To Be Filled in By PURCHASER

Line No.	No. of Packages	Size of Package	Name of Item
1			
2			
3			
4			
5			
6			
7			
8			
9			
10			

To Be Filled in By SUPPLIER

National Drug Code	Packages Shipped	Date Shipped

◄ **LAST LINE COMPLETED** *(MUST BE 10 OR LESS)*

Signature of **PURCHASER** or Attorney or Agent

Date Issued | DEA Registration No.

Schedules | Name and Address of Registrant

Registered As a

No. of This Order Form

FIGURE 5-8   DEA Form 222 is used to order Schedule II drugs and can be completed online through the DEA website.

fraud, and abuse within the healthcare industry. As a result, laws have been passed to control three types of illegal conduct:

1. *False billing claims.* Fraudulently billing for services not performed is prohibited.

2. *Kickbacks.* Giving financial incentives to a healthcare provider for referring patients or for recommending services or products is prohibited under the federal Anti-Kickback Law and by state laws.

3. *Self-referrals.* Referring patients to any service or facility where the healthcare provider has financial interests is prohibited by the Federal Ethics in Patient Referral Act and other federal and state laws.

Violations of laws against healthcare fraud and abuse can result in imprisonment and fines, the loss of professional licensure, the loss of healthcare facility staff privileges, and exclusion from participating in federal healthcare programs like Medicare and Medicaid.

Occupational Safety and Health Administration

The Occupational Safety and Health Administration (OSHA), a division of the U.S. Department of Labor, has created federal laws to protect healthcare workers from health hazards on the job. Medical personnel may accidentally contract a dangerous or even fatal disease by coming into contact with the bodily fluids of a patient contaminated with a virus. Medical assistants also may be exposed to toxic substances in the office. OSHA regulations describe the precautions a medical office must take with clothing, housekeeping, record keeping, and training to minimize the risk of disease or injury.

Some of the most important OSHA regulations are those for controlling workers' exposure to infectious disease. These regulations are set forth in the OSHA Bloodborne Pathogens Protection Standard of 1991. A pathogen is any microorganism that causes disease. Microorganisms are microscopic living bodies like viruses or bacteria that may be present in a patient's blood or other body fluids (saliva or semen).

Of particular concern to medical workers are the human immunodeficiency virus (HIV), which causes AIDS, and the hepatitis B virus (HBV). AIDS damages the body's immune system and thus its ability to fight disease. Historically, AIDS has almost always been fatal, but better antiviral drugs have been more and more successful in keeping the virus under control. HBV is a highly contagious disease that is potentially fatal. It causes inflammation of the liver and may cause liver failure. Every year, about 8,700 healthcare workers become HBV-infected from patient-related or body substance exposures at work, and about 200 die from the disease.

OSHA requires that medical professionals in medical practices follow what are called Standard Precautions. These were developed by the Centers for Disease Control and Prevention (CDC) to prevent medical professionals from exposing themselves and others to bloodborne pathogens. Exposure can occur, for example, through skin that has been broken from a needle puncture or other wound and through mucous membranes, like those in the nose and throat. If these areas come into contact with a patient's (or coworker's) blood or body fluids, a virus could be transferred from one person to another. The chapter on *Basic Safety and Infection Control* discusses OSHA and Standard Precautions in more detail.

Health Insurance Portability and Accountability Act

On August 21, 1996, the U.S. Congress passed the Health Insurance Portability and Accountability Act (HIPAA). The primary goals of the act were to improve the portability and continuity of healthcare coverage in group and individual markets; to combat waste, fraud, and abuse in healthcare insurance and healthcare delivery; to promote the use of medical savings accounts; to improve access to long-term care services and coverage; and to simplify the administration of health insurance.

The primary purposes of HIPAA are to

- Improve the efficiency and effectiveness of healthcare delivery by creating a national framework for health privacy protection that builds on efforts by states, health systems, individual organizations, and individuals.

- Protect and enhance the rights of patients by providing them access to their health information and controlling the inappropriate use or disclosure of that information.

- Improve the quality of healthcare by restoring trust in the healthcare system among consumers, healthcare professionals, and the multitude of organizations and individuals committed to the delivery of care.

HIPAA is divided into two main sections of law: Title I, which addresses healthcare portability, and Title II, which covers the prevention of healthcare fraud and abuse, administrative simplification, and medical liability reform. Although in this text you will study Titles I and II in more detail, you also should be aware of three other titles included in HIPAA regulations: Title III—tax-related health provisions governing medical savings accounts; Title IV—application and enforcement of group health insurance requirements; and Title V—revenue offset governing tax deductions for employers providing company-owned life insurance premiums.

Title I: Healthcare Portability The issue of portability deals with protecting healthcare coverage for employees who change jobs, allowing them to carry their existing plans with them to new jobs. HIPAA provides the following protections for employees and their families:

- Increases workers' ability to get healthcare coverage when starting a new job.

- Reduces workers' probability of losing existing healthcare coverage.

- Helps workers maintain continuous healthcare coverage when changing jobs.

- Helps workers purchase health insurance on their own if they lose coverage under an employer's group plan and have no other healthcare coverage available.

The specific protections of this title include the following:

- Limits the use of exclusions for preexisting conditions.

- Prohibits group plans from discriminating by denying coverage or charging extra for coverage based on an individual's or a family member's past or present poor health.

- Guarantees certain small employers, as well as certain individuals who lose job-related coverage, the right to purchase health insurance.

- Guarantees, in most cases, that employers or individuals who purchase health insurance can renew the coverage regardless of any health conditions of individuals covered under the insurance policy.

Title II: Prevention of Healthcare Fraud and Abuse, Administrative Simplification, and Medical Liability Reform The HIPAA Standards for Privacy of Individually Identifiable Health Information (IIHI) provided the first comprehensive federal protection for the privacy of both IIHI and personal, or protected, health information. The *HIPAA Privacy*

Rule is designed to provide strong privacy protections that do not interfere with patient access to healthcare or the quality of healthcare delivery. The privacy rule is intended to

- Give patients more control over their health information.
- Set boundaries on the use and release of healthcare records.
- Establish appropriate safeguards that healthcare providers and others must achieve to protect the privacy of health information.
- Hold violators accountable, with civil and criminal penalties that can be imposed if they violate patients' privacy rights.
- Strike a balance when public responsibility supports disclosure of some forms of data—for example, to protect public health.

Before the HIPAA Privacy Rule, the personal information transferred among healthcare providers and third-party payers fell under a patchwork of federal and state laws. This meant that unless forbidden by state or local law, IIHI could be distributed, for reasons that had nothing to do with a patient's medical treatment or healthcare reimbursement, to other agencies. For example, patient information held by a health plan could be passed on to a lender, who could then deny the patient's application for a home mortgage or a credit card; or it could be given to an employer, who could use it in personnel decisions—all without patient knowledge or consent. HIPAA stopped that.

Individually identifiable health information includes

- Patient name, address, phone numbers, and e-mail address.
- Patient dates (birth, death, admission, discharge, etc.).
- Social Security number.
- Medical record numbers.
- Health plan beneficiary numbers.
- Account numbers.
- Certificate or license numbers.
- Vehicle identifiers and serial numbers, including license plate numbers.
- Device identifiers and serial numbers.
- Web Universal Resource Locators (URLs) and Internet Protocol (IP) addresses.

The core of the HIPAA Privacy Rule is the protection, use, and disclosure of *protected health information (PHI)*. Protected health information means individually identifiable health information that is transmitted or maintained by electronic or other media, like computer storage devices. The Privacy Rule protects all PHI held or transmitted by a covered entity, which includes healthcare providers, health plans, and healthcare clearinghouses. Other covered entities include employers, life insurers, schools or universities, and public health authorities. PHI can come in any form or medium, such as electronic, paper, or oral, including verbal communications among staff members, patients, and other providers. The Privacy Rule covers the following PHI:

- The past, present, or future physical or mental health or condition of an individual.
- Healthcare that is provided to an individual.
- Billing or payments made for healthcare provided.

Information that is not individually identifiable or is unable to be tied to the identity of a particular patient is not subject to the Privacy Rule.

Use and *disclosure* are the two fundamental concepts in the HIPAA Privacy Rule. It is important to understand the differences between these terms. *Use* limits the sharing of information within a covered entity. Performing any of the following actions to PHI by employees or other members of an organization's workforce means the information is being used:

- Sharing
- Employing
- Applying
- Utilizing
- Examining
- Analyzing

Disclosure restricts the sharing of information outside the entity holding the information. Performing any of the following actions so that information is transmitted outside the entity constitutes disclosure:

- Releasing
- Transferring
- Providing access to
- Divulging in any manner

Managing and Storing Patient Information Because of HIPAA, medical facilities have undergone many changes to the way they manage and store patient information. Many facilities now contract consultants that specialize in HIPAA, and large facilities like hospitals often employ a compliance officer. Patients must be given the opportunity to read the office privacy practices and receive a copy of them, signing an acknowledgment that they have received them. Should the patient refuse to sign the acknowledgment, the refusal should be documented in the medical record to prove *due diligence* and a "good faith effort" by the office to provide the patient with the privacy practices. The Privacy Rule requires the provider to perform activities including

- Notifying patients of their privacy rights and how their information is used.
- Adopting and implementing privacy procedures for its practice, hospital, or plan.
- Training employees so that they understand the privacy procedures.
- Designating an individual responsible for seeing that the privacy procedures are adopted and followed.
- Securing patient records containing IIHI so that they are not readily available to those who do not need them.

Patient Notification Since the HIPAA Privacy Rule's effective date, medical facilities have made major changes in how they inform patients of their HIPAA compliance. You may have noticed, as a patient yourself, the forms and information packets that are now provided by your healthcare providers. The first

BWW Medical Associates, PC
305 Main Street, Port Snead YZ 12345-9876
Tel: 555-654-3210, Fax: 555-987-6543
Web: BWWAssociates.com

Paul F. Buckwalter, MD
Alexis N. Whalen, MD
Elizabeth H. Williams, MD

Notice of Privacy Practices

I understand that BWW Medical Associates, PC creates and maintains medical records describing my health history, symptoms, examinations, test results, diagnoses, treatments, and plans for my future care and/or treatment. I further understand that this information may be used for any of the following:

1. Plan and document my care and treatment
2. Communicate with health professionals involved in my care and treatment
3. Verify insurance coverage for planned procedures and/or treatments for the applicable diagnoses
4. Application of any medical or surgical procedures and diagnoses (codes) to my medical insurance claim forms as application for payment of services rendered
5. Assessment of quality of care and utilization review of the health care professionals providing my care

Additionally, it has been explained to me that:

1. A complete description of the use and disclosure of this information is included in the *Notice of Information of Privacy Practices* which has been provided to me
2. I have had a right to review this information prior to signing this consent
3. BWW Medical Associates, PC has the right to change this notice and their practices
4. Any revision of this notice will be mailed to me at the address I provided to them prior to its implementation
5. I may object to the use of my health information for specific purposes
6. I may request restrictions as to the manner my information may be used or disclosed in order to carry out treatment, payment, or health information
7. I understand that it is not required that my requested restrictions be honored
8. I may revoke this consent in writing, except for those disclosures which may have taken place prior to the receipt of my revocation

At the time of the document signing, I request the following restrictions to disclosure or use of my health information: _____

_____

Printed Name of Patient or Legal Guardian   Signature of Parent or Legal Guardian

Printed Name of Witness/Title   Signature of Witness/Title

Date: _____

FIGURE 5-9   Example of a Privacy Practices notice and acknowledgment.

step in informing patients of HIPAA compliance is the communication of patient rights, conveyed through a document called Notice of Privacy Practices (NPP). This notice must

- Be written in plain, simple language.
- Include a header that reads: "This notice describes how medical information about you may be used and disclosed and how you can get access to this information. Please review carefully."
- Describe the covered entity's uses and disclosures of PHI.
- Describe an individual's rights under the Privacy Rule.
- Describe the covered entity's duties.

- Describe how to register complaints concerning suspected privacy violations.
- Specify a point of contact.
- Specify an effective date.
- State that the entity reserves the right to change its privacy practices.

See Figure 5-9 for an example of a HIPAA Privacy Notice. Procedure 5-1, found at the end of this chapter, outlines the steps in obtaining a signature for receipt of the Privacy Practices notice.

BWW Medical Associates, PC
305 Main Street, Port Snead YZ 12345-9876
Tel: 555-654-3210, Fax: 555-987-6543
Web: BWWAssociates.com

Paul F. Buckwalter, MD
Alexis N. Whalen, MD
Elizabeth H. Williams, MD

Privacy Violation Complaint

As per our Privacy Policies and Procedures, we are providing this form for individuals who feel they have a complaint regarding how their protected health information was handled by our office. You have the right to make a complaint and we may take no retaliatory actions against you because of it. We will respond to this complaint within 30 days of its receipt.

Patient Name: _____

Address: _____

DOB: _____ Date of Complaint: _____

Phone: Home _____ Cell _____ Work _____

Best time to reach you: _____

Reason for the complaint (Please be as specific as possible, attaching additional documentation as necessary): _____
_____
_____
_____
_____

_____   _____
Signature   Date

Office Use Only

Received by: _____ Date _____

Follow-up Started on (date): _____

FIGURE 5-10 Sample of privacy violation complaint form.

In addition to understanding the office obligations under HIPAA, remember, it has also given patients an increased understanding about their right to privacy regarding their health information. These rights include the following:

- The right to access, copy, and inspect their healthcare information.
- The right to request an amendment to their healthcare information.
- The right to obtain an accounting of certain disclosures of their healthcare information.

- The right to alternate means of receiving communications from providers.
- The right to complain about alleged violations of the regulations and the provider's own information policies.

Figure 5-10 gives an example of a typical privacy violation complaint form, which the office should keep on hand should a patient feel his privacy rights have been violated. As the medical assistant, you may need to assist the patient in completing this form. Procedure 5-2 at the end of this chapter provides practice in assisting with this form.

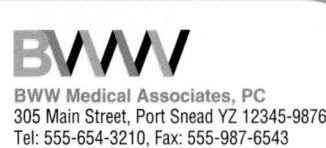

BWW Medical Associates, PC
305 Main Street, Port Snead YZ 12345-9876
Tel: 555-654-3210, Fax: 555-987-6543
Web: BWWAssociates.com

Paul F. Buckwalter, MD
Alexis N. Whalen, MD
Elizabeth H. Williams, MD

Authorization to Release Health Information

I, _____ residing at

_____ and DOB of

_____ give permission to (name of practice) _____

to release to _____ of BWW Medical Associates, PC the

following information: _____

_____

_____

Reason for the request: _____

_____

Signature of Patient or Legal Guardian _____

Printed Name of Patient or Legal Guardian _____

If Guardian, relationship to Patient _____

This authorization will expire on: _____

YOU MAY REFUSE TO SIGN THIS AUTHORIZATION. You may revoke this authorization at any time by notifying BWW Medical Associates, PC in writing. Revocation will have no effect on actions taken prior to receipt of any revocation. Any disclosure of information carries the potential for unauthorized redisclosure and the information may not be protected by federal confidentiality rules.

FIGURE 5-11　An example of an Authorization to Release Health Information form.

Sharing Patient Information　When sharing patient information, HIPAA will allow the provider to use healthcare information for *treatment, payment, and operations (TPO)*:

- *Treatment.* Providers are allowed to share information in order to provide care to patients.
- *Payment.* Providers are allowed to share information in order to receive payment for the treatment provided.
- *Operations.* Providers are allowed to share information to conduct normal business activities, like quality improvement.

If the use of patient information does not fall under TPO, then written authorization must be obtained before sharing information with anyone (Figure 5-11). Some of the core elements of an authorization form include

- Specific and meaningful descriptions of the authorized information.
- Persons authorized to use or disclose protected health information.
- Purpose of the requested information.

- Statement of the patient's right to revoke the authorization.
- Signature of the patient and date signed.

Procedure 5-3 at the end of the chapter outlines the steps to be taken to obtain an authorization to release PHI.

HIPAA Security Rule In February 2003, the final regulations were issued regarding the administrative, physical, and technical safeguards to protect the confidentiality, integrity, and availability of health information covered by HIPAA. The *Security Rule* specifies how patient information is protected on computer networks, the Internet, disks, and other storage media and extranets. However, the rapidly increasing computer use in healthcare today has created new dangers for confidentiality breaches. The Security Rule mandates that

- A security officer must be assigned the responsibility for the medical facility's security.
- All staff, including management, must receive security awareness training.
- Medical facilities must implement audit controls to record and examine staff who have logged into information systems that contain PHI.
- Organizations must limit physical access to medical facilities that contain electronic PHI.
- Organizations must conduct risk analyses to determine information security risks and vulnerabilities.
- Organizations must establish policies and procedures that allow access to electronic PHI on a need-to-know basis.

Computers are not the only concern regarding workplace security. The facility layout can propose a possible violation if not designed correctly. All facilities must take measures to reduce the identity of patient information. Some examples of facility design that can help reduce a confidentiality breach include the security of patient medical records (including charts), the reception area, the clinical station (or patient care area), and the location of fax machines.

- *Chart security.* When paper health records are used, patient charts and the information contained within them can be kept confidential by following these rules:
  1. Charts that contain a patient's name or other identifiers cannot be in view at the front reception area or nurse's station. Some offices have placed charts in plain jackets to prevent information from being seen.
  2. Charts must be stored out of view of a public area to prevent unauthorized individuals from seeing them.
  3. Charts should be placed on the filing shelves without the patient name showing.
  4. Charts should be locked when not in use. Many facilities have purchased filing equipment that can be locked and unlocked without limiting the availability of patient information.
  5. Every staff member who uses patient information must be logged and a confidentiality statement signed. Signatures of staff should be on file with the office.

- *Reception area security.* To be compliant with security rules, the following steps should be taken to secure the reception area:
  1. Log off or lock your computer or terminal, shutting off the monitor when leaving your terminal or computer.
  2. The computer must be placed in an area where patients and unauthorized personnel cannot see the screen.
  3. Many facilities are purchasing flat screen monitors to prevent visibility of the screen.
  4. Patient sign-in sheets may be used but must not include the reason or nature of the patient visit. Likewise, patient names may be called out as long as no reference to the reason for the visit is made.
  5. Call centers and reception area phone conversations must be kept confidential. Many offices put the administrative office behind sliding glass windows to allow for privacy when on the phone with other patients or offices, so that people in the reception area cannot hear phone conversations.

- *Patient care area security.* All healthcare personnel should follow these guidelines to protect PHI in patient care areas:
  1. Log off or lock computer terminals, turning off the monitor when leaving the computer station.
  2. When placing charts in exam room racks or shelves, the name of the patient or other identifiers must be concealed from view.
  3. When discussing a patient with the physician or another staff member, make sure your voice is lowered and that all doors to the exam rooms are closed. Avoid discussing patient conditions in heavy traffic areas.
  4. When discussing a condition with a patient, make sure that you are in a private room or area where no one can hear you.
  5. Avoid discussing patients in lunchrooms, hallways, or any place in a medical facility where someone can overhear you.

- *Fax security.* As a vital link among healthcare providers, insurance plans, and others, much information is exchanged over the fax machine in a medical office, particularly if the office is paper-based and does not have access to electronic communication. Private health information can be exchanged via faxes sent to covered entities, but PHI must still be safeguarded as much as possible by taking the following precautions:
  1. Use a fax cover page. State clearly on the fax cover sheet that confidential and protected health information is included. Further state that the information included is to be protected and must not be shared or disclosed without the appropriate authorizations from the patient.
  2. Keep the fax machine in an area that is not accessible by individuals who are not authorized to view PHI.
  3. Faxes received containing PHI must be stored promptly in a protected, secure area.
  4. Always confirm the accuracy of fax numbers to minimize the possibility of faxes being sent to the wrong person. Call recipients to confirm the fax was received.

5. Program the fax machine to print a confirmation for all faxes sent and staple the confirmation sheet to each document sent.

6. Train all staff members to understand the importance of safeguarding PHI sent or received via fax.

- *Copier security.* Medical assistants should follow these guidelines to protect PHI at the copier:

  1. Do not leave confidential documents anywhere on or near the copier where others can read the information.

  2. Shred copies containing PHI when no longer needed—do not discard copies in a trash container.

  3. If a paper jam occurs, after removing the paper causing the jam, shred it if PHI is contained within the document.

- *Printer security.* To maintain the confidentiality of printed materials, follow these guidelines:

  1. Do not print confidential material on a printer shared by other departments or in an area where others can read the material.

  2. Do not leave the printer unattended while printing confidential material.

  3. Before leaving the printing area, make sure all computer disks, CDs, DVDs, or "jump drives" containing confidential information and all printed material have been collected.

  4. Be certain that the print job is sent to the correct printer location.

  5. Shred any discarded printouts—do not throw them in a trash container.

Violations and Penalties Each staff member is responsible for adhering to HIPAA privacy and security regulations to ensure that PHI is secure and confidential. If PHI is abused or confidentiality is breached, the medical facility can incur substantial penalties or even the incarceration of staff. Violations of HIPAA law can result in both civil and criminal penalties.

- *Civil penalties* for HIPAA privacy violations can be up to $100 for each offense, with an annual cap of $25,000 for repeated violations of the same requirement.

- *Criminal penalties* for the knowing, wrongful misuse of individually identifiable health information can result in penalties ranging from $50,000–$250,000 in fines and between 1 and 10 years in prison.

Administrative Simplification The main key to the set of rules established for HIPAA administrative simplification is standardizing patient information throughout the healthcare system with a set of transaction standards and code sets. The codes and formats used for the exchange of medical data are referred to as *electronic transaction records.* Regulated transaction information receives a transaction set identifier. For example, a healthcare claim would receive an identifier of ASC X12N 837 version 5010—a standard transaction code given to any facility that submits an electronic healthcare claim to an insurance company.

Standardized code sets are used for encoding data elements. The following books are used for the standardized code sets for all healthcare facilities:

- *ICD-9-CM/ICD-10-CM.* This book is used to identify diseases and conditions. The transition to the ICD-10 version is planned for October 1, 2014.

- *CPT 4.* This book is used to identify physician services or procedures.

- *HCPCS.* This book is used to identify health-related services and procedures, like pharmaceuticals or hearing and vision services that are not included in the CPT manual.

▶ Confidentiality Issues and Mandatory Disclosure   LO 5.6

Related to law, ethics, and quality care is the issue of when a healthcare worker, including a medical assistant, can disclose information and when it must be kept confidential. The incidents that doctors are legally required to report to the state were outlined earlier in the chapter. A doctor can be charged with criminal action for not following state and federal laws.

Ethics and professional judgment are always important. Consider the question of whether to contact the partners of a patient who has a sexually transmitted infection (STI—formerly STD) and whether to keep the patient's name from those people. The law says that the physician must instruct patients on how to notify possibly affected third parties and give them referrals to get the proper assistance. If the patient refuses to inform involved outside parties, then the doctor's office may offer to notify current and former partners. The Caution: Handle with Care section addresses this issue.

In general, the patient's ethical right to confidentiality and privacy is protected by law. Only the patient can waive the right to confidentiality. A physician cannot publicize a patient case in journal articles or invite other health professionals to observe a case without the patient's written consent. Most states also prohibit a doctor from testifying in court about a patient without the patient's approval. When a patient sues a physician, however, the patient automatically gives up the right to confidentiality.

Listed below are six principles for preventing improper release of information from the medical office.

1. When in doubt about whether to release information, it is better not to release it.

2. It is the patient's right, not the physician's, to keep patient information confidential. If the patient wants to disclose the information, it is unethical for the physician not to do so.

3. All patients should be treated with the same degree of confidentiality, whatever the healthcare professional's personal opinion of the patient might be.

4. You should be aware of all applicable laws and of the regulations of agencies like public health departments.

CAUTION: HANDLE WITH CARE
Notifying Those at Risk for Sexually Transmitted Infection

Few things are more difficult for a patient with an STI than telling current and former partners about the diagnosis. In fact, some patients elect not to do so. When patients refuse to alert their partners, the medical office can offer to make those contacts. Often that responsibility lies with the medical assistant.

You are most likely to encounter such a situation if you are a medical assistant working in a family practice, an OB/GYN practice, or a clinic. So, becoming familiar with all facets of the situation—from ensuring patient confidentiality to handling potentially difficult confrontations—will help you best serve the patient.

The first step is to get the appropriate information from the patient who has contracted the STI. Because the patient may be sensitive about revealing former and current partners, help him feel more comfortable. First, spend some time talking about the STI. How much does the patient know about it? Educate him about implications, including the probable short- and long-term effects of the infection. Explain how the STI is transmitted. Alert the patient as to precautions to take so he will not continue to transmit the infection to others. Help the patient understand why it is important for people who may have contracted the infection from him to be told they may have it.

Then, offer to contact the patient's former and current partners. Fully explain each step in the notification process, assuring the patient that his name will not be revealed under any circumstances. Answer any questions and address any concerns about the notification process. If the patient is still reluctant to provide information, give him some time to think about it away from the office and follow up periodically with a phone call.

Once the patient agrees to reveal names, write down the names and other information, and preferably phone numbers. To make sure you have correct information, read it back to the patient, spelling each person's name in turn and reciting the phone number or address. Write down the phonetic pronunciations of any difficult names. Tell the patient when you will make the notifications.

You now are ready to contact these individuals. Professionals who work with STI patients recommend guidelines for contacting current and former partners to alert them about potential exposure to an STI. Note that these guidelines are applicable only to STIs other than AIDS.

Determine how you will contact each individual: in writing, in person, or by phone.

1. If you use U.S. mail, mark the outside of the addressed envelope "Personal." On a note inside, simply ask the person to call you at the medical office. Do not put the topic of the call in writing.

2. If you make the contact in person, ask where you can talk privately. Even if the person appears to be alone, others may still be able to overhear the conversation.

3. If you use the phone, identify yourself and your office and ask for the specific individual. Do not reveal the nature of your call to anyone but that person. If pressed, tell the person who answers the phone that you are calling regarding a personal matter.

Once on the phone or alone with the person, confirm that you are talking to the correct person. Mention that you wish to talk about a highly personal matter and ask if it is a good time to continue the discussion. If not, arrange for a more appropriate time. Inform the individual that she has come in contact with someone who has an STI and recommend that she visit a doctor's office or clinic to be tested for the infection.

Be prepared for a variety of reactions, from surprise to anger. Respond calmly and cooly. Expect to respond to questions and statements such as

- Who gave you my name?
- Do I have the disease?
- Am I really at risk? I haven't had intercourse recently (or) I've only had intercourse with my spouse.
- I feel fine. I just went to my doctor recently.

Let the person know that you cannot reveal the name of the partner because the information is strictly confidential. Assure the person that you will not reveal her name to anyone either. Explain that exposure to the disease does not mean a person has contracted it. Encourage the person to get tested to know for sure.

Tell the person that she is still at risk, even if she hasn't had intercourse recently or has had it only with a spouse. Let the person know that someone with whom she came in close contact at some point has contracted the disease. Even if the person says, "I feel fine," she may still have the infection. Again, stress the importance of getting tested.

Provide your name and phone number for contact about further questions. Recommend local offices and clinics for testing, and provide phone numbers. If the person will come to your office, offer to make the appointment.

Finally, document the results of your call. Log in the original patient's file the date that you completed notification. Include any pertinent details about the notification. Alert the patient when all people on the list have been notified.

5. When it is necessary to break confidentiality and when there is a conflict between ethics and confidentiality, discuss it with the patient. If the law does not dictate what to do in the situation, the attending physician should make the judgment based on the urgency of the situation and any danger that might be posed to the patient or others.

6. Get written approval from the patient before releasing information. For common situations, the patient should sign a standard release-of-records form.

The AMA has several standard forms for authorization of disclosure and includes disclosure clauses in many other forms. For example, the consent-to-surgery form includes a clause about consenting to picture taking and observation during the surgery. When using a standard form, cross out anything that does not apply in that particular situation. Medical practices often develop their own customized forms.

▶ Ethics LO 5.7

Medical ethics is a vital part of medical practice and following an ethical code is an important part of your job. Ethics deals with general principles of right and wrong, as opposed to requirements of law. A professional is expected to act in ways that reflect society's ideas of right and wrong, even if such behavior is not enforced by law. Often, however, the law is based on ethical considerations.

Bioethics: Social Issues

Bioethics deals with issues that arise related to medical advances. For many people, bioethical issues are particularly sensitive and highly personal issues. This may be true for you on a personal level as well. Remember, that as a medical assistant, you must remain nonjudgmental at all times regarding patient healthcare dilemmas and decisions. Here are three examples of bioethical issues.

1. A treatment for Parkinson's disease was developed that uses fetal tissue. Some women, upon learning about this treatment, might get pregnant just to have an abortion and sell the fetal tissue. Is this ethical?

2. If a couple cannot have a baby because of a medical condition of the mother, using a surrogate mother is an option some couples choose. The surrogate mother is artificially inseminated with the sperm of the husband and carries the baby to term. The couple then raises the child. Ethically speaking, who is the real mother, the woman who bears the child or the woman who raises the child? If the surrogate mother wants to keep the baby after it is born, does she have a right to do so?

3. When a liver transplant is needed by both a famous patient who has had a history of alcohol abuse and a woman who is a recipient of public assistance, what criteria are considered when determining who receives the organ? Who makes the

decision? Ethically, treating physicians should not make the decision of allocating limited medical resources. Decisions regarding the allocation of limited medical resources should consider only the likelihood of benefit, the urgency of need, and the amount of resources required for successful treatment. Nonmedical criteria like ability to pay, age, social worth, perceived obstacles to treatment, patient's contribution to illness, or the past use of resources should not be considered.

Practicing appropriate professional ethics has a positive impact on your reputation and the success of your employer's business. As a result, many medical organizations have created guidelines for the acceptable and preferred manners and behaviors, or etiquette, of administrative medical assistants and physicians.

The principles of medical ethics have developed over time. The Hippocratic oath, in which medical students pledge to practice medicine ethically, was developed in ancient Greece (see www.nlm.nih.gov/hmd/greek/greek_oath.html). It is still used today and is one of the original bases of modern medical ethics. Hippocrates, the 4th century B.C. Greek physician commonly called the "father of medicine," is traditionally considered the author of this oath, but its authorship is actually unknown.

Among the promises of the Hippocratic oath are to use the form of treatment believed to be best for the patient, to refrain from harmful actions, and to keep a patient's private information confidential.

The AMA defines ethical behavior for doctors in *Code of Medical Ethics: Current Opinions with Annotations* (Chicago: American Medical Association, 1996). Medical assistants as well as doctors need to be aware of these principles, some of which are included in italics here and explained as follows:

A physician shall be dedicated to providing competent medical service with compassion and respect for human dignity.

This concept means that medical professionals will respect all aspects of the patient as a person, including intellect and emotions. The doctor must decide what treatment would result in the best, most dignified quality of life for the patient, and the doctor must respect a patient's choice to forgo treatment.

A physician shall deal honestly with patients and colleagues and strive to expose those physicians deficient in character or competence or who engage in fraud or deception.

Medical professionals, including medical assistants, should respect colleagues, but they also must respect and protect the profession and public welfare enough to report colleagues who are breaking the law, acting unethically, or unable to perform competently. Dilemmas may arise where one suspects, but is not able to prove, for instance, that a coworker has a substance abuse problem or another problem that is affecting performance. Ignoring such a situation in medical practice could cost someone's life as well as lead to lawsuits.

In terms of billing, a doctor should bill only for direct services, not for indirect ones like referrals. The doctor also should not bill for services that do not really pertain to the practice of medicine, such as dispensing drugs.

It is also unethical for the doctor to influence the patient about where to fill prescriptions or obtain other medical services when the doctor has a personal financial interest in any of the choices.

A physician shall respect the law and also recognize a responsibility to seek changes in requirements that are contrary to the patient's best interests.

Several legal or employer requirements have come under scrutiny as being contrary to a patient's best interests. Among them are discharging patients from the hospital after a certain time limit for certain procedures, which may be too soon for many patients. Insurance company payment policies have sometimes been criticized as unfair. So have health maintenance organization (HMO) financial policies that may conflict with a doctor's treatment preference.

A physician shall respect the rights of patients, of colleagues, and of other health professionals and shall safeguard patient confidences within the constraints of law.

As previously mentioned, the Patient Care Partnership: Understanding Expectations, Rights and Responsibilities, originally established by the American Hospital Association in 1973 and revised in 1992, lists ethical principles protecting the patient. Some states have even passed this code of ethics into law. Among a patient's rights are the right to information about alternative treatments, the right to refuse to participate in research projects, and the right to privacy.

A physician shall continue to study; apply and advance scientific knowledge; make relevant information available to patients, colleagues, and the public; obtain consultation; and use the talents of other health professionals when indicated.

Keeping up with the latest advancements in medicine is crucial for providing high-quality, ethical care. Most states require doctors to accumulate "continuing education units" to maintain a license to practice. These units are earned by means of educational activities like courses and scientific meetings. As discussed in *The Profession of Medical Assisting* chapter, medical assistants who are certified by the AAMA, RMA, or CMAS have similar requirements by the sponsoring certification board to earn CEUs to maintain their credentialed status.

A physician shall, in the provision of appropriate patient care, except in emergencies, be free to choose whom to serve, with whom to associate, and the environment in which to provide medical services.

Ethically, doctors can set their hours, decide what kind of medicine to practice and where, decide whom to accept as a patient, and take time off as long as a qualified substitute performs their duties. Doctors may decline to accept new patients because of a full workload. In an emergency, however, a doctor may be ethically obligated to care for a patient, even if the patient is not of the doctor's choosing. The doctor should not abandon that patient until another physician is available.

A physician shall recognize a responsibility to participate in activities contributing to an improved community.

This ethical obligation also holds true for the allied health professions. In addition to knowing the physician's codes of ethics, medical assistants should follow the code of ethics for their certifying body, be it the AAMA or the AMT. See the Points on Practice feature for the AAMA's Code of Ethics and the AMT's Standards of Practice (Figure 5-12).

▶ Legal Medical Practice Models   LO 5.8

There are five basic types of medical practice:

- Sole proprietorship
- Partnership
- Group practice
- Professional corporation
- Clinics

Laws governing the various types of practice vary, but medical office personnel should be aware of the laws that apply to their employers' practice management models.

Sole Proprietorship

This type of practice is often referred to as a "solo practice." In this type of practice, a physician practicing alone assumes all the benefits for and liabilities of the business. Sole proprietorship practice management is no longer a popular option, as a result of the increased expenses and decreased insurance reimbursements. So, more physicians are joining group practices or professional corporations.

Partnership

When two or more physicians decide to practice together, they may form a partnership, based on a legal contract that specifies the rights, obligations, and responsibilities of each partner. Advantages of partnerships include sharing the workload, expenses, profits, and assets. A disadvantage is that each partner has equal liability for acts of misconduct, losses, and deficits of the practice, unless specified as a contingency in the contract.

Group Practice

Group practice is a medical practice model in which three or more licensed physicians share the collective income, expenses, facilities, equipment, records, and personnel for the practice. Physicians in

POINTS ON PRACTICE

AAMA Code of Ethics

The Code of Ethics of the AAMA shall set forth principles of ethical and moral conduct as they relate to the medical profession and the particular practice of medical assisting.

Members of the AAMA dedicated to the conscientious pursuit of their profession, and thus desiring to merit the high regard of the entire medical profession and the respect of the general public which they serve, do pledge themselves to strive always to:

A. Render service with full respect for the dignity of humanity;

B. Respect confidential information obtained through employment, unless legally authorized or required

by responsible performance of duty to divulge such information;

C. Uphold the honor and high principles of the profession and accept its disciplines;

D. Seek to continually improve the knowledge and skills of medical assistants for the benefit of patients and professional colleagues; and

E. Participate in additional service activities aimed toward improving the health and well-being of the community.

AMT Standards of Practice

AMT seeks to encourage, establish, and maintain the highest standards, traditions and principles of the practices which constitute the profession of the Registry. Members of the AMT Registry must recognize their responsibilities, not only to their patients, but also to society, to other health care professionals, and to themselves. The following standards of practice are principles adopted by the AMT Board of Directors, which define the essence of honorable and ethical behavior for a health care professional:

1. While engaged in the Arts and Sciences, which constitute the practice of their profession, AMT professionals shall be dedicated to the provision of competent service.

2. The AMT professional shall place the welfare of the patient above all else.

3. The AMT professional understands the importance of thoroughness in the performance of duty, compassion with patients, and the importance of the tasks, which may be performed.

4. The AMT professional shall always seek to respect the rights of patients and of health care providers, and shall safeguard patient confidences.

5. The AMT professional will strive to increase his/her technical knowledge, shall continue to study, and apply scientific advanced in his/her specialty.

6. The AMT professional shall respect the law and will pledge to avoid dishonest, unethical or illegal practices.

7. The AMT professional understands that he/she is not to make or offer a diagnosis or interpretation unless he/she is a duly licensed physician/dentist or unless asked by the attending physician/dentist.

8. The AMT professional shall protect and value the judgment of the attending physician or dentist, providing this does not conflict with the behavior necessary to carry out Standard Number 2 above.

9. The AMT professional recognizes that any personal wrongdoing is his/her responsibility. It is also the professional health care provider's obligation to report to the proper authorities any knowledge of professional abuse.

10. The AMT professional pledges personal honor and integrity to cooperate in the advancement and expansion, by every lawful means, of American Medical Technologists.

American Medical Technologists
10700 W. Higgins Road, Suite 150
Rosemont, Illinois 60018
Phone: (847) 823-5169 – Fax: (847) 823-0458
Email: mail@amt1.com – www.amt1.com

FIGURE 5-12 AMT Standards of Practice

group practice may be engaged in the same specialty, calling themselves, for example, Associates in Cardiology, or they can be several physicians offering similar specialties, like OB/GYN and pediatrics.

Professional Corporations

A corporation is a body formed and authorized by state law to act as a single entity. Physicians who form corporations are shareholders and employees of the organization. Forming a corporation has financial and tax advantages, and the fringe benefits for employees may be greater than in a sole proprietorship or partnership.

In forming a corporation, the incorporators and owners have limited liability in case lawsuits are filed. Sometimes medical practices are "managed" by for-profit corporations that are either formed by outside business interests or subsidiary corporations organized by hospitals. Physicians are hired as salaried employees with bonus options. The management corporation provides the facility, office personnel, employee benefits, human resource services, and operating expenses.

Clinics

Patients can be admitted to clinics for special circumstances and research. In many cases, clinics are hard to distinguish from large medical facilities.

Clinics are broad in their range of specialties and subspecialties, and often have sophisticated medical equipment and renowned medical practitioners. Clinics may be housed inside of a hospital or be free-standing. Urgent care centers, also known as walk-in clinics, exist so that patients will have the option of being seen without an appointment.

In-store clinics are becoming more prevalent. Housed in large major chain stores and sometimes in chain pharmacies, they offer smaller medical services like vaccinations, flu shots, and eye exams.

Employment Law

Many medical assistants find themselves promoted into supervisory and managerial positions. Knowledge of employment and labor laws like those involving civil rights, sexual harassment, employment of the disabled, fair labor laws, and family medical leave are important to all employees, but particularly so for those who oversee other employees. Labor and employment laws are covered in detail in the *Practice Management* chapter.

PROCEDURE 5-1 Obtaining Signature for Receipt of Privacy Practices Notice

Procedure Goal: To follow HIPAA guidelines and obtain the patient's signature that he or she has received and understands the office privacy policies.

OSHA Guidelines: This procedure does not involve exposure to blood, body fluids, or tissue.

Materials: Preprinted receipt of privacy practices information form (see Figure 5-9), pens, and a copy machine.

Method: Procedure steps.

1. Explain to the patient the office privacy policy regarding protected health information.
   RATIONALE: Some patients understand the spoken word more easily than the written word.

2. Ask the patient to read the policy carefully and to feel free to ask any questions he or she may have regarding the policy. Answer any questions that may arise.

   RATIONALE: Patients must have a thorough understanding in order to acknowledge receipt of the privacy policy.

3. When the patient's questions have been answered, witness the patient (or guardian) sign and print his or her name. Note any restrictions that may be placed on the document.
   RATIONALE: Restrictions must be noted so inadvertent release of information does not occur.

4. Print your name and sign the document as witness, including your title.

5. Date the document when all signatures have been completed.

6. Make a copy of the document to file in the patient medical record and give the original to the patient.
   RATIONALE: It is important that copies of all signed documents are in the patient's record in case of any legal proceedings that may arise.

PROCEDURE 5-2 Completing a Privacy Violation Complaint Form

Goal: To assist the patient in completing a Privacy Violation Complaint form if she feels her PHI has been compromised.

OSHA Guidelines: This procedure does not involve exposure to blood, body fluids, or tissue.

Materials: Privacy Violation Complaint form (see Figure 5-10), pens, private room to complete form, and a copy machine.

Method: Procedure steps.

1. Explain to the patient that all formal complaints must be made in writing.
   RATIONALE: This provides legal documentation in case it is ever needed in court.

2. Ask the patient if she feels assistance will be needed completing the form. If not, the patient may complete

the form on her own. Answer any questions she may have regarding completion of the form.

3. When the patient completes the form, read it carefully, making sure it is complete and legible and the information regarding the breach of privacy is clear.
   RATIONALE: In order to address the alleged breach, a thorough understanding of the complaint is needed.

4. If the patient requires that any copies be made for documentation backing the claim, make the copies, returning any originals to the patient.

5. Make sure the patient signs and dates the complaint.

6. As the person receiving the complaint, sign the document as indicated and date it.

7. Explain to the patient that the office will respond to the complaint within 30 days of today's receipt.

8. Make a copy of the document for the patient and keep the original for the office files.
   RATIONALE: Copies of all legal documents must be kept on file.

PROCEDURE 5-3   Obtaining Authorization to Release Health Information

Goal: To follow HIPAA guidelines when obtaining the patient's protected health information without violating confidentiality regulations.

OSHA Guidelines: This procedure does not involve exposure to blood, body fluids, or tissue.

Materials: Preprinted Authorization to Release Health Information form (see Figure 5-11), pens, and a copy machine.

Method: Procedure steps.

1. Explain to the patient the need for the requested medical information.
   RATIONALE: In order for the consent to be valid, the patient must understand the need for the release of information.

2. Obtain the name and address of the practice to which the authorization is to be mailed.

3. Fill in the patient's name, address, and DOB as required.

4. Enter the physician's or practitioner's name from your practice who is requesting the PHI.

5. Enter the information that is being requested.
   RATIONALE: Only the required information may be requested and released to the practice.

6. Complete the reason for request area, explaining why the patient is requesting the information be sent to your office.
   RATIONALE: To comply with HIPAA guidelines, a reason for the record release is necessary.

7. Enter an expiration date for the authorization, giving a reasonable amount of time for the request to be fulfilled.

8. Prior to signing the release, go over with the patient the information contained within the release, answering any questions that may arise. Be sure the patient understands the request may be withdrawn (in writing) at any time.

9. Witness the patient (or guardian) signature and date; if necessary, be sure the guardian relationship area is completed.

10. Sign and date the document as witness, including your title.

11. Make a copy of the document to file in the patient medical record and, if requested, give a copy to the patient as well.
    RATIONALE: The release is a legal document and must be kept with the patient medical record.

12. Make a notation in the medical record of the document signing and note the date the authorization is mailed.
    RATIONALE: If the records are not received in a timely manner, the office will need to be contacted.

SUMMARY OF LEARNING OUTCOMES

LEARNING OUTCOMES	KEY POINTS
5.1 **Differentiate between laws and ethics.**	A law is a rule of conduct or action prescribed or formally recognized as binding or enforced by local, state, or federal government. Ethics are standards of behavior or concepts of right or wrong beyond what the legal consideration is in any given situation.

| --- | --- |
5.2 **Identify the responsibilities of the patient and physician in a physician-patient contract, including the components for informed consent that must be understood by the patient.**	Physician responsibilities in a patient-physician contract include using due care, skill, judgment, and diligence in treating the patient; staying informed of the current diagnosis and treatment; performing to the best of the physician's ability; and providing complete information and instructions to the patient. Regarding informed consent, the physician must provide the following information: proposed treatment modes; why the treatment is necessary; risks of the proposed treatment; alternative treatments available; risks of the alternatives; and the risks if all treatment is refused. Patient responsibilities in a patient-physician contract include following instructions given by the provider and cooperating as much as possible; giving relevant information to the provider; following physician instructions for treatment; and paying fees for services provided.
5.3 **Explain the four Ds of negligence required to prove malpractice and the four Cs of malpractice prevention.**	The four Ds of malpractice are duty—it must be proven that a patient-physician relationship exists; derelict—it must be proven that the physician failed to comply with standards of the profession; direct cause—it must be proven that any damages were directly caused by the physician's breach of duty; and damages—it must be proven that the patient suffered an injury. The four Cs of medical malpractice prevention are caring—the most important asset; communication—which earns respect and trust; competence—which proves your abilities by maintaining and updating your knowledge; and charting—which documents all aspects of patient interaction.
5.4 **Relate the term *credentialing* and the importance of the FDA and DEA to administrative procedures performed by medical assistants.**	The term *credentialing* refers to the approval process a healthcare provider must go through to be allowed to bill Medicare and other insurance carriers for providing medical services to patients under their insurance plans. Often, the medical assistant is in charge of submitting the required paperwork and documentation for the provider to gain this approval. The Food and Drug Administration (FDA) approves drugs and medications for use on humans. It also regulates whether drugs are prescription-based or accessible OTC. The Drug Enforcement Agency (DEA) is responsible for controlling and overseeing the prescribing of controlled substances. Physicians must obtain and renew their license with the DEA in order to prescribe controlled substances.
5.5 **Summarize the purpose of the following federal healthcare regulations: HCQIA, False Claims Act, OSHA, and HIPAA.**	Congress enacted HCQIA in 1996 because they found that there was an increasing occurrence of medical malpractice and a need to improve the quality of medical care. The False Claims Act allows individuals to bring civil *qui tam* actions on behalf of the U.S. government for false claims made to the federal government. OSHA created federal laws to protect healthcare workers from health hazards on the job. Title I of HIPAA was created so that employees could still have access to health insurance coverage when leaving employment for any reason. Title II was created to protect patients' individually identifiable personal information as well as their personal health information. It also allows patients access to their medical information on request and allows them to limit the sharing of that information. Additionally, patients on written request must be allowed to see a record of how their PHI has been shared and with whom.

LEARNING OUTCOMES	KEY POINTS
5.6 Identify the six principles for preventing improper release of information from the medical office.	The six rules for preventing improper release of information include the following: (1) When in doubt about whether to release information, it is better not to release it. (2) It is the patient's right, not the physician's, to keep patient information confidential. (3) All patients should be treated with the same degree of confidentiality. (4) Be aware of all applicable laws and of the regulations of agencies involved with confidentiality. (5) When it is necessary to break confidentiality and when there is a conflict between ethics and confidentiality, discuss it with the patient. The physician may need to make the final decision. (6) Get written approval from the patient before releasing information.
5.7 Discuss the importance of ethics in the medical office.	Ethics reflect the general principles of right and wrong. A professional, particularly a medical professional, is expected to follow especially high ethical standards.
5.8 Explain the differences among the practice management models.	There are five basic types of practice management models: (1) sole proprietorship (one physician), (2) partnership (two or more physicians), (3) group practice (three or more physicians), (4) professional corporation (a body formed and authorized by state law to act as a single entity; physicians are stakeholders and employees of the organization), and (5) clinics.

CASE STUDY CRITICAL THINKING

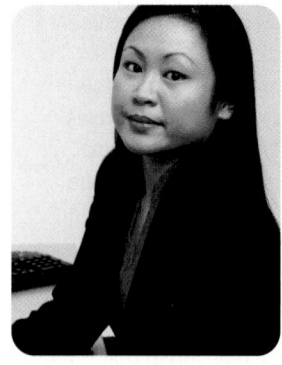

Recall Cindy Chen from the beginning of the chapter. Now that you have completed the chapter, answer the following questions regarding her case.

1. How will you respond to the extern's concerns?

2. Once Cindy becomes a phlebotomist, how should the information regarding her HIV-positive status be handled? Will the situation change should she develop AIDS?

EXAM PREPARATION QUESTIONS

1. (LO 5.1) A standard of behavior with a concept of right and wrong beyond the legal considerations is called
 a. Civil law
 b. Moral values
 c. Medical ethics
 d. Etiquette
 e. Ethics

2. (LO 5.1) The two types of law that pertain to healthcare professionals are
 a. Contract law and agency law
 b. Civil law and criminal law
 c. Civil law and medical law
 d. Litigation and malpractice
 e. Contract law and medical negligence

3. (LO 5.2) The physician's responsibility within the physician-patient contract includes all of the following EXCEPT:
   a. Setting up a practice within the boundaries of his or her license to practice medicine
   b. Setting up an office where he or she chooses and to establish office hours
   c. Whether he/she will specialize
   d. Deciding which services he or she will provide and how those services will be provided
   e. Treating every patient seeking care

4. (LO 5.3) Cases in which a person believes that a medical professional did not perform an essential action or performed an improper one, thus harming the patient, may result in
   a. Charges of slander
   b. Charges of medical negligence
   c. Charges of abandonment
   d. Charges of defamation
   e. Charges of fraud

5. (LO 5.3) Under the _____ words uttered to a patient by the medical assistant can be said to be the responsibility of the employer-physician.
   a. Law of agency
   b. Employee contract
   c. Civil law
   d. Criminal law
   e. Ethical considerations

6. (LO 5.4) The process used by various organizations, including insurance carriers, to ensure that healthcare providers are appropriately qualified to provide services and meet all the necessary requirements to do so is called
   a. Arbitration
   b. *Qui tam*
   c. Credentialing
   d. Subpoena
   e. Tort

7. (LO 5.5) Which of the federal acts passed by Congress was passed to improve the quality of medical care nationwide?
   a. HIPAA Title I
   b. HIPAA Title II
   c. OSHA
   d. HCQIA
   e. False Claims Act

8. (LO 5.6) Incidents and diseases, although normally considered confidential, that must be reported to federal, state, or local agencies come under the heading of
   a. Medical ethics
   b. HIPAA security rule
   c. STIs and AIDS
   d. Mandatory disclosure
   e. Civil law

9. (LO 5.7) Issues relating to medical advances come under the heading of
   a. Ethics
   b. Bioethics
   c. Religious freedoms
   d. Misfeasance
   e. Malfeasance

10. (LO 5.8) Which practice model provides the most legal protection for the physicians who form the practice?
    a. Sole proprietorship
    b. Partnership
    c. Group practice
    d. Professional corporation
    e. Clinics

CASE STUDY

PATIENT INFORMATION

Patient Name	Gender	DOB
Shenya Jones	Female	11/3/19XX

Attending	MRN	Allergies
Elizabeth Williams, MD	124-86-564	cinnamon, peanuts

Shenya Jones, a 34-year-old female, arrives at the office with a swelling and a red pustule on her face. She states the problem started two days ago as a small pimple near her nose. It became irritated, then became extremely swollen and painful overnight. Now this morning there was yellow drainage noted at the site and the swelling has increased. The area of drainage is approximately 1 cm in diameter. The upper lip, side of the face, and nose are all swollen. She rates the pain in her face as 7 out of 10. The physician thinks the condition may be impetigo or Methicillin-resistant Staphylococcus aureus (MRSA), a type of skin infection that is resistant to the common antibiotics used to treat it.

Keep Shenya in mind as you study this chapter. There will be questions at the end of the chapter based on the case study. The information in the chapter will help you answer these questions.

LEARNING OUTCOMES

After completing Chapter 6, you will be able to:

6.1 Describe the components of a medical office safety plan.

6.2 Identify OSHA's role in protecting healthcare workers.

6.3 Describe basic safety precautions you should take to reduce electrical hazards.

6.4 Illustrate the necessary steps in a comprehensive fire safety plan.

6.5 Summarize proper methods for handling and storing chemicals used in a medical office.

6.6 Explain the principles of good ergonomic practice and physical safety in the medical office.

6.7 Illustrate the cycle of infection and how to break it.

6.8 Summarize the Bloodborne Pathogens Standard and Universal Precautions as described in the rules and regulations of the Occupational Safety and Health Administration (OSHA).

6.9 Describe methods of infection control including those for preventing healthcare-associated infections.

6.10 Describe Centers for Disease Control and Prevention (CDC) requirements for reporting cases of infectious disease.

KEY TERMS

alcohol-based hand disinfectants (AHD)

asepsis

carrier

endogenous infection

engineered safety devices

ergonomics

exogenous infection

fomite

general duty clause

hazard label

healthcare-associated infections (HAI)

Material Safety Data Sheet (MSDS)

Occupational Safety and Health Administration (OSHA)

pathogen

personal protective equipment (PPE)

reservoir host

Standard Precautions

susceptible host

vector

work practice controls

III. C (1)   Describe the infection cycle, including the infectious agent, reservoir, susceptible host, means of transmission, portals of entry, and portals of exit

III. C (2)   Define asepsis

III. C (3)   Discuss infection control procedures

III. C (4)   Identify personal safety precautions as established by the Occupational Safety and Health Administration (OSHA)

III. C (6)   Compare different methods of controlling the growth of microorganisms

III. C (7)   Match types and uses of personal protective equipment (PPE)

III. C (8)   Differentiate between medical and surgical asepsis used in ambulatory care settings, identifying when each is appropriate

III. C (11) Describe Standard Precautions, including:
  a. Transmission based precautions
  b. Purpose
  c. Activities regulated

III. C (12) Discuss the application of Standard Precautions with regard to:
  a. All body fluids, secretions and excretions
  b. Blood
  c. Non intact skin
  d. Mucous membranes

III. C (13) Identify the role of the Centers for Disease Control (CDC) regulations in healthcare settings

III. P (1)   Participate in training on Standard Precautions

III. P (2)   Practice Standard Precautions

III. P (3)   Select appropriate barrier/personal protective equipment (PPE) for potentially infectious situations

III. P (4)   Perform handwashing

IX. C (13)   Discuss all levels of governmental legislation and regulation as they apply to medical assisting practice, including FDA and DEA regulations

XI. C (1)   Describe personal protective equipment

XI. C (2)   Identify safety techniques that can be used to prevent accidents and maintain a safe work environment

XI. C (3)   Describe the importance of Material Safety Data Sheets (MSDS) in a healthcare setting

XI. C (4)   Identify safety signs, symbols and labels

XI. C (7)   Describe fundamental principles for evacuation of a healthcare setting

XI. C (8)   Discuss fire safety issues in a healthcare environment

XI. C (9)   Discuss requirements for responding to hazardous material disposal

XI. C (10)   Identify principles of body mechanics and ergonomics

XI. C (11)   Discuss critical elements of an emergency plan for response to a natural disaster or other emergency

XI. P (1)   Comply with safety signs, symbols and labels

XI. P (2)   Evaluate the work environment to identify safe vs. unsafe working conditions

XI. P (3)   Develop a personal (patient and employee) safety plan

XI. P (5)   Demonstrate proper use of the following equipment:
  a. Eyewash
  b. Fire extinguishers
  c. Sharps disposal containers

XI. P (7)   Explain an evacuation plan for a physician's office

XI. P (8)   Demonstrate methods of fire prevention in the healthcare setting

XI. P (11)   Use proper body mechanics

ABHES

4. **Medical Law and Ethics**
   Graduates:
   f. Comply with federal, state, and local health laws and regulations

9. **Medical Office Clinical Procedures**
   Graduates:
   b. Apply principles of aseptic techniques and infection control
   i. Use standard precautions

10. **Medical Laboratory Procedures**
   Graduates:
   c. Dispose of biohazardous materials

Introduction

Accidents can happen anywhere, at any time. Daily newspaper and TV headlines feature all kinds of accidents, from sports injuries and car wrecks to house fires and factory explosions. The healthcare setting is no stranger to accidents, which can occur in the physician's front office, laboratory, exam room, or hallway. Patients and staff members can fall or cut themselves and be exposed to numerous safety hazards. As a medical assistant, you have an important responsibility to remove or correct hazards—physical, chemical, and biohazardous—that might cause injury to patients, physicians, or staff members. This responsibility constitutes an integral part of a risk management plan. In this chapter, you will learn basic office safety including the components of a safety plan, OSHA Hazard Communication, electrical, fire, and chemical safety. You also will be introduced to infection control theory and methods, including

- The cycle of infection
- OSHA Bloodborne Pathogens Standard
- Methods of infection control
- Transmission of disease from healthcare workers
- Infectious disease reporting guidelines

The Medical Office Safety Plan   LO 6.1

Minimizing risk to patients, physicians, and staff by creating a safe environment in the medical office is essential. Both the administrative and clinical areas in an office environment contain many potential hazards. Having an established, routinely updated safety plan is a good first step in hazard awareness. Awareness and understanding of potential dangers facilitates the removal or correction of these hazards.

Every medical office must have a comprehensive written safety plan that is easily accessible to all employees and updated annually. Every employee is responsible for becoming familiar with and following the safety plan's policies and procedures. This plan must contain but is not limited to

- OSHA Hazard Communication
- Electrical safety
- Fire safety
- Emergency action plan
- Chemical safety
- Bloodborne pathogen exposure
- Personal protective equipment
- Needlestick prevention

Occupational Safety and Health Administration   LO 6.2

The **Occupational Safety and Health Administration (OSHA)** was created within the Department of Labor as a result of legislation passed in 1970 (the Occupational Safety and Health Acts) to protect employee safety in the workplace.

OSHA's duties include the creation and enforcement of both general safety standards and standards for specific industries and operations. In general, if a specific standard exists, its guidelines must be followed; but if no specific standard has been developed, the **general duty clause** takes effect. This clause requires an employer to maintain a workplace free from hazards that are recognized as likely to cause death or serious injury. For example, all employers are expected to ensure that all exits are clear of obstacles and unlocked when the building is occupied. If an employer blocks a fire exit, a fire breaks out, and employees are injured because they are unable to safely leave the building, the employer has violated the general duty clause. OSHA also acts to enforce guidelines developed by the Centers for Disease Control and Prevention (CDC), in particular the guidelines for Standard Precautions. Copies of these guidelines can be obtained from many sources, including local OSHA offices; the CDC in Atlanta, Georgia; many industrial organizations throughout the country; and the Internet.

OSHA Hazard Communication

In order to further promote employee safety within the workplace, the Hazard Communication Standard requires that employees receive training in workplace hazards, including how to interpret documentation about hazardous substances that pose an exposure threat. Hazardous materials must be correctly labeled and employees must have access to this information, including the measures they can take to protect themselves against harm from these substances.

Biohazard Labels All containers used to store waste products, blood, blood products, or other specimens that may be contaminated with bloodborne pathogens are considered biohazardous. They must be clearly marked with the biohazard symbol, as shown in Figure 6-1. The biohazard symbol label must be bright orange-red and clearly lettered so that no one can mistake the meaning of the warning. Labels should be securely attached to containers.

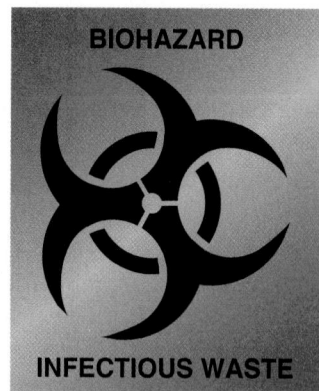

FIGURE 6-1 The biohazard symbol identifies material that has been exposed to potentially contaminated substances such as blood, blood products, or other body fluids. This symbol is used wherever there is a possibility of exposure to biohazardous substances.

BIOHAZARDS PRESENT!!!

NO EATING
NO DRINKING
NO SMOKING
NO MOUTH PIPETTING

DO NOT APPLY COSMETICS OR LIP BALM
DO NOT MANIPULATE CONTACT LENSES

FIGURE 6-2 The biohazard warning sign alerts personnel to the presence of potentially contaminated substances and advises them about safety guidelines.

In addition to individual biohazard labels that identify particular containers, warning signs must be posted in the laboratory itself. These signs, such as the one shown in Figure 6-2, identify the presence of biohazardous material and list important safeguards to follow.

Material Safety Data Sheets You can find information about hazardous chemicals or other substances by referring to the **Material Safety Data Sheets (MSDSs)**. Every hazardous chemical must have a copy of the MSDS, which you are required to keep in your facility at all times. Websites like www.msds.com provide a searchable database of MSDSs. You also may find information on the product website for your specific chemical. Currently, each MSDS must contain the following information about the product it describes:

- Substance name, as it appears on the container label.
- Chemical name(s) of each ingredient.
- Common name(s) of each ingredient.
- Chemical characteristics of the product (boiling point, specific gravity, melting point, appearance, odor).
- Physical hazards posed by the product (fire, vapor pressure).
- Health hazards posed by the product (carcinogenicity [ability to cause cancer], routes and methods of entry, signs and symptoms of exposure).
- Guidelines for safe handling of the substance.
- Emergency and first-aid procedures to be followed in the event of exposure.

Hazard Labels In addition to the MSDS, each hazardous substance must be identified with a hazard label. A **hazard label** is a shortened version of the MSDS that is permanently affixed to the substance container. OSHA requires that a hazard label display the name of the material contained, either trade or chemical, and a brief statement of the chemical's hazardous effects. OSHA does not specify a system of colors or numbers that require special training to identify a product. If you encounter a label with a color-coded, numbered

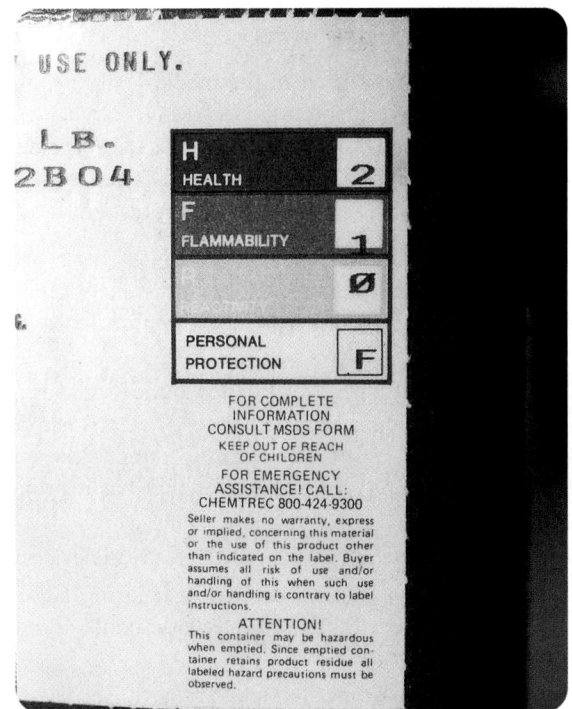

FIGURE 6-3 A hazard label is a condensed version of the MSDS and displays important information about a substance. It must be permanently affixed to the substance container.

system, consult the manufacturer for a description of the specific labeling system. Different manufacturers use slightly different labeling systems. A sample hazard label is shown in Figure 6-3.

Updates to OSHA's Hazard Communication Standard

In order to improve safety in the workplace, OSHA has published their final rule on Hazard Communication. This final rule is designed to standardize the labeling systems and safety information for hazardous materials. The goal of this new standard is to transition from the workers' "right to know" to the workers' "right to understand" the workplace hazards they may encounter. Required final implementation of this rule is June 1, 2016. Employee training on the new label elements and SDS format must begin December 1, 2013. A summary of the major changes to the Hazard Communication Standard are as follows:

- *Hazard classification*: Chemical manufacturers and importers are required to determine the hazards of the chemicals they produce. This includes the health and physical hazards and classification of chemical mixtures.
- *Labels*: All labels must include a signal word, pictogram, hazard statement, and precautionary statement for each hazard class and category. Labels must have a red border.
- *Material Safety Data Sheets*: These are simply called Safety Data Sheets and are standardized. The format will include 16 sections and must follow a uniform format including section numbers and headings.

▶ Electrical Safety

LO 6.3

Because the equipment used in the medical office can make the office especially vulnerable to electrical hazards, it is critical that you know how to respond to an electrical accident. In addition to familiarizing yourself with the location of circuit breakers and emergency power shutoffs, practice these safeguards, which reduce electrical hazards:

- Avoid using extension cords. If they must be used, be sure the circuit is not overloaded. Tape extension cords to the floor to avoid tripping.
- Frayed electrical wires, overloaded outlets, and improperly grounded plugs present a danger of electric shock and fire. Contact a licensed electrician to remedy these problems. Repair or replace equipment that has a broken or frayed cord.
- Dry your hands before working with electrical devices.
- Do not position electrical devices near sinks, faucets, or other sources of water. Be sure electrical cords do not run through water.

▶ Fire Safety

LO 6.4

Fire is a safety hazard anywhere, but it is especially likely where there is sophisticated, high-voltage medical equipment such as an X-ray machine. Any electrical instrument in the exam room, however, is a potential fire hazard. Other potentially hazardous items are gas tanks and flammable chemicals. As discussed below, you should practice fire safety by taking action to prevent it and knowing what action to take in the event of a fire.

Fire Prevention

Be aware of anything that might cause a fire in the exam room, examples of which are outlined in the following bullets. If you cannot correct the situation yourself, report the hazard to your supervisor.

- Extremely flammable materials, including alcohol and some disinfectants. Supplies such as paper table coverings also can ignite and spread flames quickly in the event of a fire. Check to make sure that all flammable items are stored and disposed of properly to minimize fire danger. Also, keep flammable liquids away from any heat source. If you are not sure whether a chemical is flammable, read the manufacturer's label or Material Safety Data Sheet.
- Smoking. Smoking should not be permitted anywhere in a medical facility. In addition to causing health problems, smoking is a fire hazard. "No Smoking" signs should be posted prominently throughout the office.
- Inoperative smoke detectors. Make sure that smoke detectors throughout the office are working properly. Replace batteries promptly. If smoke detectors are wired into the building's electrical system, report any malfunction to the building manager. If possible, alarms should have sound and visual modes.

Working in the physician's office laboratory may sometimes require that you use a flame. These special precautions are essential in such circumstances:

- If you must use an open flame, extinguish it immediately after use.
- When using an open flame, keep your hair, clothing, and jewelry away from the flame source.
- If you must use a chemical in a procedure that requires an open flame, double-check the MSDS to identify the fire risk level for that chemical. If necessary, bring a fire extinguisher to the area in which you will be working.
- Never lean over an open flame.
- Never leave an open flame unattended.
- Turn off gas valves immediately after use. If you must use an open flame in the vicinity of a gas valve, always double-check to be sure the gas is off. Make sure there is adequate ventilation.

In Case of Fire

Despite the precautions that you and your coworkers take, a fire may break out. Be prepared to use fire safety equipment and to evacuate the building safely. The paragraphs that follow provide specific information on using fire safety equipment and carrying out emergency action plans and drills.

Using Safety Equipment The number of fire extinguishers in the office depends on the office's size and its number of rooms. Regardless of the total number of extinguishers, you should locate an all-purpose fire extinguisher in or close to each exam room. The office manager or safety officer should have the fire extinguisher professionally serviced once a year to ensure its effectiveness. It is important that each employee learns how to use a fire extinguisher. Procedure 6-1 describes the proper method for handling a fire emergency. OSHA recommends that employees know the "PASS" system:

- Pull the pin.
- Aim at the base of the fire.
- Squeeze the trigger.
- Sweep side to side.

Posters with the "PASS" acronym are available from OSHA.

If there is a fire blanket in the exam room, be sure that you know how to use it and that it is stored for easy access in an emergency. To use a fire blanket to smother burning clothing, wrap the victim in the blanket and roll him on the floor. You also can contact your local fire department for more information about fire safety training.

Emergency Action Plans and Drills

Every employee must be prepared to take appropriate action during a fire emergency. An emergency action plan that outlines the employees' responsibilities is needed in order to reduce panic in an emergency and to reduce the likelihood of severe bodily injury. Participation in periodic fire drills is an essential part of this plan. The other important components

FIGURE 6-4 An evacuation route is clearly outlined on a map and posted throughout the office.

of an effective emergency action plan are outlined in the paragraphs that follow.

Name of the person or persons responsible for reporting the fire and overseeing the entire operation. Ideally, two people are responsible for this task—a primary and a secondary. In the event the person with primary responsibility is out of the office, the person who is second on the list takes primary responsibility for reporting and overseeing.

Building evacuation routes. Maps of the office floor plan should be located throughout the office and marked with the current location and nearest exit. The route between the current location and the nearest exit should be highlighted or outlined on the map. See Figure 6-4. All exits should have a well-lit and easy-to-see exit sign. Halls leading to the exit should have emergency lighting so they remain lit in the event of a power failure. Halls also should be clutter free at all times. Exit routes should be large enough to accommodate all evacuees, including those with disabilities.

Evacuation procedure. Several employees should be responsible for ensuring that patients and staff are appropriately evacuated from the building. Patients in exam and procedure rooms may have special needs. Large medical practices may need to create different zones within the office. Each zone should have two individuals in charge of that specific area. Zones in the patient reception areas might be handled differently than zones in the clinical areas. Those responsible for evacuation should be the last to leave and should perform a quick search of bathrooms, break rooms, and other areas to ensure everyone has left the building. Two employees should be responsible for removing the book containing the MSDS and handing it over to the first responders at the scene. Having designated areas outside the building to assemble the evacuees makes accounting for employees and patients easier.

A plan for accounting for all employees and patients after the evacuation is completed. Conduct a head count or roll call of all employees. To account for patients in the office, use the check-in roster. Give the name of any missing employee or patient to the person in charge. Quick action is a matter of life or death if someone is trapped in the building during a fire emergency.

Emergency action plan drills. Practice the emergency action plan on a regular basis and conduct unannounced drills so that each individual better understands his role. Having an emergency action plan drill allows for evaluation and refinement of the plan. You don't want to find out your plan doesn't work in the middle of a true emergency.

Local emergency contacts. Dialing 911 is the most common way to report an emergency; there may be other internal numbers if your facility is large. A list of fire and EMS numbers should be readily available at all times and updated regularly. The contact list also should include the name and number of the person (such as the officer manager or the safety officer) who may have additional information regarding individual employee duties.

Developing and maintaining a relationship with local emergency authorities is vital. Trained fire personnel can often identify hidden workplace hazards and advise you in correcting them. Most local fire departments will come to your office and assess for fire hazards at your request.

▶ Chemical Safety   LO 6.5

A number of chemicals are used in a physician's office, and although most of these are found in the clinical lab area, they may be delivered to your office through the administrative office. If you are responsible for accepting a shipment containing chemicals, you must handle the package appropriately and make sure it is delivered to the proper person in the office.

If laboratory personnel are not present when the order arrives, you must make certain that the chemical is properly stored. The MSDS is a good source of information regarding proper chemical storage and handling; consult the MSDS and the packing slip on the container if you have questions.

If you are working in the lab, familiarize yourself with the MSDS and hazard label of every chemical you will use during a procedure. If the MSDS indicates the need for special equipment or conditions to use a chemical safely, be sure you meet the requirements before beginning to work with the substance. General precautions as you prepare include the following:

- Store caustic chemicals and other hazardous substances below eye level to reduce the risk of upsetting the container and spilling the substance into your eyes.
- Wear protective gear to prevent harm to your skin or damage to your clothing. (Be sure to properly remove the protective gear before leaving the laboratory.)
- Always carry chemical containers with both hands as you gather supplies.
- Make sure you work in a properly ventilated area.

When you are ready to begin work, adhere to these guidelines:

- If you must smell the chemicals you are using, do not hold them directly under your nose. Instead, hold them a few inches away and fan air across them and toward your nose.
- Work inside a fume hood if the chemical vapor is hazardous.
- Wear a personal ventilation device when working with certain chemicals, as specified by the MSDS.
- Never combine chemicals in ways not specifically required in test procedures.
- Mouth pipetting is prohibited at all times.
- If you are combining acids with other substances, always add the acid to the other substance. Adding substances to the acid increases the risk of splashing.
- If you encounter a spill of an unknown chemical substance, do not pour any other chemicals on it. Clean it up following strict hazardous waste control procedures. Never touch an unknown substance with your bare hands.

If there is an eyewash station in your lab, OSHA recommends that you know where it is and be able to find it with limited or no vision. See Figure 6-5. All employees who may incur splashes or splatters should be trained in its use. The eyewash station should be checked monthly to make sure it is working properly. Procedure 6-2 demonstrates the proper use of an eyewash station.

▶ Ergonomics and Physical Safety LO 6.6

The medical office is a busy place, and it is sometimes easy to ignore basic safe practice when rapidly faced with multiple tasks. However, unsafe practice can have long-lasting effects on your health and quality of life. Protecting yourself from ergonomic and physical hazards ultimately reduces office costs by limiting unnecessary sick time. A safe employee is a valuable employee.

FIGURE 6-5 Eye wash station.

Ergonomics

Scientists study the way people work; this study is known as **ergonomics**. People who perform repetitive tasks often develop work-related musculoskeletal disorders. Workplace injuries also may be the result of poor posture while performing a task such as leaning over to lift a patient from a wheelchair instead of bending your knees or positioning your arms too far above the computer keyboard when keying information. Good ergonomic practice (sometimes called body mechanics) is designed to reduce the likelihood of injury at work. The CDC's National Institute for Occupational Safety and Health (NIOSH) has specific recommendations for reducing work-related musculoskeletal injuries. These include

- Do not overextend your reach when attempting to grasp supplies. Use only approved equipment, such as stepladders or stools, to reach high shelves. Do not climb onto chairs, desks, or tables to reach anything.
- When lifting an object, squat close to the object. Keep your back straight but not rigid. Lift the item by pushing up with your legs, not by pulling with your back. Hold the load firmly with both hands, close to your body. If necessary, put on a back-support belt before attempting to move heavy loads.

- When transferring a patient, always bend at the knees to lift and ask for assistance if you are not sure you can lift or move the patient by yourself. When performing the transfer, move the patient's wheelchair as close to the exam table as possible to reduce the distance the patient must be moved. Remove the wheelchair footrests if possible. Have the patient help as much as possible. If a transfer device is available, use it. Transfer devices include gait belts, sliding boards, pivot discs, and sling-type transfer equipment.
- Adjust your seat to the correct position to prevent back strain.
- If you are using a computer, take frequent breaks to reduce eyestrain and hand cramping.

Your employer has the responsibility to provide a safe work environment, including equipment designed to reduce injury and workstations that adjust to the worker. Many employers offer training seminars for reducing work-related injuries. It is your responsibility to follow safe practice when using equipment or performing tasks where there is a possibility of work-related injury.

Physical Safety

There are many ways to ensure physical safety in the medical office. You must understand and apply all the appropriate safeguards. Because accidents can happen, however, post emergency numbers in multiple locations throughout the office. Once each quarter, make sure the numbers are accurate and up-to-date.

Some safeguards come under the heading of common sense, meaning their application requires no special knowledge. These include

- Walk, do not run, in the office.
- Prevent falls by wiping or mopping up spills immediately.
- Clear the floor of dropped objects.
- If the floor is carpeted, make sure there are no snags or tears that could cause someone to trip and fall.
- Spilled medications, chemicals, and other substances pose a threat to young children, who may ingest anything they find on the floor. Destroy and dispose of medications that are accidentally dropped on the floor.
- Be careful when carrying objects through the facility, especially when approaching blind corners.
- Close all cabinets, closet doors, desks, and worktable drawers.
- Routinely inspect the furniture in the exam room and reception area. Make sure there are no rough edges or sharp corners on the examining table, countertop, chairs, or other furniture.
- Electrical cords and medical and office equipment cables should run along the walls and be taped or fastened down securely.
- Never use damaged equipment or supplies, such as cracked or chipped glassware.

Being aware of the laboratory environment will help you protect your health and well-being. So, other safeguards to practice in the laboratory include

- Do not eat or drink in the laboratory, and do not store food there. Never use laboratory supplies, such as beakers or flasks, for eating or drinking.

FIGURE 6-6 First-aid kit.

- Do not put anything in your mouth while working in the laboratory. (Some people have a habit of chewing on the end of their pencils, for example.)
- Do not apply makeup or lip balm or insert contact lenses in the laboratory.
- Familiarize yourself with the location of the first-aid kit. If you are responsible for the kit in your area, check it weekly to make sure it is adequately stocked with supplies and that expiration dates on medications have not passed. See Figure 6-6.
- Familiarize yourself with the location and operation of the emergency eyewash and shower stations.

Additionally, in your efforts to promote safe practice in the laboratory, always wear appropriate protective gear and clothing. Use heat-resistant mitts or gloves to prevent burns. Wear sturdy, low-heeled, closed-toe shoes with rubber soles to prevent injury if you drop or spill something and to avoid slipping. Do not wear dangling jewelry or loose clothing that could get caught in laboratory equipment. Keep hair pulled back or covered for the same reason.

When you work with laboratory equipment, always follow manufacturers' guidelines. For example, wait for centrifuges to stop spinning before you open them.

Many laboratory materials and supplies require special handling and precautions, which include:

- Do not attempt to grasp bottles, jars, or other containers if your hands or the containers are wet.
- Close containers immediately after use.
- Clean up spills immediately.
- Clean up broken glass with a broom. Do not handle the debris. If the material is biohazardous, use tongs or forceps to pick up the glass. Package the pieces in a sturdy container with a label identifying the contents.

Special Safety Precautions Some patients, such as children and people with disabilities, may be particularly susceptible to accidents in your office. You need to take special precautions to ensure their safety.

Children Follow these precautions when assisting children:

- Keep sharp instruments out of the reach of children.
- Store toxic items in high cabinets.
- Keep all medications and objects out of the reach of young children because children are likely to pick up items and put them in their mouths and could choke or be poisoned.
- Keep children's toys and books in the reception area or exam room picked up and stored safely when not in use.
- Toys should be washable and made of safe materials.
- Sanitize toys that children put in their mouths daily; sanitize other toys weekly.
- If well children and sick children use the same reception area or exam room, sanitize and disinfect toys after sick children play with them.
- Periodically check toys for sharp edges that might cause cuts.
- Ensure toys do not have small parts or pieces that could cause choking if swallowed.

Patients with Physical Disabilities Patients with disabilities are more likely than other patients to fall. Some patients may use walkers or canes for support, whereas others may simply be unsteady on their feet. Follow these recommendations when assisting patients with physical disabilities:

- Provide assistance as needed with disrobing prior to an exam or redressing afterward.
- Never leave severely disabled patients alone in an exam room. Check office policies for guidelines regarding appropriate chaperones for patients with disabilities.

In addition, keep in mind that patients with vision impairments may have difficulty seeing obstacles, stairs, and other potential hazards. Safe flooring and handrails in the reception area, bathroom, hallways, and exam room help ensure the safety of patients with impaired mobility or vision.

▶ The Cycle of Infection

LO 6.7

As a medical assistant, your role in helping to create and maintain a safe and healthy environment for both patients and employees is key. This role includes understanding how infections occur and are transmitted in the population and practicing all necessary infection control precautions. To understand how infections are spread, you need to understand the cycle of infection.

Five elements make up the cycle of infection (Figure 6-7) These five parts must all be present for infection to occur:

1. Reservoir host
2. Means of exit
3. Means of transmission
4. Means of entrance
5. Susceptible host

FIGURE 6-7 The cycle of infection must be broken at some point to prevent the spread of disease.

Reservoir Host

The infection cycle begins when the **pathogen** invades the reservoir host. The **reservoir host** is an animal, insect, or human whose body is capable of sustaining the growth of a pathogen. Many pathogens require a reservoir host to provide nutrition and a place to multiply.

The presence of the pathogen in the reservoir host may cause an infection in the host. At times, however, the host avoids full infection. A human **carrier** is a reservoir host who is unaware of the presence of the pathogen and so spreads the disease. The carrier exhibits no symptoms of infection. A human host also may have a subclinical case, which is a manifestation of the infection that is so slight that it is unnoticeable. The host experiences only some of the symptoms of the infection or milder symptoms than in a full case. A wide range of diseases can be manifested subclinically.

An infection in the reservoir host may be either endogenous or exogenous. An **endogenous infection** is one in which an abnormality or malfunction in routine body processes has caused normally beneficial or harmless microorganisms to become pathogenic. A bladder infection caused by *Escherichia coli* bacteria (commonly known as *E. coli*) is an endogenous infection. *E. coli* are beneficial bacteria normally found in the intestinal tract, but when introduced into the bladder via the urethra, *E. coli* can cause a bladder infection. An **exogenous infection** is one that is caused by the introduction of a pathogen from outside the body. A wound infection that occurs as the result of a healthcare worker transferring staph bacteria from her hands to a surgical site is an example of an exogenous infection.

CAUTION: HANDLE WITH CARE

Respiratory Hygiene and Cough Etiquette

With the recent increase in widespread respiratory disease outbreaks like Severe Acute Respiratory Syndrome (SARS) and H1N1 influenza, the CDC identified the need to establish a set of guidelines to protect patients and their families in the healthcare setting. These guidelines include

- Educating healthcare workers, patients, and their families about cough etiquette.
- Posting cough etiquette signs.
- Posting signs reminding patients to report flu symptoms.

- Controlling the source of transmission by covering coughs with a tissue and properly disposing of the tissue.
- Coughing or sneezing into your elbow or sleeve if no tissue is available.
- Using proper hand hygiene consistently.
- Separating patients with respiratory infections so they are at least three feet away from other patients in waiting areas or asking them to wear a mask.

Means of Exit

The next step in the cycle of infection is the pathogen's exiting from the reservoir host. Common routes of exit include

- Through the nose, mouth, eyes, or ears
- In feces or urine
- In semen, vaginal fluid, or other discharge through the reproductive tract
- In blood or blood products from open wounds

Means of Transmission

To reproduce after it has exited from the reservoir host, the pathogen must spread to another host by some means of transmission, either direct or indirect. Direct transmission occurs when the pathogen moves immediately from one host to another (through contact with the infected person or with the discharges of the infected person, such as saliva or blood).

Indirect transmission is possible only if the pathogen is capable of existing independently of the reservoir host. In this case, the pathogen survives until a new host encounters it and the pathogen takes up residence in that new host.

Airborne Transmission Pathogens can be transmitted to a new host through the air. For example, microorganisms may enter the respiratory tract of a new host by inhalation. Respiratory diseases such as influenza, or flu, are often transmitted this way.

Pathogens may be inhaled from a variety of sources, such as soil particles or secretion droplets from a sneeze or cough. When people inhale contaminated soil particles, fungal diseases may be contracted. If contaminated droplets are inhaled, diseases including influenza, chickenpox, and tuberculosis may be contracted. Because pathogens can spread relatively rapidly through airborne transmission, they may cause large epidemics among susceptible people.

Bloodborne Transmission Pathogens also can enter a new host through contact with blood or blood products. Bloodborne pathogens may be transmitted in a variety of ways:

- Indirectly—when pathogens are transferred through blood transfusions, needlesticks, or improperly sterilized dental equipment.

- Directly—when the contaminated blood of one person comes into contact with another person's broken skin or mucous membrane, or when a pregnant woman transmits a disease to her fetus across the placenta.

Transmission during Pregnancy or Birth If a mother becomes infected during her pregnancy, she can pass on pathogens to the fetus. An infection may be transmitted while the fetus is in the mother's uterus, which may result in damage to the fetus. This transmission is a form of bloodborne transmission.

Some bloodborne infections that produce only mild symptoms in the mother may be devastating to the fetus (for example, rubella). Other infections, such as herpes, gonorrhea, syphilis, or streptococcal infections, may infect the baby during passage through the birth canal. An infection that is present in a child at the time of birth is said to be congenital.

Foodborne Transmission A new host may be exposed to pathogens by ingesting contaminated food or liquids. Food can become contaminated when it is handled by an infected person who has poor hygiene habits, such as a customer at a self-service salad bar who did not wash his hands. The amount of contamination needed in a food to make someone ill varies. People who produce less stomach acid may become infected with a smaller dose of pathogens than those with higher acid production because stomach acid kills many microorganisms. An example of a pathogen transmitted by ingestion is a strain of *E. coli*, which can cause severe food poisoning.

Vector-Borne Transmission A living organism that carries microorganisms from an infected person to another person is known as a **vector.** The most common carriers are insects such as fleas, flies, mosquitoes, and ticks.

- Fleas carry the organism responsible for plague. Though the number of cases in the United States is very low, plague has been identified as a possible bioterrorism agent.
- Common houseflies carry pathogens from garbage and feces on their bodies and feet. When they land on food, they mechanically transfer these microorganisms to the food.

- Mosquitoes are carriers of several diseases of importance in the United States. They carry the organisms responsible for West Nile Virus and malaria.
- Ticks carry the microorganisms responsible for Lyme disease and Rocky Mountain spotted fever.

Transmission by Touching Direct or indirect contact through touch is another method of transmitting infection. Direct transmission occurs through contact with an infected person's mucous membranes. Sexually transmitted diseases are spread through the direct contact of one mucous membrane with another (in the penis, vagina, urethra, mouth, or anus) during sexual activity.

Indirect transmission occurs through contact with **fomites**. A fomite is any inanimate reservoir of pathogenic microorganisms. Examples of fomites include drinking glasses, door knobs, shopping cart handles, pencils, and almost any surface or object that can temporarily hold microorganisms. So, any object that can be contaminated by an infected person and then can transmit the infective agent to a susceptible host is considered a fomite.

Means of Entrance

Just as the pathogen needs a means of exit from the reservoir host, it also needs a means of entrance into the new host. Pathogens can enter a new host through any cavity lined with mucous membrane, such as the mouth, nose, throat, vagina, or rectum. They also can enter through the ears, eyes, intestinal tract, urinary tract, reproductive tract, or breaks in the skin. Most pathogens can take advantage of any means of exit and entry. For example, the droplets from an infected child's sneeze can land on a toy in a common play area. The next child to pick up the toy can transfer the infected droplets to his own nose, spreading the infection.

Susceptible Host

A final requirement must be met for the infection cycle to remain intact. The person into whom the pathogen has been transmitted must be an individual who has little or no immunity to infection by that organism. This individual is called a **susceptible host**.

Susceptibility is determined by a variety of factors—some related to the host, some to the pathogen, and some to the environment. Factors related to the host include the following:

- Age
- Genetic predisposition to certain illnesses
- Nutritional status
- Other disease processes
- Stress levels
- Hygiene habits
- General health

Factors related to the pathogen include the number and concentration of pathogens, the strength (virulence) of the pathogen, and the point of entry. Environmental factors, such as the host's living conditions and exposure to hazardous substances, also affect susceptibility.

Once a new host has been infected, the cycle can continue. This host becomes the reservoir host and eventually transmits the pathogen to yet another host.

Environmental Factors in Disease Transmission

The climate, food, water, animals, insects, and people in a community may greatly influence the types and courses of infection that exist there. In a highly dense population, the infection rate may be higher than in a low-density population because pathogens spread more quickly from person to person when people are in closer proximity. Proximity is one reason for the increase in respiratory disease during seasons when people are indoors for long periods.

Animals can also play a role in infection, as infections related to pathogens are found in domestic and wild animals. Unpasteurized milk from an infected cow may cause disease. Some pathogens can infect both animals and people. Butchers, hunters, and people in occupations dealing with animals may be at greater risk than other individuals for infection by those pathogens.

The environment affects the incidence of diseases carried by insects. Whether a potentially disease-carrying insect is in a certain area depends on whether that area has the appropriate climate and environment the insect needs to live. For instance, ticks may carry Rocky Mountain spotted fever or Lyme disease.

Economic and political factors also influence the pattern of infection transmission. They help determine the cleanliness of an area, the availability of medical care, and people's knowledge about preventing infection. Other factors that influence infection transmission include the availability of transportation, urbanization, population growth rates, and sexual behavior.

Breaking the Cycle

The principles of **asepsis** must be applied to break the cycle of infection and its spread. Asepsis is the condition in which pathogens are absent or controlled. For example, killing all microorganisms by sterilizing a suture removal kit or reducing the number of microorganisms on your hands by thoroughly washing them are types of aseptic practice. In medical settings, where many people are hosts to pathogens and many others are susceptible, asepsis can break the cycle by preventing the transmission of pathogens.

Specific measures to help break the cycle of infection include:

- Maintaining strict housekeeping standards to reduce the number of pathogens present.
- Adhering to government guidelines to protect against diseases caused by pathogens.
- Educating patients in hygiene, health promotion, and disease prevention.

▶ OSHA Bloodborne Pathogens Standard and Universal Precautions LO 6.8

You must know the laws that require basic practices of infection control, also called infection prevention, in a medical office and how to apply these laws in your office. Federal regulations related to infection control and asepsis were developed by the

Department of Labor's Occupational Safety and Health Administration and described in the OSHA Bloodborne Pathogens Standard of 1991. These laws protect healthcare workers from health hazards on the job, particularly from accidentally acquiring infections. They also help protect from health hazards patients and any other people who may come into the medical office.

OSHA Bloodborne Pathogens Standard

To ensure that biohazardous materials do not endanger people or the environment, laws set forth in the OSHA Bloodborne Pathogens Standard of 1991 dictate how you must handle infectious or potentially infectious waste generated during medical or surgical procedures. According to these rules, any potentially infectious waste materials must be appropriately discarded or held for processing in biohazardous waste containers. These wastes include

- Blood products
- Body fluids
- Human tissues
- Cultures
- Vaccines (special preparations administered to produce immunity)
- Table paper, linen, towels, and gauze containing body fluids
- Used scalpels, needles, sutures with needles attached, and other sharp instruments (known as sharps)
- Specula
- Inoculating loops
- Used gloves, disposable instruments, cotton swabs, and disposable applicators

Many medical offices today use only disposable paper gowns, drapes, coverings, and towels. Some offices, however, use cloth linens, which must be laundered. Certain rules apply to the laundering of cloth linens that are soiled with potentially infectious materials.

Medical offices use outside, licensed waste management services approved by the Environmental Protection Agency (EPA) to dispose of medical waste. A waste management service can provide instructions for preparing items before they are taken away.

The disposition and handling of contaminated sharps are of special concern because these instruments can easily puncture the skin and expose you to extremely dangerous viruses. Used sharps must never be bent, broken, recapped, or otherwise tampered with. After use, place them in a rigid, leakproof, puncture-resistant biohazardous waste container for sharps. Procedure 6-3 demonstrates the correct method for using a biohazardous sharps container. Disposable and reusable sharps are kept in separate containers. Metal basins containing disinfectant are often used to store reusable sharps until they can be processed. The outside waste management company may supply containers for the disposable items, sterilize them on its premises, and discard them in the city trash dump or incinerate them. See the Caution: Handle with Care section

	TABLE 6-1	Infectious Waste Disposal: Penalties for Not Following Regulations, as Set Forth by OSHA	
Type of Violation	**Characteristics of Violation**	**Penalties for Violation**	
Other than serious violation	Direct relationship to job safety and health but would probably not result in death or serious physical harm.	Fine of up to $7,000 (discretionary).	
Serious violation	Substantial probability that death or serious physical harm could result; employer knew, or should have known, of the hazard.	Fine of up to $7,000 (mandatory).	
Willful violation	Violation committed intentionally and knowingly.	Fine of up to $70,000 with a $5,000 minimum; if violation resulted in death of employee, additional fine and/or up to 6 months' imprisonment.	
Repeated violation	Substantially similar (but not the same) violation found upon re-inspection; not applicable if initial citation is under contest.	Fine of up to $70,000.	
Failure to correct prior violation	Initial violation was not corrected.	Fine of up to $7,000 for each day the violation continues past the date it was supposed to stop.	

on the next page for a discussion of the guidelines you must follow when disposing of biohazardous waste and potentially infectious laundry waste.

OSHA's laws for hazardous waste disposal, as well as other OSHA regulations about measures to prevent the spread of infection, provide a margin of safety, ensuring that medical facilities meet at least the minimal criteria for asepsis. These laws include requirements for training personnel, keeping records, housekeeping, wearing protective gear, and other measures.

Although federal laws exist, individual states have some discretion in applying them. You should become familiar with the laws in your state to ensure that you are helping your medical office comply. Any outside cleaning service used by the office also should be made aware of these standards. Penalties for failing to comply with regulations can be severe (see Table 6-1).

To be in compliance with the Bloodborne Pathogens Standard, an employer must meet these requirements:

- A written OSHA Exposure Control Plan must be created and updated annually or whenever procedures that require exposure to potentially contaminated material are added or changed. The plan must be available to all employees and to authorized OSHA authorities.
- Training must be provided to all employees describing the documentation mandated by the standard. This documentation includes the symptoms, methods of transmission, and epidemiology of infectious diseases caused by bloodborne pathogens. Employees must also be instructed in the use of personal protective equipment, Universal Precautions, and engineering controls designed to prevent exposure. Procedures to follow in the event of exposure or emergency

Proper Use of Biohazardous Waste Containers and Handling of Infectious Laundry Waste

Biohazardous waste containers are available in a variety of designs. Frequently, more than one design is used in the clinical setting. These containers are often provided by outside sterilization and waste management companies. Examples of biohazardous waste containers include

- Bags or containers that are red or have a biohazardous waste label (for any material contaminated with blood or body fluids, such as used dressings or gloves).
- Boxes with biohazardous waste labels (sometimes lined with red bags and used for disposable gowns, examination table covers, and similar items that may be contaminated with blood or body fluids).
- Rigid, leakproof, and puncture-proof sharps containers that are red or have a biohazardous waste label (for lancets, needles, and other sharp objects).

Every biohazardous waste container has a lid that you must replace immediately after use. In addition, you may not overfill the container, and you must replace it when it is two-thirds full. All biohazardous waste containers must have a fluorescent orange or orange-red label with the biohazard symbol and the word *BIOHAZARD* in a contrasting color (Figure 6-8). Red bags or red containers may be substituted for containers with biohazardous waste labels.

You must follow these guidelines when handling biohazardous waste:

- Always wear gloves.

- Place biohazardous waste in the appropriate biohazardous waste container immediately or as soon as possible.
- Keep biohazardous waste containers close to the place where the waste material is generated.
- Keep the containers closed when not in use, close them before removing them from the area of use, and keep them upright to avoid any spills.
- If outside contamination of the primary container occurs, place that container in a secondary container to prevent leakage during handling, processing, storage, and transport.
- Drop—do not push—intact contaminated needles into the biohazardous waste container for sharps (Figure 6-9).
- To avoid accidental puncture wounds, never break off, recap, reuse, or handle needles after use.
- If there is a danger of biohazardous waste puncturing the primary container, place that container in a secondary container.
- Do not open, empty, or clean reusable sharps containers by hand.
- When they are two-thirds full, discard disposable sharps containers in large biohazardous waste containers.

Spills of hazardous chemicals or biohazardous materials can happen anywhere in the office. Immediately clean up spills or splashes of potentially contaminated material. Depending on the material, you may need to use special hazardous waste control products. Be sure to dry the area if appropriate, or clearly indicate that the area is still wet. When cleaning up spills, take the following measures:

- Place material in a biohazardous waste bag.

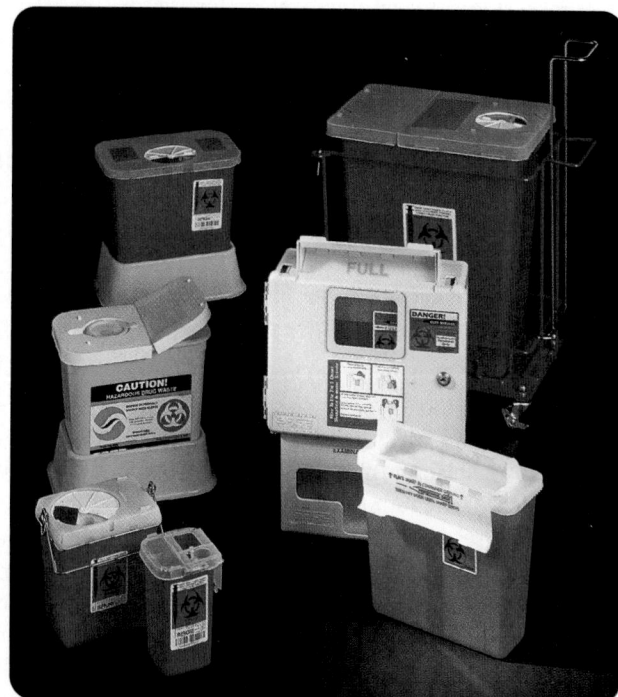

FIGURE 6-8 All biohazardous sharps containers must be rigid, leakproof, and labeled with the biohazard symbol.

FIGURE 6-9 A sharps disposal container is a receptacle for used needles, lancets, specimen slides, transfer pipettes, and other disposable pointed or edged instruments, supplies, and equipment.

- Ensure that the bag is leakproof on the sides and bottom and can be closed tightly.
- Place the plastic bag in a cardboard box also marked with the biohazard symbol.

The outside waste management agency will pick up the box for incineration before disposing of it in a public landfill. Procedure 6-4 demonstrates the proper disposing of biohazardous waste.

Potentially infectious laundry waste also must be handled in a specific manner. OSHA has issued these regulations for handling this type of waste:

- Place contaminated laundry in a red laundry bag that is marked with the biohazard symbol, or recognizable to facility employees as contaminated material to be handled using Standard Precautions.
- Pack any laundry to be transported so that it does not leak in transit.
- Have the laundry washed in a designated area onsite or at a professional laundry facility.

Any laundry service the medical office uses should abide by all OSHA regulations. For example, anyone handling laundry must wear gloves and handle contaminated materials as little as possible.

situations also must be part of the training. New employee training is required before the worker can perform a task that might pose a risk of occupational exposure and then on a yearly basis. Additional training is required when a new task or procedure is introduced that may change the employees' occupational exposure risk.

- The employer must make the hepatitis B vaccine available at no charge to all employees who are at risk for occupational exposure. Employees must either receive the vaccination or decline it in writing. The employer must maintain documentation of vaccinations and refusals. Employees who initially decline the vaccine are free to reverse their decision at any point during their employment.

Universal Precautions

OSHA requires medical professionals to follow specific "universal blood and body fluid precautions" as set forth by the Department of Health and Human Services' Centers for Disease Control and Prevention. These Universal Precautions prevent healthcare workers from exposing themselves and others to infections. Following Universal Precautions means assuming that all blood and body fluids are infected with bloodborne pathogens. Universal Precautions apply to

- Blood and blood products
- Human tissue
- Semen and vaginal secretions
- Saliva from dental procedures
- Cerebrospinal, synovial, pleural, peritoneal, pericardial, and amniotic fluids, which bathe various internal structures in the body
- Other body fluids, if visibly contaminated with blood or of questionable origin in the body

Breast milk, although not on the list of fluids covered by Universal Precautions, is generally treated as such because it has been shown that mothers can pass along the human immunodeficiency virus (HIV) to their infants through breast milk.

Healthcare facilities now use **Standard Precautions**, which are a combination of Universal Precautions and rules to reduce the risk of disease transmission by means of moist body substances (known as Body Substance Isolation [BSI] guidelines). Standard Precautions apply to

- Blood
- All body fluids, secretions, and excretions except sweat
- Nonintact skin
- Mucous membranes

Standard Precautions are used in healthcare facilities for the care of all patients. They are an important measure for preventing the transmission of disease in the healthcare setting.

As mentioned earlier, some types of pathogens can be transmitted when the host's infected blood comes in contact with another person's skin. Skin that has been broken from a needle puncture or other wound and mucous membranes, such as those lining the nose and throat, are the areas that need the most protection. If a patient's (or coworker's) blood or body fluids come in contact with such areas, pathogens can be transferred from the patient's body to that of the medical worker.

OSHA outlines the routine safeguards to take when performing each medical procedure or task, depending on that task's level of risk. The degree of risk is determined by how much exposure to potentially infectious substances you are likely to encounter. When a procedure is explained, particular icons will be used to represent each of the OSHA guidelines. Figure 6-10 shows these icons.

FIGURE 6-10 These icons will appear at the beginning of each Procedure to let you know which OSHA guidelines you should follow. They represent (A) handwashing, (B) gloves, (C) mask and protective eyewear or face shield, (D) laboratory coat or gown, (E) reusable sharps container, (F) sharps disposal, (G) biohazardous waste container, and (H) disinfection.

OSHA divides tasks into the following three categories.

1. Category I tasks are those that expose a worker to blood, body fluids, or tissues or tasks that have a chance of spills or splashes. These tasks always require specific protective measures.

2. Category II tasks do not usually involve risk of exposure. Because they may involve exposure in certain situations, however, OSHA requires that precautions be taken.

3. Category III tasks do not require any special protection. These tasks, such as taking a patient's blood pressure, involve no exposure to blood, body fluids, or tissues. (Observe patients for open wounds before you touch them to perform such tasks.)

Category I Tasks A Category I task you might perform would be assisting with a minor surgical procedure in the office, such as the removal of a cyst. This procedure requires that you wash your hands before and after the procedure and that you wear protective gloves, a mask and protective eyewear or a face shield, and protective clothing. After the procedure, you must follow the guidelines for dealing with disposable and nondisposable sharp equipment and decontaminating work surfaces.

Category II Tasks A Category II task you might perform would be giving mouth-to-mouth resuscitation to a patient. Because blood is usually not visible in such situations, the task is not classified as Category I. Gloves are still recommended, however, although you may not have time to get them in an emergency. Because you will be exposed to saliva in such a procedure, OSHA recommends using disposable airway equipment and resuscitation bags (shown in Figure 6-11), which medical offices are required to supply.

OSHA recommends taking these precautions to decrease the risk of transmitting infectious diseases through mouth-to-mouth resuscitation. Of particular concern to healthcare workers are HIV, which causes AIDS, and the hepatitis B virus (HBV).

AIDS damages the body's ability to fight disease and is ultimately fatal in most instances. Hepatitis B is a highly contagious and potentially fatal disease that causes inflammation of the liver and sometimes liver failure. Healthcare workers become infected with these viruses at work every year. Hepatitis B infection occurs far more frequently on the job than does HIV infection.

FIGURE 6-11 Resuscitation bags are used when a person requires mouth-to-mouth resuscitation. You must use one of these bags or another barrier device when performing mouth-to-mouth resuscitation.

Category III Tasks A Category III procedure you may perform is giving a patient medicated nose drops. This task involves tilting the patient's head and holding the dropper above the patient's nostril. Although you must perform aseptic handwashing before and after the procedure, there are no other protective requirements. Some Category III tasks require no precautions. Examples of these tasks are instructing a patient in how to use a heating pad or how to take care of a cast for a broken leg.

Written Exposure Plan

In order to reduce the risk of bloodborne pathogen exposure, OSHA requires that every medical facility have a written exposure control plan (ECP). Employees who are at risk of bloodborne exposure must have access to the ECP. This plan must be reviewed with new employees at the onset of employment and with all employees on an annual basis. A written copy of the plan must be made available if an employee requests it. The ECP must include the following:

- Determination of employee exposure
- Implementation of exposure control methods including Universal Precautions, engineering and work practice controls, personal protective equipment, and housekeeping
- Hepatitis B vaccination
- Post-exposure evaluation and follow-up
- Communication of hazards to employees and hazard training
- Recordkeeping
- Procedures for evaluating circumstances surrounding exposure incidents

Exposure Incidents

The OSHA Bloodborne Pathogens Standard also specifies what to do in case of an exposure incident. An exposure incident is one in which a worker, despite all precautions, has reason to believe that he has come in contact with a substance that may transmit infection. Contact may occur when a medical worker accidentally sticks himself with a used needle. A puncture exposure incident is the most common kind of exposure.

The basic rules covering exposure incidents apply to all serious infections, such as HBV and HIV. The rules covering HBV also include vaccination.

When an exposure incident occurs, the physician or employer must be notified immediately. This prompt action is extremely important because quick and proper treatment can help prevent the development of many diseases, such as hepatitis B. Timely action also can prevent the worker from exposing other people to a potentially acquired infection. Reporting the incident helps to prevent the same type of accident from happening again.

After such an exposure, the employer must offer the exposed employee a free medical evaluation. The employer must refer the employee to a licensed healthcare provider who can counsel the employee about what happened as well as about how to prevent the spread of any potential infection. The healthcare provider also takes a blood sample and prescribes appropriate treatment. If the employee does not want to participate in the medical evaluation and treatment, he has the right to refuse it. If this occurs, the employee's refusal should be documented.

If an employee who has not received the HBV vaccination and is not known to be immune is exposed to any infected person, especially someone who is HBV-positive or at high risk, it is recommended that the employee be tested for HBV and receive the vaccination if necessary. This vaccination may prevent infection. When the source person's HBV status is unknown and the person does not wish to be tested, the employee should be tested. If the source person agrees to be tested, the law requires that the employee be informed of the test results. The employee may agree to give blood but not to be tested. In such a case, the blood sample must be kept for 90 days in case the employee later develops symptoms of HBV or HIV infection and decides to be tested then.

The healthcare provider who performs the postexposure evaluation must give the employer a written report stating whether HBV vaccination was recommended and received and that the employee was informed of the results of any blood tests. Any additional information must be kept confidential.

Other OSHA Requirements

OSHA also requires that all healthcare workers who have occupational exposure to blood or other potentially infectious materials have the opportunity to receive the HBV vaccine, free of charge, as needed throughout employment. Within 10 days of a medical worker's starting a job, the doctor or employer is required to offer the worker the opportunity to receive this vaccination. The vaccine is recommended for all healthcare workers *unless*

- They have received it in the past;
- A blood test shows them to be immune to the virus; and/or
- There are medical reasons for which the vaccine is contraindicated.

In most cases, the employee is permitted to decline the vaccination if he signs a form accepting all the conditions. (A few employers require HBV vaccination as a condition for employment.) Even if the healthcare worker declines the vaccination when beginning employment, he still has the opportunity to receive the free vaccine and any necessary booster shots throughout his employment.

Needlestick Safety and Prevention Act

Needlestick Safety and Prevention Act In response to the Needlestick Safety and Prevention Act, which was signed into law in November 2000, OSHA revised the Bloodborne Pathogens Standard. The additional provisions to the standard are

- Healthcare employers must evaluate new safety-engineered control devices on an annual basis and implement the use of devices that reasonably reduce the risk of needlestick injuries.
- Healthcare facilities must maintain a detailed log of sharps injuries incurred from contaminated sharps.
- Healthcare employers must solicit input from employees involved in direct patient care to identify, evaluate, and implement engineering and **work practice controls** (controlling injuries by altering the way a task is performed).

In an effort to reduce needlestick injuries, NIOSH has specific recommendations for employers and employees regarding **engineered safety devices**, devices specifically designed to isolate or remove the hazard, and work practice controls. NIOSH recommendations for employers include

Engineering Controls

- Eliminate the use of needles where safe and effective alternatives are available.
- Implement the use of engineered safety devices and evaluate their use on a regular basis.

Needlestick Prevention Programs

- Analyze sharps injuries to identify hazard trends in the workplace.
- Ensure employees are properly trained in the proper use and disposal of sharps.
- Adapt work practices that involve sharps to make them safer.
- Make safety awareness in the workplace a priority.
- Have established procedures for reporting all needlestick injuries.
- Evaluate prevention procedures and provide feedback to employees.

NIOSH recommendations for employees include

- Avoid using needles if a safe alternative exists.
- Paticipate in choosing engineered safety devices.
- Use the engineered safety devices provided by your employer.
- Do not recap needles if possible.
- Before beginning a procedure, make sure you have a means of safe sharps disposal close by and ready for use.
- Dispose of used needles promptly and appropriately.
- Promptly report all sharps-related injuries.
- Advise your employer if you see sharps hazards in the workplace.
- Participate in bloodborne pathogen training.

▶ Infection Control Methods   LO 6.9

As a medical assistant, you will take measures to eliminate the elements that must be present for disease to occur. To do so, you must have a thorough knowledge of the two types of asepsis:

- Medical asepsis, or clean technique, is based on maintaining cleanliness to prevent the spread of microorganisms and to ensure that there are as few microorganisms in the medical environment as possible. The goal of medical asepsis is to reduce/control microorganisms after they leave the body.
- Surgical asepsis, or sterile technique, depends on a completely sterile environment that eliminates all microorganisms. The goal of surgical asepsis is to keep organisms from entering the body. (See the chapter *Assisting in Surgery* for more information about surgical asepsis.)

Medical asepsis and surgical asepsis are required by law. Each individual who works in a medical setting must recognize the importance of asepsis and strictly adhere to aseptic procedures in daily routines.

Medical Asepsis

Because the medical office can be a host to many pathogens, strict, controlled asepsis is crucial. All employees in the medical office must observe and practice the principles of asepsis to ensure a safe environment for patients and staff.

You can promote asepsis through vigilant cleanliness. Every day before patients arrive, you must inspect the office for any surfaces or objects that may be dirty or contaminated. Keeping the office clean reduces the number of microorganisms on surfaces.

Office Procedures

Other physical aspects of the medical office that contribute to asepsis include

- A reception room that has designated waiting areas for well and sick people. If there is not enough space, sick patients should be led immediately to an examination room. You may need to explain this policy to well people who have been waiting so that no one thinks other patients are getting preferential treatment.
- An office that is cleaned daily.
- An office that is well lit and ventilated, has no drafts, and has a temperature of approximately 72°F.
- Furniture that is kept in good repair and is replaced when necessary.
- A strict "no eating or drinking" policy in the lab, clinical, and other patient areas.
- Trash that is emptied as necessary, at least once daily.
- An insect-free environment.
- A sign stating that any safety or health hazard be reported to the receptionist.
- A sign asking that patients use tissues for coughs or sneezes, put all waste in the trash can, and tell the receptionist if they are nauseated or have to use the restroom. (Ideally, the reception area should be equipped with a restroom for emergencies.) See Figure 6-12.

Asepsis during Medical Assistant Procedures

Many of the procedures you perform require aseptic techniques to prevent cross contamination from one place to another. For

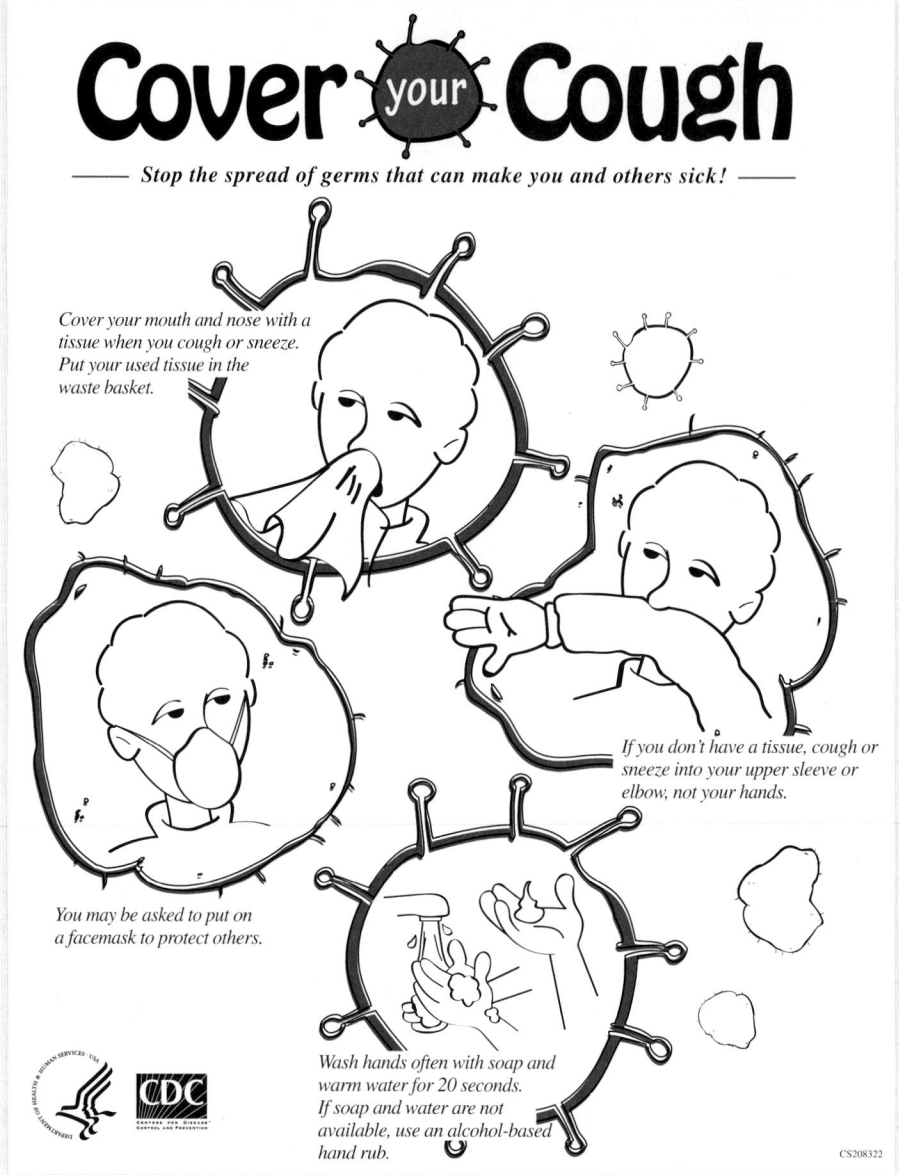

Cover your Cough

—— *Stop the spread of germs that can make you and others sick!* ——

Cover your mouth and nose with a tissue when you cough or sneeze. Put your used tissue in the waste basket.

If you don't have a tissue, cough or sneeze into your upper sleeve or elbow, not your hands.

You may be asked to put on a facemask to protect others.

Wash hands often with soap and warm water for 20 seconds. If soap and water are not available, use an alcohol-based hand rub.

CS208322

FIGURE 6-12 Posting notices like this CDC poster in patient reception areas reminds patients to use tissues and cover their coughs to reduce the spread of infectious agents.

instance, when opening a sterile container, you should rest its lid face-up instead of facedown. Placing it facedown contaminates the inside of the lid by picking up materials on the surface of the counter such as dust, dirt, blood, or body fluids, making it unsuitable to be put back on the sterile container. When administering tablets or capsules, you should pour them into the bottle cap or a cup rather than into your hand to prevent the transfer of microorganisms from your hand onto the medication. To prevent cross contamination, you also must follow guidelines about the types of protective gear to wear during a procedure. (Personal protective equipment is discussed later in this chapter.)

Hand Hygiene

Transmission by touching is the most common means of transmitting pathogens. The single most important aseptic procedure for a medical assistant is proper hand hygiene. The two most common methods of hand hygiene in the medical office are handwashing with plain or antimicrobial soap and water and hand disinfection with **alcohol-based hand disinfectants (AHD)**. Consistent hand hygiene using appropriate methods protects the patient, your co-workers, and you from healthcare-associated infections.

Handwashing Aseptic handwashing removes accumulated dirt and microorganisms that could cause infection under the right conditions. Procedure 6-5 describes how to perform aseptic handwashing. In most cases, plain soap and water are adequate. There is some evidence that overuse of antimicrobial soap leads to antibiotic-resistant pathogens. For this reason, only use antimicrobial soap after assisting with exams and procedures where body fluids are present.

Go to CONNECT to see videos about *Aseptic Handwashing* and *Applying Standard Precautions.*

Alcohol-Based Hand Rubs If water is not readily available, an alternative to handwashing is the use of alcohol-based hand disinfectants. These are gels, foams, or liquids that have an alcohol content of 60–95%. AHDs may be safely used in most circumstances; however, conditions in which they should not be used include

- When hands are visibly dirty or contaminated
- Before and after eating
- After using the bathroom
- If you suspect you have come in contact with spore-forming bacteria

A number of factors can affect the effectiveness of AHDs. These include

- The type of alcohol used
- The concentration of alcohol
- Whether the hands are wet when the product is applied
- Contact time
- Amount used

If your hands feel dry before the recommended amount of time has passed, you most likely did not use enough. You should reapply the AHD using a larger amount. Procedure 6-6 describes the proper use of an alcohol-based hand disinfectant.

Fingernail Length Fingernails are a haven for pathogens. There is ample documentation that a large number of bacteria and some yeasts can be cultured from underneath and around the nail, especially right next to the border of the skin and the nail. The CDC recommends that natural nail length does not exceed one-quarter inch.

Nail Polish and Artificial Nails The use of nail polish and artificial nails is discouraged in healthcare workers as there is enough evidence that nail polish and artificial nails harbor pathogens. Although freshly applied nail polish has not been shown to contain increased numbers of bacteria and more research is needed, polish that is chipped has a much higher bacteria count than natural unpolished or freshly polished nails.

Healthcare workers who wear artificial nails or extensions have more gram-negative bacteria on their fingers than healthcare workers with natural nails. These increases were seen both before and after handwashing. The CDC recommends that healthcare workers should not wear artificial nails or extensions when working with high-risk patients. The World Health Organization (WHO) recommends that heathcare workers should not wear artificial nails when working with any patients.

Other Aseptic Precautions

You need to make certain precautions part of your daily routine. For example, take these safeguards:

- Avoid leaning against sinks, supplies, or equipment.
- Avoid touching your face or mouth.
- Use tissues when you cough or sneeze, and always wash your hands afterward.
- Whenever possible, avoid working directly with patients when you have a cold.
- Wear gloves and a mask if you have a cold and must work with patients.
- Stay home if you have a fever, and remain there until you have maintained a normal temperature for 24 hours.

Personal Protective Equipment

Employers are required by law to supply **personal protective equipment (PPE)** at no charge to their employees. PPE is any type of protective gear worn to guard against physical hazards. Healthcare workers require many kinds of personal protective equipment to do their jobs, including gloves, masks and protective eyewear or face shields, and protective clothing (Figure 6-13). During each procedure, keep in mind that the greater your chances of exposure to blood, the more protective equipment you need to wear.

FIGURE 6-13 Healthcare workers may need to use various types of personal protective equipment including gloves, masks and protective eyewear or face shields, gowns, and other protective clothing.

Gloves You must wear gloves for all procedures that involve exposure to blood, other body fluids, or broken skin. Several kinds of gloves for different situations are described in the following bullets.

- Disposable gloves—worn once and discarded. They cannot be used if they are torn, punctured, or otherwise damaged. Both examination and sterile gloves are disposable.
- Examination gloves—worn during procedures that do not require a sterile environment.
- Sterile gloves—used for sterile procedures such as minor surgery or urinary catheterization.
- Utility gloves—used when cleaning up. They are stronger than disposable gloves and may be decontaminated and reused if they show no signs of deterioration (including discoloration) after use.

Masks and Protective Eyewear or Face Shields You must wear appropriate masks and protective eyewear or face shields for procedures in which your eyes, nose, and mouth may be exposed. These procedures are ones that have a potential for spraying or splashing blood, such as surgery or the collection or examination of blood.

Protective Clothing If you are likely to have blood or body fluids sprayed or splashed on your clothing during a procedure, you must wear a protective laboratory coat, gown, or apron. You also may wear a hair covering and/or shoe coverings for such procedures. You should always have a change of work clothing available in the event that blood or body fluids penetrate your regular clothes around or through the protective clothing.

Use of Multiple Types of PPE There may be situations that require you to wear more than one type of PPE. You may have to wear gloves, a gown, and a mask/face shield. The order in which you put these on and take them off is important. Since the gloves must go over the sleeves of the gown, the gown must go on first. The proper placement order for multiple PPE is gown, mask/face shield, and gloves. To reduce the possibility of cross contamination, remove contaminated PPE in the opposite order; that is, gloves, mask/face shield, and gown. Procedure 6-7 demonstrates the correct method for removing contaminated gloves and Procedure 6-8 demonstrates the proper method for removing a contaminated gown.

Transmission from Healthcare Workers

There may be times when a healthcare worker has a serious infection that could be transmitted to a patient. An infection acquired by a patient in a healthcare facility is known as a **healthcare-associated infection (HAI)** or what is also sometimes referred to as a nosocomial infection. The CDC uses the more current term *healthcare-associated infection*. OSHA has special recommendations for workers who perform procedures that could result in a patient's exposure to disease. Although the risk of a healthcare worker's transmitting an infection to a patient is small if OSHA standards are

followed, these additional precautions are advised for high-risk procedures. High-risk procedures include the following:

- Those that are thought to have caused the transmission of infection from a medical worker to a patient in the past;
- Those that may carry a high risk of infection, such as oral, obstetric, and gynecologic procedures; and
- Those that involve needles, especially if a needle is in a body cavity or a body space that is difficult to see and the healthcare worker's fingers are nearby (if the worker's skin is cut, the patient could be exposed to the worker's blood).

Workers who perform high-risk procedures should know their HIV and HBV status. HBV vaccination is strongly recommended. Also, workers who have skin conditions characterized by sores that secrete fluid should forgo direct patient care and the handling of equipment used for exposure-prone procedures until their condition has healed.

A member of the medical staff who is infected with HIV or HBV should not perform procedures that might result in exposure for the patient without the advice of an expert review panel. This panel could include the healthcare worker's own physician, someone with expert knowledge about the transmission of infectious disease, a medical professional with expert knowledge about the procedures in question, public health officials, and a member of the infection-control committee of the institution, if applicable.

The panel advises the worker on whether procedures may be performed. The advice includes requiring the worker to inform potential patients of the infection before the procedure. Each medical facility has policies in place outlining if and how patients will be notified of a healthcare professional's HIV or HBV status. The notification may be in writing from the panel or the healthcare worker may speak directly to the patient. It is the healthcare worker's ethical duty to protect a patient from known exposure to bloodborne pathogens. However, the panel also must protect the healthcare worker's confidentiality if possible.

Although great controversy has surrounded the subject of required testing of all healthcare workers for HIV or HBV, no recommendations are in place for such testing. The risk of infection transmission from worker to patient is not considered great enough to justify the extensive resources that mandatory testing would require.

▶ Reporting Guidelines for Infectious Diseases
LO 6.10

The CDC requires reporting of certain diseases to the state or county department of health. This information, which is forwarded to the CDC, helps research epidemiologists control the spread of infection. Table 6-2 lists diseases that must be reported to the National Notifiable Disease Surveillance System of the CDC, through your state or county health department. When you report a communicable disease, you must fill out a report form. Your state health department may have a different form for each reportable disease. You must obtain the correct form and a disease identification number from the health department

TABLE 6-2 The Notifiable Disease Surveillance System

Anthrax

Arboviral neuroinvasive and non-neuroinvasive diseases

Babesiosis

Botulism, foodborne

Botulism, infant

Botulism, other (wound and unspecified)

Brucellosis

Chancroid

Chlamydia trachomatis, genital infections

Cholera

Coccidioidomycosis

Cryptosporidiosis

Cyclosporiasis

Dengue Fever

Dengue Hemorrhagic Fever

Dengue Shock Syndrome

Diphtheria

Ehrlichiosis/Anaplasmosis

- *Ehrlichia chaffeensis*

- *Ehrlichia ewingii*

- *Anaplasma phagocytophilum*

- Undetermined

Giardiasis

Gonorrhea

Haemophilus influenzae, invasive disease

Hansen disease (leprosy)

Hantavirus pulmonary syndrome

Hemolytic uremic syndrome, post-diarrhea

Hepatitis A, acute

Hepatitis B, acute

Hepatitis B, chronic

Hepatitis B virus, perinatal infection

Hepatitis C, acute

Hepatitis C, past or present

HIV infection*

- HIV infection, adult/ adolescent (age $\geq$ 13 years)

- HIV infection, child (age $\geq$ 18 months and $<$ 13 years)

- HIV infection, pediatric (age $<$ 18 months)

Influenza-associated pediatric mortality

Legionellosis

Listeriosis

Lyme disease

Malaria

Measles

Meningococcal disease

Mumps

Novel influenza A virus infections

Pertussis

Plague

Poliomyelitis, paralytic

Poliovirus infection, nonparalytic

Psittacosis

Q fever, acute and chronic

Rabies, animal

Rabies, human

Rubella

Rubella, congenital syndrome

Salmonellosis

Severe Acute Respiratory Syndrome-associated Coronavirus (SARS-CoV) disease

Shiga toxin-producing *Escherichia coli* (STEC)

Shigellosis

Smallpox

Spotted Fever Rickettsiosis

Streptococcal toxic-shock syndrome

Streptococcus pneumoniae, invasive disease

Syphilis, all stages

Syphilis, congenital

Syphilitic stillbirth

Tetanus

Toxic-shock syndrome (other than Streptococcal)

Trichinellosis (Trichinosis)

Tuberculosis

Tularemia

Typhoid fever

Vancomycin-intermediate Staphylococcus aureus (VISA)

Vancomycin-resistant Staphylococcus aureus (VRSA)

Varicella (deaths only)

Varicella (morbidity)

Vibriosis

Viral Hemorrhagic Fevers, due to

- Ebola virus

- Marburg virus

- Arenavirus

- Crimean-Congo Hemorrhagic Fever virus

- Lassa virus

- Lujo virus

- New world arena viruses

Yellow fever

*Acquired Immunodeficiency Syndrome (AIDS) (reclassified as HIV stage III).

Source: From Centers for Disease Control and Prevention Nationally Notifiable Infectious Conditions US 2011.

every time you report a communicable disease. To fill out such a form, you need access to the following information:

- Disease identification (usually a code number as well as the name of the disease).
- Patient identification (including name, address, date of birth, sex, ethnic origin, and occupational or educational status) if required.
- Infection history (date of onset, vaccination history, laboratory results).

- Reporting-institution information (name of person completing report, title, contact information).

Each state and each medical facility have specific guidelines for filling out such a form. Procedure 6-9 describes, in general, how to notify state and county agencies about reportable diseases.

Reporting guidelines also must be followed if a worker comes in contact with a substance that may transmit infection. These guidelines, which are explained in OSHA's Bloodborne Pathogens Standard, include reporting exposure incidents to employers immediately.

PROCEDURE 6-1 Handling a Fire Emergency

Procedure Goal: To ensure safe use of a fire extinguisher during a fire emergency.

OSHA Guidelines: This procedure does not involve exposure to blood, body fluids, or tissue.

Materials: Fully charged fire extinguisher that has been professionally serviced on a yearly basis.

Method: Procedure steps.

1. In the case of an open fire or continuous smoke, pull the fire alarm or call emergency services to alert the local fire authorities.
2. Move patients out of the area.
3. Remove the fire extinguisher from its stored location.
4. Assess the fire. If it is too large, do not attempt to extinguish the fire. Leave the building immediately and wait for the fire department to arrive.
   RATIONALE: You must determine if you can easily contain the fire so that you know whether to have everyone leave the building.

If the Fire Cannot Be Easily Contained

5. Calmly and quickly ask each employee to follow the established fire plan.
6. Remove all patients to the outside of the building; ensure patient comfort and safety at all times.

If the Fire Is Small and Easily Contained

7. Hold the fire extinguisher upright.
8. **Pull** the safety pin on the fire extinguisher.

FIGURE Procedure 6-1 Step 8   To activate a fire extinguisher, pull the safety pin.

9. **Aim** at the base of the fire.

FIGURE Procedure 6-1 Step 9   You should aim at the base of the fire, not the flames. The source or fuel of the fire is at the base.

10. **Squeeze** the trigger.

FIGURE Procedure 6-1 Step 10   Once you are aiming at the base of the fire, squeeze the lever to deliver the extinguishing agent.

11. Sweep side to side until the fire is out.

FIGURE Procedure 6-1 Step 11 Sweep back and forth at the base of the fire until it is out.

12. Do not reenter the area until the fire department assesses and clears the area.

RATIONALE: A professional firefighter should assess the area to ascertain if there is a danger of the fire reigniting.

PROCEDURE 6-2 Maintaining and Using an Eyewash Station

Procedure Goal: To ensure safe use of eyewash station following a splash or splatter accident.

OSHA Guidelines:

Materials: Eyewash station. This may be plumbed or free-standing. Gloves, moisture-proof lab coat, and goggles or face mask.

Method: Procedure steps.

On a Weekly Basis

1. Check that the path to the eyewash station is clear and no more than 10 seconds from the hazard.

2. Ensure that the Eyewash sign is easily visible.

3. Make sure the covers are in place.

RATIONALE: To ensure there are no contaminants on the eyewash.

4. Ensure that the unit comes on in one second and stays on once it is activated.

5. Check the flow of the eyewash to ensure it has sufficient flow to wash the eye but is not so strong it will damage the eye tissues. Approximately 0.4 gallon per minute is required for an eyewash and 3 gallons per minute is required for an eyewash/facewash station.

6. Check that the temperature of the water is above 60°F and below 100°F.

7. Flush the system for one minute.

RATIONALE: To remove any particulate matter such as sediment from standing water that may have collected in the water line.

8. Complete the Safety Inspection record attached to the eyewash station.

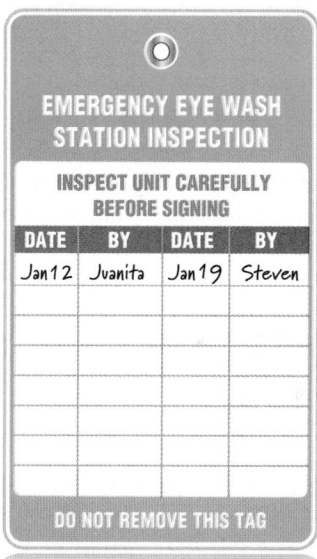

FIGURE Procedure 6-2 Step 8 The safety inspection record should be completed each week.

During a Splash or Splatter Emergency

9. Assist the victim to the eyewash station.

10. Activate the system.

11. If the eyewash is a plumbed unit, have the victim lean into the eyewash, keeping her eyes continuously open. You may have to don gloves and gown and assist the victim by holding her eye or eyes open.

12. Continuously flush the eyes for at least 15 minutes or the length of time recommended on the MSDS if applicable.

13. Alert the physician or EMS.

RATIONALE: So that the victim receives prompt and appropriate post-exposure care.

PROCEDURE 6-3 Using a Biohazardous Sharps Container

Procedure Goal: To ensure safe use of a sharps disposal unit.

OSHA Guidelines:

Materials: Approved sharps container and gloves.

Method: Procedure steps.

1. Wash your hands and put on gloves.
2. Ensure that biohazardous waste containers are close to the place where the waste material is generated. **RATIONALE:** To avoid accidental puncture wounds or exposure to biohazardous waste.
3. Hold the article by the unpointed or blunt end.
4. Drop the object directly into an approved container. (If you are using an evacuation system, do not unscrew the needle. Drop the entire system with the needle attached and the safety device engaged into the receptacle.) The container should be puncture-proof, with rigid sides and a tight-fitting lid.

RATIONALE: To avoid needlestick injuries.

5. Place sharps in appropriate biohazardous waste container immediately or as soon as possible.
6. Keep containers closed when not in use. Close them before removing them from the area or use and keep them upright to avoid spills.
7. Place the container in a secondary container if the outside of the primary container becomes contaminated.
8. Drop—do not push—intact contaminated needles into the biohazardous waste container for sharps. **RATIONALE:** To avoid accidental puncture wounds.
9. Never break off, recap, reuse, or handle needles after use. **RATIONALE:** To avoid accidental puncture wounds.
10. Do not open, empty, or clean sharps containers.
11. Discard sharps containers that are two-thirds full in large biohazardous waste containers. Depending on your office's procedures, the container and its contents may be sterilized before further disposal, or they may be collected by an authorized waste management agency.
12. Remove the gloves and wash your hands.

PROCEDURE 6-4 Disposing of Biohazardous Waste

Procedure Goal: To correctly dispose of contaminated waste products, including sharps and contaminated cleaning and paper products.

OSHA Guidelines:

Materials: Biohazardous waste containers, gloves, and waste materials.

Method: Procedure steps.

1. Wash your hands and put on gloves.
2. Carefully deposit the biohazardous materials in a properly marked biohazardous waste container.

A standard biohazardous waste container has an inner plastic liner (either red or orange and marked with the biohazard symbol) and a puncture-proof outer shell (also marked with the biohazard symbol).

3. Never "dump" the contents of one biohazardous waste container into another. **RATIONALE:** Doing so puts you at risk of exposure to biohazardous materials.
4. If the container is full, secure the inner liner and place it in the appropriate area for biohazardous waste. **RATIONALE:** Biohazardous waste must be held in an area separate from regular waste and trash.
5. Remove the gloves and wash your hands.

PROCEDURE 6-5 Aseptic Handwashing

Procedure Goal: To remove dirt and microorganisms from under the fingernails and from the surface of the skin, hair follicles, and oil glands of the hands.

OSHA Guidelines: This procedure does not involve exposure to blood, body fluids, or tissues.

Materials: Liquid soap, nailbrush or orange stick, and paper towels.

Method: Procedure steps.

1. Remove all jewelry (plain wedding bands may be left on and scrubbed).
2. Turn on the faucets using a paper towel and adjust the water temperature to moderately warm. (Sinks with knee-operated faucet controls prevent contact of the surface with the hands.)

FIGURE Procedure 6-5 Step 2   Using a paper towel to turn on the faucet reduces the possibility of cross contamination.

3. Wet your hands and apply liquid soap. Use a clean, dry paper towel to activate soap pump. Liquid soap, especially when dispensed with a foot pump, is preferable to bar soap.
    RATIONALE: There is less available area for dirt to accumulate on a liquid soap dispenser than on bar soap, and there is a smaller chance of dropping the soap dispenser into the sink or onto the floor.

4. Work the soap into a lather, making sure that all surface areas of both hands are lathered. Rub vigorously in a circular motion for 2 minutes. Keep your hands lower than your forearms so that dirty water flows into the sink instead of back onto your arms. Your fingertips should be pointing down. Interlace your fingers to clean between them, and use the palm of one hand to clean the back of the other. It is important that you wash every surface of your hands.
    RATIONALE: Microorganisms are found on every surface of the hand and if not washed away, can be transferred to the patient.

5. Use a single-use disposable nailbrush or plastic, single-use nail cleaner under running water to dislodge dirt around your nails and cuticles.
    RATIONALE: Microorganisms under the nails are not directly subjected to the running water and must be dislodged so that they can be washed away.

6. Rinse your hands well, keeping the hands lower than your forearms and not touching the sink or faucets.

FIGURE Procedure 6-5 Step 6   Keep your hands lower than your forearms and avoid touching the sink when rinsing after an aseptic handwash.

7. With the water still running, dry your hands thoroughly with clean, dry paper towels.

8. Turn off the faucets using a clean, dry paper towel. Discard the towels.

PROCEDURE 6-6 Using an Alcohol-Based Hand Disinfectant

Procedure Goal: To use an alcohol-based hand-cleansing substance to reduce pathogens on the hand surfaces and prevent recontamination.

OSHA Guidelines: This procedure does not involve exposure to blood, body fluids, or tissue.

Materials: 60–95% alcohol-based foam, gel, or liquid rub.

Method: Procedure steps.

1. Remove all jewelry (plain wedding bands may be left on).

2. Pump the recommended amount of AHD onto the palm of the hand.
    RATIONALE: You must use enough AHD to cover all surfaces of the hands and there must be enough so that it does not dry too quickly.

3. Rub the hands together vigorously ensuring the alcohol comes in contact with all surfaces, including backs of hands, between fingers, and fingernails.
    RATIONALE: Microorganisms are found on every surface of the hand and if not washed away, can be transferred to the patient.

4. Continue to rub the solution in a rotary fashion until it is evaporated and the hands are dry (10–15 seconds). Do not wave hands to hasten drying.
    RATIONALE: Once they evaporate, AHDs have no effect on pathogens.

PROCEDURE 6-7 Removing Contaminated Gloves

Procedure Goal: To remove gloves contaminated with blood, body fluids, or other potentially hazardous substances while avoiding cross contamination of your hands or other surfaces.

OSHA Guidelines: This procedure does not involve exposure to blood, body fluids, or tissue if performed correctly.

Materials: Contaminated gloves, lined trash container or biohazardous waste container.

Method: Procedure steps.

1. Using your dominant hand, grasp the palm of the glove of your nondominant hand.
2. Gently pull the glove off the nondominant hand, turning it inside out and holding it in your dominant hand.
3. Encase the removed glove completely in the dominant hand.

RATIONALE: To contain any contaminants in the glove so that they are not accidently transferred to your hands. Encasing the glove also limits the possibility of splattering contaminants by flipping the glove.

4. Place the thumb or two fingers of the ungloved hand under the cuff of the remaining glove, being careful not to touch the outside of the glove with your bare hand.
   RATIONALE: The inside of the glove is most likely not contaminated.
5. Pull the glove over your hand, turning it inside out over the other glove, leaving no outside surface exposed.
6. Throw the gloves away in the appropriate waste container.
7. Wash your hands.

PROCEDURE 6-8 Removing a Contaminated Gown

Procedure Goal: To remove a gown contaminated on the front and sleeves with blood, body fluids, or other potentially hazardous substances while avoiding cross contamination of your hands, body, or other surfaces.

OSHA Guidelines: This procedure does not involve exposure to blood, body fluids, or tissue if performed correctly.

Materials: Contaminated gloves, lined trash container or biohazardous waste container.

Method: Procedure steps.

1. Unfasten ties from the neck, then from behind your back.

2. Peel the gown down and away from neck and shoulders, touching inside of gown only.
   RATIONALE: You should always move from clean to dirty to avoid cross contamination.
3. Continue pulling the gown down from the neck and shoulders and away from your body.
4. Turn gown inside out, making sure you do not touch the outer surface of the gown.
   RATIONALE: To avoid contaminating your hands.
5. Slowly fold or roll into a bundle and discard.

PROCEDURE 6-9 Notifying State and County Agencies About Reportable Diseases

Procedure Goal: To report cases of infection with reportable disease to the proper state or county health department.

OSHA Guidelines: This procedure does not involve exposure to blood, body fluids, or tissues.

Materials: Communicable disease report form, pen, envelope, and stamp.

Method: Procedure steps.

1. Check to be sure you have the correct form. Some states have specific forms for each reportable infectious disease or type of disease. CDC forms also may be used for reporting specific diseases.

2. Fill in all blank areas unless they are shaded (generally for local health department use).
3. Follow office procedures for submitting the report to a supervisor or physician before sending it out.
4. Sign and date the form. Address the envelope, put a stamp on it, and place it in the mail.

MICHIGAN DEPARTMENT OF PUBLIC HEALTH
Division of Disease Surveillance

ENTERIC ILLNESS CASE INVESTIGATION
(Please check appropriate illness)

_____ Shigellosis   _____ Giardiasis
_____ Non-typhoid Salmonellosis   _____ Amebiasis
_____ Campylobacter enteritis

CASE INFORMATION

Name: _____ Age or Birthdate: _____ Sex: _____ Race: _____

Address: _____ Phone: _____
        (Street)   (City)   (County)   (Zip)

Occupation: _____ *High Risk: Y N
        (What)   (Where)
(If infant or student list school, nursery or day care center)

Attending   Address or   Was the patient
Physician: _____ Phone: _____ hospitalized: Y N

Hospital: _____ Dates: _____
                                   (Admission)   (Discharge)

Onset: _____ Date recovered: _____ Symptom Summary: _____
_____
_____

Suspected Causative Agent: _____
(include species or serotype if known)

HOUSEHOLD CONTACTS INFORMATION

Name	Age	Family Relationship	Occupation	*High Risk Y N	Provide date of onset for all household members with concurrent similar illness
1) _____					_____
2) _____					_____
3) _____					_____
4) _____					_____
5) _____					_____
6) _____					_____
7) _____					_____
8) _____					_____
9) _____					_____
10) _____					_____

*"High Risk" = occupation as food handler, direct patient care worker, day care center worker or person attending day care <u>or</u> who is institutionalized. Stool specimens should be obtained on "high risk" cases and "high risk" household contacts as appropriate for the illness. Results may be recorded in <u>Laboratory Information Section</u> of this form (see over).

Name of the person who completed this form: _____ County: _____

Information obtained from: _____ Date: _____

Telephone Interview: _____ Home Visit: _____ Outbreak Investigation: _____

C-30 Rev. 10/83   AUTH: Act 368, P.A. 1978

FIGURE Procedure 6-9 Step 1   Some states have specific forms for use with particular communicable diseases or diseases of a certain type. *(Continued)*

NON-HOUSEHOLD CONTACTS WITH A CONCURRENT SIMILAR ILLNESS

Name	Approximate date of onset of symptoms	Address and/or Phone	Relationship to case (Nature of contact)
1)			
2)			
3)			
4)			
5)			

ADDITIONAL EXPOSURES OR COMMENTS

Home Sewage System: Municipal   Septic Tank   Other_____

Home drinking Water Type: Municipal   Private Well   Other_____

As appropriate for the illness, ask about meals eaten away from home, stores where groceries bought, brand of poultry, meat, dairy products consumed, overnight travel, recent foreign travel, group functions, exposure to raw milk, untreated water, animals, etc. within one incubation period before onset.

(shigellosis to 7 days, salmonellosis - up to 3 days, Campylobacter enteritis - up to 10 days)

Be specific, provide place name(s) and date(s).

FOLLOW-UP FECAL CULTURE RESULTS FOR "HIGH RISK" CASE AND/OR CONTACTS.

Name or Initials	Date(s) Obtained and Findings
1)	
2)	
3)	
4)	
5)	

FIGURE Procedure 6-9 Step 1   (*Concluded*)

SUMMARY OF LEARNING OUTCOMES

LEARNING OUTCOMES	KEY POINTS
6.1 **Describe the components of a medical office safety plan.**	The medical office safety plan should include OSHA's Hazard Communication; electrical, fire, and chemical safety; emergency action plans; bloodborne pathogen exposure plans; PPE; and needlestick prevention plans.
6.2 **Identify OSHA's role in protecting healthcare workers.**	The U.S. Department of Labor created OSHA to protect the employees' safety in the workplace. Through the creation and enforcement of standards such as the Bloodborne Pathogens Standard, Hazard Communication, and the Needlestick Safety and Prevention Act, OSHA serves to protect healthcare workers from hazards.
6.3 **Describe basic safety precautions you should take to reduce electrical hazards.**	To reduce electrical hazards in the medical office, you should avoid using extension cords, repair or replace damaged cords, avoid overloading circuits, ensure that all plugs are grounded, dry your hands before using electrical devices, and keep electrical devices away from sinks or other sources of water.

LEARNING OUTCOMES	KEY POINTS
6.4 **Illustrate the necessary steps in a comprehensive fire safety plan.**	A comprehensive fire safety plan must include fire prevention strategies, actions to take in the event of a fire, building evacuation routes and plans, fire drills, and local emergency contacts.
6.5 **Summarize proper methods for handling and storing chemicals used in a medical office.**	When using chemicals in the medical office, you should always wear protective gear, carry the container with both hands, work in a well-ventilated area, never combine chemicals unless it is specifically required in the test procedures, always add acid to water if the procedure requires that you combine chemicals, and properly clean up spills immediately.
6.6 **Explain the principles of good ergonomic practice and physical safety in the medical office.**	In order to protect yourself from work-related musculoskeletal disorders at work, you must follow the principles of good body mechanics. Your physical safety at work depends on understanding and applying appropriate workplace safeguards, including never running in an office, taking care when carrying objects through the facility, closing cabinets and drawers, and following appropriate safety procedures in the lab.
6.7 **Illustrate the cycle of infection and how to break it.**	In order for an infection to occur, these five elements must be in place: a reservoir host, a means of exit, a means of transmission, a means of entrance, and a susceptible host. The most effective means of breaking the cycle of infection is by using aseptic techniques. These include maintaining strict housekeeping standards, adhering to government health guidelines, and educating patients in hygiene, health promotion, and disease prevention.
6.8 **Summarize the Bloodborne Pathogens Standard and Universal Precautions as described in the rules and regulations of the Occupational Safety and Health Administration (OSHA).**	Laws set forth in the OSHA Bloodborne Pathogens Standard of 1991 dictate how you must handle infectious or potentially infectious waste generated during medical or surgical procedures. According to these rules, any potentially infectious waste materials must be discarded or held for processing in biohazardous waste containers.
6.9 **Describe methods of infection control including those for preventing healthcare-associated infections.**	The two basic methods of infection control are medical asepsis (clean technique) and surgical asepsis (sterile technique). OSHA recommends that healthcare workers who work with high-risk patients know their HIV and HBV status, participate in a HBV vaccination program, and avoid direct patient contact if they have a skin condition characterized by sores that secrete fluid. Any healthcare worker who is HIV- or HBV-positive should not perform procedures that might expose a patient without first consulting an expert review panel.
6.10 **Describe Centers for Disease Control and Prevention (CDC) requirements for reporting cases of infectious disease.**	The CDC requires reporting of certain diseases to the state or county department of health, who then reports the information to the National Notifiable Disease Surveillance System of the CDC.

Recall Shenya Jones from the beginning of the chapter. Now that you have completed the chapter, answer the following questions regarding her case.

1. What aseptic technique practices would be most important with this patient?
2. Whom do these aseptic technique practices protect?

EXAM PREPARATION QUESTIONS

1. (LO 6.3) The general duty clause requires
   a. That every employee performs every duty in the office
   b. An employer to maintain a safe workplace
   c. That each employee follows OSHA regulations
   d. That safety plan duties be well defined

2. (LO 6.3) Which of the following requires that all employees receive workplace hazard training?
   a. Standard Precautions
   b. Emergency action plans
   c. Needlestick prevention regulations
   d. Hazard Communication Standard
   e. Bloodborne pathogens

3. (LO 6.3) The comprehensive sheet that accompanies every hazardous chemical is known as a/an
   a. Hazard label
   b. Biohazard label
   c. MSDS
   d. UL label
   e. HAI

4. (LO 6.5) The PASS system is an acronym outlining the proper use of which of the following?
   a. Fire extinguisher
   b. Chemical hood
   c. Gas-fed open flame
   d. Alcohol-based hand disinfectant
   e. Evacuation plan

5. (LO 6.9) Which of the following is the most common means of transmitting pathogens?
   a. Ingesting food
   b. Sneezing
   c. Coughing
   d. Sexual contact
   e. Touching

6. (LO 6.9) Which of the following would be considered a fomite?
   a. Mosquito
   b. Pencil
   c. Sneeze
   d. *E. coli*
   e. Mucus

7. (LO 6.11) You should empty a disposable sharps container when it is
   a. Half full
   b. Contaminated
   c. Two-thirds full
   d. Three-fourths full
   e. Never

8. (LO 6.12) Which of the following glove types may be decontaminated and reused?
   a. Utility
   b. Examination
   c. Sterile
   d. Disposable
   e. Latex

9. (LO 6.11) Which of the following would be considered a Category II task?
   a. Oral surgery
   b. Performing CPR
   c. Taking vital signs
   d. Measuring height
   e. Controlling bleeding

10. (LO 6.11) Means of controlling injuries by altering the way a task is performed is known as
    a. Universal precautions
    b. Engineering controls
    c. Personal protection
    d. Work practice controls
    e. Safety plan controls

Patient Reception

PATIENT INFORMATION	Patient Name	Gender	DOB
	Peter Smith	M	3/28/19XX
	Attending	MRN	Allergies
	Paul F. Buckwalter, MD	428-69-544	NKA

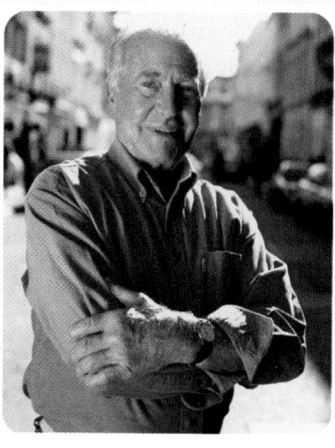

Peter Smith is a 73-year-old male with mild Type 2 diabetes. When he called to schedule today's appointment, he stated that he was feeling very anxious and fatigued and that he was having difficulty eating and sleeping. He arrives at the reception desk today, appearing "flat" in affect. After he signs in, his wife whispers to you, "I want to talk with the doctor about him, before he sees the doctor."

Keep Mr. Smith in mind as you study the chapter. There will be questions at the end of the chapter based on the case study. The information in the chapter will help you answer these questions.

ACTIVSim™

LEARNING OUTCOMES

After completing Chapter 7, you will be able to:

7.1 List the design items to be considered when setting up an office reception area.

7.2 Summarize the housekeeping tasks required to keep the reception area neat and clean.

7.3 Relate how the Americans with Disabilities and Older American Acts have helped to make physical access to the medical office easier for all patients.

7.4 Articulate the cause of most injuries to medical office workers and the four body areas where they occur.

7.5 Explain the Red Flags Rule, giving the four red flags that the reception staff should be alert to.

7.6 Implement policies and procedures for opening and closing the office.

KEY TERMS

Americans with Disabilities Act (ADA)
color family
contagious
infectious waste
medical identity theft
Older Americans Act of 1965
Red Flags Rule

III. C. (3) Discuss infection control procedures

IV. C (14) Recognize the role of patient advocacy in the practice of medical assisting

IV. P (13) Advocate on behalf of patients

IX. C (3) Describe the implications of HIPAA for the medical assistant in various medical settings

IX. C (11) Identify how the Americans with Disabilities Act (ADA) applies to the medical assisting profession

X. C (3) Discuss the role of cultural, social and ethnic diversity in ethical performance of medical assisting practice

XI. C (7) Describe fundamental principles for evacuation of a healthcare setting

XI. P (7) Explain an evacuation plan for a physician's office

5. **Psychology of Human Relations**
Graduates:

b. Identify and respond appropriately when working/caring for patients with special needs

e. Advocate on behalf of family/patients, having ability to deal and communicate with family

8. **Medical Office Business Procedures Management**
Graduates:

e. Locate resources and information for patients and employers

x. Maintain medical facility

hh. Receive, organize, prioritize, and transmit information expediently

kk. Adapt to individualized needs

10. **Medical Laboratory Procedures**
Graduates:

c. Dispose of biohazardous materials

▶ Introduction

In general, the medical office is divided into two broad, functional categories: the "back office" is the clinical area where patient care takes place and the "front office," including the reception area, is where business and nonclinical tasks take place. The facility's design and furnishings create the office environment, which is key to delivering this care, and the reception area, or point of entry, creates the first impression of the office. Is the office bright and cheerful, cool and modern, or warm and cozy? The impression created by the reception area reflects on the quality of care patients can expect to receive. A carefully designed and well-maintained patient reception area ensures a pleasant and comfortable experience for patients while they wait to receive medical care, and it sets the stage for a successful interaction between the patient and the entire medical staff.

This chapter discusses the many considerations related to the design and furnishings for this area of the medical office. The type of practice and the patient population's special needs are major influences, so you will explore the Americans with Disabilities and the Older Americans Acts, as well as the Red Flags Rule. The roles of reception staff and what they need to accomplish in these roles will also be covered.

▶ Design of the Reception Area   LO 7.1

The word *reception* means the place or event where one is greeted. In the medical office, reception describes the area where the patient enters the practice, informs the staff of his or her presence by "signing in," receives a greeting, and waits to be seen. Avoid using the term *waiting room* since waiting is only one function and the term does not have a positive association. Although the practice manager is usually responsible for

the office design, awareness of the aspects that affect the design is valuable knowledge for any medical assistant. The primary consideration in the design is the type of practice. For example, the furnishings, colors, and patient flow patterns of a pediatric office will differ from those of an internal medicine office.

Size and Schedule

After identifying the type of practice, size is the next factor. Knowledge of the number of practitioners and the number of patients anticipated daily is important. Knowing when individual physicians plan to utilize the space is equally important. For example, one surgeon in the practice may have office hours on Mondays, Wednesdays, and Fridays and perform surgeries on Tuesdays and Thursdays. Another surgeon may perform surgeries in the morning and see patients in the afternoon. Still another surgeon may do surgeries on opposite days and times. These differences in physician scheduling allow better utilization of space and relative ease in planning for the reception size. Other offices may have staggered hours where one physician will see patients between 7:00 a.m. and 3:00 p.m. and another physician in the practice will see patients from 11:00 a.m. to 7:00 p.m. This is challenging since more space is needed during the four overlap hours than the remainder of the day. Dealing with overlapping office hours and other time and space issues is often part of the medical assistant's role.

Utilization of Space

Utilization of space differs by type of practice. For example, an orthopedic office or geriatric office where a significant number of patients will need room for wheelchairs and walkers requires more open space for mobility and devices than does a cardiologist's office. There may be the false assumption that pediatric offices need a smaller reception area since the patients are smaller, but this is incorrect for a few reasons. First, a caregiver

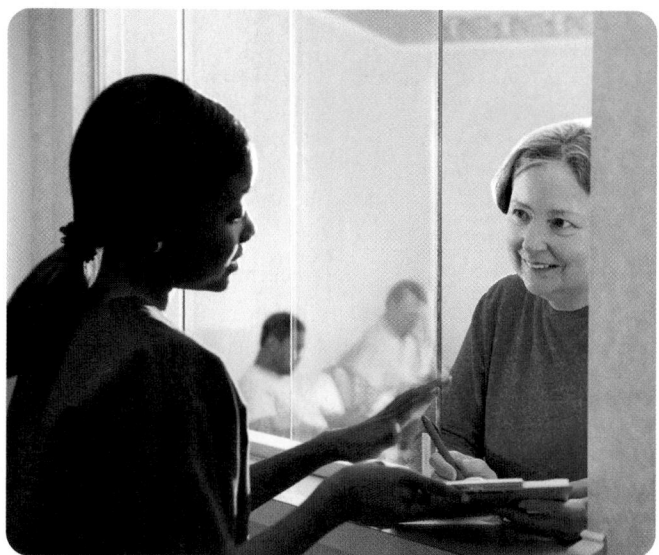

FIGURE 7-1 The receptionist's desk and window are part of every patient reception area and allow for privacy during patient check-in.

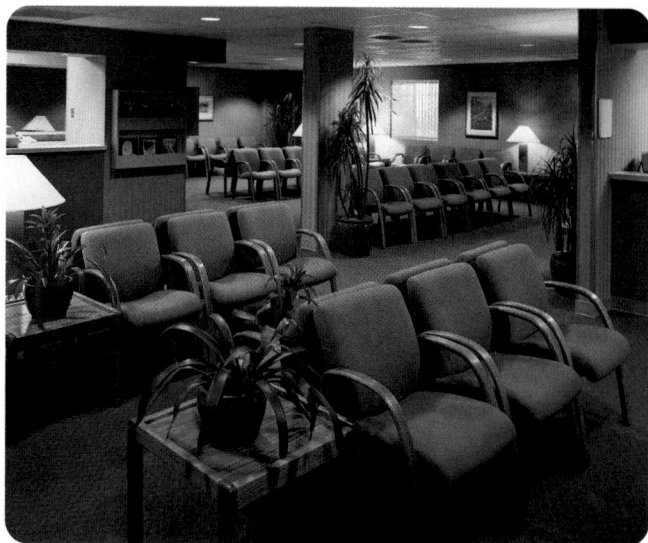

FIGURE 7-2 Decorator colors and furniture groupings make for a comfortable reception area.

always accompanies the pediatric patient. Second, children require play space. Third, pediatric offices normally have separate "well child" and "sick child" areas in an attempt to avoid cross-contamination from sick to well patients.

Overcrowding in a reception area is undesirable for patient comfort and for the potential of disease transmission. The reception area, which allows the patient to sit while waiting to be seen, is usually separated from the functional areas of the practice by a high counter and a sliding window (Figure 7-1). These areas should be HIPAA-compliant so the patient at the counter cannot overhear staff talking to or about other patients and cannot view an open computer screen or paper record.

Décor

Colors and fabrics are the primary elements that make up a room's décor. Colors can be used throughout the room—on walls, furniture, carpeting, and other items. Fabrics are used primarily on furniture and draperies.

When using several colors, it is important to decorate in color families to avoid a jarring, unprofessional look. A **color family** is a group of colors that work well together. In general, colors fall within two basic areas: cool and warm. Using all cool colors—like white, blue, and mauve—creates a more harmonious impression in the reception area than mixing cool colors with warm ones like red, orange, and hot pink. When choosing the color family, consider the mood you want to create, as studies demonstrate that the use of color affects mood. For example:

- Red increases heart rate and blood pressure.
- Blue causes the body to produce calming chemicals.
- Green is easy on the eyes and relaxing.
- Light browns are warm and inviting.
- Black and dark browns are associated with power and depression.
- White is related to cleanliness and purity.

Traditionally, the pediatric office incorporates primary colors for a lively atmosphere (although the use of red should be limited). Obstetric offices are often decorated in pastels; geriatric offices often use soft colors in beige tones. Other offices tend to use popular decorator color palettes like earth tones and jewel tones (Figure 7-2). Colors may also reflect the cultural preferences of the dominant patient population. You might also want to consider the effect of color when choosing your scrubs or other office attire.

Fabrics, too, add to the atmosphere in the room. Heavy fabrics like velvet or brocade are more formal, whereas lightweight or sheer fabrics create a soft, delicate appearance. Patterns on fabrics or wallpaper can immediately change the mood of the room. No matter what the design, fabrics should be easy to clean and maintain.

Many medical offices are carpeted for greater appeal and improved noise reduction. Carpeting, available in a variety of colors and patterns, also provides a comfortable cushion when people walk through the office. Carpeting should be easy to clean and durable enough to handle a large volume of patient traffic. Scatter rugs, which can cause injuries if someone slips on or trips over them, should be avoided.

Furnishings

Chairs should be comfortable but have a straight back to allow the patient to get up easily, especially in obstetric, geriatric, and orthopedic offices. Many attractive stain-resistant cloth fabrics are available for medical use. Choose chairs and tables with rounded—not sharp—corners to avoid injuries.

Arranging Furniture The furniture arrangement can make the office seem comfortable or uncomfortable. If furniture is too close together, patients do not have sufficient space to move around easily or to stretch their legs. They may feel cramped. To ensure that patients have adequate room, a good rule of thumb is to allow 12 square feet of space per person. By this measurement, a 120-square-foot room (10 feet by 12 feet) can accommodate 10 people comfortably.

The furniture arrangement should allow maximum floor space. Patients should be able to stretch out their legs when seated and to walk around the reception area if they wish. Placing chairs against the wall usually produces the greatest amount of floor area. Additional seating in the middle of the room can be placed back-to-back to conserve space. Seats should be grouped so that families or friends can sit together. Remember to reserve room for patients in wheelchairs and to allow enough space for wheelchairs with extended leg supports. Also, keep in mind that some patients value their privacy; placing single chairs or small groups of chairs in corners of the room offers patients some measure of privacy, if needed.

Specialty Items Accessories or specialty items can make the reception area more comfortable and inviting. The following are additional items to be considered when selecting or modifying medical office furnishings:

- Artificial plants and floral arrangements are preferred due to allergies, poisons, and the potential for microbes associated with living plants; plants should be kept dust-free.

- Lighting should be adequate for reading and completing forms and provide a pleasant atmosphere; softer lights are preferred in geriatric offices since glare is a problem for this age group. Pediatric offices tend to have brighter lighting.

- Aquariums are popular and soothing but require upkeep; some offices employ a service to care for the aquarium, others have virtual aquariums.

- Heavy objects like large aquariums should be built into a wall if possible or securely fastened and stabilized to avoid injury. Likewise, large pictures, shelving, and bookcases should be securely fastened to walls.

- Music, like color, should not increase the heart rate or blood pressure; soft music is recommended for all practices.

- Refreshment centers (coffee, tea) are not wise for pediatric practices due to the danger of hot water, or for practices where many patients are fasting in preparation for procedures. In general, avoid glass objects when possible as they can break and cause injury.

- Toys and toy pieces should be easily and frequently disinfected and be larger than would fit into a small child's mouth. Balls or other throwing toys are dangerous in the medical environment.

Although specialty pieces can enhance the room's décor, they should be kept to a minimum (Figure 7-3). Too many pieces can create a cluttered look. Try to select specialty items that will be pleasing or helpful to patients. A clock is one example. Another useful item is a coat rack, which helps prevent clutter by providing a place for coats, umbrellas, and briefcases. Avoid accessories like scented candles or potpourri that may be offensive to some people or cause allergic reactions.

Other Considerations

Lighting Most medical offices use fairly bright lighting in the reception area, allowing patients to see their surroundings easily. Subdued lighting, like that sometimes used in restaurants, could be hazardous as it may cause patients to trip

FIGURE 7-3 Specialty items like artificial plants and paintings enhance the patient reception area.

over or bump into hard-to-see objects. In addition, bright lighting is essential for reading—a common activity in the patient reception area. Bright lighting also conveys an impression of cleanliness. Be aware, however, that extremely bright light can be harsh on the eyes and create an annoying glare. A specialist, like an electrician or lighting showroom salesperson, can help determine the appropriate level of lighting for the patient reception area.

Room Temperature Patients will be uncomfortable if the reception area is too hot or too cold. In an uncomfortable setting, waiting time can seem much longer than it really is. So, maintaining an average, comfortable temperature is important.

To ensure a comfortable versus an uncomfortable temperature, keep the thermostat at a temperature that feels comfortable to you and to the office staff. You might periodically survey patients to see if they are comfortable and adjust the setting accordingly. Many elderly people feel cold because of lowered metabolisms. You may want to increase the temperature setting for a geriatric practice or if the office sees a large number of elderly patients. The room temperature in the reception area may be a bit cooler than in the examination rooms, where patients may be required to disrobe.

Music Many medical offices pipe soothing background music through speakers to the reception area as well as elsewhere in the office. Because the music is meant to calm patients, it should be chosen accordingly. Classical music, light jazz, and soft rock are appropriate choices, whereas heavy metal and rap music are not. Some offices use prepared tapes or compact discs. Others tune in to an "easy listening" local (or satellite) radio station.

Tailoring Office Magazines to Patient Interests

It is a common sight: Patients waiting their turn for an appointment select one of the many magazines in the reception area. Sometimes it is hard to choose—because every magazine is interesting or because none of them are.

As the office medical assistant, you may be responsible for selecting magazines for the office reception area. The right selection may be the difference between a pleasant wait and a tedious one for your patients. Following these guidelines will help you compile a suitable mix of magazines that will satisfy a majority of patients.

1. Patients in some practices immediately share a common ground because they fall within the category of the practice specialty, like geriatrics or pediatrics. Some magazines may be a natural fit for this category. A geriatric practice, for example, may provide publications geared toward senior citizens. A pediatric practice may offer parenting and children's magazines.

2. People waiting in a physician's office usually have an interest in their health. So, health magazines geared toward the general public are good choices. Of course, the reception area is not the place for the highly technical medical journals, with graphic pictures, that the doctor might receive, nor is it the appropriate place for religious materials of any kind.

3. Make sure the magazines cover a variety of interests. The more topics available, the greater the chance that someone will be interested in one of them. Instead of subscribing to several magazines on one topic, try to limit subscriptions to one magazine per topic, unless the topic is of special interest to most patients.

4. Choose magazines that cover topics in a general way—travel, news, sports, fashion, or entertainment. Delving into these areas too specifically—as in a tennis magazine rather than one on a variety of sports—will interest a smaller audience.

5. Magazines should be discarded after three months or if they become torn and tattered looking. When you discard a magazine, be sure to replace it with a current edition or another more current periodical.

6. The best way to determine your patients' interests is to ask them. Develop a form on which patients can indicate their hobbies, interests, and favorite types of magazines. Periodically display the form in the reception area and encourage patients to make suggestions.

Educational/Entertainment Materials

Practice-appropriate educational and entertainment materials are more likely to be read by patients if the materials are placed on tables close to the seating. While wall and countertop racks are appropriate and conserve space, keep some materials on tables for easier access by the elderly and differently abled (Figure 7-4). Magazines, newspapers, and other reading material also may be present. The publications should be relatively current and reflect the interests and languages of the populations served. Materials should be neatly arranged, tasteful, and not torn or dirty. Avoid tabloids. Some large-print editions should be available for elderly and other sight-impaired patients.

Magazines and Books Choosing the right mix of reading material to interest all patients is a challenge. You probably have been in offices that have wonderful selections, and in an equal number of offices that do not. Try to have varied types of reading material to accommodate your patients' broad range of interests. If your office sees teen and younger patients, be sure to include reading material for their interests, too.

You or someone on the office staff should be sure to screen publications for medical content so that you can alert physicians to articles that might stimulate patient questions. Make sure magazines are current. There is nothing worse than having a patient reception area full of outdated or worn magazines. The Points on Practice feature will give you "pointers" on choosing magazines to interest your patients.

(a)

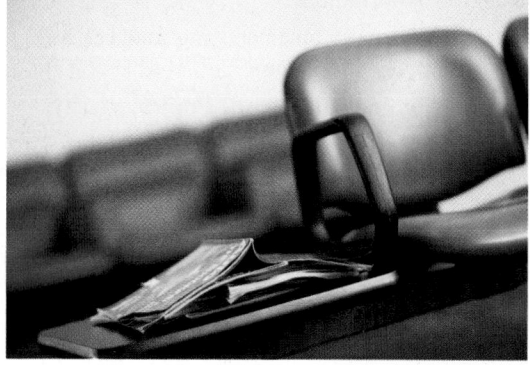

(b)

FIGURE 7-4 (a) Magazine racks save space, but do not forget to have (b) some reading material on tables for elderly or differently abled patients.

Patient Information Packet Many offices today compile a patient information packet to inform new patients about the practice. The packet can be designed in many ways, from a simple flyer to a formal folder with pockets to hold individual sheets of information. Topics covered in the packet can range from billing and insurance processing policies to biographical information on each physician in a group practice. The *Patient Education* chapter will discuss how to develop the contents of a patient information packet.

Medical Information Medical brochures are another type of reading material commonly found in the reception area. Patients may be interested in information that pertains to their general health or to specific conditions, particularly those that are treated by your physicians. Brochures on a variety of topics are available to medical offices either free of charge or for a nominal fee. These brochures are usually produced by nonprofit associations that specialize in a disease or condition (like the American Cancer Society) and by pharmaceutical companies.

Before displaying pamphlets and brochures in the reception area, read them thoroughly to ensure they provide accurate information; both you and the physicians may want to review them for medical accuracy and to prepare for any questions patients may have.

Bulletin Board Many reception areas contain bulletin boards that highlight area support group meetings and offer other current information. To encourage patients to look at the bulletin board, change the format and content frequently. Tailor items on the bulletin board to patient interests. Other, more general items for display on any physician's bulletin board might include the following:

- Office policies and procedures for patients such as no smoking or eating in the patient reception area, late or missed appointment policies, and patient payment information.
- Government reports on drug and nutrition information.
- Pamphlets or flyers from nonprofit healthcare organizations like the American Heart Association and requests from the American Red Cross or local blood bank for blood donors.
- Flyers on upcoming health fairs, including blood pressure or other health screening opportunities.
- Newspaper or magazine articles on interesting medical issues pertinent to the practice specialties.
- Community notices for food drives or similar charity events.
- Current information about practice staff and their accomplishments.

Finally, the bulletin board is an ideal place to display the office brochure. Put some extra copies of the brochure in an open envelope tacked to the bulletin board to encourage patients to take one home. To keep the bulletin board up to date, all time-sensitive materials, such as notices about a class or seminar, should be removed as soon as the date of the scheduled event has passed (Figure 7-5).

FIGURE 7-5 Keep the office bulletin board neat, current, and uncluttered so the information remains of interest to the patients.

Television and Videotapes

Although reading remains the traditional pastime in patient reception areas, watching television and DVDs is a common activity in physician offices across the country. Many patient reception areas now include a television, which can be tuned to regular or satellite news or entertainment stations or can play preselected videos. Physicians may provide informative healthcare videos of general interest to their patients or videos that meet the more specific interests of the practice. Videos are helpful for patients with limited reading ability and can also be helpful if customized for non-English speakers.

Accommodating Children

A pediatric reception area caters to a unique age group of patients. To accommodate this specialized clientele, in addition to regular chairs, child-size chairs may also be available. Playhouses or play furniture, like small tables, are also appropriate choices. The use of bright colors and storybook characters can also help to make the décor appealing to young children. It is important to make the setting feel familiar and comfortable. The reception desk may stock rolls of stickers or other inexpensive prizes to give to young patients after they have seen the doctor. Some pediatric offices have found it helpful to include two reception areas—one for well visits and one for children who are potentially **contagious**—to separate the sick children from those who are well.

Because children—even sick ones—do not usually like to sit still for long periods, you may want to consider including toys, games, videos, and books (Figure 7-6) in the pediatric reception area. If this reception area separates sick children from well children, the "well" side may include more active entertainment, like an indoor slide or playhouse, while the "sick" side may provide quieter games and activities, like books and puzzles.

Choose toys carefully. You do not want children—even well ones—to be too active in the reception area because they might

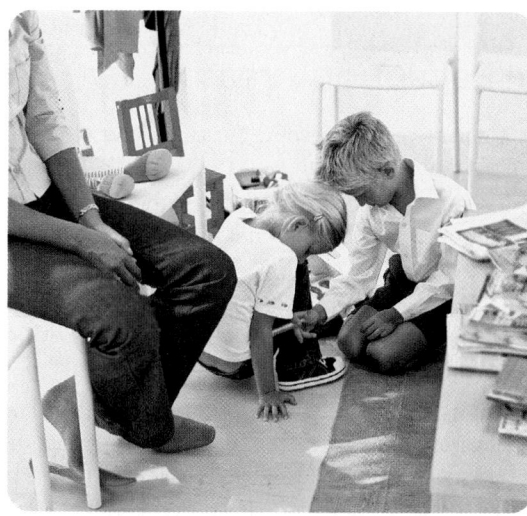

FIGURE 7-6 Toys, games, and videos that encourage quiet play are well suited for pediatric patient reception areas.

disrupt other patients and their families. Avoid balls, jump ropes, and other toys meant for outside use. Puzzles and blocks are good choices because they encourage quieter play. All toys should be easy to clean (a bleach-water solution or nonaerosol disinfectant can be used) and, for safety and health reasons, should not include stuffed animals. Stuffed animals are not appropriate because they are difficult to keep clean and can be a source of infection. Their small parts can also pose a choking hazard. You might informally ask parents and children if they like the play items or if they would prefer other types of toys. Procedure 7-1 explains how to set up a pediatric reception area.

▶ The Importance of Cleanliness   LO 7.2

No matter how tastefully it is decorated, the reception area will be unappealing if it is not clean. Patients expect a physician's office to maintain a high standard of cleanliness. The perception is that a messy or dirty reception area or patient bathroom reflects a practice that does not meet minimum standards for cleanliness. A practice with a spotless, attractive reception area reassures patients that they have chosen a practice with high standards of cleanliness. Another reminder of these high standards is the availability of alcohol-based hand rubs for patient use in the reception area (as well as in patient treatment areas) with directions for their use.

Housekeeping

Keeping the patient reception area neat and clean usually falls within the medical assistant's duties. In most cases, you will be responsible for supervising the work of a professional cleaning service. In a small medical office, you may be required to clean the area yourself, using appropriate antibacterial agents and a vacuum. Cleaning should occur daily, with emergency cleanups as needed.

Because professional services generally clean in the evening after business hours, you will probably not be present while the housekeeping staff is working. You may be asked to provide feedback to the cleaning company, however. It also may be your responsibility to outline the tasks you expect workers to complete, including any special requests.

One way of communicating with the cleaning staff is to create a Cleaning Communications Notebook. Arrange with the cleaning staff to leave the notebook open every evening in the same place. Date all entries. Write short, concise directions about any special requests for cleaning. Describe the nature of any stain so the service can best treat it. Sign each entry. Be sure to comment when something is done especially well. Like all of us, your cleaning staff likes to hear when they have done a particularly nice job.

Tasks Although housekeeping tasks vary from office to office, basic routines are applicable to areas like the patient reception room. The Caution: Handle with Care section gives more information about maintaining a clean reception area.

Whether or not the office employs a professional cleaning service, you or another staff member will need to check for cleanliness throughout the day. As patients spend time in the office, items may become soiled or be moved out of place. Taking time between patient appointments or at midday to spot-clean small areas that no longer appear "spotless" and to neaten items will help keep the patient reception area pleasing to the eye.

Equipment If you, and not a professional service, are responsible for cleaning, the person in charge of the office budget will approve the purchase of cleaning equipment and supplies. Examples of cleaning equipment include handheld and upright vacuums, mops, and brooms. Supplies include trash bags, cleaning solutions, cleaning rags, and buckets. It is a good idea to have some basic cleaning materials on hand in case an emergency cleanup job is needed during office hours. Always wear gloves when doing cleaning of any kind and use OSHA guidelines for safety. Be sure to also obtain the MSDS for any cleaning materials stored in the office and insert the sheets in the office MSDS binder.

Cleaning Stains

If furniture, carpet, or other items in the reception area become stained, it is important to remove the stains quickly. Follow these tips for stain removal:

* Try to remove the stain right away. The longer a stain remains, the more difficult it is to remove.
* Blot as much of the stain as possible before rubbing it with a cleaning solution.
* Take special precautions in handling stains involving blood, feces, and urine. Put on latex gloves before blotting or scraping up the stain.
* Wipe the area with a cleaning solution and water.
* Blood, urine, and feces may require special cleaners with an enzyme that breaks down organic waste.
* Use cold water instead of hot water because hot water often sets stains into the fabric.
* Keep all cleaning materials within easy reach for quick action when a stain occurs.

CAUTION: HANDLE WITH CARE

Maintaining Standards of Cleanliness in the Reception Area

Cleanliness is (and should be) one of a medical office's hallmarks. Not only is cleanliness required in the examination and testing rooms, it is also expected in the patient reception area. A messy patient reception area reflects badly on the practice. Patients may think, "If they don't care about this, what else do they not care about?" Maintaining standards of cleanliness helps ensure that the reception area is presentable and inviting at all times.

As a medical assistant, you may be involved—along with the physician, office manager, and other staff members—in setting the office's cleanliness standards. Standards are general guidelines. In addition to setting standards, you will need to specify the tasks required to meet each standard. You also may want to create a checklist of the tasks required to meet all of these standards.

The following list outlines standards you may want to consider. Specific housekeeping tasks for meeting those standards are included in parentheses.

1. Keep everything in its place. (Complete a daily visual check for out-of-place items. Return all magazines to racks. Push chairs back into place.)
2. Dispose of all trash. (Empty trash cans. Pick up trash on the floor or on furniture.)
3. Prevent dust and dirt from accumulating on surfaces. (Wipe or dust furniture, lamps, and artificial plants. Polish doorknobs. Clean mirrors, wall hangings, and pictures.)
4. Spot-clean areas that become dirty. (Remove scuffmarks. Clean upholstery stains.)
5. Disinfect areas of the reception area if they have been exposed to body fluids. (Immediately clean and disinfect all soiled areas.)
6. Handle items with care. (Take precautions when carrying potentially messy or breakable items. Do not carry too much at once.)

After the standards have been established, type and post them in a prominent place for the office staff (but not the patients) to see. The cleaning activities checklist may be posted, but the person responsible for cleaning the office also should keep a copy. It is everyone's duty to keep the office looking clean and presentable.

A schedule of specific daily and weekly cleaning activities also should be posted. Less frequent housekeeping duties, like laundering drapes, shampooing the carpet, and cleaning windows and blinds, can be noted in a tickler file so that they will be performed on a regular basis.

It is always a good idea to have a second staff member responsible for periodically working with the medical assistant on housekeeping responsibilities. That person also may be responsible for handling cleaning duties when the medical assistant is away from the office.

Removing Odors

Odors are particularly offensive in a medical office because people do expect (and should find) a high level of cleanliness. Because patients are in the office for a scheduled appointment, they cannot suddenly leave to escape the odor. Some odors that may occasionally be present in a medical practice include those of urine, feces, vomit, body odors, and laboratory chemicals. A good ventilating system with charcoal filters can help minimize odors. If the system has temporary high-speed blowers, they can be activated as well. Disinfectant sprays and deodorizing sprays also may help, but deodorizers should be used sparingly as more and more people are developing allergies to many of the scents used to mask odors.

One odor that can be prevented is smoke. Display "Thank You for Not Smoking" signs prominently in the patient reception area. Many offices, particularly those located in large buildings or attached to hospitals, are "nonsmoking zones." Smokers who visit these offices must leave not only the office, but the grounds, too, if they insist on smoking. This common rule is simply because not only does smoking produce an offensive odor, it also may affect the health of other patients in the reception area. People with asthma or other breathing disorders, or who are feeling unwell for any reason, are particularly sensitive to smoke and strong odors. It is up to the healthcare facility and its employees to protect their health while in the medical office and its grounds.

Infectious Waste

There may be times when you will need to clean up infectious waste. **Infectious waste,** also known as biohazardous waste, is waste that can be dangerous to those who handle it or to the environment. Infectious waste includes human waste, human tissue, and body fluids like blood and urine. It also includes any potentially hazardous waste generated in the treatment of patients, like needles, scalpels, cultures of human cells, and dressings.

Although infectious waste is not commonly generated in the patient reception area, it can happen—for example, when a patient vomits or bleeds on the rug or on furniture. If that situation should occur, you must clean up the waste promptly. Remember, infectious waste must be handled in accordance with federal law and following OSHA guidelines. Your office may choose to purchase commercially prepared hazardous waste kits for use in cleaning up spills. After cleaning infectious waste from the patient reception area, deposit it in a biohazard container. Disinfect the site to eliminate possible contamination of other patients. Refer to the chapter *Basic Safety and Infection Control* to review OSHA guidelines and Standard Precautions.

▶ Office Access for All

The path patients must take to get from the parking area or street to the office and then back out again is called the office access. Some offices have easier access than others, but ease of access is important to your patients, particularly those who are older or differently abled (see Figure 7-7).

Parking Arrangements

Although some patients walk to the medical office or take public transportation, the majority of patients will probably travel by their personal vehicles. Patients who drive to the office need a place to park.

The office can offer either on-street parking or a parking lot or parking garage. On-street parking requires patients to fend for themselves. They may have to put money into parking meters and parking spaces may be difficult to find. Both the money required and the potential problems in finding parking spots limit the ease with which patients can gain access to the office.

On the other hand, a free parking lot or parking garage improves office access. Parking lots and garages should be well lit for safety. To determine the number of parking spaces the office needs, calculate the average length of time a patient spends in the office from arrival to departure and the number of appointments scheduled during that time period. Allow one parking spot per appointment if most patients drive to the office and fewer if many use public transportation. In your count, be sure to include parking spaces for office staff. Periodically reevaluate the office's parking needs because they may change over time. All offices must also provide handicapped parking spaces for patients. Visit www.adaptiveaccess.com/handicap_parking.php for more information on handicapped parking. You will read more about patients with special needs later in the chapter.

Entrances

The entrance to the office should be clearly marked so that patients can find the office easily. The name of the practice and of the physician(s) should be on the door or beside the door.

FIGURE 7-7 All patients should have access to ample parking and easy access to the office.

Just outside the doorway should be a doormat to help control the amount of dirt tracked into the office. If the office door opens directly to the outside, people inside will feel a sudden change in temperature each time the door is opened in hot or cold weather. A foyer or double-door arrangement helps minimize the weather's effects by keeping the office at a consistent, comfortable temperature. All doorways must be wide enough to accommodate patients using wheelchairs and walkers. Hallways should be well lit and without obstructions.

Safety and Security

Safety and security are important concerns in any public building, and they are especially important for a medical office. To ensure both patient and staff safety, including protection from hazardous wiring or poorly lit hallways, there are guidelines for businesses, some of which pertain to the patient reception area. The medical office also must be secure from burglary.

Building Exits Make sure you and the office staff members are familiar with *all* building exits. It may be necessary to leave the office quickly, as during a fire, flood, or other emergency. You and other staff members must be prepared to assist and direct patients toward the exits in such a situation. Posting evacuation plans near each exit will assist staff and patients in the event of an emergency, necessitating evacuation of the building.

Ideally, the office should have at least two doorways that lead directly to the outside or to a hallway that leads to stairs (often in an emergency, elevators are inoperable). This arrangement affords patients and staff members the speediest, most direct route outside in case of an emergency. All exits must be clearly labeled with illuminated red "Exit" signs. These signs normally have a battery backup power system, which keeps them lit even during a power outage. Posting evacuation plans and displaying the nearest exits will assist staff and patients.

Having two or more exits also allows staff members to enter and leave the office during nonemergency situations without disrupting people in the patient reception area. Deliveries can also be made at the second entrance, further minimizing interruptions.

Smoke Detectors By law, a medical office is required to install smoke detectors that sound an alarm when triggered by heat or smoke. The office staff should be trained in the proper procedure if the smoke alarm sounds—including how to evacuate patients from the building efficiently. Smoke detectors must be checked regularly to ensure that they are operating properly.

Security Systems No matter where the medical office is located, a security alarm system is a wise investment, even if security personnel patrol the office building. A security alarm system offers valuable protection for the confidential patient information housed in a medical office. After the alarm system is installed, all office staff members should thoroughly familiarize themselves with it. They should be able to arm and disarm it easily and know what to do if it is accidentally activated. Each staff member should have her or his own individually assigned security access code. This number is required to authorize locking or unlocking the system. Like a credit card, bank, or other security PIN (personal identification number), it should never be shared.

Considerations for Patients with Special Needs

Some patients who come into the medical office will be disabled; that is, they were born with or have acquired a condition that limits or changes their abilities. A more positive way to refer to these patients who are differently abled is the use of the term *special needs*. For example, people who are paralyzed from the waist down have special needs; so do people who are visually impaired. This does not mean that these people cannot perform the same tasks that other people can; they may simply need special accommodations to do so. With some forethought and planning, the office can appropriately accommodate special needs patients. Ensuring wheelchair access through doors and hallways, as mentioned earlier, is just one way. Using ramps instead of steps, as shown in Figure 7-8, allows easier access not only for wheelchair users but also for others who have limited mobility. Allowing additional space in the reception area for wheelchairs, walkers, crutches, and guide dogs accommodates several types of special needs patients. Procedure 7-2, found at the end of the chapter, explains how to organize the patient reception area to meet the special needs of patients who are physically challenged. For more information on meeting the needs of the differently abled, visit the Adaptive Access website at www.adaptiveaccess.com/index.php.

Americans with Disabilities Act Individuals with special needs are often singled out for their differences and are sometimes discriminated against. For example, if a company building does not have access ramps for wheelchairs, workers in wheelchairs cannot qualify for jobs there. This would violate the **American with Disabilities Act (ADA)**, which prevents discrimination based solely on a person's physical or mental disability.

Passed in 1990, this federal act is sometimes referred to as the civil rights act for the disabled since it forbids discrimination based on physical or mental disabilities. The intent of the ADA is to provide equal access and reasonable accommodation in several important areas, including employment, facilities, sports, and education. The two sections involving medical practices are employment (discussed in the *Practice Management* chapter) and facilities. The following are required and reasonable facility accommodations:

- Handicapped parking.
- Wheelchair ramps.
- Wheelchair-accessible doors, halls, and bathrooms.
- Handrails in halls and bathrooms.
- Handicapped bathrooms including toilets, sinks, and room for a wheelchair to turn.
- Braille elevator floor indicators.
- Large-print patient forms.
- Devices to communicate with the hearing impaired, as discussed the *Telephone Techniques* chapter.

Service Animals A service animal may accompany a patient with special needs (Figure 7-9) into a medical office or facility. The dog is the most common service animal, but cats, monkeys, and even miniature ponies are in use. Service animals wear a special vest that identifies them and they should have a certification. Remember that these animals are not pets and they should not be distracted while "on duty." Service animals are well behaved and calm unless their charge appears to be threatened.

Vision and Hearing Impairments Although they should, there are still many offices that do not make special accommodations for patients with vision or hearing impairments. As a medical assistant, you can do your part in the office by posting prominent signs in the reception area with information that patients need to know. A staff member should

FIGURE 7-8 Ramps allow people using wheelchairs and other assistive devices easier access to the office.

FIGURE 7-9 Service animals should not be disturbed or distracted when working.

offer to assist patients with hearing or vision impairments as needed from the reception area to the examination room when it is their turn to see the doctor.

Patients who are hearing impaired may request the presence of a certified sign language interpreter to assist in communicating with the medical staff. If requested, federal law requires that the office provide and pay for this interpreter.

It is also helpful, but not required by law, to provide a device, also known as a telecommunications device for the deaf (TDD), for hearing-impaired patients. This specially designed telephone, formerly called a TTY (teletypewriter), looks very much like a laptop computer with a cradle for the receiver of a traditional telephone. The receiver is placed in the cradle and the hearing-impaired patient can then type the communication on the keyboard. The message can be received by another TDD or relayed through a specialty relay service.

Some states offer a relay service for patients with hearing impairments or speech disabilities. When an individual accesses this service through the TDD, the service then places the call using voice. It is important to understand that a relay service could call a medical office to make an appointment for a patient. The medical assistant needs to be careful to respond appropriately and not mistake the call as an unwanted marketing call. You will read about TDD in more detail in the *Telephone Techniques* chapter.

Older Americans Act of 1965
The fastest growing segment of the American population is the elderly. Like those who are differently abled, many elderly people face discrimination. One reason for the discrimination may be that with age come medical conditions and disorders that create physical limitations.

Congress passed the **Older Americans Act of 1965** to eliminate discrimination against the elderly. Among other benefits, the act guarantees elderly citizens the best possible healthcare regardless of ability to pay, an adequate retirement income, and protection against abuse, neglect, and exploitation.

What does the Older Americans Act mean for the medical office reception area? If the practice serves elderly patients, the office staff must be sensitive to their special needs. The patient reception area should be as comfortable as possible for patients with arthritis, failing eyesight, and other common ailments of the elderly. Make sure there are a few straight-backed chairs located near the front door and near the examination rooms. These chairs are easier to get into and out of than soft sofas and offer greater back support than low chairs or couches with sinking cushions. In addition, arms on chairs provide support when sitting and standing for patients who are unsteady.

Place reading materials within easy reach of the chairs so that elderly patients do not have to get up from their chairs for them. Have large-print books and magazines available, if possible, for patients with poor eyesight. You also might offer magnifying glasses for patients who like to use them. In addition, make sure that the print on all office signs is large and easy to read. As stated earlier, the patient reception area and restrooms should be well lit to help everyone, including elderly patients, see more clearly.

Special Situations Patients in a medical practice are usually a diverse group of people. Their interests, needs, and medical conditions can have an impact on the design of the reception area.

Patients from Diverse Cultural Backgrounds The United States has long been called a melting pot because of its mixture of people and cultures. Each culture lends its own special qualities, and together the cultures combine to create a unique blend of people called Americans.

You may work in a neighborhood that has a distinct culture or one in which many cultures are represented. To help patients feel comfortable, make the reception area reflect aspects of the local cultural backgrounds whenever possible. This effort will help patients feel more welcome.

Suppose, for example, that the medical office where you work serves many Latino patients. Posting signs in Spanish and English acknowledges the fact that both languages are spoken in that neighborhood. Providing reading materials, like newspapers and magazines, in a second language—for both adults and children—is another way to show respect and interest. Decorating the office for Spanish holidays in addition to American ones demonstrates that you care about what is important to patients. Displaying artwork created by local artists and artisans is another idea.

Patients Who Are Highly Contagious Patients may have to come into the physician's office when they are highly contagious. This fact is a concern for all patients, but it is especially critical for patients who are immunocompromised. The immune system of an immunocompromised patient is not functioning at a normal level. Because these patients do not have the normal ability to fight off disease, they are at greater risk than the average person for becoming sick. Patients undergoing chemotherapy and patients with AIDS, for example, have compromised immune systems.

To protect patients who are immunocompromised, as well as other patients and staff members, you may need to separate a highly contagious patient from the other patients in the reception area. Instead of having contagious patients wait in the reception area, for example, you might bring them directly into an examination room to wait. By screening patients for highly contagious conditions and taking such precautions, you can minimize the chances of exposing other people unnecessarily to potentially contagious conditions.

▶ Preventing Injury in the Front Office
LO 7.4

In addition to taking care of our patients, medical assistants also must be aware of their environment in the medical office and how it affects their ability to perform the job of medical assisting effectively.

The medical office environment's many work functions require many physical tasks. Examples are using the computer, carrying and unpacking boxes, filling copy machine trays, and helping patients with impairments. The associated movements are often performed using repetitive motions, like typing, lifting, bending, stooping, and sitting. In the chapter on *Basic Safety and Infection Control*, you learned how to prevent work-related injuries that can occur in the medical office. The most common office-related injuries are those occurring to office workers, including medical assistants, who spend much of their workday seated at a computer station. Common injuries or conditions involve the forearm, wrist, hand, and back. Table 7-1 contains ergonomic excerpts from an OSHA computer station checklist to use in prevention of these common injuries.

The ideal medical office environment is an efficient, safe, and caring place for patients, visitors, and staff. You will find the Caution: Handle with Care feature helpful in preventing carpal tunnel syndrome, as well as identifying the symptoms and treatments for CTS, should it occur.

TABLE 7-1   OSHA Computer Workstations Checklist
1. Head and neck to be upright, or in-line with the torso (not bent down/back).
2. Head, neck, and trunk to face forward (not twisted).
3. Trunk to be perpendicular to floor (may lean back into backrest but not forward).
4. Shoulders and upper arms to be in-line with the torso, generally about perpendicular to the floor and relaxed (not elevated or stretched forward).
5. Upper arms and elbows to be close to the body (not extended outward).
6. Forearms, wrists, and hands to be straight and in-line (forearm at about 90 degrees to the upper arm).
7. Wrists and hands to be straight (not bent up/down or sideways toward the little finger).
8. Thighs to be parallel to the floor and lower legs to be perpendicular to floor (thighs may be slightly elevated above knees).
9. Feet rest flat on the floor or are supported by a stable footrest.
10. Backrest provides support for your lower back (lumbar area).
11. Seat width and depth accommodate the specific user (seat pan not too big/small).
12. Seat front does not press against the back of your knees and lower legs (seat pan not too long).
13. Seat has cushioning and is rounded with a "waterfall" front (no sharp edge).
14. Armrests, if used, support both forearms while you perform computer tasks and they do not interfere with movement.
15. Keyboard/input device platform(s) is stable and large enough to hold a keyboard and an input device.
16. Input device (mouse or trackball) is located right next to your keyboard so it can be operated without reaching.
17. Input device is easy to activate and the shape/size fits your hand (not too big/small).
18. Wrists and hands do not rest on sharp or hard edges.
19. Top of the screen is at or below eye level so you can read it without bending your head or neck down/back.
20. User with bifocals/trifocals can read the screen without bending the head or neck backward.
21. Monitor distance allows you to read the screen without leaning your head, neck, or trunk forward/backward.
22. Monitor position is directly in front of you so you don't have to twist your head or neck.
23. Glare (for example, from windows, lights) is not reflected on your screen, which can cause you to assume an awkward posture to clearly see information on your screen.
24. Thighs have sufficient clearance space between the top of the thighs and your computer table/keyboard platform (thighs are not trapped).
25. Legs and feet have sufficient clearance space under the work surface so you are able to get close enough to the keyboard/input device.
26. Document holder, if provided, is stable and large enough to hold documents.
27. Document holder, if provided, is placed at about the same height and distance as the monitor screen so there is little head movement, or need to re-focus, when you look from the document to the screen.
28. Wrist/palm rest, if provided, is padded and free of sharp or square edges that push on your wrists.
29. Wrist/palm rest, if provided, allows you to keep your forearms, wrists, and hands straight and in-line when using the keyboard/input device.
30. Telephone can be used with your head upright (not bent) and your shoulders relaxed (not elevated) if you do computer tasks at the same time.
31. Workstation and equipment have sufficient adjustability so you are in a safe working posture and can make occasional changes in posture while performing computer tasks.
32. Computer workstation, components, and accessories are maintained in serviceable condition and function properly.
33. Computer tasks are organized in a way that allows you to vary tasks with other work activities, or to take micro-breaks or recovery pauses while at the computer workstation.

Source: www.osha.gov/SLTC/etools/computerworkstations/checklist.html (2012).

Carpal Tunnel Syndrome

As the number of computers used in the home and workplace has escalated in recent years, the number of cases of carpal tunnel syndrome also has risen dramatically. Carpal tunnel syndrome is a hand disorder often associated with computer use. The term for this condition comes from the name for a canal (the carpal tunnel) located in the wrist. Several tendons pass through this tunnel, allowing the hand to open and close.

Carpal tunnel syndrome results from repetitive motion, such as keyboarding, for hours at a time. This motion may cause swelling to develop around the tendons and carpal tunnel. The swelling compresses the nerve. The people most likely to develop this disorder are workers whose jobs require them to perform repetitive hand and finger motions.

Symptoms

The symptoms associated with carpal tunnel syndrome include

- Tingling or burning in the hands or fingers.
- Weakness or numbness in the hands or fingers.
- Hands that go to sleep frequently.
- Difficulty opening or closing the hands.
- Pain that stems from the wrist and travels up the arm.

Tips for Prevention

If you use a keyboard for extended periods, you should practice proper techniques, as outlined in the following bullets, to prevent carpal tunnel syndrome (Figure 7-10).

- While seated, hold your arms relaxed at your sides. Make sure your keyboard is positioned slightly higher than your elbows. As you input, keep your elbows at your sides, and relax your shoulders (see Figure 7-10).
- Use only your fingers to press keys and do not use more pressure than necessary. Use a wrist rest and keep your wrists relaxed and straight.
- When you need to strike difficult-to-reach keys, move your whole hand rather than stretching your fingers. When you

need to press two keys at the same time, such as "Control" and "F1," use two hands.

- Try to break up long periods of keyboard work with other tasks that do not require computer use.

Tips for Relieving Symptoms

If you have carpal tunnel syndrome symptoms, try these suggestions for relief:

- Elevate your arms.
- Wear a splint on the hand and forearm.
- Discuss your symptoms with a physician, who may prescribe medication.

FIGURE 7-10 Maintaining proper posture and hand position helps avoid straining of the neck, back, arms, and eyes when using a computer.

▶ Functions of the Reception Staff   LO 7.5

The person who works at the *front desk* is commonly called the receptionist. The receptionist's main function is to greet people, register them, give them direction, and answer the phone. In the past, people have taken the receptionist for granted, but truly, the receptionist is one of the most important people in the practice. Just as the reception area décor gives the patient his first impression of the office itself, it is the receptionist who gives the first impression of the office staff and sets the perception of the care the patient will receive from the medical staff. The multiple tasks the receptionist is responsible for provides the very basis for the patient's medical care and for the overall positive impression you wish to convey to your patients. It is

her attitude and communication skills that create this positive (or negative) first impression. This staff member, who is frequently an administrative medical assistant, should immediately acknowledge and greet the arriving patient with a smile and pleasant voice. If the receptionist is on the phone, looking up at the patient with a smile and head nod is appropriate to acknowledge the patient and let him know she will be with him shortly. This small gesture will convey that the office staff is attentive and put the patient at ease from the start of the appointment.

Patient Registration and HIPAA

Patient registration is often referred to as patient check-in or sign-in. In many offices, upon arrival, patients are asked to "sign in" to notify staff that they are there. Two commonly used forms of check-in or sign-in are the paper version and the digital or electronic version. Both may include the arrival time, the appointment time, and the practitioner's name. As you read earlier, under HIPAA, PHI (personal health information) is considered private and confidential; however, the rules do state that sign-in sheets are allowable, as long as the reason for the visit is not included on the sign-in sheet. If the physician specialty is of a confidential nature (like psychology or drug treatment), it is suggested that sign-in sheets not be used, as by the very nature of seeing the practitioner, an "assumption" about the nature of the visit can be made.

If an electronic sign-in is utilized, two methods are approved:

- Providing a digital pad (similar to electronic debit or charge).
- Use of a computer in the reception area for patients to input information.

Once the patient has signed in, the receptionist will provide him or her with appropriate forms. Returning patients may receive a copy of their information to update. Some offices will interview the patient, line-by-line, and input this information directly into the system (Figure 7-11). This method is usually more time-consuming than having the patient provide hard copy and then inputting directly from the form. Regardless of which method is used, the information given should be reviewed with the patient.

New patients receive a complete new patient registration packet that includes

- Demographic/insurance coverage form.
- Authorizations for release of information to insurance carriers, assignment of benefits, and financial responsibility.
- Notice of privacy practices.
- Health history.
- Information regarding the payment and other policies of the practice.

The forms must be completed and signed. The patient's or insured party's insurance card and a picture identifier like a driver's license are copied or scanned (Figure 7-12). The picture identifier is one method to help reduce healthcare

FIGURE 7-11 In some offices, new patients are interviewed to gather demographic information and their answers are directly inputted into the computer system.

FIGURE 7-12 Patient picture ID is either copied or scanned into the patient's record.

fraud, by preventing a friend or family member who may not have health insurance from "borrowing" another insurance card. The ID should be checked every time the patient comes into the office. You will explore medical identity theft in more detail a bit later in this chapter. From the demographic and health information provided by the patient, the medical assistant initiates a medical record or electronic health record. The record may be totally electronic or a combination of electronic health record and hard-copy financial information or electronic financial information and paper health record. The components of the medical record are covered in the *Medical Records and Documentation* and *Electronic Health Records* chapters. When all forms are completed and signed, the appropriate clinical staff member is notified that the patient is ready to be seen.

Payment

Another reception responsibility is collecting the patient's insurance copayment, which is usually done prior to the visit. The amount of the copayment, if applicable, is usually shown on the patient's insurance card. Depending on the office, acceptable payment methods are cash, check, debit, and charge cards. Third-party checks should never be accepted and any personal checks should be written for the exact amount. Cash and checks are kept in a cash drawer that is locked when the reception desk is unmanned. In some offices, the patient will return to the reception area after the visit and may make any payments due at that time. All financial transactions will be discussed in depth in the *Financial Management* chapter. Follow-up and referral appointments are often also scheduled at the front desk. Once all patient transactions are completed, the receptionist should extend a pleasant farewell to all patients.

Observation and Updates

Another function of the front desk staff is to be observant. As discussed earlier, some patients should not sit in the main reception area. These include patients who are

- Having chest pain (adults).
- Experiencing shortness of breath.
- Bleeding.

- Feeling faint (syncope), dizzy, light-headed.
- Vomiting.
- Experiencing an undiagnosed or contagious rash.

If a patient complains of any of these symptoms, or if you notice a change in a patient's status, immediately notify a member of the clinical staff, who will determine where to place the patient. If you are concerned about the condition of any patient, do not hesitate to ask the clinical staff for advice.

As mentioned earlier in the chapter, the receptionist (or any office staff member) should address spills, trash, and any potential hazards—like frayed cords, broken furniture, or tears in rugs—as quickly as possible. If the reception area becomes overcrowded, "traffic control" is required. Ensure chairs are not occupied with personal items and determine if there is room in treatment areas. Keeping patients updated if appointments are running late is another important function of the front office staff. If the wait time is significant, giving patients the option of rescheduling their appointments shows respect for the patient's time.

The Red Flags Rule

Identity theft is an increasing problem. **Medical identity theft** is using another person's name or insurance to seek healthcare. This form of identity theft results in millions of dollars in uncompensated care, and it creates the potential risk of a person receiving incorrect treatment if treatment is based on another person's medical record. On August 1, 2009, the Federal Trade Commission enacted the **Red Flags Rule.** This law requires certain businesses, including most medical offices and other healthcare facilities, to develop written programs to detect the warning signs, or red flags, of identity theft. The law applies to and defines two categories that determine if a business must comply. Both categories pertain to the majority of medical practices:

1. Creditors—entities that regularly defer payment for goods or services or arrange the extension of credit. An example of extending credit is billing patients after the service is rendered, including fees that are billed after insurance payments are received.
2. Covered account—a consumer (patient) account that allows multiple payments or transactions. Most patient records fall in this category.

Not adhering to the law may result in financial penalties. The more important issue is protection of the patients and the practice from the consequences of identity theft. The red flags include

- Suspicious documents.
  - Those with an altered or forged appearance.
  - Photo or description inconsistent with the patient's appearance.
  - Inconsistent information provided, such as date of birth, chronic medical condition.
- Suspicious personal identifying information from other sources like a Social Security number different from what you have on file.

- Suspicious activities such as mail being returned repeatedly but the patient continuing to keep appointments and maintain that address on file (this emphasizes the importance of verifying patient information at every visit), and inconsistency with physical exam and past medical treatment.
- Notifications of identity theft from patients or staff.

The Identity Theft Prevention Program

In many instances, HIPAA and medical identity theft go hand in hand. The person in the practice with the dual responsibility is generally the privacy or compliance officer. A three-pronged approach for the medical office's prevention program is recommended:

1. Prevention—implementing sound electronic and other security systems maintaining HIPAA compliance.
2. Detection—staff training on what to look for and electronic "red flagging" such as automatic on-screen identification of a difference in date of birth.
3. Mitigation—ensuring medical records of the perpetrator and the authentic patient are not co-mingled. The medical assistant should know what to look for in suspicious behaviors and both how to report such behaviors as well as how to find out if suspicious behavior by the patient has been previously reported.

▶ Opening and Closing the Office LO 7.6

You are learning that efficiency in the medical office is a result of good organization and adhering to office policies and procedures. These policies include establishing set procedures for opening and closing the facility. This is generally the responsibility of the staff member in the reception area. Following a set routine and using specially designed check sheets ensures no process is overlooked. Some offices perform specific tasks when opening the office, like restocking supplies, and other offices perform these tasks at closing. Let's take a general look at both of these procedures.

Beginning the Day

The person opening the office arrives approximately 30 minutes prior to the scheduled time for office operations to begin. Safety is a consideration. Be aware of the activity outside the office door such as persons in the parking area, elevators, or hallways. If you feel uncomfortable, notify the facility's security or await the arrival of another staff member. Laboratory specimens, like blood, obtained by staff for delivery to reference laboratories are often placed in a special container on the office door or in the vicinity. Upon arrival in the morning, ensure the specimens were picked up from the previous day. Do not completely turn your back while unlocking the door. Once inside, deactivate the security system.

The first priority is accessing the answering service or answering machine to determine if any staff member may have called in with an emergency, patients have canceled appointments, patients need a same-day appointment, or hospitals reported patients seen during the night. Convey this vital information to the correct staff member as soon as possible. The fax machine is usually the next priority: turning it on if it is not kept on at night, reviewing newly arrived faxes, distributing these faxes to the appropriate personnel, and ensuring the paper trays are full. Another task may be to turn on coffee makers for staff and patients. Some offices divide the responsibility for the administrative areas and the clinical areas. Table 7-2, Daily Checklist for Opening the Office, provides a general guideline for opening the medical office.

Ending the Day

Table 7-3, Daily Checklist for Closing the Office, includes typical duties for ending the day efficiently, which is just as important as beginning the day efficiently. It completes the day's responsibilities and sets the stage for the next day.

The person closing the office that has extended or split hours may not be the same person who opened the office. So, cooperation and good communication are essential between both staff members. Turn off equipment, like the coffeemaker and the fax machine, if that is the office policy. Check exam

TABLE 7-2 Daily Checklist for Opening the Office						
Daily Checklist for Opening BWW Medical Associates, PC W/E _____						
	M	T	W	Th	F	S
1. Security system is disarmed						
2. Voicemail/answering service messages are retrieved						
3. Messages are routed and ready for callback						
4. Fax machine is checked						
5. Computers are turned on						
6. Appointments and insurance rosters are checked						
7. Charts are pulled and paperwork is attached						
8. Equipment is working properly						
9. Rooms are supplied and ready						
10. Refrigerator temperature is checked						
11. Emergency supplies, including O_2, are checked						
12. Reception area is in order and patient education material is available						
13. Lab specimens from the day before were picked up						

TABLE 7-3 Daily Checklist for Closing the Office						
Daily Checklist for Closing BWW Medical Associates, PC W/E _____						
	M	T	W	Th	F	S
1. Computers are logged off and shut down						
2. Contaminated supplies/equipment are properly disposed of or tagged for cleaning/sterilization						
3. Areas are restocked						
4. Patient charts are pulled/reviewed for next day and all test results are available						
5. Laboratory specimens are in pick-up receptacle						
6. All office equipment is turned off (including kitchen)						
7. Reception area is neat and organized						
8. Calls are forwarded to voicemail/answering machine						
9. Medical records are secured						
10. All doors and windows are locked						
11. Security system is armed						

rooms to be sure supplies are well stocked for the next day and give the reception room one last "look" to be sure it is neat and presentable for the morning patients. Ensure that confidential information is not in view for any cleaning or security personnel that may enter the office after hours. Notify the answering service that the office is closing or turn on the answering machine. Ensure laboratory specimens are placed in the proper container for pick-up. Activate the security system (Figure 7-13).

Be alert when exiting the building for any unusual or suspicious activity. Refer to Procedure 7-3, Opening and Closing the Medical Office, for practice on these procedures. Following consistent policies and procedures guarantees that important tasks are not forgotten and, in this case, ensures that the office, its equipment, medications, and its private information remain safe and secure at all times.

FIGURE 7-13　Arming the office security system is usually the final task to end the workday.

PROCEDURE 7-1   Creating a Pediatric Reception Area

Procedure Goal: To create an appropriate environment for children in the patient reception area of a medical (pediatric) practice.

OSHA Guidelines: This procedure does not involve exposure to blood, body fluids, or tissue.

Materials: Children's books and magazines, games, toys, nontoxic crayons and coloring books, television and DVD player, children's DVDs, child- and adult-size chairs, child-size table, bookshelf, boxes or shelves, decorative wall hangings, or educational posters (optional).

Method: Procedure steps.

1. Place all adult-size chairs against the wall. Position some of the child-size chairs along the wall with the adult chairs.

2. Place the remainder of the child-size chairs in small groupings throughout the room. In addition, put several chairs with the child-size table.

3. Put the books, magazines, crayons, and coloring books on the bookshelf in one corner of the room near a grouping of chairs.

4. Choose toys and games carefully. Avoid toys that encourage active play, such as balls, or toys that require a large area. Make sure that all toys meet safety

guidelines. Watch for loose or small (smaller than a golf ball) parts. Toys should also be easy to clean.
   RATIONALE: Helps ensure safety in the patient reception area.

5. Place the activities for older children near one grouping of chairs and the games and toys for younger children near another grouping. Keep the toys and games in a toy box or on shelves designated for them. Consider labeling or color-coding boxes and shelves and the games and toys that belong there to encourage children to return the games and toys to the appropriate storage area.

6. Place the television and DVD player on a high shelf, if possible, or attach them to the wall near the ceiling. Keep children's DVDs behind the reception desk, and periodically change the video in the DVD player.
   RATIONALE: Doing so helps ensure safety in the patient reception area as DVDs and video equipment are easily damaged or destroyed by young patients. Young patients also may be harmed in trying to reach the equipment.

7. To make the room more cheerful, decorate it with wall hangings or posters.

PROCEDURE 7-2   Creating a Reception Area Accessible to Patients with Special Needs

Procedure Goal: To arrange elements in the reception area to accommodate patients with special needs.

OSHA Guidelines: This procedure does not involve exposure to blood, body fluids, or tissue.

Materials: Ramps (if needed), doorway floor coverings, chairs, bars or rails, adjustable-height tables, magazine rack, television/DVD player, large-type and Braille magazines.

Method: Procedure steps.

1. Arrange chairs to create gaps that allow substantial space along walls and near other chair groupings for wheelchairs. Keep the arrangement flexible so that chairs can be removed to allow room for additional wheelchairs if needed.
   RATIONALE: To meet all the requirements of the Americans with Disabilities Act.

2. Remove any obstacles that may interfere with the space needed for a wheelchair to swivel around completely. Also, remove scatter rugs or any carpeting that is not attached to the floor. Such carpeting can cause patients to trip and creates difficulties for wheelchair traffic.
   RATIONALE: Helps ensure safety in the patient reception area.

3. Position coffee tables at a height and location accessible to people in wheelchairs.

4. Place office reading materials, like magazines, at a height accessible to people in wheelchairs (for example, on tables or in racks attached midway up the wall).

5. Locate the television and DVD within full view of patients sitting on chairs and in wheelchairs so that they do not have to strain their necks to watch.

6. For patients who have a vision impairment, include large-type and Braille reading materials.

7. For patients who have difficulty walking, make sure bars or rails are attached securely to walls 34 to 38 inches above the floor, to accommodate requirements set forth in the Americans with Disabilities Act. Make sure the bars are sturdy enough to provide balance for patients who may need it. Bars are most important in entrances and hallways, as well as in the bathroom. Consider placing a bar near the receptionist's window for added support as patients check in.
   RATIONALE: To meet all the requirements of the Americans with Disabilities Act.

8. Eliminate sills of metal or wood along the floor in doorways. Otherwise, create a smoother travel surface for wheelchairs and pedestrians with a thin rubber covering to provide a graduated slope. Be sure that the covering is attached properly and meets safety standards.
   RATIONALE: Helps ensure safety in the patient reception area.

9. Make sure the office has ramp access.
   RATIONALE: To meet all the requirements of the Americans with Disabilities Act.

10. Solicit feedback from patients with physical disabilities about the accessibility of the patient reception area. Encourage ideas for improvements. Address any additional needs.
    RATIONALE: Doing so lets patients know that their comfort and well-being are important to you.

PROCEDURE 7-3   Opening and Closing the Medical Office

Goal: To ensure readiness and to receive and care for patients in an efficient, organized, and safe manner.

OSHA Guidelines: This procedure does not involve exposure to blood, body fluids, or tissue.

Materials: Checklist for opening and closing the office (Tables 7-2 and 7-3 may be used as samples), pen, telephone, and pad of paper.

Method: Procedure steps.

1. Using Table 7-2, Daily Checklist for Opening the Office, as a guide, simulate the functions of opening the office. Enter the week ending date.

RATIONALE: Using a checklist ensures no task is inadvertently skipped

a. Begin by disarming the security system.

b. Telephone the answering service to pick up messages or do the same using the office answering machine or voicemail system. Document any messages and notify the appropriate person of the call.

c. Conduct each task on the form, placing your initials in the column for the correct day of the week.

Daily Checklist for Opening BWW Medical Associates, PC	W/E ___					
	M	T	W	Th	F	S
1. Security system is disarmed						
2. Voicemail/answering service messages are retrieved						
3. Messages are routed and ready for callback						
4. Fax machine is checked						
5. Computers are turned on						
6. Appointments and insurance rosters are checked						
7. Charts are pulled and paperwork is attached						
8. Equipment is working properly						
9. Rooms are supplied and ready						
10. Refrigerator temperature is checked						
11. Emergency supplies, including O_2, are checked						
12. Reception area is in order and patient education material is available						
13. Lab specimens from the day before were picked up						

FIGURE Procedure 7-3 Step 1   Use a daily checklist when opening the office.

Daily Checklist for Opening BWW Medical Associates, PC	W/E 4/30/xx					
	M	T	W	Th	F	S
1. Security system is disarmed	mk					
2. Voicemail/answering service messages are retrieved	mk					
3. Messages are routed and ready for callback	mk					
4. Fax machine is checked	mk					
5. Computers are turned on	mk					
6. Appointments and insurance rosters are checked	mk					
7. Charts are pulled and paperwork is attached	mk					
8. Equipment is working properly	mk					
9. Rooms are supplied and ready	mk					
10. Refrigerator temperature is checked	mk					
11. Emergency supplies, including O_2, are checked	mk					
12. Reception area is in order and patient education material is available	mk					
13. Lab specimens from the day before were picked up	mk					

FIGURE Procedure 7-3 Step 1c   Insert your initials when each task is completed under the correct day of the week.

RATIONALE: It is important to know who performed each task in case questions arise.

2. Using Table 7-3, Daily Checklist for Closing the Office, as a guide, simulate the functions of closing the office. Enter the week ending date.

Daily Checklist for Closing BWW Medical Associates, PC	W/E					
	M	T	W	Th	F	S
1. Computers are logged off and shut down						
2. Contaminated supplies/equipment are properly disposed of or tagged for cleaning/sterilization						
3. Areas are restocked						
4. Patient charts are pulled/reviewed for next day and all test results are available						
5. Laboratory specimens are in pick-up receptacle						
6. All office equipment is turned off (including kitchen)						
7. Reception area is neat and organized						
8. Calls are forwarded to voicemail/answering machine						
9. Medical records are secured						
10. All doors and windows are locked						
11. Security system is armed						

FIGURE Procedure 7-3 Step 2   Use a daily checklist to close the office.

a. Begin with logging out and turning off the computers.

b. Use the telephone to turn on the answering machine/voicemail or notify the answering service that the office is closing.

c. Conduct each task on the form, placing your initials in the column for the correct day of the week.

RATIONALE: It is important to know who performed each task in case questions arise.

Daily Checklist for Closing BWW Medical Associates, PC	W/E 4/30/xx					
	M	T	W	Th	F	S
1. Computers are logged off and shut down	mk					
2. Contaminated supplies/equipment are properly disposed of or tagged for cleaning/sterilization	mk					
3. Areas are restocked	mk					
4. Patient charts are pulled/reviewed for next day and all test results are available	mk					
5. Laboratory specimens are in pick-up receptacle	mk					
6. All office equipment is turned off (including kitchen)	mk					
7. Reception area is neat and organized	mk					
8. Calls are forwarded to voicemail/answering machine	mk					
9. Medical records are secured	mk					
10. All doors and windows are locked	mk					
11. Security system is armed	mk					

FIGURE Procedure 7-3 Step 2c   Insert your initials when each task is completed under the appropriate day of the week.

SUMMARY OF LEARNING OUTCOMES

LEARNING OUTCOMES	KEY POINTS
7.1 List the design items to be considered when setting up an office reception area.	The size of the space you have to work with and the schedule of the physicians seeing patients must be considered first. Utilize the space to give as much room and privacy as possible. The décor should include a color family to suit the practice type. Furnishings should be comfortable, but easy to get in and out of, and easy to clean. Lighting should be appropriately bright to avoid accidental falls. Accessories like wall hangings, aquariums, coat racks, and magazine racks should complement the décor but not make the room feel cluttered. Current magazines and other reading materials on multiple topics should be available to entertain and inform the patient. TV and/or informational DVDs also may be played. If the practice sees children, special accommodations to entertain them also must be made.
7.2 Summarize the housekeeping tasks required to keep the reception area neat and clean.	Housekeeping tasks for the reception area include overseeing the professional cleaning staff (if one is employed), keeping everything in its place, disposing of trash, preventing visible dust and dirt on surfaces, spot-cleaning areas that become soiled, disinfecting areas exposed to body fluids, and handling items with care. OSHA guidelines should be followed in all aspects of keeping the office neat and clean. Standards of office cleanliness should be created and posted for all staff to see.

LEARNING OUTCOMES	KEY POINTS
7.3 **Relate how the Americans with Disabilities and Older American Acts have helped to make physical access to the medical office easier for all patients.**	The American with Disabilities Act and the Older Americans Act both prevent discrimination based solely on a person's physical or mental disability or his/her age. Both of these acts mandate accessibility for the differently abled, including, but not limited to, adequate parking for vehicles with and carrying assistive devices such as wheelchairs, ramps instead of stairs, wider doorways and hallways, well-lit areas throughout the office, large-print instructions, and Braille markings for elevators and other instructions.
7.4 **Articulate the cause of most injuries to medical officer workers and the four body areas where they occur.**	Most office-related injuries are those associated with repetitive motions, like typing, lifting, bending, stooping, and sitting. Common injuries or conditions involve the forearm, wrist, hand, and back.
7.5 **Explain the Red Flags Rule, giving the four red flags that the reception staff should be alert to.**	The Red Flags Rule was enacted to detect medical identity theft. The four red flags that all medical staff, particularly reception staff, should be alert to are suspicious documents, suspicious personal identifying information, suspicious activity like mail being returned although the patient insists the mail address is correct, and notification of identity theft by patients or staff.
7.6 **Implement policies and procedures for opening and closing the office.**	Maintaining specific policies and procedures for opening and closing the office ensures the necessary tasks are completed daily in a uniform manner. This results in an efficient and prepared medical office each day.

CASE STUDY CRITICAL THINKING

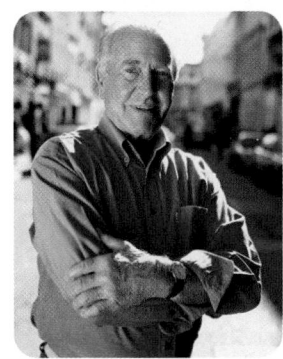

Recall Peter Smith from the beginning of the chapter. Now that you have completed the chapter, answer the following questions regarding his case.

1. How should you respond to Mrs. Smith's request that she be allowed to speak with Dr. Buckwalter privately?
2. Summarize your role as the "first person" Mr. Smith (and all patients) sees as he enters the office.

EXAM PREPARATION QUESTIONS

1. (LO 7.1) When designing the reception area for a medical practice, the first consideration should be the
  a. Color
  b. Furnishings
  c. Patient education material
  d. Type of practice
  e. Music

2. (LO 7.1) Which color family for the reception area would be best if the goal is to produce a calming effect?
  a. Reds
  b. Blues
  c. Greens
  d. Light browns
  e. Whites

3. (LO 7.2) Which federal agency produces guidelines for maintaining office cleanliness and the MSDS for cleaning solutions?
   a. HIPAA
   b. ADA
   c. OSHA
   d. FDA
   e. DEA

4. (LO 7.3) A violation of the ADA might be not permitting
   a. Smoking
   b. Pharmacy refills
   c. Charge cards
   d. Service animals
   e. Beverages in the reception area

5. (LO 7.3) Which of the following would show insensitivity to the Older Americans Act?
   a. Straight-back chairs with arms
   b. Wall-to-wall carpeting
   c. Large-print reading materials
   d. Slightly warmer reception room temperature
   e. Soft-cushioned sofas

6. (LO 7.4) Which injury may be caused by repetitive motions using a computer?
   a. Eye strain
   b. Scoliosis
   c. Arthritis
   d. Whiplash
   e. CTS

7. (LO 7.5) The receptionist's functions include all of these EXCEPT
   a. Greeting patients
   b. Registering patients
   c. Assisting with patient exams
   d. Giving directions
   e. All of the above

8. (LO 7.5) The federal law that involves medical identity theft is
   a. Red Flags Rule
   b. HIPAA
   c. Rule of Nines
   d. ADA
   e. None of the above

9. (LO 7.5) When the physician is running very late, the receptionist should
   a. Inform patients they will be seen soon
   b. Offer refreshments while the patients are waiting
   c. Cancel appointments
   d. Provide patients with the option to reschedule appointments
   e. Avoid eye contact with waiting patients

10. (LO 7.6) The best reason for consistent office closing procedures using a checklist is
   a. If someone forgets something, you will know who to blame
   b. The coffeemaker will not inadvertently be left on overnight
   c. The job will be rotated so the same person will not always have the responsibility
   d. Everyone will be able to "test" the alarm system at least once
   e. The office, its equipment, medications, and private information remain safe and secure at all times

Office Equipment and Supplies

CASE STUDY

Employee Name	Gender	Date of Hire
Miguel A. Perez	M	6/21/20XX
Position	Credentials	Supervisor
Administrative MA	CMA (AAMA)	Malik Katahri, CMM

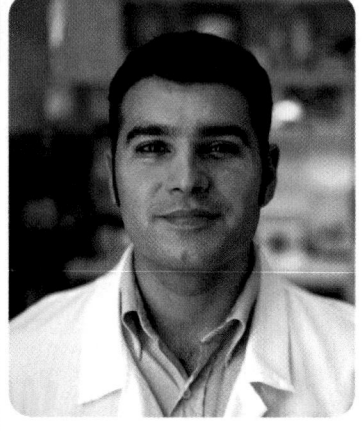

Miguel A. Perez is the CMA (AAMA) for BWW Medical Associates PC, a busy medical practice, and he is the first to arrive each morning. This morning, as Miguel walks through the office turning on the lights, he notices the fire extinguisher hanging on the wall. He makes a mental note to call the maintenance company today to notify them that the expiration date on the extinguisher is this month. They will replace the old one with a new extinguisher. Miguel continues through the quiet office and picks up three faxes in the fax machine that have come in overnight. He scans them quickly and places them in the center of his desk. He also checks the late-night pick-up specimen boxes, notes the specimens left last evening were picked up by the lab, and removes the lab reports left in the box by the lab. He switches on the copy machine, noting the number on the top of the machine, indicating the number of copies made this month. Because the office is billed based on how many copies are made each month, he will call the leasing company to report this number. Next, Miguel turns on his computer and reviews his calendar and task list for the day. He has received e-mail from another practice asking about a new referral and also an e-request for medical records. He prints out two computerized appointment listings for the day, placing one in the front office and one in the back office for easy reference. Because medical records in the office are computerized, he is grateful paper charts no longer need to be pulled. He takes a quick look around the administrative office to identify any items that need to be restocked, and he restocks the supply of pens and forms at the reception desk and makes sure the copier tray is filled with paper. He then scans the reception area to make sure it is neat and ready for the day.

Keep Miguel in mind as you study this chapter. There will be questions at the end of the chapter based on the case study. The information in the chapter will help you answer these questions.

LEARNING OUTCOMES

After completing Chapter 8, you will be able to:

8.1 Identify common types of computers.

8.2 Describe computer hardware components and explain the functions of each.

8.3 Describe the types of software applications commonly used in the medical office.

8.4 Summarize the options available for learning computer software programs.

8.5 Recall the steps involved in selecting new or upgrading existing office computer equipment.

KEY TERMS

central processing unit (CPU)

covered entity

cursor

database

digital subscriber line (DSL)

disbursement

disclaimer

hardware

icons

local area network (LAN)

optical character recognition (OCR)

purchase order

random-access memory (RAM)

8.6 Outline the basic care and maintenance required for the office computer system.

8.7 Identify several reasons why security is particularly important in the computerized office.

8.8 Recognize advances that are occurring with computers of the future.

8.9 Explain the function of other types of administrative medical office equipment.

8.10 Outline the steps to be taken in deciding whether new office equipment is needed.

8.11 Explain the difference between a maintenance contract and a service contract.

8.12 Define vital, periodic, and incidental supplies.

8.13 Outline the steps in performing a supply inventory.

8.14 List the items that should be considered when choosing a vendor for supply ordering.

KEY TERMS

read-only memory (ROM)

requisition

software

virtual private network (VPN)

wide area network (WAN)

MEDICAL ASSISTING COMPETENCIES

CAAHEP

IV. C (9) Discuss applications of electronic technology in effective communication

V. C (14) Discuss the importance of routine maintenance of office equipment

V. P (6) Use office hardware and software to maintain office systems

V. P (7) Use internet to access information related to the medical office

V. P (9) Perform routine maintenance of office equipment with documentation

V. P (10) Perform an office inventory

ABHES

7. **Basic Keyboarding/Computer Concepts**
Graduates:

b. Identify and properly utilize office machines, computerized systems, and medical software such as:
   (1) Efficiently maintain and understand different types of medical correspondence and medical reports
   (2) Apply computer application skills using variety of different electronic programs including both practice management software and EMR software

8. **Medical Office Business Procedures Management**
Graduates:

d. Apply concepts for office procedures

y. Perform routine maintenance of administrative and clinical equipment

z. Maintain inventory equipment and supplies

ll. Apply electronic technology

▶ Introduction

The modern medical office requires many different types of administrative equipment in order to function effectively and smoothly. In fact, it is fair to say that a medical office today without a computer, its related software, and other administrative equipment is like a car without gasoline. Your role as a medical assistant includes learning how to evaluate, purchase or lease, operate, and maintain this essential equipment.

Imagine how difficult it would be to function in our current culture's complex office environment without computers for claims submission, patient billing, payroll, bank deposits, and, of course, e-mail. Medical office staff also depend on copiers, fax machines, adding machines, and paper shredders to accomplish daily tasks efficiently. Going hand-in-hand with this equipment are the administrative supplies like paper and toner, as well as everyday consumable supplies like pens, pencils, highlighters, staples, paper clips, and tape.

In this chapter, you will learn about the use and maintenance of many important pieces of administrative medical office equipment. You also will become proficient in the process of keeping an inventory of not only the equipment in the medical office, but also the basic supplies needed to keep the office running efficiently.

▶ Computers
LO 8.1

Computer skills are essential for most career choices, and medical assisting is no exception. As a medical assistant, understanding the fundamentals of computers and their uses is a must. This knowledge will enable you to perform many office tasks with ease. The more you know about computers, the more easily you will be able to solve or avoid computer problems. Four basic types of computers are used today—supercomputers, mainframe computers, minicomputers, and personal computers (which include laptops, notebooks, subnotebooks, and PDAs)—and each type is suitable for a specific type of work in a particular kind of workplace.

Supercomputers

Supercomputers are the biggest, fastest, and most complex computers in use. Primarily used in research medicine—for genetic coding and for DNA and cancer research—supercomputers are considered to be the hope of tomorrow's medicine.

Mainframe Computers

Often used by government facilities and large institutions, including universities and hospitals, mainframes can process and store huge quantities of information. Large governmental service programs such as Medicare and Medicaid use mainframe computers.

Minicomputers

Minicomputers are smaller than mainframes but larger than personal computers. Minicomputers have traditionally been used in network settings. A *network* is a system that links several computers together. In this environment, a minicomputer typically functions as a server—a computer used as a centralized storage location for shared information. However, personal computers are becoming as powerful as minicomputers and may eventually replace them.

Personal Computers

Also called microcomputers, personal computers can be found in homes, offices, and schools. They are ideal for these settings because they are small, self-contained units. Because users have different needs, personal computers are available in several different types.

Desktop The most common type of personal computer in the medical office, a desktop model fits easily on a desk or other flat surface. The system unit of many desktop models is housed in a tower case, which is often placed on the floor next to the desk to allow more surface area at the workstation (Figure 8-1).

Laptop and Notebook A laptop computer is small, about the size of a magazine, and weighs only a few pounds.

FIGURE 8-1 The desktop computer is the most common computer type in the medical office.

Laptops operate either on battery power or on an AC adapter. Using laptops and notebook computers, physicians and other healthcare professionals can instantly communicate with the medical office computer, accessing data and information from other locations. With more and more offices utilizing electronic health records, laptops and notebooks are extremely popular in offices because they are mobile and can be moved between exam rooms.

Subnotebook and Tablet PC Subnotebooks, which have screens measuring 14 inches or less, are smaller than laptops but larger than handheld computers. Subnotebooks are now quickly being replaced by the tablet PC. These are slate-shaped mobile computers equipped with touchscreen and/or graphics table technology. This allows users to operate the computer with a stylus, digital pen, or simply the user's finger, instead of a keyboard or mouse.

Personal Digital Assistant (PDA) PDAs are common in medical offices and other healthcare facilities. Doctors often use them to look up medications and other reference information (Figure 8-2). They also may enter data that are transferred into a patient's chart.

Cell Phones and the Internet Cell phone use is so widespread that imagining your life without one may be near to impossible. The days of having a landline connection in your home, complete with an actual handset and separate phone for dialing, are almost a thing of the past. Cell phones are now most often used personally and not professionally. However, for research purposes, cell phone capabilities have increased exponentially in the last several years and will continue to expand. Smartphones using Android™, or a BlackBerry™, or Apple's iPhone allow users to access the Internet and perform multiple applications in addition to simply making phone calls

FIGURE 8-2 A PDA like this one can be added to the office computer network.

and sending text messages. Many "techies" believe that cell phones are the "computers of the future." Cell phones will be discussed in more detail in the *Telephone Techniques* chapter.

▶ Components of the Computer   LO 8.2

When most people talk about computer components, they are referring to the computer **hardware** or its physical components which include the monitor, keyboard, and printer. Let's look at each component in more detail here.

Hardware

Computer hardware components are responsible for performing each of four main functions: inputting data, processing data, storing data, and outputting data. In order to work, unless the office is set up with wireless capability and wireless devices are purchased, hardware devices must be connected by a cable, such as a USB or serial cable. In the paragraphs that follow, you will explore the four main types of computer hardware—input devices, processing devices, storage devices, and output devices—and their respective role in the medical office.

Input Devices For a computer to handle information like patient records, the data must first be entered, or input. Several types of input devices—keyboards, touch screens, pointing devices, modems, and scanners—may be used to enter data into the computer. After this information is entered, it can be displayed on the monitor, processed, printed, or stored.

Keyboard The keyboard is the most common input device. The main part of a keyboard resembles a typewriter, but most keyboards have several additional key types.

When you use the keyboard, it is important to position your hands properly to avoid injury. Refer to the *Patient Reception* chapter for more information on how to prevent and cope with carpal tunnel syndrome, a condition resulting from repetitive motion such as using a computer keyboard.

Pointing Device Many software programs require both a keyboard and a pointing device to enter information into the computer. The three common types of pointing devices are the mouse, the touch pad, and the touch screen.

- A *mouse*, the most common pointing device, has two or three buttons on top and sometimes a rolling ball on the bottom. A laser mouse detects movement through a laser and does not have a ball. As you move the mouse across a flat surface or mouse pad, you cause a light-sensing device on the bottom to move. This controls an arrow on the screen that points at the desired button or on-screen object. Then you push one of the buttons on the mouse to access a function, like opening a file.

- A *touch pad* is a form of pointing device common on laptops and notebooks. It is a small, flat device that is highly sensitive to the touch. To move the on-screen arrow, you simply slide your finger across the touch pad. To click on an item, you push a button similar to that on a mouse or trackball, or you tap your finger on the touch pad.

- A *touch screen* is a monitor screen that is illuminated at the touch of a pen, wand, or finger. When an object is touched on the screen, the touch itself acts as a pointing device and conveys information to the computer. Touch screens are increasingly being used in clinical and hospital settings, as they are now commonly found with notebooks, iPads, and smart phones.

Modem The term *modem* is the shortened form of the words *modulator-demodulator*. A modem is used to transfer information from one computer to another over telephone lines. Because modems allow information to be transferred both to and from a computer, they are considered input/output devices. Modems are essential for any medical office that needs to transfer files electronically, as when submitting insurance claim forms. Modems can be internal or external, as well as wireless. The three standard types of modems are cable modems, digital subscriber line modems, and fax modems.

- A cable modem is a modem that operates over cable television lines to provide fast Internet access.

- **DSL (digital subscriber line)** modems operate over telephone lines but use a different frequency than a telephone frequency. This type of modem allows computer Internet access and telephone use at the same time.

- A fax modem is an advanced type of modem that allows the computer to send and receive files much as a fax machine does. A fax modem is not quite as versatile as a regular fax machine, as the information being sent must first be input into the computer. In addition, without the use of a scanner, you cannot use a fax modem to send a patient record with handwritten notes on it.

Scanner A scanner is a device used to input printed matter and convert it into a readable format for the computer. Scanners are useful in the medical office because patient reports (from another doctor, hospital, or outside source) can be easily entered into the computer and, often, directly into the patient medical record. This makes it possible to move into a paperless medical system. Using a scanner is much faster than keying, or inputting the information with a keyboard. Three types of scanners are available:

- Handheld scanners are generally the least expensive but are more difficult to use and produce lower-quality results than the other two types.
- A single-sheet scanner feeds one sheet of paper through at a time and looks similar to a single-sheet printer.
- A flatbed scanner is the most expensive type of scanner but is the easiest to use and produces the highest-quality input. It works much like a small photocopier: the paper lies flat and still on a glass surface while the machine scans it. Today, many photocopiers are configured with a scanning capability and can transmit the images of scanned documents directly into computers.

Processing Devices There are two major processing components inside the system unit, or computer cabinet: the motherboard and the central processing unit. The *motherboard* is the main circuit board that controls the other components in the system. The **central processing unit (CPU),** or microprocessor, is the primary computer chip responsible for interpreting and executing programs. The CPU is considered the most important piece of hardware in a computer system because it interprets instructions from software programs. Without a functioning CPU, the software programs will not run.

Storage Devices One of the computer's main tasks is to store information for later retrieval. The computer uses memory to store information either temporarily or permanently. Several types of drives are used for permanent information storage.

Memory Computers use two types of memory to store data: **random-access memory (RAM)** and **read-only memory (ROM).** RAM is temporary, or programmable, memory. While you are working on a software program, such as Microsoft® Word, the computer is accessing RAM. In general, the more RAM that is available, the faster the computer will perform. As software programs become more sophisticated, they require more RAM.

ROM is permanent memory. The computer can read it, but you cannot make changes to it. An example of ROM is Windows® 7, a computer operating system. The purpose of ROM is to provide the basic operating instructions the computer needs to function.

Hard Disk Drive The hard disk drive is where information is stored permanently for later retrieval. Software programs and important data are usually stored on the hard disk for quick and easy access. The amount of hard disk space needed to store software programs is increasing rapidly. The more software programs you want to store, the larger the hard disk you will need.

Removable Drives Removable drives consist of CDs, jump drives, tape drives, zip drives, and DVDs.

- *CD-ROM drive.* CD-ROMs look just like audio compact discs, but they contain software programs. The term CD-ROM stands for "compact disc—read-only memory." A CD-ROM can include videos and sound. For instance, a CD-ROM medical dictionary may provide not only the spelling of terms, but also the spoken pronunciation of the terms, and diagrams and videos to aid in understanding. CD-ROMs also can be used to back up information from the hard drive. Multimedia refers to software that uses more than one medium—like graphics, sound, and text—to convey information (Figure 8-3).

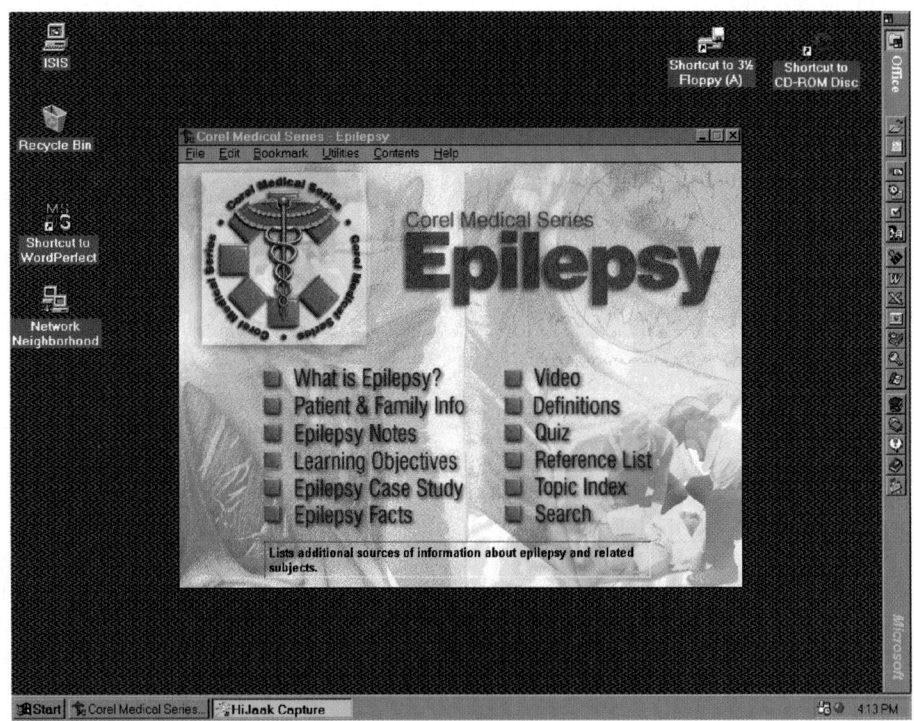

FIGURE 8-3 A multimedia program provides both visual and audio information.

- *CD burner or recorder.* Most modern computers also have a CD burner or recorder (CD-R), which allows information to be taken from one CD (or any other source) and "burned" to another CD.

- *External hard drive.* It is not uncommon in larger offices to use a separate computer hard drive as a backup, or to hire a company to back up the files nightly or weekly via the Internet, and store them in a separate facility.

- *Jump drive.* A jump drive—also called a flash drive, pen drive, key drive, memory key, flash key, or USB drive—is an externally attached drive that is small enough to be carried on a key chain, yet holds 16 gigabytes or more of data. It provides easy portability for large bodies of data, and may be used for backup operations in a medical practice when stored off-premises. Jump drives attach to the CPU via the USB ports found on the front, back, or side of the CPU device (see Figure 8-4).

- *Zip drive.* A zip drive is a high-capacity floppy disk drive developed by Iomega™. Zip diskscan hold up to 750 MB of data. Zip drives are durable, are relatively inexpensive, and may be used for backing up hard disks and transporting large files.

- *DVD.* DVD (digital video disc) is optical disc storage technology. It is similar to CD technology except it is faster and can hold more information. One double-sided, dual-layer disk can store about eight hours of high-quality video.

Output Devices Output devices are used to display information after it has been processed. A monitor and a printer are two output devices needed in the medical office.

Monitor The monitor displays currently active information, such as a word processing document, an Internet link, or e-mail. In many healthcare facilities, LCD (liquid crystal display) monitors are commonly used. LCD screens provide for better privacy than the older, bulkier models because they cannot be seen from the side. They also generate less heat than older models.

Resolution refers to the crispness of the images and is measured in dot pitch. The lower the dot pitch, the higher the resolution. For example, a monitor with a 0.26 dot pitch displays sharper images than a monitor with a 0.39 dot pitch. Using a high-resolution monitor can help you avoid eye strain. Monitors are also available in a variety of sizes to suit the needs of the user.

Printer A printer is required to produce a *hard copy*—a readable paper copy or printout of information. You will need a printer to print out correspondence, patient reports, bills, insurance claims, and other documents. Printer resolution is noted in terms of dots per inch (dpi). The higher the dpi, the better the print quality. Printer output varies, depending on the printer type and model. The two most commonly used printers are laser and ink-jet.

- Laser printers are high-resolution printers that use a technology similar to that of photocopiers. They are the fastest type of printers, produce the highest-quality output, and are now the most common type of office printer. Their cost has decreased as technology has improved.

- Ink-jet printers are nonimpact printers that form characters using a series of dots created by tiny drops of ink. Many ink-jet printers are capable of printing in both black ink and color. Because of their high-quality output and affordable prices, ink-jet printers are popular small-office use.

A current trend in printers is the "all-in-one" model (Figure 8-5), which functions not only as an ink-jet or laser printer but also as a fax machine, scanner, and photocopier. This type of machine may be convenient for a small medical office that requires each of these functions but does not have space for four separate devices. In addition, purchasing an all-in-one unit is usually more economical than purchasing the machines separately.

FIGURE 8-4   Plugging a jump drive into the USB port of a CPU.

FIGURE 8-5   An all-in-one printer-scanner-fax machine can be networked to multiple computers in the office.

▶ Software

The program or set of instructions that tells the computer what to do is known as its **software.** Computer software is generally divided into two categories: operating system and application software. The operating system controls the computer's operation. Application software allows you to perform specific tasks, such as scheduling appointments.

Operating System

When you turn on a computer, the operating system starts working, providing instructions that the computer needs to function. Examples of operating system software include Microsoft® Windows® XP, Microsoft® Windows® 7, and Linux. Most computers come pre-installed with Windows® XP or Windows® 7.

Operating system software is sometimes referred to as the platform for the system. Most medical practices use IBM-compatible personal computers, which are very suitable for businesses that use computers primarily to manipulate words. On the other hand, advertising agencies or design firms, which are extensively involved in graphics, visual images, or desktop publishing, tend to use Apple® (Macintosh-MAC) computers.

Windows This operating system employs a graphical user interface (GUI). With a GUI, menu choices are identified by **icons,** or graphic symbols (Figure 8-6). For example, the "Print" command is usually identified by a button with a tiny illustration of a printer on it. To print a document, you move the pointing device until the arrow is on the printer icon and then click the button.

Windows operating systems are easy to learn because you do not have to remember commands. Instead, you simply need to recognize the icon to know what command will be performed if you click that icon with the mouse. Another benefit of Windows is that it is a "multitasking system," so users can run two or more software programs simultaneously. You could, for example, enter patient information into a **database** (a collection of records created and stored on the computer), while a word processing program is running in the background.

Applications

Most of the software sold in stores is application software like Microsoft® Office. Microsoft® Office includes word processing (Word), presentation software (PowerPoint), spreadsheets (Excel), database management (Access), and desktop publishing (Publisher). Medical Manager®, Medware®, Medasis, and MediSoft™ are practice management applications. These software packages are specifically designed to meet the needs of a medical practice. Standard computer practice management software packages can be purchased, and custom-made practice management software can be designed to meet the needs of a particular practice. Word processing, database, and accounting software are just a few examples of the wide variety of applications available.

Optical Character Recognition Optical character recognition (OCR) software enables the conversion of images to text so they can be treated like any other type of word processing document. An OCR system includes an optical scanner for reading text and state-of-the-art software for analyzing images. An OCR system enables an article or patient file to be fed into an optical scanner, where it is transferred into an electronic computer file. It is then possible to manipulate and edit the file using a word processor.

Using Application Software

Computer software has been developed for nearly every office function imaginable. Using software, you can complete tasks with greater speed, accuracy, and ease than with a manual system. Learning how to use the software correctly, however, is the key to getting the most out of your computer system.

Word Processing In the medical office, as in any office, word processing is a common computer application. It has replaced the typewriter for writing correspondence and reports, transcribing physician notes, and performing many other functions. With word processing, a form letter can be merged with a patient mailing list to create letters that are personalized with patients' names without having to retype each letter.

Database Management A database is a collection of records created and stored on a computer. In a medical office, databases are used to store patient records such as billing information, medical chart data, and insurance company facts. These records can be sorted and retrieved in many ways and for a variety of purposes. You may be asked to find, add to, or modify information in a database. For example, you might use a database to determine all the patients covered by a particular insurance company. Microsoft Access® is a common database management software program.

FIGURE 8-6 MS Word 2007 formatting toolbar with GUI icons, pointing out the Printer icon.

Accounting and Billing Accounting and billing software is extremely useful in an office environment. It enables you to perform many tasks, including keeping track of patients' accounts, creating billing statements, preparing financial reports, and maintaining tax records. (You will learn more about billing and accounting functions in the *Insurance and Billing* and *Financial Management* chapters.)

Appointment Scheduling Instead of writing in an appointment book, you can use software to schedule appointments. Some scheduling packages allow you to enter patient preferences, like day of the week and time, and then to list available appointments based on that information. If the office system is on a network, scheduling software is particularly valuable because more than one user can access the appointment schedule at a time (Figure 8-7).

Electronic Transactions Using a computer equipped with a modem and communications software, you can perform several types of electronic transactions. This technology enables you to send and receive information instantaneously rather than waiting the days or weeks required for regular mail. Common electronic transactions include sending insurance claims and communicating with other computer users. Electronic medical records can easily be sent anywhere in seconds.

Sending Insurance Claims In the majority of medical offices, insurance claims are submitted electronically directly from the medical office to an insurance company. This procedure enables claims to be processed quickly and efficiently. (The *Insurance and Billing* chapter discusses health insurance billing procedures.)

Communicating The ability to communicate and share information with other computer users and systems is important in many medical offices. This communication may take place through electronic mail, online services, and the Internet. The Points on Practice section gives valuable ideas for saving time online.

- *Electronic mail.* Commonly known as e-mail, electronic mail is a method of sending and receiving messages almost instantly through a network. Through e-mail, it is possible to communicate with computer users in your own office, across town, or on the other side of the world. The use of e-mail in a professional context, including appropriate formats and confidentiality, is discussed in more detail in the *Written and Electronic Documents* chapter.

- *Online services.* These services, known as servers, provide a means for healthcare professionals to communicate with one another. Most online services contain forums that offer information and discussion groups focusing on a wide range of

FIGURE 8-7 SpringCharts™ screen showing office appointment schedule.

TABLE 8-1 Medical Resources on the Internet

Organization	Web Address	Description
American Medical Association	www.ama-assn.org	News announcements and press releases; articles from *JAMA* and other AMA journals; links to other medicine-related Internet sites
eMedicineHealth	www.emedicinehealth.com	Health resource center containing information about health issues and the latest treatments available
MedlinePlus®	http://medlineplus.gov	A service of the U.S. National Library of Medicine and NIH; site includes current health news; a medical encyclopedia; and directories for doctors, dentists, and hospitals
National Institutes of Health	www.nih.gov	Medical news and current events; press releases; biomedical information about health issues; scientific resources; links to Internet sites of related government agencies
National Library of Medicine	www.nlm.nih.gov	Internet site for world's largest biomedical library; research and developmental activities; connections to online medical information services
New England Journal of Medicine	http://content.nejm.org	Articles and abstracts; archives of past issues
Virtual Hospital	www.healthcare.uiowa.edu/Radiology	Information on a variety of health issues, medical resources, tutorials and multimedia textbooks
WebMD Health®	www.webmd.com	Trustworthy, credible, and timely health information written by experts in medicine, journalism, and health communications

medical topics. Healthcare workers can learn about the latest medical research and technology or exchange ideas with others in their field. In addition, some online services provide access to medical databases like MEDLINE®, created by the National Library of Medicine. Users can search MEDLINE® for records and abstracts from thousands of medical journals around the world.

- *Internet.* The Internet is a global network of computers. E-health or medical information and products are easy to access worldwide via the Internet. Many large medical facilities, universities, and other organizations—such as the National Institutes of Health (NIH) and the Centers for Disease Control and Prevention (CDC)—provide medical resources, databases, and other information on the Internet. Table 8-1 describes some popular medical resources available on the Internet.

The Internet has also become a profitable marketing tool for medical practices. Medical websites can generate more new patients than paper advertising. Within the website, doctors can include patient education, newsletters, referring provider forms, and other patient-related information. Additionally, patients can e-mail the medical office personnel to ask questions and find out other pertinent non-PHI (protected health information).

▶ Software Training

LO 8.4

Software programs may seem quite complex, especially at first. Most people need a period of training before they feel comfortable using the application. Several methods of training—some from outside sources and some provided by the software manufacturer—are available.

Classes

Many computer vendors offer training classes for the software packages they sell. In addition, community colleges and high schools sometimes offer adult education classes for a variety of applications, including word processing and communications. These classes may be at the beginner, intermediate, or advanced level.

Tutorials

Several software packages come with a *tutorial*, which is a small program designed to give users an overall picture of the product and its functions. The tutorial usually provides a step-by-step walk-through and exercises that allow you to try out your newly acquired knowledge. (See Figure 8-8.)

Documentation

Nearly all software manufacturers provide some type of documentation with their programs. Documentation is usually in the form of written instruction manuals or online help that is accessed from within the program.

Technical Support

A software company's technical support service is designed to assist you with problems that go beyond the scope of the user's guide or manual. A call to technical support is important when you encounter a problem that cannot be solved by simple problem-solving techniques. By calling a toll-free number, you can access a knowledgeable team who will listen to the description of the problem and suggest solutions over the phone.

Before calling technical support:

- Check the system for errors to the best of your ability.
- Check your manual for answers. Ask your supervisor for assistance.
- Have the software registration number available.
- Be prepared to follow the technical support personnel's instructions.
- Allow uninterrupted time to spend on the phone with the technical support person.
- Plan to call from a location that gives ready access to the problem computer.

Technical support is also helpful when you are upgrading software and can be a good source of information regarding the

FIGURE 8-8 Software programs like SpringCharts™ provide help screens and demo guides (tutorials) to assist you before you begin or when working with the software.

latest products and their applications. Some software companies automatically notify their customers of available upgrades.

▶ Selecting Computer Equipment   LO 8.5

Most medical offices are computerized, so if the decision is made to upgrade the system, you may be a part of the decision-making process in selecting equipment. As a medical assistant who will be using the system, you may be asked for your input in selecting software, adding a network, or choosing a vendor.

The first step for helping in the selection process is to learn as much as you can about hardware and software. You can get information by taking an introductory computer class at an adult school or community college; by reading computer magazines or books; or by talking to friends, relatives, or coworkers who use computers.

Upgrading the Office System

Computer hardware is changing and improving at such a rapid pace that a system seems to become outdated almost as soon as it is purchased. In addition, more advanced software is introduced every day, and this software requires more advanced hardware in order to run. So, an office system purchased only a year or two ago may need to be upgraded. Sometimes an upgrade simply requires replacement or addition of certain components. For instance, a laser printer can take the place of an ink-jet printer or a CD burner can be added. In other cases, such a solution is not possible or cost-effective, so an entirely new system must be purchased.

Selecting Software

After a decision is made regarding the type of software needed, such as an accounting program, a specific product must be chosen. To make an informed decision, you can read software reviews in computer magazines or trade publications. Check with other medical offices to get opinions on software packages. A crucial step in selecting software is to make sure the office computer system meets the minimum system requirements listed on the software box.

Adding a Network

There are several advantages to adding a network to the medical office's computer system. A computer network enables users to share software programs and files and allows more than one person to work on the same patient's information at one time. While you are working on a patient's insurance claim, for example, another medical assistant might be inputting billing information. Some medical offices are virtually paperless, using a highly sophisticated network with a notebook or desktop computer in every examination room. Doctors input information into patients' computerized records. If a doctor is in her office and a patient is waiting, a staff member at the front desk sends an e-mail message to the doctor's desktop computer and a beep sounds as an alert. Networks also allow large medical facilities to communicate with employees via e-mail. For instance, an internal memo about changes in office policies may be sent by e-mail to all employees. For networks to operate, the computer must have either a network

Working Efficiently Online

If the medical office where you work is computerized, the system most likely has a modem for sending e-mail and transferring files electronically, as well as accessing various online services and the Internet. If this access is not currently available in the office, it probably will be in the near future, and you may even be asked to help choose the service provider that is most appropriate for your office.

These services, known as *Internet service providers (ISPs)*, allow access to a network of servers that provides a means for healthcare professionals to communicate with one another.

Choosing an Online Service

Compare several services for the following features:

- The speed and accessibility of services. A cable modem or DSL through the phone line has faster speeds for communicating information than regular phone line service. Also, these services are always on and do not interfere with the telephone service at the facility.
- Free trial membership. Many services offer a free 1-month membership to try out the service. The trial periods enable office staff members to test several services to determine which one best suits their needs.
- Availability of healthcare information. Some online services provide discussion groups (commonly known as chat rooms) and resources that would be useful to the medical office. Other services may not offer as much relevant information. By comparing several services, you can determine which service best meets the needs of the practice.
- Extra fees for online information. Although access to most of the information found online is free, some online sites may charge a fee. For example, if you want to read the full text or print medical journal articles you may need to join and pay a fee to a professional association. Make sure you consider these extra fees when budgeting for needed online services.

Sending and Receiving E-mail

When using e-mail, follow these guidelines to manage your online time efficiently:

- Use computerized address books. As part of the e-mail system, most services provide an online address book for storing frequently used e-mail addresses. Instead of wasting time searching for an e-mail address in a standard card file, you simply click on the person's name in the address book and the mail is automatically sent to that person. You also can use the address book to send the same e-mail message to several people at once. If one message is being sent to several people, you can bcc (blind copy) the other recipients. By using bcc, you are protecting the privacy of other recipients' e-mail addresses.

  To use bcc effectively, insert your own e-mail address in the TO box. In the BCC box, enter the e-mail addresses of the people you wish to receive the e-mail. Each recipient will see only your name and e-mail address and no one else's, thus protecting the privacy of each person's e-mail address.
- After sending an e-mail, watch for any alert that the message did not go through. If an alert appears, check the address again and resend the e-mail.

Doing Research

Although a great deal of valuable information can be found through online services and the Internet, searching for this information can be time-consuming. To make the most of your online time, follow these tips:

- Use the favorite places feature to keep a list of favorite places, or sites that you visit frequently.
- Refine your searches. Searching for *arthritis*, for example, might produce hundreds of references that you would have to read through to determine their relevance. Narrowing your search to *juvenile rheumatoid arthritis*, on the other hand, would produce fewer references and more exact matches.
- Download files. *Download* means to transfer a file to the hard disk. Instead of reading through information while you are online, download the files to retrieve them or print to read later.

interface card or a wireless connection to the network. Networks can be run with Windows®, Novell®, or Unix® network operating systems.

Virtual Private Networks

When a group of two or more computer systems are linked together, it is known as a network system. The computers in a **local-area network** (**LAN**) are geographically close together (for example, in the same building). The computers in a **wide-area network** (**WAN**) are farther apart and are connected by telephone lines. **Virtual private networks** (**VPN**) are used to connect two or more computer systems. They are also constructed using public telephone lines and use the Internet as the medium for transporting data. VPNs use encryption and other security methods to ensure that only authorized users can access the network. This type of network makes it possible for physicians to access patient records in a secure manner from a variety of locations.

Choosing a Vendor

When purchasing computer equipment, you should look for a reputable vendor who not only offers a reasonable price but also provides training, service, and technical support. A first step might be to check with personnel in other medical offices that use a computer system. Find out which dealer they use and if they are satisfied with the system, salespeople, and support. You also can ask dealers for references from medical offices that have purchased systems from them. It is a good idea to get cost estimates from at least three vendors, and it is preferable to buy all hardware components from the same vendor.

▶ Computer System Care and Maintenance LO 8.6

Like a car, a computer needs routine care and maintenance to stay in sound condition; the computer user's manual outlines the steps required. Also, a good general rule is not to eat or drink near the computer. Crumbs and spilled liquids can damage the system components and storage devices.

Care for the System Unit

The system unit should be placed in a well-ventilated location, with nothing blocking the fan in the back of the cabinet. To keep the system's delicate circuitry from being damaged by an electrical power surge, you should use a power strip with a surge protector. You plug the computer into the power strip and then plug the power strip into the electrical outlet. If a power surge should occur, the surge protector will absorb the power, not the computer system. Basic care for the system components is outlined as follows:

- *Monitor.* A screen saver automatically changes the monitor display at short intervals or constantly shows moving images on the computer monitor or screen. All Windows® operating systems come equipped with screen savers. To protect their screens, many monitors "power down" after a certain period of inactivity. If no one uses the computer for 30 minutes, for example, the monitor screen goes blank. To resume using the computer after the screen saver has been activated or the monitor has powered down, you may need to simply touch any key or move the mouse. However, if the medical office has activated the "On resume, display logon screen" feature that is standard on Windows machines you may be required to enter your login information again. Also, adding a screen cover to a monitor when it is not in use will protect the monitor.

- *Printer.* Printer maintenance generally consists of replacing the ink cartridge or toner cartridge when required. When the cartridge needs to be changed, the ink on your printouts becomes very light and colors become faded. Some integrated computer and printer systems automatically provide a "Low Ink" message on the screen when printer cartridges need replacing. The message appears when the "Print" command is given. A graph indicates the amount of ink left in the cartridge. Ink can be ordered online through a link provided with the printer program. Replacement is usually a simple process, described in the printer manual.

- *Storage devices.* Jump drives and CD-ROMs are highly sensitive devices. Even a small "injury" may cause permanent damage or make it impossible to retrieve data. To avoid problems, handle and store these devices properly. A jump drive

should be protected when it is not attached to the computer. Always put the cap back on when it is not attached to the CPU or when you are transporting the drive to another location. When you handle a CD-ROM disc or pick it up, touch only the edges or the edge and the hole in the center; always be careful not to touch the flat service of the disc. CD-ROMs should be stored in the clear plastic case (sometimes called a jewel case) in which they are packaged. If a CD-ROM becomes dusty or smudged with fingerprints, clean it by rubbing it gently with a soft cloth. Always rub from the center to the outside. Never rub in a circular motion.

Disk Cleanup and Disk Defragmentation

Disk Cleanup Disk cleanup is a computer maintenance utility designed to free up space on your computer by removing unnecessary files on your hard drive. It compresses old files, deletes temporary Internet files, and sends some files to the recycle bin. Microsoft Windows already has this capability included in its package.

Disk Defragmentation "Defragging" physically organizes the contents of your hard disk drive to store pieces of each file closely. This also frees up space on your computer. Fragmentation occurs when the operating system cannot or will not allocate contiguous (adjacent) space to store a complete file as a unit.

▶ Security in the Computerized Office LO 8.7

Although security measures are important in any office, they are especially important in a computerized medical office. Great care must be taken to safeguard confidential files, make backup copies on a regular basis, and prevent system contamination. HIPAA laws require that privacy and security procedures are in place to prevent the misuse of health information. These procedures also must ensure confidentiality.

Safeguarding Confidential Files

Much of the information collected in a medical office is confidential. Just as with paper records, confidential information stored on the computer should be accessible only to authorized personnel. Two common ways to provide security in a computerized office are to employ passwords and to install an activity-monitoring system.

Passwords In many hospitals and physician offices, each employee who is allowed access to computerized patient files receives a password. The employee must enter the password into the computer when using the files. Access codes or passwords only allow the user into approved areas according to the individual's job description. When you receive a password, do not divulge it to anyone else. If an employee leaves or is terminated, the user account should be deleted. When you choose a password, do not use common ones such as your birthday. This is so important that many times specific guidelines for creating

Guidelines for Security and Privacy in the Computerized Office

Computer use is widespread within the typical medical practice. Though the computer is valuable for many administrative functions, it also can be a risk in terms of patient privacy and HIPAA compliance. You must follow special safeguards for computers in order to protect the patient's privacy.

- Computers are typically placed in or near the patient reception area. Keep the computer screen positioned so that it is not visible to unauthorized personnel or patients. Using screensavers can minimize the amount of time any information is visible on the screen.

- All computers should automatically log the user off after a period of inactivity. The computer should require that all users must reenter their password to regain access after an idle period.

- Always keep your computer username and password confidential. Change your password often, using a variety of numbers, symbols, and both lower- and uppercase letters.

- Consider the use of practice management software, which can track users and follow their activity within a computer system.

- Formal policies should be developed for every practice regarding the transfer and acceptance of outside protected health information. When using any computer system, always follow practice policy to assure that protected health information is being transferred in a secure and compliant manner.

a password must be followed and commonly used formats, like birthdates, will not be accepted by the password program.

Activity-Monitoring System In conjunction with passwords, most healthcare facilities use a computer system that monitors user activity. Whenever someone accesses computer records or an Internet site, the system automatically keeps track of the user's name and the files (or sites) that have been viewed or modified. In this way, if necessary, problems or security breaches can be traced back to specific employees.

Preventing System Contamination

Computer viruses constitute another important security issue in the computerized medical office. Viruses are programs written specifically to contaminate the hard disk by damaging or destroying data. They can be passed from computer to computer through shared, infected diskettes. Computer viruses also can be spread through infected files retrieved from online services, the Internet, e-mails, and electronic bulletin boards. Several software programs are available to detect and correct computer viruses. Most are fairly inexpensive but provide an invaluable service.

Antivirus Software and Firewalls There are literally hundreds of security vulnerabilities awaiting your computer system. You need to be concerned about everything on your computer from the operating system to the software applications. Antivirus software provides protection for your computer. It scans your system for viruses automatically and manually. If it finds a virus, it either destroys it automatically or alerts the user to respond by "cleaning" the file, thus destroying it. Antivirus software responds to spammers (persons that abuse e-mails by sending them in mass without permission), who often send malicious e-mails and files. If you do not know who sent you the e-mail, it is best not to open the file.

Firewalls (barriers to keep destructive forces away from your computer) also are called security protection. Firewalls are helpful in putting a stop to offensive Internet sites and potential computer hackers (a person that can get inside of a computer legally or illegally and do anything) who are trying to gain access to your computer.

Computer Disaster Recovery Plan

When any business is dependent on computer technology for daily functioning, a computer disaster recovery plan for the business must be in place. A recovery plan offers a possible solution if the primary computer system should fail or "crash," making all information on the hard drive unavailable. Disaster recovery planning can be developed within an organization, or it can be purchased as a software application or a service.

In a medical practice, it is important to discuss the computer disaster recovery plan with the staff so that everyone knows the part he or she will play if the computer system fails. As devices, systems, and networks become more complex, there are simply more things that can go wrong. As a result, these plans have become increasingly important and sophisticated.

Although a computer disaster recovery plan will vary from practice to practice, all plans should include these elements:

- *Minimizing damage to equipment.* Automatic warnings are built into computer systems to indicate when a fatal error has occurred. Warnings also provide direction to help prevent information loss and minimize damage to the computer equipment.

- *Retrieving information.* As stated earlier in the chapter, it is essential to routinely back up the office files using either an automated or manual backup system. An example of an automated system is a second computer, networked to the first, to which information is regularly backed up in the event the primary computer system fails. With this type of backup, the operation of the office can continue while the primary system

FIGURE 8-9 No matter what method is used, backing up the office computer files and storing them properly is a vital function.

is repaired or replaced. An example of a manual electronic backup system would be copying files to CDs and keeping these backups off site (Figure 8-9). An example of a paper backup system, which is less useful, is a handwritten list of patients and the procedures performed each day.

How often backups are made varies among medical offices; your supervisor will tell you the policy for your office. If the office staff is responsible for performing the backup, remember that storing the backups properly is just as important as making them. Backup files should not be stored near the original files. Ideally, they should be kept outside the medical office—perhaps at a storage site or lock box—for security in case of fire, burglary, or other office catastrophe. Backup systems are also vital. If the main system fails, the backup system will allow all the information to be retrieved and not permanently lost.

- *Guarding protected health information.* Even during an office emergency, like a computer failure, healthcare professionals are still required to carefully protect the privacy of patient records. If an electronic or manual backup system is implemented, safeguards to protect patient information must still be observed.

▶ Computers of the Future   LO 8.8

Computers are evolving at such a rapid pace that it is virtually impossible to predict the changes that will take place even in the next few years. Some important new technologies, however, have already been introduced in the medical office and will be improved in the near future. Telemedicine, CD-R and DVD-R technology, and speech recognition technology are only three examples of new computer technologies. Undoubtedly, more will be explored and developed every year.

Telemedicine

Telemedicine refers to the use of telecommunications to transmit video images of patient information, such as CT scans or even teleconferences involving multiple care providers. These images are already used to provide medical support to physicians caring for patients in rural areas. The use of telemedicine and advancements in computer technology allow medical practices to quickly access vast amounts of current medical information.

CD-R and DVD-R Technology

While CD-ROMs and DVDs can only be *read* by the computer, CD-R (compact disc–recordable) media and DVD-Rs can be read *and* written to. CD-R and DVD-R technology allows you to use compact discs like diskettes to store data and information. Recordable CDs and DVDs, however, can store much more information than diskettes can.

Speech Recognition Technology

Speech recognition technology enables the computer to comprehend and interpret spoken words through the use of a specialty software program. The user simply speaks into a microphone instead of inputting information with a keyboard or a scanner. Because every human voice is different, and the English language is vast and complex, this technology is, however, difficult to perfect. As speech recognition technology becomes more advanced, more accurate, and less expensive, it will likely gain widespread acceptance. It has a great deal of potential, including the ability to virtually eliminate the need for medical assistants to transcribe physicians' notes. There are a variety of speech recognition software applications available for use.

▶ Administrative Medical Office Equipment   LO 8.9

Using automated equipment enables you to perform a task more easily and quickly than doing it manually. For example, adding numbers on a calculator is a much faster process than doing it on paper. Many of the administrative tasks in a medical practice can be accomplished with the help of automated equipment, allowing you more time to perform other tasks.

Facsimile Machines

Critical documents, like laboratory reports and patient records, often need to be sent immediately to locations outside the office. A facsimile (fax) machine can be an efficient way to accomplish this. A fax machine scans each page of a document, translates it into electronic impulses, and transmits those impulses over the telephone line. When another fax machine receives the impulses, they are converted into an exact copy of the original document.

A fax machine in a medical office should have its own telephone line. A separate line ensures that transmission of incoming and outgoing faxes will not be interrupted and that the machine will not tie up a needed telephone line when sending or receiving information. Always keep in mind that faxed material may include protected health information. For this reason, fax machines should never be placed in patient examination rooms or reception areas where unauthorized persons may be able to view incoming or outgoing documents. Only staff members with a "need to know" should have access to faxed and other confidential information. Because of the confidential nature of many faxes, all faxes should also be sent with a fax cover sheet that contains a **disclaimer.** This disclaimer should state that the material within the fax is

BWW Medical Associates, PC
305 Main Street, Port Snead YZ 12345-9876
Tel: 555-654-3210, Fax: 555-987-6543
Web: BWWAssociates.com

Paul F. Buckwalter, MD
Alexis N. Whalen, MD
Elizabeth H. Williams, MD

FACSIMILE COVER SHEET

Date: _____

To: _____   From: _____

Fax #: _____   Fax #: _____

# of pages (including this cover sheet): _____

Message:

_____

_____

_____

_____

_____

_____

_____

The information contained in this transmission is privileged and confidential, intended only for the use of the individual or entity named above. If the reader of this message is not the intended recipient, you are hereby notified that any dissemination, distribution, or copying of this communication is strictly prohibited. If you have received this transmission in error, do not read. Please immediately respond to the sender that you have received this communication in error and then destroy or delete it. Thank you.

FIGURE 8-10 Example of a Facsimile (Fax) Cover Sheet.

intended only for the person to whom it is being sent and if the fax is received in error, to inform the sender and destroy the fax immediately (see Figure 8-10).

Benefits of Faxing A fax machine can send an exact copy of a document to a recipient within minutes. The cost for sending a fax is the same as for making a telephone call to that location. For a short document, this is usually less expensive than an overnight mail service.

In addition, many fax machines have a copier function and can be used as an extra copy machine. The telephone for the fax also may be used as an extra extension for outgoing calls, if

needed. Procedure 8-1, found at the end of the chapter, details the correct steps for using a fax machine.

Receiving a Fax Faxes can be received 24 hours a day if the fax machine is turned on and has an adequate paper supply (Figure 8-11). Newer-model fax machines have memories and can store and receive documents. If the fax machine is not already sending or receiving a fax, the fax telephone rings, or the machine buzzes briefly, signaling the start of a transmission. The transmission begins shortly thereafter, with the machine printing out the document as it is sent. When completed, the machine may print a transmission

FIGURE 8-11   Typical Office Facsimile (Fax) Machine.

report that includes the number of pages, the date and time, and the originating fax number.

Typewriters

Although typewriters are used very little in a medical practice, they may still be used to complete medical forms brought in by patients or sent from an insurance company if the office does not use electronic billing software. These forms can be completed more clearly when the information is typed instead of handwritten.

Most modern medical practices have eliminated typewriters altogether and, instead, use computers with word processing software and scanners to create and manipulate word documents.

Photocopiers

A photocopier, also called a copier or copy machine, instantly reproduces office correspondence, forms, bills, patient records, and other documents. A photocopier works by taking a picture of the document it is to reproduce and printing it on plain paper using a heat process. Photocopiers use either liquid or dry toner (a form of ink). Various kinds of paper can be used in the machine, including office stationery and colored paper. Many photocopiers accept different sizes of paper, from the standard 8- by 11-inch paper to 8- by 14-inch legal paper and even larger.

Photocopiers come in many models with varying features and speeds—from desktop machines for limited use to industrial models for continual heavy use. All styles are available through purchase or lease. Procedure 8-2, found at the end of the chapter, describes the correct method for using a photocopier machine.

FIGURE 8-12   The office copier produces hard copies of documents.

Special Features Copiers offer a wide range of special features. They may collate (assemble sets of multiple pages in order) and staple pages, punch holes, enlarge or reduce images, and produce double-sided copies (print on both sides of the page). Some also can adjust contrast and even track the cost of a job via a specific code input into the machine. Some photocopiers produce black-and-white copies as well as color copies. Some copiers can make transparencies (text and images printed on clear acetate), which physicians often use for presentations. Copiers can even be configured to electronically scan documents for electronic communications and to send and receive faxes. Many copiers can also be networked to computers and act as both printers and copiers (see Figure 8-12).

One of the more useful features of photocopiers is the "Help" function. Selecting this function displays directions in plain English that explain how to fix a paper jam or deal with other routine copier problems. Some copiers are even programmed to indicate that service is needed.

Adding Machines and Calculators

For handling tasks such as patient billing, bank deposits, and payroll, many medical practices depend on adding machines and calculators. The difference between the two types of machines is minimal. Adding machines typically plug into an outlet and produce a paper tape on which calculations are printed. Calculators are more often battery or solar powered, with memory to store figures. Calculators are portable and usually do not produce a paper tape.

Routine Calculations Both adding machines and calculators are sufficient for most routine office calculations, such as basic arithmetic functions like addition, subtraction, multiplication, and division. More contemporary models perform such specialized functions as computing percentages and storing data. Some are even computerized.

Do remember that it is easy to hit an incorrect key or to key in a number twice when using an adding machine or a calculator. So, always double-check all mathematical computations. If the machine produces a paper tape, check the numbers on the tape against the numbers you are adding. The paper tape is especially useful when adding a long series of numbers. Without a printed record, you must perform the same calculations again to make sure the total is correct.

Folding and Inserting Machines

Letter-folding equipment can help minimize the amount of time staff spends preparing large volumes of outgoing mail. Letter folders are also used for creating folded brochures. A medical practice may use folding and inserting machines for a variety of items, including invoices, newsletters, checks, statements, letters, and flyers.

Lower-end folding equipment requires letters to be fed manually. The speed of this machine is limited to the speed an individual can feed in letters, which is typically about 200 pieces per hour. An automatic feeder is required for faster folding. You will learn more about fold types and folding machines in the *Written and Electronic Documents* chapter.

Postage Meters

Every medical office uses the U.S. Postal Service. Patient bills, routine correspondence, purchase orders, and payments are just some of the items typically sent by mail. The *Medical Records and Documentation* chapter will also provide additional information on mailing correspondence.

Although some medical offices use stamps, most use a postage meter. A postage meter is a machine that applies postage to an envelope or package, eliminating the need for postage stamps (Figure 8-13). A postage meter often has two parts: the meter, which belongs to the post office, and the mailing machine, which the practice can own. The meter actually applies the postage and the mailing machine (if available) seals the envelope.

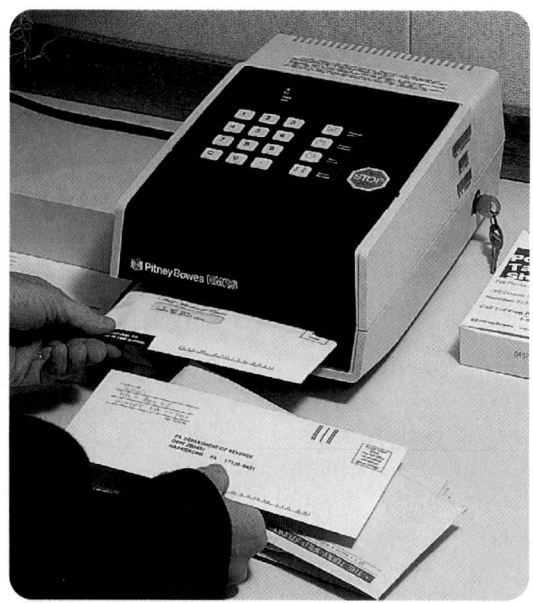

FIGURE 8-13 The postage meter is a convenient and cost-efficient way to apply postage to correspondence and packages.

Benefits of Using a Postage Meter Using a postage meter instead of purchasing stamps saves frequent trips to the post office. It also saves money for the office by providing the exact amount of postage needed for each item, instead of using a combination of stamps, which can cause you to exceed the minimum required postage. Some postage meters can even imprint envelopes with the name of your medical practice or with a message at the same time postage is applied. The message appears immediately to the left of the postal mark, at the top of the envelope.

There are many types of postage meters available, from basic models for a small office to advanced models for large businesses. The latest machines include automatic date setting, memory to program a large mailing, and display alerts for low postage or the need for ribbon replacement. Some models can apply postage to parcels without the use of labels or tape. Procedure 8-3, at the end of this chapter, describes how to use a postage meter.

Prepaying for Postage To use a postage meter, you must prepay the postage. You can take your meter to the post office to add postage, use a postage meter service, or order postage online. A service maintains the postal account for you. Although the money in each account is the property of the U.S. Postal Service, the provider manages the account and adds postage to the meter, as long as money is in your account with the service. Keeping the postage account current ensures that postage is always available and all mail is sent on a timely basis. This task may be one of your responsibilities. On any meter, you can check the amount of postage used and the amount remaining with the touch of a button. On some models, the meter must have $10 or more for the machine to apply postage to an envelope or package.

Postal Scales

Besides the postage meter, a medical practice also needs a postal scale. Postal scales are a good investment because they show both the weight and the amount of postage required. Some postage meters include an electronic scale. If you need a postal scale but one is not available, you can use any scale that weighs in ounces. When using a simple scale, you can then translate the weight into the correct postage by using a current postal rate chart, available from the U.S. Postal Service, which cuts down on mail being returned for inadequate postage.

Dictation-Transcription Equipment

Physicians usually do not type their own correspondence, patient records, or other documents. Medical assistants, although not professional medical transcriptionists, may be asked to transcribe recorded words into written text. Using dictation-transcription equipment is the most efficient way to complete this task. *Dictation* is another word for speaking; *transcription* is another word for writing. Together, they mean to transform spoken words into written form.

Dictation-transcription equipment has greatly advanced. There are now "starter kits" that are generally for smaller medical offices, as well as more advanced digital dictation and transcription kits. Speechmikes are great for physicians, as they are lightweight and when the physician speaks, the sounds are more audible to the transcriber. The standard functions of transcription equipment include controls for starting, stopping, reversing and fast-forwarding; volume, tone, and speed control; headphones; and a counter.

Larger medical facilities may provide call-in transcription services for the physician, which makes it easy to link to external databases. Doctors can dictate from remote locations and the information can be uploaded to the computer so the medical assistant can transcribe it.

Voice recognition software is available to help the physician when he or she wants to set up dictation via the computer. Specialized programs are provided for various medical specialties.

Dictating Quite often, the physician's handwriting can be confusing. Dictation is a wonderful tool that not only assists the medical assistant, but, frankly, keeps the physician out of trouble because the notes are clear and easy to read (see Figure 8-14). Using these steps can make transcribing much easier. Ask the physician to

1. Indicate the date and the type of document being dictated and provide explicit instructions about the document. For example, it is helpful to indicate that the document is a letter that needs to be produced on office stationery and mailed to a patient.
2. Spell out all names, addresses, and any unfamiliar terms.
3. Indicate punctuation by saying, for example, "comma" or "begin new paragraph."
4. Speak clearly and slowly. Neither eat while dictating nor record in a noisy environment, if at all possible.

FIGURE 8-14 Transcribing dictation requires knowledge of anatomy, physiology, and medical terminology and attention to detail.

The chapter on *Medical Records and Documentation* describes the medical transcription process in greater detail.

Check Writers

Medical practice personnel need to write checks to pay for equipment, supplies, and payroll. This common office procedure can be automated by using a check writer, which is a machine that imprints checks. Procedure 8-4, located at the end of this chapter, details the correct steps for operating a check-writing machine.

The safety advantage of using such a machine is that the name of the payee (the person receiving the check) and the amount of the check, once imprinted, cannot be altered. Numerous check-writing software packages can assist you, including QuickBooks, Checksoft, and VersaCheck.

Paper Shredders

Paper shredders cut documents into tiny pieces to make them unreadable. They are quite common in medical practices, as they allow protection of protected health information that is no longer required by the office. A paper shredder, like the one shown in Figure 8-15, is often used when confidential documents, such as patient records, need to be destroyed. The most common type of shredder cuts paper into ribbon-like strips, which differ in width, depending on the model. Other shredders cut the paper in two directions, forming small pieces. Some paper shredders offer additional options, such as an electronic eye that automatically starts the machine when paper is inserted and stops when it is done. Other features available are paper jam detection, automatic reverse, and automatic shutdown when the machine gets too hot.

How to Shred Materials A paper shredder is ready to use when it is turned on. To shred a document, insert it into the feed tray at the top of the shredder. The machine feeds the paper through hundreds of knife-like cutters, instantaneously shredding the paper. A basket attached beneath the shredder

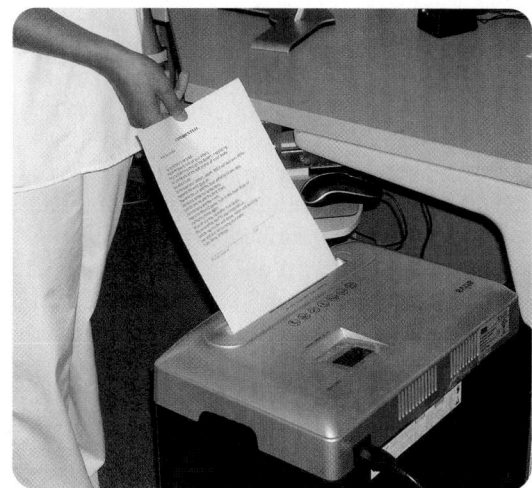

FIGURE 8-15 Using a paper shredder protects patient PHI when it is no longer needed.

Recycling in the Medical Office, Hospital, Laboratory, or Clinic

You may easily incorporate recycling procedures into the daily routine of a medical office, hospital, laboratory, or clinic. Recycling may be required by state law. Some states levy large fines for noncompliance with recycling regulations. Purchase paper products that can be recycled, or those made of postconsumer recycled materials, and take care in disposing of them. Care should be taken to ensure HIPAA compliance when recycling paper. Shredding is the most effective way to comply with HIPAA regulations.

There are two essential aspects of recycling: disposal and purchasing. To create a complete recycling program, ensure that materials are disposed of properly and that purchased products have been made from recycled materials. Your town's recycling center provides guidelines for packaging recycled materials and for a pickup schedule as well as containers for recyclable materials and a list of paper materials that can and cannot be recycled. Follow regulations from OSHA and your office policy for disposal of biohazardous materials and other medical wastes. As discussed in the *Basic Safety and Infection Control* chapter, these are disposed of in designed protective containers.

When purchasing items for recycling, look for the universal recycling symbol which has three chasing arrows (Figure 8-16).

This symbol could mean that the product or package is made up of recycled materials or that the product or package is recyclable. Unless the package is made of 100%

recycled materials, the law requires the package to display how much. Watch out for claims that do not mean anything. Claims that a product or service is "environmentally friendly," "environmentally safe," "environmentally preferable," or "eco-safe" or labels that contain environmental seals are unhelpful. These phrases alone do not provide the specific information you need to compare products, packaging, or services on their environmental merits. If you want to go "green," look for claims that give some substance and additional information that explains why the product is environmentally friendly or has earned a special seal. For more about recycling, check the website of the Federal Trade Commission (www.ftc.gov) or the Environmental Protection Agency (http://epa.gov).

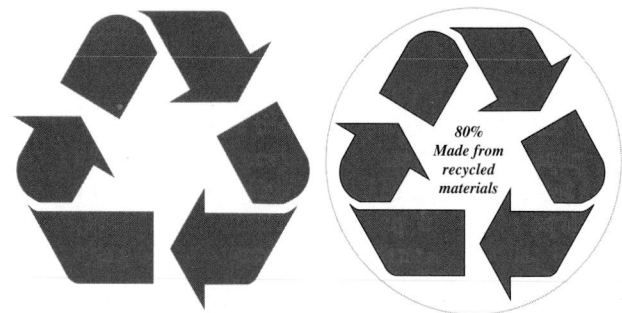

FIGURE 8-16 Check products for this symbol to determine if they are environmentally friendly.

catches the bits of paper. Different models can accommodate different amounts of paper through the cutters. Shredder baskets must be emptied periodically to allow room for additional shredded paper. Some shredders even signal when the basket is full. Avoid wearing loose-fitting clothing while operating a shredder to prevent accident or personal injury.

When to Shred Materials Medical practices need to eliminate old patient records and other sensitive materials. These items cannot simply be thrown into the trash because of confidentiality problems. The shredder is an effective disposal solution. If records have incorrect information that has been corrected on subsequent documents, the old records are shredded to prevent incorrect information from being mistakenly placed in the patient's folder. A document that has been shredded cannot be put back together. So, do not decide on your own to shred a document. The physician or office manager will set guidelines regarding when a document should be shredded. If you are not sure whether to shred a document, check with a senior staff member before beginning the process.

Shredding Vendors Many medical practices contract with a shredding company to come into the practice to

remove and then shred designated materials. Using another company for this task does not relieve the medical practice of the responsibility for the confidential materials. The healthcare provider is still considered the **covered entity** and must comply with HIPAA law. It is important to contract only with companies that also abide by HIPAA confidentiality statutes.

Microfilm and Microfiche Readers

Microfilm is a roll of film imprinted with information and stored on a reel. Film also can be stored in cartridges to protect it from being touched. Microfiche is film imprinted with information and stored in rectangular sheets. Special equipment is required to read documents stored on both of these media. See Figures 8-17 and 8-18.

Although considered to be old technology, microfilm and microfiche are still in use in many medical practices, particularly for old records that are not being converted to electronic format. Even if your office does not store records on microfilm or microfiche, you may still need to have access to a reader because back issues of medical journals and other publications are often available only in these formats.

FIGURE 8-17 Storing information on microfilm helps reduce the amount of storage space needed by the office.

FIGURE 8-18 Special equipment is used to read text stored on mcrofiche.

▶ Purchasing Decisions for Office Equipment

LO 8.10

As the office medical assistant, in addition to your possible role in making purchasing decisions for computer equipment, you also may be involved in helping to select the most appropriate office equipment. You may be asked to investigate whether the practice needs a new photocopier or whether hiring a shredding company makes sense for the office. To make a sound decision about whether the office will benefit from such a purchase, you will need to conduct thorough research, documenting your findings for further discussion.

Evaluating Office Needs

The first step in evaluating the equipment needs of a healthcare office is the research process. Make note of the equipment that is already available and consider the different tasks this equipment can perform. To obtain a complete list of office needs, ask other staff members for their ideas.

When considering the replacement of an old piece of equipment, ask what advantages the new piece of equipment offers over the current one. Create a list of equipment on hand and a list of any new products the office staff recommends. Compare the benefits offered by the new product to the capability of the currently used equipment. Many medical magazines review medical office equipment periodically and are good resources to consult in making your purchasing decisions. Go online to shop and compare products, features, and prices. Discuss with the office manager the budget for the equipment under consideration. Consider calling a supplier for more detailed information.

Contacting Suppliers Put together a list of the features you would like in your machine. Then contact suppliers who sell models that offer those features. You can call or e-mail the manufacturer directly to find out the name of a local vendor. Many manufacturers prepare brochures giving information about their products. Request that this information be sent to you.

Go online or look in the Yellow Pages for office supply stores and other companies that sell office equipment. Obtain product and pricing information on each model. For certain equipment, such as photocopiers, a sales representative will come to your office to demonstrate and discuss the product.

Evaluating Warranty Options Most products come with a warranty, which is a contract that guarantees free service and parts replacement for a certain period, usually 1 year. Warranties are valid only for specified service and repairs. They usually do not cover accidents, vandalism, acts of God (such as damage caused by floods or earthquakes), or mistreatment of the machine. In most cases, warranty repairs must be made at an authorized service center.

If you want more coverage than the warranty allows, consider buying an extended warranty. Extended warranties increase the amount of time that equipment is covered. For expensive equipment or parts, the additional cost of an extended warranty may be justified.

After you purchase a product, you must fill out the warranty card and mail it to the manufacturer. File the receipt in a safe place in the office where it can easily be retrieved.

Preparing a Recommendation After you have obtained all the information, you are ready to evaluate it. To compare and contrast the different models, construct a chart. Place the product model names in columns across the top. Down the left side, list factors that will influence the purchase decision: cost, warranty options (including the length of the warranty and the price of an extended warranty), special features, and delivery time. Then fill in the information. This chart will provide an easy-to-use summary of your research. Finally, analyze the list and choose the product that will best meet the office's needs. Meet with the physician or office manager to discuss your recommendation.

Leasing versus Buying Equipment

Once the product has been selected, there is one more decision to make: whether to lease or buy it. When buying a product, the purchaser becomes the owner. Owners are free to do with the product anything they choose, which may include selling it to someone else.

For most large pieces of office equipment, like photocopiers, there is also an option to *lease* the equipment. Leasing, or renting, usually involves an initial charge and a monthly fee. On average, the initial charge is equal to about two monthly payments. The ownership of a leased piece of equipment is retained by the leasing company.

Lease Agreement A lease is for a specified time, after which time the equipment is returned to the seller per the lease agreement (Figure 8-19). Some leases allow purchase of the equipment at the end of the rental period for an additional payment. The details of the purchase option are covered in the lease agreement.

Advantages and Disadvantages of Leasing When you lease a product, your office does not own it, but you have several advantages.

1. Leasing allows purchasers to keep more of their money. The initial cost of obtaining the machine is a fraction of the full cost of purchasing it. So the remainder of the money can earn interest in the bank or be used for other expenses. Leasing is advantageous when you do not have enough money to buy the equipment but need the services it provides. In addition, leasing allows businesses to update equipment every few years at the end of each lease period. Updating may not be as affordable if you buy equipment.

2. Often the company that leases the product is also responsible for servicing it.

3. In most cases, businesses are able to take lease payments as a tax deduction each year.

But leasing is not always the best solution—you will not own the equipment so the office will not gain any equity for the money it is spending on it. It is important to weigh the advantages of

Metropolitan Office Systems

Lease Agreement

Customer (Location)

BWW Medical Associates, PC
Full Legal Name (Please Print)

Address
305 Main Street

Port Snead   YZ   12345-9876
City   County   State   Zip

Billing Contact

Dealer:

Customer (Billing address, if different)

Full Legal Name (Please Print)

Address

City   County   State   Zip

Phone

Quantity	Description: Make, Model, and Serial Number	Quantity	Description: Make, Model, and Serial Number
1	FT 6655 Copier AA3365430358		
1	Sorter A337502010902		
1	Document Feeder A338506		
1	RT314 Large-capacity Tray		

Minimum Lease Term:	Payment Due:	Amount of Monthly Payment With Sales, Use, and Property Tax:	Advance Payment of $965.56 (Tax Included) by Check #	Documentation Fee
60 Months	__X__ Monthly ____ Quarterly ____ Annually ____ Other: $455.46	$482.78	____ First Month's Rent __X__ First and Last ____ Security Deposit (Without Tax) ____ Other	$ –0–

FIGURE 8-19 Read all lease agreements carefully before signing.

leasing against the advantages of buying equipment for your medical practice.

Whether you decide to lease or buy, always ask whether the price is firm or if there is room for negotiation. Many available discounted rates are not extended to a customer simply because the customer did not ask. Although some equipment prices are nonnegotiable, terms can sometimes be negotiated on more expensive pieces of equipment. Companies that lease office equipment are often flexible in determining the monthly payment. For example, equipment companies may accept smaller payments in the beginning of the rental or purchase agreement period and require larger payments near the end.

In a competitive market, some suppliers may match their competitors' prices. When purchasing several pieces of equipment at the same time, a supplier may be able to offer some savings on the total cost of the purchase or provide some service, such as free delivery, or an extension on the service contract.

▶ Maintaining Office Equipment LO 8.11

Office equipment (as with computers) must be regularly maintained to provide optimum service. Daily or weekly maintenance, such as cleaning the glass on the photocopier or replacing toner, can be performed by the office staff. However, more extensive maintenance should be done by the equipment supplier. Consult the equipment manual for details about the care of each piece of equipment.

Equipment Manuals

The best source of information about maintaining a piece of equipment is the manual that comes with it. This booklet gives basic information about the equipment, including how to set it up, how it works, special features, and problems you may encounter. The information in an equipment manual is extremely valuable. If the manual is lost, call the manufacturer or research the Internet to obtain another one. Equipment manuals should be stored where they can be retrieved easily. Some large pieces of office equipment provide racks or slots on the side of the equipment for manual storage.

POINTS ON PRACTICE
Equipment Manual Tips

It is helpful to write the following information on the inside front cover of the equipment manual upon initial setup. If there is a problem with the equipment that requires a maintenance call, this valuable information will be quick and easy to retrieve.

- The date of purchase or lease.
- The serial number of the equipment.
- The phone number of the company contracted to repair the equipment.

Maintenance and Service Contracts

Equipment suppliers provide standard maintenance contracts when office equipment is purchased. A maintenance contract specifies when the equipment will be cleaned, checked for worn parts, and repaired. A standard maintenance contract may include regular checkups as well as emergency repairs.

In addition, some suppliers offer a service contract, which covers services that are not included under the standard maintenance agreement, such as emergency repairs. In some cases, service contracts are combined with maintenance contracts in one document.

Make sure to keep track of all maintenance performed on your equipment. Many offices have a maintenance log, where staff members record the date and purpose of each service call. This log is helpful in identifying whether equipment should be replaced because of the need for frequent servicing.

Troubleshooting

Before calling the service supplier for service on any piece of equipment that appears to be malfunctioning, steps should be taken to determine if you can correct the problem yourself. This process is called "troubleshooting." Resolving the problem can save you the cost of a service call that may not be covered by the standard agreement.

The first step in troubleshooting is to eliminate possible simple causes of a problem. For example, if the equipment is powered by electricity, make sure that it is plugged into a functioning outlet and that it is turned on. Are all doors and other openings in their correct positions? Are all machine connections firmly in place? If you cannot discover a simple cause for the problem, it is time to test the machine to determine what it is failing to do. In the case of a malfunctioning photocopier, for example, try making a copy and note the response. Write down any error messages the machine provides.

Next, consult the equipment manual. Many manuals devote a section to troubleshooting. If you cannot find the solution after reading the manual, call the manufacturer or the place of purchase for additional assistance. Be prepared to explain the steps you have already taken toward resolving the problem.

Backup Systems

Earlier in the chapter, you read about the importance of having a backup system for the office's computer system(s) and the information contained within it. It is also important to have a "backup plan" in case of other equipment failure. Occasionally, more than one piece of equipment can be affected by a single problem. For example, if the electricity goes off, all electrical equipment will go out at once. To avoid losing important information and records, it is important to have backup systems in place.

Telephones The use of cell phones in addition to traditional phones offers a backup to communication in the event that phone service is interrupted. Cell phones are also helpful during emergency weather conditions.

Electricity An emergency generator may supply emergency power for lighting in key hallways and exam rooms.

Interior rooms and halls can quickly become very dark and hazardous when the electricity is unexpectedly cut off.

Battery Power Battery power backup is a key component of security and warning system backups. Audio warning signals sound when it is time to replace the batteries in smoke and security detectors. All batteries should routinely be replaced every six months.

Fire Extinguishers Fire extinguishers need to be serviced or replaced once a year to ensure maximum performance. The office may choose to contract with a local company to provide this annual maintenance evaluation.

Equipment Inventory

Each piece of equipment is an asset of a business. It is part of the business's net worth and should be listed on the medical practice's balance sheet. So taking inventory of office equipment provides relevant information for the practice's money manager. It also may indicate whether old equipment is due for replacement.

There are many different ways to take an office equipment inventory. Figure 8-20 shows a simple, manual example. Many offices use a master inventory, which may be in electronic format or on a single sheet to survey all equipment at a glance. The master sheet usually includes such general information as equipment name and purchase price and the quantity of each type of equipment. Many offices also keep more detailed information about each individual piece of equipment in electronic files or on a single sheet of paper. Detailed information may include the following:

- Name of the equipment, including the brand name.
- Brief description of the equipment.
- Model number and registration number.
- Date of purchase.
- Place of purchase, including contact information.
- Estimated life of the product.
- Product warranty.
- Maintenance and service contracts.

All equipment inventories should be updated periodically. Inventory software packages are becoming more effective in managing your equipment and supplies. If you decide to invest in a software inventory package, make sure you choose the package that best fits the office's needs.

▶ Maintaining Medical Office Supplies

LO 8.12

Purchasing and maintaining the office supplies and equipment in a medical office is an essential skill in managing the office. You will be responsible for evaluating and recommending equipment and supplies, taking inventory of equipment and supplies, and negotiating prices with suppliers. When managing office supplies, your goal is to achieve efficiency, which is the ability to produce the desired result with the least effort, expense, and waste.

The word *supply* refers to an expendable item, or an item that is used and then must be restocked, like examination table paper. Ideally, office supplies are stored on labeled shelves (Figure 8-21). This does not include more durable equipment that is used indefinitely—such as telephones, computers, examination tables, stethoscopes, and reflex hammers.

Determining Responsibility for Organizing Supplies

The medical assistant is often responsible for organizing office supplies. In a small practice, one medical assistant may be able to handle this responsibility alone, but a practice with several physicians may require more help to manage supplies. When two medical assistants handle this responsibility, one is often assigned to handle administrative items and the other to handle clinical (medical) supplies. In a very large practice, a third assistant might handle computer, copier, and fax supplies.

Categorizing Supplies

Most medical office supplies fall into two main categories: administrative and clinical. Examples of administrative supplies include items that are used in the office portion of the practice,

EQUIPMENT INVENTORY

ITEM	PURCHASE DATE	PURCHASE PRICE
1. TotalOffice oak desk	07/25/10	$295.00
2. TotalOffice rolling desk chair	02/19/10	$119.00
3. TotalOffice 4-drawer file cabinet	12/21/11	$150.00
4. TotalOffice 2-drawer file cabinet	08/05/11	$100.00
5. HYtech Pentium 100 computer	03/10/12	$1150.00
6. HYtech 14-inch monitor	03/10/12	$200.00

FIGURE 8-20 Typical equipment inventory including the name and quantity of each equipment type.

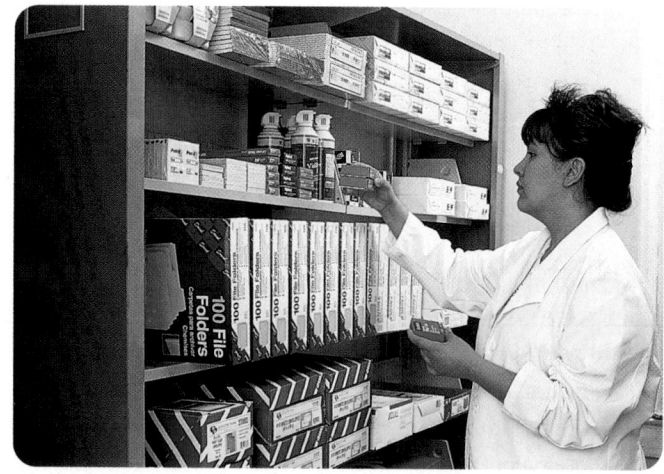

FIGURE 8-21 Keeping an up-to-date, organized inventory of supplies is crucial to a well-run office.

such as stationery, insurance forms, pens, pencils, and clipboards. Clinical supplies are medically related and include alcohol swabs, tongue depressors, disposable tips for otoscopes, and disposable sheaths for thermometers.

General supplies are used by both patients and staff. Examples of general supplies include paper towels, liquid hypoallergenic soap, and facial and toilet tissue.

The Supply List You will need to determine what items in your office are used routinely and reordered systematically.

Keep a list of these items and update it as needed. This master supply list is usually kept in the office procedures manual. Appropriate sections of this list may be posted on the cabinets where the items are stored.

One good way to help keep track of supplies is to categorize them according to their importance within the practice. You may find it helpful to identify an item as belonging to one of three categories: vital, incidental, and periodic use. Table 8-2 will help you determine vital, incidental, and periodic supplies for your office.

TABLE 8-2   Typical Supplies in a Medical Office

Administrative Supplies

Appointment books, daybooks (still used in noncomputerized offices)	Insurance manuals
Back-to-school/back-to-work slips	Local welfare department forms
Clipboards	Patient education materials
Computer supplies	Pens, pencils, erasers
Copy and facsimile (fax) machine papers	Prescription pads
File folders, coding tabs	Rubber bands, paper clips
HIPAA forms (Notice of Privacy Practices, authorization forms, disclosure logs, request to inspect/copy medical records forms, request for amendment forms, acknowledgment of request for amendment forms)	Registration forms
	Social Security forms
History and physical examination sheets/cards	Stamps
Insurance forms, disability, HMO and other third-party payers, life insurance examination forms, VA and W/C forms	Stationery, appointment cards, bookkeeping supplies (ledgers, statements, billing forms), letterhead, second sheets, envelopes, business cards, notebooks, notepads, telephone memo pads

Clinical Supplies

Alcohol swabs	Safety pins
Applicators	Silver nitrate sticks
Bandaging materials: adhesive tape, gauze pads, gauze sponges, elastic bandages, adhesive bandages, roller bandages (gauze and elastic)	Suture removal kits
	Sutures
Cloth or paper gowns and drapes	Examination table covers
Cotton, cotton swabs	Tongue depressors
Culture tubes	Topical skin freeze
50% dextrose solution	Urinalysis test strips
Disposable sheaths for thermometers	Urine containers (sterile and nonsterile)
Disposable tips for otoscopes	Injectable medications: diazepam (Valium), diphenhydramine hydrochloride (Benadryl), epinephrine (Adrenaline), furosemide (Lasix), isoproterenol (Isuprel), lidocaine (Xylocaine: 1%, 2%, and plain), meperidine hydrochloride (Demerol), morphine, phenobarbital, sodium bicarbonate, sterile saline, sterile water
Gloves: sterile and nonsterile examination	
Hemoccult test kits	
Iodine or Betadine pads	Other medications, chemicals, solutions, ointments, lotions, and disinfectants, as needed
Lancets	
Lubricating jelly	
Microscope slides and fixative	
Needles, syringes	
Nitroglycerine tablets	

General Supplies

Liquid hypoallergenic soap	Tampons and sanitary pads
Paper cups	Tissues: facial and toilet
Paper towels	

Vital Supplies These items are absolutely essential for the practice's functioning. They include paper examination table covers and prescription pads. Without these items, the physician would be unable to work in a clean examination environment or to readily prescribe medication for patients during office visits. Another type of vital supply is an item that requires a special order, such as a printed form. Special orders take time to obtain, so they must be ordered well before supplies run low.

Incidental Supplies These supplies are needed in the office but do not threaten the office's efficiency if the supply runs low. Incidental supplies include staples and rubber bands, which can be purchased quickly and easily at a local stationery store.

Periodic Supplies These supplies require ordering only occasionally. For example, if your office uses appointment books, you will order them only once or twice a year, probably in small numbers. The urgency of ordering some periodic items can depend on the size of the office. A multiphysician office, for example, would require more copy paper than a single-physician office. Another example of a periodic item might be holiday cards to send to the physician's colleagues and patients.

Storing Office Supplies

Storing office supplies requires good organizational skills and attention to detail. Many people in an office use these supplies, so the items should be stored neatly and in an orderly way. In addition, it is important to store supplies safely to prevent loss or theft, damage, or deterioration.

Location In a small medical office, supplies are generally kept near the areas where they are used. For example, administrative supplies are usually stored behind or adjacent to the reception area, while clinical supplies are stored near the examination rooms. If the practice has a laboratory, pertinent supplies are stored in or near the laboratory. Offices with separate supply rooms offer more storage space.

Small medical offices may not have ample storage space, so it may be tempting to store boxes on the floor behind the air-conditioning unit, stacked up close to the ceiling, or in potentially hazardous locations, such as near a heat source. However, it is essential that supplies be stored according to the guidelines described by TJC (The Joint Commission).

Items may not be stored on the floor; instead, they must be raised off the floor, as on a crate or shelf, to avoid contamination by water. Items stored close to the ceiling are considered a fire hazard. TJC standards require that supplies stored on the top shelf of a closet or storage area be at least 18 inches below the ceiling.

Avoid storing any boxes or supplies near a water heater, air-conditioning unit, heater, or stove. Many expendable items and their packaging are combustible and can quickly become a fire hazard. Air-conditioning units may drip water on the floor. If boxes of expensive forms are stored nearby, they can quickly become ruined as water seeps unnoticed into the packaging.

Storage Cabinets Each storage cabinet should be labeled with a list of its contents. Keep all stock of one item together.

Finding supplies is easier if you keep small items at eye level. Put large, bulky goods, like reams of stationery, on lower shelves. Label boxes and containers clearly so that all employees can readily find what they need and so that the inventory process is easier.

As you initially arrange items on storage shelves, label the shelves. Reserve enough space to completely stock each item. Do not put anything but the appropriate item in each designated space. This easy system allows for a quick review when you reorder supplies.

To reduce the risk of errors on reorders, keep each item's original label attached to it. Cover the label with clear tape, if necessary. If you must replace a worn label, do it immediately when needed, making sure the new label has the same detailed information as the old one. Bottles with pouring spouts should be labeled on the side opposite the spout to prevent the liquid from dripping onto the label. Use a laundry marking pen to label linens with the name of your office. Linen services usually premark linens with the name of the company or the practice.

Many items have a shelf life after which they are no longer usable. By not overordering and by rotating supplies—using older ones first—your office will be able to use items during their shelf life. This is true not only for perishable items like medications, but also for linens and paper, which can deteriorate. Keep in mind when stocking medications or chemicals that a more recent shipment may have an earlier expiration date than a previous shipment. So, always check expiration dates when storing supplies.

Store all items based on their expiration date. The oldest items should be stored in the front and the newer items stored in the rear of the cabinet. Be sure to rotate the inventory every time you add new stock, placing the newly received stock at the back of each shelf. Because items can sometimes expire before they are used, be sure to check every item for the expiration date before use. Discard all expired items carefully and appropriately according to TJC and OSHA standards.

Administrative Supplies In addition to such expendable items as pens, pencils, and paper clips, paper products are important to a medical office. In general, paper products should be stored flat in their original boxes or wrappings to prevent pages from bending or curling. Information booklets may be stored upright to save space. Envelopes and other paper goods with gummed surfaces must be kept dry to prevent them from sticking together.

Clinical Supplies The rules of good housekeeping and asepsis creating the germ-free environment discussed in the *Basic Safety and Infection Control* chapter, not only apply to the daily office environment that is visible to patients, physicians, and office staff, but also to storage areas for clinical supplies. These areas must be kept clean and protected from damage and exposure to the elements.

All dressings and most bandaging materials must be kept sterile, including gauze that may be used to bandage an open wound. Elastic rolled bandages, which do not touch open wounds, must be clean but not necessarily sterile.

Chemicals, drugs, and solutions should be kept in a cool, dark place because light and heat cause some substances to deteriorate. Refer to the Material Safety Data Sheet (MSDS) provided by each manufacturer for proper storage instructions. The importance of MSDS is discussed in detail in the *Basic Safety and Infection Control* chapter, but here are some basic guidelines:

- Store all liquids in their original containers. Line cabinets with plastic-coated shelf paper and wipe it frequently with a damp cloth. Do not store liquids above dry supplies.
- Store all poisons and narcotics separately from each other and from all other products.
- Narcotics must be stored securely out of sight in a locked cabinet.
- Never store strong acids near alkaline solutions or flammable items near sources of heat. Solutions that will be stored for a considerable length of time should have a small amount of space at the top of the bottle to allow for heat expansion.
- Some liquids should be stored in the refrigerator.
- Again, check each item for specific storage instructions. If storage space is limited, consider eliminating some items—especially bulky ones that are rarely used or items that a patient can purchase at surgical supply stores.
- Clinical refrigerators may be needed to store certain clinical supplies that require refrigeration. Never store food items and clinical items in the same refrigerator. A clinical refrigerator must be kept at a constant temperature to properly maintain the chemical integrity of lab supplies. Monitoring and recording the date and temperature of the clinical refrigerator should be completed once a week or per office protocol. Refer to each MSDS for storage details on each substance.

▶ Taking a Supply Inventory   LO 8.13

As you discovered earlier, the responsibility of maintaining office supplies often falls to the medical assistant. It is a job that requires careful planning, attention to detail, and basic math skills. Accurate inventory activity ensures that the office never runs out of much-needed supplies.

Understanding Your Responsibilities

Generally, you will be responsible for overseeing the flow of supplies bought and used, calculating the budget for supplies, selecting supplies and vendors, following correct purchasing and payment procedures, and storing the goods properly.

All efficient offices will have a process for everyone within the practice to record their supply needs. The process may be as simple as a notebook stored at the front desk or a supply list positioned in a key location. As a supply need in the office is noted, it can be recorded on the supply list by anyone for the next order. Then, the medical assistant who is compiling the order should check all the inventory cards, reorder reminder cards, and supply lists before ordering.

Go to CONNECT to see videos about *Establishing and Conducting the Supply Inventory* and *Receiving Supplies*.

The Inventory Filing System

To oversee the flow of inventory efficiently, you will need a filing system. See Procedure 8-5 at the end of this chapter for a step-by-step overview. This system consists of several elements:

- The list of supplies (discussed earlier in the chapter).
- An itemized inventory.
- An inventory card or record page for each item.
- A list of the names and addresses of current vendors.
- A file of current catalogs from vendors (including some vendors not currently used, for comparison shopping).
- A wish list of brands or items that the office does not currently use but may want to try in the future.
- Files for *invoices*, or bills from vendors, and completed order forms.
- Reorder reminder cards to indicate when an in-stock item should be reordered.
- Color-coded, removable self-adhesive flags to indicate "Need to Order" or "On Order."
- An inventory and ordering schedule.
- Order forms for each vendor (may be multicopy forms, fax forms, electronic forms, or e-mail forms).

The Inventory Card or Record Page The inventory card or record page for each item or category of items may be a 4-by-6-inch index card, a page in a loose-leaf binder, or a spreadsheet stored in the computer system (Figure 8-22). These methods make it easy to group together the items that need to be ordered at any given time. Records help you monitor how quickly items are used and how much should be ordered each time.

Of course, some information may change. As you become more proficient at monitoring inventory or as the practice grows or diminishes in size, you may find that quantities, vendors, or reorder quantities need to be adjusted. With the help of the doctor or office manager, you will be able to determine the ideal quantity of each item to have on hand, depending on the size of the practice, the available storage space, and the ordering schedule.

Be sure to check the storage areas regularly, preferably at specific times, and to count the items on hand. When the supply of an item begins to run low, you (or another staff member) should flag the inventory card or record page to indicate the need to reorder it at the next regular ordering time.

Color-coded, removable self-adhesive flags on the inventory card or record page are an efficient way to track inventory. A red flag, for example, might indicate that a supply needs to be ordered. A yellow flag might be substituted when the item has been ordered.

Reorder Reminder Cards Reorder reminder cards (Figure 8-23) are usually brightly colored cards inserted directly into stock on the supply shelf to indicate when it is time to reorder an item. For example, if you have determined that four boxes of staples is a sufficient quantity to keep on hand

(ITEM NAME) _Exam Table Paper 21"_

ORDER QUANTITY _____12_____ REORDER POINT _____4_____

ORDER	QTY	REC'D	UNIT COST	PRICE	PREPAID	ON ACCT.	ORDER	QTY	REC'D	UNIT COST	PRICE	PREPAID	ON ACCT.
1/4	12	1/8	$12.25	$147.00	check 1214	X							
2/5	12	2/9	$12.25	$147.00	check 2110	X							

INVENTORY COUNT

	JAN.	FEB.	MAR.	APR.	MAY	JUNE	JULY	AUG.	SEPT.	OCT.	NOV.	DEC.
DATE _____	7	10										
DATE _____												

ORDER SOURCE

Smith Physician's Supply Co.

493 Carlton Avenue

South Union, NJ 07422

908-899-6123   Contact: Martin Kohn

UNIT PRICE

_12 - $147.00_

_36 - $441.00_

FIGURE 8-22 An inventory spreadsheet may be created manually or computer generated.

REORDER TAG

When you reach this inventory point, it's time to reorder.

PRODUCT
_____

ORDER NO.
_____

WASHINGTON BUSINESS SUPPLIES
121 Main Street, Houston, TX 41414
(619)587-8700

FIGURE 8-23 Reorder reminder cards are typically brightly colored cards inserted within the current supply stock reminding you when it is time to reorder the item.

and your office supply orders are filled in 2 business days, you might place the reorder reminder card between the third and fourth boxes of staples. The reorder quantity on the inventory card or record page for staples would indicate "four boxes."

The reorder reminder cards also remind other staff members to tell you when an item is in short supply. In some offices, the medical assistant labels the reminder card with the supply item's name and bar code number, such as "staples 002345." This method allows any staff member to pull the card when the last box of staples before the reminder card is taken from the supply shelf. The staff member can then place the card in a "To Be Ordered" envelope. Some offices can reorder simply by scanning the bar code. Staff members in some offices request supplies by writing them in an order book or on an order list.

Inventory Reminder Kits Some mail-order supply vendors sell inventory kits, complete with cards and tabs or flags. Computerized inventory systems are also available. Because shelves still need to be checked and counts logged on to the computer, smaller offices generally do not benefit as much as larger ones from a computerized inventory system.

Scheduling Inventory and Ordering

Establish a regular schedule for counting the office supplies, such as taking inventory every 1 or 2 weeks. Estimating when you will probably need to reorder a particular item—and putting that date on your calendar or in your appointment book—is also helpful. You and the physician can determine how often storage areas should be checked.

Established Ordering Times You should have established ordering times, such as the same day each week or month, after inventory is taken. For example, you might take inventory the first Tuesday of every month and order supplies the first Thursday of every month.

A regular schedule for taking inventory and ordering helps all staff members remember when they must give their requests to you. Although you may need to adjust the ordering time occasionally, try to stick to the schedule to avoid the expense and inconvenience of rush orders.

When to Order Ahead of Schedule When you take inventory and the spare supply of an item has not been reached but is close to the placement of the reorder reminder card, you must decide whether you should reorder then or wait until the next regular ordering time. You will probably find it is more efficient to go ahead and order rather than wait. Ordering early assures you that the supply will not be depleted before the next regular ordering time. Make sure you consider your storage capacity, as this could limit your purchases.

Ordering ahead of schedule can be especially important if there is a large demand for a particular product and manufacturers' production levels have not caught up with that demand. This situation can occur if there has been an outbreak of a particular flu or virus, or if the Food and Drug Administration has determined that a certain product is harmful, resulting in higher demand for an alternative product.

Unanticipated Shortage of a Supply Item If the supply of an item reaches the reorder reminder card, and there is still a long time before the next regular ordering time, place the order immediately so that you do not risk running out of the item.

To help you oversee inventory effectively, finish one container before opening a new one. Keep all stock of the same item in one place, as the need to count inventory of an item in more than one location or container increases the likelihood of errors. If an item is kept in more than one location, as in the case of multiple exam rooms, inventory is best maintained per room.

As a medical assistant, you want to be sure that there are always sufficient quantities of supplies to keep the office running efficiently. It is unwise to stock spare supplies in too great a quantity, however, because the administrative budget is not likely to support such expenditures. In addition, spare quantities of supplies can be a storage problem.

▶ Ordering Supplies
LO 8.14

Ordering supplies requires a procedure to deal with vendors and to order and check supplies. You can avoid common purchasing mistakes by understanding the most efficient way to order supplies for your office.

Locating and Evaluating Supply Vendors

A vendor will most likely already be in place when you join a practice. You should, however, be aware of competitors' prices, services, and other incentives intended to attract your office as a customer. Sometimes the incentives, such as bonus supplies with certain purchases, can represent sizable savings. Remember also that your time has a dollar value to the practice and services that save you time are worth comparing when evaluating vendors.

Obtaining recommendations from other medical offices is a good way to locate reputable office-supply dealers who sell items at reasonable prices. Reputable vendors fulfill orders accurately with quality items, deliver products in good condition, and charge fair prices. Keep in mind when evaluating vendors that the physician may have preferences for certain trade names or vendors.

Gathering Competitive Prices The costs of maintaining a medical practice are continually rising. Saving money on supplies through careful purchasing strategies is one way to help your physician/employer reduce spending. The medical assistant is often largely responsible for comparison pricing, ordering, and establishing and maintaining relationships with vendors. Your awareness of the most up-to-date information about vendors and supplies is valuable to your physician/employer. Discuss prices with the physician, who in turn may want to discuss them with an accountant.

Setting Up a Supply Budget The average medical practice spends 4% to 6% of its annual gross income on administrative, clinical, and general supplies. If an office is spending more than 6%, it may be time to reevaluate the office spending practices. Remember, though, that any budget is only a guide. A budget is meant to serve your office, not the reverse. You and your physician/employer may need to adjust the supply budget based on prices and discounts available from vendors.

Comparing Vendors To collect competitive data from vendors, contact them by telephone or in writing to request catalogs and other forms of product information. If you are not in charge of routing mail, make sure that supply-related mail, such as product catalogs and sale notices, is routed to you. Catalogs usually include basic information such as the dealer's name, address, and telephone number; order numbers for items; and vendor policy (see Figure 8-24). When investigating a vendor, obtain the following information:

- Prices—costs for supplies, delivery, and any other services; special discounts; minimum quantities applicable; and bonus supplies with purchases.

ORDERING INFORMATION

BY PHONE

Call our toll-free number:
(800) BIBBERO
(800-242-2376)
Monday through Friday,
6:00 a.m. – 5:00 p.m. (PT)

BY WEB

www.bibbero.com

BY MAIL

Complete order form and mail to:
Bibbero Systems, Inc.
1300 N. McDowell Blvd.
Petaluma, CA 94954-1180

BY FAX

Complete enclosed order form and transmit via fax to:
(800) 242-9330.
Our fax line is open 24 hours a day.

SHIPPING POLICY

Most in-stock items normally ship the same day (exclusive of file cabinets, file storage, office accessories and furnishings).

FREE DELIVERY

Free delivery on pre-paid orders totaling $300.00 or more, shipping within the Continental U.S.

Thank you for reviewing our catalog. We are confident that you will be pleased with both our products and our service. If you are in a hurry for product or samples, CALL us toll-free at (800) BIBBERO, FAX us at (800) 242-9330, or visit our web site. Our Customer Service Department is always happy to assist you.

If ordering by mail or fax, fill out the enclosed order form located at the back of this catalog. Either return it in the enclosed postage-paid envelope or fax it to us.

For items requiring custom imprinting, please include the following information, either typed or hand printed: name, specialty, address, city/state/zip, telephone number, and state license number (when required).

Don't see what you are looking for in our catalog? Submit a sample or provide specifications for any folder, divider, patient registration form, clinical form, health history questionnaire, etc., and we will promptly provide you with a quote. We can print single or multiple part forms, custom imprint folders, and manufacture a wide range of chart dividers.

Please Note: All custom printed orders are subject to an overrun or underrun variance of 10%.

Most orders for in-stock items received by 2:00 p.m. (PT) are normally shipped the same day (excluding cabinets, file storage, office accessories and furnishings). Out-of-stock items are automatically backordered. Personalized stationery items normally ship in 5–7 working days, after proof approval. Custom printed orders normally leave our plant within 7–10 working days, after proof approval. If certain items require an extended ship time, such as those listed above, delivery time will be quoted when order is received.

Custom printing or personalization on a rush basis is available on most products for an additional charge.

Some combined stock and custom printed items can be shipped together if requested in advance. All orders are shipped via the most economical, expeditious method to your locale. Items ordered together may not ship from the same locations or be received at the same time.

Common carriers are used for large volume orders. Overnight, 2nd and 3rd Day delivery services are available upon request.

All orders prepaid by check, Visa, MasterCard or American Express totaling $300.00 or more will be shipped freight free via surface transport within the Continental U.S. This offer excludes file cabinets, file storage, office accessories and furnishings and special order items. We regret that the high cost of shipping outside the contiguous 48 states prohibits us from extending our freight free policy; however, we will use the most economical shipping methods available to your location.

TERMS

Full payment is due upon receipt of merchandise. Accounts are considered overdue after thirty (30) days and are subject to a 1% monthly service charge. A service charge of $10.00 will be applied to all returned checks. For information regarding special financial arrangements, please contact our Credit Department at (800) 242-2376.

GUARANTEE!

Your satisfaction Guaranteed!

We guarantee our stock products. If you wish to return something, call to obtain a return authorization number and return shipment instructions. Most of our stock items can be returned within 60 days of purchase for full credit, exchange or a refund of your purchase price, with prior return authorization. After 60 days, your return is subject to a 20% restocking charge. Call our Customer Service Department at (800) 242-2376 for your return authorization number. Dymo® Products can be returned within 30 days of receipt with prior return authorization. Opened or unpackaged items are subject to a 15% or $15.00 restocking charge, which ever is greater. For disposable products located in our Clinical Supplies section, opened packages are subject to a 15% re-stocking charge with prior return authorization. Personalized items, custom printed items, custom manufactured or special order items, file cabinets, high density filing systems and opened and unlocked software are not returnable.

Items damaged in transit will be replaced as quickly as possible. Note any visible damage to the cartons on the bill of lading or delivery receipt and keep the original packaging in case items within are damaged.

Please Note: Self-adhesive products have a limited shelf life. Store in a cool, dry place.

Please Note: All custom printed orders are subject to an overrun or underrun variance of 10%.

We accept Visa, MasterCard and American Express for all your purchases.

BIBBERO SYSTEMS, INC.®

FIGURE 8-24 Examine supply catalogs and websites closely to obtain the best value for the office.

- Quality—product descriptions, illustrations, trade names, recommendations for use, durability, and guarantees.
- Service—availability of products, delivery time and procedures, sales representative availability, and damaged goods policy.
- Payment policies.

Competitive Pricing and Quality

Part of your responsibility in managing office supplies is to stay informed about the pricing and quality of competitors to your vendors. Savings can add up quickly, and ongoing comparison pricing can save the practice hundreds of dollars a year.

Unit Pricing Because many medical items come in a variety of package sizes, you need to be aware of how much the office is actually paying per item. To calculate an item's unit price, divide the total price of the package by the quantity, or number, of items. For example, if a package of 12 pens costs $12, the unit price, or price per pen, is $1 ($12 divided by 12 pens). If another vendor provides the same type of pen in a package of 18 for $17.10, the unit price is 95 cents ($17.10 divided by 18 pens). The second set of pens is the better buy.

Unit prices are generally lower at larger quantities. So, it makes sense to place one large order for a nonperishable item to cover the office until the next ordering time. Generally, however, you should not order more than a year's supply of any one item, particularly if the item is custom printed. Addresses, insurance codes, or additions to medical staff can change. When placing quantity discount orders, always consider the following factors:

- Whether the supply can be used within a reasonable time;
- The possibility of spoilage or deterioration;
- The amount of storage space in the office; and
- Whether the doctor will continue to use the item.

Avoid overspending by not ordering more of an item than is reasonable or necessary.

Rush Orders Unexpected rush orders usually cost the office more money than regularly scheduled orders. (In some cases, a vendor may not charge extra to a steady customer, but these cases would be exceptions.) To avoid rush orders, be aware of approximately how long the vendor takes to deliver an order. You can obtain this information from the vendor policy and by keeping accurate records of your own experience with deliveries.

Mail-Order Companies Using large, established mail-order companies often saves money for the medical office, but there may be less control over orders and a greater potential for hidden costs. The neighborhood pharmacy may also offer discounts, but ordering from wholesalers or directly from the manufacturer is usually more economical. The Points on Practice section on the next page provides helpful information about cost-efficient ordering by telephone, by fax, or through an online service.

Purchasing Groups Purchasing groups are groups of practices that order supplies together to obtain a quantity discount. For example, several medical offices associated with a nearby hospital may order through the hospital. In return for this convenience, the physicians pay dues and guarantee the vendors a certain amount of business. Some programs require members to spend a certain percentage of their supply budget through the group. Groups also may require that members not disclose the group's prices to other physicians. Large medical practices that participate in these groups usually save an average of 20% on supplies. The savings are not usually significant for small offices.

Group Buying Pools If a medical office wants to use local vendors instead of, or in addition to, a purchasing group or if it is too small to benefit from a purchasing group, it can still pool resources with other area offices to qualify for quantity discounts. Even if the offices are ordering different items, discounts are based on the total order and savings can range from 10% to 20%. Under this arrangement, the offices must usually take responsibility for distributing the items among themselves. A buying pool is convenient for medical practices that are in the same building or office complex (Figure 8-25).

Cost Controls Medical practices are increasingly interested in saving money and controlling costs in general. Physician reimbursement is constantly being reevaluated. As a result, more than ever, physicians are interested in controlling the operating costs of their practices. Managing expenses within the practice is a very important responsibility for the medical assistant. What may seem to be just a small reduction in cost to the practice can actually result in a substantial reduction to office expenses over the course of a year. As a medical assistant, it is your job to constantly look for ways to reduce costs within the practice without sacrificing quality.

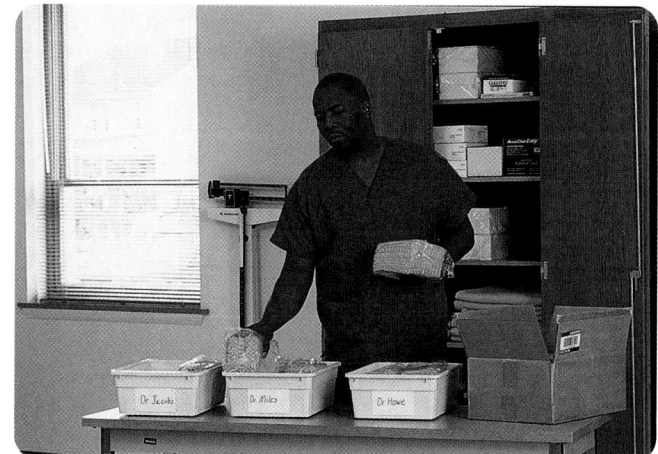

FIGURE 8-25 Ordering jointly with other practices can cut down on costs for everyone.

Ordering by Telephone, Fax, or Online

You may occasionally purchase office supplies at a local office supply store, but usually you will order them without even leaving your office. Three common ways to do so are by telephone, by fax machine, and through an online service. The following tips are included to help you make sure that every order—no matter which option you choose—is successfully placed.

Ordering by Telephone

1. Clear communication is a must when ordering by telephone. Speak slowly and enunciate your words carefully to make sure you are understood. It is also a good idea to spell each word of the practice name and the address to ensure proper delivery. Use expressions like "S as in Sam, P as in people" to clarify your spelling.

2. Ask the representative taking your order to repeat the order. Check that every item is included with the appropriate price, quantity, style, and color.

3. Confirm the expected delivery date so that you will know if something is late. Also confirm how payment will be made, to prevent unexpected delays.

4. Record the name and telephone number of the person who takes the order in case there is a problem with the order. Get an order number (or confirmation number) in case you have to call back with a question or a change in your order.

FIGURE 8-26 Read online information just as carefully as you read a printed catalog.

5. If possible, avoid placing telephone orders on Mondays and Fridays, when call volume is typically high.

Ordering by Fax

1. When ordering by fax, use the form provided by the vendor if one is available. This form uses the format to which the supply company is accustomed and will speed your order's processing.

2. Type your order, or write it neatly and legibly, to prevent miscommunication. Fill out the form completely. Make sure you indicate quantities, descriptions, and prices (including shipping) for each item you order.

3. Proofread your order before you send it. Checking the accuracy of the order now will save time later.

4. Follow up by telephone to make sure your order was received and understood, and to confirm the delivery date and payment requirements.

Ordering Online

1. Ordering online requires a computer and a modem connection to the Internet or to an online service. Before ordering online, make sure you are fully familiar with the equipment and the process, or have your supervisor or the supply company's sales representative oversee your initial orders.

2. Type your name and address accurately.

3. If pictures of supplies are not available online, consult the company's printed catalog or CD-ROM catalog. If you do not have access to a catalog, read the online text descriptions carefully, checking trade names and specifications, to select the appropriate merchandise (Figure 8-26). If you have questions, call the supply company.

4. When you have completed the selections, the online service will display your order for you to confirm. Check that all the information is accurate, including your name, address, and telephone number.

5. If you have an account with the company, you may type in your account number to place the order. Otherwise, you may wish to arrange to make payment on delivery. If you prefer to pay by credit card, first make sure that the company is reputable and that it uses a security system that prevents your number from being read by anyone unauthorized to do so.

If, despite your best efforts, your order is processed incorrectly, take appropriate action immediately. Although ordering by telephone, by fax, or online is convenient, it still requires additional time to package items that must be returned.

By law, orders that you place must be fulfilled within a reasonable time. The Federal Trade Commission (FTC) monitors purchases by telephone, fax, and online services to protect consumers. The FTC requires supply companies to provide merchandise within 30 days or to give you the option of canceling the order and receiving a full refund.

Benefits of Using Local Vendors

There are many potential vendors, including local dealers, mail-order companies, and nearby pharmacies. Try to establish good credit and business relationships with reputable local vendors. Although these companies usually charge a little more than mail-order companies, spending most of the office's supply budget through one favored local dealer often results in discounts, special service in the event of an emergency, and information about upcoming sales and specials. Local dealers also may offer more personal assistance—perhaps even a salesperson's help with taking inventory—to compete with larger vendors whose business is based primarily on catalog sales. The extra service may be worth the higher cost.

Buying from local vendors also can provide a public relations benefit for physicians; it means keeping business in the community. However, specialty items may need to be ordered from other vendors. For example, letterhead should be ordered from a reliable printer, whether that printer is located in the community or out of state.

Payment Schedules

Another factor that affects the cost of supplies is the payment schedule. Many vendors do not charge for handling if an order is prepaid. Others offer a discount for enclosing a check with an order. Some delay billing for 30 to 90 days, allowing the physician to keep the money in the bank, collecting interest for a longer period.

The vendor's invoice usually describes payment terms. Two examples of payment terms are

- "Net 30": This means you have 30 days in which to pay the total amount.
- "1% 10 Days Net 30": This means that you will get a savings of 1% of the total price by paying within 10 days.

Copies of all bills and order forms for supplies should be kept on file for at least 7 years in case the practice is audited by the Internal Revenue Service (IRS).

Ordering Procedures

Ordering procedures for supplies vary from office to office but always involve these tasks: completing paperwork, checking orders received, correcting errors in shipments, and making payment.

Order Forms Before ordering merchandise, you should inquire about a vendor's ordering options, discuss them with the physician, and determine which method is best for the office. Many vendors now have ordering capability through telephone, fax, e-mail, and online as well as traditional written order forms. Always be sure to keep a copy of each order you submit.

Before you place an order, gather all the necessary information, such as correct names of items, item numbers, and order and account numbers. This information helps to ensure the order's accuracy. Immediately after placing the order, note all order information on the inventory card or record page for that item.

Purchase Requisitions You will need to follow any special ordering procedures established in your medical office. The specific procedures and the medical assistant's level of authority vary from one office to another. Sometimes placing an order requires a **requisition** (a formal request from a staff member or doctor), which is given to the medical assistant who does the actual ordering. The doctor's approval may be necessary for large purchases—for example, for orders that total more than $300. Recurring orders may not require the doctor's approval, but you may need to get approval before ordering a new brand or quantities of a particular item over a certain amount.

In a group practice where doctors order different items and several staffers are in charge of ordering, procedures for ordering can be complicated. One common way to simplify matters is to use a **purchase order**—a form that authorizes a purchase for the practice. Figure 8-27 shows a sample purchase order. Purchase orders are usually preprinted with consecutive numbers. The medical assistant submits approved purchase orders to the vendor for fulfillment. This method is most often used for expensive items, such as office equipment, but some large practices also use purchase orders for supplies.

Checking Orders Received When the shipment of supplies arrives, record on the inventory card or record page the

date received and the quantity of each item. Check the shipment against the order form to make sure the correct items—in the correct sizes, styles, packaging, and quantity—have been delivered.

Then check the contents against the packing slip (a description of the package contents) enclosed in the package. This checking takes time, but catching even one error is worth the time taken. If several people on a staff have ordering responsibility, they can share the task. The employee should write on the package slip the date items were received; check off each item as you verify and initial.

Correcting Errors All errors in a shipment should be reported immediately to the vendor so that the records can be corrected and missing supplies can be delivered. When you call to report errors, be sure you have all the paperwork in front of you. You will need the invoice number, order date, name of the person who placed the order, name of the person who took the order, and a list of questions or a description of the complaint. If a catalog was used in ordering, have it open to the appropriate page. Always record the name and title of the person you speak with when reporting the error.

Invoices Typically, the vendor sends an invoice to the medical office, either accompanying the merchandise or separately. This invoice also should be checked carefully against the original order and the packing slip. It is a good idea to staple the order list, packing list, and a copy of the invoice

PURCHASE ORDER #2532

Submitted by: _____

Order Number: _____

Date Ordered: _____

Date Required: _____

SHIP TO: BWW Medical Associates, PC
305 Main Street
Port Snead, YZ 12345-9876

PHONE: 555-654-3210

NO	ITEM	DESCRIPTION/MODEL	COLOR	SIZE	QUANTITY	PRICE EACH	TOTAL
1							
2							
3							
4							
5							
6							
7							
8							
						TOTAL	

Approved: _____   Date: _____

FIGURE 8-27 Typical purchase order form.

together for the office records to verify all items were received. See Figure 8-28. Be sure to check the arithmetic, too. Then sign or stamp the invoice to confirm that the order was received. If an item you order is temporarily out of stock, the vendor usually sends an invoice stamped "Back Ordered." Later, when the item is back in stock, the vendor will ship it to your office.

It is also a good habit to record the check number, date, and amount of payment on the invoice. You may initial it or have the doctor initial it. By keeping a copy of the paid invoice with the attached order slip and packing slip in the office records, it will be easy to track the items included within each invoice. This step makes verifying payments easier and decreases the chance of inadvertently paying an invoice twice.

Disbursements An invoice is paid with a **disbursement** (payment of funds) to a vendor. Disbursements may be made in cash or by check or money order. Usually, you will write a check to the vendor and have the physician sign it. Be sure to show the physician the original order, packing slip, and invoice. On the front of the check, record the invoice number. Finally, mail the check to the vendor with the vendor's copy of the invoice. File the office copy of the invoice, along with the original order and the packing slip, according to your inventory filing system.

If you make a cash disbursement, obtain a receipt to keep on file. If you are the one responsible for maintaining the practice's financial records and presenting them to the accountant, you also may be responsible for recording the payment information in the office's accounting books.

Avoiding Common Purchasing Mistakes

Even the most watchful professional can make purchasing mistakes. The best you can do is to educate yourself about common mistakes and try to avoid them. For example, be aware of the possibility of dishonest telephone solicitations. A caller may claim to be a sales representative for the manufacturer of the office photocopier, offering bargains on paper or toner. The caller may require advance payment to be sent to a post office box. The bargains may never arrive.

The best way to deal with these solicitations is to tell the caller that your office does not purchase supplies by telephone. If a telephone offer appears to be legitimate and to offer substantial savings, ask for the name and telephone number of the firm so that you can return the call at a more convenient time. This will give you time to verify the number with the telephone company and check the firm's name with the Better Business Bureau.

Another disreputable tactic some vendors use is bait and switch, meaning the price of one item is lowered to attract the customer, but that item is always "sold out" and the customer is encouraged to buy a more expensive one. A vendor may also mislead you by raising the price of an item you have been ordering without informing you. Always confirm the current

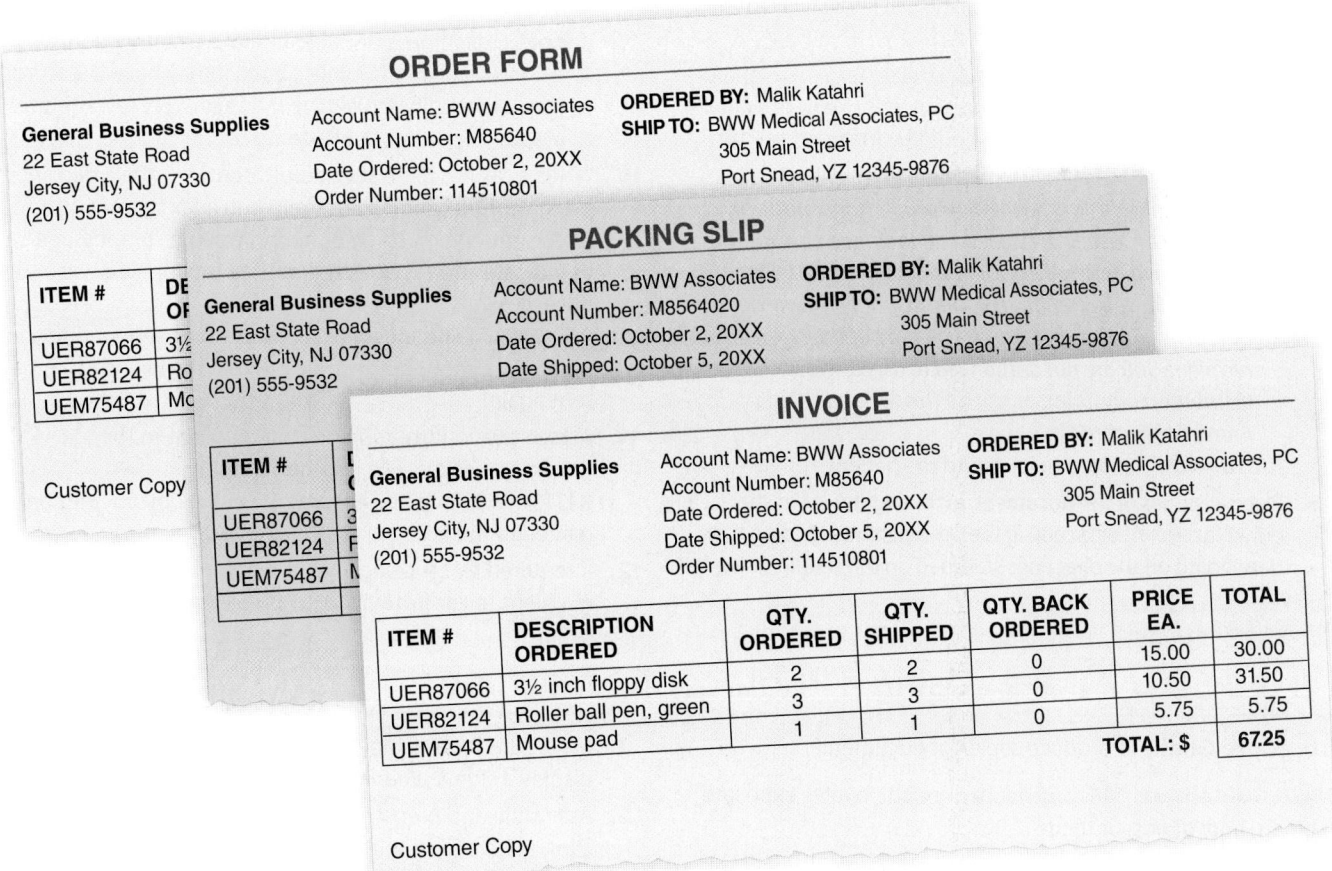

FIGURE 8-28 Fill out purchase orders clearly and carefully to avoid having to return items.

price, check invoices as they come in, and record everything in the item's file. Having your inventory card or record page open while ordering will prompt you to notice and question price changes. If there is an honest error, a reputable firm will readily and courteously correct it.

Problems also can be avoided by carefully supervising a new vendor's sales representative until a comfortable, professional rapport has been established. Discuss your inventory system with representatives, and ask them questions about their procedures.

PROCEDURE 8-1 Using a Facsimile (Fax) Machine

Procedure Goal: To correctly prepare and send a fax document, while following all HIPAA guidelines to guard patient confidentiality.

OSHA Guidelines: This procedure does not involve exposure to blood, body fluids, or tissue.

Materials: Fax machine, fax line, cover sheet with statement of disclaimer, area code and phone number of fax recipient, document to be faxed, telephone line, and telephone.

Method: Procedure steps.

1. Prepare a *cover sheet*, which provides information about the transmission. Cover sheets can vary in appearance but usually include the name, telephone number, and fax number of the sender and the receiver; the number of pages being transmitted; and the date of the transmission. Preprinted cover sheets also can be used.
   RATIONALE: The fax should clearly identify where it originated and to whom it is being sent. If another recipient receives the fax in error, he will know who to notify regarding the error.

2. All cover sheets must carry a disclaimer statement to guard the patient's privacy. A *disclaimer* is a statement of denial of legal liability. A disclaimer should be included on the cover sheet and may read something like this:

   This fax contains confidential or proprietary information that may be legally privileged. It is intended only for the named recipient(s). If an addressing or transmission error has misdirected the fax, please notify the author by replying to this message. If you are not the named recipient, you are not authorized to use, disclose, distribute, copy, print, or rely on this fax and should immediately shred it.

   RATIONALE: This step helps guard the patient's privacy.

3. Place all pages of the document, including the cover sheet, either facedown or faceup in the fax machine's sending tray, depending on the directions stamped on the sending tray.

4. If the pages are placed facedown, write the area code and fax number on the back of the last page.

5. Dial the receiving fax machine's telephone number using either the telephone attached to the fax machine or the numbers on the fax keyboard. Include the area code for long-distance calls.

6. When using a fax telephone, listen for a high-pitched tone. Then press the "Send" or "Start" button and hang up the telephone. This step completes the call circuit in older-model fax machines. Your fax is now being sent. Newer fax machines do not require this step.
   RATIONALE: This step completes the call circuit in older-model fax machines.

7. If you use the fax keyboard, press the "Send" or "Start" button after dialing the telephone number. This button will start the call.

8. Watch for the fax machine to make a connection. Often a green light appears as the document feeds through the machine.

9. If the fax machine is not able to make a connection, as when the receiving fax line is busy, it may have a feature that automatically redials the number every few minutes for a specified number of attempts.

10. When a fax has been successfully sent, most fax machines print a confirmation message. When a fax has not been sent, the machine either prints an error message or indicates on the screen that the transmission was unsuccessful.
    RATIONALE: This message confirms to the sender that the fax has been sent or indicates that the fax needs to be sent again.

11. Attach the confirmation or error message to the documents faxed. File appropriately.
    RATIONALE: This step ensures thorough documentation related to the fax.

12. If required by office policy, the sender should call the recipient to confirm the fax was received.

PROCEDURE 8-2 Using a Photocopier Machine

Procedure Goal: To produce copies of documents.

OSHA Guidelines: This procedure does not involve exposure to blood, body fluids, or tissue.

Materials: Copier machine, copy paper, and documents to be copied.

Method: Procedure steps.

1. Make sure the machine is turned on and warmed up. It will display a signal when it is ready for copying.

2. Assemble and prepare your materials, removing paper clips, staples, and self-adhesive flags.
   RATIONALE: This step helps avoid loose items getting caught in the copier and provides for optimum efficiency.

3. Place the document to be copied in the automatic feeder tray as directed, or upside-down directly on the glass. The feeder tray can accommodate many pages; you may place only one page at a time on the glass. Automatic feeding is a faster process, and you should use it when you wish to collate or staple packets. Page-by-page copying is best if you need to copy a single sheet or to enlarge or reduce the image. To use any special features, such as making double-sided copies or stapling the copies, press a designated button on the machine.

4. Set the machine for the desired paper size.
   RATIONALE: The copier will select the paper size automatically if the size is not selected. This could result in a waste of paper.

5. Key in the number of copies you want to make and press the "Start" button. The copies are made automatically.

6. Press the "Clear" or "Reset" button when your job is finished.
   RATIONALE: The machine is now ready for the next user and will not perform unwanted functions on the next document.

7. If the copier becomes jammed, follow the directions on the machine to locate the problem (for example, there may be multiple pieces of paper stuck inside the printer) and dislodge the jammed paper. Most copy machines will show a diagram of the printer and the location of the problem.

PROCEDURE 8-3 Using a Postage Meter

Procedure Goal: To correctly apply postage to an envelope or package for mailing, according to U.S. Postal Service guidelines.

OSHA Guidelines: This procedure does not involve exposure to blood, body fluids, or tissue.

Materials: Postage meter, addressed envelope or package, and postal scale.

Method: Procedure steps.

1. Check that there is postage available in the postage meter.
   RATIONALE: For the postage meter to function, there must be money in your postal account. Contact the company that manages your account or your local post office for more information.

2. Verify the day's date.
   RATIONALE: U.S. Postal Service guidelines prohibit mailing envelopes and packages that are postmarked with an incorrect date.

3. Check that the postage meter is plugged in and switched on before you proceed.

4. Locate the area where the meter registers the date. Many machines have a lid that can be flipped up, with rows of numbers underneath. Months are represented numerically, with the number "1" indicating the month of January, "2" indicating February, and so on. Check that the date is correct. If it is incorrect, change the numbers to the correct date.

5. Make sure all materials have been included in the envelope or package. Weigh the envelope or package on a postal scale. Standard business envelopes weighing up to 1 oz require the minimum postage (the equivalent of one first-class stamp). Oversize envelopes and packages require additional postage. A postal scale will indicate the required postage.

6. Key in the postage amount on the meter and press the button that enters the amount. For amounts over $1, press the "$" sign or the "Enter" button twice.
   RATIONALE: This feature verifies large amounts, catching errors in case you mistakenly press too many keys.

7. Check that the amount you typed is the correct amount. Envelopes and packages with too little postage will be returned by the U.S. Postal Service. Sending an envelope or package with too much postage is wasteful to the practice.

8. While applying postage to an envelope, hold it flat and right side up (in order to read the address). Seal the envelope (unless the meter seals it for you). Locate the plate or area where the envelope slides through. This feature is usually near the bottom of the meter. Place the envelope on the left side and give it a gentle push toward the right. Some models hold the envelope in a stationary position. (If the meter seals the envelope for you, it is especially important that you insert it correctly to allow for sealing.) The meter will grab the envelope and pull it through quickly.

9. For packages, create a postage label to affix to the package. Follow the same procedure for a label as for an envelope. Affix the postmarked label on the package in the upper-right corner.

10. Check that the printed postmark has the correct date and amount and that everything written or stamped on the envelope or package is legible.

PROCEDURE 8-4 Using a Check-Writing Machine

Procedure Goal: To produce a check using a check-writing machine.

OSHA Guidelines: This procedure does not involve exposure to blood, body fluids, or tissue.

Materials: Check-writing machine, blank checks, office checkbook, or accounting system.

Method: Procedure steps.

1. Assemble all equipment.

2. Turn on the check-writing machine.

3. Place a blank check or a sheet of blank checks into the machine.

4. Key in the date, the payee's name, and the payment amount. The check-writing machine imprints the check with this information, perforating it with the payee's name. The perforations are actual little holes in the paper that prevent anyone from changing the name on the check.

5. Turn off the check-writing machine.

6. A doctor or another authorized person then signs the check.

RATIONALE: The check is not valid without the proper signature.

7. To complete the process, record the check in the office checkbook or accounting system.
   RATIONALE: To maintain accurate records, all financial transactions must be promptly and accurately recorded.

PROCEDURE 8-5 Step-by-Step Overview of Inventory Procedures

Procedure Goal: To set up an effective inventory program for a medical office.

OSHA Guidelines: This procedure does not involve exposure to blood, body fluids, or tissue.

Materials: Pen, paper, file folders, vendor catalogs, index cards or loose-leaf binder and blank pages, reorder reminder cards, and vendor order forms.

Method: Procedure steps.

1. Discuss and define with your physician/employer the extent of your responsibility in managing supplies. Know whether the physician's approval or supervision is required for certain procedures, whether any systems have already been established, and if the physician has any preference for a particular vendor or trade-name item. If your medical practice is large, determine which medical assistant is responsible for each aspect of supply management.

2. Know what administrative and clinical supplies should be stocked in your office. Create a formal supply list of vital, incidental, and periodic items and keep a copy in the office's procedures manual.

3. Start a file containing a list of current vendors with copies of their catalogs.

4. Create a wish list of brands or products the office does not currently use but might like to try. Inform other staff members of the list so that they can make entries.

5. Make a file for supply invoices and completed order forms. (Keep these documents on file for at least 3 years.)
   RATIONALE: Keep completed documents for future reference as well as for legal protection, if needed.

6. Devise an inventory system of index cards, loose-leaf pages, or a computer spreadsheet for each item. List the following data for each item on its card:
   • Date and quantity of each order.
   • Name and contact information for the vendor and sales representative.
   • Date each shipment was received.
   • Total cost and unit cost, or price per piece for the item.
   • Payment method used.
   • Results of periodic counts of the item.
   • Quantity expected to cover the office for a given period of time.

   • Reorder quantity (the quantity remaining on the shelf that indicates when reorder should be made).

7. Have a system for flagging items that need to be ordered and those that are already on order. For example, mark their cards or pages with a self-adhesive tab or note. Make or buy reorder reminder cards to put into the stock of each item at the reorder quantity level.
   RATIONALE: Having a system in place makes your job easier and also will make it easier for anyone else taking over the task at a later date.

8. Establish with the physician a regular inventory-taking schedule. Every 1 to 2 weeks is usually sufficient. As a backup system for remembering to check stock and reorder, estimate the times for these activities. Mark them on your calendar or create a tickler file on your computer.
   RATIONALE: A regular schedule means inventory and ordering will not be forgotten.

9. Order at the same times each week or month, after inventory is taken. However, if there is an unexpected shortage of an item and more than a week or so remains before the regular ordering time, place the order immediately.

10. Fill in the vendor's order form (or type a letter of request). Order by telephone, by fax, by e-mail, or online. Online ordering will expedite the order. Follow procedures that have been approved by the physician or office manager. When placing an order, have all the necessary information at hand, including the correct name of the item and the order and account numbers. Record the order information in the inventory file for that item. Be sure to obtain from the vendor an estimated arrival time for the order and mark that date and order number on your calendar.

11. When ordering online, save the website to "Favorites" for easy, one-click future access. Select the website and establish an account with the company. To establish an account, you will need to give information about your office practice, including the name of the practice, the contact name, the address, the phone number, an e-mail address, and a payment source. Ask about adding the practice to any special contact lists for promotional materials and discounts.

12. When you receive the shipment, record the date and the amount received on the item's inventory card or record page. Check the shipment against the original order and

the packing slip inside the package to ensure that the right items, sizes, styles, packaging, and amounts have arrived. Initial each item on the packing slip as a record that the correct item and amount were received. If there is any error, immediately call or e-mail the vendor, with the catalog page and the inventory card or record page at hand.
RATIONALE: Items should be unpacked and checked immediately so that if a problem is discovered, it will be relatively easy to prove that the error or problem is with the shipment and not caused by office personnel.

13. Check the invoice carefully against the original order and the packing slip, making sure that the amount of the bill matches the items listed on the invoice and the packing list, and ensure that the bill has not already been paid. Sign or stamp the invoice to show that the order was received.

14. Write a check to the vendor to be signed by the physician. (Check-writing procedures are described in the *Financial Management* chapter.) Be sure to show the physician the original order, packing slip, and invoice. Record the check number, date, and amount of payment on the invoice and initial it or have the physician do so. Write the invoice number on the front of the check.
RATIONALE: Writing the invoice number on the check will ensure that the payment is posted to the correct account. Writing the check number and date on the invoice will be useful for future reference if there is a payment dispute.

15. Mail the check and the vendor's copy of the invoice to the vendor within 30 days and file the office copy of the invoice with the original order and packing slip.

SUMMARY OF LEARNING OUTCOMES

LEARNING OUTCOMES	KEY POINTS
8.1 **Identify common types of computers.**	Common types of computers include mainframes, minicomputers, desktop computers, laptops, notebooks, subnotebooks, PDAs, and some types of cell phones.
8.2 **Describe computer hardware components and explain the functions of each.**	Computer hardware components include the monitor, which allows information contained in the system to be seen; the keyboard, which allows for inputting of information; and the printer, which produces "hard copies" of information.
8.3 **Describe the types of software applications commonly used in the medical office.**	Software components include both the operating system that controls the computer and applications that run on the operating system. Software applications commonly used in the medical office include operating system software such as Microsoft Windows XP, Microsoft Windows 7, and Linux. Application software commonly used in medical offices includes word processing, database management, spreadsheets, practice management, electronic transfer, scheduling, and desktop publishing.
8.4 **Summarize the options available for learning computer software programs.**	Options available for learning computer software programs include classes, tutorials, manuals, documentation, and online learning with online software "Help" features.
8.5 **Recall the steps involved in selecting new or upgrading existing office computer equipment.**	Learn as much as you can about the hardware and software being considered. Consider the office needs now and in the future. What is the existing hardware and/or software capable of and can it meet the needs now and in the future? Will an upgrade suffice or will new equipment or software save the office money in the long run? These are the most important considerations.
8.6 **Outline the basic care and maintenance required for the office computer system.**	The system unit should be placed in a well-ventilated location and a power strip with a surge protector should be used to protect the circuitry. Use screen savers and power-down capabilities when the system is not in use. Protect storage devices with appropriate covers when not in use. Never eat or drink near computers. Follow maintenance directions provided with all equipment.

LEARNING OUTCOMES	KEY POINTS
8.7 **Identify several reasons why security is particularly important in the computerized office.**	Great care must be taken to safeguard confidential files, make backup copies on a regular basis, and prevent system contamination. HIPAA laws require that privacy and security procedures are in place to prevent the misuse of health information. These procedures also must ensure confidentiality.
8.8 **Recognize advances that are occurring with computers of the future.**	Telemedicine, CD-R and DVD-R technology, and speech recognition technology are three examples of new computer technologies.
8.9 **Explain the function of other types of administrative medical office equipment.**	Other administrative medical office equipment includes faxes to send information; photocopiers to copy information; typewriters, adding machines, and calculators to perform business functions; folding/inserting machines and postage meters to efficiently prepare mail; dictation-transcription machines for clear medical records; check writers to assist with accounts payable; and paper shredders for confidentiality.
8.10 **Outline the steps to be taken in deciding whether new office equipment is needed.**	The first step in evaluating the equipment needs of a healthcare office is the research process. Consider office needs and ask about advantages of new equipment versus existing equipment, comparing the benefits of each. Compare products, features, and prices, calling the suppliers for more information as needed. Do not forget to review the warranties.
8.11 **Explain the difference between a maintenance contract and a service contract.**	A maintenance contract specifies when the equipment will be cleaned, checked for worn parts, and repaired. A standard maintenance contract may include regular checkups as well as emergency repairs. A service contract may cover emergency repairs not covered under standard maintenance.
8.12 **Define vital, periodic, and incidental supplies.**	Vital supplies are items that are absolutely essential for the practice's functioning. Incidental supplies are needed in the office but do not threaten the office's efficiency if the supply runs low. Periodic supplies are those supplies that require ordering only occasionally, like appointment books.
8.13 **Outline the steps in performing a supply inventory.**	Review Procedure 8-5 for an outline on performing a supply inventory.
8.14 **List the items that should be considered when choosing a vendor for supply ordering.**	Obtaining recommendations from other medical offices is a good way to locate reputable office-supply dealers who sell items at reasonable prices. Reputable vendors fulfill orders accurately with quality items, deliver products in good condition, and charge fair prices. Compare vendors on price, quality, timeliness, and how they handle customer problems and complaints.

CASE STUDY CRITICAL THINKING

Recall Miguel from the beginning of the chapter. Now that you have completed the chapter, answer the following questions regarding his case.

1. Why is it important that Miguel keep track of the usage of the various types of administrative equipment and supplies used by BWW Medical Associates?

2. Why is it important for Miguel to stay current with communications coming into the office via fax and e-mail?

1. (LO 8.2) Which of the following items is NOT a pointing device?
   a. Mouse
   b. Trackball
   c. Touch pad
   d. Touch screen
   e. Keyboard

2. (LO 8.1) Which of the following are considered personal computers?
   a. Desktops
   b. Laptops
   c. PDAs
   d. All of the above
   e. All but c

3. (LO 8.2) Which of the following is the smallest storage drive?
   a. Zip drive
   b. Jump drive
   c. CD-ROM
   d. DVD-ROM
   e. Diskettes

4. (LO 8.3) Which software program would be most helpful if you want to produce a report on your patients with a family history of breast cancer?
   a. Database management
   b. Spreadsheet
   c. Communication
   d. Appointment scheduling
   e. Word processing

5. (LO 8.2) Many copiers are now capable of multiple tasks. Which of the following is NOT one of those tasks?
   a. Copying
   b. Faxing
   c. Calculations
   d. Scanning
   e. Collating

6. (LO 8.9) Which of the following is a financial reason for considering a postage meter?
   a. It saves on trips to the post office
   b. It cuts down on the different types of stamps needed in the office
   c. Calculating postage for larger articles, including packages, is easier
   d. It saves money by calculating and printing the exact postage needed
   e. All of the above

7. (LO 8.9) What is the most important reason to have paper-shredding capabilities for the medical office?
   a. Decreases waste by cutting paper into small strips
   b. Destroys "mistakes" made in a medical record
   c. Destroys unneeded documents containing PHI
   d. Increases readily available packing material
   e. Destroys records of patients who leave the practice

8. (LO 8.12) When managing office supplies, the goal is to achieve
   a. Efficiency
   b. Organization
   c. Resourcefulness
   d. Independence
   e. All of the above

9. (LO 8.12) Expendable items are those that are
   a. Able to be thrown away
   b. Used and must be restocked
   c. Used indefinitely
   d. Restored and reused
   e. Vital to the running of the office

10. (LO 8.12) Examples of clinical supplies are
    a. Needles, syringes, and lubricating jelly
    b. Paper cups and toilet tissue
    c. Rubber bands, stamps, and file folders
    d. Patient education materials and insurance forms
    e. Paper drapes and HIPAA forms

Go to CONNECT to see activities about *Creating Pick-Lists for Ordering Supplies* and *Creating a Reminder for Ordering Supplies.*

PATIENT INFORMATION

Patient Name	Gender	DOB
Shenya Jones	F	11/03/19XX

Attending	MRN	Allergies
Elizabeth H. Williams, MD	124-86-564	Peanuts and cinnamon

Shenya Jones, 34-year-old female, arrives at the office with swelling and a red pustule on her face. She states that the problem started two days ago as a small pimple near her nose. It became irritated, and then extremely swollen and painful overnight. This morning, she noticed yellow drainage at the lesion site and the swelling has increased. The area of drainage is approximately 1 cm in diameter. Her upper lip, side of the face, and nose are all swollen. The examination and treatment areas need to be prepared before you bring her to the back office.

Keep Shenya in mind as you study this chapter. There will be questions at the end of the chapter based on the case study. The information in the chapter will help you answer these questions.

LEARNING OUTCOMES

After completing Chapter 9, you will be able to:

9.1 Describe the layout and features of a typical examination room.

9.2 Differentiate between sanitization and disinfection.

9.3 List steps to prevent the spread of infection in the exam and treatment rooms.

9.4 Describe the importance of temperature, lighting, and ventilation in the exam room.

9.5 Identify instruments and supplies used in a general physical exam and tell how to arrange and prepare them.

KEY TERMS

accessibility

consumable

disinfection

fixative

general physical examination

lubricant

occult blood

sanitization

spores

sterilization

CAAHEP

III. C (3) Discuss infection control procedures

III. C (6) Compare different methods of controlling the growth of microorganisms

IX. C (11) Identify how the Americans with Disabilities Act (ADA) applies to the medical assisting profession

IX. C (13) Discuss all levels of governmental legislation and regulation as they apply to medical assisting practice, including FDA and DEA regulations

XI. P (2) Evaluate the work environment to identify safe vs. unsafe working conditions

ABHES

9. Medical Office Clinical Procedures
Graduates:
  b. Apply principles of aseptic techniques and infection control
  k. Prepare and maintain examination and treatment area

10. Medical Laboratory Procedures
Graduates:
  c. Dispose of biohazardous materials

▶ Introduction

The care and maintenance of the medical office's examination and treatment areas are duties of the medical assistant. Preventing accidents by following physical safety guidelines discussed in the *Basic Safety and Infection Control* chapter are just the beginning of such duties. The medical assistant must perform specific tasks to prepare and maintain the rooms, equipment, and supplies. These tasks include knowing the equipment and supplies and practicing infection control at all times.

▶ The Exam Room   LO 9.1

The exam room is the area where the physician observes the patient, listens to the patient's description of symptoms, performs a general physical exam, and dispenses treatment. A physician performs a **general physical examination** to confirm a patient's health or diagnose a medical problem. Figure 9-1 shows a typical exam room.

FIGURE 9-1 You are responsible for making sure the exam room is clean and orderly.

Number and Size of Rooms

The number of exam rooms in a medical office depends on the number of physicians who work there and on each physician's patient load. Ideally, each physician in a medical office has at least two exam rooms for her or his exclusive use. A minimum of two rooms per physician enables the medical assistant to prepare one room while the physician examines a patient in the other room.

The customary size for an exam room is 8 by 12 feet—large enough to accommodate the physician, the patient, and one assistant comfortably, yet small enough that instruments and supplies will be within easy reach. Doors and interior walls should be soundproofed to ensure privacy for patients. Some exam rooms have dressing cubicles in one corner, while others have screens behind which the patient may disrobe. Regardless of a room's layout, you should provide privacy for patients whenever they need to disrobe and put on gowns.

A rack for the patient's medical records usually hangs on the wall directly outside the exam room or on the outside of the door. A light or other device like colored tabs on the wall or door may be used to signal that the room is occupied.

Furnishings

Furnishings should be arranged for efficiency, physician convenience, and patient comfort. The examining table is the exam room's key piece of equipment and should be positioned in the center of the room or extending out from the wall. This arrangement allows the physician and an assistant to attend to the patient on at least three sides. The examining table usually contains a pullout step for the patient to use when getting onto the table. It also may contain drawers for storing instruments and table coverings. Examining tables are usually adjustable to enable the patient to assume the various positions the physical exam may require. The physician will probably tell you beforehand if you need to adjust the table in a particular way. Most exam rooms also have a sink, a countertop, and a writing surface large enough to spread out the patient's records. Shelves, cupboards, and drawers store routine supplies like dressings, adhesive tape, and bandages. The exam room also may include the following items:

- One or more chairs for the patient and family member.
- A rolling stool for the physician.
- A weight scale with height bar (there may not be a scale in every room).
- A metal wastebasket with a lid.
- Biohazardous waste containers for disposal of biohazardous materials (biological agents that can spread disease to living things).
- Puncture-proof containers for disposal of biohazardous sharps.
- A high-intensity lamp.
- Wall brackets for hanging instruments such as a blood pressure cuff.

Special Features

The Americans with Disabilities Act of 1990 (ADA) requires that businesses, services, and public transportation provide "reasonable accommodations" for individuals with disabilities. To comply with this act, at least one exam room in a medical office must have features that make the area accessible to patients who use wheelchairs or who have visual or other types of physical impairments. **Accessibility** refers to the ease with which people can move in and out of a space.

The ADA accessibility guidelines require the following:

- A doorway at least 36 inches (915 mm) wide to allow a person in a wheelchair to pass through.
- A clearance space in rooms and hallways that is 60 inches (1525 mm) in diameter to allow a person in a wheelchair to make a 180-degree turn.
- Stable, firm, slip-resistant flooring.
- Door-opening hardware that can be grasped with one hand and does not require the twisting of the wrist to use.
- Door closers adjusted to allow time for a person in a wheelchair to enter or exit through the door.
- Grab bars in the lavatory.

▶ Sanitization and Disinfection LO 9.2

Specific measures to achieve medical asepsis and prevent the spread of pathogenic microorganisms must be followed in the medical office. In addition to the basic measures outlined in *Basic Safety and Infection Control,* sanitation and disinfection must be performed.

Sanitization

Sanitization is the scrubbing of instruments and equipment with special brushes and detergent to remove blood, mucus, and other contaminants or media where pathogens can grow. Sanitization is used to clean items that touch only healthy, intact skin. For other equipment, sanitization is the first step before disinfection and sterilization. Examples of instruments and equipment that you can sanitize and reuse without further disinfection or sterilization include the following:

- Blood pressure cuff.
- Ophthalmoscope (an instrument containing a mirror and lenses used to examine the interior of the eye).
- Otoscope (an instrument used for inspecting the ear).
- Penlight.
- Reflex hammer.
- Stethoscope.
- Tape measure.
- Tuning fork.

Collecting Instruments for Sanitization Sanitize instruments as soon as possible after use. If you cannot sanitize them immediately, place them in a sink or container filled with water and a neutral-pH detergent solution so that blood and tissue will not dry on the instrument.

In a surgical setting, use a special receptacle of disinfectant solution for collecting contaminated instruments. In an examination setting, place instruments in a sink or a container that can be transported to a sink. Take care when placing instruments in sinks or basins, as you can damage pieces of equipment if you drop them carelessly into a receptacle. Nicks or scratches can affect their function and can provide opportunities for bacterial contamination.

When you are ready to begin the sanitization procedure, put on properly fitting, intact utility gloves. They are the barrier between your skin and any infectious material on the instruments and equipment to be cleaned. When you work with instruments that may be contaminated with blood, body fluids, or tissue, you may want the additional protection of a mask, eye protection, or protective clothing.

Separate the sharp instruments from all other equipment (Figure 9-2). This reduces the risk of blunting sharp edges or points, damaging other equipment, and injuring yourself.

Scrubbing Instruments and Equipment Begin by draining the disinfectant or detergent solution in which the

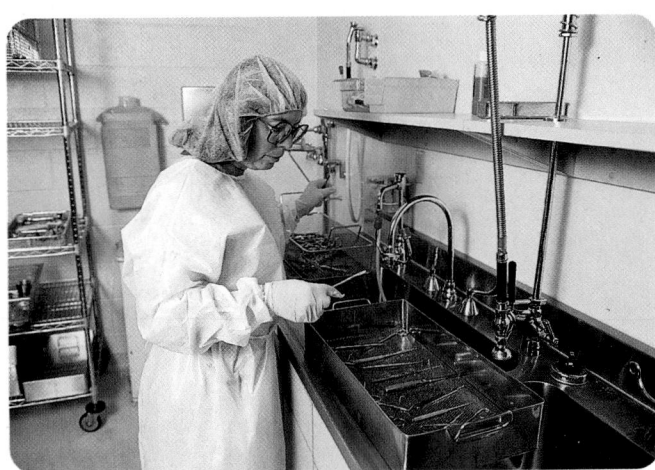

FIGURE 9-2 When working with instruments and equipment, separate pointed or sharp-edged instruments from all others.

FIGURE 9-3 Clean all areas of an instrument, using a brush for hard-to-reach surfaces.

equipment was soaking. Rinse each piece of equipment in hot running water and handle only one item at a time (by its handles where applicable). Scrub each item using hot, soapy water and a small plastic scrub brush. Never use metal brushes or steel wool, which can scratch and damage instruments. Pay careful attention to hinges, ratchets, and other nooks and crannies where contaminated material may collect (Figure 9-3). Use different-sized brushes to clean all areas of each item, along with a low-sudsing, neutral-pH detergent specially formulated to dissolve blood and blood products for medical instruments and equipment. Equipment and instrument manufacturers provide guidelines for sanitizing various types of products. For example, stainless steel items must be sanitized differently from chrome-plated instruments. Follow manufacturers' guidelines when working with their products.

After scrubbing all surfaces and removing all visible stains and residue, rinse instruments individually and place each one on a clean towel. Roll the instrument in the towel to remove moisture, dry it thoroughly, and examine it closely to be sure it is operating correctly. Check that all moving parts operate smoothly and that surfaces are free from nicks, scratches, and other imperfections. Instruments that need only to be sanitized can be returned to trays or bins for storage. Wrap items that require disinfection and **sterilization** (complete destruction of all living organisms) in a clean covering and set them aside for those processes. The process of sterilization is discussed in the chapter *Assisting in Surgery*.

Rubber and Plastic Products To sanitize rubber and plastic products, you may need to soak them only for a short period or not at all. Be sure to follow manufacturers' guidelines, as some rubber and plastic products fade or discolor if left in a detergent solution.

Ultrasonic Cleaning Delicate instruments and those with moving parts should be sanitized using ultrasonic cleaners. Ultrasonic cleaning involves placing instruments in a special bath. The cleaner generates sound waves through a cleaning solution, loosening contaminants. Ultrasonic cleaning is safe for even very fragile instruments. Follow the manufacturer's guidelines and Procedure 9-1, Performing Sanitization with an Ultrasonic Cleaner, at the end of this chapter when performing ultrasonic cleaning.

Disinfection

Sanitization is often only the beginning of the microorganism elimination process. After sanitization, some instruments and equipment require only disinfection before being used again. Disinfection of other items, however, is merely the second step in infection control, performed before the sterilization process.

Disinfection is a process that destroys most microorganisms; however, it cannot kill all microorganisms. Bacterial **spores** (thick-walled, reproductive bodies capable of resisting harsh conditions) and certain viruses have been known to survive disinfection with strong chemicals and boiling water. It is essential to understand this limitation of disinfection when you work with instruments and equipment. To destroy microorganisms, a disinfectant solution must reach every surface of an instrument. You must wear gloves when handling instruments during disinfection procedures because instruments requiring disinfection are considered to be contaminated.

Disinfection is usually sufficient for instruments that do not penetrate a patient's skin or that come in contact only with a patient's mucous membranes or other surfaces not considered sterile. Instruments and equipment that you can disinfect and reuse without sterilization include the following:

- Enamelware
- Endotracheal tubes (tubes used to establish an artificial airway through the nose, mouth, or direct tracheal route)
- Glassware
- Laryngoscopes (tubes equipped with lighting used to examine the interior of the larynx through the mouth)
- Nasal specula (instruments used to enlarge the opening of the nose to permit viewing)

Note that you must sterilize any instrument or piece of equipment before another use, including those just listed, if there is visible contamination with blood or blood products, even if disinfection is commonly considered sufficient. Sterilization is the only reliable measure you can take to eliminate bloodborne pathogens.

Using Disinfectants Disinfectants are cleaning products—used primarily on inanimate materials—applied to instruments and equipment to reduce or eliminate infectious organisms. In contrast, cleaning products used on human tissues as anti-infection agents are called *antiseptics*.

There are no clear visual indications that an item has been properly and completely disinfected. To ensure the optimum effectiveness of disinfectants, follow manufacturers' guidelines carefully when using them. Other factors also may have an impact on a disinfectant's effectiveness. For example, if the disinfectant solution has been used many times, it may not be as powerful as a fresh solution. When wet items are put in the disinfectant bath, the surface moisture may dilute the solution. Traces of the soap used in the sanitization process can alter the chemical makeup of the disinfectant, making it nonlethal to pathogens. Evaporation also can alter the solution's chemical makeup.

Choosing the Correct Disinfectant Manufacturers' guidelines are the most accurate and up-to-date sources of information about the type of disinfectant to use on a given product. Generally, disinfect instruments and equipment by using one or more of the following agents:

- Germicidal soap products
- Alcohol
- Chlorine and chlorine products
- Formaldehyde
- Glutaraldehyde
- Hydrogen peroxide
- Iodine and iodine compounds
- Acid products

Each of these disinfectants has advantages and disadvantages. Before using any disinfectant product or procedure, it is important to understand some general guidelines about disinfectant use as well as specific concerns with each approach. Review Table 9-1 for more details about example disinfectants. Keep in mind, selection and use of disinfectants may change since products may become available that were not in existence as of this writing. Review new products carefully to be sure they are approved by the FDA (Food and Drug Administration) and the EPA (Environmental Protection Agency).

Handling Disinfected Supplies After disinfecting equipment, handle it with care to prevent contaminating any surface that may later come in contact with a patient. Use sterile transfer forceps, or sterilizing forceps, to

TABLE 9-1	Disinfectants		
Product	**Description**	**Example Uses**	**Advantages/Disadvantages**
Germicidal soap products	The germ-killing additive may increase effectiveness.	Items that do not come in contact with a patient's mucous membranes.	The scrubbing and rinsing steps are most important.
Alcohol (70% isopropyl)	Used to clean instruments and equipment that would be damaged by immersion in soap and water or other disinfectant solutions.	• Oral and rectal thermometers • Scissors • Stethoscopes	Corrosive product that can cause damage to instruments with long-term use and to skin when used excessively.
Chlorine and chlorine compounds (bleach)	Effective in a 10% bleach solution.	• Used to disinfect surfaces and soak rubber equipment before sanitization • Decontamination of blood spills	Ventilation may be necessary because the fumes should not be inhaled for a prolonged period.
Formaldehyde	• Used as a preservative in a 10% solution • Used as a germicidal and sporicidal agent in a 5% solution • Must be used at room temperature because its effectiveness is reduced in cooler environments	• Preservation of anatomic specimens • Sterilization of surgical instruments	• Irritating fumes and pungent odor • Corrosive and an irritant to body tissue • Rinse clean items thoroughly with distilled or sterile water before using on patients
Glutaraldehyde (Cidex, Cidex Plus, and Glutarex)	• Used in chemical sterilization processes and as a high-level disinfectant • Immersing instruments or equipment in a bath of glutaraldehyde for 10 to 30 minutes is sufficient for disinfection	Respiratory therapy and spirometry equipment	Any chemical used in this "cold disinfection" method must be rated as a sterilant and registered with the EPA.
Hydrogen peroxide	Available in a 3% solution.	• Soft contact lenses • Spot-disinfection of fabrics	Must be stored in a dark container.
Iodine and iodine compounds	• 2% or greater solutions used as disinfectants • Weaker than 2% solutions used as antiseptics	• Skin antiseptic • Disinfection of blood culture bottles	• Somewhat corrosive • Effectiveness is limited by the presence of blood products, mucus, or soap
Acid products	Includes phenol (carbolic acid)	• Laboratory surfaces • Used as pre-cleaner before sterilization	Extremely corrosive and toxic to tissue and should be used with care.

remove items from whatever disinfection unit is used. Always wear gloves to handle disinfected items and make sure you store disinfected equipment in a clean, moisture-free environment.

Preparation of the Exam and Treatment Areas   LO 9.3

A medical assistant must maintain the examination and treatment areas. The treatment room is basically an exam room that includes additional equipment and supplies and is used for procedures like suturing a wound or excising an abscess. Medical offices may or may not have a special treatment room. All areas of the medical office should be clean and well-organized. A clean exam and treatment area is extremely important in preventing the spread of infectious diseases to patients and healthcare workers.

Infection Control
People with a variety of contagious diseases visit medical offices every day. The potential for the spread of infection is thus higher in medical offices than in most other places. For that reason, you must be especially careful to follow infection-control procedures at work. You can safeguard the health of staff members and patients by

- Making hand hygiene a priority.
- Keeping the examining table clean.
- Disinfecting all work surfaces.

Hand Hygiene Clean hands are the first step in preventing infection transmission in the exam room and treatment area. Follow the steps for aseptic hand washing and the use of alcohol-based hand cleaners as outlined in the procedures in the *Basic Safety and Infection Control* chapter. Review Table 9-2 for hand hygiene guidelines. After performing hand hygiene, use a clean paper towel to handle faucets or doorknobs to help you avoid contaminating your clean hands with microorganisms.

Examining Table The disposable paper that covers the examining table provides a barrier to infection during an exam. Always change the covering after each use (Figure 9-4). Your office might use precut lengths, or you might need to tear off a piece from a roll of paper.

Cover pillows with fresh paper. Also, provide tissues or special wipes for patients who need to wipe away excess **lubricant** (a water-soluble gel used during an exam of the rectum or vaginal cavity) after certain procedures.

When you remove the used covering from the examining table, roll it up quickly and carefully with the contaminated side on the inside. You should have a small, tight bundle of paper when you finish. Crumpling the paper haphazardly or shaking it in the air stirs up dust and microorganisms and can spread infection.

Dispose of used paper coverings soiled by body fluids, especially blood, in a biohazardous waste container. (Refer to the

TABLE 9-2	Hand Hygiene

Recommended Practices

- Wash your hands at the beginning of the workday.
- Wash your hands with soap and water whenever they are visibly contaminated with blood or other body fluids.
- If your hands are not visibly contaminated, you can use an alcohol-based hand rub.
- Wash your hands at the end of the workday before leaving the facility.

Indications for Hand Hygiene

- Before putting on and after removing gloves
- Between patient contacts
- Between different procedures on the same patient
- After touching blood, body fluids, secretions, excretions, and contaminated objects
- After restroom visits, eating, combing hair, handling money, and any other time hands get contaminated
- After contact with a patient's skin
- After contact with wound dressings (bandages)
- After contact with inanimate objects near a patient
- Before eating, applying cosmetics, or manipulating contact lenses
- Before and after handling clean or sterile supplies
- After blowing your nose, sneezing, or coughing
- After touching soiled items such as exam table coverings or clothing

Basic Safety and Infection Control chapter for specific guidelines for disposing of hazardous items.) Used coverings with no visible fluids may be disposed of according to the procedures established by your office. Place soiled linen cloths and pillowcases in biohazard-labeled bags to be sent to a laundry for cleaning.

Surfaces You are responsible for disinfecting work surfaces in the exam room, including the examining table, sink, and countertop. As discussed earlier, disinfection involves exposing all parts of a surface to a disinfectant like

FIGURE 9-4 When you remove the cover from the examining table, roll it up tightly and quickly. Then dispose of it immediately.

a 10% solution of household bleach in water or a product approved by the EPA. The EPA's mission is to protect human health and the environment.

Surfaces must be disinfected at the following times:

- After an exam or treatment during which surfaces have become visibly contaminated with tissue, blood, or other body fluids;
- Immediately following accidental blood or body fluid spills or splatter; and
- At the end of your work shift.

Routinely clean and disinfect the patient lavatory toilet and sink, and inspect and disinfect reusable receptacles like wastebaskets. In most offices, these tasks are performed once a day. Follow the schedule established by your office. Procedure 9-2 at the end of this chapter describes how to disinfect work surfaces, floors, and equipment in the exam room. Replace protective coverings on equipment or surfaces that were exposed to blood, other body fluids, or tissue during the exam.

Go to CONNECT to see an activity about *Guidelines for Disinfecting Exam Room Surfaces.*

Storage During the exam, you may need to collect biohazardous specimens, like blood or urine, from the patient for testing. These specimens must be handled and stored properly because they have the potential to be biohazards. Exposure that can spread disease may occur through the following routes:

- Inhalation (breathing)
- Ingestion (swallowing)
- Transcutaneous absorption (absorption through a cut or crack in the skin)

Occupational Safety and Health Administration (OSHA) regulations require storing biohazardous materials separately from food and beverages. Do not place food and beverages in refrigerators, freezers, or cabinets where blood or other potentially infectious materials are present or put specimens in a refrigerator otherwise used to store food and beverages.

It is dangerous to put food or beverages in the laboratory refrigerator for several reasons. If a biohazardous substance is not clearly labeled and you are in a hurry, you might accidentally ingest it. There is always the possibility that containers of biohazardous substances might leak or spill or that residue from the hazardous material might not have been thoroughly cleaned from the outside of containers. This residue could contaminate food or beverages.

OSHA regulations also require that a warning label containing the biohazard symbol be clearly and securely posted on the outside of refrigerators, freezers, and cabinets where biohazardous materials are stored. The government also recommends keeping the laboratory refrigerator and the refrigerator for the employees' personal use in separate rooms. These measures help prevent employees from accidentally putting food and beverages in the wrong place.

OSHA regulations prohibit medical personnel from doing any of the following activities in a room where potentially infectious materials are present:

- Eating
- Drinking
- Smoking
- Chewing gum
- Applying cosmetics
- Handling contact lenses
- Chewing pencils or pens
- Rubbing eyes

These work practice controls, like all OSHA regulations, represent safeguards to protect workers against the health hazards of bloodborne pathogens.

Testing kit and specimen storage often involves refrigeration as a means of preservation. Adequate preservation requires maintaining careful temperature control in a refrigerator. Read the Caution: Handle with Care: Refrigerator Temperature Control section for more information on preventing spoilage by controlling refrigerator temperature.

Putting the Room in Order

After ensuring that the examining table is clean, all surfaces are properly disinfected, and all necessary items are stored, take time to straighten the exam room and put things in order. A neatly arranged room boosts patient confidence and supports the impression of a well-run office. It also contributes to the physical safety of patients and staff. Tasks include the following:

- Putting the rolling stool in its place.
- Pushing in the examining-table step.
- Returning supplies to containers.
- Securing sample medications and solutions, prescription pads if used, and other items that may have been left out.

Housekeeping

Medical offices usually contract with a janitorial service for after-hours cleaning. These services perform general cleaning tasks like emptying wastebaskets, vacuuming carpets, scrubbing floors, dusting furniture, washing windows, and cleaning blinds. To be sure the service cleans and sanitizes all areas adequately, work with your employer to develop and implement a cleaning schedule. Take into account the types of surfaces to be cleaned, the type of contamination present, and the tasks or procedures to be performed.

You may be responsible for assigning housekeeping chores to janitorial workers. If so, you will need to monitor their work and let the service know if there are any lapses in cleanliness. You also may do some housekeeping chores yourself, like damp dusting an open shelf. Because dust harbors bacteria and allergens, it is important to keep the exam rooms as dust-free as possible.

Refrigerator Temperature Control

Health inspectors visit medical facilities periodically to check that health and safety standards are being upheld. One of the first things they check is the temperature of refrigerators. To prevent spoilage or deterioration of testing kits, blood specimens, and other stored materials, the laboratory refrigerator temperature should be maintained between 36°F and 46°F (2°C and 8°C). Keep a thermometer in the refrigerator to monitor the temperature. See Figure 9-5.

Similar guidelines apply to the refrigerator in the employee area. Food spoils quickly in a refrigerator if the temperature is not low enough. The temperature of the food refrigerator should be maintained between 32°F and 40°F (0°C and 4.4°C). In addition to monitoring the temperature, make sure food is not stored in the refrigerator too long. All food containers, including brown bags containing lunches, should be dated and thrown out when their freshness has expired. You can prevent bacteria growth by wiping up food spills immediately and cleaning the interior and exterior of the refrigerator routinely.

Follow office procedures for the routine cleaning of both laboratory and food refrigerators and for the proper temperature maintenance of refrigerated contents while the refrigerator interiors are cleaned. Specimens, for example, must be kept at a specific temperature at all times. For documentation purposes, keep a log of dates when the laboratory refrigerator is cleaned.

FIGURE 9-5 A temperature monitor is used to maintain a temperature within the refrigerator that prevents spoilage and deterioration of laboratory and food items.

▶ Room Temperature, Lighting, and Ventilation
LO 9.4

No patient wants to sit in an unkempt exam room. Nor do patients feel comfortable in a cold, dimly lit, or stuffy room. Adjusting the temperature, lighting, and ventilation is part of keeping the exam room in good order and fit for use.

Room Temperature

Because patients may be wearing only a thin paper gown or drape while in the exam room, you must be sure the exam room is warm enough. Set the thermostat to maintain the temperature at approximately 72°F and make sure there are no drafts from windows or doors. Patients often feel anxious while waiting for the physician; a warm room can help them relax.

Lighting

Good lighting is required to make accurate diagnoses, to correctly carry out medical procedures, and to read orders and instructions. A well-lit room also helps prevent accidents. Adjust room lights and blinds or drapes as necessary in preparation for an exam. If there is an exam lamp with a movable arm, be sure the arm is positioned appropriately. Replace all burned-out light bulbs as soon as possible.

Ventilation

The air in the exam area should smell fresh and clean. Periodically, you may have to deal with offensive odors from urine, vomitus, body odors, or laboratory chemicals. First you must eliminate the source of the odor, especially if the source is potentially infectious or toxic. Then you can take steps to remove the odor.

Some exam rooms have a ventilation system with an odor-absorbing filter. If the rooms in your office do not, you may be able to turn on a high-speed blower to vent room air to the outside. In some cases, an open window and a fan may be sufficient to freshen the air. Remember to check the room temperature after using fresh-air approaches to odor control.

If necessary, you can temporarily mask unpleasant odors with a room deodorizer or spray. Some sprays also help kill germs. Be careful that the room deodorizer you choose does not have a strong odor.

▶ Medical Instruments and Supplies
LO 9.5

Physicians require various instruments and supplies to perform an exam or procedure. Instruments are tools or implements physicians use for particular purposes. Disposable instruments are often referred to as supplies. You must maintain all instruments and supplies needed in the exam room. This responsibility involves the following three tasks:

- Ordering and stocking all supplies needed for exams and treatment procedures.
- Keeping the instruments sanitized, disinfected, or sterilized (as appropriate) and in working order.
- Ensuring all instruments and supplies are placed where the physician can easily reach them.

Instruments Used in a General Physical Exam

Many of the instruments physicians use are made of reusable fine-grade stainless steel. Some of these instruments may have disposable parts. Physicians also use a number of disposable instruments, like curettes and needles, because these instruments are both convenient and sanitary. Place any such items contaminated with blood or other body fluids in biohazardous waste containers.

These commonly used instruments are shown in Figure 9-6:

- An anoscope is used to open the anus for an exam. Although not always used for the general physical examination, a stool specimen is usually obtained in order to check for blood.

- An exam light provides an additional source of light during the exam. It is usually on a flexible arm to permit light to be directed to the area being examined.

- A laryngeal mirror reflects the inside of the mouth and throat for exam purposes.

- A nasal speculum is used to enlarge the opening of the nose to permit viewing. This type of speculum may consist of a reusable handle with a disposable speculum tip, or it may be a disposable one-piece unit.

- An ophthalmoscope is a lighted instrument used to examine the inner structures of the eye.

Anoscope

Examination light

Reflex hammer

Laryngeal mirror

Nasal speculum

Ophthalmoscope

Otoscope

Tuning fork

Sphygmomanometer

Stethoscope

Thermometer

Penlight

Tape measure

Vaginal speculum

FIGURE 9-6 These instruments may be used in a general physical exam.

- An otoscope is used to examine the ear canal and the tympanic membrane. The otoscope consists of a light source, a magnifying lens, and an ear speculum. An otoscope also may be used to examine the nostrils and the anterior sinuses. Like a nasal speculum, an otoscope may have disposable tips.
- A penlight is a small flashlight used when additional light is necessary in a small area. It also may be used to check pupil response in the eye.
- A reflex hammer—used to check a patient's reflexes—has a hard-rubber triangular head.
- A sphygmomanometer, or blood pressure cuff, is a piece of equipment used to measure blood pressure.
- A stethoscope is used to listen to body sounds. It is described in more detail in the *Vital Signs and Measurements* chapter.
- A tape measure is a long, narrow strip of fabric, marked off in inches and sometimes in centimeters, used to measure size or development of an area or part of the body.
- A thermometer is used to measure body temperature.
- A tuning fork tests patients' hearing.
- A vaginal speculum is used to enlarge the vagina to make the vagina and the cervix accessible for visual exam and specimen collection. This instrument is used only for a female when an examination and testing of the female reproductive system is done.

Inspecting and Maintaining Instruments Prior to the exam, make sure all instruments are sanitized, disinfected, or sterilized (as appropriate) and in good working order. For example, test the otoscope and ophthalmoscope to make sure the lights work. Place all rechargeable batteries in a battery charger when the instruments are not in use.

Medical instruments are expensive and are designed to work in precise ways. Read the manufacturers' directions so you are familiar with the care and maintenance of various instruments. Routinely check instruments for chipping and rusting, and report to the physician any instruments that need repair or replacement.

Arranging Instruments The physician must be able to find and reach instruments easily during an exam. You can assist by placing instruments in the same place for every exam or by arranging them in the order the physician will use them.

Physicians usually begin a general physical exam by examining the patient's head and face and working down the body. They may want instruments placed in that order. Other physicians may have individual preferences about how they want instruments arranged. In any case, make certain you know each physician's preferences.

With the exception of the stethoscope, which most physicians carry with them, instruments are kept in one of three places during an exam:

- Mounted on the wall (sphygmomanometer, some otoscopes and ophthalmoscopes);
- Set out on the countertop (penlight, reflex hammer, tape measure, tuning fork, thermometer, some otoscopes and ophthalmoscopes); or

TABLE 9-3	General Guidelines for Cleaning Instruments.	
Process	**Guidelines***	**Instruments**
Sanitization	• Use detergent, or as indicated by the manufacturer • Applies to instruments that do not touch the patient or that touch only intact skin • Disinfect these instruments after sanitization if they have come in contact with blood or body fluids	• Ophthalmoscope • Otoscope • Penlight • Reflex hammer • Sphygmomanometer • Stethoscope • Tape measure • Tuning fork
Disinfection	• Use only EPA-approved chemical or a 10% bleach solution to kill infectious agents outside the body • Applies to instruments that touch intact mucous membranes but do not penetrate the patient's body surfaces	• Laryngeal mirror • Nasal speculum
Sterilization	• Use an autoclave or approved method to kill all microorganisms • Applies to instruments that penetrate the skin or contact normally sterile areas of the body	• Anoscope • Curette • Needle (reusable) • Syringe (reusable) • Vaginal speculum

*Keep in mind, these guidelines are general. Each office may have its own methods and schedule for cleaning instruments, depending on the office's specialty.

- Set on a clean (or sterile, if appropriate) towel or tray (anoscope, laryngeal mirror, nasal speculum, vaginal speculum).

Preparing Instruments You must prepare some instruments before they can be used. For example, you may need to warm a vaginal speculum by holding it under warm water just prior to the exam. You might warm the mirrored end of the laryngeal mirror with water or over an alcohol lamp. You also can spray it with a special spray that prevents fogging. Any time you will be handling instruments, you must first wash your hands. If the instruments are sterile, you also must wear sterile gloves.

Cleaning Instruments After the exam, put used instruments in a container and take them to the cleaning area. Always handle instruments carefully because mishandling can alter their precision. Dispose of supplies in the appropriate containers and use approved procedures for sanitizing, disinfecting, and sterilizing reusable instruments and equipment. Refer to Table 9-3 for general guidelines on cleaning instruments.

Supplies for a General Physical Exam

Supplies for a general physical exam may be either disposable or consumable. Figure 9-7 shows various types of supplies.

Disposable supplies are items that are used once and discarded. These include

- Cervical scraper (a plastic or wooden scraper used to obtain samples of cervical secretions used for female exams only)

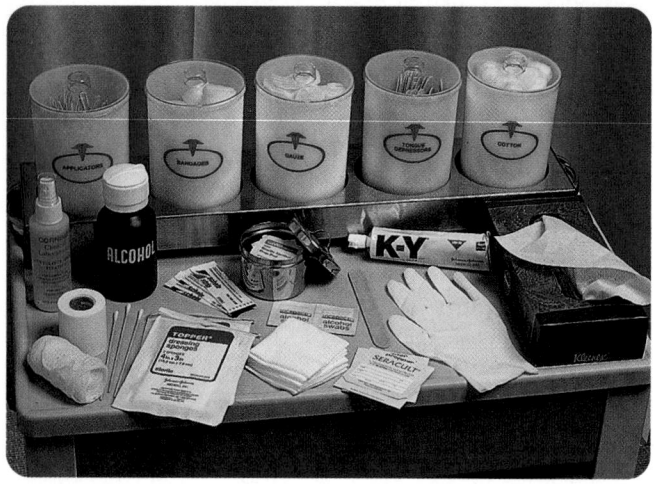

FIGURE 9-7 These supplies may be used in a general physical exam.

FIGURE 9-8 Arrange the instruments for a general physical exam so that they are convenient for the doctor.

- Cotton balls
- Cotton-tipped applicators
- Curettes
- Disposable needles
- Disposable syringes
- Gauze, dressings, and bandages
- Glass slides
- Gloves, both sterile and exam (nonsterile) types
- Paper tissues
- Prepared paper slides used to test the stool for the presence of **occult blood** (blood not visible to the naked eye)
- Specimen containers
- Tongue depressors

Consumable supplies are items that can be emptied or used up in an exam. These items include the following:

- **Fixative** (a chemical spray used for preserving a specimen obtained from the body for pathologic exam)
- Isopropyl alcohol (for cleansing skin)
- Lubricant

As they do with instruments, physicians may have a preferred arrangement of supplies for the general physical exam. Figure 9-8 shows a typical arrangement of instruments. Certain supplies, like needles, medications, and prescription blanks, if used, should be kept in a locked cabinet away from patient access.

Storing Supplies You can use the cabinets and drawers in the exam room to store nonperishable supplies. Store every item in its own place so you can find it quickly. Consider color-coding or labeling drawers and cabinets so you can easily locate items. Store supplies that come in various sizes, like bandages, according to size and routinely straighten and clean the insides of all exam room cabinets and drawers.

Restocking Supplies To be sure you have a sufficient quantity of items on hand, order new supplies well in advance of needing them. A good guideline to follow is to order a new supply when the first half of a box, tube, or bottle has been used up. A recordkeeping system will help you determine which supplies you need to restock most frequently and how long it takes for new supplies to arrive. Keep track of the following information in order to develop such a system:

- The types of supplies your office uses.
- The quantities of each type of supply used in a given amount of time, such as a month.
- The frequency with which you must reorder particular supplies.
- The names of various suppliers, along with the amount of time it takes to receive your orders.

PROCEDURE 9-1 Performing Sanitization with an Ultrasonic Cleaner

Procedure Goal: To decontaminate items safely and effectively using an ultrasonic cleaner.

OSHA Guidelines:

Materials: Ultrasonic cleaner, contaminated items and instruments, ultrasonic cleaning fluid, and manufacturer's directions.

Method: Procedure steps.

1. Review the manufacturer's directions for safe operation of the ultrasonic cleaner.
2. Fill the container of the ultrasonic cleaner with water. Look for the fill line on the machine. In some cases, you may use distilled water.

3. Add the directed amount of ultrasonic cleaning fluid. Typically, only a small amount of fluid is used. Check the directions.

4. Plug in and turn on the ultrasonic cleaner. Some cleaners require a warm-up period. Check the instructions.

5. Separate instruments and equipment made of different metals.
   RATIONALE: Different metals may fuse together during the cleaning process, making them useless.

6. Separate instruments with sharp points.
   RATIONALE: To avoid injury.

7. Open hinges on instruments and equipment.
   RATIONALE: Contaminated materials can become trapped between two surfaces.

8. Place instruments and equipment in the ultrasonic cleaner, but do not overfill.

9. Close the lid, turn on the machine or timer, and wait for the cycle to be completed.

10. Rinse each instrument or piece of equipment in cool running water and then distilled or demineralized water as policy dictates.
    RATIONALE: Ultrasonic cleaning fluid may cause damage to instruments or equipment.

11. Dry each instrument or piece of equipment.

12. Prepare each item for storage or further disinfection or sterilization.

13. Replace ultrasonic cleaning solution according to office policy and manufacturers' guidelines.
    RATIONALE: Cleaning solution can be used for several cleaning baths but must be replaced as needed to maintain effectiveness.

PROCEDURE 9-2   Guidelines for Disinfecting Exam Room Surfaces

Procedure Goal: To reduce the risk of exposure to potentially infectious microorganisms in the exam room.

OSHA Guidelines:

Materials: Utility gloves, disinfectant (10% bleach solution or EPA-approved disinfecting product), paper towels, dustpan and brush, tongs, forceps, and a clean sponge or heavy rag.

Method: Procedure steps.

1. Wash your hands and don utility gloves.

2. Remove any visible soil from exam room surfaces with disposable paper towels or a rag.
   RATIONALE: Removing visible soil first allows for better penetration of the disinfectant.

3. Thoroughly wipe all surfaces with the disinfectant.

4. In the event of an accident involving a broken glass container, use tongs, a dustpan and brush, or forceps to pick up shattered glass, which may be contaminated.
   RATIONALE: Using your fingers to pick up broken glass puts you at risk for exposure to bloodborne pathogens.

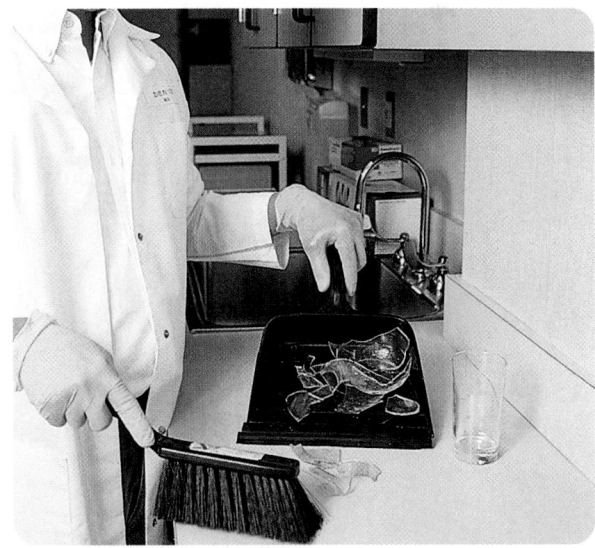

FIGURE Procedure 9-2 Step 4   Because broken glass may be contaminated, never pick it up directly with your hands. Use a brush and dustpan, tongs, or forceps to clean it up.

5. Remove and replace protective coverings, like plastic wrap or aluminum foil, on equipment if the equipment or the coverings have become contaminated. After removing the coverings, disinfect the equipment and allow it to air-dry. (Follow office procedures for the routine changing of protective coverings.)

6. When you finish cleaning, dispose of the paper towels or rags in a biohazardous waste receptacle. (This step is especially important if you are cleaning

surfaces contaminated with blood, body fluids, or tissue.)

7. Remove the gloves and wash your hands.

8. If you keep a container of 10% bleach solution on hand for disinfection purposes, replace the solution daily to ensure its disinfecting potency.

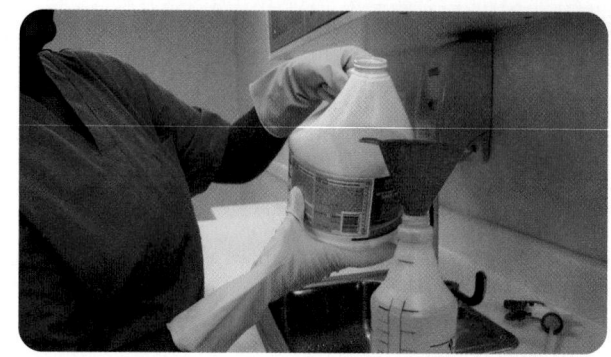

FIGURE Procedure 9-2 Step 8   Replace the bleach solution each day to ensure its disinfecting potency.

LEARNING OUTCOMES	KEY POINTS
9.1 **Describe the layout and features of a typical examination room.**	A typical examination room is about 8 by 12 feet, large enough to accommodate the physician, the patient, and one assistant. Instruments and equipment in the room should be easily accessible.
9.2 **Differentiate between sanitization and disinfection.**	Sanitization is the scrubbing of instruments and equipment with special brushes and detergent to remove blood, mucus, and other contaminants or media where pathogens can grow. Disinfection uses special cleaning products applied to instruments and equipment to reduce or eliminate infectious organisms.
9.3 **List steps to prevent the spread of infection in the exam and treatment rooms.**	Steps involved in preventing the spread of infection in the examination room include covering the examination table with a paper cover and changing the cover between each patient. It is also important to disinfect all surfaces that come in contact with blood or body fluids after each patient and at the beginning and end of the day.
9.4 **Describe the importance of temperature, lighting, and ventilation in the exam room.**	A comfortably warm, well-lit, and properly ventilated room will help the patient feel comfortable and more relaxed during his examination.
9.5 **Identify instruments and supplies used in a general physical exam and tell how to arrange and prepare them.**	A variety of instruments and supplies are used in a general physical examination. To ensure the examination room always has the necessary instruments and supplies, the medical assistant should order and stock all supplies needed for examinations and treatment procedures; keep the instruments sanitized, disinfected, or sterilized and in working order; and place all instruments and supplies where the physician can easily reach them.

Recall Shenya from the beginning of the chapter. Now that you have completed the chapter, answer the following questions regarding her case.

1. What needs to be done before Shenya is brought back into the exam room?

2. Shenya is diagnosed with community-acquired MRSA (a highly contagious microorganism). What measures should you take to ensure there is no transfer of infection?

3. After Shenya's examination, you will need to use an ultrasonic cleaner for sanitization. Describe how you would proceed and what source you would use if you had questions about the cleaner you are using.

E X A M P R E P A R A T I O N Q U E S T I O N S

1. (LO 9.1) The ADA requires that door-opening hardware can be grasped with one hand and
   a. Can be locked securely
   b. Is marked with reflective tape
   c. Does not require twisting the wrist to open
   d. Does not catch completely
   e. Opens automatically

2. (LO 9.5) Which of the following is considered a disposable supply?
   a. Glass slides
   b. Lubricant
   c. Fixative
   d. Isopropyl alcohol
   e. Nasal speculum

3. (LO 9.2) Which of the following may be sanitized and reused without further disinfection or sterilization?
   a. Curette
   b. Otoscope
   c. Laryngeal mirror
   d. Anoscope
   e. Vaginal speculum

4. (LO 9.1) Which of the following would you be *least* likely to find in an examination room?
   a. High-intensity lamp
   b. Medications
   c. Biohazardous sharps container
   d. Rolling stool
   e. Metal wastebasket with lid

5. (LO 9.2) Which disinfectant would *least* likely be corrosive or require ventilation when in use?
   a. Alcohol
   b. Bleach
   c. Hydrogen peroxide
   d. Formaldehyde
   e. Iodine

6. (LO 9.3) In which of the following situations would alcohol-based hand cleaner most likely be acceptable for use?
   a. After cleaning up a blood spill
   b. After changing the paper on the exam table
   c. After assisting with suturing
   d. After your break
   e. After helping a patient in the restroom

7. (LO 9.3) At which of the following times do you need to disinfect surfaces in the exam room?
   a. Immediately before an accidental blood or body fluid spill or splatter
   b. At the beginning of your shift
   c. After assisting with a wound dressing
   d. During a patient examination
   e. After each patient examination

8. (LO 9.4) A patient vomits in exam room 2. Which of the following would be your best course of action?
   a. Immediately call the housekeeping department to clean it up
   b. Spray the room with deodorizer and leave it empty for at least 15 minutes
   c. Clean up the vomit and then open the window or spray a room deodorizer
   d. Clean up the vomit, then turn off the ventilation system so the odor does not permeate the entire office
   e. Turn on the ventilation system and spray deodorizer

9. (LO 9.5) What instrument would be used to look inside the ear?
   a. Ophthalmoscope
   b. Anoscope
   c. Nasal speculum
   d. Vaginal speculum
   e. Otoscope

10. (LO 9.5) Which of the following consumable supplies is used to preserve a specimen obtained during an exam?
    a. Lubricant
    b. Alcohol
    c. Hydrogen peroxide
    d. Fixative
    e. Bleach

Written and Electronic Documents

C A S E   S T U D Y

PATIENT INFORMATION

Patient Name	Gender	DOB
Valarie Ramirez	F	8/4/19XX

Attending	MRN	Allergies
Paul F. Buckwalter, MD	829-78-462	Penicillin

When asked, she states that she did not get a flu shot this year. After a physical exam, Dr. Buckwalter orders a CBC and chest X-ray and gives her a prescription for antibiotics. Dr. Buckwalter will be in touch with her when the lab and X-ray results are in.

Keep Valarie in mind as you study this chapter. There will be questions at the end of the chapter based on the

Valarie Ramirez, a 33-year-old female, arrives at the clinic with complaints of "a cold that won't go away." She states that she has had body aches, a cough, and fever for at least 3 days and feels like she is getting worse rather than better.

case study. The information in the chapter will help you answer these questions.

L E A R N I N G   O U T C O M E S

After completing Chapter 10, you will be able to:

10.1 Explain why well-written documents are important to the image of the medical practice.

10.2 Describe the types of document supplies that will be used in a medical office.

10.3 Outline the general guidelines to effective writing.

10.4 List and explain the purpose of different types of documents used in a medical office.

10.5 Explain why it is important to have a signed written consent from the patient for e-mail communications.

10.6 Describe the tasks involved in editing and proofreading a document.

10.7 Outline the steps for preparing a completed letter for mailing.

10.8 Explain the differences among the different types of mail services offered by the USPS.

10.9 Describe the steps involved in processing incoming mail.

K E Y   T E R M S

annotate

body

clarity

complimentary closing

concise

editing

full-block letter style

inside address

modified-block letter style

optical character reader (OCR)

proofreading

salutation

signature block

simplified letter style

subject line

template

IV. C (8) Recognize elements of fundamental writing skills

IV. C (9) Discuss applications of electronic technology in effective communication

IV. P (10) Compose professional/business letters

7. **Basic Keyboarding/Computer Concepts**
   Graduates:
   a. Perform basic keyboarding skills, including:
      (2) Typing medical correspondence and basic reports
   b. Identify and properly utilize office machines, computerized systems, and medical software such as:
      (1) Efficiently maintain and understand different types of medical correspondence and medical reports
      (2) Apply computer application skills using a variety of different electronic programs including both practice management software and EMR software

8. **Medical Office Business Procedures Management**
   Graduates:
   a. Perform basic clerical functions
   d. Apply concepts for office procedures
   hh. Receive, organize, prioritize, and transmit information expediently
   jj. Perform fundamental writing skills including correct grammar, spelling, and formatting techniques when writing prescriptions, documenting medical records, etc.
   ll. Apply electronic technology

11. **Career Development**
    Graduates:
    b. Demonstrate professionalism by:
       (3) Maintaining confidentiality at all times
       (8) Being courteous and diplomatic

▶ Introduction

Communication skills—verbal, nonverbal, and written—are important in nearly every profession. Consider, just for a moment, the way you communicate verbally, nonverbally, and in writing, and what this may say about you to your audience. Now, consider what your communication skills may say to others about the office where you work as a medical assistant. Written documents—whether they are produced on traditional paper format or in an electronic format—are tangible demonstrations of the office staff's ability to communicate and conduct business.

The community as a whole may often evaluate an entire medical practice by the work of one employee. When a letter, form, or document is carelessly prepared and sent into the community, the physician may be judged as "careless." However, when a letter or other business correspondence is constructed in a neat, concise, and well-organized fashion, the physician is often judged to be organized and competent. The skill demonstrated in the creation of a simple business document reflects on the medical skills of the physician and the practice. So, it is fair to say that professional image is conveyed in all written correspondence.

Because written documents also serve as legal records, all paper and electronic documents must be prepared with great care and attention to detail. The medical assistant's administrative role includes the creation of consistently accurate and clear documents.

In this chapter, you will learn how to write effectively. You will develop skills in composing business documents using different writing styles and formats. You will also learn how to professionally manage all forms of correspondence commonly used in an ambulatory care setting.

▶ Professionalism and Document Preparation
LO 10.1

As in any business, correspondence from healthcare professionals to patients and colleagues must be handled carefully, with appropriate attention to content and presentation. By learning how to create, send, and receive correspondence and other types of documents, you can ensure positive, effective communication between your office and others. Well-written, neatly prepared correspondence is one of the most important means of communicating a professional image for the medical office (Figure 10-1).

FIGURE 10-1 Well-written correspondence is vital to the professional reputation of a medical practice.

▶ Selecting Document Supplies LO 10.2

The first step in preparing professional-looking documents is choosing the right supplies. Many offices already have most of these supplies on hand. However, you may be responsible for selecting and ordering such supplies. You may need to make decisions about letterhead paper, envelopes, labels, invoices, and statements.

Letterhead Paper

Letterhead refers to formal business stationery on which the physician (or office) name and address are printed at the top, along with the names of all the associates in the practice. In most cases, the office phone and fax numbers are listed along with the office website information and an e-mail address. Letterhead is used for all professional, written correspondence coming from the office, but it is important to note that letterhead is used only for the first page of a letter. If a letter is more than one page, all the additional pages are printed on plain paper (the same color and bond as the letterhead).

Letterhead paper can be cotton fiber bond (sometimes called rag bond) or sulfite bond. Cotton fiber bond is usually more expensive than other types of paper. Cotton bond contains a watermark—an impression or pattern that can be seen when the paper is held up to the light—that indicates that the paper is of high quality. The most popular cotton bond used for letterhead is 25% cotton because it is economical, but all higher grades can be used. Sulfite bond paper begins as wood pulp, which is treated with peroxide or hypochlorite to bleach it a paler color. Further chemical processes give sulfite paper a brilliant white appearance, making it a favorite for producing photographs. Businesses, including medical practices, use sulfite paper for portfolios, folders, and other items that need an attractive and durable paper.

The two most common letterhead paper sizes are standard and legal. Standard or letter-size paper is 8½ × 11 inches and is used for most general business documents. Legal size is 8½ × 14 inches and, as the name indicates, is used for legal and especially lengthy documents.

Formal invitations or announcements, like those announcing an office opening, may be engraved or embossed. Embossing involves a process where the letters are pressed into the paper and often set in black, gold, or silver.

Envelopes

Envelopes are used for correspondence, invoices, and statements. Typically, business letterhead and matching envelopes are printed together on higher-quality paper. Although the letterhead format for statements and invoices may be the same, these documents and their envelopes are usually printed on a lower-quality paper.

Familiarize yourself with the many types of envelopes used in the medical office.

- The most common envelope size used for correspondence is the No. 10 envelope (also called business size). It measures 4½ by 9½ inches.

- Envelopes used for invoices and statements can range from No. 6 (3⅝ by 6½ inches) to No. 10. These envelopes usually have a transparent window that allows the address on the invoice or statement to show through, saving time and reducing the potential for errors involved in retyping the address.

- Smaller payment return envelopes—preaddressed to the physician's office—are often included along with the statement, for the patient's convenience.

- Tan Kraft envelopes, or clasp envelopes, are available in many sizes and are used to send large or bulky documents.

- Padded envelopes are used to send documents or materials, like slides, that may be damaged in the normal course of mail handling.

- The stock and quality of the envelope should always match the stationery. An office typically has two grades of envelopes with a return address. One is a less expensive stock and quality of paper with a block format return address printed in black, used for everyday documents like insurance inquiries. The second is a more expensive stock and quality of paper with a block format return address printed in black or a dark color, used for professional correspondence.

- Data mailers are produced by a computer and used by larger businesses and hospitals for batch mailings of items like paychecks, appointment reminders, and some invoices. The envelopes are opened by tearing off perforated sides, peeling the envelope apart, or utilizing a pull tab.

Labels

Address labels, printed from a computerized mailing list, can make the process of addressing envelopes for bulk mailings much speedier. For example, you may have to send a notice of a change in office hours or a quarterly office newsletter to a large number of patients in a practice.

You may choose to set up a system for frequently used labels. Many practices write insurance inquiries and other business letters to the same addresses repeatedly. For fast and easy access, it is helpful to print out labels of the same address a full page at a time. Pages of labels can then be stored in alphabetized folders near the transcription desk. Excel databases can also be set up to print labels and to insert names and addresses in standardized formats known as **templates**.

Invoices and Statements

Several different types of invoices and statements are currently used. The term *invoice* is usually used when billing for products. Because a physician provides a service, most medical bills are referred to as statements. The different types of statements include

- Preprinted statements.
- Computer-generated invoices and statements.
- Superbills or encounter forms (discussed in *Patient Billing and Collections*).

▶ Effective Writing
LO 10.3

Written communication is much like holding a conversation in person. The recipient will form a fairly quick impression of the physician or the office based on the appearance of the document and the way the message in the document makes the recipient feel, be it a letter, patient instructions, or even an e-mail message. So, all written communication must be clear and well written, and must politely and concisely convey the appropriate information to the recipient. To create effective, professional correspondence that reflects well on the practice, be sure that you use clear and **concise** language, the active voice, and an appropriate style. Following are some general guidelines to help you write more effectively.

- Before you write, know the type of person to whom you are writing. Consider him to be your audience. Is the letter to a physician, a patient, a vendor, or fellow staff members? Decide if the tone should be formal or more relaxed.
- Know the purpose of the letter before you begin and make sure your letter accurately conveys that purpose.
- Be concise. Use short sentences. Be brief. Be specific.
- Do not use unnecessary words. Use the simplest way to say what you mean.
- Show **clarity** in your writing; state your message so that it can be understood easily.

- Use the active voice whenever possible. Voice shows whether the subject of a sentence is acting or is being acted upon. Here is an example of the active voice:

    "Dr. Huang is seeing 18 patients today."

    Here is an example of the same sentence, written in the passive voice:

    "Eighteen patients will be seen by Dr. Huang today."

    Note that the active voice is more direct and livelier to read.
- Use the passive voice, however, to soften the impact of negative news:

    "Your account will be turned over to a collection agency if we do not receive payment promptly."

    It would sound harsher to say:

    "We will turn over your account to a collection agency if we do not receive payment promptly."
- Always be polite and courteous.
- Always check spelling and the accuracy of dates and monetary figures.
- Always check your grammar. Do not use slang.
- Avoid leaving "widows and orphans" or dangling words and phrases. These are words and short phrases at the end or beginning of paragraphs that are left to sit alone at the top or bottom of a page or column or separated from the rest of the thought. Do not start a paragraph at the bottom of a page if the rest of the sentence must be continued on the next page.

Grammar

Although seldom a popular topic in today's text-messaging culture, excellent grammar is essential for every medical assistant who composes professional documents. Let's look at Table 10-1 for a quick review of the parts of speech.

There are also basic rules of writing that should be followed when composing professional documents. Table 10-2 summarizes these rules.

TABLE 10-1	The Parts of Speech	
Part of Speech	**Description**	**Example**
Nouns	Describe a person, place, thing, concept, thought, or idea. *Proper nouns* describe specific persons, places, or things.	Massachusetts, town, medical assistant, Dr. Whalen, freedom, kindness
Pronouns	Replace nouns by referring back to them.	He, she, it, they, him, her, us, them, theirs, you, yours, ours, mine
Verbs	Action verbs describe movement. Linking verbs express a condition or state. Linking verbs also express the senses.	Walk, type, speak, laugh Is, are, am, be, being, was Hear, smell, taste, touch, feel
Adjectives	Describe nouns and pronouns or explain which one, how many, or what kind. Adjectives also include *articles*.	Playful cat, talented artist, 15 medical records, tasty apple "A,""an," and "the"
Adverbs	Describe verbs, adjectives, or other adverbs and explain when, where, how, and to what extent.	Extremely thirsty, always cheerful, bitter taste
Prepositions	Connecting words demonstrating a relationship between nouns, pronouns, or other words.	at, by, from, on, to, in, of, into, with
Conjunctions	Join words or phrases together.	and, or, nor, but
Interjections	Show strong feeling or emotion. Often followed by an exclamation point or comma if used in professional writing.	Help! Ouch! Call 911!

TABLE 10-2	**Basic Rules of Writing**
Word Division	Divide: • According to pronunciation • Compound words between the two words from which they derive • Hyphenated compound words at the hyphen • After a prefix • Before a suffix • Between two consonants that appear between vowels • Before –ing unless the last consonant is doubled; in that case, divide before the second consonant Do not divide: • Suffixes like –sion, –tial, and –gion • A word so that only one letter is left on a line
Capitalization	Capitalize: • All proper names • All titles, positions, or indications of family relation when preceding a proper name or in place of a proper noun (not when used alone or with possessive pronouns or articles) • Days of the week, months, and holidays • Names of organizations and membership designations • Racial, religious, and political designations • Adjectives, nouns, and verbs that are derived from proper nouns (including currently copyrighted trade names) • Specific addresses and geographic locations • Sums of money written in legal or business documents • Titles, headings of books, magazines, and newspapers

Plurals	• Add *s* or *es* to most singular nouns (plural forms of most medical terms do not follow this rule)
	• With medical terms ending in *is*, drop the *is* and add *es*:
	    metastasis/metastases
	    epiphysis/epiphyses
	• With terms ending in *um*, drop the *um* and add *a*:
	    diverticulum/diverticula
	    atrium/atria
	• With terms ending in *us*, drop the *us* and add *i*:
	    calculus/calculi
	    bronchus/bronchi
	(Two exceptions to this are virus/viruses and sinus/sinuses)
	• With terms ending in *a*, keep the *a* and add *e*:
	    Vertebra/vertebrae

Possessives	To show ownership or relation to another noun: • For singular nouns, add an apostrophe and an *s* • For plural nouns that do not end in an *s*, add an apostrophe and an *s* • For plural nouns that end in an *s*, just add an apostrophe
Numbers	Use numerals: • In general writing, when the number is 11 or greater • With abbreviations and symbols • When discussing laboratory results or statistics • When referring to specific sums of money • When using a series of numbers in a sentence Tips: • Use commas when numerals have more than three digits. • Do not use commas when referring to account numbers, page numbers, or policy numbers. • Use a hyphen with numerals to indicate a range.

Because certain information in an office is used repeatedly, commonly used paragraphs and even entire letter formats, or *templates*, are often used in many practices. These templates or bodies of text are saved in the computer for quick and easy repeated access. With very few keystrokes, the material can be selected and displayed almost immediately. Then, minor changes specific to the requirements of the specific document or letter can be made. When making changes to a template, make sure to read the document carefully once you have completed your work to ensure that all necessary changes have been made.

It is also helpful to use the cut, copy, and paste features in word processing software to quickly piece together a document that uses sentences or paragraphs from other documents. Large and small bodies of text can easily be moved or copied from document to document, instead of rekeying information. These features help to save time for the medical assistant.

▶ Medical Office Documents and Correspondence   LO 10.4

As a medical assistant, you will be responsible for preparing routine documents and correspondence at the physician's request. You may transcribe some documents from the doctor's dictation and compose others from notes.

The purpose of most patient correspondence is to explain, clarify, or give instructions or other information. Correspondence includes:

- Letters of referral.
- Letters about scheduling, canceling, or rescheduling appointments.
- Patient reports for insurance companies.
- Instructions for examinations or laboratory tests.
- Answers to insurance or billing questions.
- Cover letters or form letters to order supplies, equipment, or magazine subscriptions.

Parts of a Business Letter

Figure 10-2 illustrates the parts of a typical business letter. Details about format may vary from office to office. Specific characteristics of the parts included in a typical business letter are discussed here.

Letterhead The letterhead is the preprinted portion of formal business stationery.

Dateline The dateline consists of the month, day, and year. It should begin about three lines below the preprinted letterhead text on approximately line 15. The month should always be spelled out, and there should be a comma after the day.

Inside Address The **inside address** contains all the necessary information for the letter's correct delivery. The inside address spells out the name and address of the person to whom the letter is being sent. In general, you should

- Key, or type, the inside address on the left margin, two to four spaces down from the date. It should be two, three, or four lines in length.
- Include a *courtesy title* (Dr., Mr., Mrs., and so on) and the intended recipient's full name. Note: If Dr. is used, do not put MD after the name. For example, either of these forms is acceptable: Dr. John Smith; John Smith, MD. This form is *not* acceptable: Dr. John Smith, MD. Generally, the John Smith, MD format is used for the inside address and the Dear Dr. Smith format is used for the salutation.
- Include the intended receiver's title on the same line with the name, separated by a comma, or on the line below it.
- Include the company name, if applicable.
- Use numerals for the street address, except the single numbers one through nine, which should be spelled out—for example, Two Markham Place.
- Spell out numerical names of streets if they are numbers less than ten.
- Spell out the words *Street*, *Drive*, and so on.
- Include the full city name; do not abbreviate.
- Use the two-letter state abbreviation recommended by the U.S. Postal Service (USPS). These abbreviations are easily found online by searching for "USPS state abbreviations."
- Leave one space between the state and the zip code; include the zip + 4 code, if known.

Attention Line An attention line is used when a letter is addressed to a company but sent to the attention of a particular individual. If you do not know the individual's name, call the company directly to inquire about the appropriate contact person's name. A colon between the word *Attention* and the person's name is optional. Place two lines below Inside Address (if using).

Salutation When addressing a person by name, use a **salutation**—a written greeting such as "Dear"—followed by Mr., Mrs., or Ms., and the person's last name. The salutation should be keyed at the left margin on the second line below the inside address. A colon should follow. When you do not know the name, it is becoming common practice to use the business title or department in the salutation, as in "Dear Sir," "Dear Laboratory Director," or "Dear Claims Representative." This also avoids confusion if you do not know the gender of a person with aname such as Pat or Chris.

Subject Line A **subject line** is sometimes used to bring the subject of the letter to the reader's attention. The subject line is not required, but, if it is used, it should be keyed on the second line below the salutation. The subject line may be flush with the left margin, indented five spaces, or centered to the page. The subject line should be limited to two or three words and should be keyed in all capital letters to capture the reader's attention. Some offices use "RE:" (short for regarding) instead of the word Subject.

Letterhead	**BWW**
	BWW Medical Associates, PC
	305 Main Street, Port Snead YZ 12345-9876
	Tel: 555-654-3210, Fax: 555-987-6543
	Web: BWWAssociates.com

Paul F. Buckwalter, MD
Alexis N. Whalen, MD
Elizabeth H. Williams, MD

Dateline

November 14, 20XX

CERTIFIED MAIL

Inside Address

Mr. Hunter Boyd
4080 Magnolia Point Drive
Port, Snead YZ 12345

Salutation

Dear Mr. Boyd:

Subject Line

SUBJECT: RESCHEDULING OF APPOINTMENT

Body

Unfortunately, Dr. Buckwalter will not be in the office on December 5, 20XX, and we must reschedule your appointment for that date. Please call our office at your earliest convenience to arrange for a new appointment date and time.

Your health is of great concern to us and we apologize for any inconvenience this rescheduled appointment may cause you.

Complimentary Closing

Sincerely,

Signature Block

Malik Katahri, cmm

Malik Katahri
Office Manager

Identification Line

MK: mp

Notations

Enc: Appointment calendar

C: Miguel A. Perez, Scheduling Coordinator

FIGURE 10-2 Knowing the parts of a typical business letter enables medical assistants to create written documents that reflect well on the office.

Body The **body** of the letter begins two lines below the salutation or subject line. The text is single-spaced with double-spacing between paragraphs.

If the body contains a list, set the list apart from the rest of the text. Leave an extra line of space above and below the list. For each item in the list, indent 5 to 10 spaces from each margin. Single-space within items, but leave an extra line between items. A bulleted list has a small, solid, round circle before each item.

Complimentary Closing The **complimentary closing** is placed two lines below the last line of the body. Capitalize only the first word of the closing. "Sincerely" is a common closing. "Very truly yours" and "Best regards" are also acceptable closings in business correspondence. A comma is placed after the complimentary closing.

Signature Block The **signature block** contains the writer's name on the first line and the writer's business title on the second line. The block is aligned with the complimentary closing and typed three to four lines below it, to allow space for the signature.

Identification Line The letter writer's initials followed by a colon or slash and the typist's initials are sometimes included in the letter. These initials are called the *identification line*. This line is typed flush left, two lines below the signature block.

Notations Notations include information such as the number of enclosures (be sure to note what is enclosed) that are included with the letter and the names of other people who will be receiving copies of the letter (sometimes referred to as c:). If there are enclosures, a notation should appear flush left, one or two lines below the identification line (or one or two lines below the signature block if no identification line is present). You may abbreviate the word *Enclosure* by typing "Enc," "Encl," or "Encs" (with or without

punctuation, depending on the style of the letter you are writing). The copy notation, "c," appears after the enclosure notation and includes one or more names or initials.

Letter Format

Follow these general formatting guidelines for all letters.

- The margin is the space around the edges of a form or letter that is left blank. The standard setting for margins in business correspondence is one inch (left and right margins) for 8½ inch-wide paper.
- Roughly center the letter on the page according to the length of the letter. For shorter letters, you can use wider margins and start the address farther down the page. For longer letters, use standard margins but start higher up on the page.
- Single-space the body of the letter. Double-space between paragraphs or parts of the letter.
- Use short sentences (no more than 20 words on average).
- Include at least two to three sentences in each paragraph.

BVVV

BWW Medical Associates, PC
305 Main Street, Port Snead YZ 12345-9876
Tel: 555-654-3210, Fax: 555-987-6543
Web: BWWAssociates.com

Paul F. Buckwalter, MD
Alexis N. Whalen, MD
Elizabeth H. Williams, MD

May 28, 20XX

Mr. Shawn Collins
234 Deerfield Drive
Port Snead YZ 12345

Dear Mr. Collins:

Congratulations! Your lab results have come back and, overall, your screenings are great. However, we are a bit concerned about your cholesterol screening result, which is 225. Generally, we like to see our patients with levels under 200.

Please call our office to schedule an appointment with Kaylyn, our clinical medical assistant, to obtain information on diet and exercise programs to help you try to lower your cholesterol number naturally. At that time, she will make an appointment for you to return for a second screening in six months. Also, please check out our website at BWWAssociates.com for delicious low-fat/low-sodium recipe ideas that are easy to prepare and great for the whole family.

As always, if you have any questions at any time, please call the office.

Sincerely,

Elizabeth H. Williams MD

Elizabeth H. Williams, MD

EHW/mp

FIGURE 10-3 Example of a block-style letter. Note that all lines begin at the left margin.

- Divide long paragraphs of more than 10 lines of type into shorter ones.

As stated previously in the discussion on supplies, for multipage letters, use letterhead for the first page and matching plain bond paper for the subsequent pages. Use a 1-inch margin at the top and include a heading with the addressee name, date, and page number on all subsequent pages. The text of the letter should continue about three lines below the heading.

Letter Styles

Four common letter styles are used for different purposes. Your office is likely to have a preferred style in place. Let's take a look at each of these styles individually.

Full-Block Style The **full-block letter style**, also called block style, is typed with all lines flush left. Figure 10-3 shows an example of the block letter style. This style may include a subject line two lines below the salutation.

Block-style letters are quick and easy to write because there are no indented paragraphs to slow the typist. Block style is one of the most common formats used in the medical office.

Modified-Block Style The **modified-block letter style** is similar to full block but differs in that the dateline, complimentary closing, signature block, and notations are aligned and begin at the center of the page or slightly to the right of center (Figure 10-4). This type of letter has a traditional, balanced appearance.

Modified-Block Style with Indented Paragraphs This style is identical to the modified-block style except that the paragraphs are indented one-half inch (Figure 10-5).

Simplified Style The **simplified letter style** is a modification of the full-block style. Figure 10-6 shows an example of the simplified letter style. The salutation is omitted,

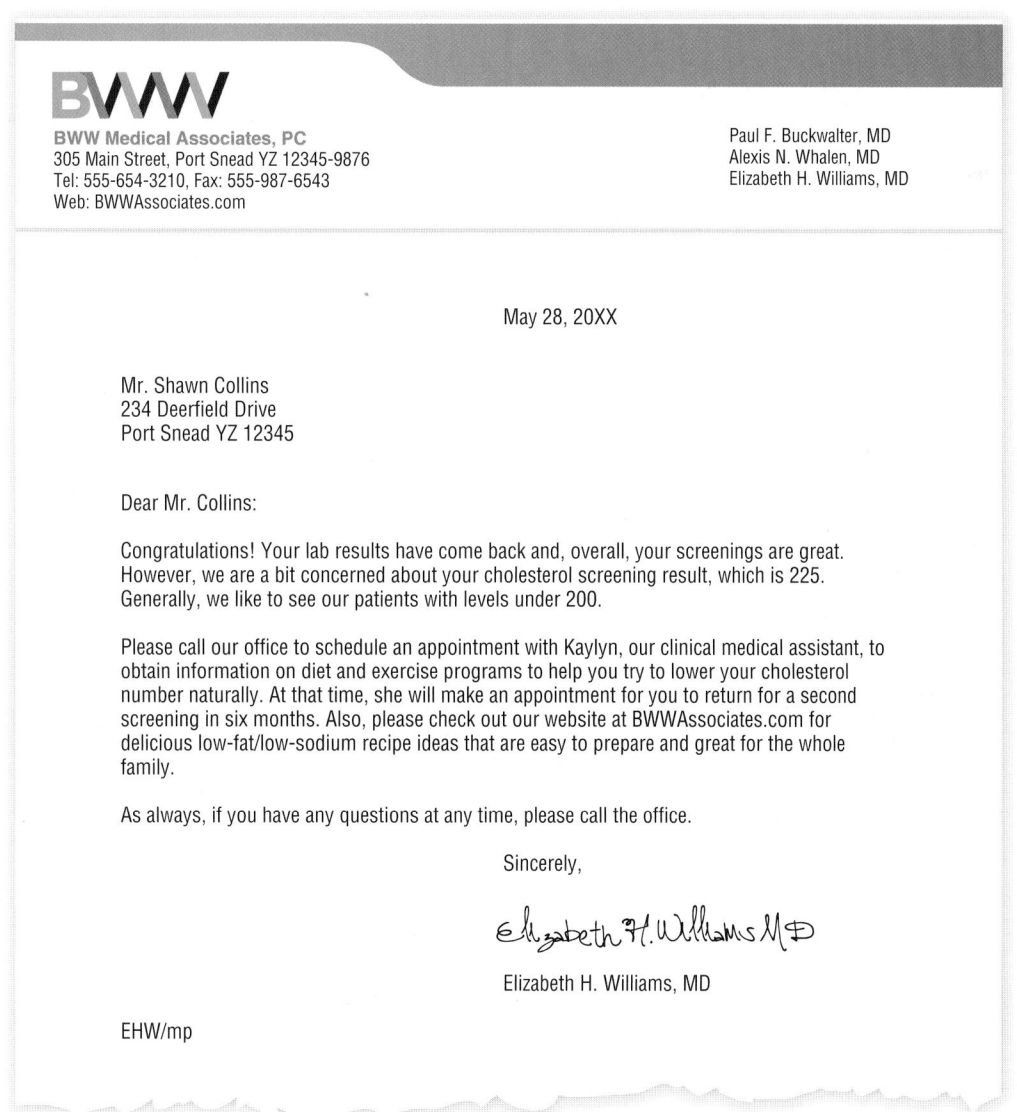

FIGURE 10-4 Example of a modified-block style letter. Note that the date line, complimentary closing, signature block, and notations begin slightly to the right of center.

BWW Medical Associates, PC
305 Main Street, Port Snead YZ 12345-9876
Tel: 555-654-3210, Fax: 555-987-6543
Web: BWWAssociates.com

Paul F. Buckwalter, MD
Alexis N. Whalen, MD
Elizabeth H. Williams, MD

May 28, 20XX

Mr. Shawn Collins
234 Deerfield Drive
Port Snead YZ 12345

Dear Mr. Collins:

Congratulations! Your lab results have come back and, overall, your screenings are great. However, we are a bit concerned about your cholesterol screening result, which is 225. Generally, we like to see our patients with levels under 200.

Please call our office to schedule an appointment with Kaylyn, our clinical medical assistant, to obtain information on diet and exercise programs to help you try to lower your cholesterol number naturally. At that time, she will make an appointment for you to return for a second screening in six months. Also, please check out our website at BWWAssociates.com for delicious low-fat/low-sodium recipe ideas that are easy to prepare and great for the whole family.

As always, if you have any questions at any time, please call the office.

Sincerely,

Elizabeth H. Williams MD

Elizabeth H. Williams, MD

EHW/mp

FIGURE 10-5 Example of a modified-block style letter with indented paragraphs. Except for the indented paragraphs, it is identical to the modified-block style.

eliminating the need for a courtesy title. A subject line in all-capital letters is placed between the address and the body of the letter. The subject line summarizes the letter's main point but does not actually use the word *subject*. All text is typed flush left. The complimentary closing is omitted, and the sender's name and title are typed in capital letters in a single line at the end of the letter. Note that this letter style always uses open punctuation, so it is both easy to read and quick to type. In most medical office situations, however, the simplified letter style may be too informal.

Punctuation Styles

Two different punctuation styles are used in correspondence: open punctuation and mixed punctuation. Once a style is selected, be sure that you remain consistent and true to the chosen style throughout the letter.

Open Punctuation This style uses no punctuation after the following items when they appear in a letter:

- The word *Attention* in the attention line
- The salutation
- The complimentary closing
- The signature block
- The enclosure and copy notations

Mixed Punctuation This style includes the following punctuation marks used in specific instances:

- A colon after *Attention* in the attention line.
- A colon after the salutation.
- A comma after the complimentary closing.
- A colon or period after the enclosure notation.
- A colon after the copy notation.

Now that you have a basic understanding of letter styles and formats, including punctuation styles, Procedure 10-1 at the end of the chapter outlines the steps for creating a professional business letter using word processing software.

BWW Medical Associates, PC
305 Main Street, Port Snead YZ 12345-9876
Tel: 555-654-3210, Fax: 555-987-6543
Web: BWWAssociates.com

Paul F. Buckwalter, MD
Alexis N. Whalen, MD
Elizabeth H. Williams, MD

May 28, 20XX

Mr. Shawn Collins
234 Deerfield Drive
Port Snead YZ 12345

LAB RESULTS

Congratulations! Your lab results have come back and, overall, your screenings are great. However, we are a bit concerned about your cholesterol screening result, which is 225. Generally, we like to see our patients with levels under 200.

Please call our office to schedule an appointment with Kaylyn, our clinical medical assistant, to obtain information on diet and exercise programs to help you try to lower your cholesterol number naturally. At that time, she will make an appointment for you to return for a second screening in six months. Also, please check out our website at BWWAssociates.com for delicious low-fat/low-sodium recipe ideas that are easy to prepare and great for the whole family.

As always, if you have any questions at any time, please call the office.

Elizabeth H. Williams MD

Elizabeth H. Williams, MD

FIGURE 10-6 The simplified letter is considered by some to be the most readable style for correspondence.

Interoffice Memoranda (Memos)

Interoffice memoranda (memos) are periodically used by medical offices, clinics, and hospitals. Most word processing software has templates for formatting interoffice memos. Memos generally facilitate informal written communication within an office.

The heading for a memo generally consists of the following components, written in all caps, followed by a colon:

TO:

FROM:

DATE:

SUBJECT:

Figure 10-7 reveals what a typical office memo looks like. Refer to Procedure 10-2 at the end of the chapter to review the steps for creating an interoffice memo.

In many large practices today, printed memos have been replaced by "e-mail blasts" to reach all employees simultaneously. You will explore e-mail and other electronic communications next.

▶ Written Communication Using Electronic Format
LO 10.5

It is no secret that electronic communication has taken the United States by storm. Can you answer *yes* to more than two of the followings statements?

- I have multiple personal e-mail accounts.
- I have a Facebook account and use it daily.
- I use a cell phone for texting.
- I "tweet" at least once a day.
- I use other forms of electronic communication.
- I use online banking and also pay my bills online.

Now, answer the following questions, true or false.

- I have mailed a letter to someone in the past 2 weeks.
- I pay my bills by writing a check and mailing it.

Electronic communication is the preferred method of communication for many people. For the newest generation, many

INTEROFFICE MEMO

TO: All Staff
FROM: Malik Katahri, Office Manager
DATE: December 14, 20XX
RE: Patient PHI

It has come to my attention that a computer screen was left on while it contained patient protected health information. Worse yet, the computer is in a location where patients and visitors could view it. This is unacceptable.

We all must be very aware of what we are doing at all times and shut off computer screens, even if we are leaving the computer "just for a minute." Better yet, log off the computer prior to leaving the station. Remember, patient information is to be revealed only on a "business need-to-know basis" and it should NEVER be revealed because someone was temporarily distracted.

FIGURE 10-7 Typical office memorandum format.

would rather communicate via text message or on Facebook rather than by phone or instead of in-person, face-to-face contact. For this reason, professional, grammatically correct writing (in both electronic and paper format) is largely unused by an increasingly large segment of the population. This cannot hold true for electronic communications coming from a medical office, however. Here, the information is simply too important not to be presented clearly and concisely at all times, regardless of the format.

Electronic Media and E-mail to Patients

According to HIPAA law, transmissions that are physically moved from one location to another using magnetic tape, disk, compact disk, or any other portable computer drive are considered electronic media. When used to transport patient information, the portable device and the information it contains must be handled in the same confidential manner as patient paper records. All patient information, regardless of the form, is protected by HIPAA law and is to be guarded by the healthcare provider. The same holds true for e-mail transmissions to and from patients. One word of caution regarding e-mail communications with patients: e-mail is not considered a secure method of communication. As with cell phone communication, information can be *intercepted* and so received by someone who was not the intended recipient. Before undertaking e-mail communication with a patient, be sure to have a signed written consent for e-mail communication on file. Figure 10-8 gives an example of an e-mail consent form.

Once the signed consent is on file, the patient chooses the provider she wishes to communicate with. Depending on the office, by choosing a specific provider, the patient often also agrees to receive e-mail communication from members of that physician's staff, including, but not limited to, nurses, medical assistants, and administrative personnel. The office electronic

health record, or EHR program makes this communication easier in many larger offices. Several EHR programs include an e-mail component. The beauty of these types of programs is that the patient's e-mail address becomes part of her medical chart and is then readily accessible to medical staff members that have access to the patient's chart. Figure 10-9 gives an example of a typical e-mail screen from an EHR program.

Procedure 10-3, found at the end of this chapter, outlines the steps for creating a professional e-mail message. In addition to e-mail messages, many EHR programs also contain templates for completion of electronic letters in often-used formats. Procedure 10-4 at the end of the chapter gives a basic outline of how one of these programs works.

Interoffice E-mail

As more and more offices—medical and nonmedical—increase their e-mail use, e-mail and Internet etiquette and rules have become increasingly more important. For example, most offices with Internet access now have written policies regarding e-mail, spelling out the "dos" and "don'ts" concerning use of the practice's e-mail system. The American Medical Informatics Association and Health E-mail (a nonprofit physician outreach program) are two professional organizations that have established policies relating to e-mail. And larger offices with IS (information systems) departments even audit e-mail and Internet usage. Always remember that when you are using the office computer system, no Internet site you access, and no e-mail that you send or receive, is private; it belongs to the office and the practice owners have the right to monitor and even limit the access you have to the computer system. A good rule of thumb to follow regarding any e-mail from you coming from your office computer is, "Would I be OK with my supervisor seeing this e-mail?" If the answer is not an emphatic "Yes," do not send it.

BWW Medical Associates, PC
305 Main Street, Port Snead YZ 12345-9876
Tel: 555-654-3210, Fax: 555-987-6543
Web: BWWAssociates.com

Paul F. Buckwalter, MD
Alexis N. Whalen, MD
Elizabeth H. Williams, MD

Consent to Use E-mail Communication

BWW Medical Associates pledges to use all reasonable measures to protect the private health information of our patients. This includes any information that may be transmitted to or from our office via e-mail. We cannot, however, guarantee the security or confidentiality of information shared via e-mail and we will not accept any liability for disclosure of confidential information that is not caused by professional misconduct on the part of a member of our office team. In order to honor your request to use e-mail communication, we require written consent regarding the following conditions:

- All e-mail messages to or from the patient regarding diagnosis or treatment of a medical condition will become part of the patient's permanent health record. As with any part of the health record, authorized office personnel, including billing and coding professionals in our office, will have access to the information contained within the e-mail message.

- We will forward no e-mail messages, nor the information contained within them, to any third parties, including insurance carriers, without the patient's express written consent, unless otherwise authorized or required by law.

- Because we cannot guarantee that e-mail messages will be received or read within any particular time frame, e-mail is not to be used for transmitting any time-sensitive material or information. E-mail is also not to be used for transmitting information regarding any medical emergency.

- It remains the patient's responsibility to schedule and keep any medically necessary appointments.

I have read and understand the outlined risks associated with e-mail communication between BWW Medical Associates and me. I agree to the conditions and instructions listed above, as well as to any further instructions or limitations BWW Medical Associates may impose regarding e-mail communications. All of my questions have been answered and I understand I may withdraw this consent in writing, at any time.

_____   _____
Patient Signature   Date

_____   _____
Patient Name   Patient E-mail Address

FIGURE 10-8 E-mail consent form.

Managing E-mail

E-mail management, while helpful on a personal level, is imperative on a professional level. Most offices limit the amount of storage each user has, so it is important to manage the documents you send, receive, keep, and delete, so that documents and e-mails that may be needed later are not inadvertently "lost in the system." The following management tools will help you to manage your Inbox and your saved e-mails.

- Check your office e-mail regularly, emptying any unwanted e-mails.

- Do not open unidentifiable e-mails, even if they appear to be sent from someone you trust.

If there is no subject line topic, contact the sender by simply hitting reply (without opening the contents) to see if they actually sent it or if it is SPAM (unwanted, potentially virus-carrying e-mail) that may damage your computer, or, worse, the entire office system. The office should have up-to-date antivirus software running, but always be very cautious of unsolicited e-mails.

- Set up subfolders for e-mails that have to be kept for an indefinite period of time.

- Set time limits for deleting or retaining messages.

- Save all e-mail responses that contain PHI (protected health information).

FIGURE 10-9 Incoming e-mail message from patient.

Source: Screen captures of SpringCharts™ Electronic Health Records software are reprinted with permission from Spring Medical Systems, Inc. All rights reserved.

▶ Editing and Proofreading LO 10.6

Editing and proofreading take place after you create the first draft of any document, on paper or in electronic format. **Editing** involves checking a document for factual accuracy, logical flow, conciseness, clarity, and tone. **Proofreading** involves checking a document for grammatical, spelling, and formatting errors. When possible, ask another person to proofread your work as well. *Never* skip over the very important steps of editing and proofreading!

Tools for Editing and Proofreading

Reference books can help you prepare letters that appear professional. Keep the following tools available.

Dictionary An up-to-date dictionary gives you more than just definitions of words. A dictionary tells you how to spell, divide, and pronounce a word and what part of speech it is, such as a noun or adjective. A dictionary can be accessed on the Internet or in book form.

Medical Dictionary It is nearly impossible for even the most experienced healthcare professional to be familiar with every medical term and its correct spelling. So, a medical dictionary will serve as a handy reference for terms with which you are unfamiliar or about which you would like more information. Like a regular dictionary, a medical dictionary can also be accessed on the Internet or in book form. However, a medical dictionary in book form may not have the most updated terms. Like other medical reference books, a medical dictionary needs to be replaced periodically. Becoming familiar with some of the prefixes and suffixes commonly used in medical terms can help you understand the meanings of many words. Appendix II at

the end of this textbook lists some common medical prefixes and suffixes.

Thesaurus A thesaurus provides synonyms, or similar words to a word you are using. It helps you avoid repetition in your writing and helps you find a word for an idea you have in mind. A thesaurus can be found in word processing programs, in print, and online.

Physicians' Desk Reference (PDR) The *PDR* is a dictionary of medications. Published yearly, it provides up-to-date information on both prescription and nonprescription (also known as over-the-counter or OTC) drugs. Consult the *PDR* for the correct spelling of a particular drug or for other information about its usage, side effects, contraindications, and other information.

English Grammar and Usage Manuals These manuals answer questions concerning grammar and word usage. They usually contain sections on punctuation, capitalization, and other details of written communication.

Word Processing Spelling Checkers Most word processing programs used in medical offices have built-in spelling checkers. There are also programs designed specifically to check spelling in medical documents. These spelling checkers include most common medical terms that would not be found in a regular software program. Always keep in mind that spell check alone should not be relied on as the only means of checking a document, as it may not detect all spelling errors. Spell checkers will not find correctly spelled words that are used incorrectly and this type of mistake will reflect negatively on the practice. For example, if you type the word *form* instead of *from*, spell checkers will not recognize this as incorrect because *form* is also a correctly spelled word.

Spelling checkers do pick up many spelling errors and often give suggestions for correct spellings. If you indicate the choice you meant to input, the program automatically replaces the misspelled word. You may be able to add words—like medical terms—that are not currently recognized by the spelling checker in your computer. A word of caution is important here! Before you add the word to the computer's dictionary, be sure to look up the exact spelling in a medical dictionary. The computer will recognize only the spelling you add. If you place the *wrong* spelling in the computer, your spelling checker will not correct it.

When you type e-mails, take special care to use correct grammar and punctuation. Spelling checkers are available in most e-mail programs and should be used once you have finished writing the e-mail, before you hit "Send." Note that the e-mail spelling checker does not automatically point out mistakes as you type.

Some software packages offer grammar-checking and style-checking features. These programs can identify certain problems, but the person using them still must know basic grammar and style rules in order to correct errors.

Editing Process

The editing process ensures that a document is accurate, clear, and complete; free of grammatical errors; organized logically; and written in an appropriate style. It is a good idea to leave some time between the writing and editing stages so that you can look at the document in a fresh light. As you edit, you must examine language usage, content, and style.

Language Usage Learn basic grammar rules (refer to Tables 10-1 and 10-2). When in doubt, refer to a grammar handbook or reference manual. Make sure all sentences are complete. Continually ask yourself, "Is this the best way to convey what I want to say? Do my word choices reflect the overall tone of the document?" For example, in a business letter, you would avoid choosing phrases that are too casual such as "Thanks a million" or "Take it easy." These expressions are informal and inappropriate for a business letter.

Content A business letter should contain all the necessary information the writer intends to convey. If you are editing someone else's letter and something appears to be missing, check with the writer. She or he may have omitted information by mistake.

The content of a letter should follow a logical thought pattern. Create a clean, concise letter by

- Stating the purpose of the letter in the first sentence.
- Discussing one topic at a time.
- Changing paragraphs when you change topics.
- Listing events in chronological order.
- Sticking to the subject.
- Selecting words carefully.
- Reading over what you have written before printing.

Style Use a writing style that is appropriate to the reader. A letter written to a patient is likely to require a different style than one written to a physician. Consider medical terms, for example. In writing to a patient to confirm her surgery date, you might say, "The surgery to remove your gallbladder is scheduled for Friday, May 8, at 7 a.m." However, when confirming the same surgery with the physician, you would state, "Mrs. Stark's cholecystectomy is scheduled for Friday, May 8, at 7 a.m."

Proofreading

Proofreading means to thoroughly check a document for errors. After editing a document, again, put it aside for a short time before proofreading it. Ideally, after you proofread the document, also have a coworker proofread your work. Someone else will often notice errors that you may have missed. The three types of errors that can occur when preparing a document are formatting, data, and mechanical.

Formatting Errors These errors involve the positioning of the various parts of a letter. They may include errors in indenting, line length, or line spacing. To avoid these errors, take the following two steps:

1. Scan the letter to make sure that the indentions are consistent, that the spacing is correct, and that the text is centered from left to right and top to bottom.
2. Follow the office style consistently throughout the document.

Data Errors Data errors involve mistyping monetary figures, like the balance on a patient statement. Mistyped monetary figures can potentially have huge repercussions for the office, the insurance company, and the patient. So, be sure to verify the accuracy of all figures by checking them twice or by having another coworker check them.

Mechanical Errors Mechanical errors are errors in spelling, punctuation, spacing between words, and division of words. Make sure that your word processing spelling checker has medical terminology included; otherwise, medical terms may be overlooked. Mechanical errors also include reversing words or characters, typing them twice, or omitting them altogether. Here are some tips to help you avoid mechanical errors.

- Learn basic spelling, punctuation, and word division rules. When in doubt, be sure to check a manual on English usage. Review Table 10-2, which outlines some basic rules concerning the mechanics of writing. Table 10-3 lists some of the most commonly misspelled medical terms and other words.
- Check carefully for transposed (misplaced) characters or words.
- Avoid dividing words at the end of a line. Most word processing programs automatically wrap words to the next line, so if you are writing on a computer, word division should not present a problem.

TABLE 10-3	Commonly Misspelled Medical Terms and Other Words		
Medical Terms			
abscess	diluent	larynx	pleurisy
aerobic	dissect	leukemia	pneumonia
anergic	eosinophil	leukocyte	polyp
anesthetic	epididymis	malaise	prescription
aneurysm	epistaxis	menstruation	prophylaxis
anteflexion	erythema	metastasis	prostate
arrhythmia	eustachian	muscle	prosthesis
asepsis	fissure	neuron	pruritus
asthma	flexure	nosocomial	psoriasis
auricle	fomites	occlusion	psychiatrist
benign	glaucoma	ophthalmology	pyrexia
bilirubin	glomerular	oscilloscope	respiration
bronchial	gonorrhea	osseous	rheumatism
calcaneus	hemocytometer	palliative	roentgenology
capillary	hemorrhage	parasite	serous
cervical	hemorrhoids	parenteral	specimen
chancre	homeostasis	parietal	sphincter
choroid	humerus	paroxysm	sphygmomanometer
chromosome	ileum	pericardium	squamous
cirrhosis	ilium	perineum	staphylococcus
clavicle	infarction	peristalsis	surgeon
curettage	inoculate	peritoneum	vaccine
cyanosis	intussusception	pharynx	vein
defibrillator	ischemia	pituitary	venereal
desiccation	ischium	plantar	wheal
Other Words			
absence	apparatus	changeable	definite
accept	apparent	characteristic	dependent
accessible	appearance	cigarette	description
accommodate	appropriate	circumference	desirable
accumulate	approximate	clientele	development
achieve	argument	committee	dilemma
acquire	assistance	comparative	disappear
adequate	associate	complement	disappoint
advantageous	auxiliary	compliment	disapprove
affect	balloon	concede	disastrous
aggravate	bankruptcy	conscientious	discreet
all right	believe	conscious	discrete
a lot	benefited	controversy	discrimination
already	brochure	corroborate	dissatisfied
altogether	bulletin	counsel	dissipate
analysis	business	courtesy	earnest
analyze	category	defendant	ecstasy

effect	it's	pleasant	secretary
eligible	labeled	possession	seize
embarrass	laboratory	precede	separate
emphasis	led	precedent	similar
entrepreneur	leisure	predictable	sizable
envelope	liable	predominant	stationary
environment	liaison	prejudice	stationery
exceed	license	preparation	stomach
except	liquefy	prerogative	subpoena
exercise	maintenance	prevalent	succeed
exhibit	maneuver	principal	suddenness
exhilaration	miscellaneous	principle	supersede
existence	misspelled	privilege	surprise
fantasy	necessary	procedure	tariff
fascinate	noticeable	proceed	technique
February	occasion	professor	temperament
fluorescent	occurrence	pronunciation	temperature
forty	offense	psychiatry	thorough
grammar	oscillate	psychology	transferred
grievance	paid	pursue	truly
guarantee	pamphlet	questionnaire	tyrannize
handkerchief	panicky	rearrange	unnecessary
height	paradigm	recede	until
humorous	parallel	receive	vacillate
hygiene	paralyze	recommend	vacuum
incidentally	pastime	referral	vegetable
indispensable	persevere	relieve	vicious
inimitable	persistent	repetition	warrant
insistent	personal	rescind	Wednesday
irrelevant	personnel	résumé	weird
irresistible	persuade	rhythm	
irritable	phenomenon	ridiculous	
its	plagiarism	schedule	

▶ Preparing Outgoing Mail   LO 10.7

After you have created, edited, and proofread a letter, you need to prepare it for mailing. This preparation includes having the letter signed, preparing the envelope, and folding and inserting the letter into the envelope. Your letter will then be ready for postage to be calculated and affixed.

Signing Letters

After your letter is complete—it has been proofread and the envelope and enclosures have been prepared—it is ready for signing. Some physicians authorize other staff members to sign for them. If you have been authorized to sign letters, you should sign the doctor's name and place your initials after the doctor's signature.

If the physician prefers to sign all letters, you should place the letter on her desk in a file folder marked "For Your Signature." If the letter is of an urgent nature, give it to the doctor as soon as possible. Otherwise, you can collect several letters in the folder and present the entire group for signing at one time. However, all prepared work should be given to the physician at the end of the day. Make sure that all enclosures are included with the letter and that they remain with the letter when it is returned to you with the physician's signature.

Using a Letter Folding and Inserting Machine

Large offices and hospitals often have letter-folding equipment, which can help minimize the amount of time staff spends preparing large volumes of outgoing mail. Letter folders are also used for creating folded brochures. In addition to folding letters, a medical practice may use folding and inserting machines for a variety of items, including invoices, newsletters, checks, statements, letters, and flyers.

Lower-end folding equipment requires letters to be fed manually. The speed of this machine is limited to the speed at which an individual can feed in letters, which is typically about 200 pieces per hour. An automatic feeder is required for faster folding. Letter-folding machines can make many different types of folds, including standard business letter folds (c-fold), accordion folds (z-fold), single folds, right-angle folds, and brochure folds (Figure 10-10). Most machines can fold more than one sheet of paper together but do not allow stapled pages to be fed and folded.

Many special features are available that may help the processing of mail and brochures. Batch counters and stackers help to prevent a letter folding machine from folding more sheets than desired. A jogger helps align stacks of paper and dissipates or removes static electricity. Some machines are better designed for certain types of paper, like glossy or carbonless paper. Inserters are used to insert a folded document into an envelope.

Manually Folding a Letter

A business letter is folded twice into horizontal thirds to fit easily into a prepared standard business envelope. Be sure to include any enclosures that have been noted within the letter at the time it is being folded. See Figure 10-11 for more detailed instructions on how to manually fold and insert a business letter into an envelope.

Letters and invoices must be folded neatly before they are inserted into the envelopes. The proper way to fold a document depends on the type of envelope into which the letter will fit.

- With a small envelope, fold the enclosure in half lengthwise and insert it.
- With a regular, business-size envelope, fold the letter in thirds. Fold the bottom third up first, then the top third down, and insert the letter.

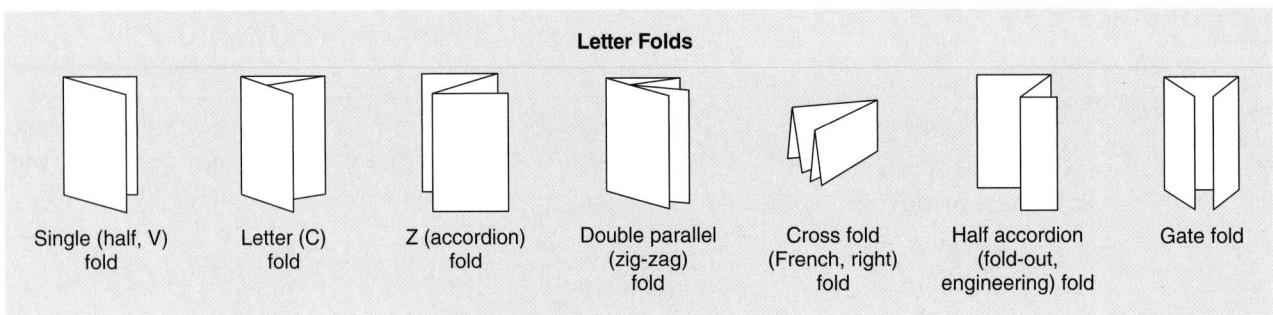

FIGURE 10-10 Examples of different folds available with folding machines.

FIGURE 10-11 Correct folding of a business letter.

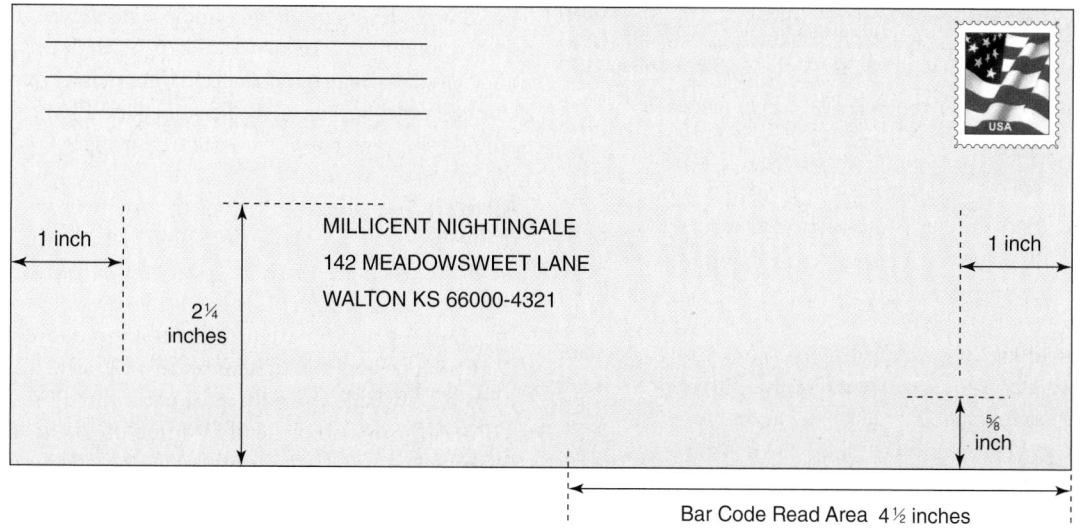

FIGURE 10-12 Correct address format and placement to allow processing by USPS electronic equipment.

- With a window envelope, use an accordion fold. Fold the bottom third up. Then, fold the top third back so the address appears in the window, and insert the enclosure.

Preparing the Envelope

To ensure the quickest delivery of mail, the USPS has issued several guidelines for preparing envelopes. The USPS uses electronic **optical character readers (OCRs)** to help speed mail processing. OCRs read the last two lines of an address and sort the mail accordingly. To take advantage of this technology, envelopes must be no smaller than 3½ by 5 inches and no larger than 6 by 11½ inches. They must be addressed in a specific format that can be read by the OCR, following USPS guidelines for addressing envelopes.

Address Placement The address must be placed in a certain location on the envelope for reading by the OCR (Figure 10-12). The area the OCR can read has the following characteristics:

- It is bordered by a 1-inch margin on both the left and right sides of the envelope.
- It has a ⅝-inch margin on the bottom. The top of the city/ state/zip code line (the last line in the address block) must be no higher than 2 inches from the bottom edge of the envelope.
- An area 4½ inches wide in the bottom right corner of the envelope should be left clear. The OCR reads the address and prints a bar code that corresponds to the zip code in this area.

Two Delivery Addresses Sometimes a location may have two delivery addresses, a post office box and a street address. The mail is delivered to the address that appears directly above the city-state-zip. If the two addresses have different zip codes, the zip must be the one of the actual delivery point (Figure 10-13).

Address Format When you type an address, follow these format guidelines:

- Type or machine-print (for example, by computer) the address. (The OCR cannot read handwriting.) The OCR cannot read fancy script fonts.
- Single-space the lines and use the block format. Use only one or two spaces between numbers and words in the address. Do not punctuate as it is difficult for scanners to read.
- Use only USPS-approved abbreviations for location designations, as presented in Table 10-4 on the next page.
- Put the addressee's name on the first line of the address block, the department (if any) on the second line, and the company name on the third line. If the letter is to go to someone's attention at a company, put the company name on the first line and "Attention:" before the address begins.
- The line above the city, state, and zip code should contain the street address or post office box number. Include suite or apartment numbers on the same line as the street address.

FIGURE 10-13 When both street address and PO Box are listed, delivery is dependent upon the information on line 3, or directly above the city-state-zip.

TABLE 10-4	USPS Abbreviations		
Word	**Abbreviation**	**Word**	**Abbreviation**
Avenue	AVE	Junction	JCT
Boulevard	BLVD	Lane	LN
Center	CTR	North	N
Circle	CIR	Parkway	PKY
Corner	COR	Place	PL
Court	CT	Plaza	PLZ
Drive	DR	South	S
East	E	Street	ST
Expressway	EXPY	West	W
Highway	HWY		

- The last line of the address must include the city, state, and zip code. Use the zip + 4 code whenever possible.

- Include the hyphen in the zip + 4 code, for example, 08520-6142.

- Obtain current zip codes by logging on to the USPS Web page at http://zip4.usps.com.

- Type any special notations (such as SPECIAL DELIVERY, CERTIFIED, or REGISTERED) two lines below the postage in all-capital letters. This information should appear outside the area the OCR can read.

- Type any handling instructions (such as PERSONAL or CONFIDENTIAL) three lines below the return address. This information should also be outside the area the OCR can read.

- Letters going to foreign countries should have the name of the country on the last line of the address block in all-capital letters.

- Some letters may be appropriate for interoffice or company mail systems. These letters are usually placed in a large envelope with multiple address lines. The envelope can be reused many times by crossing out the previous name and address and using the next line. Place interoffice mail in a specially designated area or basket for pickup. Be sure not to mix it with outgoing mail.

▶ Mailing Options
LO 10.8

Not too long ago, there was one option for delivering correspondence or documents from one location to the other—the U.S. Post Office. Today, aside from electronic delivery options, there are multiple ways to deliver correspondence and documents from one location to the other. Let's explore some of these options.

Mailing Equipment and Supplies

The proper equipment and supplies will help you handle the mail efficiently and cost-effectively. In addition to letterhead, blank stationery for multipage letters, and envelopes described earlier in the chapter, you will need some standard supplies. The USPS provides forms, labels, and packaging for items that need special attention, like airmail, Priority Mail, Express Mail, certified mail, or registered mail. Private delivery companies, like United Parcel Service (UPS) and Federal Express (FedEx), also provide shipping supplies to their customers.

Airmail Supplies In the past, any piece of mail that was transported by air was designated as airmail. Today, nearly all first-class mail outside a local area is routinely sent by air. However, airmail services are still available for some packages and for most mail going to foreign countries.

If you are sending an item by airmail, attach special airmail stickers, available from the post office, on all sides. (The word *AIRMAIL* can also be neatly written on all sides.) Special airmail envelopes for letters can be purchased from the USPS.

Envelopes for Overnight Delivery Services For correspondence or packages that must be delivered by the next day, a number of overnight delivery services are available through the USPS and private companies. Most companies require the use of their own envelopes and mailing materials. Make sure you keep adequate supplies on hand.

Postal Rates, Scales, and Meters Postal rates and regulations change periodically, and every medical office should have a copy of the latest guidelines—available from the USPS. The *Office Equipment and Supplies* chapter describes postal scales and meters.

Posting Mail

As stated previously, before you begin posting mail, make sure the envelope or package is complete with all noted enclosures and materials included. After inserting the document(s) in the appropriate envelope (or package in the appropriate container), apply the proper postage and place the postmarked envelope or package in the area of your office designated for mail pickup.

U.S. Postal Service Delivery

The USPS offers a variety of domestic and international delivery services for letters and packages. As a result of a comprehensive USPS Transformation Plan in 2002, many new services were added to the post office, making it much better able to compete with other mail and package delivery services. Following are some of the services you will most likely use in the medical office setting.

Regular Mail Service Regular mail delivery includes several classes of mail as well as other designations like Priority Mail and Express Mail. The class or designation determines how quickly a piece of mail is delivered.

First-Class Mail Most correspondence generated in a medical office—letters, postcards, and invoices—is sent by first-class mail. Items must weigh 11 ounces or less to be considered first-class. (An item over 11 ounces that requires quick delivery must be sent by Priority Mail, which is discussed later in this section.) The cost of mailing a first-class item is based on its weight. The standard rate is for items 1 ounce or less that are no larger than 6⅛ inches high, 11½ inches wide, and ¼ inch thick. Additional postage is required for items that are heavier or larger. Postage for postcards is less than the letter rate. First-class mail is forwarded at no extra cost.

Second-Class Mail Most medical offices do not use second-class mail. This class of mail is designed for the delivery of newspapers and periodicals only.

Media Mail (Third-Class Mail) Media mail is also known as book rate mail. Like second-class mail, it is not often used in medical offices. Media mail is used for the mailing of books, catalogs, and other printed material that weighs less than 16 ounces. This class of mailing is available only to authorized mailers and it is only forwarded if it contains a special endorsement.

Parcel Post This type of mail was formerly called Fourth-Class Mail. It is used for items that weigh at least one pound but not more than 70 pounds and that do not require speedy delivery. Rates are based on weight and distance. There is a special fourth-class rate for mailing books, manuscripts, and some types of medical information.

Bound Printed Matter Formerly called Special Fourth-Class Mail, this is a rate applied to promotional advertising, directories, and other types of advertisements. No personal correspondence is allowed. Bulk rates are available for a minimum of 300 pieces.

Priority Mail Priority class is useful for heavier items that require quicker delivery than is available for Fourth-Class Mail. Any first-class item that weighs between 11 ounces and 70 pounds requires Priority Mail service. Although the rate for Priority Mail varies with the item's weight and the distance it must travel, the USPS offers a flat rate for all material that can fit into its special Priority Mail envelopes and boxes. The USPS guarantees delivery of Priority Mail items in 2 to 3 business days.

Express Mail Express Mail is the quickest USPS service. Different types are available, including next-day and second-day delivery. Express Mail deliveries are made 365 days a year. Rates vary, depending on the weight and the specific service. A special flat-rate envelope is also available. Items sent by Express Mail are automatically insured against loss or damage. You can drop off packages at the post office or arrange for pickup service.

Special Postal Services The USPS offers a variety of special mail delivery services in addition to the regular classes of mail. These services may require an additional fee above and beyond postage costs.

Online Postage Postage can now be purchased online by using USPS-approved software. This software makes it possible for customers to purchase products via the Internet.

Pitney Bowes has software called ShipStream™; however, you may search the Internet for other USPS-approved software. USPS.com also sells postage online as well as other shipping and mailing supplies.

Special Delivery Use special delivery if you want an item delivered as soon as it reaches the recipient's post office. Delivery of the item is typically made before the regularly scheduled mail delivery. This service is available within certain distance limits and during certain hours.

Certified Mail Certified mail offers a guarantee that the item has been received. The item is marked as certified mail and requires the postal carrier to obtain a signature on delivery (Figure 10-14). The signature card is then returned to the sender. The card should be added to the patient's file. This documentation is evidence that the document was not only mailed but also received. The receiver's name is clearly printed along with the signature. The certified mail signature card becomes a legal document, which may be important in court.

Return Receipt Requested You may request a return receipt (for a small additional fee) to obtain proof that an item was delivered. The receipt indicates who received the item and when. This type of mail service is very important when a medical practice requires proof that a letter was received. When returned to the office, the return receipt should be carefully added to the patient's record. It may become an important legal document—required at a later date in a court of law.

Registered Mail Use registered mail to send items that are valuable, irreplaceable, or otherwise important. Registered mail provides the sender with evidence of mailing and delivery. It also provides the security that an item is being tracked as it is transported through the postal system. Because of this tracking process, delivery may be slightly delayed.

To register a piece of mail, take it to the post office and indicate the full value of the item. Both first-class mail and Priority Mail can be registered.

Delivery Confirmation Delivery confirmation is a service that, for an added fee, tracks your mail with a tracking number by the delivery date and signature.

International Mail The USPS offers both surface (via ship) and airmail service to most foreign countries. Information on rates and fees is available from the post office.

There are various types of international mail, which are similar to the domestic classes. The USPS also provides international Express Mail and Priority Mail services, along with special mail delivery services like registered mail, certified mail, and special delivery.

Tracing Mail If a piece of registered or certified mail does not reach its destination by the expected time, you can ask

Back side of signature card

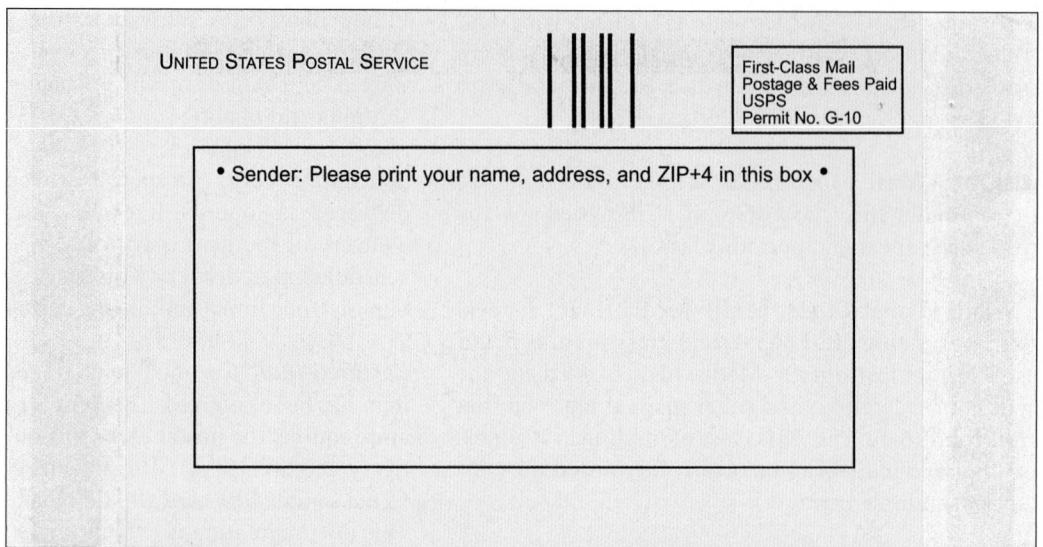

Front side of signature card

Certified mail receipt

FIGURE 10-14 Certified mail with return receipt guarantees receipt of correspondence or package sent to the addressee.

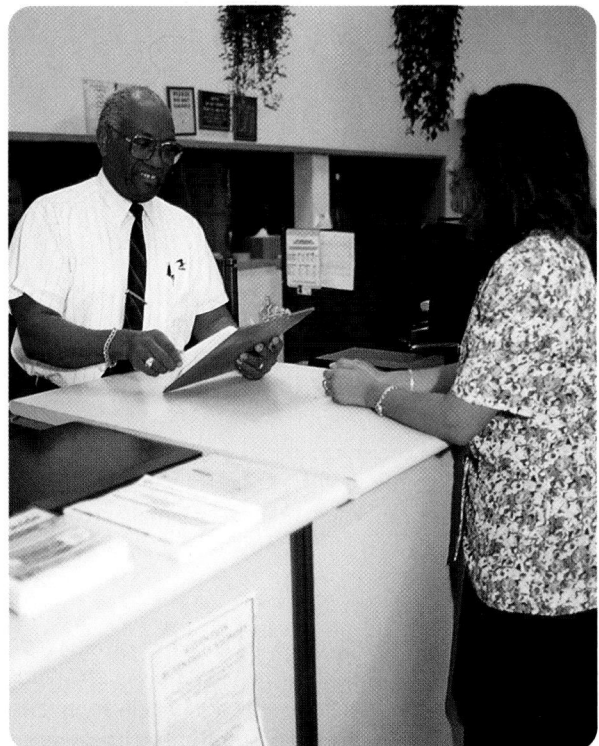

FIGURE 10-15 Items sent by registered or certified mail can be traced by the USPS if delivery is not made as expected.

the post office to trace it (Figure 10-15). You will need to present your original receipt for the item. You can also trace mail on the Internet through a UPC symbol that is scanned at the post office.

Other Delivery Services

In addition to the USPS, other companies provide mail and package delivery services around the globe. UPS, FedEx, and DHL are three of the largest and most popular of these companies; DHL is the newest of the three.

All three services deliver packages and provide overnight letter and express services. Packages can be dropped off at drop-off locations (which can be found online or in the phone book) or at drop boxes (often located near post offices), or they can be picked up at your office. Fees depend on the service(s) provided, such as ground or air, and also may vary between companies. Each company also offers express delivery services with rates varying according to weight, time of delivery, and whether you use office pickup or drop the package off at one of the company's local branches. Packages sent using any of these private companies are automatically insured against theft or damage.

Messengers or Couriers Before e-mail and options like FedEx and UPS were widely used, local messenger or courier services were popular for deliveries made within a local area. Except for interoffice couriers that are still used by some large organizations—like hospitals with multiple satellite locations—fewer courier services are now available for hire. Such courier services are listed in the telephone book's Yellow Pages.

▶ Processing Incoming Mail LO 10.9

Mail is an important connection between the office and other professionals and patients. An office often has an established procedure for handling the mail. It is best to set aside a specific time of the day to process all the incoming mail at once rather than trying to do a little bit at a time. Although it sounds simple, processing mail involves more than merely opening envelopes. In general, it involves the following steps: sorting, opening, recording, annotating, and distributing.

Sorting and Opening

The first step in processing mail is to sort it. Always sort the mail in an uncluttered area to avoid mixing it with other paperwork. As you sort, place any personal or confidential mail aside. Unless you have special permission, never open personal mail addressed to another person. Instead, carefully place it on the addressee's desk, unopened. Sort the remaining mail according to priority. Follow a regular sorting procedure each time to avoid missing any steps. Procedure 10-5, found at the end of this chapter, outlines suggested steps for sorting and opening the mail. The Points on Practice section on the next page discusses how to recognize urgent incoming mail.

Recording

Keep a log of each day's mail. This daily record lists the mail received and indicates follow-up correspondence and the date correspondence is completed. This method helps in tracing items and keeping track of correspondence.

Annotating

Because you will be reading much of the incoming mail, you also may be encouraged to **annotate** it. To annotate means to underline or highlight key points of the letter or to write reminders, comments, or suggested actions in the margins or on self-adhesive notes. An example of annotating is including "please sign here" next to where a signature should be. Annotating may involve pulling a patient's chart or any previously received, related correspondence from a file and attaching it to the letter.

Distributing

Once you have reviewed the mail and made any necessary annotations, then sort the letters into separate batches for distribution. These batches might include correspondence that requires the physician's attention, payments to be directed to the billing supervisor, and correspondence that requires your attention. Each batch should be presented to the appropriate person in a file folder or arranged with the highest-priority items on top. You may be given specific instructions on how to distribute magazines, newspapers, and advertising circulars.

How to Spot Urgent Incoming Mail

How can you tell if a piece of incoming mail is urgent? First-class mail marked "Urgent" tells you that it requires immediate attention. Here are some other signals to look for (Figure 10-16).

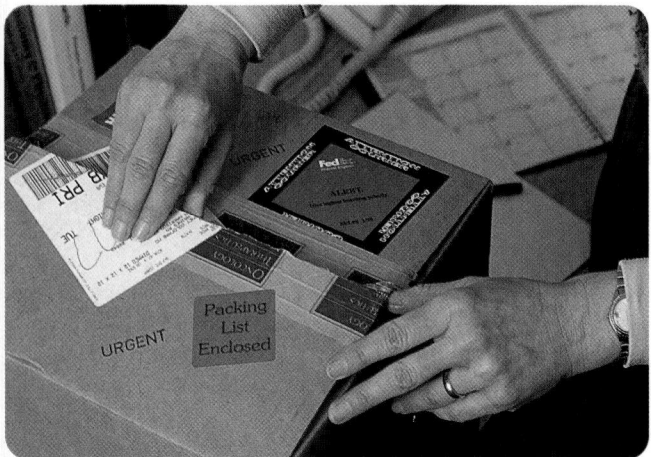

FIGURE 10-16 Packages and correspondence marked "Urgent" receive priority when received by the office.

Overnight Mail

Any package that has been sent by an overnight carrier or by USPS Express Mail should be considered urgent and should be opened immediately.

Certified Mail

Certified mail requires your signature on delivery. The sender used certified mail to be sure that the item would be sent to the proper person.

Registered Mail

Items sent by registered mail typically are valuable, irreplaceable, or otherwise important. Registered mail provides the sender with evidence of mailing and delivery.

Special Delivery

An item sent by special delivery is likely to be delivered sometime before the normal mail delivery—possibly even on a Sunday or holiday. The sender requested special delivery to ensure that the item would be delivered promptly after it was received at the addressee's post office.

Handling Drug and Product Samples

Many physicians receive a number of drug and product samples in the mail. Handling procedures vary from office to office. Samples of nonprescription products, like hand creams or cough drops, may be placed in the patient treatment area for patient distribution, as directed by the physician.

The physician may ask that you put samples of any new prescription drugs in the consultation room for him to evaluate. Store all other drug samples in a locked cabinet reserved solely for such samples. Sort and label the samples by category, such as antibiotics, sedatives, pain-killers, and so on. Never give samples to patients or use them yourself unless directed by the

physician. If the doctor directs you to give samples to a patient, make sure to write this information in the patient's chart and date the entry.

When a box of samples is outdated, you should properly dispose of them, following all state and DEA regulations. You will most likely use the disposal company that handles your biomedical waste to dispose of unused, outdated sample medications. Flushing samples down the sink or toilet is no longer allowed as this can pollute the environment. And samples should never be placed in the trash where unauthorized individuals could take the medications. Your local pharmacy may also have a program for disposing of outdated medications.

PROCEDURE 10-1 Creating a Professional Letter

Procedure Goal: To follow standard procedure for constructing a business letter.

OSHA Guidelines: This procedure does not involve exposure to blood, body fluids, or tissue.

Materials: Word processor or personal computer, letterhead paper, dictionaries or other professional tools.

Method: Procedure steps.

1. Format the letter according to the standard office procedure. Use the same punctuation and style throughout.
   RATIONALE: Consistency in format creates a professional-looking document.

2. Start the dateline three lines below the last line of the printed letterhead. (Note: Depending on the letter's length, it is acceptable to start between two and six lines below the letterhead.)
   RATIONALE: The letter should be centered both vertically and horizontally on the page for visual appeal.

3. Two lines below the dateline, type in any special mailing instructions (such as REGISTERED MAIL, CERTIFIED MAIL, and so on).

4. Three lines below any special instructions, begin the inside address. Type the addressee's courtesy title (Mr., Mrs., Ms.) and full name on the first line. If a professional title is given (M.D., RN, Ph.D.), type this title after the addressee's name instead of a courtesy title.

RATIONALE: A professional title is used when available in professional correspondence. Never use both a courtesy title and a professional title at the same time.

5. Type the addressee's business title, if applicable, on the second line. Type the company name on the third line. Type the street address on the fourth line, including the apartment or suite number. Type the city, state, and zip code on the fifth line. Use the standard two-letter abbreviation for the state, followed by one space and the zip code.

6. Two lines below the inside address, type the salutation, using the appropriate courtesy title (Mr., Mrs., Ms., Dr.) prior to typing the addressee's last name.
   RATIONALE: The salutation uses a courtesy title. Do not include the professional title or the addressee's first name in the salutation.

7. Two lines below the salutation, type the subject line, if applicable.

8. Two lines below the subject line, begin the body of the letter. Single-space between lines. Double-space between paragraphs.

9. Two lines below the body of the letter, type the complimentary closing.

10. Leave three blank lines (return four times) and begin the signature block. (Enough space must be left to allow for the signature.) Type the sender's name on the first line. Type the sender's title on the second line.
    RATIONALE: Adequate space must be left for the signature. If the signer has a long signature, more than three blank lines may be left. Typing the name allows the addressee to understand who sent the letter if the sender's signature is not legible.

11. Two lines below the sender's title, type the identification line. Type the sender's initials in all capitals and your initials in lowercase letters, separating the two sets of initials with a colon or a forward slash.

12. One or two lines below the identification line, type the enclosure notation, if applicable.

13. Two lines below the enclosure notation, type the copy notation, if applicable.

14. Edit the letter.
    RATIONALE: Make appropriate changes to clarify the meaning of the letter.

15. Proofread and spell-check the letter.
    RATIONALE: Every letter must be read again to assure there are no errors.

PROCEDURE 10-2 Writing an Interoffice Memo

Procedure Goal: To follow standard procedure for writing an interoffice memo.

OSHA Guidelines: This procedure does not involve exposure to blood, body fluids, or tissue.

Materials: Word processor or personal computer, plain paper, dictionaries or other professional references as needed.

Method: Procedure steps.
1. Gather all necessary materials and documents needed to compose the memo.
2. Decide whether the memo will be created "free-hand" or by using an existing template.
   RATIONALE: If a template is to be used, it must be pulled up using the appropriate computer or EHR software prior to keying the document.

3. If using a template, fill in the headings as listed with the appropriate information. If the memo is being created free-hand, use the headings DATE:, TO:, FROM:, and RE: or SUBJECT:. Fill in each heading with the appropriate information.

4. Double- or triple-space after the memo headings or, if using a template, move to the body area of the memo and begin typing the information to be included in the memo.

5. Single-space the information within the memo and double-space between paragraphs. Use either the block or indented paragraph format, depending on office policy.

6. Spell-check and proofread the document carefully, correcting errors as necessary.
   RATIONALE: All professional documents must be perfect to reflect well on the writer and the office.

PROCEDURE 10-3 Composing a Professional E-mail Message

Procedure Goal: To follow standard procedure for writing a professional e-mail message.

OSHA Guidelines: This procedure does not involve exposure to blood, body fluids, or tissue.

Materials: Computer with e-mail (Internet) capabilities, dictionary or other professional references as needed.

Method: Procedure steps.
1. Verify that the patient's medical record contains a signed "Consent to Use E-mail" form, allowing communication by this method.

   RATIONALE: Because e-mail is not a secure form of communication, the office must have written approval to use this form of communication with the patient.

2. Use a classic easy-to-read font such as Times New Roman at 12–14 pt. Use black ink only.
   RATIONALE: Larger, crisp fonts are easy to read. Black ink lends a professional appearance.

3. If responding to a patient e-mail, open the e-mail and choose "Reply." If composing a new message, choose "New" to open a new e-mail document. Carefully enter the patient's e-mail address.

RATIONALE: It is imperative that the correct person receives the e-mail.

4. Add the e-mail address to the office address book for easy reference, if it is not saved in the office EHR program.

5. If answering a patient e-mail, you may keep the subject line from the original message. If you are writing a new e-mail, enter a descriptive subject line.

   RATIONALE: The subject line gives the receiver an idea of what the email pertains to.

6. Insert a salutation, using the patient's surname as you would with an ordinary letter.

7. Compose the body of the message, aligning the information with the left margin.

8. Double-space at the end of the message and enter your name, including a signature line with the practice information, and a phone number.

   RATIONALE: It is important that the patient can easily reach you by methods other than e-mail if needed.

Including the office information and phone number makes this easier for the patient.

9. Spell-check and proofread the message carefully for any errors.

   RATIONALE: Even though e-mail is considered less formal, you still represent the office and the document must be professional in tone and free of errors.

10. Click "Send" and wait for the message informing you the message has been sent.

11. If the message is returned as undeliverable, verify the e-mail address was entered correctly. If necessary, correct the address and attempt delivery again.

12. If the message is returned a second time as undeliverable, contact the patient by phone or an alternate communication method to be sure that he or she receives the required information.

PROCEDURE 10-4 Composing an Electronic Patient Letter

Procedure Goal: To create and send an electronic letter to a patient.

OSHA Guidelines: This procedure does not involve exposure to blood, body fluids, or tissue.

Materials: EHR software program with letter templates, information necessary to compose the letter, dictionary or other professional references as needed.

Method: Procedure steps

1. After verifying that there is a signed "Consent to Use e-mail" in the patient's record, access the *New* menu in the appropriate screen of the software program. Choose *New Letter Template.*

2. In the *RE:* window, key the subject line, such as "Welcome to BWW Medical Associates, PC."

   RATIONALE: The name gives the recipient an idea of what is included in the e-mail message.

3. In the Text box, key the body of the letter. Begin the letter with an introductory statement, such as, "Welcome to BWW Medical Associates, and thank you for choosing us for your healthcare needs. We look forward to working with you."

   Enter all pertinent information required for the letter. If continuing a "welcome to the practice" letter, be sure to include the practice name, address, phone numbers, and website information, as well as names of the medical staff, office personnel, and office hours.

4. When you complete the letter, give the template an easily identifiable name, such as *Welcome New Patient Letter.*

RATIONALE: This makes it easy for all users to identify each template.

5. Open the EHR software and enter the appropriate patient's medical record. Select the *New* menu and choose the letter template you just created. Because you are in the patient's medical record, most software programs will automatically enter the patient's address in the inside address section of the letter. The standard greeting and closure also should be inserted from the medical record. Check to be sure the information listed is correct.

   RATIONALE: Even though this is an electronic letter, the professional format remains the same as a written letter mailed to the patient. All information must be correct.

6. Add a signature to the letter's signature block by using the "Sign" icon within the EHR program. Choose the correct provider/staff member from the drop-down list and verify that the correct signature is inserted.

7. If the signed "Consent to use E-mail Communication" is in the patient's chart, the letter may be sent by clicking "Send." If the consent is not signed, print the letter and send it to the patient via USPS.

   RATIONALE: Without a signed consent, e-mail is not an approved communication between the patient and medical office.

8. Be sure to click "Save" or "Done" depending on the EHR software used, so that the template is saved for future use.

PROCEDURE 10-5 Sorting and Opening Mail

Procedure Goal: To follow a standard procedure for sorting, opening, and processing incoming office mail.

OSHA Guidelines: This procedure does not involve exposure to blood, body fluids, or tissue.

Materials: Letter opener, date and time stamp (manual or automatic), stapler, paper clips, and adhesive notes.

Method: Procedure steps.

1. Check the address on each letter or package to be sure that it has been delivered to the correct location.

2. Sort the mail into piles according to priority and type of mail. Your system may include the following:
   - Top priority. This pile will contain any items that were sent by overnight mail delivery, in addition to items sent by registered mail, certified mail, or special delivery. (Faxes and e-mail messages are also top priority.)
   - Second priority. This pile will include personal or confidential mail.
   - Third priority. This pile will contain all first-class mail, airmail, and Priority Mail items. These items should be divided into payments received, insurance forms, reports, and other correspondence.
   - Fourth priority. This pile will consist of packages.
   - Fifth priority. This pile will contain magazines and newspapers.
   - Sixth priority. This last pile will include advertisements and catalogs.

3. Set aside all letters labeled "Personal" or "Confidential." Unless you have permission to open these letters, only the addressee should open them.

4. Arrange all the envelopes with the flaps facing up and away from you.

5. Tap the lower edge of the envelope to shift the contents to the bottom. This step helps to prevent cutting any of the contents when you open the envelope.

6. Open all the envelopes.
   RATIONALE: It is more efficient to open all the envelopes first and then remove the contents.

7. Remove and unfold the contents, making sure that nothing remains in the envelope.

8. Review each document and check the sender's name and address.
   - If the letter has no return address, save the envelope, or cut the address off the envelope, and tape it to the letter.
   - Check to see if the address matches the one on the envelope. If there is a difference, staple the envelope to the letter and make a note to verify the correct address with the sender.

9. Compare the enclosure notation on the letter with the actual enclosures to make sure that all items are included. Make a note to contact the sender if anything is missing.

10. Clip together each letter and its enclosures.

11. Check the date of the letter. If there is a significant delay between the date of the letter and the postmark, keep the envelope.
    RATIONALE: It may be necessary to refer to the postmark in legal matters or cases of collection.

12. If all contents appear to be in order, you can discard the envelope.

13. Review all bills and statements.
    - Make sure the amount enclosed is the same as the amount listed on the statement.
    - Make a note of any discrepancies.

14. Stamp each piece of correspondence with the date (and sometimes the time) to record its receipt. If possible, stamp each item in the same location, such as the upper-right corner.
    RATIONALE: It may be necessary to refer to the date in legal matters or in cases of collection.

SUMMARY OF LEARNING OUTCOMES

LEARNING OUTCOMES	KEY POINTS
10.1 Explain why well-written documents are important to the image of the medical practice.	Well-written, neatly prepared documents are one of the most important means of communicating a professional image for the medical practice.
10.2 Describe the types of document supplies that will be used in a medical office.	Document supplies used in a medical office include letterhead and matching plain bond paper; matching envelopes for professional correspondence; lesser bond envelopes of varying sizes for other types of correspondence; padded envelopes and data mailers; and labels and statements.
10.3 Outline the general guidelines to effective writing.	Know the type of person to whom you are writing. Know the purpose of the letter and be concise, brief, and specific in meeting that purpose, using clarity in the writing. Use active voice whenever possible, being polite and courteous. Check spelling, grammar, and accuracy. Avoid leaving "widows and orphans."

LEARNING OUTCOMES	KEY POINTS
10.4 List and explain the purpose of different types of documents used in a medical office.	The different types of documents and correspondence used in a medical office include letters of referral; letters about scheduling, canceling, or rescheduling appointments; patient reports for insurance companies; instructions for examinations or laboratory tests; answers to insurance or billing questions; and cover letters or form letters to order supplies, equipment, or magazine subscriptions. Also, internal documents like memos may be used to provide staff information.
10.5 Explain why it is important to have a signed written consent from the patient for e-mail communications.	All patient information, regardless of the form, is protected by HIPAA law and is to be guarded by the healthcare provider. E-mail is not considered a secure method of communication because information can be *intercepted* and received by someone who is not the intended recipient. Before undertaking e-mail communication with a patient, a signed written consent for e-mail communication must be on file.
10.6 Describe the tasks involved in editing and proofreading a document.	Editing involves checking a document for factual accuracy, logical flow, conciseness, clarity, and tone. Proofreading involves checking a document for grammatical, spelling, and formatting errors.
10.7 Outline the steps for preparing a completed letter for mailing.	After you have created, edited, and proofread a letter, it must be prepared for mailing. This preparation includes having the letter signed, preparing the envelope, and folding and inserting the letter into the envelope. Be sure to include any enclosures noted in the letter when folding it for insertion into the envelope.
10.8 Explain the differences among the different types of mail services offered by the USPS.	The mail delivery options offered by the USPS include special delivery, certified mail, return receipt requested, registered mail, and delivery confirmation.
10.9 Describe the steps involved in processing incoming mail.	The steps involved in processing incoming mail include sorting and opening, recording, annotating, and distributing.

C A S E   S T U D Y   C R I T I C A L   T H I N K I N G

Recall Valarie from the beginning of the chapter. Now that you have completed the chapter, answer the following questions regarding her case.

1. Valarie's lab results and chest X-ray come back showing no acute pathology. You are to compose a letter to her per Dr. Buckwalter stating her results are normal and she should call the office for a flu shot when she feels better.

2. You have a "Consent to use E-mail Communication" on file for this patient. Draft a short e-mail to her about her lab and chest X-ray results, requesting she contact the office by phone or e-mail to set up an appointment to receive a flu shot.

1. (LO 10.4) The _____ is the space around the edges of a form or letter that is left blank.
   a. Dateline
   b. Courtesy title
   c. Letterhead
   d. Margin
   e. Indentation

2. (LO 10.4) The complimentary closing is placed how many lines below the last line of the body?
   a. 2
   b. 6
   c. 4
   d. 3
   e. 5

3. (LO 10.8) What type of USPS mail service should be utilized to verify that the patient has received the document?
   a. Registered
   b. Certified
   c. Special delivery
   d. Certified with return receipt
   e. Mail tracing

4. (LO 10.6) Which of the following is spelled correctly?
   a. Professor
   b. Proffessur
   c. Profesur
   d. Profesor
   e. None of the above

5. (LO 10.3) Which of the following is an example of a linking verb?
   a. Ran
   b. See
   c. Be
   d. Feel
   e. Type

6. (LO 10.9) Marking incoming mail to note important points for the recipient is called
   a. Opening
   b. Sorting
   c. Recording
   d. Annotating
   e. Distributing

7. (LO 10.4) Which letter format places the date, complimentary close, and signature block just to the right of center?
   a. Block
   b. Modified block
   c. Modified block with indented paragraphs
   d. Simplified
   e. All of the above

8. (LO 10.5) Why is written consent required before using e-mail to communicate with a patient?
   a. The patient may not have a computer.
   b. You must be sure you have a current e-mail address.
   c. Parents may restrict e-mail use for their teenagers.
   d. If the patient is not expecting e-mail from the office, it may be considered SPAM.
   e. E-mail is not a secure form of communication.

9. (LO 10.4) Which document format is most often used for interoffice communication?
   a. Simplified letter style
   b. Block letter style
   c. E-mail
   d. Memo
   e. Any of the above is appropriate for interoffice communication

10. (LO 10.1) Better bond paper embossed with the practice name, address, and phone number is called
    a. Bonded
    b. Letterhead
    c. Envelope
    d. Label
    e. Lettering

Go to CONNECT to see activities on *Creating a Letter Template* and *Using a Letter Template*.

11 Medical Records and Documentation

C A S E   S T U D Y

PATIENT INFORMATION	Patient Name	Gender	DOB
	Mohammad Nassar	M	5/17/20XX
	Attending	MRN	Allergies
	Elizabeth H. Williams, MD	423-90-687	NKA

Mohammad Nassar is a 15-year-old male who is new to the practice and comes to the office today for his annual physical examination. He has a known past medical history of asthma, which has been relatively stable until recently. He states when he arrives that he has been experiencing an increasing need for his rescue inhaler in the last several days. His mother has brought him to the appointment, but Mohammad has asked that she remain in the reception area during his appointment. She does give you a list of Mohammad's current asthma medications and the previously completed new patient documents.

Keep Mohammad (and his mother) in mind as you study this chapter. There will be questions at the end of the chapter based on the case study. The information in the chapter will help you answer these questions.

L E A R N I N G   O U T C O M E S

After completing Chapter 11, you will be able to:

11.1 Explain the importance of patient medical records.

11.2 Identify the documents that comprise a patient medical record.

11.3 Compare SOMR, POMR, SOAP, and CHEDDAR medical record formats.

11.4 Recall the six Cs of charting, giving an example of each.

11.5 Describe the need for neatness, timeliness, accuracy, and professional tone in patient records.

11.6 Illustrate the correct procedure for correcting and updating a medical record.

11.7 Describe the steps in responding to a written request for release of medical records.

K E Y   T E R M S

audit
CHEDDAR
demographics
documentation
noncompliant
objective
patient record/chart
Problem Oriented Medical Record (POMR)

review of systems
sign
Subjective, Objective, Assessment, Plan (SOAP)
Source Oriented Medical Record (SOMR)
subjective
symptom
transcription

IV. P (1) Use reflection, restatement and clarification techniques to obtain a patient history	**3. Medical Terminology** d. Recognize and identify acceptable medical abbreviations
IV. P (2) Report relevant information to others succinctly and accurately	**4. Medical Law and Ethics** Graduates:
IV. P (8) Document patient care	a. Document accurately
IV. P (9) Document patient education	b. Institute federal and state guidelines when releasing medical records or information
V. C (6) Describe various types of content maintained in a patient's medical record	**8. Medical Office Business Procedures Management** Graduates:
V. C (12) Identify types of records common to the healthcare setting	b. Prepare and maintain medical records
V. P (3) Organize a patient's medical record	d. Apply concepts for office procedures
IX. C (2) Explore the issue of confidentiality as it applies to the medical assistant	gg. Use pertinent medical terminology
IX. C (3) Describe the implications of HIPAA for the medical assistant in various medical settings	**11. Career Development** Graduates:
IX. C (14) Describe the process to follow if an error is made in patient care	b. Demonstrate professionalism by: (3) Maintaining confidentiality at all times
IX. P (7) Document accurately in the patient record	

▶ Introduction

In your career as a medical assistant, you will play a major role in documenting in and maintaining patient health (or medical) records. These records detail the evaluation, management, and treatment given to the patient. Patient records are critical to the patient's care. Without accurate and complete patient records, medical care can easily be compromised with the potential for (unintentional) harm to the patient.

Patient health records have many sections that describe individual facets of every patient, including

- Personal information or data.
- Physical and mental conditions.
- Medical history.
- Current medical care.
- Future medical care if the patient is referred to other physicians or for further testing.

In this chapter, you will learn how to carefully manage patient records with the understanding that if the medical care is not documented, in a legal sense, the medical care did not occur at all.

▶ The Importance of Medical Records

LO 11.1

Patient medical (or health) **records**, also known as **charts**, contain important information about a patient's medical history and present condition. Patient records serve dual roles as communication tools and legal documents. They also play a role in patient and staff education and may be used for quality control and research. Traditionally, patient records have existed in a paper format, but more and more offices are adopting electronic health records in lieu of the traditional paper format. This chapter will focus on the paper record format and the next chapter, *Electronic Health Records*, will focus on the electronic format. Regardless of which format is used, the medical record is initiated by the medical assistant or another staff member and is consistently updated whenever the patient has contact with the office. As stated in the *Legal and Ethical Issues* chapter, it is important to remember that although the medical facility owns the physical record (electronic or paper), the patient owns the information contained within that record as his personal health information. So, the patient has control over who may access that information.

The patient chart provides physicians and other medical care providers with all the important information, observations, and opinions recorded about a patient. The healthcare professional can read the complete patient medical history and information about previous treatments and outcomes. With the patient's permission, the information in the records also can be sent to other physicians or healthcare specialists if the patient needs further treatment, changes physicians, or moves to a new location. The information recorded in the medical chart provides a "map" or plan to follow for the continuity of patient care. It also serves as supporting documentation for billing and coding purposes and as a legal document, it is admissible in a court of law. All medical records should include the following general information about the patient:

- Address and phone number.
- Occupation.

- Medical history.
- Current complaint or condition.
- Healthcare needs.
- Medical treatment plan or services received.
- Radiology and laboratory reports (when performed).
- Response to care.

Standard paper patient records are usually assembled for new patients well before their actual use. The medical assistant is responsible for making sure adequate patient records are prepared and available to meet the practice's needs.

Legal Guidelines for Patient Records

In addition to being essential documents for patient care management and treatment, patient records are also important for legal reasons. As a general rule, if information is not documented, no one can prove that an event or procedure took place. Medical records are used in lawsuits and malpractice cases to support a patient's claim of malpractice against a doctor, and also to support the doctor in defense against a claim. As stated in the *Legal and Ethical Issues* chapter, legally, medical records must be retained for 7 years (for pediatric records, 7 years from the age of majority, which in most states is age 18). Remember, however, that because the Federal False Claims Act requires patient financial records to be kept for 10 years, many legal experts suggest that medical records also should be kept for 10 years. This is because the medical record backs up the information within the financial record.

All medical care, evaluations, and instructions the physician gives to the patient must be documented. **Documentation** is the process of recording information in the medical record. Because every patient chart is a legal document, every entry must be clear, accurate, legible, dated, signed and, per HIPAA guidelines, written in blue ink. Before making any entry, always consider how the patient record would present if it were called into a court of law for review. Never insert an opinion in a patient medical record. For instance, you would not write in a medical record, "The patient appears to be drunk." Instead, "The patient's balance is unsteady and there appears to be the smell of alcohol on his breath" would be appropriate. If you are unsure how to document a situation appropriately, speak to the physician or your supervisor for appropriate guidance. In this case, you might wish to relay your observations to the physician and allow him to make the appropriate documentation.

As discussed in the *Legal and Ethical Issues* chapter, it is also very important to document when a patient is noncompliant. **Noncompliant** is the medical term used to describe a patient who does not follow the medical advice he or she receives. After a clear record has been made of the directions given to a patient for optimum health, it is essential to record the level of patient compliance. For example, after you have instructed a patient on how to collect a 24-hour urine specimen, you may write in her chart, "Patient stated she understood all directions regarding collection of 24-hour urine specimen. Written instructions also given to patient." If it is determined that a patient did *not* follow the medical instructions or advice, it is then essential to chart this as well. The physician may wish to withdraw from the care of a patient because of the patient's noncompliance. However, without proper and accurate documentation of the patient's noncompliance, the physician may not be able to withdraw care without becoming legally liable. Additionally, documented noncompliance can be used in the physician's defense in a malpractice suit if it can be proven that, due to patient noncompliance, the physician was not solely responsible for inadequate medical care or results. Please refer to the *Legal and Ethical Issues* chapter for further details on noncompliance and proper steps for withdrawal from patient care.

Standards for Records

Records that are complete, accurate, and well documented can be convincing evidence that a doctor provided appropriate care. On the other hand, altered, incomplete, inaccurate, or illegible records may imply that the care provided by the physician is below standard.

It is important to understand that the physicians in a practice are not the only people who document (or chart) in the practice medical records. However, it is equally important to remember that under *respondeat superior* (see the *Legal and Ethical Issues* chapter), if an employee of the practice charts inappropriately or inaccurately in a patient's medical record, in a court of law, the physician will also be held responsible for that action. For instance, if an MA documents an erroneously high glucose level and the patient is given too much insulin based on that result and then ends up in insulin shock, the physician will be held responsible. All records, both medical and financial, are the physician's responsibility. As the office medical assistant, you are responsible to the patient and the physician for both the medical and administrative procedures you perform and the accurate recording of those procedures.

Additional Uses of Patient Records

Patient records serve as ongoing references about individual patients' medical care. They also provide valuable information for patient education, quality of treatment, and research.

Patient Education Patient health records can be used to educate patients about their own conditions and treatment plans. The physician can point out how test results have changed or how the patient's general health has improved or worsened. The physician can also emphasize the importance of following treatment instructions. The medical assistant may also use some of this information to educate the patient about his condition or its management. Records can also be used to educate the healthcare staff about unusual medical conditions, patient progress, or treatment plan results.

Quality of Care Patient medical records are frequently used to evaluate the quality of care and treatment a facility or specific physician provides. Auditing groups, such as peer review organizations or The Joint Commission (TJC), may review medical records to monitor whether the care provided and the fees charged meet accepted standards. Records also provide statistics for healthcare analysis and future healthcare plans and policy decisions.

Research Medical records also play an important role in medical research. For example, a medical research team may be testing a new antihypertensive drug with volunteers who fit a certain medical category—perhaps men between the ages of 45 and 54 who have high blood pressure. Carefully kept records are valuable sources of data about patient responses, behavior, symptoms, side effects, and outcomes.

Information in charts may spur researchers to begin a study. For example, the records may show that 80% of all patients taking a particular heart medication experience dizziness. Researchers can investigate why this reaction might be happening.

▶ Contents of Patient Medical Records   LO 11.2

As the office medical assistant, you will fill out a record for each new patient who comes to the office. Although each medical office has its own forms and physical chart type, in general, all medical records must contain certain standard information. This standard chart information covers a variety of carefully detailed notes and facts about a patient, from his medical history to the physician's diagnosis and comments on follow-up care. Let's look at each form in more detail here.

Patient Registration Form

When a new patient makes an appointment with the office, certain basic **demographic** information—specific information required of a population—must be obtained; in this case, the basic information required of all patients seen in the medical practice. Very often, the first document a new patient completes is the registration form. Depending on practice policy, the registration form may be mailed to the patient prior to the first visit with the expectation that the patient will complete it prior to the visit and bring it with her at the time of her first appointment. Some facilities have the patient complete their registration online before their first appointment. Other offices request the patient to arrive for the first appointment 15–20 minutes early and complete the registration form at that time. Although the format may vary from office to office, the information requested in the registration form itself is fairly uniform and generally includes

- Date of current (first) visit.
- Patient's legal name and physical address (P.O. box may be listed as the mailing address, but the physical address is also required).
- Phone numbers including area code (home, cell, work). E-mail address also may be requested, but written permission must be received prior to e-mailing the patient.
- Patient's date of birth (DOB), sex, marital status, and Social Security number.
- Medical insurance information, employer name/address, and patient occupation.

- Emergency contact name, relationship, and phone number.
- Primary care physician (if specialty office) and referral source.

The completed registration form (with front and back copies of the patient's insurance card) is the base document for each patient's financial record. Patient financial and medical records are separated into two distinct records and are filed separately as well. Because of the importance of this "base" demographic document, review it carefully when the patient returns it to you to be sure it is filled out completely and properly. Each time the patient returns to the office, query the patient whether her address, phone, and/or insurance information has changed since her last visit, so that the office information is always current. Figure 11-1 is an example of a patient registration form.

Go to CONNECT to see a video about *Registering a New Patient.*

Patient Medical History

The medical history form, the second part of the registration process, contains the patient's past medical history (including illnesses, surgeries, known allergies, and current medications), family medical history, and social and occupational history (including diet, exercise, smoking, and use of alcohol or drugs). Usually, the history form also includes a section for the patient to describe the history of the condition or complaint that is the reason for her visit. This section is known as the *history of present illness* or HPI. Medicare and managed care plans now require that the patient's complaint be entered into the medical record. This primary problem is also known as the *chief complaint*, and it should be recorded in the medical records using the patient's own words, if at all possible. The patient medical history form—similar to the patient registration form—serves as the base document for the patient's medical record. Because of this, it should contain as much information about the patient's medical history as possible. In some offices, the medical assistant reviews the medical history form with the patient to make sure it is complete. If this task is part of your job, be sure to perform this initial interview in a private location. See Figure 11-2. Make sure there are no blanks and, if you are assisting the patient with filling out the document, be sure to use his own words as much as possible. For example, when asking the patient about alcohol consumption, you might document, "Patient states that . . .," filling in the blanks using the exact words of the patient. When the interview is completed, be sure to ask the patient, "Is there anything else you would like me to share with the physician for you?" Be sure to document any positive responses. If the patient brought any medical documents with him from previous healthcare providers, including lab, X-ray, or test results, be sure to attach them to the patient's medical record for the physician's review.

In most offices, the physician will use the medical history form as the "springboard" for a discussion with the patient as

BWW Medical Associates, PC
305 Main Street, Port Snead YZ 12345-9876
Tel: 555-654-3210, Fax: 555-987-6543
Web: BWWAssociates.com

Paul F. Buckwalter, MD
Alexis N. Whalen, MD
Elizabeth H. Williams, MD

Patient Registration

Patient Information

Name: _____ Today's date: _____

Address: _____

City: _____ State: _____ Zip code: _____

Telephone (Home): _____ (Work): _____ (Cell): _____

Birthdate: _____ Age: ____ Sex: M F   Marital status: M S W D

Social security number: _____ Employer: _____ Occupation: _____

Primary physician: _____

Referred by: _____

Person to contact in emergency: _____

Emergency telephone: _____

Special needs: _____

Responsible Party

Party responsible for payment: Self   Spouse   Parent   Other

Name (If other than self): _____

Address: _____

City: _____ State: _____ Zip code: _____

Primary Insurance

Primary medical insurance: _____

Insured party: Self   Spouse   Parent   Other

ID#/Social security no.: _____ Group/Plan no.: _____

Name (If other than self): _____

Address: _____

City: _____ State: _____ Zip code: _____

Secondary Insurance

Secondary medical insurance: _____

Insured party: Self   Spouse   Parent   Other

ID#/Social security no.: _____ Group/Plan no.: _____

Name (If other than self): _____

Address: _____

City: _____ State: _____ Zip code: _____

FIGURE 11-1 Typical patient registration form.

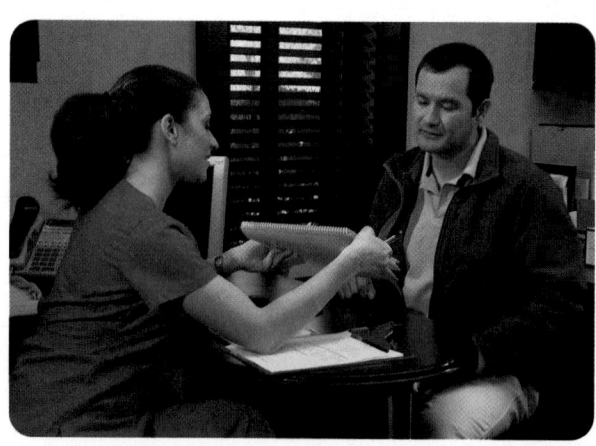

FIGURE 11-2 Perform the initial patient interview in a private location.

to the reason for her appointment, and to get to know a little bit about each new patient. See Figure 11-3.

Physical Examination Form

Many times, a form is used to record the patient **review of systems**, often abbreviated ROS, and the results of a general physical examination. The review of systems is an "inventory" of the body obtained by the healthcare provider through a series of questions. The purpose of this review is to identify any signs or symptoms the patient may be experiencing that may reveal information about an illness or condition. As an "oral examination," the ROS should not be confused with the actual physical exam. The use of a physical examination form ensures consistency in the examination format and minimizes the risk of "forgotten documentation." In most offices, the physician will perform both the ROS and the physical examination, but as the medical assistant, you may perform and document the patient's vital signs (temperature,

---

BWW

BWW Medical Associates, PC
305 Main Street, Port Snead YZ 12345-9876
Tel: 555-654-3210, Fax: 555-987-6543
Web: BWWAssociates.com

Paul F. Buckwalter, MD
Alexis N. Whalen, MD
Elizabeth H. Williams, MD

Patient Medical History

Name: _____ Age: _____ Sex: _____ MS: S M W D

Address: _____

Occupation: _____

Reason for visit: _____

History of present illness: _____

Allergies: _____

Current medications: _____

Cigarettes _____ Alcohol _____ Drugs _____

Past medical history:
Surgeries and dates: _____

Illnesses/Immunizations:
Chickenpox _____ Measles _____ Rubella _____ Mumps _____ DTP _____ TD _____ Polio _____

Whooping cough _____ Flu _____ Pneumonia _____ Hepatitis B _____

Other _____

Females: Age first period _____ LMP _____ # pregnancies _____ # children _____

Family history:

Relationship	Age if Alive	Medical Issues	Age at Death	Cause of Death
Mother				
Father				
Brothers				
Sisters				

Have you or an immediate family member (mother, father, sister, brother, grandparent) been diagnosed with:

Cancer _____ Location _____ Whom _____ Hypertension _____

Thyroid disorder _____ Heart disease _____ GI disorder _____ Blood disorder _____

Depression _____ Nervous disorder _____ Asthma _____ Migraines _____

FIGURE 11-3 Example of a patient medical history form.

pulse, BP, respiration, and height and weight) on the physical examination form for the physician. Figure 11-4 shows a typical ROS and physical examination form.

Results of Laboratory and Other Tests

Test results include findings from tests performed in the office and those received from other physicians, hospitals, independent laboratories, or other outside sources. Some offices use a laboratory summary or flow sheet to help the doctor detect significant changes more easily.

Test results received from sources outside the practice are best organized in sections within a specific section of the medical record designed for this purpose. You will learn more about arranging information within the medical chart a bit later in the chapter.

BWW

BWW Medical Associates, PC
305 Main Street, Port Snead YZ 12345-9876
Tel: 555-654-3210, Fax: 555-987-6543
Web: BWWAssociates.com

Paul F. Buckwalter, MD
Alexis N. Whalen, MD
Elizabeth H. Williams, MD

Review of Systems and Physical Examination
ROS

HEENT _____

CV _____

Resp _____

GI _____

GU _____

MS _____

Integ _____

Neuro _____

Psych _____

Endo _____

Allergic/Immuno _____

Physical Examination

T_____ P_____ BP_____ R _____ HT_____ WT _____

Appearance _____ Skin _____ Mucus membrane _____

Eyes _____ Vision _____ Pupils _____ Fundus _____

Ears _____ Nose _____ Throat _____

Chest _____ Breasts _____

Heart _____

Lungs _____

Abdomen _____

Genitalia _____

Rectum _____

Pelvic _____

Extremities _____ Pulses _____

Lymph nodes _____ Neck _____ Axilla _____ Inguinal _____ Abd _____

Neuro _____

FIGURE 11-4 Review of Systems and Physical Examination form.

Documents from Other Sources

Incoming records from other sources also must be entered and stored in the patient's medical record. If a patient has requested documents from another physician or hospital to be sent to your office, a copy of the patient's written request authorizing the release of these records to your office from its original source also must be included in the medical record.

Diagnosis and Treatment Plan

The patient's diagnosis must be recorded in the medical record, along with the physician's proposed treatment plan. The treatment plan may include treatment options, the final treatment plan, instructions to the patient, and any medications prescribed. The physician (or other healthcare provider such as the nurse practitioner or physician assistant) also may include any specific comments or impressions regarding the patient and his care on record. All of this information is recorded for every patient visit in documents known as progress notes. See Figure 11-5.

Operative Reports, Follow-up Visits, and Telephone Calls

Continuation of the record lasts as long as the patient is under the doctor's care. All procedures, surgeries, follow-up care, notes, phone calls, and all other patient contacts by the office staff should be recorded in the patient's medical record. Multiple progress notes also may be added to the medical record as needed. A discussion on charting methods will follow later in the chapter. Dependent upon office policy, phone calls and between-visit contacts may be inserted in the record in chronological order, or a log of telephone contacts may be kept separately in the patient record.

Hospital Discharge Summaries

The hospital discharge summary generally includes information that summarizes the reason the patient entered the hospital; tests, procedures, and operations performed in the hospital; medications administered to the patient; and the disposition (outcome) of the case. Elements of the summary may include the following:

- Date of admission.
- History of present illness (HPI).
- Date of discharge.
- Admitting diagnosis.
- Surgeries, procedures, or hospital course (treatment obtained in the hospital).
- Complications (if any).
- Patient instructions for follow-up care after hospital discharge.
- Discharging physician's signature.

PROGRESS NOTES

Patient Name _Sylvia Gonzales_   Date of Birth _9/1/XX_   MRN _341-73-792_

Prob. No. or Letter	Date	Subjective	Objective	Assess	Plans
1	11/11/XX	Patient states, "I have had a fever and a sore throat for the past two days"			
			Vital signs: T 101.1 P 96 R 24 BP 124/76 Weight: 155 Height: 5' 7"		
			General: patient seems alert. HEENT: sclera clear. Pharynx red with pus pockets noted. Heart: regular w/o murmur Lungs: clear to auscultation and percussion. Abdomen: negative for tenderness		
				Strep throat	
					1. prescription for Amoxicillin, 1 tsp q8h for 10 days
					2. schedule appointment for three weeks from today's date for repeat testing

Alexis N. Whalen, MD (Attending Physician)

Kaylyn R. Haddix, RMA (AMT)

Date: November 11, 20XX

FIGURE 11-5   Typical progress note using SOAP format.

Consent Forms

As discussed in the *Legal and Ethical Issues* chapter, signed informed consents must be obtained when any procedure is being performed on a patient. An example of such a form is shown in Figure 11-6. In order for any consent to be considered "informed," the patient must understand the treatment offered and the possible outcomes or side effects of the treatment. The patient also should be informed of the possible outcome if the patient receives no treatment, as well as be informed of any alternative treatments and possible risks. Once the patient signs the consent form, he may withdraw consent at any time prior to the treatment being carried out.

Correspondence with or about the Patient

All written correspondence from the patient or from other providers, laboratories, or independent healthcare agencies must be kept in the patient's medical record. Each piece of correspondence should be marked or stamped with the date the medical office received the document.

Information Received by Fax

Some information—like laboratory results, physician comments, or correspondence—may be received by fax transmission if the information is required rapidly. If possible, request that an original be mailed to the office as a final record.

Dating and Initialing You must be careful not only to date everything you put into the patient chart, but also to initial each entry. This system makes it easy to identify who in the practice is responsible for each entry. In many practices, the physician initials or stamps reports before they are filed to prove that the physician has seen them prior to filing.

Go to CONNECT to see a video about *Initiating a Paper-Based Patient Medical Record.*

BWW

BWW Medical Associates, PC
305 Main Street, Port Snead YZ 12345-9876
Tel: 555-654-3210, Fax: 555-987-6543
Web: BWWAssociates.com

Paul F. Buckwalter, MD
Alexis N. Whalen, MD
Elizabeth H. Williams, MD

CONSENT TO OPERATION, ADMINISTRATION OF ANESTHETICS, AND RENDERING OF OTHER MEDICAL SERVICE

Patient: _____ DOB: _____

1. I authorize and direct _____ with the associates and assistants of his/her choice to perform upon myself the following procedure:

_____

_____

If any unforeseen conditions arise in the course of this procedure or in the post-procedure period, calling on their judgment for other procedures or surgery, I further request and authorize them to do whatever is deemed advisable for my health and well being.

2. The risks and alternative aspects of autologous blood transfusions (receiving my own blood donated prior to surgery), designated blood transfusions (donated in advance by family/friends for my use), or homologous blood transfusions (from the general donor population) have been explained to me. I understand autologous and designated transfusions can be accommodated only for nonemergency surgeries.

6. I certify that I understand the above consent to surgery and that the explanations referred to have been made to me.

Signature _____ Date: _____

Witness _____ Date: _____

FIGURE 11-6 An informed consent form must be completed and signed by the patient prior to any procedure being performed.

Maintaining Confidentiality

As always, every patient's personal health information, whether coming into the office or being transmitted to another location, is covered by the HIPAA privacy and security rule and must be kept confidential. As per HIPAA, patients have the following specific rights regarding their PHI (protected health information) and their medical records:

1. *The right to notice of privacy practices.* Because it is unlikely that your patients will be reading federal laws, the law states that it is your responsibility to give them a copy of the laws that protect them concerning their PHI. Patients must receive a written notice of privacy practices on their first visit to a healthcare provider. They should sign a form stating they have received this information. This signed form must be carefully filed in the patient's medical record.

2. *The right to limit or request restriction on their PHI and its use and disclosure.* This means that patients can limit how your office uses their medical information and how much of that information is shared. For example, a patient with a history of sexually transmitted infection may not wish to have that information released to the orthopedic physician who is setting his broken arm. It is not necessary. In general, only the minimal amount of patient information should be released to meet the current needs of the patient. This is called the "Need to Know" general rule.

3. *The right to confidential communications.* This means that patients can request to receive PHI in a manner other than during a medical appointment. For example, your patients may request that you call them at a variety of different numbers, including home, work, or cell phone number. The patient does not have to explain the request. The law says you must make a reasonable effort to communicate with the patient in a confidential manner as the patient requests.

4. *The right to inspect and obtain a copy of their PHI.* This means that patients have a right to request and receive a copy of their own medical records. There are a few exceptions to this rule; however, in general, the medical assistant receives and processes all patient requests for medical records. It is important to always follow the protocols established in your office for medical record copying. It is considered an acceptable practice to act on a request within 30 days of the request and to charge a reasonable fee to cover the expense for copying supplies and labor.

5. *The right to request an amendment to their PHI.* Patients have the right to request an amendment to their PHI. The request may be denied if the healthcare provider receiving the request is not the original recorder of the PHI, or if the PHI is believed to be accurate and complete. Healthcare providers have the right to require that a request to amend a record be made in writing. All requests for amendment and response must be carefully documented and filed in the medical chart.

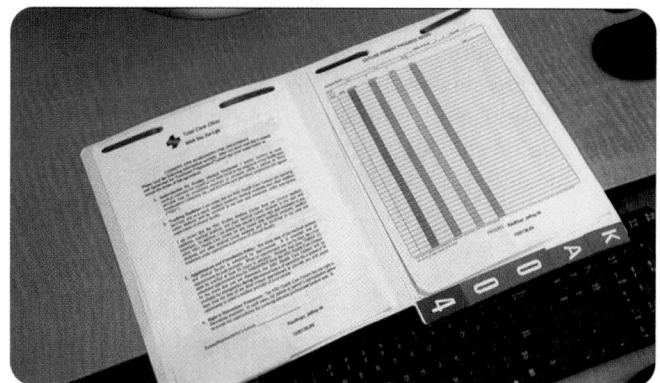

FIGURE 11-7 A newly assembled paper patient medical record.

6. *The right to know if their PHI has been disclosed and why.* Providers are required to keep a written record of every disclosure made of a patient's PHI. You must also keep a written record of any request by the patient for this information and the response of the healthcare provider. This information is usually filed in the patient's medical record. When making a disclosure of information, always record the date of the disclosure, the name and address of the person receiving the PHI, a brief summary of the information released, and the purpose of the disclosure.

The HIPAA privacy and security rule as it relates to all aspects of patient care, including the care and protection of patient medical records, is covered in detail in the *Legal and Ethical Issues* chapter. Now that you have learned about the forms that may be found in a medical record, Procedure 11-1, found at the end of the chapter, will outline how to assemble a new patient paper medical record. See Figure 11-7.

▶ Types of Medical Records   LO 11.3

The process of documenting information in medical records can be accomplished using several methods and formats. You should be familiar with the different approaches to documenting patient information and learn to be comfortable using each approach. The most common methods are the source-oriented (conventional) and problem-oriented medical records.

Source-Oriented Medical Records

In the **Source Oriented Medical Record** (sometimes called the conventional method) or **SOMR** approach, patient information is arranged within the chart or medical record according to who supplied the data—the patient, treating physician, specialist, hospital, lab, or other location. If a specific form is used to attach these documents to the medical record, it often contains a space for patient remarks, followed by a section for the physician's comments.

These records describe all problems and treatments on the same form in simple chronological order. For example, a patient's broken wrist would be recorded on the same form as her stomach ulcer. Although easy to initiate and maintain, this system presents some difficulty in tracking the progress of a specific ailment. For instance, in order for anyone to find information on the patient's stomach ulcer, the approximate time frame of the diagnosis would need to be known so that the chronological record can be searched. Another downfall of this type of record can occur if the patient has a recurrence of a problem. Because of the chronologic nature of the record, if the patient develops a second stomach ulcer 2–3 years down the road, the first episode and the second one will be filed in separate locations, causing more searching to locate the related "past medical history."

Problem-Oriented Medical Records

One way to overcome the disadvantages of the source-oriented approach is to use the **Problem Oriented Medical Record (POMR)** system. This approach, developed by Lawrence L. Weed, MD, makes it easier for the physician to keep track of a patient's progress. The information in a POMR includes the following items: database; problem list; educational, diagnostic, and treatment plan; and progress notes. Let's take a look at each of these components in a bit more detail.

Database The database includes a record of the patient's past medical history; information gained in the initial interview with the patient (for example, "Patient unemployed for the second time in past 12 months"); all findings and results from the physical examinations (such as "Pulse 105 bpm, BP 210/80"); and any tests, X-rays, and other procedure results.

Problem List Each condition or diagnosis a patient has is listed separately and given its own number, including the date of onset. Each "problem" is then identified by its number throughout the record. Work-related, social, or family problems that may be affecting the patient's health also may be listed in this problem list. For instance, the problem list for the example patient who is unemployed might include, "Severe stomach pain, worse at night and after eating, has begun since the patient became unemployed for the second time."

You can alert the doctor to the fact that the patient has lost two jobs within 1 year. Such radical life changes can often provoke strong physical (and psychological) reactions. In this patient's case, the elevated blood pressure may be related to the job losses, and stress may be causing the stomach pain.

When you document problems, be careful to distinguish between patient signs and symptoms. **Signs** are objective, or external, factors—like blood pressure, rashes, or swelling—that can be seen or felt by the doctor or measured by an instrument. **Symptoms** are subjective, or internal, conditions felt by the patient—like pain, headache, or nausea—but are not necessarily apparent in a physical examination. Together, signs and symptoms help clarify a patient's problem and can help lead to a diagnosis.

Educational, Diagnostic, and Treatment Plan Each problem should have a detailed educational, diagnostic, and treatment summary in the record. The summary contains diagnostic workups, treatment plans, and instructions for the patient. Here are two examples.

Problem 1. Elevated BP, 2/2/xx [date of entry]

P 105, R 25. BP recorded at 210/80 by MA; 180/90 by MD.

Suggested patient should start on Atenalol, but he wants to try stress management first (see problem 2).

Recheck BP in one week.

Problem 2. Stomach Pain, 2/2/XX [date of entry]

Upper GI exam negative, CBC normal.

Prescribed over-the-counter antacid, 2 tablets by mouth t.i.d. after each meal.

Set up appointment for patient with R. Neil, Ph.D., at the stress-management clinic (Broughten Professional Center) for Monday, February 4, at 4:30 p.m.

Patient's anxiety is high. Recheck in 1 week.

Progress Notes Progress notes are entered for each problem listed in the initial record. The documentation always includes—in chronological order—the patient's condition, complaints, problems, treatment, and responses to care. Using the same two problems, here are two examples.

Problem 1. Elevated BP, 2/9/XX

Patient began stress reduction class. Through them, also began looking for employment, seeking assistance through local community college. Feeling more positive. BP down to 130/82. P 90 and regular R 20. Explained to patient that BP is still borderline, but considering the dramatic reduction, will hold off on medication. Gave patient low-fat/low-salt diet and asked him to return for recheck in 4 weeks.

Problem 2. Stomach Pain, 2/9/XX

Patient enrolled in stress-reduction class. Reports stomach pain has diminished; "I can eat without pain; only a little discomfort at night." Reduced antacid to one tablet by mouth two times daily after meals. Anxiety much reduced. Recheck anxiety level in 4 weeks.

SOAP Documentation

Many medical records, like the POMR format, emphasize the **Subjective, Objective, Assessment, and Plan (SOAP)** approach to documentation, which provides an orderly series of steps for dealing with any medical case. Information is documented in the record in the following order.

1. **S: Subjective** data come from the patient; the patient describes his or her signs and symptoms and supplies any other opinions or comments about the current problem.
2. **O: Objective** data come from the physician, examinations, and test results.

3. **A:** Assessment is the diagnosis or impression of a patient's problem.
4. **P:** Plan of action includes treatment options, chosen treatment, medications, tests, consultations, patient education, and follow-up.

Regardless of whether your office keeps SOMR or POMR charts, the SOAP format for documentation can still be used. It is a popular documentation model because it allows each type of data to be located within each documented note easily, instead of searching the entire entry. Figure 11-8 shows an example of the SOAP note format using a preprinted form. The shaded columns noting where the subjective, objective, assessment, and plan information are to begin makes finding specific information easier for the user.

Note that in Figure 11-8, abbreviations such as RLQ (right lower quadrant), F (Fahrenheit), BP (blood pressure), and T (temperature) are used. If you choose to use abbreviations when charting in a medical record, use only approved medical abbreviations. To reduce confusion in medical records, abbreviations are being used less often, except for those that are very clear in meaning. Currently, TJC (The Joint Commission) does not produce an approved list of abbreviations, but it does state that the following should NOT be used when charting:

- The symbols ">" and "<"
- All abbreviations for medication names
- Apothecary units
- The symbol "@"
- The abbreviation "cc"
- The abbreviation "μg"

Before charting in the office medical record, check the policies and procedures manual to see if your office has specific abbreviations that are not to be used in the patient medical records. The purpose of the patient medical record is that information be documented so that all who have access to the information clearly know what is being documented. If you are questioning if an abbreviation may be misunderstood, it is better to write out the word for the sake of clarity. See Appendix II at the end of the book for a list of the common abbreviations used in medical records.

CHEDDAR Format

The **CHEDDAR** format of medical records documentation takes the SOAP format further, breaking it down into smaller components. CHEDDAR stands for

1. **C:** Chief complaint, presenting problems, subjective statements.
2. **H:** History; past medical, family, and social histories as well as the history of presenting problem (HPI) and any other contributing information.
3. **E:** Examination, including extent of body systems examined.
4. **D:** Details of problem and complaints.
5. **D:** Drugs and dosage—for example, a list of current medications including dosage and frequency.

PROGRESS NOTES

Patient Name: Mohammad Nassar   Date of Birth: 05/17/XX   MRN: 423-90-687

Prob. No. or Letter	Date	Subjective	Objective	Assess	Plans
1	6/16/XX	Patient complaining of pain in RLQ. Has been running fever between 100.5 F and 101.3F since Sunday morning. Has queasy feeling in stomach and has been unable to eat since yesterday morning.	BP 125/76. T 101.2F. Abdominal exam reveals rebound tenderness and tenderness in RLQ	Appendicitis	1. Immediate admission 2. Emergency appendectomy

Elizabeth H. Williams MD

FIGURE 11-8 Example of SOAP note using preprinted form.

PROGRESS NOTES

| Patient Name | _Sylvia Gonzales_ | Date of Birth | _9/1/XX_ | MRN | _341-73-792_ |

Prob. No. or Letter	Date	C H E D D A R
1	11/11/XX	Patient states, "I have had a fever and a sore throat for the past two days"
		Patient was healthy and well until two days ago when she noted the onset of fever and sore throat. Past history includes strep pharyngitis.
		Vital signs: T 101.1 P 96 R 24 BP 124/76 Weight: 155 Height: 5'7"
		General: patient seems alert. HEENT: sclera clear. Pharynx red with pus pockets noted. Heart: regular w/o murmur Lungs: clear to auscultation and percussion. Abdomen: negative for tenderness.
		Other than sore throat and fever with noted temperature elevation, patient has no other complaints.
		Patient takes no daily medication except for a multi-vit. She is given an Rx for Amoxicillin 250 mg 1 tab q8h for 10 days.
		Strep Pharyngitis.
		Schedule follow-up appointment for three weeks from today for repeat throat culture.

Elizabeth H. Williams MD (Attending Physician)

Maria A. Perez, CMA

Date: November 11, 20XX

Form OMB-1243

FIGURE 11-9 Typical chart note using the CHEDDAR format.

6. **A**: Assessment of the diagnostic process and the impression (diagnosis) made by the physician.
7. **R**: Return visit information or referral, if applicable.

Figure 11-9 shows you an example of a medical record note using the CHEDDAR format.

▶ Documentation and the 6 Cs of Charting
LO 11.4

Now that you have an understanding of the basic formats used in documentation or "charting," let's discuss the types of information that will require your new expertise.

Updating Medical Forms

You have already learned that you may be asked to assist new patients with completion of the patient registration and medical history forms. You also will be updating these forms as inevitable changes take place in the lives of your patients—new addresses, changes in marital status, the birth or adoption of a child, and changes in insurance coverage. All of these changes require updates to the patient registration information. In order to make such changes in a paper record, generally you retrieve the chart from the files and cross out the old information, using one line with a note stating the information has changed. You then add the date and your initials. Depending on the extent of the change, the new information may simply be written by hand as near as possible to the original location or, more likely, a note is made to see the "updated" registration sheet. On the new sheet, the current date will be given, the updated information will be neatly typed into the required spaces, and the new registration sheet will be inserted into the appropriate location of the medical record.

Documenting Test Results

Every time a patient has an X-ray or a lab test, or a letter arrives from a specialist about the patient, it must be inserted in the medical record. Be sure to follow the office policy in placing these items in the same location in each medical record and always in reverse chronological order—which means the most current result will always be on top. If your office uses a lab flow sheet, you also may be required to record the results on a separate test summary sheet in the chart. When doing so, be extremely careful to record the results accurately and in the correct location—the patient's health and treatment will depend upon it.

Examination Preparation and Vital Signs

As the office medical assistant, you will often prepare each patient for his or her examination. You will record vital signs, any medication(s) the patient is currently taking, and any responses to treatment. Before you leave a patient, always remember to ask, "Is there anything else you would like the doctor to know?" The patient may be more comfortable sharing further information with you than with the doctor. You will document the vital signs, medication information, and any treatment response in the medical record. If the patient does make any additional comments, document these as well and remember to use the patient's own words if at all possible. Refer to Figure 11-10 for a sample chart note.

Follow-Up

After you record the initial interview, any background information, vital signs, and subjective information (chief complaint),

the physician will decide what entries will be made regarding examination, diagnosis, treatment options and plans, including comments or observations about each case. You will then maintain the patient record by performing some or all of the following duties:

- Transcribe notes the doctor dictates about the patient's progress, follow-up visits, procedures, current status, and other necessary information. Transcription does not occur in all practices using paper records because a transcription service is often responsible for this task.
- Post laboratory or examination results in the medical record or on the summary sheet.
- Record telephone calls from the patient and calls that the doctor or other office staff members make to the patient.
  - Telephone calls can be an important part of good follow-up care. Calls must be dated and the content of the conversations must be documented (Figure 11-11).
  - You must initial the entry. Even if the doctor did not reach the patient, the call should be recorded and dated. State whether the doctor got an answer, left a message on an answering machine or with a person, and so on. Legally, if an item is not in the record, it did not happen.
- Record any medical instructions or discharge instructions the doctor gives to the patient.
- At the physician's request, counsel or educate the patient regarding the treatment regimen or home care procedures

---

PROGRESS NOTES

Patient Name _Beals_ _Bentley_ _Rian_ Date of Birth _11/29/XX_ Chart # _896-25-789_
  Last First Middle

T: 101.1 P. 96 and reg. R 16. BP 100/60.

Prob. No. or Letter	Date	Subjective	Objective	Assess	Plans
	9/01/XX	3 y/o male arrives with mom, Lexus, who states Bentley has been running slight temp x2 days. Still playful, but complaining of bilateral ear pain. When asked directly, patient states, "My ears hurt." Mom states Bentley did have ear infection once as an infant.			
					KH, RMA (AMT)

FIGURE 11-10 Chart note update started by medical assistant in preparation for patient examination.

PROGRESS NOTES

Patient Name ___Beals___ ___Bentley___ ___Rian___   Date of Birth __11/29/XX__ Chart # __896-25-789__
              Last   First   Middle

T: 101.1 P. 96 and reg. R 16. BP 100/60.

Prob. No. or Letter	Date	Subjective	Objective	Assess	Plans
	9/01/XX	3 y/o male arrives with mom, Lexus, who states Bentley has been running slight temp x2 days. Still playful, but complaining of bilateral ear pain. When asked directly, patient states, "My ears hurt." Mom states Bentley did have ear infection once as an infant.			
					KH, RMA (AMT)
			Playful 3 y/o male who appears slightly flushed. HEENT examination without findings except for bilateral inflamed TMs with slight serous drainage.		
				Bilateral serous otitis media.	
					Amoxil oral suspension™ 150 mg PO q8h. Mom to call in one week to report on progress.
					Alexis N. Whalen, MD

9/8/XX Telephone Call. Lexus Beals called in as requested to report on Bentley's BOM. States he is much improved and no longer complaining of ear pain. Temperature is also back to normal. Told her to call office if symptoms return, otherwise we will see Bentley for his scheduled CPE in January. MAP, CMA (AAMA)

FIGURE 11-11 Completed chart note including telephone call from patient in follow-up.

the patient must follow. This information must be entered into the record, dated, and initialed. For patient convenience, many offices have preprinted instruction sheets for patients to refer to once they arrive home.

The Six Cs of Charting

To maintain accurate patient records, always keep these six Cs in mind when filling out and maintaining charts: Client's (patient's) words, Clarity, Completeness, Conciseness, Chronological order, and Confidentiality.

1. *Client's words.* Be careful to record the patient's exact words rather than your interpretation of them. For instance, if a client says, "My right knee feels like it's thick or full of fluid," write that down. Do not rephrase the sentence to say, "Client says he's got fluid on the knee." Often the patient's exact words, no matter how odd they may sound, provide important clues for the physician in making a diagnosis.

2. *Clarity.* Use precise descriptions and accepted medical terminology when describing a patient's condition. For instance, "Patient got out of bed and walked 20 feet without shortness of breath" is much clearer than "Patient got out of bed and felt fine."

3. *Completeness.* Fill out completely all the forms used in the patient record. Provide complete information that is readily understandable to others whenever you make any notation in the patient chart.

4. *Conciseness.* While striving for clarity, also be concise, or brief and to the point. Abbreviations and specific medical terminology can often save time and space when recording information. For instance, you can write, "Patient got OOB and walked 20 ft w/o SOB." OOB and SOB are standard abbreviations for "out of bed" and "shortness of breath," respectively. Every office staff member should use the same abbreviations to avoid misunderstandings. Refer to Appendix II, which lists some common medical abbreviations.

5. *Chronological order.* All entries in patient records must be dated to show the order in which they are made. This factor is critical, not only for documenting patient care but also in case there is a legal question about the type and date of medical services.

6. *Confidentiality.* Always remember that the information in patient records and forms is confidential and is considered to be PHI. Only the patient, attending physicians (or other caregivers like physician assistants and nurse practitioners), and the medical assistant (who needs the record to tend to the patient and/or to make entries into the record)

are allowed to see the medical record without the patient's written consent. Never discuss the information in a patient record, forward it to another office, fax the information, or share it with anyone except the people in the office directly involved in caring for the patient, unless you have the patient's written permission to do so. Refer to the *Legal and Ethical Issues* chapter for detailed information about PHI and patient confidentiality, including HIPAA laws and regulations.

▶ Appearance, Timeliness, and Accuracy of Records   LO 11.5

Complete medical records will do no one any good if they cannot be understood. They also must be written neatly and legibly; contain up-to-date information; and present an accurate, professional record of a patient's case.

Neatness and Legibility

A medical record is useless if it is difficult (or impossible) to read. Make sure that every word and number in the record is clear and legible. For this reason, if an office uses paper medical records, the records are usually transcribed. Let's look at the transcription process.

Medical Transcription Your knowledge of abbreviations, medical terminology, and medical coding will be invaluable if you are asked to transcribe a physician's notes or dictation. **Transcription** means transforming spoken notes into accurate written form. These written notes are then entered into the patient medical record. As with all parts of the medical record, they are part of the patient's continuing (and confidential) case history and often include findings, treatment stages, prognoses, and final outcomes. Always date and initial all transcription pages. With the advent of voice recognition software, transcription can be done pretty much automatically by the computer, which will type based on the words spoken by the physician. These notes still need to be proofread carefully, until the software recognizes the physician's voice and accent and its dictionary contains the words—particularly medical terms—used most often by the physician.

Regardless of how the transcription occurs, transcribed material will contain the six Cs and, as such, should be accurate and complete, using appropriate grammar, correct spelling, and accurate medical abbreviations and terminology. As always, when dealing with abbreviations, if there is any doubt as to the meaning or use of an abbreviation, use the standard rule of thumb in healthcare: "When in doubt, spell it out." Use the medical dictionary and the medical computer spelling check function to verify the spelling or meaning of words. Ask the physician only if you cannot find something in a reference source. In order to be efficient, above-average typing or word processing speed and accuracy are also important.

Keep a library of medical, secretarial, and transcription reference books and medical terminology texts near the transcription workstation. Abbreviations can save time, but you should use only those that are accepted as standard. Reference books will help you find the correct word quickly and easily and help you apply proper grammar, style, and usage to the copy. Refer to the *Office Equipment and Supplies* chapter for the procedure on using a dictation machine.

Handwritten Notes If handwritten entries are used in the medical record, follow these tips to keep charts neat and easy to read.

- Use a good-quality pen that will not smudge or smear.
- HIPAA requires that all original documents be maintained in the patient's medical record. Blue ink is considered the best choice for charting for several reasons. It is easy to confuse an original written in black ink with a copy. Blue ink will copy as black, making the original and copy look different, reducing the possibility of error. Blue ink is also more difficult to match, making any additions to the medical record easy to spot, which can cut down on fraudulent entries.
- Use highlighting pens to call attention to specific items like allergies. Be aware, however, that unless the office has a color copier, most colored ink will photocopy black or gray. Because highlighting-pen marks may not be visible on a photocopy, many offices use brightly colored stickers to list allergies within and on the medical record.
- Make sure all handwriting is legible. Take time to write names, numbers, and abbreviations clearly.
- Make any corrections to the chart by following Procedure 11-2, Correcting Paper Medical Records.

Timeliness

Medical records should be kept up-to-date and be readily available when a doctor or another healthcare professional needs to see them. Follow these guidelines to ensure that a doctor can readily find the most recent information on a patient when it is needed.

- Record all exam and test results as soon as they are available.
- If you forget to enter a result into the record when it is received, record both the original date of receipt and the date the report was entered into the record.
- To document telephone calls, record the date and time of the call, who initiated it, the information discussed, and any conclusions or results. Depending on office policy, the call may be recorded directly into the record or a note may be made referring the reader to a separate telephone log, kept elsewhere within the medical record.
- Establish a procedure for retrieving a file quickly in case of emergency. Should the patient be in a serious accident, for example, the emergency doctor will need the patient's pertinent medical history immediately.

Accuracy

The physician must be able to trust the accuracy of the information in the medical records. Make an accuracy check of all data entered within the medical record a priority. To ensure accurate data, follow these guidelines.

- Never guess at or assume knowledge of names, procedures, medications, findings, or any other information about which there is some question. Always check all the information carefully. Make the extra effort to ask questions of the physician or senior staff member to verify information if there is any doubt as to its accuracy.
- Double-check the accuracy of findings and instructions recorded in the chart. Have all numbers been copied accurately? Are instructions for taking medication clear and complete?
- Make sure the latest information has been entered into the chart (and in the appropriate location) so that the physician has an accurate picture of the patient's current condition.

Professional Attitude and Tone

Part of creating timely and accurate records is maintaining a professional tone in your writing when recording information. As stated earlier, whenever possible, record information from the patient using his own words, particularly when recording the chief complaint (the reason for the visit). Also record the physician's observations and comments and any laboratory or test results. Never record your personal, subjective comments, judgments, opinions, or speculations about a patient's words, problems, or test results. You may call attention to a particular problem or observation, for example, by attaching a note to the chart, but do not, however, make such comments a permanent part of the patient's medical record.

▶ Correcting and Updating Medical Records
LO 11.6

In legal terms, medical records are regarded as having been created in "due course." All information in the medical record should be entered at the time of a patient's visit and not days, weeks, or months later. Information corrected or added some time after a patient's visit can be regarded as "convenient" and may damage the physician's position in a lawsuit. Untimely medical record submissions also can jeopardize a patient's care. For instance, if a medication is given to a patient but not charted appropriately in a timely fashion, the patient could inadvertently be given another dosage of the same medication, potentially causing an overdose.

Using Care with Corrections

If changes to the medical record are not done correctly, the record can become a legal problem for the physician and the practice. A physician may be able to more easily explain poor or incomplete documentation than to explain a chart where the original documentation appears to have been altered. Always be extremely careful to follow the appropriate procedures for correcting patient records.

Mistakes in medical records are not uncommon. The best defense is to correct the mistake immediately or as soon as possible after the original entry was made. To correct any mistake in a medical record, carefully draw a single line through the error, making sure that the original entry is still legible. Write

or type the corrected information above or below the original entry or even in the margin, as close as possible to the original entry. If there is not enough room near the error to make the full correction, make a notation near the error as to where in the chart the correction may be found. When making the correction, note the date and reason for the correction and initial the completed correction. If at all possible, have another staff member witness the correction and also initial it as witness. See Figure 11-12.

Go to CONNECT to see a video about *Correcting the Patient Medical Record.*

Updating Patient Records

All additions to a patient's record—test results, observations, diagnoses, procedures—should be done so there can be no interpretation of deception on the physician's part. In a note accompanying the material, the physician should explain why the information is being added to the record. The material may simply be the physician's recollections or observations regarding a patient visit that occurred in the past. Each item added to the record must be dated and initialed. As the office medical assistant, you may be asked to act as a third-party witness of these additions to paper records.

Most hospitals, clinics, and larger medical practices have detailed guidelines for late entries and corrections to patient charts. You must follow these guidelines carefully to avoid potential legal problems. See Procedure 11-3 at the end of this chapter for a list of steps for adding information to a paper patient record. Throughout the textbook, you will find procedures requiring you to document (chart) the procedure you just learned. This will allow you to continue to practice the charting techniques you have learned in this chapter—feel free to refer back here at any time to refresh your memory on proper techniques.

▶ Responding to Release of Records Request
LO 11.7

As you learned in the *Legal and Ethical Issues* chapter, all physical medical records, including X-rays, test results, and medical notes created by the physician, are considered the property of the practice. Although the information belongs to the patient, the law may require the physician to release the record, as in the case of a patient with a contagious disease or when a court subpoenas the records. Under no circumstances should you release patient information to insurance companies over the telephone. This information should be released in writing only after the patient has signed a written release statement. Under HIPAA, release of information over the telephone will likely be problematic.

Additionally, any request to release medical records should be approved by the physician.

Procedures for Releasing Records

Physicians often receive requests from lawyers, other physicians, insurance companies, government agencies, and the patient himself for copies of all or part of his medical record. Follow these steps for releasing medical information.

PROGRESS NOTES

Patient Name <u>Beals</u>   <u>Bentley</u>   <u>Rian</u>   **Date of Birth** <u>11/29/XX</u>   **Chart #** <u>986-25-789</u>
Last   First   Middle

T: 101.1 P. 96 and reg. R 16. BP 100/60.

Prob. No. or Letter	Date	Subjective	Objective	Assess	Plans
	9/01/XX	This 3 y/o male arrives with mom, Lexus, who states Bentley has been running slight temp x2 days. Still playful, but complaining of bilateral ear pain. When asked directly, patient states, "My ears hurt." Mom states Bentley did have ear infection once as an infant. *KH, RMA/AMT*	Playful 3 y/o male who appears slightly flushed. HEENT examination without findings except for bilateral inflamed TMs with slight serous drainage.	Bilateral serous otitis media.	Amoxicillin 250 mg b.i.d. x 7 days, Mom to call in one week to report on progress. *Alexis N. Whalen, MD*

9/8/XX Telephone Call. Lexus Beals called in as requested to report on Bentley's BOM. States he is much improved and no longer complaining of ear pain. Temperature is also back to normal. Told her to call office if symptoms return, otherwise we will see Bentley for his scheduled CPE in ~~January~~. MAP, CMA (AAMA) Date Error please see below

9/9/XX Correction to documentation of 9/8/XX. Patient's scheduled CPE is in June, not January as previously recorded. MAP, CMA (AAMA)

FIGURE 11-12   Example of a corrected medical record.

1. Obtain a signed and newly dated release from the patient authorizing the *transfer* of specific information—from his or her medical record to another party outside the physician's office. Please note that *verbal consent in person or over the telephone is not considered a valid authorization.* The signed and dated authorization should be filed in the patient's medical record. Refer to Figure 5-11 in the *Legal and Ethical Issues* chapter for an example of an authorization to release (transfer) health information form.

2. Make photocopies of the requested original material. Copy and send only those portions of the record covered by the release and usually only records originating from your facility. Unless the patient specifically requests that you do so, you should not release records that were obtained from other sources, such as consultations or tests done in a hospital. Do not send original documents. (If a record will be used in a court case, however, you must submit the original unless the judge specifies that a photocopy is acceptable.) In the past, originals of X-rays were often required because copies could not be made, but often today CDs can be made of X-rays and even MRIs and CT scans that will often be acceptable to the person requesting the records. If you must

send the originals, the recipient should be asked to sign a statement of responsibility for the original records until they are returned to the office. Document in the patient's medical record who has possession of the original documents, the date the recipient received the originals, and the date they are returned. Do request that the recipient return the original documents as soon as possible. Remember to follow up with the recipient until the originals have been returned and placed in the patient's file.

3. Call the recipient to confirm that all materials were received. Avoid faxing confidential records. Unless the recipient has a locked and password-protected fax mailbox, there is no way to tell who will have access to documents sent by fax.

Go to CONNECT to see a video about *PHI Authorization to Release Health Information.*

Special Cases It may not always be immediately clear who has the right to sign the authorization to release medical records form. When a couple divorces, for example, both parents are still considered legal guardians of their children, and either one can sign a release form authorizing transfer of medical records. If a patient dies, the patient's next of kin or legally authorized representative, such as the executor of the estate, may see the records or authorize their release to a third party. When you are in doubt regarding who is authorized to sign, *always* ask your supervisor before releasing confidential, protected health information.

Confidentiality

When children reach age 18, most states consider them adults with the right to privacy. No one, not even their parents, may see their medical records without the child's written consent. States extend this right to privacy to emancipated minors who are under the age of 18 and living on their own, or are married, a parent, or in the armed services. Confidentiality is often extended to minors seeking care for STIs, birth control, and drug or alcohol counseling. In these instances, the minor is considered a "mature minor" and her treatment cannot be discussed with her parents without her permission, even though the parents may still be held responsible for payment of such treatment through insurance or self-payment unless the patient pays for treatment at the time of service. Refer to the information regarding minors and their access to medical care in the *Legal and Ethical Issues* chapter for more detailed information.

The main legal and ethical principle to keep in mind is that you must protect each patient's right to privacy at all times.

Auditing Medical Records

The auditing of medical records is a great housekeeping tool. To **audit** a record means to examine and review a group of patient records for completeness and accuracy—particularly as related

---

CHART REVIEW FORM

Patient name: _____ Date of service: _____

Teaching physician: _____ CPT code: _____

ICD-9 codes:(1) _____ (2) _____ (3) _____ (4) _____

Please review the medical record for the following elements:

1. Was the medical record for this service found? ○ Yes ○ No
2. Is the medical record legible? ○ Yes ○ No
3. Is the attending/teaching physician's note written by the billing physician? ○ Yes ○ No
4. Does the date of service billed agree with the date of the progress note? ○ Yes ○ No
5. If a resident was involved in providing this service, review teaching physician ○ Yes ○ No
   documentation and answer the following questions:
   A. Does this service meet the primary care exception? ○ Yes ○ No
   B. Does the medical record demonstrate teaching physician involvement? ○ Yes ○ No
   C. Does the teaching physician's note link to the resident's note? ○ Yes ○ No
6. Does the documentation support the ICD-9 codes billed? ○ Yes ○ No
7. Does the documentation support the level of service billed? (Use lower portion of this page to evaluate.) ○ Yes ○ No

Level of service evaluation

History
(To qualify for a given level, all three elements must be met or exceeded.)

History of present illness (HPI)	Review of systems (ROS)	Past, family and/or social history (PFSH)	Type of history
Brief	N/A	N/A	Problem-focused
Brief	Problem pertinent	N/A	Expanded PF
Extended	Extended	Pertinent	Detailed
Extended	Complete	Complete	Comprehensive

Physical exam
(See page 18 in HCFA's "Documentation Guidelines for Evaluation and Management Services" for definitions.)

Problem-focused	Expanded PF	Detailed	Comprehensive

Medical decision making
(To qualify for a given level, two of the three elements must be met or exceeded.)

Number of diagnoses or management options	Amount and/or complexity of data to be reviewed	Risk of complications and/or morbidity or mortality	Type of decision making
Minimal	Minimal or none	Minimal	Straightforward
Limited	Limited	Low	Low complexity
Multiple	Moderate	Moderate	Moderate complexity
Extensive	Extensive	High	High complexity

Time-based codes
If more than 50 percent of the face-to-face time with the patient was spent in counseling or coordination of care, indicate the total time.

Counseling/coordination of care time:_____ minutes

Total face-to-face time:_____ minutes

CPT code: _____

Developed by Ronald Bradshaw, MD, CPA. Copyright © 2000 American Academy of Family Physicians. Physicians may photocopy or adapt for use in their own practices; all other rights reserved. "Using Peer Review for Self-Audits of Medical Record Documentation." Bradshaw RW. *Family Practice Management*. April 2000:28-32, http://www.aafp.org/fpm/20000400/28usin.html.

FAMILY PRACTICE
MANAGEMENT

FIGURE 11-13 Medical record audit tool.

Source: Compliments of American Academy of Family Physicians.

to their ability to back up the charges sent to health insurance carriers for reimbursement. There are two types of audits: internal and external. The medical assistant, and generally the medical office manager, and others that handle medical records for a medical office, should periodically perform audits to verify that the medical documentation meets required minimum standards. Many medical offices are now hiring compliance specialists to do internal auditing of their charts.

Internal Audits The medical staff can perform internal audits. Records are chosen randomly. Audits should be done both before billing is submitted (*prospective*) and after billing is submitted (*retrospective*). The audit schedule of how often audits should be performed should be determined by the medical office, based on the findings of the audits themselves. Many offices perform biannual audits, while others prefer quarterly audits. If an office finds many charts are "failing" the internal audits, medical staff training should take place and internal audits should be performed more frequently until the medical records meet the required standards. A sample chart review form created by Ronald Bradshaw, MD, CPA, can be found at www.aafp.org/fpm/2000/0400/fpm20000400p28-rt1.pdf. See Figure 11-13 for a copy of this medical record audit tool.

External Audits Government entities (such as Medicare and Medicaid), managed care organizations (MCOs), and private insurance carriers perform external audits. The number of government (and private) audits has increased greatly in the past decade, as federal programs and private payers seek to recover possible overpayments. External auditors may want to investigate the medical records further by interviewing the staff members, patients, and all physicians who participated in the patient's care. If the medical record does not back up the charges sent to the payer, the provider (physician and office) may be found guilty of fraudulent billing practices. At the very least, the charges considered as fraudulently obtained will need to be returned to the payer and/or to the patient. If federal programs like Medicare and Medicaid are involved, more severe penalties may be incurred, including large financial penalties, loss of the ability to participate in federal programs, jail, and loss of the physician's medical license. More about medical billing and fraudulent practices will be discussed in the chapters on insurance, coding, and billing.

PROCEDURE 11-1 Preparing a New Patient Paper Medical Record

Procedure Goal: To assemble a new patient paper medical record.

OSHA Guidelines: This procedure does not involve exposure to blood, body fluids, or tissue.

Materials: File folder, labels as appropriate (alphabet, numbers, dates, insurance, allergies, etc.), forms (patient registration, medical history, advance directives, physician progress notes, laboratory forms), and a hole punch.

Method: Procedure steps.
1. Carefully create a chart label according to practice policy. This label may include the patient's last name followed by the first name, or it may be a medical record number for those offices that utilize numeric or alphanumeric filing.
   RATIONALE: The label must be correct to help avoid filing errors.
2. Place the chart label on the right edge of the folder, extending the label the length of the tab on the folder.

3. Place the date label on the top edge of the folder, updating the date according to practice policy. (The date is usually updated annually, if the patient has come into the office within the last year.)
   RATIONALE: This makes it easy to identify current patient records for retrieval and identify records for purging if the patient has not been seen for a specified amount of time (often, three years).
4. If alpha or numeric filing labels are utilized, place a patient name label on the chart according to practice policy.
5. Punch holes in the appropriate forms for placement within the patient's medical record.
6. Place all the forms in appropriate sections of the patient's medical record.
   RATIONALE: Consistency in document placement assures that items can be found quickly when required.

PROCEDURE 11-2 Correcting Paper Medical Records

Procedure Goal: To follow standard procedures for correcting a paper medical record.

OSHA Guidelines: This procedure does not involve exposure to blood, body fluids, or tissue.

Materials: Patient file, other pertinent documents that contain the information to be used in making corrections (for

example, transcribed notes, telephone notes, physician's comments, correspondence), and a good ballpoint pen.

Method: Procedure steps.
1. Corrections and additions should be made so the original information remains readable, so there can be no suggestion of intent to conceal information. Draw a single line through the information to be replaced.

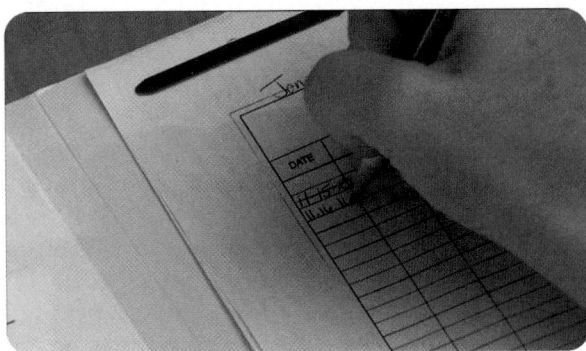

FIGURE Procedure 11-2 Step 1 Corrections should be made using a single line through the error so it can still be read.

RATIONALE: The single line ensures that the original entry can still be seen, avoiding future potential charges of a "cover-up."

2. Write or type in the correct information above or below the original line or in the margin. The location in the chart for the new information should be clear. If a separate sheet of paper or another document is required for the correction or addition, clearly note in the record "See attached document A" or use similar wording to indicate where the corrected information can be found.
   RATIONALE: It is important that information within the chart may be readily found at all times to allow for excellent patient care.

3. Place a note near the correction or addition stating why it was made (for example, "error, wrong date; error, interrupted by phone call"). Make sure you initial and date the correction. This indication can be a brief note in the margin or an attachment to the record. Do not make any changes or additions in a record without noting the reason for them.
   RATIONALE: By noting the reason as well as the correction, you clearly indicate that the correction is intentional and necessary.

4. Enter the date and time, and initial the correction or addition.
   RATIONALE: No correction to a medical chart is complete or acceptable without these elements.

5. If possible, have another staff member or the physician witness and initial the correction to the record when you make it.

PROCEDURE 11-3 Entering (Adding) Information into a Paper Medical Record

Procedure Goal: To document continuity of care by creating a complete, accurate, timely record of the medical care provided to a patient in your medical facility.

OSHA Guidelines: This procedure does not involve exposure to blood, body fluids, or tissue.

Materials: Patient medical record, pertinent documents (test results, X-ray results, telephone notes, correspondence, etc.), blue ballpoint pen, notebook, keyboard, and transcription equipment.

Method: Procedure steps.

1. Verify that you have the correct chart for the documents to be filed. Carefully check the patient's name, DOB, and medical record number (if available) as verification.
   RATIONALE: The patient's medical record is a legal document. You must be certain that documentation takes place in the correct medical record.

2. Transcribe any dictated notes as soon as possible and enter them into the patient record. If notes are handwritten, be sure they are filed in the correct location within the medical record.
   RATIONALE: Records must be kept up-to-date to maintain patient continuity of care.

3. Spell out the names of disorders, diseases, medications, and other terms the first time you enter them into the patient record, followed by the appropriate abbreviation. For example: "congestive heart failure (CHF)." Thereafter, you may use the abbreviation alone.
   RATIONALE: Follow the six Cs of documentation, one of which is clarity. There can be no confusion due to the use of abbreviations.

4. Enter only what the doctor has dictated. Do *not* add your own comments, observations, or evaluations. Use self-adhesive flags or other means to call the doctor's attention to something you have noticed that may be helpful to the patient's case. Date and initial each entry.
   RATIONALE: As a legal document, there is no place for personal comments or observations as part of the permanent patient medical record.

5. Follow office procedure to record routine or special laboratory, X-ray, or other test results. These results may be posted in a particular section of the file or on a separate test summary form. If you use the summary form, make a note in the file that the results were received and recorded. Place the original report in the patient's file if required to do so by office policy. Date and initial each entry. File all correspondence and hospital records in the appropriate area of each chart, using reverse chronological order so that the most recent record is on top. Be sure that each document is initialed or stamped by the physician as having been seen, prior to filing it within the patient's chart.
   RATIONALE: In order for the record to be useful for any medical professional using it, all documents must be filed using a consistent, easily understandable method such as POMR.

6. Make a note in the record of all telephone calls to and from the patient. Date and initial the entries. These entries also may include the doctor's comments, observations, changes in the patient's medication, new instructions to the patient, and so on. If calls are recorded in a separate telephone log, note in the patient's record the time and date of the call and refer to the log. It is particularly important to record such calls when the patient resists or refuses treatment, skips appointments, or has not made follow-up appointments.

   RATIONALE: As a legal representation of the patient's medical care, it is equally important to log the patient's response and responsibility toward his own medical care, plan, and treatment.

7. Make notations in the medical record of any immunizations and vaccines that have been given to the patient. Notations should be posted in the patient's immunization record inside the medical chart.

Input them into your state's public health database as well. Immunization records are kept indefinitely as a permanent part of the patient's medical history.

8. Read over the entries for omissions or mistakes. Ask the doctor to answer any questions you may have.

   RATIONALE: It is imperative that all parts of the medical record contain the six Cs of medical charting and are free of errors and omissions.

9. Make sure that you have dated and initialed each entry.

10. Be sure that all documents are included in the file and within the appropriate location so they may be located easily when needed.

11. Return the patient's medical record to its appropriate location in the filing system as soon as possible.

    RATIONALE: If the medical record is perfectly maintained but cannot be found, it does neither the physician nor the patient any good.

SUMMARY OF LEARNING OUTCOMES

LEARNING OUTCOMES	KEY POINTS
11.1 Explain the importance of patient medical records.	Medical records are legal documents that give a complete, concise, chronological history of a patient's past medical history, current medical issues, treatment plan, and treatment outcome. Additionally, they act as a communication tool between care providers. The patient medical record provides physicians and other healthcare providers with all the important information, observations, and opinions that have been recorded about a patient.
11.2 Identify the documents that comprise a patient medical record.	The records that comprise the patient medical record include, but are not limited to, the following: patient registration form, medical history form, physical exam form, laboratory and other test results, records from physicians or hospitals, physician diagnosis and treatment plan, operative reports, hospital discharge summaries, follow-up notes, records of telephone calls, signed informed consents, and correspondence with or about the patient.
11.3 Compare SOMR, POMR, SOAP, and CHEDDAR medical record formats.	SOMR files documents in the medical record in strict chronological order. POMR files the same documents according to numbered problems found on the patient problem list. SOAP notes organize medical record documentation according to subjective, objective, assessment, and plan. The CHEDDAR format breaks down this information even further into chief complaint, history, exam, details, drugs, assessment, and return visit plan.
11.4 Recall the 6 Cs of charting, giving an example of each.	The six Cs of charting are client's words, clarity, completeness, conciseness, chronological order, and confidentiality.
11.5 Describe the need for neatness, timeliness, accuracy, and professional tone in patient records.	Neatness, legibility, accuracy, and professional tone are musts in maintaining medical records. Remember that patient medical records are legal documents. They must be kept up-to-date and should be easy to read. Make sure you project a professional tone when recording information. Always check for accuracy and never guess at information. Personal thoughts and observations should never be a permanent part of the patient medical record.

LEARNING OUTCOMES	KEY POINTS
11.6 Illustrate the correct procedure for correcting and updating a medical record.	The proper way to make corrections in a medical record is to draw a single line through the error so that the original entry is still legible. Make the correction as close as possible to the original entry, noting the reason for the correction, and initial the correction. Any additions to a medical record also should be made as soon as the need for the addition is noted, and the reason for the addition or change also should be clearly documented.
11.7 Describe the steps in responding to a written request for release of medical records.	In order to release any confidential medical information, express written permission from the patient must be received. Unless it is impossible to do so, copies should be made and the originals should remain in the office. If originals must be released, a statement of responsibility should be signed by the receiver and should be noted in the patient's chart. Follow-up should take place until the original records are returned to the office and to the patient's record. Only release records that are expressly requested and authorized by the patient.

CASE STUDY CRITICAL THINKING

Recall Mohammad from the beginning of the chapter. Now that you have completed the chapter, answer the following questions regarding his case.

1. As a new patient, which documents should be completed prior to Mohammad being seen by the physician? What documents should he have brought with him, if available?

2. Your office uses a SOAP format for medical records. After Dr. Williams completes her exam, explain where each of the new documents or pieces of information obtained during Mohammad's exam will be filed using the SOAP format.

EXAM PREPARATION QUESTIONS

1. (LO 11.1) The process of recording information in a patient's medical record is called
   a. Auditing
   b. SOAP
   c. CHEDDAR
   d. Documentation
   e. Demographics

2. (LO 11.1) Which of the following are possible uses for patient medical records?
   a. Research
   b. Quality of care (quality control)
   c. Patient education
   d. b and c only
   e. a, b, and c

3. (LO 11.2) Which document serves as the "base" for the patient medical record?
   a. The registration form
   b. The patient medical history form
   c. The physical examination form
   d. The patient demographic form
   e. The patient review of systems

4. (LO 11.2) Which of the following documents from other sources frequently become part of a patient's medical record?
   a. X-rays, CT scan, and MRI results
   b. Lab results from private labs or hospitals
   c. Hospital discharge summaries
   d. Hospital operative notes
   e. All of the above

5. (LO 11.3) Which filing system uses the patient problem list as the source for filing within the patient medical record?
   a. POMR
   b. SOMR
   c. SOAP
   d. CHEDDAR
   e. All of the above

6. (LO 11.3) Which of the following patient details would be filed under "O" using the SOAP documentation method?
   a. "I have the flu"
   b. Nausea
   c. BP 160/92
   d. Influenza
   e. Rest, fluids, ibuprofen; f/u in 5 days by phone

7. (LO 11.4) Which of the 6 Cs means "getting to the point"?
   a. Clarity
   b. Completeness
   c. Chronological
   d. Confidentiality
   e. Conciseness

8. (LO 11.5) In order to "trust" the information in the medical record, documentation must be _____ at all times.
   a. Timely
   b. Chronological
   c. Transcribed
   d. Accurate
   e. Professional in tone

9. (LO 11.6) Which of the following is necessary when correcting or making additions to a paper medical record?
   a. Draw a single line through the error
   b. Make the correction as close as possible to the original entry
   c. Note the reason for the correction and sign and date the correction
   d. A witness should also initial the entry
   e. a–c are required; d is advisable

10. (LO 11.7) Why are internal chart audits advisable for every medical office?
   a. To verify that the medical record "backs up" the charges being billed
   b. To give staff members practice reading physician handwriting
   c. To assure that all members of the staff are current with all patient medical issues
   d. To be sure that all possible charges are being submitted to the insurance carrier
   e. None of the above

Go to CONNECT for an activity about *Updating a Patient's Chart.*

Electronic Health Records

PATIENT INFORMATION		
Patient Name	**Gender**	**DOB**
Ken Washington	M	12/1/19XX
Attending	**MRN**	**Allergies**
Paul F. Buckwalter, MD	891-12-743	Sulfa

Ken Washington is a 61-year-old who arrives for his routine follow-up visit for his known diagnosis of hypertension. He mentions today that he has had occasional weakness in his left arm. While you are checking him in, you notice him looking at the computer monitor on your desk. The monitor is displaying the screen saver for the new EHR program recently installed at the office. He asks, "What is EHR?"

Keep Mr. Washington in mind as you study the chapter. There will be questions at the end of the chapter based on the case study. The information in the chapter will help you answer these questions.

LEARNING OUTCOMES

After completing Chapter 12, you will be able to:

12.1 List four medical mistakes that will be greatly decreased through the use of EHR.

12.2 Differentiate among electronic medical records, electronic health records, and personal health records.

12.3 Contrast the advantages and disadvantages of electronic health records.

12.4 Illustrate the steps in creating a new patient record and correcting an existing record using EHR software.

12.5 Describe some of the capabilities of EHR software programs.

12.6 Explain how you might alleviate a patient's security fears surrounding the use of EHR .

KEY TERMS

customized

electronic health record (EHR)

electronic medical record (EMR)

personal health record (PHR)

V. C (11) Discuss principles of using Electronic Medical Record (EMR)

V. P (5) Execute data management using electronic healthcare records such as the EMR

IX. C (2) Explore issue of confidentiality as it applies to the medical assistant

IX. C (3) Describe the implications of HIPAA for the medical assistant in various medical settings

IX. P (7) Document accurately in the patient record

7. Basic Keyboarding/Computer Concepts
Graduates:
a. Perform basic keyboarding skills including:
   (2) Typing medical correspondence and reports
b. Identify and properly utilize office machines, computerized systems, and medical software such as:
   (1) Efficiently maintain and understand different types of medical correspondence and medical reports
   (2) Apply computer application skills using variety of different electronic programs including both practice management software and EMR software

8. Medical Office Business Procedures Management
Graduates:
b. Prepare and maintain medical records
d. Apply concepts for office procedures
ll. Apply electronic technology

11. Career Development
Graduates:
b. Demonstrate professionalism by:
   (2) Exhibiting a positive attitude and a sense of responsibility
   (3) Maintaining confidentiality at all times

Introduction

Has your primary care physician (PCP) ever referred you to a specialist and in the specialist's office, you spent the first 15 minutes filling out a medical history form so the medical staff had "the same medical history" that they have on file at your PCP's office? Have you ever been asked about any medication allergies or your surgical history and you just could not remember the name of the new drug you developed an allergy to, or the year you had your appendix removed? Now, imagine that before you even arrive at the office, the medical staff already has that information at their fingertips, thanks to their new electronic health record (EHR) system. All you need to do is review the information with the specialist to verify that everything is correct to the best of your knowledge. Welcome to the world of electronic health records.

A Brief History of Electronic Medical Records
LO 12.1

In the early 1990s, it became apparent that paper medical records could no longer meet patients' or healthcare providers' needs. The increasing need for coordination of care (consider how many physicians you see), rising healthcare costs (15% of the U.S. gross national product), and the rather alarming increase in medical errors fueled this realization. Medical errors are the 8th leading cause of patient death in the United States. Most of these errors can be traced to communication problems, including

- Lost or misfiled paper records.
- Mishandled or "forgotten" patient messages.
- Inaccurate or unreadable information in a paper medical record.
- Mislabeled or unreadable laboratory or prescription orders.

Because of this, President George W. Bush signed an executive order in August 2006 to promote the overall efficiency and quality of healthcare in America. At the base of this order was the promotion of the electronic health record, with a goal of most Americans having access to electronic health records by 2014. The overall goal of this order was to decrease medical errors through record legibility and record uniformity, and to increase information available among patients, medical providers, and the insurance carriers who pay for that care. Meeting this overall goal would help to control the rising cost of healthcare to both the patient and the insurance carriers, including government-funded programs like Medicare and Medicaid. Although implementation can be expensive, the electronic record (see Figure 12-1) is quickly becoming the physician's most important business and legal record.

FIGURE 12-1 Example of a Patient's Electronic Chart from SpringCharts EHR program.

Source: Screen captures of SpringCharts™ Electronic Health Records software are reprinted with permission from Spring Medical Systems, Inc. All rights reserved.

▶ Electronic Records   LO 12.2

The terms *electronic medical record* and *electronic health record* are seemingly used interchangeably, but they are defined differently by the National Alliance for Health Information Technology (NAHIT). The **electronic medical record (EMR)** is an electronic record of health-related information for an individual patient that is created, compiled, and managed by providers and staff members located within a *single* healthcare organization. If that same information on an individual patient is created, managed, and gathered in a manner that conforms to nationally recognized *interoperability standards*, so that it can be utilized by members of more than one healthcare organization, it is known as an **electronic health record (EHR)**. These

EHRs are the federal government's ultimate goal. Because any provider with an interoperable EHR system will have access to a patient's information—no matter where the information originated—there will be increased patient continuity of care, reduction in medical errors, and, ultimately, decreased healthcare costs.

One of the offshoots of EHRs that is less understood by both physicians and patients is the **personal health record (PHR)**. A personal health record is basically an electronic version of the comprehensive medical history and record of a patient's lifelong health that is collected and maintained by the individual patient. This record may then be shared with providers at the patient's discretion. See Table 12-1, which outlines the basic differences between PHRs and EHRs.

TABLE 12-1	**Basic Differences between Electronic Health Records and Personal Health Records**	
Description	**EHR**	**PHR**
Record ownership/management	EHR files are owned and managed by providers or facilities.	PHR files are owned and updated by the individual.
Legal document?	EHRs are legal documents regulated by state and federal laws.	PHRs are not legal records and have no legal regulations.
Information access	EHR access is controlled by the provider with patient authorization.	PHR access is controlled by the patient.
Providers involved	In general, EHRs contain information related to treatment by one provider.	PHRs contain treatment information from multiple providers.
Data entry	EHR data are entered by providers or their staff.	PHR data are entered by the patient.
Information users	EHR is used by the medical office or facility.	PHR is used by the individual patient.

In this era of employers, government, and insurance plans asking patients to take a much more active role in their healthcare, the PHR is a natural response to this need. PHRs may be stored and maintained on secure Internet sites where the information may be efficiently managed by the patient and shared with providers as the patient wishes. Keep in mind that no matter what form a patient record takes, protected health information (PHI) is involved. As covered by HIPAA laws, PHI cannot be disclosed without patient express written permission unless allowed by federal or state statute. Refer to the *Medical Records and Documentation* chapter for more detailed information regarding HIPAA and PHI.

▶ Advantages and Disadvantages of EHR

LO 12.3

The federal government has mandated electronic health records for eligible Medicare providers with very few exceptions by 2015, even including financial incentives (until 2014) for providers who demonstrate "meaningful use" of EHRs for Medicare or Medicaid patients. Step 1 of meaningful use requires the provider to use all major functions of a certified EHR program. The provider must document the percentage of visits, diagnoses, prescriptions, immunizations, and other pertinent health information electronically; use the EHR clinical support tools; share patient information; and report quality measures and public health information. Step 2 is proposed to include all of step 1 and adds that EHR must be used to send and receive clinical information such as lab orders and reports. The proposal for step 3, which is not yet completed, states that in addition to continuing with steps 1 and 2, the provider will participate in clinical decision support for national, high-priority conditions, enrolling patients in PHR, accessing comprehensive patient data, and improving population health.

Figure 12-2 shows these steps and the timeline from the Centers for Medicare and Medicaid Services (CMS). Included with this mandate is the use of electronic prescribing (e-prescribing) to transmit prescriptions electronically to pharmacies, which also has its own financial incentives for providers.

Qualified providers for Medicare are defined as follows: *A Medicare EP is a doctor of medicine or osteopathy, a doctor of dental surgery or dental medicine, a doctor of podiatric medicine, a doctor of optometry, or a chiropractor, who is legally authorized to practice under state law.*

Qualified providers for Medicaid are defined in this way: *Eligible providers (EP) are physicians (primarily doctors of medicine and doctors of osteopathy), dentists, nurse practitioners, certified nurse midwives, and physician assistants practicing in a Federally Qualified Health Center (FQHC) led by a physician assistant or Rural Health Clinic (RHC) that is so led.*

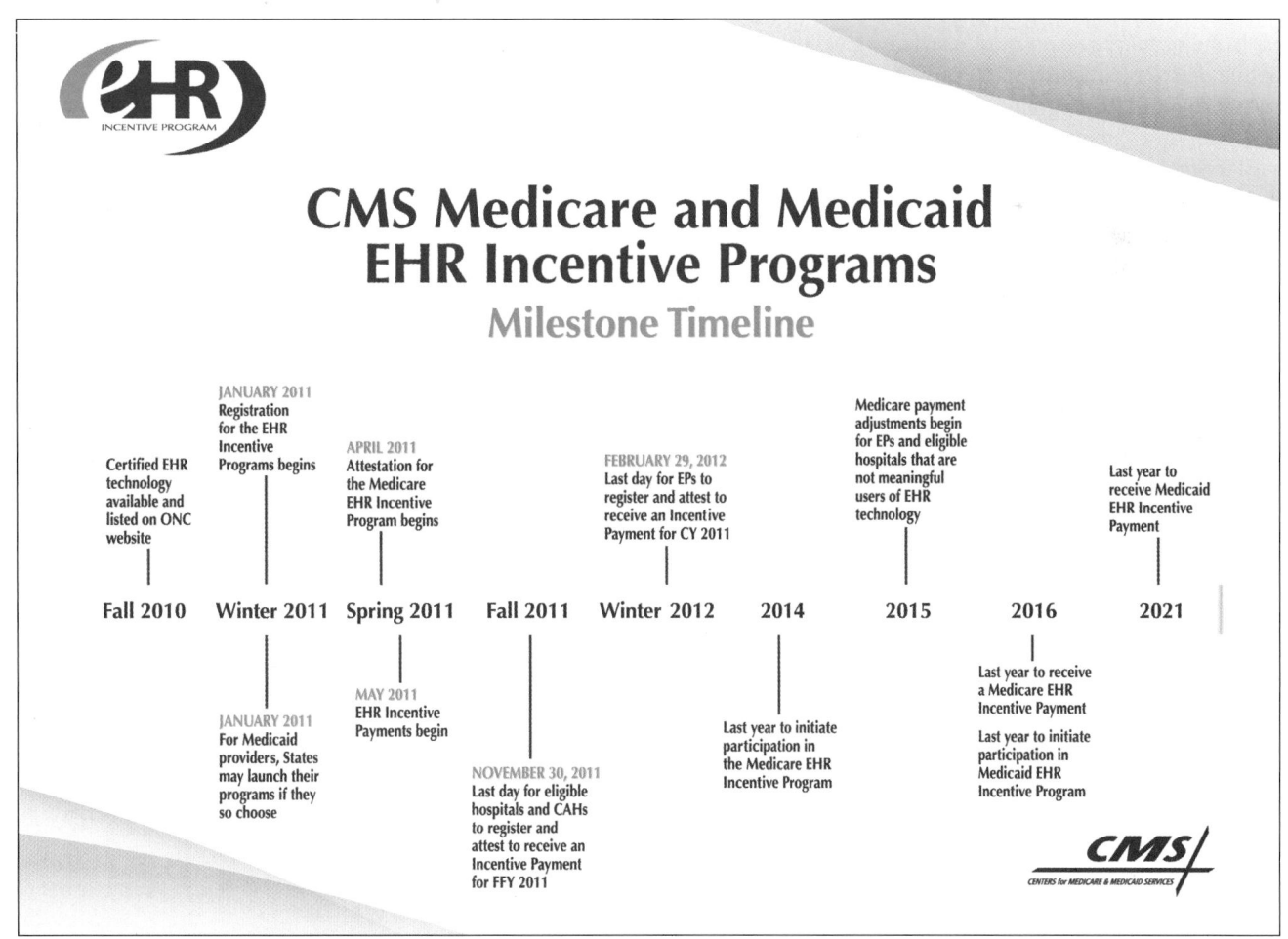

FIGURE 12-2 CMS EHR incentive timeline for Medicare and Medicaid.

If a provider is eligible for both programs—Medicare *and* Medicaid—he must choose only one. No one may participate in both incentive programs. Eligible providers must also meet specific criteria outlined by each program regarding the volume threshold (percentage of the practice that consists of Medicare or Medicaid patients) and must demonstrate *meaningful use* of the EHR program for each quarter the provider participates in the program.

The incentives for participation in an EHR program are considerable, and the earlier a provider joins the program and attests to meaningful use, the more money he will earn from the program. The maximum amount an EP can earn from the Medicare program is $44,000 and the maximum total incentive payment from the Medicaid program is $63,750. Even with these incentives, a great number of providers are still not taking advantage of these programs. In fact, the latest figures from the CDC show that only 10% of physicians report a fully functioning (interoperable) EHR program and another 20% report having some type of basic EHR program in their office. With an estimated 404,000 eligible providers in the United States as of 2011, CMS predicts that 10–36% will adopt EHR by the end of 2011, 15–44% will adopt by 2013, and 21–53% will be using EHR by 2015. EHR use is growing, partially due to the stimulus program, but it is not growing as quickly as the federal government would like.

Disadvantages of EHR Programs

Cost is the primary reason most providers give for not implementing electronic records in their offices. The estimated cost to establish an EHR program is $44,000 per full-time provider (FTP) with an estimated maintenance cost of $8,500 per year per FTP. Some physicians simply do not have the initial financial outlay available, or feel the time needed to recoup the initial cost to implement the program justifies the initial financial outlay. Aside from financial concerns, other reasons listed for not implementing electronic health records include

- Staff training requirements.
- Possible need for full-time or part-time IT staff member.
- Possible damage to system and to software and/or required upgrades.

Advantages of EHR Programs

- Fewer lost medical records (charts do not require pulling or refiling).
- Eliminated (or reduced) transcription costs.
- Increased readability/legibility of charts.
- Ease of chart access for multiple users.
- Chart availability outside of office hours.
- Increased access to patient education materials.
- Decreased duplication of test orders.
- More efficient transfer of records.
- More efficient billing processes using electronic billing methods.
- Greatly decreased storage needs.

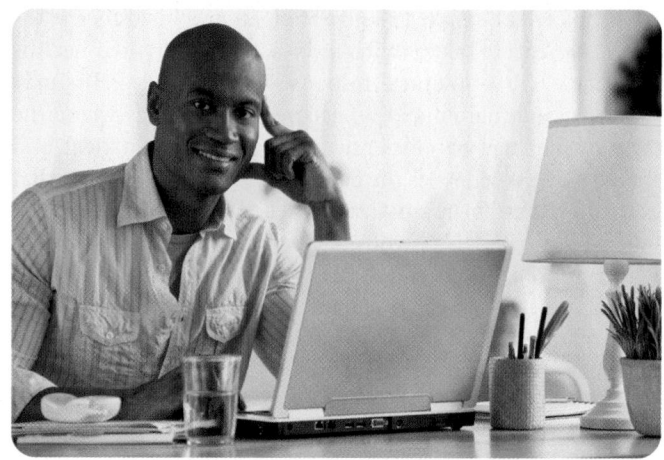

FIGURE 12-3 Electronic health records and a laptop computer combined with Internet access provide physicians with easy record access no matter where they are.

Additional Advantages of EHR

In addition to the advantages listed above, a fully functioning EHR program presents other advantages. If a physician is at home and needs to access a patient's record, he can access the EHR program from any computer (using his secure access code and password) at any time, review or update the file, and save it to the central computer again. See Figure 12-3.

Computerized records also can be used in teleconferences, where people in different locations can look at the same record on their individual computer screens at the same time. Computer access to patient records is also helpful for healthcare providers with satellite offices in different cities or different parts of a city, or may be used by a physician who is covering a practice while the patient's usual doctor is out of town.

▶ Working with an Electronic Health Record   LO 12.4

By now, you are beginning to understand some of the EHR's advantages. As a medical assistant concerned with patient care and patient confidentiality, you should also understand that the basic rules for working with a medical record do not change when that record is electronic instead of paper. The way you work with the record may change, but the way you treat a record does not. You may refer back to the chapter *Written and Electronic Documents* regarding the basic rules of working with a patient medical record.

Creating a New Patient Record Using EHR Software

Keep in mind that even though EHR programs will eventually be required to communicate with each other and they are similar in many ways, there will be differences. With practice and time, you will become an expert in your office's EHR program. All programs will have a type of template that will require completion for

 Building a Patient Face Sheet

FIGURE 12-4   Screen Print from SpringCharts. Fields outlined in red are required fields.

Source: Screen captures of SpringCharts™ Electronic Health Records software are reprinted with permission from Spring Medical Systems, Inc. All rights reserved.

each new patient. Included in that template will be *required fields,* like the patient's name, date of birth, address, next of kin, sex, and insurance information (Figure 12-4). This information is sometimes part of a face sheet. However, the way you complete these fields will vary with each software package. Procedure 12-1 at the end of this chapter outlines the basic procedure for creating a new patient record using an EHR program.

Go to CONNECT to see a video about *Creating a New Patient Record Using an EHR Program.*

Correcting an Electronic Health Record

As you learned in the previous chapter, when correcting a paper medical record, you neatly draw a line through the error and make the correction as close to the original entry as possible. Obviously, once information is saved in an electronic format, a line cannot be drawn through it. In fact, because electronic medical records are legal documents, once information has been saved, it cannot be changed in any way (which is why you want to double-check your work prior to clicking "save"). When an error or omission is found in an electronic

record, an addendum to the omitted or incorrect information is made as soon as possible once the error or omission is noted. If an error is noted in a previous entry, many programs do allow a note to be inserted at the original entry, telling the user to look at a further entry in the record for the corrected information. Procedure 12-2, found at the end of this chapter, outlines basic steps to make an addendum using an EHR program. The Points on Practice feature outlines other important information about using EHR programs.

▶ Other Functions of EHR Programs   LO 12.5

In addition to the obvious advantages of electronic health records, all interoperable EHR programs have numerous other capabilities. Let's look at some of the common options for EHR programs.

Tickler Files

Computerized records can also be useful as tickler files (files that need periodic attention). For example, they can alert staff members about patients who are due for yearly checkups and patients who require follow-up care. Some hospitals have begun to use electronically scanned images of patient thumbprints or

Working with Electronic Health Records

Electronic health records (EHRs) are essentially computer-based or digital recordings of patient information that is accessible by authorized personnel both within the office where the information originated and also outside the original practice's scope. You also may hear electronic health records referred to as computer records, electronic medical records (EMRs), electronic charts, and computer health records, but, in general, these terms refer to records that are accessible only within the originating provider's office. Paper records can be lost and information is frequently not consistent in content or layout. In addition, if the records are not typed or transcribed, handwriting is often illegible. EHRs provide a multitude of solutions to the problems found with paper records, including

- *Access*. Healthcare providers can access electronic records at various locations, including the laboratory, pharmacy, and even the medical records department.
- *Availability*. Information is immediately available, so healthcare providers do not have to wait for the paper document to get written and sent. The data are entered and then immediately viewed at any electronic record location.
- *Security*. Electronic records provide security through special passwords for each individual entering the records. Passwords can be set to open access to only the parts necessary for the type of healthcare provider.
- *Safety*. Sophisticated programs help prevent patient identification errors by including a photo of each patient as part of the patient record.

- *Extra features*. Electronic software programs can alert the healthcare provider to abnormal test results or the need for routine tests to be performed. More sophisticated programs can document health trends, provide voice recognition, and convert notes to complete sentences.

As a medical assistant working with electronic records, you should keep the following in mind:

- Become familiar with the software and hardware used at your facility. Make sure you are not focused on the computer when you are with the patient. Becoming comfortable with the system you are using will help you to focus on the patient. If necessary, take notes and enter them in the computer when the patient is not present until you become comfortable.
- Retrieve the patient record carefully just as you would a paper record. Make sure you have identified the patient with at least two identifiers such as the name, date of birth, and/or medical record number.
- Keep your password information secure. Change the password on a regular basis or as directed by the healthcare facility.
- Secure the computer that maintains the electronic records and keep a backup of electronic files.
- Check your entries carefully before hitting the enter button. An EHR is a legal document just like a paper chart. What is written in the chart occurred and what is omitted from the chart did not occur.

photos to keep track of records. This also assists with patient security by identifying the patient at the time of each visit, which can cut down on insurance fraud. This system saves time and helps maintain patient record security. (Review the *Office Equipment and Supplies* chapter for more information on computer use in the medical practice.)

Specialty Specific

Once you become accustomed to reading a medical record and documenting in it, you will begin to notice there are similarities in many of the records within any specific specialty. Cardiologists use certain terms like *cardiomegaly, congestive heart failure, echocardiogram*, and *hypertension* in many of their medical records. On the other hand, an OB/GYN would seldom use those terms, but you would see terms and abbreviations like *LMP, gravida, para*, and *C-section* in these records. Similarly, when dictating or producing a physical exam or writing up an operative summary, physicians, like all of us, are creatures of habit and frequently use the same phrases time and time again. Recognizing this, EHR software programs may be **customized** to suit a specific specialty and style of a physician's office. Often, templates or "checkoffs" are available, so with a few simple clicks of the mouse, the physician may add entire sentences or

phrases, instead of typing the same information repetitively—saving time and cutting down on errors.

Electronic Schedulers

When working with a paper appointment book, only one user at a time may make appointments. If a staff member is using the appointment book and a patient calls about an appointment, the patient on the phone must wait for the appointment book to be free before he can be assisted. Ever forget the date of an appointment? In a traditional paper book, the scheduler must go page by page in order to find the forgotten appointment—inefficient at best! Electronic schedulers (Figure 12-5) have several advantages over the traditional appointment book. Multiple users may use them at any time. Depending on the software package you are using, if you need to find a patient's appointment, you can search by the patient's name or even look up the patient's record and the date of the next appointment in the record. In addition to these tasks, electronic schedulers can keep a listing of patients who want an earlier appointment if one becomes available and allow you to search for appointments by time frame needed or by appointment type needed (like a complete physical or a BP check).

One disadvantage of electronic schedulers is the fact that if the computer is down, appointments cannot be made and

FIGURE 12-5 Electronic scheduler program using SpringCharts.

Source: Screen captures of SpringCharts™ Electronic Health Records software are reprinted with permission from Spring Medical Systems, Inc. All rights reserved.

the day's schedule is not accessible. So, it is always a good idea to print out a copy of each day's schedule at the beginning of the day. Some offices also keep a "backup" appointment book handy in case of power failure. Some EHR scheduler programs also include appointment reminder and confirmation programs to automatically remind patients of their appointments. These programs then give patients the option to either confirm attendance or change the appointment by phone or online. Procedure 12-3 outlines the procedure for creating an electronic scheduler appointment matrix. Procedure 12-4 outlines the procedure for booking a patient appointment using an electronic scheduler.

Eligibility Verification and Referral Management

It is always wise—before performing any procedure—to verify the patient's insurance coverage. Many EHR programs make this process easier by assisting with online insurance verification. In addition to verifying coverage, most programs also allow for capturing the patient's demographic information at the same time.

Many managed care programs require the patient's PCP to provide any specialist with a referral before the specialist can see the patient and before most procedures can be performed. Most EHR software programs not only allow the physicians to

readily share information about the patient via the software package, but they also allow for electronic transmission of referrals among the PCP, the specialist, and the insurance plan involved. In addition, the number of visits allowed by the referral, the time frame involved, as well as the number of visits left on any given day can be tracked within the patient's medical record.

Billing and Coding Software

Many EHR programs include billing and coding software programs, allowing for electronic coding of medical records, and electronic claims submission to insurance carriers. Depending on the software program being used, the procedure and diagnosis codes may be automatically chosen by the software program based on the medical record or may be coded and inserted manually by the office medical coder (Figure 12-6). Alerts to the system may be added, so if a charge does not match a diagnosis code, a flag is produced. An example would be a patient skin biopsy, but the only diagnosis for the visit is hypertension. Even if an electronic coding program is being used, an experienced coder should perform random internal coding audits several times a year to ensure that coding is being performed correctly. Once coding is completed, the electronic claim is submitted to the insurance carrier.

FIGURE 12-6   Screen print showing diagnosis with coding for patient office visit using SpringCharts.

Source: Screen captures of SpringCharts™ Electronic Health Records software are reprinted with permission from Spring Medical Systems, Inc. All rights reserved.

Once the insurance carrier has paid the claim, most programs also include a patient billing component so the administrative staff can then produce a billing statement for the patient. This statement lists the total amount of the charges, the amount paid by the insurance plan, deductibles, and the copayment or coinsurance balance due from the patient. You will learn more about medical billing and coding in the chapters covering these subjects found later in this text.

Report Generators

Most EHR programs also include a report writer. The types of reports that may be produced include:

- Patient statistics.
- Patient demographics.
- Office A/R (accounts receivable) and A/P (accounts payable).
- Office statistics (including the number of individual procedures done during a specified time frame).
- Revenue generated by specific procedures.
- Other tracking mechanisms to assist the office business manager in tracking both profitable and nonprofitable procedures for the practice.
- Patient and insurance carrier aging reports to see who is or who is not paying the office claims and statements promptly.

Electronic Prescriptions

With Medicare and Medicaid offering e-prescribing incentives, virtually all EHR programs include prescription writers. These programs allow entry of prescriptions, which may be transmitted directly to the pharmacy or printed and given to the patient. Lists of the most common medications (and dosages) prescribed by the physician also may be kept in the program. Because the program communicates with the patient's individual medical record, any allergies can cause a flag for an ordered prescription; possible medication interactions will do the same.

Ancillary Order Integration

Many EHR programs also include ancillary programs for labs, X-rays, and other diagnostic and therapeutic services. Orders can be submitted to the lab or ancillary office electronically at the time the patient appointment is made. Once the testing is complete, the results of the test(s) are transmitted back to the office as soon as they are available, allowing for immediate upload to the patient's medical record. This greatly cuts down on patient and physician wait time for results. Additionally, results may be faxed, scanned, or e-mailed as necessary.

Patient Access

Most patients today are technically quite savvy. In fact, many prefer most communication to occur through electronic means instead of spending time on hold, or waiting for someone at the office to be free to make an appointment or provide routine information. Recognizing this, many EHR packages and offices provide patient portals so that a patient may access routine information and perform routine tasks, like making an appointment, accessing a child's immunization record, or even paying a balance on his or her account, online through the office patient portal.

▶ Security and Confidentiality and EHR

LO 12.6

When medical records are kept electronically, it is essential that the facility have policies in place to ensure security and confidentiality of records. As already discussed, all users of the EHR program will have individual access codes and passwords. The access code will only allow each user access to the areas of the record to which the user is entitled, based on his or her job description. Additionally, these access codes insert a date and time stamp within the medical record, including the user's initials, so that office administration and the patient (if requested) may know who is accessing each medical record.

The office also should have a written procedure in place to document when someone requests information from the patient file, if the patient has given permission to release that information, and when it was released. When requested by the patient, this listing must be provided as part of the HIPAA privacy and security act. Protecting the confidentiality of patient records in computer files is the greatest concern of electronic health records. Electronic healthcare records should be kept just as secure as paper healthcare records are kept.

Remember too, that whether you are documenting by hand or electronically, accuracy is always important. Careful key entry is essential to maintaining accurate electronic health files, to protect both the patient and the medical office. In addition, processes must be in place so that electronic files are backed up on a regular basis to avoid accidental data loss.

Reassuring Others about EHR Confidentiality and Security

As the office medical assistant, it will often be part of your job to reassure patients and other staff members that the office EHR program and the information it contains are confidential and secure. There are several ways you can do this.

- Be knowledgeable about all the confidentiality and security aspects of the office EHR program.
- Never display negativity about the new program, even when things don't go "exactly right" when you are using it. Remember, there is a learning curve with every new process. Remain patient and interested in the process.
- Suggest the office create a pamphlet or flyer for the patients regarding the office EHR program and assist in preparing the document for the patients.
- When working in the program, show the patient his own medical record and how information is entered, maintained, and saved, including the backup process. Explain the security systems that are in place in easy-to-understand terms to reassure the patient that his medical information is accurate, safe, and secure.
- Explain the office access process to the patients, including the fact that they may view the list of people or companies (like insurance carriers) who have accessed their information, when the access took place, and why.

Overall, the benefits of electronic health records far outweigh the consequences and with the federal government stepping in to mandate the conversion to EHR, change is inevitable. As the office medical assistant, always be willing to learn any new process, including EHR, assist others with their learning process; and help the patients understand that EHR will only improve the healthcare they receive from your office.

Go to CONNECT to see a video about *Electronically Order and Track Medical Test Results.*

PROCEDURE 12-1 Creating a New Patient Record Using EHR Software

Procedure Goal: To create a new patient record using EHR software.

OSHA Guidelines: This procedure does not involve exposure to blood, body fluids, or tissue.

Materials: Initial patient forms (patient information, advance directives, physician notes, referrals, and laboratory orders).

Method: Procedure steps.

1. Open the New Patient window of the EHR program as directed by the software vendor.
2. Enter the patient's full name as directed, being careful to enter the name in the correct order.
   RATIONALE: It is important to enter the patient name in the correct order as directed by the software program or the information may not be "filed" correctly.

3. If the patient has a family member who also comes to the practice, you may be able to use a shortcut to copy the patient's address from the existing patient information; otherwise, carefully enter the patient's demographic information, including address, phone number, birth date, etc.
   RATIONALE: This is a legal record. The information must be entered correctly.
4. Follow the software directions for completing each screen including the patient's insurance, guarantor, and employer information.
5. Depending on office policy, you also may enter the patient's medical history information. Open the software program's medical history screen and carefully key in the information required for each screen.

6. Carefully inspect all information for accuracy and save the new patient record as directed by the software program instructions.
   RATIONALE: This information will become part of the patient's permanent medical record. Proofread all information and verify accuracy before striking "Save."

7. Depending on office policy, information from a hard-copy medical record may be scanned into the EHR or a manual file created to maintain it. Follow your office procedure for filing this information.
   RATIONALE: All patient information must be readily available for healthcare providers when required for patient care.

PROCEDURE 12-2 Making an Addition or Addendum (Correction) to an Electronic Health Record

Procedure Goal: To follow standard procedures for correcting or making an addendum to an electronic health record.

OSHA Guidelines: This procedure does not involve exposure to blood, body fluids, or tissue.

Materials: Access to the patient's EHR, and other pertinent documents containing the information to be used in making corrections (for example, handwritten notes, telephone notes, physician comments, correspondence, or test results).

Method: Procedure steps.

1. Open the patient record requiring the correction or addendum following the software program instructions.
   RATIONALE: Be sure to open the correct records or another correction will be required later.

2. Following the software program instructions, obtain the *Edit* feature of the software program for this health record.

3. When the pop-up window appears, stating the record is *not editable* but asking if an addendum (or change) is required, answer *Yes.*
   RATIONALE: Once the provider has signed a health record, it is locked and not editable for other changes.

4. The program will now automatically date and time stamp the new entry with the current date and time, as well as initial stamp the entry with the current user's initials when the save feature is used.
   RATIONALE: This is a security feature. The date and time the addition was added and the identity of the person making the change are automatically inserted.

PROCEDURE 12-3 Creating an Appointment Matrix for an Electronic Scheduling System

Procedure Goal: Using an electronic scheduling system, indicate the days and times when the office is not scheduling appointments.

OSHA Guidelines: This procedure does not involve exposure to blood, body fluids, or tissue.

Materials: Electronic scheduling program; physician schedule of meetings, conferences, vacations, and other times of unavailability, including staff meetings and hours when patients are not seen.

Method: Procedure steps.

1. Using the physician schedule of availability as the base for the matrix, confer with the physician or office manager to assure that no additional schedule changes are planned.
   RATIONALE: The matrix is the base for all appointments and must adequately reflect physician availability.

2. Open the office appointment scheduler per the program format.

3. Block the dates and times when the general office or physician will not be available for patient appointments, using the physician and office schedules as guides.
   RATIONALE: It is important that appointments are booked only when the physician is available to see patients to avoid rescheduling and inconveniencing patients.

4. Choose the appropriate option if the time frame is repeatedly unavailable.
   RATIONALE: This option allows "one click" to block out repeated time frames, saving time.

5. Enter a reason that the time is not available for future reference. The office program may use color coding to assist with this process.

6. If cluster scheduling is used for the office, most schedulers allow you to specify what types of appointments may be entered; again, the scheduler may use color coding to outline specific types of appointments.
   RATIONALE: With a glance, the person scheduling appointments can readily see what types of appointments are available for patients.

7. Many programs will allow you to specify specific time frames necessary for different types of appointments and these may be set up now also. For instance, physical exams for new patients may require 45 minutes, and visits for a BP check or a typical sick visit may be set up for 15 minutes. If the program allows, set up these matrixes now, too.
   RATIONALE: This is another option to make it easier for the appointment scheduler to choose the correct appointment for each patient.

PROCEDURE 12-4 Scheduling a Patient Appointment Using an Electronic Scheduler

Procedure Goal: Utilizing the previously created matrix, book patient appointments, applying the correct amount of time for each appointment.

OSHA Guidelines: This procedure does not involve exposure to blood, body fluids, or tissue.

Materials: Electronic scheduler and template outlining time frames for patient appointment types.

Method: Procedure steps.

1. Establish the type of appointment required by the patients, particularly noting if the appointment is for a new patient or an established patient.
   RATIONALE: In general, new patient appointments take longer time frames than do existing patient appointments.

2. If needed, consult the office template for the amount of time required for the patient appointment. Keep in mind the reason for the appointment, as that may affect timing.
   RATIONALE: If a patient is required to be fasting, for example, the appointment should be made earlier in the day and not in the afternoon.

3. When possible, schedule appointments earlier in the day first, and then move to later time frames. Do ask if the patient has a preferred time frame and, if possible, honor the request.

4. Following the electronic scheduler instructions, use the search option to find the next available appointment for the time frame required for the patient's appointment. Once the patient agrees to the appointment offered, enter the patient's name, phone number, and reason for the appointment. Save the appointment per software instructions.
   RATIONALE: It is helpful to the office staff to have an idea why the patient is being seen. The phone number is helpful in case the appointment needs to be rescheduled or the patient needs to be reached for any reason.

5. Repeat the appointment information to the patient, giving any necessary instructions regarding preparation for the appointment.
   RATIONALE: For some appointments, it is important that the patient be prepared correctly (i.e., fasting) or the appointment may need to be rescheduled.

SUMMARY OF LEARNING OUTCOMES

LEARNING OUTCOME	KEY POINTS
12.1 List four medical mistakes that will be greatly decreased through the use of EHR.	Medical mistakes that will be greatly decreased or eliminated with EHR include lost or misfiled paper records, mishandled or "forgotten" patient messages, inaccurate or unreadable information in a paper medical record, and mislabeled or unreadable laboratory or prescription orders.
12.2 Differentiate among electronic medical records, electronic health records, and personal health records.	The electronic medical record is an electronic record of health-related information for an individual patient that is created, compiled, and managed by providers and staff members located within a *single* healthcare organization. An electronic health record is created, managed, and gathered in a manner that conforms to nationally recognized *interoperability standards*, so that members of more than one healthcare organization can utilize it. A personal health record is an electronic version of the comprehensive medical history and record of a patient's lifelong health that is collected and maintained by the individual patient.
12.3 Contrast the advantages and disadvantages of electronic health records.	Advantages of EHR include fewer lost medical records, elimination of transcription costs, increased readability/legibility of charts, ease of chart access for multiple users, chart availability outside of office hours, increased access to patient education materials, decreased duplication of medical tests, more efficient records transfer, more efficient billing processes using electronic billing methods, and decreased need for storage space. Disadvantages include cost, need for training, possible need for F/T or P/T IT personnel, and need for computer hardware/software upgrades or changes.

LEARNING OUTCOMES	KEY POINTS
12.4 **Illustrate the steps in creating a new patient record and correcting an existing record using EHR software.**	The same rules apply with EHR as for paper-based medical records when initiating or documenting in a patient's electronic health record. Follow the basic steps in Procedure 12-1 for setting up a new patient EHR and 12-2 for correcting or making an addition in an existing patient's electronic health record.
12.5 **Describe some of the capabilities of EHR software programs.**	Aside from housing patient electronic health records, many EHR programs also can perform the following functions: tickler files, specialty-specific software, electronic scheduler, eligibility verification and referral management, billing and coding capabilities, report generation, electronic prescriptions and ancillary order integration, and a patient access portal.
12.6 **Explain how you might alleviate a patient's security fears surrounding the use of EHR.**	Be knowledgeable on all aspects of the office EHR program and never display a negative attitude about it. Assist in preparing written information for the patients regarding the EHR program, including how the patient's medical information will remain confidential and secure. When the patient is in the office, offer to show the patient his EHR and demonstrate adding information, explaining how the information is entered, maintained, and kept secure. Understand and be able to explain the backup process for the EHR program. Understand the office access policy as it pertains to HIPAA and explain it to the patients.

C A S E   S T U D Y   C R I T I C A L   T H I N K I N G

Recall Ken Washington from the beginning of the chapter. Now that you have completed the chapter, answer the following questions regarding his case.

1. How will you explain the benefits of using electronic health records to Ken Washington?

2. The screen Ken Washington has seen displays only the screen saver for the new EHR program. What precautions should be taken to ensure patients do not see another patient's information on the computer monitor?

E X A M   P R E P A R A T I O N   Q U E S T I O N S

1. (LO 12.1) Medical errors in the United States are calculated to be the _____ leading cause of patient death.
   a. 2nd
   b. 4th
   c. 6th
   d. 8th
   e. 10th

2. (LO 12.2) Patient electronic health information created in a format meeting *interoperability standards* is defined as being in a(n) _____ format.
   a. EMR
   b. EHR
   c. PHR
   d. a or b
   e. None of the above

3. (LO 12.2) An individual's lifelong health record is a(n)
   a. EMR
   b. EHR
   c. PHR
   d. Any of the above
   e. None of the above

4. (LO 12.3) Which government insurance plan offers EHR incentive programs?
   a. Medicare
   b. Medicaid
   c. TRICARE
   d. a and b
   e. b and c

5. (LO 12.3) Medicare and Medicaid use the term EP to describe providers who may participate in the EHR incentive programs. What does EP stand for?
   a. Educated provider
   b. Educated physician
   c. Eligible person
   d. Educated person
   e. Eligible provider

6. (LO 12.4) Many EHR programs use the term _____ for a correction made to an electronic health record.
   a. Deletion
   b. Error
   c. Addendum
   d. Omission
   e. Correction

7. (LO 12.5) Which of the following other functions of the EHR program will be most helpful to the administration when reviewing the financial health of the practice?
   a. Report generator
   b. Ticker file
   c. Billing/coding
   d. Electronic scheduler
   e. Specialty-specific programs

8. (LO 12.5) Which of the other functions of the EHR program would be most helpful to the staff who schedules appointments for patients with specialists?
   a. Billing coding
   b. Specialty-specific programs
   c. Ancillary order integration
   d. Electronic prescriptions
   e. Insurance verification

9. (LO 12.6) Which item below maintains each user's ability to work in certain areas of a patient's electronic health record?
   a. Password
   b. Access code
   c. Confidentiality
   d. HIPAA
   e. None of the above

10. (LO 12.6) Which of the following will not reassure patients about the privacy and security of the office EHR system?
   a. Showing the patient how information is entered in his medical record
   b. Being knowledgeable about the security of the office EHR system
   c. Sharing "computer frustrations" with the patient
   d. Explaining how the backup system for the EHR program works
   e. Assisting in the creation of a pamphlet for the patients regarding the new office EHR system

Go to CONNECT to see EHR activities about *Adding a New Patient, Editing a Patient Record,* and *Archiving a Patient Record.*

Access the OLC to practice in a live EHR program. Refer to the EHR Appendix IV at the back of the book for more information and directions.

Telephone Techniques

L E A R N I N G   O U T C O M E S

After completing Chapter 13, you will be able to:

13.1 Explain the purpose of the telecommunications equipment commonly found in the medical office.

13.2 Relate the five Cs of effective communication to telephone communication skills.

13.3 Define the following terms involved in making a good impression on the telephone: telephone etiquette, pitch, pronunciation, enunciation, and tone.

13.4 Describe how to appropriately handle the different types of calls coming into the medical practice.

13.5 Summarize the purpose of the office routing list with regard to call screening.

13.6 Carry out the procedure for taking a complete telephone message.

13.7 Outline the preparation required prior to making outgoing calls and the skills used in making the phone call.

K E Y   T E R M S

automated voice response unit

enunciation

etiquette

interactive pager

pitch

pronunciation

telecommunications device for the deaf (TDD)

telephone triage

IV. P (7) Demonstrate telephone techniques

IV. A (1) Demonstrate empathy in communicating with patients, family and staff

IV. A (7) Demonstrate recognition of the patient's level of understanding in communication

VII. A (2) Demonstrate sensitivity in communicating with both providers and patients

IX. C (2) Explore issue of confidentiality as it applies to the medical assistant

IX. C (3) Describe the implications of HIPAA for the medical assistant in various medical setttings

8. **Medical Office Business Procedures Management**
   Graduates:

   bb. Are impartial and show empathy when dealing with patients

   ee. Use proper telephone techniques

   hh. Receive, organize, prioritize, and transmit information expediently

11. **Career Development**
    Graduates:

    b. Demonstrate professionalism by:
       (2) Exhibiting a positive attitude and a sense of responsibility
       (3) Maintaining confidentiality at all times
       (8) Being courteous and diplomatic
       (9) Conducting work within scope of education, training, and ability

▶ Introduction

Most offices have policies and procedures for routing calls that come into the office. You will learn which types of calls you may handle and which should be directed to clinical medical personnel or the physician. You will learn to triage (prioritize) calls so that emergencies are handled correctly. Of equal importance, you will learn how to take a complete telephone message, how to be prepared when placing calls, how to leave effective and HIPAA-compliant messages for patients, and how to handle difficult telephone calls, including those from angry patients with complaints and from callers who will not identify themselves.

Finally, in addition to using the telephone correctly, you will learn how other communication devices are used in the medical office, including setting up and using automated telephone menu equipment, voicemail, answering services and machines, TDDs, cell phones, and pagers.

▶ Telecommunications Equipment LO 13.1

When thinking about telecommunications equipment in the medical office, the first item that naturally comes to mind is the office telephone system. In addition to the office telephone line(s), you will also explore how cell phones, beepers, answering machines, voicemail, and answering services play vital roles in the medical office's management.

Telephone System

The telephone is one of the most important pieces of communication equipment in the medical practice. Not only is it the primary instrument patients use to communicate with the office, but it is also the primary means of communication among providers, hospitals, laboratories, and other businesses important to the practice.

Advances in technology and the advent of the Internet are dramatically changing voice communications. Technologies like Voice over Internet Protocol (VoIP), also known as Internet Voice, allow the integration of voice and data communication through the computer and Internet service. This means that medical practices have the option of using the computer for Internet access and telephone conversations.

Multiline Phones

Few practices can function with just one or two telephone lines. Most modern medical offices have a telephone system that includes several telephones and multiple lines for incoming or outgoing calls, an intercom system, and the ability to transfer calls, leave voicemail, and put calls on hold (Figure 13-1). The larger the practice, the greater the demand on the phone system. Larger practices often need complex communications systems to handle all their needs.

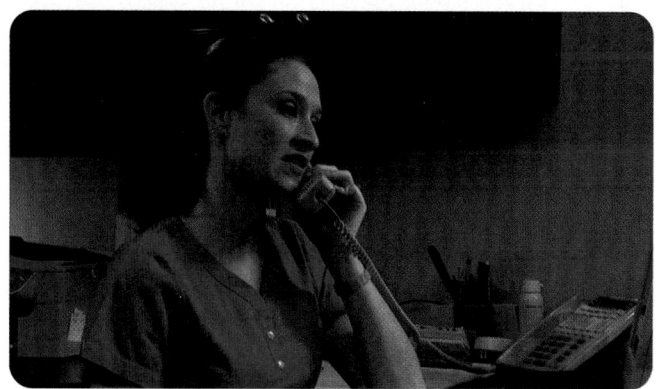

FIGURE 13-1 Most modern medical offices have multiline phones that are capable of multiple functions.

Call Routing

The telephone system can be set up so that all incoming calls ring on all the telephones in the office, but the more common setup in most practices is that one or more "main phones" receive all calls. The receptionist(s) then routes calls to the appropriate telephone extensions.

The **automated voice response unit** is quickly becoming a popular alternative to the traditional phone system, which requires someone to answer each call. Instead, this unit automatically answers all calls. A recorded voice offers the caller various options for routing the call. Once the caller selects an option, the system automatically routes the call to another detailed menu or to the designated department or person. The use of automated voice response units can provide greater flexibility for the medical staff, as well as offer enhanced service to the patient, providing direct access to the type of assistance required. However, the use of more than three menu levels may be frustrating to callers if they "get lost in the system." When medical offices use these units, the first option should always be instructions for the caller if the call is regarding an emergency. There also should be an option for the caller to "dial zero at any time to reach the operator." This is especially true for offices with many elderly patients who can easily become frustrated when they "cannot get to a live person." The Points on Practice section on these automated systems provides tips on their use.

Other Automated Telephone Options

In very busy practices, many practices opt to use an automated system to place routine reminder calls to patients. Medical assistants spend a great deal of time on the telephone calling patients to remind them of appointments, calling patients about no-shows, and leaving other types of messages.

Physicians feel that they can make better use of staff time by using automated phone systems. In fact, the system often pays for itself in less than a year. In addition to reminding patients of upcoming appointments, it can allow them to leave messages for staff. Automated phone systems can offer much more than just financial benefits: They can conduct patient surveys and give patient test results through a privacy mechanism (patient inputs his or her password). The phone system also can assist in managing referrals from the managed care organizations requiring them, and it can assist with preventive care by giving direct access to nurses for minor problems and concerns.

Voicemail and the Office Phone

An automated menu is often used in conjunction with voicemail—a form of answering machine. If the office is closed or the person the patient is calling is on the phone or away from her desk, voicemail answers the call and the caller can leave a message. The advantage of a voicemail system is that the caller never receives a busy signal. Another advantage is that voicemail

---

POINTS ON PRACTICE

Routing Calls Through an Automated Menu

An automated menu system answers calls for the office and separates requests into categories so that the appropriate staff member may deal with each call efficiently. Someone who calls an automated system hears a recorded message identifying the business. The message gives the caller a list of options from which to choose. The caller selects an option by pressing the corresponding button on her telephone or by speaking the number of the option. For example, the voice response may say, "Press or say 1 for appointments. Press or say 2 for prescription renewals. Press or say 3 for referrals."

How does an automated menu system save time and effort in a medical office? You do not have to answer calls as they come in but can instead reserve a block of time in which to listen and respond to messages. This system allows you to complete other work without interruption. Though this practice is efficient, it is a policy that needs to be approved by the office manager and physicians within the practice before it is implemented. Some medical offices maintain a philosophy that places the importance of a patient call (as the customer and the reason for the office in the first place) above all other office tasks. Always ask the supervisor in charge of the office how you should use the automated system.

To set up an automated system, you need to plan specific categories from which patients can choose. Categories may include but are not limited to:

- Making and changing appointments
- Billing questions
- Medical questions of clinical personnel
- Reporting patient emergencies
- Receiving calls from other physician offices

When the caller presses the code for a patient emergency, the call rings in the office because it needs to be answered immediately. You or other staff members should respond to calls in the other categories in a timely fashion. Questions for doctors or nurses can be routed immediately to the appropriate voicemail, bypassing the front office lines.

A variety of telephone vendors can set up automated menu systems. When choosing an automated telephone system, be careful that callers do not become lost in the process. It is a good idea to set up a system that allows callers to return easily to the main menu or to request a live operator's assistance. Following up on messages promptly also will help callers feel comfortable with your voicemail system. You should check for messages at least once every hour.

is a more secure system, in that each person on a voicemail system has a unique password to retrieve only her messages.

Answering Machine

If the office phone system does not include voicemail, many offices use a telephone answering machine to answer calls after office hours, on weekends and holidays, and when the office is closed for any reason. A typical recorded message announces that the office is closed and states the usual business hours. In addition, the message must always indicate how the caller can reach the covering physician in the case of an emergency.

Answering Service

Instead of, or in addition to, an answering machine, many medical offices use an answering service. Unlike answering machines, answering services provide actual people who answer the telephone. They take messages and communicate them to the physician on call, who is responsible for handling emergencies that may occur when the office is closed—at night or on weekends or holidays. Upon receiving a message from the answering service, the physician returns the patient's call and decides on the course of action.

Answering services can be used in a number of ways. The medical office may use an answering machine to record calls of a routine nature and give the number of the answering service to call in emergencies. Alternatively, the answering service may have a direct connection to the physician's office, picking up calls after a certain number of rings day or night or during specific hours. This ensures that calls do not get missed if the office is very busy and the staff cannot get to the phone.

Some answering services specialize in medical practices. These medical specialty services ask the medical practice to give specific directives for the triage of calls. Although most answering services provide satisfactory, sometimes even outstanding, service, it is good practice to check up on the service every so often by calling it during its coverage hours. This quality check ensures that the service meets office standards and expectations. Always ask any service for references before signing a contract for service.

Cellular (Cell) Phones—Personal and Business Use

Cell phones today are as common as people wearing shoes. In fact, cell phone use is so widespread, many people no longer have a "land line." Instead, they depend solely on their cell phones, not only for calls, but for texting, directions, and many online apps (applications) for information and communication. Physicians, medical practice employees, and patients may all be carrying their own personal cell phones into the medical office. With all that technology available at a button's touch, cell phone etiquette is a key concern. Generally, it is appropriate to turn off all personal cell phones while inside a medical office. In fact, it is not unusual for offices to have signs posted, requesting that cell phones be shut off when entering the office or at least when patients are in the treatment areas. The patients should be shown this same consideration by the physician and medical staff. Cell phone calls from outside the practice are usually an interruption in the communication among the physician, the staff, and the patient, who, as the *customer* of the practice, should have your

full attention. More important, personal cell phone use should be avoided within the office, as it can interfere with other electronic equipment that may be functioning inside the medical practice.

However, cell phones do play an important part in the business functioning of the medical office. Physicians may use a cell phone to respond quickly to a message from staff or a hospital. Office staff may use personal cell phones in an emergency when traditional phone systems fail. Some medical practices even issue a cell phone to key employees who conduct business for the practice outside the office. In addition, patients may use their cell phones to call for a taxi after an appointment. If your medical office allows staff and patient cell phone use, make sure it is clearly noted in which areas cell phone use is permitted, and for employees, when personal cell phones may be used. In most offices, personal cell phones may only be used during break times; at other times, they must be turned off or left in vibrate mode.

Pagers (Beepers)

Physicians often need to be reached when they are out of the office, so in addition to a cell phone, many also carry pagers (also known as beepers). Pagers are small electronic devices that give the user a signal to indicate that someone is trying to reach him. Although generally considered outdated technology, pagers are still used in some areas, particularly in rural areas, where cell phone signals are not as reliable.

Technology of Paging Like a cell phone, each paging device is assigned a telephone number. When the number is called, the pager picks up the signal and beeps, buzzes, or vibrates to indicate a call has been made. Most pagers have a window that displays either the caller's telephone number or a short message, so the receiver can return the call. Pagers also may store the telephone number so that the receiver can return several calls without having to write down the numbers.

Calling a Pager Many telephone messages can wait until the physician returns to the office or calls in for messages. When a message needs to be delivered immediately, and a cell phone is not an option, paging is an efficient response. A list of pager (and cell phone) numbers for each physician in the practice should be kept in a prominent place in the office, such as by the main telephone or switchboard. Make sure you know where these numbers are kept. The paging process is as simple as making a telephone call.

1. Look up the telephone number for the pager of the physician you need to contact.
2. Dial the telephone number for the pager.
3. You will hear the telephone ringing and the call picked up. Listen for a high-pitched tone, which signals the connection between the telephone and the pager.
4. To operate most pagers, dial the telephone number you wish the physician to call, followed by the pound sign (#). (Some pager services have an operator and work much like an answering service. Give the operator a message and the operator will contact the physician.)

5. Listen for a beep or a series of beeps signaling that the page has been transmitted. Then hang up the phone. The physician will call the number at his earliest convenience.

Interactive pagers (I-pagers) are designed for two-way communication. The individual carrying the pager is paged in much the same way as the traditional pager. The pager can be set on "Audio" or "Vibrate" to alert the carrier that a message is coming in. However, the interactive pager screen displays a printed message and allows the physician to respond by way of a mini keyboard.

The physician can respond to the printed page by typing a return message, which is relayed back to the office in real time. The office computer and the physician enter into a conversation much like e-mail or an Internet chat room. Many problems can be handled quickly and efficiently in this manner. Additionally, because the I-pager can function silently, the physician can communicate with her office while in a restaurant without disturbing others or compromising patient confidentiality.

Each interactive pager has its own wireless Internet address. The user types in the receiving party's e-mail address and creates a message on a monitor screen. The interactive pager indicates on the screen when the message has been sent, received, or read. I-pagers can communicate with other I-pagers as well, and they have broadcast capability, meaning the sender can send to more than one receiver at a time. For this reason, I-pagers can be very helpful for practices with multiple physicians, especially where cell phone service is not always reliable.

I-pagers can also send messages to traditional telephones. The message is typed into the pager and the system "calls" the telephone number. When answered, an electronic voice reads the message to the individual who has answered.

Patient Courtesy Phone

The widespread use of cell phones has pretty much eliminated the need, but a few medical offices still have a patient courtesy phone, usually located in the reception area, that provides an outside local phone line strictly for patient use. Long-distance calls are usually blocked from this phone. The addition of such a line leaves office lines free for business calls while providing a line of communication for patients to call for transportation or to contact work or family as needed. It is helpful to post a sign near the phone to indicate guidelines for its use, and calls are usually limited to less than five minutes.

Telecommunications Devices for the Deaf

If your office has a significant number of patients with hearing impairments, it may be equipped with a **telecommunications device for the deaf,** known as a TDD (formerly known as a TTY—teletypewriter). A TDD is a specially designed telephone that looks very much like a laptop and may have a cradle for a telephone receiver (Figure 13-2). To call the office, the patient places the telephone receiver (if it has one) in the cradle and, instead of speaking, types his message using the TDD keyboard. If the office has a TDD, the message will be received in type format (similar to e-mail) on the TDD screen.

FIGURE 13-2 Telecommunications device for the deaf (TDD).

If the office does not have TDD equipment, the message may still be received through the use of a telecommunications relay service (TRS). When a patient utilizes a TRS, a specialty relay operator will receive the patient's written message through TDD equipment and then read the message to you when you answer the office phone. When a relay operator is used, the operator will identify herself as a relay operator for the patient utilizing the service. She will read the typed information from the patient. When the message is completed, she will say "go ahead" as your signal that it is your turn to reply. You will reply to the patient by speaking to the operator , and she will then enter your reply into the TDD device so the patient can read it. You will also use the key term *go ahead* when your message is completed.

TDD devices are becoming more common in the United States and throughout the world. Keep in mind that keying information takes longer than speaking and be patient with the process. As with text messaging, certain abbreviations are commonly used with a TDD. Table 13-1 lists some of them for your reference. Procedure 13-1 at the end of the chapter outlines the procedure for using a TDD.

TABLE 13-1	Abbreviations Commonly Used with TDD Devices
Abbreviation	**Meaning**
GA	Go ahead
SK	Stop keying
SKSK	Call complete
Q	Question
BEC	Because
U	You
UR	Your
PLS	Please
NBR	Number
TMW	Tomorrow
AM	Morning
PM	Night

Effective Telephone Communication

LO 13.2

When you answer the telephone, you may be the first contact a person has with the practice. The impression you leave can be either positive or negative. Your job is to ensure that it is positive.

Good telephone management leaves callers with a positive impression of you, the physicians, and the practice. Poor telephone management can result in negative feelings, misunderstandings, and an overall unfavorable impression. The image you present over the phone should convey the message that the staff is caring, attentive, and helpful. Showing concern for each patient's welfare is a quality that patients rate highly when evaluating healthcare professionals. In addition, you must sound professional and knowledgeable when handling telephone calls. Using proper telephone management skills will help keep patients informed and ensure their satisfaction with the medical practice.

Communication Skills

Excellent communication skills are important in telephone management because they help project a positive image and thus satisfy the patient's needs and expectations. Individuals who are adept at effective communication employ the following communications skills:

- Display tact and sensitivity.
- Show empathy.
- Give respect.
- Appear genuine.
- Display openness and friendliness.
- Refrain from passing judgment or stereotyping others.
- Are supportive.
- Ask for clarification and feedback.
- Use paraphrasing to ensure an understanding of what others are saying.
- Are receptive to each patient's needs.
- Know when to speak and when to listen.
- Exhibit a willingness to consider other viewpoints and concerns.

As a medical assistant, you should also apply the five Cs of communication to be as effective when using the telephone as you are when having a face-to-face conversation with someone. Get to know and use the five Cs of effective communication in all forms of communication:

- *Completeness.* The message must contain all necessary information.
- *Clarity.* The message must be legible and free from ambiguity.
- *Conciseness.* The message must be brief and direct.
- *Courtesy.* The message must be respectful and considerate of others.
- *Cohesiveness.* The message must be organized and logical.

Guidelines for Using the Telephone Effectively

The following guidelines will help you use the telephone effectively and professionally:

- Answer the phone promptly, by the second or third ring.
- Hold the telephone to your ear, or use a headset to hold the earpiece securely against your ear. Do not cradle the telephone with your shoulder; doing so can cause muscle strain.
- Hold the mouthpiece about an inch away from your mouth and leave one hand free to write with.
- When answering the phone, greet the caller first with the practice name, then with your name. If accepting a call routed by an automated answering system or forwarded to you by someone else, always identify yourself by name.
- Acknowledge the caller. Demonstrate your willingness to assist the caller by asking, "Ms. Jones, how may I help you?"
- Be courteous, calm, and pleasant no matter how hurried you are.
- Identify the nature of the call and devote your full attention to the caller. Do not attempt to "multitask" while on the phone.
- At the end of the call, allow the caller to hang up first to be sure any questions have been answered. Always say goodbye and use the caller's name.

Following HIPAA Guidelines

As you learned in the *Legal and Ethical Issues* chapter, HIPAA is the act concerned with the privacy and confidentiality of patient information, including information communicated via the telephone. Healthcare providers are allowed to disclose patient information for the purpose of treatment, payment, and healthcare operations (known as TPO) only. Any use of this information outside of these reasons requires a written authorization from the patient, except in emergency situations or in cases of information required by government agencies for compliance issues. As a general rule, patient information should not be revealed over the phone unless you are speaking directly to the patient or have written consent from the patient to speak to another person about his condition. Always follow your office policy and procedures manual with regard to disclosing patient information.

Telephone Etiquette

LO 13.3

Proper telephone **etiquette** means handling all calls politely and professionally using good manners. Confidence in your role of providing quality patient care includes the ability to communicate effectively not only in person, but also on the telephone. Your professionalism and caring attitude must come through the phone to the caller.

Your Telephone Voice

Customer service is critical when using the telephone. After all, your voice is representing the medical office. You must present your message effectively and professionally. Because you cannot rely on body language or facial expressions to help you

FIGURE 13-3 Smiling comes over the phone, making patients feel you want to help them.

FIGURE 13-4 Using a hands-free headset allows you to speak directly into the mouthpiece, keeping your hands free to complete a task such as booking an appointment for a patient.

communicate over the telephone, it is important to make the most of your telephone voice. Use the following tips to make your voice pleasant and effective.

- Speak directly into the receiver. Otherwise, your voice will be difficult to understand.
- Smile. The "smile" in your voice will convey your friendliness and willingness to help (Figure 13-3).
- Visualize the caller and speak directly to that person.
- Convey a friendly and respectful interest in the caller.
- Be helpful and alert.
- Use language that is nontechnical and easy to understand. Never use slang.
- Speak at a natural pace, not too quickly or too slowly.
- Use a normal conversational tone.
- Try to vary your pitch while you are talking. **Pitch** is the high or low level of your speech. Varying the pitch of your voice allows you to emphasize words and makes your voice more pleasant to listen to.
- Make the caller feel important.

Pronunciation Proper **pronunciation** (saying words correctly) is one of the most important telephone skills. If you are unsure how to pronounce the name of the person on the phone, ask him to repeat it for you. This demonstrates respect for the person and shows him that he has your undivided attention. When clarifying the spelling of a name, verify letters that sound alike by repeating the letter and include a word that begins with that letter. Examples include D as in dog, V as in Victor, and M as in Mary.

Enunciation **Enunciation** (clear and distinct speaking) is the opposite of mumbling. Good enunciation helps the person you are speaking to understand you, which is especially important when you are trying to convey medical information.

Speaking clearly over the telephone is very important because the speaker cannot be seen. Correct interpretation of the message is determined by hearing the words precisely. Activities like chewing gum, eating, or propping the phone between the ear and shoulder hinder proper enunciation. Many offices today provide the medical assistant and/or the receptionist with a wireless headset. These hands-free devices allow you to use your hands freely while on the phone, eliminating the need to hold the phone between your ear and shoulder. See Figure 13-4. The Points on Practice feature discusses hands-free headsets in more detail.

Tone Because you are not face-to-face with the caller, the most important measurements of good telephone communication are voice quality and tone. Always speak with a positive and respectful tone.

POINTS ON PRACTICE
The Wireless Headset

The wireless headset, also called a hands-free headset, is popular in offices, including the medical office. It allows the user to speak on the phone while using her hands to schedule an appointment, look up information on the computer, or locate the physician for an emergency phone call. Because the headset eliminates the need to hold the handset between the ear and the shoulder while attempting to multitask, it reduces office-related neck, back, and shoulder pain.

One word of caution when using these headsets in the medical office: Always keep HIPAA and patient confidentiality in mind if you must walk about the office while on the phone with a patient. Anything you say will be heard by anyone within listening range. Although tempting, do not walk around the office while on the phone with a patient unless an emergency demands that you do so.

Making a Good Impression

In a sense, your telephone duties include public relations skills. How you handle telephone calls will have an impact on the medical practice's public image.

Exhibiting Courtesy Show common courtesy by projecting an attitude of helpfulness. Always use the person's name during the conversation and apologize for any errors or delays. When ending the conversation, be sure to ask the caller if there is anything else you can do for him and thank him before hanging up.

Giving Undivided Attention Do not try to answer the telephone while continuing to carry out another task. Before answering the phone, complete any conversations occurring in the office or excuse yourself while you answer the phone. Once you make sure that the call is not for an emergency, ask the caller if you may either put him on hold for a moment or call him back shortly. By interrupting the patient in the office briefly and giving the caller the option as to how he would like his call handled, both patients receive the undivided attention they deserve.

Putting a Call on Hold Although you should try not to put a caller on hold, there will be times when it is unavoidable. Calls may come in on another line, or a situation in the office may prevent you from devoting your full attention to the caller. Sometimes you may have to check a file or ask someone else in the office a question on behalf of the caller. Before putting a call on hold, however, always let the caller state the reason for the call. This step is essential so that you do not inadvertently put an emergency call on hold. Never answer the phone, "Dr. Buckwalter's office, please hold," and immediately put the call on hold. You must ask permission to put the caller on hold and wait for the response.

Your medical office may have a standard procedure for placing a call on hold. Typically, you will ask the caller the purpose of the call, state why you need to place the call on hold, and explain how long you expect the wait to be. Ask the caller if she would like to hold or if she would prefer you to return her call. If she requests a return call, ask her if there is a time that is best for the return call. If she decides to wait on hold and if you cannot end the task at hand quickly, return to the caller every 2 to 3 minutes asking her if she wishes to remain on hold. An excessive wait on hold makes people feel they have been "forgotten" or are "unimportant." Checking in with them and giving options minimizes these negative thoughts and feelings.

If you know you can return to the line shortly, put the caller on hold and complete your current task or call. If you need to answer a second call, get the second caller's name and telephone number and, unless this call includes an emergency situation, put the call on hold until you have completed the first call. You can then return to the second call. If possible, ask a coworker to assist with the second call, minimizing wait time for both callers.

Returning Patient Calls Some people do not like to hold and will request that you call them back. Obtain the caller's name and phone number, taking the time to repeat both to avoid errors. Return the call in a reasonable amount of time or as close as possible to the time requested by the caller, and give the patient your undivided attention. Be sure to apologize for the inconvenience and thank the caller for her patience.

Remembering Patient Names When patients are recognized by name, they are more likely to have positive feelings about the practice. Using a caller's name during a conversation makes the caller feel important. If you do not recognize a patient's name, it is better to ask, "Has it been some time since you've been in the office?" rather than to ask if the patient has been to the practice before.

Checking for Understanding When communicating by telephone, you do not have visual signals to convey the caller's feelings and level of understanding of the information you are discussing. If a call is long or complicated, summarize what was said to be sure that both you and the caller understand the information. Ask if the caller has any questions about what you have discussed. You may even want to have the caller repeat any instructions to make sure she understands. If a situation requires a lengthy conversation, it might be best to have the patient come into the office or to follow up the phone call with a written summary of the discussion. Do not forget to document the call in the patient's medical record.

Communicating with Empathy Whenever information is conveyed over the telephone, feelings are also communicated. When dealing with a caller who is nervous, upset, or angry, try to show empathy (an understanding of the other person's feelings). Communicating with empathy helps the caller feel more positive about the conversation and the medical office.

Ending the Conversation It is not useful to let a conversation run on if you can effectively complete the call sooner. Before hanging up, however, take a few seconds to complete the call so that the caller feels properly cared for and satisfied. You can complete the call by summarizing the important points of the conversation and thanking the caller. Let the caller hang up first.

Occasionally, you will encounter the patient who simply will not hang up. Often these patients are merely lonely and your friendliness and helpfulness ease their loneliness. In this case, you may find that you must politely but firmly explain that another patient (or the physician) needs your assistance and you must complete the call. When you put the receiver down, never slam it—even if the caller has already hung up. Remember, all your actions reflect the medical practice's professional image. Patients in the reception area may see (and hear) you when you are talking on the telephone.

▶ Types of Incoming Calls   LO 13.4

In dealing with incoming telephone calls, you will encounter a variety of questions and requests from numerous people. Many incoming calls are from patients. You also will receive calls from various people, including attorneys, physicians, pharmaceutical sales representatives, and other salespeople.

Calls from Patients

Patients call the medical office for a variety of reasons, including rescheduling appointments and requesting prescription renewals. If you will be discussing clinical matters over the telephone, it is a good idea to pull the patient's chart. If the office uses EHR technology, this may be as simple as accessing his medical record on the computer screen. If paper records are used, you may need to ask him to hold for a moment while you retrieve the record. The information in the chart will often enable you to address any problems quickly. Pulling the chart also allows you to document the conversation immediately.

Always keep in mind that the physician is legally responsible for your actions, including relaying information to patients over the telephone. The office policy manual typically specifies what you may and may not discuss with patients. If you are uncertain about giving particular information to a patient, it is best to discuss the situation with the physician or have the physician return the patient's call.

Appointment Scheduling Follow office procedures for making or changing appointment times over the telephone. Ask the patient to provide his name, a telephone number where he can be reached during the day, and the reason for the visit. Repeat the information back to the patient to verify all information before ending the call. (Scheduling appointments is discussed in the *Schedule Management* chapter.)

Billing Inquiries If a patient calls about a billing problem, you will need to pull the patient's billing information and possibly the medical record as well. With this information, you can compare the charges with the actual services performed.

If a patient claims to have been overcharged, check to see if the correct fee was charged. If you find that an error was made, apologize and tell the patient the office will send a corrected statement. Ask the patient to wait for the new statement before sending payment. If in fact the proper fee was charged, it may be helpful to speak to the physician before responding to the patient. The physician may be able to tell you if there were special circumstances regarding the visit or charge in question. Allowing the patient to pay the bill in installments is usually an acceptable option. The details on arranging for payment plans is discussed in the *Patient Billing and Collections* chapter.

Many offices use billing services instead of taking care of the insurance submission and monthly patient billing in the office. In that case, the patient may have called the billing service about charges and has now been referred to the office to dispute either the performance of a procedure or its cost. In this case, you may not have access to information about individual charges and may need to refer the patient to the office manager. Be aware that the patient may be upset about his bill and now is being referred to yet another person. Listen patiently to the patient and take notes regarding his complaint, remaining tactful and understanding to his concerns and possible frustration that an answer does not appear to be a simple process. No matter what your office policy is, if a patient is dissatisfied, document all appropriate comments and relay the information to the physician or office manager. If a bill has not been paid, ask if there are special circumstances affecting the patient's ability to pay. Always give this information to the physician or office manager. Figure 13-5 gives an example of appropriate documentation of such a call.

Requests for Laboratory or Radiology Reports If a patient calls the office requesting the results of a test, obtain the patient's chart to see if the report has been received. If it has not, suggest that the patient call back in a day or two. If the need for the result is urgent, you may call the laboratory or radiology office to obtain the results over the phone.

In some offices, you may be authorized to give laboratory results by telephone if they are normal, or negative, so the patient does not have to wait for results to be mailed or for a return phone call from the physician. Make a note on the patient's chart if you provide any information about test results. If a test result is abnormal, the physician will need to speak with the patient. In such a case, tell the patient that the office has received the results and that the physician will call as soon as possible. Then place the patient's chart and the telephone

---

Patient Name: Shenya Jones   **Date:** 2/26/XX

TC: Patient called stating bill appears to contain an error. She was charged for a urinalysis during her last visit, but states she was unable to produce a specimen for such testing. Review of medical record reveals no urinalysis was done. Patient is informed the charge will be removed from her bill. Insurance company will be notified so payment for lab can be refunded.———*M. Katahri, Office Manager*

FIGURE 13-5   Medical record documentation of a patient telephone call.

| **Patient Name:** | Sylvia Gonzales | | **Date:** | 5/12/XX |

TC: Patient called inquring about FBS result performed 5/10/XX. Reading of 130 given to patient. Per Dr. Whalen, patient is to remain on current insulin dosage. ——————— *M. Perez, CMA (AAMA)*

FIGURE 13-6   Typical chart note documenting patient receipt of lab results by phone.

message on the physician's desk. See Figure 13-6 for a chart note example of such a telephone call.

Questions About Medications   One of the most common types of calls from patients involves questions about medications. A patient may ask about using a current prescription or may want to renew an existing one.

Prescription Renewals   Calls for prescription renewals may come from the patient's pharmacy or from the patient. A pharmacist usually calls to check before dispensing refills if more than a year has passed since the original prescription was written. If the physician has indicated in the patient's medical record that renewals are approved, you may authorize the pharmacy to renew a prescription. In any other case, only the physician may authorize renewals. If the physician authorizes a renewal, you may be asked to telephone it in to the patient's pharmacy. Procedure 13-2 at the end of this chapter outlines the instructions for renewing a precription by telephone. All renewals must be documented in the patient's medical record, with the date and the initials of the person authorizing the renewal. See Figure 13-7.

Go to CONNECT to see a video on how to *Manage a Prescription Refill.*

Old Prescriptions   Patients may call to ask if they can use a medication that was prescribed for a previous condition. In these instances, recommend that the patient come in for an appointment. Explain why the medication should not be used: it may be old and no longer effective, the current problem may not be the same as the previous one, the medication

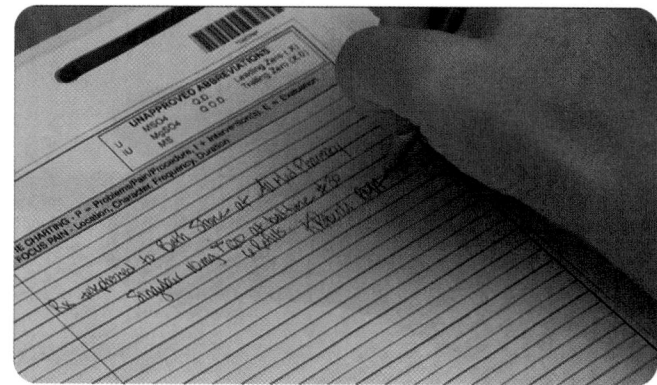

FIGURE 13-7   Documenting prescription refill.

may not be helpful, and using the medication may mask the symptoms of the current problem, making a diagnosis (and so identifying the proper treatment) more difficult.

If the patient does not want to make an appointment, relay the information to the physician. The physician will probably want to speak with the patient. Again, briefly document the conversation in the patient medical record.

Progress Reports   Physicians often ask patients to call the office to let them know how a prescribed treatment is working. If a patient has a satisfactory progress report to make to the doctor, it is not necessary that the patient speak to the physician. It is important that the medical assistant relay the information to the doctor and log the call in the patient's medical record immediately. You also may be responsible for making routine follow-up calls to patients to verify that they are following treatment instructions. See Figure 13-8 for an example of a patient's progress report made by

| **Patient Name:** | Mohammad Nassar | | **Date:** | 5/28/XX |

TC: Mohammad called in today to report that the addition of Flovent® to his medication regime is having a positive effect. He has used his rescue inhaler x2 in 3 days. Next appt in one week for recheck.
K. Haddix, RMA (AMT)

FIGURE 13-8   Patient progress note called in by telephone and documented in medical record.

FIGURE 13-9 Telephone message from a patient using SpringChart's EHR program.

Source: Screen captures of SpringCharts™ Electronic Health Records software are reprinted with permission from Spring Medical Systems, Inc. All rights reserved.

telephone. Figure 13-9 shows a similar patient update phone call documented using an EHR program.

Requests for Advice Sometimes patients call the office about problems or symptoms they are having. Although a patient may ask you for your medical opinion, as a medical assistant, you are not licensed to give medical advice of any kind. Explain that you are not trained to make a diagnosis or licensed to prescribe medication. Stress that the patient must see the physician. Listen attentively to the patient. If the patient is in real distress, try to schedule an appointment that day or as soon as possible.

If the patient cannot come into the office, assure her that the physician will return the call or that you will call back after discussing the problem with the physician. Write down the patient's symptoms completely, accurately, and immediately. In many instances, the physician may be able to suggest simple emergency relief measures that you can relay to the patient. Occasionally, a patient will want to speak only with the physician, not other staff members. You must honor this request.

In some cases, the physician may feel that a patient's symptoms warrant immediate attention and will insist on seeing the patient before prescribing any treatment. If the patient refuses to come to the office, note the reason on the chart and suggest a visit to the emergency room or to a nearby physician or urgent care center. As discussed in the *Legal and Ethical Issues* chapter, it is important to document such conversations completely in the patient's chart, including the refusal of treatment. It is always appropriate and professional to offer to take a message to have the physician return the call. Figure 13-10 gives an example of such documentation.

Complaints Even when an office provides the highest quality care, complaints still occur. When a patient calls

---

Patient Name: Ken Washington   **Date:** 3/1/XX

TC: Patient called today stating he has had severe headaches over the last week. Advil is not helping. Requesting refill of Imitrex® as the meds he has have expired. Dr. Buckwalter requested pt come in for BP check. Pt refused stating he does not have time. Dr. Buckwalter informed of pt refusal. He will call pt.
M. Perez, CMA (AAMA)

FIGURE 13-10 Chart note documenting patient refusal of treatment request.

with a complaint, such as a medication that does not appear to be working, it is important to listen carefully, without interrupting. Take careful notes of all the details and read them back to the caller to ensure that you have written them down correctly. Let the caller know the person to whose attention you will bring the complaint and, if possible, when to expect a response.

Always apologize to the caller for any inconvenience the problem may have caused, even if the problem occurred through no fault of the office. Make sure the proper person receives the information about the complaint.

Sometimes a patient who calls with a complaint is angry. Responding to this type of call can be difficult and uncomfortable. Your first priority is to stay calm and try to pacify the caller. Follow these guidelines when dealing with an angry caller.

- Listen carefully and acknowledge the patient's anger. By understanding the problem, you will be better able to work toward a solution.
- Remain calm and speak gently and kindly. Do not act superior or talk down to the patient. Do not interrupt the patient. Do not return the anger or blame.
- Let the patient know that you will do your best to correct the problem. This message will convey that you care.
- Take careful notes and be sure to document the call.
- Do not become defensive.
- Never make promises you cannot keep.
- Follow up promptly on the problem.
- Any time a staff member has a difficult time with a patient, it is important to inform the physician, even when the situation is resolved. Always inform the physician immediately if an angry patient threatens legal action against the office.

Other Calls

Besides calls from patients, a medical office receives many other types of calls. For example, family members and friends of patients may call the physician at the office. However, the use of the office telephone is never appropriate for personal calls. The physician will let you know how to handle these calls.

Remember, a patient's information is confidential. HIPAA requires medical providers to obtain authorization from the patient before any information can be disclosed. This is usually in the form of a written, patient-signed authorization indicating what type of information may be given out and to whom. The following are guidelines for managing calls from attorneys, other physicians, and salespeople.

Attorneys Refer to the procedures listed in the office policies and procedures manual regarding how to handle calls from attorneys. Follow the office guidelines closely and ask the physician or practice manager how to proceed if you receive a call that does not fall within the guidelines. Remember, never release any patient information to an outside caller unless the physician has asked you to do so.

Other Physicians Patients at your practice may be referred to surgeons, specialists, and other physicians for consultations. Consequently, you may receive calls from those physicians or from their offices. Route those calls to the physician if the caller requests that you do so. Always remember to ask if the call is about a medical emergency. Also keep in mind that you may not give out any patient information—even to another physician—unless you have a written, signed release from the patient. The exception to this rule is information requested by physicians to whom you have referred the patient for care. Because of the referral, there is a contract involved for continuity of care. You may release medical information specific to the care that the physician has been asked to provide.

Salespeople As a medical assistant, you will probably be the contact for salespeople, unless the office policy manual states that another staff member should handle this duty. On the telephone, ask the salesperson to send you information about any new products or equipment. Pharmaceutical sales representatives may want to meet with the physician. Forward such messages to the physician with a request to let you know when to schedule the appointment. Many physicians see pharmaceutical sales representatives on certain days at specific times. Sometimes they limit the number of representatives they will see in one day or one week. Make sure you know your office policy and each physician's preferences.

Conference Calls Periodically, physicians may need to have a conference call with several individuals. For example, the physician, the nurse, and the medical assistant may need to talk with the insurance company representative at the same time. Telephone conferencing is an ideal setup in this case. Most of today's telephone equipment has features for establishing and joining conference calls.

▶ Managing Incoming Calls LO 13.5

Screening Calls

Even if your office uses an automated answering unit, it is likely that part of your responsibility as the office medical assistant will be screening calls. Screening involves deciding which calls should be put through immediately and which calls are better handled by taking a message and allowing a callback at a more convenient time. The Points on Practice section on the next page describes some guidelines for screening calls. The procedure will remain basically the same, whether the calls come directly to you as you answer the phone or are directed to you by a telephone answering system.

Routing Calls

Incoming phone calls can generally be separated into three distinct groups: calls dealing mainly with administrative issues; emergency calls that require immediate action by the physician; and calls relating to clinical issues that require the attention of the physician, physician assistant, nurse practitioner, office

POINTS ON PRACTICE
Screening Incoming Calls

Each medical office has its own policy about how to screen incoming calls before transferring them to the appropriate person. Calls come not only from patients but also from other physicians, hospital personnel, pharmacists, insurance company personnel, sales representatives, and family members and friends of patients. Here are some general tips for screening calls.

Find out who is calling. A polite way to do this is to say, "May I ask who is calling?" Another option is, "May I tell Dr. Williams who is calling?"

Ask what the call is in reference to. When a caller asks to speak with the physician, you should ask the purpose of the call. Depending on the answer, you may determine that you or someone else in the office can handle the situation without disturbing the physician. The response may be as simple as solving a billing problem or clarifying instructions. Remember to consider the scope of practice for each member of the healthcare team when you transfer a call. Emergency calls should be transferred to the physician right away.

Decide whether the call should be put through. Although most calls are routed to the appropriate person, any callers who refuse to identify themselves should not be put through. In such a case, suggest that the caller write a letter to the physician and mark it "Personal."

Determine what to do if the matter is personal. The physician may ask you to take a message in these instances. Inform the caller that the physician will return the call as soon as possible.

TABLE 13-2 Symptoms and Conditions Requiring Immediate Medical Assistance

- Unconsciousness
- Lack of breathing (apnea) or difficulty breathing (dyspnea)
- Severe bleeding
- Pressure or pain in the abdomen that will not go away
- Severe vomiting or bloody stools
- Poisoning
- Injuries to the head, neck, or back
- Choking
- Drowning
- Electrical shock
- Snake bites
- Vehicle collisions
- Allergic reactions to foods or insect stings
- Chemical or foreign objects in the eye
- Fires, severe burns, or injuries from explosions
- Human bites or any deep animal bites
- Heart attack. Symptoms include chest pain or pressure; pain radiating from the chest to the arm, shoulder, neck, jaw, back, or stomach; nasuea or vomiting; sweating; weakness; shortness of breath; pale or gray skin color.
- Stroke. Symptoms include seizures, severe headache, slurred speech, and sudden inability or difficulty in moving a body part or one side of the body.
- Broken bones. Symptoms include being unable to move or bear weight on the injured body part. The injured part is very painful or looks misshapen.
- Shock. Symptoms include paleness; feeling faint and sweaty; weak, rapid pulse; cold, moist skin; confusion or drowsiness.
- Heatstroke (sunstroke). Symptoms include confusion or loss of consciousness; flushed skin that is hot and may be moist or dry; strong, rapid pulse.
- Hypothermia (drop in body temperature during prolonged exposure to cold). Symptoms include becoming increasingly clumsy, unreasonable, irritable, confused, and sleepy; slurred speech; slipping into a coma with slow, weak breathing and heartbeat.

If someone calls the office on behalf of a patient who is experiencing any of these symptoms or conditions, you may instruct the caller to dial 911 to request an ambulance. Procedure 13-4 at the end of the chapter describes the steps for handling emergency calls. If in the office, the physician should be called to the telephone immediately to offer assistance.

---

nurse, or clinical medical assistant. Procedure 13-3 at the end of this chapter will provide the outline for you to practice screening and routing calls.

Calls Requiring the Physician's Attention Certain calls will require the doctor's personal attention. These include the following:

- Emergency calls that include serious or life-threatening medical conditions, such as severe bleeding, a reaction to a drug, injuries, poisoning, suicide attempts, loss of consciousness, severe burns, or whatever your medical office deems an emergency; Table 13-2 lists symptoms and conditions that require immediate help.
- Calls from other doctors.
- Patient requests to discuss test results, particularly abnormal results.
- Reports from patients concerning unsatisfactory progress.
- Requests for prescription renewals (unless previously authorized in the patient's chart).
- Personal calls.

Most physicians have a set time, such as a half hour in the late morning or at the end of the day, for returning nonemergency patient calls. If a patient prefers to discuss symptoms with the physician, you may tell the patient to expect a phone call from the physician at this set time. If the physician does not have a set time for returning phone calls, do not make a commitment as to the time of the return phone call.

In many practices, some of these calls may be handled by others on the staff, such as a nurse practitioner or physician assistant. For example, a nurse practitioner may be able to order a renewal of a regular prescription, provide advice for the care of a sprain, or answer well-baby questions or questions about the side effects of a drug.

Calls Handled by the Medical Assistant

The most common calls to a medical office involve administrative and clinical issues. Depending on the practice, the office manager or someone in the billing department may handle some administrative calls. The calls handled by the medical assistant may include:

- Appointments (scheduling, rescheduling, canceling).
- Questions concerning office policies, fees, and hours.
- Billing inquiries.
- Insurance questions.
- Other administrative questions.
- X-ray and laboratory reports.
- Reports from hospitals regarding a patient's progress.
- Reports from patients concerning their progress.
- Requests for referrals to other doctors.
- Requests for prescription renewals, where prior approval for refills is noted in the chart.
- Complaints from patients about administrative matters.

The Routing List

Each medical office has a standard policy that documents how incoming telephone calls are to be routed and handled. A routing list, like the one shown in Figure 13-11, specifies who is responsible for the various types of calls in the office and how the calls are to be handled. For example, the routing list indicates which calls should be put through to the doctor immediately and which ones can be returned later.

The routing procedure may simply identify the general title of the person responsible for handling a call. When more than one person in the office have the same title, however, the name of the individual who has that particular responsibility should be specified.

Telephone Triage

Some physicians delegate some of the clinical decision making that is done over the telephone to other experienced staff members. In these instances, **telephone triage** is used to decide what action to take. The word *triage* refers to the screening and sorting of emergency incidents. Performing triage correctly is an important skill.

Using Triage Guidelines

Proper office staff training is vital in providing safe, sound, and cost-effective medical care over the telephone. An increasing number of medical practices are preparing guidelines for the telephone staff to follow when patients call the office with specific medical problems or questions.

Guidelines are often written for common questions, such as how to deal with sniffles and fevers during cold and flu season or how to make a child with chickenpox more comfortable. Members of the telephone staff must realize, however, that their responsibility is to determine whether a caller

HANDLING INCOMING TELEPHONE CALLS			
	Route to doctor immediately	Take message for doctor	Route to nurse or assistant
Emergencies: bleeding, drug/allergic reaction, difficulty breathing, injury, pain, poisoning, shock, unconsciousness, incoherence or hysteria	X		
Calls from other physicians	if possible		
Patient progress report		X	
Patient request for laboratory report		X (if abnormal)	Kaylyn (if normal)
Patient questions re medication		X	
Patient questions re billing or insurance			Miguel
Patient complaints			Kaylyn
Appointments			Kaylyn
Prescription renewals or refills		X	
Office business			Miguel
Personal business		X	
Salespeople			Miguel

FIGURE 13-11 The routing list identifies the staff member responsible for each type of incoming call.

needs additional medical care. They cannot diagnose or treat the patient's problem.

Office guidelines outline the specific information the telephone staff must obtain from the patient. In general, this information is the same type as that obtained during an office visit and should include the patient's age, the patient's symptoms, when the problem began, and the patient's level of anxiety about the problem.

Categorizing Problems and Providing Patient Education After the patient information is obtained, the guidelines help the staff categorize the problem according to severity. The medical assistant then decides whether the problem can be handled safely with advice over the telephone, the patient needs to come into the office, or the problem requires immediate attention at an emergency room. For instance, if a caller is having chest pains, you would be performing a type of triage by instructing him to go to the emergency room immediately, preferably by ambulance.

If a problem is deemed appropriate for telephone management, the guidelines may include recommendations for nonprescription treatment that may relieve symptoms and anxiety. This information falls under the category of patient education. Advise the caller that recommendations are based on the symptoms and are not a diagnosis. Remember, only the doctor is authorized to make a diagnosis and prescribe medication. Ask the caller to repeat any instructions you give and tell the patient to call back within a specified time if symptoms do not improve or worsen. Be sure to document in the medical record the critical elements of the conversation that relate to the patient's health status.

▶ Taking Complete and Accurate Phone Messages

LO 13.6

Always have paper or telephone message pad (Figure 13-12) and pen near the telephone so that you are prepared to write down messages. Proper documentation protects the physician if the caller takes legal action. A record of telephone calls also should be included in a patient's file or electronic health record as part of a complete medical history. Because of their importance as part of the patient's legal health record, messages should never be taken on pieces of scrap paper, which are easily misplaced or accidentally discarded.

Documenting Calls

Documenting telephone calls is essential in a medical office, and several options are available to assist the administrative medical assistant with taking a complete message every time. You can use the previously mentioned telephone message pads, a manual telephone log book, or an electronic (computerized) telephone log. Again, remember that many calls (for example, those concerning clinical problems or referrals) and the actions or decisions they lead to must be documented in patients' charts. Every entry into a patient's chart

FIGURE 13-12 Using a telephone message pad ensures that no important information is omitted when the message form is filled out completely.

is considered a legal document, so the information must be accurate and legible.

Telephone Message Pads You can use preprinted telephone message pads, which often come in brightly colored paper, to record the following information:

- Date and time of the call.
- Name of the person for whom you took the message.
- Caller's name, or the patient's name if different from the caller.
- Caller's telephone number (always include the area code and extension, if any).
- A description or an action to be taken, including comments like "Urgent," "Please call back," "Wants to see you," "Will call back," or "Returned your call."
- The complete message, such as "Dr. Stephenson wants to reschedule the committee meeting."
- Name or initials of the person taking the call.

Figure 13-13 shows an example of a completed preprinted telephone message.

The Manual Telephone Log Some medical offices use spiral-bound, perforated message books with carbonless forms to record messages (refer to Figure 13-12). The top copy, or original, of each message is given to the appropriate person and a copy is kept in the book for future reference in the event that the original is misplaced or accidentally destroyed.

TELEPHONE MESSAGE

BWW
BWW Medical Associates, PC

For: _Kaylyn Haddix_

Patient calling as requested with update. She is feeling much

better after 3 days on Abx. Temperature is back to normal. No more

sore throat; body aches and pains are less.

Name of Caller: _Shenya Jones_

Name of Patient (if not caller): _____

Date/Time Called: _4/12/20XX @ 11:15 a.m._

Message Taken by: _M.Perez, CMA(AAMA)_

FIGURE 13-13 It is important that messages be filled out as completely as possible.

The Electronic Telephone Log Some medical offices use an electronic or computer-based system to record messages. The message is keyed in as it is received, creating an automatic backup copy for the office record. A copy of the message can be stored in an electronic record, printed out, or e-mailed as needed.

Tips for Ensuring Accurate Messages The following suggestions will help you provide accurate documentation for incoming messages:

- Always have a pen and paper on hand.
- Jot down notes as the information is given.
- Verify information, especially the spelling of patient or caller names and the correct spelling of medications.
- Obtain the patient's full name and date of birth if pulling the chart is necessary, in case there are two patients with the same name.
- Verify the correct callback number.
- When taking a phone message for the physician, never make a commitment on behalf of the physician by saying, "I'll have the physician call you." A more appropriate response would be, "I will give your message to the physician."

Maintaining Patient Confidentiality

When you are on the phone with a patient discussing confidential information, be aware of the people around you and the volume of your voice when verifying such information. If necessary, move to a private office for such conversations so that patient confidentiality will not be inadvertently breached. When leaving patient messages for the physician containing confidential information, insert the message in a folder marked "Confidential" so it cannot readily be seen by others.

▶ Placing Outgoing Calls   LO 13.7

You will often be required to place outgoing calls on behalf of the medical office. You may need to return calls, obtain information, provide patient education, pick up messages from the answering service or voicemail, or arrange patient consultations with other physicians. If you are making a long-distance call, it is important to determine the time zone and the time of day in the location you are calling before you place the call. Time zones can be determined by checking the front of the phone book, going online, or speaking with a telephone operator. For information on time zones, go to www.time.gov.

Locating Telephone Numbers

The medical office should have at least one telephone directory, or telephone book, for the local calling area and perhaps additional directories for surrounding areas. Use these books, an Internet phone directory such as www.anywho.com/ (by AT&T), the company website, or call for directory assistance to locate telephone numbers for outside calls. The office also may have a card file, a list, or an electronic record of commonly used telephone numbers, or these numbers may be listed in the office policies and procedures manual. If you are calling a patient, the telephone number should be in the patient's chart.

If you need to find a long-distance telephone number, many offices use the directory assistance service. You can reach this service by dialing 1-[area code]-555-1212. You also can search the Internet for free "411" services. Use directory assistance only when you have exhausted other options, however, because most long-distance carriers charge a fee each time you use the service. If you are required to call out of the country, you will need to use an international dialing code. These codes, as well as area codes and long-distance numbers, can be located through the Internet and through directory assistance. Two websites that are helpful for finding information on area codes are www.lincmad.com/areacodemap.html and www.nanpa.com.

Applying Your Telephone Skills

You can apply the telephone skills you use for answering incoming calls when placing outgoing calls. Here are additional tips for handling outgoing calls:

- Plan before you call. Have all the information you need in front of you before you dial the telephone number. Plan what you will say and decide what questions to ask so you will not have to call back for additional information.

- Double-check the telephone number. If in doubt, look it up in the telephone directory. If you do dial a wrong number, be sure to apologize for the mistake.
- Allow enough time, at least a minute or about eight rings, for someone to answer the telephone. When calling patients who are elderly or physically disabled, allow additional time.
- Identify yourself. After reaching the person to whom you placed the call, give your name and state that you are calling on behalf of the doctor or practice.
- Ask if you have called at a convenient time and whether the person has time to talk with you. If it is not a good time, ask when you should call back.
- Be ready to speak as soon as the person you called answers the telephone. Do not waste the person's time while you collect your thoughts.
- If you are calling to give information, ask if the person has a pencil and piece of paper available. Do not begin with dates, times, or instructions until the person is ready to write down the information.

Reaching Voicemail or an Answering Machine On occasion, it is important to leave a message on a patient's answering machine or on his voicemail. It is now required by HIPAA law that you use these pieces of equipment correctly and confidentially to guard the patient's private medical information. The goal in calling a patient's home is to speak directly to the patient or to leave a message with enough information to get the patient to call back. It is unlawful to disclose confidential patient information to anyone but the patient. HIPAA requires that you *never* leave any information if you are unsure of the phone number dialed. As a medical assistant, you cannot ensure that only the intended patient will receive any message left on an answering machine or voicemail. To guard the patient's privacy, *state only the following information*:

- The name of the individual for whom the message is intended.
- The date and time of the call.
- The name of your office or practice (see caution below).
- Your name as the contact person in the office (see caution below).
- The phone number of your office or practice.
- The hours the office is open for a return call.

A word of caution: Leave the name of the practice only if it does not reveal the purpose of the call. For instance, you would not state, "Please call Tiffany Heath from the STD Clinic." An example of an appropriate substitute would be, "Please call Tiffany Heath from Dr. Greene's office at 413-788-0001, Monday through Friday between 8 a.m. and 5 p.m."

Alternatively, when patients sign the Office Privacy Agreement, a release may be added inquiring if messages may be left on an answering machine or voicemail and if there are any restrictions to that permission. A second release also may be added asking if there is anyone at the home number to whom the office may speak and the relationship of that person to the patient. Each release should be signed and dated by the patient.

Improper or careless use of a patient's answering system or voicemail (or fax machine) can be viewed as abusive behavior in the eyes of the law. It is imperative that the patient's right to privacy be carefully guarded at all times. If in doubt whether a patient's privacy might be violated by leaving a verbal (or written message) on a machine, it is best to leave no message at all but to attempt to reach the patient at a different time. Further information regarding this topic can be accessed on the HIPAA website, www.hipaa.org.

Retrieving Messages from the Answering System or Service

If callers are allowed to leave messages on an answering machine or a voicemail system, the medical assistant is usually responsible for retrieving these messages at the start of each day and, if the office closes for a lunch break, to check for messages after this break as well. Never use the speakerphone setting when retrieving messages from an answering machine, as a patient may leave personal information in a message that might be heard by others in the office. This could be considered a breach of patient confidentiality.

When an answering service is used, it is a good idea to call the service to retrieve messages at a set time (or multiple times, if the service or system is employed during office hours) each day. In doing so, you ensure that messages are not missed. When calling the service to retrieve messages, as when taking any message, verify the information for correctness and completeness before ending the call. Procedure 13-5, located at the end of this chapter, describes how to do this.

Arranging Conference Calls

It may be necessary for you to schedule conference calls with patients, hospital personnel, or other doctors to discuss tests or surgical results. When dealing with several people, suggest several time slots in case someone is not available at a particular time. Also keep in mind the various time zones in the country. Make sure that all the conference call participants are given the proper time in their time zone to expect the call. As mentioned earlier in this chapter, the office phone system will likely have an option allowing you to set up a conference call.

Additionally, there are services that provide "call-in conferencing." The host will provide a number and the time for you or your physician to call in as a participant, or your office may host the call. All of the participants are given a code and are asked to identify themselves as they call into the system. They will ask for an e-mail address to confirm the information, time, date, and passcodes that will be given to each individual. More information on free conference calling services can be found online. Two such services can be found at www.freeconference.com and www.freeconferencecalling.com.

PROCEDURE 13-1 Using a Telecommunications Device for the Deaf (TDD)

Procedure Goal: To properly communicate with the hearing-impaired patient using a TDD.

OSHA Guidelines: This procedure does not involve exposure to blood, body fluids, or tissue.

Materials: Telephone, TDD (if available), patient chart for documentation, and a pen.

Method: Procedure steps.

Answering a Call with a TDD

1. Answer the phone as usual. If you hear a rapid clicking sound, you know you have a TDD call. You may hear no sound at all; do not hang up, as it may still be a TDD call.
   RATIONALE: It is important to listen carefully, so as to not hang up on the patient.

2. If you know (or believe) this is a TDD call, place your phone receiver on the TDD as directed.

3. Type your normal office greeting: "BWW Medical Associates, this is Miguel. How may I help you?"
   RATIONALE: It is important to always identify the practice and then yourself, so the caller knows he has reached the correct party.

4. When you complete your message, type "GA," which stands for "Go Ahead." This tells the patient you have completed your message and it is his turn to respond.

5. Give the patient time to type his response. When you see "GA" at the end of his message, it is your turn to respond.

6. When the patient receives all of the information required, he will type "Bye, SK," which stands for Good-Bye, Stop Keying.

7. If you agree the call is completed, you may also reply "Bye, SK." This will give the patient the opportunity to be the one to end the call.

8. When you receive a response of SKSK (Stop Keying, Stop Keying), the conversation is complete and you may hang up and turn off the TDD.
   RATIONALE: As with a hearing/speaking patient, it is important to let the person initiating the call also be the person to end the call. This way, you know you have answered all questions and provided all needed information to the caller.

Making a Call with a TDD

1. Turn on the TDD.

2. Dial the patient's phone number on your standard telephone and listen for the phone to ring.

3. When you hear the TDD sound, place the phone receiver on the TDD as directed.

4. After the patient types a greeting and "GA" appears on the TDD display, identify yourself and proceed with the conversation.
   RATIONALE: It is important to always identify yourself and where you are calling from when making any call.

5. Remember to type "GA" when you complete your message so the patient knows it is his turn to respond.
   RATIONALE: This is the only way the patient will know you have completed your communication and it is his turn to respond.

6. Even though you were the one to initiate the call, you should still allow the patient to make the decision that the call is completed by keying "SKSK."
   RATIONALE: You are providing a service to the patient. It is important to make sure that all information has been received and understood by him by letting him end the call.

PROCEDURE 13-2 Renewing a Prescription by Telephone

Procedure Goal: To ensure a complete and accurate prescription is received by the patient.

OSHA Guidelines: This procedure does not involve exposure to blood, body fluids, or tissue.

Materials: Telephone, appropriate phone numbers, message pad or prescription refill request form, pen, and patient chart with prescription order.

Method: Procedure steps.

1. Take the message from the call or the message system. For the prescription to be complete, you must obtain the patient's name, date of birth, phone number, pharmacy name and/or phone number, medication, and dosage.

2. Follow your facility policy regarding prescription renewals. Typically, the prescription is usually called into the pharmacy the day it is requested. An example policy may be posted at the facility and may state,

"Nonemergency prescription refill requests must be made during regular business hours. Please allow 24 hours for processing."

3. Communicate the policy to the patient. You should know the policy and the time when the refills will be reviewed. For example, you might state, "Dr. Williams will review the prescription between patients and it will be telephoned within one hour to the pharmacy. I will call you back if there is a problem."
   RATIONALE: Letting the patient know the policy demonstrates good communication skills and will result in less misunderstandings as to when the prescription will be available for pickup.

4. Obtain the patient's chart or reference the electronic chart to verify you have the correct patient and that the patient is currently taking the medication. Check the patient's list of medications, which are usually part of the chart.

5. Give the prescription refill request and the chart to the physician or prescriber. Do not give a prescription refill request to the physician without the chart or chart access information. Wait for an authorization from the physician before you proceed.
RATIONALE: All prescription refills must be authorized by the physician.

6. Once the physician authorizes the prescription, prepare to call the pharmacy with the renewal information. Be certain to have the physician order, the patient's chart, and the refill request in front of you when you make the call. The request should include the name of the drug, the drug dosage, the frequency and mode of administration, the number of refills authorized, and the pharmacy's name and phone number. Note: You cannot call in Schedule II or III medications; these are medication that have the greatest possibility of abuse. Renewals can be called in for Schedule IV and V medications.

7. Telephone the pharmacy. Identify yourself by name, the practice name, and the doctor's name.
RATIONALE: Only an identified representative from a medical practice can authorize a prescription refill.

8. State the purpose of the call. (Example: "This is Miguel Perez from BWW Medical Associates. I am calling to request a prescription refill for a patient.")

9. Identify the patient. Include the patient's name, date of birth, address, and phone number.

RATIONALE: It is essential that the correct drug be prescribed for the correct patient according to the physician's order.

10. Identify the drug (spelling the name when necessary), the dosage, the frequency and mode of administration, and any other special instructions or changes for administration (such as "take at bedtime").
RATIONALE: Accuracy and complete information are essential for medication administration.

11. State the number of refills authorized.

12. If leaving a message on a pharmacy voicemail system set up for physicians, state your name, the name of the doctor you represent, and your phone number before you hang up.
RATIONALE: If the pharmacist has any questions, he must be able to reach the physician.

13. Document the prescription renewal in the chart after the medication has been called into the pharmacy. Include the date, the time, the name of the pharmacy, and the person taking your call. Also include the medication, dose, amount, directions, and number of refills. Sign your first initial, last name, and title. An example of charting is as follows:

5/03/XX Rx telephoned to Beth Stone at Noname Pharmacy: Zyrtec 10 mg, one tablet daily at bedtime, #30, 6 refills _____
_____ M.A. Perez, CMA (AAMA)

PROCEDURE 13-3 Screening and Routing Telephone Calls

Procedure Goal: To properly screen incoming telephone calls.

OSHA Guidelines: This procedure does not involve exposure to blood, body fluids, or tissue.

Materials: Telephone, telephone pad, pen or pencil, appointment book or computerized scheduling software (computer), and office routing list.

Method: Procedure steps.
Use the office routing list to route calls appropriately.

1. Make sure all of the materials are within reach of the telephone equipment.

2. Answer the telephone promptly within two to three rings.

3. Identify the medical office and identify yourself. Make sure you know office procedure for answering the phone in your facility even if a telephone answering system is employed to route calls to you. For example: "BWW Medical Associates, this is Malik, how may I help you?"

4. If the caller does not identify himself, ask him to do so and the number he is calling from, and write down this information. Find out the reason for the call. Is it

an emergency? (Refer to Table 13-2.) If so, follow office policy.
RATIONALE: As soon as you make certain a call is an emergency, it is important for the patient's welfare that you follow the office protocol for these situations.

5. If you can handle the call, take care of the query. Listen carefully to what the caller has to say, paying particular attention to tone and feeling.
RATIONALE: If the caller's query is within your scope of practice and job description, it is up to you to take care of the patient's problem or request as quickly and professionally as possible.

6. If this is a call that needs to be transferred to someone (per the routing list), tell the caller to whom and to what number you will be transferring the call. Make sure you write down the caller's name and phone number in case the call is accidentally dropped. If the other staff member does not answer promptly or is on another line, ask the caller if he would like to be transferred to the staff member's voicemail (if available) or would like to leave a message.

HANDLING INCOMING TELEPHONE CALLS			
	Route to doctor immediately	Take message for doctor	Route to nurse or assistant
Emergencies: bleeding, drug/allergic reaction, difficulty breathing, injury, pain, poisoning, shock, unconsciousness, incoherence or hysteria	X		
Calls from other physicians	if possible		
Patient progress report		X	
Patient request for laboratory report		X (if abnormal)	Kaylyn (if normal)
Patient questions re medication		X	
Patient questions re billing or insurance			Miguel
Patient complaints			Kaylyn
Appointments			Kaylyn
Prescription renewals or refills		X	
Office business			Miguel
Personal business		X	
Salespeople			Miguel

FIGURE Procedure 13-3 Step 6   Use the office routing list to route calls appropriately.

PROCEDURE 13-4 Handling Emergency Calls

Procedure Goal: To determine whether a telephone call involves a medical emergency and to learn the steps to take if it is an emergency call.

OSHA Guidelines: This procedure does not involve exposure to blood, body fluids, or tissue.

Materials: Office guidelines for handling emergency calls; list of symptoms and conditions requiring immediate medical attention; telephone numbers of area emergency rooms, poison control centers, and ambulance transport services; and telephone message forms or a telephone message log.

Method: Procedure steps.

1. When someone calls the office regarding a potential emergency, remain calm.
   RATIONALE: This attitude will help calm the caller and enable you to gather necessary information in the most efficient manner.

2. Obtain the following information, taking accurate notes:
   a. The caller's name.
   b. The caller's telephone number and the address from which the call is being made.
   RATIONALE: It may be necessary for you to put the call on hold or to hang up so you can call for medical assistance. Before you do so, however, be sure to read the information back to the caller to ensure that you have written it down correctly. If you deem the call a medical emergency, ask another medical assistant to dial 911 and give the information you have written down.
   c. The caller's relationship to the patient (if it is not the patient who is calling).
   d. The patient's name (if the patient is not the caller).
   e. The patient's age.

f. A complete description of the patient's symptoms.
g. If the call is about an accident, a description of how the accident or injury occurred and any other pertinent information.
h. A description of how the patient is reacting to the situation.
i. Treatment that has been administered.

3. Read back the details of the medical problem to verify them.
   RATIONALE: Details are necessary to determine whether or not an emergency exists and the steps you need to take next.

4. If necessary, refer to the list of symptoms and conditions that require immediate medical attention to determine if the situation is indeed a medical emergency.

If the Situation Is a Medical Emergency

1. Put the call through to the doctor immediately, or handle the situation according to the established office procedures.
   RATIONALE: Medical emergencies take precedence over all other matters.

2. If the doctor is not in the office, follow established office procedures. These may involve one or more of the following:
   a. Transferring the call to the nurse practitioner or other medical personnel, as appropriate;
   b. Instructing the caller (if not the patient) to hang up and dial 911 to request an ambulance for the patient;
   c. Instructing the patient to be driven to the nearest emergency room;
   d. Instructing the caller to telephone the nearest poison control center for advice and supplying the caller with its telephone number; and/or
   e. Paging the doctor.

7. If you need to take a message, make sure you repeat the information that is given to you, especially the name of the person and his phone number. Take a complete message.
   RATIONALE: If the message is not complete, the person receiving it may not take the appropriate action or the patient may end up needlessly being directed to multiple people.

If the Situation Is Not a Medical Emergency

1. Handle the call according to established office procedures.
2. If you are in doubt about whether the situation is a medical emergency, treat it like an emergency. You must always alert the doctor immediately about an emergency call, even if the patient declines to speak with the doctor.
   RATIONALE: It is better to be overly cautious than to let an emergency go untreated. The doctor should be the one to decide how to handle these situations.

PROCEDURE 13-5 Retrieving Messages from an Answering Service or System

Procedure Goal: To follow standard procedures for retrieving messages from an answering service or system.

OSHA Guidelines This procedure does not involve exposure to blood, body fluids, or tissue.

Materials: Telephone message pad, manual telephone log, or electronic telephone log.

Method Procedure steps.

1. Set a regular schedule for calling the answering service (system) to retrieve messages.
   RATIONALE: A regular schedule ensures the procedure will not be forgotten and calls will not be missed.
2. Call at the regularly scheduled time(s) to see if there are any messages.
3. If calling a service, identify yourself and state that you are calling to obtain messages for the practice.
   RATIONALE: Most services have a list of people at the office who are allowed to pick up messages.
4. If calling an answering system, when the call is answered, you will enter the passcode for the office.
   RATIONALE: The passcode is given only to staff members allowed to retrieve messages.
5. For each message, write down all pertinent information on the telephone message pad or telephone log, or key it into the electronic telephone log. Be sure to include the caller's name and telephone number, time of call, message or description of the problem, and action taken, if any.

FIGURE Procedure 13-5 Step 5 Write down all pertinent information to take a complete message.

   RATIONALE: Always take a complete message for the convenience of the caller and the person receiving the message.
6. If calling an answering service, repeat the information, confirming you have the correct spelling of all names and the complete, correct information.
   RATIONALE: This step ensures you have the information correct.
7. If calling an answering system, be sure you listen carefully and replay messages if necessary to get complete information given within each message.
   RATIONALE: This step ensures you have complete and correct information.
8. When you have retrieved all messages, route them according to office policy.

LEARNING OUTCOMES	KEY POINTS
13.2 Relate the five Cs of effective communication to telephone communication skills.	The five Cs of effective communication are important in all types of communication and the telephone is no exception. All forms of communication are more easily understood using these principles: completeness of the message, clarity of the message, conciseness of the information, courtesy when delivering the message, and cohesiveness (logic and organization) of the message.
13.3 Define the following terms involved in making a good impression on the telephone: telephone etiquette, pitch, pronunciation, enunciation, and tone.	Telephone etiquette means to handle all calls professionally and politely using good manners. Pitch is the high or low level of your voice, projecting interest in what you are saying. Pronunciation is saying words correctly and enunciation is saying them clearly. Tone projects how you are feeling; in the office, your tone should always be positive and respectful.
13.4 Describe how to appropriately handle the different types of calls coming into the medical practice.	The medical assistant may receive calls from patients, attorneys, and others. Always refer to the office policies and procedures manual regarding how to handle incoming calls appropriately. Remember, always be courteous to the caller.
13.5 Summarize the purpose of the office routing list in regards to call screening.	Screening calls categorizes the importance of the call in regard to how quickly the patient's problem or question needs to be handled. The routing list is a guideline for the entire staff to recognize which types of calls should go to each member of the medical staff, following office protocol as to the duties and scope of practice for each team member.
13.6 Carry out the procedure for taking a complete telephone message.	In addition to complete information from the caller regarding what the call is about, each complete telephone message should contain the following information: date and time of the call; name of the person for whom the message was taken; the caller's name and name of the patient (if different from the caller); the caller's telephone number with area code; a description or action to be taken; a complete and concise message; and the name or initials of the person taking the message.
13.7 Outline the preparation required prior to making outgoing calls and the skills used in making the phone call.	Prior to placing an outgoing call, be sure to have all necessary information in front of you, including the name of the person to be reached and the correct phone number. Dial the number carefully, identifying yourself when the phone is answered, asking for the person you need to reach. As always, use the five Cs of communication to complete the exchange.

CASE STUDY CRITICAL THINKING

Recall Shenya Jones from the beginning of the chapter. Now that you have completed the chapter, answer the following questions regarding her case.

1. How should you best handle the situation of the two ringing phone lines while still responding to Shenya's request for an appointment?

2. Shenya is obviously upset. When you return to her, how might you handle her request for an appointment, considering the packed schedule?

1. (LO 13.1) Which of the following is NOT a common function of many of today's multiline phones?
   a. Transfer options
   b. Hold
   c. Voicemail
   d. Intercom
   e. Voice recognition

2. (LO 13.1) What is the main reason pagers are not used as often in medical offices?
   a. Physicians hate carrying them
   b. Improved healthcare means fewer "emergencies"
   c. Cell phones
   d. It is becoming harder to find signals for pagers
   e. c and d

3. (LO 13.2) Which of the following is NOT one of the five Cs of effective communication?
   a. Compassion
   b. Clarity
   c. Conciseness
   d. Cohesiveness
   e. Completeness

4. (LO 13.2) Which of the following is an appropriate statement for answering the office telephone?
   a. "Doctor's office, Jayden speaking."
   b. "Jayden here, this is BWW Medical Associates."
   c. "BWW Medical Associates, Jayden, hold please."
   d. "BWW Medical Associates; this is Jayden. How may I help you?"
   e. Any of the above are acceptable

5. (LO 13.3) The term for speaking clearly and distinctly is
   a. Tone
   b. Enunciation
   c. Etiquette
   d. Pronunciation
   e. Clarity

6. (LO 13.4) Which of the following are common reasons patients call the office?
   a. Appointment requests
   b. Billing inquiries
   c. Lab or X-ray reports
   d. Compliments to the medical staff
   e. a, b, and c

7. (LO 13.5) Deciding how emergent a patient's problem is and how it may best be handled is a procedure known as
   a. Screening
   b. Routing
   c. Triage
   d. Paging
   e. Etiquette

8. (LO 13.5) _____ is the term used when a call is transferred to an appropriate person based on the caller's request.
   a. Screening
   b. Routing
   c. Triage
   d. Paging
   e. Etiquette

9. (LO 13.6) Taking an effective message involves which of the following items?
   a. Date and time of call
   b. Whom the call is for
   c. Name and phone number of caller
   d. Message and action to be taken
   e. All of the above and more

10. (LO 13.7) When placing a call to a patient with medical information, if you reach the patient's answering machine, what should you do?
    a. Leave a complete message . . . it is the patient's private answering machine.
    b. Leave your name, the name of the practice, and your phone number so the patient may call back.
    c. Leave your name and phone number, stating there is a medical issue that requires discussion.
    d. Leave the practice name only if the reason for the call is not easily identifiable, your name, and your phone number. If unsure, try calling back at another time.
    e. Leave your name and number with no message.

Go to CONNECT to see activities on *Documenting a Patient Call, Sending an Internal Message Regarding a Patient, Processing an Internal Message Regarding a Patient, Creating a Non-Patient-Related Message, Archiving a Message,* and *Sending an Urgent Message.*

Patient Education

PATIENT INFORMATION

Patient Name	Gender	DOB
Sylvia Gonzales	F	9/1/19XX

Attending	MRN	Allergies
Alexis N. Whalen, MD	341-73-792	Penicillin

A 51-year-old female, Sylvia Gonzales, is at the office for a 3-month return check for newly diagnosed Type II diabetes. She appears overweight and is snacking on a bag of potato chips and chocolate milk when you bring her back into the exam room. She states she has taken the medication she was given for her "sugar" and she knows the doctor wants to do a special "sugar test" this time. Her medication list includes Januvia 100 mg daily, which is a medication to help lower her blood sugar.

Keep Sylvia Gonzales in mind as you study the chapter. There will be questions at the end of the chapter based on the case study. The information in the chapter will help you answer these questions.

LEARNING OUTCOMES

After completing Chapter 14, you will be able to:

14.1 Identify the benefits of patient education and the medical assistant's role in providing education.

14.2 Describe factors that affect learning and teaching.

14.3 Implement teaching techniques.

14.4 Choose reliable patient education materials used in the medical office.

14.5 Explain how patient education can be used to promote good health habits.

14.6 Describe the types of information that should be included in the patient information packet.

14.7 Describe the benefits and special considerations of patient education prior to surgery.

KEY TERMS

consumer education
factual teaching
modeling
participatory teaching

philosophy
return demonstration
screening
sensory teaching

IV. C (7) Identify resources and adaptations that are required based on individual needs, i.e., culture and environment, developmental life stage, language, and physical threats to communication

IV. C (9) Discuss applications of electronic technology in effective communication

IV. P (4) Explain the general office policies

IV. P (5) Instruct patients according to their needs to promote health maintenance and disease prevention

IV. P (9) Document patient education

IV. P (12) Develop and maintain a current list of community resources related to patients' health-care needs

V. P (5) Execute data management using electronic healthcare records such as the EMR

V. P (7) Use internet to access information related to the medical office

IX. C (3) Describe the implications of HIPAA for the medical assistant in various medical settings

IX. P (2) Perform within scope of practice

1. **General Orientation**
   e. Define scope of practice for the medical assistant, and comprehend the conditions for practice within the state that the medical assistant is employed

2. **Anatomy and Physiology**
   Graduates:
   a. Comprehend and explain to the patient the importance of diet and nutrition; effectively convey and educate patients regarding the proper diet and nutrition guidelines; identify categories of patients who require special diets or diet modifications

8. **Medical Office Business Procedures Management**
   Graduates:
   e. Locate resources and information for patients and employers
   cc. Communicate on the recipient's level of comprehension
   dd. Serve as liaison between physician and others
   hh. Receive, organize, prioritize, and transmit information expediently
   ii. Recognize and respond to verbal and nonverbal communication
   kk. Adapt to individualized needs
   ll. Apply electronic technology

9. **Medical Office Clinical Procedures**
   Graduates:
   p. Advise patients of policies and procedures
   q. Instruct patients with special needs
   r. Teach patients methods of health promotion and disease prevention

11. **Career Development**
   Graduates:
   b. Demonstrate professionalism by:
      (9) Conducting work within scope of education, training, and ability

▶ Introduction

Health education should be a lifelong pursuit for all of us. The ultimate goal of all medical professionals is to encourage and teach healthy habits and behaviors to all patients. People first have to understand what is good for them, and then they have to make a decision to follow that advice. In patient education, the medical assistant shares health information and encourages patients to make good health decisions.

In this chapter you will learn about patient education. Understanding your role and scope of practice related to patient education is necessary. Then you will develop skills in recognizing and overcoming roadblocks to education. You will become more comfortable with teaching and demonstrating

procedures to others. Most importantly, you will begin to recognize the incredible responsibility of the medical assistant to correctly lead others to their highest level of health.

▶ The Educated Patient

LO 14.1

Patient education is an essential process in the medical office. It encourages patients to take an active role in their medical care. It results in better compliance with treatment programs. When patients are suffering from illness, disease, or injury, education can often help them regain their health and independence more quickly. Simply put, patient education helps patients stay healthy. Educated patients are more likely to comply with instructions if they understand the "why" behind

Patient Education and Scope of Practice

A medical assistant must be competent and knowledgeable before he or she can provide patient education. If a physician asks you to perform education, the content of that education must be approved by that physician. You must understand the content in order to teach it, but you should not go beyond the content you have been asked to teach. In addition, while performing education, you must not make any judgments or answer any questions that require a diagnosis, assessment, or evaluation.

the instructions. Also, educated patients are more likely to be satisfied clients of the practice.

Patients benefit from education, but the medical office benefits as well. Preoperative instruction to surgical patients, for example, lessens the chance that procedures will have to be rescheduled because surgical guidelines were not followed. Educated patients will also be less likely to call the office with questions. Thus, the office staff will have to spend less time on the telephone.

Patient education takes many forms and includes a variety of techniques. It can be as simple as answering a question that comes up during a routine visit. Patient education may involve printed materials or patient participation. No matter what type of patient education is used, the goal is the same—to help patients help themselves attain better health.

As a medical assistant, you play a role in the process of patient education, primarily because of your constant interaction with patients in the office. The amount and type of education you provide will be decided by your place of employment and scope of practice. See Caution Handle with Care: Patient Education and Scope of Practice. As a medical assistant, even if you are not providing the education, you should be aware of the patient's educational needs and ability to understand. In addition, being a role model by practicing good health behaviors is important.

▶ Learning and Teaching   LO 14.2

In order to provide patient education, it is necessary to understand the process of learning. Learning is the acquiring of new knowledge, behaviors, or skills, which are also known as the *domains of learning*. Knowledge, the cognitive domain, includes the theoretical or practical understanding of a subject and the ability to recall it. Behavior, the affective domain, is how one approaches learning. It includes feelings, values, appreciation, enthusiasms, motivations, and attitudes. Skills, the psychomotor domain, include physical movement, coordination, and use of motor skills to complete a task. See Figure 14-1.

Sensory = Behaviors
(affective domain)

Factual = Knowledge
(cognitive domain)

Participatory = Skills
(psychomotor domain)

FIGURE 14-1   Learning occurs through the three domains: cognitive, affective, and psychomotor. Teaching is accomplished by factual, sensory, and participatory techniques.

To better understand these domains, let's use the example of our patient, Sylvia Gonzales, who just found out she is diabetic. In order for her to be able to manage her diabetes and have the best outcome for her health, she will need to learn through all three of the domains.

- *Cognitive (knowledge)*: Sylvia will need to understand and recall the basic information about diabetes, including the effects of diet, exercise, and treatments. The information can come in many formats, as discussed later in this chapter. This information must be available to the person who is doing the teaching, or the patient would need to find the information herself.
- *Affective (behaviors)*: Sylvia must have the desire or be motivated to make a change in order to improve her health. Once she appreciates the need, is motivated, and has a positive attitude, she will then be able to make the change. This is part of the learning process. If she does not have the desire to learn about diabetes or is not motivated to improve her health, she will not make any change. Being aware of a patient's level of motivation and encouraging the patient are important parts of the teaching process.
- *Psychomotor (skills)*: Once Sylvia has the basic knowledge and correct behavior, she will be able to learn and perform the skills necessary to improve her condition and keep her diabetes under control. This may include eating better foods, increasing exercise, and taking any medications that might be prescribed. These are all skills that are done as part of the learning process.

For learning to occur, all three domains of learning must be considered during the teaching process. The patient, Sylvia, must be provided the information, she must be motivated and have a desire to learn the information, and then she must perform the skills or "do" what is necessary to improve her condition.

▶ Teaching Techniques   LO 14.3

Patient education can take many forms. Any instructions—verbal, written, or demonstrative—that you give to patients are types of patient education. When providing education, three types of teaching can occur: **factual, sensory,** and **participatory.** These three types of teaching correspond to the three domains of learning.

The combination of these teaching methods gives the patient an overall understanding because it encourages learning through all three of the domains of learning.

Factual Teaching

Factual teaching informs the patient of details of the information that is being taught. For example, when preparing a patient for surgery, you should tell the patient what will happen during the surgery, when it will happen, and why the procedure is necessary. Factual information provided to a patient before surgery can also include restrictions on diet or activity that may be necessary both before and after surgery. Factual information is usually supported with written materials so the patient can refer to the information as needed at a later date.

Sensory Teaching

Sensory teaching provides patients with a description of the physical sensations they may have as part of the learning or procedure involved. This learning relates to how the person is affected, that is, the affective domain. For example, prior to surgery you might need to explain how much pain or what other sensations, such as numbness or tingling, the patient may feel. All five senses may be involved: feeling, seeing, hearing, tasting, and smelling.

Participatory Teaching

Participatory teaching includes demonstrations of techniques that may be necessary to show that something has been learned. For example, as part of preoperative teaching, aspects of postoperative care include cleaning the wound, changing the dressing, and applying ice packs. A new diabetic might need to be taught how to check his blood sugar. During this phase of teaching, you need to first describe the technique to the patient and then demonstrate it. The patient should then repeat the demonstration for you. This practice is called **return demonstration.** If any aspects of the technique are unclear to the patient, you should demonstrate the technique again. The patient should be capable of performing the procedure properly. This process of teaching a new skill by having the patient observe and imitate is called **modeling**.

Verifying Patient Understanding

The key to the success of any educational process is verifying that patients have actually understood the information. A good way to check for understanding is to have patients explain in their own words what they have learned. This is a form of feedback. In addition, have them engage in return demonstrations.

Cultural and Educational Barriers

Some practices serve patients who cannot read well or who do not speak or understand English. It may be necessary to create educational materials written in very simple terms that present information through pictures and charts. The information also may need to be translated into one or more languages. Patients must understand the office's policies and procedures as well as any other educational information provided.

One-on-one explanations may be required for these patients. However, printed materials should still be taken home. Family members or friends may be able to read the materials for them, reinforcing what they learned in the office. When demonstrating a procedure to patients, keep in mind any physical limitations they may have and adjust the procedure accordingly. Make sure patients understand the instructions by asking them to perform the procedure for you.

It is important to match the learning materials to the patient's needs and to her level of understanding. Consider the patient's cultural background, age, medical condition, emotional state, learning style, educational background, disabilities, religious background, and readiness to learn when providing new materials. Review the Points on Practice: Respecting Patients' Cultural Beliefs. Keep in mind that patients can refuse treatment and information. If this occurs, notify the doctor and document the event in the patient's chart.

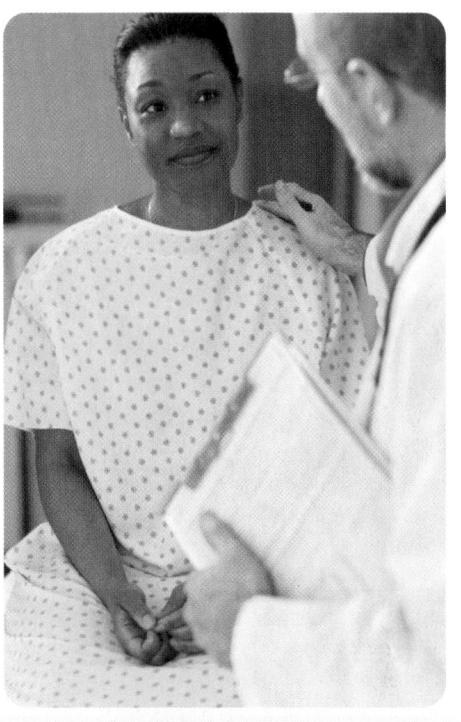
▶ Patient Education Materials   LO 14.4

Most formal types of patient education involve some printed information. They may also include visual materials, such as videotapes, DVDs, and Internet sites. Patient education materials inform patients and enable and encourage them to become involved in their own medical care.

Printed Materials

Printed educational materials come in a variety of formats. They can be as simple as a single sheet of paper, or they can be several sheets that are folded or stapled together to form a booklet.

Brochures, Booklets, and Fact Sheets Many medical offices have materials available that explain procedures performed in the medical office or give information about specific diseases and medical conditions. For example, women who have had a cesarean section delivery may be given a fact sheet describing simple exercises they can do in bed to help regain strength in the abdominal muscles. Many educational aids are prepared by pharmaceutical companies and are provided free of charge to medical offices. Others may be written by the physician or members of the office staff. You may be asked to help prepare some of these materials.

Electronic health record systems provide the ability to create or import informational materials for patients. Spring-Charts™ is one example of an electronic health record system that allows you to generate the information sheet and then save it as an RTF (rich text format) document on the computer (Figures 14-2 and 14-3). On the Internet, you can also find patient information sheets that you import directly into SpringCharts™. Using electronic health records allows you to save multiple information sheets and access and modify them quickly and easily.

Whenever written materials of any kind are given to a patient, it must be noted in the patient's chart. Be sure to document exactly which brochure or leaflet was distributed. Using electronic health records, you can create and document patient receipt of pertinent information quickly and easily. See Procedure 14-1, Creating Electronic Patient Instructions, at the end of this chapter.

Educational Newsletters A popular patient education tool is the medical office newsletter. Newsletters contain timely, practical healthcare tips. Regular newsletters can also offer updates on office policies, information about new diagnostic tests or equipment, and news about the office staff. Newsletters are often written by the doctor or office staff. Some publishing companies and medical groups also offer newsletters that can be customized to a particular practice, using the Internet or software programs such as Microsoft® Publisher.

Community-Assistance Directory Patients often require the assistance of health-related organizations within the community. For example, an elderly patient may need

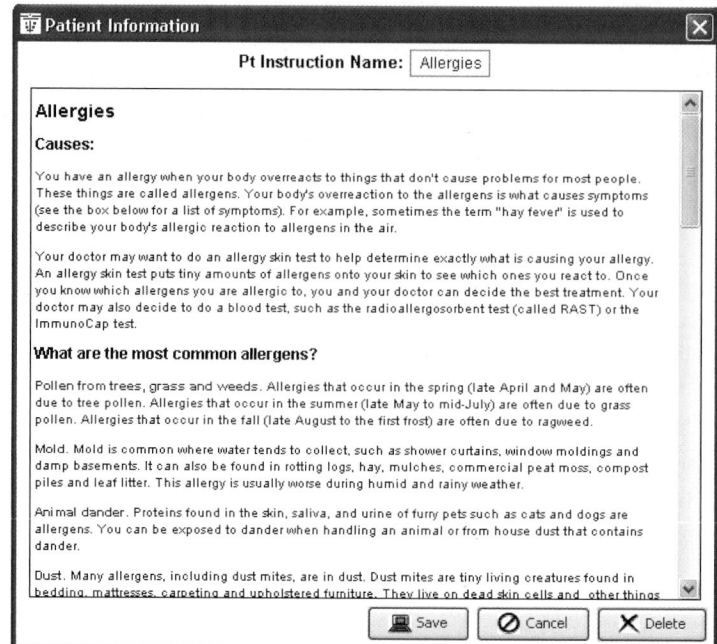

FIGURE 14-2 A patient information sheet, such as this one, can be developed quickly and easily using an electronic health record system such as SpringCharts™.

Source: Screen captures of SpringCharts™ Electronic Health Records software are reprinted with permission from Spring Medical Systems, Inc. All rights reserved.

FIGURE 14-3 When using electronic health records, you can import or create your own patient instruction sheets.

Source: Screen captures of SpringCharts™; Electronic Health Records software are reprinted with permission from Spring Medical Systems, Inc. All rights reserved.

the services of a visiting nurse or a meals-on-wheels food program. Other patients may need the services of a day-care center, speech therapist, or weight clinic.

There are many community resources available in your local area that provide needed services to patients. The medical facility often works with outside resources such as laboratories, home healthcare agencies, and social service agencies. It is beneficial to the patient if the medical assistant is familiar with services that could assist with his or her care. Good customer service is founded on providing or researching services that can assist in the goal of patient health and well-being.

The first step in developing a community resource library is to gather a listing of local agencies. You will need the correct name, address, Web address, phone number, contact person, and directions for submitting a referral for each resource listed. It may take some research on your part to locate and organize this information. The Internet and phone directory can be useful tools. Contact the community resource and request

information such as brochures, newsletters, and referral applications. Type up an inventory sheet or Excel spreadsheet of your resources and make sure that all appropriate departments have a copy. A filing drawer can be used to organize and maintain the informational material regarding each resource. A written community resource directory prepared by the office that is accessible to staff and patients is a valuable aid for referring patients to appropriate agencies. See Procedure 14-2, Identifying Community Resources, at the end of this chapter.

Visual Materials

Many patients are better able to comprehend complicated medical information when it is presented in a visual format. When using visual educational materials, it is usually best to provide corresponding written materials that patients can keep for reference.

POINTS ON PRACTICE
EHR and Patient Education

Utilizing an electronic health record system opens the door to a vast amount of electronic patient information from the Internet that can easily be imported and formatted. Creating the patient information packet or patient instruction sheets and searching the Internet for new patient information is all at your fingertips. The ability to develop patient education materials with EHR, although it may take some learning time, will help you advance in your career as a medical assistant. It will also help you provide the latest education materials to your patients.

DVDs or Videotapes DVDs are often used to educate patients about a variety of topics and to instruct them in self-care techniques. The use of DVDs is especially effective when teaching about complex subjects and procedures. Examples of helpful DVDs used in patient education include those on breast self-examination, dressing change, and infant care.

Seminars and Classes Many physicians conduct or arrange educational seminars or classes for their patients. For example, an obstetrician might offer classes in childbirth preparation for patients and their partners. Other seminars and classes may be conducted depending on the type of medical practice.

Libraries and Patient Resource Rooms Most public libraries have an assortment of books, magazines, and electronic databases pertaining to health and medical topics. Hospitals may provide patient resource rooms, which include a variety of educational materials—such as books, brochures, and videotapes—for public use. Some hospitals provide patient education materials on demand through televisions in patient rooms. A medical librarian is a healthcare team member and, if available, a good contact to assist you with obtaining and providing patient education materials.

Associations Thousands of health organizations and associations can be contacted for information about preventive healthcare and virtually every known disease or disorder. The names, addresses, telephone numbers, and websites of these organizations are provided in several directories, which are available online or at most libraries. Table 14-1 provides a sample list of patient resource organizations.

TABLE 14-1	Patient Resource Organizations
Organization	**Web Address**
Alzheimer's Disease Education and Referral Center	www.alzheimers.org
American Academy of Pediatrics	www.aap.org
American Cancer Society	www.cancer.org
American Diabetes Association	www.diabetes.org
American Dietetic Association	www.eatright.org
American Heart Association	www.americanheart.org
Arthritis Foundation	www.arthritis.org
Asthma and Allergy Foundation of America	www.aafa.org
Centers for Disease Control and Prevention Department of Health and Human Services	www.cdc.gov
National AIDS Hotline	www.sfaf.org
National Cancer Institute, NCI Public Inquiries Office	www.cancer.gov
National Clearinghouse for Alcohol and Drug Information	www.ncadi.samhsa.gov
National Health Information Center	www.health.gov/nhic
National Kidney Foundation	www.kidney.org
National Organization for Rare Disorders	www.rarediseases.org
President's Council on Physical Fitness and Sports Department	www.fitness.gov

Search the Internet to obtain the latest contact information for each organization.

Online Health Information The Internet is a widely used source of medical information. It will be helpful to suggest specific, reputable websites for patients to research. Website addresses should be checked for credibility before using them or referring your patients to them. See Procedure 14-3, Locating Credible Patient Education Information on the Internet, at the end of this chapter. You may need to obtain assistance and approval from the physician, a medical librarian, or other medical staff members. Developing a list of reputable sites to suggest to patients as part of patient education is a must.

Once you are comfortable with types of learning and teaching as well as the educational materials available, you should be ready to start patient education. Begin by creating a patient education plan. This plan includes identifying the education needs of the patient, creating an outline, collecting resources for teaching, carrying out the teaching, and then evaluating the effectiveness. Keep in mind that education is an ongoing process. However, the patient education plan gives you a place to start. See Procedure 14-4, Developing a Patient Education Plan, at the end of this chapter.

▶ Promoting Health and Wellness through Education LO 14.5

Maintaining or improving your health is the best way to protect yourself against disease and illness. It is also part of being a good role model in your position as a medical assistant. **Consumer education**—education that is geared, in both content and language, toward the average person—has helped Americans become more aware of the importance of good health. As a result, many people are beginning to take greater responsibility for their own health and well-being.

There are many ways to achieve good health. You can develop healthy habits, take steps to protect yourself from injury, and take preventive measures to decrease the risk of disease or illness. Patient education in the medical office should help patients achieve these goals.

Healthy Habits
Patient education can be used to promote good health habits by teaching patients the importance of

- Good nutrition, including limiting fat intake and eating an adequate amount of fruits, vegetables, and fiber.
- Regular exercise.
- Adequate rest (7 to 8 hours of sleep a night).
- Avoiding smoking and drug use.
- Limiting alcohol consumption.
- Safe-sex practices.
- A balanced lifestyle of work and leisure activities (moderation).
- Safety practices.

Whenever possible, these guidelines should be recommended to patients of all ages. Good health should be a top priority in life. Although it is best to incorporate healthy behavior before illness develops, remind patients that it is never too late to work toward improving their health.

Protection from Injury

Many accidents happen because people fail to see potential risks and do not develop plans of action. Following safety measures at home, at work, at play, and while traveling can help prevent injury. A discussion of ways to avoid accidents and injury should be part of the educational process. See the Educating the Patient feature Tips for Preventing Injury to help patients avoid injury at home and at work.

Another essential aspect of educating patients about injury prevention is teaching them about the proper use of medications. A prescription includes specific instructions for taking the medication. Emphasize to the patient that these instructions must be followed exactly. In addition, the patient must not change the dosage or mix medications of any kind without first checking with the physician. Patients who do not adhere to these rules run the risk of potentially dangerous side effects. Tell patients to report to the physician any unusual reactions experienced when taking medications. Patients also must be cautioned to never share their medications with anyone else, no matter how tempting it may be to "help" a family member or friend.

When providing a patient with a new prescription, always ask the patient if he has told the doctor about all the medications he is already taking, including herbs, vitamins, and over-the-counter (OTC) medications. If the patient tells you that he has not, immediately inform the physician before the patient leaves the office. Some medications taken together or with certain foods can interfere with how well the drug works or cause side effects or adverse reactions. The physician needs to know about all drugs as well as herbal preparations and OTC medications that the patient is taking.

EDUCATING THE PATIENT

Tips for Preventing Injury

To avoid accidents and injury, teach patients to use common sense and follow these guidelines:

At Home

- Install smoke detectors, carbon monoxide detectors, and fire extinguishers.
- Keep all medicines, chemicals, and household cleaning solutions out of the reach of children.
- Purchase products in childproof containers. Lock or attach childproof latches to all cabinets, medicine chests, and drawers that contain poisonous items.
- Keep chemicals in their original containers and store them out of children's reach.
- Install adequate lighting in rooms and hallways.
- Install railings on stairs.
- Use nonskid backing on rugs to help prevent falls, or remove rugs altogether.
- In the bathroom, use nonskid mats or strips that stick to the tub floor.
- Stay with young children when they are in the bathroom.
- Do not rely on bath seats or rings as a safety device for babies and children.
- Set the water temperature on the water heater at 120°F.
- Never use appliances in the bathtub or near a sink filled with water.
- Practice good kitchen safety: Store knives and kitchen tools properly. Unplug small appliances when not in use. Wipe up spills immediately.

- When cooking, take care to turn all handles of pots and pans inward, toward the cooking surface, to avoid spills and burns.
- Shorten long electrical cords and speaker wires, or secure them with electrical tape. Avoid plugging too many electrical appliances into the same outlet.
- Exercise caution when using electrical appliances. Use outlet covers when outlets are not in use.
- To reach high places, use proper equipment, such as stepladders, not chairs.
- Use child safety gates at the top of stairwells.

At Work

- Use appropriate safety equipment and protective gear, as required.
- Lift heavy objects properly: Bend at the knees, not at the waist. As you straighten your legs, bring the object close to your body quickly. That way, strong leg muscles do the lifting, not weaker back muscles.
- Never attempt to move furniture on your own. Request that a member of the office building maintenance staff be engaged to do so.
- Use surge protectors on computer and other electronic equipment to prevent overloading outlets.
- Make sure hallways, entrance areas, work areas, offices, and parking lots are well lit.
- If your job involves desk work, practice proper posture when sitting. Do not sit for long periods of time. Get up and stretch, or walk down the hall and back.

Preventive Measures

Preventive healthcare is an area in which patient education plays a vital role. Patients need to know that they can decrease their chances of getting certain illnesses and diseases by taking preventive measures and avoiding certain behaviors. Preventive techniques can be described on three levels: *health-promoting behaviors, screening,* and *rehabilitation.*

Health-Promoting Behaviors The first level of disease and illness prevention involves adopting the health-promoting behaviors described in the section titled Healthy Habits. This primary level of prevention also includes educating patients about the symptoms and warning signs of disease.

Screening The second level of disease prevention is screening. **Screening** involves the diagnostic testing of a patient who is typically free of symptoms. Screening allows early diagnosis and treatment of certain diseases. Examples of screening tests include colonoscopy, mammography, and Pap smears for women and prostate examinations for men.

Annual screening is important to health maintenance. Although the requirements may differ according to the age and condition of the patient, annual screenings usually include routine blood work, urinalysis, chest x-ray, ECG (electrocardiogram), and a physical examination (PE).

Rehabilitation The third level of disease prevention involves the rehabilitation and management of an existing illness. At this level the disease process remains stable, but the body will probably not heal any further. The objective is to maintain functionality and avoid further disability. Examples of this level of prevention include stroke rehabilitation programs, cardiac rehabilitation, and pain management for conditions such as arthritis.

▶ The Patient Information Packet   LO 14.6

When patients come to the medical practice, they need to learn not only about health and medical issues but also about the medical office itself. The patient information packet explains the medical practice and its policies. Unlike most other patient education materials, the patient information packet deals mainly with administrative matters rather than with medical issues.

The patient information packet may be as simple as a one-page brochure or pamphlet. It may be a multipage brochure or a folder with multiple-page inserts. In some practices, the patient information packet is available online or through the EHR system for review or printing.

Benefits of the Information Packet

The patient information packet is a simple, effective, and inexpensive way to improve the relationship between the office and the patients. It provides important information about the practice and the office staff. This information helps patients feel more comfortable with the qualifications of the healthcare professionals involved in their care. The packet may help clarify the roles that each office staff member has in patient care.

The information packet also informs patients of office policies and procedures. Patients will learn the doctor's office hours, how to schedule appointments, the office's payment policies, and other administrative details. This information helps limit misunderstandings about these procedures.

The patient information packet also benefits the office staff. It is both an excellent marketing tool and an aid to running the office more smoothly. Providing patients with a prepared information packet saves staff time by answering a number of potential patient inquiries. The information packet is also a good way to acquaint new office staff members with office policies.

Contents of the Information Packet Regardless of the material the information packet contains, it must be written in clear language so that patients are able to read and understand it. All materials should be written at a sixth-grade reading level to accommodate the greatest number of patients. Information should not be presented in a technical medical style. Because you may be responsible for developing portions of the information packet, you should be familiar with the contents of a typical packet.

Introduction to the Office A brief introduction serves to welcome the patient to the office. It may be helpful to summarize the office's philosophy of patient care. The office's **philosophy** means the system of values and principles the office has adopted in its everyday practices.

Physician's Qualifications The packet commonly contains information about the physician's professional qualifications and training. It includes details about education, internship, and residency. It may list credentials such as board certification or board eligibility in a certain medical specialty. It also may list the physician's membership in professional societies. The information packet for a group practice may contain a paragraph or a page for each physician.

Description of the Practice The information packet should include a brief description of the practice, particularly if it is a specialty practice. Explaining the types of examinations or procedures that are commonly performed in the office as well as a list of any special services the office provides, such as physical examinations for employment, workers' compensation cases, or other occupational services, would be helpful. Be sure to make medical terms and specialties clear by avoiding the use of initials. Spell out everything the first time the reference is made and place the appropriate initials in parentheses.

Introduction to the Office Staff Many patients are not familiar with the qualifications and duties of the various members of the office staff. It is a good idea, therefore, to identify the staff positions according to their responsibilities and duties. Patients need to understand that some duties commonly thought to be a nurse's responsibilities may also be performed by a medical assistant. It may be helpful to include the professional credentials and licenses of key staff members.

Office Hours This section should list the exact days and hours the office is open, including holidays. In addition, patients need to know what to do if an emergency occurs outside regular office hours. Tell the patient what number to call first (for example, the answering service, 911, or the hospital emergency room) and what to do next. Include the telephone number and address of the emergency room at the hospital with which the doctor is affiliated. Assure patients that the doctor or a physician partner can be reached at all times through the answering service. Some practices have multiple offices, and the physicians rotate from office to office on a regular schedule. List all office addresses and phone numbers along with directions to all office sites.

Appointment Scheduling This section of the packet should explain the procedure for scheduling and canceling appointments. You might suggest that patients can benefit by scheduling routine checkups and visits as far in advance as possible. Also note if certain times of the day are reserved for sudden or unexpected office visits.

In this section, encourage patients to be on time for appointments. Explain the problems that result from late or broken appointments. If the office charges a fee for breaking an appointment without advance notice, mention it here. Be careful to address these sensitive areas with a positive, nonthreatening tone. The office's written material should simply state the office policies and the problems that can result when the policies are not followed.

Telephone Policy Providing the office's telephone policies in the information packet can help reduce the number of unnecessary calls to the office and thus save time for the office staff. Explain which procedures can be handled over the telephone and which cannot. Explain procedures such as calling in for prescription renewals or laboratory test results. If the physician returns patients' calls at a certain time of day, mention that policy in this section. Some practices bill patients for telephone calls in which medical advice is given but not for follow-up calls. For example, if a parent of a child who was vomiting uncontrollably called the physician to get immediate medical advice, the call might be billed. If the physician called to inform a patient of test results, however, the call would not be billed. It is important that patients know about these policies, particularly because many insurance plans do not cover charges for medical advice given over the phone, so the patient will be responsible for these charges.

Some offices (particularly pediatric offices) schedule a certain time of the day for patients (or parents and guardians) to call the physician for answers to their questions. This type of policy benefits both the office and the patients. The patients (or parents) have the assurance that they can speak with the physician about their concerns, and the office is spared interruptions during other times of the day.

Payment Policies Inform patients of the office's policies regarding payment and billing. State whether payment is expected at the time of a visit or whether the patient can be billed. List accepted forms of payment (for example, cash, personal checks, and credit cards). It is not common practice to mention specific fees in an information packet.

Insurance Policies List the major insurance carriers accepted by your office, or state that "most major insurance plans are accepted." Advise patients to bring proof of insurance coverage and a picture ID if this is their first visit to the office. A copy of this ID should be made and inserted in the patient's medical chart. State whether the office submits insurance claim forms directly to the insurance company or whether the patient has this responsibility. If the office or a billing service bills the insurance carrier, also include information regarding whether claims are submitted manually, using paper claims, or electronically. Generally, there is no charge for submission of the first insurance claim form; but if the office charges for submission of secondary insurance forms, this should be stated. Outline the practice's policy for handling Medicare coverage, including whether or not the office accepts assignment on Medicare claims. If the office does not submit insurance claims directly, explain that the staff will help patients fill out insurance forms when necessary and will provide the appropriate paperwork (usually a superbill) containing dates of service and procedure and diagnosis codes for attachment to the claim form.

Patient Confidentiality Statement The information packet must include a copy of the office privacy policy. Complete information regarding the privacy policy and HIPAA regulations can be found in the *Legal and Ethical Issues* chapter. An important first step of HIPAA compliance is informing the patient of his or her rights. These rights are communicated through the Notice of Privacy Practices (NPP) (discussed in the *Legal and Ethical Issues* chapter), which must adhere to certain specifications.

The information packet also must state that no information from patient files will be released without a signed authorization from the patient. Each patient who receives a copy of the privacy notice must sign a document stating that he received the privacy notice and had the opportunity to have his questions about the notice answered. This document should remain in the patient's medical file.

Other Information The patient information packet may include the practice's policy on referrals. It may provide information about access to available community health resources or agencies. It also may include special instructions for common office procedures (for example, whether the patient needs to fast before a procedure or to avoid certain foods).

Distributing the Information Packet

For the information packet to be effective, you must make sure that new patients receive and read it. One way is to hand the packet to new patients at the time of their first office visit and briefly review the contents with them. Explain that they can find answers to many questions in the packet. Encourage patients to take the packet home, read the information, and keep it handy for future reference, but be sure to obtain the signed documentation that the patient has received and read the privacy notice for your files.

BWW Medical Associates, PC
305 Main Street, Port Snead YZ 12345-9876
Tel: 555-654-3210, Fax: 555-987-6543
Web: BWWAssociates.com

Paul F. Buckwalter, MD
Alexis N. Whalen, MD
Elizabeth H. Williams, MD

Consent for Treatment

I voluntarily give my permission to the healthcare providers of BWW Medical Associates, PC and such assistants and other healthcare providers as they may deem necessary to provide medical services to me. I understand by signing this form, I am authorizing them to treat me for as long as I seek care from BWW Medical Associates, PC or until I withdraw my consent in writing.

_____
Signature of Patient or Guardian

_____
Date

_____
Printed Name of Patient or Guardian

_____
Relationship to Patient

Statement of Financial Responsibility/Assignment of Benefits

I acknowledge that I am legally responsible for all charges in connection with the medical care and treatment provided by BWW Medical Associates, PC and Associates. I assign and authorize payments to BWW Medical Associates, PC. I understand my insurance carrier may not approve or reimburse my medical services in full due to usual and customary rates, benefit exclusions, coverage limits, lack of authorization, or medical necessity. I understand I am responsible for fees not paid in full, co-payments, and policy deductibles and co-insurance except where my liability is limited by contract or State or Federal law.

_____
Signature of Patient or Guardian

_____
Date

_____
Printed Name of Patient or Guardian

_____
Relationship to Patient

A duplicate or faxed copy of this form is considered the same as the original document.

FIGURE 14-4 Sample patient consent for treatment form.

When new patients make an appointment, many offices send them a copy of the information packet if there is enough time before the appointment to get it to them by regular mail. (It is a nice gesture to include a detailed map or written directions to the office for new patients who are not familiar with the area.) In some cases, the patient is referred to the practice's website to review the patient information packet, complete patient registration forms, as well as obtain directions. Patients can review the packet and the consent for treatment form before coming to the office (Figure 14-4). Additional copies of the packet should be placed in an accessible area in the office so that patients can take them home.

▶ Patient Education Prior to Surgery

When a patient undergoes a surgical procedure, patient education is vital to a successful outcome. Although exact instructions vary according to the procedure, their purpose is to prepare the patient for the procedure and to aid the patient during the recovery period.

Providing Patient Education

Patients must receive information from the physician (not the medical assistant) about the need for surgery and its nature.

Educating and preparing patients for surgery may be your responsibility. You should provide support and explanations to patients. You must verify that they understand any information they may have been given by other members of the healthcare team. Preoperative instruction may include discussion of postoperative care issues, such as temporary dietary restrictions or surgical wound care.

Determining whether patients have all the information they need before surgery is essential from both an educational and a legal standpoint. All patients who are undergoing a surgical procedure must first sign an informed consent form. This legal document provides specific information about the surgical procedure, including its purpose, the possible risks, and the expected outcome. The informed consent form, along with documentation of all preoperative instructions, must be put in the patient's chart. (See Figure 14-5.)

BWW

BWW Medical Associates, PC
305 Main Street, Port Snead YZ 12345-9876
Tel: 555-654-3210, Fax: 555-987-6543
Web: BWWAssociates.com

Paul F. Buckwalter, MD
Alexis N. Whalen, MD
Elizabeth H. Williams, MD

Patient Surgical Consent Form

Your surgeon for this procedure is: _____

I hereby authorize and request the surgeon, along with any assistants he/she feels are necessary, to perform upon me the following operation(s):

_____

I understand that the nature and purpose of the above mentioned procedure(s) is/are to:

_____

I also authorize the surgeon to do any therapeutic procedure or investigation that in his/her judgment may be advisable for my well-being.

The nature of the planned operation has been thoroughly explained to me by my surgeon and I have decided to proceed with this form of therapy over other alternative methods. The risks, benefits, and alternatives, including doing nothing, have been explained to me. I understand that the practice of medicine and surgery is not an exact science and I acknowledge that no guarantees have been made about the results of the operation or procedure planned. Furthermore, the risks and complications inherent in the operation have been explained to me and I accept these.

I further give permission to have such anesthetics administered to me as the surgeon or the anesthetist deems necessary or advisable.

Pictures may be taken of the treatment site for record purposes. I understand that these photographs/videos will be the property of the attending physician.

 ☐ I DO agree to allow these pictures to be used for publication or teaching purposes.
 ☐ I DO NOT agree to allow these pictures to be used for publication or teaching purposes.

If I agree, I understand that my name and identity will be kept confidential and protected.

I agree to keep the office of the surgeon informed of my post-operative progress and I agree to cooperate with instructions given for my post-operative care.

Patient or Legal Guardian (Signature)	_____
Patient or Legal Guardian (Please Print)	_____
Surgeon as Witness (Signature)	_____
Surgeon as Witness (Please Print)	_____
Date	_____
	Year Month Day

I hereby acknowledge receiving a copy of the post-operative instructions which have been reviewed with me. I understand the advice and restrictions given and agree to abide by them. I will notify my doctor immediately if any unusual bleeding, respiratory problems, or acute pain occurs after my discharge from this surgical facility.

Patient (Signature) _____   Witness (Signature) _____

Patient (Please Print) _____   Witness (Please Print) _____

Date _____
  Year   Month   Day

FIGURE 14-5 Sample patient surgical consent form.

Preoperative Education

Preoperative education increases patients' overall satisfaction with their care. It helps reduce patient anxiety and fear, use of pain medication, complications following surgery, and recovery time. Letting the patient know what to expect during the surgery and afterward allows the patient to emotionally and educationally prepare for all aspects of the surgical procedure. The use of effective teaching techniques is essential to ensure patient understanding. Make sure the patient has a patient instruction sheet and can repeat the expectations back to you.

It may be difficult for a patient to visualize exactly what will take place in some surgical procedures. For example, think of arthroscopy of the knee. When told that the doctor will insert a viewing instrument into the knee, patients probably have no idea of the size of this scope. As a result, they may be particularly fearful of the procedure. An anatomical model, diagram, or photo is useful to show exactly what will happen and ease patients' fears. For example, an anatomical model may help a patient who is having surgery on his ear see how the surgical procedure will help correct his problem. (See Figure 14-6.)

Helping Relieve Patient Anxiety

When you provide preoperative education, be aware that the fear and anxiety of patients who are about to undergo a surgical procedure can adversely affect the learning process. Consequently, allow extra time for repetition and reinforcement of material.

Always consider your choice of words carefully, stressing the positive rather than the negative whenever possible. Involving family members in the educational process is often

FIGURE 14-6 An anatomical model can help patients visualize what will happen during surgery.

beneficial, particularly if the patient is especially apprehensive about the surgery. Provide patients with contact information in case they have additional questions after they leave. Present your instructions and explanations in straightforward language that they can understand. Remember to be reassuring but to not "promise" a specific result for which the physician may be held liable if the expected result is not the actual result. Remember to verify that they understand everything. This will also help to reduce their anxiety level. Procedure 14-5 will guide you through the process of outpatient surgery teaching.

PROCEDURE 14-1   Creating Electronic Patient Instructions

Goal: To create and administer patient instructions electronically.

OSHA Guidelines: This procedure does not involve exposure to blood, body fluids, or tissue.

Materials: An electronic health records software program (such as SpringCharts™) that includes a patient instructions feature.

Method: Procedure steps.

1. Search the EHR to find the button or icon to create patient instructions. (Check the Help button or review the training manual.)

2. Determine if you will need to write your own or can select from a previously created list of patient instructions. Select the correct button to proceed. (See Figure 14-3 for an example using SpringCharts™; EHR.)

3. Create new instructions by either of the following methods:

   a. Type your patient instructions directly in the open window or a word processing program. This will depend on the EHR you are using. (See Figure 14-2 for an example of the open window taken from SpringCharts™.)

   b. Open the Web browser and navigate to a credible Internet site for patient instruction. (Review Procedure 14-3 before selecting this option.) If available on the site, select the "printer friendly" version. Highlight the information you want to use from the website, place your cursor at the beginning of the text, and, with your left mouse button depressed, drag the cursor to the end of the instruction page. Right-click on any highlighted area and choose Copy. Click in the patient instruction window or in the word processing program and, using the keypad, press the [Ctrl] and [V] keys. Close the Web page and return to the EHR.

4. Import instructions by opening a previously created document saved as an .RTF or other word processing file type. Import the document according to the manufacturer's instructions.

5. Use existing instructions by selecting them from a list within the EHR or a file folder on your computer. Check the specific directions for the EHR program you are using. An example of how to enter the existing patient instructions from SpringCharts™ is shown in the figure on the next page.

FIGURE Procedure 14-1 Step 5   Select the "Patient Instructions" link on the drop-down menu.

Source: Screen captures of SpringCharts™ Electronic Health Records software are reprinted with permission from Spring Medical Systems, Inc. All rights reserved.

6. Record in the EHR the instructions that you provided to the patient. In most programs this occurs when you generate the instructions and they become a permanent record in the patient's chart. An example charting entry using SpringCharts™ is shown below.

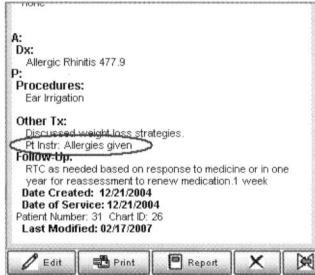

FIGURE Procedure 14-1 Step 6   As seen, here, once patient instructions have been given to the patient, they should be documented.

Source: Screen captures of SpringCharts™ Electronic Health Records software are reprinted with permission from Spring Medical Systems, Inc. All rights reserved.

PROCEDURE 14-2 Identifying Community Resources

Goal: To create a list of useful community resources for patient referrals.

OSHA Guidelines: This procedure does not involve exposure to blood, body fluids, or tissue.

Materials: Computer with Internet access, phone directory, printer.

Method: Procedure steps.

1. Determine the needs of your medical office and formulate a list of community resources. The specific needs of your patients will help you formulate your list. Being able to help patients find outside assistance when necessary is the goal.

2. Use the Internet to research the names, addresses, Web addresses, and phone numbers of local resources such as state and federal agencies, home healthcare agencies, long-term nursing facilities, mental health agencies, and local charities. Use the phone directory to assist in locating local agencies such as Meals on Wheels;

Alcoholics Anonymous; shelters for abused individuals; hospice care; Easter Seals; Women, Infants, and Children (WIC); and support groups for grief, obesity, and various diseases.

3. Contact each resource and request information such as business cards and brochures. Some agencies may send a representative to meet with you regarding their services. If patients can access information easily, they are more likely to take advantage of the services available to them.

4. Compile a list of community resources with the proper name, address, phone number, e-mail address, and contact name. Include any information that may be helpful to the office.

5. Update and add to the information often because outdated information will only frustrate you and your patients, creating even more anxiety.

6. Post the information in a location where it is readily available. Maintain an electronic record for easy reference.

PROCEDURE 14-3 Locating Credible Patient Education Information on the Internet

Goal: To determine the credibility of patient education information on the Internet.

OSHA Guidelines: This procedure does not involve exposure to blood, body fluids, or tissue.

Materials: Computer with Internet access.

Method: Procedure steps.

1. Open your Internet browser and locate a search engine. Search engines vary in the way they search so you may want to use more than one search engine for different results.

2. Search the topic. Be specific when entering the search term. For example, if you want to know about the proper diet for high cholesterol, you should type, "high

cholesterol diet." For different or more medical sites, try using different terms; instead of "high cholesterol" try "hyperlipidemia."

3. Select a site from the list of results and evaluate the source.

   a. Click the "about us" link to find out who developed the site. Sites should have an active link available to contact the Webmaster and verify the source.

   b. Sites developed by professional organizations, educational institutions, or a branch of the federal government are generally better than those developed by an individual or a commercial company.

4. Review the "about us" page to determine the quality of the information.

   a. Review the mission statement or other detailed information about the developer.

   b. Look for information about the writers or authors of the site. Make sure they are medical professionals.

5. Check the content of the site.

   a. Avoid sites that have sensational writing or make claims that are too good to be true.

   b. Make sure the language of the information is at a level that you can understand. Avoid sites that use lots of technical jargon for patient instruction.

6. Make sure the information is current by checking the copyright or by checking with the contact information on the site. Medical information changes frequently, so check the date and avoid information over five years old.

7. Avoid websites that are potentially biased. For example, if the site is written by a pharmaceutical company, the site will only present information about the medication manufactured by that company. There may be alternative medications. Sites written by individuals are interesting, but may be biased as well.

8. Protect your privacy. If the sites require you to register, review their Privacy Policy. They may be able to share your or your patient's information with other companies.

9. Once you have evaluated the site and decide to use it, you may want to have your supervisor or licensed practitioner review and approve the information you will be providing to the patient.

PROCEDURE 14-4 Developing a Patient Education Plan

Goal: To create and implement a patient teaching plan.

OSHA Guidelines: This procedure does not involve exposure to blood, body fluids, or tissue.

Materials: Pen, paper, various educational aids (such as instructional pamphlets and brochures), and/or visual aids (such as posters, videotapes, or DVDs).

Method: Procedure steps.

1. Identify the patient's educational needs in order to provide instruction at the patient's point of need. Consider the following:

   a. The patient's current knowledge.

   b. Any misconceptions the patient may have.

   c. Any obstacles to learning (loss of hearing or vision, limitations of mobility, language barriers, and so on).

   d. The patient's willingness and readiness to learn (motivation).

   e. How the patient will use the information.

   RATIONALE: All instruction must begin at the patient's point of need.

2. Using the various educational aids available, develop and outline a plan that addresses all the patient's needs. Include the following areas in the outline:

   a. What you want to accomplish (your goal).

   b. How you plan to accomplish it.

   c. How you will determine if the teaching was successful.

   RATIONALE: Developing an educational plan ensures that all patient needs will be addressed.

3. Write the plan. Try to make the information interesting for the patient.

4. Before carrying out the plan, share it with the physician to get approval and suggestions for improvement.

5. Perform the instruction. Be sure to use more than one teaching method. For instance, if written material is being given, be sure to explain or demonstrate the material instead of simply telling the patient to read the educational materials.

6. Document the teaching in the patient's chart for continuity of care and to maintain a legal record.

   RATIONALE: All patient education must be documented in the patient's medical chart for continuity of care and as a legal record.

7. Revise your plan as necessary to make it even more effective. To be an effective teacher, you must evaluate the methods you use.

PROCEDURE 14-5 Outpatient Surgery Teaching

Goal: To inform a preoperative patient of the necessary guidelines to follow prior to surgery.

OSHA Guidelines: This procedure does not involve exposure to blood, body fluids, or tissue.

Materials: Patient chart, surgical guidelines.

Method: Procedure steps.

1. Review the patient's chart to determine the type of surgery to be performed and then ask the patient what procedure is being performed.

RATIONALE: This confirms the patient's knowledge of the procedure.

2. Tell the patient that you will be providing both verbal and written instructions that should be followed prior to surgery.

3. Inform the patient about policies regarding makeup, jewelry, contact lenses, wigs, dentures, and so on.

4. Tell the patient to leave money and valuables at home.

5. If applicable, suggest appropriate clothing for the patient to wear for postoperative ease and comfort.

6. Explain the need for someone to drive the patient home following an outpatient surgical procedure.
   RATIONALE: Driving after even simple surgery can be very dangerous. Surgery can be canceled if a patient does not identify a responsible driver before surgery occurs.

7. Tell the patient the correct time to arrive at the office, surgery center, or hospital for the procedure.

8. Inform the patient of dietary restrictions. Be sure to use specific, clear instructions about what may or may not be ingested and at what time the patient must abstain from eating or drinking. Also explain these points:
   a. The reasons for the dietary restrictions.
   b. The possible consequences of not following the dietary restrictions.
   RATIONALE: Surgery can be canceled if the patient has not followed dietary instructions.

9. Ask patients who smoke to refrain from or reduce cigarette smoking during at least the 8 hours prior to the procedure. Explain to the patient that reducing smoking

improves the level of oxygen in the blood during surgery.

10. Suggest that the patient shower or bathe the morning of the procedure or the evening before.

11. Instruct the patient about medications to take or avoid before surgery. For example, patients may need to stop taking a daily aspirin or vitamin E before surgery to reduce the risk of bleeding.
    RATIONALE: Surgery can be canceled if the patient has not followed medication instructions.

12. If necessary, clarify any information about which the patient is unclear.

13. Provide written surgical guidelines and suggest that the patient call the office if additional questions arise.
    RATIONALE: Patients may not understand or remember verbal instructions. Written instructions can be taken home and reviewed again.

14. Document the instructions in the patient's chart for continuity of care and as a legal record.
    RATIONALE: All patient education must be documented in the patient's medical chart for continuity of care and as a legal record.

Example Documentation:

> Surgical instructions for arthroscopic left knee surgery provided. Dietary, medication, and driving restrictions explained to the patient. Informed consent signed and placed on chart. Patient did not have questions. Written instructions sent home with the patient. _____
> _____ *Kaylyn Haddix RMA (AMT)*

SUMMARY OF LEARNING OUTCOMES

LEARNING OUTCOMES	KEY POINTS
14.1 Identify the benefits of patient education and the medical assistant's role in providing education.	Patients benefit from patient education because it can help them regain their health and independence more quickly. The medical office also benefits because patients will be less likely to call the office with questions and, therefore, the office staff can spend less time on the telephone. Educated patients take a more active role in their medical care.
14.2 Describe factors that affect learning and teaching.	Learning occurs in three domains: knowledge, behaviors, and skills. The patient must be able to recall the information, have the right attitude and be motivated to learn, and then implement the skills needed to demonstrate that the knowledge is retained.
14.3 Implement teaching techniques.	Teaching methods and formats are adjusted for the best possible result depending on patient need and level of understanding. The best possible education plan comes from knowing your patient and his needs and abilities, as well as the goal of the instruction. Always assess your instruction at its completion and revise the plan as needed.

LEARNING OUTCOMES	KEY POINTS
14.4 Choose reliable patient education materials used in the medical office.	The types of patient education materials in medical offices include brochures, booklets, fact sheets, newsletters, DVDs, Internet-based sites, and community-assistance directories. Using already-completed print or electronic patient instruction sheets, ensuring that Internet sources are credible, and obtaining assistance from other healthcare team members are all methods of ensuring reliability of educational materials.
14.5 Explain how patient education can be used to promote good health habits.	Patient education promotes good health by teaching patients the importance of developing healthy habits such as eating properly and exercising regularly.
14.6 Describe the types of information that should be included in the patient information packet.	The contents of the patient's information packet should include an introduction to the medical office, the physician's qualifications, a description of the practice, an introduction to the staff, office hours, appointment scheduling, telephone policies, payment and insurance policies, a confidentiality statement, and other pertinent information.
14.7 Describe the benefits and special considerations of patient education prior to surgery.	Educating patients prior to surgery is vital to a successful outcome and involves instructing them on proper procedures before surgery and also having the patient sign a surgical consent.

CASE STUDY CRITICAL THINKING

Recall Sylvia Gonzalez from the beginning of the chapter. Now that you have completed the chapter, answer the following questions regarding her case.

1. What might be important to consider when creating an educational plan for Sylvia?

2. What factors could block effective patient education?
3. Why are good listening skills an important part of teaching?
4. What do you consider behaviors that indicate you are "talking down" to a patient?

EXAM PREPARATION QUESTIONS

1. (LO 14.6) A benefit of the patient information packet is that it
   a. Promotes better compliance with treatment programs
   b. Helps patients feel more comfortable with the qualifications of the healthcare professionals who are caring for them
   c. Can answer a treatment question that may come up during an office visit
   d. Encourages patients to help themselves achieve better health
   e. Ensures patient compliance

2. (LO 14.3) Which of the following types of teaching gives patients a description of the physical sensations they may have during the procedure?
   a. Factual
   b. Sensory
   c. Participatory
   d. Modeling
   e. Media

3. (LO 14.4) Which of the following is the most difficult way to create electronic patient instructions?
   a. Type the instructions directly into the open window
   b. Import the instructions from the Internet
   c. Use previously created instructions
   d. Print the instructions directly from the Internet
   e. Use preprinted instructions

4. (LO 14.1) Which of the following is the *least* likely patient benefit of patient education?
   a. Patients are less likely to call the office
   b. Patients take a more active role in their medical care
   c. Office staff are not interrupted as often by patient phone calls
   d. Patients will not need as much medication
   e. Patients are more likely to understand instructions

5. (LO 14.2) Which of the following is an example of the psychomotor learning domain?
   a. The patient is willing to read the brochure
   b. The patient performs his own blood glucose test
   c. The medical assistant tells the patient how she is going to feel during a procedure
   d. The medical assistant provides the patient with a patient information package
   e. The patient searches the Internet for information about his condition

6. (LO 14.4) When checking an Internet site for credibility, which of the following is probably *not* necessary?
   a. Use caution if the site uses a sensational writing style
   b. Look for the author of the information you plan to use
   c. Check the date of the document you plan to use
   d. Click links on the site to make sure they are not broken and are kept up-to-date
   e. Ensure that the site is listed on at least two search engines

7. (LO 14.6) Which of the following would *least* likely be in the patient information packet?
   a. Office policies and hours
   b. Patient instruction sheet regarding common tests done at the practice
   c. Patient instruction sheet about healthy living
   d. List of the physicians with their qualifications
   e. Patient confidentiality statement

8. (LO 14.7) What visual tool is especially helpful when performing preoperative education?
   a. Anatomical model
   b. Printed information sheet
   c. Line drawing
   d. Class or seminar
   e. Sensory teaching

9. (LO 14.5) Which of the following is a healthy habit that should be part of patient teaching?
   a. Adequate rest (4 to 5 hours of sleep a night)
   b. Limiting fruits, vegetables, and fiber
   c. The use of cigarettes in moderation
   d. Balancing lifestyle of work and leisure activities (moderation)
   e. Exercising about 15 minutes per day

10. (LO 14.5) Your patient has a history of cardiovascular disease. Which of the following is *least* likely a screening procedure that would be done?
    a. Blood work
    b. Colonoscopy
    c. Chest x-ray
    d. ECG
    e. Cardiac rehabilitation

Go to CONNECT to see activities on *Administrating Patient Educational Material* and *Creating Patient Educational Material.*

Managing Medical Records

EMPLOYEE INFORMATION

Employee Name	Gender	Date of Hire
Malik Katahri	M	04/20/xx

Position	Credentials	Supervisor
Office Manager	CMM	BWW Physicians

Malik and the office staff have been discussing the pros and cons of converting to a numeric filing system or possibly doing away with paper records totally and moving toward a more progressive EHR program. The physicians are reluctant to commit to an EHR program related to the financial outlay and staff training time required.

Keep Malik in mind as you study this chapter. There will be questions at the end of the chapter based on the case study. The information in the chapter will help you answer these questions.

Malik Katahri is the office manager for BWW Medical Associates, P.C. The number of patients the office sees is growing at an amazing rate and although good for the practice, it is taxing the current alphabetic filing system.

LEARNING OUTCOMES

After completing Chapter 15, you will be able to:

15.1 Identify the common equipment used to file and store paper medical records.

15.2 Outline the security and safety measures that should be employed when working with paper medical records.

15.3 List the common filing supplies used in the medical office.

15.4 Contrast the methods used for various filing systems and how color-coding can assist with the filing systems.

15.5 Recall the steps in the filing process.

15.6 Compare active, inactive, and closed files and how to set up a records retention program for the office.

KEY TERMS

active file
alphabetic filing system
closed file
compactible file
cross-referenced
file guide
inactive file
indexing
indexing rules
lateral file
middle digit

numeric filing system
out guide
records management system
retention schedule
sequential order
terminal digit
tickler file
unit
vertical file

V. C (5)   Identify systems for organizing medical records

V. C (7)   Discuss the pros and cons of various filing methods

V. C (8)   Identify both equipment and supplies needed for filing medical records

V. C (9)   Describe indexing rules

V. C (10) Discuss filing procedures

V. P (4)   File medical records

V. P (8)   Maintain organization by filing

V. A (1)   Consider staff needs and limitations in establishment of a filing system

IX. C (3) Describe the implications of HIPAA for the medical assistant in various medical settings

8. Medical Office Procedures Management
   Graduates:
   b. Prepare and maintain medical records
   d. Apply concepts for office procedures

11. Career Development
   b. Demonstrate professionalism by:
     (3) Maintaining confidentiality at all times
     (4) Being cognizant of ethical boundaries
     (9) Conducting work within scope of education, training, and ability

▶ Introduction

One important administrative function of the medical assistant is the careful management of the patient medical records. The information contained in these records is the most valuable information in a medical office. For a practice to operate smoothly and efficiently, it is critical that these records be organized in a way that makes them easily retrievable. Maintaining a well-organized, easy-to-use **records management system** (the way patient records are created, filed, and maintained) is essential to providing good patient care.

You learned about management of EHR in the *Electronic Health Records* chapter. In this chapter, you will explore the various options for handling large volumes of paper medical records and learn how to develop an organized approach to maintaining these critical files. As you read, watch for helpful tips to locate and access patient records quickly and efficiently.

▶ Filing Equipment   LO 15.1

Filing equipment generally refers to the place where records, or files, are housed. Although there are various types of equipment, two of the most common options are shelves and cabinets. The choice of whether to use filing shelves or filing cabinets is often made according to space considerations and personal preference. Although it is unlikely that you will be involved in the purchase of filing equipment because most medical offices already have filing systems in place, you may need to purchase more equipment as the number of patients in the practice grows or if the physicians decide to open a satellite office. In either case, you will need to determine how much office space is available for the files and the number of patient files to be stored. This information will help you figure out how many cabinets or shelves to purchase as well as the type of filing equipment necessary. Remember, the records being housed within the filing system are virtually the medical history of each patient, so the

filing equipment should be fireproof and secure to protect the personal health information.

Filing Shelves

Files can be kept on shelves, which resemble traditional shelves, as shown in Figure 15-1. Many shelf systems have doors that slide from side to side or slide out from above the files. These

FIGURE 15-1   Medical records kept on shelves are easily accessible and can be kept secured in a separate room.

doors can be locked for security. Other shelf systems have no front covers. Some file units are on wheels for ease of transporting a shelf system. Filing shelves are often long, sometimes extending the full length and height of an office wall or room. An advantage of keeping files on shelves is that it allows several people to retrieve and return files at the same time.

Filing Cabinets

Filing cabinets are sturdy pieces of office furniture, usually made of metal or wood. They contain a series of pullout drawers in which files are hung. Filing cabinets, unlike shelves, are best used by one person at a time because the drawer setup provides limited maneuvering room. In addition, cabinets require more floor space than filing shelves. About twice the depth of the file drawer is needed to allow it to fully open. Cabinets are used less often in larger offices, since only one drawer can be safely opened at a time because the weight of an open drawer can make the files dangerously top heavy. Consequently, only one person at a time can be pulling medical records.

Unlike shelves, which are horizontal in design, filing cabinets can stand vertically or horizontally. A **vertical file** features pullout drawers that usually contain a metal frame or bar equipped to handle letter-size or legal-size documents. Hanging file folders are hung on this frame, with identifying names facing out. Vertical files may have two, three, four, or six drawers.

Horizontal filing cabinets, called **lateral files**, often feature doors that flip up and pullout drawers. Depending on the length and width of the drawer, files can be arranged in 2–3 rows alphabetically or numerically, with separators placed between each row. Lateral files require more wall space but do not extend as far into the room as vertical file drawers.

Compactible Files

Many offices have limited space in which to house filing cabinets or shelves. These offices may choose to use a variation of shelf filing, called **compactible files**. Compactible files are kept on rolling shelves that slide along permanent tracks in the floor.

When not in use, these files can be stored close together—even one on top of another—to conserve space. When needed, they can be rolled out into an open area so that the staff can easily use them. Compactible files can be moved manually or automatically with the touch of a button.

Rotary Circular Files

Rotary circular files are another option to consider when space is limited. These files are stored in a circular fashion, similar to a revolving door, and are accessed by rotating the files. They also can be operated either manually or electronically.

Plastic or Cardboard Tubs or Boxes

Very small offices may use plastic or cardboard storage boxes for their files. The medical records are placed in hanging files within the storage box. Because of the number of boxes needed to store files in this manner, it is inefficient and not advised for larger practices.

When not in use, all storage units must be locked in a secure storage area to protect patient confidentiality. Additionally,

open storage bins collect dust and are inappropriate for storage in a dirty warehouse storage area. TJC (The Joint Commission) also requires (and will check during any inspection) that all storage containers be stored off the floor, either on shelves or on platforms, to avoid potential water damage.

In addition to potential security concerns, storage boxes are often stacked to save space, which can make it very difficult to locate files. TJC also requires that nothing be stacked within 18 inches of the ceiling. Keep in mind that although "portable," any type of storage box is usually very heavy once filled. Care should be taken to avoid injury when moving storage containers holding paper records.

Labeling Filing Equipment

Regardless of which type of filing equipment your office uses, files should be clearly labeled on the outside of the drawer so that you do not have to open doors or drawers to know the contents. Labeling allows you to go directly to the appropriate place when retrieving a file. When labeling storage boxes, use a permanent marker to write on the top and on the front of the box. Writing directly on the box, instead of using self-sticking labels, minimizes the chances that the label will be lost or unreadable. The label should clearly list the range of files contained within the drawer or shelf. For example, if the drawer includes all the files of patients whose last names begin with the letters A, B, C, and D, the drawer should be labeled "A–D."

▶ Security and Safety Measures LO 15.2

All filing systems must be secured under HIPAA privacy and security regulations. HIPAA states that there must be a "reasonable safeguard" to protect health information from any disclosure, whether intentional or unintentional. Using locking, fireproof filing cabinets to store patient records is an important element of this requirement. *Never* place patient records in an unsecured filing system. Additionally, both staff and patients must be safe when using and being around the office filing system.

Medical Record Security

Today's filing cabinets come with a lock and key. Cabinets that are not in a separate room should be locked every night when the office is being closed for the day. To protect filing shelves in a separate room, you can lock the file room. Security of the keys to that room then becomes an important issue. The number of staff members who have keys to that room should be limited—perhaps to just the physician(s) and the office manager. When the office manager comes into the office each morning, she can unlock the files. Because the files remain open during the day, it is important to make sure they are not placed in areas where unauthorized people can obtain access to them. Posting a sign on the file room door stating "Authorized Personnel Only" helps ensure that files remain secure. To ensure office security after hours, some practices install alarm systems.

Keys and locks bring a measure of security only when they are *used*. Do not become lazy and neglect to lock filing cabinets and file rooms when leaving the office for the day. Security survey teams will always ask to see the keys to any locked door or cabinet and ask the staff to demonstrate that they work. Within a medical office, conducting regular security drills at the same time that fire drills are held will aid staff in staying sharp and aware of security risks.

Equipment Safety

Safety is an important consideration for all filing systems. For example, if the bottom drawer in a vertical file is left open, someone can easily trip over it. Shelving can be dangerous if staff members need to climb a ladder to retrieve files from the highest level.

Safety guidelines for each piece of equipment should be posted prominently in the office. Make sure that every staff member knows where the rules are posted. Then, make sure that everyone follows the rules to prevent possible injury. Refer to the *Patient Reception* chapter for detailed information on ergonomics and preventing injuries in the medical office.

▶ Filing Supplies   LO 15.3

Once you have chosen your filing equipment, the next step is selecting filing supplies. Figure 15-2 features an assortment of filing supplies commonly used by medical practices.

File Folders

The most basic filing supply is the file folder, often referred to as a manila folder. This folder is made of heavy paper folded in half to form a pocket that can hold papers. File folders come in two sizes: letter size, which is 8½ by 11 inches, and legal size, which is 8½ by 14 inches.

Tabs The tapered rectangular or rounded extension at the top or side of the folder is called the tab. Tabs may extend the full length of the folder, as with straight-cut folders, but more often they are cut to extend partway across a folder.

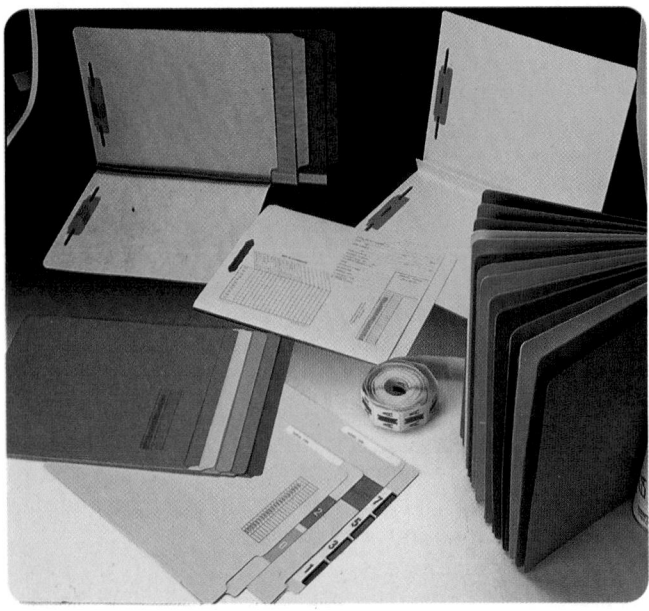

FIGURE 15-2 Medical offices use a wide assortment of filing supplies.

Using folders with a variety of tab locations makes it easier to read the names on the tabs. The most common type of folder for medical charts is the third-cut folder. Tabs are one-third the width of the folder and appear at the left side, center, or right side.

Labels Labels are often used on the folder tabs to identify the individual folder's contents. You can write directly on the tab area in pen or pencil, but it is critical that each label be printed very clearly, so it is more desirable to type or print the chart label. This method is consistently easier to read and lends a more professional appearance. Printed labels can easily be created using a label template available with most word processing software programs, like Microsoft Word.

No matter what filing system your office uses, it is important to be consistent in preparing file labels. If all the files are labeled with the patient's last name, followed by the patient's first name and middle initial (for example, Brown, Emma L.), each label must then follow this format. If the alphabetic filing system is used, be sure that you spell each patient's name correctly on the label.

Hanging File Folders

File folders cannot be suspended inside filing cabinet drawers. In order to keep medical records neat and orderly, they must be placed inside hanging file folders. These hanging file folders resemble regular file folders, but have metal or plastic hooks on both sides at the top that hook onto the metal bars inside the drawers. Like file folders, hanging folders come in letter and legal size.

Plastic tabs—either colored or clear—serve to identify the contents of hanging file folders and contain inserts labeled (using type or print) to correspond with the folders' contents. All inserts should be prepared in a consistent and legible style, similar to that of the medical charts.

Binders

Some offices keep patient records in three-ring binders rather than in file folders. The binders are labeled on the outside spine. Documents are three-hole-punched and then placed inside the binder. Binders are stronger than a file folder but require more storage space and so may not be functional for most medical offices. Inactive patient records can be transferred to a file folder for off-site storage. The binder can then be used again. Binders are especially effective for practices that see patients repeatedly, resulting in very large medical records.

File Guides

To identify a group of file folders in a file drawer, you may use **file guides**, which are heavy cardboard or plastic inserts to separate the contents so individual files can be found easily. For example, if a drawer contains the files for patients whose last names begin with the letters A through C, the guides might separate A from B and B from C.

Out Guides

Another filing supply is an **out guide**. An out guide is a marker made of stiff material. It is used as a placeholder when a file has been removed from the filing system. Many out guides include a clear pocket that can hold the name of the file that belongs in that place or the name of the individual who took the file, and its return due date. Other out guides contain a lined sheet of paper where you can write who has the chart and the date it was taken on the out guide, and then cross it out when the file is returned. Out guides can be used for both shelf and cabinet filing.

Although out guides are not essential, they are extremely helpful in ensuring that files are returned to their proper places. Out guides also save time, as they make it obvious when a file is missing and where it is to be returned. Out guides work best when the entire staff, including the physicians, makes a dedicated effort to use the system.

File Sorters

File sorters are large accordion-style folders with tabs in which records can be stored temporarily, until the patient records can be returned to their proper placement in the cabinet or shelf. Other file sorters made of metal, wood, or plastic may sit on a desk and have multiple slots for temporary placement of patient records.

▶ Filing Systems   LO 15.4

A filing system is the method by which files are organized. A variety of filing systems may be used, but every system places patient records in some sort of **sequential order**—one after another in a pattern, or sequence, that can be predicted. Find out which filing system your office is using and follow it exactly, as any deviation can result in lost or misplaced records. Never make any changes in the filing system without first consulting the physicians and other staff members in the practice.

Alphabetic Filing System

One of the common filing systems for maintaining patient files in sequential order is the **alphabetic filing system**. It is simple and easy to use. In the alphabetic filing system, files are arranged in alphabetic order (last name, first name, middle initial). Each patient's medical record is labeled with the patient's last name, followed by the first name and the middle initial (if any). Let's look at this example, consisting of four patient names, filed alphabetically:

Williams, Louis R.

Wilson, Michelle A.

Wilson, T. Andrew.

Wilson, Thomas A.

The specific rules to follow when filing personal names alphabetically are called **indexing rules** (Table 15-1). These rules are used as guidelines for the sequencing of files based on current business practice. They define a consistent method for the ordering of filed materials. The Association of Records, Managers, and Administrators monitors and updates these suggested methods periodically. In this way, the best, most efficient management of paper records is continually being reevaluated. From time to time, individual medical practices may choose to deviate from some of these accepted practices. However, indexing rules are the norm for most medical practice filing systems.

Indexing rules define each part of a person's name or title as a **unit**. The rules then describe the order to display and manage each unit in an alphabetized system. These rules are designed to keep alphabetizing simple and consistent. Although considered simple, you must know the exact spelling of a patient's name to retrieve a file. You also must know the rules of indexing. Check out the Points on Practice feature for common indexing rules and examples on correct filing order when indexing names that are very similar.

Chronological Filing

A chronological filing system is based on dates. Chronological filing is a type of numeric arrangement that uses numeric dates as the indexing units. The most common order of units is year, month, and day, as in 13-11-06 to denote the sixth of November 2013. It is also common practice to order the most current dates first with the files that follow in decreasing date order.

In a medical practice, filing chronologically is one method used to file documents *within* a patient's chart. The most recent files (by date) are inserted so they are on top of documents with earlier dates in the file folder. This is known as *reverse chronologic order*.

Numeric Filing

A **numeric filing system** organizes files by numbers instead of by names. In this system, each patient name is assigned a number. New patients are assigned the next unused number in sequence. Then, instead of being filed by name, the files are arranged in numeric order—1, 2, 3, 4, and so on. The resulting files are sequential by the order in which patients have come to the practice.

Only the numbers are indicated on the files. Patient names are recorded elsewhere. This system used to be applied primarily when patient information was highly confidential—as in the case of HIV-positive patients; but with HIPAA treating all patient information as protected, more and more offices are converting to numeric filing systems.

The numeric system can be expanded to indicate the location of files. For example, if the last three numbers represent the patient's number, the number 113306 may represent the file of the 306th patient, which can be found in the eleventh filing cabinet in the third drawer.

A numeric system must include a master list of patient names and their corresponding medical record numbers (MRN). If the office is not computerized, to ensure confidentiality, the office manager should keep the master list in a secure place. The physician should hold a duplicate copy, which must also be kept under lock and key. To find a patient's file number using a computer system, you would click the "Open Patient Chart" button (Figure 15-3) and enter the first few letters of the patient's last name. Then scroll through the names and find the required patient. Choose that patient (usually by highlighting the patient name) and press the "Enter" key. The computer would then provide the medical record number for that patient.

TABLE 15-1 Indexing Rules of Alphabetic Filing of Personal Names

In alphabetizing, treat each part of a patient's name as a separate unit and look at the units in this order: last name, first name, middle initial, and any subsequent names or initials last. Disregard punctuation. Follow the "nothing before something" rule—an initial will come before a full name spelled out.

Name	Unit 1	Unit 2	Unit 3	Unit 4
Stephen Jacobson	Jacobson	Stephen		
Stephen Brent Jacobson	Jacobson	Stephen	Brent	
B. T. Jacoby	Jacoby	B	T	
C. Bruce Hay Jacoby	Jacoby	C	Bruce	Hay
D. Jones	Jones	D		
David Jones	Jones	David		
Kwong Kow Ng*	Ng	Kwong	Kow	
Philip K. Ng	Ng	Philip	K	

Treat a prefix, such as the "O" in O'Hara, as part of the name, not as a separate unit. Ignore variations in spacing, punctuation, and capitalization. Treat prefixes—such as De La, Mac, Saint, and St.—exactly as they are spelled.

Name	Unit 1	Unit 2	Unit 3	Unit 4
A. Serafino Delacruz	Delacruz	A	Serafino	
Victor P. De La Cruz	DeLaCruz	Victor	P	
Irene J. MacKay	MacKay	Irene	J	
Walter G. Mac Kay	MacKay	Walter	G	
Kyle N. Saint Clair	SaintClair	Kyle	N	
Peter St. Clair	StClair	Peter		

Treat hyphenated names as a single unit. Disregard the hyphen

Name	Unit 1	Unit 2	Unit 3	Unit 4
Victor Puentes-Ruiz	PuentesRuiz	Victor		
Jean-Marie Vigneau	Vigneau	JeanMarie		

A title, such as Dr. or Major, or a seniority term, such as Jr. or 3d, should be treated as the last filing unit to distinguish names that are otherwise identical.

Name	Unit 1	Unit 2	Unit 3	Unit 4
Dr. George B. Diaz	Diaz	George	B	Dr
Major George B. Diaz	Diaz	George	B	Major
George B. Diaz, M.D.	Diaz	George	B	MD
James R Foster Jr.	Foster	James	R	Jr
James R Foster Sr.	Foster	James	R	Sr
Sister Theresa**	Sister	Theresa		

*In the case of foreign or Asian names, when unsure of first- and last-name order, many offices cross-reference the file with a "dummy record" at the alternate location stating, "see Ng, Kwong Kow."

**"Sister Theresa" and similar names, where there is no clear first or last name, are "filed as written."

Source: Adapted from William A. Sabin, *The Gregg Reference Manual, 11th ed.* (Columbus, OH: Glencoe/McGraw-Hill, 2011).

FIGURE 15-3 The toolbar for the SpringCharts™ EHR program highlighting the Open Patient Chart icon.

Source: Screen captures of SpringCharts™ Electronic Health Records software are reprinted with permission from Spring Medical Systems, Inc. All rights reserved.

Indexing Rules

Rule 1: Individual Names

The last name is the first indexing unit, the first name is the second unit, and the middle name is the third unit. If an initial is used instead of a name, the single initial is viewed as the entire unit.

Name	Unit 1	Unit 2	Unit 3	Unit 4
D. Jones	Jones	D		
David Jones	Jones	David		
David R. James Jones	Jones	David	R	James

Rule 2: Business Names

As written (on letterhead) each word is a unit. If "The" is used as the first word, it is considered the last unit.

Name	Unit 1	Unit 2	Unit 3	Unit 4
Jones Hearing Supplies	Jones	Hearing	Supplies	
The Jones Hearing Supplies	Jones	Hearing	Supplies	The

Rule 3: Hyphenations and Abbreviations

All hyphenated names are considered to be one unit (i.e., Terry-Jones, Sheila); an abbreviated name is combined to form the unit. An abbreviated name, such as Wm. for William, is filed as Wm, without the use of a period.

Name	Unit 1	Unit 2	Unit 3	Unit 4
St. Mary, William	StMary	William		
St. Mary, Wm.	StMary	Wm		
Terry-Jones, Sheila	TerryJones	Sheila		

Rule 4: Titles and Seniority Terms

Titles are normally disregarded unless they are used to distinguish between two patients with the same name. If there are patients with the same name and a title precedes the name, use it as the fourth unit. Seniority terms such as Jr. or Sr. may be indexed as the last unit. It is important to remember that if a male child has exactly the same name as his father, he is considered Jr. until his father dies. He is a "III" if his father and his grandfather have the same name. If "II" or "III" is used as a seniority title, the basic rule states that numbers come before letters, so David Jones III would be filed before David Jones Jr.

Name	Unit 1	Unit 2	Unit 3	Unit 4
David C. Jones	Jones	David	C	
Rev. David C. Jones	Jones	David	C	Rev
David Jones Jr.	Jones	David	Jr	
David Jones Sr.	Jones	David	Sr	

Rule 5: Prefixes

If the last name has a prefix such as Mc, Van, or de; the prefix is part of the last name. It starts the first indexing unit. The prefixes Mc and Mac are usually filed in alphabetical order as part of the last name.

Name	Unit 1	Unit 2	Unit 3	Unit 4
Elias DeLongino	DeLongino	Elias		
Drew MacDreamy	MacDreamy	Drew		
Drew McDreamy	McDreamy	Drew		
Elias D. Van Collins	VanCollins	Elias	D	

Rule 6: Names of Married Women

A woman may retain her maiden name as her last name instead of taking her husband's surname; she also may use both names and hyphenate them (see Rule 3—hyphenation). She will always keep her first and middle name as part of her original name. A married woman's name may take several forms.

Name	Unit 1	Unit 2	Unit 3	Unit 4
Mrs. David (Cynthia M.) Jones	Jones	Cynthia	M	
Mrs. Gisele Marie Jones	Jones	Gisele	Marie	
Mrs. Gisele M. Monagan-Jones	MonaganJones	Gisele	M	

Rule 7: Identical Names

If two names are identical, make sure you index them first under their names; location is next (city as the first unit, state as the second unit, street is the third unit, and street number listed lowest to highest is the fourth and final unit). This rule is used for businesses and individuals.

Terminal digit filing is often the filing system of choice for numeric filing systems. This type of filing allows for the storage of an endless number of files with only a minimal amount of searching needed to obtain the correct files. Numbers are assigned in small groups of two or three numbers, similar to a social security number. Each group of numbers is then read from right to left, starting with the last unit as the primary index. Filing is done numerically, starting with the lowest number and moving to the highest. For example, all files ending in 000 are filed first. They are then followed by files ending in 001, etc. See Table 15-2 for an example.

Middle digit filing is similar to terminal digit filing but instead uses the middle group of numbers as the primary index, followed by the left-hand number and then the right-hand one. See Table 15-3 to view the same medical record numbers filed using the middle digit system.

TABLE 15-2	MRNs Filed in Terminal Digit Order*		
Medical Record Number	Unit 1	Unit 2	Unit 3
002-25-565	565	25	002
001-25-566	566	25	001
001-24-667	667	24	001
002-24-667	667	24	002

*Showing each filing unit.

TABLE 15-3	MRNs Filed in Middle Digit Order*		
Medical Record Number	Unit 1	Unit 2	Unit 3
001-24-667	24	001	667
002-24-667	24	002	667
001-25-566	25	001	566
002-25-565	25	002	565

*Showing each filing unit.

Numeric, terminal digit, and middle digit filing can all be used in combination with color-coding to add even more information to the filing system.

Color-Coding

Color-coding is used when there is a need to distinguish files within a filing system. For example, you may wish to find at a glance all the new patients in the office, all patients on Medicare, or all patients whose last names begin with the letters WI. Coding by color can help you do so quickly and easily. Color-coding may be done in a variety of ways using colored file folders, colored labels, plastic tabs, and/or stickers.

Using Classifications To make the best use of color, you must first identify the classifications that are important to your office. For example, it may be important to identify all new patients easily, or those on Medicare. Once a classification is selected, the decision must be made as to what method of coding will be used (folder, labels, or stickers). Then, a different color must be chosen to denote each classification. For example, all new patients may be kept in red folders, or plain manila folders may be used, but a red sticker or red filing label is attached to the charts of new patients.

An office that uses colored charts to denote specific patient demographics might look something like this: Patients under the age of 18 have blue charts; patients over the age of 65 have red charts; and patients with diabetes have green charts, with a pink sticker added for those who are on insulin. In an emergency situation, such as when a patient with diabetes passes out while in the office, the color-coding could give staff quick and vital information at a glance.

After a color-coding system is finalized, the codes should be prominently posted on a chart in the file room so that all staff members are aware of them. This chart will help to ensure that records are filed correctly. Remember, update color-coded files consistently, coding new ones and revising older ones as a patient's status changes.

Using Color in an Alphabetic Filing System Another way to use color-coding is in conjunction with alphabetic filing systems. After files are organized alphabetically, each letter of the alphabet is assigned a color. Then the first two (or three) letters of each patient's last name are color-coded, usually with colored stickers.

The colored tabs are attached to the top of straight-edged or tabbed file folders. For example, if the letter S is coded as light blue and the letter M is coded as light green, all names starting with SM—like Smith—would have light-blue and light-green colored stickers on the tabs of their medical charts. The name Snyder would be filed under a different color combination, such as light blue (for S) and peach (for N). See Figure 15-4. Because the colors will be the same in each segment of the file drawer, a color-coded system makes it easy to tell at a glance if files are filed correctly (refer back to Figure 15-1).

Using Color in a Numeric Filing System Color can be used in a similar way with numeric systems. The numerals 1 to 9 may each be assigned a distinct color. As with the alphabetic system, color-coding helps identify numeric files that are out of place. When using color with numeric filing systems, most offices color the primary index or "key unit" for each chart. If the key unit is three numbers, then all three numbers of the key unit will use a colored tab to identify each file. For example, recall our medical record numbers from Table 15-2 for terminal digit filing, as shown in part (a). If #5 is blue, #6 is red, and #7 is yellow, our chart tabs for filing would look as shown in part (b).

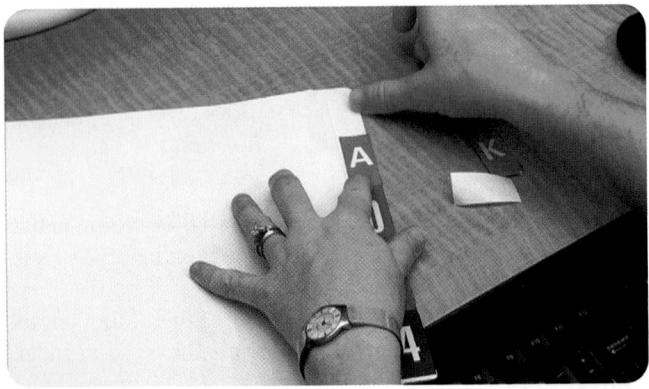

FIGURE 15-4 Colored stickers for both letters and numbers help identify charts rapidly.

002-25-565		5	6	5
001-25-565		5	6	5
001-24-667		6	6	7
002-24-667		6	6	7
(a)		(b)		

Procedure 15-1, at the end of this chapter, explains how to use your knowledge of alphabetic and numeric filing and color-coding to set up a patient records system.

Supplemental Files

Occasionally, you may need to set up additional files to supplement the medical records filing system. For example, you may wish to keep some information separate from the primary file, such as older patient records or the required separate filing system for patient financial and insurance information. In these cases, you set up supplemental files, which allow you to keep this additional information about each patient without cluttering up the primary filing cabinets or making it difficult to find information.

Supplemental files are usually created using the same system as the primary files, but they are kept in a different location. Depending on frequency of use, they may be stored in a less-accessible, but equally secure, area of the office. If you are keeping supplemental files, it is important to distinguish their content from that of the primary files. For example, all medical information—like patient diagnosis and treatment—will be kept in the primary files, but the financial, insurance, and billing information for each patient will be kept in a separate billing filing system. This designation will help you and other office staff members know exactly where to go to retrieve specific information.

Tickler Files

To avoid losing track of important dates, many medical practices use tickler files. A **tickler file** is a date-ordered reminder file. Think of your smartphone or home calendar; many of us record important activities and reminders, creating an informal tickler file for our personal activities. Any office activity that needs to be scheduled ahead of time can be noted and a reminder placed in the file. For example, reminders to order supplies or send patient checkup cards can be entered. When the task has been completed, the note can be crossed off the list or removed from the file and thrown away. In computerized offices, many office software packages include calendars and "tickler files" with pop-up reminders of meetings and other activities. Regardless of how it is set up, the person involved with the activity should regularly check the tickler files at a minimum of once a week—preferably daily. This is important because tickler files only work if they are used regularly.

You can organize tickler files in a variety of ways. The common manual method, discussed in Procedure 15-2 at the end of this chapter, is to allot one file folder to each month of the year or to use a three-ring binder separated with tabs for each month. Tickler files also can be organized by day of the week or week of the month. This method is most useful if there are responsibilities that occur regularly on a certain day of the week or in a certain week within the month. If you find there are so many notes in a monthly folder that it becomes cumbersome, organizing files by the week should make this easier.

Computerized tickler files are usually in the form of a calendar. When the computer is turned on, it lists, for example, "Things to Do Today" with the tickler information posted for that date. Reminders can be set for tasks that must be completed on a regular basis—daily, weekly, or monthly—or on a one-time basis.

▶ The Filing Process
LO 15.5

Pulling and filing patient records and filing individual documents may be among your responsibilities as a medical assistant. Some practices require that records be returned to the files as soon as they are no longer in use. Other practices schedule a specific time at the end of each day to file the current day's records and pull those for the next day.

Records waiting to be filed should be placed temporarily in a file return area. To protect patient privacy, this place should be in a secure area of the office. Clear rules should designate who may handle these files and under what conditions.

The Steps in Filing

Essentially, you will be filing three types of items: new patient records, individual documents that belong in existing patient records, and patient records that are being returned to the filing system. There are five steps involved in filing: inspecting, indexing, coding, sorting, and storing.

Inspecting The first step in the filing process is to make sure the item is ready to be filed. Inspect the document or patient medical record for a mark, notation, or stamp indicating that it is ready to be filed. For example, it may be initialed by the physician or stamped with the word *File* on a self-adhesive flag attached to the upper-right corner. Some offices have staff members simply place folders ready for filing in a specially designated box or bin.

Remove paper clips, rubber bands, and any extraneous material that does not need to be filed. Staple loose papers to keep them together, per office protocol. Documents are less bulky when stapled than when held together by clips or rubber bands.

If the document to be filed is much smaller than standard size, it may become lost in the file or even fall out. To prevent this, you may want to use special paper containing self-adhesive areas that allow smaller documents to be attached to a standard size sheet, or even "shingling" (layering) the smaller document to save space and avoid lost documents. When small documents have wording on both sides of the paper, they can be placed in standard-size clear plastic sheet protectors and then filed.

Indexing Another term for naming a file is **indexing**. Names should be chosen carefully as that is how the file will be known, retrieved, and replaced. Traditionally, patient names have been used as the file names for patient records, but today, this is often replaced with a numeric name or index. Most offices that use a numeric system use computer software to create new patient medical record numbers. Part of the indexing process will be to verify that the color-coding (if used) is correct and that any stickers or labels are securely fastened to the file. If colored files are used to denote patient diagnosis or insurance type, indexing is also the time to verify if any changes need to be made to the patient's file related to their current demographic.

Note that some files can logically be placed in more than one location. Such files should be **cross-referenced**, or filed in two or more places, with each place noted in each file. When cross-referencing a file, you may create a cross-reference form that gives the correct location to look for the file. For instance, an elderly woman might refer to herself as Mrs. John Smith. If you cannot remember her legal name, in the area where *Smith, John, Mrs.* would be located, you would place a mock folder that reads "Smith, John, Mrs., SEE Smith, Christine." You would then place the form under any heading where it is possible to look for that file. You may wish to attach it to a blank file folder, cutting the file folder in half so it consists of only one sheet, so that no documents are mistakenly filed within it.

Coding When you put an identifying mark or phrase on a document to ensure that it is placed in the correct file, that is known as coding. To code a document, simply write the patient's name, MRN, or the subject title of the file folder on the document. Alternatively, you can underline or highlight key words on the document itself. This step can be skipped when returning patient documents to their medical record or returning the records themselves to their properly filed location.

Sorting If you have more than one document or medical record to be filed, you must sort the files (documents) that have accumulated. Sort them in the order in which they are kept—such as alphabetically or numerically. Sorting saves you time later when you return the files to their proper places. If you will not be filing the items immediately, store them in a temporary location, like a file sorter.

Storing The final step in the filing process is to store the files in the appropriate filing equipment. Documents should be stored neatly within their file folders in the proper sequence.

Careful attention to file storage will make your job easier. Make sure the charts (folders) are in good condition. Replace them whenever they appear damaged or torn to prevent file contents from spilling out during the retrieval and filing process. If a file contains too many documents and becomes too bulky, divide it into two or more folders and label each one (for example, Glass, Ann M.—Folder 1 of 2; Glass, Ann M.—Folder 2 of 2). Also, be sure when labeling records that consist of more than one chart that the content of each chart is clear (Folder 1 of 2, records prior to 2011; Folder 2 of 2, records from 2011 forward). Replace any labels that are no longer legible.

Filing Guidelines

There are specific rules for each filing system, as well as general guidelines, or helpful hints, that are applicable to any system. Following these guidelines will help you file more efficiently (Figure 15-5).

- Each time you pull or file a patient record, glance at its contents. You should be familiar with the typical contents and the order of a patient record folder to help avoid filing errors.

FIGURE 15-5 Filing on a regular basis keeps the task from becoming overwhelming and reduces the incidence of lost files.

- Keep files neat. Make sure that documents fit neatly into the file folders. Papers should not extend beyond the edge of the folder. Do not place too many papers in each file folder. Folders should stay closed when laid on a flat surface.

- When inserting documents into folders already in place in the drawer, lift the folders up and out of the drawer; otherwise, this can lead to misfiling of documents. Attempting to force documents into a folder inside the drawer can damage the documents.

- Do not crowd the file drawer. Leave extra space to allow for leafing through the files and for retrieving and replacing files easily. Where possible, use a combination of uppercase and lowercase letters to label folders. This format is easier to read than labels written completely in capital letters.

- Choose file guides with a different tab position than your folders to help them stand out. Do not place guides so close together that they hide one another. A good rule of thumb is to position guides at least 5 inches apart.

- If you are unsure whether to cross-reference a file, do it. It is better to err on the side of providing too many cross-references than too few.

- File regularly so that you are not overwhelmed with too many records or documents.

- Store only files in filing cabinets or on filing shelves.

- Do not store office equipment or supplies where files belong.

Evaluating the Office Filing System

The filing system you have probably does an adequate or better-than-average job of fulfilling the practice's needs. Otherwise, retrieving and filing patient records would have become annoyingly inefficient. It is always beneficial to see where improvements can be made, however. Even a good filing system can be enhanced to increase office efficiency and save staff members valuable time.

Here are some simple guidelines for evaluating your filing system.

1. How well do you think your filing system meets your needs? Rate it on a scale of 1 to 10, with 10 representing the best. Survey staff members to determine their ratings and calculate a composite number. *Based on this feedback, does your filing system seem to do a poor, adequate, or exceptional job?*

2. Note the type of system you use—for example, alphabetic or numeric. Then list the various reasons why files are retrieved from the system. *Would another system, a combination of systems (such as alphanumeric), or the addition of color-coding save time or offer other benefits?*

3. Survey the office staff to determine whether there have been difficulties in retrieving or filing or problems with lost or misplaced files. Solicit suggestions for improvement. *If there have been problems, what steps could you take to avoid future difficulties?* (You might even ask your local office-supply representative for ideas.)

4. Consult personnel at other, similar medical practices to determine which filing system works for them. Compare and contrast their systems with yours. *How would their systems work in your office?*

Before making any major changes to your filing system, evaluate each idea in terms of the time and effort it will require and the benefits it will deliver. For example, changing from an alphabetic to a numeric system may provide a relatively small benefit to your office but require a great deal of time to prepare new files and refile current documents. In that case, implementing a numeric system is probably not worthwhile.

If you do make changes to your system, make sure that all staff members are retrained on how to file documents. It is well worth the extra time required at the start to prevent having to locate misplaced files in the future.

- Train all staff members who will retrieve and replace files to make sure they have a thorough understanding of the system. Update them on any changes.
- Periodically evaluate your office's filing system. The Points on Practice section will help you with this task.

Locating Misplaced Files

Even in the best filing systems, there is a chance of temporarily misplacing or even losing a patient medical record. No matter how good a system is, errors will still be made. If a file is misplaced, here are steps you can take to try to locate it.

1. Determine the last time you or anyone else in the practice knew the file's location.

2. Go to that location and retrace the steps of the last person who handled the file. Look for the file along the way.

3. Look in the filing cabinet where the file belongs. Check neighboring files. Possibly, the file was simply put in the wrong place. Look inside other, thicker files to determine if the missing file was accidentally placed inside another file.

4. Check underneath the files in the drawer or shelf to see if the file slipped out.

5. Check the pile of items to be filed or the file sorter envelope.

6. Consider possible cross-references or similar indexes (for example, similar patient names) for the file. Check those headings to see if the file was accidentally placed there.

7. Check with other staff members to determine if they have seen the file.

8. Check to make sure the missing file was not filed under the patient's *first* name instead of the last.

9. Stand back from the file cabinet and view the *top* of the folders, looking at only the first three letters of the last names. A misfiled file will stand out.

10. If using a color-coded system, look for the color of the misfiled chart.

11. Even though files should always be kept in a secure area, occasionally individuals who are not part of the office staff, such as visiting physicians, may be in the area and may inadvertently pick up a file with their own materials. If you think someone could have taken the file, call the person immediately.

12. Ask another staff person to complete steps 1 through 7 to double-check your search.

13. Straighten the office, taking care to check through all piles of information where a file could be lodged.

14. Check those charts that have been pulled for next day's appointments to see if misplaced charts have been accidentally pulled.

15. Check the physician's desk (and office).

If the misplaced file is not found within a reasonable time—24 to 48 hours—it may be considered lost. Losing a file has potentially devastating consequences as it contains the patient's medical history, test results, and treatments. It may not be possible to duplicate the information within the file, but you can try to recreate it in a new medical record.

To do this, meet with the physician and clinical staff members to review the information needed. Record their recollections of information in the file. Note on the medical record that it is a duplicate and that the information is not official.

Consult with other offices and departments who may have records related to the file. Contact laboratories, hospitals, and other providers to request copies of documents previously included in the lost file. Place copies of those records in the new medical record, or excerpt information given to you. If the physician considers it appropriate, tell the patient whose file has been misplaced about its status and the steps you have taken to re-create it, including the offices and facilities that have been contacted to obtain information needed to recreate the medical record.

Limiting Medical Record Access

As stated earlier, the information in a patient's medical record is on a "business need to know." In computerized offices, your access ID and password will restrict the information you are allowed to see. Some offices using paper records restrict the number of people who can retrieve and return files, adding an extra measure of security to the practice. To obtain a file, staff members must fill out a requisition slip with their name, the name of the patient, and the reason for the request.

A record of who has the file is kept either in a notebook or on index cards in a card file. It also may be placed on the out guide, which is kept in the same location as the record until the record itself is returned to the filing system.

Unless required by court order, original patient medical records should not leave the practice. Photocopies can be made, if necessary. Review the *Legal and Ethical Issues* chapter regarding release of patient information.

▶ Active, Inactive, and Closed Files LO 15.6

No office has unlimited space. So, you need to understand the differences between active, inactive, and closed files. In your role as medical assistant, you may regularly need to transfer inactive and closed files from the office filing area to a storage area.

Active versus Inactive Files

At any given time, there are files that you use frequently, called **active files**, and files that you use infrequently or not at all, called **inactive files**. What constitutes an active, as opposed to an inactive, file? It depends on your individual practice. In a cardiologist's office, a patient who has not been seen for a year may be considered inactive, while in a dental office, a year may simply indicate one missed appointment.

A third category of files, called **closed files**, are files of patients who have died, have moved away, or for some other reason no longer come to the office. Although closed files could be moved immediately to storage, they are usually treated in the same manner as inactive files. That is, they are kept in the office for a certain length of time to make sure that there are no requests for the information in the file.

The length of time inactive and closed files are kept or retained is 7 to 10 years. All medical records must be retained for 7 years; but because the Federal False Claims Act requires financial records be kept for 10 years and medical records provide the medical necessity information for the billing records, many legal experts suggest also keeping medical records for 10 years (see the *Legal and Ethical Issues* chapter). Ultimately, it is the physician who will determine when a patient file is deemed inactive or closed. You and the physician (or office manager) can meet regularly (once a month or once a quarter) to review these files.

Basic Storage Options

Before you can transfer files to storage, you need to determine how and where they will be stored. The design and layout of file storage should make even older stored files easily accessible so that they can be periodically evaluated for retention or elimination.

There are many ways to store inactive files. For example, they can be stored in their original paper state or transferred into another format, such as onto a computer disk or into microfilm or microfiche. Files can even be electronically coded with bar codes for immediate retrieval with a computer system. Regardless of the medium chosen for storing and preserving documents, keeping related material together and retrieving it should be made as easy as possible. Inactive files contain PHI and must be kept just as secure as active files.

Paper Storage If the practice chooses to store files in their original form, they will likely be stored in boxes labeled with their contents. Choose boxes that are uniform in size so they will stack well and have lift-off lids for easy access to contents.

Although paper files are bulky to store and require roughly the same amount of space as they occupied while in the office, these files preserve the original documents. Access to these documents can be important when providing evidence of medical treatment in legal proceedings. However, if paper files start to become brittle, they should be transferred to another storage medium.

Computer Storage If storage space is limited, there are a number of paperless options for storing files, which include recordable CDs or DVDs, jump or flash drives, and external hard drives. To store records or information electronically, the office needs a computer system that can transfer documents to some type of electronic or digital format and then read them when they are retrieved from storage. (Refer to the *Office Equipment and Supplies* and the *Electronic Health Records* chapters for electronic storage options.)

The easiest way to transfer documents directly into the computer is to use a scanner, which copies a document into a document on the computer's hard drive. This process saves countless hours of rekeying documents into the computer. Most scanners can also copy graphics and handwritten notes. The document is then labeled and saved. Documents that were originally created using the computer can also be transferred to CD, DVD, or external hard drive and then deleted from the computer system's internal hard drive. The chosen storage device is then dated and stored in labeled file boxes or other containers. The *Electronic Health Records* chapter provides more detailed information about electronic document creation and storage options.

Other paperless storage options include microfilm, microfiche, and film cartridges. When considering transferring files to these formats, explore microfilm services, which index and transfer files for a fee. Using a service helps ensure that files are correctly indexed and thus easily found later on. Always have the microfilm service sign a confidentiality agreement. The *Office Equipment and Supplies* chapter covers these media in more detail.

Retaining Files in the Office

Every office will develop a length of time appropriate for the long-term storage of files. Most practices develop a records retention program.

Typically the physician decides—based on the potential need for the information—how long to keep inactive or closed patient files in the office before sending them to storage. Working with the physician and/or office manager, you should prepare a retention schedule. A **retention schedule** specifies how long to keep different types of patient records in the office after files have become inactive or closed. The schedule also details when files should be moved to a storage area and how long they should be kept in storage before being destroyed. The retention schedule should be posted in the file room to make certain that all staff members are aware of it.

Although the doctor decides how long to keep inactive or closed patient records in the office, there are legal requirements for retaining certain types of information that determine how long these documents must be stored. The *Legal and Ethical Issues* chapter should be reviewed for the legal guidelines regarding retention of various types of records found in the medical office. For the most updated and complete list of required record retention periods according to HIPAA law, go to the HIPAA advisory website (www.hhs.gov/ocr/hipaa). This guide is updated annually. State and local retention requirements can be obtained from offices with which you regularly conduct business, like insurance companies, state and local agencies, and medical associations. If you do business in more than one state, follow the schedule that requires the longest retention time for materials. Also, if your state's (retention or other) requirements are more stringent than HIPAA laws, follow your state requirements.

When counting years in a retention schedule, remember not to count the year in which the document was produced but to begin counting with the following year. This way, documents produced near the end of a calendar year will be tracked more efficiently. Procedure 15-3 summarizes the steps for setting up a records retention program.

When records are to be eliminated, they cannot simply be thrown away, as even old records hold confidential information about patients. So, these must be completely destroyed by shredding. Be careful not to destroy records prematurely because they often cannot be re-created. It is vital that you retain a list of documents that have been destroyed.

Storage Facilities

You may wish to store files in a remote area of your office building, like an unused closet or office. Check to make sure that the area is secure, accessible, and safe for storing files (for example, do not store files where hazardous materials are stored). The practice may have to pay additional rent if the space is not within the confines of its office suite.

If there is no space in the building, consider a neighboring building, perhaps one in the same office complex. Many buildings rent space that can be used to store records. If you pursue this option, you will be responsible for managing the storage of records, including transporting them to the space, positioning them, and retrieving them as needed.

Certain storage facilities, called commercial records centers, will do some of the work for you. For a monthly fee, these centers typically house and manage stored documents. When evaluating commercial records centers, inquire about whether they will retrieve and/or deliver boxes or files and whether there is an on-site work area if someone needs to review the files at the storage location.

Maintain a separate list of files stored off-site. This list can save a wasted trip to the storage site if a needed file is not housed there. The list also provides a valuable record if files are damaged or destroyed. Remember, always update the list as new files are moved into storage and old files are taken out of storage and destroyed.

Storage Safety

No matter where you store files, you must consider the issue of safety as well as security. Beware of general storage facilities that are not specially equipped for document management. For example, these facilities may not address safety concerns by taking precautions for fire or floods—an absolute necessity for medical records. So, it is wise to evaluate the storage site and to take some basic precautions.

- Choose a site with moderate temperatures year-round and adequate ventilation.
- Select waterproof storage containers that can also withstand intense heat. When possible, use metal or plastic boxes that are designated as fireproof and waterproof. Cardboard boxes, although often used for storage, are not as strong or durable. If cardboard storage boxes are used, they need to be placed on shelving well off the floor to avoid water damage.
- Choose a site equipped with a smoke alarm, sprinkler system, and fire extinguishers.
- Select a site that is above ground and away from flood hazards. One way to find out if a site is susceptible to flooding is to inquire whether the facility has flood insurance, a requirement for sites at risk.
- Choose a site that is kept locked, is regularly patrolled, or has an alarm system, to prevent theft or vandalism.
- Remove old, brittle files as soon as possible or transfer them into another format. They can then be placed in file storage again.

- Ask for references from people at other offices who have stored files at the site. Talk to these people about what they like and dislike about the storage facility and any problems they have had in storing or retrieving documents.

- If you are storing files in another form—on computer disk or microfiche—inquire about any special precautions the site owner takes to ensure safety.

Taking the time to thoroughly research storage options ultimately saves time and effort as you manage stored files.

PROCEDURE 15-1 Creating a Filing System for Paper Medical Records

Procedure Goal: To create a filing system that keeps related materials together in a logical order and enables office staff to store and retrieve medical records efficiently.

OSHA Guidelines: This procedure does not involve exposure to blood, body fluids, or tissue.

Materials: Vertical or horizontal filing cabinets with locks, tabbed file folders, labels, file guides, out guides, filing sorters.

Method: Procedure steps.

1. Evaluate which filing system is best for your office—alphabetic or numeric. Make sure the doctor approves the system you choose.
   RATIONALE: The purpose of a filing system is to provide accessibility of all medical records for the entire staff.

2. Establish a style for labeling files and make sure that all file labels are prepared in this manner.

3. Avoid writing labels by hand. Use a keyboard, label maker, or preprinted adhesive labels.

4. Set up a color-coding system to distinguish the files (for example, use blue for the letter A, red for B, yellow for C, and so on). Create a chart, suitable to be hung in a professional file room, that uses the color-coding system.

5. Use file guides to divide files into sections.

6. Use out guides as placeholders to indicate which files have been taken out of the system. Include a charge-out form to be signed and dated by the person who is taking the file.
   RATIONALE: Out guides allow for quick and easy identification of a missing file and its location.

7. To keep files in order and to prevent them from being misplaced, use a file sorter to hold those patient records that will be returned to the files during the day or at the end of the day.

8. Develop a manual that explains the filing system to new staff members. Include guidelines on how to keep the system in good order.
   RATIONALE: A filing system only works when all office personnel use it consistently.

PROCEDURE 15-2 Setting Up an Office Tickler File

Procedure Goal: To create a comprehensive office tickler file designed for year-round use.

OSHA Guidelines: This procedure does not involve exposure to blood, body fluids, or tissue.

Materials: 12 manila file folders or 3-ring binder with 12 separators, 12 file labels, pen or typewriter, paper.

Method: Procedure steps.

1. Write or type 12 file labels, 1 for each month of the year. Abbreviations are acceptable. Do *not* include the current calendar year, just the month.

2. Affix one label to the tab of each file folder.

3. Arrange the folders so that the current month is on the top of the pile. Months should follow in chronological order.

4. Write or type a list of upcoming responsibilities and activities. Next to each activity, indicate the date by which the activity should be completed. Leave a column after this date to indicate when the activity has been completed. Use a separate sheet of paper for each month.
   RATIONALE: Each sheet should clearly indicate when the activity has been completed and by whom. Each sheet should be filed within the appropriate month's folder.

5. File the notes by month in the appropriate folders.
   RATIONALE: This will create a neat and orderly way to collect tickler notes for each month.

6. Place the folders in order, with the current month on top, in a prominent place in the office, such as in a plastic box mounted on the wall near the receptionist's desk.

7. Check the tickler file at least once a week on a specific day, like every Monday. Assign a backup person to check it in case you happen to be out of the office.

8. Complete the tickler activities on the designated days, if possible. Keep notes concerning activities in progress. Be sure to note when activities are completed and by whom.
   RATIONALE: Keep a record of responsibilities and completed activities in case a question concerning the activity or responsibility comes up at a later date.

9. At the end of the month, place that month's file folder at the bottom of the tickler file. If notes are remaining in that month's folder, move them to the current month's folder.
   RATIONALE: Incomplete activities must be moved to the new month to be sure they are not overlooked.

10. Continue to add new notes to the appropriate tickler files.
    RATIONALE: To provide for continual update to the tickler system.

PROCEDURE 15-3 Developing a Records Retention Program

Procedure Goal: To establish a records retention program for patient medical records that meets office needs, as well as legal and government guidelines.

OSHA Guidelines: This procedure does not involve exposure to blood, body fluids, or tissue.

Materials: Updated guide for record retention as described by federal and state law (go to the HIPAA advisory website), file folders, index cards, index box, paper, pen or typewriter.

Method: Procedure steps.

1. List the types of information contained in a typical patient medical record in your office. For example, a file for an adult patient may include the patient's case history, records of hospital stays, and insurance information.

2. Research the state and federal requirements for keeping documents. Contact your appropriate state office (such as the office of the insurance commissioner) for specific state requirements, like rules for keeping records of insurance payments and the statute of limitations for initiating lawsuits. If your office does business in more than one state, be sure to research all applicable regulations. Consult with the attorney who represents your practice.

3. Compile your research results in a chart. At the top of the chart, list the different kinds of information your office keeps in patient records. Down the left side of the chart, list the headings "Federal," "State," and "Other." Then, in each box, record the corresponding information.

4. Compare all the legal and government requirements. Indicate which one is for the longest period of time.
   RATIONALE: Retaining all records for the longest period of time required by the laws governing your organization will assure that you are in compliance with all laws.

5. Meet with the physician (or office manager) to review the information. Working together, prepare a retention schedule. Determine how long different types of patient records should be kept in the office after a patient leaves the practice and how long records should be kept in storage. Although retention periods can vary based on the type of information kept in a file, it is often easiest to choose a retention period that covers all records. Determine how files will be destroyed when they have exceeded the retention requirements. Usually, records are destroyed by paper shredding. Purchase the appropriate equipment, or contract with a shredding company as necessary.
   RATIONALE: Shredding complies with HIPAA privacy rules regarding protected health information (PHI).

6. Put the retention schedule in writing and post it prominently near the files. In addition, keep a copy of the schedule in a safe place in the office. Review it with the office staff.

7. Develop a system for easily identifying files under the retention system. For example, for each file deemed inactive or closed, prepare an index card or create a master list containing the following information:
   - Patient name and Social Security number.
   - Contents of the file.
   - Date the file was deemed inactive or closed and by whom.
   - Date the file should be sent to inactive or closed file storage (the actual date will be filled in later; if more than one storage location is used, indicate the exact location to which the file was sent).
   - Date the file should be destroyed (the actual date will be filled in later).

   Have the card signed by the physician (or office manager) and by the person responsible for the files. Keep the card in an index box or another safe place. This is your authorization to destroy the file at the appropriate time.

8. Use color-coding to help identify inactive and closed files. For example, all records that become inactive in 2013 could be placed in green file folders or have a green sticker with "13" placed on them and moved to a supplemental file. Then, in January 2015, all of these files could be pulled and sent to storage.

9. One person should be responsible for checking the index cards once a month to determine which stored files should be destroyed. Before retrieving these files from storage, circulate a notice to the office staff stating which records will be destroyed. Indicate that the staff must let you know by a specific date if any of the files should be saved. You may want to keep a separate file with these notices.

10. After the deadline has passed, retrieve the files from storage. Review each file before it is destroyed. Make sure the staff members who will destroy the files are trained to use the equipment properly. Develop a sheet of instructions for destroying files. Post it prominently with the retention schedule, near the machinery used to destroy the files.
    RATIONALE: To guard patient confidentiality and follow all HIPAA laws governing the protection of patient information.

11. Update the index card, giving the date the file was destroyed and by whom.

12. Periodically review the retention schedule. Update it with the most current legal and governmental requirements. With the staff, evaluate whether the current schedule is meeting the needs of your office or whether files are being kept too long or destroyed prematurely. With the physician's approval, change the schedule as necessary.

LEARNING OUTCOMES	KEY POINTS
15.1 **Identify the common equipment used to file and store paper medical records.**	Filing shelves, filing cabinets (horizontal and vertical), compactable files, and rotary files are all commonly used to store paper medical records. A very small office might opt to use storage bins for its medical records, but because of bulk, storage concerns, as well as weight and safety issues when moving the units, this method is ill advised for most practices.
15.2 **Outline the security and safety measures that should be employed when working with paper medical records.**	HIPAA requires that filing shelves or cabinets should be fireproof and locked when the office is closed. If files are kept in a file room, the room should be locked when not in use with only a minimal number of staff members possessing the key. Filing systems must be safe for those using them and instructions on their proper use should be posted and understood by all staff members using them. All staff should be instructed on proper body mechanics regarding all tasks in the medical office to avoid work-related injuries.
15.3 **List the common filing supplies used in the medical office.**	Filing supplies used in the medical office include tabbed file folders, labels, hanging file folders, binders, tabs with inserts for labeling, file guides, out guides, and file sorters.
15.4 **Contrast the methods used for various filing systems and how color-coding can assist with the filing systems.**	Alphabetic filing is the traditional filing system for medical offices. Using the filing rules found in Table 15-1 and the indexing rules in the Points on Practice feature, medical records are filed alphabetically using each patient's last name, first name, and middle initial as the first 3 filing units. Color-coding can enhance this process when each letter is assigned a different color and the first 2–3 letters of each patient's last name are attached to the chart using colored labels so filing errors stand out. Numeric systems are used more often because of the confidentiality they provide. These systems use a series of numbers assigned to each patient (medical record number), which are then filed by the terminal digit or middle digit format. As with alphabetic filing, color can be used in a similar way with numeric filing by assigning each number 0–9 a distinct color so that filing mistakes stand out more readily.
15.5 **Recall the steps in the filing process.**	The steps in the filing process include inspecting, indexing (naming), coding, sorting, and storing.
15.6 **Compare active, inactive, and closed files and how to set up a records retention program for the office.**	Active records are those that are used frequently. Infrequently used records are known as inactive records. Closed files are those of patients who, for whatever reason, no longer come to the office. Procedure 15-3 outlines the procedure to be used in creating an office medical records retention program.

Recall Malik Katahri from the beginning of the chapter. Now that you have completed the chapter, answer the following questions regarding his case.

1. What are some of the advantages of changing the filing system from an alphabetic-based system to a numeric system?

2. Would there be advantages to staying with the current system? How might you convince the physicians that electronic records would solve the filing "dilemma," making the financial outlay worthwhile? (Using information from the *Electronic Health Records* chapter may be helpful when answering this question.)

EXAM PREPARATION QUESTIONS

1. (LO 15.1) Which of the following are commonly used in medical offices as storage units for medical records?
   a. Filing shelves
   b. Filing cabinets
   c Compactible files
   d. Rotary circular files
   e. All of the above

2. (LO 15.2) Which of the following does not follow recommended security guidelines for medical records?
   a. Locking the records in a separate room
   b. Using locking shelves
   c. Using locking file cabinets
   d. Giving everyone in the office a key to the file room
   e. Posting a sign next to the file room stating, "Authorized Personnel Only"

3. (LO 15.3) Which of the following supplies are commonly used as the medical record?
   a. File folders (hanging)
   b. File folders
   c. File tabs
   d. File sorters
   e. File guides

4. (LO 15.4) Which of the following lists the correct unit order for patient Quin Kwan Po MD?
   a. 1. MD   2. Po   3. Kwan   4. Quin
   b. 1. Quin   2. Kwan   3. Po   4. MD
   c. 1.Po   2. Quin   3. Kwan   4. MD
   d. 1. Po   2. Kwan   3. Quin   4. MD
   e. b, c, and d may be used with cross-references to each

5. (LO 15.4) Which of the following lists the correct filing order for the names listed?
   a. Beals, Bentley Rian/Beals, Jazmyn/Beals, Kim/Beals, Lexus
   b. Johnson, B. James/Johnson, Bradley/Johnson, Bryan/Johnsen, Calvin
   c. Stark, Eleanor/Stark, Elinor/Stark-Ward, Eliner/Stark-Ward, Eleanor
   d. Whalen, Mari/Whalen, Mari L./Whalen, Mary Lou/Whalen, Mari Lou

   e. Smith, James J. II/Smith, James J. III/Smith, James J. Sr./Smith, James J. Jr.

6. (LO 15.4) Which of the following numeric sequences are correct using middle digit filing?
   a. 010 333 285 / 001 333 285 / 010 333 284 / 123 334 219
   b. 001 333 262 / 010 333 285 / 010 333 284 / 123 334 219
   c. 001 333 262 / 010 333 284 / 010 333 285 / 123 334 219
   d. 123 334 219 / 010 333 285 / 010 333 284 / 001 333 262
   e. 010 333 284 / 010 333 285 / 001 333 262 / 123 334 219

7. (LO 15.4) Which of the following numeric sequences uses terminal digit filing?
   a. 010 333 285 / 001 333 285 / 123 334 285 / 010 334 285
   b. 001 333 285 / 010 333 285 / 010 334 285 / 123 334 285
   c. 123 334 285 / 010 334 285 / 010 333 285 / 001 333 285
   d. 010 334 285 / 010 333 285 / 001 333 285 / 123 334 285
   e. 010 333 285 / 010 334 285 / 001 333 285 / 123 334 285

8. (LO 15.4) If names are absolutely identical, what is the address order that is used to choose the filing order?
   a. State, city, street name, street number
   b. City, state, street number, street name
   c. Street name, street number, city, state
   d. City, state, street name, street number
   e. Each office may choose the order that works best for them

9. (LO 15.5) The filing term that means you are *naming* the document in order to file it correctly is
   a. Inspecting
   b. Indexing
   c. Coding
   d. Sorting
   e. Storing

10. (LO 15.6) Which of the following describes the records of patients who have moved across the country?
   a. Active
   b. Inactive
   c. Closed
   d. Retained
   e. "Old patients"

16

Schedule Management

CASE STUDY

<table>
<tr><td rowspan="3">PATIENT INFORMATION</td><td>Patient Name</td><td>Gender</td><td>DOB</td></tr>
<tr><td>John Miller</td><td>M</td><td>12/5/19XX</td></tr>
</table>

Patient Name	Gender	DOB
John Miller	M	12/5/19XX
Attending	**MRN**	**Allergies**
Paul F. Buckwalter, MD	082-09-981	Bee stings

John Miller is a 65-year-old patient with a history of hypertension, type 2 diabetes mellitus, history of MI (myocardial infarction) 4 years ago, and a confirmed current diagnosis of CHF (congestive heart failure). He is taking glyburide 2.5 mg daily, Captopril 25 mg twice a day, and HCTZ 25 mg a day. You notice when he arrives today that he is significantly short of breath. When asked, he states, "Have been doing OK until I fell down yesterday. I was carrying a box of stuff to take to the Salvation Army and lost my footing." He then shows you abrasions of his right elbow and left knee. After his examination, Dr. Buckwalter speaks to Mr. Miller's cardiologist and then asks you to book a cardiac catheterization. Mr. Miller is a Medicare patient, but he is covered under a Medicare (managed care) replacement plan instead of the traditional Medicare plan.

Keep Mr. Miller in mind as you study this chapter. There will be questions at the end of the chapter based on the case study. The information in the chapter will help you answer these questions.

LEARNING OUTCOMES

After completing Chapter 16, you will be able to:

16.1 Describe how the appointment book is key to the continuity of patient care.

16.2 Identify how to properly apply a matrix to an appointment book.

16.3 Compare different types of appointment scheduling systems.

16.4 Identify ways to organize and schedule patient appointments.

16.5 Model how to handle special scheduling situations.

16.6 Explain how to schedule appointments that are outside the medical office.

16.7 Implement ways to keep an accurate and efficient physician schedule.

KEY TERMS

advance scheduling
cluster scheduling
double-booking system
itinerary
locum tenens
matrix
minutes
modified-wave scheduling

no-show
open-hours scheduling
overbooking
time-specified scheduling
underbooking
walk-in
wave scheduling

V. C (1)   Discuss pros and cons of various types of appointment management systems

V. C (2)   Describe scheduling guidelines

V. C (3)   Recognize office policies and protocols for handling appointments

V. C (4)   Identify critical information required for scheduling patient admissions and/or procedures

V. P (1)   Manage appointment schedule, using established priorities

V. P (2)   Schedule patient admissions and/or procedures

8. Medical Office Business Procedures Management

Graduates:

   c.   Schedule and manage appointments

   f.   Schedule inpatient and outpatient admissions

  dd.   Serve as liaison between physician and others

  ll.   Apply electronic technology

11. Career Development

Graduates:

Demonstrate professionalism by:

  (1) Exhibiting dependability, punctuality, and a positive work ethic

  (3) Maintaining confidentiality at all times

  (8) Being courteous and diplomatic

▶ Introduction

As a medical assistant, you will need to know all aspects of how to create and utilize an appointment book and/or electronic scheduler. In this chapter you will learn how to identify the different types of scheduling systems, how each is used, and which type of system will work best for each type of practice. You also will learn how to handle many types of scheduling situations within the medical office, including patient appointments, emergencies, pharmaceutical representatives, and the scheduling of patient appointments with other medical facilities. Legal aspects of the appointment book are discussed and proper documentation is stressed. Additional topics include appointment cards, reminder mailings, reminder calls, and recall notices for patients.

▶ The Appointment Book   LO 16.1

Time is of great value for everyone involved—the physician, the patient, and the office staff. Scheduling appointments in an organized fashion shows respect for everyone's time and creates an efficient patient flow. If the schedule is changed for any reason, the medical assistant must update the appointment book or scheduler and make sure that everyone involved is aware of the change. A well-managed appointment book, regardless of whether it is an actual book or an electronic format within a computer system, is key to patient continuity of care and presents the office in a positive, professional manner, ultimately keeping all parties involved on task and on time.

The office schedule depends on physician preferences and habits, the facilities available, and patient need. Although most patients understand that they may have to wait in the reception area before they are seen by the physician, few patients are willing to wait more than 20 minutes. Offices that routinely have long waiting times can find themselves with dissatisfied

patients, which can lead to other problems (such as *former* patients). You may find that some patients will get creative in an attempt to avoid waiting. They may deliberately arrive after their scheduled appointment time to avoid waiting or come in earlier in hopes of being seen before their scheduled appointment time. Still others may avoid the schedule entirely and walk in expecting to be seen. All of these behaviors, if accommodated, can throw the office schedule off track. Other patients may become resentful and decide to seek medical care with a competing practice.

Even in a well-run office, however, unexpected events can disrupt the schedule. Some patients may unexpectedly require the physician to spend more time with them than was originally scheduled and patients who are ill will need to be added to the schedule, sometimes with little or no notice. Still others will forget appointments or arrive later than scheduled. For these reasons, making an office schedule flow smoothly can be a challenge. A schedule that "plans for the unexpected" combined with excellent communication between the physician, staff, and patients will allow a medical practice to run smoothly despite these obstacles.

Computerized Scheduling

Computerized scheduling systems are becoming more common in medical offices because they have several advantages over handwritten systems (Figure 16-1). As more practices become compliant with electronic health record regulations, the advantages seem to outweigh the disadvantages. Some of the advantages of computerized scheduling include

1. It enables locking out selected areas for designated purposes, such as last-minute or emergency visits.

2. It allows information to be accessed from multiple areas within the office.

FIGURE 16-1 Screen from the Electronic Scheduling Program from SpringCharts.

Source: Screen captures of SpringCharts™ Electronic Health Records software are reprinted with permission from Spring Medical Systems, Inc. All rights reserved.

3. It helps staff to identify problem patients for cancellations, no-shows, and late arrivals.

4. It provides a "search" for upcoming appointments to ensure that proper follow-up care is given.

5. It provides reports on overall scheduling practices.

6. It adds color-coding as a visual aid to identify areas designated for certain types of appointments.

7. It allows searches for requested day or time availability.

Online Scheduling

The online scheduling option (e-scheduling) is slowly gaining acceptance, but it is not recommended for all office types. Online scheduling allows patients to schedule themselves or request an appointment via the Internet. Cost and security have been the barriers to many offices; however, new security measures ensure protection of patient data online and as more programs become available, costs are also becoming more reasonable. Adding an online scheduler to the practice takes some time and requires staff training, but it can be a convenience for your patients, particularly if many of them are computer-savvy.

Before adopting an e-scheduler, assess the practice needs, survey patients regarding web access and potential for usage, and be diligent in your research about available products, particularly regarding privacy issues. One of the frontrunners in e-scheduling is Compass Scheduling, found at www.compassscheduling.com.

▶ Applying the Matrix LO 16.2

Before you begin scheduling appointments, you need to prepare the appointment book or electronic scheduler. The first step is establishing the **matrix,** or basic outline of times the physician

is and is not available to see patients. To create the matrix, block off times within the schedule during which the doctor is not available to see patients. In a paper format, drawing an "X" through the unavailable time slots with a brief explanation is standard practice to avoid errors. The type of appointment book used—whether it uses 10- or 15-minute units—will determine how many "blocks" are crossed out for each designation. Electronic schedulers often use colors to designate the reason the provider is out; they may also place an "X" in the time frames selected. For example, the schedule will show when the doctor is away for the following reasons:

- Hospital rounds
- Surgery/procedures
- Lunch
- Vacation days
- Holidays
- Personal appointments for the physician
- Scheduled meetings (for example, pharmaceutical company or in-service meetings)

The day's schedule is then built around the established matrix. Should the physician or office manager direct that a meeting has been canceled and patients should be seen during a time that had been blocked out, the "X" should be removed and patients scheduled as usual. Some offices prefer the "X" remain and the initials of the person approving the new schedule be added to the appointment time frame. See Figure 16-2 for an example of a matrix for a multiphysician office. For a single-physician schedule with appointments in 15-minute increments, see Figure 16-3.

The same concept is true for the format of an electronic scheduler; if the matrix needs to be changed because the provider will be available to see patients, the time frame is unblocked and patients are then scheduled as usual. This is demonstrated in Figure 16-4. Procedure 16-1 provides the opportunity to practice completing an appointment matrix using an appointment book and Procedure 16-2 outlines the procedure when using an electronic scheduler. Both procedures can be found at the end of this chapter.

Required Patient Information

When the matrix has been established, you can begin scheduling appointments. Some practices enter the information into both traditional paper appointment books and computerized systems. Then, if the computer fails to work for some reason, the office has the book for reference. Some doctors who have been in practice for many years are used to the appointment book method and do not want to give it up for a computer system. Other offices are completely computerized. Per your office policy, you should obtain the following patient information in order to efficiently book a patient appointment regardless of the system used:

- Patient's full name. Obtain the correct spelling of the patient's name.
- Daytime telephone numbers. Repeat phone numbers to ensure accuracy.

APPOINTMENT RECORD

12 November Tuesday				**13** November Wednesday		
Dr. Buckwalter	Dr. Williams	DOCTOR	Dr. Buckwalter	Dr. Williams		

Dr. Buckwalter	Dr. Williams	DOCTOR	Dr. Buckwalter	Dr. Williams
		AM		
Surgery		8:00		
		8:15	Surgery	
		8:30		
		8:45		
		9:00		
		9:15		
		9:30		
		9:45		
		10:00		
		10:15		
		10:30		
		10:45		
		11:00		
		11:15		
		11:30		
		11:45		
	Lunch	12:00		
		12:15		
		12:30		
		12:45		
		PM		
		1:00		
		1:15		
		1:30		
		1:45		
		2:00		
		2:15		
		2:30		
		2:45		
		3:00		
		3:15		
		3:30		
		3:45		
		4:00		
		4:15		
		4:30		
Staff Meeting at		4:45		Conference
Mercy General		5:00		
		5:15		
		5:30		
		5:45		

REMARKS & NOTES

FIGURE 16-2 The first step in appointment scheduling is to establish the matrix—defining when the physician is available to see patients.

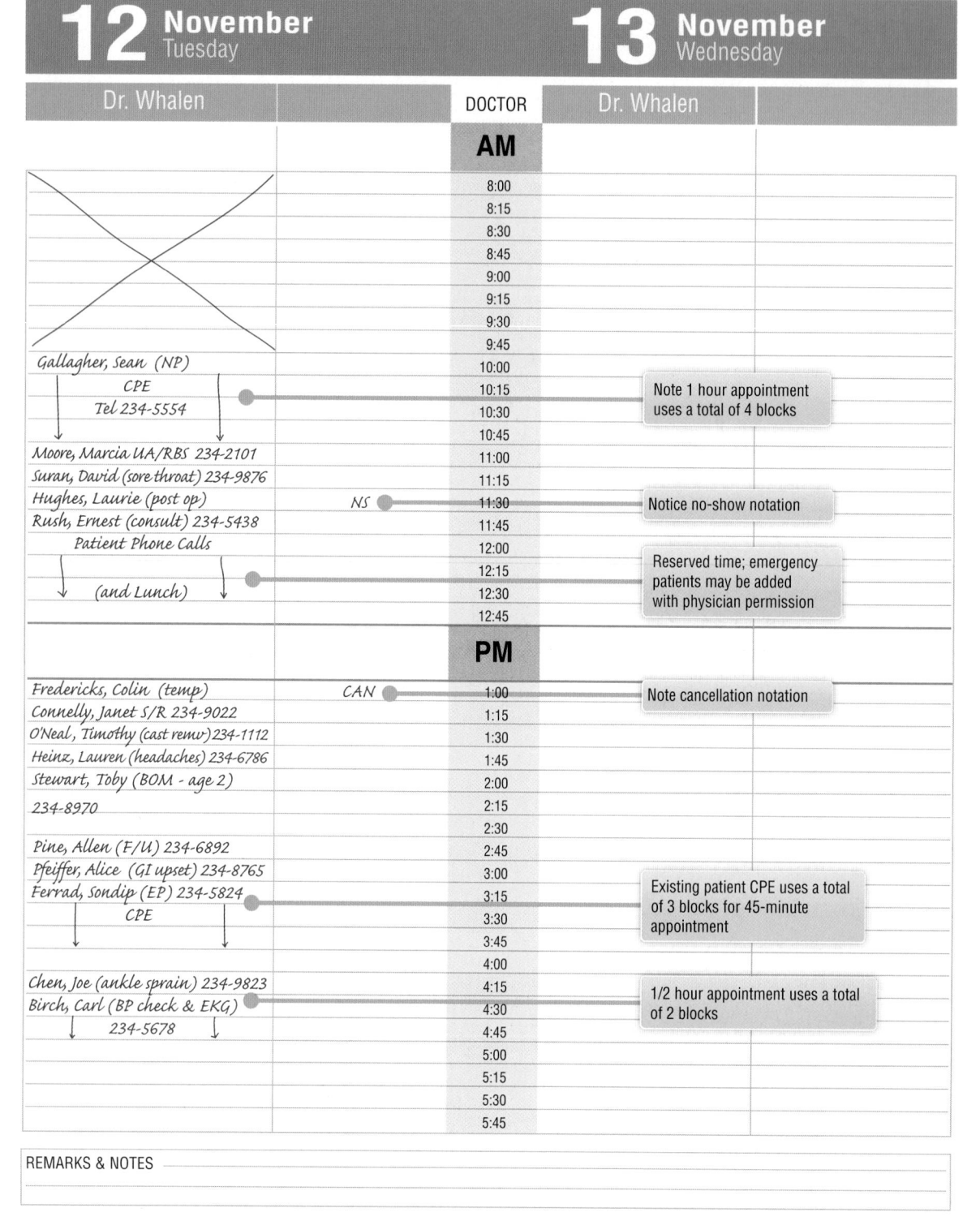

FIGURE 16-3 Single-physician appointment book using 15-minute appointment blocks with explanation for time allotted for each appointment.

FIGURE 16-4 Electronic scheduler for the SpringCharts Program. Note the section identified as B as unavailable to see patients.

Source: Screen captures of SpringCharts™ Electronic Health Records software are reprinted with permission from Spring Medical Systems, Inc. All rights reserved.

- Purpose of the visit. Use a brief description and utilize approved abbreviations when possible without disclosing the patient's diagnosis or violating HIPAA. Do not create your own abbreviations as this can lead to errors or misunderstandings regarding the reason for the patient appointment.

Abbreviations in Appointment Scheduling

If you are the person who maintains the appointment book, you will find that certain procedures and conditions occur frequently. Usage of the abbreviation will depend on the office specialty. Only approved universal medical abbreviations should be used. To save space and time when entering information, use the abbreviations found in Table 16-1.

Standard Appointment Times

If you are to schedule appointments efficiently, you must have a guideline of how long visits are expected to take. Working with the physician(s) in your practice, create a list of standard appointment times. Also indicate in the list how much time to allow for tests that are commonly performed in the practice. This list, which should be kept near the appointment book or programmed into the electronic scheduling system, helps you identify which openings are appropriate for the appointment type or

procedure involved. This list is intended as a guide only, as each patient visit is unique. The list will also assist you in choosing an appropriate appointment book or scheduler, as most are based on 10-, 15-, or 30-minute increments. The lengths and types of tests and procedures will depend on the practice policy and procedure manual. Table 16-2 lists the typical lengths of common office appointments and procedures.

The Appointment Book as a Legal Record

The appointment book is considered a legal record. Some experts advise keeping old appointment books for at least three years. Because the appointment book could be used as evidence in legal proceedings, entries must be clear and easy to read. Management consultants suggest that because the appointment book is a legal document, the schedule should be written in blue ink, although many offices still prefer black ink. In spite of this, many offices that still use the paper method use pencils to record the initial entry. If pencil is used, at the end of each day you should write directly over the penciled entries in ink to create a permanent document.

Never erase a name or use correction fluid to blot the name out. Instead, as with any medical record draw a single line through the name and beside it write in the reason such as

TABLE 16-1 Common Abbreviations Used in Appointment Scheduling

Abbreviation	Description
BP	blood pressure check
can/cx	cancellation
CDE or CPE	complete diagnostic exam/ complete physical exam
c/o	complains of
cons	consultation
CP	chest pain
ECG/EKG	electrocardiogram
FBS	fasting blood sugar
FU or f/u	follow up
I&D	incision and drainage
inj	injection
lab	laboratory studies
minor surg	minor surgery
N&V	nausea and vomiting
NP	new patient
NS	no-show patient
P&P	pelvic (exam) and pap (smear)
Pap	Pap smear
pt	patient
PT	physical therapy
RBS	random blood sugar
re	recheck
ref	referral
RS	reschedule
Rx	prescription
Sig	sigmoidoscopy
S/R	suture removal
surg	surgery
US or U/S	ultrasound

TABLE 16-2 Typical Appointment Times for Specific Appointment Types

Appointment Type or Procedure	Time Frame Allotted
Complete physical examination (existing/new patient)	30 minutes/60 minutes
New patient visit	30–45 minutes
Follow-up appointment	5–15 minutes
Emergency office visit	15–20 minutes
Prenatal examination	15 minutes
Pelvic exam and Pap smear	15–30 minutes
Minor (in-office) surgery (e.g., mole removal)	30 minutes
Suture removal	10–20 minutes

"NS" or "can". You may also write the date, time of the new appointment if known, with "RS" (rescheduled) and the new date, and reason (if known) why the appointment was missed or canceled, then initial the entry. This information also should be documented in the patient's medical record to track possible compliance issues. (Complete information on patient documentation is found in the *Medical Records and Documentation* chapter.)

▶ Appointment Scheduling Systems

LO 16.3

There are several popular appointment scheduling systems. The method chosen usually depends on the type of practice and physician preferences. No matter which method your office uses, it should be regularly reviewed to see whether it is meeting its goals: a smooth flow of patients and minimal waiting time.

Open-Hours Scheduling

In the **open-hours scheduling** system, patients arrive at their own convenience with the understanding that they will be seen on a first-come, first-served basis. The only thing that may alter this is an emergency. Depending on how many patients have arrived ahead of them, they may have a considerable wait. The open-hours system eliminates the problems caused by broken appointments because there are no assigned appointment times, but it increases the possibility of inefficient downtime for the physician and office staff should there be no patients in the office. In addition to possible long wait times, if paper medical records are used, the medical assistant cannot retrieve patients' charts before they arrive. Although still used by emergency departments, urgent care centers, and some rural practices, most private practices have replaced this system with scheduled appointments.

Even though appointments are not booked ahead of time with an open-hours system, a matrix must still be established so the staff will know when a physician is unavailable to see patients. Additionally, for legal (as well as tracking) reasons, an open-hours system still requires the use of an appointment book or electronic scheduling system to record patients as they arrive in the office.

Time-Specified Scheduling

Time-specified scheduling (also called stream scheduling) assumes a steady stream of patients all day long at regular, specified intervals. Once the matrix has been applied and physician availability has been established, it can be determined how many slots or blocks should be used for each appointment type (refer to Table 16-2). Most minor medical problems, such as sore throats, earaches, or blood pressure follow-ups, usually require only 10- to 15-minute appointment slots. More time may be required for appointments such as physical exams, which usually require 60 minutes, or new patient visits, which usually require 30 minutes. When a visit requires more time, you simply assign the patient additional back-to-back slots. Using arrows or parentheses on both sides of the appointment entry will allow you to easily see the length of existing appointments and the remaining open time slots. Refer back to Figure 16-2 for an example of a completed schedule for a single physician and Figure 16-3 for a similar schedule using an electronic scheduling system.

Wave Scheduling

Wave scheduling works effectively in larger medical facilities that have enough departments and personnel to provide services to several patients at the same time. This method of scheduling is based on the reality that some patients will arrive late and that others will require more or less time than expected with the physician. Wave scheduling has the flexibility to allow for appointments that require more time than anticipated or for patients who miss appointments. The goal is to begin and end each hour with the overall office schedule on track. You determine the number of patients to be seen each hour by dividing the hour by the length of the average visit. If the average is 15 minutes, for example, you schedule four patients for each hour. An example of wave scheduling would be

10:00 A.M.	Mohammad Nassar	555-5683	Sore throat
10:00 A.M.	Shenya Jones	555-7322	Low back pain
10:00 A.M.	John Miller	555-4673	FU B/P
10:00 A.M.	Raja Lautu	555-2854	B12 inj

You ask all four patients to arrive at the beginning of the hour and have the physician see them in the order of their actual arrival. The main problem with wave scheduling is that patients may realize they have appointments at the same time as other patients. The result may be confusion and possibly annoyance or anger.

Modified-Wave Scheduling

The wave system can be modified in several ways. With **modified-wave scheduling,** as shown in Figure 16-5, patients might be scheduled in 15-minute increments. Another option is to schedule four patients to arrive at planned intervals during the first half hour, leaving the second half hour unscheduled. Appointments that are anticipated to require more time should be scheduled at the beginning of the hour. Appointments that are expected to be less time-consuming should be scheduled in 10- to 20-minute time slots. This method allows time for catching up before the next hour begins.

Double-Booking

With a **double-booking system,** two or more patients are purposely scheduled for the same appointment slot. Unlike the wave or modified-wave system, however, the double-booking system assumes that both patients will actually be seen within the scheduled period.

This type of system is especially useful when one patient can be managed by the nurse practitioner or physician assistant for an immunization or blood pressure check and the other patient is seen at the same time by the physician. Double-booking can also be helpful if a patient calls with a problem and needs to be seen that day but no appointments are available. You may double-book this patient with an already-scheduled patient.

In such cases you should explain to the caller that he might have to wait a bit before being seen by the physician. To avoid these circumstances, some offices purposely leave one or two appointment slots open each morning and each afternoon to accommodate these "urgent" appointments.

Cluster Scheduling

Cluster scheduling groups similar appointments together on a specific day or for a specific block of time during the day or week (also called categorization scheduling). Cluster scheduling is often used for appointments such as blood sugar screenings, school physicals, and the like; for instance, Wednesdays after 3 p.m. might be set aside for school physicals as it would be a more convenient time for parents. Cluster schedules are also helpful in offices where specialized equipment or services (such as physical therapy or ultrasound) are available only at certain times.

Advance Scheduling

In some specialties patients might be booked weeks or months in advance, as for annual gynecologic examinations. In such practices **advance scheduling** is used. It is still advisable to leave a few slots open each day, however, for patients who call with unexpected or unusual problems.

Combination Scheduling

Some practices combine two or more scheduling methods. For example, they might use cluster scheduling for new patients and double-booking for quick follow-ups such as sore throats, hypertension, or a new medication.

▶ Organizing and Scheduling Appointments LO 16.4

As you determine patient needs and office availability when arranging appointments, always keep in mind that you are representing the office. How you interact with patients will have either a positive or negative impact depending on your actions and choices. Being polite and courteous while maintaining a professional manner is key. Try to be as accommodating as possible to the patient but at the same time uphold the policies and protocols of the office.

As discussed earlier in the chapter, patient status (new or existing patient) and chief complaint must be clearly identified prior to scheduling any appointment, as this will dictate the length of time the physician will spend with the patient.

New Patients

Patients who have never been seen in the practice or have not been seen by the practice in three or more years are considered to be new patients. A convenient decision tree to help define patients as new or existing is found in the *Procedure Coding* chapter—Figure 19-4. Appointments for new patients are most often arranged over the telephone. Be sure to obtain all the necessary information, including the correct spelling of the person's name, home address, daytime telephone number,

APPOINTMENT RECORD

12 November Tuesday

Dr. William		DOCTOR		
		AM		
Auerbach, Conrad	Sinclair, Monica	8:00		
FU	FU	8:15		
		8:30	Purdy, Marianne	Ganzalez, Hector
		8:45	↓ INJ	↓ INJ
Molini, Francesca	Jacobson, Eloise	9:00		
BP	LAB	9:15		
		9:30	Buffer	Sherbert, Philip
		9:45		↓ LAB
Willis, Nina	Smith, Marshall	10:00		
	FU	10:15		
		10:30	Chandler, Larry	MacDonald, Liam
		10:45	↓ GI	↓ GI
Buffer	Ward, Sylvia	11:00		
	UTI	11:15		
		11:30	Campbell, Joel	Ramoson, Katrina
		11:45	↓ FU	↓ PMS
		12:00		
		12:15		
		12:30		
		12:45		
		PM		
Gibble, Cora	Bunsen, Elmer	1:00		
ECG	SOB	1:15		
		1:30	Moskowitz, Matthew	Cheng, Amy
		1:45	↓ ECG	↓ BP
Silverstein, Sidney	Burns, Laura	2:00		
SOB	ECG	2:15		
		2:30	↓ Buffer	↓ Osborne, Jonathan ↓
		2:45		BP
Warren, Mary	Harris, Noel	3:00		
CP	CP	3:15		
		3:30	McDermott, Elizabeth	Corbin, Allicia
		3:45	↓ FU	↓ FU
Buffer	Warner, Steve	4:00		
	RE	4:15		
		4:30	Thompson, Will	Stein, Merle
		4:45	↓ CPE	↓ CPE
Cabrisi, Claudia	Velone, Tina	5:00		
US	US	5:15		
		5:30	Tucker, Bob	Kapoor, Fatima
		5:45	↓ CONS	↓ CONS

REMARKS & NOTES

FIGURE 16-5 Modified wave schedule: two patients are booked each half hour.

and date of birth. The patient's insurance information as well as the full name of the guarantor (if not the patient) and his or her relationship to the patient also should be obtained at this time. With so many insurance plans available, this has become increasingly important because it is impossible for any office to accept every insurance type. Even if the insurance is accepted by the office, verification of coverage should be done prior to the patient being seen in the practice. Obtaining this information also will allow you to remind the patient that if any copayment is required by his insurance plan, the payment is expected at the time of the visit. For more information on insurance coverage and the verification process, please refer to the *Insurance and Billing* chapter.

When arranging the appointment, keep in mind that the matrix will dictate availability of some types of appointments. When scheduling an appointment for a new patient, ask the patient to arrive 15–30 minutes early to allow time for filling out the required "new patient forms," if they have not been sent to the patient prior to the appointment. Information regarding these forms may be found in the *Medical Records and Documentation* chapter. Upon arrival, the new patient also should be given the HIPAA guidelines for your office while his or her chart is being prepared for the visit. As discussed in the *Legal and Ethical Issues* chapter, a signed receipt of the HIPAA privacy practices is now a requirement for all patients seen in the practice.

Established Patients

Established patients are those that have been seen by the practice within the last 3 years. Many times, return appointments for existing patients are made at the time they are being checked out from a current appointment. It is always good practice to ask patients returning to the reception area if they need to schedule another appointment. It is helpful for patients who are followed routinely to have appointments scheduled in a set pattern whenever possible. For instance, if a patient needs monthly B$_{12}$ injections, scheduling the appointments for the first Tuesday of each month at 3 p.m. will be easier for the patient to remember than a different day or time each month. Scheduling patients while they are still in the office also allows you to give them an appointment card to remind them of the appointment so they can enter it in their schedule or on the "home calendar." If the patient's visit is being made by phone and is not for the immediate future, you also may ask her if she would like an appointment card mailed to her. Remember to remind existing patients, also, that any copayment is due at the time of the appointment. Procedure 16-3 at the end of the chapter outlines the procedure to utilize when booking patient appointments.

Go to CONNECT to see a video about *Scheduling Appointments.*

Appointment Confirmations and Reminders

It seems today that everyone is busy with hectic schedules. It is often difficult for patients to remember their next appointment, especially if they arrange it far in advance. To help patients keep track of their appointments, you can use several types of appointment reminders.

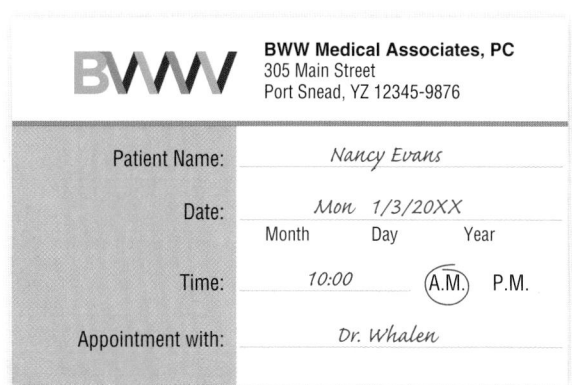

	BWW Medical Associates, PC
BWW	305 Main Street
	Port Snead, YZ 12345-9876

Patient Name:	Nancy Evans		
Date:	Mon	1/3/20XX	
	Month	Day	Year
Time:	10:00	(A.M.)	P.M.
Appointment with:	Dr. Whalen		

FIGURE 16-6 Typical appointment card given to patients to remind them of upcoming appointments.

Appointment Cards In many offices when making a return appointment at check-out, the medical assistant completes and gives the patient an appointment reminder card, like the one shown in Figure 16-6.

To reduce the chance of error, enter the appointment in the appointment book or scheduler first, then fill out the card. Otherwise, when the patient takes the appointment card, you have to rely on your memory when entering the appointment in the book and in a busy office this often can lead to errors. Refer to Procedure 16-4 at the end of the chapter for the steps in completing an appointment card.

Encounter Forms/Superbills As the patient leaves the office, he or she is often given paperwork to return to the front desk. This form, commonly known as the superbill or encounter form, lists services performed, diagnoses, health insurance, and demographic information regarding the patient, as well as account balance. This *super document* also can serve as a receipt if payments are made at the time of the visit. Most superbills, like the one shown in Figure 16-7, also include an area to insert information regarding the patient's next appointment.

Reminder Mailings When making a follow-up appointment in person, ask the patient to address a postcard to himself on which you have written the next appointment's date and time. This postcard serves as a backup in case the patient loses the original appointment reminder card. Place the postcard in the tickler file under the day when it should be sent (usually a week or two before the appointment). Reminder mailings also can be sent to patients who make appointments over the telephone. In this case, of course, you must address the postcard for the tickler file yourself. Although reminder mailings are useful when appointments are made many months in advance or for geriatric patients, they can become costly for the practice and should be limited when possible.

Confirmation Calls Depending on office policy and available time, you might also call patients 1 or 2 days before their appointments to confirm the scheduled time. This technique can be especially helpful for patients with a history of late arrivals or for **"no-shows"** (patients who do not

BWW Medical Associates, PC
305 Main Street, Port Snead YZ 12345-9876, Tel: 555-654-3210, Fax: 555-987-6543

☐ PRIVATE ☐ BLUECROSS ☐ IND. ☐ MEDICARE ☐ MEDI-CAL ☐ HMO ☐ PPO

PATIENT'S LAST NAME		FIRST		ACCOUNT #	BIRTHDATE / /	SEX ☐ MALE ☐ FEMALE	TODAY'S DATE / /
INSURANCE COMPANY		SUBSCRIBER			PLAN #	SUB. #	GROUP

ASSIGNMENT: I hereby assign my insurance benefits to be paid directly to the undersigned physician. I am financially responsible for non-covered services. SIGNED: (Patient, or Parent, if Minor) DATE: / /	RELEASE: I hereby authorize the physician to release to my insurance carrers any information required to process this claim. SIGNED: (Patient, or Parent, if Minor) DATE: / /

✔	DESCRIPTION	M/Care	CPT/Mod	DxRe	FEE	✔	DESCRIPTION	M/Care	CPT/Mod	DxRe	FEE	✔	DESCRIPTION	M/Care	CPT/Mod	DxRe	FEE
	OFFICE CARE						PROCEDURES						INJECTIONS/IMMUNIZATIONS				
	NEW PATIENT						Tread Mill (In Office)		93015				Tetanus		90718		
	Brief		99201				24 Hour Holter		93224				Hypertet	J1670	90782		
	Limited		99202				If Medicare (Set up Fec)		93225				Pneumococcal		90732		
	Intermediate		99203				Physician Interpret		93227				Influenza		90724		
	Extended		99204				EKG w/Interpretation		93000				TB Skin Test (PPD)		86585		
	Comprehensive		99205				EKG (Medicare)		93005				Antigen Injection-Single		95115		
							Sigmoidoscopy		45300				Multiple		95117		
	ESTABLISHED PATIENT						Sigmoidoscopy, Flexible		45330				B12 Injection	J3420	90782		
	Minimal		99211				Sigmoidos. , Flex. w/Bx.		45331				Injection, IM		90782		
	Brief		99212				Spirometry, FEV/FVC		94010				Compazine	J0780	90782		
	Limited		99213				Spirometry, Post-Dilator		94060				Demerol	J2175	90782		
	Intermediate		99214										Vistaril	J3410	90782		
	Extended		99215										Susphrine	J0170	90782		
	Comprehensive		99215				LABORATORY						Decadron	J0890	90782		
							Blood Draw Fee		36415				Estradiol	J1000	90782		
	CONSULTATION-OFFICE						Urinalysis, Chemical		81005				Testosterone	J1080	90782		
	Focused		99241				Throat Culture		87081				Lidocaine	J2000	90782		
	Expanded		99242				Occult Blood		82270				Solumedrol	J2920	90782		
	Detailed		99243				Pap Handling Charge		99000				Solucortef	J1720	90782		
	Comprehensive 1		99244				Pap Life Guard		88150-90				Hydeltra	J1690	90782		
	Comprehensive 2		99245				Gram Stain		87205				Pen Procaine	J2510	90788		
	Dr.						Hanging Drop		87210								
	Case Management		98900				Urine Drug Screen		99000				INJECTIONS - JOINT/BURSA				
													Small Joints		20600		
	Post-op Exam		99024										Intermediate		20605		
							SUPPLIES						Large Joints		20610		
													Trigger Point		20550		
													MISCELLANEOUS				

DIAGNOSIS:	ICD-9									
__ Abdominal Pain	789.0	__ Gout	274.0	__ C.V.A. - Acute	436.	__ Electrolyte Dis.	276.9	__ Herpes Simplex	054.9
__ Abscess (Site)	682.9	__ Asthma	493.90	__ Cere. Vas. Accid. (Old)	438	__ Fatigue	780.7	__ Herpes Zoster	053.9
__ Adverse Drug Rx	995.2	__ Asthmatic Bronchitis	493.90	__ Cerumen	380.4	__ Fibrocys. Br. Dis	610.1	__ Hydrocele	603.9
__ Alcohol Detox	291.8	__ Atrial Fib.	427.31	__ Chestwall Pain	786.59	__ Fracture (Site)	829.0	__ Hyperlipidemia	272.4
__ Alcoholism	303.90	__ Atrial Tachi.	427.0	__ Cholecystitis	575.0	__ Open/Close		__ Hypertension	401.9
__ Allergic Rhinitis	477	__ Bowel Obstruct.	560.9	__ Cholelithiasis	574.00	__ Fungal Infect. (Site)	110.8	__ Hyperthyroidism	242.9
__ Allergy	995.3	__ Breast Mass	611.72	__ COPD	492.8	__ Gastric Ulcer	531.90	__ Hypothyroidism	244.9
__ Alzheimer's Dis.	290.1	__ Bronchitis	490	__ Cirrhosis	571.5	__ Gastritis	535.0	__ Labyrinthitis	386.30
__ Anemia	285.9	__ Bursitis	727.3	__ Cong. Heart Fail.	428.9	__ Gastroenteritis	558.9	__ Lipoma (Site)	214.9
__ Anemia - Pernicious	281.0	__ Cancer, Breast (Site)	174.9	__ Conjunctivitis	372.30	__ G.I. Bleeding	578.9	__ Lymphoma	202.8
__ Angina	413.9	__ Metastatic (Site)	199.1	__ Contusion (Site)	924.9	__ Glomerulonephritis	583.9	__ Mit. Valve Prolapse	424.0
__ Anxiety Synd.	300.00	__ Colon	153.9	__ Costochondritis	733.99	__ Headache	784.0	__ Myocard. Infarction (Area)	410.9
__ Appendicitis	541	__ Cancer, Rectal	154.1	__ Depression	311.	__ Headache, Tension	307.81	__ M.I., Old	412
__ Arterioscl. H.D.	414.0	__ Lung (Site)	162.9	__ Dermatitis	692.9	__ Migraine (Type)	346.9	__ Myositis	729.1
__ Arthritis, Osteo.	715.90	__ Skin (Site)	173.9	__ Diabetes Mellitus	250.00	__ Hemorrhoids	455.6	__ Nausea/Vomiting	787.0
__ Rheumatoid	714.0	__ Card. Arrhythmia (Type)	427.9	__ Diabetic Ketosis	250.1	__ Hernia, Hiatal	553.3	__ Neuralgia	729.2
__ Lupus	710.0	__ Cardiomyopathy	425.4	__ Diverticulitis	562.11	__ Inguinal	550.9	__ Nevus (Site)	216.9
		__ Cellulitis (Site)	682.9	__ Diverticulosis	562.10	__ Hepatitis	573.3	__ Obesity	278.0

DIAGNOSIS: (IF NOT CHECKED ABOVE)

SERVICES PERFORMED AT: ☐ Office ☐ E.R. ☐ CLAIM CONTAINS NO ORDERED REFERRING SERVICE	REFERRING PHYSICIAN & I.D. NUMBER

RETURN APPOINTMENT INFORMATION: 5 - 10 - 15 - 20 - 30 - 40 - 60 [DAYS] [WKS.] [MOS.] [PRN]	NEXT APPOINTMENT M - T - W - TH - F - S DATE / / TIME:	ACCEPT ASSIGNMENT? AM ☐ YES PM ☐ NO	DOCTOR'S SIGNATURE

INSTRUCTIONS TO PATIENT FOR FILING INSURANCE CLAIMS:	☐ CASH	TOTAL TODAY'S FEE	
1. Complete upper portion of this form, sign and date. 2. Attach this form to your own insurance company's form for direct reimbursement. **MEDICARE PATIENTS - DO NOT SEND THIS TO MEDICARE. WE WILL SUBMIT THE CLAIM FOR YOU.**	☐ CHECK #_____	OLD BALANCE	
	☐ VISA	TOTAL DUE	
	☐ MC		
	☐ CO-PAY	AMOUNT REC'D. TODAY	

FIGURE 16-7 This encounter form has an appointment block included at the bottom left.

call to cancel and do not come to the appointment). Writing patients' phone numbers next to their names in the appointment book makes it convenient for you to make appointment reminder calls. Procedure 16-5 at the end of the chapter outlines the steps in making appointment confirmation (or reminder) calls. Many offices that utilize electronic phone systems program the system to make reminder calls, freeing the office staff from this task. Be aware of patients who do not wish to be contacted by phone or to have messages left. Having the patient fill out a verbal contact agreement at his first visit can limit HIPAA violations. Figure 16-8 provides an example of a HIPAA-compliant verbal agreement form.

If patients agree that messages may be left on voice mail or answering machines, be sure this information is added to the verbal agreement form.

Recall Notices Some offices book appointments no more than a few weeks in advance; others may not have the next year's schedule available when a patient is ready to book a return appointment. In either case, you need a way to make sure patients do not forget to call for appointments that are 6 months—or even a year—away from their last appointments.

BWW

BWW Medical Associates, PC
305 Main Street, Port Snead YZ 12345-9876
Tel: 555-654-3210, Fax: 555-987-6543
Web: BWWAssociates.com

Paul F. Buckwalter, MD
Alexis N. Whalen, MD
Elizabeth H. Williams, MD

Patient Name: _____   MRN: _____

VERBAL RELEASE OF INFORMATION

BWW Medical Associates is allowed to give verbal information or updates on your medical condition to you and your Power of Attorney for Healthcare/Legal Representative as listed in your medical record.

If you wish others, such as relatives or friends WHO ASK about your condition, to have the right to be verbally informed about your condition, please list the names of those individuals and their relationship to you.

Name: _____   Relationship: _____

Name: _____   Relationship: _____

Name: _____   Relationship: _____

Name: _____   Relationship: _____

Additionally, should verbal messages need to be relayed to me via phone when I am not available to take the call, messages may be left for me on the available voice mail or answering device at the following phone numbers:

Phone Number: _____ (Please circle)   Home   Cell   Work

Phone Number: _____ (Please circle)   Home   Cell   Work

Phone Number: _____ (Please circle)   Home   Cell   Work

- I understand that BWW Medical Associates will continue to rely on the information contained within this form as current unless I request a change in writing.

- I understand that I may revoke this verbal agreement authorization at any time.

- I understand that if I choose to revoke this authorization, I must do so in writing and present my written revocation to the Privacy Officer at BWW Medical Associates. The revocation will NOT apply to information that has already been disclosed prior to the receipt of the written revocation.

_____   _____
Signature of Patient or Guardian   Date

FIGURE 16-8   Example of Verbal Release of Information agreement.

Suppose, for example, that the physician tells a patient she should have an annual breast examination. How can you help her remember to call to schedule one at the appropriate time? One way is to use a system of recall notices. In a tickler file, enter the patient's name under the month when she should call the office. When the time arrives, send a form letter reminding her that she will soon be due for a breast examination and asking her to call for an appointment. Many EHR software programs offer such reminder programs as part of the software package.

E-mail Notifications With more practices trying to accommodate all patient groups, a newer approach to appointment scheduling is through the use of e-mail. Patients sign up (and sign the appropriate release to allow communication via e-mail) and are assigned passwords by the office. The patient may request an appointment as long as it is not needed immediately. The office returns a confirmation e-mail of the scheduled appointment. When a scheduled appointment is approaching, an automatically generated notification goes out to the patient's e-mail address reminding him of the appointment. This is not suitable for all patients or all types of appointments. Some appointment types will still need to be handled by the office staff either by phone or in person because of the amount of information that needs to be relayed regarding the appointment and/or patient preparation for the appointment.

▶ Special Scheduling Situations LO 16.5

In most cases scheduling is routine; however, critical thinking, creativity, and flexibility are necessary for scheduling some special cases. These special situations often involve patients, but they also may involve physicians. Here are just a few of the special situations that may arise.

Patient Scheduling Situations

On some days all patients will keep their appointments and arrive on time. On many other days, however, patients may walk in without appointments, arrive late for scheduled appointments, or miss appointments entirely. Being able to anticipate needs and being prepared for these possibilities allow you to handle them more efficiently, keeping the office schedule running smoothly.

Emergencies Your training as a medical assistant will help you recognize the signs of an emergency. In some instances you will refer the caller to the nearest hospital emergency room or instruct the caller to call emergency medical services (EMS) for an ambulance. The procedure you will follow will depend on office policies and procedures (refer to the *Telephone Techniques* chapter). In other instances you will ask the caller to come to the office right away so you can "work" him into the schedule. It is vital that the physician see an emergency patient before patients who are already in the reception area or on the schedule. It is best to explain to waiting patients that there has been an emergency (without

POINTS ON PRACTICE
Scheduling Emergency Appointments

As a multiskilled medical assistant, you will be well-prepared to tell the difference between acute conditions that are emergencies and those that are not. Guidelines on types of emergencies to be seen in the office and types to be referred elsewhere vary. If you have any doubt, check with the office manager or interrupt the physician to ask for instructions.

Even with allotted "open" times built into the daily schedule, emergencies are still disruptive to most practices. Your ability to stay calm, respond quickly, and remain flexible will be of great comfort to the patient seeking care and to others in the reception area. Read the following story to see how an emergency situation can be handled skillfully.

The Situation

It is 4:15 p.m. in a busy family practice. The telephone rings. The caller is the father of a 10-year-old boy. Kaylyn, the medical assistant, can hear the panic in his voice. His son Kyle has injured his knee while playing football with friends. Kyle cannot straighten the knee and it is quite swollen.

Kaylyn consults the practice orthopedist, who suspects torn cartilage. The physician tells Kaylyn to have Kyle's dad wrap ice in a towel, apply it to Kyle's knee, and bring him in immediately. Kaylyn relays this advice to the father and asks

him how soon he can get to the office. "It will take about 25 minutes," he replies.

The office schedule includes a time opening at 4:30, but based on the father's estimate, Kyle cannot possibly arrive until 4:40. Kaylyn notes that Mrs. Griffin, a good-natured retiree, is scheduled to come in for her weekly blood pressure check at 4:45 p.m. Her appointment is the last scheduled appointment of the day.

The Solution

Mrs. Griffin lives about 5 minutes from the office. Kaylyn calls her home and explains that there has been an emergency. She offers Mrs. Griffin three choices: she can come in at 4:30 and be seen then; she can arrive at the usual time and expect to wait; or she can be rescheduled for tomorrow due to an opening in the schedule. "No problem," Mrs. Griffin says cheerfully. "I'll come right over."

Mrs. Griffin arrives at 4:35. At 4:40, Kyle hobbles in, supported by his father. Kaylyn greets them and offers Kyle a chair on which to prop his foot.

Mrs. Griffin's blood pressure check is complete at 4:45. Kyle waits only 5 minutes before he is seen.

Thanks to Kaylyn's quick thinking, the office stays on schedule—essentially by switching one appointment for another and accommodating both patients with minimal interruptions.

giving details). This announcement helps them understand and accept the delay and also gives them an opportunity to reschedule their appointments if they are unable to wait. Read the Points on Practice feature on scheduling emergency appointments, which contains a mock emergency appointment scenario.

Referrals If your practice includes specialists, it is a common occurrence that other physicians will refer their patients to the practice for second opinions or special consultations. A patient seeking a second opinion before deciding on surgery, often at the request of his or her insurance carrier, should be fit into the schedule as soon as possible. Other referred patients also should be seen as soon as possible, both as a professional courtesy to the referring doctor and as good business practice.

Many offices maintain a listing of preferred physicians and facilities that they would like their patients to see and use. This list should contain the physician or facility names, specialty, address, and their phone numbers. When arranging a referral, try to give the patient two names to choose from, along with the referral phone numbers and addresses.

When choosing the referral names of either physicians or facilities, be sure that the facility accepts the patient's insurance and that all of the paperwork required by the insurance company has been completed. Some insurance carriers require a specific paper referral form be filled out. Most others today utilize an area of their website as a type of point of service (POS), where the medical office enters the information into the insurance company database and an authorization is returned on the spot. Some smaller carriers may require a phone request in which the medical office speaks to a customer service representative or enters specific information into an automated voice response telephone system. Regardless of the method used, all referrals should be documented in the patient's medical record, including the authorization number given (if applicable) by the insurance carrier, authorizing the referral.

Go to CONNECT to see a video about *Requesting Prior Authorization.*

Fasting Patients Some procedures and tests require patients to fast or refrain from eating or drinking anything beginning the night before. Schedule these patients as early in the day as possible to show consideration for their needs. When scheduling appointments that require the patient to fast, be sure to inform the patient of the need to fast and when the fasting should start, including the fact that the test may not be completed if the patient does not fast.

Patients with Diabetes Similar to fasting patients, patients with diabetes can use extra consideration when you schedule their appointments. In general, patients who take insulin must eat meals and snacks at regular times. This routine keeps their blood sugar from dropping too low—a condition that can result in confused thinking or even loss of consciousness. Therefore, you might want to avoid scheduling patients with diabetes for slots in late morning. If the schedule is running late by the time these patients arrive, they will be waiting in your reception area at a time when they really need to eat.

Late Arrivals If the practice has patients who are routinely late and gentle reminders to be on time have not helped, you might try booking them toward the end of the day. Even if a patient arrives late for a late-afternoon appointment, the doctor has already seen most of the day's patients and the late patient will not disrupt the schedule. Document late arrivals or missed appointments in the patient's chart. With documentation, patients who are habitually late can be called to discuss the reasons for their chronic tardiness. The goal of the discussion should be to find a solution so that patients can make their appointments on time and the schedule will run smoothly.

Walk-Ins From time to time, a patient may arrive without an appointment and still expect to see the doctor. These people are called **walk-ins.** Office policies on how to handle walk-ins vary. If the person is experiencing an emergency, handle the situation as you would handle any emergency. Otherwise, you might politely explain that the doctor is fully booked for the day and offer to schedule an appointment in the usual manner. If an office PA or NP is available, suggest to the patient that this practitioner may be able to be of assistance. If, by chance, the doctor is available and willing to see the walk-in, you should still ask the person to call to schedule appointments in the future, as this is the usual policy for the practice. If your physician's office has a policy of no walk-ins, post a sign in the patient check-in area stating that patients are seen by appointment only.

Cancellations When patients call to cancel appointments, try to reschedule the appointment while they are on the telephone. If patients say they will call later to reschedule, note this information in the appointment book and thank them for the notice.

You should also write "canceled" in the appointment book, drawing a single line through the patient's name. To avoid confusion, cancel the first appointment *before* entering the patient's rescheduled appointment. Remember that the appointment book is a legal record. If you forget to cross out the name at the time of the first appointment, it may later seem that the doctor saw the patient twice. It is also important to note the cancellation in the patient's medical record. This notation can protect the practice from possible legal action. For example, a patient whose surgical incision becomes infected cannot blame the doctor if the patient canceled a scheduled appointment for a dressing change.

You may be able to fill slots created by cancellations by calling patients who have appointments scheduled for later in the day or week. Some patients may be willing to come in earlier than planned. When you make appointments, you can ask patients if they would be interested in coming in earlier if openings occur. Placing the names of interested patients in a tickler file or on a cancellation list can save time later.

Missed and Wrong-Day Appointments It is important for legal reasons to document a no-show in the appointment book and patient medical record. Always inform the physician of any missed appointments in case the patient's condition requires a follow-up. The physician may want you to call the patient with a polite reminder that the patient has missed an appointment and needs to reschedule. There may have been a misunderstanding about the time, or the patient may simply have forgotten the appointment. Some offices, especially ones that use computerized scheduling systems, send out form letters when patients miss appointments.

If failure to keep the appointment could endanger the patient's health, mention this possibility to the patient. The physician also may wish to speak to the patient about the health issues possible due to repeated missed appointments. Some practices limit the number of times that a patient can miss, cancel, or repeatedly not show up for appointments, as this can lead to liability issues for the physician. Because of potential legal issues, it bears repeating to always document any missed or canceled appointments in the patient medical record.

Periodically, physicians charge for missed appointments, especially if patients habitually miss their appointments. These missed appointment charges are for missed business opportunities and not for services rendered. If your office implements this policy, make sure that you let patients know in advance before you start charging them for missed appointments. Most offices with this policy have the policy posted near the reception desk. Some offices also opt for a notation on the appointment cards that states patients will be charged for appointments that are canceled with less than 24 hours' notice.

Sometimes a patient may show up on the wrong day for her appointment. If the patient lives in the local area, rescheduling makes sense. But if the patient made special transportation arrangements or traveled from a long distance, it is good business practice to try to work the patient into the schedule for that day. If the patient provides an appointment card verifying the appointment for that day, but she is not on the schedule, the office is obligated to honor the appointment if the physician is in the office. When in doubt about the best course of action, consult with the doctor or office manager.

Physician Scheduling Situations

Not all scheduling problems result from patients. Sometimes physicians disrupt the office schedule as well. They may be called away on an emergency, may be delayed at the hospital, or may simply arrive late.

Some physicians are occasionally late for appointments, while others are frequently late, either when arriving in the morning or when returning from lunch or a scheduled meeting. If this situation occurs in your office, it may be handled in several ways.

Speaking to the physician directly about the problem may be helpful in resolving the situation. You also might use the staff meeting to mention that the morning or afternoon schedule often seems to get off to a late start and ask if anyone has suggestions for improving this situation. The physician may recognize that she is the cause of the problem and decide to resolve it.

If the physician does not take responsibility for the problem, however, you may need to adjust the office schedule to handle the situation. Suppose, for example, that the first patient appointment slot is at 8:30 a.m., but the physician usually does not arrive until 8:35 a.m. You could simply avoid scheduling patients between 8:30 and 8:45 a.m. If a physician is often 15 minutes late returning from lunch or from meetings, you might leave open the first appointment slot after the scheduled arrival time in an attempt to avoid long wait times for patients, keeping satisfied clients.

▶ Scheduling Outside Appointments LO 16.6

You may be responsible for arranging patient appointments outside the medical office. These appointments may include

- Consultations with or referrals to other physicians
- Laboratory work
- Radiology (x-ray, CT scans, MRI)
- Other diagnostic tests (EKG, stress testing)
- Hospital stays
- Inpatient and outpatient surgeries

Scheduling Outpatient Procedures

Always verify the patient's insurance coverage before choosing the facility or physician for the patient's referral or other service. Today, a patient's insurance coverage may dictate both where a procedure may be performed as well as the physician allowed to provide the service. A prior approval or referral from the insurance carrier also may be required. The medical assistant is often the person responsible for knowing not only the preferred physicians and facilities of the physician, but also the physicians and facilities allowed by specific insurance carriers. Obtaining referrals and prior authorizations also will often be your responsibility. (Refer to the *Insurance and Billing* chapter for more information on this topic.)

Once a facility and provider have been agreed upon by the physician, patient, and insurance carrier, document any referrals or prior authorization numbers (again, refer to the *Insurance and Billing* chapter). If the procedure is elective, ask the patient if there is a preferred date and time. If the request fits into the provider and facility schedule, try to accommodate the patient's preference, as this gesture allows the patient to have some small sense of control over a situation that is likely anxiety-provoking.

Before calling the surgery center, laboratory, or outpatient department required for the procedure, be sure that you have the patient's medical record; the exact name of the procedure to be performed; the approximate amount of time required (if your physician is performing the service); the diagnosis; and the patient's insurance information, date of birth, phone number, and home address. Give this information to the scheduler, keeping in mind the patient's preferred time frame if it can be accommodated. Once an appointment time has been agreed upon, ask the scheduler for any patient instructions, carefully documenting them to relay to the patient. If paperwork will be sent to the patient from the facility, be sure the patient also understands this.

When arrangements have been made, inform the patient orally and also provide him with written instructions, asking for and answering any questions the patient may have. Be sure he understands any pre-procedure instructions and the fact that if the pre-procedure instructions are not followed perfectly, the procedure may need to be rescheduled or repeated. Remember to note in the patient's chart the date and time of the procedure as well as instructions provided to the patient. Procedure 16-6, found at the end of the chapter, outlines the procedure for booking an outpatient surgical appointment.

Go to CONNECT to see a video about *Scheduling Outpatient Surgical Appointments.*

Reserving an Operating Room

If the doctor in your office plans to perform surgery at a hospital, you will need to call the operating room scheduler to reserve the facility. As when booking an outpatient procedure, you will first give the preferred dates and times, the type of surgery, and the length of time the doctor will need the operating room. After the day and time are set, provide the scheduler with all relevant patient information. Relay any requests from the doctor, such as the blood type and units of blood that may be needed. It also may be your responsibility to make arrangements for surgical assistants, an anesthetist, and a hospital bed for the patient following surgery. Make sure that all health insurance requirements such as referrals and prior authorizations are met and copies of forms and authorization numbers are filed appropriately. As when scheduling outpatient procedures, be sure the patient receives all necessary oral and written instructions and information regarding pre- and post-surgical care and that all questions are answered. Procedure 16-7, found at the end of the chapter, outlines the steps for booking an inpatient surgical appointment.

Go to CONNECT to see a video about *Scheduling Inpatient Surgical Appointments.*

▶ Maintaining the Physician's Schedule

LO 16.7

The schedules of busy physicians are not limited to office visits with patients. Physicians also need to attend professional meetings, travel to conferences, present speeches to colleagues, complete paperwork, and perform other duties. Your job is to help the physicians in your practice to make the most efficient use of their time.

One way to assist the physician with his schedule is to avoid overbooking appointments with patients. **Overbooking** (scheduling more patients than can reasonably be seen in the time allowed) creates stress for the physician and the staff and makes it difficult to maintain a timely schedule.

The opposite problem, **underbooking**—leaving large, unused gaps in the schedule—does not make the best use of the physician's time. Of course, you have no control over patients who cancel or do not show for appointments, but, as mentioned previously, there are ways to decrease this, such as calling patients to remind them of their appointments a day or two ahead of the scheduled appointment. If you cannot reschedule another patient for the empty slot, the physician can use the time to catch up on telephone calls to patients or to attend to other matters.

At times you will have to cancel appointments because the physician has been delayed or called away by an emergency. Apologize to waiting patients on behalf of the physician and offer them a choice. Explain that they can wait in the office (give an estimated waiting time), leave to run errands and return later, or reschedule their appointments for another day. Documentation should be noted in the patient's chart that because of an emergency in the office, the appointment had to be rescheduled by the office so the patient is not held at fault for the cancellation. Be sure to write the date of the rescheduled appointment in the chart as well. Always make sure patients who need immediate attention are seen by another physician if available, staying within office policies.

Visits Outside the Office

Some physicians provide care outside of the office—in patient homes, in nursing homes, or during rounds within the hospital when their patients have been admitted.

House Calls Physicians may want to check on home-bound or nonambulatory patients as part of their follow-up care. Although not as common as it once was, house calls are a valuable service that physicians can provide to patients who can no longer easily make it to the doctor's office for their appointments. Many insurance companies allow the physician to bill for these services with restrictions that vary depending on the plan. Supplies required for visits vary depending on the type and location of the visit, but general supplies that should be kept in a medical bag include the following:

- Blood pressure cuff
- Stethoscope
- Specimen containers
- Otoscope
- Ophthalmoscope
- Prescription pad
- Pen light
- Thermometer
- Gloves, face shield

Hospital Rounds Historically, physicians typically visited their own patients when they became hospitalized. Today, more and more hospitals are turning this responsibility over to a physician specialist known as a hospitalist. A hospitalist does not hold office hours and does not maintain a practice, but only sees patients while they are hospitalized. If your office or the hospital where your physicians have privileges utilize hospitalists, they will report to the physician on the patient's progress and findings while an inpatient.

Nursing Home Visits Some physicians check on their patients even when they are receiving around-the-clock care from a skilled nursing facility. Usually the physician has seen these patients for years and stays involved with their care because of the long-standing relationship or because the patient will be returning home after a rehabilitation stay and will need follow-up care.

"Mouse Calls" With all of the new technology available to them, physicians are learning new ways to communicate with their patients. In their daily schedule, time is often allotted for physicians to return phone calls, which today can also include "mouse" calls—physicians answering e-mail inquiries from their patients. These also can be "virtual visits" covered by some insurance plans. Be sure that the appropriate releases are in the patient's file before the physician undertakes this type of communication with the patient.

Scheduling Pharmaceutical Sales Representatives

Drug manufacturers often send pharmaceutical sales representatives into medical offices with printed information about new drugs as well as free samples that can be given to patients. This is an added benefit for your patients but can be time-consuming as the representatives will want to market their products. The representatives are required to obtain signatures from the physicians in order to leave the samples behind, and for this reason, some doctors do not want to meet with pharmaceutical representatives. Other doctors are willing to spend a few minutes if time permits and if the products are likely to be useful to their patients. Some doctors set aside certain times or days during the week when they will meet with pharmaceutical representatives. Others prefer that the representative leave a business card with the products represented, and if the physician is interested, he will call and arrange for an appointment at a mutually agreeable time. When a pharmaceutical representative who is unknown to you comes into the office, ask for a business card and check with the physician or business manager before scheduling an appointment (Figure 16-9).

Making Travel Arrangements

You may be responsible for arranging transportation and lodging when physicians attend meetings, speaking engagements, and other events out of town. You may be responsible for contacting the airlines, car rental agencies, hotels, or other services yourself or you may use an online service such as Orbitz® or work through a travel agent. No matter which method is used to

FIGURE 16-9 Pharmaceutical sales representatives who cannot see the physician often leave a business card listing the medications from their company.

make travel arrangements, always request confirmation documents of travel and room reservations.

Before the day of departure, obtain an itinerary from the travel agent or online service, or create one yourself. An **itinerary** is a detailed travel plan, listing dates and times of flights and events, locations of meetings and lodgings, and telephone numbers. Give several copies to the physician and keep one for the office (Figure 16-10).

You also may be responsible for scheduling and confirming professional coverage of the practice during the physician's absence. In larger practices and more urban areas, physicians in the same or a nearby practice often provide coverage while the physician is away. This coverage may be important for legal reasons, most importantly so the physician cannot be charged with "abandoning" his patients. If a local physician is not readily available, a **locum tenens** (Latin for "one occupying the place of another"), or substitute physician, may be hired to see patients while the regular physician is unavailable. You may have more than one *locum tenens* on call, depending on the practice. In some areas special firms provide these services and other temporary medical and nursing assistance. Before hiring *locum tenens* physicians, you may want to contact some of the major insurance carriers providing health insurance coverage for your patients to find out their credentialing and claim requirements so that the services provided by the *locum tenens* physicians will be considered covered services.

Paul F. Buckwalter, MD
Travel Itinerary

BWW Medical Associates, PC
305 Main Street, Port Snead YZ 12345-9876
Tel: 555-654-3210, Fax: 555-987-6543
Web: BWWAssociates.com

Client Information

Traveler's Name	Paul F. Buckwalter, MD
Address	560 Williamsburg Ct., Port Snead, YZ
Telephone Number	555-279-0098
Fax Number	555-987-6543
E-Mail Address	
Travel Dates	May 5 – 9, 20XX

Departure Flight

Date	May 5, 20XX
Airline	United International
Flight Number	567
From	Port Snead, YZ
Departure Time	6:45 am
Departure Terminal/Gate	56C
To	Los Angeles, CA
Arrival Time	9:45 am Pacific time
Length of Flight	5 hours
Class	First Class
Seat Number	12a
Status	confirmed

FIGURE 16-10 Typical travel itinerary.

Monday – May 5, 20XX

• Morning:

8:00 – 8:45	Physician Recruiter
9:00 – 10:00	Formal interview with Team, facilitated by Recruiter
10:00 – 11:00	Medical Director
11:00 – 12:00	Tour of UCLA including department with Area Manager

• Afternoon:

12:30 – 1:30	Lunch with physician(s) from another department with similar interests
2:00 – 3:00	One (1) hour with Department Chair and/or Physician Area Manager
4:00 – 6:00	One-on-one interviews with department or other physicians
	Informal time in interviewing department, as appropriate

• Evening:

7:00 – until	Dinner* ** (or private dinner on their own)

Planning Meetings

Another of your duties may be to assist the physician in setting up meetings for professional societies or committees. To do so, you will need to know how many people are expected to attend, how long the meeting will last, and the purpose of the meeting. In addition, ask the doctor if a meal is to be served.

Some groups always meet at the same location, but if there is no established meeting place, you must choose and reserve one. Select a location with an adequately sized meeting room, sufficient parking, and, if needed, food services. Be sure also to arrange for necessary audiovisual (AV) equipment, such as a microphone, podium, or projector.

Many conference centers and hotels have an on-site catering manager or conference manager to assist you with these arrangements. When the facility has been booked, mail an invitation to all those expected to attend the meeting. On the invitation, provide the topic, names of the speakers, date, time, place, and admission costs or fees associated with the event if applicable.

With direction from the physician, you also may be responsible for creating the meeting's agenda, as discussed in more detail in the *Practice Management* chapter. After the meeting, you also may be asked to prepare the **minutes,** the report of what was discussed and decided upon at the meeting.

Scheduling Time with the Physician

You and the physician should meet on a scheduled basis to discuss any irregularities or changes in the day-to-day workings of the office. These meetings may be held between you and the physician alone or include the office manager. If items are not pressing or "private," many discussions may be included in regularly scheduled office meetings. Topics discussed may include practice finance items such as insurance premiums, taxes, and other financial matters, as well as professional licenses and renewal requirements for the medical staff. These items are discussed in further detail in the *Practice Management* chapter.

PROCEDURE 16-1 Creating an Appointment Matrix

Procedure Goal: To create an appointment matrix to indicate the days and the hours the physician is not scheduling patients.

OSHA Guidelines: This procedure does not involve exposure to blood, body fluids, or tissue.

Materials: Appointment book; pencil or pen; physician schedule of meetings, conferences, vacations, staff meetings, and other times of unavailability when patients are not seen.

Method: Procedure steps.

1. Using the physician schedule of availability as the base for the matrix, confer with the physician or office manager to ensure that no additional schedule changes are planned.
   RATIONALE: The matrix should be as complete as possible to avoid the need to reschedule appointments.

2. Indicate within each area the reason why the time is being closed to appointments, such as lunch, hospital rounds, AAMA meeting, etc.
   RATIONALE: Allows for all users to be aware of provider location both in and outside of the office.

3. If the office utilizes cluster scheduling for certain appointments such as physical exams, blood sugar testing, etc., these time frames also must be set apart. Following office policy, such as using brackets, note the appropriate appointment type to be scheduled during this time frame.
   RATIONALE: It is important for all users to know what type of appointments can be booked in each time frame.

PROCEDURE 16-2 Creating an Appointment Matrix for an Electronic Scheduling System

Procedure Goal: Using an electronic scheduling system, indicate the days and times when the office is not scheduling patients.

OSHA Guidelines: This procedure does not involve exposure to blood, body fluids, or tissue.

Materials: Appointment book; pencil or pen; physician schedule of meetings, conferences, vacations, staff meetings, and other times of unavailability when patients are not seen.

Method: Procedure steps.

1. Using the physician schedule of availability as the base for the matrix, confer with the physician or office manager to ensure that no additional schedule changes are planned.

2. Open the office appointment scheduler per the program format.

3. Block the dates and times when the general office or physician will not be available for patient appointments using the physician and office schedules as guides.
   RATIONALE: The matrix should be as complete as possible to avoid the need to reschedule appointments.

4. Choose the appropriate option if the time frame is repeatedly unavailable.

5. Enter a reason that the time is not available for future reference. The office program may use color-coding to assist with this process.
   RATIONALE: Allows for all users to be aware of provider location both inside and outside of the office.

6. If cluster scheduling is used for the office, most schedulers allow you to specify what types of appointments may be entered; again, color-coding may be used by the scheduler to outline specific types of appointments.
   RATIONALE: It is important for all users to know what type of appointments can be booked in each time frame.

7. Many programs will allow you to specify time frames necessary for different types of appointments and these may be set up now also. For instance, physical exams for new patients may require 45 minutes and visits for BP and typical sick visits are set up for 15 minutes. If the program allows, set up these matrixes now also.
   RATIONALE: This ensures that the proper amount of time will be allotted for each patient's appointment.

PROCEDURE 16-3 Scheduling Appointments

Procedure Goal: Utilizing the previously created matrix, book patient appointments applying the correct amount of time for each appointment.

OSHA Guidelines: This procedure does not involve exposure to blood, body fluids, or tissue.

Materials: Appointment book and pen or pencil, or electronic scheduler (with appropriate matrix) template, outlining time frames for patient appointment types.

Method: Procedure steps.

1. Establish the type of appointment required by the patient, particularly if this is a new patient or a returning patient.
   RATIONALE: New patients typically require a longer appointment time than do returning existing patients.

2. If necessary, consult the template for the amount of time required for the patient appointment. Keep in mind the reason for the appointment when scheduling (i.e., is the patient required to be fasting).
   RATIONALE: Some appointments are best scheduled at certain times of the day depending on patient preparation, and equipment or personnel availability.

3. When possible, schedule appointments earlier in the day first and then move to later time frames. Do ask the patient if he/she has a preferred time frame in mind and, if at all possible, accommodate the request.
   RATIONALE: Open appointments later in the day allow space for unexpected appointments required at a later time.

4. When using an appointment book, enter the patient name, phone number, and reason for the appointment in the appropriate space, blocking out additional blocks of time if necessary to accommodate a longer appointment time.

5. If an electronic scheduler is used, use the search option to find the next available appointment for the time frame required for the appointment. Enter the patient name, phone number, and reason for the appointment.

6. Repeat the appointment information to the patient giving any necessary instructions regarding preparation for the appointment, such as early arrival for blood tests, completion of paperwork, etc. Also, this is a good time to remind patients about any copayments that will be due at the time of the appointment.
   RATIONALE: Patients respond best when they know what is expected ahead of time.

PROCEDURE 16-4 Completing the Patient Appointment Card

Procedure Goal: To accurately complete a patient appointment card for the patient's next visit.

OSHA Guidelines: This procedure does not involve exposure to blood, body fluids, or tissue.

Materials: Appointment book or electronic scheduler, pen, and appointment card.

Method: Procedure steps.

1. After entering the patient's appointment in the appointment book or electronic scheduler, repeat the appointment date and time to the patient to verify accuracy.

2. Complete the patient appointment card entering the appointment date and time on the card. If the practice has multiple providers, there may also be a place for the appropriate physician name to be entered and you should do so.
   RATIONALE: If patients see multiple providers, it is not unusual for them to forget a provider's name.

3. Repeat appointment information to patient one more time when giving the card to him/her, again verifying the information.

PROCEDURE 16-5 Placing Appointment Confirmation Calls

Procedure Goal: To decrease the number of no-show patients by making appointment confirmation calls 24–48 hours prior to the scheduled appointment.

OSHA Guidelines: This procedure does not involve exposure to blood, body fluids, or tissue.

Materials: Office appointment book, electronic scheduler, or listing of patients scheduled to be seen tomorrow or the next day with their home phone numbers.

Method: Procedure steps.

1. Starting with the first appointment of the day, call the patient listed.

2. If the phone is answered, ask for the patient. If you reach the patient, give your name and the name of the practice and state that you are confirming the patient's appointment for the applicable date and time.

3. Remind the patient of any special instructions regarding the appointment such as fasting, bringing in medical record or registration information, and copayments due.
   RATIONALE: It is important that the patient come to the appointment prepared or any testing may need to be postponed.

4. If the patient is not available, leave your name and phone number asking that the patient return your call.

RATIONALE: Unless the person answering the phone has been listed by the patient as someone to whom you may give confidential information, you must speak directly with the patient to avoid breach of patient confidentiality.

5. If a voice mail or answering machine system is reached, follow the practice confidentiality rules of leaving only your name and phone number, asking the patient to call you back, unless you have permission from the patient to leave more explicit information on voice mail.

RATIONALE: Unless you have express written permission from the patient to leave a message on an answering machine or voice mail, confidentiality regulations require you not leave explicit information.

6. Thank the patient for his/her time, stating you will see him/her at the stated date and time.

7. Allow the patient to hang up first, so if there are questions, you may answer them.

RATIONALE: This allows the patient to have all questions or issues addressed adequately.

PROCEDURE 16-6 Scheduling Outpatient Surgical Appointments

Procedure Goal: To schedule an outpatient surgical procedure.

OSHA Guidelines: This procedure does not involve exposure to blood, body fluids, or tissue.

Materials: Patient medical record, scheduling form, calendar, telephone, pen.

Method: Procedure steps.

1. Obtain detailed information regarding the procedure to be performed from the physician and patient medical record. Information should include the name of procedure to be performed, the amount of time the outpatient surgical suite will be needed, and the reason (diagnosis) for the procedure.

RATIONALE: Without this information, you will be unable to efficiently book the required appointment.

2. From the patient's medical record, you will need the patient's full name, DOB, allergies, current medications, address, phone number, and insurance information.

RATIONALE: This information will be needed by the facility booking the procedure.

3. Place a call to the appropriate surgery center or outpatient surgical unit at the requested facility. Have the name of the surgeon, assistant, or PA (if they will be used) available, as well as the patient's and physician's preferred dates for the procedure.

4. When the appointment scheduler answers the phone, identify yourself, the practice, and the procedure you need to schedule, as well as the preferred dates.

5. When a date for the procedure is agreed upon by the patient, give the scheduler the patient's name, address, phone number, DOB, gender, and insurance information including the prior authorization number if needed. Also give the patient's diagnosis as required for medical necessity.

RATIONALE: This information will be needed by the facility for booking and billing purposes.

6. Inquire as to any pre-procedure testing that may need to be done as well as any patient preparation required prior to the procedure, including patient arrival time.

RATIONALE: This information will need to be relayed to the patient for adequate preparation for the procedure.

7. Confirm the appointment date and time prior to hanging up. If necessary, book any pre-procedure testing for the patient and document these appointments in the patient instructions and appropriate office form(s) such as the surgical check-off sheet and/or within the patient's medical record.

RATIONALE: Always document any patient-related information in the patient's medical record.

8. Provide the patient with written instructions from the physician as well as all information obtained while booking the appointment. The patient also should be informed that he should arrange for someone to drive him to and from this appointment.

9. Go over the written dates and instructions with the patient, asking the patient if there are any questions, answering them if possible and if not, asking a clinical member of the team to do so.

RATIONALE: It is important that the patient thoroughly understand the reason for the procedure and all pre-procedure instructions to be adequately prepared for the procedure.

10. Give a copy of instructions and information to the patient and keep a copy in the patient record. Remind the patient to feel free to call the office at any time with any questions or concerns.

RATIONALE: Written instructions will back up what has been relayed to the patient and serve as a reminder for the patient.

PROCEDURE 16-7 Scheduling Inpatient Surgical Appointments

Procedure Goal: To schedule an inpatient surgical procedure.

OSHA Guidelines: This procedure does not involve exposure to blood, body fluids, or tissue.

Materials: Patient medical record, scheduling form, calendar, telephone, pen.

Method: Procedure steps.

1. Obtain detailed information regarding the procedure to be performed from the physician and patient medical record. Information should include the name of the procedure to be performed, the amount of time the outpatient surgical suite will be needed, and the reason (diagnosis) for the procedure.

RATIONALE: Without this information, you will be unable to efficiently book the required appointment.

2. From the patient's medical record, you will need the patient's full name, DOB, allergies, current medications, address, phone number, and insurance information.
   RATIONALE: This information will be needed by the facility booking the procedure.

3. Place a call to the appropriate surgical unit at the requested hospital. Have the name of the surgeon, assistant, or PA (if they will be used) available, as well as the patient's and physician's preferred dates for the procedure.

4. When the appointment scheduler answers the phone, identify yourself, the practice, and the procedure you need to schedule, as well as the preferred dates.

5. When a date for the procedure is agreed upon by the patient, give the scheduler the patient's name, address, phone number, DOB, gender, and insurance information including the prior authorization number if needed. Also give the patient's diagnosis as required for medical necessity.
   RATIONALE: This information will be needed by the facility for booking and billing purposes.

6. Inquire as to any pre-procedure testing that may need to be done as well as any patient preparation required prior to the procedure, including patient arrival time.
   RATIONALE: This information will need to be relayed to the patient for adequate preparation for the procedure.

7. Confirm the appointment date and time prior to hanging up. If necessary, book any pre-procedure testing for the patient and document these appointments in the patient instructions and appropriate office form(s) such as the surgical check-off sheet and/or within the patient's medical record.
   RATIONALE: Always document any patient-related information in the patient's medical record.

8. Provide the patient with written instructions from the physician as well as all information obtained while booking the appointment. The patient also should be informed that he should arrange for someone to drive him to and from the hospital.

9. Go over the written dates and instructions with the patient, asking the patient if there are any questions, answering them if possible and if not, asking a clinical member of the team to do so.
   RATIONALE: It is important that the patient thoroughly understand the reason for the procedure and all pre-procedure instructions to be adequately prepared for the procedure.

10. Give a copy of instructions and information to the patient and keep a copy in the patient record. Remind the patient to feel free to call the office at any time with any questions or concerns.
    RATIONALE: Written instructions will back up what has been relayed to the patient and serve as a reminder for the patient.

SUMMARY OF LEARNING OUTCOMES

LEARNING OUTCOMES	KEY POINTS
16.1 **Describe how the appointment book is key to the continuity of patient care.**	The appointment book or electronic scheduler and its matrix, when used properly, allow the office staff to respect the time of both the physician and the patient, by keeping an efficient and timely flow of patients throughout the day.
16.2 **Identify how to properly apply a matrix to an appointment book.**	To create a matrix, in either an appointment book or an electronic scheduler, you must know the usual schedule of physician availability to see patients as well as the times the physician (or practice) will not be open to see patients. The latter times should be X'd out with a short reason given as to why the time is unavailable. Follow the instructions for the electronic scheduler to block out the appropriate time frames.
16.3 **Compare different types of appointment scheduling systems.**	The most commonly used types of scheduling systems are open-hours, time-specified, wave, modified-wave, double-booking, cluster, and advance scheduling. It is also common for offices to use any combination of the above as best suits each practice.
16.4 **Identify ways to organize and schedule patient appointments.**	When organizing and scheduling patient appointments, always maintain a positive, professional image as a representative of the office. The patient's status as a new or established patient should be considered as well as patient preference whenever possible. The goal is to accommodate the patient as much as possible, while maintaining an efficient office schedule. Appointments should be confirmed through appointment cards, phone calls, e-mail notification (when permitted by the patient), and mailing of recall notices.

LEARNING OUTCOMES	KEY POINTS
16.5 Model how to handle special scheduling situations.	Handling special scheduling situations requires critical thinking skills and creativity. Scheduling situations can arise if the physician is running late or if a patient requires an emergency appointment. Other scheduling problems also may include a patient who does not show, arrives late, or arrives on the wrong day. Documentation of any patient-related appointment issues should be recorded in the patient's medical record for legal purposes.
16.6 Explain how to schedule appointments that are outside the medical office.	Outside appointments may need to be made to laboratories, for radiology services, for in- and outpatient surgeries, for hospital stays, or for other diagnostic tests. In order to efficiently book such appointments, you will require the patient's demographic and health insurance information along with the procedure or service to be performed and the reason for the service. Preferred dates and times also should be noted. If referrals or prior authorizations are required, you also may be required to obtain these so that the procedure/service is eligible for payment by the patient's insurance plan.
16.7 Implement ways to keep an accurate and efficient physician schedule.	As the office medical assistant, your duties will include maintenance of the office schedule. The physician's schedule should ensure an even flow of patients throughout the day. Errors or overbooking may require you to rearrange appointments as necessary and to accommodate emergency appointments with minimal interruptions to the already-established schedule. If the schedule is consistently overbooked or patient wait time becomes consistently too long, it will be your responsibility to find the cause(s) and corrections for the issues and present these to the physician or office manager.

CASE STUDY CRITICAL THINKING

Recall John Miller from the beginning of the chapter. Now that you have completed the chapter, answer the following questions regarding his case.

1. What information will you need before you can book the cardiac catheterization?

2. Explain the process for scheduling this procedure.

EXAM PREPARATION QUESTIONS

1. (LO 16.1) The appointment book and its format are dependent on all of the following items EXCEPT
   a. Physician preference
   b. Facilities available
   c. Patient need
   d. Physician habits
   e. Office location

2. (LO 16.2) When should you apply the matrix to your appointment book?
   a. On the first day of the new year
   b. When you first get it, if possible
   c. When scheduling appointments
   d. After appointments have been made
   e. At the beginning of every quarter

3. (LO 16.3) This type of scheduling groups similar appointments together on a certain day of the week or for certain times of day, which may be helpful with equipment and staffing.
   a. Time-specified
   b. Wave
   c. Open-hour
   d. Cluster
   e. Modified-wave

4. (LO 16.3) Which type of scheduling is also called *stream scheduling*?
   a. Time-specified
   b. Wave
   c. Open-hour
   d. Cluster
   e. Modified-wave

5. (LO 16.4) In terms of scheduling, the term "no-show" means
   a. The patient has passed away
   b. The patient is no longer coming to the office
   c. The patient does not call or show up for his scheduled appointment
   d. The patient comes to his appointment but then leaves before seeing the doctor
   e. The patient shows up early for his appointment

6. (LO 16.5) What is the best approach for handling the cancellation of an appointment by a patient?
   a. Send the patient a letter pointing out she canceled a necessary appointment
   b. Attempt to schedule another patient in the canceled slot
   c. Schedule other activities in those canceled slots
   d. Encourage the physician to take time off
   e. Remind the patient of the importance of follow-up care and if possible schedule her for another appointment while she is still on the phone

7. (LO 16.6) Why should the insurance company be contacted prior to scheduling an appointment outside of the office?
   a. To pay for services
   b. As a courtesy
   c. Because the test is physician ordered
   d. To give them the confirmation number
   e. To determine if the service is covered and obtain an authorization number

8. (LO 16.6) When scheduling an appointment for an abdominal CAT scan, what steps should be taken?
   a. Have all information from the physician regarding the appointment and access to the patient's medical record
   b. If possible book the appointment when the patient is present to ascertain a convenient time for the patient.
   c. After making the appointment, repeat the information, writing it down for the patient
   d. Give the patient oral and written instructions, answering any questions
   e. All of the above

9. (LO 16.7) Two ways the medical assistant can assist the physician with his in-office schedule are to
   a. Avoid overbooking
   b. Avoid underbooking
   c. Double-book appointments when possible
   d. a & b
   e. b & c

10. (LO 16.7) All of these appointments take place outside of the physician office EXCEPT
   a. House calls
   b. Nursing home visits
   c. Mouse calls
   d. Hospital visits
   e. ED visits

Go to CONNECT to see *activities* on the following topics: *Scheduling an Existing Patient, Scheduling a New Patient, Setting Up a Secondary Schedule, Scheduling Events and Blocking Time, Charting a No Show, Finding Appointments for Established Patients,* and *Finding Appointments for New Patients.*

Insurance and Billing

PATIENT INFORMATION			
Patient Name	**Gender**		**DOB**
Sylvia Gonzales	F		09/01/19XX
Attending	**MRN**		**Allergies**
Alexis N. Whalen MD	341-73-792		Penicillin

Sylvia Gonzales is a 51-year-old female with recently diagnosed Type 2 diabetes mellitus. She states that she has been faithful in taking the new medication the doctor has prescribed for her "sugar." She knows she is having a special "sugar test" done during her visit today. Her medications include Januvia 100 mg daily. Dr. Whalen has ordered a fasting blood sugar (FBS) and hemoglobin A_1C test to be done today. The FBS result is 106 and the hemoglobin A_1C result is 7.0. Mrs. Gonzales is encouraged to continue with her weight-loss program through the local hospital's diabetes clinic and receives a return appointment for 3 months from now. Mrs. Gonzales has insurance through her husband, Juan (DOB 6/24/XX), and also has coverage through her own employer. Her husband's insurance is a traditional fee-for-service plan and her coverage is an HMO plan in which BWW Medical Associates participates.

Keep Sylvia Gonzales in mind as you study this chapter. There will be questions at the end of the chapter based on the case study. The information in the chapter will help you answer these questions.

LEARNING OUTCOMES

After completing Chapter 17, you will be able to:

17.1 Define the basic terms used by the insurance industry.

17.2 Compare fee-for-service plans, HMOs, and PPOs.

17.3 Outline the key requirements for coverage by the Medicare, Medicaid, TRICARE, and CHAMPVA programs.

17.4 Describe allowed charge, contracted fee, capitation and the formula for RBRVS.

17.5 Outline the tasks performed to obtain the information required to produce an insurance claim.

17.6 Produce a clean CMS-1500 health insurance claim form.

17.7 Explain the methods used to submit an insurance claim electronically.

17.8 Recall the information found on every payer's remittance advice.

KEY TERMS

allowed charge
birthday rule
capitation
clearinghouse
coinsurance
copayment
deductible
dual coverage
elective procedure
explanation of benefits (EOB)
explanation of payment (EOP)
fee-for-service
fee schedule
health maintenance organization (HMO)
preauthorization
preferred provider organization (PPO)
premium
remittance advice (RA)
resource-based relative value scale (RBRVS)
third-party payer

VII. C (1)	Identify types of insurance plans
VII. C (2)	Identify models of managed care
VII. C (3)	Discuss workers' compensation as it applies to patients
VII. C (4)	Describe procedures for implementing both managed care and insurance plans
VII. C (5)	Discuss utilization review principles
VII. C (6)	Discuss referral process for patients in a managed care program
VII. C (7)	Describe how guidelines are used in processing an insurance claim
VII. C (8)	Compare processes for filing insurance claims both manually and electronically
VII. C (9)	Describe guidelines for third-party claims
VII. C (10)	Discuss types of physician fee schedules
VII. C (11)	Describe the concept of RBRVS
VII. P (1)	Apply both managed care policies and procedures
VII. P (2)	Apply third party guidelines
VII. P (3)	Complete insurance claim forms
VII. P (4)	Obtain precertification, including documentation
VII. P (5)	Obtain preauthorization, including documentation
VII. P (6)	Verify eligibility for managed care services
VII. A (1)	Demonstrate assertive communication with managed care and/or insurance providers
VII. A (3)	Communicate in language the patient can understand regarding managed care and insurance plans
IX. C (6)	Describe liability, professional, personal injury, and third party insurance

4. Medical Law and Ethics

Graduates:

a. Document accurately

f. Comply with federal, state, and local health laws and regulations

8. Medical Office Business Procedures Management

Graduates:

r. Apply third-party guidelines

s. Obtain managed care referrals and pre-certification

u. Prepare and submit insurance claims

v. Use physician fee schedule

ee. Use proper telephone techniques

hh. Receive, organize, prioritize, and transmit information expediently

11. Career Development

Graduates:

Demonstrate professionalism by:

b.(8) Being courteous and diplomatic

▶ Introduction

Insurance claims are a critical part of the reimbursement process. Accurate claims sent to payers ensure that medical practices receive the maximum appropriate payment for the services they provide. Patients are also concerned with their healthcare plans, asking, "How much will my insurance pay?" "How much will I owe?" "Why are this doctor's fees different from my previous doctor's fees?"

As the office medical assistant, you will handle questions like these every day. Not only must you correctly prepare healthcare claims, but you also will review each patient's insurance coverage, explain the physician's fees, estimate what services are covered by payers, prepare the claims to be submitted for these charges, and then understand the payment explanation when it is returned with the payment from the payer. This chapter prepares you for these tasks by explaining the types of healthcare insurance plans available to patients today, how payers calculate their payments for services provided, how to transmit complete and accurate claims. Finally—because, ultimately, the patient is responsible for the cost of the treatment received—you also will learn how to calculate the patient's financial responsibility for the treatment and his/her responsibility for care not covered by the insurance carrier.

▶ Basic Insurance Terminology   LO 17.1

The first step in understanding insurance is learning some basic terminology used by the insurance industry. Medical insurance, also known as health insurance, is a written contract in the form of a policy between a policyholder and a health plan (insurance carrier). The policyholder may also be called the insured, the member, or the subscriber. Under the insurance policy, the policyholder pays a **premium** (usually monthly)—the charge for keeping the insurance policy in effect. In exchange, the health plan provides *benefits*—payments for medical services—for a specified time period. The policy may cover *dependents* of the policyholder, like a spouse or children. The contract also may specify a lifetime maximum benefit, which is a total sum the health plan will pay out over the patient's lifetime.

There are actually three participants under insurance contracts. The patient (policyholder) is the *first party* and the physician who provides medical services is the *second party*. A patient-physician contract is created when a physician agrees to treat a patient who seeks medical services. This is an implied contract. The patient signs a written financial contract as the party legally responsible for paying for services. The patient may have a policy (written contract) with a health plan, the *third party*, who agrees to carry the risk of paying for those services and therefore is called a **third-party payer.**

Depending on the type of health plan, the policyholder may pay a **deductible**—a fixed dollar amount that must be paid by the insured for charges of providers, or "met" once a year, in addition to the premium, before the third-party payer begins to cover medical expenses. The patient also may have to pay **coinsurance**—a fixed percentage of covered charges after the deductible is met. The coinsurance rate represents the health plan's percentage of the charge followed by the insured's percentage, such as 80-20. This means the insurance carrier would pay 80% of allowed charges and the patient would be responsible for the remaining 20%. If the patient belongs to a managed care health plan, like a health maintenance organization (HMO), instead of paying coinsurance, the patient is responsible for a per-visit **copayment**—a fixed fee collected at the time of the visit. The health plan then pays an agreed-upon contracted payment for the charges with any balance being adjusted off by the service provider per its *preferred provider* contract with the health plan.

Some expenses, like routine eye examinations or dental care, may not be covered under the insured's contract. These noncovered expenses are called *exclusions*. Although many insurance plans offer prescription drug benefits, be aware that such benefits often require the use of drugs listed on the plan's *formulary* (a list of approved brands). If a prescription for a nonformulary medication is written, the pharmacy or health plan case manager will usually contact the physician, asking if a substitution of a formulary drug can be made. If not, the patient may be responsible for a large portion, if not all, of the prescription's cost.

Many procedures and surgeries done today are "planned" procedures; that is, done at the convenience of the physician or surgeon and the patient. This type of procedure is known as an **elective procedure**. Many of these procedures are covered by third-party payers but only if certain rules prior to performance of these procedures are followed. **Preauthorization**, or precertification, describes the process of the provider contacting the insurance plan to see if the proposed procedure is a covered service under the patient's insurance plan. Specific information for the particular patient's case is also given to the insurance carrier. If the insurance plan agrees the patient requires the procedure—in other words, it is *medically necessary*—they will issue a prior authorization number approving the need for the service or procedure. The prior authorization does not, however, mean they agree to pay for the service. This requires the next step of *predetermination*, in which the insurance plan informs the physician of the maximum amount they will pay for the procedure to be performed. Once preauthorization is given, remember that the documentation about the care given must "back up" the procedure codes submitted to the insurance carrier or the charges may still be denied.

▶ Private Health Plans   LO 17.2

All insurance companies have their own rules about benefits and procedures. Most even have their own printed and/or online manuals that must be kept handy in the office for reference. Most insurance plans also have websites and toll-free numbers available for providers to answer questions. Do not be afraid to use these tools. If the first answer you receive does not sound correct, hang up and call back. You will more than likely get a different representative. Ask your question again. If you get the same answer the second time, it is more likely to be correct. Always get the name and extension number of the representative you speak with and document the call. Many companies also give you a call reference number in case a similar issue arises later. Keep all of this information with the patient's financial or insurance record for further reference. In order to refer back to the original call, you will need to give the insurance company that original reference number.

In the United States, the majority of individuals with insurance are covered by group policies, usually through their employers. Some people (often the self-employed) have individual plans. Many others are covered under a government plan (Medicare, Medicaid, TRICARE), which will be discussed later. Still others—over 49.9 million Americans (according to the U.S. Census Bureau figures for 2010)—have had no health insurance. The federal government through the Obama administration has changed that. On March 23, 2010, President Barack Obama signed into law a massive healthcare overhaul bill. The core of this new law, which will take several years to fully phase in (2014 is the goal), is the extension of insurance coverage to all Americans who now lack healthcare coverage. Also included in the law are bans on the ability of private insurance carriers to impose lifetime limits on coverage, denial of coverage for pre-existing conditions, and policy cancellations when an insured person becomes ill. Parents will also be allowed to keep their children covered under the family policy until age 26.

Traditionally, every insurance plan issued each of their providers an identification number, similar to the policy number given to each subscriber. Since the advent of HIPAA, although individual insurers may still issue individual ID numbers, every physician and provider who submits a claim to an insurance carrier must now use a specific provider number, known as a National Provider Identifier (NPI), from the *Centers for Medicare and Medicaid Services (CMS)*. During the transition period, while providers obtained their NPIs, certain non-NPI numbers and two-character identifiers (Table 17-1) were allowed. Now that all providers have an NPI, these non-NPI numbers and their identifiers are used only for certain payers who still require them.

Fee-for-Service and Managed Care Plans

There are two major types of health plans: traditional fee-for-service plans and managed care plans. **Fee-for-service** plans, the oldest and most expensive type, repay policyholders for healthcare costs due to illnesses and accidents. The policy lists the covered medical services. The physician who provides the

TABLE 17-1	National Uniform Claim Committee (NUCC) Non-NPI Qualifiers
Qualifier	**Description**
0B	State License Number
1B	Blue Shield Provider Number
1C	Medicare Provider Number
1D	Medicaid Provider Number
1G	Provider UPIN Number
1H	CHAMPVA Identification Number
E1	Employer's Identification Number
G2	Provider Commercial Number
LU	Location Number
N5	Provider Plan Network Identification Number
SY	Social Security Number (may not be used for Medicare)
X5	State Industrial Accident Provider Number
ZZ	Provider Taxonomy Number

service controls the amount charged for services, but the insurance carrier controls the amount paid for each service.

Managed care organizations (MCOs) control both the financing and delivery of healthcare to policyholders. They enroll policyholders, and they also enroll physicians and other care providers to provide services for their members at reduced rates. This allows them to control all aspects of the care provided to their members, including the providers their members may see; the fees those providers may charge the MCO; and the co-payment charge the physician may bill the patient. Many people who are insured through their employers are covered by some form of managed care plan.

Physicians who enroll with managed care plans are called *participating physicians.* They have contracts with the MCOs that stipulate not only the physician fees, but also the credentials they must have and their responsibilities to the patients and to the MCO itself. Most MCOs also publish their participating physicians' names in booklets and on their website so policyholders can easily choose a participating provider from the list.

Managed care plans pay their participating physicians in one of two ways—by either contracted fees or a fixed prepayment called **capitation**. In most plans, the primary care physician, or PCP, is reimbursed using the capitation method, which involves payment of a fixed amount per patient who signs up with a particular PCP. The physician is paid for each patient enrolled in her practice, regardless of whether she sees that patient multiple times during the month or not at all. In addition to these capitated payments, the PCPs will be paid additional contracted fees for certain other services they provide for the patient such as labs and immunizations. In most managed care plans, specialists are paid in a negotiated fee-for-service manner. These fees are usually less than those paid by private fee-for-service plans, but more than those paid by the government health plans. Providers and insurance carriers negotiate these contracts and fee schedules on a periodic basis.

As shown in Figure 17-1, more than half of all health plans are **preferred provider organizations (PPOs)**. A PPO is a managed care plan that establishes a network of providers to perform

Distribution of health plan enrollment for covered workers, by plan type, 1988–2011

FIGURE 17-1 Distribution of health plan enrollment for covered workers by plan type 1988–2011.

Source: Kaiser/HRET Survey of Employer-Sponsored Health Benefits, 1999-2011; KPMG Survey of Employer-Sponsored Health Benefits, 1993, 1996; The Health Insurance Association of America (HIAA), 1988.

services for plan members. In exchange for the PPO sending them patients, the physicians agree to charge discounted fees. In most PPOs, plan members may also choose to receive care from doctors or providers outside the network. However, if they do, they are responsible for paying a higher percentage of the charges for these visits and may also be subject to a deductible they would not be responsible for if they saw in-network providers.

Another common type of managed care system, covering 17% of those with private healthcare insurance, is a **health maintenance organization (HMO)**. Physicians with HMO contracts are often paid a capitated rate, or they may be employees of the organization who are paid salaries. Patients who enroll in an HMO pay premiums and usually also pay a copayment, often $15 to $35, at the time of the office visit. No other fees are required for any covered service a member needs. In HMOs, patients must usually choose from a specific group of healthcare providers. If they seek services from a provider who is not in the health plan, the HMO does not pay for the care. Patients also pay for excluded services—those not included in the plan as covered services.

An important aspect of cost control used by managed care organizations is a process known as *utilization review* (UR). In this process, committee members who have training similar to that of the physician providing the medical care review individual cases to be sure that all services provided were medically necessary and that there was appropriate use of medical resources. Should UR find that services were not medically necessary, payment can be denied at a loss to the practice, as the patient cannot be billed for services considered not medically necessary.

Commercial Payers

Blue Cross and Blue Shield Although many people think Blue Cross and Blue Shield (BCBS) is one large corporation, it is actually a nationwide federation of nonprofit and for-profit service organizations that provide prepaid healthcare services to BCBS subscribers. Each state's organization operates under its own state laws, and covered services and benefits for BCBS plans can vary greatly from state to state and plan to plan.

Private Commercial Carriers There are too many private commercial payers to list, and rules and regulations among the carriers vary as much as the covered services and the fees allowed for those covered services. Aetna, CIGNA, and Travelers are common commercial carriers.

In addition to health insurance, two other special types of insurance—liability insurance and disability insurance—are available to cover medical expenses. *Liability insurance* covers injuries caused by the insured or that occurred on the insured's property. If an individual (or company) has home, business, automobile, or health liability insurance, the injured person can claim benefits under the insured's policy. To obtain specific details about the individual policy's coverage, contact the liability insurance company.

Disability insurance may be offered to employees (at employee expense), provided by an employer for its employees, or purchased privately by self-employed individuals. Disability insurance is activated when the insured is injured or disabled for non-work-related reasons. Disability insurance is not health insurance and does not cover medical expenses. When an insured person cannot work, and can provide the insurance carrier with documentation as to the medical reason he or she cannot work, the insurance company pays the insured a prearranged monthly amount to assist with the insured's normal daily expenses. There are two types of disability policies. Short-term policies offer coverage for shorter periods of time, usually 7 (consecutive) days to 6 months, and long-term disability policies may last for 1 year or more depending on policy stipulations.

▶ Government Plans LO 17.3

Government plans are generally designed to offer healthcare to retirees, low-income and disadvantaged individuals, and active or retired military personnel and their families. Some of these plans maintain many of the features of managed care plans.

Medicare

The largest federal program providing healthcare is *Medicare*, which provides health insurance for citizens aged 65 and older. Patients under the age of 65 also may be eligible, including those who are dependent widows aged 50 to 65, the disabled, the blind, and workers of any age who have chronic kidney disease requiring dialysis or end-stage renal disease (ESRD) requiring transplant. Kidney donors are also eligible for Medicare. The Medicare program is managed by CMS. Two websites are available to obtain more information regarding Medicare: www.medicare.gov (supplies patients and beneficiaries with information) and www.cms.gov (includes provider and claims information for both Medicare and Medicaid). Medicare is divided into two main parts—Part A and Part B.

Part A Medicare Part A is the hospital benefit, which is billed by hospitals (or other healthcare facilities) and financed through contributions collected from the Federal Insurance Contributions Act (FICA) tax on income earned by workers and the self-employed. Currently, the FICA tax for workers is 6.2% and 12.4% for the self-employed up to a wage maximum of $94,200. You will learn more about FICA tax deductions in the *Practice Management* chapter. Medicare Part A pays most of the costs for the following individuals:

- Patients who are admitted as inpatients for up to the 90-day benefit period. A benefit period begins the day a patient is admitted to the hospital and ends when that patient has not been hospitalized or placed in a skilled nursing facility for a period of 60 continuous days after discharge.

  The 90-day benefit period is divided into two parts. The initial benefit period is 60 days where, after the patient pays a deductible, hospital coverage is at 100%. After the first 60 days, the patient enters into a 30-day period called coinsurance days. During this 30-day period, the patient must pay an additional per-day payment, or coinsurance. If the hospital stay extends beyond the 30 coinsurance days, the patient may use up to 60 lifetime reserve days, which also include a per-day charge. It is important to note these 60 lifetime reserve days are not renewable. Once they are used up during the patient's lifetime, they are no longer available. If the patient is admitted to the hospital again for longer than 90 days, after the reserve days are exhausted, the patient will be responsible for all charges after the 90th day.

- A patient who has been admitted to a skilled nursing facility (SNF) after inpatient hospitalization. Coverage is for no more than 100 days in each benefit period—usually 1 calendar year.
- A patient who is receiving medical care at home.
- A patient receiving hospice care either at home or in a hospice facility. Terminally ill patients with a prognosis (prediction) of 6 months or less to live are eligible for hospice care. Hospice programs provide *palliative care* including pain relief and support for terminal patients and their family members.
- A patient who requires psychiatric treatment. Currently, Medicare covers only 190 days of psychiatric hospitalization in a patient's lifetime.
- A patient who requires respite care. In certain clearly and narrowly defined circumstances, Medicare provides for a respite, or short break, for the person who cares for a terminally ill patient at home. The terminally ill patient is moved to a care facility for the respite.

Anyone who receives Social Security benefits is automatically enrolled in Part A and does not have to pay a premium. Individuals aged 65 or older who are not eligible for Social Security benefits may enroll in Part A, but they must pay premiums for the coverage.

Part B Medicare Part B covers a portion (usually 80%) of the allowed charges for a wide range of outpatient procedures and supplies. For example, it covers physician services, outpatient hospital services, diagnostic tests, clinical laboratory services, and outpatient physical and speech therapy as long as these services are considered medically necessary. Individuals entitled to Part A benefits automatically qualify for Part B benefits. In addition, U.S. citizens and permanent residents over the age of 65 are also eligible. Part B is a voluntary program; eligible persons may or may not take part in it. However, those desiring Part B must enroll because coverage is not automatic. The Medicare beneficiary has a 6-month time frame to apply, beginning 3 months prior to his 65th birthday until 3 months after it. If the deadline is missed, the beneficiary must wait until open enrollment, which is from January 1–March 31 of each year. If the Medicare B enrollment takes place more than 12 months after the initial enrollment period, there is a permanent 10% increase in the premium for each year the beneficiary was eligible to enroll but did not. Unlike Part A, Part B coverage is not premium-free. Starting in 2007, the Medicare Part B premium is based on the beneficiary's income. The cost ranges

between $0 and $211.90 per month, and the premium usually increases annually. Each Medicare enrollee receives a health insurance card that lists the beneficiary's name, sex, effective dates for Part A and Part B coverage, and Medicare number. CMS assigns the Medicare number, which usually consists of the Social Security number followed by an alpha or alphanumeric suffix. The suffix indicates how the beneficiary is eligible for Medicare. The three most common suffixes are as follows:

- Suffix "A" is attached to the patient's own social security number because it was his income making him eligible for Medicare.
- Suffix "B" is attached to the social security number of the spouse because the patient (who usually has not paid enough into the system to be eligible under her own number) is eligible because of her spouse's contributions.
- Suffix "D" is attached to the social security number of a spouse who is deceased. This benefit type has commonly been known as "widow's benefits".

See Table 17-2 for an overview of Medicare A and B premium, deductible, and benefit differences as of 2012.

Medicare Part C and Part D Medicare Part C, introduced in 1997, provides several plan choices for individuals called Medicare Advantage plans. These include PPOs, HMOs, private fee-for-service (PFFS) plans, special needs plans, and Medicare medical savings account plans (MSA). The MSA plan started in 2007.

In 2003, the legislature passed the Medicare Part D prescription drug plan and coverage began January 1, 2006. All Medicare beneficiaries can enroll in a prescription drug plan through the Medicare Prescription Drug plan, Medicare Advantage, or other Medicare plans, and through employers and unions. Figure 17-2 is the Medicare Part D Coverage Determination Request Form.

Medicare Plan Options Medicare beneficiaries can choose from a number of insurance plan options, including fee-for-service and Medicare Advantage plans consisting of different types of managed care plans.

Fee-for-Service—The Original Medicare Plan The Medicare fee-for-service plan allows the beneficiary to choose any licensed physician certified by Medicare. Each time the beneficiary receives outpatient services, a fee is billable. Medicare generally pays part of this fee and part is due from the beneficiary. Once the patient meets the annual deductible, if the patient sees a participating provider, Medicare pays 80% of approved charges directly to the provider and the patient is responsible for the remaining 20% and any disallowed charges. Providers who accept the Medicare-allowed charge as payment in full are known as those who "accept assignment." These providers cannot charge the patient more than this allowed charge, regardless of the original fee. A Medicare beneficiary may

TABLE 17-2 Comparison of Medicare A and B Premiums, Deductibles, and Benefits

Medicare Plan	Premium	Deductible	Benefit Period	Patient Coinsurance
Medicare A	None	Yes/per admission		
Hospitalization			Days 1–60	$0—Medicare pays 100%
			Days 61–90	$289/day
			Days 91–150 (includes 60 lifetime reserve days)	$566/day
			After 150 days	100%—No Medicare benefit
Skilled Nursing Facility (Patient must have been hospitalized at least 3 days and be admitted to approved SNF within 30 days of hospital discharge)			Days 1–20	$0—Medicare pays 100%
			Days 21–100	$144.50/day
			After 100 days	100%—No Medicare benefit
Home Healthcare (includes P/T home nursing and aide services, durable medical equipment (DME), and supplies)			Unlimited, as long as Medicare criteria are met and services are *medically necessary*	$0 for home health service 20% of allowed charges for DME
Hospice Services (Palliative care for the terminally ill and family members)			Patient elects hospice care and physician certifies need for hospice	$0 except for outpatient medication and inpatient hospital care
Blood				First 3 pints per year
Medicare B (Outpatient Medical)	Yes	Yes/per year	January 1–December 31	20% of approved charges
Outpatient Mental Health				50% of approved charges
Outpatient Laboratory				$0 of approved charges (Medicare pays 100%)
Home Healthcare (includes P/T home health nursing and aides, PT/OT/ST/DME supplies and services)				$0 for home care (Medicare covers 100%) 20% for DME
Blood				First 3 pints and 20% of approved charges
Ambulatory Surgery				20% of predetermined charge after deductible

choose a provider who does not participate in the Medicare program and who does not accept assignment. In that case, the provider does not have to accept the Medicare allowable as payment in full and may charge the patient up to the "limiting charge"—usually defined as 115% of the nonparticipating allowable fee—as described by Medicare. This usually results in an increased out-of-pocket expense for the patient.

To help with the responsibility of the 20% coinsurance, individuals enrolled in the Original Medicare B Plan often buy additional insurance called a *Medigap* plan. While coverage of these plans varies from policy to policy, the core benefits common to all Medigap plans include reimbursement of the patient's Part B deductible and picking up the 20% balance of the Medicare-allowed charge. If Medicare does not pay a claim, Medigap is not required to pay the claim either. Although private insurance carriers offer Medigap plans, federal and state laws regulate coverage and standards. In exchange for Medigap coverage, the policyholder pays a monthly premium. A number of different options labeled A through J are available. Monthly premiums vary widely across the different plan levels as well as within a single plan level, depending on the insurance company selected. In 2009, CMS changed how claims were processed through Medicare contracting reform. At the forefront of these changes was the creation of Medicare

Administrative Contractor (MAC) Jurisdictions for claims processing. Table 17-3 outlines the jurisdictions for Medicare medical claims and the states contained within each. At the time of this writing, MACs are undergoing redistricting. DME (durable medical equipment) claims are separated from medical claims and are submitted to MACs set up specifically for DME.

Medicare Managed Care Plans Medicare managed care plans charge a monthly premium and a small copayment for each office visit, but not a deductible. Like private payer managed care plans, Medicare managed care plans often require patients to select a primary care physician (PCP) who oversees and manages the patient's medical care through *referrals.* Usually, patients are also required to use a specific network of physicians, hospitals, and facilities. Some plans allow members the option of receiving services from providers outside the network, but the member's portion of the charges will be higher. Medicare MCOs offer coverage for services not reimbursed in the Original Medicare Plan, like physical examinations and immunizations.

Medicare Preferred Provider Organization Plan In the Medicare preferred provider organization (PPO) plan, patients pay less when they use doctors within a network, but they may choose to go outside the network for additional

Medicare Part D Coverage Determination Request Form

This form <u>cannot</u> be used to request:
- Medicare non-covered drugs, including barbiturates, benzodiazepines, fertility drugs, drugs prescribed for weight loss, weight gain or hair growth, over-the-counter drugs, or prescription vitamins (except prenatal vitamins and fluoride preparations).
- **Biotech or other specialty drugs for which drug-specific forms are required. [See <Part D plan website.>] OR [See links to plan websites at http://www.cms.hhs.gov/PrescriptionDrugCovGenIn/04_Formulary.asp]**

Patient Information	Prescriber Information
Patient Name:	Prescriber Name:
Member ID#:	NPI# (if available):
Address:	Address:
City: / State:	City: / State:
Home Phone: / Zip:	Office Phone #: / Office Fax #: / Zip:
Sex (circle): M F / DOB:	Contact Person:

Diagnosis and Medical Information

Medication:	Strength and Route of Administration:	Frequency:
☐ New Prescription OR Date Therapy Initiated:	Expected Length of Therapy:	Qty:
Height/Weight:	Drug Allergies:	Diagnosis:
Prescriber's Signature:		Date:

Rationale for Exception Request or Prior Authorization
FORM CANNOT BE PROCESSED WITHOUT REQUIRED EXPLANATION

☐ Alternate drug(s) contraindicated or previously tried, but with adverse outcome (eg, toxicity, allergy, or therapeutic failure)

→ Specify below: (1) Drug(s) contraindicated or tried; (2) adverse outcome for each; (3) if therapeutic failure, length of therapy on each drug(s);

☐ Complex patient with one or more chronic conditions (including, for example, psychiatric condition, diabetes) is stable on current drug(s); high risk of significant adverse clinical outcome with medication change

→ Specify below: Anticipated significant adverse clinical outcome

☐ Medical need for different dosage form and/or higher dosage

→ Specify below: (1) Dosage form(s) and/or dosage(s) tried; (2) explain medical reason

☐ Request for formulary tier exception

→ Specify below: (1) Formulary or preferred drugs contraindicated or tried and failed, or tried and not as effective as requested drug; (2) if therapeutic failure, length of therapy on each drug and adverse outcome; (3) if not as effective, length of therapy on each drug and outcome

☐ Other:_____ → Explain below

REQUIRED EXPLANATION:_____

_____

_____

Request for Expedited Review

☐ REQUEST FOR EXPEDITED REVIEW [24 HOURS]

→ BY CHECKING THIS BOX AND SIGNING ABOVE, I CERTIFY THAT APPLYING THE 72 HOUR STANDARD REVIEW TIME FRAME MAY SERIOUSLY JEOPARDIZE THE LIFE OR HEALTH OF THE MEMBER OR THE MEMBER'S ABILITY TO REGAIN MAXIMUM FUNCTION

Information on this form is protected health information and subject to all privacy and security regulations under HIPAA.

FIGURE 17-2 Medicare Part D Coverage Determination Request Form.

costs, such as a higher copayment or higher coinsurance. Patients do not need a PCP, and referrals are not required.

Medicare Private Fee-for-Service Plan Under a Medicare private fee-for-service plan, patients receive services from the provider they choose, as long as Medicare has approved the provider or facility. A private insurance company contracting with Medicare to provide services to beneficiaries operates this plan. The plan sets its own rates for services, and physicians are allowed to bill patients the amount of the

TABLE 17-3	Medicare MAC Jurisdictions for Medical Claims
A/B MAC Jurisdiction Number	**States Included in Each Jurisdiction**
1	American Samoa, California, Guam, Hawaii, Nevada, and Northern Mariana Islands
2	Alaska, Idaho, Oregon, and Washington
3	Arizona, Montana, North Dakota, South Dakota, Utah, and Wyoming
4	Colorado, New Mexico, Oklahoma, and Texas
5	Iowa, Kansas, Missouri, and Nebraska
6	Illinois, Minnesota, and Wisconsin
7	Arkansas, Louisiana, and Mississippi
8	Indiana and Michigan
9	Florida, Puerto Rico, and U.S. Virgin Islands
10	Alabama, Georgia, and Tennessee
11	North Carolina, South Carolina, Virginia, and West Virginia
12	Delaware, District of Columbia, Maryland, New Jersey, and Pennsylvania
13	Connecticut and New York
14	Maine, Massachusetts, New Hampshire, Rhode Island, and Vermont
15	Kentucky and Ohio

charge not covered by the plan. A copayment may or may not be required.

Recovery Audit Contractor Program In 2008, CMS announced aggressive new steps to find and prevent waste, fraud, and abuse in Medicare. Since then, CMS has been working closely with beneficiaries and providers, consolidating its fraud detection efforts, strengthening its oversight of medical equipment suppliers and home health agencies, and launching the national recovery audit contractor (RAC) program. Contracts have been awarded to four permanent RACs, each of which audits one-fourth of the country, designed to guard the Medicare Trust Fund by fighting fraud, waste, and abuse in the Medicare program. The recovery audit program's goal is to identify improper payments—overpayments or underpayments—made on claims of healthcare services provided to Medicare beneficiaries. Overpayments can occur when healthcare providers submit claims that do not meet Medicare's coding or medical necessity policies. Underpayments can occur when healthcare providers submit claims for a simple procedure, but the medical record reveals that a more complicated procedure was actually performed. Healthcare providers subject to review include hospitals, physician practices, nursing homes, home health agencies, durable medical equipment suppliers, and any other provider or supplier that bills Medicare Parts A and B. For further information, go to www.cms.hhs.gov/RAC/.

Medicaid

Medicaid, also run by CMS, is a health-benefit program designed for low-income, blind, or disabled patients; needy families; foster children; and children born with birth defects. Medicaid is a health cost assistance program, *not* an insurance program. The difference between an assistance program and a health insurance program is this: the government provides assistance programs to the recipient (or patient) at no charge, while the subscriber (or patient) pays for health insurance programs through premiums. The federal government provides funds to all 50 states to administer Medicaid (covering specified mandated services), and then each state adds its own funds (for additional optional services). Every state has a program to assist with medical expenses for citizens who meet its qualifications. Such programs may have different names and slightly different rules, but they provide basically the same assistance, which includes

- Physician services
- Emergency services
- Laboratory services and X-rays
- Skilled nursing facility (SNF) care
- Early diagnostic screening and treatment for minors (aged 21 and younger)
- Vaccines for children

Accepting Assignment Any physician who agrees to treat Medicaid patients also agrees to accept the established Medicaid payment for covered services as payment in full. This agreement is called *accepting assignment*. If the physician's fee is higher than the Medicaid payment, the patient cannot be billed for the difference. The physician can, however, bill the patient for services Medicaid does not cover. Note that, as a federally funded assistance program, Medicaid is known as the *payer of last resort*, meaning that if both a private insurance plan and Medicaid cover a patient, the private plan must be billed before Medicaid. It is considered fraud to knowingly bill Medicaid if another insurance company provides medical coverage for a patient.

Dual Coverage or Medi/Medi Elderly or disabled patients who have Medicare and who cannot pay the difference between the charges submitted and the Medicare payment may qualify for Medicare and Medicaid—formerly known as Medi/Medi, this is now more commonly known as **dual coverage**. In such cases, Medicare is the primary payer and Medicaid is the secondary payer. The patient with dual coverage is never billed for a balance unless a noncovered service is provided (and the patient is notified in advance in writing of this fact), or Medicare/Medicaid states that the patient may be billed.

State Guidelines Medicaid benefits can and often do vary greatly from state to state. Eligibility is based on how much income the patient reported for the previous month. It is important to understand the Medicaid guidelines in your state so the Medicaid reimbursement to your office is prompt and trouble-free. Here are some suggestions:

- Do not submit a claim to Medicaid without verification of Medicaid benefit eligibility. Doing so may constitute fraud.

You should contact Medicaid to verify eligibility every time the patient is seen in the office.

- Ensure that the physician signs all claims, unless claims are submitted electronically (the physician's signature is kept on file). Send the completed and signed claims to the state's Medicaid-approved contractor (which pays on behalf of the state) or to the state department that administers Medicaid (for example, the state department of social services or public health). Check with your state Medicaid office if you are unsure where to send the claim.

- Unless the patient has a medical emergency, Medicaid often requires authorization before services are performed, which must be obtained from the state Medicaid office in advance. If the patient is seen on an emergency basis, it is not unusual for the Medicaid office to require that they be notified as soon as possible of any emergency treatment given to the patient. Not meeting these requirements can result in claim denial.

- Check the time limit (deadline) on claim submission with your state's Medicaid office. It can be as short as 2 months or as long as 1 year from the date of service. Claims submitted after this time limit will be denied or rejected. The patient cannot be held responsible for the charges; they will need to be adjusted off the account as a loss of income to the practice.

- Treat Medicaid patients with the same professionalism and courtesy you extend to other private-pay patients. Simply because a patient qualifies for Medicaid assistance does not mean the patient is in any way inferior to those with private insurance.

TRICARE and CHAMPVA

The U.S. government provides healthcare benefits to families of current military personnel, retired military personnel, and veterans through the TRICARE and CHAMPVA programs. TRICARE and CHAMPVA patients are most commonly seen at a military-related facility.

Run by the Defense Department, TRICARE (formerly known as CHAMPUS, or Civilian Health and Medical Program for Uniformed Services) is not a health insurance plan. Rather, it is a healthcare benefit for families of uniformed personnel and retirees from the uniformed services, including the Army, Navy, Marines, Air Force, Coast Guard, Public Health Service, and National Oceanic and Atmospheric Administration (Figure 17-3). TRICARE offers families three choices of healthcare benefits:

1. TRICARE Prime, a health maintenance organization.
2. TRICARE Extra, a managed care network of healthcare providers families can use on a case-by-case basis without a required enrollment
3. TRICARE Standard, a fee-for-service plan.

Another program, TRICARE for Life, is aimed at Medicare-eligible military retirees and Medicare-eligible family members. TRICARE for Life offers the opportunity to receive healthcare at a military treatment facility to individuals aged 65 and older who are eligible for both Medicare and TRICARE.

Under TRICARE for Life, enrollees in TRICARE who are aged 65 and older can continue to obtain medical services at military hospitals and clinics as they did before they turned 65. As a general rule, TRICARE for Life acts as a secondary payer

FIGURE 17-3 TRICARE covers healthcare services for family members of military personnel and military retirees at facilities such as the military base hospital pictured here.

to Medicare; Medicare pays first and TRICARE pays the remaining out-of-pocket expenses.

CHAMPVA is the acronym for Civilian Health and Medical Program of the Veterans Administration and it covers the expenses of the families (dependent spouses and children) of veterans with total, permanent, service-connected disabilities. It also covers surviving spouses and dependent children of veterans who died in the line of duty or as a result of service-connected disabilities.

TRICARE and CHAMPVA Eligibility As with any healthcare plan, you must verify TRICARE eligibility. All TRICARE patients should have a valid identification card. To receive TRICARE benefits, eligible individuals must be enrolled in the Defense Enrollment Eligibility Reporting System (DEERS)—a computer database.

Eligibility for CHAMPVA is determined by the nearest Veterans Affairs medical center. Contact this center if any questions arise. Patients can choose the doctor they wish after CHAMPVA eligibility is confirmed.

Unlike Medicaid-participating providers who must accept all Medicaid patients once they agree to participate, TRICARE- and CHAMPVA-participating providers have the option of deciding whether to accept patients on a case-by-case basis. Make sure you know the policy of the physicians in your office regarding this issue.

State Children's Health Insurance Plan

Originally enacted in 1997, the State Children's Health Insurance Plan (SCHIP) was reenacted in 2009 and is now more commonly known simply as CHIP. The plan allows states to provide health coverage to uninsured children in families whose incomes are too high to qualify for Medicaid but too low to afford private insurance. States have raised eligibility levels to provide coverage to more families. Check your state's requirements for this plan through its website.

Workers' Compensation

Workers' compensation insurance covers employment-related accidents or diseases. Federal law requires employers to purchase and maintain a certain minimum amount of workers' compensation insurance for their employees. Workers' compensation laws vary from state to state, but, in most states, this insurance includes these benefits:

- Basic medical treatment.
- A weekly amount paid to the patient for a temporary disability, which compensates workers for loss of income until they can return to work.
- A weekly or monthly sum paid to the patient for a permanent disability.
- Rehabilitation costs to restore an employee's ability to work again.
- Death benefits for survivors.

Not all medical practices accept workers' compensation cases. Every procedure or treatment deemed necessary must be approved in order for payment to be made. Prior to treating a patient who states her care is related to a work-related illness or injury, call the employer to verify this information. When contacting the employer, speak to the office manager or human resources department. Be sure to get the name and extension of the person who verifies information for you. Give the verifier the patient's name and ask if the treatment is to be covered by workers' compensation. If the answer is yes, be sure to get the date of the original injury or illness and a brief description of the event causing the illness or ask the verifier if a workers' compensation case has been opened by the employer with the insurance carrier and obtain the case number. If a case has not been opened, ask the employer to report the incident. Until this

report—known as the Employer's First Report of Illness or Injury—is received from the employer, the insurance carrier will not open a case, which means you will not be paid. Obtain the name, address, and phone number of the insurance carrier and carefully document this information. After completing the call to the employer and receiving permission to treat the patient, call the insurance carrier and verify that the employer has an active workers' compensation policy with them.

Records management of workers' compensation varies by state. If you see a patient privately and then she comes to you for a work-related illness or injury, be sure to keep the medical and financial records of the private care and the care related to the workers' compensation case separate. Because the employer and insurer have contracted with the physician to provide care, they have the right to see any and all treatment and applicable financial records related to the workers' compensation claim without patient consent. It is up to the office to maintain the patient's confidentiality related to any care provided to her that is not related to the workers' compensation claim and keeping separate files makes it easier to do so.

Procedure 17-1, found at the end of the chapter, outlines the steps for verifying a patient's workers' compensation coverage.

▶ Fee Schedules and Charges   LO 17.4

Physicians establish a list of their usual fees—charged to most of their patients most of the time under typical conditions—for procedures and services they frequently perform. These fees are listed on the office **fee schedule**. Figure 17-4 shows a sample of an office fee schedule.

BWW Medical Associates, PC
Multi-Specialty Fee Schedule

SERVICES RENDERED	CPT	FEE	SERVICES RENDERED	CPT	FEE
Initial OV	99204	$100.00	EKG with Interp	93000	$80.00
Follow-up Visit	99214	$65.00	24-Hour Holter Monitor	93224	$300.00
LCMDM Consultation	99241	$120.00	Sigmoidoscopy	45330	$800.00
HCMDM Consultation	99245	$180.00	Spirometry	94010	$35.00
Hospital Admission	99223	$150.00	Throat Culture	87081	$25.00
Hospital Consultation	99253	$150.00	Flu Immunization	90724	$25.00
ER Visit	99284	$150.00	Pneumococcal Immunization	90732	$25.00
Hospital Visit	99232	$125.00	Allergy Injection, Single	95115	$25.00
Urinalysis w/ Micro	81000	$25.00	Allergy Injection, Multiple	95117	$60.00
Culture	87086	$45.00	Hemoccult x 3	82270	$30.00
CBC	85025	$60.00	Tetanus Injection	90718	$20.00
Venipuncture	36415	$35.00	Screening Mammography	77057	$425.00

FIGURE 17-4 The practice fee schedule shows the charge for each service provided by the practice.

Medicare Payment System: RBRVS

Third-party payers set the fees they are willing to pay providers; these fees are often less than the physician's fee schedule. Most payers base their fees on the amounts Medicare allows because the Medicare method of fee setting takes into account important factors other than only the usual fees.

The payment system Medicare uses is called the **resource-based relative value scale (RBRVS)**. The RBRVS establishes the relative value units for services, replacing the providers' consensus on fees (the "usual" or historical charges) with amounts based on resources (what each service really costs to provide).

An RBRVS fee has three parts and uses the formula RVU × GAF × CF. Listed below is an explanation for each part of this formula:

1. The national uniform relative value unit (RVU). The relative value of a procedure is based on three cost elements: the physician's work, the practice cost (overhead), and the cost of malpractice insurance. For example, the relative value unit for a simple office visit, say, to administer a flu shot, is much lower than the relative value for a complicated encounter like planning a patient's treatment of uncontrolled diabetes.

2. A geographic adjustment factor (GAF). A GAF is used to adjust each relative value to reflect a geographical area's relative costs, such as office rent and utilities.

3. A nationally uniform conversion factor (CF). A uniform CF is a dollar amount used to multiply the relative values to produce a payment amount. It is used by Medicare to make adjustments according to changes in the cost-of-living index.

When RBRVS fees are used, providers receive considerably lower payments than when usual fees are used. Each part of the RBRVS—the relative values, the geographic adjustment, and the conversion factor—is updated each year by CMS. The Medicare fee schedule (MFS) is also published each year by CMS in the *Federal Register* at www.cms.hhs.gov/FeeScheduleGenInfo/.

Payment Methods

Most third-party payers use one of three methods for reimbursing physicians:

1. Allowed charges
2. Contracted fee schedule
3. Capitation

Allowed Charges Most payers set an **allowed charge**—the maximum amount the payer will pay any provider—for each procedure or service. The term *allowed charge* has many equivalent terms, including *maximum allowable fee, maximum charge, allowed amount, allowed fee,* or *allowable charge.*

The physician's usual charge is often greater than a plan's allowed charge. If the physician participates in the plan, only the allowed charge will be the basis for the payer's payment. The plan's contract with the provider governs whether the provider is permitted to bill a patient for the part of a usual charge the payer does not cover. Billing a patient for the difference between a higher usual fee and a lower allowed charge is called *balance billing.* Under most contracts, participating providers may not bill the patient for the difference. Instead, the provider must write off the difference, meaning the difference between the fee charged and the allowed charge is subtracted from the patient's bill and never collected. The common term for this write-off is *adjustment.*

For example, Medicare-participating providers may not collect any amount greater than the Medicare-allowed charge from the Medicare fee schedule. Medicare is responsible for paying 80% of this allowed charge (after patients have met their annual deductible) and patients (or their secondary insurance) are responsible for the other 20%.

Here is an example of a Medicare billing. A Medicare-participating provider reports a usual charge of $200 for a service and the Medicare-allowed charge is $84. The provider must write off the difference between the two charges. The patient is responsible for 20% of the allowed charge, not of the provider's usual charge:

Provider's usual fee:	$200.00
Medicare-allowed charge:	$ 84.00
Medicare pays 80%	$ 67.20
Patient pays 20%	$ 16.80

The total the provider can collect is $84. The provider must write off the difference between the usual fee and the allowed charge, or $116.00 in this example. Remember, in this example, it is assumed the patient has paid her annual deductible; otherwise, her coinsurance would be higher.

Contracted Fee Schedule Some payers, particularly PPOs, establish fixed fee schedules with their participating physicians. The plan's terms determine what percentage of the charges, if any, the patient owes and what percentage the payer covers. Participating providers can typically bill patients their usual charges for procedures and services not covered by the plan.

Capitation The fixed prepayment for each plan member in capitation contracts is determined by the managed care plan that initiates contracts with providers. The plan's contract with the provider lists the services and procedures covered by the capitation rate. For example, a typical contract with a primary care provider might include the following services:

- Preventive care, including well-child care, adult physical exams, gynecological exams, eye exams, and hearing exams.
- Counseling and telephone calls.
- Office visits.
- Medical care, including medical care services such as therapeutic injections and immunizations, allergy immunotherapy, electrocardiograms, and pulmonary function tests.
- The local treatment of first-degree burns, the application of dressings, suture removal, the excision of small skin lesions, and the removal of foreign bodies or cerumen from the external ear.

These services are covered in the capitation rate for each plan member who selects a particular PCP. The patient is often responsible for a fixed copayment at the time of the visit, but no other charges will be incurred unless the visit includes a noncovered service, which can be billed to the patient using the physician's usual rate. Plans often require the provider to notify the patient in advance that a service is not covered and to state the fee for which the patient will be responsible. It is always a good idea to have the patient sign a waiver of liability—a notification in writing that he will be responsible for any noncovered charges, and the expected amount, prior to performing any such procedure.

Calculating Patient Charges

In addition to premiums, patients may be obligated to pay deductibles, copayments, coinsurance, excluded and over-limit services, and balance billing (only if allowed by the insurance plan).

All payers require patients to pay for excluded (noncovered) services. Physicians generally can charge their usual fees for these services. Likewise, in managed care plans that set limits on the annual (or other period) usage of covered services, patients are responsible for usage beyond the allowed number. For example, if one preventive physical examination is permitted annually, additional preventive examinations are denied by the payer and become the patient's responsibility.

Communicating with Patients About Charges

When patients have office visits with a physician who participates in the plan under which they have coverage, like a Medicare-participating (PAR) provider, they generally sign an assignment of benefits statement. When this occurs, the provider agrees to prepare healthcare claims for patients, to receive payments directly from the payers, and to accept a payer's allowed charge. Patients are billed for charges that payers deny or do not pay. When patients have encounters with nonparticipating (nonPAR) providers, the procedure is usually different. To avoid the difficulty of collecting patient payments at a later date, practices may require that the patient either (1) assigns benefits directly to the practice or (2) pays in full at the time of services.

Patients often call the office regarding statements they receive from the practice. For example, suppose a patient receives a bill for $100 from your practice. She calls to say that she has paid her deductible for the year, so her insurance company should have paid 80% of the charges. You call the patient's insurance company and, after confirming coverage, learn that her deductible increased to $200 this year and she still has to pay $100 to meet her deductible. If she pays the $100 bill in full, her deductible will then be met. Alternatively, many insurance carrier websites now include a calculator that, based on the CPT (procedure) code and ICD (diagnosis) codes you enter, will calculate the payment to expect from the insurer, and the probable patient balance, as well as give you information as to the deductible amount and balance still owed by the patient. You now can call the patient to explain these facts to her.

To estimate patients' responsibility for charges, you should check with the payer to find out

- The patient's deductible amount and whether it has been paid in full, the covered benefits, and coinsurance or other patient financial obligations.
- The payer's allowed charges for the services the provider anticipates providing.

Patients should always be reminded of their financial obligations under their plans, including claim denials, according to practice procedures. The practice's financial policy regarding payment for services is usually either displayed on the reception area wall or included in the new patient information packet. The policy should explain what is required of the patient and when payment is due. For example, the policy may state the following:

- For unassigned claims: Payment for the physician's services is expected at the time of your appointment, unless you have made other arrangements with our practice manager.
- For assigned claims: After your insurance company processes your claim, you will be billed for any amount that is your responsibility. You are responsible for any part of the charges that are denied or not paid by the carrier. Patient payments are expected to be paid in full within 30 days of the statement date, unless prior arrangements have been made.
- For managed care members: Copayments must be paid prior to seeing the practitioner.

It is also good practice to notify patients in advance of the probable cost of procedures that are not going to be covered by their plan. For example, some private plans as well as Medicare do not pay for services like chiropractic care and some preventative services. Patients should be asked to sign a document known as a waiver of liability, which should specify why the service will not be covered and the cost of the procedure, *before* the service is provided.

The Advance Beneficiary Notice of Noncoverage or ABN (CMS-R-131) is a notice given to Medicare beneficiaries to convey that Medicare is not likely to provide coverage in a specific case (Figure 17-5). "Notifiers" include physicians, providers (including institutional providers like outpatient hospitals), practitioners, and suppliers paid under Part B (including independent laboratories), and hospice providers and religious nonmedical healthcare institutions (RNHCIs) paid exclusively under Part A.

The ABN must be verbally reviewed with the beneficiary or his or her representative and any questions raised during that review must be answered before it is signed. The ABN must be delivered far enough in advance that the beneficiary or representative has time to consider the options and make an informed choice. Employees or subcontractors of the notifier may deliver the ABN. ABNs are never required in emergency or urgent care situations. Once all blanks are completed and the form is signed, the beneficiary or representative receives a copy. In all cases, the notifier must retain the original notice on file.

(A) **Notifier(s):**
(B) **Patient Name:** _____ *(C)* **Identification Number:** _____

ADVANCE BENEFICIARY NOTICE OF NONCOVERAGE (ABN)

NOTE: If Medicare doesn't pay for *(D)*_____ below, you may have to pay.

Medicare does not pay for everything, even some care that you or your health care provider have good reason to think you need. We expect Medicare may not pay for the *(D)*_____ below.

(D) _____	*(E)* Reason Medicare May Not Pay:	*(F)* Estimated Cost:

WHAT YOU NEED TO DO NOW:

- Read this notice, so you can make an informed decision about your care.
- Ask us any questions that you may have after you finish reading.
- Choose an option below about whether to receive the *(D)*_____ listed above.
  Note: If you choose Option 1 or 2, we may help you to use any other insurance that you might have, but Medicare cannot require us to do this.

(G) OPTIONS: **Check only one box. We cannot choose a box for you.**

☐ **OPTION 1.** I want the *(D)*_____ listed above. You may ask to be paid now, but I also want Medicare billed for an official decision on payment, which is sent to me on a Medicare Summary Notice (MSN). I understand that if Medicare doesn't pay, I am responsible for payment, but **I can appeal to Medicare** by following the directions on the MSN. If Medicare does pay, you will refund any payments I made to you, less co-pays or deductibles.

☐ **OPTION 2.** I want the *(D)*_____ listed above, but do not bill Medicare. You may ask to be paid now as I am responsible for payment. **I cannot appeal if Medicare is not billed**.

☐ **OPTION 3.** I don't want the *(D)*_____ listed above. I understand with this choice I am **not** responsible for payment, and **I cannot appeal to see if Medicare would pay.**

(H) Additional Information:

This notice gives our opinion, not an official Medicare decision. If you have other questions on this notice or Medicare billing, call **1-800-MEDICARE** (1-800-633-4227/**TTY**: 1-877-486-2048).

Signing below means that you have received and understand this notice. You also receive a copy.

(I) **Signature:**	*(J)* **Date:**

According to the Paperwork Reduction Act of 1995, no persons are required to respond to a collection of information unless it displays a valid OMB control number. The valid OMB control number for this information collection is 0938-0566. The time required to complete this information collection is estimated to average 7 minutes per response, including the time to review instructions, search existing data resources, gather the data needed, and complete and review the information collection. If you have comments concerning the accuracy of the time estimate or suggestions for improving this form, please write to: CMS, 7500 Security Boulevard, Attn: PRA Reports Clearance Officer, Baltimore, Maryland 21244-1850.

Form CMS-R-131 (03/08)   Form Approved OMB No. 0938-0566

FIGURE 17-5   Advance Beneficiary Notice of Noncoverage.

Source: Centers for Medicare and Medicaid Services.

▶ The Claims Process: An Overview   LO 17.5

From the time the patient enters a physician's office until the time the insurer pays the practice for that office visit and associated services, several steps are carried out. In brief, the physician's office performs the following services:

- Obtains patient information.
- Delivers services to the patient and determines the diagnosis and fee.
- Records charges and codes, records payment from the patient, and prepares and submits the healthcare claim.

- Reviews the insurer's processing of the claim, remittance advice, and payment.

In offices that use electronic billing, medical assistants use the medical billing program to support administrative tasks such as:

- Gathering and recording patient information.
- Verifying patients' insurance coverage.
- Recording procedures and services performed.
- Recording applicable diagnosis and codes for each procedure performed.
- Filing insurance claims and billing patients.
- Reviewing and recording payments.

Billing programs streamline the important process of creating and following up on healthcare claims sent to payers and bills sent to patients. For example, a large medical practice with a group of providers and thousands of patients may receive a phone call from a patient who wants to know the amount owed on an account. With a billing program, the medical assistant can key the first few letters of the patient's last name and the patient's account data will appear on the screen. The outstanding balance can then be communicated to the patient. Billing programs are also used to exchange health information about the practice's patients with health plans. Using *electronic data interchange* (EDI), similar to the technology behind ATMs, information is sent quickly and securely between the medical practice and the insurance carrier.

Obtaining Patient Information

You will need certain information to be able to complete insurance claims and bill correctly for the patients of the medical practice where you work. This information is usually completed on a patient registration form, as discussed in the *Medical Records and Documentation* chapter.

Basic Facts When the patient first arrives, obtain or verify the following personal information:

- Patient Name (be sure to get the correct spelling of the patient's *legal* name).
- Current home address.
- Current home telephone number.
- Date of birth (month, day, and the four digits of the year).
- Social Security number.
- Next of kin or person to contact in case of an emergency.

Obtain the following insurance information:

- Current employer (may be more than one).
- Employer address and telephone number.
- Insurance carrier and effective date of coverage.
- Insurance group plan number.
- Insurance identification number.
- Name of subscriber or insured.

Obtain the following release signatures:

- Patient's signature on a form authorizing release of information to the insurance carrier.
- Patient's signature on a form for assignment of benefits.

Eligibility for Services After verifying the patient's personal and insurance information, copy or scan the front and back of the patient's insurance card and obtain the release signatures for inclusion in the patient's financial record. Without the signed authorization to release information, you do not have legal permission to give the insurance carrier information regarding the patient's diagnosis and treatment. And without the assignment of benefits signature, the insurance carrier may send the payment for services to the patient instead of to the office. Also, verify the effective date of insurance coverage; the insurance carrier will not cover services performed before this date. To reduce possible payment problems, remember to inform the patient (in writing) before a service is performed if there is a possibility it may not be covered. By signing the waiver, the patient agrees to accept responsibility for payment should the insurer not pay for the service. Be sure to retain the original waiver of liability in the patient's financial record and provide a copy to the patient for his records.

Obtaining Prior Authorization In today's office, prior authorization can often be performed on the insurance carrier's website or initiated over the phone. When calling the insurance company, have the patient's insurance group number and ID number available, as well as the name, address, phone number, and date of birth for identification purposes. If the patient is not the subscriber (insured), you should have the subscriber's name and birth date available and the relationship between the patient and the subscriber. You also will need the name and CPT (procedure) code of the planned procedure and the diagnosis and ICD (diagnosis) code as the reason for the procedure to document medical necessity. New in 2012 is the standard prior authorization request form accepted by many payers for providers who do not have access to electronic technology to obtain prior authorizations. This new standard form may be viewed in Figure 17-6 and is accepted by payers either via fax or U.S. mail.

If you call the insurance carrier, ask for or select the prior authorization department. You will likely be speaking to a nurse case manager who will take down the information regarding the planned procedure. She may give authorization over the phone and, if so, carefully write down the authorization number and place it in the patient's chart for further reference. Should the insurance plan website give you the ability to obtain prior authorization online, you will complete the authorization form as directed inserting the above information. The authorization will be given either immediately or within 24 hours and an authorization will be sent to the office via secure e-mail or USPS. Keep this authorization in the patient's record as proof of receipt. As always, note the authorization

Standardized Prior Authorization Request Form

COMPLETE ALL INFORMATION ON THE "STANDARDIZED PRIOR AUTHORIZATION FORM".
INCOMPLETE SUBMISSIONS MAY BE RETURNED UNPROCESSED.

Please direct any questions regarding this form to the *plan* to which you submit your request for claim review.

The Standardized Prior Authorization Form is not intended to replace payer specific prior authorization procedures, policies and documentation requirements. For payer specific policies, please reference the payer specific websites.

Health Plan:	Health Plan Fax #:	*Date Form Completed and Faxed:

Service Type Requiring Authorization[1, 2, 3] (*Check all that apply*)

Ambulatory/Outpatient Services	Ancillary	Dental	Durable Medical Equipment
☐ Surgery/Procedure (SDC) ☐ Infusion or Oncology Drugs	☐ Acupuncture ☐ Chiropractic ☐ IVF/ART ☐ Non-Participating Specialist	☐ Adjunctive Dental Services ☐ Endodontics ☐ Maxilliofacial Prosthetics ☐ Oral Surgery ☐ Restorative	☐ Prosthetic Device ☐ Purchase ☐ Renal Supplies ☐ Rental
Home Health/Hospice	**Inpatient Care/Observation**	**Nutrition/Counseling**	**Outpatient Therapy**
☐ Home Health (Please circle: SN, PT, OT, ST, HHA, MSW) ☐ Hospice ☐ Infusion Therapy ☐ Respite Care	☐ Acute Medical/Surgical ☐ Long Term Acute Care ☐ Acute Rehab ☐ Skilled Nursing Facility ☐ Observation	☐ Counseling ☐ Enteral Nutrition ☐ Infant Formula ☐ Total Parental Nutrition	☐ Occupational Therapy ☐ Physical Therapy ☐ Pulmonary/Cardiac Rehab ☐ Speech Therapy
Transportation ☐ Non-emergent Ground ☐ Non-emergent Air	☐ Other—please specify:		

Provider Information (**Denotes required field*)

*Requesting Provider Name and NPI#:	*Phone:	Fax:
*Servicing Provider Name and NPI# (and Tax ID if required): ☐ *Same as Requesting Provider*	*Phone:	Fax:
*Servicing Facility Name and NPI#: ☐ *Same as Requesting Provider*	*Phone:	Fax:
*Contact Person:	*Phone:	Fax:

Member Information (**Denotes required field*)

*Patient Name:	*☐ Male ☐ Female	*DOB:
*Health Insurance ID#: *If other insurance, please specify:*	*Patient Account/Control Number:	
Address:	Phone:	

Diagnosis/Planned Procedure Information (**Denotes required field*)

*Principal Diagnosis Description: ICD-9 Codes:	*Principal Planned Procedure (Description and CPT/HCPCS Code): # of Units Being Requested: ☐ Hours ☐ Days ☐ Months ☐ Visits ☐ Dosage
Secondary Diagnosis Description: ICD-9 Codes:	Secondary Planned Procedure (Description and CPT/HCPCS Code): # of Units Being Requested: ☐ Hours ☐ Days ☐ Months ☐ Visits ☐ Dosage
*Service Start Date:	*Service End Date:

[1] Please attach plan specific templates that are required for supporting clinical documentation.
[2] Not all services listed will be covered by the benefits in a member's health plan product.
[3] This form does not replace payer specific prior authorization requirements.

Clear Form

Massachusetts Administrative Simplification Collaborative–Standardized Prior Authorization Request Form V1.1   May 2012

FIGURE 17-6   Standardized Prior Authorization Request Form from Healthcare Administrative Solutions.

number for insertion in block 23 of the CMS-1500 claim form when submitting the procedure for payment. Procedure 17-2 at the end of this chapter outlines the steps for obtaining prior authorization.

Coordination of Benefits This refers to legal clauses in insurance policies that prevent payment duplication by restricting insurance company payments to no more than 100% of the covered benefits' cost. In many families, the husband and wife are both wage earners, so they and their children are frequently eligible for health insurance benefits through both employers' plans. In such cases, the two insurance companies coordinate their payments to pay up to 100% of a procedure's cost. A payment of 100% includes the policyholder's deductible and coinsurance or copayment. The *primary* plan is the policy that pays benefits first. The *secondary*, or supplemental, plan pays the deductible and coinsurance or copayment. A policyholder's primary plan is always his employer group health plan. If both a husband and wife have insurance through their employers, the husband's plan is his primary plan and the wife's insurance plan is her primary plan. To determine the primary plan for dependents who are covered by two or more medical plans, in many states, the **birthday rule** is followed. It states that the insurance policy of the policyholder whose birthday comes first in the calendar year is the primary payer for all dependents.

For example, if a husband's birthday is July 14 and his wife's birthday is June 11, following the birthday rule, the wife's insurance plan is the primary payer for their children and the husband's is the secondary payer. If a husband and wife were born on the same day, the policy that has been in effect the longest is the primary payer. Be sure to check with your state's insurance commission to see if the birthday rule applies in your state. Table 17-4 lists widely used coverage guidelines.

Delivering Services to the Patient

To ensure claims processing accuracy, any services the physician or other healthcare team members deliver to the patient in the office must be entered into the patient record, along with referrals to outside physicians or specialists.

Physician's Services The physician who examines the patient notes the patient's symptoms, a diagnosis, a treatment plan (including prescribed medications), and if and when the patient should return for a follow-up visit—all in the medical record. After completing the visit, the physician writes the diagnosis, treatment, and sometimes the fee on an encounter form (superbill) (Figure 17-7) or charge slip (Figure 17-8) and instructs the patient to give you the superbill or charge slip before leaving. If the patient has a per-visit copayment, it is usually collected at the time the patient is leaving the office.

Medical Coding Today, the superbills used by most offices are preprinted with common procedures and procedure

TABLE 17-4	Guidelines for Determining Primary Insurance Coverage

- If the patient has only one policy, it is primary.
- If the patient has coverage under two plans, the plan covering the employee for the longest period of time is primary. However, if an active employee has a plan with the present employer and is still covered by a former employer's plan as a retiree or a laid-off employee, the current employer's plan is primary.
- If the patient is also covered as a dependent under another insurance policy, the patient's plan is primary.
- If an employed patient has coverage under the employer's plan and additional coverage under a government-sponsored plan, the employer's plan is primary. An example of this is a patient enrolled in a PPO through employment who is also covered by Medicare.
- If a retired patient is covered by the plan of the spouse's employer and the spouse is still employed, the spouse's plan is primary, even if the retired person has Medicare.
- If the patient is a dependent child covered by both parents' plans and the parents are not separated or divorced (or have joint custody of the child), the primary plan is determined by which parent has the first birth date in the calendar year (the birthday rule).
- If two or more plans cover the dependent children of separated or divorced parents who do not have joint custody of their children, the children's primary plan is determined in this order:
  1. The plan of the custodial parent.
  2. The plan of the spouse of the custodial parent (if the parent has remarried).
  3. The plan of the parent without custody.

codes. If the charges are not preprinted, there is a space next to each procedure where the current charge may be inserted. For a procedure not listed on the superbill, a blank space at the bottom can be completed with the procedure name, procedure code, and charge. It is critical to verify that the procedure checked off on the form was actually completed by comparing the superbill to the medical record. This step ensures the patient is not inadvertently charged for a procedure that did not take place. Also, be sure the appropriate diagnosis code(s) are checked off proving medical necessity for the procedures performed. If your office uses a charge slip instead of a superbill, you will need to translate the procedures listed on the charge slip into charge codes for the insurance carrier. This topic is covered in the *Diagnosis Coding* and *Procedure Coding* chapters.

Referrals and Authorizations for Other Services You may be asked to secure authorization from the insurance company for additional procedures. If so, contact the insurance company to explain the reason for the procedure(s) and obtain an authorization number using the previously described procedures. Enter this authorization number in the billing program for inclusion on claims related to this procedure.

Frequently, you will be asked to arrange an appointment for required services, particularly if the physician believes they are urgently needed. For example, a physician may send a patient

BWW Medical Associates, PC

305 Main Street, Port Snead YZ 12345-9876, Tel: 555-654-3210, Fax: 555-987-6543

☐ PRIVATE ☐ BLUECROSS ☐ IND. ☐ MEDICARE ☐ MEDI-CAL ☐ HMO ☐ PPO

PATIENT'S LAST NAME	FIRST	ACCOUNT #	BIRTHDATE / /	SEX ☐ MALE ☐ FEMALE	TODAY'S DATE / /
INSURANCE COMPANY	SUBSCRIBER		PLAN #	SUB. #	GROUP

ASSIGNMENT: I hereby assign my insurance benefits to be paid directly to the undersigned physician. I am financially responsible for non-covered services. SIGNED: (Patient, or Parent, if Minor) DATE: / /	RELEASE: I hereby authorize the physician to release to my insurance carrers any information required to process this claim. SIGNED: (Patient, or Parent, if Minor) DATE: / /

✔	DESCRIPTION	M/Care	CPT/Mod	DxRe	FEE	✔	DESCRIPTION	M/Care	CPT/Mod	DxRe	FEE	✔	DESCRIPTION	M/Care	CPT/Mod	DxRe	FEE
	OFFICE CARE						PROCEDURES						INJECTIONS/IMMUNIZATIONS				
	NEW PATIENT						Tread Mill (In Office)		93015				Tetanus/Diphtheria		90718		
	Brief		99201				24 Hour Holter		93224				MMR		90707		
	Limited		99202				If Medicare (Set up Fec)		93225				Pneumococcal		90732		
	Intermediate		99203				Physician Interpret		93227				Influenza		90656		
	Extended		99204				EKG w/Interpretation		93000				TB Skin Test (PPD)		86580		
	Comprehensive		99205				EKG (tracing only)		93005				Antigen Injection-Single		95115		
							Sigmoidoscopy		45300				Multiple		95117		
	ESTABLISHED PATIENT						Sigmoidoscopy, Flexible		45330				B12 Injection	J3420	90782		
	Minimal		99211				Sigmoidos. , Flex. w/Bx.		45331				Injection, IM		90782		
	Brief		99212				Spirometry, FEV/FVC		94010				Compazine	J0780	90782		
	Limited		99213				Spirometry, Post-Dilator		94060				Demerol	J2175	90782		
	Intermediate		99214										Vistaril	J3410	90782		
	Extended		99215										Susphrine	J0170	90782		
	Comprehensive		99215				LABORATORY						Decadron	J0890	90782		
							Blood Draw Fee		36415				Estradiol	J1000	90782		
	CONSULTATION-OFFICE						Urinalysis, Chemical		81000				Testosterone	J1080	90782		
	Focused		99241				Throat Culture		87081				Lidocaine	J2000	90782		
	Expanded		99242				Occult Blood		82270				Solumedrol	J2920	90782		
	Detailed		99243				Pap Handling Charge		99000				Solucortef	J1720	90782		
	Comprehensive 1		99244				Pap Life Guard		88150-90				Hydeltra	J1690	90782		
	Comprehensive 2		99245				Gram Stain		87205								
	MCR Pts - use E/M codes						Hanging Drop		87210				INJECTIONS - JOINT/BURSA				
	Case Management		98900				Urine Drug Screen		80100				Small Joints		20600		
													Intermediate		20605		
	Post-op Exam		99024				SUPPLIES						Large Joints		20610		
													Trigger Point		20552		
													MISCELLANEOUS				

DIAGNOSIS:

		ICD-9										
___ Abdominal Pain	789.0	___ Gout	274.0	___ C.V.A. - Acute	436.	___ Electrolyte Dis.	276.9	___ Herpes Simplex	054.9
___ Abscess (Site)	682.9	___ Asthma	493.90	___ Cere. Vas. Accid. (Old)	438	___ Fatigue	780.7	___ Herpes Zoster	053.9
___ Adverse Drug Rx	995.2	___ Asthmatic Bronchitis	493.90	___ Cerumen	380.4	___ Fibrocys. Br. Dis	610.1	___ Hydrocele	603.9
___ Alcohol Detox	291.8	___ Atrial Fib.	427.31	___ Chestwall Pain	786.59	___ Fracture (Site)	829.0	___ Hyperlipidemia	272.4
___ Alcoholism	303.90	___ Atrial Tachi.	427.0	___ Cholecystitis	575.0	___ Open/Close		___ Hypertension	401.9
___ Allergic Rhinitis	477	___ Bowel Obstruct.	560.9	___ Cholelithiasis	574.00	___ Fungal Infect. (Site)	110.8	___ Hyperthyroidism	242.9
___ Allergy	995.3	___ Breast Mass	611.72	___ COPD	492.8	___ Gastric Ulcer	531.90	___ Hypothyroidism	244.9
___ Alzheimer's Dis.	290.1	___ Bronchitis	490	___ Cirrhosis	571.5	___ Gastritis	535.0	___ Labyrinthitis	386.30
___ Anemia	285.9	___ Bursitis	727.3	___ Cong. Heart Fail.	428.9	___ Gastroenteritis	558.9	___ Lipoma (Site)	214.9
___ Anemia - Pernicious	281.0	___ Cancer, Breast (Site)	174.9	___ Conjunctivitis	372.30	___ G.I. Bleeding	578.9	___ Lymphoma	202.8
___ Angina	413.9	___ Metastatic (Site)	199.1	___ Contusion (Site)	924.9	___ Glomerulonephritis	583.9	___ Mit. Valve Prolapse	424.0
___ Anxiety Synd.	300.00	___ Colon	153.9	___ Costochondritis	733.99	___ Headache	784.0	___ Myocard. Infarction (Area)	410.9
___ Appendicitis	541	___ Cancer, Rectal	154.1	___ Depression	311.	___ Headache, Tension	307.81	___ M.I., Old	412
___ Arterioscl. H.D.	414.0	___ Lung (Site)	162.9	___ Dermatitis	692.9	___ Migraine (Type)	346.9	___ Myositis	729.1
___ Arthritis, Osteo.	715.90	___ Skin (Site)	173.9	___ Diabetes Mellitus	250.00	___ Hemorrhoids	455.6	___ Nausea/Vomiting	787.0
___ Rheumatoid	714.0	___ Card. Arrhythmia (Type)	427.9	___ Diabetic Ketosis	250.1	___ Hernia, Hiatal	553.3	___ Neuralgia	729.2
___ Lupus	710.0	___ Cardiomyopathy	425.4	___ Diverticulitis	562.11	___ Inguinal	550.9	___ Nevus (Site)	216.9
		___ Cellulitis (Site)	682.9	___ Diverticulosis	562.10	___ Hepatitis	573.3	___ Obesity	278.0

DIAGNOSIS: (IF NOT CHECKED ABOVE)

SERVICES PERFORMED AT: ☐ Office ☐ E.R. ☐	☐ CLAIM CONTAINS NO ORDERED REFERRING SERVICE	REFERRING PHYSICIAN & I.D. NUMBER

RETURN APPOINTMENT INFORMATION: 5 - 10 - 15 - 20 - 30 - 40 - 60 [DAYS] [WKS.] [MOS.] [PRN]	NEXT APPOINTMENT M - T - W - TH - F - S DATE / / TIME:	AM PM	ACCEPT ASSIGNMENT? ☐ YES ☐ NO	DOCTOR'S SIGNATURE

INSTRUCTIONS TO PATIENT FOR FILING INSURANCE CLAIMS:	☐ CASH	TOTAL TODAY'S FEE	
1. Complete upper portion of this form, sign and date. 2. Attach this form to your own insurance company's form for direct reimbursement. **MEDICARE PATIENTS - DO NOT SEND THIS TO MEDICARE. WE WILL SUBMIT THE CLAIM FOR YOU.**	☐ CHECK #	OLD BALANCE	
	☐ VISA	TOTAL DUE	
	☐ MC ☐ CO-PAY	AMOUNT REC'D. TODAY	

INSUR-A-BILL ® BIBBERO SYSTEMS, INC. • PETALUMA, CA • UP. SUPER. © 6/94 (BIBB/STOCK)

FIGURE 17-7 A superbill (encounter form) can be used as a charge slip and invoice and contains the information required to submit a health insurance claim.

DATE	DESCRIPTION–CODE	CHARGE	PAYMENT	CURRENT BALANCE

521-234-0001

Tax ID No. 11-0004004

BWW Medical Associates, PC
305 Main Street,
Port Snead, YZ 12345-9876

99205	Office Visit, New Patient	36425	Venipuncture	59025	NST
99215	Office Visit, Established Patient	57454	Colposcopy with Biopsy	54150	Circumcision
99213	Office Visit, Established, Brief	57511	Cryosurgery	58300	IUD Insertion
88155	Pap	58100	Endometrial Biopsy	57170	Diaphragm Fitting
84703	Urine Pregnancy Test	56600	Vulva Biopsy		

NAME _____ DX _____ No. 0005807

FIGURE 17-8 A charge slip shows the services performed for a patient and the charge for those services.

to a specialist's office for evaluation on the same day the patient visits your office. If the patient is a member of a managed care program, prior to making the required appointment, you will need to verify with the insurance plan that the insurance company allows the specialist requested. If so, a referral also may be needed. Depending on the insurance plan and your office capabilities, this referral may be completed in writing or via the insurance plan's website. Without this referral, the specialist's charges may not be covered.

Patient Checkout

As stated earlier, everyone who receives services from a physician in the practice is ultimately responsible for paying the practice for those services. When the patient brings you the superbill at the end of the visit, you may perform one or more of the following procedures, depending on your practice's policy:

- Prepare and transmit a healthcare claim on behalf of the patient directly to the insurance company.
- Accept payment from the patient for the full amount. The patient will submit a claim to the insurance carrier for reimbursement. With offices increasingly submitting electronic claims, this option is becoming less common.
- Accept an insurance copayment or coinsurance from the patient and credit the account appropriately.

You now have all the information needed to prepare the healthcare claim for submission to the insurance carrier.

▶ Preparing and Transmitting the Healthcare Claim

LO 17.6

Healthcare claims are a critical communication between medical offices and payers on behalf of patients. Processing claims is a major task in most offices, and the numbers can be huge. For example, a 40-physician group practice with 55,000 patients served annually typically processes 1000 claims (or more) daily!

Filing Limits In order for claims to be processed, they must be considered "clean"—free of errors. The first item the insurance carrier is going to review when receiving the claim is the date of service, as the clock for timely filing begins on this date. Time limits for filing claims vary from company to company. For example, some insurers will not pay a claim unless it is filed within 60 or 90 days from the date of service, while others, like Medicare, will allow up to a year for claim submission. In the typical medical practice, claims are transmitted within a few business days after the date of service. Many large practices file claims every day or several times a week to ensure that missing the filing limit never happens. The issue of clean claims and other errors that cause the most problems for submitters will be discussed later in the chapter.

Electronic Claims Transmission

The electronic claim transaction is the HIPAA Healthcare Claim or Equivalent Encounter Information, commonly referred to as the "HIPAA (or 4010) claim" or simply the "837P (P for physician claim)." Its official name is *X12 837 Health Care Claim*. As of January 1, 2012, a new version of this 837 claim was mandated, known as the "5010." If you hear someone refer to a "5010 claim," they are speaking of the current format for electronic claims submission.

As of October 2003, Medicare mandated the X12 837 transaction for all Medicare claims except those from very small practices. Third-party payers may continue to accept paper transactions. Practices that elect to use paper claims must have two versions of their medical billing software: one to capture the necessary data elements for HIPAA-compliant electronic

Medicare claims and another version to generate CMS-1500 paper claims. Also, under HIPAA regulations, only medical offices that do not handle any other HIPAA-related transactions may still use paper claims. Because most insurance carriers accept electronic claims and the process for submitting electronic claims has become more streamlined and cost efficient, even smaller offices are submitting electronic claims, which, in general, are paid within a week or two instead of the usual 6–8 weeks for paper claim reimbursement.

Preparing Electronic Claims The information entered on electronic claims is called data elements. Many elements, like the patient's personal and insurance information, are entered in the billing program before or at the time of the patient appointment, based on the patient registration form and on payer information and requirements. After the appointment is concluded, the claim is completed when the medical assistant keys the billing transactions—the services, charges, and payments—as detailed on the superbill (encounter form) into the billing claims software program. Once all the claims for the day are prepared, or often at a specified time each day, the software program is programmed to prepare claims for editing ("scrubbing") and transmission.

Follow these tips when entering data in medical billing programs:

- Enter data in all capital letters.
- Do not use prefixes for people's names, such as Mr., Ms., or Dr.
- Unless required by a particular insurance carrier, do not use special characters like hyphens, commas, or apostrophes.
- Use only valid data in all fields; avoid words such as "same."

The X12 837 transaction requires many data elements, and all must be correct. Most billing programs or claim transmission programs automatically reformat data such as dates into the correct formats. These data elements are reported in five major sections:

1. Provider
2. Subscriber (the insured or policyholder)
3. Patient (who may be the subscriber or another person)
4. Claim details
5. Services

Not all data elements are required. Some are considered situational and are required only when a certain condition applies. When it does apply, then that data element also becomes required. For example, if a claim involves pregnancy, the date of the last menstrual period is required. If the claim does not involve pregnancy, that date should not be reported.

One of the provider elements required for electronic claims is the provider *taxonomy code*—a 10-digit number representing a physician's medical specialty. Physicians select the taxonomy code that most closely matches their education, license, or certification. The code is reported on claims because payment for some services is impacted by the particular specialty of the doctor performing them and by payers' contracts. For example, nuclear medicine is usually a higher-paid specialty than internal medicine. An internist who also has a specialty in nuclear medicine would report the nuclear medicine taxonomy code when billing for that service and use the internal medicine taxonomy code when reporting internal medicine claims.

Before the HIPAA mandate for standard transactions, some payers required additional records, like their own information sheet, when providers billed them. Some payers also used their own coding systems. The HIPAA Electronic Health Care Transactions and Code Sets (TCS) mandate means that all health plans are required to accept the standard claim submitted electronically, although the information required by each payer may vary. Be sure to follow each payer's specifications when submitting claims.

Other standard transactions also support the claim process—such as advising the office of claim status and payment—and apply to the treatment, payment, and operations (TPO) information exchanged between medical offices and health plans. Each electronic transaction has both a title and a number. Each number begins with X12—the number of the EDI format—followed by a unique number that stands for the transaction. Here are some examples of titles and numbers medical assistants may encounter while processing X12 837 healthcare claims:

Number	Title
X12 276/277	Claim status inquiry and response
X12 270/271	Eligibility inquiry and response
X12 278	Referral authorization inquiry and response
X12 835	Payment and remittance advice
X12 820	Health plan premium payments
X12 834	Enrollment in and withdrawal from a health plan

Paper Claim Completion

As stated previously, regardless of the office's billing method, the patient's demographic and billing information is usually updated at the patient's office visit and entered into the office medical billing program. Then the program is instructed to print the data on a CMS-1500 paper form (also called the CMS-1505 because of the form's 2005 update), shown in Figure 17-9. This claim may be mailed or faxed to the third-party payer.

Because of the HIPAA mandate regarding electronic claims submission, the paper claim is not as widely used as previously; however, the information it contains is very similar to the X12 837. The CMS-1500 contains 33 form locators, which are numbered blocks. Blocks 1–13 refer to the patient information and the patient and guarantor insurance coverage information. Blocks 14–33 contain information about the provider and the transaction information, including the patient's diagnoses, procedures, and charges.

The following instructions provide step-by-step guidance in completing a CMS-1500 paper form, which you can practice with Procedure 17-3, Completing the CMS-1500 Claim Form, found at the end of this chapter. Figure 17-10 is an example of a completed Medicare claim that includes a secondary payer.

FIGURE 17-9 The CMS-1500 is the paper professional health insurance claim form.

HEALTH INSURANCE CLAIM FORM

1500

APPROVED BY NATIONAL UNIFORM CLAIM COMMITTEE 08/05

		PICA								PICA		

1. MEDICARE [X] (Medicare #) MEDICAID ☐ (Medicaid #) TRICARE CHAMPUS ☐ (Sponsor's SSN) CHAMPVA ☐ (Member ID#) GROUP HEALTH PLAN ☐ (SSN or ID) FECA BLK LUNG ☐ (SSN) OTHER ☐ (ID)

1a. INSURED'S I.D. NUMBER (For Program in Item 1)
000 11 2345 A

2. PATIENT'S NAME (Last Name, First Name, Middle Initial)
WARD   ELEANOR   M

3. PATIENT'S BIRTH DATE MM 02 DD 02 YY 1929 SEX M ☐ F [X]

4. INSURED'S NAME (Last Name, First Name, Middle Initial)

5. PATIENT'S ADDRESS (No., Street)
305   MAIN STREET

6. PATIENT RELATIONSHIP TO INSURED
Self ☐ Spouse ☐ Child ☐ Other ☐

7. INSURED'S ADDRESS (No., Street)

CITY
FUNTON STATE XY

8. PATIENT STATUS
Single ☐ Married ☐ Other [X]
Employed ☐ Full-Time Student ☐ Part-Time Student ☐

CITY STATE

ZIP CODE 12345-6789 TELEPHONE (Include Area Code) (521) 628 3270

ZIP CODE TELEPHONE (Include Area Code) ( )

9. OTHER INSURED'S NAME (Last Name, First Name, Middle Initial)
WARD   ELEANOR   M

10. IS PATIENT'S CONDITION RELATED TO:

11. INSURED'S POLICY GROUP OR FECA NUMBER
NONE

a. OTHER INSURED'S POLICY OR GROUP NUMBER
625743289

a. EMPLOYMENT? (Current or Previous)
☐ YES [X] NO

a. INSURED'S DATE OF BIRTH MM DD YY SEX M ☐ F ☐

b. OTHER INSURED'S DATE OF BIRTH MM 02 DD 02 YY 1929 SEX M ☐ F [X]

b. AUTO ACCIDENT? PLACE (State)
☐ YES [X] NO

b. EMPLOYER'S NAME OR SCHOOL NAME

c. EMPLOYER'S NAME OR SCHOOL NAME

c. OTHER ACCIDENT?
☐ YES [X] NO

c. INSURANCE PLAN NAME OR PROGRAM NAME

d. INSURANCE PLAN NAME OR PROGRAM NAME
MEDEX

10d. RESERVED FOR LOCAL USE

d. IS THERE ANOTHER HEALTH BENEFIT PLAN?
[X] YES ☐ NO If yes, return to and complete item 9 a-d.

READ BACK OF FORM BEFORE COMPLETING & SIGNING THIS FORM.

12. PATIENT'S OR AUTHORIZED PERSON'S SIGNATURE I authorize the release of any medical or other information necessary to process this claim. I also request payment of government benefits either to myself or to the party who accepts assignment below.

SIGNED SIGNATURE ON FILE DATE

13. INSURED'S OR AUTHORIZED PERSON'S SIGNATURE I authorize payment of medical benefits to the undersigned physician or supplier for services described below.

SIGNED SIGNATURE ON FILE

14. DATE OF CURRENT: MM DD YY ◄ ILLNESS (First symptom) OR INJURY (Accident) OR PREGNANCY(LMP)

15. IF PATIENT HAS HAD SAME OR SIMILAR ILLNESS. GIVE FIRST DATE MM DD YY

16. DATES PATIENT UNABLE TO WORK IN CURRENT OCCUPATION MM DD YY FROM TO MM DD YY

17. NAME OF REFERRING PROVIDER OR OTHER SOURCE
WHALEN MARI LOU

17a. ZZ 201400000X
17b. NPI 423 543 6543

18. HOSPITALIZATION DATES RELATED TO CURRENT SERVICES MM DD YY FROM TO MM DD YY

19. RESERVED FOR LOCAL USE

20. OUTSIDE LAB? ☐ YES [X] NO $ CHARGES

21. DIAGNOSIS OR NATURE OF ILLNESS OR INJURY (Relate Items 1, 2, 3 or 4 to Item 24E by Line)

1. 482 . 9
2. 496 .
3. ____ . ____
4. ____ . ____

22. MEDICAID RESUBMISSION CODE ORIGINAL REF. NO.

23. PRIOR AUTHORIZATION NUMBER

24. A. DATE(S) OF SERVICE From MM DD YY	To MM DD YY	B. PLACE OF SERVICE	C. EMG	D. PROCEDURES, SERVICES, OR SUPPLIES (Explain Unusual Circumstances) CPT/HCPCS MODIFIER	E. DIAGNOSIS POINTER	F. $ CHARGES	G. DAYS OR UNITS	H. EPSDT Family Plan	I. ID. QUAL.	J. RENDERING PROVIDER ID. #
1 05 10 20xx	05 10 20xx	11		99213 25	1	80 00	1		NPI	9876543210
2 05 10 20xx	05 10 20xx	11		71020	1	120 00	1		NPI	9876543210
3 05 10 20xx	05 10 20xx	11		82805	2	65 00	1		NPI	9876543210
4 05 10 20xx	05 10 20xx	11		85025	1	40 00	1		NPI	9876543210
5									NPI	
6									NPI	

25. FEDERAL TAX I.D. NUMBER SSN ☐ EIN [X]
222518600

26. PATIENT'S ACCOUNT NO.

27. ACCEPT ASSIGNMENT? (For govt. claims, see back)
[X] YES ☐ NO

28. TOTAL CHARGE
$ 305 00

29. AMOUNT PAID
$

30. BALANCE DUE
$

31. SIGNATURE OF PHYSICIAN OR SUPPLIER INCLUDING DEGREES OR CREDENTIALS (I certify that the statements on the reverse apply to this bill and are made a part thereof.)

SIGNED Alexis N. Whalen, MD DATE 15/12/xx

32. SERVICE FACILITY LOCATION INFORMATION

a. NPI b.

33. BILLING PROVIDER INFO & PH # 555-654-3210
BWW Medical Associates
305 Main Street
Port Snead YZ 12345-6789

a. 1002003001 b.

NUCC Instruction Manual available at: www.nucc.org

APPROVED OMB-0938-0999 FORM CMS-1500 (08/05)

FIGURE 17-10 Completed CMS-1500 claim form for a Medicare patient with secondary insurance coverage.

HIPAA laws are equally important when working with patient financial information and when working with patient PHI in the medical record. Remember, keep access to patient medical and financial records confidential at all times, including the information contained within a paper or electronic health or claim file.

Completing the CMS-1500 Form In this section, let's complete the CMS 1500 claim form block by block. Here is how to complete blocks 1–13, the patient and insured's information:

Block 1   Place an X in the appropriate insurance box.

Note: Each box is slightly to the left of the insurance plan it represents.

1. MEDICARE	MEDICAID	TRICARE CHAMPUS	CHAMPVA	GROUP HEALTH PLAN	FECA BLK LUNG	OTHER
(Medicare #)	(Medicaid #)	(Sponsor's SSN)	(Member ID#)	(SSN or ID)	(SSN)	(ID)

Block 1a   Insert the insured's ID number exactly as it appears on the insurance card.

1a. INSURED'S I.D. NUMBER   (For Program in Item 1)

Block 2   Enter the patient's name in this order: last, first, middle initial (if used).

2. PATIENT'S NAME (Last Name, First Name, Middle Initial)

Block 3   Enter the patient's birth date in the 8-digit format: XX/XX/XXXX. Place an X in the box representing the patient's sex.

3. PATIENT'S BIRTH DATE   MM | DD | YY   SEX   M   F

Block 4   Enter the insured's name in this order: last, first, middle initial (if used). If the insured is the patient, enter SAME; if Medicare, leave blank; if TRICARE, enter the Sponsor's name.

4. INSURED'S NAME (Last Name, First Name, Middle Initial)

Block 5   Enter the patient's street address, city, state, zip code, and phone number.

5. PATIENT'S ADDRESS (No., Street)

Block 6   Enter an X for the patient's relationship to the insured. If the patient is the insured, use Self; if Medicare, leave blank; if TRICARE, enter the patient's relationship to the Sponsor.

6. PATIENT RELATIONSHIP TO INSURED
Self   Spouse   Child   Other

Block 7   Enter the insured's street address, city, state, zip code, and phone number.

7. INSURED'S ADDRESS (No., Street)

Block 8   Use an X to note the patient's marital status as single, married, or other. Note whether the patient is employed or a F/T or P/T student.

8. PATIENT STATUS
Single   Married   Other
Employed   Full-Time Student   Part-Time Student

Block 9a–d   *Note: Block 9 is used for the* secondary *insurance information and block 11 is used for the primary insurance information. You may find it easier to complete blocks 11 and 10 first, and then come back to block 9.*

9   If the patient has a *secondary* policy, enter the name (last, first, middle initial) of the insured for this *secondary* policy.

9a   Enter the *secondary* policy's group number or individual policy ID number. For a Medigap plan, enter the word "Medigap" before the ID number.

9b   Enter the date of birth of the insured for the *secondary* policy using the 8-digit format (XX/XX/XXXX) and mark the box for the insured's sex with an X.

9c   Enter the employer or school name of the insured for this *secondary* plan. If this is a Medigap plan, enter the plan address here.

9d   Enter the name of this *secondary* insurance plan. If this is a Medigap plan, enter the 9-digit CMS-assigned PAYERID.

9. OTHER INSURED'S NAME (Last Name, First Name, Middle Initial)
a. OTHER INSURED'S POLICY OR GROUP NUMBER
b. OTHER INSURED'S DATE OF BIRTH   MM   DD   YY   SEX   M   F
c. EMPLOYER'S NAME OR SCHOOL NAME
d. INSURANCE PLAN NAME OR PROGRAM NAME

Block 10a–c   Place an X in the correct Yes or No box in each area to indicate whether the patient's condition is related to employment, auto accident, or other accident. If auto accident is answered Yes, insert the two-letter abbreviation for the state in which the accident occurred. (*Note: If any of these questions are answered yes, a workers' compensation, automobile, or other liability insurer may be responsible for the charges.*)

10. IS PATIENT'S CONDITION RELATED TO:
a. EMPLOYMENT? (Current or Previous)   YES   NO
b. AUTO ACCIDENT?   YES   NO   PLACE (State)
c. OTHER ACCIDENT?   YES   NO

Block 10d   If the secondary payer is Medicaid, some states require insertion of the abbreviation *MCD* followed by the Medicaid number here instead of in block 9. Check your state's regulations. For other payers, if attachments are required with the claim, insert the word *ATTACHMENT* here.

```
10d. RESERVED FOR LOCAL USE
```

Block 11a–d *Block 11 is used for the* primary *insurance information. Many administrative assistants and billers find it easiest to complete block 11 before completing blocks 9 and 10.*

11 Enter the group number for the primary insurance plan. If Medicare is the primary payer, enter the word NONE here and leave 11a–d blank. (The word NONE tells Medicare it is the primary payer. Without its presence, Medicare assumes it is the secondary payer.)

11a For primary payers other than Medicare, enter the insured's date of birth (XX/XX/XXXX) and sex.

11b Enter the primary insured's employer or school name (if this information is completed, Medicare is NOT the primary payer).

11c Enter the insurance plan name.

11d Place an X in the appropriate box indicating if there is a secondary payer or not. If Yes is chosen, then blocks 9a–d will be completed; if No is chosen, blocks 9a–d will be left blank.

```
11. INSURED'S POLICY GROUP OR FECA NUMBER

a. INSURED'S DATE OF BIRTH          SEX
    MM   DD   YY
                            M         F
b. EMPLOYER'S NAME OR SCHOOL NAME

c. INSURANCE PLAN NAME OR PROGRAM NAME

d. IS THERE ANOTHER HEALTH BENEFIT PLAN?
    YES      NO    If yes, return to and complete item 9 a-d.
```

Block 12 The patient or authorized representative signs here, giving the provider permission to release his/her medical information to the insurance carrier.

Block 13 The patient or authorized representative signs here, authorizing the insurance carrier to send payment directly to the provider.

```
READ BACK OF FORM BEFORE COMPLETING & SIGNING THIS FORM.
12. PATIENT'S OR AUTHORIZED PERSON'S SIGNATURE  I authorize the release of any medical or other information
necessary to process this claim. I also request payment of government benefits either to myself or to the party who
accepts assignment below.

SIGNED_____  DATE_____

13. INSURED'S OR AUTHORIZED PERSON'S SIGNATURE  I authorize payment of medical benefits to the
undersigned physician or supplier for services described below.

SIGNED_____
```

Here's how to complete blocks 14–33, the provider's information:

Block 14 Enter the date of the current illness, injury, or pregnancy using the 8-digit format.

```
14. DATE OF CURRENT:    ILLNESS (First symptom) OR
    MM   DD   YY         INJURY (Accident) OR
                         PREGNANCY(LMP)
```

Block 15 Enter the date the patient was first seen for the illness or injury using the 8-digit format; for Medicare, leave this block blank.

```
15. IF PATIENT HAS HAD SAME OR SIMILAR ILLNESS.
    GIVE FIRST DATE    MM   DD   YY
```

Block 16 Enter the dates the patient is or was unable to work using the 8-digit format (this information could signal a workers' compensation case if work-related).

```
16. DATES PATIENT UNABLE TO WORK IN CURRENT OCCUPATION
       MM   DD   YY              MM   DD   YY
   FROM                    TO
```

Block 17 Enter the name of the referring physician, laboratory, or other source. Some payers will require the treating physician's name here, if there was no referring physician. Check the individual insurer's guidelines.

Block 17a–b Some insurers require provider identifiers other than the NPI.

17a If required, enter the approved two-digit qualifier from Table 17-1 with the provider identifier next to it; otherwise leave blank.

17b Enter the referring provider NPI number.

```
17. NAME OF REFERRING PROVIDER OR OTHER SOURCE    17a.
                                                  17b. NPI
```

Block 18 If applicable, enter the dates the patient was hospitalized during this claim.

```
18. HOSPITALIZATION DATES RELATED TO CURRENT SERVICES
       MM   DD   YY              MM   DD   YY
   FROM                    TO
```

Block 19 Block 19 is used for varying information depending on insurance carrier; check carrier instructions as to information requested here. If non-NPI identifiers are requested, be sure to use the appropriate qualifier from Table 17-1. Leave blank if no information is required.

```
19. RESERVED FOR LOCAL USE
```

Block 20 If the office is billing for services provided by an outside laboratory, place an X in the Yes box and enter the amount being billed for the lab and enter the laboratory name, address, and NPI in block 32. If only labs performed in your office are being billed, enter an X in the No box.

```
20. OUTSIDE LAB?              $ CHARGES
       YES      NO
```

Block 21 Enter the multidigit ICD-9-CM codes indicating the patient diagnoses. (You will learn more about diagnosis coding in the *Diagnostic Coding* chapter). Enter the codes in spaces 1–4 in descending order of importance. Do NOT use decimal points when inserting the diagnosis codes.

```
21. DIAGNOSIS OR NATURE OF ILLNESS OR INJURY (Relate Items 1, 2, 3 or 4 to Item 24E by Line)

1. ____ . ____                    3. ____ . ____

2. ____ . ____                    4. ____ . ____
```

Block 22 For Medicaid claims, enter the Medicaid resubmission code and original reference number if applicable; for all other payers, leave blank.

22. MEDICAID RESUBMISSION CODE	ORIGINAL REF. NO.

Block 23 If required, enter the prior authorization number received by the payer for the procedure performed (if prior authorization is required and not received, or if authorization is received, but the number is not present on the claim, the claim will be denied).

23. PRIOR AUTHORIZATION NUMBER

Block 24a–j The six service lines here are used to enter the services provided to the patient. They are divided horizontally between shaded and nonshaded areas to accommodate NPI and non-NPI identifiers if required. The NPI is inserted in the nonshaded areas and the non-NPI information is inserted in the shaded areas. Follow individual payer requirements for use of these shaded areas.

24a Enter the dates of service using the 8-digit format. If the service is provided on one date, enter the same date twice.

24b Enter the two-digit place of service code from Table 17-5. Keep a listing nearby for handy reference.

24c EMG stands for emergency services. If the insurer requires this information, and the service was provided on an emergency basis, enter a Y for yes. If service was not provided on an emergency basis or if the insurer does not require the information, leave blank. For Medicare, leave blank.

24d Enter the appropriate CPT or HCPCS code with modifier, one per line, to represent each service provided. (You will learn more about CPT and HCPCS coding in the *Procedure Coding* chapter.)

24e Enter the reference number 1, 2, 3, 4 from block 21 to represent the diagnosis code associated with each procedure or service performed. This identifies the

TABLE 17-5 Place of Service Codes for CMS-1500 Form

Code	Place of Service
11	Office
12	Home
21	Inpatient Hospital
22	Outpatient Hospital
23	Emergency Department—Hospital
24	Ambulatory Surgical Center
25	Birthing Center
26	Military Treatment Facility
31	Skilled Nursing Facility
32	Nursing Facility
33	Custodial Care Facility
34	Hospice

medical necessity for the service provided (known as code linkage; you will learn more about this in the *Diagnostic Coding* chapter).

24f Enter the fee charged for each service provided.

24g Enter the days or units for each service provided. For instance, if the patient had three 15-minute (15 minutes = 1 unit) physical therapy treatments, enter 3. Even if the unit is one, the number 1 must be entered.

24h EPSDT stands for Early, Periodic, Screening, Diagnosis, and Treatment. It is for Medicaid programs. If the procedure is related to EPSDT for a Medicaid patient, enter Y; otherwise leave blank.

24i If the payer requires a non-NPI identifier, enter its qualifier (Table 17-1) in the shaded area. If it is not required, leave blank.

24j If a non-NPI qualifier was entered in the shaded area, enter the appropriate non-NPI identifier in the shaded area. If it is not required, leave the shaded area blank. Enter the provider's NPI number in the nonshaded area.

24. A. DATE(S) OF SERVICE From MM DD YY To MM DD YY	B. PLACE OF SERVICE	C. EMG	D. PROCEDURES, SERVICES, OR SUPPLIES (Explain Unusual Circumstances) CPT/HCPCS | MODIFIER	E. DIAGNOSIS POINTER	F. $ CHARGES	G. DAYS OR UNITS	H. EPSDT Family Plan	I. ID. QUAL.	J. RENDERING PROVIDER ID. #
1								NPI	
2								NPI	
3								NPI	
4								NPI	
5								NPI	
6								NPI	

Block 25 Enter the provider's Tax ID number. Place an X in the box identifying it as SSN (Social Security Number) or EIN (Employer Identification Number).

25. FEDERAL TAX I.D. NUMBER   SSN EIN

Block 26 Enter the patient's account number (if used by your office).

26. PATIENT'S ACCOUNT NO.

Block 27 Place an X in the Yes box to indicate the provider is accepting assignment on the claim (the check will be issued directly to the provider). Place an X in the No box to indicate the provider is not accepting assignment on the claim (the check will be issued to the patient).

27. ACCEPT ASSIGNMENT?
(For govt. claims, see back)
YES   NO

Block 28 Enter the total charges for the claim by totaling charges from column 24f in lines 1–6.

Block 29 Enter any amount paid by a primary payer. If this is a primary claim, leave blank. For Medicare claims, leave blank.

Block 30 Subtract block 29 from block 28. Enter the difference in block 30 as the amount due. For Medicare claims, leave blank.

28. TOTAL CHARGE   29. AMOUNT PAID   30. BALANCE DUE
$ $ $

Block 31 The physician or provider should sign and date the form here.

31. SIGNATURE OF PHYSICIAN OR SUPPLIER INCLUDING DEGREES OR CREDENTIALS
(I certify that the statements on the reverse apply to this bill and are made a part thereof.)

SIGNED   DATE

Block 32 Enter the name and address of the facility providing the services if different from the billing provider. If the billing provider and the service facility provider are the same or if the service took place in the patient's home, leave block 32 blank.

32a Enter the servicing provider's NPI.

32b If required by the insurer, enter the servicing provider's appropriate two-digit qualifier followed by the non-NPI identifier required.

32. SERVICE FACILITY LOCATION INFORMATION

a. NPI   b.

Block 33 Enter the billing provider's name, address (no post office boxes), city, state, 9-digit zip code, and phone number. As of January 1, 2012, post office boxes are no longer accepted for the provider address and the zip code must consist of the full 9 digits given by the U.S. Postal Service.

33a Enter the billing provider's NPI.

33b If required by the insurer, enter the billing provider's appropriate two-digit qualifier, followed by the non-NPI identifier required.

33. BILLING PROVIDER INFO & PH #   (   )

a. NPI   b.

Although the basic information required to complete the CMS-1500 claim is the same for every provider and insurance plan, you will find that instructions for completing the claim form vary among insurance carriers. So follow the individual carrier's instructions carefully to obtain a clean claim with every submission. Procedure 17-3 provides an outline for completing the CMS-1500 claim.

Go to CONNECT to see a video about *Completing the CMS-1500 Form.*

▶ Transmitting Electronic Claims   LO 17.7

Although hospitals and large practices have been using the X12 837 healthcare claims for quite some time now, smaller offices are still using paper claims for many of their claims submissions. Although even larger practices that have been using electronic claims processing consistently may be hesitant about choosing an electronic health records (EHR) software program, they will find health claims filing to be more efficient with EHR, as many of these programs can streamline the overall claims process. For example, with an EHR program, there is no need to repeatedly handwrite, type, or produce a computer-generated claim. The electronic claim template contains the instructions on placement of the information within the electronic claim. This information is pulled from the patient record automatically with a few of the medical assistant's simple keystrokes, which queue the claim for processing. At the time of transmission, all queued "clean" claims are transmitted with a few basic computer commands.

Practices handle electronic claims transmission—also called electronic media claims, or EMC—in a variety of ways. Some practices transmit claims themselves; others hire outside vendors to handle this task for them.

Three major methods are used to transmit claims electronically: direct transmission to the payer, clearinghouse use, and direct data entry.

Transmitting Claims Directly

In the direct transmission approach, medical offices and payers exchange transactions directly, using the necessary information systems—including a translator and communications technology—to conduct electronic data interchange (EDI).

Using a Clearinghouse

Many offices whose medical billing software vendors do not have translation software must use a **clearinghouse** in order to send and receive data in the correct EDI format.

Clearinghouses can translate nonstandard formats into standard formats and many also "scrub" the claims "clean" prior to submission to ensure each claim meets coding and payer claim standards so the claim will be paid rapidly. Clearinghouses also apply software checks to claims they receive and transmit back reports of errors or missing information to the provider so claims can be corrected before they even reach the payer. To ensure that the standard format is compliant, the clearinghouse must receive all the required data elements from the physician, as clearinghouses are prohibited from creating or modifying data content.

Medical offices may use a clearinghouse to transmit all their claims, or they may use a combination of direct transmission and a clearinghouse. For example, they may send claims directly to Medicare, Medicaid, and a few other major commercial payers and use a clearinghouse to send claims to other smaller payers.

Using Direct Data Entry

Some payers offer online direct data entry (DDE), which uses an Internet-based service into which employees can key the standard data elements. Although the data elements must meet the HIPAA standards requirements regarding content, EDI formatting is not required. Instead, the elements are loaded directly in the health plans' computer. One drawback is that each claim must be hand-keyed into the system each time the patient is seen, unlike the office billing software, which keeps the patient's prior information within its database.

Generating Clean Claims

Although healthcare claims, whether submitted electronically or by paper, require many data elements and are complex, it is often simple errors that prevent you from generating "clean" claims—those accepted for processing by the payer. Claims should be carefully checked for common errors (see Table 17-6) before transmission or printing. Prior to submitting any insurance claim, make sure you have access to the insurance carrier's most recent claim submission manual. Following the instructions in that manual carefully will result in clean claims the majority of times.

If you receive a paper query from an insurance carrier or electronic notification of claim rejection for any reason (including those shown in Table 17-6), provide the missing or corrected information or, if required, submit a new claim

TABLE 17-6 Common Errors Preventing Clean Claims

- Missing or incomplete service or billing provider name, address, and identification for the services rendered, including invalid zip codes or state abbreviations.
- Missing Medicare assignment indicator or benefits assignment indicator.
- Missing part of the name or the identifier of the referring provider.
- Missing or invalid subscriber or patient information, including misspelling of names.
- Missing or invalid information regarding secondary insurance plans.
- Missing payer name and/or payer identifier, required for both primary and secondary payers.

with corrected information. For instance, if any facility information is missing, insert the missing information and submit a corrected claim. If a provider number is missing, obtain the correct provider number from the referring or treating physician's office and submit a corrected claim with the appropriate ID number. Do note that most errors are errors of omission and if claims are checked carefully prior to submission, most errors can be caught, resulting in clean claims the first time around.

Claims Security

Most medical offices use computer networks in which personal computers are connected to a local area network (LAN), so users can exchange and share information and hardware. The LAN is linked to remote networks like the Internet by a router that determines the best route for data (which includes electronic patient data) to travel across the network. Packets of data traveling between the LAN and the Internet—like electronic claims—must usually pass through a firewall, a security device that examines information (for example, e-mails) that enters and leaves a network, determining whether to forward the information to its destination.

The HIPAA rules set standards for protecting individually identifiable health information when it is maintained or transmitted electronically. Medical offices use a number of security measures to protect the confidentiality, integrity, and availability of this information, including

- Access control, passwords, and log files to keep intruders out.
- Backups (saved copies of files) to replace items after damage to the computer.
- Security policies to handle violations that do occur.

Refer to the *Legal and Ethical Issues* chapter for further information regarding all HIPAA and confidentiality standards, including those for electronic transmissions.

▶ Insurer Processing Claims and Payments

LO 17.8

The Claims Register

If claims are transmitted electronically, the billing program or the clearinghouse will create a log of transmitted claims to allow you to track the progress of the submitted charges. If your office submits paper claims, you should create and maintain a claims register like the one shown in Figure 17-11. Procedure 17-4, at the end of the chapter, outlines the steps for creating a claims register.

Your transmitted claim for payment will undergo a number of reviews by the insurer. Currently, much of the review process occurs electronically.

Review for Medical Necessity

The insurance carrier reviews each claim to determine whether the procedures provided and the accompanying diagnoses are compatible and whether the treatment is medically necessary, as explained further in the *Diagnostic Coding* and *Procedure Coding* chapters.

| Patient Name | Insurance Company | Claim Filing | | Insurance Response Pd, Denied, Rejct, Suspd, Info Req | Date Resubmitted | Payment | | Patient Balance | Date Patient Billed |
		Date	Amount	Date		Date	Amount		
Smith, Peter	Aetna	1/4/XX	182 50	Info Req	1/6/XX	1/25/XX	85 25	25.12	2/2/XX

FIGURE 17-11 After submitting each claim, track it in an insurance claims register similar to this one.

Review for Allowable Benefits

The claims department also compares the fees the physician has charged with the benefits provided by the patient's health insurance policy. This review determines the amount of deductible and/or coinsurance the patient owes. The amount the patient owes the practice is known as patient liability.

Payment and Remittance Advice

After reviewing and accepting the claim, the insurer pays a benefit, either to the practice or to the subscriber (patient), depending on whether an assignment of benefits was signed and on the policy of the insurance carrier. With the payment, the insurer sends a **remittance advice (RA)** or an **explanation of payment (EOP)**, sometimes called an **explanation of benefits (EOB)**. If the payment is made electronically, the RA will also be received electronically. In this case, the RA is known as an electronic remittance advice (ERA) or electronic explanation of benefits (EEOB). A patient who receives the payment receives an RA summary containing only his information and the practice receives a practice RA that typically contains information for multiple patients at one time. Each insurance plan has its own EOP (RA) format and you will learn those of your office's most popular payers. Because many patients may be included on each EOP (RA), you may find it easiest to use a ruler to read each line of a paper RA and check off each line as you credit each patient's account. If a secondary insurance carrier requires a copy of a patient's primary insurance EOP, remember to black out any information on the EOP that does not pertain to the patient information required by the insurance carrier, to protect the information of the other patients on the EOB. The RA or the EOP explains the medical claim. For each service submitted to an insurer, the RA or EOP form gives the following information:

- Name of the insured and identification number.
- Patient name.
- Claim number.
- Date of service, place of service, and procedure code for service provided.
- Amount billed by the practice.
- Amount allowed.
- Amount of patient liability (coinsurance, copayment, deductible, or noncovered services).
- Amount paid.
- A notation of any services not covered and an explanation of why they were not covered (for example, many insurance plans do not cover routine vision screenings and only a certain dollar amount of well-baby visits for infants).

Reviewing the Insurer's RA and Payment

Verify all information on the RA, line by line, using your records for each patient represented on the RA. As stated earlier, in a large practice, you will frequently receive payments and RAs for multiple patients at one time. An example of a Medicare RA, or Medicare Remittance Advice, is shown in Figure 17-12.

If all numbers on the RA agree with your records, you can make the appropriate entries in the insurance tracking log for claims paid. In a small practice, the insurance tracking log is used to track filed claims, using such information as patient name, date the claim was filed, services the claim reflects, notations about the claim results, and any balance due from the patient. Larger practices tend to track claims in the computer billing program in a file called, for example, "Unpaid Claims." If you do not hear from a payer about a claim or the payment does not appear to match your records, you will need to trace the claim or place a query with the insurance company.

When a claim is rejected or denied, the RA states the reason. You will need to review the claim, examining all procedural and diagnosis codes for accuracy, and compare it with the patient's insurance information. In order to receive payment for the claim, you will often need to contact the insurance company by telephone to find out how to resolve the claim problem and then submit a corrected claim to obtain payment.

Callout labels:
- Name of Patient (subscriber) and ID NO.
- Claim NO.
- Dates and types of services (coded)
- Medicare pays 80% of this amount
- Medicare pays 100% of this amount
- Amount paid by medicare to doctor
- Notation for services not covered
- The 20% medicare copayment
- Amount allowed according to policy
- Amount billed by provider
- Physician performing services
- Number of claims included in statement
- Total amount of check paid to provider
- Number of check enclosed

		1	2		3	4	5	6	7	8	9	10	11	12
PATIENT	INSURANCE CLAIM CONTROL NO.	PROCEDURE CODE	NO SVCS / WHEN FROM MO DAY — TO MO DAY / SERVICE CODES PL TYP		AMOUNT BILLED	AMOUNT APPROVED	AMOUNT APPLIED TO DEDUCTIBLE	CO-INSURANCE	MEDICARE PAYS 80% OF THIS AMOUNT	SERVICES PAID IN FULL	WITHHELD FOR OFFSET	MEDICARE PAID PATIENT	MEDICARE PAID PROVIDER	MEDICARE DOES NOT PAY FOR THESE SERVICES
MARY DOE 123-45-6789A	11311101414-00	99214	001 0909 0909 11 1 1		55.57	55.57								
		81000	001 0909 0909 6 11 5		4.37	4.37								
		78730	001 0909 0909 6 11 4		76.80	76.80								
		CLAIMS TOTALS			136.74	136.74	0.00	26.47	132.37	4.37	0.00	0.00	110.27	

PAYMENT FOR THE LABORATORY TEST IS BASED ON A FEE SCHEDULE. A COPY OF THIS CLAIM DETERMINATION WILL BE FORWARDED TO THE BENEFICIARY'S SUPPLEMENTAL INSURER WITHIN THE NEXT 30 DAYS. QUESTIONS REGARDING PAYMENT OF SUPPLEMENTAL BENEFITS SHOULD BE DIRECTED TO THAT INSURER. PAYMENT FOR THIS SERVICE IS BASED ON THE MEDICARE FEE SCHEDULE.

		1	2		3	4	5	6	7	8	9	10	11	12
JANE JONES 555-44-3211A	11311101415-00	99244	001 0905 0905 6 11 3		131.03	131.03								
		81000	001 0905 0905 6 11 5		4.37	4.37								
		52000	001 0905 0905 6 11 2		150.68	150.68								
		78730	001 0905 0905 6 11 4		76.80	76.80								
		CLAIMS TOTALS			362.88	362.88	0.00	71.71	358.51	4.37	0.00	0.00	291.17	
JACK SMITH 987-65-4321A	11311101436-00	99214	001 0912 0912 6 11 1		55.57	55.57								
		81000	001 0912 0912 6 11 5		4.37	4.37								
		78730	001 0912 0912 6 11 4		76.80	76.80								
		CLAIMS TOTALS			136.74	136.74	0.00	26.47	132.37	4.37	0.00	0.00	110.27	

Summary:

TOTAL	NUMBER OF CLAIMS	AMOUNT BILLED	AMOUNT APPROVED	AMOUNT APPLIED TO DEDUCTIBLE	CONINSURANCE	MEDICARE PAYS 80% OF THIS AMOUNT	AMOUNT OF 80% PAYMENT	SERVICES PAID IN FULL	WITHHELD FOR OFFSET	MEDICARE PAID PATIENT	MEDICARE PAID PROVIDER
PAGE-CHECK-	3	636.36	636.36	0.00	124.65	623.25	498.60	13.11	0.00	0.00	511.71

SUMMARY ► PROVIDER NUMBER: 000412000   WEEK ENDING: 10/11/12   CHECK NUMBER: 047507806   DATE PAID: 10/15/12

Elizabeth Williams, MD
305 Main Street,
Port Snead,YZ 12345-9876

FIGURE 17-12 The payer sends a remittance advice to explain payment made to the medical practice.

PROCEDURE 17-1 Verifying Workers' Compensation Coverage

Procedure Goal: To verify workers' compensation coverage before accepting a patient.

OSHA Guidelines: This procedure does not involve exposure to blood, body fluids, or tissue.

Materials: Telephone, paper, and a pen.

Method: Procedure steps.

1. Call the patient's employer and verify that the accident or illness occurred on the employer's premises or at an employment-related work site.

2. Obtain the employer's approval to provide treatment. Be sure to write down the name and title of the person giving approval, as well as his phone number.
   RATIONALE: Without approval, treatment costs may not be covered.

3. Ask the employer for the name of its workers' compensation insurance company. (Employers are required by law to carry such insurance. It is a good policy to notify your state labor department about any employer you encounter that does not have workers' compensation insurance, although you are not required to do so.)
   If the employer has not done so, remind them to report the incident to the W/C carrier, using the First Report of Injury or Illness, and to the state labor department within 24 hours of the incident.
   RATIONALE: Without this form on file, the claims will not be approved for payment.

4. Contact the insurance company and verify that the employer does indeed have an active policy in good standing with the company.
   RATIONALE: The insurance company will not pay for services without a valid policy.

5. Obtain the claim number assigned to the case from the insurance company. This claim number is placed on all claims and submitted paperwork.
   RATIONALE: All invoices must include the claim number in order for the practice to receive payment.

6. When the patient begins treatment, create a patient record. If the patient is already an active patient with the practice, create separate medical and financial records for the workers' compensation–related treament.
   RATIONALE: This is the legal procedure to protect patient confidentiality with regard to private medical care. Confidentiality does not exist with regard to care related to workers' compensation cases because the employer and its insurer are paying for the patient's medical care.

PROCEDURE 17-2 Submitting a Request for Prior Authorization

Procedure Goal: To submit a request for prior authorization.

OSHA Guidelines: This procedure does not involve exposure to blood, body fluids, or tissue.

Materials: Patient medical chart with planned procedure and CPT code, diagnosis and ICD code for proof of medical necessity, and patient financial record or the following information: patient name, address, DOB, subscriber name and relationship to patient if not the same, insurance policy group, and ID numbers.

Method: Procedure steps.

1. Place a call to the insurance carrier or access the website if available.

2. When you reach the nurse manager for the patient's policy, explain that you would like to obtain prior authorization for the requested procedure. She will ask a series of questions regarding the patient, procedure, and diagnosis. Answer these questions using the assembled materials from the patient's medical and financial records.
   RATIONALE: The more information available regarding the proposed procedure and the reason for it, the easier it is to obtain prior authorization.

3. If obtaining authorization via the insurance carrier's website, access the website utilizing your user ID and password. Enter the prior authorization area of the website and enter the required information using the assembled materials from the patient's medical and financial records.
   RATIONALE: The more information available regarding the proposed procedure and the reason for it, the easier it is to obtain prior authorization.

4. When prior authorization is obtained, carefully record the authorization number and the name and extension number of the person issuing the authorization (if obtained over the phone). If the authorization is obtained via a website, print out the authorization documentation.
   RATIONALE: If authorization is received, but the authorization number is not on the claim form or is incorrect, payment may still be denied.

5. Place the authorization number and/or documentation in the patient medical and financial record for further reference, as it will be required when submitting the patient's health insurance claim.

PROCEDURE 17-3 Completing the CMS-1500 Claim Form

Procedure Goal: To complete the CMS-1500 claim form correctly.

OSHA Guidelines: This procedure does not involve exposure to blood, body fluids, or tissue.

Materials: Patient record, CMS-1500 form, typewriter, computer or pen, and patient ledger card or charge slip.

Method: Procedure steps. *Note: The numbers below correspond to the numbered fields on the CMS-1500.*

Patient Information Section

1. Place an *X* in the appropriate insurance box.

   a. Enter the insured's insurance identification number as it appears on the insurance card.

2. Enter the patient's name in this order: last name, first name, middle initial (if any).

3. **a.** Enter the patient's birth date using an 8-digit format.

   b. Indicate the patient's sex: male or female.

4. If the insured and the patient are the same person, enter SAME. If not, enter the policyholder's name.

5. Enter the patient's mailing address, city, state, and zip code.

6. Enter the patient's relationship to the insured. If they are the same, enter SELF.

7. Enter the insured's mailing address, city, state, zip code, and telephone number. If this address is the same as the patient's, enter SAME. For Medicare, leave blank.

   RATIONALE: Medicare patients are always the insured and the patient.

8. Indicate the patient's marital, employment, and student status by placing an *X* in the appropriate boxes.

   RATIONALE: Commercial insurers may deny the claim without this information.

9. Enter the last name, first name, and middle initial of any other insured person whose policy might cover the patient. If the claim is for Medicare and the patient has a Medigap policy, enter the patient's name again.

   RATIONALE: This is the block for the secondary insurance. The primary insurer will want to know who carries the secondary coverage.

   a. Enter the policy or group number for the other insured person.

   b. Enter the date of birth and sex of the other insured person (listed in field 9).

   c. Enter the other insured's employer or school name.

   d. Enter the other insured's insurance plan or program name. If the plan is Medigap and CMS has assigned it a nine-digit number called PAYERID, enter that number here.

   RATIONALE: The PAYERID tells Medicare the coverage is a Medigap plan.

10. Place *X*s in the appropriate YES or NO boxes in a, b, and c to indicate whether the patient's place of employment, an auto accident, or other type of accident precipitated the patient's condition. If an auto accident is responsible, for PLACE, enter the two-letter state postal abbreviation for the location of the accident.

    RATIONALE: If any of these boxes is marked "Yes," another insurance plan is likely liable for the charges (W/C, auto insurance, or other liability plan).

11. Enter the insured's policy group number. For Medicare claims, fill out this section only if there is other insurance primary to Medicare; otherwise, enter NONE and leave fields a–d blank.

    a. Enter the insured's date of birth and sex as in field 3, if the insured is not the patient.

    b. Enter the employer's name or school name here. This information will determine if Medicare is the primary payer.

    RATIONALE: If there is an employer listed, Medicare will not be the primary payer; a private group health plan (GHP) will be primary.

    c. Enter the insurance plan or program name.

    d. Place an *X* to indicate YES or NO related to another health benefit plan.

    RATIONALE: If the answer is "No," there is no other insurance coverage and block 9a–d will remain blank.

12. The patient or an authorized representative signs and dates the form here. If a representative signs, have the representative indicate the relationship to the patient. If signatures are on file, this may be noted by inserting "Signature on File."

    RATIONALE: Without a signature authorizing release of information, you do not legally have the patient's permission to submit this information to the insurance carrier.

13. Have the insured (the patient or another individual) sign here. If signatures are on file, this may be noted by inserting "Signature on File."

    RATIONALE: Without this signature, the insurance carrier may send payment for the physician's services to the patient.

Physician Information Section

14. Enter the date of the current illness, injury, or pregnancy using 8 digits, if not the same as the date of service.

15. Enter the date the patient was first seen for illness or injury. Leave it blank for Medicare.

    RATIONALE: Information is used to determine "preexisting conditions," which is information not required by Medicare.

16. Enter the dates the patient is or was unable to work. This information could signal a workers' compensation claim.

17. Enter the name of the referring physician, clinical laboratory, or other referring source.

    a. Depending on insurance carrier instructions, enter an approved 2-digit qualifier (refer to Table 17-1) in the small space and the appropriate referring provider identifier next to it. If the carrier requires only the NPI, leave this box blank.

    b. Enter the referring provider NPI number.
    RATIONALE: All payers require the NPI number.

18. If the patient was hospitalized during this encounter, enter the dates here.

19. Use the payer's current instructions for this field. In many cases, it may be left blank.

20. Place an *X* in the YES box if a laboratory test was performed outside the physician's office and enter the test price if you are billing for these tests. Place an *X* in the NO box if the test was done in the physician's office that is billing the insurance company.

21. Enter the ICD code number for each diagnosis or nature of injury. Enter up to four codes in order of importance.
    RATIONALE: The diagnosis codes prove medical necessity for the services provided.

22. Enter the Medicaid resubmission code and original reference number if applicable.

23. Enter the prior authorization number if required by the payer.

24. The six service lines in block 24 are divided horizontally to accommodate NPI and other proprietary identifiers per insurance carrier instructions. Otherwise, use the nonshaded areas only if the payer requires just the NPI for claims submission.

    a. Enter the date of each service, procedure, or supply provided. Add the number of days for each and enter them, in chronological order, in field 24g.

    b. Enter the two-digit place-of-service code (see Table 17-5).

    c. EMG stands for emergency care. Check with the insurer to see if this information is needed. If it is required and emergency care was provided, enter Y; if it is not required or care was not on an emergency basis, leave this field blank.

    d. Enter the CPT/HCPCS codes with modifiers for the procedures, services, or supplies provided.
    RATIONALE: These codes tell the payer what services were provided to the patient.

    e. Enter the diagnosis code (or its reference number—1, 2, 3, or 4—depending on carrier regulations) that applies to that procedure, as listed in field 21.
    RATIONALE: Each "pointer" tells the payer which diagnosis (or diagnoses) is the reason the service was provided, showing medical necessity for treatment.

    f. Enter the dollar amount of the fee charged.

    g. Enter the days or units for the number of times the service was performed.

h. This field is Medicaid-specific for early periodic screening diagnosis and treatment programs. For all other payers, leave this field blank.

i. (shaded) If required by the insurance carrier, enter the appropriate non-NPI identifier here. If not required, leave this area blank.

j. If the carrier requires a non-NPI number, enter the PIN identified in 24i in the shaded area. Use the nonshaded area below this to enter the provider's NPI in 24j.
RATIONALE: The NPI identifies the physician providing the service.

25. Enter the physician's or care provider's federal tax identification number or Social Security number and enter an *X* in the box identifying which number is listed.
    RATIONALE: This information is required for tax purposes.

26. Enter the patient's account number assigned by your office, if applicable.

27. Place an *X* in the YES box to indicate the physician will accept Medicare or TRICARE assignment of benefits.
    RATIONALE: This block tells the payer if you are a participating provider.

28. Enter the total charge for the service.

29. Enter the amount already paid by any primary insurance company or the patient, if it pertains to his deductible.

30. Enter the balance due to your office. For primary Medicare claims, leave this field blank.

31. Have the physician or service supplier sign and date the form here. In most cases, because claims are filed electronically, the signature is on file and the typed name of the provider is acceptable in this block.

32. Enter the name and address of the organization or individual who performed the services. If service was provided in the provider's office or the patient's home, leave this field blank.

    a. If block 32 is completed, enter the NPI for the service facility.

    b. If block 32 is completed and if required by the insurance carrier, enter the appropriate two-digit qualifier immediately followed by the identification number being used. Do not place any spaces or punctuation between the qualifier and the identification number.

33. List the billing physician's or supplier's name, address, zip code, and phone number.

    a. Enter the billing provider's NPI.

    b. If required by the insurance carrier, enter the non-NPI qualifier in field 33b, immediately followed by the identification number being used. Do not place any spaces or punctuation between the qualifier and the identification number.

PROCEDURE 17-4 Tracking Insurance Claims Submissions

Procedure Goal: To create and use a spreadsheet to track insurance claims submissions.

OSHA Guidelines: This procedure does not involve exposure to blood, body fluids, or tissue.

Materials: CMS-1500 claims prepared for submission or record of CMS-1500 claims submitted electronically; spreadsheet or grid for handwritten record with pen; or computer with software program such as MS Excel, allowing for the creation of a spreadsheet.

Method: Procedure steps.

1. Using Figure 17-10 as a guide, create columns with the following (or similar) headings: Patient Name (and/or account number); Insurance Company; Date of Submission and Amount of the Claim; Insurance Response and Date of Response; Date of Resubmission; Date of Payment; Payment Amount; Patient Balance; and Date of Patient Billing.

2. Using the list of claims submitted, complete the blanks for patient name, insurance company, date of submission, and amount of the claim.

3. When the RA (EOB) is received, complete the date and response columns, including whether the claim is paid, rejected, or denied or a request was made for more information.
   RATIONALE: This allows you to follow up in the future once correction or requested information is submitted to the insurance carrier.

4. If resubmission is required, enter the date of resubmission.

5. If payment is received, enter the date of receipt and the amount of the payment.
   RATIONALE: This information tells you the insurance carrier has met its obligation.

6. Record patient balance (if any) and the date the patient is billed.
   RATIONALE: You now can track the remaining balance owed by the patient.

SUMMARY OF LEARNING OUTCOMES

LEARNING OUTCOMES	KEY POINTS
17.1 Define the basic insurance terms used by the insurance industry.	The following are terms used by insurance companies, knowledgeable medical assistants, medical billers, and coders: premium, benefit, lifetime maximum, deductible, coinsurance, copayment, exclusions, formulary, elective procedure, precertification, and preauthorization.
17.2 Compare fee-for-service plans, HMOs, and PPOs.	Fee-for-service plans are traditional plans where after a yearly deductible is met, the insurance plan pays for a percentage of the charges and the patient is responsible for the other percentage (often 80% insurance plan and 20% patient). HMOs are prepaid plans that pay the providers either by capitation or by contracted fee-for-service with patients choosing a PCP, seeing preferred providers, and paying a fixed per-visit copay. A PPO is a managed care plan that establishes a network of providers to perform services for plan members. Members may seek out-of-network care, but their costs will be higher.
17.3 Outline the key requirements for coverage by the Medicare, Medicaid, TRICARE, and CHAMPVA programs.	Medicare provides health insurance for citizens aged 65 and older as well as for certain disabled workers, disabled widows of workers, and patients with long-term disability related to chronic kidney disease on dialysis and end-stage renal disease requiring transplant. Medicaid is a health benefit plan for low-income, blind, or disabled patients; needy families; foster children; and children born with birth defects. TRICARE is a healthcare benefit for families of uniformed personnel and retirees from the uniformed services. CHAMPVA covers the expenses of the families of veterans with total, permanent, service-connected disabilities as well as expenses for surviving spouses and dependent children of veterans who died in the line of duty or as a result of service-connected disabilities.

LEARNING OUTCOMES	KEY POINTS
17.4 Describe allowed charge, contracted fee, capitation and the formula for RBRVS.	An allowed charge is the maximum dollar amount an insurance carrier will base its reimbursement on—it is also the maximum amount a participating provider is allowed to collect. A contracted fee is a negotiated fee between the MCO and the provider. Capitation is a fixed prepayment paid to the PCP in most plans. RBRVS stands for resource-based relative value scale. Its formula is RVU $\times$ GAF $\times$ CF.
17.5 Outline the tasks performed to obtain the information required to produce an insurance claim.	The claims process includes obtaining patient information, delivering services to the patient and determining the diagnosis and fee, recording charges and codes, documenting payment from the patient, and preparing the healthcare claims.
17.6 Produce a clean CMS-1500 health insurance claim form.	Using the step-by-step instructions within the chapter and Procedure 17-3, and given a completed encounter form (superbill) with all necessary information, the student should produce a legible, clean, and acceptable CMS-1500 claim form.
17.7 Explain the methods used to submit an insurance claim electronically.	The three methods used to submit claims electronically are a claims submission directly to the payer's website via an electronic data interchange, the use of a clearinghouse to "scrub" and submit claims to the payer for the provider, and the use of direct data entry or DDE.
17.8 Recall information found on every payer's remittance advice.	Although the format may vary from payer to payer, all RAs (EOBs) contain the following information: name of the insured and identification number; patient name; claim number, date of service, place of service, and code for the service provided; amount billed; amount allowed; amount of subscriber liability; amount paid; and a notation of any services not covered and an explanation of why they were not covered.

CASE STUDY CRITICAL THINKING

Recall Sylvia Gonzales from the beginning of the chapter. Now that you have completed the chapter, answer the following questions regarding her case.

1. Which insurance plan will be primary for Mrs. Gonzales if the state she lives in uses the birthday rule?

2. If Mr. Gonzales' insurance is primary, explain how the payment will be calculated by the insurance carrier for today's office visit and two lab tests.

3. If the HMO plan is considered primary, what will Sylvia's portion of the charges consist of?

EXAM PREPARATION QUESTIONS

1. (LO 17.1) A fixed-dollar amount the subscriber must pay or "meet" each year before the insurer begins to cover expenses is the
   a. Copayment
   b. Deductible
   c. Premium
   d. Coinsurance
   e. Lifetime maximum

2. (LO 17.1) Depending upon the type of plan, the patient's portion of the medical charges after the insurance has paid is known as the
   a. Copayment
   b. Deductible
   c. Coinsurance
   d. Premium
   e. a or c

3. (LO 17.2) Most specialists are paid by MCOs using which of the following methods?
   a. Fee-for-service
   b. Capitation
   c. Copayment
   d. Coinsurance
   e. Negotiated per-service fees

4. (LO 17.3) The national health insurance plan for Americans age 65 and older is
   a. Medicaid
   b. Medicare
   c. TRICARE
   d. CHAMPVA
   e. Workers' compensation

5. (LO 17.3) The appropriate definition for Medicaid plans is
   a. Health insurance plan
   b. Welfare
   c. Health benefit plan
   d. Liablity plan
   e. Health insurance benefit

6. (LO 17.4) RBRVS consists of which components?
   a. RVU
   b. GAF
   c. CF
   d. All of the above
   e. Some of the above

7. (LO 17.5) Which of the following is NOT performed by the medical practice when preparing a healthcare claim for payment and reviewing the insurance payment?
   a. Submitting the employer's first report of illness or injury
   b. Obtaining patient information
   c. Delivering services to the patient and determining the diagnosis and fee
   d. Recording charges and codes, recording payment from the patient, and preparing and submitting the healthcare claim
   e. Reviewing the insurer's processing of the claim, remittance advice, and payment

8. (LO 17.6) Why is it important that each procedure on the CMS-1500 be matched with a diagnosis code?
   a. It proves the procedure was performed
   b. It keeps the coder employed
   c. It increases the reimbursement amount
   d. It proves medical necessity for the procedure
   e. It truly does not matter

9. (LO 17.7) Which of the following is the most common method for medical practices to submit electronic medical claims to third-party payers?
   a. Paper claims via U.S. mail
   b. DDE
   c. Direct submission
   d. Clearinghouse
   e. None of the above

10. (LO 17.8) Which of the following documents provides information regarding the payer's payment (or denial) of charges received?
    a. RA
    b. EOB
    c. a and b
    d. Claims register
    e. 1505

Go to CONNECT to see activities about *Setting up a Doctor's PIN Numbers*, *Verifying a Patient's Insurance Coverage*, *Creating a Patient Referral Form*, and *Creating a Routing Slip for Billing*.

Diagnostic Coding

CASE STUDY

<table>
<tr><td rowspan="4">PATIENT INFORMATION</td><td>Patient Name</td><td>Gender</td><td>DOB</td></tr>
<tr><td>Cindy Chen</td><td>F</td><td>7/15/19XX</td></tr>
<tr><td>Attending</td><td>MRN</td><td>Allergies</td></tr>
<tr><td>Alexis N. Whalen, MD</td><td>324-86-542</td><td>NKA</td></tr>
</table>

Cindy Chen, a 28-year-old female complaining of inability to sleep and nervousness, arrives at the office. She tested positive for HIV in 2005, although she has been asymptomatic on antiviral drugs. Currently, she lives with her aunt and is going to school to become a phlebotomist. During her interview, she says she thinks her nervousness may be due to upcoming exams and the recurrent sore throat and tiredness she has been experiencing in the last several months.

Keep Cindy Chen in mind as you study this chapter. There will be questions at the end of the chapter based on the case study. The information in the chapter will help you answer these questions.

LEARNING OUTCOMES

After completing Chapter 18, you will be able to:

18.1 Recall the six ways that ICD codes are used today.
18.2 Describe the conventions used by ICD-9-CM.
18.3 Outline the steps to code a diagnosis using ICD-9-CM.
18.4 Explain the purpose and usage of V codes and E codes.
18.5 Name the appendixes found in ICD-9-CM.
18.6 Compare ICD-9-CM and the ICD-10-CM.
18.7 Summarize the ICD-10-CM general coding guidelines.
18.8 Illustrate unique coding applications for neoplasms, diabetes mellitus, fractures, R codes, poisonings, and Z codes.

KEY TERMS

Alphabetic Index
categories
chapters
chief complaint (CC)
conventions
cross-reference
diagnosis (Dx)
diagnosis code
E code
etiology
International Classification of Diseases

morbidity
mortality
primary diagnosis
principal diagnosis
secondary diagnosis
subcategories
Tabular List
V code
World Health Organization (WHO)

VII. C (12) Define Diagnosis-Related Groups (DRGs)

VIII. C (3) Describe how to use the most current diagnostic coding classification system

VIII. P (2) Perform diagnostic coding

VIII. A (1) Work with physician to achieve the maximum reimbursement

3. **Medical Terminology**
   Graduates:
   d. Recognize and identify acceptable medical abbreviations

4. **Medical Law & Ethics**
   Graduates:
   f. Comply with federal, state, and local health laws and regulations

8. **Medical Office Business Procedures Management**
   Graduates:
   t. Perform diagnostic and procedural coding

▶ Introduction

Patients who come to the medical office have a variety of reasons for seeking medical care. Each of those reasons results in at least one diagnosis. The word *diagnosis*, when split into its component word parts, means "the condition of complete knowledge" (osis–condition, dia–complete, gnos–knowledge). When submitting claims to insurance carriers to receive reimbursement for the care the patient receives, this knowledge must be converted into numeric and alphanumeric codes, known as ICD codes. ICD stands for **International Classification of Diseases**. As this chapter is being written, the United States is preparing to transition from ICD-9-CM (ICD-9th Edition, Clinical Modification) to the next edition, known as ICD-10-CM (ICD-10th Edition, Clinical Modification), scheduled for October 1, 2014.

With the passage of the Medicare Catastrophic Coverage Act of 1988, diagnosis coding became mandatory for Medicare claims (using ICD-9) and shortly thereafter, its use was also mandated for Medicaid and commercial insurance carriers. Just as you learn medical terminology to communicate with all members of the healthcare team, as a medical assistant, it is equally important to learn the *language* of coding—in this chapter, ICD-9 and ICD-10, and in the following chapter, the language of CPT and HCPCS procedural coding. Because insurance carriers pay claims based on the codes assigned to describe the information within the medical record (not on the medical record itself), it is vitally important that you have an understanding of what the codes mean and how to choose the correct code based on the information found on the encounter forms and within the patient medical record.

▶ The Reasons for Diagnosis Codes LO 18.1

Patients present physicians with a description of their medical problem, called their **chief complaint (CC)**, which is documented at each visit. To diagnose a patient's condition, the physician follows a complex decision-making process based on the patient's statements, an examination, and the physician's evaluation of this information. The physician establishes a **diagnosis (Dx)** that describes the primary condition for which a patient is receiving care. Additional conditions or symptoms that affect the patient's management are called *coexisting conditions,* or *comorbidities.* These conditions may be related or totally unrelated to the primary condition, but if they currently affect the patient's condition or treatment, they also must be noted in the chart, coded, and reported to the insurance carrier. The diagnoses listed on a healthcare claim form should prove medical necessity for the treatment provided.

The diagnosis is communicated to the third-party payer through a **diagnosis code** on the healthcare claim. Until October 1, 2014, diagnosis codes used in the United States are found in the 9th edition of the clinical modification of the ICD reference, more commonly referred to as the ICD-9-CM, or simply ICD-9. Also available on CD-ROM, this code set is based on a system maintained by the **World Health Organization (WHO)** of the United Nations. Scheduled for release on October 1, 2014, in the United States is the 10th edition of the clinical modification of ICD, which will be referred to as ICD-10-CM, or simply ICD-10.

The Health Insurance Portability and Accountability Act (HIPAA) mandates ICD code use in the healthcare industry for reporting patients' diseases, conditions, or their signs and symptoms if no actual diagnosis has been assigned. The codes are updated every year on October 1, which explains why ICD-10 will be effective October 1, 2014, instead of in January when the new procedure codes come out. It is important to remember that the edition of diagnosis codes being used is based on the date of service (DOS), not on the date the claim is submitted. For instance, when completing claims on October 1, 2014, you will use 2013 ICD-9 codes on a claim for services provided on September 30, 2013. However, for a claim reporting services provided on October 1, 2014, the new 2014 ICD-10 codes would be used. Medical office must always have the current year's coding reference books and should update office forms and computer programs containing diagnosis (and procedure) codes because using outdated codes will result in denied claims.

ICD-9-CM was originally created for the classification of patient **morbidity** (sickness) and **mortality** (death) statistics and to provide access for medical research, education, and administration. Today, however, ICD-9 (and soon ICD-10) codes are increasingly important and they are used for the following reasons:

- Facilitation of payment for medical services.
- Evaluation of utilization patterns (patient use of healthcare facilities).
- Study of healthcare costs.
- Research regarding quality of healthcare.
- Prediction of healthcare trends.
- Planning for future healthcare needs.

Keep in mind as you learn coding that just as whatever you document in a patient's health record becomes part of his/her permanent record, so does any code you assign to the patient for receipt by the insurance carrier. It also may be part of statistical reporting for communicable diseases, pregnancies, cancer diagnosis, and so on, so it is extremely important that you understand the information you are coding and the descriptions of the codes you are assigning.

▶ An Overview of ICD-9   LO 18.2

The ICD-9-CM consists of two parts: the Tabular List, known as Volume 1, and the Alphabetic Index, known as Volume 2 (found at the beginning of the manual (Figure 18-1)). ICD-9 also contains an edition for hospitals called Volume 3, which consists of the tabular and alphabetic listings of procedures performed primarily in hospitals.

The correct procedure when using the ICD reference is to look up the diagnosis description in the **Alphabetic Index** (Volume 2) and then verify the code given by cross-referencing it in the **Tabular List** (Volume 1). In order to use both indices easily, you must understand the *conventions* used in both indices. Let's take a look at these now.

Conventions

A list of abbreviations, punctuation, symbols, typefaces, and instructional notes appears at the beginning of the ICD-9. These items, called **conventions**, provide guidelines for using the code set. Here are some important conventions:

- NOS. This abbreviation means "not otherwise specified," or "unspecified." It is used when a condition is not described in enough detail to choose a more specific code. In general,

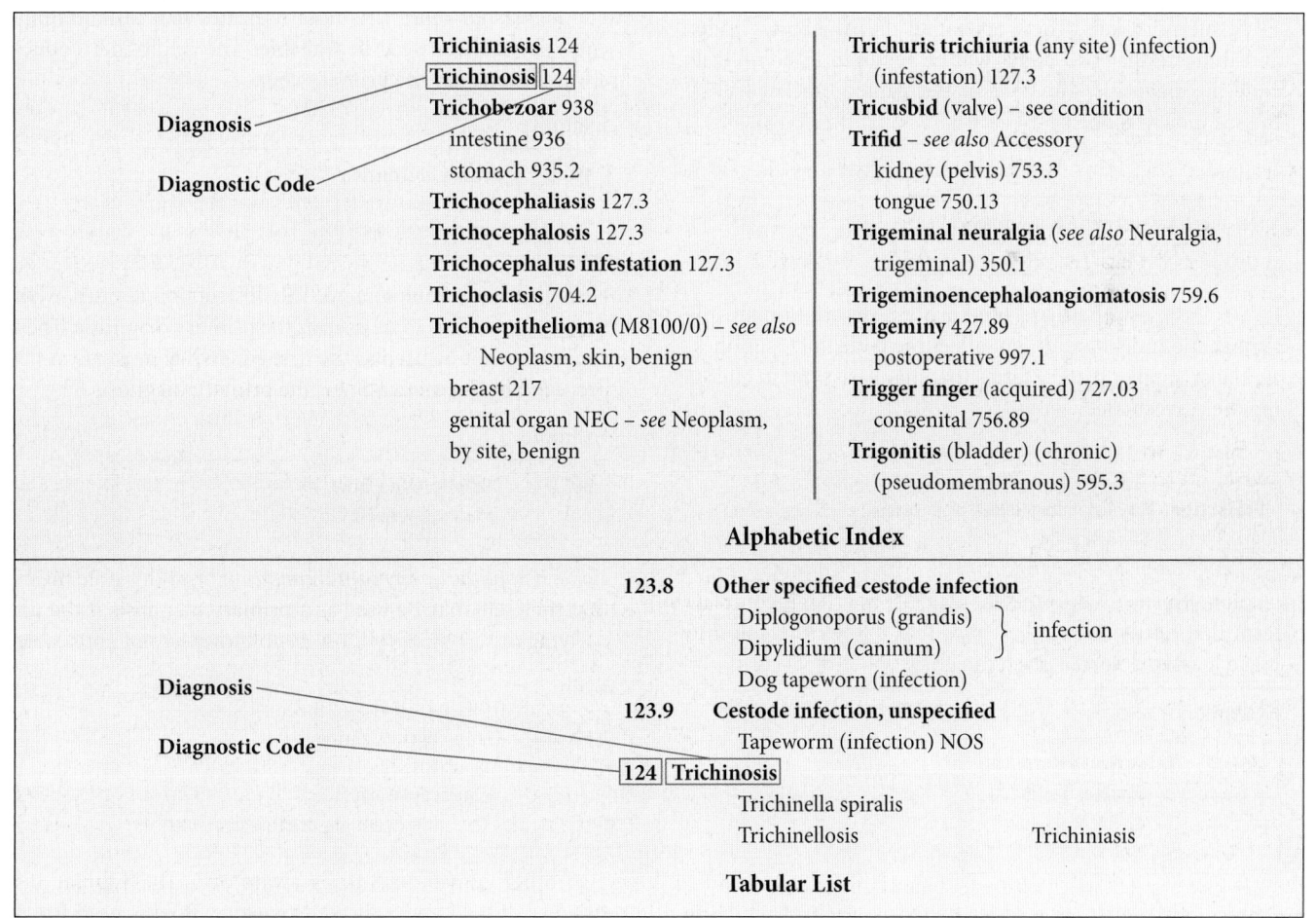

FIGURE 18-1   ICD Alphabetic Index and Tabular List.

Source: International Classification of Diseases, Ninth Revision, Clinical Modification, 2012, Volumes 1, 2, and 3.

codes with NOS should be avoided unless no other option is available. The physician should be asked for more specific information to help select a more specific code, if possible. Most of the NOS codes end with the number 9.

Example:

038.9	**Unspecified septicemia**
	Septicemia NOS

- NEC. This abbreviation means "not elsewhere classified." It is used when the ICD-9 does not provide a code specific enough for the patient's condition. Only use these codes when you are sure a more specific code does not exist. In general, the NEC codes end with the number 8.

Example:

244.8	**Other specified acquired hypothyroidism**
	Secondary hypothyroidism NEC

- [ ] Brackets. These are used around synonyms, alternative wordings, or explanations.

Example:

482.2	**Pneumonia due to Hemophilus influenza [H. influenzae]**

- [ ] Slanted brackets. These appear in the Alphabetic Index and indicate that two codes will be required to completely code the diagnosis. The code in the slanted bracket will be the secondary code.

Example:

Fleischer (-Kayser) ring (corneal pigmentation)
275.1 *[371.14]*

- ( ) Parentheses. These are used around descriptions in the Alphabetic Index that do not affect the code, that is, nonessential or supplementary terms that may assist you in choosing the correct code.

Example:

Fleischer (-Kayser) ring (corneal pigmentation)
275.1 *[371.14]*

- : Colon. This is used in the Tabular List after an incomplete term that needs one of the terms that follows the colon to make it assignable to a given category.

Example:

009.2	**Infectious diarrhea**
	Diarrhea:
	dysenteric
	epidemic

- } Brace. This encloses a series of terms, each of which is modified by the statement that appears to the right of the brace.

Example:

308.0	**Predominant disturbance of emotions**
	Anxiety
	Emotional crisis } as acute reaction to exceptional
	Panic state [gross] stress

- *Includes.* This note indicates that the entries following it further define the content of a preceding entry.

Example:

249	**Secondary diabetes mellitus**
	INCLUDES diabetes mellitus (due to) (in) (secondary with):
	drug-induced or chemical-induced infection

- *Excludes.* These notes, which are boxed and italicized, indicate that an entry is not classified as part of the preceding code. The note may also give the correct location of the excluded condition to assist you in locating the correct code.

Example:

246.2	**Cyst of thyroid**
	EXCLUDES cystadenoma of thyroid (226)

- *Use additional code.* This note indicates that an additional code should be used, if available. The additional code is always listed after the primary code.

Example:

599.6	**Urinary obstruction**
	Use additional code to identify urinary incontinence
	(635.6, 788.30-788.39)

- *Code first underlying disease.* This instruction appears when the category is not to be used as the primary diagnosis. These codes may not be used as the first code; they must always be preceded by another code for the primary diagnosis.

Example:

362.0	**Diabetic retinopathy**
	Code first diabetes (249.5, 250.5)

- *Code, if applicable, any causal condition first.* This note means that the code may be used as a primary diagnosis if the underlying or "causal condition" is unknown or not applicable.

Example:

590.0	**Chronic pyelonephritis**
	Chronic pyelitis
	Chronic pyonephrosis
	Code, if applicable, any causal condition first

Two other conventions to be aware of in the Tabular List are the use of bold and italicized typeface. Bold is used for all codes and titles in the Tabular List. Italicization is used for all exclusion notes and to identify codes that are not used to describe the primary diagnosis; they are only used as secondary diagnoses.

The Alphabetic Index includes two notations you should also be aware of:

- *Omit Code* is used to let you know that the medical term should not be coded as a diagnosis.

Example:

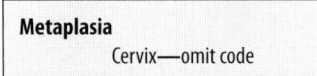

- *See Condition.* When found in the Alphabetic Index, it is meant to refer you to a different "main term" for the condition. For instance, if you look up the term *Cervix* in the Alphabetic Index, you will be directed to *See condition.* Cervix is not a diagnosis; it is a location. Keep in mind that the diagnosis (and its main term) is "what is wrong with the patient." The location will be used as a subterm. If the patient has a diagnosis of cervical cancer, you would then look up neoplasm, cervix—neoplasm (new growth–cancer) being the main condition.

Example:

Cervix—See Condition

- *See also.* If the diagnosis for the patient is cervical inflammation, the main term is *inflammation.* When you look up *inflammation, cervix* (subterm for the location of the inflammation), you are directed to 616.0, but you are also directed to *See also* "Cervicitis."

Example:

Inflammation
Cervix (uteri) (See also Cervicitis) 616.0

The direction "See condition" is a directive; you must do so to locate the code. "See also" is a suggestion; you might find a better code for the diagnosis you are coding. In the case of "cervicitis," you will find multiple codes available depending on what is causing the cervicitis. Follow all directions in ICD-9. It will make you a better coder and, in many cases, increase the reimbursement for the provider because you are giving the insurance carrier the most specific information available for the medical necessity for the services provided. Read the Coding Guidelines in the beginning of the manual. Broken out by section, these guidelines give very specific instructions on how to code each of the 17 chapters of the ICD-9 manual and the best use of E codes and V codes. Read and highlight this area of the manual as you learn to code—you will be glad you did.

The Alphabetic Index

As stated earlier, when coding, the Alphabetic Index is your starting point (after you read the guidelines). It contains all the medical terms necessary to locate codes in the Tabular List—including common terms that are not found in the Tabular List. The index is organized by condition. To use the Alphabetic Index, think about what is wrong (the problem) and not where the problem occurred. For example, you would find the term *wrist fracture* by looking under *fracture* (the condition) and then, below it, *wrist* (the location), rather than by looking under *wrist* to find *fracture.* In fact, if you look up the word *wrist*, you will be told "See also condition," telling you to look up the problem with the wrist.

The assignment of the correct code begins with looking up the medical term that describes the patient's condition in the Alphabetic Index. The following example illustrates the index's format. Each main term is printed in boldface type and is followed by its code number. For example, if the diagnostic statement is "the patient presents with blindness," the main term *blindness* is located in the Alphabetic Index.

Blindness (acquired) (congenital) (both eyes)
369.00
with deafness V49.85
blast 921.3
    with nerve injury—see Injury, nerve, optic
Bright's—see Uremia
color (congenital) 368.59
    acquired 368.55
    blue 368.53
    green 368.52
    red 368.51
    total 368.54
concussion 950.9
cortical 377.75

Any other terms that are needed to select correct codes are printed and indented after the main term. These terms, called *subterms*, may show the cause or source of the disease, or describe a particular type or body site for the main term. In this shortened example, the main term *blindness* is followed by five additional terms, each indicating a different type—such as color blindness—for this medical condition. Additionally, when coding color blindness, note that each of its subterms, which denote the actual type of color blindness, has its own code. When cross-referencing with the Tabular List, you will note that the main code of 368 represents a visual disturbance. The fourth digit (after the decimal point) of 5 represents color vision deficiencies, and the fifth digit changes to indicate the type of color blindness.

Other helpful terms, in parentheses, known as *nonessential terms*, also may be shown. Nonessential terms are those that assist you in choosing the correct code, but it is not mandatory that they be present within the code description. In the example, any of the terms *acquired, congenital,* and/or *both eyes* may be in the diagnostic statement, such as "the patient presents with blindness acquired in childhood."

Cross-references of *see* or *see also* are used frequently in ICD. If the cross-reference *see* appears after a main term, you *must* look up the term that follows the word *see* in the index. The *see* reference means that the main term where you first looked is not correct; another category must be used. In the previous example regarding color blindness, to code *Bright's*, you are instructed to *See* the term *Uremia* to locate the correct code. The reference *see also* is a suggestion that you may find more information looking under a different term.

The Tabular List

The Tabular List for ICD-9 consists of 17 chapters of disease descriptions and codes. It also contains a chapter for services provided for patients who seek care but are not considered ill, like patients with a family history of a disease, or those who are seen for an annual physical to prevent illness—known as V codes—and a chapter for the causes of illnesses and injuries, known as E codes. ICD-9 also includes five appendixes. Table 18-1 outlines the list of chapters in the Tabular List for ICD-9.

Very simply, the Tabular List contains very specific information in numeric sequence, to back up, or expand on, the information found in the Alphabetic Index. Once you find the condition you believe is needed—your "start point"—in the Alphabetic Index, then locate in the Tabular List the code given by the Alphabetic Index to obtain the "final destination." This is the exact code, including any fourth or fifth digits required to give you the most specific, accurate diagnosis code available for the information you are given in the medical record.

Code Structure ICD-9-CM diagnosis codes are made up of three, four, or five digits. The system uses three-digit categories, known as *rubrics*, for diseases, injuries, and symptoms. Many of these categories are divided into four-digit codes known as subcategories. Some codes are further subdivided into five-digit codes that are known as subclassifications. For example:

415	**Acute pulmonary heart disease**
	[three digits]
415.1	**Pulmonary embolism and infarction**
	[four digits; more specific]
415.11	**Iatrogenic pulmonary embolism and infarction**
	[five digits; most specific]

When listed in the ICD-9, four- and five-digit diagnosis codes must be reported on claims because they represent the most specific diagnosis documented in the patient medical record. This is known as coding to the highest level of specificity and payers require it. For example, CMS rules state that a Medicare claim will be rejected when the most specific code available is not used. In the above example, it would be incorrect to use code 415 or 415.1 because code 415.11 is available and so, as the most specific code, it must be used. Always keep in mind that the minimum code contains 3 digits, but if a fourth digit is available, it must be used, and if a fifth digit is available, it also must be used. The fourth and fifth digits are preceded by a decimal point. When placing diagnosis codes on the CMS-1500 form, however, the decimal points are omitted. More on this is covered in the *Insurance and Billing* chapter.

V Codes and E Codes These codes are used for very specific purposes, outlined here.

- **V codes** identify encounters for reasons other than illness or injury, such as annual checkups, immunizations, and normal childbirth. The descriptions for V codes are found throughout the main portion of the Alphabetic Index. V codes can be used either as primary codes for an encounter or as additional codes. You should be aware that some insurance carriers, like Medicare, do not cover V codes, so the charges associated with them may become the patient's responsibility.

- **E codes** identify the external causes of injuries and poisoning. E (for external) codes are used for injuries resulting from various environmental events, such as transportation accidents, accidental poisoning by drugs or other substances, falls, and fires. E codes are often used in collecting public health information and, more importantly, to identify who is responsible for paying the claim (worker's comp, author insurance, liability). Some beginning coders find it easy to remember that if a diagnosis makes you question "How did that happen?" at least one E code will be required to answer the question. An E code is never used alone as a diagnosis code. It always supplements the code that identifies the injury or condition itself. You might find it helpful to imagine that in addition to "external," the E also stands for "extra," so you will not be tempted to let an E code stand by itself. The alphabetic descriptions for E codes are found at the end of the Alphabetic Index in two sections. Section 2 is the alphabetic Table of Drugs and Chemicals, which is used to identify drugs and chemicals responsible for poisonings. Immediately following this, in Section 3, is the Alphabetic Index for all E codes.

TABLE 18-1	Tabular List of Chapters for ICD-9-CM.	
Classification of Diseases and Injuries		
Chapter		**Categories**
1	Infectious and Parasitic Diseases	001–139
2	Neoplasms	140–239
3	Endocrine, Nutritional, and Metabolic Diseases, and Immunity Disorders	240–279
4	Diseases of the Blood and Blood-Forming Organs	280–289
5	Mental Disorders	290–319
6	Diseases of the Central Nervous System and Sense Organs	320–389
7	Diseases of the Circulatory System	390–459
8	Diseases of the Respiratory System	460–519
9	Diseases of the Digestive System	520–579
10	Diseases of the Genitourinary System	580–629
11	Complications of Pregnancy, Childbirth, and the Puerperium	630–679
12	Diseases of the Skin and Subcutaneous Tissue	680–709
13	Diseases of the Musculoskeletal System and Connective Tissue	710–739
14	Congenital Anomalies	740–759
15	Certain Conditions Originating in the Perinatal Period	760–779
16	Symptoms, Signs, and Ill-Defined Conditions	780–799
17	Injury and Poisoning	800–999
Supplementary Classifications		
V Codes—Supplementary Classification of Factors Influencing Health Status and Contact with Health Services		V01–V91.99
E Codes—Supplementary Classification of External Causes of Injury and Poisoning		E800–E999

Both V and E codes are alphanumeric. For example, the code for a complete physical examination of an adult is V70.0. The code for a fall from a ladder is E881.0. The same rule for specificity applies to E and V codes regarding fourth and fifth digits; if a fourth or fifth digit is available, it must be utilized or the insurance carrier will reject the code.

▶ Coding with ICD-9
LO 18.3

You may think that if your office uses a superbill or an EHR program to select codes, you will not need to understand coding. This is simply not true. Every diagnosis and procedure checked off on the encounter form must be verified in the medical record. EHR programs do not understand *medical necessity*—figuring out which diagnoses best explain why a specific procedure was performed. With the limited room on an encounter form, it is very possible that the most specific diagnosis code available for the patient's condition is not listed on the encounter form. It may be your responsibility to locate the "best code for the job." If the physician uses a SOAP note format when charting (see the *Medical Records and Documentation* chapter), you can locate the diagnosis in the assessment area. If a more "free-hand" approach or "narrative" style note is used, a little detective work may be needed.

> **Example #1, from a Patient Medical Record:**
>
> CC: *Chest and epigastric pain; feels like a burning inside. Occasional reflux.*
>
> Exam: *Abdomen soft, flat without tenderness. No bowel masses or organomegaly.*
>
> Dx: *Peptic ulcer.*

The diagnosis is peptic ulcer.

Now, decide what the main term is for the condition or the diagnosis. For the diagnosis in the above scenario, the main term is *ulcer*. The word *peptic* (stomach) describes the type of ulcer and is considered a subterm. Because there is an exact diagnosis, the pain and reflux will not be coded in outpatient facilities like physician offices. Inpatient facilities such as hospitals have different rules and the symptoms would be coded.

> **Example #2, from a Patient Medical Record:**
>
> The diagnosis is sebaceous cyst. Look under *cyst*, the condition, and not *sebaceous*, the descriptive subterm. If you do look up *sebaceous*, you will see it is followed by instructions in parentheses that say "(*see also* Cyst, sebaceous)." Be sure to follow all cross-reference instructions.

Once you find the description, locate the code given for that description; it is usually to the right of the description or just below it. Verify the code in the Tabular Index and be sure to read all instructions in this section because there are often more specific instructions in the Tabular List that will help you find the right code or affirm that you have the correct code; here are some examples.

1. For the first diagnosis of peptic ulcer, the main 3-digit code for peptic ulcer is 533. The fourth digit, 9, indicates that the ulcer is not specified as acute or chronic and there is no mention of hemorrhage or perforation. The fifth digit, 0, is chosen because there is no mention of obstruction. The final code for the peptic ulcer is 533.90.

2. In the second scenario, the sebaceous cyst, the main code is 706, which denotes diseases of the sebaceous glands. The fourth digit, 2, indicates that the "disease" is a sebaceous cyst. In this example, there is no fifth digit, so the final code for a sebaceous cyst is 706.2.

In both of these cases, the level of specificity of each diagnosis was greatly increased by the addition of the "optional" fourth and fifth digits. As you can see, these digits truly are not optional at all. Lastly, do not forget to look for instructions such as *Code also* and *Code first underlying condition*, as well as *includes* and *excludes* notes that assist you in deciding on the correct code or codes.

Additional Guidelines for ICD-9 Coding

Now that you understand that you must first look up the main term and then the subterm in the Alphabetic Index, and then confirm the code in the Tabular List (a step that can never be skipped), let's look at some further guidelines that will make your coding more specific and efficient.

Acute versus Chronic Conditions An acute (including subacute for coding purposes) condition is defined as one that is of sudden onset or a more long-standing (chronic) condition that has suddenly worsened. There are times, such as with bronchitis, where the patient has both the acute form (466.0) and the underlying chronic form (491.9). When this occurs and both codes must be reported, the acute code is always listed first, followed by the code for the chronic form of the condition.

Combination Codes A combination code is one in which two diagnoses are included in one code. This may be a diagnosis with an associated secondary process (known as a manifestation) or a diagnosis with an associated complication. When a combination code is available, it must be used in place of the two single codes. An example of this is cholelithiasis (gallstones), code 574.20, with acute cholecystitis (gallbladder inflammation), code 575.0. However, because they are being diagnosed together, when you look up *cholecystitis* and see the subterm "with," you will find a direction stating that should the cholecystitis be associated with calculus (stones) in the gallbladder—See Cholelithiasis. When you do so, you will note that cholelithiasis with cholecystitis, acute, is coded at 574.0 with a notation for a fifth digit. Just above this is a box indicating that the fifth digit 0 is used if there is no mention of obstruction and 1 is used if there is obstruction. As we have no mention of obstruction in the description, the final code will be 574.00. See Figure 18-2.

Multiple Coding There are many instances when one code does not fully describe the patient's diagnosis. This often occurs when a disease or condition is the result (manifestation) of another condition. Most complications of

FIGURE 18-2   **(a)** Alphabetic Index for cholecystitis directing you to cholelithiasis. **(b)** Alphabetic Index showing the final code for acute cholecystitis with cholelithiasis (checkmark indicates the need for 5th digit). **(c)** Tabular List for 574.00 verifying correct description of calculus of gallbladder with acute cholecystitis.

Source: International Classification of Diseases, Ninth Revision, Clinical Modification, 2012, Volumes 1, 2, and 3.

diabetes mellitus fall under this category. Diabetes, as the underlying condition, is coded first (250.xx), followed by the manifestation, for instance, gangrene (785.4). Regardless of whether you look up gangrene, diabetic or diabetes, with gangrene, you will see the 250.7x code listed first with 785.4 for the gangrene in parentheses as the secondary code. Figure 18-3 outlines combination coding using the diagnosis of gangrene due to diabetes.

As this case outlines, no matter how you look up the code in the Alphabetic Index or check it in the Tabular List, you are directed which code to use first. The only information you don't have is what digit to use in the fifth position for the diabetes code. At the beginning of the diabetes section of the Alphabetic Index (Figure 18-3a) and at the beginning of the Tabular List of code 250, you will find the box represented in Figure 18-4 to assist you.

Note that diabetes codes always require a fifth digit. Be sure not to inadvertently "drop" the fourth digit prior to adding the fifth digit. So, code 250.3 is not juvenile diabetes uncontrolled; it is the rubric for diabetes with other coma and still requires one of the above numbers to complete the code.

Coding Unclear Diagnoses

Physicians frequently do not have an exact diagnosis documented. Terms such as *probable, suspected, likely, questionable, possible,* or *rule out* flag a diagnosis as being uncertain. Outpatient coding rules require that unclear diagnosis be coded using the symptoms that lead the patient to seek care, until an absolute diagnosis is made. The rules are different for inpatient coding.

Example:

Diagnosis: Nonproductive cough and fever,
Rule out bronchitis
Outpatient diagnosis: Cough (786.2)
Fever (780.60)

A similar situation occurs with "impending" or "threatened" conditions. If the condition actually occurs, code it as a confirmed diagnosis. If it did not occur, check to see if a code exists for the threatened condition and if it exists, use it. If it does not exist, code the underlying conditions or symptoms as if the condition did not exist.

Diabetes, diabetic (brittle) (congenital) (familial)
(mellitus) (severe) (slight) (without complication) 250.0 ☑

> *Note — Use the following fifth-digit subclas-*
> *sification with category 250:*
>
> 0   *type II or unspecified type, not stated*
>   *as uncontrolled*
>
> *Fifth-digit 0 is for use for type II patients,*
> *even if the patient requires insulin*
>
> 1   *type I [juvenile type], not stated as*
>   *uncontrolled*
>
> 2   *type II or unspecified type, uncon-*
>   *trolled*
>
> *Fifth-digit 2 is for use for type II patients,*
> *even if the patient requires insulin*
>
> 3   *type I [juvenile type], uncontrolled*

with

    coma (with ketoacidosis) 250.3 ☑
       due to secondary diabetes 249.3 ☑
       hyperosmolar (nonketotic) 250.2 ☑
          due to secondary diabetes 249.2 ☑
    complication NEC 250.9 ☑
       due to secondary diabetes 249.9 ☑
    specified NEC 250.8 ☑
       due to secondary diabetes 249.8 ☑
    gangrene 250.7 ☑ [785.4]
       due to secondary diabetes
          249.7 ☑ [785.4]

(a)

Gangrene, gangrenous (anemia) (artery) (cellulitis (dermatitis) (dry) (infective) (moist)
(pemphigus) (septic) (skin) (stasis) (ulcer)
785.4

with

    arteriosclerosis (native artery) 440.24
       bypass graft 440.30
          autologous vein 440.31
          nonautologous biological 440.32
    diabetes (mellitus) 250.7 ☑ [785.4]
       due to secondary diabetes
          249.7 ☑ [785.4]
abdomen (wall) 785.4
adenitis 683
alveolar 526.5
angina 462
    diphtheritic 032.0
anus 569.49
appendices epiploicae — *see* Gangrene,
    mesentery
appendix — *see* Appendicitis, acute
arteriosclerotic — *see* Arteriosclerosis, with,
    gangrene
auricle 785.4
Bacillus welchii (*see also* Gangrene, gas) 040.0
bile duct (*see* also Cholangitis) 576.8
bladder 595.89
bowel — *see* Gangrene, intestine
cecum — *see* Gangrene, intestine
Clostridium perfringens or welchii (*see also*
    Gangrene, gas) 040.0
colon — *see* Gangrene, intestine
connective tissue 785.4
cornea 371.40
corpora cavernosa (infective) 607.2
    noninfective 607.89
cutaneous, spreading 785.4
decubital (*see* also Ulcer, pressure) 707.00 [785.4]
diabetic (any site) 250.7 ☑ [785.4]
    due to secondary diabetes 249.7 ☑ [785.4]

(b)

§ ☑5th   **250.7**   **Diabetes with peripheral circulatory disorders**
    [0-3]   Use additional code to identify manifestation, as:
             diabetic:
               gangrene (785.4)
               peripheral angiopathy (443.81)
         DEF: Blood vessel damage or disease, usually in the feet, legs,
         or hands, as a complication of diabetes.
         AHA: 1Q, '96, 10; 3Q, '94, 5; 2Q, '94, 17; 3Q, '91, 10, 12; 3Q '90,
         15; **For code 250.70:** 1Q, '04, 14
         E10.51 Type 1 DM w/diab periph angiopathy w/o   1-10
         gangrene

(c)

785.4   Gangrene   CC
        Gangrene:
           NOS
           spreading cutaneous
        Gangrenous cellulitis
        Phagedena
        Code first any associated underlying condition
        EXCLUDES   *gangrene of certain sites* — *see* Alphabetic
                        Index
                       gangrene with atherosclerosis of the
                        extremities (440.24)
                       gas gangrene (040.0)

        DEF: Gangrene: necrosis of skin tissue due to bacterial
        infection, diabetes, embolus and vascular supply loss.
        DEF: Gangrenous cellulitis: group A streptococcal infection;
        begins with severe cellulitis, spreads to superficial and deep
        fascia; produces gangrene of underlying tissues.
        CC Excl: 338.0-338.4, 440.24, 780.91-780.99, 785.4,
        799.81-799.89
        AHA: 1Q, '04, 14; 3Q, '91, 12; 3Q, '90, 15; M-A, '86, 12
        196 Gangrene not elsewhere classified   1-10

(d)

FIGURE 18-3   **(a)** Alphabetic Index for diabetes, gangrene; **(b)** Alphabetic Index for gangrene, diabetic; **(c)** Tabular List for code 250.7x. **(d)** Tabular List for code 785.4.

Source: International Classification of Diseases, Ninth Revision, Clinical Modification, 2012, Volumes 1, 2, and 3.

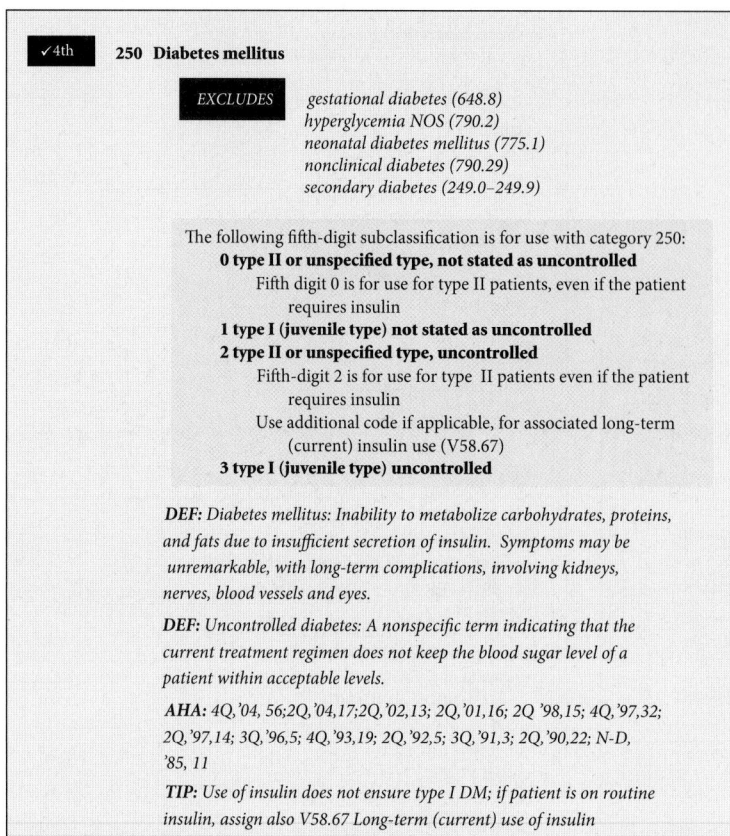

FIGURE 18-4 Fifth-digit subclassifications for category 250 (diabetes mellitus).

Source: International Classification of Diseases, Ninth Revision, Clinical Modification, 2012, Volumes 1, 2, and 3.

Example:

| **Diagnosis:** Hemorrhage in early pregnancy with threatened abortion |
| **CPT:** 640 Hemorrhage in early pregnancy |
| 640.0 Threatened abortion |

Use code 640.0 as it describes exactly the diagnosis given.

Principal versus Primary Diagnosis

The **principal diagnosis** is defined by the Uniform Hospital Discharge Data Set (UHDDS) as "that condition established after study to be chiefly responsible for occasioning the admission of the patient to the hospital for care." Outpatient coding does not generally use principal diagnoses; instead, it uses the **primary diagnosis**, defined as the main reason for the patient's visit. The **secondary** (or subsequent) **diagnoses** are other conditions that are also affecting the patient at the time of the visit and so are coded after the primary diagnosis. Procedure 18-1 at the end of this chapter outlines the steps for locating an ICD-9-CM code.

Diagnosis Related Groups and IP Coding

Unlike outpatient claims where payment is often based on the procedure performed, IP claims are paid based on a system known as *Diagnosis-related groups* or DRGs. There are over 700 DRGs which are based on four elements: Principal diagnosis; other diagnoses; significant procedures performed; and the age, sex and discharge status of the patient. As a medical assistant, you will probably never assign a DRG, but the information you give to the admitting clerk regarding the patient's condition on admission can affect the DRG assigned, so you must be thorough and accurate in the information you give regarding your patients.

▶ V Codes and E Codes   LO 18.4

As stated earlier, V codes are defined by ICD-9-CM as Supplementary Classification of Factors Influencing Health Status and Contact with Health Services. This is a very long title for codes that describe patients who are not currently ill but come to the office for reasons including history of an illness (personal or family); preventative medicine (like immunizations and physical exams); employment, school, and camp examinations; well-baby care; contraception; screenings; after care (like post surgical care); carrier status; organ donor; testing for status; and so on. The official title for E codes is Supplementary Classification of External Causes of Injury and Poisoning. As stated earlier, these are "extra" codes that tell the insurance company how an illness or injury came about. If you see a friend coming down the hall on crutches and he tells you he broke his ankle, your first question will logically be, "How did you do that?"—there is an E code for whatever explanation he gives you! E codes also include burns, poisonings, and other exposure incidences.

V Codes

Because the patient is basically "healthy," V codes are generally used in the outpatient setting. Examples of common V codes include the following:

- V04.81: Influenza vaccination (remember this is a diagnosis, not a procedure code)
- V58.11: (Encounter for) Chemotherapy treatment
    (The patient does have cancer, but the reason for the visit today is the chemotherapy administration. This will be followed by the appropriate code for the neoplasm being treated.)
- V14.0: History (personal) of allergy to penicillin
- V30.00: Vaginal delivery of single, live-born newborn (status of the newborn child)

V codes are coded via the same Alphabetic Index as the other ICD-9 codes. For the above examples, the key terms *vaccination, encounter, history,* and *delivery* will be italicized in the Alphabetic Index. Their Tabular List for verification is located directly after the injury and poisoning codes (800–999). Procedure 18-2 outlines the procedure for locating a V code.

E Codes

Because coding external cause (E) codes can be complicated, let's simply focus on getting acquainted with the basic concepts first. Some of the major categories of E codes include transport accidents; poisonings and adverse effects; accidental falls; accidents from fire and flames; accidents due to natural and environmental factors; late effects of accidents; assaults or self-injury; assaults or purposely inflicted injury and suicide; or self-inflicted injury. Both the Table of Drugs and Chemicals and the Alphabetic Index for E codes are found at the end of the main Alphabetic Index for ICD-9 codes. Now, let's discuss some specifics for the general use of E codes.

General Use of E Codes E codes are used with any diagnosis code from 001–V84.4, except for CMS (Medicare), which does not require E codes on its claim forms. In general, E codes are only used for the initial treatment for the acute illness or injury, and not for subsequent visits. The exception to this rule is treatment for acute fractures. In this case, use the E code for as long as acute treatment of the fracture is taking place. Use as many E codes as necessary to completely explain how the incident occurred. For instance, if a patient accidentally overdoses on a combination of alcohol and Valium, at least two E codes will be necessary to explain the overdose of both substances. Another example may relate to your friend with the broken ankle. It is possible that two E codes may be applicable. If he was at work and fell from scaffolding while painting a house, two codes would be necessary—fall from scaffolding (E881.1) and a place of occurrence code denoting that the accident took place at a private residence (E849.0). Place of occurrence codes are found under the key term of

Accident. All accidents occurring while using machinery or any type of motorized vehicle (including boats, motorcycles, ATVs, heavy machinery, etc.) require an E code describing the vehicle involved in the accident. Many of these codes require a fifth digit that describes the person injured—driver (1); passenger (2); motorcyclist (3); passenger of motorcycle (4); rider of animal (5); pedal cyclist (6); pedestrian (7); other specified person (8); or unspecified person (9). As with all other diagnosis codes, if a fourth or fifth digit is available, it must be used, so watch for the notes in the Tabular List (√4th or √5th) so you do not forget them and code incorrectly, resulting in possible claim rejection or denial.

Poisonings and Adverse Effects The Table of Drugs and Chemicals is located directly after the Alphabetic Index. The table consists of a row for each drug name and then six columns with the following titles: Poisoning, Accident, Therapeutic Use, Suicide Attempt, Assault, and Undetermined. Refer to the poisoning column when the medical record states "poisoning," "overdose," "wrong substance given or taken," or "intoxication." The poisoning codes (960–989) will be listed first. You then will stay in the same row but move to the column that describes how the poisoning occurred. Remember, if it is not in the medical record, it did not occur. You can only code what is described in the record. The following definitions will be helpful when deciding which column to use when choosing the E code:

- Accidental poisoning (E850–E869). This column is used for accidental overdose, wrong substance given or taken, drug taken by mistake, accidental drug usage, and accidents in drug usage in a medical facility.
- Therapeutic use (E930–E949). This column is used when the correct substance is properly administered in the correct dosage but caused a poisoning or other adverse effect.
- Suicide attempt (E950–E952). This column is used only when there is documentation of self-inflicted injury or poisoning.
- Assault (E961–E962). Documentation indicates that the injury or poisoning was inflicted by another person with the intent to injure or kill the patient.
- Undetermined (E980–E982). These codes are to be used when the intent of the poisoning or injury cannot be determined.

Examples:

#1	Diagnosis:	Hives (urticaria) due to newly diagnosed Penicillin allergy (taken as prescribed)
	ICD-9 Codes:	708.9 (allergic urticaria) and E930.0 (Penicillin therapeutic use) (There was no poisoning, so no code is used from the poisoning column)
#2	Diagnosis:	Vomiting due to intentional overdose of Valium
	ICD-9 Codes:	787.03 (vomiting), 969.4 (Valium poisoning), E950.3 (intentional OD = suicide attempt)

Burns Coding burns typically requires three codes: the degree of the burn (if there are multiple burns, they are sequenced with the highest degree first); the extent (percentage of the body burned); and the E code for how the burn occurred. To code burns, first use the key term *Burn*, then find the indented subterm for the burn location, and, finally, use the subclassification for the extent of the burn (1st, 2nd, or 3rd degree). Locations with multiple burn degrees are coded to the highest extent of the burn. Once that code is completed, return to the key term *Burn* and subterm *Extent*. Using the Rule of Nines, found in the Tabular List at the beginning of the 948 section, calculate the percentage of the body burned. Finally, locate the E code description from the Alphabetic Index for External Cause Codes and verify it in the Tabular List.

Example:

Diagnosis:	Patient presents with 1st and 2nd degree burns to right hand and wrist from boiling water
ICD-9 Codes:	944.20 (2nd degree burn hand and wrist), 948.10 (less than 10% of body surface burned and fifth digit 0 for less than 10% at 3rd degree), and E924.0 (burn by hot liquid)

Always remember that E codes are never the primary or first diagnosis listed. When used, they are listed after the primary (or secondary) diagnosis to which they relate. More than any other type of diagnosis code, E codes require practice to get perfect. Procedure 18-3 found at the end of the chapter outlines how to use E codes.

▸ Appendixes of ICD-9　　　　LO 18.5

The appendixes of the ICD-9 manual contain helpful research and technical information. Appendix A is the Morphology of Neoplasms. As you remember from your A&P and terminology classes, the term *morphology* means to change or develop. This table defines the development or changing nature of diagnosed neoplasms (new growths), most of which are malignant or cancerous. These codes, sometimes referred to as "M" codes (as they always begin with that letter), are not reported on insurance claim forms. They are used with "O" codes developed by WHO for tracking of oncology diagnoses. Administrative medical assistants and other coders can assign M codes while coding diagnoses, but certified tumor registrars are responsible for assigning the M codes based on the diagnosis code assigned. M codes are noted in the Alphabetic Index in parentheses.

Example:

Paget's disease (osteitis deformans) 731.0
　　with infiltrating duct carcinoma of the breast
　　(M8541/3)—See Neoplasm, breast, malignant

In the above example, in order to code Paget's disease with breast cancer, you would look up neoplasm, breast, malignant. The instructions also direct you to the morphology code of M8541/3. In looking at Appendix A, you will find that code M8541/3 reads "Paget's disease with infiltrating duct carcinoma of the breast." The M code itself defines the type of cancer and the digit after the forward slash (/) represents the morphology (behavior) of the neoplasm as listed below:

/0	Benign
/1	Uncertain whether benign or malignant. Borderline malignancy
/2	Carcinoma in situ
	Intraepithelial (within epithelial cells)
	Noninfiltrating (cancer that has not spread to other nearby areas)
	Noninvasive (cancer that has not spread outside of the original site)
/3	Malignant, primary site
/6	Malignant, metastatic (or secondary) site
/9	Malignant, uncertain whether primary or metastatic site

When coding malignant neoplasms, the primary site is the location where the cancer originated. The secondary or metastatic site(s) describes the area where the cancer or malignancy has spread.

Appendix B formerly contained the glossary of Mental Disorders. It was officially deleted on October 1, 2004.

Appendix C is the Classification of Drugs by American Hospital Formulary Service Number and the ICD-9 Equivalent. These are equivalent codes between the AHA Formulary and ICD-9. The Formulary number is in the left column, the description is in the middle, and the ICD-9 code is in the right column.

Example:

AHFS	Description	ICD-9-CM
8:12.16	The Penicillins	960.0

Appendix D is the Classification of Industrial Accidents According to Agency. It lists the 3-digit categories for occupational hazards divided into the following subcategories:

1. Machines
2. Means of Transport and Lifting Equipment
3. Other Equipment
4. Materials, Substances and Radiations
5. Working Environment
6. Other Agencies, Not Elsewhere Classified
7. Agencies Not Classified for Lack of Sufficient Data

Again, these codes are not placed on insurance claims; instead they are used by state and federal agencies to summarize industrial accidents.

Appendix E consists of a listing of the Three Digit Categories used by ICD-9-CM, labeled for the chapter each represents. An example is shown here:

17. INJURY AND POISONING	
Fracture of skull (800–804)	
800	Fracture of vault of skull
801	Fracture of base of skull
802	Fracture of face bones
803	Other and unqualified skull fractures
804	Multiple fractures involving skull or face with other bones

A Basic Comparison of ICD-9-CM and ICD-10-CM

LO 18.6

The ICD was originally introduced in 1893 by The International Statistical Institute as the first International List of Causes of Death, requiring physicians to better track a patient's diagnosis and medical care. The responsibility of ICD was taken over by WHO in 1948 when morbidity causes were added in the sixth edition. ICD-9, introduced in 1975, does not allow the addition of new, more precise diagnoses that have developed over the years. There are approximately 14,200 codes in the ICD-9-CM, while the new ICD-10-CM contains over 68,000 codes. This allows greater specificity for diagnosis classifications and provides expansion for new codes. This is particularly important relating to *code linkage*—between ICD diagnosis codes and the CPT procedure codes to prove the *medical necessity* of a patient's procedure or treatment (refer to the *Insurance and Billing* chapter for more information). You will learn more about CPT in the *Procedure Coding* chapter. At this time, many other countries in the world have adopted at least some version of ICD-10-CM. As with any change or update in the medical office, such as the claim update from the 4010 to the 5010 format or from paper medical records to an EHR program, the transition from ICD-9 to ICD-10 presents challenges to medical assisting students and to medical offices. The student must learn both systems instead of only one system, as in the past. The medical offices must not only learn the new system but also accommodate both systems during an overlap period. Table 18-2 shows basic comparisons of the two systems.

Additionally, remember that ICD-9 also includes volume 3, containing procedures performed primarily in the hospital-based setting. Because of the increase in the number of diagnoses and hospital-based procedures, ICD-10 will include a totally separate volume for hospital procedure codes called ICD-10-PCS.

ICD-10 Information

As you can see from Table 18-2, by converting to ICD-10, we jumped from 14,200 diagnosis codes available with ICD-9 to 68,000 possibilities with ICD-10. Because of this increase in codes, the number of chapters also increased from 17 with the two additional chapters for V- (18) and E- (19) codes to 21 chapters for ICD-10.

Alphabetic and Numeric Indexes

Like ICD-9, the 10th edition of ICD contains the Alphabetic (Alpha) Index of the diseases, conditions, and related terms. When coding in ICD-10, as with ICD-9, you will still begin with the Alpha Index, which may direct the coder to a related term such as "pain." Once the term is identified in the Alpha Index, just like in ICD-9, it directs the coder to the lists of appropriate codes in the Tabular (numeric) List. The ICD-10 Tabular List incorporates 21 **chapters** with the alphanumeric range for each as listed in Table 18-3. A **category** has

TABLE 18-2	Basic Comparison of ICD-9-CM and ICD-10-CM Codes	
Feature	**ICD-9**	**ICD-10**
Number of codes	14,200	68,000
Format	3–5 characters. First character may be alpha or numeric; 2–5 are numeric	3–7 characters. First character alpha (uppercase); 2 and 3 are numeric; 4–7 may be alpha or numeric
Specificity	Limited	Expanded
Laterality	None	Has laterality
Decimal point	After 3rd character; not always used	Decimal must be used after third character
Placeholder	0 as 4th digit is present when 5th digit is required	"x" used as placeholder for a nonexistent digit when 6th or 7th digit is required for code specificity
Combination codes	Some	Expanded number of combination codes
External causes of morbidity and mortality including poisonings	E codes	Instead of a separate section, external causes are included as V01–Y99 codes
Factors influencing health status	V codes	Instead of a separate section, health status codes are included as Z00–Z99 codes

TABLE 18-3	Chapter, Description, and Code Ranges for ICD-10-CM	
Chapter	**Description**	**Code Range**
1	Certain infectious and parasitic diseases	A00–B99
2	Neoplasms	C00–D49
3	Diseases of the blood and blood-forming organs and certain disorders involving the immune mechanism	D50–D89
4	Endocrine, nutritional, and metabolic diseases	E00–E89
5	Mental and behavioral disorders	F01–F99
6	Diseases of the nervous system	G00–G99
7	Diseases of the eye and adnexa	H00–H59
8	Diseases of the ear and mastoid process	H60–H95
9	Diseases of the circulatory system	I00–I99
10	Diseases of the respiratory system	J00–J99
11	Diseases of the digestive system	K00–K95
12	Diseases of the skin and subcutaneous tissue	L00–L99
13	Diseases of the musculoskeletal system and connective tissue	M00–M99
14	Diseases of the genitourinary system	N00–N99
15	Pregnancy, childbirth, and the puerperium	O00–O9A
16	Certain conditions originating in the perinatal period	P00–P96
17	Congenital malformations, deformations, and chromosomal abnormalities	Q00–Q99
18	Symptoms, signs, and abnormal clinical and laboratory findings; not elsewhere classified	R00–R99
19	Injury, poisoning, and certain other consequences of external causes	S00–T88
20	External causes of morbidity	V01–Y99
21	Factors influencing health status and contact with health services	Z00–Z99

TABLE 18-4 Example of Greater Specificity Available with ICD-10 vs. ICD-9

ICD-9 (limited specificity)	ICD-10 (expanded specificity)
Code: 233.0 Carcinoma in situ breast (vague as to cancer type)	Code: D05.01 Lobular carcinoma in situ of right breast OR Code: D05.11 Intraductal carcinoma in site of right breast

TABLE 18-5 Example of ICD-10 Placeholder, Which Is Not Available in ICD-9

ICD-9-CM	ICD-10-CM
910.0 Face, neck, and scalp; abrasion or friction burn without mention of infection	S00.01 Abrasion of scalp (code noted to √x7th)
910.1 Face, neck, and scalp; abrasion or friction burn, infected	S00.01xA Abrasion of scalp, initial encounter S00.01xD Abrasion of scalp, subsequent encounter S00.01xS Abrasion of scalp, sequela

TABLE 18-6 Example of an ICD-10 Combination Code

ICD-9-CM	ICD-10-CM
995.92 Severe sepsis and 785.52 Septic shock	R65.21 Severe sepsis with septic shock

3 characters and a **subcategory** has 4–5 characters, with the final code consisting of up to 7 characters. The use of these characters will become clearer as examples are provided later in the chapter.

Characters and Specificity

Although there are similarities between ICD-9 and ICD-10, perhaps the most striking difference is the way the ICD-10 code looks in comparison to an ICD-9 code. The change in the look is directly related to the need to expand the specificity of many of the diagnosis codes and so a new format was required. All ICD-10 codes begin with an alpha character. The number of possible characters has increased from 3–5 in ICD-9 to 3–7 in the ICD-10 edition. Again, the intent of the ICD-10 is to provide a more precise clinical picture of the patient and enhanced trending analysis. Table 18-4 provides an example of the increased specificity of the new coding system using the diagnosis of breast cancer.

From the example in Table 18-4, some of the limitations of ICD-9 can be clearly seen. For example, code 233.0, which consists of only 4, all-numeric characters, only tells us the patient has carcinoma in situ of the breast—it does not tell us the type of cancer, nor does it tell us which breast is affected. In order to choose the most specific code in ICD-10, which consists of 6 characters, you would need to know both the type of cancer affecting the patient and which breast was affected (replacing the 5th digit 1 for the above ICD-10 codes with a 2 would mean the patient's cancer is affecting the left breast).

Placeholders

The ICD-9 did not incorporate a placeholder in anticipation of new codes. If a 5th digit was required, a 4th digit was present and had to be used before adding the "optional" 5th digit. The ICD-10 uses an "x" to hold a place for future expansion of the code's specificity. An example is illustrated in Table 18-5. Note the instruction of √x7th—our base code (only contains 5 characters).

In looking at Table 18-5, it is clear that ICD-10 Chapter 19 "S" (injury) codes require a 7th-digit to explain the encounter determination:

- "A" designates an initial encounter.
- "D" designates a subsequent encounter.
- "S" designates sequel.

If the "x" placeholder and 7th digit are not present, the code will not be accepted. Also note that just like in ICD-9, these "optional characters" are not optional. You must also be careful when adding characters that you do not "drop" the "x" placeholder. For example, if you dropped the "x" placeholder in coding the initial encounter for a scalp abrasion, you would end up with S00.01A—a code that does not exist in ICD-10 and would be rejected. You must be very detail-oriented to code efficiently and accurately.

Combination Codes

The ICD-9-CM accommodates only a relatively small number of combination codes, often requiring the use of multiple codes to completely code a condition, illness, or injury. The ICD-10-CM contains many more combination codes, greatly cutting down on the need for multiple codes for a single diagnosis. An example of a combined code appears in Table 18-6.

In some cases, multiple codes are also used with ICD-10 coding when appropriate. One example is coding for pregnancy and prenatal visits, which often require more than one code to describe completely.

▶ Basic Coding Guidelines for ICD-10   LO 18.7

The basic rules for coding with ICD-10 remain similar to those of ICD-9. Many of the same conventions are used in ICD-10 to assist the coder in finding and choosing the correct code. Although coding manuals and coding software are publisher specific and may include color-coding and formatting assists, the conventions are universal. The general steps "walk" you through the coding structure to locate the correct code. They may be compared to putting together the pieces of a puzzle. Let's review the basic guidelines for ICD coding:

- Locate the term in the Alphabetic Index.
- Refer to the notes under the appropriate heading.
- Read and follow the terms in the parentheses and brackets.

TABLE 18-7   Common Conventions found in ICD-10-CM

Convention	Meaning	Example
Code First/Use Additional Code	The underlying condition must be listed first and any manifestation caused by this condition is listed second. In the Alphabetic Index, the manifestation code is listed in brackets.	F02 Dementia in other diseases classified elsewhere Code first underlying physiological condition, such as: Alzheimer's (G30.-)
NEC (Not elsewhere classifiable)	In the index, this means "other specified." When a specific code is not available, you are directed to an "other specified" code.	Dislocation of foot, specified site NEC S93.33- (the dash means an additional digit will be given in the tabular index to complete the code.)
NOS (Not otherwise specified)	The provider has not given enough information to choose a more specific code.	A04.9 Bacterial intestinal infection, unspecified
Code Also	Instruction that two codes may be required, if enough information is provided, in order to completely code the scenario; but sequencing information is not given.	J44 Other chronic obstructive pulmonary disease *Code also type of asthma, if applicable (J45.-)*
See and See Also	*See* follows a main term in the Alpha Index and instructs that another term should be investigated. *See also* is also in the Alpha Index and indicates that another term may be helpful in choosing the correct description.	Amentia —See also Retardation, mental Dilatation cardiac (acute) (chronic) see also Hypertrophy, cardiac
Default codes	Codes listed next to a main term. It represents the condition commonly associated with the main term or the unspecified code for that condition.	K37 Appendicitis (If no other information about the patient's condition is given, this default code will be used.)
Includes	Terms/conditions listed may be included with the diagnosis.	J36 Peritonsillar abscess Includes: abscess of tonsil peritonsillar cellulitis quinsy
Excludes1	The code is excluded and should never be used at the same time as the code above the Exclude1 note. The two conditions cannot occur together.	E11 Type 2 diabetes Excludes1: gestational diabetes(O24.4-) type 1 diabetes (E10.-)
Excludes2	The condition is excluded as not part of the condition represented by the code, but if the patient actually has both conditions, both may be coded.	J03 Acute tonsillitis Excludes2: chronic tonsillitis (J35.0)
[] Brackets	Brackets are used in the alphabetic index and indicate manifestation (secondary) codes.	Disease, diseased Alzheimer's G30.9 [F02.80]
() Parentheses	Parentheses are used in both indices enclosing supplemental or "nonessential" information, which will not affect the code selection.	Discord (with) boss Z56.4 classmates Z55.4
: Colon	A colon is used after an incomplete term that requires one or more of the modifiers that follow it to allow the code to be assigned.	J33 Nasal polyp Use additional code to identify: exposure to environmental tobacco smoke (Z77.22) exposure to tobacco smoke in the perinatal period (P96.81)
, Comma	Words following a comma are essential modifiers and must be present in the diagnosis in order to use the code.	K40.0 Bilateral inguinal hernia, with obstruction, without gangrene

- Proceed to the Tabular List number(s) as directed by the Alphabetic Index.
- Follow instructional terms to direct you to the appropriate code.
- Use caution with chapter categories that have an alphabetical character that may be mistaken for a numerical character, like the letter "O" for Chapter 15, Pregnancy, Childbirth, and the Puerperium (may be mistaken for the number "0").
- Assign the appropriate code using the highest degree of specificity.
- Assign an additional appropriate code for other signs and symptoms that may not be routinely associated with the condition or disease process.

To follow these steps, it is also necessary to understand the terms, abbreviations, and symbols found in Table 18-7.

As you will discover, the importance of the medical record is emphasized throughout this text. To accurately code a diagnosis, the coder must first obtain an accurate diagnostic description from the medical record. The ICD-10 requires more detailed physician documentation to attain the level of description required by the new system. Like the ICD-9, NEVER code directly from the Alpha Index (Figure 18-5). All codes must be verified in the Tabular List to be sure descriptions are correct and all notes are followed. Always select the code that corresponds to the medical record documentation.

FIGURE 18-5 The first "page" of the ICD-10-CM Alphabetic Index.

Source: ICD-10-CM, The Official Draft Code Set, 2010 Draft by Ingenix.

▶ Synopsis of ICD-10 Coding Guidelines by Chapter

LO 18.8

The majority of ICD-10-CM codes follow the general guidelines. However, unique coding applications also exist. These include but are not limited to neoplasms, diabetes mellitus, fractures, pregnancy, external causes of morbidity and mortality, R codes, poisonings, and expanded Z codes (formerly V codes). A synopsis of guidelines for the ICD-10 chapters that require unique coding applications follows.

Chapter 1: Certain Infectious and Parasitic Diseases (A00–B99)

In an outpatient setting, requesting a confirmatory serology or culture for HIV is not enough to code HIV positivity. Only the diagnostic statement such as "known HIV" or "positive HIV" is adequate from the provider. When no definitive diagnosis or manifestation of HIV is present and the patient has an inconclusive serology, code R75, inconclusive laboratory evidence of human immunodeficiency virus, should be assigned. Patients who have had a positive serology or culture and have developed an HIV-related illness should be assigned code B20 on every encounter. Patients who are HIV positive but asymptomatic in status should be assigned code Z21. This code should be assigned for all patients with the diagnostic statement of positive HIV. When a patient presents with any signs or symptoms while being seen for HIV testing, code only the signs and symptoms. If counseling is provided during the same encounter, an additional counseling code out of Z71.7 may be reported.

Chapter 2: Neoplasms (C00–D49)

Chapter 2 of ICD-10-CM deals with neoplasms and is very similar to the ICD-9. To assign a proper code, documentation of the neoplasm must state whether it is benign, malignant, in situ, or of uncertain behavior. These are presented in the Table of Neoplasms and are listed by anatomic location such as an adenoma (a tumor of a gland). Once the site of the neoplasm is identified, any additional instructions for coding must be observed. An additional code, like one identifying exposures to carcinogenic (cancer-causing) substances that may be the underlying cause of the patient's cancer diagnosis, may be required. Two examples of carcinogens as underlying causes are exposure to tobacco smoke (Z77.22) or exposure to tobacco smoke in the perinatal period (P96.81).

The correct coding and sequencing of neoplasms is critical. As when coding in ICD-9, if the treatment is directed at the primary neoplasm, that code is used as the principal (or primary) diagnosis. If the neoplasm has metastasized and the patient's treatment is for the secondary site, then the secondary neoplasm would become the primary diagnosis. If chemotherapy, radiation therapy, or immunotherapy—although each is generally considered a procedure and not a diagnosis—is the primary reason for medical care, it is coded first, followed by the code for the malignancy being treated.

Chapter 4: Endocrine, Nutritional, and Metabolic Diseases (E00–E89)

Chapter 4 contains the codes for diabetes mellitus. The documentation and the assignment of codes within this ICD-10 chapter are very similar to those in the ICD-9. Codes for diabetes mellitus are combination codes that include the type of diabetes:

- Type 1—insulin-dependent diabetes (IDDM), sometimes referred to as juvenile diabetes
- Type 2—noninsulin-dependent diabetes (NIDDM)

In addition to the type of diabetes, the body system affected by diabetes and the condition affecting the anatomical structure are included. When the type of diabetes is not documented in the medical record (and the physician cannot be queried), then the patient should be assigned a code for type 2 diabetes mellitus. The coding and sequencing rules for diabetes mellitus remain the same for ICD-10 as for ICD-9. As shown in Figure 18-6, any underlying condition must be sequenced first. If the diabetes causes a complication (like retinopathy—disease of the retina), code the diabetes first and code the retinopathy second. If documentation supports the patient's use of insulin, then assignment of code Z79.4 should be sequenced after the diabetes diagnosis is coded completely.

Chapter 5: Mental and Behavioral Disorders (F01–F99)

When patients experience pain, whether acute or chronic, it should be documented if the pain is exclusively psychological. Pain that is associated with and is exclusively psychological should

Diabetes mellitus (E08-E13)

E08 Diabetes mellitus due to underlying condition

Code first the underlying condition, such as:
    Congenital rubella (P35.0)
    Cushing's syndrome (E24.-)
    Cystic fibrosis (E84.-)
    Malignant neoplasm (C00-C96)
    Malnutrition (E40-E46)
    Pancreatitis and other diseases of the pancreas (K85-K86.-)
Use additional code to identify any insulin use (Z79.4)
Excludes1: drug or chemical induced diabetes mellitus (E09.-)
    gestational diabetes (O24.4-)
    neonatal diabetes mellitus (P70.2)
    type 1 diabetes mellitus (E10.-)
    type 2 diabetes mellitus (E11.-)

E08.0 Diabetes mellitus due to underlying condition with hyperosmolarity
    E08.00 Diabetes mellitus due to underlying condition with hyperosmolarity without nonketotic hyperglycemic-hyperosmolar coma (NKHHC)
    E08.01 Diabetes mellitus due to underlying condition with hyperosmolarity with coma
E08.1 Diabetes mellitus due to underlying condition with ketoacidosis
    E08.10 Diabetes mellitus due to underlying condition with ketoacidosis without coma

FIGURE 18-6 Diabetes mellitus codes with underlying conditions using ICD-10.
Source: ICD-10-CM, The Official Draft Code Set, 2010 Draft by Ingenix.

be assigned code F45.41: pain disorder with related psychological factors, followed by the appropriate code from the category G89.

Chapter 6: Diseases of the Nervous System (G00-G99)

The nervous system chapter in ICD-10 no longer includes the eye and ear; they have each been given individual chapters (7 and 8); otherwise, the coding from the nervous system has changed very little since ICD-9. As stated above, code G89 is used for pain diagnoses. This code may be used as a first-listed diagnosis when the reason for the encounter is the treatment of the pain. If the patient is seen for a definitive diagnosis (like cancer) and pain is also noted, then the definitive diagnosis should be listed first, followed by the most specific pain code possible. If malignant neoplasm is the underlying cause of the pain, the appropriate pain code is G89.3.

Chapter 9: Diseases of the Circulatory System (I00-I99)

ICD-10, like ICD-9, uses the hypertension table in the Alpha Index and the rules for coding hypertension have not changed. Primary hypertension, also known as essential hypertension, is coded as I10. When hypertension is caused by an underlying condition (secondary hypertension), two codes are required—the first to identify the underlying **etiology** (cause) and the second to code the hypertension. A patient who has elevated blood pressure may not necessarily have a diagnosis of hypertension. This is known as transient hypertension, and the code R03.0 should be assigned.

Chapter 10: Diseases of the Respiratory System (J00-J99)

Coding within the respiratory system has also changed very little between ICD-9 and ICD-10. It should be noted, however,

that positive laboratory documentation is not required in order to code either avian or H1N1 influenza as a diagnosis. When the physician's documentation states "suspected or probable" avian influenza or H1N1 influenza, codes should be assigned as if the condition exists (J09.0 category). Documentation of any another type of influenza should be assigned codes from the J10 category. Figure 18-7 shows the difference in the Tabular List between Avian influenza codes and descriptions and

J09.098 Influenza due to identified avian influenza virus with other manifestations
    Influenza due to identified avian influenza virus encephalopathy
    Influenza due to identified avian influenza virus myocarditis
    Influenza due to identified avian influenza virus otitis media
J09.1 Influenza due to identified novel H1N1 influenza virus
    2009 H1N1 [swine] influenza virus
    Novel 2009 influenza H1N1
    Novel H1N1 influenza
    Novel influenza A/H1N1
    Swine flu
    J09.11 Influenza due to identified novel H1N1 influenza virus with respiratory manifestations
        Acute influenzal upper respiratory infection due to identified novel H1N1 influenza virus
        Influenzal laryngitis due to due to identified novel H1N1 influenza virus
        Influenzal pharyngitis due to due to identified novel H1N1 influenza virus
        Influenzal pleural effusion due to due to identified novel H1N1 influenza virus
        Code also any associated pneumonia (J12-J18)

(a)

J10 Influenza due to other influenza virus
Influenza due to unspecified influenza virus
Code first any associated lung abscess (J85.1)
Use additional code to identify the virus (B97.-)
Excludes2: Hemophilus influenzae [H.influenzae] infection NOS (A49.2)
    Hemophilus influenzae [H. influenzae] laryngitis (J04.0)
    Hemophilus influenzae [H. influenzae] meningitis (G00.0)
    Influenza due to avian influenza virus (J09.0-)
    Influenza due to novel H1N1 influenza virus (J09.1-)
    Influenza due to swine flu (J09.1-)
J10.1 Influenza due to other influenza virus with respiratory manifestations
    Acute influenzal upper respiratory infection due to other influenza virus
    Influenza NOS
    Influenzal laryngitis due to other influenza virus
    Influenzal pharyngitis due to other influenza virus
    Influenzal pleural effusion due to other influenza virus
    Code also any associated pneumonia (J12-J18)
J10.8 Influenza due to other influenza virus with other manifestations
    J10.81 Influenzal gastroenteritis
        Excludes1: "intestinal flu" [viral gastroenteritis] (A08.-)
    J10.89 Influenza due to other influenza virus with other manifestations
        Influenzal encephalopathy
        Influenzal myocarditis
        Influenzal otitis media

(b)

FIGURE 18-7 (a) Tabular List for influenza due to avian influenza virus and (b) Tabular List for influenza due to other influenza virus.
Source: ICD-10-CM, The Official Draft Code Set, 2010 Draft by Ingenix.

those for Influenza due to other influenza virus. Note that manifestations of avian and H1N1 virus are included in the code descriptions.

Chapter 13: Diseases of the Musculoskeletal System and Connective Tissue (M00–M99)

This chapter contains the categories for fractures, which are coded quite differently in the ICD-10 than in ICD-9. Laterality for fractures is new and designated as follows:

- unilateral—4th digit "1"
- laterality designated by—5th digit:
  - 0—unspecified
  - 1—right
  - 2—left

Another major change in ICD-10 is the addition of a 7th character designating the type of encounter for which the patient is being seen. Pathological fractures due to osteoporosis include this 7th character. Shown in Figure 18-8 are the six capital letters used for this mandatory 7th character.

For the purposes of these 7th-character extensions, the term *initial* means an active fracture that is still healing, *subsequent* defines follow-up after the active fracture care, and *sequela* refers to care after the injury has healed, but there are now different issues related to the initial injury that must be attended to. To better understand the coding concepts within this section, let's take a look at Figure 18-9 for a patient who has age-related osteoporosis with a current pathological fracture of the right shoulder. Based on the information in Figure 18-9, the code would be M80.011; however, because of the information you received on the necessary 7th characters (Figure 18-8), you know that if the patient had a subsequent visit for the fracture as a routine checkup for a healing fracture, you would use the code M80.011D.

M80 Osteoporosis with current pathological fracture
Includes: osteoporosis with current fragility fracture
Note: fragility fracture is defined as a fracture sustained with trauma
            no more than a fall from a standing height or less that occurs
            under circumstances that would not cause a fracture in a
            normal healthy bone
Use additional code to identify major osseous defect, if applicable
(M89.7-)
Excludes1:collapsed vertebra NOS (M48.5)
            pathological fracture NOS (M84.4)
            wedging of vertebra NOS (M48.5)
Excludes2:personal history of (healed) osteoporosis fracture (Z87.310)
The appropriate 7th character is to be added to each code from
category M80:
            A   initial encounter for fracture
            D   subsequent encounter for fracture with routine healing
            G   subsequent encounter for fracture with delayed healing
            K   subsequent encounter for fracture with nonunion
            P   subsequent encounter for fracture with malunion
            S   sequela

FIGURE 18-8 Codes and the 7th characters for osteoporosis with pathological fracture.
Source: ICD-10-CM The Official Draft Code Set 2010 Draft by Ingenix.

M80.01 Age-related osteoporosis with current pathological fracture, shoulder
M80.011 Age-related osteoporosis with current pathological fracture, right shoulder
M80.012 Age-related osteoporosis with current pathological fracture, left shoulder
M80.019 Age-related osteoporosis with current pathological fracture, unspecified shoulder

FIGURE 18-9 Tabular List for subclassification M80.01 Age-related osteoporosis with current pathological fracture, shoulder.
Source: ICD-10-CM, The Official Draft Code Set, 2010 Draft by Ingenix.

Chapter 14: Diseases of the Genitourinary System (N00–N99)

ICD-10 provides for four stages of chronic kidney disease (CKD). Code N18.1 is the beginning stage; N18.2, mild CKD; N18.3, moderate CKD; and N18.4, severe CKD. If end-stage renal disease (ESRD) is documented, use code N18.6. This code will be used alone, even if both chronic kidney disease and end-stage renal disease are documented. Keep in mind that kidney transplant (Z94.0–kidney transplant status) may not totally restore kidney function so both Z94.0 and a code for chronic kidney disease, if still present, may be coded.

Chapter 15: Pregnancy, Childbirth, and the Puerperium (O00–O9A)

Similar to the ICD-9 that requires a 5th digit (the highest specificity for the system) when coding pregnancies, the ICD-10 often requires a 7th digit (the highest specificity for the system). With many codes, the 7th digit specifies the trimester of the pregnancy in which the condition occurs. Read these descriptions carefully. If the patient is in a different trimester than the one stated, you must look for a different code. With codes describing pregnancy conditions related to multiple gestation, the 7th digit specifies the number of fetuses in utero. Maternity coding can be complicated, but thorough reading of the medical record documentation and understanding of the coding guidelines specific to this chapter will allow optimal confidence in coding.

Chapter 17: Congenital Malformations, Deformations, and Chromosomal Abnormalities (Q00–Q99)

Codes from this chapter are used exclusively when a patient's medical record documents that the diagnosis or condition is congenital or chromosomal in nature. Codes Q00–Q99 may be listed as either primary or secondary diagnoses, depending on the guidelines given within the coding instructions. Diseases and conditions found within this section include hydrocephalus, spina bifida, atrial septal defect, limb malformations and deformities, cleft lip/palate, Trisomy 21 (Down syndrome), and many others.

Chapter 18: Signs, Symptoms, and Abnormal Clinical and Laboratory Findings (NEC) (R00–R99)

Chapter 18, Signs, Symptoms and Abnormal Clinical and Laboratory Findings (NEC), R00–R99, is primarily used to code for the following types of conditions:

TABLE 18-8 Excerpt from ICD-10 Table of Drug and Chemicals for the substance Sulfonazide

Substance	Poisoning Accidental	Poisoning Intentional	Poisoning Assault	Poisoning Undetermined	Adverse Effect	Underdosing
Sulfonazide	T37.1x1	T37.1x2	T37.1x3	T37.1x4	T37.1x5	T37.1x6

- Cases that do not have a more specific diagnosis after all the findings are analyzed.
- Transient signs and symptoms at the initial encounter with undetermined cause.
- Provisional diagnosis in a patient not returning for further care.
- Cases without a definitive diagnosis referred elsewhere.
- Cases in which a definitive diagnosis could not be determined.
- Additional information that represents a significant but currently asymptomatic medical problem (such as an asymptomatic HIV-positive patient).

There are multiple combination codes available in this chapter. Watch for them and follow guidelines for their use. If a combination code is available, it must be used to avoid "unbundling" the code.

Chapter 19: Injury, Poisoning, and Certain Other Consequences of External Causes (S00–T88)

With the exception of the new 7th-character extension used in ICD-10, coding from this chapter is very similar to coding with ICD-9. As in ICD-9, the table format for poisonings is also used in ICD-10. You will also note that because poisoning codes require very specific codes, the "x" placeholder is often found in the 5th position, the sixth digit of 1–6 describes how the poisoning took place, and then a 7th digit of A (initial), D (subsequent), or S (sequelae) is used to describe the type of encounter. An illustration for the substance "sulfonazide" is in Table 18-8.

Note that the table does not give you the 7th-digit options. This is a perfect example of why you must always verify codes in the Tabular List to obtain the entire correct code. If a 7th digit is required and is not in place, the insurance carrier will not accept the code. For any of the above poisoning codes for sulfonazide to be complete, the letter, A, D, or S will have to be added to the code describing the encounter as initial, subsequent, or a sequela.

Burns and Corrosions Burns are classified by three factors: depth of the burn (first-degree, second-degree, or third-degree), the extent (total body area—based on the rule of nines), and the agent (fire, thermal, or appliance). Burns that are caused by a corrosive material are coded the same as any burn with the additional code for the corrosive material being sequenced first.

Chapter 20: External Causes of Morbidity and Mortality (V00–Y99)

Codes within this chapter identify who, what, when, and where an accident or injury occurred. They are used for data

in determining research and prevention strategies for injuries. These codes may be used as secondary codes to describe health conditions and are applicable for categories A00–T88.9 and Z00–Z99. Figure 18-10 shows some of the categories for these secondary codes, previously referred to as E codes in ICD-9. The use of these codes should completely identify the patient's cause of injury. An example would be a sprained ankle while playing football. The cause of the injury is a fall, the activity is football, and the location is the playground at the time of injury. When assigning multiple external cause codes, the code indicating the cause or intent, or medical misadventure, is reported before the code for the place, activity, or external status codes. When reporting multiple causes of injuries, codes for child and adult abuse take priority over all other external cause codes. Read the guidelines carefully.

Chapter 21: Factors Influencing Health Status and Contact with Health Services (Z00–Z99)

The unique ICD-9 V codes (used to code for healthcare encounters other than injury or illness, such as prenatal care or administration of immunizations) were replaced by Chapter 21, Factors Influencing Health Status and Contact with Health

V10–V19	Pedal cyclist injured in transport accident
V20–V29	Motorcycle rider injured in transport accident
V30–V39	Occupant of three-wheeled motor vehicle injured in transport accident
V40–V49	Car occupant injured in transport accident
V50–V59	Occupant of pick-up truck or van injured in transport accident
V60–V69	Occupant of heavy transport vehicle injured in transport accident
V70–V79	Bus occupant injured in transport accident
V80–V89	Other land transport accidents
V90–V94	Water transport accidents
V95–V97	Air and space transport accidents
V98–V99	Other and unspecified transport accidents
W00–X58	Other external causes of accidental injury
W00–W19	Slipping, tripping, stumbling and falls
W20–W49	Exposure to inanimate mechanical forces
W50–W64	Exposure to animate mechanical forces
W65–W74	Accidental drowning and submersion
W85–W99	Exposure to electric current, radiation and extreme ambient air temperature and pressure
X00–X08	Exposure to smoke, fire and flames
X10–X19	Contact with heat and hot substances
X30–X39	Exposure to forces of nature
X52, X58	Accidental exposure to other specified factors
X71–X83	Intentional self-harm
X92–Y08	Assault
Y21–Y33	Event of undetermined intent
Y35–Y38	Legal intervention, operations of war, military operations, and terrorism
Y62–Y84	Complications of medical and surgical care
Y62–Y69	Misadventures to patients during surgical and medical care

FIGURE 18-10 Sample from the Tabular List of external cause code ranges for ICD-10.

Source: ICD-10-CM, The Official Draft Code Set, 2010 Draft by Ingenix.

Services, Z00–Z99 in ICD-10. In addition to incorporating the traditional ICD-9 V codes, this category is greatly expanded to include, but is not limited to, the following reasons for health-care encounters:

- Chemo, radiation, and immunotherapy.
- After care.
- Administrative exams (such as a sports physical).
- Family history if the patient may be at risk for like illness.
- Personal history if the patient's habits or past illnesses or condition place him at risk.

Diagnosis coding can be intimidating. Like learning anything new, take it a little bit at a time, and remember, practice does make perfect. Read all guidelines carefully. Don't be afraid to ask questions—particularly if you do not understand terminology—so that you are capable of choosing the most appropriate code. Coding takes concentration, an in-depth knowledge of A&P and medical terminology, and, most importantly, an "inquiring mind" to get to the heart of the patient's diagnosis and make sure that the codes truly describe what is wrong with each patient. Procedure 18-4 at the end of this chapter outlines the steps in coding from the ICD-10-CM manual.

Go to CONNECT to see a video about *Locating an ICD-10-CM Code.*

PROCEDURE 18-1 Locating an ICD-9-CM Code

Procedure Goal: To analyze diagnoses and locate the correct ICD code.

OSHA Guidelines: This procedure does not involve exposure to blood, body fluids, or tissue.

Materials: Patient record, charge slip or superbill, and ICD-9-CM manual.

Method: Procedure steps.

1. Locate the patient's diagnosis on the superbill (encounter form) or elsewhere in the patient's chart. If it is found on the superbill, verify documentation in the medical chart.
   RATIONALE: The medical record documentation must back up all diagnosis codes used for billing.

2. Find the diagnosis in the ICD-9's Alphabetic Index. Look for the condition first, then locate the indented subterms that make the condition more specific. Read all cross-references to check all the possibilities for a term, including its synonyms and any eponyms.

3. Locate the code from the Alphabetic Index in the ICD-9's Tabular List.

RATIONALE: All codes must be verified in the Tabular List to be sure the most accurate code is chosen.

4. Read all information to find the code that corresponds to the patient's specific disease or condition. Study the list of codes and descriptions. Be sure to pick the most specific code available. Check for the symbol that shows that fourth (and) fifth digits may be required.
   RATIONALE: The 4th and 5th digits allow for specificity. If they are given, they must be used or the insurance carrier will not accept the code for payment.

5. Be sure that all necessary codes are chosen to completely describe each diagnosis. Check for instructions stating an additional code is needed. If more than one code is needed, be sure instructions are followed and the codes are listed in the correct order.
   RATIONALE: In order to accurately code the patient's condition, all applicable codes must be chosen and recorded as instructed by the ICD manual.

6. Carefully record the diagnosis code(s) on the insurance claim and proofread the numbers.

PROCEDURE 18-2 Locating a V Code

Procedure Goal: To analyze the patient record (or encounter form) and decide whether a V code is an appropriate diagnosis code.

OSHA Guidelines: This procedure does not involve exposure to blood, body fluids, or tissue.

Materials: Patient record, charge slip or superbill, and ICD-9-CM manual.

Method: Procedure steps.

1. Locate the patient's diagnosis. This information may be found on the superbill (encounter form) or elsewhere in the patient's chart. If it is on the superbill, verify documentation in the medical chart.

   RATIONALE: All information billed to the insurance carrier must be backed up by the patient medical record.

2. If the reason for the patient encounter relates to a physical exam, immunization, well-child visit, or other visit where there is no diagnosis or condition of illness found, a V code will be used to code the reason for the visit (diagnosis).

3. Find the diagnosis in the ICD-9's Alphabetic Index. Look for the condition first and then locate any indented subterms that make the condition more specific. Read all cross-references.

   RATIONALE: Subterms assist in locating codes with the greatest specificity.

4. Locate the code from the Alphabetic Index in the V code area of the ICD-9's Tabular List.

5. Read all descriptive information to find the code that corresponds to the patient's specific reason for today's visit. Be sure to pick the most specific code available. Check for the symbol that shows that a fourth and (possibly) a fifth digit is required.
   RATIONALE: Fourth and fifth digits are required to record the most specific code available.

6. Be sure that that no other codes are required to describe the patient's reason for the visit. Check for instructions stating an additional code is needed. If more than one code is needed, be sure instructions are followed and the codes are listed in the correct order.
   RATIONALE: The patient's condition must be coded so all information about the diagnosis is included in the coded diagnoses. If codes are listed in the wrong order, the insurance carrier may reject them.

7. Carefully record the diagnosis code(s) on the insurance claim and proofread the numbers.

PROCEDURE 18-3 Locating an E Code

Procedure Goal: To analyze the patient record (or encounter form) and decide whether an E code is required to completely code the encounter.

OSHA Guidelines: This procedure does not involve exposure to blood, body fluids, or tissue.

Materials: Patient record, charge slip or superbill, and ICD-9-CM manual.

Method: Procedure steps.

1. Locate the patient's diagnosis. This information may be found on the superbill (encounter form) or elsewhere in the patient's chart. If it is on the superbill, verify documentation in the medical chart.
   RATIONALE: All information billed to the insurance carrier must be backed up by the patient medical record.

2. If the patient's diagnosis begs the question "How did that happen?" an E code is required to give the insurance carrier as much information as possible.
   RATIONALE: Without the E code, the payer does not know how the injury or illness occurred.

3. After coding the diagnosis of the condition requiring treatment, open the ICD-9 manual to the External Cause Alphabetic Index or, if necessary, use the Table of Drugs and Chemicals. Find the appropriate description in the

ICD-9's Alphabetic Index, looking for the condition first, and then locate any indented subterms that make the condition more specific. Read all cross-references.
   RATIONALE: Subterms assist in locating codes with the greatest specificity.

4. Locate the code from the Alphabetic Index in the E code area of the ICD-9's Tabular List.

5. Read all descriptive information to find the code that corresponds to how the patient's current condition came about. Choose the most specific code available. Check for the symbol that shows that a fourth and (possibly) a fifth digit are required; many E codes require these.
   RATIONALE: Fourth and fifth digits are required to record the most specific code available.

6. Carefully record the diagnosis code(s) on the insurance claim and proofread the numbers.

7. E codes are always secondary, so be sure that the primary diagnosis code is listed first. Check for instructions stating an additional code(s) is needed. If more than one code is needed, be sure instructions are followed and the codes are listed in the correct order.
   RATIONALE: The coding order is important. Insurers may deny claims if codes are not placed in the appropriate order.

PROCEDURE 18-4 Locating an ICD-10-CM Code

Procedure Goal: To analyze diagnoses and locate the correct ICD code.

OSHA Guidelines: This procedure does not involve exposure to blood, body fluids, or tissue.

Materials: Patient record, charge slip or superbill, and access to ICD-10-CM codes on the CMS website: www.cms.hhs.gov/ICD10/01_Overview.asp, or access to a draft copy of the 2010 ICD-10-CM manual.

Method: Procedure steps.

1. Locate the patient's diagnosis. This information may be found on the superbill (encounter form) or elsewhere in the patient's chart. If it is on the superbill, verify documentation in the medical chart.
   RATIONALE: The medical record must back up all diagnoses chosen.

2. Find the diagnosis in the ICD-10 Alpha Index. Look for the condition first, then locate the indented subterms that make the condition more specific. Read all cross-references to check all the possibilities for a term, including its synonyms and any eponyms.
   RATIONALE: Cross-references give additional information, making coding easier.

3. Following the directions in the Alpha Index, locate the code or code range from the Alpha Index in the ICD's Tabular List.

4. Read all information and instructions carefully to find the code that exactly corresponds to the patient's specific

disease or condition. Carefully study the list of codes and descriptions. Be sure to pick the most specific code available.

RATIONALE: ICD-10 was created to allow for code expansion and greater specificity.

5. Watch for instructions advising of the need for additional codes as well as instructions regarding coding sequence and need for 6th and 7th digits or placeholders.

RATIONALE: Placeholders and the additional digits supply the specificity required by insurance carriers for payment.

6. Document the chosen codes carefully, remembering sequencing instructions.

RATIONALE: Transposing characters on the correctly chosen code will make it incorrect for the payer, and sequencing can mean the difference between payment and denial.

SUMMARY OF LEARNING OUTCOMES

LEARNING OUTCOMES	KEY POINTS
18.1 Recall the six ways that ICD codes are used today.	ICD codes are used to facilitate payment for medical services, evaluate utilization patterns (patient use of healthcare facilities), study healthcare costs, research quality of healthcare, predict healthcare trends, and plan for future healthcare needs.
18.2 Describe the conventions used by ICD-9-CM.	The conventions used in ICD include NOS; NEC; brackets; slanted brackets; parentheses; colon; brace; includes and excludes notes; instructions to *use additional code, code first underlying disease*, and *code, if applicable, any causal condition first*. Additionally, bold and italics are used in both the Alphabetic Index and Tabular List. Instructions to *omit code, see condition*, and *see also* are found exclusively in the Alphabetic Index.
18.3 Outline the steps to code a diagnosis using ICD-9-CM.	To choose an ICD code, check the encounter form (superbill) and/or patient medical record for all applicable diagnoses. Find the key term in the Alphabetic Index and then search for any applicable subterms. Once the code has been located, verify its description in the Tabular List, again reading all applicable notations for other coding options and instructions. Document each code carefully using instructions as to code sequencing on the CMS-1500 claim form.
18.4 Explain the purpose and usage of V codes and E codes.	V codes are defined as *Supplementary Classification of Factors Influencing Health Status and Contact with Health Services.* They are used for patients who, though not ill, are seeking healthcare. They are used for exams (V70.0), counseling (V61.10), donors (V59.01), and so on. E codes are defined as *Supplementary Classification of External Causes of Injury and Poisoning.* They are used to explain how an illness or injury came about. Examples of E codes include cyclist accident (E826.1), accidental poisoning by antibiotics (E856), and exposure to laser radiation (E926.4).
18.5 Name the appendixes found in ICD-9-CM.	The following appendixes are found in ICD-9-CM: Appendix A is the Morphology of Neoplasms. Appendix B formerly contained the Glossary of Mental Disorders; it was officially deleted on October 1, 2004. Appendix C is the Classification of Drugs by American Hospital Formulary Service Number and the ICD-9 Equivalent. Appendix D is the Classification of Industrial Accidents According to Agency. Appendix E consists of a listing of the Three Digit Categories used by ICD-9-CM.

LEARNING OUTCOMES	KEY POINTS
18.6 Compare ICD-9-CM and the ICD-10-CM.	ICD-10-CM is intended to provide a more precise clinical picture of the patient and enhanced trending analysis for data reporting. The number of codes increases from under 15,000 in the ICD-9 to 68,000 in the ICD-10 and the characters change from 3–5 numerical (with the exception of the E and V codes) to 3–7 alphanumeric. Both the 9th and 10th revisions contain the Alphabetic Index of the diseases, conditions, and related terms. The ICD-10 Tabular List incorporates 21 chapters (versus ICD-9 with 17 chapters) with a corresponding range of codes. Many codes use an "x" as a placeholder for future expansion, which was not possible with ICD-9.
18.7 Summarize the ICD-10-CM general coding guidelines.	The technique of coding with ICD-10 is very similar to that of coding with ICD-9-CM. The diagnosis or symptom is located first in the Alphabetic Index and all notes considered. You then move to the Tabular List as instructed in the Alpha Index. After following terms, abbreviations, and symbols, the appropriate code with the highest specificity supported by medical record documentation is selected.
18.8 Illustrate unique coding applications for neoplasms, diabetes mellitus, fractures, R codes, poisonings, and Z codes.	The majority of ICD-10 CM codes follow the general guidelines. However, unique coding applications do exist and chapter guidelines must be followed. These include but are not limited to the chapters on neoplasms, diabetes mellitus, fractures, R codes, poisonings, and the new Z codes.

C A S E   S T U D Y   C R I T I C A L   T H I N K I N G

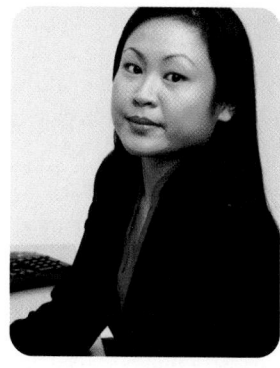

Recall Cindy Chen from the beginning of the chapter. Now that you have completed the chapter, answer the following questions regarding her case.

1. How would you code Cindy's HIV-positive status using (a) ICD-9? (b) ICD-10?
2. What other diagnosis codes would you use related to Cindy's symptoms, using each coding system?

E X A M   P R E P A R A T I O N   Q U E S T I O N S

1. (LO 18.1) Which organization maintains and updates the ICD system?
   a. AMA
   b. AAMA
   c. WHO
   d. TJC
   e. BWW

2. (LO 18.2) The Alphabetic Index for ICD-9-CM is organized by
   a. The part of the body involved
   b. Symptoms the patient displays
   c. Codes found in the Tabular List
   d. The condition
   e. The alphabet

3. (LO 18.2) _____ provide coding guidelines for using the ICD code set.
   a. Abbreviations
   b. Punctuation
   c. Chapter openers
   d. Notes
   e. Conventions

4. (LO 18.3) Matching a procedure with the diagnosis describing why the procedure was done is known as
   a. Reasonable doubt
   b. Medical necessity
   c. Proof of need
   d. Rationale
   e. A requirement

5. (LO 18.3) Which diagnosis gives the primary reason for the patient's outpatient visit?
   a. Primary diagnosis
   b. Principal diagnosis
   c. Secondary diagnosis
   d. Probable diagnosis
   e. V code diagnosis

6. (LO 18.4) Which diagnosis code type can never "stand alone"?
   a. A principal diagnosis
   b. A V code
   c. An E code
   d. A primary diagnosis
   e. A supplemental diagnosis

7. (LO 18.5) Which is the description for Appendix A of ICD-9?
   a. Three Digit Categories used by ICD-9-CM
   b. Classification of Drugs by American Hospital Formulary Service
   c. Glossary of Mental Disorders
   d. Classification of Industrial Accidents According to Agency
   e. Morphology of Neoplasms

8. (LO 18.6) The primary reason for the ICD-10 update is:
   a. There are more diagnoses to choose from
   b. It works better with EHR programs
   c. It provides greater specificity for diagnosis classifications
   d. It provides room for expansion for new codes
   e. c & d

9. (LO 18.7) Which coding convention is NOT new in ICD-10?
   a. Includes 1 & 2
   b. Excludes 1 & 2
   c. Default Code
   d. See/See Also
   e. Placeholders

10. (LO 18.8) Which ICD-10 chapter replaces the V codes found in previous versions of ICD?
    a. Chapter 21
    b. Chapter 20
    c. Chapter 10
    d. Chapter 5
    e. Chapter 1

www.mhhe.com/BoothMA5e

Go to CONNECT to see EHR activities on *Activating an ICD-9 Code* and *Using an ICD-9 Code*.

Procedure Coding

PATIENT INFORMATION

Patient Name	Gender	DOB
Raja Lautu	F	8/3/19XX

Attending	MRN	Allergies
Elizabeth H. Williams, MD	224-86-564	Benzalkonium Chloride, Sulfa

Raja Lautu is a 42-year-old woman who had a (screening) digital mammogram with CAD (computer-aided detection) performed recently as part of her physical examination. When the mammogram revealed a small density in the right breast, an ultrasound of this breast was ordered with stereotactic breast biopsy. Considering Raja's family history reveals that both her mother and maternal aunt have had breast cancer, she is understandably nervous about this development.

Keep Raja in mind as you study this chapter. There will be questions at the end of the chapter based on the case study. The information in the chapter will help you answer these questions.

LEARNING OUTCOMES

After completing Chapter 19, you will be able to:

19.1 List the sections of the CPT manual, giving the code range for each.
19.2 Describe briefly each of the CPT's general guidelines.
19.3 List the types of E/M codes within the CPT.
19.4 List the areas included in the Surgical coding section.
19.5 Locate a CPT code using the CPT manual.
19.6 Explain how to locate a HCPCS code using the HCPCS coding manual.
19.7 Explain the importance of code linkage in avoiding coding fraud.

KEY TERMS

add-on code
bundled codes
concurrent care
consultation
counseling
critical care
Current Procedural Terminology (CPT)
downcoding
E/M code
established patient

global period
HCPCS Level II codes
Healthcare Common Procedure Coding System (HCPCS)
modifier
new patient
panel
procedure code
unbundling
upcoding

VIII. C (1) Describe how to use the most current procedural coding system

VIII. C (2) Define upcoding and why it should be avoided

VIII. C (4) Describe how to use the most current HCPCS coding

VIII. P (1) Perform procedural coding

VIII. A (1) Work with physician to achieve the maximum reimbursement

7. Basic Keyboarding/Computer Concepts

Graduates:

b. (2) Apply computer application skills using variety of different electronic programs including both practice management software and EMR software

8. Medical Office Business Procedures/Management

Graduates:

t. Perform diagnostic and procedural coding

hh. Receive, organize, prioritize, and transmit information expediently

Introduction

In the previous chapter, you were introduced to diagnosis coding—the reason(s) why the patient sought healthcare. In this chapter, you will explore the language of procedural coding. You will learn how to translate the medical terms for the procedures and services provided to patients into code numbers selected from standardized procedural coding systems. These codes, when placed correctly on the healthcare claims introduced in the *Insurance and Billing* chapter, explain to third-party payers the services patients received from the provider.

After you study the concepts of procedure or CPT codes, you will explore the "linking" of diagnosis codes with procedure codes to explain the *medical necessity* of each procedure or service performed. Finding the correct codes can require detective work! The reward is accurate procedure codes that, when combined with accurate and appropriate diagnosis codes, bring the maximum appropriate reimbursement to the physicians in your medical office.

The CPT Manual   LO 19.1

After an office or clinic visit, hospital or nursing home visit, inpatient or outpatient consultation, or even a house call, each procedure and service performed on or for a patient is reported on healthcare claims using a **procedure code**. These codes represent medical procedures, such as surgery and diagnostic tests, as well as medical services, like physical examinations to evaluate a patient's condition. Medical assistants often choose these procedure codes—based on the information provided by the physician on the encounter form, or from within the patient medical chart or electronic health record—and use them to report physicians' services.

Current Procedural Terminology (CPT)

The most commonly used system of procedure codes is found in the **Current Procedural Terminology** or simply **CPT**, a reference manual published by the American Medical Association (AMA). CPT is the HIPAA-required code set that translates descriptions for physicians' and other providers' healthcare-related procedures into 5-digit codes.

Like ICD, the CPT manual is updated yearly; new codes are used for services provided beginning January 1 of each new year. In each edition, newly developed procedures are added and old ones are revised or, if obsolete, deleted. These changes are also available in an electronic file for computerized medical offices. As with ICD codes, remember that the choice of which set of codes to use is based on the date of service, not the date of the claim. If claims are submitted January 2, 2014, and the date of service was December 23, 2013, CPT codes from 2013 would be used; for services provided on January 2, 2014, the 2014 edition of the CPT codes would be used.

Medical offices should always have the current year's CPT available for reference and keep forms up to date. Like ICD codes, if current codes are not used, medical claims are often denied. Previous editions of each coding manual should be kept for at least several months after the new edition is released for use with claims for dates of service in the prior year, and for reference in case questions arise regarding previously submitted claims.

Organization of the CPT Manual

CPT codes are organized into six main sections:

Section	Range of Codes
Evaluation and Management	99201–99499
Anesthesiology	00100–01999 99100–99140
Surgery	10021–69990
Radiology	70010–79999
Pathology and Laboratory	80048–89356
Medicine (except for anesthesia)	90281–99199 99500–99602

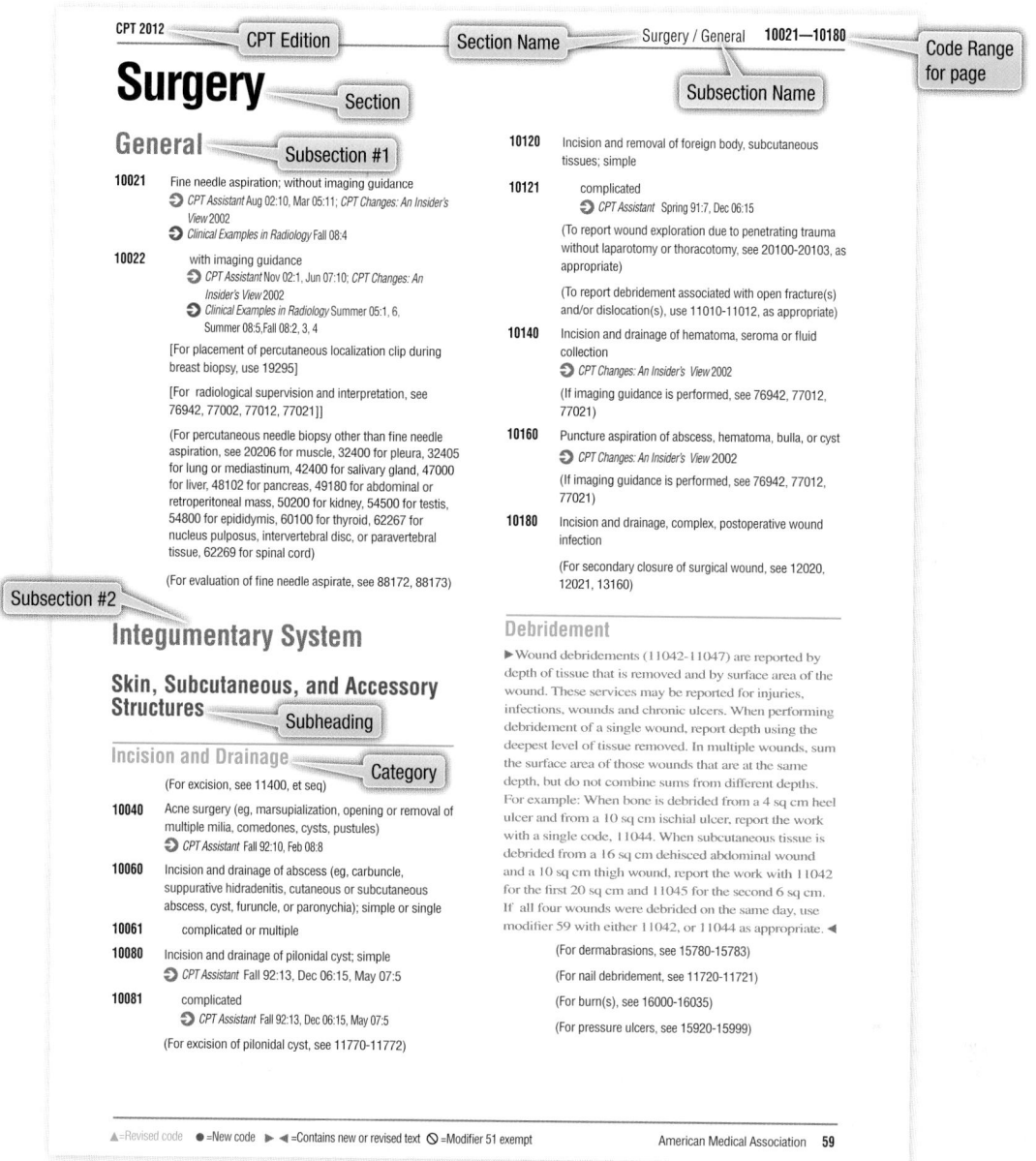

FIGURE 19-1 CPT manual page showing edition, section, subsection, subheading, and category names as well as the code range on the page.

In looking at the section numbers above, you will note that except for the Evaluation and Management section, the sections are listed in numeric order by code range. Because Evaluation and Management (or E/M codes) are used so frequently, they are placed in the front of the manual for easy reference.

The Introduction to the CPT manual gives the user important general instructions for the use of CPT. In this section, you will also find helpful information regarding common prefixes, suffixes, and word roots found within the manual. CPT is also full of helpful illustrations of the human body. A descriptive list of illustrations and the page number where each can be found is also in the Introduction. In addition, pay close attention to the guidelines found at the beginning of each new section, as these provide important overall information for coding in each section. The CPT sections are divided into categories, which, in turn, are further divided into headings according to the type of test, service, or body system. Code number ranges included on a particular page are found in the upper-right corner so a code can be located quickly after using the index (see Figure 19-1).

Note that each page also gives you other important information, including

- Section name. The section is the name used by CPT to denote each chapter. In Figure 19-1, the section name is Surgery.

- Subsection name. The subsection is the area within the section detailing the body system you are in. In Figure 19-1, the first subsection is General. Note that the next subsection for Surgery—Integumentary System—starts part way down the page.

- Subheading. The subheading describes the body area for the body system you are looking at. Figure 19-2 shows the subheading of Skin, Subcutaneous, and Accessory Structures.

Integumentary System

Subsection #2 on page

Skin, Subcutaneous, and Accessory Structures

Subheading

Incision and Drainage

Category

(For excision, see 11400, et seq)

10040   Acne surgery (eg, marsupialization, opening or removal of multiple milia, comedones, cysts, pustules)
> CPT *Assistant* Fall 92:10. Feb 08:8

10060   Incision and drainage of abscess (eg, carbuncle, suppurative hidradenitis, cutaneous or subcutaneous abscess, cyst, furuncle, or paronychia); simple or single

10061   complicated or multiple

10080   Incision and drainage of pilonidal cyst; simple
> CPT *Assistant* Fall 92:13, Dec 06:15, May 07:5

10081   complicated
> CPT *Assistant* Fall 92:13, Dec 06:15, May 07:5

(For excision of pilonidal cyst, see 11770-11772)

FIGURE 19-2   Surgery subsection for the Integumentary System.

- Category. The category describes the procedure area. In Figure 19-2, you will find the Incision and Drainage (or I&D) category.

▶ General CPT Guidelines

LO 19.2

As stated earlier, each CPT section contains guidelines for that particular section. Now, let's discuss the general guidelines, found at the beginning of the manual and followed throughout.

CPT Code Format

CPT codes are 5-digit numeric codes. Most codes are stand-alone codes with the complete description listed next to the appropriate code. The exception to this rule is the code description containing a semicolon, which is then followed by a code with an indented description. An indented description means that you refer back to the previous code description, reading the information prior to the semicolon and adding the indented code information after the colon to complete the description. Let's look at the following example:

Example:

| 25500 | Closed treatment of radial shaft fracture; without manipulation |
| 25505 | with manipulation |

To read the full description for code 25505, read code 25500 up to the semicolon and then substitute the description for 25505 after the semicolon. Following these instructions, the full description for 25505 is: *Closed treatment of radial shaft fracture; with manipulation.*

Add-on Codes

A plus sign (+) is used for **add-on codes**. These codes are used to describe procedures done in addition to a "main" procedure. For example, in Figure 19-3, you will note that code 11001 has a plus sign in front of it with a description of *each additional 10% of body surface, or part thereof* (List separately in addition to code for primary procedure).

CPT code 11001 is also an indented code, meaning it is related to the code immediately preceding it (code 11000). The description for code 11000 is *Debridement of extensive eczematous or infected skin; up to 10% of body surface.* In putting the two codes together, you would be telling the insurance carrier that up to 20% of the body surface was debrided. Example #1 shows you the correct coding when 20% of the body surface area is debrided and Example #2, when 25% (up to 30%) of the body is debrided.

Example #1: Debridement of 20% of body surface area.

Code 11000	(debridement of first 10% of body surface)
	And
Code 11001	(debridement of second 10% of body surface area or part thereof)

11000—11043   Surgery / Integumentary System

—— *Coding Tip* ——

Use of Depth and Surface Area For Reporting Debridement of Wounds

When performing debridement of a single wound, report depth using the deepest level of tissue removed. In multiple wounds, sum the surface area of those wounds that are at the same depth, but do not combine sums from different depths.

CPT Coding Guidelines, Debridement

11000   Debridement of extensive eczematous or infected skin; up to 10% of body surface
> CPT *Assistant* May 99:10

(For abdominal wall or genitalia debridement for necrotizing soft tissue infection, see 11004-11006)

+ 11001   each additional 10% of the body surface, or part thereof (List separately in addition to code for primary procedure)
> CPT *Assistant* May 99:10 CPT *Changes: An Insider's View* 2009

(Use 11001 in conjunction with 11000)

FIGURE 19-3   Add-on code 11001 for use exclusively with primary code 11000.

Example #2: Debridement of 25% of body surface area.

Code 11000	(debridement of first 10% of body surface)
	And
Code 11001	(debridement of second 10% of body surface area)
	And
Code 11001	(debridement for the next 5% as the description states "next 10% or part thereof")

Appendix D in the CPT manual contains a complete listing of all add-on codes in the manual.

As stated previously, also be alert for indented codes. For these codes, you will read the description of the "parent code" up to the semicolon and then replace the information following the semicolon with the information found in the indented code description. In Figure 19-1, codes 10022, 10061, 10081, and 10121 are all examples of indented codes. Add-on codes are never reported alone. They are always used with the primary code.

Symbols Used in CPT

The CPT manual uses instructional symbols to give repetitive information without adding multiple pages. Refer to Table 19-1 for examples of each symbol.

- *Blue triangle*. This symbol tells the user the code description has been revised in some way from last year. Note in Table 19-1 that code 22520 has a blue triangle next to it; this indicates the code description has changed from the 2011 CPT manual's description. This information could be important, as the change could mean the procedure performed by the physician may now require a different code. It could also

mean something as simple as the placement of a comma or semicolon has changed.

- *Red dot*. The symbol denotes a new code for this edition of the CPT. In Table 19-1, note that code 20527 is a new procedure code as of 2012 CPT.
- *The # sign*. The # (pound) sign, introduced in 2010, is used to denote codes that are out of numeric sequence. Referring to Table 19-1, (indented) code 27337 "works with" code 27327. It is followed by code 27328—causing it to be out of numeric order.

Example:

27327	Excision, tumor, soft tissue of thigh or knee area, subcutaneous; less than 3 cm
27337	3 cm or greater
27328	Excision, tumor, soft tissue of thigh or knee area, subfascial (eg, intramuscular); less than 5 cm

This was done so code numbers would not be "reshuffled" every year. If the pound sign were not used and codes were to remain in numeric order, for code 27327 to have an indented code, code 27328 would have to be used. Code 27328 had previously been assigned its description. To keep all codes in numeric order, all codes from 27328 with its new description and all other codes on this page would have to be assigned new descriptions. This is a lot of work and very confusing with constantly changing code descriptions on a yearly basis. Note that each code is also found in red, in its "proper numeric place" with directions telling the coder in what code range to locate the out-of-sequenced code.

TABLE 19-1	**Common CPT Symbols, Descriptions, and Examples**		
Symbol	**Meaning**	**Example**	
▲	Code description has changed since last revision	22520	Percutaneous vertebroplasty (bone biopsy included when performed), 1 vertebral body, unilateral or bilateral injection; thoracic
●	New code since last revision	20527	Injection, enzyme (e.g., collagenase), palmar fascial cord (i.e., Dupuytren's contracture)
#	Codes are out of numeric sequence	27337	3 cm or greater
		27328	Excision, soft tissue of thigh or knee area, subfascial (e.g., intramuscular); less than 5 cm
►◄	Text between triangles is new or revised	29581	Application of multi-layer compression system; leg (below knee), including ankle and foot ►(Do not report 29581 in conjunction with 29540, 29580, 29582, 36475, 36478, 97140)◄
⊘	Multiple procedures performed or add-on code which does not require multiple procedure modifier of 51	20974 ⊘	= Modifier 51 Exempt Electrical simulation to aid bone healing; noninvasive (nonoperative)
⚡	FDA approval pending	90664	Influenza virus vaccine, pandemic formulation, live for intranasal use
⊙	Moderate (conscious) sedation is included in the procedure	44385	Endoscopic evaluation of small intestinal (abdominal or pelvic) pouch; diagnostic, with or without collection of specimen(s) by brushing or washing (separate procedure)

- *Triangles pointing toward each other.* Triangles pointing toward each other with text between them denote new or revised text information. Traditionally, these arrows were green, but you will also see them used for the out-of-sequence coding information. See code 29581 in Table 19-1.

Example:

> ▲ 29581   Application of multi-layer compression system; leg (below knee), including ankle and foot
> ● *CPT Changes: An Insider's View* 2010, 2012
>
> ▶ (Do not report 29581 in conjunction with 29540, 29580, 29582, 36475, 36478, 97140) ◀

- *Circle with diagonal line.* This symbol is noted in Table 19-1 as "Modifier 51 Exempt." As you will learn shortly, modifier 51 is used when multiple procedures are performed in the same session. Modifier 51 exempt codes are those to which the multiple procedure modifier does not apply. Appendix E of the CPT manual lists the modifier 51 exempt codes. Additionally, modifier 51 is never appended to a designated add-on code.
- *Lightning bolt.* The lightning bolt is used to denote vaccines pending FDA approval. Appendix K in the CPT manual lists the vaccines affected by this symbol. When the vaccines are approved, they will be listed on the AMA site at www.ama-assn .org/ama/pub/category/10902.html and then in subsequent CPT editions.
- *Bull's-eye.* The bull's-eye symbol denotes moderate (conscious) sedation and means it is understood that conscious sedation is necessary for the procedure performed and so is included in the procedure; it cannot be billed separately. Many endoscopy procedures include this symbol.

Example:

> 44385   Endoscopic evaluation of small intestinal (abdominal or pelvic) pouch; diagnostic, with or without collection of specimen(s) by brushing or washing (separate procedure)

Because this code includes sedation as part of the procedure, administered by the physician performing the procedure, there will be no separate charge for the anesthesia. The CPT manual's Appendix G lists all codes that include moderate (conscious) sedation.

Whenever you are coding, always watch carefully for these symbols. Their instructions are explicit and must be followed to ensure correct procedural coding.

Modifiers

One or more two-digit **modifiers** (up to three per procedure) may be assigned to the five-digit main code. Modifiers are written in column 24D on the CMS-1500 Claim Form (see Figure 17-9). The use of a modifier shows that one or more special circumstance applies to the service or procedure the physician performed. For example, in the surgery section, the modifier 62 indicates that two surgeons worked together, each performing part of a surgical procedure during an operation. Each

physician will be paid part of the amount normally reimbursed for that procedure code. The CPT's Appendix A explains the proper use of each modifier. Some section guidelines also discuss the use of modifiers within the individual section's coding information. Table 19-2 gives a brief overview with examples of common CPT modifiers.

Category II Codes, Category III Codes, and Unlisted Procedure Codes

Category II codes are optional, supplemental tracking codes used to track healthcare performance measures, like programs and counseling to avoid tobacco use (Code 4000F or 4001F if medication is instituted to assist patient). Category III codes are "temporary" CPT codes for emerging technology, services, and procedures. An example of a category III code is 0051T Implantation of a total replacement heart system (artificial heart) with recipient cardiectomy. If available, these codes should be used instead of the *unlisted codes* found throughout the CPT manual. Category II and III codes are both found directly after the last of the Medicine codes in the CPT manual.

When no code is available to completely describe a procedure, a code for an unlisted procedure is selected. Unlisted procedure codes are used for new services or procedures that have not yet been assigned codes in CPT. When these codes are used, which is rare, a procedure or service description (usually from the medical record) is sent with the claim submission. Some payers, including Medicare and Medicaid, prefer the use of HCPCS codes (when available) instead of the unlisted procedure codes used with CPT. Check with individual payers to learn each payer's preferences.

Coding Terminology

Before you begin coding, you must have a basic understanding of common terminology used throughout the CPT manual. Some of these terms are defined in the following paragraphs.

Bundled codes consist of any code that includes more than one procedure in its description. Read code descriptions carefully, as it is unethical (and often considered fraudulent) to intentionally unbundle procedures into component codes when a bundled procedure code is available. For instance, all therapeutic procedures include diagnostic codes unless noted otherwise, so if a diagnostic knee arthroscopy (29870) is turned into a therapeutic arthroscopy (29871), only the therapeutic arthroscopy will be reported because it is understood that a diagnostic procedure must have taken place in order for the therapy to have taken place.

Concurrent care is described as similar care being provided by more than one physician. This frequently occurs when a patient is hospitalized and multiple specialists are caring for the patient. The services provided may be similar, but because of the differing specialties, the care is not considered to be duplication of services.

Critical care is provided to unstable, critically ill patients. Constant bedside attention is needed in order to code critical care, so the physician's documentation must be explicit regarding the time spent with the patient. The time need not

TABLE 19-2   Common CPT Modifiers

Modifier	Description	Example
22	**Increased Procedural Services.** When the work required to complete the service is much more than usually required, modifier 22 may be added to the CPT code. Medical record documentation will be required. This modifier may not be attached to E/M code.	Because of extreme scarring and previous surgeries, lysis of adhesions (CPT 58740) requires almost twice the normal time frame. Code 58740-22.
23	**Unusual Anesthesia.** Once in a while, a procedure that normally does not require anesthesia or anesthetic, because of unusual situations, will require general anesthesia.	Excision of subcutaneous tumor of neck because of patient age of 4, requires general anesthesia. Code 11424-23.
24	**Unrelated E/M Service by the same physician during a post-operative period.** The patient may require the services of the physician for treatment of an unrelated condition during a global surgical period.	The patient is one week post-op laparoscopic cholecystectomy. During post-op check, patient states asthma appears to be in exacerbation. Code 99024 for post-op visit. Code 99213-24 for E/M visit for asthma.
25	**Significant, Separately Identifiable E/M Service by the Same Physician on the Same Day of the Procedure or Other Service.** While in the office for a specific procedure, the patient may require an E/M service above and beyond that normally provided during usual pre- and/or post-procedure period.	Patient comes in for a previously scheduled mole removal (11401). Prior to procedure, physician notes BP is elevated. When procedure is completed, BP is still noted to be elevated. Physician makes adjustment to patient's anti-hypertensive medication and counsels diet adjustments. Code 11401. Code 99212-25
26	**Professional Component.** Some procedures (like radiology) contain a combination of professional and technical components. If the physician provides only the professional component, modifier 26 is added.	Screening mammography, bilateral (CPT 77057). Hospital performs the mammogram; physician provides interpretation. Code 77057-26.
TC	**Technical Component.** This is the HCPCS modifier that is the "reverse" of modifier 26. It designates the provision of the technical component only.	Screening mammography, bilateral (CPT 77057). Hospital performs the mammogram; physician provides interpretation. Hospital Code 77057-TC.
32	**Mandated Services.** Service (like a consult) is required by insurance carrier, governmental, or regulatory agency.	Insurance carrier requires a second opinion prior to an elective surgical procedure. Physician performs consult regarding need for surgery. Code 99242-32.
47	**Anesthesia by Surgeon.** Surgeon provides and administers anesthesia other than local anesthesia. Modifier is appended to the surgical procedure.	Procedure performed is shoulder manipulation under regional anesthesia by orthopedic surgeon. Code 23700-47.
50	**Bilateral Procedure.** Modifier used if procedure is not defined as bilateral but procedure is performed on both sides of the body.	Procedure: Bilateral knee arthroscopy. Code 29870-50.
51	**Multiple Procedures.** When the same provider performs multiple procedures (other than E/M, PT, and Rehab or supply provision) in the same session, the first procedure is listed as usual and subsequent procedures should include the addition of modifier 51.	Code 15877. Suction-assisted lipectomy; trunk. Code 15879-51. Suction-assisted lipectomy; lower extremity.
52	**Reduced Services.** Due to circumstances, service is reduced or eliminated by the physician.	Exploratory laparotomy for removal of malignant neoplasm, but cancer is widely metastasized so procedure is halted. Code 49000-52.
53	**Discontinued Procedure.** Similar to modifier 52, except in this case, the procedure is discontinued due to patient condition becoming endangered.	Patient is undergoing diagnostic colonoscopy when significant PVCs become evident and uncontrollable. Procedure is halted. Code 45330-53.
54	**Surgical Care Only.** Surgeon provides only the surgical care with other physician(s) providing pre- and post-op care.	Total abdominal hysterectomy with bilateral salpingo-oophorectomy (TAH-BSO) surgery only. Code 58150-54.
55	**Postoperative Management Only.** Physician provides postoperative care only.	Total abdominal hysterectomy with bilateral salpingo-oophorectomy (TAH-BSO) postoperative care only. Code 58150-55.
56	**Preoperative Management Only.** Physician provides preoperative care only.	Total abdominal hysterectomy with bilateral salpingo-oophorectomy (TAH-BSO) preoperative care only. Code 58150-56.
57	**Decision for Surgery.** During an E/M service, decision is made that surgery is required.	Patient in office for biopsy results. Decision is made that treatment option includes mastectomy. Code 99214-57.

(continued)

TABLE 19-2 *(concluded)*

Modifier	Description	Example
58	**Staged or Related Procedure or Service by the Same Physician during the Postoperative Period.** Circumstances may include staged (planned) procedure, procedure being more extensive than originally thought, or therapy following original procedure.	Patient has breast biopsy, which has a post-op period. During this period, mastectomy is decided upon and performed. Code 19302-58.
59	**Distinct Procedural Service.** Used when the secondary procedure is identified as *different session, different procedure/surgery, different site or organ system. Separate incision/excision, separate lesion, separate injury or area of injury when injuries are extensive.* (Note, some Medicare codes have edits that state certain procedures cannot be performed together regardless of use of 59 modifier.)	Medical records indicate that colonoscopy with polyp removal using snare (45385) and colonoscopy with hot biopsy forceps (45384) were done in same session. Code 45385. Code 45384-59.
62	**Two Surgeons.** Modifier indicates that two surgeons performed a procedure that normally is performed by one surgeon, each performing distinct aspects of the procedure.	Two surgeons work as a team for spinal cord exploration and decompression. Code 63075-62. Code 63077-62.
66	**Surgical Team.** As with modifier 62, this modifier is used when a team of surgeons is required for a complicated procedure.	Patient requires a heart-lung transplant. Team includes cardiac surgeon, thoracic surgeon, perfusionist, and anesthesiologist. Code 33935-66.
76	**Repeat Procedure or Service by Same Physician.** Procedure is performed and complication requires repeat or related service. Used to explain this is not a duplicate service but is medically necessary.	Patient undergoes arteriovenous anastomosis (36821), but anastomosis does not hold and requires repeat procedure. Code 36821-76.
77	**Repeat Procedure by Another Physician.** As with modifier 76, a second procedure is required, but in this case, a different physician provides the service.	Patient undergoes arteriovenous anastomosis (36821), but anastomosis does not hold and requires repeat procedure; performing physician is not available. Code 36821-77.
78	**Unplanned return to the OR by the same Physician following Initial Procedure for Related Procedure during the Postoperative Period.** Complications related to the initial procedure are most often the reason for the return to surgery.	Patient undergoes implantation of central venous access device (36558), which clots off later in the day, requiring declotting. Code 36593-78.
79	**Unrelated Procedure or Service by the Same Physician during the Postoperative Period.** Usually, patient undergoes a primary procedure and, for an unrelated issue, requires a second surgery or procedure during the post-op period.	Patient undergoes laparoscopic cholecystectomy (47562). Two weeks later, experiences acute appendicitis episode and undergoes emergency appendectomy. Code 44970-79.
80	**Assistant Surgeon.** Surgeon acts as assistant to primary surgeon. (A physician assistant may function in this role.)	Surgeon performs total knee replacement with assistant surgeon. Code 27447-80.
81	**Minimum Assistant Surgeon.** This modifier is used only when minimal assistance during surgery is required.	Patient undergoing 4-vessel CABG. Second physician asked to assist only in stabilizing patient during procedure. Code 33536-81. Code 33518-81.
82	**Assistant Surgeon (when qualified resident surgeon is not available).** This modifier is used only in teaching hospitals where resident surgeons are normally available.	Patient undergoing 4-vessel CABG. Second physician asked to assist only in stabilizing patient during procedure because the surgical resident is assisting with another procedure. Code 33536-82. Code 33518-82.
90	**Reference (Outside) Laboratory.** Modifier is used when physician is billing for services provided by an outside laboratory. (Not allowed by Medicare.)	Provider office bills for comprehensive metabolic panel performed by "Allied Labs" and then reimburses the lab. Code 80053-90.
91	**Repeat Clinical Diagnostic Laboratory Test.** This modifier is used when serial (multiple) labs are required on the same day to monitor the patient's condition.	After surgery, the patient appears to be in acute renal failure, requiring monitoring of kidney function Code xxxxx-91.
92	**Alternative Laboratory Platform Testing.** Modifier 92 is used for disposable kit testing such as HIV testing.	Patient is tested for HIV using disposable test at hospital bedside. Code 86701-92.
99	**Multiple Modifiers.** Used when more than three modifiers are applicable to CPT code being used and the payer only accepts one modifier per code.	Medical Insurance Inc. accepts only one modifier per line, requiring modifier 99 be used and applicable modifiers are listed in block 19 of the CMS form. Procedure performed: Bilateral (50) mastectomy with assistant surgeon (80). Code 19307-99.

Note: You can see the complete listing of all modifiers in the *Current Procedural Terminology* manual, Appendix A.

Source: American Medical Association, *Current Procedural Terminology*, 2012 Professional Edition, copyright 2012.

be continuous, but the time is added together so that critical care codes chosen are based on the sum total of the critical care given during one particular date. Unlike emergency care codes, which can only be used when the patient's care is provided in an emergency department, the patient need not be in a critical care or intensive care bed in order for the codes to be used, but his condition must be critical in nature.

Consultations are provided at the request of other healthcare providers. A service can only be considered a consultation if the 3Rs are present: *request* (from another physician), *record* (documentation) findings and recommendations, and *report* to the referring physician. If the consulting physician takes over the care of the patient, then he is no longer considered a consulting physician, but a treating physician. As of January 2010, Medicare stopped accepting consultation codes; comparable inpatient and outpatient E/M service codes are to be used instead. Many commercial payers also have begun denying consultation codes, so again, it is important to know each payer's rules and regulations before submitting claims to the payers.

Counseling is considered part of E/M (evaluation and management) services, but if a complete history and physical exam does not take place (making an E/M code inappropriate), counseling codes may be used. These codes may be used when discussing with the patient and family questions or concerns regarding one or more of the following: diagnostic results and recommendations; prognosis, risks, and benefits of options; instructions for treatment and/or follow-up; importance of compliance; risk factor reduction; and patient/family education.

Downcoding is the term used when the insurance carrier bases reimbursement on a code level lower than the one submitted by the provider. This can occur for several reasons:

- The coding system used by the insurer does not match that used by the provider. This can occur if the provider uses a HCPCS code the insurer does not recognize. Always verify the code set accepted by the payer.

- If a workers' compensation carrier bases payment on an RVS (relative value system), the carrier may convert a CPT code to the lowest-paying code within the system. Again, check with the payer as to the system in use.

- If a payer requests backup documentation (medical records) on a case and finds the documentation does not "back up" the level of code used on the claim. This is by far the most common cause of downcoding in medical offices. Be sure your provider's documentation always is specific enough to back up the level of code used.

Unbundling, as stated above in the bundling definition, is defined as breaking a bundled code into its component parts for higher reimbursement and is not allowed. Code 77055 is defined as mammography, unilateral. Without research, you might think a bilateral mammography would be coded by adding modifier 50, but this is not the case. Code 77056 is an indented code with the description of mammography, bilateral—this code without a modifier is used for bilateral mammography.

Upcoding refers to coding a procedure or service at a higher level than that provided to receive a higher level of reimbursement. Other terms for this process are *code creep, overcoding,*

and *overbilling*, and all are fraudulent practices when done knowingly or repeatedly.

It is important to remember that insurers, particularly federally funded ones like Medicare and Medicaid, assume that if they are being billed, those doing the billing are appropriately trained to bill services following all appropriate guidelines. Ignorance (i.e., "I didn't know") is not considered an excuse when these payers are repeatedly billed excessive amounts for procedures. So, it is imperative that each provider's documentation in the patient medical record is clear and concise and backs up (or proves) the level of service being billed actually occurred.

▶ Evaluation and Management Services LO 19.3

To diagnose conditions and plan treatments, physicians use a wide range of time, effort, and skill for different patients and circumstances. Evaluation and management codes (**E/M codes**) are often considered the most important of all CPT codes because all physicians in any medical specialty can use them. Table 19-3 gives the E/M breakdown by type with code range.

TABLE 19-3	E/M Code Breakdown with Code Ranges
E/M Type	**Code Range**
Office/Other Outpatient Services	New Pt 99201–99202 Est. Pt 99211–99215
Hospital Observation Services	99217–99220
Hospital Inpatient Services	99221–99239
Consultations	OutPt 99241–99245 InPt 99251–99255
Emergency Department Services	99281–99288
Critical Care Services	99291–99292
Nursing Facility Services	99304–99318
Domiciliary, Rest Home (Boarding Home), or Custodial Care Services	New Pt 99324–99328 Est. Pt 99334–99337
Domiciliary, Assisted Living Facility, or Home Care Plan Oversight Services	99339–99340
Home Services	New Pt 99341–99345 Est. Pt 99347–99350
Prolonged Services	99354–99360
Case Management Services	99363–99368
Care Plan Oversight Services	99374–99380
Preventative Medicine Services (includes counseling services)	New Pt 99381–99387 Est. Pt 99391–99397 Other 99420–99429
Non-Face-to-Face Physician Services	99441–99444
Special Evaluation and Management Services	99450–99456
Newborn Care Services	99460–99465
Inpatient Neonatal Intensive Care Services and Pediatric and Neonatal Critical Care Services	99466–99480
Other Evaluation and Management Services	99499

Source: American Medical Association, *Current Procedural Terminology,* 2012 Professional Edition, copyright 2012.

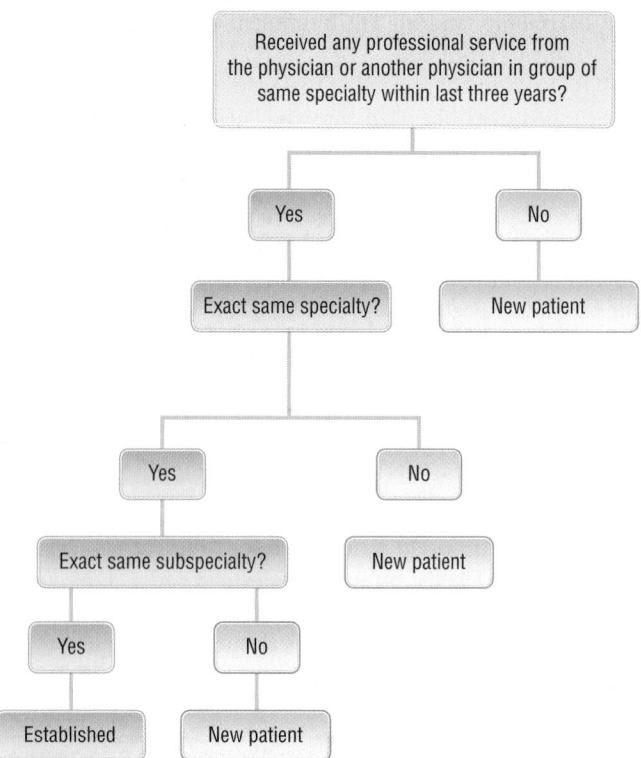

FIGURE 19-4 Decision tree for new versus established patient.

Many E/M codes are divided based on the patient status of **new patient** versus **established patient**. This is simply because, in many cases, a physician will need to spend more time with a new patient, getting to know him and his history, than will be necessary with a patient who has been coming to the practice for several years and whose history is well-known. The general rule of thumb is if a patient has been seen by a physician of the same specialty in the same practice within 3 years, he is an existing patient. If the patient has not been seen in the practice within the last 3 years, he is considered a new patient.

Figure 19-4 shows an example of a new versus established patient decision tree.

In addition to being the most important codes in the CPT manual, the E/M codes are considered by many the most difficult to code because of the many factors that must be considered when choosing an E/M Code. Let's examine the various components that must be considered when choosing an E/M code. As with any coding exercise, practice is the most important factor when learning procedure (or diagnostic) coding.

Key Factors in Determining Level of Service

The E/M section guidelines explain how to code different levels of these services. Three key factors documented in the patient's medical record help determine the level of service:

1. The extent of the patient history taken.
2. The extent of the examination conducted.
3. The complexity of the medical decision making.

Let's look briefly at each of these key factors.

Patient History The elements of a history include the chief complaint (CC); history of present illness (HPI); review of systems (ROS); and past, family, and/or social history (PFSH). When coding, the history is described using one of the following terms:

- Problem-focused—limited to the chief complaint and a brief history of the present problem.
- Expanded problem-focused—includes the chief complaint, a brief history of the current problem, and a "problem-pertinent" review of systems.
- Detailed—still focuses on the chief complaint but includes an extensive history of the current problem and an extended review of systems and pertinent past, family, and/or social history.
- Comprehensive—the most complex of the histories; all four components of CC, HPI, ROS, and PFSH are documented.

Physical Exam The elements of the physical exam include the same terminology but relate to the level of examination performed. The physical exam has three elements:

1. The constitutional exam includes any of the following: BP sitting or lying, pulse, respirations, temperature, height, weight, and general appearance.
2. Body areas (BA) include head (including face), neck, chest (including breasts and axillae), abdomen, genitalia, groin and buttocks, back, and each extremity.
3. Organ systems (OA) include the following systems: ophthalmologic (eyes), otolaryngologic (ears, nose, throat, and mouth), cardiovascular, respiratory, GI (gastrointestinal), GU (genitourinary), musculoskeletal, integumentary (skin), neurologic, psychiatric, and hematologic/lymphatic/immunologic (blood, lymph, immunity).

Physical exam terms include

- Problem-focused—exam is limited to the body area or organ system directly related to the chief complaint. (1 BA or OS)
- Expanded problem-focused—limited exam of the affected body area or organ system and any other symptomatic or related BA or OS. (2–7 limited BA or OS)
- Detailed—includes an extended exam of the affected body area and any other related, symptomatic BA or OS. (2–7 extended BA or OS)
- Comprehensive—the most extensive exam; includes either a complete single-specialty exam or a complete multisystem examination. (8+ BA or OS)

Medical Decision Making The most important key component in establishing an E/M code is the medical decision making (MDM) and it is probably the most difficult to document. It is based on the complexity of the decision making by the provider about the patient's care and diagnosis. The three elements that must be documented to establish MDM are: number of diagnoses or management options (minimal, limited, multiple, or extensive); amount or complexity of data to be reviewed (none or minimal,

TABLE 19-4 Medical Decision-Making Elements for E/M Codes

Elements	Straightforward	Low	Moderate	High
Number of diagnostic or management options	Minimal	Limited	Multiple	Extensive
Amount or complexity of data to be reviewed	Minimal/None	Limited	Moderate	Extensive
Risk of complication or death	Minimal	Low	Moderate	High

limited, moderate, or extensive); and risk of complication or death if condition is untreated (minimal, low, moderate, or high). Here we outline the complexity levels of medical decision making:

- Straightforward MDM—there are minimal diagnosis and management options with no or a minimal amount or complexity of data to be reviewed and minimal risk to the patient of complication or death if the condition is left untreated.
- Low-complexity MDM—there are a limited number of diagnoses and management options with a limited amount/complexity of data to be reviewed and low risk of complication or death if the patient is not treated.
- Moderate-complexity MDM—there are multiple diagnoses and management options with a moderate amount and complexity of data to review. If not treated, the condition presents a moderate risk of complication or death to the patient.
- High-complexity MDM—the physician has extensive diagnosis and management options with an extensive amount and complexity of data for review. The patient is at high risk for complication and/or death if not treated.

Some medical assistants and billers/coders like to use a grid similar to Table 19-4 to assist with the MDM decision-making process when assigning E/M codes.

Three Contributory Factors in Assigning Codes

In addition to these three key components, some E/M codes take three *contributory factors*, listed as follows, into consideration when codes are assigned:

1. Counseling. This component is only considered critical for E/M codes when counseling is the reason for the encounter and constitutes 50% or more of the total time of the visit.
2. Coordination of care. The time the physician uses to coordinate patient care with other healthcare agencies like home care or nursing home care.
3. Nature of the presenting problem. This is another term for the severity of the patient's chief complaint.
   - A minimal complaint may not require the presence of a physician, but service is provided under the physician's supervision such as a BP reading or dressing change.
   - A self-limited complaint is a minor problem that will run a "known" course and is transient in nature. A problem

with a good prognosis when the patient is compliant also may be considered self-limiting.

- Low-severity complaints are those with a low risk of morbidity and mortality (death) if there is no treatment. Full recovery is expected.
- Moderate-severity complaints have a moderate risk of morbidity and mortality if there is no treatment. Prognosis is uncertain and there is increased risk of impairment.
- High-severity complaints are those of high to extreme risk. Risk of death is moderate to high and there is a high risk of prolonged functional impairment.

Finally, *time* is listed as a component to some codes after being incorporated in 1992 to assist with code choice. The times listed are considered averages and unless the code choice, such as with face-to-face contact codes, is based on time, time should not be considered a critical factor when choosing an E/M code. As noted in Table 19-3, the location of the service is also important because different E/M codes apply to services performed in a physician's office or other outpatient location, a hospital inpatient room, a hospital emergency department, a nursing facility, an extended-care facility, or a patient's home.

Appendix C of the CPT code manual lists clinical examples of each E/M code type to assist you in choosing appropriate E/M codes for your provider.

▶ Surgical Coding LO 19.4

Figure 19-5 illustrates an encounter form listing codes from the integumentary part of the surgical section. Many insurance carriers cover the surgical procedures found in CPT as part of a *surgical package.* Included in most surgical packages are the preoperative exam and testing; the surgical procedure itself, including local or regional anesthesia if used; and routine follow-up care for a set period of time. Payers assign a fee to each of these packaged codes that pays for all the services provided in this package. If using anesthesia other than local anesthesia, the anesthesiologist billing for his services would use an anesthesia code.

The period of time covered for follow-up care is called the **global period.** For example, the global period for repairing a tendon might be set at 15 days. A global period for major surgery like an abdominal hysterectomy might be set at 90 days. During the global period, any care provided related to the surgical procedure is included in the surgical fee and cannot be billed separately; remember, any attempt to do so is called *unbundling* and is considered fraud. As discussed earlier, if a patient is seen for an unrelated problem, the service or procedure may be billed separately using a modifier 24 for E/M services, or modifier 79 for an unrelated surgical procedure taking place in a global period. After the global period ends, additional services related to the initial surgery can be reported separately for payment.

As shown in Figure 19-5, to make the coding process more efficient, most medical offices list frequently used procedures and their applicable CPT codes on superbills or encounter

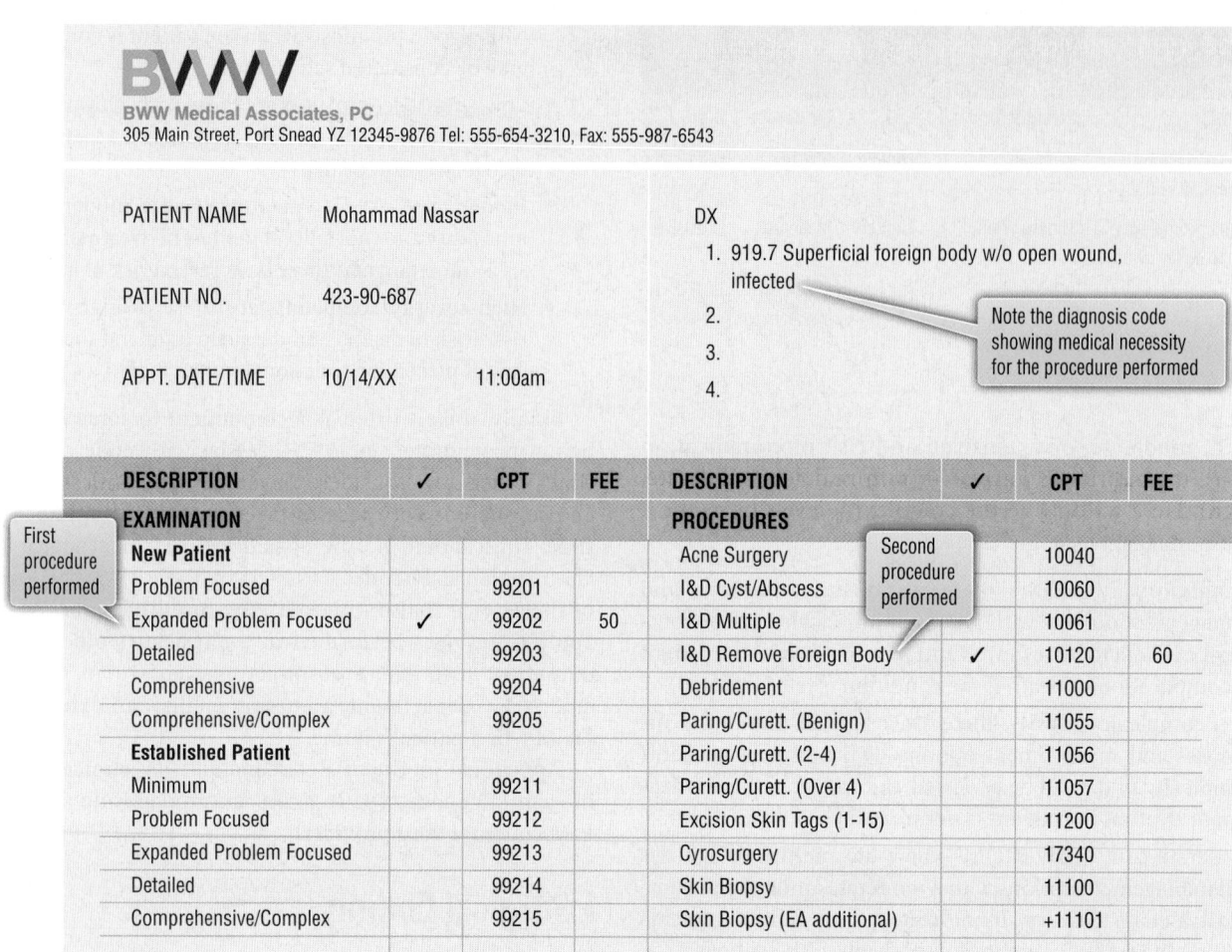

FIGURE 19-5 Superbill (encounter form) with procedures and diagnosis proving medical necessity for procedure performed.

forms. After seeing the patient, the physician checks off the appropriate procedures or services and the patient returns the form to the medical assistant at the front desk. The medical assistant then inputs the information into the facility computer system, if the office is computerized. If the office uses a manual system, the administrative medical assistant will put the office copy of the completed superbill in a designated area so it can be used to quickly and efficiently complete the CMS-1500 form for submission to the patient's insurance carrier. If superbills are used in the office, the office must remember to update both the ICD and CPT codes on the superbills and in any computer programs when the new codes are available each year (October for ICD codes and January for CPT codes). See Figure 19-6 for an example of an electronic superbill produced by the Spring-Charts PrimeSuite EHR program.

Let's look at each subsection of the surgery chapter with a brief overview of coding guidelines for each area.

Integumentary System

Integumentary subheadings are skin, subcutaneous, and accessory structures; nails; pilonidal cyst; introduction; repair (closure); destruction; and breast. These are further subdivided by the procedures done within each subheading, such as I&D, excision, paring, biopsy benign and malignant lesions, and so on. Many codes in this section are based on size and location; choose carefully. Carefully read instructions regarding closure of any removed or repaired lesion. Simple closure is often included in the main code, so you will often only be coding closures if they are intermediate (layered) or complex (greater than layered). The instructions within the integumentary section give great information as to how to choose the correct closure type. Read everything carefully and follow the instructions exactly.

Musculoskeletal System

The musculoskeletal subheadings begin with general and then start with the head and work their way down to the foot and toes. You will find this to be true for the rest of the CPT manual. Codes start from the top of the body and work their way down within each section and subsection. Casts and strappings as well as endoscopy and arthroscopy are also found in this chapter. Probably the most common codes from this section include the fracture codes. Here are a couple of straight-forward rules:

FIGURE 19-6 Screenprint of electronic superbill (encounter form) from SpringCharts EHR program.

Source: Screen captures of SpringCharts™ Electronic Health Records software are reprinted with permission from Spring Medical Systems, Inc. All rights reserved.

- A fracture treatment is closed unless stated otherwise; that is, treatment occurs without opening the skin. Open treatment means that surgery occurred to repair the fracture. Percutaneous treatment (fixation) immobilizes the fracture with hardware (pins) inserted using X-ray guidance.

- Be careful with cast and strapping codes. Fracture repair assumes cast application and includes it. Cast application and removal for fractures are coded only when the physician applying or removing the cast did not initially treat the patient's fracture.

- Last, any therapeutic procedure (like arthroscopy) includes the diagnostic procedure, so if a diagnostic procedure becomes a therapeutic (surgical) procedure, in the end, only the therapeutic procedure will be coded.

Respiratory System

The most important item to remember when coding the respiratory system is to code to the furthest extent of the procedure. For instance, many endoscopy procedures for the respiratory system begin with the nose and proceed further into the respiratory system. If the procedure results in a laryngoscopy, the scope passes through the trachea, so the code includes scoping of the trachea, which is not coded separately, as the description for code 31515 states *with or without tracheoscopy, for aspiration.* Be sure to also read information regarding the approach for the procedure. Many procedures can be done via a scope (scopy) or as an open procedure using an incision (tomy); these procedures are very different, so be cautious when coding similar procedures using different approaches. Be alert also for *incision* codes (cutting into—suffix tomy) versus *excision* codes

(removal—suffix ectomy) and for the suffix *plasty,* signifying a repair procedure like rhinoplasty. Your anatomy and terminology knowledge will be invaluable when coding.

Cardiovascular System

As you might expect, cardiology coding consists of some of the more complicated coding scenarios. Often, in order to completely code cardiovascular surgery, codes from the cardiovascular surgery section, medicine section (for nonsurgical services), and radiology section (for diagnostic or visualization assistance) will all be necessary. When coding bypass procedures, read instructions carefully. You must know not only whether veins or arteries (or both) are used in the bypass, but also the correct coding sequence; the right codes in the wrong order will also hold up a claim. Injection codes will be used for diagnostic and therapeutic procedures and you will also find embolectomy and thrombectomy codes in this section. Nonsurgical cardiography procedures include ECGs, Holter monitors, and exercise tests. The echocardiography area includes all cardiac ultrasound procedures as well as vascular Doppler procedures for noncardiac vascular areas, such as the extremities. Read *everything* and make sure to code procedures completely, using as many codes as necessary.

Hemic/Lymphatic Systems and Mediastinum and Diaphragm

These two short subsections of the surgery section include procedures on the spleen, bone marrow, and lymph nodes as well as surgical procedures related to the mediastinum and diaphragm. Coding in these sections is pretty straightforward *if* you read carefully.

Digestive System

The most common procedures found in the upper digestive system are incisions and excisions followed by repairs. The lower digestive system (stomach, intestines, rectum) include these as well as endoscopies (and laparoscopies). As always, remember that therapeutic procedures include diagnostic procedures unless you are specifically instructed within the chapter that two codes may be used. You will also find procedures on the liver, pancreas, biliary tract, abdomen, and peritoneum in this chapter.

Urinary System

The most "intense" coding in the urinary system revolves around the kidneys and renal function and treatment, including services for renal transplantation. In addition to kidney procedures, you will find diagnostic (including urodynamics) and therapeutic procedures for the ureters, bladder, and urethra. Again, as with the respiratory and digestive system, many procedures may be done laparoscopically as well as through an open incision, so read notes and code descriptions carefully to be sure to choose the correct approach.

Male Genital System

Because of the many repair codes associated with it, the subheading Penis is the largest within the male genital section. Other procedure codes found throughout this chapter include excision, incision, biopsy, destruction (of lesions) including laser surgery (treatment for BPH and prostate cancer), and brachytherapy (radiotherapy). The two codes for intersex surgery (male to female and female to male) are also found in this section.

Female Genital System/Maternity and Delivery

Medical assistants and coders either use this section extensively or almost never, as the codes found here are used almost exclusively by OB/GYN providers. This chapter is set up from "the outside in," starting with the introitus (vaginal opening) moving to the ovaries within the pelvis, with a separate subsection devoted to labor and delivery. This chapter has definitions and specialized guidelines too numerous to cover here, so if you find yourself coding for the specialty of OB/GYN, read the entire chapter carefully, taking notes and highlighting important information. Seeking the assistance of an experienced OB/GYN coder will be very helpful when you start out.

Endocrine System

Another short section, the endocrine system codes include those for procedures on the thyroid, parathyroid, thymus, adrenal glands, pancreas, and carotid body. Procedures include incisions, excisions, and laparoscopies.

Nervous System

Codes describing procedures on the brain, spinal cord, and peripheral nerves are all found in this section. Anatomic sites create the subheadings, which are subdivided by the procedure performed. Because of the complicated nature of coding procedures related to this delicate system, multiple specialized guidelines are found within this chapter. The approach again is an important consideration when coding surgery on the brain (anterior, middle, or posterior cranial fossa), as is the definitive procedure that describes the procedure done to the lesion and the reconstruction or repair necessary at the end of the surgery. Lumbar punctures, CSF (cerebrospinal fluid) shunt procedures for hydrocephalus treatment, and all treatments for spinal column and cord defects and peripheral nerve repair and destruction are found in this chapter.

Eye and Ocular Adnexa

This chapter covers everything from everyday eye exams and removal of a foreign body from the external eye to enucleation surgery to remove the contents of the eye socket. Many of the procedures found here are highly specialized and require careful reading of instructions and guidelines. The codes are divided by anterior and posterior segments, ocular adnexa, and conjunctiva (including the lacrimal system). Procedures include incisions, excisions, repairs, destruction, and reconstructions.

Auditory System

The auditory system section is divided by the external ear diagnostics and treatments, middle ear diagnostics and treatments, and then the inner ear diagnostics and treatments, followed by temporal bone procedures. An operating microscope is necessary for many procedures and code descriptions must be read carefully to avoid unbundling, as some procedures include this component and others allow a separate code for its use. Procedures include incisions (including "tubing" or tympanostomy), excisions, introductions, and repairs (tympanoplasty).

Radiology

The radiology section includes diagnostic radiology (imaging), diagnostic ultrasound, radiologic guidance, mammography, bone and joint procedures, radiation oncology, and nuclear medicine.

Many diagnostic radiology procedures use modifiers 26 (professional component only) and TC (technical component only); however, read descriptions carefully. When a code states, includes "radiologic supervision and interpretation," as with code 77031, the code is all-inclusive and modifiers cannot be used. There are many instructions throughout this chapter leading you to correct code usage. Read all includes and excludes instructions carefully.

Laboratory Procedures

Organ- or disease-oriented **panels** listed in the pathology and laboratory section of the CPT include tests frequently ordered together. An electrolyte panel, for example, includes tests for carbon dioxide, chloride, potassium, and sodium. Each element of the panel has its own procedure code. However, when the tests are performed together, the code for the panel must be used rather than the separate procedure codes. To code a panel correctly, the physician must order each test listed within the panel and there must be a need for each of them. If a panel is appropriate but one or two laboratory tests are also ordered that are not included in the panel, code the panel and then the additional tests separately.

If each test in a panel or procedure in a surgical package is listed separately, it will cause unbundling of the panel or package. The review performed by the insurance carrier's claims department will "rebundle" the services under the appropriate code, which could delay payment. Remember—when unbundling is done intentionally or repeatedly to receive more payment than is correct, you and the practice can be investigated for fraud.

Medicine and Immunizations

Injections and infusions of immune globulins, vaccines, toxoids, and other substances require two codes—one for giving the injection and one for the particular vaccine or toxoid that is given. An E/M code is not used along with the codes for immunization unless a significant evaluation and management service is also performed (like a yearly physical exam) and documented appropriately by the doctor. Modifier 59 would be appended to the E/M code in this case, indicating the need for both procedures.

▶ Using the CPT Manual LO 19.5

Now that you have a basic understanding of the CPT manual's format, its conventions, and its sections, including where to find section guidelines and instructions, it is time to actually use the CPT manual. Remember, when choosing E/M codes you must know whether the patient is a new or established patient and where the services took place. Use all of the information you have studied, and the chapter guidelines, to assist you in locating the correct codes.

The next step is to find the procedures and services provided by the office. As with diagnosis codes, these may be found on the superbill. However, remember to check the patient's chart to verify that documentation on the procedures and services exists within the medical chart (if it is not written down, it did not happen). When coding E/M codes, you may find it easiest to go directly to the E/M section in the front of the CPT manual to choose the correct code. For all other procedures, you will need to use the alphabetic listing of procedures found in the back of the CPT manual.

The number or number range in the index to the right of the description represents the coding possibilities for the description. If a hyphen is between two codes, this indicates a code range and each code in the range will need to be checked in the numeric index to choose the correct code. Code numbers with commas between them indicate there is more than one location possibility. Again, all codes will have to be checked. In some cases, the patient's medical record may show an abbreviation, an *eponym* (a person or place for which a procedure is named), or a synonym. For example, the record might state, "treated for bone infection." In the CPT's index, the entry for "Infection, Bone," is followed by the instruction "See Osteomyelitis." The greater your knowledge of anatomy and physiology and terminology, the easier it will be for you to code. Let's look at a couple of examples.

Once you decide on the appropriate CPT code(s), the next step is to check for any applicable modifiers. The use of modifiers can greatly enhance your reimbursement and can cut down on claim inquiries from the insurance carrier, but the ability to use modifiers correctly and proficiently will require practice. As discussed earlier, Appendix A of the CPT manual contains all CPT modifiers, and many of the section guidelines also contain information regarding the use of modifiers within that section. This is not an optional step. Modifier use is required if one is available for the situation.

Once all procedures and services have been assigned a CPT code and modifier as needed, carefully enter the 5-digit code(s) and modifiers in block 24d of the CMS-1500 form as you learned in the *Insurance and Billing* chapter. Remember that the primary procedure—often this is the most labor-intensive one or the principal reason for the patient's encounter—is listed first and is matched with the appropriate diagnosis code, often the primary diagnosis, to demonstrate medical necessity for the insurance carrier. After the principal procedure is listed, enter all other procedures provided to the patient during this date of service and match each with its appropriate diagnosis to verify its medical necessity as well.

Procedure 19-1, found at the end of this chapter, outlines the correct steps for locating a CPT code.

Go to CONNECT to see a video about *Locating a CPT Code*.

The HCPCS Coding Manual LO 19.6

The **Healthcare Common Procedure Coding System**, commonly referred to as **HCPCS** (pronounced hick-picks), was developed by the Centers for Medicare and Medicaid Services (CMS) for use in coding services for Medicare patients. Today, in addition to Medicare, Medicaid and private insurance programs also accept some HCPCS codes. To avoid claim denials due to an invalid or unacceptable code, be sure to check with the insurance carrier to see if they accept HCPCS codes and, if so, which ones. The HCPCS coding system has two levels:

1. HCPCS Level I codes are more commonly known as CPT codes.
2. **HCPCS Level II Codes**, issued by CMS, are called national codes and cover many supplies, such as sterile trays, drugs, injections, and DME (durable medical equipment). If CPT and HCPCS have identical descriptions, the HCPCS Level I (CPT) code should be used. However, if CPT has a generic description and HCPCS has a more specific description, HCPCS Level II should be used. Level II codes also cover services and procedures not included in the CPT. For instance CPT has one (generic) code to cover the supplies and materials used for in-office procedures (99070), whereas the HCPCS manual lists very specific codes for each item supplied.

The HCPCS codes for Level II have five characters, either numbers, letters, or a combination of both. At times, there are also two-character modifiers, either two letters or a letter with a number. These modifiers are different from the CPT modifiers but may be used with CPT codes as well as with Level II codes. For example, HCPCS modifiers may indicate social worker services (HO) or equipment rentals (KH). Appendix 2 of the HCPCS manual gives a complete list of all HCPCS modifiers.

Examples of Level II codes are listed here:

Code Number	Description
A0225-QN	Ambulance service, neonatal transport, base rate, emergency transport, one way, furnished directly by the provider of services
E0781	Ambulatory infusion pump, single or multiple channels…
G0008	Administration of influenza virus vaccine
G0104	Colorectal cancer screening; flexible sigmoidoscopy
Q0091	Screening Papanicolaou (Pap) smear; obtaining, preparing, and conveyance of cervical or vaginal smear to laboratory
V5298	Hearing aid, not otherwise specified

In medical offices where the HCPCS system is used, regulations issued by CMS are reviewed to determine the correct code and modifier for use on each payer's claims. Medical assistants who code with the HCPCS manual find its steps for coding mimic those of CPT, except that the Alphabetic Index is found in the front of the manual with the alphanumeric index found toward the back.

As with all coding procedures, the first step is to locate the description of the service, procedure, or item in the Alphabetic Index. Once this is located, note the code(s) or code range given and move to that area of the alphanumeric index to verify the description. Choose the code description that exactly matches the service, procedure, or item supplied as documented in the medical record. If you are coding medications supplied to the patient, you will find it easiest to locate the drug name in the Table of Drugs found in Appendix 1 of HCPCS. This table will list the unit, route of administration, and the appropriate "J" code. Even though only one code is given, do not skip the step of verifying the information in the alphanumeric index.

Once all CPT and HCPCS codes are located and verified, enter them in block 24d of the CMS-1500 form if your office is not computerized. Otherwise, enter the codes in the appropriate area of the office medical billing software so the information may be transmitted to the health insurance carrier electronically. Procedure 19-2, at the end of the chapter, outlines the steps for locating a HCPCS code. Procedure 19-3 outlines the procedure for entering CPT (HCPCS) and ICD codes into an electronic system using the SpringCharts program.

Coding Compliance LO 19.7

Physicians have the ultimate responsibility for proper documentation and correct coding as well as for compliance with regulations, but many expect their medical assistants to have working knowledge of this, too. Medical assistants help ensure maximum appropriate reimbursement for reported services by submitting correct healthcare claims. These claims, and the process used to create them, must comply with the rules imposed by federal and state law and with payer requirements.

Code Linkage

As you learned in the *Insurance and Billing* chapter, clean claims are those in which each reported service is connected to a diagnosis that supports the procedure as necessary to investigate or treat the patient's condition. Insurance company representatives analyze this connection between the diagnostic and the procedural information, called code linkage, to evaluate the medical necessity of the reported charges. Correct claims also comply with many other government agency regulations.

The possible consequences of inaccurate coding and incorrect billing include

- Denied claims
- Delays in processing claims and receiving payments
- Reduced payments
- Fines and other sanctions
- Loss of hospital privileges
- Exclusion from payers' programs
- Prison sentences
- Loss of the physician's license to practice medicine

To avoid errors, the codes on healthcare claims are checked against the medical documentation. A code review, also known as a coding audit, checks these key points:

- Are the codes appropriate to the patient's profile (age, gender, condition; new or established), and is each coded service billable?
- Is there a clear and correct link between each diagnosis and procedure?
- Have the payer's rules about the diagnosis and the procedure been followed?
- Does the documentation in the patient's medical record support the reported services?
- Do the reported services comply with all regulations?

Insurance Fraud

The majority of those involved in the delivery of healthcare are trustworthy people devoted to patients' welfare. However, some people are not. For example, according to the Department of Health and Human Services (DHHS), in one year alone, the federal government recovered more than $1.3 billion in judgments, settlements, and other fees in healthcare fraud cases. Fraud is an act of deception used to take advantage of another person or entity (refer to the *Legal and Ethical Issues* chapter). For example, it is fraudulent for people to misrepresent their credentials or to forge another person's signature on a check.

Claims fraud occurs when physicians or others falsely represent their services or charges to payers. For example, a provider may bill for services that were not performed (phantom billing), overcharge for services, or fail to provide complete services under a contract. A patient may exaggerate an injury to get a settlement from an insurance company or ask the medical assistant to change the date a service was actually provided so the service is covered by a health plan policy that is no longer active.

A number of coding and billing practices are fraudulent. Investigators reviewing physicians' billings look for patterns like these:

- Reporting services that were not performed.

    Example: A lab bills Medicare for a general health panel (CPT 80050) but fails to perform one of the tests in the panel.
- Reporting services at a higher level than was carried out.

    Example: After a visit for a flu shot, the provider bills the encounter as an evaluation and management service plus an injection.
- Performing and billing for procedures not related to the patient's condition and therefore, not medically necessary.

    Example: After reading an article about Lyme disease, a patient is worried about having worked in her garden over the summer and requests a Lyme disease diagnostic test. Although no symptoms or signs have been reported, the physician orders and bills for the Lyme disease test, stating an exposure had occurred.
- Billing separately for services bundled in a single procedure code (unbundling).

    Example: When a physician orders a comprehensive metabolic panel (CPT 80053), the provider bills for the panel as well as for a quantitative glucose test, which is included in the panel.
- Reporting the same service twice.

    Example: The office submits a claim the same day the patient is in the office for a urinalysis, but the patient was unable to produce a specimen. When the patient returns later in the week with the specimen, a second claim is submitted for the urinalysis.

Note that HIPAA calls for penalties for giving remuneration to anyone eligible for benefits under federal healthcare programs. The forgiveness or waiver of copayments may violate the policies of some payers; others may permit forgiveness or waiver if they are aware of the reasons for the forgiveness or waiver, such as the patient's inability to pay (be sure to have documentation of such inability to avoid charges of discrimination). Routine forgiveness or waiver of copayments or deductibles constitutes fraud when billing federal programs like Medicare or TRICARE. The physician practice should ensure that its policies on copayments are consistent with applicable law and with the requirements of its agreements with payers.

Compliance Plans

To avoid the risk of fraud, medical offices have a compliance plan to uncover compliance problems and correct them. A compliance plan is a process for finding, correcting, and preventing illegal medical office practices. Its goals are to

- Prevent fraud and abuse through a formal process to identify, investigate, fix, and prevent repeat violations relating to reimbursement for healthcare services provided;
- Ensure compliance with applicable federal, state, and local laws, including employment laws and environmental laws as well as antifraud laws; and
- Help defend physicians if they are investigated or prosecuted for fraud by showing the desire to behave compliantly and thus reduce any fines or criminal prosecution.

When a compliance plan is in place, it demonstrates to payers like Medicare that honest, ongoing attempts have been made to find and fix weak areas of compliance with regulations. The development of this written plan is led by a compliance officer and committee with the intention to (1) audit and monitor compliance with government regulations, especially in the area of coding and billing; (2) develop consistent written policies and procedures; (3) provide for ongoing staff training and communication; and (4) respond to and correct errors. Although coding and billing compliance are the compliance plan's major focus, it covers all areas of government regulation of medical practices, such as equal employment opportunity (EEO) regulations (for example, hiring and promotion policies) and OSHA regulations (for example, fire safety and handling of hazardous materials like bloodborne pathogens). For further information, go to www.oig.hhs.gov/fraud/docs/complianceguidance/thirdparty.pdf.

PROCEDURE 19-1 Locating a CPT Code

Procedure Goal: To locate correct CPT codes using the CPT manual.

OSHA Guidelines: This procedure does not involve exposure to blood, body fluids, or tissue.

Materials: Patient record, superbill or charge slip containing procedure(s) performed, and a CPT manual.

Method: Procedure steps.

1. Find the services listed on the superbill (if used) and in the patient's record.
   RATIONALE: Only documented services and procedures may be coded for submission to the insurance carrier.

   a. Check the patient's record to see which services were documented. For E/M procedures, note whether the patient is a new or established patient and then look for clues as to the location of the service and the extent of history, examination, and medical decision making that were involved.
   RATIONALE: To code E/M services correctly, all of this information is required.

2. Look up the procedure code(s) in the Alphabetic Index of the CPT manual.

   a. Verify the code number in the numeric index, reading all notes and guidelines for that section.
   RATIONALE: All codes must be verified in the Tabular Index; never code only from the Alphabetic Index.

   b. If a code range is noted, look up each code in the range and choose the correct code given in the Tabular Index. If the correct description is not found, start the process again. Use the same process if multiple codes are given, looking each one up in the numeric index until you find the correct code description.
   RATIONALE: The Tabular Index gives specific information and direction not found in the Alphabetic Index.

3. Determine appropriate modifiers.

   a. Check section guidelines and Appendix A to choose a modifier if needed to explain a situation involving the procedure being coded, such as bilateral procedure, surgical team, or a discontinued procedure.
   RATIONALE: Modifiers give the payer specific information about the procedure, which may affect payment for that procedure.

4. Carefully record the procedure code(s) on the healthcare claim or, if the office is computerized, enter the codes into the office billing system for placement on an electronic health claim form. Usually, the primary procedure—the one that is the primary reason for the encounter or visit—is listed first.

5. Match each procedure with its corresponding diagnosis. The primary procedure is often (but not always) matched with the primary diagnosis.
   RATIONALE: This code-linking provides the payer with the medical necessity for each procedure—the reason why the service or procedure was needed.

PROCEDURE 19-2 Locating a HCPCS Code

Procedure Goal: To locate correct HCPCS codes using the HCPCS manual.

OSHA Guidelines: This procedure does not involve exposure to blood, body fluids, or tissue.

Materials: Patient record, superbill or charge slip containing procedure(s) performed, and HCPCS manual.

Method: Procedure steps.

1. Locate the service, supplies, and equipment requiring a HCPCS code from the encounter form or from the patient's record. If an encounter form is used, verify procedure completion in the medical record.
   RATIONALE: Only services, supplies, and equipment documented as provided may be billed to the insurance carrier.

2. Use the Alphabetic Index in the beginning of the manual to locate the section in which the category of codes is found.

3. Find the code or code range listed, reading descriptions carefully. Do not code from the Alphabetic index.
   RATIONALE: The Tabular Index includes further information on each code so the correct code may be chosen.

4. Look up the code or each code in the code range listed in the Tabular Index. Read descriptions carefully.
   RATIONALE: The Tabular Index includes further information on each code so the correct code may be chosen.

5. Make sure the code is valid for the type of insurance the patient carries.
   RATIONALE: If the insurance carrier does not accept HCPCS codes, the equivalent CPT code will need to be used instead of HCPCS.

6. Enter the correct code(s) on the superbill or encounter form (if necessary) and, if the office uses a computerized billing program, in the patient's computerized record so it can be used for billing purposes. Otherwise, place the HCPCS code in block 24d of the 1500 claim form for submission to the insurance carrier. Match each HCPCS code with the appropriate diagnosis code to demonstrate medical necessity.
   RATIONALE: This code-linking provides the payer with the medical necessity for each procedure—the reason why the service or procedure was needed.

PROCEDURE 19-3 Entering CPT/HCPCS and ICD Codes into an EHR Program

Procedure Goal: To enter procedure and diagnosis codes into the SpringCharts EHR/Billing Program.

OSHA Guidelines: This procedure does not involve exposure to blood, body fluids, or tissue.

Materials: Paper or electronic superbill, patient's medical record, and a computer with SpringCharts EHR program loaded.

Method: Procedure steps.

1. Open the appropriate patient's record in the EHR Program.
2. Click **Assessment.**
3. Click **Add Diagnosis** and then **Search.**
4. Key in the first few words of the diagnosis, such as **Type II Diabetes.**
5. Based on the information on the superbill or in the medical record, choose the correct diagnosis for the patient's visit.

RATIONALE: This proves the medical necessity for the patient's visit.

6. When the diagnosis is chosen, click **OK.**
7. Click **Plan** and then **Search.**
8. Click **Search for Code.**
9. Locate the correct description/code for the procedure performed in the **Procedure Code Search** field.
10. Strike the **tab** key to confirm your entry.
11. Click **Search** and choose the **procedure** you just found.
12. Click ***Category.**
13. Choose the correct service category for the procedure performed.
14. Click **OK.**
15. Confirm the entries are correct and saved in the **Orders** section.

SUMMARY OF LEARNING OUTCOMES

LEARNING OUTCOMES	KEY POINTS
19.1 List the sections of the CPT manual, giving the code range for each.	The sections for the CPT manual are Evaluation and Management, Anesthesiology, Surgery, Radiology, Pathology and Laboratory, and Medicine, with code ranges from 00100–99602.
19.2 Describe briefly each of the CPT's general guidelines.	A CPT code is a 5-digit code representing the service provided to the patient. The CPT manual general guidelines include the following symbols, each of which represents important information about the code being described: blue triangle, red dot, # sign, triangles facing each other, circle with a diagonal through it, lightning bolt, bull's-eye, as well as add-on codes and modifiers. Always begin coding by looking up the description in the Alphabetic Index and verifying in the Tabular (numeric) List. Carefully read all guidelines and information surrounding the codes.
19.3 List the types of E/M codes within the CPT.	The E/M code types include office and other outpatient services; hospital observation; hospital inpatient; consultations; ED services; critical care, nursing facility, domiciliary, and rest home services; domiciliary and assisted-living services; home care plan oversight; home services; prolonged services; case management; care plan oversight; preventative medicine; non-face-to-face physician services; special E/M; newborn care, neonatal ICU, and critical care services; and other E/M services.
19.4 List the areas included in the Surgical coding section.	Surgical coding sections include integumentary, musculoskeletal, respiratory, cardiovascular, digestive, urinary, male and female genital systems, endocrine, nervous, eye and ear, radiology, pathology and lab, and medicine.
19.5 Locate a CPT code using the CPT manual.	Student answers will vary depending upon the information (encounter forms or mock medical records) they are given to practice coding with the CPT manual. They should be able to select an accurate code for simple, straightforward coding scenarios.

LEARNING OUTCOMES	KEY POINTS
19.6 **Explain how to locate a HCPCS code using the HCPCS coding manual.**	Student answers will vary depending upon the information (encounter forms or mock medical records) they are given to practice coding with the HCPCS manual. They should be able to select an accurate code for simple, straightforward coding scenarios.
19.7 **Explain the importance of code linkage in avoiding coding fraud.**	Code linkage demonstrates the medical necessity of services provided to the patient by accurately linking each procedure code to its appropriate diagnosis. All procedures, services, and diagnoses must be documented in the patient's medical record to be used on any health insurance claim form.

CASE STUDY CRITICAL THINKING

Recall Raja Lautu from the beginning of the chapter. Now that you have completed the chapter, answer the following questions regarding her case.

1. What is the correct CPT code for the physical examination that was performed on Raja?

2. Code the screening bilateral mammogram using both the CPT and HCPCS coding references. Which payer will require the HCPCS code instead of the CPT?

3. Using the CPT manual, code the ultrasound of the breast and the breast biopsy. Include any necessary modifiers.

EXAM PREPARATION QUESTIONS

1. (LO 19.1) All of the following are sections of the CPT manual EXCEPT
   a. Anesthesiology
   b. E/M
   c. Surgery
   d. Pathology and lab
   e. Integumentary

2. (LO 19.1) Which area gives instructions on how to code within a specific chapter?
   a. Appendix A
   b. Section notes
   c. Guidelines
   d. Modifiers
   e. Index

3. (LO 19.2) Which of the following CPT conventions indicates the code is new to the current edition?
   a. Triangle
   b. Plus sign
   c. Lightning bolt
   d. Red dot
   e. Bull's-eye

4. (LO 19.2) Which of the following CPT conventions indicates the code description is revised?
   a. Blue triangle
   b. Plus sign
   c. Lightning bolt
   d. Red dot
   e. Bull's-eye

5. (LO 19.3) The _____ codes are considered to be the most important of the CPT codes.
   a. Level II
   b. E/M
   c. Add-on
   d. Unlisted procedure
   e. Surgical

6. (LO 19.3) For reporting purposes, CPT considers a patient "new" if he or she has not received professional services within the past _____ year(s).
   a. One
   b. Two
   c. Three
   d. Four
   e. Five

7. (LO 19.4) Which of the following are components of a surgical package?
   a. Preoperative work-up
   b. Surgery itself
   c. Usual postoperative follow-up
   d. All of the above
   e. b and c only

8. (LO 19.5) Which of the following is the correct code for vaginal hysterectomy (255 g) including removal of fallopian tubes and ovaries with appendectomy?
   a. 58291, 44950
   b. 58291, 44950-51
   c. 58260, 44955
   d. 58262, 44950-51
   e. 58262, 44955

9. (LO 19.6) What is the correct HCPCS code for a folding walker with wheels?
   a. E0143
   b. E0141
   c. E0149
   d. E0148
   e. E0144

10. (LO 19.7) The "key" to showing medical necessity for a procedure or service is
    a. A working compliance plan
    b. Using appropriate ICD codes
    c. Upcoding
    d. Downcoding
    e. Accurate code linkage

Go to CONNECT to see activities about *Adding a CPT Code* and *Using a CPT Code & Test Code*

Patient Billing and Collections

PATIENT INFORMATION		
Patient Name	**Gender**	**DOB**
Nancy Evans	F	1/29/19XX
Attending	**MRN**	**Allergies**
Elizabeth H. Williams, MD	654-88-099	Amoxicillin

Nancy Evans is a 71-year-old female who has been referred to the neurologist because of a possible diagnosis of Alzheimer's disease. The charges for today total $360.00. Her husband reminds you that she has Medicare and a Medigap plan that picks up her 20% coinsurance after Medicare. You inform Mr. Evans that the office is a participating provider with Medicare. You bill Medicare and find out from the RA (remittance advice) that Nancy has $122.65 left on her deductible for this year.

Keep Nancy Evans in mind as you study this chapter. There will be questions at the end of the chapter based on the case study. The information in the chapter will help you answer these questions.

LEARNING OUTCOMES

After completing Chapter 20, you will be able to:

20.1 Describe accounts receivable and accounts payable and the common payment methods accepted in medical practices today.

20.2 Identify the different types of documents used as statements to bill patients and how these documents are used in *cycle billing.*

20.3 Compare open-book, written-contract, and single-entry accounts and the purpose of creating an accounts receivable aging.

20.4 Explain the purposes of the following credit and collections acts: ECOA, FCRA, FDCPA, and TLA.

20.5 Relate the required components of a Truth in Lending Statement to credit practices in the medical office.

20.6 Summarize two common types of problem collection accounts in the medical office.

KEY TERMS

accounts payable (A/P)
accounts receivable (A/R)
age analysis
class action lawsuit
credit
credit bureau
cycle billing
damages
disclosure statement
guarantor
open-book account
single-entry account
skip
statement
statute of limitations
Truth in Lending Statement
written-contract account

VI. C (4)   Discuss precautions for accepting checks

VI. C (6)   Differentiate between accounts payable and accounts receivable

VI. C (9)   Explain both billing and payment options

VI. C (10)   Identify procedures for preparing patient accounts

VI. C (11)   Discuss procedures for collecting outstanding accounts

VI. C (12)   Describe the impact of both the Fair Debt Collection Act and the Federal Truth in Lending Act of 1968 as they apply to collections

VI. P (2)   Perform accounts receivable procedures, including:
- b. Perform billing procedures
- c. Perform collection procedures
- h. Post collection agency payments

VI. P (3)   Utilize computerized office billing systems

VI. A (1)   Demonstrate sensitivity and professionalism in handling accounts receivable activities with clients

VII. A (2)   Demonstrate sensitivity in communicating with both providers and patients

8. **Medical Office Business Procedures Management**

   Graduates
- i.   Perform billing and collections procedures
- k.   Perform accounts receivable procedures
- ee.   Use proper telephone techniques
- hh.   Receive, organize, prioritize, and transmit information expediently

11. **Career Development**

   Graduates
- b.   Demonstrate professionalism by:
  - (1) Exhibiting dependability, punctuality, and a positive work ethic
  - (3) Maintaining confidentiality at all times
  - (7) Expressing a responsible attitude

▶ Introduction

Medical assisting is a multifaceted career. As such, a medical assistant may be required to take on many duties in the medical office that are administrative in nature. Medical practices have customers who have various payment arrangements like third-party payer payments (usually insurance carriers) followed by balance billing of the patient, patients who require payment plans, and others who have large outstanding balances. A proper understanding and administration of billing—for all of these patient situations, as well as payment collection methods—is therefore required.

▶ Patient Payments in the Office   LO 20.1

Once the health insurance claims have been filed and the insurance pays its portion of the patient's charges, the patient will be held accountable for his portion of the fees. In any business, basic administrative functions involve managing accounts receivable and accounts payable. **Accounts receivable (A/R)** is the term for income, or money, owed to the business (think "able to be received"). **Accounts payable (A/P)** is the term for money owed by the business (in this case, "able to be paid"). In a medical practice, accounts receivable represent the money patients (and insurance companies) owe in return for medical services. Accounts payable describe the money the medical practice must pay out to run the practice. You will learn more about accounts payable in the *Financial Management* chapter. Billing and collections are vitally important tasks because

they convert the practice's accounts receivable into income, or cash flow, from which the accounts payable can be paid. Unless billing and collections are carried out effectively, a practice might have plenty of money due in accounts receivable but not enough cash on hand to pay its accounts payable, including staff salaries!

There are methods of improving billing and collection procedures to increase income for the practice. You will need to know about standard payment, billing, and collection procedures as well as credit arrangements and common problems in collecting payment. Patients who have insurance (third-party payer) often request that the office submit a claim to the insurance carrier and then bill them for the balance, and most offices do so. It makes good business sense, however, if a patient belongs to a managed care organization (MCO) with a known copayment for each visit that this charge should be collected at each visit. And most medical offices require this. (Refer to the *Insurance and Billing* chapter for more information.) Immediate patient payment not only brings income into the practice faster, but it saves the cost of preparing and mailing **statements** (patient bills) and collection of past-due accounts. Many offices post a small sign at the reception desk that states, for example, "Payment is requested when services are rendered unless other arrangements are made in advance." As the medical assistant, you are responsible for collecting these payments. If the patient cannot pay all or part of the charges at the time of the visit, it may be your responsibility to bill for the physician's services and possibly to extend credit utilizing payment plans for larger patient-due balances.

Accepting Patient Payment

When the patient comes to you at the completion of his visit with the superbill (refer to the *Insurance and Billing* chapter), you enter the charges for the services provided (if they are not preprinted on the form) and ask for payment. There are several effective yet diplomatic ways to request payment. Two examples are, "For today's visit, the total charge is $50. How would you like to pay for that today?" and "The charge for your laboratory work today is $80. Would you like to pay for that now?" The first example is the preferred method because, in the second example, asking the patient if he would like to pay for the service now leaves him open to say, "No, bill me," which will slow your cash flow and cost the practice the expense of sending a billing statement. Computerized offices post the payments to the patient's account using the office billing software. Offices that use a manual, paper system often use a pegboard or write-it-once system that allows you to record the payment on the patient ledger card and produce a receipt for payment simultaneously. You will learn more about both electronic billing systems and the pegboard system in the *Financial Management* chapter.

To encourage patients to pay for treatment at the time of service, most practices accept several forms of patient payment, including cash, check, and debit and credit cards. Giving the patient these options encourages payment at the time of service.

Cash If the patient chooses to pay in cash, count the money carefully to be sure you have received the proper amount. Next, record the payment on the patient's ledger card or, with a computerized system, credit the patient's account as per system instructions and give the patient a receipt. All of these tasks are discussed in detail in the *Financial Management* chapter.

Once the money is posted to the account, a computerized billing program gives you the option of printing a receipt that you can give to the patient. If the office uses superbills, one of the copies can be given to the patient as the receipt. If your office does not use either of these methods, prepare a cash receipt manually, as shown in Figure 20-1. Be sure that whatever method is used, the office also retains a copy of the receipt. Then place the money in the cash drawer or cash box.

Check If your office accepts checks, always ask for proof of identity if you do not know the person writing the check to avoid the accidental acceptance of fraudulent checks. The check should be completed fully and correctly. Many offices have a stamp with the office name on it for patient convenience and to ensure that the practice name is spelled correctly. Unless the patient has made previous arrangements, the check should be made out for the full amount owed. Verify that the check is dated for the current date and signed when accepting it. Endorse it immediately and place it with other checks for the day's deposit. If a check is returned for nonsufficient funds (NSF), notify the patient immediately requesting payment in full by another method. Many offices subsequently insist that the patient be seen on a cash-only basis, unless the patient can produce a valid credit card (assuming the office takes credit cards). The office is also allowed to charge the patient an additional fee for the expense of processing the NSF check. You will learn more about this process in the *Financial Management* chapter.

Debit Card Many patients now use debit cards instead of paying by cash or check. A debit card looks like a credit card but immediately transfers the funds from the patient's bank account to the practice account. The advantage to the practice is that if there are insufficient funds in the account, the transaction will be refused and other arrangements can be made immediately. Debit cards, like credit cards, are read through electronic readers (Figure 20-2) and the patient inputs a PIN (personal identification number) verifying his or her wish that funds be transferred.

Credit Card Many medical practices accept credit cards, such as Visa or MasterCard. This payment method offers advantages for both the practice and the patient. For the practice, it provides prompt payment from the credit card company, thus increasing cash flow. It also reduces the amount of time and money spent on preparing and mailing statements, thus decreasing expenses. For the patient,

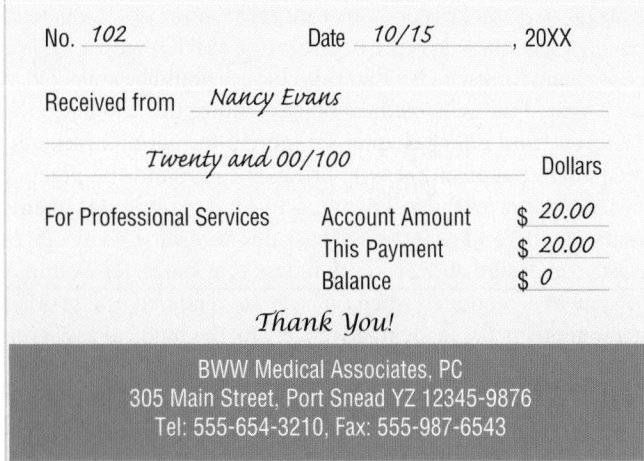

No. *102*   Date *10/15* , 20XX

Received from *Nancy Evans*

Twenty and 00/100   Dollars

For Professional Services   Account Amount $ *20.00*
This Payment $ *20.00*
Balance $ *0*

Thank You!

BWW Medical Associates, PC
305 Main Street, Port Snead YZ 12345-9876
Tel: 555-654-3210, Fax: 555-987-6543

FIGURE 20-1 A receipt such as this may be used when the patient makes a payment while in the office.

FIGURE 20-2 Swiping a debit or credit card produces instant payment authorization from the financial institution or credit card company.

it is convenient and allows a large bill to be paid in several smaller amounts, usually once a month.

Credit cards have one major disadvantage for the practice—cost. The credit card company deducts a percentage of each transaction for its collection service, usually between 1% and 5%. If a patient charges $100 in services on a credit card, for example, the practice receives only $95 to $99. The credit card company keeps the difference. Some banks are also beginning to charge a similar fee for the convenience of accepting debit cards as well. A disadvantage for patients is the accrued interest charges on unpaid balances.

If the practice accepts credit card payments, the American Medical Association (AMA) suggests several guidelines.

- Do not set higher fees for patients who pay by credit card.
- Do not encourage patients to use credit cards for payment.
- Do not advertise outside the office that the practice accepts credit cards.

If a patient chooses to pay by credit card, process the transaction carefully to ensure that the credit card company charges the patient correctly. Check the expiration date on the front of the credit card. If the card has expired, it cannot be used for payment. Swipe the card through an electronic reader or record it through the use of a credit card machine that mechanically records the information on the card. To operate a credit card machine, place the credit card in the machine and place a credit card voucher on top of it. Slide the imprint arm firmly to the right and back across the machine. Remove the voucher from the machine. Write in the date and circle the type of credit card, such as Visa or MasterCard, after it is removed from the machine. Return the credit card to the patient.

Next, obtain the authorization code from the credit card company. Some offices have devices that read the magnetic strip on the credit card and automatically transmit the information to the credit card company electronically (Figure 20-2). If your office has such a device, type in the amount to be charged on its keypad. Then, the credit card company issues an authorization code, which appears on the device's screen.

If your office does not have such a device, call the credit card company for the authorization code. Give the operator the patient's credit card number and the amount of the payment. The operator then gives you the authorization code.

Write the authorization code in the box marked "Authorization" on the credit card voucher. Initial the voucher in the appropriate box. Then, fill in the services provided and the amount of the charges. Enter the total charges in the box marked "Total."

Give the receipt to the patient to sign. Compare the patient's signature on the receipt with the signature on the back of the credit card (they should be identical). Keep one copy of the receipt for the office. Give the other copy (and the credit card) to the patient.

When the payment comes in from the credit card company, they will have deducted their fee from the funds being deposited in the office account. When posting these payments to the individual patient account, you will need to adjust (write off) the amount withheld by the credit card company so the patient is not inadvertently billed for this charge. You will learn more about posting payments and adjustments (and all transactions) in the *Financial Management* chapter.

Online Payments Many hospitals and larger practices that accept credit and debit card payments are also now accepting payments online through their websites or via the patient's online banking program. The payment is then directed into the office checking account with notification to the practice so the patient's account can be credited appropriately.

Payment Responsibility

The person with financial responsibility for the patient is known as the **guarantor**, the person who "guarantees" payment. In most cases, any patient who is 18 or over is legally considered to be his own guarantor. This is true even if someone else (such as a spouse or parent) is the insured person (the person who carries the insurance for the family). As with every rule, there are some exceptions to this rule. A few are listed here.

Responsibility for Minors When a child's parents are married, either parent may consent to treatment for the minor child. Both parents are responsible for payment for the minor's treatment, although usually only one is listed on the patient's account as the guarantor. If you must send a bill for services provided to a minor child, it should be addressed to the guarantor to ensure payment. Emancipated minors are the exception to this process. If you have been shown legal proof of emancipation, any bills will be addressed to the emancipated minor; because of the emancipation process, the minor is legally responsible for her bills.

The legal and financial arrangements of a divorced couple are private. Unless you have legal documentation stating otherwise (retain a copy of this document in the patient financial record), you should assume that the parent bringing the patient to the office has consent ability and payment responsibility. Unless you have documentation otherwise, it should be made clear to the parents that payment is due at the time of the visit, regardless of which parent brings the child to the office. Refer to the *Legal and Ethical Issues* chapter for a more in-depth discussion on this topic.

Elderly Patients and Patients with Disabilities Sometimes when elderly patients or patients with disabilities are brought in for medical care, you may be asked to send the bill to another party such as an adult child. Because of HIPAA confidentiality laws, you cannot send a patient's bill to another person without first obtaining written consent to do so from the patient and the person accepting responsibility for payment. If the patient has been found to be incompetent, you should request proof of legal guardianship (keeping a copy in the patient's financial file) prior to sending a bill to the guardian.

Professional Courtesy Although much less common than in the past, a doctor may treat some patients free of charge or for just the amount covered by the patient's insurance. This practice is known as professional courtesy. These patients often include other doctors and their families, the practice's staff members and their families, other healthcare professionals, and clergy members. If the patient is part of a managed care organization or has Medicare, the provider must collect any copayment or deductible as part of the contracted agreement with the insurance carrier. It is considered fraud to consistently not collect copayments or deductibles if the collection of such payments is stipulated in the provider-insurer contract.

Follow the office policy regarding provision of professional courtesy. If you are unsure, check with the physician or office manager before making such adjustments to any patient's account.

▶ Standard Billing Procedures   LO 20.2

In today's practice, most offices receive payments from insurance carriers and then find they must bill the patient for any balance due. As the medical assistant, part of your duties may include preparing these patient billing statements. You also may have to manage related billing responsibilities, such as establishing and maintaining billing cycles.

Preparing Statements

Part of the medical assistant's job may be to prepare statements to mail to patients who do not pay when services are rendered or who make only a partial payment. Figure 20-3 shows a statement with an itemized list of services. You can obtain most of the information for the statement from the patient ledger

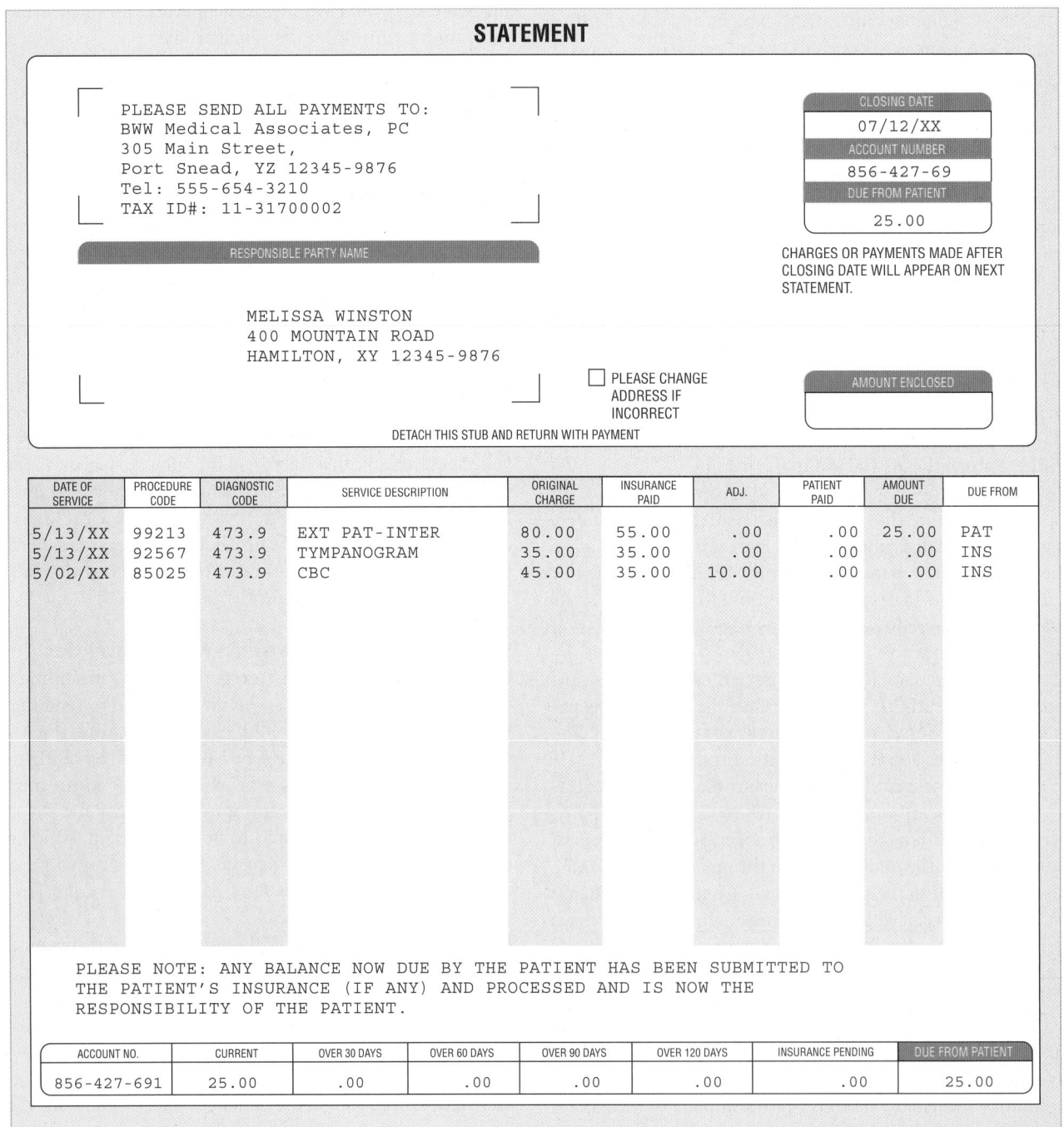

FIGURE 20-3   The patient billing statement should list all services and their charges, any payments made, and the amount now due.

card or from the patient's computerized account. Regardless of the format used, all statements should include the following information:

- Practice name, address, and telephone number (usually preprinted on the statement or prepared by the computer program).
- Patient's name and address.
- Guarantor's name (if different from the patient).
- Balance (if any) from the previous month(s).
- Itemized list of services and charges, by date, for the current month.
- Payments from the patient or insurer during the month.
- Total balance due.

Whatever billing procedure you use, enclose a self-addressed envelope with the statement to encourage prompt payment. Some offices have found that using a lightly colored return envelope, such as pale yellow, actually encourages faster payment because the color stands out against the usual white envelopes, jogging the patient's memory to "pay that one."

Manual Statements If the office wishes to produce manual statements, a template can be made on the computer in a format similar to Figure 20-3. Each procedure should be listed using abbreviations for common procedures, such as OV for office visit. Be sure that an explanation of the abbreviations appears on the statement, usually at the bottom. Also include the CPT codes for the procedures performed. Some statements also include the diagnosis code attached to each procedure. Using an itemized list of services provided on statements is standard practice in most medical offices as it decreases the number of patient calls asking, "Why am I being billed?" After completing the statement, fold it in thirds and mail it in a typewritten or window business envelope.

The Patient's Ledger Card as a Statement A common alternative to typing up statements, especially in smaller, noncomputerized offices, is to photocopy the patient's ledger card and fold the photocopy so that the patient's address shows through the window in a window envelope. If your practice uses ledger cards for this purpose, be sure there are no stray marks or comments on the card and that the copy is clean and easy to read.

Computer-Generated Statements If the practice utilizes an electronic billing program, statements similar to Figure 20-3 will be produced by the program, either automatically at certain times during the month after insurance payments have been made and a patient balance remains or on demand with a few simple keystrokes. Follow the instructions in the software procedure manual. You can then fold the printouts and mail them in window envelopes with a return payment envelope.

Using an Independent Billing Service Large practices may have both their insurance and patient billing procedures handled by an independent billing service. In addition to billing the insurance plan, the billing service may rapidly copy ledger cards or produce computer-generated statements listing the practice business office address for patients with balances due. The statements are then mailed to patients, usually with an envelope for sending payment directly to the provider's office.

Using the Superbill as a Statement

As stated earlier in the chapter, many paper-based practices still use the superbill (encounter form), which lists the charges and procedure codes (CPT) for services rendered on that day, including appropriate diagnoses and codes (ICD). As a carbonless form, when the charges and any payments are entered on the superbill, an automatic receipt and first statement are generated all at the same time, saving time and money. Some offices even give the patient a return envelope if there is a balance on the account to encourage prompt payment, as this is considered the first bill received by the patient. Procedure 20-1, located at the end of the chapter, will give you practice billing with a superbill.

Managing Billing Cycles

Smaller practices send out their statements monthly, usually at the end of the month. Larger practices tend to spread the billing process out over the month in a process known as **cycle billing**. In cycle billing the accounts are split into groups and statement mailing dates are staggered.

For example, you may bill on the fifth of the month for patients whose last names begin with A through D. Then, on the tenth of the month, you may bill patients whose names begin with E through H, and so on. Using cycle billing not only staggers the workload throughout the month, it also tends to spread out the payments coming into the office, giving the office a more even cash flow.

▶ Standard Collection Procedures LO 20.3

Although many patients pay a statement within the standard 30-day period, some do not. When a patient does not pay his bill during the standard period, you need to take steps to collect the payment. For example, you may need to call or write the patient to determine the reason for nonpayment or to set up a payment arrangement.

Whether you use telephone calls, notes, or letters, there are laws, such as each state's statute of limitations, as well as professional standards and guidelines to direct your efforts in collecting overdue payments from patients.

Statute of Limitations

The **statute of limitations** is a state law that sets a time limit on when a collection suit on a past-due account can legally be filed.

The time limit varies with the type of account and the state in which the debt was incurred.

Open-Book Account An account that is left open to charges that are made on an intermittent basis is known as an **open-book account**. Most of a physician's long-standing patients have this type of account. An open-book account uses the last payment date or the date of the last charge for each illness as the start date to determine the time limit for that specific debt.

Written-Contract Account As it sounds, a **written-contract account** is one in which the physician and patient sign an agreement regarding the treatment and the payment agreement. For this type of an account, the payment agreement often states that the patient will pay the bill in more than four installments. Some states allow longer time limits for these accounts than for open-book accounts. Written-contract accounts are regulated by the Truth in Lending Act, discussed later in this chapter.

Single-Entry Account An account consisting of only one charge is referred to as a **single-entry account**. For example, someone vacationing in your area might come in for treatment of a cold. This person's account would list only one office visit. If the vacationer did not become a regular patient, the account would be considered a single-entry account. Some states impose shorter time limits on single-entry accounts than on open-book accounts.

Using Collection Techniques

Individual practices have their own ways of approaching the task of account collections. Most begin the process with statements, then telephone calls, and finally letters.

Initial Telephone Calls When calling a patient (or sending a letter) about collections, be friendly and sympathetic. Call the patient at home unless you have specific permission to call her at work. The first phone call to the patient should occur if payment has not been received after 30–45 days. Because the patient received a receipt or superbill at the time of the visit, any statement mailed after that is essentially the second notice of payment due. The first mailed statement usually contains a message that is friendly in tone such as, "Your prompt payment is appreciated." When you call, assume that the patient forgot to pay or was temporarily unable to pay. You should ask the patient for the full amount due but have a minimum amount you would accept in mind (for instance half). If the patient states that she cannot afford full payment, ask her what amount she feels could be sent and if the amount is acceptable, obtain a date you can expect to receive the payment. If you do not receive the payment within 24 hours of the stated date, a phone call may be made and another statement sent. The message on this statement will be more urgent in tone because the patient

did not respond to your phone call and the tone of any subsequent communication will be still more urgent.

Follow-up Statements and Collection Letters Once an account is 60 days past due, it is advisable to send an initial letter of inquiry. Usually this letter still has a friendly, "we want to help" tone, giving the patient options to take care of his obligation, but makes it clear that the patient must take some sort of action. Figure 20-4 shows an example of such a letter.

If an account is 90 days past due, your collection letter can contain stronger wording. For example, it might say, "Please let us know when you plan to pay the $250 past-due balance. We have sent you three monthly reminders. If you cannot pay in full now, please contact us at (number) to make payment arrangements. We want to be understanding but need your cooperation."

If an account is 120 days or more past due, you can send a final letter. It might state, "Every courtesy has been extended to you in arranging for payment of your long overdue account. Unless we hear from you by (date), the account will be given to (name of collection agency) for collection." Be sure to note the cutoff date on the patient's ledger card. By law, you cannot threaten to send an account to a collection agency unless it will actually be sent on that cutoff date. Therefore, you must be sure you are ready to do so before you send such a letter. This collection letter should be mailed by certified mail with return receipt so you have proof that the letter was sent and that the intended recipient received the letter.

If the patient does not respond with payment prior to the date stated in the letter, the physician will have no choice but to turn the account over to the office collection agency. We will discuss collection agencies later in the chapter.

Preparing an Age Analysis

Age analysis is the process of classifying and reviewing past-due accounts by age from the first date of billing. A monthly age analysis, such as that shown in Figure 20-5, helps you keep on top of past-due accounts and determine which ones need follow-up.

Computer billing programs will prepare an age analysis for you, but you can also prepare one by hand if your office is not computerized. Offices that use ledger cards to track patient accounts often have a procedure to track how long since the last payment has been received. For instance, color-coded tags may be placed on the cards—yellow denoting 30 days past due; green, 60 days past due; red, 90 days past due; and black, 120 days past due. By pulling the ledger cards by color grouping, an age analysis can be completed easily either on graph paper or by using a spreadsheet. Include the patient's name, balance due, date of charges, date of most recent payment, and how long each part of the balance has been "waiting" on the A/R. It also may be helpful to insert a column at the end for action the office has taken in attempting to collect this debt. Procedure 20-2, at the end of the chapter, outlines this process.

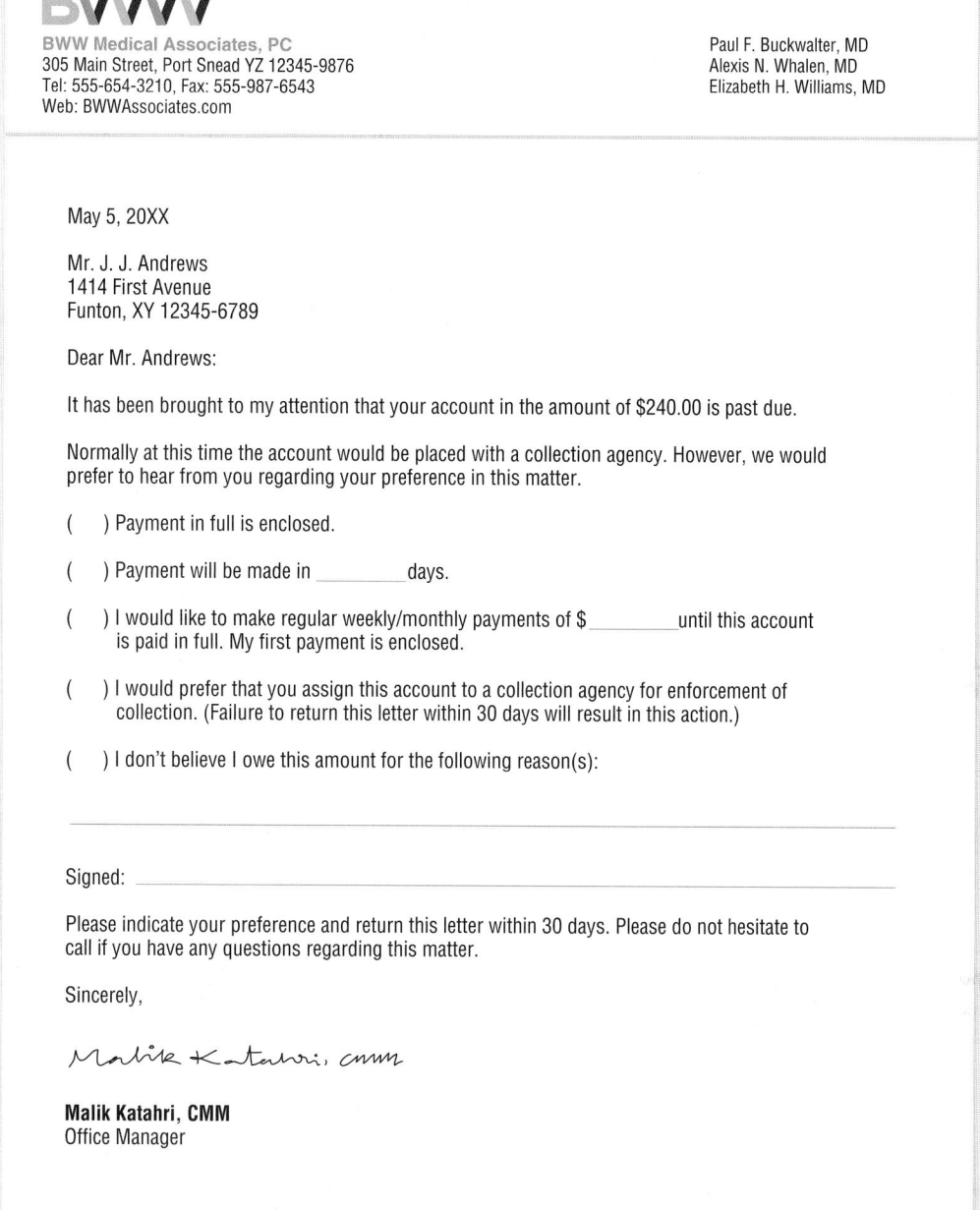

FIGURE 20-4 Most offices use a collection letter similar to this so the patient can simply make a choice and sign the letter and return it to the office.

▶ Laws That Govern Credit and Collections

LO 20.4

Federal and state laws govern debt collection. Table 20-1 outlines the penalties for violating laws that regulate credit and debt.

Fair Debt Collection Practices Act of 1977

This act (also called Public Law 95-109) governs the methods that can be used to collect unpaid debts. Its goal is to eliminate abusive, deceptive, or unfair debt collection practices, such as threatening to take action that is illegal or that is not actually planned. It is this law that states that if you threaten to turn an account over to a collection agency if a payment is not made by the 15th of the month, you must actually do so.

Following are guidelines for sending letters and making calls requesting payment from patients. For further information, visit www.ftc.gov/bcp/edu/pubs/consumer/credit/cre27.pdf.

- Do not call the patient before 8 a.m. or after 9 p.m. Calling outside those hours can be considered harassment.

Patient	Balance	Date of Charges	Most Recent Payment	30 days	60 days	90 days	120 days	Remarks
Black, K.	120.00	5/24	5/24			75.00	45.00	3rd Notice
Brown, R.	65.00	8/30	8/30	65.00				
Green, C.	340.00	8/25						Medicare filed
Jones, T.	500.00	6/1	6/30		125.00	125.00	250.00	3rd Notice
Perry, S.	150.00	7/28	7/28	75.00	75.00			1st Notice
Smith, J.	375.00	6/15	7/1			375.00		2nd Notice
White, L.	200.00	6/24	7/5	20.00	30.00	150.00		2nd Notice

Accounts Receivable–Age Analysis Date: October 1, 20XX

FIGURE 20-5 An age analysis organizes accounts by how long each has been on the A/R.

TABLE 20-1	**Laws That Govern Credit and Collection Procedures**	
Law	**Requirements**	**Penalties for Breaking the Law**
Equal Credit Opportunity Act (ECOA) www.ftc.gov/bcp/edu/pubs/consumer/credit/cre15.shtm	• Creditors may not discriminate against applicants on the basis of sex, marital status, race, national origin, religion or age. • Creditors may not discriminate because an applicant receives public assistance income or has exercised rights under the Consumer Credit Protection Act.	• If an applicant sues the practice for violating the ECOA, the practice may have to pay **damages** (money paid as compensation), penalties, lawyers' fees, and court costs. • If an applicant joins a class action lawsuit against the practice, the practice may have to pay damages of up to $500,000 or 1% of the practice's net worth, whichever is less. (A **class action lawsuit** is a lawsuit in which one or more people sue a company that wronged all of them the same way.) • If the Federal Trade Commission (FTC) receives many complaints from applicants stating that the practice violated the ECOA, the FTC may investigate and take action against the practice.
Fair Credit Reporting Act (FCRA) www.ftc.gov/os/statues/fcra/htm	• This act requires credit bureaus to supply correct and complete information to businesses to use in evaluating a person's application for credit, insurance, or a job.	• If one applicant sues the practice in federal court for violating the FCRA, the practice may have to pay damages, punitive damages (money paid as punishment for intentionally breaking the law), court costs, and lawyers' fees. • If the FTC receives many complaints from applicants stating that the practice violated the FCRA, the FTC may investigate and take action against the practice.
Fair Debt Collection Practices Act (FDCPA) www.ftc.gov/bcp/edu/pubs/consumer/credit/cre27.pdf	• This act requires debt collectors to treat debtors fairly. It also prohibits certain collection tactics such as harassment, false statements, threats, and unfair practices.	• If one debtor sues the practice in a state or federal court for violation of the FDCPA, the practice may have to pay damages, court costs, and lawyers' fees. • If the debtor joins a class action suit against the practice, the practice may have to pay damages of up to $500,000 or 1% of the practice's net worth, whichever is less. • If the FTC receives many complaints from debtors stating that the practice violated the FDCPA, the FTC may investigate and take action against the practice.
Truth in Lending Act (TLA) www.occ.treas.gov/handbook/til.pdf	• This act requires creditors to provide applicants with accurate and complete credit costs and terms, clearly and obviously.	• If one applicant sues the practice in a federal court for violation of the TLA, the practice may have to pay damages, court costs, and lawyers' fees. • If the FTC receives many complaints from applicants stating that the practice violated the TLA, the FTC may investigate and take action against the practice.

- Do not make threats or use profane language. For example, do not state that an account will be given to a collection agency in 7 days if it will not be.
- Do not discuss the patient's debt with anyone except the person responsible for payment. If the patient is represented by a lawyer, discuss the problem only with the lawyer, unless the lawyer gives you permission to talk to the patient.
- Do not use any form of deception or violence to collect a debt. For example, do not pose as a government employee or other authority figure to try to force a debtor to pay.

Telephone Consumer Protection Act (TCPA) of 1991

This act protects telephone subscribers from unwanted telephone solicitations, commonly known as telemarketing. The act prohibits autodialed calls to emergency service providers, cellular and paging numbers, and patients' hospital rooms. It prohibits prerecorded calls to homes without prior permission of the resident and it prohibits unsolicited advertising via fax machine.

These regulations do not apply to people who have an established business relationship with the telemarketing firm or people who have previously given the telemarketing firm permission to call. The law also does not apply to telemarketing calls placed by tax-exempt nonprofit organizations, such as charities.

Although most provisions of this federal law do not apply to medical practices, you should be aware of the law. One way to avoid an unknowing violation of this law is to limit your calls to patients to the hours between 8 a.m. and 9 p.m. (some states, however, have exceptions for the TCPA provisions). Do not use an automated dialing device for calls to patients regarding their accounts; always place the calls yourself. For more information on this act, visit the American Teleservices Association website: www.ataconnect.org/public/aboutata/index.php.

Observing Professional Guidelines for Finance Charges and Late Charges

According to the AMA, it is appropriate to assess finance charges or late charges on past-due accounts if the patient is notified in advance. Advance notice may be given by posting a sign at the reception desk, giving the patient a pamphlet describing the practice's billing practices, and/or including a note on the statement.

The physician must adhere to federal and state guidelines that govern these charges. The physician also should use compassion and discretion when assigning charges, especially in hardship cases. Because of the nature of medical care, many offices choose not to assess finance or late charges to patient accounts.

Using Outside Collection Agencies

If in-house collection efforts do not result in payment, the practice may wish to select a collection agency to manage the account. Because collection agencies keep a percentage of any funds they collect for their clients (usually between 40% and 60% of the collected amount), the office staff should use all reasonable methods to collect unpaid balances prior to sending an account to collection. Because of the humanitarian and ethical standards of the medical profession, physicians must be careful to avoid collection agencies that use harsh or harassing collection techniques. The Points on Practice feature outlines points to be considered when selecting an outside collection agency.

Once an agency is chosen and accounts are deemed eligible for referral to the agency (after the appropriate notice outlined above has been given), the following information must be given to the agency regarding each account:

- Full name of patient and the last known address.
- Occupation and business name and address.
- Name of spouse, if any.
- Total amount of the debt.
- Date of the last activity (payment or charge) on the account.
- Description of actions taken to collect the debt.
- Response(s) received to collection attempts.

Once an account has been turned over to the collection agency, all communication between the patient and the office concerning her debt must cease. All inquiries must be referred to the collection agency. If a payment is received after the account has been turned over, follow the procedure outlined in the agreement with the agency—some agencies allow the office to deposit the check and send them their percentage, and others ask you to return the check to the patient with the request that the patient call the agency. Procedure 20-3, at the end of the chapter, outlines the steps in turning an account over to a collection agency and posting a payment from them for a collection account.

Because the debt is now the responsibility of the collection agency, it is important to note all accounts that have been turned over to them. For computerized accounts, a comment may be made to the account or the patient's name and account number may be "color-coded," denoting collection proceedings have begun. As stated earlier in the chapter, for practices that use ledger cards, the color-coded tabs used for aging may also be used to denote collection proceedings (often black tabs are used for this purpose).

Lastly, it should always be the decision of the practice (and not the collection agency) whether to pursue legal action regarding an account or to adjust the debt off the books. All collection agencies should make a monthly report to the office documenting the activity on the accounts they are working. Give the collection agency a set amount of time to collect the debt, such as 60–90 days. After that time, the practice should decide how to best deal with the account.

When an account is deemed "uncollectable" by the physician or the office manager, the balance may be written off to "relieve" the AR of money that will not be received. This topic will be discussed in more detail in the *Financial Management* chapter.

Insuring Accounts Receivable

To protect the practice from lost income because of nonpayment, the practice may buy accounts receivable insurance. Policies can pay when a large number of patients (or one large account or insurance plan) do not pay and the physician must absorb the lost income. Some policies also protect the practice in the event that its A/R records are destroyed and so the individual records may no longer be available. It will not pay to recreate the records but it will allow for at least some recoupment of at least some of the outstanding A/R. Accounts receivable insurance can protect the practice cash flow and help ensure that the practice will have sufficient income to cover expected expenses.

▶ Credit Arrangements   LO 20.5

Sometimes a doctor or practice agrees to extend credit to a patient who is unable to pay immediately. This situation is common when a patient's medical bills are high. By extending **credit**, the doctor gives the patient time to pay for services, which are provided on trust. If the doctor knows the patient well, she may offer credit without checking the patient's credit history. However, to avoid charges of discrimination under the Equal Credit Opportunity Act (ECOA), you will normally perform a credit check prior to extending credit.

Following Laws Governing Extension of Credit

When you help the physician decide whether to grant credit to a patient, you must comply with certain laws governing extension of credit.

Equal Credit Opportunity Act The Equal Credit Opportunity Act states that credit arrangements may not be denied based on a patient's sex, race, religion, national origin, marital status, or age. Credit also cannot be denied because the patient receives public assistance or has exercised rights under the Consumer Credit Protection Act, such as disputing a credit card bill or a credit bureau report.

Under ECOA, the patient has a right to know the specific reason that credit was denied. Some reasons might include having too little income or not being employed for a certain period of time. Vague reasons about not meeting minimum standards or not receiving enough points on a credit-scoring system are not acceptable. In order to comply with ECOA, a credit check is required on any patient the practice is considering for extension of credit.

Performing a Credit Check To perform a credit check, be sure you have the patient's most current information including the patient's address, telephone number, and Social Security number as well as the name, address, and telephone number of the patient's employer. With this information you can verify employment and generate a credit bureau report.

Employment Verification Explain to the patient that you will be calling his employer to verify employment. Many employers have a designated person to handle such calls. The patient may be able to give you that name before you call the place of employment. After calling, record the updated information on the patient's registration card, along with any credit references obtained from the patient.

Credit Bureau Report A **credit bureau** is a company that provides information about the creditworthiness of someone seeking credit. If a patient's credit history is in question, you may request a report from a credit bureau, a sample of which is shown in Figure 20-6. A credit bureau collects information about an individual's payment history on credit cards, student loans, and similar accounts. The three leading national credit bureaus are TRW Inc., Equifax Inc., and Trans Union Credit Information Company. If the practice decides not to extend credit based on the credit report, the Fair Credit Reporting Act states that you must inform the patient in writing that credit was denied based on the credit report. You also must provide the name and address of the credit bureau, but you are not required to discuss the information obtained from the report. The patient may contest the credit report and have any inaccurate information

corrected. Once the information has been corrected, the provider may then decide to extend credit to the patient.

Extending Credit If the doctor decides to extend credit, two common arrangements are made: the unilateral agreement and the mutual (bilateral) agreement.

Unilateral Agreement If the patient offers to pay the debt over a period of months, and the physician agrees, the patient will be billed every month for the full amount owed and should make whatever payment is possible each month. This type of arrangement is considered a unilateral agreement and is not regulated by the Truth in Lending Act.

Mutual Agreement The second option is the mutual or bilateral agreement between physician (practice) and patient. They might agree that the patient will be billed for the full amount owed each month and will pay a minimum amount each month. If the physician does not assess finance charges, and if the total number of payments is four or fewer, this

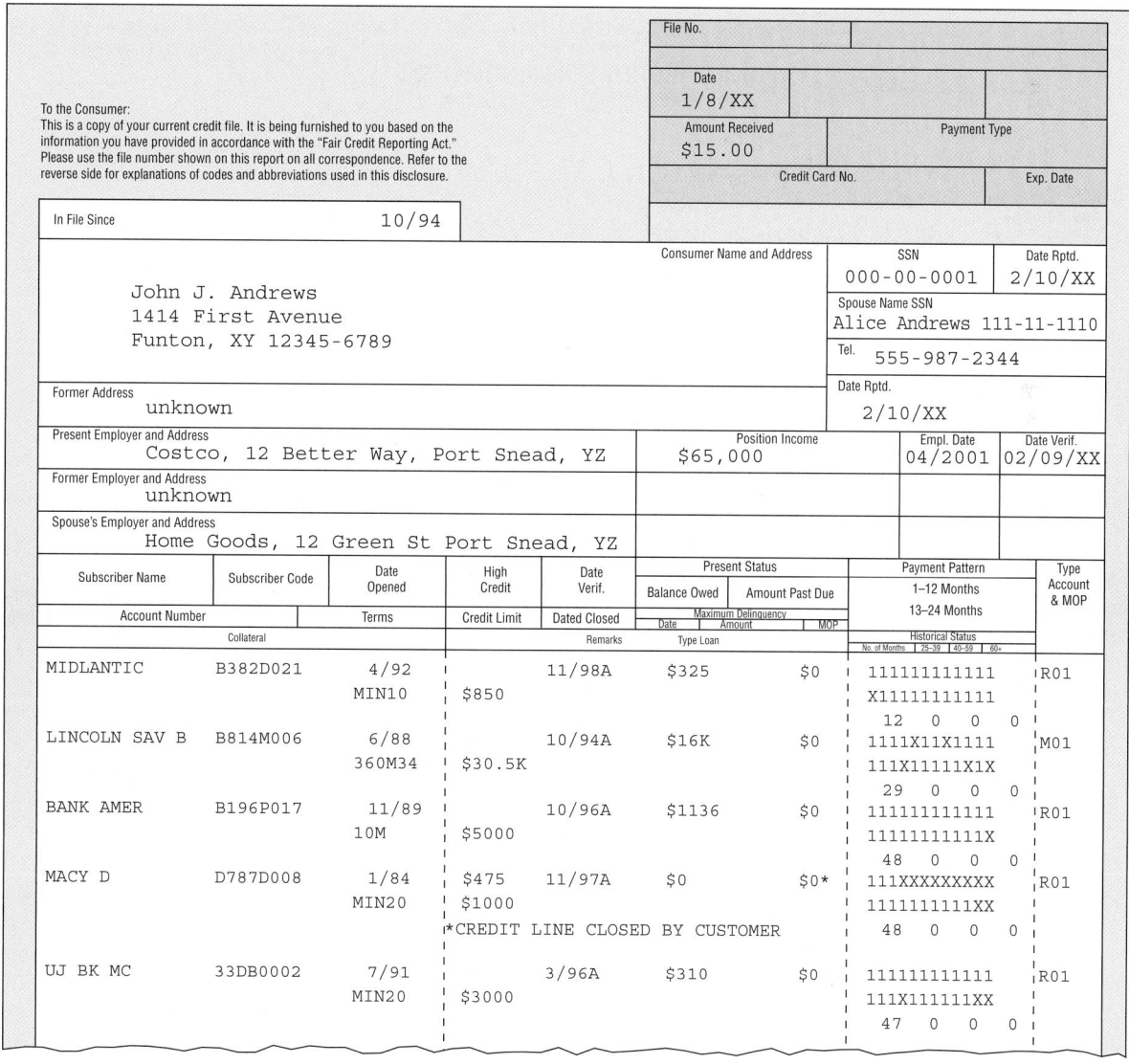

FIGURE 20-6   Credit reports can be used to help the practice decide whether to extend credit on a case-by-case basis.

type of agreement is also not covered by the Truth in Lending Act. If the physician and patient make a bilateral agreement that includes more than four payments, or if the practice assesses finance charges, the agreement is subject to the requirements of the Truth in Lending Act.

Truth in Lending Act

The Truth in Lending Act comes under Regulation Z of the Consumer Credit Protection Act. This act covers credit agreements that involve more than four payments. It requires the practice and patient to discuss, sign, and retain copies of a **disclosure statement** (frequently called a federal **Truth in Lending Statement**), which is a written description of the agreed terms of payment (Figure 20-7). According to the Truth in

Lending Act, a disclosure statement must meet the following two requirements:

1. The agreement must be discussed with the patient when the terms are first determined. The practice and the patient must agree on the payment terms.
2. Both the physician (or his representative) and the patient must sign the document to indicate mutual agreement on the written terms.

Further, a disclosure statement must include the following six pieces of information:

1. The amount of total debt (the amount for which the patient is receiving credit).

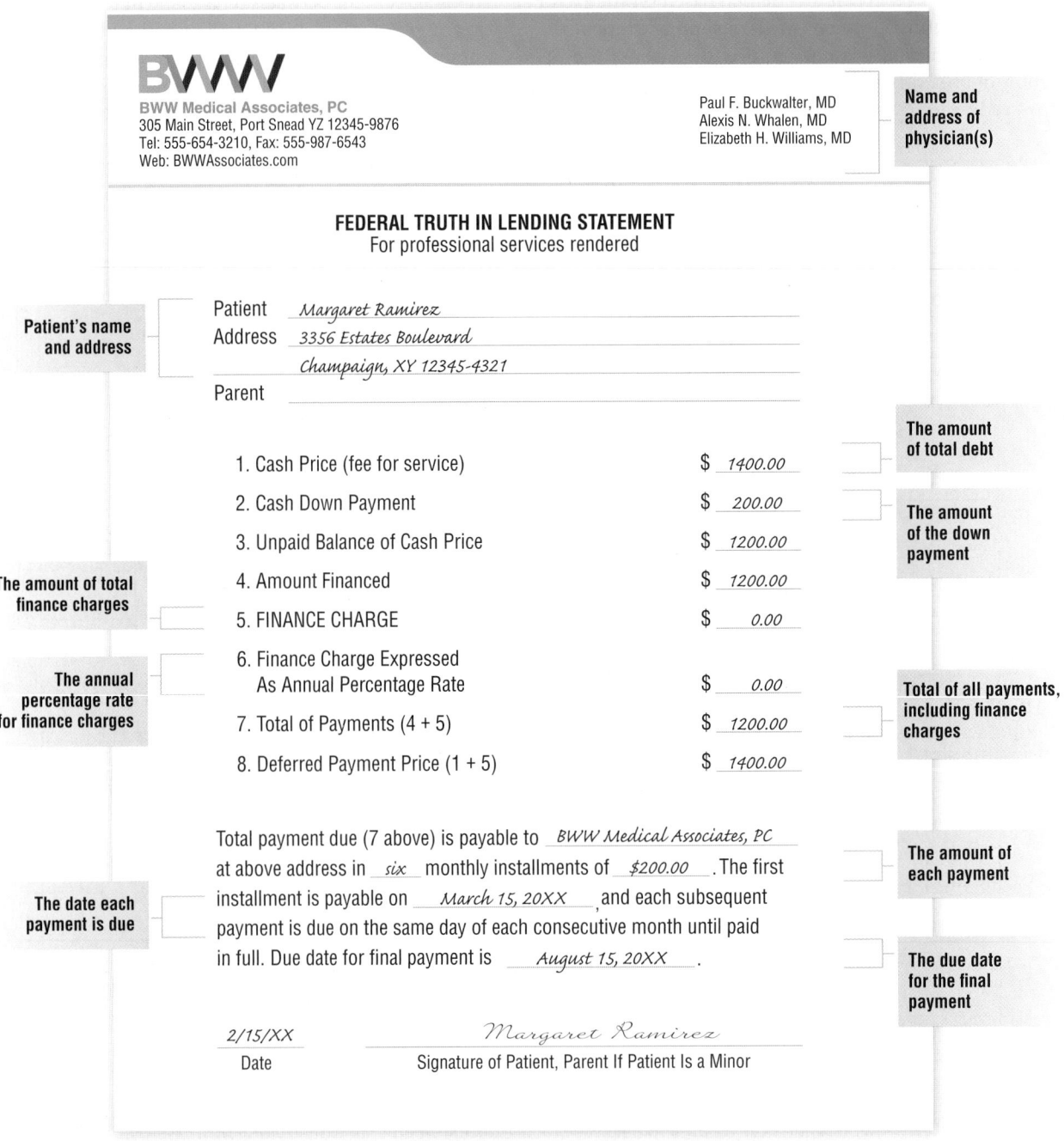

FIGURE 20-7 Typical Truth in Lending Statement completed and signed by the patient.

2. The amount of the down payment.

3. The amount of each payment (which may be weekly or monthly or for another period) and the date it is due. (Frequently the total number of payments to be made after the down payment is also included.)

4. The due date for the final payment and the amount of the final payment if different from the other payment amounts.

5. The interest rate, if interest is to be paid, expressed as an annual percentage.

6. The total finance charges, if any. (If interest is charged, the total amount of interest accrued during the course of the debt will be entered here.)

The practice and the patient should each keep a copy of the signed disclosure agreement. Procedure 20-4, at the end of the chapter, outlines the steps in creating and completing a Truth in Lending Statement (Agreement). Under the Truth in Lending Act, the patient is billed only for the monthly amount agreed upon and not the total amount of the debt. To avoid mailing a monthly statement, some offices create a master document, given to the patient at the time of the agreement signing, that outlines each month's due date and the amount due, with a running total of the new balance once the payment is made. Figure 20-8 is an example of such a document.

BWW

BWW Medical Associates, PC
305 Main Street, Port Snead YZ 12345-9876
Tel: 555-654-3210, Fax: 555-987-6543
Web: BWWAssociates.com

Paul F. Buckwalter, MD
Alexis N. Whalen, MD
Elizabeth H. Williams, MD

February 15, 20XX

Margaret Ramirez
3356 Estates Boulevard
Champaign XY 12345-4321

RE: Monthly Payment Agreement

Dear Ms. Ramirez:

As outlined in the Truth and Lending Statement signed in our office today, for your convenience we have outlined below your monthly payment schedule.

Amount Financed: $1200.00

Monthly Payments: $200.00

Date of Payment	Current Balance
3/15/20XX	$1000.00
4/15/20XX	$ 800.00
5/15/20XX	$ 600.00
6/15/20XX	$ 400.00
7/15/20XX	$ 200.00
8/15/20XX	$ 0.00

If for any reason, you cannot make the agreed-upon monthly payment as outlined above, please call me immediately so a new arrangement may be made.

As always, we thank you for choosing BWW Medical Associates, PC for your health care needs.

Sincerely,

Malik Katahri, cmm

Malik Katahari, CMM
Office Manager

MK/map

FIGURE 20-8 Patient letter outlining the Truth in Lending Agreement, including the payment dates and the amount of each payment.

▶ Common Collection Problems LO 20.6

Collection problems come in many forms, but there are two common collection problems encountered by medical practices. The first is patients who cannot pay—also called hardship cases—and the second is patients who have moved without leaving a forwarding address and therefore have not received a statement.

Hardship Cases

A physician may decide to treat some patients without charge—or at a deep discount—simply because they cannot pay. These patients may be poor, uninsured, underinsured, or elderly and on a limited income. They may be patients who have suffered a severe financial loss or family tragedy. Medical ethics require physicians to provide care to individuals who need it, regardless of their ability to pay. Nevertheless, free treatment for hardship cases is at the physician's discretion.

Providing free care must be undertaken very carefully because, under the ECOA, if a patient is given free or reduced-fee treatment based on her inability to pay and another patient under similar circumstances is treated, she also must be extended the same financial consideration or a charge of discrimination may be levied against the physician. Some providers treat such patients for urgent problems and then refer the patients to federally funded clinics that are allowed to provide free or reduced-fee services related to their government funding.

Patient Relocation and Address Change

Sometimes a patient account remains unpaid because the patient has moved without leaving a forwarding address and has not received the statement. These patients are known as **skips**. Obviously, reaching such a patient about payment issues will provide a challenge.

Remember, you cannot discuss a debt with anyone except the person responsible for the charges. When you make a telephone call for collection, however, you may ask a third party for the patient's new address or phone number if known. If the third party states the new address is not known, do not call again unless there is reason to believe that the third party has learned of the person's address or phone number since the first inquiry. If the patient had given permission to e-mail him, you may also try that avenue. Ask the post office for a forwarding address. If these avenues do not locate the patient, he may be labeled a skip and then referred to the office collection agency. Be sure to keep the returned statement and envelope stamped by the post office as "addressee unknown" or "no forwarding address" to prove a reasonable attempt to collect the debt.

PROCEDURE 20-1 Using the Superbill as Bill/Receipt

Procedure Goal: To complete a superbill accurately for use as the patient first bill or receipt.

OSHA Guidelines: This procedure does not involve exposure to blood, body fluids, or tissue.

Materials: Superbill, patient ledger card, patient information sheet, fee schedule, pen.

Method: Procedure steps.

1. From the patient ledger card and information sheet, fill in the patient data, such as name, sex, date of birth, and insurance information.

2. Fill in the date of service. If there are multiple practice locations, circle the location where the service is taking place.

3. Attach the superbill to the patient's medical record and give them both to the physician.
   RATIONALE: The physician must have the superbill to enter the services performed during the visit.

4. At the end of the visit, accept the completed superbill from the patient. Make sure that the doctor has indicated the procedures performed and an appropriate diagnosis for each.
   RATIONALE: Ensures medical necessity for the insurance carrier to allow for payment.

5. If the physician has not already recorded the charges, refer to the fee schedule for procedures that are marked. Then fill in the charges next to those procedures.
   RATIONALE: Each procedure must have a charge for accurate billing.

6. In the appropriate blanks, list the total charges for the visit and the previous balance (if any).

7. Calculate the subtotal.

8. Fill in the amount and type of payment (cash, check, money order, debit or credit card) made by the patient during this visit.
   RATIONALE: This information ensures accurate posting to the patient's account.

9. Calculate and enter the new balance.

10. If not already on file, have the patient sign the authorization-and-release section of the superbill.
    RATIONALE: Without these signatures there is no authorization to share information with the insurance carrier, nor is there agreement for the payer to pay the service provider directly for the services provided.

11. Keep a copy of the superbill for the practice records. Give the original to the patient along with one copy to file with the insurer.

PROCEDURE 20-2 Preparing an Age Analysis

Procedure Goal: To create and examine an age analysis of practice accounts.

OSHA Guidelines: This procedure does not involve exposure to blood, body fluids, or tissue.

Materials: Computer, patient accounts, ledger cards (if a manual system is used), accounts receivable age analysis form or template (Figure 20-5), policy and procedure manual, pen.

Method: Procedure steps.

1. Using the reporting section of your billing computer program, create an age analysis report for patients and insurance companies. This also can be done manually by pulling patient ledger cards, noting balances due and dates of last payments. Use Figure 20-5 as a guide to create a spreadsheet for your findings.
   RATIONALE: If the office billing is computerized, pulling an aging report from the system is efficient and reliable.

2. Review the accounting report. Check the report—highlight each account for proposed actions according to your office policy.
   RATIONALE: Efforts to collect outstanding accounts become more urgent as accounts age and it becomes more difficult to collect the outstanding balance.

3. Mark the accounts that are under 31 days as "No action to be taken at this time."
   RATIONALE: Accounts of this age are considered current.

4. Bills that are unpaid at more than 31 days should be marked as "Contact or follow up with insurance company."
   RATIONALE: Patients frequently wait for the insurance carrier to pay its portion before they pay the patient balance.

5. Accounts that are 31–60 days old should be marked according to your office policy. An initial phone call may be made inquiring as to payment arrangements.

RATIONALE: The older an account becomes, the more difficult it is to collect. These accounts are at "prime time" to be collected.

6. Accounts that are 61–90 days old should be marked according to your office policy. Make notations such as "Account Past Due." A follow-up phone call and/or more insistent statement message letter for payment may be in order.
   RATIONALE: Collecting accounts aged less than 91 days have a better success rate than those that are older.

7. Accounts that are 91–120 days old should be marked according to your office policy. A last phone call to attempt discussing the account and more insistent collection statement/letter should be sent.

8. For accounts older than 120 days, make sure you review previous collection attempts. At this point, after discussion with the physician, a letter stating the account will be turned over to the collection agency will take place with a specific date listed in the letter. This letter should be mailed by certified, return receipt mail.
   RATIONALE: After 120 days without a payment, it is unlikely the patient will pay the bill without a more aggressive course of action.

9. Record all actions that have been taken beside each account.
   RATIONALE: This diary provides a written record of all attempts to collect the debt.

10. Finally, write follow-up letters to patients and document any agreements that you and the patient have discussed via telephone. Be sure to keep a copy of any correspondence mailed to the patient in the financial record.
    RATIONALE: All documentation will be necessary should any legal action be taken regarding this debt.

PROCEDURE 20-3 Referring an Account to a Collection Agency and Posting the Payment from the Agency

Procedure Goal: To follow the correct procedure in turning an account over to a collection agency and posting the payment from them when received.

OSHA Guidelines: This procedure does not involve exposure to blood, body fluids, or tissue.

Materials: Computer, patient accounts, ledger cards (if a manual system is used), patient's financial record containing demographic information, collection agency's phone number, pen.

Method: Procedure steps.

1. Make sure all attempts that have been made to collect the debt per office policy have been documented, including return receipt from letter sent to patient stating account would be turned over to the collection agency by a specific date (today).

RATIONALE: To avoid charges of harassment, once a threat of collection proceedings has been made, the account must be turned over on the specified date.

2. Verify that the following information is in the patient's financial file to be turned over to the collection agency:
   - Last known phone number and address for the patient.
   - Employer (if any) name and phone number.
   - Name of spouse, if applicable.
   - Total amount of debt, with last payment amount and date.
   - If there has been no payment, the last date a service was provided.
   - Description of office actions to collect debt.
   - Any patient response to those actions.

RATIONALE: This information is required by the collection agency prior to their taking over the account.

3. Place a call to the agency, identifying yourself and the office, and explain you are calling to turn accounts over to them.

4. For each account to be turned over, supply the information listed in step 2.

5. When a payment arrives from the agency, each account will be identified with the total amount of the debt collected. The agency will also deduct their fee from this amount.
RATIONALE: The agency will collect its fee up front from the payment received per contracted agreement with the practice.

6. When posting the payment, post the actual amount of the payment sent to the office from the collection agency to the patient's account, not the full amount of the payment made by the patient.
RATIONALE: The agency kept a portion of the payment as their fee; it will not be posted to the patient's account.

7. Make an adjustment (write-off) on the patient's account in the amount kept by the agency as their fee.
RATIONALE: You cannot add the fee charged by the collection agency to the patient's account. It is a "cost of doing business."

8. Subtract both the payment and the adjustment from the patient's balance. If the payment is noted by the agency as being the full payment on the account, the payment and adjustment should result in a zero balance on the patient's account.

PROCEDURE 20-4 Completing a Truth in Lending Statement (Agreement)

Procedure Goal: To create an accurate and complete Truth in Lending Statement.

OSHA Guidelines: This procedure does not involve exposure to blood, body fluids, or tissue.

Materials: Computer, paper, patient financial record, the name of the procedure or service to be financed, total cost of procedure or service to be financed, amount of down payment, number of payments, amount of each payment, date of month for each payment, pen.

Method: Procedure steps.

1. Create a document (or use a template) similar to that of Figure 20-7 to use as the Truth in Lending Statement.

2. Make sure the following information is included:
   - Patient name and address.
   - Price for service or procedure.
   - Amount of down payment received.
   - Unpaid balance.
   - Amount financed.
   - Finance charge (if applicable).
   - Finance charge as a percentage rate (if applicable).

   - Total amount to be financed.
   - Number of payments and the amount of each.
   - Date payments are due, including final payment date.

3. Once template is completed, fill in the information for the patient's agreement. Make calculations carefully and check your work.
RATIONALE: For the TLS to be valid, all information must be included and accurate.

4. After going over the statement with the patient, have the patient sign and date the agreement.
RATIONALE: Without the patient's signature the agreement is not valid.

5. Give a copy of the signed agreement to the patient and keep a copy in the patient's financial record for future reference.

6. If desired, a master document, such as that found in Figure 20-8, may be created outlining the agreement and listing the actual date and payment amount for each month of the agreement.
RATIONALE: This document avoids the need for mailing a monthly statement for the agreed-upon amount to the patient.

SUMMARY OF LEARNING OUTCOMES

LEARNING OUTCOMES	KEY POINTS
20.1 **Describe accounts receivable and accounts payable and the common payment methods accepted in medical practices today.**	Accounts receivable refers to the money that is owed to the practice (able to be received). Accounts payable refers to the money that the practice owes other vendors (able to be paid). Common payment methods accepted by medical practices include cash, check, and debit and credit cards.
20.2 **Identify the different types of documents used as statements to bill patients and how these documents are used in *cycle billing*.**	Common statement documents include the use of superbills, typed or computer-produced itemized statements, and copies of ledger cards. In cycle billing the accounts are split in groups and statement mailing dates are staggered.

LEARNING OUTCOMES	KEY POINTS
20.3 **Compare open-book, written-contract, and single-entry accounts and the purpose of creating an accounts receivable aging.**	An open-book account is the account type most commonly found in a medical practice, consisting of periodic charges and payments added as needed when patients are seen in the practice. A written-contract account is used when the physician and patient sign a contract for a specific service or procedure. A single-entry account is one used for patients when it is expected they will be seen only once, such as for a relative visiting the area on vacation. An age analysis is the process of classifying and reviewing past-due accounts by age from the first date of billing. It helps you keep on top of past-due accounts and determine which ones need follow-up.
20.4 **Explain the purposes of the following credit and collections acts: ECOA, FCRA, FDCPA, and TLA.**	ECOA is the Equal Credit Opportunity Act. It prohibits discrimination based on sex, marital status, race, national origin, religion, or age. Applicants also cannot be discriminated against for receiving public assistance income or exercising their rights under the Consumer Credit Protection Act. The Fair Credit Reporting Act (FCRA) requires credit bureaus to supply correct and complete information to businesses to use in evaluating a person's application for credit, insurance, or a job. The Fair Debt Collections Practices Act (FDCPA) requires debt collectors to treat debtors fairly and prohibits certain collection tactics, including harassment, false statements, threats, and unfair practices. The Truth in Lending Act (TLA) requires creditors to provide applicants with accurate and complete credit costs and terms.
20.5 **Relate the required components of a Truth in Lending Statement to credit practices in the medical office.**	The Truth in Lending Statement must include the following elements: the amount of total debt, the amount of the down payment, the amount of each payment and the date due, the due date for the final payment, the interest rate (if any) expressed as an annual percentage rate, and the total finance charges (if any).
20.6 **Summarize two common types of problem collection accounts in the medical office.**	The two most common types of collection problems in the medical office are hardship cases, who simply cannot afford to pay their debt, and accounts known as skips, where the debtor moved and left no valid forwarding information so it is not possible to bill the patient.

CASE STUDY CRITICAL THINKING

Recall Nancy Evans from the beginning of the chapter. Now that you have completed the chapter, answer the following questions regarding her case.

1. How much of the $360 bill for the neurology consult services will be Nancy's responsibility? (Refer to the *Insurance and Billing* chapter if necessary.)
2. What is the best way to bill Nancy for this balance?
3. Why is this way the preferred method?

1. (LO 20.1) Billing and collections is important to the medical practice because
   a. It keeps the A/R up
   b. It keeps the front office staff busy
   c. It produces cash flow for the office
   d. It increases the office A/P
   e. It proves how important the practice is to the community

2. (LO 20.1) Which of the following is a diplomatic way to ask a patient for payment?
   a. "I need $50 for today's visit."
   b. "For today's visit, the total charge is $50. How would you like to pay for that?"
   c. "That will be $50. What is your check number?"
   d. "Your charge for today's visit is $50. We take cash, check, credit, and debit cards."
   e. Either b or d would be acceptable

3. (LO 20.2) Which of the following pieces of information should be included on a patient statement?
   a. The patient's income
   b. The balance from the previous month and an itemized list of charges
   c. The patient's credit card information
   d. The patient's occupation and place of employment
   e. b, c, and d

4. (LO 20.2) Which of the following would not be acceptable for use as a patient statement?
   a. A completed superbill
   b. A handwritten statement
   c. A computer-generated statement
   d. A "clean" copy of the office ledger card
   e. A typed statement

5. (LO 20.3) Which of the following account types is most common in the medical office?
   a. Open-book accounts
   b. Single-entry accounts
   c. Accounts involving Truth in Lending Statements
   d. Skip accounts
   e. Written-contract accounts

6. (LO 20.3) What is the most important reason for running an age analysis of the patient accounts?
   a. It allows you to see "deadbeats" at a glance
   b. It allows you to track the "high dollar" accounts
   c. It tracks delinquent insurance payments
   d. It allows you to track past due accounts so the patients may be contacted
   e. It lets the physician know how much money is owed to the practice

7. (LO 20.4) Which of the following laws govern(s) credit policies in medical practices?
   a. ECOA
   b. FCRA
   c. FDCPA
   d. TLA
   e. a, b, and d

8. (LO 20.4) Which of the following laws govern(s) collection policies in medical practices?
   a. ECOA
   b. FCRA
   c. FDCPA
   d. TLA
   e. a, b, and d

9. (LO 20.5) Under what conditions is a Truth in Lending Agreement (Statement) required?
   a. When the physician informally agrees that the patient can pay a bill in installments
   b. If a bilateral agreement of less than four installments is reached
   c. When the patient pays at the time of service
   d. When a finance charge is to be assessed by the practice
   e. All of the above require a TLS

10. (LO 20.6) Which credit and collections act requires that if a physician decreases or forgives a patient's debt, he must do the same for another patient in a similar situation?
    a. ECOA
    b. FCRA
    c. FDCPA
    d. TLA
    e. HIPAA

Financial Management

PATIENT INFORMATION	Patient Name	Gender	DOB
	Sylvia Gonzales	F	9/1/19XX
	Attending	**MRN**	**Allergies**
	Alexis N. Whalen, MD	341-73-792	Penicillin

Sylvia Gonzales is a 51-year-old female with type 2 diabetes. She is returning today after starting Januvia 100 mg daily and is in a fasting state so that FBS (fasting blood sugar) and hemoglobin A1C blood tests may be done as CLIA-waived tests, in the office. Dr. Whalen has encouraged Ms. Gonzales to lose some weight, arranging for an appointment with a nutritionist, and has also requested a follow-up 15-minute appointment in 3 months. As you check out Ms. Gonzales, you explain that there is a $25 previous balance on her account after the insurance paid its portion of her last visit. She gives you a check for this balance. Today's charges total $175.00, which will be submitted to her insurance carrier.

Keep Sylvia in mind as you study the chapter. There will be questions at the end of the chapter based on the case study. The information in the chapter will help you answer these questions.

McGraw Hill ACTIVSim™

L E A R N I N G   O U T C O M E S

After completing Chapter 21, you will be able to:

21.1 Summarize the importance of and how to establish good bookkeeping and banking practices.

21.2 Compare single-entry, double-entry, and write-it-once bookkeeping systems.

21.3 Outline patient-related financial transactions.

21.4 Identify negotiable instruments and the items that must be present for a check to be negotiable.

21.5 Describe the different types of check endorsements and the steps in creating a bank deposit.

21.6 Carry out the process of reconciling the office bank statement.

21.7 List several advantages to electronic banking.

21.8 Implement setting up, classifying, and recording disbursements in a disbursements journal.

K E Y   T E R M S

ABA number
accounting
bookkeeping
cash flow statement
cashier's check
certified check
check
counter check
endorsement
journalizing
limited check
money order

negotiable
payee
payer
power of attorney
reconciliation
third-party check
tracking
traveler's check
voucher check
write-it-once (pegboard) system

VI. C (1) Explain basic bookkeeping computations

VI. C (2) Differentiate between bookkeeping and accounting

VI. C (3) Describe banking procedures

VI. C (4) Discuss precautions for accepting checks

VI. C (5) Compare types of endorsement

VI. C (6) Differentiate between accounts payable and accounts receivable

VI. C (7) Compare manual and computerized bookkeeping systems used in ambulatory healthcare

VI. C (8) Describe common periodic financial reports

VI. C (10) Identify procedure for preparing patient accounts

VI. C (13) Discuss types of adjustments that may be made to a patient's account

VI. P (1) Prepare a bank deposit

VI. P (2) Perform accounts receivable procedures, including:
  - a. Post entries on a day sheet
  - d. Post adjustments
  - e. Process a credit balance
  - f. Process refunds
  - g. Post non-sufficient fund (NSF) checks
  - h. Post collection agency payment

VI. A (1) Demonstrate sensitivity and professionalism in handling accounts receivable activities with clients

4. Medical Law and Ethics

Graduates:
  - f. Comply with federal, state, and local health laws and regulations

8. Medical Office Business Procedures Management

Graduates:
  - g. Prepare and reconcile a bank statement and deposit record
  - h. Post entries on a day sheet
  - j. Perform accounts payable procedures
  - k. Perform accounts receivable procedures
  - m. Post adjustments
  - n. Process credit balances
  - o. Process refunds
  - p. Post non-sufficient funds (NSF)
  - q. Post collection agency payments
  - w. Use manual or computerized bookkeeping systems
  - ll. Apply electronic technology

▶ Introduction

Often, when you ask someone why he or she entered the medical field, you will hear, "I want to be involved with patient care." Excellent patient care is at the heart of every medical office, but what is behind this heart, the true backbone of the practice? Financial management. Without current, sound financial practices and management in place, a medical practice cannot succeed. A physician may have a thriving practice and be loved by her patients, but without employees who understand and perform sound business and financial management procedures, the practice will fail and ultimately close. In this chapter, you will explore the practices necessary to keep a successful medical practice thriving.

▶ The Medical Practice as a Business

LO 21.1

A medical practice is a business. If it is to prosper, its income must exceed its expenses. In other words, it must produce a profit. The process of communicating the income and expenses of a business and its financial health is known as **accounting**. The practice's finances must be watched closely to be sure that expenses do not exceed income. Part of this process is the systematic recording of business transactions, known as **bookkeeping**. As the office medical assistant, recording daily business transactions may be part of your responsibility. Your records, along with other financial records, will later be analyzed by an accountant or by a more experienced medical assistant to monitor the practice's financial health. In addition to bookkeeping, banking is another key responsibility of many medical assistants. To fulfill these administrative responsibilities, you need an understanding of basic accounting systems and the procedures surrounding banking and financial management.

Importance of Accuracy

Whenever you perform bookkeeping or banking procedures, strive for 100% accuracy. Because bookkeeping records form a chain of information, an undetected error at the first link will be carried through all other links in the chain. You might compare this to a set of dominoes: if one domino is not perfectly balanced, it will affect all those that come after it, collapsing the entire bunch. Undetected errors in the medical office can result in billing a patient twice for the same visit, omitting bank deposits, or making improper payments to suppliers. These actions can result in lost money—and patients—for the practice. Establishing procedures that are consistently carried out will help ensure accuracy and also help avoid forgetting a potentially important step in the procedure.

Establishing Procedures

Here are some general suggestions to assist you in maintaining accuracy in bookkeeping and banking procedures for your medical practice.

- Be organized. Maintain the practice's bookkeeping and banking records and written procedures in a logical and organized way.

- Be consistent. Always handle the same kinds of transactions in exactly the same way. For example, endorse all checks with the same information, regardless of who wrote them or when you will be depositing them. Using a preprinted bank stamp is helpful for consistency with this procedure.

- Use markers. Make check marks as you work to avoid losing your place if you are interrupted. For example, place a red check mark on each checkbook entry as you check it against the bank statement when you reconcile the office checkbook with the bank statement.

- Write clearly. Always use the same type and pen color and clear, easy-to-read handwriting. If more than one person performs bookkeeping and banking tasks, each person should initial her part of the procedure to identify her work. It is recommended that as few people as possible perform these tasks, however, to minimize possible duplication or accidental "skipping" of steps because "Judy and Michaela each mistakenly thought the other had performed the bank reconciliation." You may use pencil for trial balances and worksheets, but you should use pen for final bookkeeping entries.

- Check your work. Frequently review your work to detect and correct any errors. To correct errors, draw a straight line through the incorrect figure and write the correct figure above it. Never erase errors or delete them with correction fluid or tape. As with medical records, the office financial records are legal documents and every entry, even corrected ones, needs to be readable at all times.

- Use straight columns. Keep all columns of figures straight, so that decimal points align correctly. This makes totaling of figures easier and also looks neat and professional.

Using set procedures, even as more and more of these procedures become computerized, will help you organize your work, help ensure accuracy, and make you a more valuable member of the practice staff because others will trust that your work will be concise and accurate.

▶ Medical Office Accounting Methods

LO 21.2

Patient accounting methods within a medical practice may be computerized or manual, but more and more offices are turning to computerized patient accounting systems. Three types of manual accounting systems may be used by medical practices that are not computerized: single-entry, double-entry, and pegboard system (also known as the write-it-once system). All accounting systems record income, *charges* (money owed to the practice), *disbursements* (money paid out by the practice), and

other financial information. The choice of system is based on the size and complexity of the practice. Even if your office is computerized, it is important to have a basic understanding of each of these systems, as you will find that computerized systems work in the same manner. Not only that, but if the office computer system goes down for any reason, you will still need to have a mechanism to track any transactions that take place during the "computer down time."

Electronic Bookkeeping

Offices that utilize a computerized bookkeeping system enjoy several important benefits over traditional manual bookkeeping methods. With computerized bookkeeping, you save time because

- The computer performs repetitive tasks.

- The computer automatically performs mathematical calculations within the software.

- Built-in tax tables are available that calculate tax liabilities for you.

Many bookkeeping software programs or practice management software programs are available on the market and perform the same tasks that are performed manually. Understanding these tasks is an essential part of managing books on a computer as well as with a manual system. The practice in which you work may already have a computerized bookkeeping program in place, which you will learn as the office medical assistant. It is also a good idea to stay current on new software programs as they become available by reading computer software magazines or joining your local medical assisting organization, which often keeps members updated on new trends in the market. If you learn about a more efficient way to use the practice's current financial management software or discover a new software program that you feel might be helpful to your office, gather the pertinent information and make a recommendation to the physician or office manager regarding your proposal.

Manual Bookkeeping Systems

Traditionally, there were two types of accounting systems: single-entry and double-entry. In the single-entry system, a transaction is listed once (each) in the patient ledger, the daily log, and the checkbook. Although simple to use, this system is not self-balancing and errors may easily go undetected. In the double-entry system, all entries are listed twice, based on the accounting formula of Assets = Capital + Liabilities. An asset is anything owned by the company (or practice). Capital is the portion of the asset that is paid for and a liability is the amount of money owed by the practice on the asset. To better understand this formula, consider the new ECG machine purchased by the practice in the example shown below. The cost of the machine is $15,000 and the office made a down payment of $5000.

Example:

$15,000 (Asset) = $5000 (capital) + $10,000 (liability)

Every month, when a payment is made, the asset amount will remain the same, but the capital amount will increase and the liability amount will decrease. However, both sides of the equation will continue to balance.

Write-It-Once or Pegboard System Most medical offices using a manual bookkeeping system use the **pegboard** (or **write-it-once**) **system,** which contains a formula to check your work. The write-it-once system uses the same bookkeeping forms as the single- and double-entry systems, but the day sheet, also called the daily log, has pre-punched holes on the right or left side of the log. There are similar holes in the shingled (layered) charge sheets that are placed in designated areas on top of the day sheet, which has been placed on the pegboard. Each charge sheet is made with no-carbon-required (NCR) paper, so when the patient ledger card is placed between the day sheet and charge sheet and an entry is made, it appears on all three documents at the same time—hence the term "write-it-once." You will examine this system in more detail later in the chapter.

Bookkeeping Forms Regardless of the type of bookkeeping method used, each of these systems uses similar forms and records to maintain the bookkeeping system. Each form is discussed in further detail in the following paragraphs.

Daily Log The daily log is also known as a general ledger, day sheet, or daily journal, depending on the practice. Regardless of the name used, it is a chronological list of each patient's charges, any payments made on the account, and any adjustments on the account (like the difference between the charge billed to the insurance carrier and the "allowed charge" that the payment is based on). See Figure 21-1. In the daily log, you record the name of each patient seen that day. Across from the name, you record the service provided (using the proper procedure codes), the fee charged, and the payment (if any) received. This process is called **journalizing**. You then post (copy) the charges, adjustments, and payments from the daily log to patient ledger cards. Using a daily or monthly cash control sheet, you record checks and cash received as well as deposits made each day.

In most offices, medical assistants maintain the daily log. You can obtain the information needed to post transactions from the charge slip, which may also be called the encounter form or superbill. (Note: A charge slip is the original record of all of the doctor's charges and services performed on that day for an individual patient.) Because some charge slips include the areas for payment and next appointment information, the term *superbill* is often used. Typically, a charge slip/receipt includes duplicate (and sometimes triplicate) copies underneath to use for bookkeeping purposes—one copy for the patient, one for the medical office, and one for the business office, if that is a separate entity. Remember, you need to track charges *and* receipts for payment, for each patient, regardless of the bookkeeping method used. If the physician also performs house calls or visits to nursing homes, records of these visits must also be accounted for, so additional copies of charge slips may be sent with the physician for his use when visiting these outside facilities.

As a medical assistant, it is also your job to record any night calls or other unscheduled visits in the daily log. Simply check with the physician each morning to determine if a charge slip needs to be generated to record the proper fees. If the physician has not noted the charge amount on a charge slip/receipt or record of outside visits, you may have to apply the appropriate fees according to the agreed-upon fee schedule for your office.

In addition to payments made by patients while in the office, other payments will come into the office by mail from both insurance companies and patients. These payments also must be recorded in the daily log for proper tracking of accounts receivable (A/R). When payment is sent from an insurance company, it is usually in the form of a check (or electronic payment) and will have an explanation of benefits (EOB) or remittance advice (RA) attached that will display the amount paid on each patient's behalf. You must post the amount indicated to each individual patient account and record any adjustment that may be required according to the contract the practice has with the insurance company.

If extra columns are available, and if it is part of office policy, you also may record additional financial information in the daily log. For example, in addition to showing the total amount charged to the patient, you might show a breakdown of that total into the amounts generated by different physicians in a group practice or by different functions of the office, such as the laboratory or X-ray department.

At the end of each day, total the charges and receipts in the daily log and post these totals to the monthly summary of charges

Date: 4/15/XX

Patient	Service	Charge	Payment	Adj	Cur. Bal	Prev. Bal	MD
Washington, Ken	99212, 93000	150.00	25.00		125.00	0.00	PFB
Ramirez, Valarie	99213	80.00			190.00	110.00	PFB
Lautu, Raja	99384	145.00	20.00		160.00	35.00	EHW
Chen, Cindy	99215, 36415	210.00		25.00	185.00	0.00	ANW
Matthews, Chris	99212	65.00	65.00		0.00	0.00	ANW
TOTALS		**650.00**	**110.00**	**25.00**	**660.00**	**145.00**	

FIGURE 21-1 The daily log is used to record all patient-based financial activity in the office for each day.

and receipts. To double-check your totals, perform the following steps, outlined in Procedure 21-1 at the end of this chapter:

- Ensure that the day's total cash and check receipts are the same as the day's total bank deposit.
- Ensure that the sum of the day's charges for each type of service is the same as the total of the day's charges.

Patient Ledger Cards Another bookkeeping task is preparing a *patient ledger card* for each patient. This card includes the patient's name, address, home and work telephone numbers, the name of the guarantor (the one who is responsible

for payment of the charges if different from the patient), health insurance information, Social Security number, employer's name, and any special billing instructions. Figure 21-2 shows an example of a patient ledger card.

You will use the patient ledger card to record charges incurred by the patient, payments received, adjustments made, and the resulting balance owed to the doctor as described in Procedure 21-1. Because these cards document the financial transactions of the individual patient account, they are sometimes called *account cards*. In some practices that perform manual billing procedures, they are photocopied for use as monthly statements.

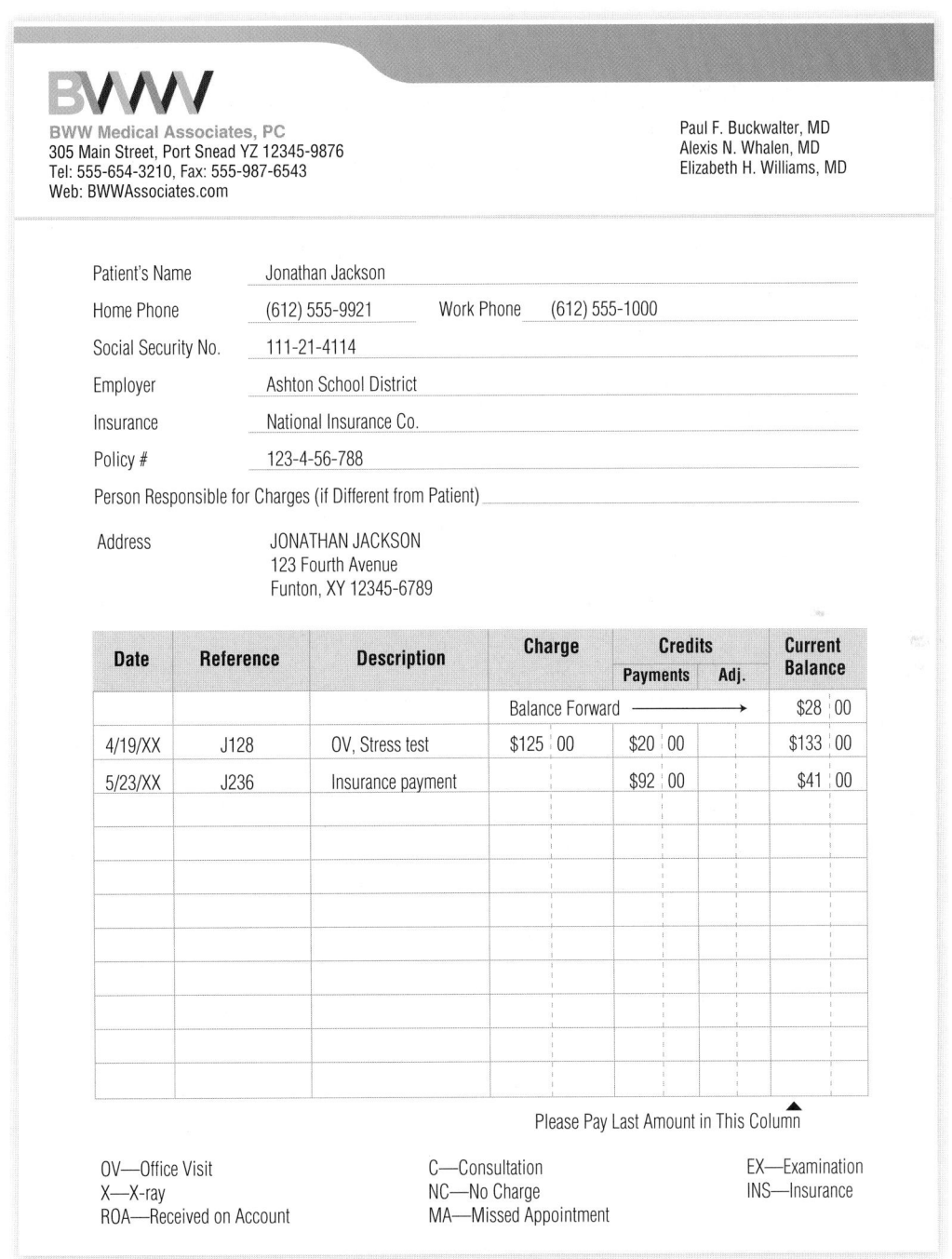

FIGURE 21-2 A patient ledger card shows an individual patient's charges, adjustments, receipts, and balance due.

The information for the patient ledger cards comes from the daily log and includes the information found on the superbill (charge slip). It is best to complete all the cards at the end of each business day. If this is not possible, you may complete them as time permits during the next business day. To prevent duplicate or omitted postings, put a small check mark next to each entry in the daily log after you post it to the proper ledger card. Take great care when posting because errors posted on the patient's ledger card will be reflected on the patient billing statements. To ensure accuracy, add up the total charges and receipts from the ledger cards and make sure the information matches the total charges and receipts in that day's daily log.

When working with patient financial records, including patient ledger cards, keep in mind that each patient's financial records must be kept just as confidential as his or her medical record information. Regardless of whether you are working with paper financial records or using an electronic system, just as with medical information, be sure that only those staff members with a "need to know" are allowed access to any patient's financial information. More about these practices is covered in the *Patient Billing and Collections* chapter.

Bookkeeping Records Regardless of whether the office bookkeeping system is computerized or manual, the records kept on the office finances remain the same. Let's look at each of these records here.

Accounts Receivable Each day, you must update the accounts receivable record, which shows the total owed to the practice (the amount able to be received but not yet received). Total up the items on the accounts receivable record and then total up the outstanding balances on the patient ledger cards. The two numbers should match. If they do not, recheck your work to find the cause of the discrepancy.

Accounts Payable Accounts payable are the amounts the practice owes to vendors (the amount able to be paid but not yet paid). If your responsibilities include accounts payable, keep careful records of equipment and supplies ordered and compare orders received against the invoices. In the checkbook register, keep detailed and accurate records of accounts paid.

Record of Office Disbursements This record is a list of the amounts paid for items like medical supplies, office rent, office utilities, employee wages, postage, and equipment over a certain period of time. It shows the **payee** (the person who will receive the payment), the date, the check number, the amount paid, and the type of expense. Figure 21-3 is an example of a disbursement record.

Record of Office Disbursements
April 20XX

DATE	PAYEE	CK. NO.	TOTAL AMOUNT	RENT	UTILITIES	POSTAGE	LAB./X-RAY	MEDICAL SUPPLIES	OFFICE SUPPLIES	WAGES	INSURANCE	TAXES	TRAVEL	MISC.
01	Philips' Med. Suppl.	1778	125.00					125.00						
01	Postage	1779	16.85			16.85								
02	Medi Path	1780	32.50				32.50							
02	Quik Service Co.	1781	82.40						82.40					
02	Philips' Med. Suppl.	1782	92.00					92.00						
02	Jean Medina	1783	77.06							77.06				
05	State Dept. of Rev.	1784	189.16									189.16		
06	General Insurance	1785	165.92								165.92			
07	Postage	(Cash)	5.19			5.19								
07	Micah Smith	(Cash)	15.00										15.00	
08	IRS	1786	419.41									419.41		
12	Quik Service Co.	1787	124.00						124.00					
13	City Laundry	1788	75.00											75.00
13	National Insurance	1789	189.00								189.00			
14	Broyer Assoc.	1790	1500.00	1500.00										
14	Postage	(Cash)	12.11			12.11								
15	City Gas Co.	1791	125.00		125.00									
19	Jean Medina	1792	85.92							85.92				
19	Postage	(Cash)	8.95			8.95								
21	Philips' Med. Suppl.	1793	85.00					85.00						
23	Medi Path	1794	67.90				67.90							
24	Micah Smith	(Cash)	10.00										10.00	
24	Elena Paxson	1795	126.00							126.00				
27	Postage	1796	17.32			17.32								
28	Johnson Assoc.	1797	123.45				123.45							
	Total		3770.14	1500.00	125.00	60.42	223.85	302.00	206.40	288.98	354.92	608.57	25.00	75.00

FIGURE 21-3 The office disbursements journal is a record of payments made by the office, showing who was paid, when the payment was made, and the amount paid.

A checkbook register may be used to record office disbursements. As an alternative, a disbursement journal or the bottom section of the daily log may also be used to record office disbursements. For income tax purposes, this record should include only office expenses. The doctor's personal expenses should not be listed here.

Summary of Charges, Receipts, and Disbursements

Charges, receipts, and disbursements are usually summarized at the end of each month, quarter, or year depending on your office policies and procedures (Figure 21-4). The summary is used to compare the current period's income and expenses with any previous period's income and expenses.

By analyzing summaries, a physician (or practice manager) can see which functions of the practice are profitable, the total amount charged for services, the payments received for services, the total cost of running the office, and a breakdown of expenses into various categories. Based on this information, the practice can make vital business decisions. For example, after analyzing monthly summaries, it may decide to budget expenses differently, collect payments more promptly, cut unprofitable services, or expand profitable services.

Although an accountant may prepare these reports, an experienced administrative medical assistant can prepare them. If you are asked to prepare them, follow these guidelines.

- Every business day, post the total charges and receipts from the daily log to the appropriate line and column of the monthly summary.
- Each business day, also post the disbursements from the record of office disbursements to the appropriate lines and columns of the monthly summary.
- At the end of the month, total the columns on the monthly summary.
- At the end of each quarter, post the charges, receipts, and disbursements for each of the previous 3 months to the quarterly summary. Then, total each column.
- At the end of the year, post the charges, receipts, and disbursements for each of the previous 12 months (or 4 quarters) to the annual summary. Then, total each column.

Remember, the total charges and total receipts in any summary should be almost the same. They may not be identical because some bills may not have been fully collected.

Quarterly Summary of Charges, Receipts, and Disbursements, 20XX

MONTH	1 CHARGES	2 RECEIPTS	3 DISBURSE-MENTS	4 WAGES	5 RENT & UTILITIES	6 OFFICE EXPENSES	7 GENERAL MEDICAL	8 X-RAY/LAB.	9 TAXES	10 PERSONAL	11 MISC.
Jan.	15400.00	14800.00	6218.14	3349.50	1625.00	129.86	93.45	241.86	589.02	100.00	89.45
Feb.	18255.00	18950.00	7050.40	3872.80	1683.08	235.00	118.72	266.00	611.20	186.60	77.00
Mar.	13850.00	13250.00	6530.14	3666.10	1702.85	43.85	243.11	187.02	577.00	88.11	22.10
Subtotal	47505.00	47000.00	19798.68	10888.40	5010.93	408.71	455.28	694.88	1777.22	374.71	188.55
Apr.											
May											
June											
Subtotal											
July											
Aug.											
Sept.											
Subtotal											
Oct.											
Nov.											
Dec.											
Subtotal											
Grand Total											

FIGURE 21-4 Depending on office policy, the monthly, quarterly and/or yearly summary of office charges, receipts, and disbursements is used to summarize the office financial health.

▶ In-Office Patient Transactions   LO 21.3

Many patient-related financial transactions take place within the office on a daily basis. Some examples include patients with appointments incurring charges and making payments, payments from patients and insurance carriers requiring payment posting and adjustments, and even the occasional "bounced check." In this section, you will explore these transactions in more detail.

Starting the Business Day

At the beginning of each day, place a daily log sheet on the pegboard. Then, place the stack of superbills (charge slips/receipts) on the pegs, aligning the top line of the first superbill with the daily log top line. Because the superbills are layered one over the other from top to bottom, alignment of the first will align all others. The superbills are prenumbered. This numbering promotes good cash control and theoretically prevents embezzlement. Figure 21-5 shows the setup for the pegboard system.

Patient Process

As each patient comes into the office, place the patient's ledger card under the next available superbill, aligning the card's first blank line with the carbon strip on the superbill. Write the date, the patient's name, and the patient's previous balance on the charge slip section. The information will automatically be recorded in the daily log and on the patient ledger card. Most pegboard sheets also contain a column just to the right of the superbill where the preprinted number of the patient's superbill may be recorded on the day sheet as a checks and balances entry.

Attach the Superbill to the Patient Chart

Remove the superbill and attach it to the patient chart so it is ready for the doctor to check off both the services provided and the applicable diagnoses for the day's visit. After examining the patient, the doctor checks off or fills in the appropriate

charges and diagnoses on the superbill, indicates when the next appointment is needed, and gives the superbill to the patient to return to the front desk on the way out.

Patient Checkout

When the patient returns the completed superbill you again place the ledger card between the superbill and the daily log, checking to ensure proper alignment. On the superbill, enter the date, procedure (or code), charges, payments, new balance, and the date and time of the next appointment (if any). As you write this information, it should be automatically transferred onto the ledger card and daily log. Finally, tear off the receipt and give it to the patient. You can now return the patient ledger card to the file.

Payments after the Patient Visit

If you receive payments sometime after the patient visit, either by mail or in person, record them on the patient ledger card and day sheet as you normally would. Record charges for doctor visits to hospitalized patients or other out-of-office visits in the same way. If required, you can use the pegboard system to record bank deposits and petty cash disbursements in the daily log, but you will need the appropriate disbursement journal and overlapping forms.

In the *Patient Billing and Collections* chapter, we discussed the use of collection agencies to collect accounts that are greatly overdue. When you receive payments from the collection agency, they will list the total amount collected from the patient, the amount deducted from their fee, and the amount being forwarded to the office. When posting this payment, insert the amount received from the agency in the paid column. Use the adjustment column to insert the portion of the payment that was paid to the collection agency for their services. Subtract both amounts from the patient's balance to obtain the current balance. If the payment was considered payment in full, be sure to take the full balance on the account as an adjustment to bring the patient's balance to zero. Follow your office procedure regarding this account once the payment is made. Once a patient goes to collection, some offices also send a letter of discontinuation of services due to nonpayment, giving the patient 30 days to locate a new healthcare provider.

Returned Checks

If a patient's check does not clear due to nonsufficient funds (NSF), you must adjust the account accordingly. NSF payments are first deducted from the office checking account. The patient's account is then updated with a negative payment (noted in parentheses in the payment column) for the amount of the check, adding that amount back to the patient balance. An office fee also may be charged for the inconvenience of dealing with the NSF check. Any fees your office charges for NSF must be clearly stated and in plain view for patients to see. In addition, if the bank imposes a fee on the office, these bank fees also should be passed to the patient to recoup the loss for the practice and marked on the patient's ledger. Depending on office policy, the patient may now be seen on a *cash-only* basis by the practice. Procedure 21-2, at the end of this chapter, explains the procedure for posting an NSF payment.

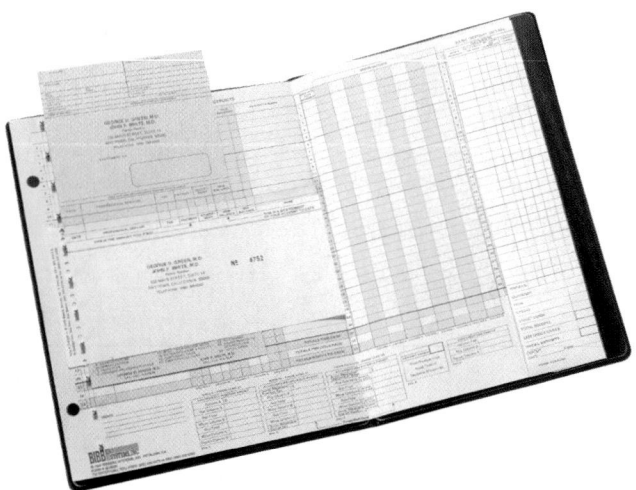

FIGURE 21-5   Using the pegboard system, shown here with a correctly aligned ledger card and superbill on the pegboard.

Refunding an Overpayment (Credit Balance)

Periodically, the combination of insurance payments and patient payments exceeds the allowed charges. This is called an overpayment. Sometimes this happens when patients feel they have not met their annual deductible, pay their balance, and then the insurance carrier also makes a payment on the patient's behalf. After posting the payments, the account balance will be a negative number, which is called a *credit balance*. When this happens, the medical office owes the patient money. In some medical offices, if this amount is small, they leave it in place so that the next scheduled visit's new charges will be applied against this amount. Procedure 21-3, at the end of this chapter, outlines the procedure for processing a credit balance.

Go to CONNECT to see a video about *Posting Charges, Payments, and Adjustments.*

Many times, instead of leaving a credit balance on the books, the office will need to refund the overpayment amount to the patient. This refunded amount is noted in the patient's account, bringing the balance to zero. When this happens, you will create a letter explaining how the overpayment occurred and enclose the check for the refund amount. Procedure 21-4, at the end of this chapter, outlines the steps for processing refunds to patients.

Uncollectable Accounts

In every office, despite the best collection efforts by the staff and even an outside collection agency, there will be patients who simply will not, or cannot, pay their medical bills. These accounts are known as *uncollectable*. In most offices the medical assistant and office manager or physician will meet monthly to discuss these accounts. When it is agreed that the money owed is never going to be collected, the practice manager or physician will give approval to adjust the remaining balance off the account. This practice *relieves* the AR of these funds that will never be brought into the practice. An adjustment is made on the account for the full balance due, bringing the current balance to zero. Be sure to note the account with the name of the person giving approval for this adjustment and if it is office policy, also send the patient a registered letter informing him that they have 30 days to find a new physician because of the nonpayment of his account.

End of the Day

At the end of each day, total and check the calculations in all columns. If you find an error, correct it immediately by drawing a line through it and making a new entry on the next available writing line. Remember to make the correction on the patient ledger card also and to issue a new receipt to the patient. To balance a pegboard system or patient ledger card, after adding the figures in each column, use the following formula for the column totals:

$$\text{Previous balance} + \text{Today's charges} - (\text{Payments} + \text{Adjustments}) = \text{New accounts receivable total}$$

Banking and Negotiable Instruments

LO 21.4

In addition to the financial practices outlined above, your administrative responsibilities also may include handling the practice's banking. Because a practice may use traditional (manual) or electronic (computerized) banking methods, you should be familiar with both. Regardless of which method you use, remember to keep all banking materials secure because they represent the finances of the practice. For example, to prevent theft of checks, always put the checkbook in a securely locked place when it is not in use. Also, file deposit receipts promptly. If they are lost, you have no proof that a deposit was made. Lack of proof could cost the practice thousands of dollars. Because you will be responsible for office funds, it is important that protocols be in place and consistently followed. Be sure you are clear regarding the procedure to be followed and to whom within the practice you should report suspected lost or stolen funds.

Banking Tasks

Common banking tasks in the medical office practice include

- Writing checks
- Accepting checks
- Endorsing checks
- Making deposits
- Reconciling bank statements
  - Recordkeeping of bank accounts
  - Balancing of individual accounts

Because many manual banking procedures revolve around the writing and receipt of checks, you must first have a thorough understanding of the terminology surrounding this common "piece of paper."

Checks

A **check** is a bank draft or order for payment (Figure 21-6). The person who writes the check is called the **payer**. By writing a check, the payer directs the bank to pay a sum of money on demand to the payee. In order to be considered **negotiable** (legally transferable from one person to another), a check must

- Be written and signed by the payer or maker;
- Include the amount of money to be paid, considered a promise to pay a specified sum;
- Be made payable to the payee (the person named on the check) or bearer;
- Be made payable on demand or on a specific date; and
- Include the name of the bank that is directed to make payment.

Types of Checks and Other Negotiable Papers In addition to personal checks from patients and business checks from insurance companies and other offices, you

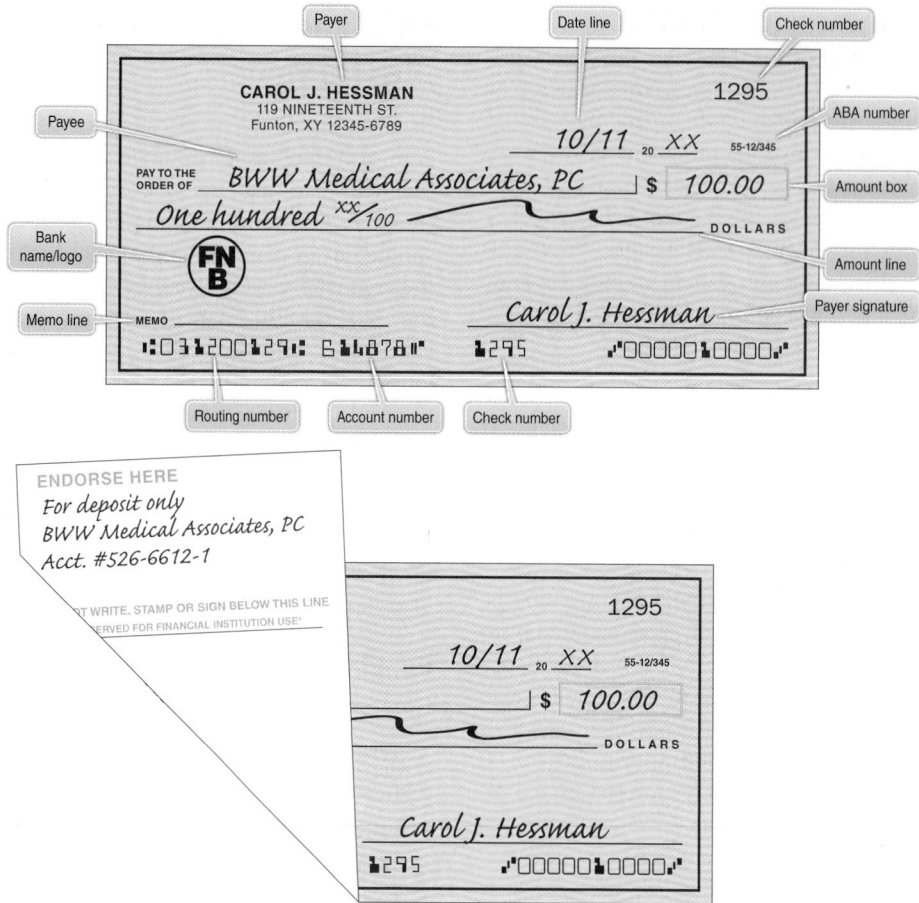

FIGURE 21-6 Parts of a check with an example of a restrictive endorsement.

may also receive or even use the following types of checks in the medical office.

- **Cashier's check**—a check issued from the bank's account and signed by a bank representative. It is usually purchased by individuals who do not have checking accounts or for use in purchases where large sums are required, such as a down payment for a car or house, when the payee wants a guarantee that the check will not be returned for insufficient funds.
- **Certified check**—a personal or business check that is written and signed by the payer, brought to the bank the check will be drawn on, and stamped "CERTIFIED" by the bank. This stamp means the bank has already drawn the money from the payer's account and set it aside to guarantee that the check will be paid when submitted. Many banks no longer use certified checks, having replaced them with cashier's checks.
- **Voucher check**—a business (or personal) check with a perforated stub attached for recordkeeping. Instead of using a checkbook register, before writing out the check, the stub is completed with all of the payee information for the user's records. Voucher checks come in various styles and often in a 3-ring binder format.
- **Limited check**—a check that is valid for redemption during a specific time frame, often only 30–90 days and usually used for payroll. Some accounts will also limit the amount of checks written as well as the valid time frames.

- **Counter check**—a special bank-issued check that allows the depositor to withdraw funds from his account only. It states, "PAY TO THE ORDER OF MYSELF ONLY." This may be used when the physician wants to draw off of the account in absence of his or her checkbook; similar to a withdrawal slip.
- **Traveler's check**—a check preprinted in established denominations of $10, $20, $50, and $100. These checks must be signed at the location where they were purchased. When using a traveler's check, it must be signed in the presence of the payee and the signatures must match in order for them to be valid for redemption.
- **Money order**—another kind of guaranteed payment. Money orders are purchased in banks or from other vendors for a small fee, using cash. They are often used by people without checking accounts who wish to have a receipt of payment for their records.

Check Codes The face (front) of every check contains two important items: the American Banking Association (ABA) number and the magnetic ink character recognition (MICR) code (refer back to Figure 21-6). The **ABA number** appears as a fraction, such as 60-117/310, on the upper edge of all printed checks. It identifies the geographic area and specific bank on which the check is drawn.

Found at the bottom of a check, the MICR code consists of numbers and characters printed in magnetic ink, which can be read by MICR equipment at the bank. This code enables checks to be read, sorted, and recorded by computer.

Parts of a Check The checks you encounter both personally and in your office contain many important features that should be inspected upon receipt to ensure prompt payment. Refer back to Figure 21-6 to familiarize yourself with the location of each item.

- *Payer*—account holder's legal name, usually preprinted with address and possibly other information like phone numbers and e-mail addresses.
- *Date line*—date that is written in by the payer, stating that the funds are available as of this date.
- *Check number*—indicates the number in a series.
- *ABA number*—preprinted numbers appearing as a fraction, such as 55-12/345, identifying the geographic area and specific bank on which the check is drawn.
- *Payee*—the name written on the "pay to the order of" line to whom the payer wishes the funds to be paid.
- *Amount box*—box in which the check's numerical amount should be entered.
- *Amount line*—line where the check's dollar amount is written out in words and the cents are usually put into a fraction over one hundred followed by a line to reduce the ability for someone to write in information. If there is a discrepancy between the amount box and the amount line, the amount line is the amount used when paying out the funds.
- *Bank information*—information that identifies the processing facility or the city and state of the account holder's branch bank that the funds are coming from and may list the logo, address, e-mail, or any other special branch information.
- *Memo line*—line that can be left blank but should be filled in to ensure that the payment is credited to the correct account. This can be done by entering any account information, which is extremely helpful when the payer is someone other than the patient such as the spouse or parent.
- *Payer signature line*—line where the payer MUST sign the check in order for the funds to be legally drawn.
- *Routing number*—9-digit MICR numbers that route the check back to the issuing bank and should match the bank name and ABA fraction code number.
- *Account number*—part of the MICR numbers that indicates the payer's account within the bank.
- *Check number*—part of the MICR numbers that identify and refer back to the check number at the top right of the check.
- *MICR recording area*—space for bank use only to record the branch and amount of the check.

Accepting Checks Before accepting any check, review it carefully. First, be sure the check has the correct date, amount, and signature and that no corrections have been made. Refer once more to Figure 21-6, which shows a correctly written and endorsed check. Do not accept a **third-party check** (one made out to the patient rather than to the practice) unless it is from a health insurance company. Also, do not accept a check marked "Payment in Full" unless it actually does pay the complete outstanding balance. You may accept a check signed by someone other than the payer if the person who signed the check has power of attorney. **Power of attorney** gives a person the legal right to handle financial matters for another person who is unable to do so. Frequently, power of attorney is granted to a patient's spouse, son, or daughter.

Be sure to follow your practice's policy when accepting a check. For example, if a patient is new or unfamiliar, office policy may require you to request patient identification and to compare the signature on the identification with the signature on the check. Many offices will not accept post-dated checks because they are then responsible for holding the check until the date the bank will accept the check. Policy also may require that you not accept a check for more than the amount due because cash will be due back to the patient and then if the check is returned for insufficient funds, the office will be out not only the amount of the check, but also the amount of the cash given to the patient.

Checking Account Types

It is not uncommon for a physician to have at least three different types of checking accounts: a personal account, a business account for office expenses, and an interest-earning account. The interest-earning account will be used for paying special expenses, like property taxes and insurance premiums. As a medical assistant, most of your banking tasks will involve the business checking account. You may sometimes, however, make payments from, or transfer money to and from, the interest-earning account, as directed.

▶ Preparing a Bank Deposit   LO 21.5

Endorsing Checks

Once a check has been presented for payment and received by the office, it should be inspected and then immediately endorsed or accepted for payment. There are four principal types of **endorsement**:

- Blank endorsement. A blank endorsement consists simply of the payee's signature. Once this endorsement is made, anyone who has possession of the check may cash it, so it should only be signed when the check is being cashed or deposited immediately, not prior to arriving at the bank.
- Restrictive endorsement. A restrictive endorsement specifies how the check may be redeemed. In the case of the medical office, the endorsement is often made by a stamp and "restricts" redemption of the check to depositing it in the office checking account. Refer back to Figure 21-6 for an example of this type of endorsement.
- Special endorsement. A special endorsement may also be called a third-party endorsement, as the payee of the check signs it over to another person. For example, if an insurance check is sent to Sylvia Gonzales, our case study patient, instead of the office, she could sign it over to the office like this:

Pay to the order of BWW Medical Associates, PC
Sylvia Gonzales

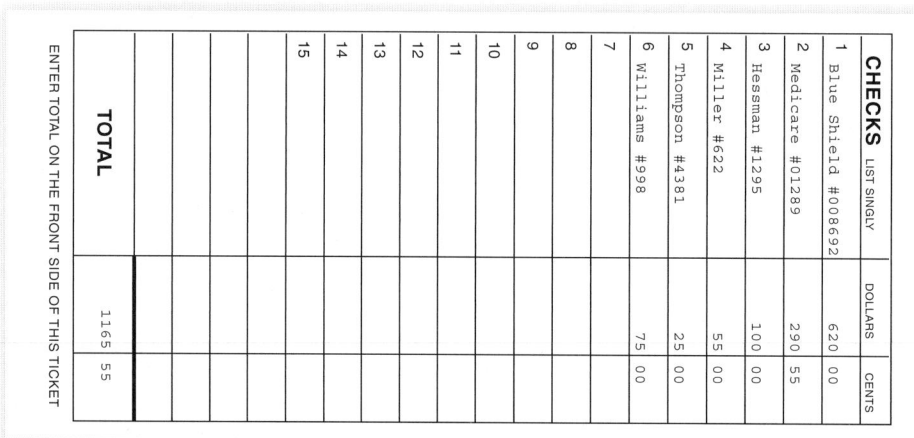

FIGURE 21-7 A correctly completed deposit slip.

By endorsing the check in this manner, Sylvia ensures that only BWW Medical Associates can redeem this check.

- Qualified endorsement. Attorneys, who may accept a check on behalf of their client but have no personal claim on the transaction, most often use qualified endorsements. In this case, the attorney might endorse the check "without recourse," which disclaims any future liability regarding this transaction.

If, after reading about the types of endorsements, you think the best type of endorsement is a restrictive endorsement, you would be correct. A restrictive endorsement prevents the check from being cashed if it is lost or stolen because the only way the check can be redeemed is by deposit into the specified account; if you do not use a restrictive endorsement for your personal checking account, do you think you might consider doing so now?

No matter what type of endorsement is chosen, always be sure to make all endorsements in ink, using a pen or rubber stamp. Place the endorsement in the 1.5-inch area indicated on the back of the check. Most personal and business checks have a number of lines or a shaded area preprinted on the checks for this purpose. (Refer to Figure 21-6.) Leave the rest of the back of the check blank for the bank's use.

Completing the Deposit Slip
After endorsing the check, post the payment to the patient ledger card and to the daily log or day sheet. Then put the check with

others to be deposited. Even if your office does not make daily deposits, it is a good idea to have a deposit slip started at the beginning of the day, adding each check to the deposit slip by hand or electronically as you receive it, as shown in Figure 21-7. In this way, you will have a running list of checks (and cash) to be deposited and can compare this to the day sheet at any time to verify the amount of the payments received by the office. The account number is printed on deposit slips in MICR numbers that match those on the checks. As mentioned, these numbers enable checks and deposit slips to be read, sorted, and recorded by computer.

Banks will accept a list of deposited items on something other than the bank-provided deposit slip if the bank's deposit slip is attached. For example, if you are depositing 50 checks, you may create a computer printout listing the payers' names, check numbers, amount of each check, and total. You can then attach the printout to a deposit slip with the total written on the deposit slip. Another method is to attach a calculator or adding machine tape listing the individual check amounts and including the total amount.

Making the Deposit
Plan to deposit checks and cash into the practice's bank account in person at the bank, as described in Procedure 21-5 at the end of this chapter. Make sure you are aware of your surroundings when making deposits because of safety issues. Always obtain a deposit receipt from the bank.

Again, depending on practice size, the frequency of deposits may be limited to several days a week; however, it should be done as often as possible to reduce theft, loss, bounced checks, and inaccurate recordings.

Electronic Deposits

With the advent of electronic claims submission, many payers and offices prefer to receive their insurance payments electronically as well. Electronic funds transfers, or EFTs, may be set up between the office and many insurance carriers, greatly decreasing the amount of time it takes to receive payment from the insurance carriers via U.S. mail. Even smaller offices that still submit paper claims to insurance carriers may be able to receive their insurance payments electronically. The office will receive notification from the insurance carrier of any payment (deposit) sent to the office checking account along with the EOB (explanation of benefit), also known as the RA (remittance advice), explaining which patient accounts the payment pertains to. You can learn more about remittance advices, both electronic and paper, in the *Insurance and Billing* chapter.

▶ Reconciling the Bank Statement LO 21.6

Another important administrative task that often is part of the medical assistant's role is the banking task of reconciling the bank statement. **Reconciliation** involves comparing the office financial records, the checkbook or disbursements journal, with the bank records (statement) to ensure that they are consistent with each other and accurate. In most practices, this task is performed once a month when the practice receives the monthly checking account statement from the bank, either in the mail or electronically if the office utilizes the bank's electronic banking services. Figure 21-8 shows an example of a typical bank statement.

When reconciling the checkbook with the bank statement, keep in mind one thought: "the bank needs to 'know'"

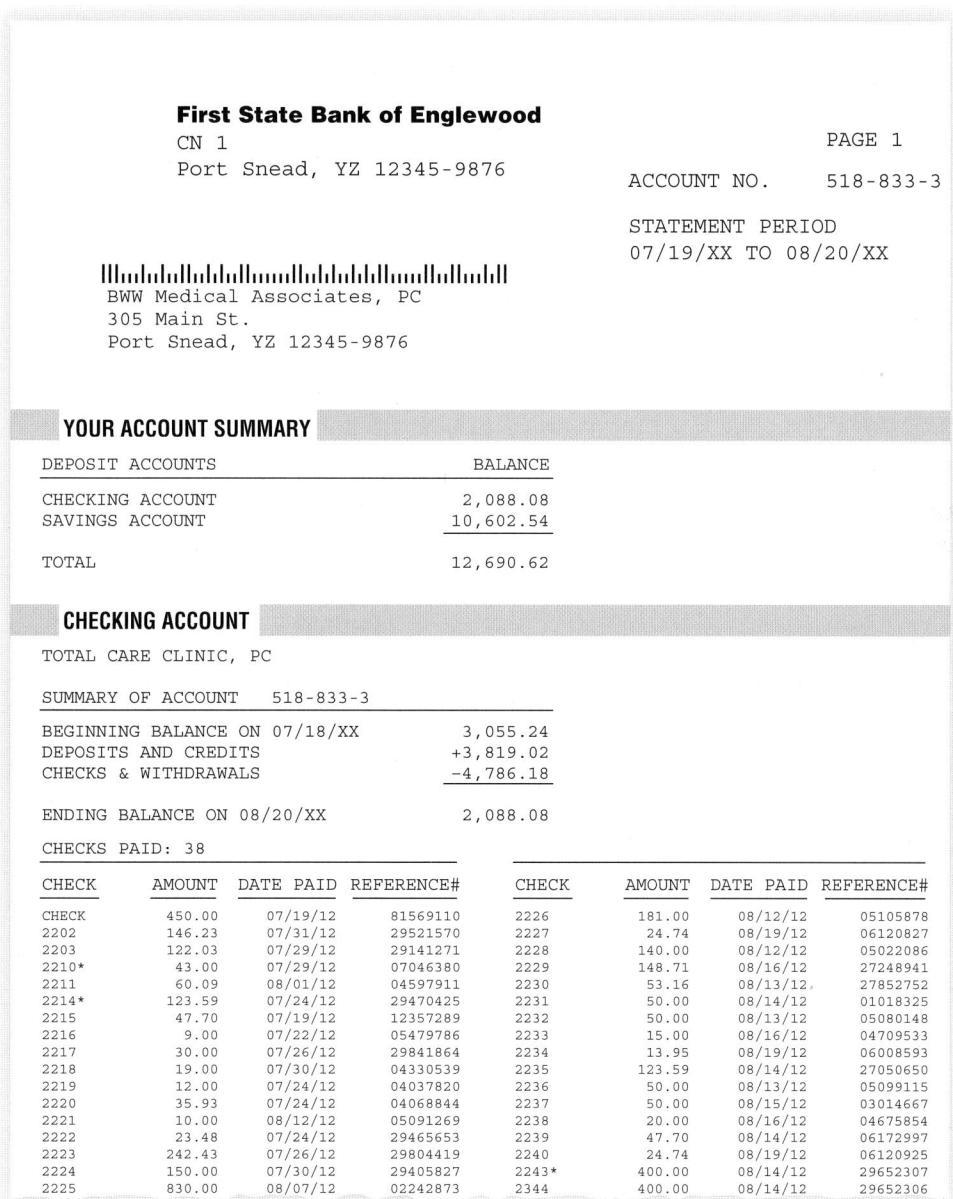

FIGURE 21-8 A typical bank statement used to reconcile the office checking account.

everything I know regarding what I have paid and deposited and I, in comparing the bank statement to the checking account, need to be sure that I have recorded everything that the bank knows." Let's look at a simple scenario:

When the bank statement comes in, you immediately block out some quiet time to take care of the reconciliation. In comparing the deposits and payments recorded by the bank as completed, you note a $2,000 deposit made two days ago, which is not yet recorded, and three checks you sent out totaling $800, which also have not yet been redeemed. These items are not yet "known" by the bank. You also notice that the automatic payment of $500 for quarterly payroll taxes has not been recorded in the checkbook. The bank statement shows a balance of $10,900. The office checkbook shows a balance of $12,600.

Bank Statement		Checkbook	
Balance	10,900.00		12,600.00
(deposit)	+ 2,000.00	(autopay)	− 500.00
	12,900.00		12,100.00 √
(outstanding	− 800.00		
checks)	12,100.00 √		

Once the deposit that has not cleared is added to the bank statement balance and the outstanding checks are subtracted, the new balance is $12,100. At the same time, when the auto-payment is subtracted from the checkbook balance, its balance is also $12,100. You have successfully reconciled the bank statement. Figure 21-9 shows you an example of a reconciliation worksheet. The complete reconciliation process is explained in Procedure 21-6 at the end of the chapter.

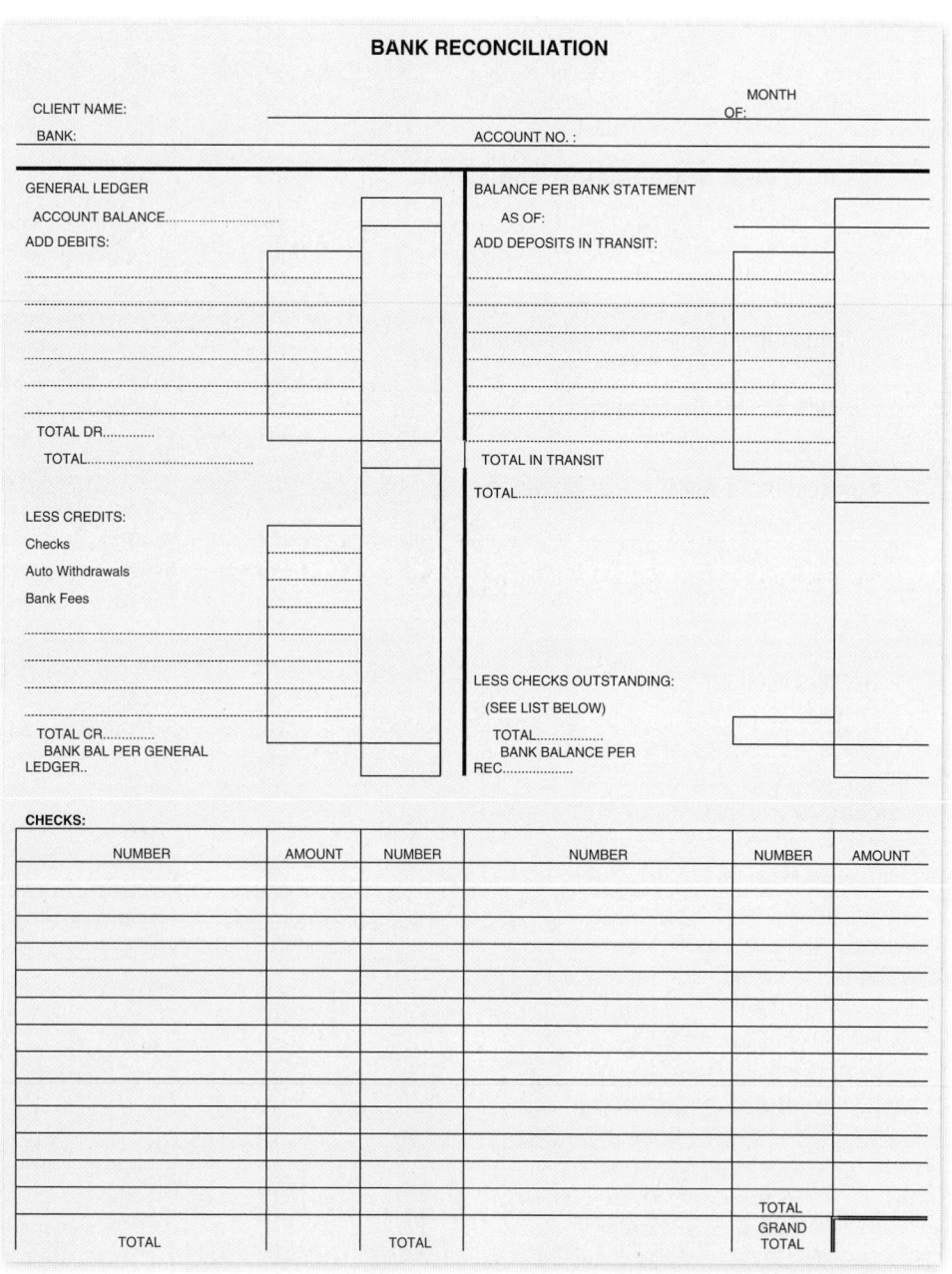

FIGURE 21-9 A typical reconciliation worksheet to aid in reconciling the checkbook to the bank statement.

Electronic Banking

LO 21.7

Compared with traditional banking methods, electronic banking has several advantages. Electronic banking can improve productivity, cash flow, and accuracy. The use of electronic banking can also speed up many banking tasks. If your medical office uses electronic banking, your basic tasks will be the same as in an office that uses traditional banking methods. How these tasks are performed, however, may be quite different. When you use electronic banking, you are still responsible for recording and depositing checks, just as if you were using traditional methods, but you will see these differences:

- Rather than your recording each check in a paper checkbook and determining the new balance, the computer software calculates the new balance for you.
- Rather than your reconciling the office bank statement on paper, the computer software does it automatically.
- Rather than putting the checkbook and banking forms in a securely locked place at the end of the day, you use a computer password for security.

Many medical office software programs are available today and each one has a different interface, uses different menus, and prompts you for information in different ways. However, certain general concepts apply to all. All software will allow you to record deposits, pay bills, display the checkbook (and account balances), and reconcile the bank statement. For specific information, consult the user's manual that comes with computer software used by your individual practice. Before electing to "sign up for electronic banking," check with the current bank used by the office to see what safeguards and protections they offer regarding the information the office is transferring electronically. Electronic banking can speed up processes for the office, but it is extremely important that the office remain in control of how that information is protected and who has access to the information. If the bank currently used by the office does not use appropriate safeguards for electronic banking procedures, the office may want to consider changing financial institutions.

Record Deposits

If you select "Record Deposits," a message on the computer screen prompts you to enter information about each check to be deposited that day. This information usually includes the check writer's name and the amount of the check. The check's ABA number also may be requested. After you enter this information, the computer gives you a chance to double-check it. If all the information is correct, you continue entering and checking the other checks, one at a time. You can then select a command to print a deposit slip that contains the information you have just entered. To make the deposit, place the cash and checks in a deposit bag along with the computerized deposit slip and the bank's deposit slip.

Pay Bills

The bill pay function allows you to log checks that you write into a computerized checkbook register. For each check you want to write, a message on the computer screen should prompt you for information, such as the payee and the amount of the check. The computer also should give you a chance to verify and correct this information before moving on to the next check or printing the actual checks. More and more programs, depending upon the bank the office uses, also allow for electronic bill pay. Recording these payments in the electronic (or paper) checkbook register is the same as when writing a check, except instead of recording the check number, you will record the transaction number assigned by the bank as proof the payment has been sent.

Some software programs automatically assign the next available check number to each new check you enter. To double-check that the computer-assigned check numbers match those on the actual checks, print a list of the checks you have entered and compare it with the checks before mailing them.

Display the Checkbook

The checkbook display function allows you to review the electronic checkbook register. Although you cannot change information that appears in the register—unless your software program and your bank allow total electronic banking—you can print it out so you can be sure the checks have been recorded properly and you can check your latest balance.

If you select "Display Checkbook" from the "Banking" menu, the computer displays a list of all checks that have been entered into the register. Information includes check number, date, payee, and amount. Scrolling up and down reveals all the checks in the register. This area also will reveal any auto withdrawals or auto deposits that have been made up until the current date (one of the advantages of electronic banking), and the balance and current statement may be checked at any time, not just once a month when the bank statement arrives.

Balance Checkbook

The "Balance Checkbook" option electronically reconciles the monthly bank statement. After you enter the appropriate date or dates, the computer screen displays all the checks and deposits that were logged into the register in the order they were posted.

The next screen highlights each check or deposit that has not been seen on a previous bank statement. You are prompted to indicate whether that item appears on the current statement, usually using Y for yes and N for no. After the computer queries these items, it may ask you to enter any items that appear on the current bank statement but are not in the checkbook, such as service charges.

Finally, a message on the screen prompts you to enter the current account balance from the bank statement. Then, the computer reconciles the bank statement. It will alert you if the system balance does not agree with the balance on the bank statement. If the balance does not agree, recheck the information you entered for possible errors. If you have rechecked your work and a coworker has also acted as a "second set of eyes" and has verified no errors or omissions, yet the balances still do not agree, call the bank to determine if a bank error has been made.

Accounts Payable and Managing Disbursements

LO 21.8

Accounts payable (A/P) are the practice expenses, and accounts receivable reflect the practice income. This section focuses on accounts payable and the process of making those payments, known as disbursements. A basic accounting principle to bear in mind is that when a practice's income exceeds its expenses, it has a profit, commonly called "being in the black." If a practice's expenses exceed its income, it has a loss, known as "being in the red."

Because of this relationship between income and expenses, most practices try to reduce expenses by controlling accounts payable. As the office medical assistant, you play an important role in helping control accounts payable in order to maximize profits.

Accounts payable fall into three main groups:

- Payments for supplies, equipment, and practice-related products and services;
- Payroll, which may be the largest of the accounts payable; and
- Taxes owed to federal, state, and local governments and agencies.

A practice's accounting system usually consists of several elements. These elements include the daily log, patient ledger cards, the checkbook, the disbursements journal, the petty cash record, and the payroll register. In this chapter, you are focusing on the first four elements. You will explore the petty cash record and payroll register in the *Practice Management* chapter.

As discussed earlier in this chapter, the daily log and patient ledger cards are used primarily for accounts receivable. The disbursements journal (as well as the petty cash record and payroll register) is used primarily in accounts payable.

Go to CONNECT to see a video about *Managing Petty Cash.*

Disbursements

A disbursement is any payment the physician's office makes for goods or services. One of the most common disbursements is payment for office supplies. Other disbursements include payments for equipment, dues, rent, taxes, salary, and utilities. No matter what type of disbursement you make on behalf of the practice, you must keep accurate records of the purchase and the payment.

Recording Disbursements You may record disbursements in a check register, in a disbursements journal, or on the bottom section of the daily log. If you use a disbursements journal, follow these steps to record disbursements:

1. When beginning a new journal page, give each column a heading to reflect the type of expense, such as utilities or rent. Procedure 21-7, at the end of this chapter, outlines how to set up a disbursements journal.

2. For each check, fill in the date, payee's name, check number, and check amount in the appropriate columns.

3. Determine the expense category of the check.

4. Record the check amount in the column for that type of business expense.

5. If you must divide a check between two or more expense columns, record the total in the check amount column. Then record the amount that applies to each type of expense in the appropriate column. The total amount listed in the check amount column must equal the sum of the amounts listed in the expense columns.

Writing Checks

Virtually all disbursements are made by check, although electronic payments are becoming more and more common. Paying by check gives the practice complete, accurate records of all financial transactions. If your office uses electronic banking, including bill pay, the transaction number given by the bank, at the time the bill is paid, should be recorded, in place of the check number, in the disbursements journal and checkbook for future reference.

Before writing a check, make sure the checking account balance is up-to-date and large enough to cover the check you want to write. Enter the date, check number, payee information, and reason for the payment on the check stub and then subtract the amount of each check from the previous balance, enter the new balance, and carry that balance forward to the next stub. Do this step before writing the check so the payment entry is not accidentally omitted from the disbursements journal. The same information holds true when electronic banking is utilized. Be sure to record the payment in the disbursements journal or online checkbook prior to sending the payment.

If you use a pegboard system for your checkbook/disbursements journal, you will automatically record the date, check number, payee, and check amount on the check register as you write out the check because of the carbonless paper that is on the back of the check itself. You must note the reason for payment and the new balance manually, however. Record that information in the appropriate spaces on the register.

If you make an error when completing a check, write VOID in ink across the front of the check in large letters so it cannot be used again. Then file the voided check in numerical order with the returned checks.

After filling out the check properly, detach it from the checkbook and give it to the doctor to sign, along with the invoice to be paid. Mark the date, check number, and amount paid on the invoice. Make a copy of the invoice for your records. Keep these copies with supporting documents, like order forms or packing slips, in a paid-invoice file. Then, mail the check and the original invoice to the payee in a neatly hand-addressed or typewritten envelope. If you use a window envelope, be sure the payee's address shows through the window.

Recording disbursements in columns for each type of expense allows you to total and track expenses by category. **Tracking** (watching for changes) is important because it helps control expenses. Before tracking, check your calculations by performing a trial balance:

1. Total the check amount column.

2. Calculate the total for each expense column.

3. Add together all the expense column totals. The combined expense column total should match the total in the check amount column.

4. If the amounts do not match, recheck every entry until you find the error. When you find it, draw a line through it and record the correct information neatly above it or to the side.

5. When the two amounts match (or balance), carry forward all column totals to the disbursements journal for the next month. Remember to prepare summaries and perform balances at the end of every month, quarter, and year.

If your office uses an office management software package, trial balances and financial summaries are created with a few keystrokes. Remember, however, computer programs are only as good as the information entered into the programs. If you make a keystroke error when entering information, the trial balance and/or financial summary will contain errors. Always enter financial information—whether you write it by hand or key it into a computer program—with great care.

Understanding Financial Summaries

The physician or practice manager may periodically analyze the practice's income and expenses. Financial summaries provide an easy-to-read report on the business transactions for a given period, such as a month, quarter, or a year.

In the past, it was necessary to have an accountant to prepare financial summaries. But with more offices utilizing practice management software, creating these reports, using the software package or templates, is a relatively simple process once the procedure is understood. A medical assistant with a basic understanding of the information contained within financial summaries will be an asset in helping the practice to remain financially stable. Following are some of the records found in most financial statements.

Statement of Income and Expense Also called a profit-and-loss statement, a statement of income and expense highlights the practice's profitability. It shows the physician the practice's total income and then lists and subtracts all expenses.

Cash Flow Statement A **cash flow statement** shows how much cash is available to cover expenses, to invest, or to take as profit. The cash flow statement begins with the cash on hand at the beginning of the period and shows the income and disbursements made during that period. It concludes with the new amount of cash on hand at the end of the period.

Trial Balance The physician or practice manager may review trial balances periodically to ensure that the books balance. As described earlier in this chapter, the combined expense column total should match the total in the check amount column. If the amounts do not match, recheck every entry until you find the error and the column amounts balance.

Although not considered by many to be as "glamorous" as patient care, the medical assistant who focuses and excels in the administrative procedures for the practice—particularly its financial practices—and takes an interest in controlling expenses while maintaining quality care for the patients of the practice will be an outstanding asset to any practice in the "business of medicine."

PROCEDURE 21-1 Posting Charges, Payments, and Adjustments

Procedure Goal: To post charges, payments, and adjustments to the patient account.

OSHA Guidelines: This procedure does not involve exposure to blood, body fluids, or tissue.

Materials: Daily log sheets, patient ledger cards, and check register or computerized bookkeeping system; summaries of charges, receipts, and disbursements.

Method: Procedure steps.

1. Create a ledger card (patient account) for each new patient and maintain a ledger card for each existing patient. Include the following information on each ledger card:
   a. Patient name
   b. Patient address
   c. Patient home and work phone numbers
   d. Insurance carrier with policy number and guarantor information

2. Update the ledger card every time the patient incurs a charge or makes a payment. Be sure to adjust the account balance after every transaction. In a computerized system, a patient record contains the same information as a ledger card. This record also must be maintained and updated.
   RATIONALE: The information on each patient's ledger card must match that of the daily log.

3. Use a new log (day) sheet each day. For each patient seen that day:

   a. Record the following: patient name, the relevant charges, and any payments received.
   b. Calculate any necessary adjustments and new balances.
   c. When using a computerized system, enter the patient's name or account number, the relevant charges, along with any payments received and adjustments made in the appropriate areas. The computer program will calculate the new balances.
   RATIONALE: Each day's transactions must be accurately and promptly recorded.

4. Record all deposits accurately in the check register.

5. File the deposit receipt—with a detailed listing of checks, cash, and money orders deposited—for later use in reconciling the bank statement.

6. The deposit amount should match the amount of money collected by the practice for that day.
   RATIONALE: If the receipts for the day and the deposit for the day match, you have balanced for the day.

7. Prepare or, if using a computerized program, print a summary of charges, receipts, and disbursements every month, quarter, or year, as directed. Double-check all entries and calculations from the monthly summary before posting them to the quarterly summary. Also, double-check the entries and calculations from the quarterly summary before posting them to the yearly summary.
   RATIONALE: Double-checking all entries ensures mistakes are found and corrected as soon as possible.

PROCEDURE 21-2   Posting a Nonsufficient Funds (NSF) Check

Procedure Goal: To post a nonsufficient funds (NSF) check amount and any applicable fees to the patient account.

OSHA Guidelines: This procedure does not involve exposure to blood, body fluids, or tissue.

Materials: Computer, returned check, patient ledger, calculator (optional), daily log sheet.

Method: Procedure steps.

1. Locate the patient's account on the computer or pull the patient's ledger card for manual processes.
   RATIONALE: To make sure that you have the correct patient (account) for the NSF check.

2. Use your medical facility code for NSF check (if used) and using today's date, create a new charge log for the patient. Use the code and the description *Check returned by bank* in the description column.

3. In the payment/adjustment column, place the amount of the check in parentheses to indicate that the amount is debited as an *adjustment*. Add the amount of the returned check to the old balance and enter it in the *current balance* column.
   RATIONALE: This negative payment/adjustment will increase the patient's amount due by the amount of the NSF check. The parentheses remind you to add the payment to the balance, instead of subtracting it as you usually would do.

4. On the next line, also using today's date, enter the medical facility's code for the NSF charge allowed by the office. Enter the charge amount in the *charge column* and add this amount to the patient's current balance.
   RATIONALE: The office has the right to charge the patient for the inconvenience of dealing with an NSF check.

PROCEDURE 21-3   Processing a Payment Resulting in a Credit Balance

Procedure Goal: To process a payment that results in a credit balance on the patient account.

OSHA Guidelines: This procedure does not involve exposure to blood, body fluids, or tissue.

Materials: Daily log or day sheet, patient ledger card, computer, calculator, patient explanation of benefits (EOB) or remittance advice (RA) if applicable, and patient or insurance payment.

Method: Procedure steps.

1. Locate the patient's account in the computer or pull the patient's ledger card for paper-based systems.
   RATIONALE: Patient financial records are legal documents, so you must be sure to post financial information to the correct account.

2. Post the total amount of the payment received to the patient's account by writing (or keying) the remittance amount in the paid column.

3. Subtract the payment amount from the previous balance and insert the new balance in the balance column. If the balance created is a *credit* balance, insert the figure in the current balance column within parentheses.
   RATIONALE: Inserting figures in parentheses tells the office staff that the balance is owed *by* the practice (credit balance), not *to* the practice (debit balance).

4. Review the account thoroughly, checking to see if any more receipts are expected on the patient's account.
   RATIONALE: Some patients have multiple insurance plans and more than one insurance payment may be expected on the account.

5. If a credit balance is verified, adjust the credit balance off the patient's account by issuing a refund (see Procedure 21-4).

PROCEDURE 21-4   Processing Refunds to Patients

Procedure Goal: To process a patient refund due to a credit balance.

OSHA Guidelines: This procedure does not involve exposure to blood, body fluids, or tissue.

Materials: Payment (check); ledger card; computer; calculator; Remittance Advice (RA) or Explanation of Benefits (EOB), if applicable.

Method: Procedure steps.

1. Calculate and determine the amount to be refunded (from Procedure 21-3). If the amount to be refunded

is determined by the EOB or RA, verify the amount listed.
   RATIONALE: If the patient made a payment and the insurance plan directs the office to return the patient's payment, that amount must be refunded to the patient.

2. Record the check number and amount in the disbursements journal or checkbook and write a check to the patient for the amount to be refunded.
   RATIONALE: Always record transactions in the checkbook first, so this step is never forgotten.

3. Ask the physician or business manager to sign the check so that it can be given or mailed to the patient.

4. Post the refund as a negative payment (credit) to the patient's ledger card or to the patient's account if a computerized system is being used. Using parentheses around the figure is a common way to record the credit.

5. Make a copy of the check, retaining a copy in the patient's financial record. Give or mail the check to the patient. If the check is being mailed, be sure to verify the patient's address prior to mailing and utilize certified return receipt mail to be sure the patient receives the check.

PROCEDURE 21-5 Making a Bank Deposit

Procedure Goal: To prepare cash and checks for deposit and to deposit them properly into a bank account.

OSHA Guidelines: This procedure does not involve exposure to blood, body fluids, or tissue.

Materials: Bank deposit slip and items to be deposited, such as checks, cash, and money orders.

Method: Procedure steps.

1. Divide the bills, coins, checks, and money orders into separate piles.

2. Sort the bills by denomination, from largest to smallest. Then, stack them—portrait side up— in the same direction. Total the amount of the bills and write this amount on the deposit slip on the line marked "currency" or cash.
   RATIONALE: The bank will require bills to be sorted for ease of counting by the teller to verify deposit information.

3. If you have enough coins to fill coin wrappers, put them in wrappers of the proper denomination. If not, count the coins and put them in the deposit bag. Total the amount of coins and write this amount on the deposit slip on the line marked "Coin."
   RATIONALE: If there are enough coins to fill denomination wrappers, the bank will require this to be done.

4. Review all checks and money orders to be sure they are properly endorsed with a restrictive endorsement. List each check on the deposit slip, including the check number and amount.

RATIONALE: Without a proper endorsement, the bank will not accept a check for deposit.

5. List each money order on the deposit slip. Include the notation "money order" or "MO" and the name of the writer.

6. Calculate the total deposit (total of amounts for currency, coin, checks, and money orders). Write this amount on the deposit slip on the line marked "Total." If you do not use deposit slips that record a copy for the office, photocopy the deposit slip for your office records.
   RATIONALE: Deposit slips must be kept in case there is ever a discrepancy between the office and bank records. The deposit slip is proof of deposit.

7. Record the total amount of the deposit in the office checkbook register.

8. If you plan to make the deposit in person, place the currency, coins, checks, and money orders in a deposit bag. If you cannot make the deposit in person, put the checks and money orders in a special bank-by-mail envelope or put all deposit items in an envelope and send it via registered mail.
   RATIONALE: If a deposit absolutely must be mailed, registered mail provides insurance for the amount of the deposit and proof of receipt by the bank.

9. Make the deposit in person or by mail.

10. Obtain a deposit receipt from the bank. File it with the copy of the deposit slip in the office for later use when reconciling the bank statement.

PROCEDURE 21-6 Reconciling the Bank Statement

Procedure Goal: To ensure that the bank record of deposits, payments, and withdrawals agrees with the practice record of deposits, payments, and withdrawals.

OSHA Guidelines: This procedure does not involve exposure to blood, body fluids, or tissue.

Materials: Previous month's bank statement, current month's bank statement, reconciliation worksheet (if not part of current bank statement), deposit receipts, red pencil, check stubs or checkbook register, returned checks or listing of checks returned.

Method: Procedure steps.

1. Check the closing balance on the previous month's statement against the opening balance on the current

month's statement. The balances should match. If they do not, call the bank.
   RATIONALE: If the ending balance from last month does not match the beginning balance of this month, there may be a problem with the bank's system.

2. Record the closing balance from the current statement on the reconciliation worksheet (Figure 21-9). This worksheet usually appears on the back of the bank statement.
   RATIONALE: This is the starting point for adjusting the bank balance as needed to accomplish reconciliation.

3. Check each deposit receipt against the bank statement.
   a. Place a red check mark in the upper-right corner of each receipt recorded on the statement.

b. Also place a check mark next to each deposit recorded in the checkbook to be sure none was skipped in this record.

4. Total the amount of deposits that do *not* appear on the statement. Add this amount to the closing balance from the bank on the reconciliation worksheet.
RATIONALE: These deposits are in transit, but the amount must be added to the bank balance in order for reconciliation to occur.

5. Compare each redeemed check with the bank statement, making sure that the amount on the check agrees with the amount on the statement.

a. Place a red check mark in the upper-right corner of each redeemed check recorded on the statement.

b. Also, place a check mark on the check stub or check register entry.

c. Any checks that were written but do not appear on the statement and were not returned as redeemed are considered "outstanding" checks. You can find these easily on the check stubs or checkbook register because they have no red check mark next to them.

6. List each outstanding check separately on the worksheet, including its check number and amount. Total the outstanding checks and subtract this total from the bank statement balance.
RATIONALE: These checks will eventually be honored by the bank. In order to balance the checkbook and bank statement, these outstanding checks must be subtracted from the bank balance. (You cannot add the amount back to your checkbook because the money will not be returned to the account.)

7. Record the ending balance found in the office checkbook in the appropriate area of the reconciliation worksheet.
RATIONALE: This is the starting point for adjusting the checkbook balance as needed to accomplish reconciliation.

8. If the statement shows that the checking account earned interest, add this amount to the checkbook balance.
RATIONALE: You did not know the interest amount prior to today, so now it must be added to the bank balance both in the checkbook and on the reconciliation worksheet.

9. If the statement lists such items as service charge, check printing charge, or automatic payment, subtract them from the checkbook balance and add these charges to the checkbook register itself.
RATIONALE: In order to balance with the bank statement, you must now enter the information you did not know until now, both in the checkbook register and on the reconciliation worksheet.

10. Compare the new checkbook balance with the new bank statement balance. They should match. If they do not, repeat the process, rechecking all calculations. Double-check the addition and subtraction in the checkbook register. Review the checkbook register to make sure you did not omit any items. Ensure that you carried the correct balance forward from one register page to the next. Double-check that you made the correct additions or subtractions for all interest earned and charges incurred.

11. If you have double-checked your work and the balances still do not agree, ask a coworker to check your figures. If the coworker also finds no error or omission, call the bank to determine if a bank error has been made. Contact the bank promptly because the bank may have a time limit for corrections and may otherwise consider the bank statement correct if you do not point out an error within a specified time. Check with your individual bank for their policy.
RATIONALE: Always ask a "fresh set of eyes" to look at the reconciliation prior to calling the bank. If anyone looks at figures for too long, it is not unusual to see "what you want to see," instead of what is really there.

PROCEDURE 21-7 Setting Up the Disbursements Journal

Procedure Goal: To set up the office disbursements journal.

OSHA Guidelines: This procedure does not involve exposure to blood, body fluids, or tissue.

Materials: Disbursements journal (either paper or electronic), pen (if journal is in a paper format), listing of the headings required for the disbursements journal.

Method: Procedure steps.

1. Write in or key column headings for the basic information required for each check: date, payee's name, check number, and check amount.
RATIONALE: This information is needed for accounting purposes.

2. Enter column headings for each type of business expense, such as utilities, payroll, and taxes.

3. Write in column headings (if space is available) for deposits and the account balance.

4. Record the data from completed checks under the appropriate column headings.
RATIONALE: The amount spent on each type of business expense is entered and tracked for income and expense reports. The practice manager will know exactly where money is being made or lost.

5. Be sure to subtract payments from the balance and add deposits to it.
RATIONALE: Allows for a running tally of income and expenses, including the current balance.

LEARNING OUTCOMES	KEY POINTS
21.1 **Summarize the importance of and how to establish good bookkeeping and banking practices.**	Procedures to be established to help maintain consistency in financial practices include being organized and consistent. Write clearly and use markers to keep track of your current location. Check your work frequently and correct any errors using the approved method of drawing one line through the error and correcting the information directly above that location. All entries must be kept readable at all times. Finally, keep all figure columns straight so that decimal points line up. Following through on these procedures can help ensure that your work will be concise and accurate.
21.2 **Compare single-entry, double-entry, and write-it-once bookkeeping systems.**	The single-entry accounting system—although easy to use because each entry is written once on the patient ledger, on the daily log, and in the checkbook—contains no checks and balances for accuracy. The double-entry system, based on assets = capital + liabilities, has checks and balances but can be cumbersome and complicated. The write-it-once system is popular with manual offices because it allows all transactions to be recorded in one procedure, using carbonless forms on all necessary documents. Many computerized office management software packages are based on the write-it-once concept.
21.3 **Outline patient-related financial transactions.**	Patient-related financial transactions include starting the day, patient process, attaching the superbill to the patient chart, patient checkout, after visit payments, returned checks, refunds, uncollectable accounts, and end of day procedures.
21.4 **Identify negotiable instruments and the items that must be present for a check to be negotiable.**	A negotiable instrument is one that is legally transferable from one person to another. To be negotiable, a check must be written and signed by the payer or maker, include the amount of money to be paid, be made payable to the payee or bearer, be made payable on demand or on a specific date, and include the name of the bank that is directed to make payment.
21.5 **Describe the different types of check endorsements and the steps in creating a bank deposit.**	The types of check endorsements are blank, restrictive, special, and qualified. To make a bank deposit, follow the steps outlined in Procedure 21-5.
21.6 **Carry out the process of reconciling the office bank statement.**	Following the guidelines outlined in Procedure 21-6, the student should successfully be able to reconcile a mock bank statement with a mock office checkbook.
21.7 **List several advantages to electronic banking.**	The computer software calculates each new balance for you. It can reconcile the monthly bank statement automatically and, instead of locking up bank forms and the office checkbook, a computer password and security system are used to keep the information safe and confidential.
21.8 **Implement setting up, classifying, and recording disbursements in a disbursements journal.**	Following Procedure 21-7, the student should set up a mock disbursements journal consisting of several columns of expenses. Once set up, given a list of several "bills" to be paid, the student should document the check information and record the disbursement amount in the correct column(s) of the journal.

Recall Sylvia Gonzales from the beginning of the chapter. Now that you have completed the chapter, answer the following questions regarding her case.

1. How will you post today's charges and payment to balance the patient's account?

2. Explain how you will prepare the patient's check for deposit in the office checking account.

EXAM PREPARATION QUESTIONS

1. (LO 21.1) Which of the following is NOT a procedure to be followed when setting up bookkeeping or banking systems?
   a. Be organized in your work area
   b. Be consistent in your procedure
   c. Use markers, jotting an "x" as you work to avoid losing your place
   d. Write clearly in pen, using the same color ink
   e. Check your work carefully

2. (LO 21.2) Which accounting system uses the formula *assets = liability + capital*?
   a. Bookkeeping
   b. Single-entry
   c. Journalizing
   d. Pegboard system
   e. Double-entry

3. (LO 21.2) When using the pegboard or write-it-once system, the daily log is also known as the
   a. Day sheet
   b. Pegboard
   c. Journal
   d. Disbursements journal
   e. Ledger card

4. (LO 21.2) The form that contains a single patient's financial information and record or transactions is called the patient
   a. Day sheet
   b. Check
   c. Pegboard
   d. Daily log
   e. Ledger card

5. (LO 21.8) If you make an error when completing a check, you should
   a. Use correction fluid to cover up the incorrect amount and write in the correct amount
   b. Tear up the check and throw it away
   c. Write VOID in ink across the front of the check and file it in numerical order with the returned checks
   d. Scratch out the error and fill in the correct amount above it
   e. a or d

6. (LO 21.4) Business (or personal) checks with stubs attached are known as
   a. Counter checks
   b. Voucher checks
   c. Limited checks
   d. Traveler's checks
   e. Cashier's checks

7. (LO 21.5) The best endorsement to use on a daily basis when preparing checks for the office deposit is the _____ endorsement.
   a. Blank
   b. Special
   c. Third-party
   d. Restrictive
   e. Qualified

8. (LO 21.6) The term _____ is used when comparing the bank statement balance to the checkbook balance to be sure no transaction has been missed.
   a. Balancing
   b. Checks and balances
   c. Trial balance
   d. Profit and loss statement
   e. Reconciliation

9. (LO 21.7) All of the following tasks can be completed by electronic banking EXCEPT:
   a. Recording deposits
   b. Paying bills
   c. Explaining the profit and loss statement
   d. Displaying the checkbook
   e. Reconciling the checkbook

10. (LO 21.8) A payment made by the office for goods or services purchased is known as
   a. Disbursement
   b. Accounts payable
   c. Accounts receivable
   d. Liability
   e. Capital

Organization of the Body

CASE STUDY

John Miller, a 65-year-old male, arrives at the clinic complaining of his shoes not fitting and feeling like he cannot take a deep breath. During the patient interview, he also states he is having intermittent pain in his chest. He has not taken his blood pressure medication for two weeks. He is hoping to get this medication renewed. The physician wants to evaluate his congestive heart failure and orders a chest X-ray. You know from your study of anatomy that the X-ray will provide an image of the structures in the thoracic cavity.

Keep John in mind as you study this chapter. There will be questions at the end of the chapter based on the case study. The information in the chapter will help you answer these questions.

LEARNING OUTCOMES

After completing Chapter 22, you will be able to:

22.1 Explain the importance of understanding both anatomy and physiology when studying the body.

22.2 Illustrate body organization from simple to more complex levels.

22.3 Describe the locations and characteristics of the four main tissue types.

22.4 Describe the body organ systems, their general functions, and the major organs contained in each.

22.5 Use medical and anatomical terminology correctly.

22.6 Explain anatomical position and its relationship to other anatomical positions.

22.7 Identify the body cavities and the organs contained in each.

22.8 Relate a basic understanding of chemistry to its importance in studying the body.

22.9 Name the parts of a cell and their functions.

22.10 Summarize how substances move across a cell membrane.

22.11 Distinguish the stages of cell division.

22.12 Explain the uses of these genetic techniques: DNA fingerprinting and the polymerase chain reaction.

22.13 Describe the different patterns of inheritance and common genetic disorders.

KEY TERMS

anatomical position
anatomy
cells
chemistry
chromosome
cytokinesis
electrolytes
gene
ions
matter

meiosis
metabolism
mitosis
molecule
organ
organelle
organism
organ systems
physiology
tissue

CAAHEP

I. C (1) Describe structural organization of the human body

I. C (2) Identify body systems

I. C (3) Describe body planes, directional terms, quadrants, and cavities

I. C (4) List major organs in each body system

I. C (5) Describe the normal function of each body system

I. C (7) Analyze pathology as it relates to the interaction of body systems

I. C (8) Discuss implications for disease and disability when homeostasis is not maintained

I. C (9) Describe implications for treatment related to pathology

IV.C (10) Diagram medical terms, labeling the word parts

IV.C (11) Define both medical terms and abbreviations related to all body systems

ABHES

2. **Anatomy & Physiology**

b. Identify and apply the knowledge of all body systems, their structure and functions, and their common diseases, symptoms, and etiologies

3. **Medical Terminology**

Graduates:

a. Define and use entire basic structure of medical words and be able to accurately identify in the correct context; i.e., root, prefix, suffix, combinations, spelling, and definitions

b. Build and dissect medical terms from roots/suffixes to understand the word element combinations that create medical terminology

c. Understand the various medical terminology for each specialty

Introduction

The human body is complex in its structure and function. Think of your own body for a moment. If you were to choose just one body part—say your eyes—consider everything about how they look, how they function, how they are connected to the rest of your face, and how your skull supports them. Consider what happens to your eyes when you smile, cry, glimpse bright sunlight, or when a misguided insect or piece of dirt makes its way into them and you have to rub one or the other eye with your finger and you end up scratching it accidentally, causing temporarily blurred vision.

Of course, the eyes are just one example. You have your entire body to deal with. This chapter provides an overview of the human body. It introduces you to the way the body is organized from the chemical level all the way up to the organ system level. You will learn important terminology used to describe body positions and parts. You will also explore how diseases develop at the genetic and organism levels.

The Study of the Body   LO 22.1

Anatomy is the scientific term for the study of body structure. For example, the heart may be described as a hollow, cone-shaped organ that is an average of 14 centimeters long and 9 centimeters wide. Understanding anatomy allows us to understand the normal position of body structures and how to describe these positions precisely and correctly. **Physiology** is the term for the study of the function of the body's organs. For example, the physiology of the heart can be described by saying that the heart pumps blood into blood vessels to transport nutrients throughout the body. Anatomy and physiology are commonly studied together because they are intimately related. For example, the anatomy of the heart (a hollow, muscular organ)

allows it to do its function (pump blood into tubular blood vessels). If the heart was not hollow, it could not allow blood to flow into it. If the heart was not muscular, it could not pump blood.

Knowledge of anatomy and physiology will help you grasp the meaning of diagnostic and procedural codes, and help you understand the clinical procedures you will perform and assist with as a medical assistant. Understanding anatomy and physiology can also make it easier to see how and why certain diseases develop. Diseases develop in the body when homeostasis—the relative consistency of the body's internal environment—is not maintained. Body conditions that must remain within a stable range include body temperature, blood pressure, and the concentration of various chemicals within the blood. Individual cells must also maintain homeostasis. For example, if chemicals within a cell change the deoxyribonucleic acid (DNA) or genetic makeup of the cell, that cell can become cancerous.

Go to CONNECT to see an animation about *Homeostasis*.

Organization of the Body   LO 22.2

The body's structure can be divided into different levels of organization. The chemical level is the simplest level. It refers to the billions of atoms and molecules in the body. Atoms are the simplest units of all matter, and many are essential to life. **Matter** is anything that takes up space and has weight. The four most common atoms in the human body are carbon, hydrogen, oxygen, and nitrogen. **Molecules** are made up of atoms that bond together. Proteins and carbohydrates are examples of molecules that consist of hundreds of atoms.

Molecules join together to form **organelles,** which can be thought of as cell parts. Organelles combine to form cells

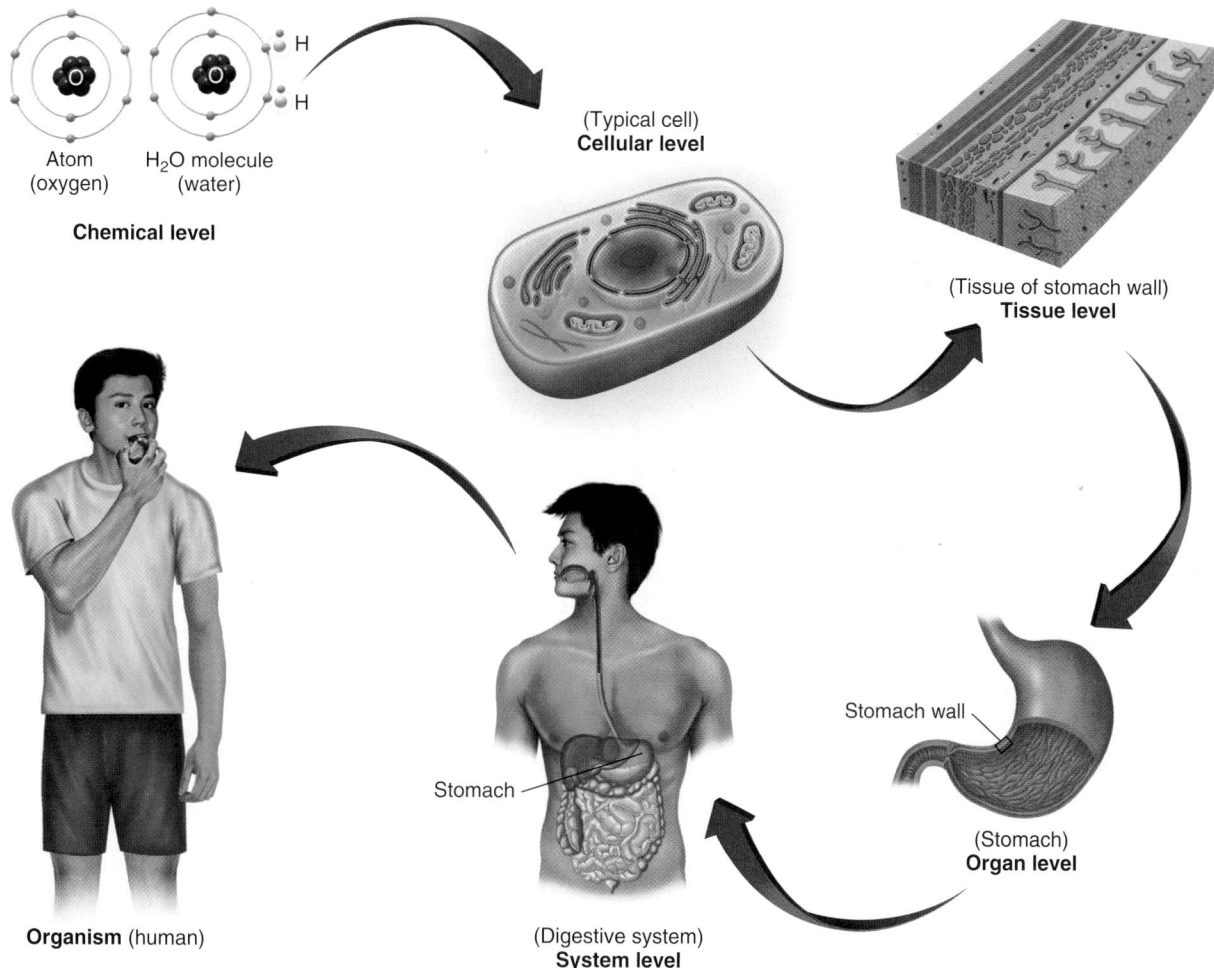

FIGURE 22-1 The human body is organized in levels, beginning with the chemical level and progressing to the cellular, tissue, organ, system, and organism (whole body) levels.

The labels in the figure are:

Atom (oxygen) H_2O molecule (water)   **Chemical level**

(Typical cell) **Cellular level**

(Tissue of stomach wall) **Tissue level**

Stomach wall

(Stomach) **Organ level**

Stomach

Organism (human)

(Digestive system) **System level**

---

such as leukocytes (white blood cells), erythrocytes (red blood cells), neurons (nerve cells), and adipocytes (fat cells). **Cells** are considered to be the smallest living units in the body. When the same types of cells organize together, they form **tissues.** Two or more tissue types combine to form **organs,** and organs arrange to form **organ systems.** Finally, organ systems combine to form an **organism.** Figure 22-1 illustrates the organization of the body's organ systems.

▶ Major Tissue Types

LO 22.3

Tissues are groups of cells that have similar structures and functions. The four major tissue types in the body are epithelial, connective, muscle, and nervous tissue. These are explained more fully in the following paragraphs.

Epithelial Tissue

When you think of epithelial tissue, think of a covering, lining, or gland. Epithelial tissue covers the body and most organs in the body. It lines the body's tubes, such as blood vessels and the esophagus, and the body's hollow organs, such as the stomach

and heart. This type of tissue also lines body cavities, such as the thoracic cavity and the abdominopelvic cavity.

Glandular tissue is also classified as a type of epithelial tissue. It is composed of cells that make and secrete (give off) substances. If a gland secretes its product into a duct, as with a sweat or oil (sebaceous) gland, it is called an *exocrine gland*. If a gland secretes its product directly into surrounding tissue fluids or blood, it does not have ducts and it is called an *endocrine gland*. The pancreas and thyroid are considered endocrine glands because they release their hormones directly into the bloodstream.

Epithelial tissues are avascular, which means they lack blood vessels. However, these tissues have a nerve supply and are very mitotic, meaning they divide constantly. In addition, the cells within epithelial tissues are packed together tightly. Epithelial tissues have many different functions, depending on their location in the body. For example, those covering the body protect against invading pathogens and toxins. Those that line the digestive tract secrete a variety of enzymes needed for digestion. They often possess microvilli, which allow the body to absorb nutrients. Epithelial tissues lining the respiratory tract have

FIGURE 22-2 Epithelial tissue lining the respiratory tract.

cilia and goblet cells. The goblet cells produce mucus that traps small particles that enter the respiratory tract. The cilia constantly push the mucus and trapped particles away from the lungs (see Figure 22-2). Epithelial cells within the kidneys act as filters that help to remove waste products from blood.

Connective Tissue

Connective tissues are the most abundant tissues in the body. The cells of connective tissues are not packed together tightly. Instead, a matrix separates the cells. Think of the matrix simply as the matter between the cells of connective tissue. It contains fibers, water, proteins, inorganic salts, and other substances. The components of the matrix vary, depending on the type of connective tissue. Connective tissues generally have a rich blood supply, except for cartilage and some dense connective tissues that contain a very poor blood supply.

Many different cell types are located in connective tissues; the most common are fibroblasts, mast cells, and macrophages. Fibroblasts make fibers, and mast cells secrete substances like heparin and histamine that promote inflammation when tissue is damaged. Macrophages are cells that destroy unwanted material, like bacteria or toxins.

The following sections discuss the body's different connective tissues in more detail.

Blood This tissue is composed of red blood cells, white blood cells, platelets, and plasma. Plasma is the matrix of blood. Unlike other connective tissues, this matrix does not contain fibers. Blood transports substances throughout the body. Blood and its cell functions will be discussed in depth in a later chapter.

Osseous (Bone) Tissue The matrix of osseous tissue contains mineral salts that make it a very hard tissue. Contrary to popular belief, bone tissue is a living tissue—it is metabolically active.

Cartilage The matrix of cartilage is rigid, although it is not as hard as osseous tissue. Cartilage gives shape to structures such as the ears and nose. It also protects the ends of long bones and forms the discs between the vertebrae of the neck and spine.

Dense Connective Tissue The matrix of dense connective tissue is packed with tough fibers that make it a soft but very strong tissue. Ligaments, tendons, and joint capsules have large amounts of this tissue type. Ligaments connect bones to bones, tendons connect muscles to bones, and joint capsules surround moveable joints in the body. Dense connective tissues also make up a large part of the skin's dermis. When skin is damaged, this tissue "fills in" the damaged space and forms a scar.

Adipose (Fat) Tissue Within adipose tissue, unique cells—adipocytes—store fats. This tissue type stores energy for body cells, cushions body parts and organs, and insulates the body against excessive heat or cold (see Figure 22-3).

Muscle Tissue

Muscle is a specialized type of tissue that contracts and relaxes. The three types of muscle tissue are: skeletal, visceral (smooth), and cardiac.

FIGURE 22-3 Adipose tissue.

FIGURE 22-4   Skeletal muscle tissue.

FIGURE 22-5   Nervous tissue.

Skeletal Muscle Tissue   As its name suggests, skeletal muscle tissue is attached to the skeleton. This type of tissue is voluntary because we can consciously control its movement. For example, we can consciously decide to contract the skeletal muscles attached to our arm bones and make them move. It is also referred to as striated because the cells of this muscle tissue type have striations or stripes in their cytoplasm (see Figure 22-4).

Visceral Muscle Tissue   This smooth muscle tissue is located in the walls of hollow organs (except the heart), the walls of blood vessels, and the dermis of skin. It is involuntary—we cannot consciously control its movement. For example, you do not consciously decide when the visceral muscle of your stomach contracts. This tissue is also called *smooth muscle* because its cells do not have striations in their cytoplasm.

Cardiac Muscle Tissue   This specialized muscle tissue is located in the wall of the heart. Like skeletal muscle tissue, cardiac muscle is striated. Like smooth muscle tissue, it is not under voluntary control; it is involuntary.

Nervous Tissue

Nervous tissue is located in the brain, spinal cord, and peripheral nerves. This tissue specializes in sending impulses or electrical messages to the neurons, muscles, and glands in the body (see Figure 22-5). Nervous tissue contains two types of cells: neurons and neuroglial cells. Neurons are the largest cells and they transmit impulses. Although neuroglial cells are smaller, they are more abundant and act as support cells for the neurons. They do not transmit impulses.

Go to CONNECT to see an animation about *Cells and Tissues.*

▶ Body Organs and Systems
LO 22.4

Organs are structures formed by the organization of two or more different tissue types that work together to carry out specific functions. For example, the heart is made of cardiac muscle tissue, connective tissue, and epithelial tissue. These tissues work together to carry out the heart's function—to effectively pump blood into blood vessels. Organ systems are formed when organs join together to carry out vital functions. For example, the heart and blood vessels unite to form the cardiovascular system. The organs of the cardiovascular system circulate blood throughout the body to ensure that all body cells receive enough nutrients. See Figure 22-6 for a summary of the human body's organ systems, their general functions, and the organs within each.

▶ Understanding Medical Terminology
LO 22.5

Unlike the English language in which word meanings often seem to have no rhyme or reason—like the overly used "whatever" and various difficult-to-translate modern slang phrasings—medical terminology often can be broken down into word parts that make the meaning concrete and easy to understand. All medical terms must have a word root that contains the base meaning for the term, and a suffix at the end of the term that alters the word root's meaning. In the term *appendectomy,* for example, the word root *append* refers to the "appendix" and is combined with the suffix *-ectomy,*

Integumentary System

Serves as a sense organ for the body, provides protection, regulates temperature, prevents water loss, and produces vitamin D precursors. Consists of skin, hair, nails, and sweat glands.

- Hair
- Skin

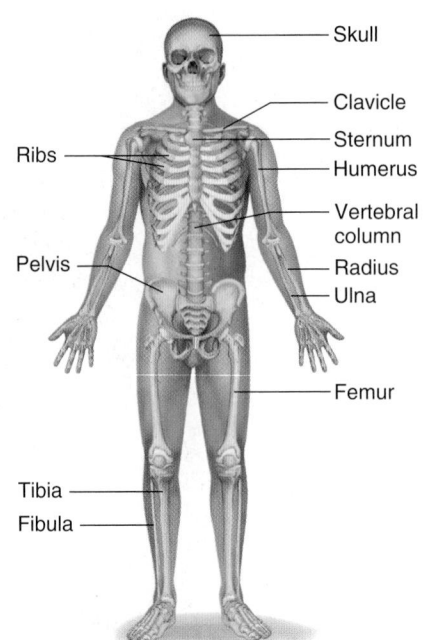

Skeletal System

Provides protection and support, allows body movements, produces blood cells, and stores minerals and fat. Consists of bones, associated cartilages, ligaments, and joints.

- Skull
- Clavicle
- Sternum
- Humerus
- Ribs
- Vertebral column
- Pelvis
- Radius
- Ulna
- Femur
- Tibia
- Fibula

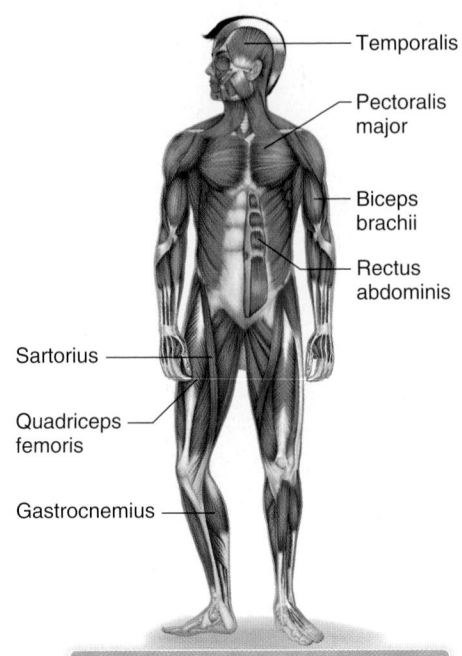

Muscular System

Produces body movements, maintains posture, and produces body heat. Consists of muscles attached to the skeleton by tendons.

- Temporalis
- Pectoralis major
- Biceps brachii
- Rectus abdominis
- Sartorius
- Quadriceps femoris
- Gastrocnemius

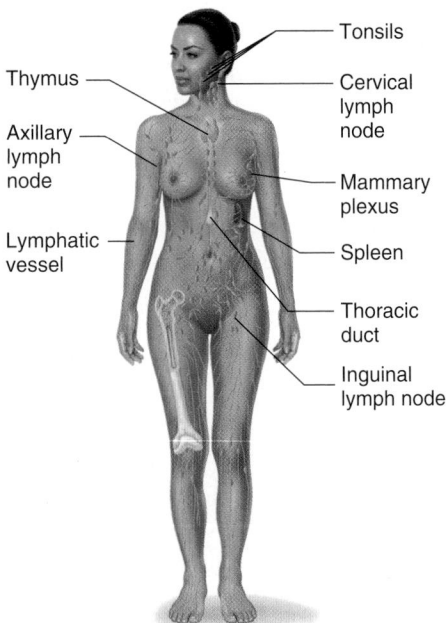

Lymphatic System

Removes foreign substances from the blood and lymph, combats disease, maintains tissue fluid balance, and absorbs fats from the digestive tract. Consists of the lymphatic vessels, lymph nodes, and other lymphatic organs.

- Tonsils
- Thymus
- Cervical lymph node
- Axillary lymph node
- Mammary plexus
- Lymphatic vessel
- Spleen
- Thoracic duct
- Inguinal lymph node

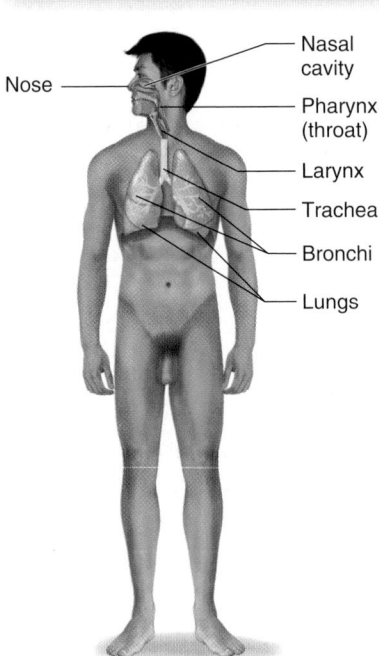

Respiratory System

Exchanges oxygen and carbon dioxide between the blood and air and regulates blood pH. Consists of the lungs and respiratory passages.

- Nasal cavity
- Nose
- Pharynx (throat)
- Larynx
- Trachea
- Bronchi
- Lungs

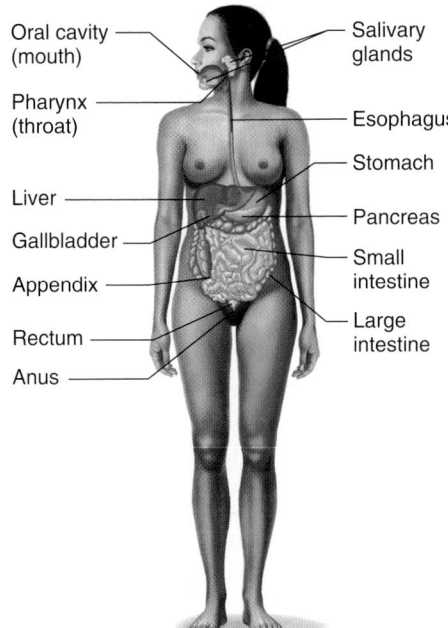

Digestive System

Performs the mechanical and chemical processes of digestion, absorption of nutrients, and elimination of wastes. Consists of the mouth, esophagus, stomach, intestines, and accessory organs.

- Oral cavity (mouth)
- Salivary glands
- Pharynx (throat)
- Esophagus
- Stomach
- Liver
- Pancreas
- Gallbladder
- Small intestine
- Appendix
- Large intestine
- Rectum
- Anus

FIGURE 22-6a Organ systems of the body.

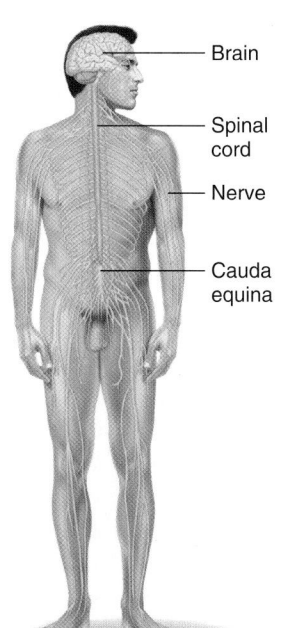

Brain

Spinal cord

Nerve

Cauda equina

Nervous System

A major regulatory system that detects sensations and controls movements, physiologic processes, and intellectual functions. Consists of the brain, spinal cord, nerves, and sensory receptors.

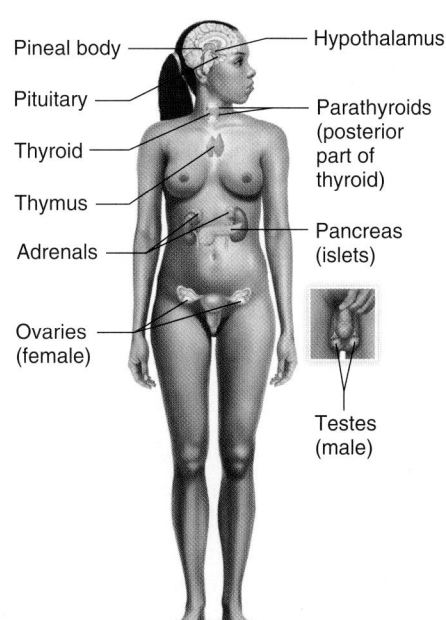

Pineal body

Pituitary

Thyroid

Thymus

Adrenals

Ovaries (female)

Hypothalamus

Parathyroids (posterior part of thyroid)

Pancreas (islets)

Testes (male)

Endocrine System

A major regulatory system that influences metabolism, growth, reproduction, and many other functions. Consists of glands, such as the pituitary, that secrete hormones.

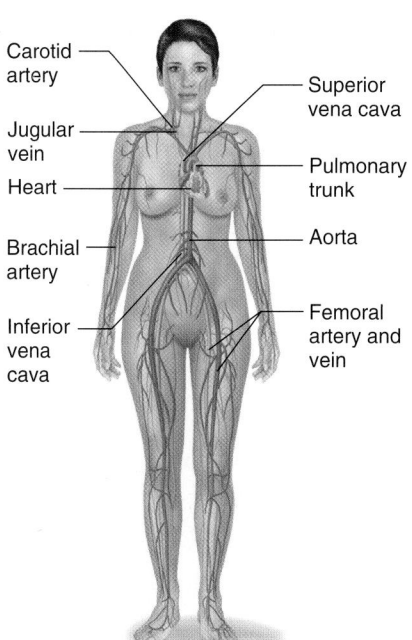

Carotid artery

Jugular vein

Heart

Brachial artery

Inferior vena cava

Superior vena cava

Pulmonary trunk

Aorta

Femoral artery and vein

Cardiovascular System

Transports nutrients, waste products, gases, and hormones throughout the body; plays a role in the immune response and the regulation of body temperature. Consists of the heart, blood vessels, and blood.

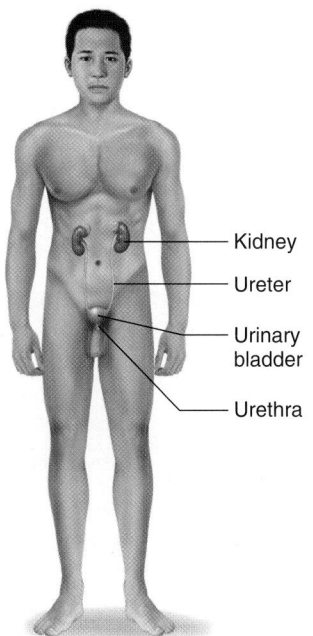

Kidney

Ureter

Urinary bladder

Urethra

Urinary System

Removes waste products from the blood and regulates blood pH, ion balance, and water balance. Consists of the kidneys, urinary bladder, and ducts that carry urine.

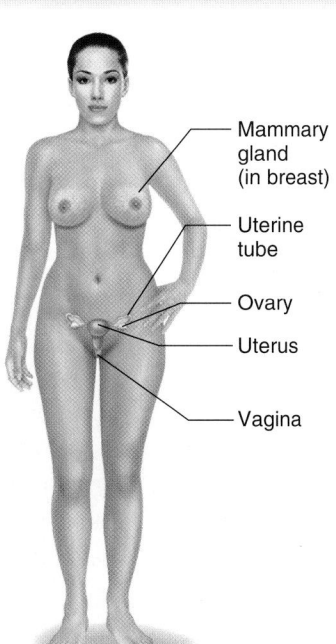

Mammary gland (in breast)

Uterine tube

Ovary

Uterus

Vagina

Female Reproductive System

Produces oocytes and is the site of fertilization and fetal development; produces milk for the newborn; produces hormones that influence sexual function and behaviors. Consists of the ovaries, vagina, uterus, mammary glands, and associated structures.

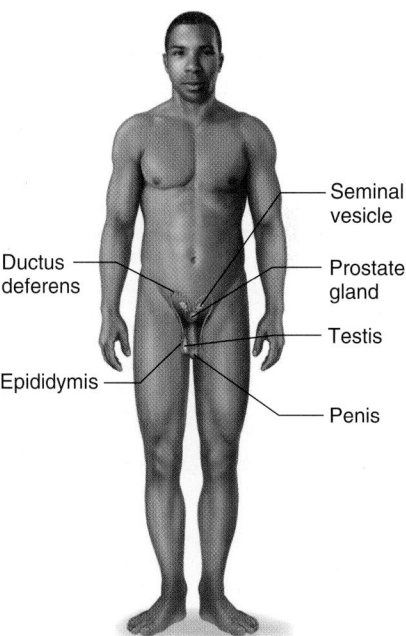

Ductus deferens

Epididymis

Seminal vesicle

Prostate gland

Testis

Penis

Male Reproductive System

Produces and transfers sperm cells to the female and produces hormones that influence sexual functions and behaviors. Consists of the testes, accessory structures, ducts, and penis.

FIGURE 22-6b (concluded)

which means "surgical removal." So, *appendectomy* means "surgical removal of the appendix." The word parts' meanings stay consistent, making it easier to learn new terms containing already understood word parts. Using your new knowledge, if you are told that the word root *hyster* means "uterus," you can easily see that *hysterectomy* means "surgical removal of the uterus."

In addition to word roots and suffixes, some terms also contain a prefix, which comes at the beginning of the term and, like the suffix, alters the term's meaning. Let's take the terms *premenstrual* and *postmenstrual*. In defining terms, the general rule is to start with the suffix, then add the prefix (if present), and finally the word root(s). For example:

- The suffix *-al* means "pertaining to"
- The prefix *pre-* means "before"
- The prefix *post-* means "after"

The word root *menstru* refers to the menstrual period. Putting them together, *premenstrual* means "pertaining to *before* the menstrual period" and *postmenstrual* is "pertaining to *after* the menstrual period."

For terms in which the suffix begins with a consonant, a combining vowel—often an "o"—is used between the word root and the suffix to ease pronunciation. An example of this would be the term *tracheotomy*. The word root *trache* (windpipe) is being joined to the suffix *-tomy* (to cut into). The letter "o" is inserted between the two to make pronunciation easier. Unlike prefixes and suffixes, combining vowels do not change the meaning of the term. Appendix I contains commonly used word roots, suffixes, and prefixes. Table 22-1 summarizes information on understanding medical terminology.

TABLE 22-1 Understanding Medical Terminology

Word Part	Description	Term Using Word Part	Term Meaning
Word root	Base meaning of the term	Colostomy	Colo = colon; -stomy = to cut (or create) a new opening
			Colostomy: to cut a new opening for the colon
Suffix	Ending of term; alters meaning of the word root	Cardiology	Cardi = heart; -logy = knowledge of Cardiology: knowledge (specialty) of the heart (with the combining vowel "o" between the two to ease pronunciation)
Prefix	Beginning of the term; alters the meaning of the word root	Tachycardia	Tachy- = rapid; cardi = heart; -ia = condition of Tachycardia: condition of rapid heart (beat)
Combining vowel	Placed between word root and suffix to ease pronunciation	Cardiologist	Cardi = heart; o = combining vowel to ease pronunciation; -logist = specialist in knowledge of Cardiologist: specialist in the knowledge of the heart

▶ Anatomical Terminology

Anatomical terms describe the location of body parts and various body regions. To correctly use these terms, it is assumed that the body is in the anatomical position. For example, picture yourself in the **anatomical position:** your body is standing upright and facing forward, and your arms are at your sides with the palms of your hands facing forward. Even if patients are lying down, for consistency and correct communication when you use anatomical terms, always refer to patients as if they are in the anatomical position. (Figure 22-9 demonstrates the anatomical position.)

Directional Anatomical Terms

The directional anatomical terms that identify the position of body structures compared to other body structures are: *superior* (*cranial*), *inferior* (*caudal*), *anterior* (*ventral*), *posterior* (*dorsal*), *medial, lateral, proximal, distal, superficial,* and *deep.* For example, the eyes are medial to the ears but lateral to the nose. See Table 22-2 and Figure 22-7 for an explanation and illustration of these important directional terms.

Anatomical Terms That Describe Body Sections

Sometimes in order to study internal body parts, it helps to imagine the body as being divided into sections. Medical professionals often use the following terms, defined in the bullets, to describe how the body is divided into sections: sagittal, midsagittal, transverse, and frontal (coronal).

- A *sagittal plane* divides the body into left and right portions.
- A *midsagittal plane* runs lengthwise down the midline of the body and divides it into equal left and right halves.

TABLE 22-2 Directional Anatomical Terms

Term	Definition	Example
Superior (cranial)	Above or close to the head	The thoracic cavity is superior to the abdominal cavity.
Inferior (caudal)	Below or close to the feet	The neck is inferior to the head.
Anterior (ventral)	Toward the front of the body	The nose is anterior to the ears.
Posterior (dorsal)	Toward the back of the body	The brain is posterior to the eyes.
Medial	Close to the midline of the body	The nose is medial to the ears.
Lateral	Farther away from the midline of the body	The ears are lateral to the nose.
Proximal	Close to a point of attachment or to the trunk of the body	The knee is proximal to the toes.
Distal	Farther away from a point of attachment or from the trunk of the body	The fingers are distal to the elbow.
Superficial	Close to the surface of the body	Skin is superficial to muscles.
Deep	More internal	Bones are deep to skin.

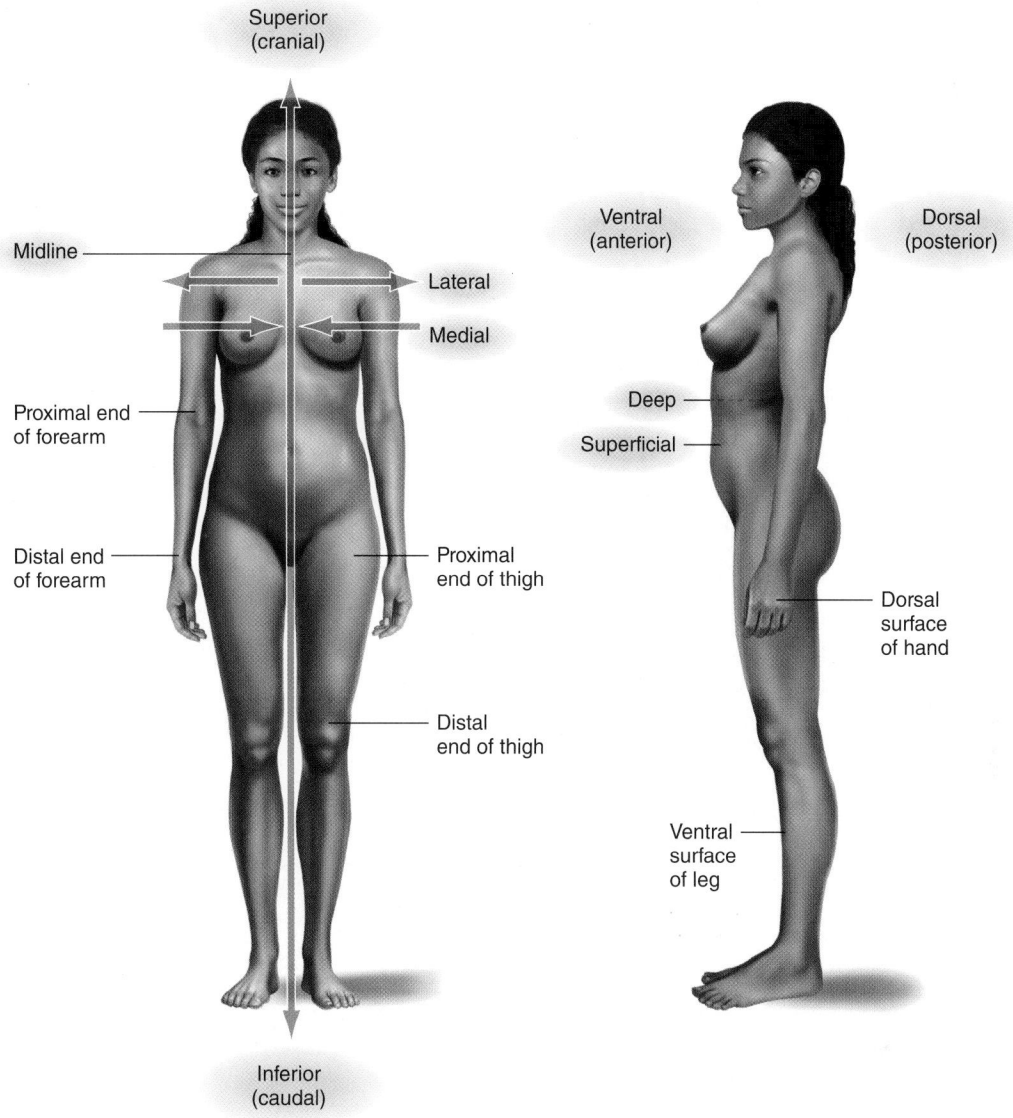

FIGURE 22-7 Directional terms provide mapping instructions for locating organs and body parts.

- A *transverse plane* divides the body into superior (upper) and inferior (lower) portions.
- A *frontal*, or *coronal*, plane divides the body into anterior (frontal) and posterior (rear) portions.

Figure 22-8 illustrates these planes.

Anatomical Terms That Describe Body Parts

Many other anatomical terms describe different regions or parts of the body. For example, the term *brachium* refers to the arm and the term *femoral* refers to the thigh. Figure 22-9 illustrates many of the common anatomical terms that describe body parts.

▶ Body Cavities and Abdominal Regions

LO 22.7

Body cavities house and protect the internal organs. The largest body cavities are the dorsal cavity and the ventral cavity. The dorsal cavity is divided into the cranial cavity (which houses the brain) and the spinal cavity (which contains the spinal cord). The ventral cavity is divided into the thoracic cavity and the abdominopelvic cavity. The muscle called the *diaphragm* separates the thoracic and abdominopelvic cavities. The thoracic cavity contains the:

- Lungs
- Heart

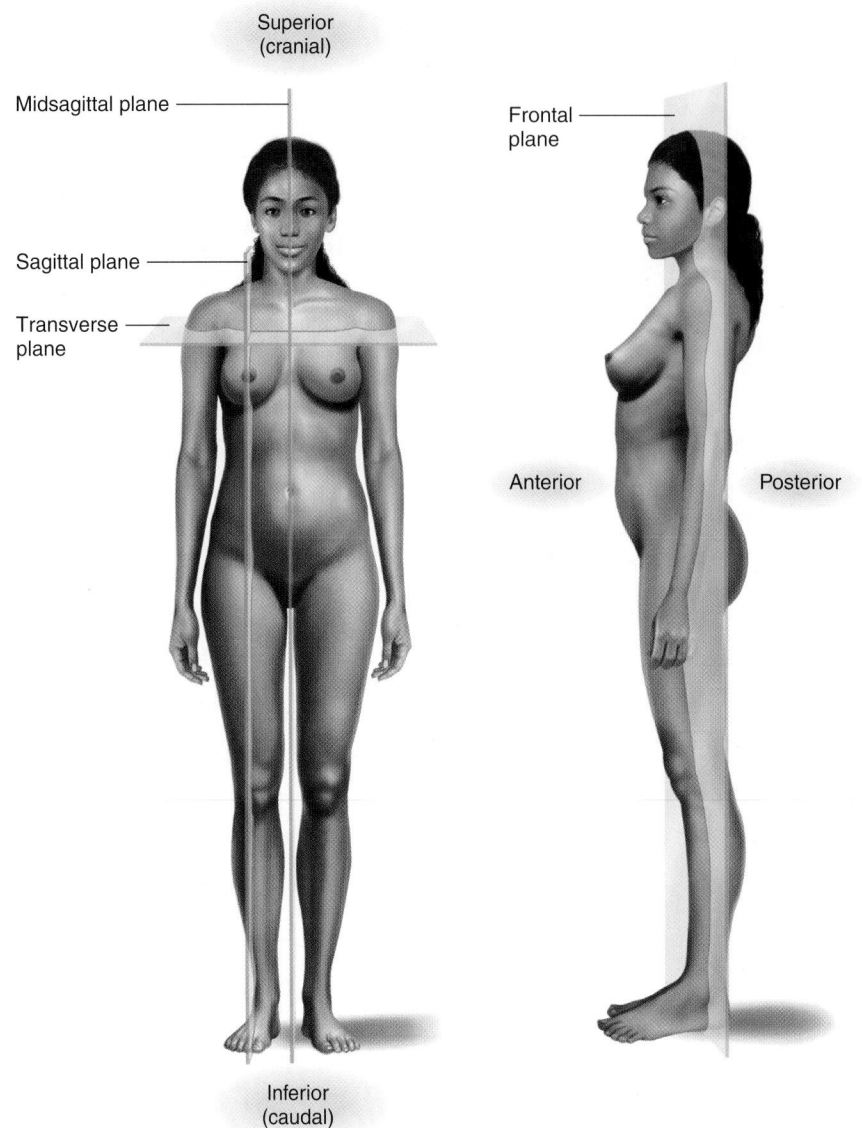

Midsagittal plane

Sagittal plane

Transverse plane

Superior (cranial)

Inferior (caudal)

Frontal plane

Anterior   Posterior

FIGURE 22-8   Spatial terms are based on imaginary cuts or planes through the body.

- Esophagus
- Trachea

The abdominopelvic cavity is divided into a superior abdominal cavity and an inferior pelvic cavity. It contains the:

- Stomach
- Small and large intestines
- Gallbladder
- Liver
- Spleen
- Kidneys
- Pancreas

The bladder and internal reproductive organs are located in the pelvic cavity, which is depicted in Figure 22-10. The abdominal

area is further divided into nine regions or four quadrants, which are illustrated in Figure 22-11.

▶ Chemistry of Life   LO 22.8

Now that you have studied how the body is organized structurally, you need to learn about its chemical structure. **Chemistry** is the study of what matter is made of and how it changes. It is important to have a basic understanding of chemistry when studying anatomy and physiology because body structures and functions result from chemical processes that occur within body cells or fluids.

Go to CONNECT to see an animation about *Basic Chemistry (Organic Molecules)*.

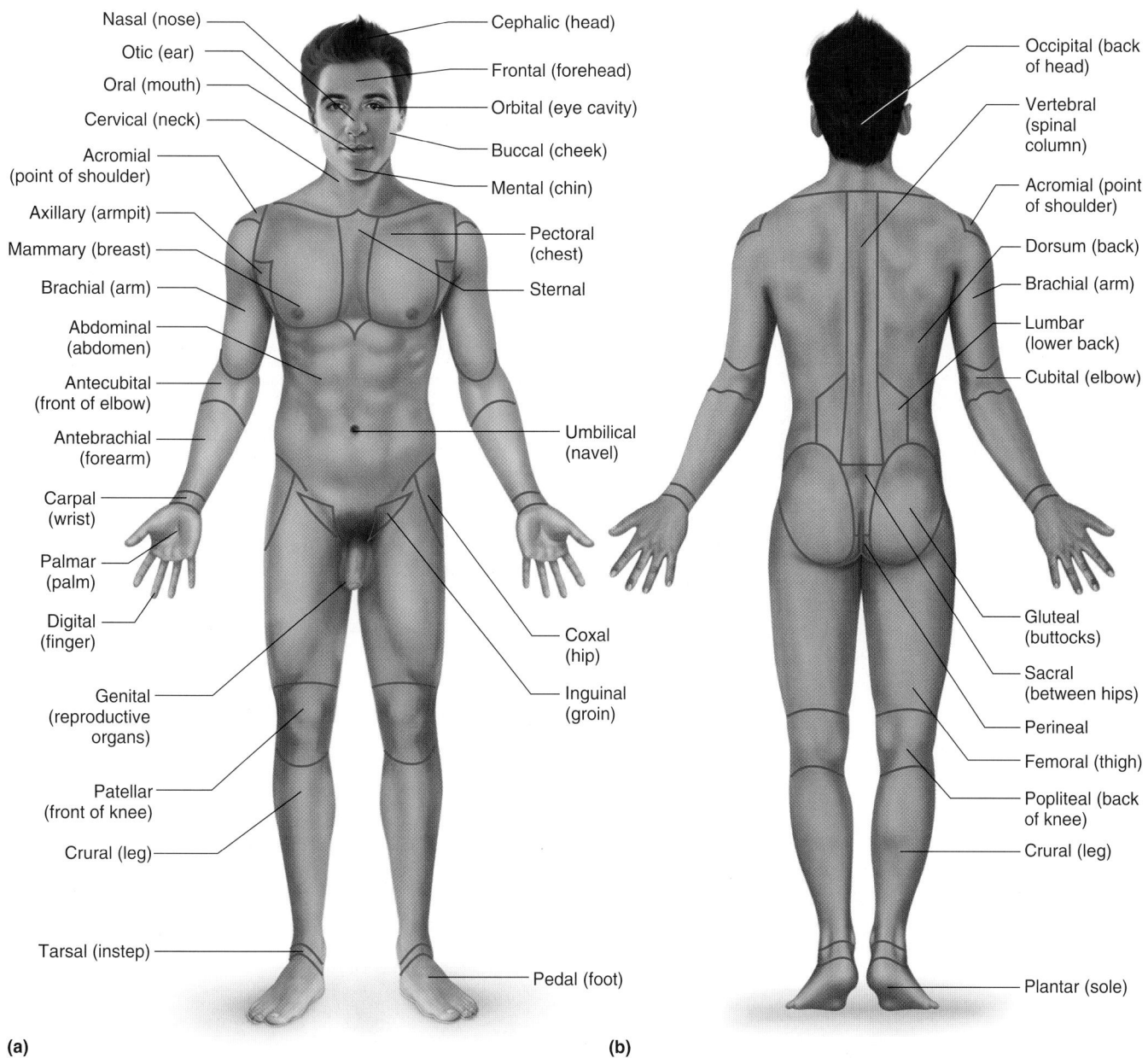

FIGURE 22-9 Numerous anatomical terms describe regions of the body: (a) anterior view and (b) posterior view.

Anterior view labels (a):

Nasal (nose) · Otic (ear) · Oral (mouth) · Cervical (neck) · Acromial (point of shoulder) · Axillary (armpit) · Mammary (breast) · Brachial (arm) · Abdominal (abdomen) · Antecubital (front of elbow) · Antebrachial (forearm) · Carpal (wrist) · Palmar (palm) · Digital (finger) · Genital (reproductive organs) · Patellar (front of knee) · Crural (leg) · Tarsal (instep)

Cephalic (head) · Frontal (forehead) · Orbital (eye cavity) · Buccal (cheek) · Mental (chin) · Pectoral (chest) · Sternal · Umbilical (navel) · Coxal (hip) · Inguinal (groin) · Pedal (foot)

Posterior view labels (b):

Occipital (back of head) · Vertebral (spinal column) · Acromial (point of shoulder) · Dorsum (back) · Brachial (arm) · Lumbar (lower back) · Cubital (elbow) · Gluteal (buttocks) · Sacral (between hips) · Perineal · Femoral (thigh) · Popliteal (back of knee) · Crural (leg) · Plantar (sole)

(a) (b)

As you learned earlier in the chapter, the chemical level is the lowest level of organization. The building blocks of every living organism are the same chemical elements that make up all matter, liquids, solids, and gases. When two or more atoms are chemically combined, a molecule is formed. A compound is formed when two or more atoms of different elements are combined. Molecules of oxygen (O_2) and hydrogen (H_2) are not compounds because they are made up of only one element. Water is an example of a molecule, which is composed of two hydrogen atoms and one oxygen atom. Water is a compound because its molecules are made up of atoms of two different elements—hydrogen and oxygen. Water is critical to both chemical and physical processes in human physiology,

and it accounts for approximately two-thirds of a person's body weight.

Metabolism is the overall chemical functioning of the body. The two processes of metabolism are anabolism and catabolism. In anabolism, small molecules combine to form larger ones (for example, when amino acids combine to form proteins). In catabolism, larger molecules are broken down into smaller ones (for example, when stored glycogen is converted to glucose molecules for energy).

Electrolytes

When put into water, some substances release **ions,** which are either positively or negatively charged particles. These

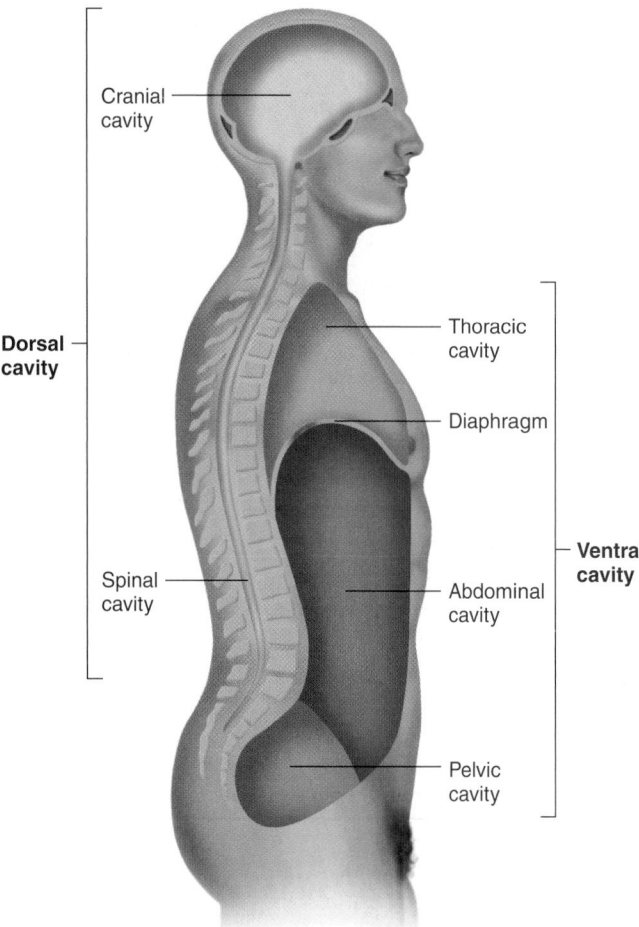

FIGURE 22-10 The two main body cavities are dorsal and ventral.

substances are called **electrolytes.** For example, when you put NaCl in water, it releases two electrolytes: the sodium ion (Na) and the chloride ion (Cl). Electrolytes are critical because the movements of ions into and out of body structures regulate or trigger many physiologic states and activities in the body. For example, electrolytes are essential to fluid balance, muscle contraction, and nerve impulse conduction. Exercising makes you sweat, causing fluid and electrolyte loss. Drinking a sports drink after exercising helps you maintain fluid balance because sports drinks contain water and electrolytes such as sodium and potassium.

Acids and Bases Acids are substances that release hydrogen ions (H^+) in water. Many acids, such as lemon juice and vinegar, have a sour taste. Bases are are substances that release hydroxyl ions (OH-) in water. A basic substance may also be referred to as an alkali. Many basic substances are slippery and bitter to the taste. Laundry detergents, bleach, dish soaps, and many other household cleaning agents are examples of basic substances.

Testing Acids and Bases In the clinical setting, litmus paper, liquid pH indicator test kits, or a pH meter is often used to determine if a substance is acidic or basic. An acidic substance will turn blue litmus paper red, and a basic substance will turn red litmus paper blue. The pH scale runs from 0 to 14. If a solution has a pH of 7, the solution is neutral, which means it is neither acidic nor basic. If a solution has a pH less than 7, the solution is acidic. If a solution has a pH greater than 7, it is basic, or alkaline. The more acidic a

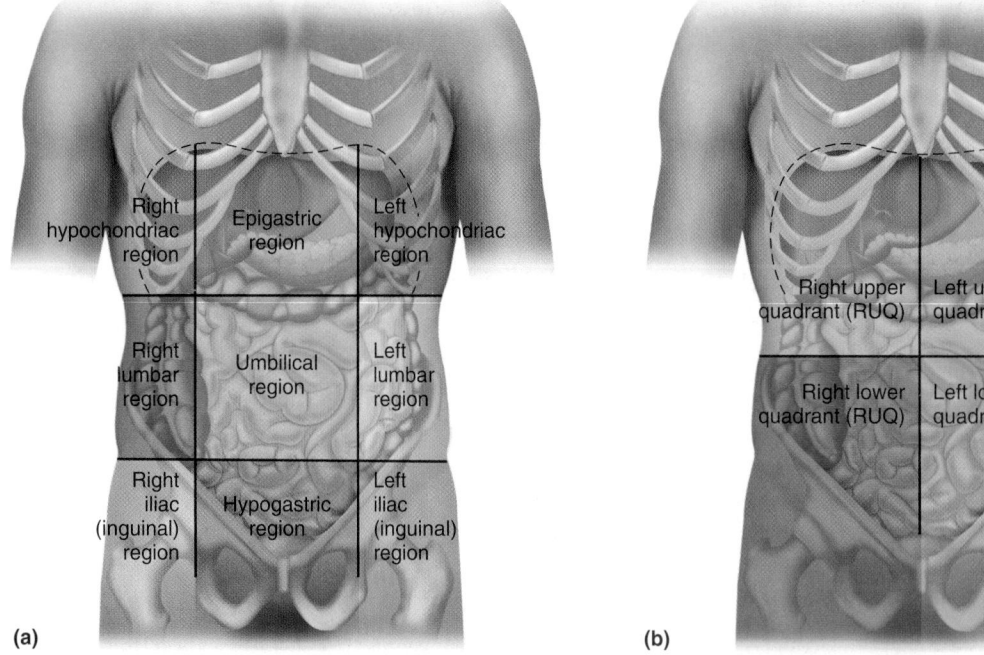

FIGURE 22-11 (a) The abdominal area divided into nine regions and (b) the abdominal area divided into four quadrants.

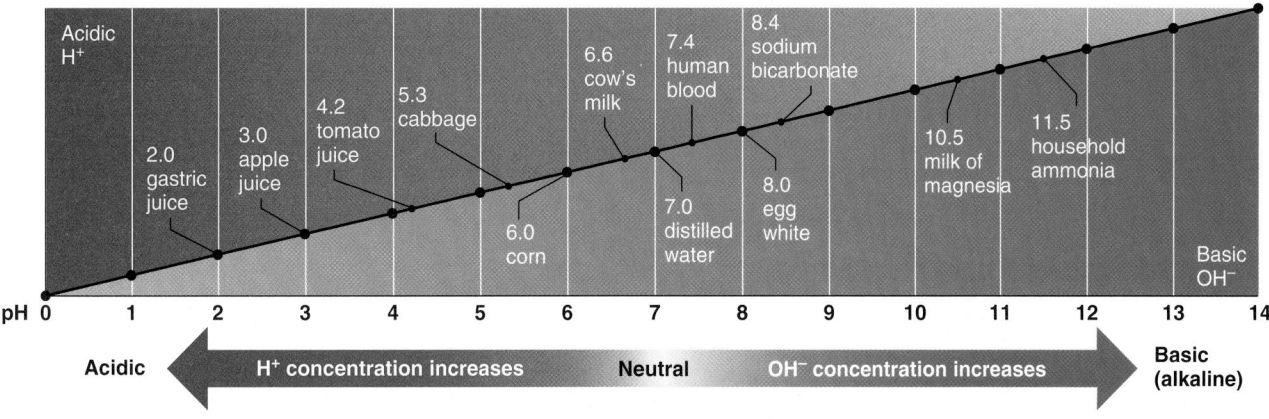

FIGURE 22-12 pH scale. As the concentration of hydrogen ions (H⁺) increases, a solution becomes more acidic, and the pH decreases. As the concentration of hydroxl ions (OH⁻) increases, a solution becomes more basic and the pH increases.

solution is, the higher the concentration of hydrogen ions it contains. The pH values of some common substances are shown in Figure 22-12.

Go to CONNECT to see an animation about *Fluid and Electrolyte Imbalances.*

Biochemistry

Biochemistry is the study of matter and chemical reactions in the body. Matter can be divided into two large categories: organic and inorganic matter. Organic matter contains carbon and hydrogen, and its molecules tend to be large. Inorganic matter generally does not contain carbon and hydrogen; these molecules tend to be small. Examples of inorganic substances are water, oxygen, carbon dioxide, and salts such as sodium chloride. Water is the most abundant inorganic compound in the body. The four major classes of organic matter in the body are carbohydrates, lipids, proteins, and nucleic acids. These are outlined in the following sections.

Carbohydrates Body cells depend on carbohydrate molecules to make energy. The carbohydrate most commonly used by the body cells is glucose. A type of carbohydrate commonly found in potatoes, pastas, and breads is starch, which is broken down into glucose when needed.

Lipids Lipids are fats. Three types of lipids are found in the body: triglycerides, phospholipids, and steroids. Triglycerides store energy for cells, and phospholipids primarily make cell membranes. Butter and oils are composed of triglycerides, and the body stores these molecules in adipose tissue (fat). Steroids are very large lipid molecules that make cell membranes and some hormones. Cholesterol is an example of an essential steroid for body cells.

Proteins Proteins have many functions in the body. Many proteins act as structural materials for the building of solid body parts. Other proteins act as hormones, enzymes, receptors, and antibodies.

Nucleic Acids DNA (deoxyribonucleic acid) and RNA (ribonucleic acid) are two examples of nucleic acids. DNA contains the genetic information of cells, and RNA makes proteins. Nucleic acids are made up of nucleotides, which are discussed later in this chapter.

▶ Cell Characteristics   LO 22.9

Chemicals react to form the complex substances that make up cells, the basic unit of life. The human body is composed of millions of cells. There are many kinds of cells, and each type has a specific function. Most cells have three main parts: cell membrane, cytoplasm (liquid matrix containing each cell's organelles), and the nucleus. Figure 22-13 shows the structure of a composite cell.

Cell Membrane

The cell membrane is the outer limit of a cell. It is very thin and selectively permeable, which means that it allows some substances to pass through it while preventing other substances from passing through. Think of a fence and gate at an amusement park; people who have a ticket can enter through the gate, those who do not have a ticket are kept behind the fence. The cell membrane is composed of two layers of phospholipids, different types of proteins, cholesterol, and a few carbohydrates.

Cytoplasm and Its Organelles

The cytoplasm is the "inside" of the cell. Mostly made up of water, proteins, ions, and nutrients, the cytoplasm houses organelles that perform many cell functions, and therefore body system functions. These organelles, described below, include: cilia, the flagellum, ribosomes, the endoplasmic

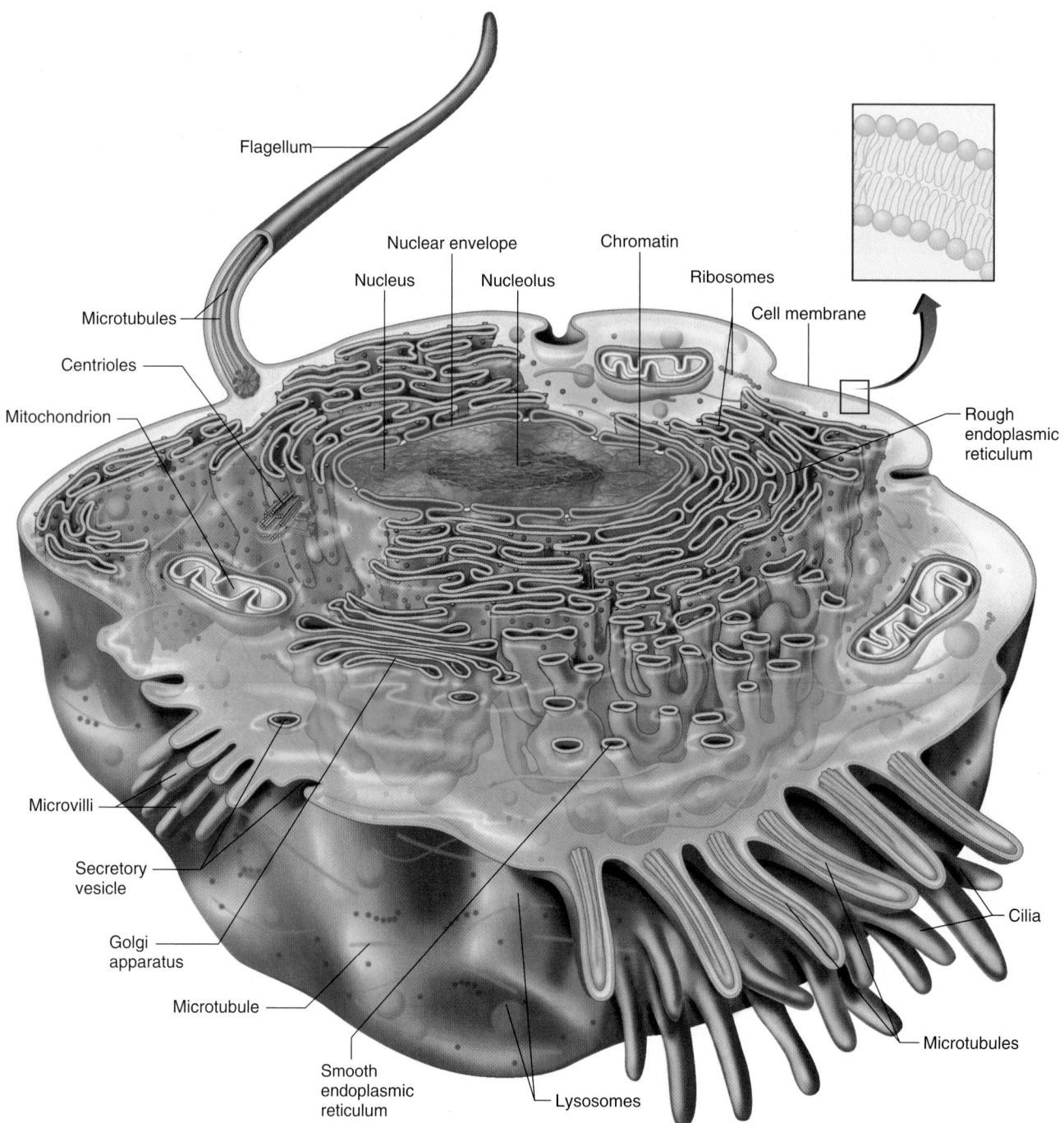

FIGURE 22-13   A composite cell drawing showing the structures that are common to many cell types. Not all types of cells have all of these structures.

reticulum, mitochondria, the Golgi apparatus, lysosomes, and centrioles.

- Many cells contain hair-like projections on the outside of the cell membrane called *cilia*. Cilia assist with propelling matter throughout the body tracts, including the respiratory system. Cells with cilia are often found in the mucous membranes.

- A flagellum is a tail-like structure found on the human sperm cell and provides its "swimming" type of locomotion.

- Ribosomes, in conjunction with RNA molecules, are responsible for protein synthesis. Amino acids are connected together to form proteins through a specialized process

involving different types of RNA molecules. The ribosome supports the protein chain as it is formed.

- The endoplasmic reticulum comes in two forms—smooth and rough. The rough endoplasmic reticulum is named for the presence of ribosomes on its surface, which give it a bumpy or rough appearance. Both types of endoplasmic reticulum form networks or passageways to transport substances throughout the cytoplasm.

- Mitochondria—the centers for cell respiration—provide energy for the cell. There may be only one mitochondrion in a cell or many, depending on how much energy each cell type requires.

- The cell's Golgi apparatus is known to process and sort proteins from the ribosome and to synthesize or produce carbohydrates. It is also thought to prepare and store secretions for discharge from the cell.
- The organelles known as lysosomes perform the cell's digestive function.
- The centrioles—two cylindrical organelles near the nucleus—are essential to cell division as they equally distribute chromosomes to the resultant "daughter" cells.

Nucleus

The nucleus of a cell is typically round and located near the center of a cell. It is enclosed by a nuclear membrane that contains nuclear pores, which allow larger substances to move into and out of the nucleus. It contains **chromosomes,** which are thread-like structures made up of DNA.

▶ Movement Through Cell Membranes

LO 22.10

The selectively permeable cell membrane controls what moves into and out of a cell. Selective permeability means there is some selection or choice in what substances cross the membrane. Some substances like oxygen and water move across the cell membrane without the use of energy. These movements are called *passive mechanisms*. Sometimes the cell has to use energy to move a substance across its membrane in movements known as *active mechanisms*. Large molecules like glucose and proteins move across the cell membrane by active transport.

Diffusion

Diffusion is the movement of a substance from an area of high concentration of that substance to an area of low concentration of the same substance; it can be described as the spreading out of a substance. Substances that easily diffuse across the cell membrane include gases such as oxygen and carbon dioxide.

Osmosis

Osmosis is the diffusion or movement of water across a semipermeable membrane, such as a cell membrane. A semipermeable membrane lets water and other solvent liquids through but nothing else. Remember, water will always try to diffuse or move toward the higher concentration of solutes (solids in solution).

Filtration

In filtration, some type of pressure, such as gravity or blood pressure, forces substances across a membrane that acts like a filter. Filtration separates substances in solutions. For example, you could separate sand from water by pouring the sand/water mixture through a filter. In the body, capillaries in the kidneys act as filters to separate components of blood.

Active Transport

In active transport, substances move across the cell membrane with the help of carrier molecules, from an area of low concentration of the substance to an area of high concentration of the substance. In other words, substances are gathered together, which is the opposite of diffusion. These molecules create channels in the cell membrane or otherwise change the membrane so large substances can pass through. Think of these carrier or transport molecules as tiny doormen opening the door for large substances to enter an already crowded room. Some substances that move across the cell membrane through active transport include sugars, amino acids, and potassium, calcium, and hydrogen ions.

▶ Cell Division

LO 22.11

Cells can become damaged, diseased, or worn out, and replacements must be made. Also, new cells are needed for normal growth. Cells reproduce by cell division, a process that involves splitting the nucleus, through **mitosis** or **meiosis,** and splitting the cytoplasm, called **cytokinesis.**

A cell that carries out its normal daily functions and is not dividing is said to be in *interphase*. For example, if a liver cell is in interphase, it is making liver enzymes, detoxifying blood, and processing nutrients. During interphase, a cell prepares for cell division by duplicating its DNA and cytoplasmic organelles. For most body cells, each daughter cell will have an exact copy of the DNA and organelles in the original mother cell. Sometimes when the DNA is duplicated, errors called *mutations* occur. These mutations will be passed on to the descendants (daughter cells) of that cell and may or may not affect the cells in harmful ways. Mutations can be simple changes in the DNA sequence or complete deletions of a gene or part of a gene. Think about this book as a gene; a simple mutation might be a misspelled word or the loss of a sentence, a chapter, or even the whole book.

Mitosis

Following interphase, a cell may enter mitosis—a part of cell division in which the nucleus divides. During this process, the cell membrane constricts to divide the cell's cytoplasm. This causes the organelles of the original cell to be distributed almost evenly into the two new cells. The stages of mitosis are listed here and pictured in Figure 22-14.

- *Prophase* occurs when the centrioles that have replicated just prior to the onset of mitosis move to opposite ends of the cell. As they separate, they create spindle fibers between them.
- During *metaphase,* the chromosomes line up in the middle of the cell between the centrioles on these spindle fibers.
- During *anaphase,* the centromeres divide, pulling the chromatids (now chromosomes) toward the centrioles at opposite sides of the cell.
- The final stage is called *telophase.* As the chromosomes reach the centrioles, each with its complete set, cytokinesis or division of the cytoplasm takes place and mitosis is complete.

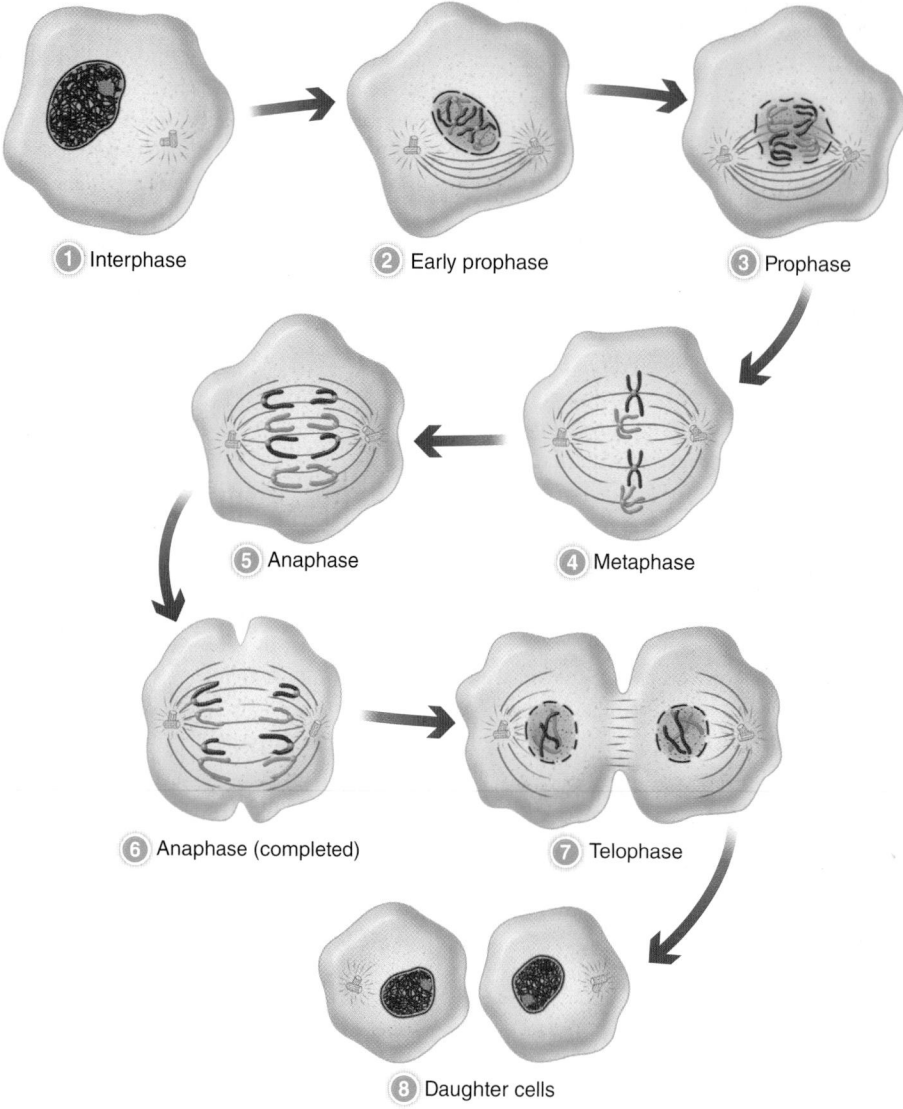

① Interphase

② Early prophase

③ Prophase

④ Metaphase

⑤ Anaphase

⑥ Anaphase (completed)

⑦ Telophase

⑧ Daughter cells

FIGURE 22-14   Cell mitosis.

Remember, during mitosis, the nucleus makes a complete copy of all 23 of its chromosome pairs (46 chromosomes altogether). As the cell divides, each new cell receives a complete set of chromosome pairs. The resulting cells are identical to each other.

Meiosis

Meiosis is reproductive cell division. It takes place only in the reproductive organs when the male and female sex cells are formed. During meiosis, the nucleus copies all 23 chromosome pairs, but two divisions take place. The four cells that are formed each contain only one of each chromosome pair, for a total of 23 chromosomes. This type of cell division must occur so that when the sex cells combine during fertilization, the resulting cell contains the usual number of chromosomes (46).

BODYANIMAT3D
POWERED BY
McGraw Hill connect®

Go to CONNECT to see an animation about *Meiosis vs. Mitosis.*

▶ Genetic Techniques

LO 22.12

DNA is the primary component of genes and is found in the nucleus of most cells within the body. A **gene** is a segment of DNA that determines a body trait. Genetic techniques involve using or manipulating genes.

The chemical structure of every person's DNA is the same. The unique sequence of the *nucleotides* (groups of molecules that form the basic unit of DNA) determines an individual's characteristics. As an illustration, take the statement "my cat has blue eyes." Think of each letter as one nucleotide. If you change the letter "c" in the statement to an "r" you have an entirely different statement; "my rat has blue eyes." Many genetic differences—excessively large muscles in sheep for instance—are caused by changes in just a few nucleotides. One DNA molecule contains hundreds or thousands of genes. Each gene occupies a particular location on the DNA molecule, making it possible to compare the same gene in a number of different samples. Two widely used genetic techniques in the clinical setting are the polymerase chain reaction (PCR) and DNA fingerprinting.

Polymerase Chain Reaction

The polymerase chain reaction (PCR) is a quick, easy method for making millions of copies of any fragment of DNA. This technique has been revolutionary in the study of genetics and has very quickly become a necessary tool for improving human health.

PCR can produce millions of gene copies from tiny amounts of DNA, even from just one cell. This method is especially useful for detecting disease-causing organisms that are impossible to culture, such as many kinds of bacteria, fungi, and viruses. For example, it can detect the AIDS virus sooner than other tests—during the first few weeks after infection. PCR is also more accurate than standard tests. The technique can detect bacterial DNA in children's middle ear fluid, which indicates an infection, even when culture methods fail to detect bacteria. Other diseases diagnosed through PCR include Lyme disease, stomach ulcers, viral meningitis, hepatitis, tuberculosis, and many sexually transmitted infections (STIs), including herpes and chlamydia.

PCR is also leading to new kinds of genetic testing because it can easily distinguish among the tiny variations in DNA that all people possess. This testing can diagnose people who have inherited disorders or who carry mutations that could be passed to their children. PCR is also used in tests that determine who may develop common disorders such as heart disease and various types of cancer. This knowledge helps individuals take steps to prevent those diseases.

DNA Fingerprinting

A DNA "fingerprint" refers to the unique sequences of nucleotides in a person's DNA and is the same for every cell, tissue, and organ of that person. Consequently, DNA fingerprinting is a reliable method for identifying and distinguishing among human beings to establish paternity and identify suspects in criminal cases (see Figure 22-15).

FIGURE 22-15 DNA fingerprinting can be used to establish paternity or identify a suspect in a criminal investigation.

It is also used to diagnose genetic disorders such as cystic fibrosis, hemophilia, Huntington's disease, familial Alzheimer's, sickle cell anemia, thalassemia, and many others. Detecting genetic diseases early, or in utero, allows patients and medical staff to prepare for proper treatment. Researchers also use this information to identify DNA patterns associated with genetic diseases.

▶ Heredity and Common Genetic Disorders   LO 22.13

Heredity is the transfer of genetic traits from parent to child. When a sperm cell and an ovum (egg) unite, a cell called a *zygote* forms. The zygote has 46 chromosomes, or 23 chromosomal pairs. One half of each pair comes from the sperm, and the other half from the ovum. The first 22 pairs, which are the same size and shape, are called *homologous chromosomes*, also known as *autosomes*. The 23rd pair are called *sex chromosomes*. If the sex chromosomes are an X chromosome and a Y chromosome, the child is a male. If the sex chromosomes are both X chromosomes, the child is a female. Although the sex chromosomes determine a child's gender, they also determine other body traits. However, the autosomes determine most body traits such as eye color or freckles.

Each chromosome possesses many genes. Homologous chromosomes carry the same genes that code for a particular trait, but the genes may be of different forms, which are called *alleles*. Many times only one allele is actually expressed as a trait even if another allele is present. The allele that is always expressed over the other is a dominant allele. The one that is not expressed is recessive. The only way a recessive allele can be expressed is if no dominant allele is present.

Detached earlobes are an example of a trait determined by a dominant allele. If a child inherits a dominant allele for this trait from one parent but inherits the recessive allele from the other parent, the child will have detached earlobes. If the child inherits recessive alleles from both parents, then he or she will have attached earlobes. See Figure 22-16.

Most traits in the body are determined by multiple alleles. For example, hair color, height, skin tone, eye color, and body build are each determined by many different genes. *Complex inheritance* is the term that describes inherited traits that are determined by multiple genes. It explains why different children within the same family can each have different characteristics.

Sex-linked traits are carried on the sex chromosomes, X and Y. The Y chromosome is much smaller than the X chromosome and does not carry many genes. So, if the X chromosome carries a recessive allele, it is likely to be expressed because there is usually no corresponding allele on the Y chromosome. For example, the presence of a recessive allele that is always found on the X chromosome determines red–green color blindness. This disorder (like most sex-linked disorders) primarily affects males because the corresponding Y chromosome does not have any allele to prevent the expression of the recessive allele. Genetic influences are known to contribute to many thousands of different health conditions.

A. Attached Earlobe

B. Detached Earlobe

FIGURE 22-16 Heredity determines whether your earlobes are (a) attached or (b) detached.

PATHOPHYSIOLOGY

Common Genetic Disorders

In addition to your understanding of the human body's anatomy and physiology, as a medical assistant it is very important to be able to recognize and comprehend the associated causes, characteristics, and available treatments of common genetic disorders. These genetic disorders, and their respective causes, signs and symptoms, and treatments are described below.

ALBINISM is a condition in which a person is born with little or no pigmentation in the skin, eyes, or hair. Albinism affects all races; in most cases there is no family history of it.

Causes. At least six different genes are involved with pigment production. This condition develops when a person inherits one or more faulty genes that do not produce the usual amounts of a pigment.

Signs and Symptoms. In addition to lack of pigment people with the condition experience visual problems and sun-sensitive skin.

Treatment. Although there is no cure, treatments are available to help the symptoms. Prenatal testing for the condition is available.

CYSTIC FIBROSIS is a life-threatening disease that mainly affects the lungs and pancreas. This disease is one of the most common inherited life-threatening disorders among Caucasians in the United States.

Causes. Inheritance is autosomal recessive, so if both parents are carriers, there is a 25% chance that each child born to them will develop cystic fibrosis.

Signs and Symptoms. Patients with this disorder have increasing problems with breathing. Thick secretions eventually block passages in the airways, and these secretions may become infected.

Treatment. There is no cure, but treatments are available to help patients live with the complications associated with this disorder. Newborn babies are commonly screened for the disease because the sooner treatment begins, the healthier the child can be. Parents are also commonly screened for the gene to determine the likelihood of having a child with cystic fibrosis.

DOWN SYNDOME, also called *Trisomy 21*, is a disorder that causes intellectual disabilities and physical abnormalities.

Causes. This disorder occurs when a person has three copies of chromosome 21 instead of two. This condition can be diagnosed through prenatal tests such as amniocentesis. The risk of having a child with Down syndrome increases with the mother's age.

Signs and Symptoms. The signs of Down syndrome include a flat facial profile, protruding tongue, oblique slanting eyes, abundant neck skin, short broad hands, and poor muscle tone. Heart, digestive, hearing, and visual problems are also common in people with this condition. Learning difficulties are common in Down syndrome and can range from moderate to severe.

Treatment. There is no cure, but support programs and the treatment of health problems allow many patients with Down syndrome to live a relatively normal life.

FRAGILE X SYNDROME is the most common inherited cause of learning disability. All races and ethnic groups seem to be affected equally by this syndrome.

Causes. In this disorder, one of the genes on the X chromosome is defective and makes the chromosome susceptible to breakage. This sex-linked disorder affects boys more severely than girls. It is estimated that approximately 1 in 300 females is a carrier for this disorder.

Signs and Symptoms. Mental impairment, learning disabilities, attention deficit disorder, a long face, large ears, and flat feet are some of the signs and symptoms. Fragile X syndrome can be easily diagnosed using prenatal tests such as amniocentesis.

Treatment. There is no cure, but some treatments and support groups are available to patients with this disorder.

HEMOPHILIA is a group of inheritable blood disorders. Each condition may be mild to severe.

Causes. In each type of hemophilia, an essential clotting factor is low or missing. Most types are X-linked recessive disorders; therefore, this disorder primarily affects males. Carriers of the gene can be identified with a blood test, and prenatal tests can diagnose the condition in the fetus.

Signs and Symptoms. Symptoms include easy bruising, spontaneous bleeding, and prolonged bleeding. Repeated bleeding in the joints leads to arthritis and permanent joint damage.

Treatment. Treatment includes injections of the missing clotting factors, often Factor VIII.

KLINEFELTER'S SYNDROME is a chromosomal abnormality that affects males.

Causes. Males with this disorder have an extra X chromosome.

Signs and Symptoms. Tall stature, pear-shaped fat distribution, small testes, sparse body hair, and infertility are the most common signs and symptoms. Thyroid problems, diabetes, and osteoporosis are also common in patients with this syndrome.

Treatment. There is no cure, but treatments such as testosterone replacement therapy can decrease the risk of osteoporosis and produce more male characteristics.

PHENYLKETONURIA (PKU) develops if a person cannot synthesize the enzyme that converts phenylalanine to tyrosine. Phenylalanine is an essential amino acid, but too much of it can be harmful, so the body regularly converts it to tyrosine.

Causes. This condition is inherited as an autosomal recessive disorder.

Signs and Symptoms. If phenylalanine builds up in the blood, it can lead to irreversible damage to organs, including the brain.

Treatment. Phenylalanine is found in many proteins, so meats and other protein-rich foods must be avoided. Early detection of PKU is important to prevent developmental delays. There is no cure for PKU, but special diets allow a person to lead a normal life. Most newborns are tested for PKU, and prenatal diagnosis is also available.

SUMMARY OF LEARNING OUTCOMES

LEARNING OUTCOMES	KEY POINTS
22.1 Explain the importance of understanding both anatomy and physiology when studying the body.	Knowledge of anatomy (the study of the body's structure) and physiology (the study of the body's function) is important when learning to assign diagnostic and procedural codes and perform clinical procedures. Since the structure of an organ is related to its function, it is necessary to learn both.
22.2 Illustrate body organization from simple to more complex levels.	The body organization levels from simplest to most complex are: chemical, cellular, tissue, organ, organ system, and organism.
22.3 Describe the locations and characteristics of the four main tissue types.	Epithelial tissues cover and line, or are glandular tissues. Connective tissue contains a matrix between its cells. Muscle tissue is specialized tissue that contracts and relaxes; there are three types of muscle tissue. Nervous tissue sends signals to the neurons, muscles, and glands and is located in the brain, spinal cord, and nerves.
22.4 Describe the body organ systems, their general functions, and the major organs contained in each.	The body organ systems include: integumentary, skeletal, muscular, lymphatic, respiratory, digestive, nervous, endocrine, cardiovascular, urinary, and reproductive systems. Each system has its particular set of organs and vessels to function in the capacities outlined within the chapter.

LEARNING OUTCOMES	KEY POINTS
22.5 **Use medical and anatomical terminology correctly.**	Knowledge and use of anatomical and medical terminology are important for medical personnel to communicate with each other in a consistent manner.
22.6 **Explain anatomical position and its relationship to other anatomical positions.**	In anatomical position, the body is erect, facing forward with arms at the sides and palms facing forward. All other body positions are defined based on their relation to anatomical position.
22.7 **Identify the body cavities and the organs contained in each.**	The dorsal cavity consists of the cranial cavity, which contains the brain, and the spinal cavity, which contains the spinal cord. The ventral cavity is composed of the thoracic cavity, the abdominal cavities, and, below the abdominal cavity, the pelvic cavity. The body's organs are contained within these cavities.
22.8 **Relate a basic understanding of chemistry to its importance in studying the body.**	It is important to have a basic understanding of chemistry when studying anatomy and physiology because body structures and functions result from chemical processes that occur within body cells or fluids.
22.9 **Name the parts of a cell and their functions.**	The main components of a cell are: cell membrane, cilia, flagella (may be present), ribosomes, endoplasmic reticulum, mitochondria, Golgi apparatus, lysosomes, and centrioles. Each has its own specialized function in the life of a cell.
22.10 **Summarize how substances move across a cell membrane.**	Cells use both active and passive mechanisms to transport substances across the cell membrane. Passive mechanisms include diffusion, osmosis, and filtration. Active transport uses carrier molecules.
22.11 **Distinguish the stages of cell division.**	A cell at rest is said to be in interphase. During mitosis, prophase, metaphase, anaphase, and telophase occur. Reproductive cell division is known as meiosis and takes place only in the reproductive cells.
22.12 **Explain the uses of these genetic techniques: DNA fingerprinting and the polymerase chain reaction.**	Genetic techniques allow the identification of individuals through the unique sequences of nucleotides found within DNA. Polymerase chain reactions allow millions of copies from just a fragment of DNA. DNA fingerprinting is used in paternity testing and in identifying suspects in criminal cases.
22.13 **Describe the different patterns of inheritance and common genetic disorders.**	Dominant traits occur through alleles. If a dominant allele is received from a parent, the trait will appear in the child. Complex inheritance is more common and is determined by multiple genes given by both parents. Sex-linked traits are carried on the sex chromosomes. There are many genetic disorders that affect the body including albinism, cystic fibrosis, Down syndrome, Fragile X, hemophilia, Klinefelter's syndrome, and phenylketonuria.

Recall John Miller from the beginning of the chapter. Now that you have completed the chapter, answer the following questions regarding his case.

1. What organs are found in the thoracic cavity?
2. What structure separates the thoracic and abdominopelvic cavities?

1. (LO 22.3) Which of the following are characteristics of skeletal muscle?
   a. Smooth and voluntary
   b. Striated and involuntary
   c. Striated and voluntary
   d. Smooth and involuntary
   e. None of the above

2. (LO 22.13) The clinical name referring to Down syndrome is
   a. Hemophilia
   b. Trisomy 21
   c. Klinefelter's syndrome
   d. Fragile X syndrome
   e. Phenylketonuria

3. (LO 22.5) Which word part does not change the meaning of a medical term but aids in pronunciation?
   a. Word root
   b. Prefix
   c. Suffix
   d. Combining vowel
   e. All of the above

4. (LO 22.7) Which abdominal region is named for its location under the stomach?
   a. Hypogastric
   b. Epigastric
   c. Hypochondriac
   d. Umbilical
   e. Iliac

5. (LO 22.8) Acids release which type of ion in water?
   a. Cl^-
   b. OH^-
   c. H^+
   d. Na^+
   e. K^+

6. (LO 22.9) Which of the following organelles are responsible for protein synthesis in the cell?
   a. Ribosomes
   b. Nucleus
   c. Mitochondria
   d. Golgi apparatus
   e. Centrioles

7. (LO 22.6) Which plane divides the body into right and left portions?
   a. Transverse
   b. Lateral
   c. Sagittal
   d. Frontal
   e. Coronal

8. (LO 22.5) The medical term meaning wrist is
   a. Tarsal
   b. Palmar
   c. Radial
   d. Brachial
   e. Carpal

9. (LO 22.11) An error in DNA duplication is known as a/an
   a. Mitosis
   b. Mutation
   c. Allele
   d. DNA fingerprint
   e. Chain reaction

10. (LO 22.6) The term meaning close to the point of attachment is
    a. Distal
    b. Superficial
    c. Medial
    d. Proximal
    e. Superior

Analyze the following medical terms, presented throughout the chapter. Using a medical dictionary (or Appendix I) place a / mark between each word part. Define each word part and then define the whole word.

EXAMPLE: append/ectomy = append means "appendix" + ectomy means "surgical removal"
Appendectomy means "surgical removal of the appendix."

1. anterior
2. caudal
3. cranial
4. distal
5. dorsal
6. femoral

7. frontal
8. inferior
9. lateral
10. medial
11. midsagittal
12. posterior

13. proximal
14. sagittal
15. superficial
16. superior
17. transverse
18. ventral

23

The Integumentary System

CASE STUDY

Patient Name	Gender	DOB
Jones, Shenya	Female	11/03/19XX

Attending	MRN	Allergies
Elizabeth H. Williams, MD	124-86-564	cinnamon, peanuts

The area of drainage is approximately 1 cm in diameter. The upper lip, side of the face, and nose are all swollen. She rates the pain in her face as a 7 out of 10. The physician thinks the condition may be impetigo or methicillin-resistant *Staphylococcus aureus* (MRSA), a type of skin infection that is resistant to the common antibiotics used to treat it. A wound culture is obtained.

Shenya Jones, a 34-year-old female, arrives at the office with a swelling and a red pustule on her face. She states the problem started two days ago as a small pimple near her nose. It became irritated then became extremely swollen and painful overnight. This morning there was yellow drainage noted at the site and the swelling has increased.

Keep Shenya in mind as you study this chapter. There will be questions at the end of the chapter based on the case study. The information in the chapter will help you answer these questions.

LEARNING OUTCOMES

After completing Chapter 23, you will be able to:

23.1 Describe the functions of skin.
23.2 Describe the layers of skin and the characteristics of each layer.
23.3 Explain the factors that affect skin color.
23.4 Summarize types of common skin lesions.
23.5 Describe the accessory organs of skin along with their structures and functions.
23.6 Explain the process of skin healing, including scar production.
23.7 Describe the common diseases and disorders of the skin.

KEY TERMS

alopecia
apocrine gland
arrector pili
dermis
eccrine gland
epidermis
follicle
hypodermis
keratin
keratinocyte

melanin
melanocyte
nail bed
oxygenated
sebaceous
sebum
stratum basale
stratum corneum
subcutaneous
sudoriferous

I. C (4) List major organs in each body system

I.C (5) Describe the normal function of each body system

I. C (6) Identify common pathology related to each body system

I. C (7) Analyze pathology as it relates to the interaction of body systems

I. C (9) Describe implications for treatment related to pathology

I. C (12) Describe the relationship between anatomy and physiology of all body systems and medications used for treatment in each

IV. C (11) Define both medical terms and abbreviations related to all body systems

2. **Anatomy & Physiology**
Graduates:

b. Identify and apply the knowledge of all body systems; their structure and functions; and their common diseases, symptoms, and etiologies

c. Assist the physician with the regimen of diagnostic and treatment modalities as they relate to each body system

3. **Medical Terminology**
Graduates:

b. Build and dissect medical terms from roots/suffixes to understand the word element combinations that create medical terminology

c. Understand the various medical terminology for each specialty

▶ Introduction

The integumentary system consists of skin and its accessory organs. Skin is the body's outer covering and its largest multifunctioning organ. The accessory organs of skin are hair follicles, nails, and skin glands. Consider what you see of your own skin when you stand undressed facing a full-length mirror. In fact, pretty much everything you see in the reflection is skin, or its accessory organs. Now, imagine that your skin accounts for approximately 15% of your entire body weight.

▶ Functions of the Integumentary System   LO 23.1

People are often interested in the appearance of their skin—the color, the texture, the presence or absence of freckles, lines, wrinkles, puffiness, redness—but rarely consider its functions. The integumentary system serves many important purposes, including:

- *Protection.* As long as skin is intact, it is the body's first line of defense against bacteria and viruses. It also protects underlying structures from ultraviolet (UV) radiation and dehydration.

- *Body temperature regulation.* Skin plays a major role in regulating body temperature. When a person is hot, dermal blood vessels dilate, which is why a person's skin becomes pinkish. Because the dermal blood vessels are dilated, more blood than normal passes through the skin. This is beneficial because blood carries a lot of the body's heat. When the blood gets close to the body's surface (to skin), the heat can escape. On the other hand, if a person is cold, the dermal blood vessels constrict, preventing the heat in blood from escaping.

- *Vitamin D production.* When exposed to sunlight, the skin produces a molecule that is turned into vitamin D. The body needs vitamin D for calcium absorption.

- *Sensation.* The skin is packed with sensory receptors that can detect touch, heat, cold, and pain.

- *Excretion.* Small amounts of waste products, such as water and salts, are lost through skin when a person perspires. This is why hydration is so important when exercising or during exposure to high temperatures, as the amount of perspiration increases and higher amounts of water and salts are lost.

▶ Skin Structure   LO 23.2

The skin is a complex organ that consists of three layers. The **epidermis** (top layer) and the dermis (middle layer) sit on a third layer called the subcutaneous layer or hypodermis (see Figure 23-1).

Epidermis

The epidermis is the most superficial layer of skin. It is made up of many layers of tightly packed cells and can be divided into two major sublayers: the stratum corneum and the stratum basale.

The **stratum corneum** is the most superficial layer of the epidermis. Most of the cells in this layer are dead and very flat. Because they have accumulated keratin, the cells in this layer stick together and form an impermeable layer for skin. Most bacteria, viruses, and water cannot penetrate the stratum corneum.

The **stratum basale,** also known as the *stratum germinativum,* is the deepest layer of the epidermis. The cells in this layer are constantly dividing (or germinating), and constantly pushing older cells up toward the stratum corneum.

Epidermis

Dermis

Subcutaneous layer

Hair shaft
Sweat gland pore
Sweat
Stratum corneum
Stratum basale
Capillary
Dermal papilla
Basement membrane
Tactile (Meissner's) corpuscle
Sebaceous gland
Arrector pili muscle
Sweat gland duct
Lamellated (Pacinian) corpuscle
Hair follicle
Sweat gland
Nerve cell process
Adipose tissue
Blood vessels
Muscle layer

FIGURE 23-1 Section of skin.

The most common cell type in the epidermis is the **keratinocyte**. This cell makes and accumulates **keratin**, which is a durable protein that makes the epidermis waterproof and resistant to bacteria and viruses. Another cell type of the epidermis is the **melanocyte**, which makes the pigment **melanin**. Melanin is deposited throughout the layers of the epidermis. This pigment absorbs UV radiation from sunlight and prevents the radiation from harming structures in the skin's underlying layers.

Dermis

The **dermis** lies below the epidermis and is the most complex skin layer; it contains all the major tissue types, including epithelial tissue, connective tissues, muscle tissue, and nervous tissue. The dermis, which binds the epidermis to the subcutaneous tissue, also contains:

- Sudoriferous (sweat) glands
- Sebaceous (oil) glands
- Hair follicles
- The arrector pili muscles
- Collagen fibers, elastin fibers, nerve fibers, and many blood vessels

Subcutaneous Layer

The **subcutaneous** layer of skin, or **hypodermis**, is largely made of adipose and loose connective tissue. This layer also contains blood vessels and nerves. The adipose or fat tissue acts as a storage facility. It also cushions and insulates the underlying structures and organs. The amount of adipose tissue varies from body region to body region, and from person to person.

▶ Skin Color

LO 23.3

The amount of melanin in the skin's epidermis is what most determines skin color. Melanin can range in color from yellowish to brownish. The more melanin a person has in the skin, the darker the skin color. All people have about the same number of melanocytes, regardless of skin color. What varies from person to person is how active the melanocytes are in producing melanin. For example, a person with dark skin has very active melanocytes. Sunlight, UV lamps, and X-rays stimulate melanin production. This is why your skin darkens when you go to a tanning bed or to the beach for the day. Patients undergoing radiation therapy often have tanned skin in the treatment area.

As you studied in *Organization of the Body*, your inherited characteristics come from your parents. So, your skin color—meaning the activity of the melanocytes—is directly related to the genes you received from your parents. As the gene pool is varied between ethnic backgrounds, it is also varied within families, which explains the differences in skin color not only among races but also within families.

Another factor that determines skin color is the amount of **oxygenated** blood in the skin's dermis. Oxygen is carried by a pigment called *hemoglobin* in the red blood cells (RBCs). *Oxygenation* refers to the amount of oxygen dissolved in the hemoglobin. Well-oxygenated hemoglobin is bright red, while poorlyoxygenated hemoglobin is darker red. A person with a rich supply of oxygenated blood will have skin that is a pinkish hue. When the supply of oxygen in the blood is low, the skin looks rather pale or bluish. A bluish color of skin is called *cyanosis*.

▶ Skin Lesions

LO 23.4

The term *skin lesion* may be generally defined as any variation in the skin (see Figure 23-2). Many of us have them; even a freckle is a lesion because it is a skin variation. Other lesions, such as ulcers and tumors, are more troublesome types of lesions. Skin lesions are classified into three major categories: primary, secondary, and vascular.

- Primary lesions such as macules and vesicles originate from disease or body changes.

- Secondary lesions, which include ulcers and keloids, are caused by a reaction to external traumas like scratching or rubbing, the healing process, or primary lesions.

- Vascular lesions are anomalies of the blood vessels and include telangiectasias, which are small dilated blood vessels on the skin's surface, and ecchymoses, commonly called bruises.

Table 23-1 lists some of the common types of skin lesions.

FIGURE 23-2 Types of skin lesions.

TABLE 23-1	Common Skin Lesions and Descriptions
Lesion Name	**Description**
Bulla	A large blister or cluster of blisters
Cicatrix	A scar, usually inside a wound or tissue
Crust	Dried blood or pus on the skin
Ecchymosis	A black and blue mark or bruise
Erosion	A shallow area of skin worn away by friction or pressure
Excoriation	A scratch; may be covered with dried blood
Fissure	A crack in the skin's surface
Keloid	An overgrowth of scar tissue
Macule	A flat skin discoloration, such as a freckle or a flat mole
Nodule	A large pimple or small node (larger than 6 cm)
Papule	An elevated mass similar to but smaller than a nodule
Petechiae	Pinpoint skin hemorrhages that result from bleeding disorders
Plaque	A small, flat, scaly area of skin
Purpura	Purple-red bruises, usually the result of clotting abnormalities
Pustule	An elevated (infected) lesion containing pus
Scale	Thin plaques of epithelial tissue on skin's surface
Tumor	A swelling of abnormal tissue growth
Ulcer	A wound that results from tissue loss
Vesicle	A blister
Wheal	Another term for hive

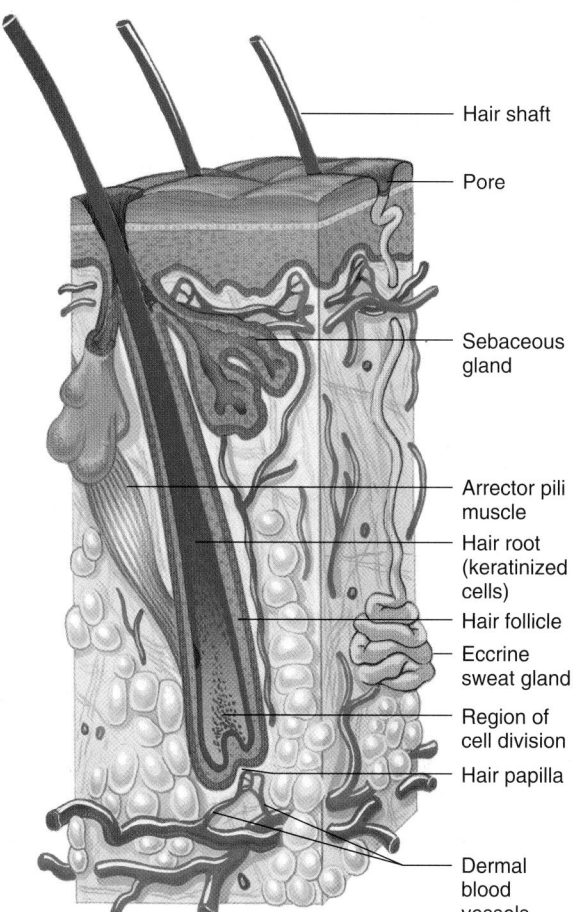

FIGURE 23-3 The hair follicle extends into the dermis.

▶ Accessory Organs

LO 23.5

The skin's accessory organs include hair follicles, **sebaceous** (oil) glands, nails, and sudoriferous (sweat) glands. Technically, breasts are considered an accessory organ of the integumentary system, but because they are more closely associated with the female reproductive system, they will be discussed in *The Reproductive Systems* chapter.

Hair Follicles

Hair **follicles** are tube-like depressions in the skin's dermis, which are made of epithelial tissue. Their function is to generate hairs (see Figure 23-3). Cells called *keratinocytes* make up most of the hair follicle. As hair follicles produce new keratinocytes, old ones are pushed toward the skin's surface. The old keratinocytes stick together to produce a hair. The portion of the hair embedded in the skin is called the *root*, and the portion of the hair extending from the surface of skin is called the *shaft*.

Melanocytes are also found in hair follicles. They produce and distribute pigments to create hair color. A person develops gray hair when these melanocytes produce less pigment than normal.

When a hair follicle goes into a resting cycle, the hair falls out. Most of the time, the hair follicle will begin a growing cycle again and produce a new hair. However, sometimes hair follicles completely die, and **alopecia** (baldness) develops.

Arrector pili muscles are attached to most hair follicles. When a person is cold or nervous, these muscles pull on hair follicles and cause hairs to stand erect. These muscles also pull on fibers in the skin's dermis, causing goose bumps (see Figure 23-3).

Sudoriferous Glands

Most **sudoriferous** (sweat) glands are located in the skin's dermis. However, their ducts open onto the skin's epidermis. There are two types of sweat glands—eccrine and apocrine.

- **Eccrine glands** are the most numerous sweat glands. They produce a watery type of sweat and are activated primarily by heat. Once sweat is deposited onto skin, it evaporates and carries heat away from the body. Eccrine sweat glands are most concentrated on the forehead, neck, and back.

- **Apocrine glands** produce a thicker type of sweat that contains more proteins than the type of sweat produced by eccrine sweat glands. Apocrine glands are most concentrated in areas of skin with coarse hair, such as the armpit and groin areas. They become active during puberty and are primarily activated by nervousness, pain, or stress, but they can also be activated by heat. Remember the last time you watched a scary movie that really frightened you? These glands were responsible for producing your cold sweat. Bacteria often break down the proteins in the sweat produced by apocrine glands. As the proteins are digested, the bacteria release a foul-smelling waste product that is responsible for the smell of body odor.

CAUTION: HANDLE WITH CARE

Preventing and Treating Scars

One of the skin's major functions is to protect your underlying tissues from injury and infection. Whether skinning your knees as a child or cutting yourself in the kitchen while preparing food, you have most likely injured your skin at some time in your life. Your skin responds to this injury by forming a scab and then a scar. Many scars simply retract and go away in time. The size and extent of the scar depends on the following:

- *Extent of the wound.* Deep or jagged wounds may produce a larger scar.
- *Wound location.* Wounds over mobile areas like the knees and elbows often have larger scars because they are constantly under tension.

It is important that you seek medical attention for wounds that:

- Bleed profusely
- Are larger than ½ inch deep or wide
- Are located on the face
- Are caused by a rusty tool or nail
- Are jagged in appearance
- Are caused by an animal bite
- Show signs of infection

These basic tips may help prevent the formation of lasting scars:

- Wash wounds with mild soap and water and clean out any debris left in the wound.
- Do not use harsh soaps, hydrogen peroxide, or alcohol to clean a wound, as these can damage tissues and delay healing.
- Cover the wound to keep out bacteria, dirt, and debris to reduce the possibility of infection.

- Keep the wound moist by applying an antibiotic ointment. This keeps the bandage from sticking to the wound and may reduce the likelihood of infection.
- Do not pick or pull at a scab. This reopens the wound and may cause infection or larger scar formation.
- Use medical honey. Honey has antibacterial properties and has been found to accelerate healing. Special medical products are available for hard-to-heal wounds.

If a scar forms, numerous treatments are available. These include:

- *Sunscreen.* Protecting a newly healed wound from UV radiation by using sunscreen with an SPF of 30 or higher helps reduce scar thickening and hyperpigmentation.
- *Silicone gel sheeting.* Studies show that covering a wound with a silicone gel sheet reduces healing time and scar formation. These sheets may be used for surgical and nonsurgical wounds.
- *Dermabrasion.* This procedure literally "sands" the surface of the skin and scar and is most often used for raised scars.
- *Surgical scar repair.* A large or hyperpigmented scar can be reduced in size by removing it surgically. Scar reduction surgical procedures include:
  - Z-plasty—a specialized plastic surgical technique that alters the pull on a tightened scar by lengthening it
  - Scar shaving—a technique for shaving off a raised scar
  - Scar removal—making an elliptical incision around the scar and removing it, which results in a scar that is thinner than the original scar.

EDUCATING THE PATIENT

Preventing Acne

Acne vulgaris, commonly known as acne, is an inflammatory condition of the skin follicles and sebaceous glands. It results in comedos (blackheads and whiteheads), as well as papules and pustules. They occur mainly on the face, but they can also occur on the neck, back, and chest. Acne often appears in adolescence from the surge of sex hormones that increase the amount of sebum the sebaceous glands produce. Excess sebum and dead skin cells clog the pores where bacteria then accumulates, causing the pimples. These pimples may rupture or leak, and as the bacteria then infect the adjacent skin areas, they cause the characteristic skin inflammation. Patients may find the following instructions helpful in controlling their acne.

- Use *noncomedogenic* (non-pore-clogging) skin care products.
- Wash your face twice a day.
- Keep your hands away from your face.
- Remove all makeup daily.
- Use makeup or lotion that contains sunscreen.
- Wash your hair frequently because oils from hair can end up on your face.

Seek a dermatologist's care for severe cases; these cases may require oral antibiotics (tetracycline) or other prescription medications (retinol).

Sebaceous Glands

Sebaceous glands—more commonly called *oil glands*—produce an oily substance called **sebum**. Sebum is secreted onto hairs to keep them soft and pliable, and it is eventually deposited onto skin to keep it soft as well. Sebum also prevents bacteria from growing on skin (see Figure 23-1).

Nails

Nails protect the ends of the fingers and toes. They are formed by epithelial cells with hard keratin, which is more permanent than the softer keratin found in your skin. For this reason, the nails must be cut because they do not slough off by themselves as your skin cells do. The portion of a nail that you can see is the nail body, and the portion embedded in skin is the nail root. The nail root contains active keratinocytes that constantly divide to produce nail growth. The white half-moon-shaped area at the base of a nail is called a *lunula*. The lunula also contains very active keratinocytes. Beneath each nail is a layer called the **nail bed**, which holds the nail down to underlying skin and provides nutrients to the nail from the blood supply under the nail bed (see Figure 23-4). Extending from the nail bed beyond the fingertip is the free edge of the nail. This is the part that you cut and file so your nails look neat and trimmed.

▶ Skin Healing

LO 23.6

When skin is injured, it becomes inflamed. Redness, swelling, localized warmth, and pain are characteristics of inflammation. An inflamed area looks red because nearby blood vessels dilate. The inflamed area also swells because the dilated blood vessels "leak" and fluids seep into spaces between cells. Inflamed areas are often painful because the excess fluid activates pain receptors. However, inflammation promotes healing because more blood travels to the area, and this extra blood carries more nutrients needed for skin repair. It also carries defensive cells to clear up the cause of inflammation.

BODYANIMAT3D
POWERED BY
connect

Go to CONNECT to see an animation about *Inflammation*.

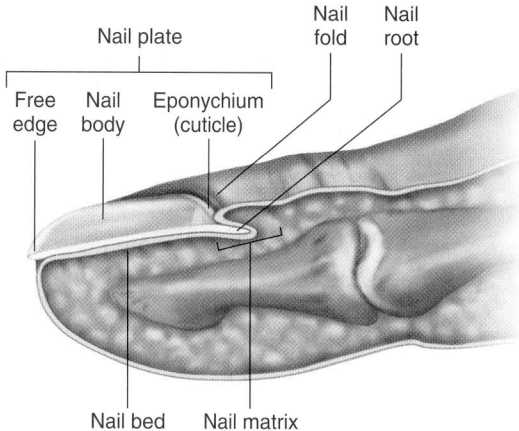

FIGURE 23-4 Anatomy of a nail.

When structures and blood vessels of the dermis are injured, a blood clot initially forms. A scab, which is basically clotted blood and other dried tissue fluids, eventually replaces the blood clot. The scab is normally replaced by collagen fibers that bind the edges of the wound together. Collagen fibers are whitish and serve as the major component of scars. Sometimes skin scars are replaced with new skin, but if the wound is extensive, a scar will persist. Scars can be merely a cosmetic nuisance, or they can cause problems with underlying structures. For example, a large scar over a joint can cause loss of movement in that joint.

EDUCATING THE PATIENT
Cancer Warning Signs

The thought of being diagnosed with cancer is scary to everyone. Awareness of the warning signs can help patients know when to seek medical care. Always stress to patients the importance of *preventive medicine* and regular physical examinations. The American Cancer Society has put together seven cancer warning signs for adults, using the acronym ***CAUTION***:

C — Change in bowel or bladder habits
A — A sore that will not heal
U — Unusual bleeding or discharge
T — Thickening or lump in the breast or elsewhere
I — Indigestion or difficulty with swallowing
O — Obvious change in a wart or mole
N — Nagging cough or hoarseness

Common Diseases and Disorders of the Skin

Burns

Although many of the skin conditions discussed in this chapter can be extremely serious and even life-threatening (such as skin cancer), the skin is also prone to burns. In fact, burns are a leading cause of accidental death in the United States, where there are approximately 150 burn care centers devoted to this very type of skin injury.

It is also important to note that an estimated 450,000 people seek medical treatment for burn injuries each year; 45,000 require hospitalization; and more than 3,500 patients die annually from burn injuries. Worldwide, more than a million people each year suffer from burn injuries that cause significant or permanent disability.

The extent of the affected body surface area and the severity (degree) of a burn are the most important factors in predicting the risk of death associated with burn injuries. The rule of nines is a quick way to estimate the extent of body surface area affected by burns. This method divides the body into 11 areas, each accounting for 9% of the total body surface. The genital area accounts for 1%. (See Figure 23-5.)

Rule of Nines. Following are the 11 body areas of the rule of nines with their percentages:

- Head   9% (front and back, 4.5% each)
- Right arm   9% (front and back, 4.5% each)
- Left arm   9% (front and back, 4.5% each)
- Front of right leg   9%
- Front of left leg   9%
- Back of right leg   9%
- Back of left leg   9%
- Front of body   18% (both areas) trunk is two areas
- Back of body   18% (both areas) trunk is two areas
- Genital area   1%

Total body area = 100%

FIGURE 23-5   Using the rule of nines aids in estimating the extent of burns.

(a) First degree

Partial thickness

(b) Second degree

Full thickness

(c) Third degree

FIGURE 23-6 The degrees of burn severity includes (a) superficial (first-degree) burns, (b) partial-thickness (second-degree) burns, and (c) full-thickness (third-degree) burns.

Burn Severity. The severity of burns indicates the thickness of the injury (see Figure 23-6). The following terms are used to report burn severity:

- *Superficial (first-degree).* These burns involve only the epidermis and are characterized by pain, redness, and swelling. Unless they are extensive, they do not require medical attention and usually heal well.
- *Partial-thickness (second-degree).* These burns involve the epidermis and dermis. Pain, redness, swelling, and blisters

characterize them. Medical staff should treat any partial-thickness burn that affects 1% or more of the body surface. A body surface area of 1% is about the size of a person's hand. Shock is likely to develop in partial-thickness burn injuries that affect 9% or more of the body surface. These burns can be life-threatening, depending on their extent.

- *Full-thickness (third-degree).* These burns involve all layers of skin and often underlying structures such as muscles and bones. The skin frequently looks black or charred, which is known as *eschar*. Full-thickness burns always require medical attention regardless of the extent or the size of the burn area.

General Guidelines for Treating Burns

- Anything sticking to the burn should be left in place.
- Do not apply butter, lotions, or ointments to the burn. Only use ointments prescribed by a doctor or recommended by a pharmacist.
- Cool the burn with large amounts of cool water. Avoid ice or extremely cold water.
- Cover the burn with a sterile sheet. However, do not cover burns to the face.
- Contact emergency medical personnel for serious burns.
- With burns to the mouth and throat, check the airways for swelling. Burns to the head are always more serious than burns to other body parts. They almost always require emergency medical treatment.

Skin Cancer and Common Skin Disorders

Skin is vulnerable to many disorders because it is the most exposed of all body organs. The following sections discuss skin cancer and common skin disorders.

Skin Cancer

Skin cancer develops from cells in the skin's epidermis. It is more common in people who have light-colored skin and who have had excessive exposure to sunlight. It can occur anywhere on the body, but it is most likely to appear on skin that is readily exposed to sunlight. The two most common types of skin cancer are basal cell carcinoma and squamous cell carcinoma, but the most deadly type is malignant melanoma (see Figure 23-7).

(a)

(b)

(c)

FIGURE 23-7 Types of skin cancer: (a) squamous cell carcinoma, (b) basal cell carcinoma, and (c) malignant melanoma.

BASAL CELL CARCINOMA accounts for approximately 90% of all skin cancers in the United States. Fortunately, it progresses slowly and rarely spreads to other body parts. It is derived from cells of the stratum basale of the epidermis.

Signs and Symptoms. These include changes on the skin and a new growth or sore on the skin that does not heal. Its appearance may be waxy, smooth, red, pale, flat, or lumpy, and it may or may not bleed.

Treatment. Several forms of treatment are available:

- *Curettage and electrodessication.* In curettage, a sharp instrument is used to scoop out the cancerous lesion. Electrodessication uses electrical currents to minimize bleeding as well as to kill any remaining cancer cells.
- *Mohs surgery.* The cancerous lesion is shaved off one layer at a time. Each layer is sent to the histology lab for evaluation until no tumor is detected in the last layer removed.
- *Cryosurgery.* Freezing is used to kill cancer cells.
- *Laser therapy.* A beam of light destroys cancer cells.

SQUAMOUS CELL CARCINOMA is much less common than basal cell carcinoma but is more likely to spread to surrounding tissues. It arises from flat cells of the epidermis and is most likely to appear on the face, lips, ears, and the backs of the hands. The signs and symptoms and the treatments for this type of cancer are the same as for basal cell carcinoma.

MALIGNANT MELANOMA, cancer that arises from melanocytes, is the most aggressive of the skin cancers. It is also the fastest-growing skin cancer, with rates increasing 5% to 7% per year. The lifetime risk of developing malignant melanoma is one in 75. It appears to be more prevalent in females, but males, when diagnosed, seem to have a poorer prognosis. Melanoma can occur anywhere on the body but most often appears on the trunk, head, and neck in men and on the arms and legs in women.

Signs and Symptoms. A mole that itches or bleeds is a common symptom. New moles may develop near it, or it may change to have any signs of the ABCDE rule:

- *Asymmetry.* The mole should not be asymmetrical. It should look equal in size from side to side.
- *Border.* The border of the mole should not be irregular. The edges should not blur into nearby normal tissue.
- *Color.* The mole should be even. It should not darken or lighten or contain a mixture of colors.
- *Diameter.* The mole should not grow larger than 6 mm, about the diameter of a pencil eraser.
- *Evolving.* The mole has been changing in size, shape, color, or appearance, or growing in an area of previously normal skin. In an existing mole, the texture of the mole may change and become hard, lumpy, or scaly. Although the skin may feel different and may itch, ooze, or bleed, melanoma usually does not cause pain.

Treatment. The treatment depends on the staging of this cancer. Melanoma has five different stages, which are described below from the least to the most serious:

- Stage 0. Malignancy is found only in the epidermis.
- Stage I. Malignancy has spread from the epidermis to the dermis, and has a thickness of 1 to 2 millimeters.
- Stage II. Malignancy has a thickness of 2 to 4 millimeters and may be ulcerated.
- Stage III. Malignancy has spread to one or more nearby lymph nodes.
- Stage IV. Malignancy has spread to other body organs or other lymph nodes far away from the original melanoma site.

Available treatments for melanoma include the following:

- Surgery to remove the melanoma
- Lymph node biopsy to determine if the cancer has spread
- Removal of cancerous lymph nodes
- Chemotherapy for advanced stages of cancer
- Radiation therapy for advanced stages of cancer
- Immunotherapy to boost the patient's immune system

Common Skin and Hair Disorders

ALOPECIA is a disorder that specifically targets hair and results in hair loss.

Causes. Most of the time, alopecia is inherited. Other common causes include hormonal changes, chemotherapy, stress, burns, and fungal infections of the skin.

Signs and Symptoms. Loss or lack of hair on the scalp or other areas of the body. Alopecia is more commonly called *baldness*.

Treatment. If a result of heredity, this disorder is not curable. Hair transplants and some drugs, such as Rogaine, may slow down hair loss. Hair loss caused by other factors, such as chemotherapy, is often temporary, but the hair may grow back a different color or texture.

CELLULITIS is an inflammation of connective tissues in skin and primarily occurs on the face and legs.

Causes. This skin disease is caused by staphylococcal and streptococcal bacteria.

Signs and Symptoms. Skin appears red and tight and is often painful. The inflammation may trigger a fever.

Treatment. Treatment includes oral and topical antibiotics. In serious cases, intravenous (IV) antibiotics and hospitalization may be required.

DERMATITIS is a general term defined as inflammation of skin or a rash. It has many causes and is a sign of many types of skin disorders. A common type of dermatitis is contact dermatitis, which results from contact with allergens or irritants. If you have ever had poison ivy, you had a type of contact dermatitis. Another common form of dermatitis is eczema.

ECZEMA is one type of chronic dermatitis that has acute phases characterized by a blistered rash that itches severely. Eczema often appears in childhood but is also commonly seen in adults.

Causes. Causes of eczema are mostly unknown, but it is thought to be a type of allergy or the result of an often unknown underlying inflammatory condition. Environmental irritants, stress, diet, and medications can exacerbate or worsen the signs and symptoms of this disease.

Signs and Symptoms. The rashes of eczema are red, scaly, and itchy.

Treatment. Treatments include topical steroids and other types of anti-inflammatory drugs. Antibiotics may be needed for any secondary infections that develop. Avoiding known factors that trigger eczema, such as stress, is also helpful.

FOLLICULITIS, sometimes called "swimmer's rash," is an inflammation of hair follicles.

Causes. This disorder usually results from shaving or excess rubbing of skin areas. It may also be caused by bacteria and fungi, which may develop from prolonged wearing of wet swimwear or using undertreated hot tubs.

Signs and Symptoms. Follicles become red and itchy and often look like pimples.

Treatment. Treatments include regular cleansing of skin, topical antibiotics, and the use of electric razors instead of razor blades. Wearing wet swimwear for prolonged periods of time should also be avoided.

HERPES SIMPLEX types 1 and 2 are the most common types of herpes simplex.

Causes. Herpes simplex types 1 and 2 are both caused by a virus. Herpes simplex type 1 causes cold sores. It is very contagious and is spread through saliva. Herpes simplex type 2, known as *genital herpes*, is sexually transmitted.

Signs and Symptoms. Herpes simplex type 1 causes painful sores on the lips, mouth, and face. Herpes simplex type 2 normally causes painful sores on genital areas.

Treatment. There is no cure for herpes simplex, and its skin lesions usually recur throughout life. However, antiviral drugs such as acyclovir (Zovirax®) prevent frequent outbreaks. Patients should also be instructed to get adequate rest and nutrition, and control stress as much as possible.

HERPES ZOSTER is a disorder commonly known as *shingles*.

Causes. Herpes zoster is caused by the *Varicella* viruswhich also causes chickenpox. After a person has chickenpox, the virus becomes dormant in the spine's dorsal nerve root but can become active again later in life to cause shingles.

Signs and Symptoms. Herpes zoster causes a painful blistering rash usually on one side of the body following the *dermatome*—the skin area along the pathway of the affected nerve root. Shingles usually starts as a tingling or pain on the torso or neck, followed by a rash that eventually blisters.

Treatment. Some antiviral medications, such as Zovirax®, shorten the duration of the disease, and pain medications assist with pain control. Recovery is usually complete, but recurrences of the disease do occur. Some patients suffer from the complication known as *post-herpetic pain syndrome*, where nerve pain continues even though the rash is no longer present. It is uncertain whether the chickenpox vaccine prevents herpes zoster. The vaccine Zostavax® by Merck Pharmaceuticals is a preventive alternative for patients 60 years of age and older with a history of having had chickenpox. Patients considering Zostavax should know that it is advertised as reducing the risk of developing shingles; it does not guarantee that shingles will not occur.

IMPETIGO causes the formation of oozing skin lesions that eventually crust over. It is highly contagious for those who come in contact with the lesions or the exudates (exuded substances) from them.

Causes. This disease is caused by staphylococcal and streptococcal bacteria.

Signs and Symptoms. The skin develops itchy, oozing lesions that eventually crust over with a distinctive honey-colored crust from the drying exudates.

Treatment. This condition is treated with antibiotics. Instructing the patient to wash the lesions two to three times a day with soap and water will help remove the exudates and decrease the spread to other skin areas.

PEDICULOSIS is more commonly known as *lice* and comes in three forms: head lice (*pediculosis capitis*), body lice (*pediculosis corporis*), and pubic lice (*pediculosis pubis*).

Causes. All forms are caused by parasitic lice and are associated with overcrowded conditions and often with poor hygiene. Pubic lice are also spread by sexual contact.

Signs and Symptoms. Skin itches and can become irritated from scratching. Head lice are also identifiable by the dandruff-like nits that cannot be shaken off.

Treatment Prescription medications and shampoos are often necessary. For head lice, some patients find equal success with over-the-counter (OTC) treatments such as *Nix*®.

PSORIASIS is a common chronic, inflammatory skin condition.

Causes. This skin disorder is most likely an inherited autoimmune disorder.

Signs and Symptoms. Patients with psoriasis have recurring episodes of itching and redness with outbreaks of distinctive silvery, scaly skin lesions. Some people also have joint pain with this condition.

Treatment. Mild cases are treated with anti-inflammatory drugs and therapeutic ointments such as creams with vitamins A and D, hydrocortisone creams, and retinoids. Some patients also experience relief with controlled UV ray treatments. Severe cases may require hospitalization.

RINGWORM is a fungal skin infection, commonly occurring in three forms: *tinea corporis* (body), *tinea capitis* (scalp), and *tinea pedis* (feet), which is commonly known as athlete's foot.

Causes. All forms of ringworm are caused by fungi called *dermatophytes*.

Signs and Symptoms. Flat, circular lesions that may be dry and scaly or moist and crusty are the hallmarks of ringworm.

Tinea capitis is characterized by small papules that may cause small, patchy areas of baldness.

Treatment. Topical and oral antifungal agents are used to treat all forms of ringworm. The spread is contained by not sharing sheets, towels, and other personal care items.

ROSACEA is a skin disorder that commonly appears as facial redness, predominantly over the cheeks and nose.

Causes. Rosacea results from dilation of small facial blood vessels, but the cause of this dilation is unknown. It occurs most frequently in fair-skinned people.

Signs and Symptoms. Redness and acne-like symptoms on the face are the most common symptoms.

Treatment. Although it is not curable, rosacea is usually managed well with topical cortisone or antibiotic creams. In severe cases, electrolysis may be useful in destroying large or dilated blood vessels.

SCABIES is a highly contagious skin condition.

Causes. Scabies is caused by an itch mite that burrows beneath skin and lays its eggs. Sometimes the burrows of the mites can be seen and look like red pencil marks.

Signs and Symptoms. Redness and severe itching, especially at night, are usually the only symptoms of scabies.

Treatment. Most cases are easily treated with prescription medications such as Elimite, which is left on the skin for 6 to 10 hours and followed by a bath. Antipyretic (anti-itching) or steroid creams may control the itching. Because scabies is contagious, it is wise to treat an entire family if one member is infected.

WARTS (verrucae) are harmless skin growths that can appear almost anywhere on the body surface but most commonly occur on the hands, feet, and face.

Causes. These growths are caused by a virus.

Signs and Symptoms. Warts vary greatly in appearance; they can be smooth, flat, rough, raised, dark, small, or large.

Treatment. Warts are often removed with OTC medications but can also be treated through surgery, lasers, freezing, or burning.

SUMMARY OF LEARNING OUTCOMES

LEARNING OUTCOMES	KEY POINTS
23.1 Describe the functions of skin.	The functions of skin include protection, body temperature regulation, vitamin D production, sensation, and excretion.
23.2 Describe the layers of skin and the characteristics of each layer.	The topmost layer of the skin is the epidermis. The dermis is the complex middle layer. The innermost layer attaching the skin to muscle is the subcutaneous layer.
23.3 Explain the factors that affect skin color.	The amount of melanin affects and determines skin color. The amount of oxygen-carrying hemoglobin in the blood also affects skin color.
23.4 Summarize types of common skin lesions.	Skin lesions are split among three main types: primary lesions such as macules and vesicles; secondary lesions, which include ulcers and keloids; and vascular lesions, which involve blood vessels and include telangiectasias and ecchymoses.
23.5 Describe the accessory organs of skin along with their structures and functions.	The accessory organs of skin include hair follicles, arrector pili muscles, sebaceous glands, sudoriferous glands, and keratin-filled nails.
23.6 Explain the process of skin healing, including scar production.	Injured skin becomes inflamed from dilating blood vessels that leak and cause swelling. A blood clot is formed, which is replaced by a scab, which is then replaced by collagen fibers that produce scar tissue.
23.7 Describe the common diseases and disorders of the skin.	Common diseases and disorders of the skin include alopecia, cellulitis, dermatitis, eczema, folliculitis, herpes simplex, herpes zoster, impetigo, pediculosis, psoriasis, ringworm, rosacea, scabies, and warts.

Recall Shenya Jones from the beginning of the chapter. Now that you have completed the chapter, answer the following questions regarding her case.

1. Considering the structures of the skin, what most likely was the cause of the original pimple on this patient's skin?

2. How could Shenya have prevented this skin infection?

EXAM PREPARATION QUESTIONS

1. (LO 23.2) Which protein gives skin its protective quality?
   a. Melanin
   b. Vitamin D
   c. Keratin
   d. Hemoglobin
   e. Collagen

2. (LO 23.4) Which of the following lesions is a vascular lesion?
   a. Tumor
   b. Macule
   c. Ecchymosis
   d. Wheal
   e. Plaque

3. (LO 23.7) The patient has burned his left arm front and back from elbow to fingertips as well as his left chest and abdomen (approximately half of his trunk). Using the rule of nines, what percentage of his body is burned?
   a. 27%
   b. 18%
   c. 13.5%
   d. 9.5%
   e. 22.5%

4. (LO 23.5) The medical term for hair loss is
   a. Folliculitis
   b. Alopecia
   c. Pediculosis
   d. Impetigo
   e. Excoriation

5. (LO 23.4) Which medical term is more commonly known as a *hive*?
   a. Cicatrix
   b. Vesicle
   c. Pustule
   d. Wheal
   e. Erosion

6. (LO 23.4) Varrucae is another term meaning
   a. Bruises
   b. Warts
   c. Nodules
   d. Wrinkles
   e. Moles

7. (LO 23.1) Which of the following is not a function of skin?
   a. Temperature regulation
   b. Protection
   c. Excretion
   d. Sensation
   e. Vitamin B production

8. (LO 23.7) Scabies is caused by
   a. Fungi
   b. Lice
   c. Mites
   d. Bed bugs
   e. Bacteria

9. (LO 23.2) The most superficial layer of the epidermis is the
   a. Stratum basale
   b. Stratum corneum
   c. Stratum germinativum
   d. Stratum dermis
   e. Stratum keratin

10. (LO 23.5) The part of the nail that holds it down to the underlying tissues and provides nutrients to the nail is the
    a. Lunula
    b. Nail bed
    c. Cuticle
    d. Free edge
    e. Nail root

Analyze the following medical terms, presented throughout the chapter. Using a medical dictionary (or Appendix I) place a / mark between each word part. Define each word part and then define the whole word.

EXAMPLE: chemo/therapy = chemo means "chemical" + therapy means "treatment"
Chemotherapy means "treatment with chemicals"

1. cellulitis
2. cyanosis
3. dermatitis
4. dermatome
5. epidermis

6. folliculitis
7. hemoglobin
8. hypodermis
9. keratinocyte
10. lunula

11. melanocyte
12. pediculosis
13. sebaceous
14. subcutaneous
15. sudoriferous

The Skeletal System

CASE STUDY

Patient Name	Gender	DOB
John Miller	Male	12/5/19XX

Attending	MRN	Allergies
Paul F. Buckwalter, MD	082-09-981	Bee Stings

John Miller is a 65-year-old patient returning to the clinic for a follow-up visit. He has a history of hypertension, diabetes type II, myocardial infarction (heart attack, 2008), and a recent confirmed diagnosis of congestive heart failure. He is taking glyburide, captopril, and HCTZ. When he arrives at the clinic, you notice he is breathing with difficulty.

Mr. Miller states, "I was doing okay until I fell down yesterday. I was carrying a box of stuff to take to the Salvation Army and lost my footing." The patient shows you an abrasion on his left knee and his right elbow. He says his knee is popping and his elbow does not bend as much as it did before he fell. He is concerned that the bursitis in his knee might flare up. He also wonders why his elbow does not bend.

Keep John in mind as you study this chapter. There will be questions at the end of the chapter based on the case study. The information in the chapter will help you answer these questions.

McGraw Hill ACTIVSim™

LEARNING OUTCOMES

After completing Chapter 24, you will be able to:

24.1 Describe the structure of bone tissue.
24.2 Explain the functions of bones.
24.3 Compare intramembranous and endochondral ossification.
24.4 Describe the skeletal structures and one location of each structure.
24.5 Locate the bones of the skull.
24.6 Locate the bones of the spinal column.
24.7 Locate the bones of the rib cage.
24.8 Locate the bones of the shoulders, arms, and hands.
24.9 Locate the bones of the hips, legs, and feet.
24.10 Describe the three major types of joints and give examples of each.
24.11 Describe the common diseases and disorders of the skeletal system.

KEY TERMS

appendicular
articulations
axial
clavicle
diaphysis
epiphysis
femur
fibula
metacarpal
metatarsal
ossification

patella
pectoral girdle
pelvic girdle
radius
scapula
sternum
suture
temporal mandibular joint (TMJ)
ulna

CAAHEP

I. C (1) Describe structural organization of the human body

I. C (5) Describe the normal function of each body system

I. C (6) Identify common pathology related to each body system

I. C (7) Analyze pathology as it relates to the interaction of body systems

I. C (9) Describe implications for treatment related to pathology

I. C (10) Compare body structure and function of the human body across the life span

I. C (12) Describe the relationship between anatomy and physiology of all body systems and medications used for treatment in each

IV. C (11) Define both medical terms and abbreviations related to all body systems

ABHES

2. Anatomy & Physiology

Graduates:

b. Identify and apply the knowledge of all body systems; their structure and functions; and their common diseases, symptoms, and etiologies

c. Assist the physician with the regimen of diagnostic and treatment modalities as they relate to each body system

3. Medical Terminology

Graduates:

b. Build and dissect medical terms from roots/suffixes to understand the word element combinations that create medical terminology

c. Understand the various medical terminology for each specialty

Introduction

Imagine that you are walking along a bustling city sidewalk, and someone behind you calls your name. As you pause and turn your head to see who it is, you catch a glimpse of your profile in the reflection of a coffee shop window. You stand taller than you think you are, with one leg in front of the other as if pivoting. You bring your right hand up to your forehead and quickly rub your brow, then let it drop to your side. Your friend then appears beside you and the two of you hug. Although it may seem as if your body is simply made of only the surface features you can see reflected in this window, dressed for the day in nice clothing and hugging your friend, of course, there is much more to this picture. After all, your bones are behind this picture, scattered all throughout your body to provide it with the structure and support you need for daily functioning.

In this chapter, you will learn about the bones of the body, their structure, and how the joints of the body work. The skeletal system is composed of 206 bones as well as joints and related connective tissues. Now, picture this many bones hiding within that person—*you!*—reflected earlier in the coffee shop window.

The skeleton has two major divisions—the **axial** skeleton and the **appendicular** skeleton (see Figure 24-1). These divisions differ in the following ways:

- The axial skeleton contains 80 bones, including the bones of the skull, vertebral column, and rib cage. It supports the head, neck, and trunk, and it protects the brain, spinal cord, and the organs in the thorax. The hyoid bone, which anchors the tongue, is also included in the axial skeleton.

- The body's other 126 bones belong to the appendicular skeleton, which includes the bones of the arms, legs, **pectoral girdle,** and **pelvic girdle.** The pectoral girdle attaches the arms to the axial skeleton, and the pelvic girdle attaches the legs to the axial skeleton.

Bone Structure
LO 24.1

Bones contain various kinds of tissues, including osseous tissue, blood vessels, and nerves. Osseous tissue can be compact or spongy (see Figure 24-2). At the microscopic level, spongy or cancellous bone has more spaces within it than compact bone does. Spongy bone looks a lot like a natural sea sponge with the spaces filled with *red bone marrow.* Compact bone looks solid, like granite or marble. However, the following structures within these bones can be observed with a microscope:

- *Osteons,* also known as the *Haversian system,* are elongated cylinders that run up and down the bone's long axis. Each osteon has a central canal that contains blood vessels and nerves.

- *Bone matrix,* made of inorganic salts, collagen fibers, and proteins, is the substance between bone cells. Bone cells are called *osteocytes.* The primary salt of the matrix is calcium phosphate, which makes bone matrix very hard.

- *Lamella* are layers of bone surrounding the canals of osteons.

- *Lacunae* are holes in the matrix of bone that hold osteocytes.

- *Canaliculi* are tiny canals that connect lacunae to each other and allow osteocytes to spread nutrients to each other.

All bones are made up of both compact and cancellous bone. They are classified according to their shape (see Figure 24-3), as described below:

- *Long bones* are located primarily in the arms and legs. Examples include the **femur** (thighbone, see Figure 24-4) and the

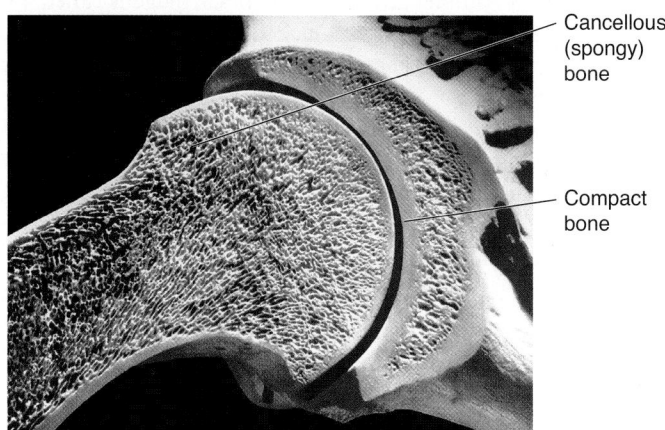

FIGURE 24-1 Major bones of the skeleton: (a) anterior view and (b) posterior view. The axial skeleton is shown in orange and the appendicular skeleton is shown in yellow.

Labels (anterior view):
Cranium — Skull
Face — Skull
Hyoid
Clavicle
Scapula
Sternum
Humerus
Ribs
Vertebral column
Coxa
Radius
Ulna
Carpals
Metacarpals
Femur
Patella
Tibia
Fibula
Tarsals
Metatarsals
Phalanges

Labels (posterior view):
Vertebral column
Sacrum
Coccyx
Phalanges
Femur

(a)　　　　(b)

FIGURE 24-2 Cross-section of bone showing compact and cancellous (spongy) bone tissue.

Cancellous (spongy) bone
Compact bone

humerus (upper arm bone). Long bones have the following parts (see Figure 24-5):

- **Diaphysis**—the shaft of a long bone. It is tubular and consists of a thick collar of compact bone that surrounds the central medullary cavity.

- **Epiphysis**—the expanded end of a long bone. It consists of a thin layer of compact bone surrounding cancellous bone. Long bones have an epiphysis at both ends.

- *Articular cartilage*—the cartilage that covers the epiphyses of long bones. It cushions bones and absorbs stress during bone movements.

- *Medullary cavity*—the canal that runs through the center of the diaphysis. In adults, it contains *yellow bone marrow* (mostly fat).

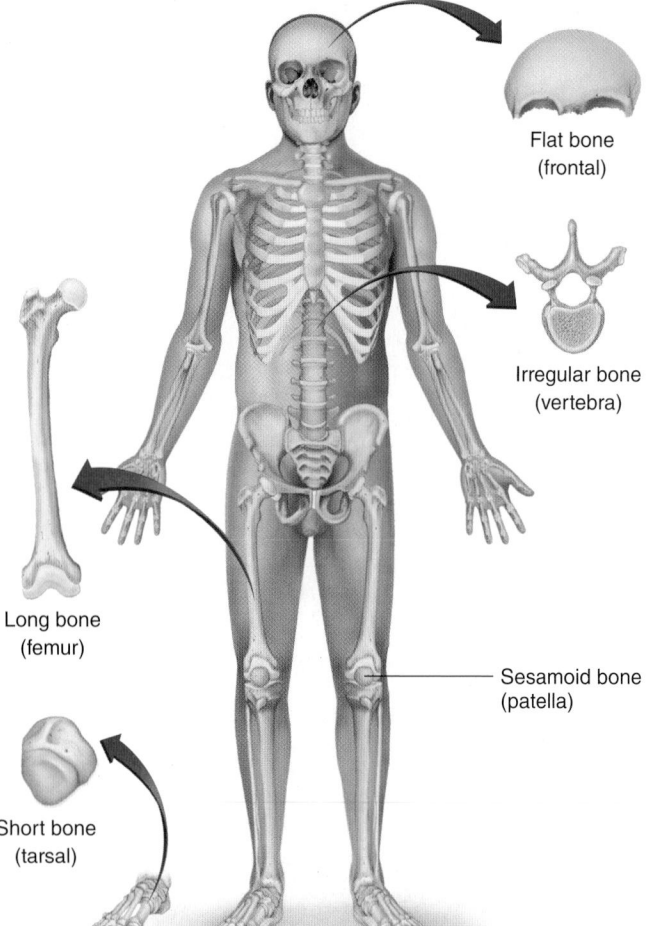

FIGURE 24-3 Classification of bone by shape: Five different classes of bone are recognized according to shape—long, short, flat, irregular, and sesamoid.

- *Periosteum*—a membrane that surrounds the diaphysis. It contains bone-forming cells, dense fibrous connective tissue, nerves, and blood vessels.
- *Endosteum*—a membrane that lines the medullary cavity and the holes of cancellous bone. It contains bone-forming cells.
- *Short bones* are located in the wrists and ankles. Examples include the carpals (wrist bones) and some of the tarsals (ankle bones).
- *Flat bones* are primarily located in the skull and rib cage. Examples include the ribs and frontal bone.
- *Irregular bones* include the vertebrae and the pelvic girdle bones.
- *Sesamoid bones* are small, rounded bones usually found next to joints or embedded in a tendon. An example is the patella or kneecap.

Gender Differences in Skeletal Structure

You may wonder how physicians, pathologists, and archeologists can tell if a skeleton is male or female. Table 24-1 outlines some of the skeletal differences between the sexes.

▶ Functions of Bones   LO 24.2

Bones have many functions. Without bones, the body would be more like a glob of jelly and not capable of very much. Bones give shape to body parts such as the head, legs, arms, and trunk. They also support and protect soft structures in the body. For example, the skull protects the brain. Bones also function in body movement because skeletal muscles attach to them, allowing you to create willful or voluntary movements.

The red marrow within cancellous bone produces new blood cells in a process called *hematopoiesis*. Blood cells have a limited life span so they need to be replaced. Red blood cells, for example, need replacing as often as every 90 to 120 days. Your red marrow is actively making more blood cells 24 hours a day. Bones also store calcium for the body. Every cell in the body needs calcium, so the body must have a large supply readily available.

▶ Bone Growth   LO 24.3

Bones grow through a process called **ossification.** The two types of ossification are intramembranous and endochondral.

In *intramembranous* ossification, bones begin as tough, fibrous membranes. Eventually, bone-forming cells called *osteoblasts* turn the membrane to bone. Except for the lower jaw bone, the bones of the skull are formed by intramembranous ossification.

In *endochondral* ossification, bones start out as cartilage models. Eventually, the osteoblasts form a bone collar around the diaphysis of the cartilage model. Think of a sculptor who first builds a framework or model of soft material before applying sculpting clay over the framework. Eventually, when the clay hardens, either through drying or firing in a kiln, there is more hard material than there is soft framework. Then bone is formed in the diaphysis of the bone. This area is called the *primary ossification center*. Later, the epiphyses turn to bone (secondary ossification centers), and the medullary cavity and spaces in cancellous bone are formed. The cells that form holes in bone are called *osteoclasts*. As long as a bone contains some cartilage between an epiphysis and the diaphysis, it can continue to grow in length. This plate of cartilage is called an *epiphyseal disk* or *growth plate*. Once the cartilage is gone, bone growth stops. For most people, bone growth stops between the ages of 18 and 25.

Even after bone growth stops, osteoclasts and osteoblasts continually remodel bone tissue. Throughout life, osteoclasts break down bone when the body needs more calcium in the blood, and osteoblasts replace the bone when there is excess calcium in the blood.

Building Better Bones

Many factors influence bone health, including diet, exercise, and a person's overall lifestyle. You can help patients improve or maintain their bone health by teaching them about behaviors that will support it.

FIGURE 24-4   Bone structures: (a) bone structures of the femur and (b) bone structures of the tibia and fibula.

Bone-Healthy Diet Good nutrition is essential for proper bone growth during childhood and the teen years. It is equally important in adulthood in order to maintain healthy bones. Bone-building nutrients are found in dairy products, broccoli, kale, spinach, salmon, sardines, egg yolks, whole grains, and fruits—especially bananas and oranges. Calcium and vitamin D are particularly important for healthy bones. Without vitamin D, the bloodstream cannot absorb calcium from the digestive tract. Without calcium, bone tissue will slowly wear away. Supplements can always be taken if a person's diet does not include adequate amounts of calcium and vitamin D.

Bone-Healthy Exercises Weight-bearing and strength-training exercises are best for bone health. When your muscles contract, they pull on your bones. This tension stimulates bones to thicken and strengthen. Lifting weights is an

effective way to increase the tension on bones. Other activities such as jogging, walking briskly, or playing a sport regularly will also stimulate your bones to increase in density.

Bone-Healthy Lifestyle A person with a bone-healthy lifestyle avoids smoking and alcohol. Smoking rids the body of calcium, which is necessary for bone growth. Alcohol prevents calcium absorption in the digestive tract. Smokers are almost twice as likely to develop osteoporosis as nonsmokers.

Bone Tests

Bone density tests and bone scans are currently the most useful tools in determining bone health. Bone density tests are painless procedures used to determine the density of a person's bones. Because osteoporosis shows no symptoms in early stages, it is important to have these tests done when your doctor

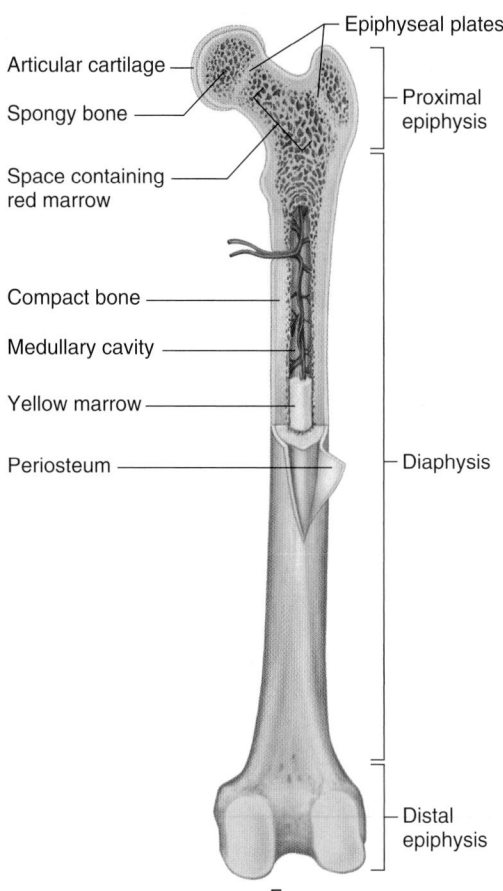

FIGURE 24-5 Parts of a long bone.

Labels:
- Epiphyseal plates
- Articular cartilage
- Spongy bone
- Space containing red marrow
- Compact bone
- Medullary cavity
- Yellow marrow
- Periosteum
- Proximal epiphysis
- Diaphysis
- Distal epiphysis
- Femur

recommends them. Bone scans help diagnose the causes of bone pain, arthritis, bone infections, and bone cancers. These scans use radioactive tracers that are injected into the patient and concentrate in bone tissue.

▶ Bony Structures   LO 24.4

The skeletal bones act as your body's rigid foundation. By design, they are not perfectly smooth or perfectly rounded. Bones have projections and processes for muscle and ligament

attachment. For bones to come together at joints or **articulations,** there are depressions and hollows. In addition, blood vessels and nerves need openings within bones for entrances and exits. Each of these structures has a specific name and design. Table 24-2 lists some of these common structures and directs you to the appropriate figures throughout this chapter.

▶ The Skull   LO 24.5

Skull bones are divided into two types: cranial and facial bones. Cranial bones form the top, sides, and back of the skull (see Figure 24-6). Facial bones form the face (see Figure 24-7). The skull bones of an infant are not completely formed. The "soft spots" felt on an infant's skull are actually *fontanels*, which are tough membranes that connect the incompletely developed bones. These structures allow the infant's skull to be somewhat moldable to assist with delivery through the birth canal. As the fontanels close, the sutures of the skull are formed.

The major cranial bones are the following:

- The *frontal bone* forms the anterior portion of the cranium. It is also called the forehead bone.
- *Parietal bones* form most of the top and sides of the skull.
- The *occipital bone* forms the back of the skull. The large hole at the base of the occipital bone is called the *foramen magnum*. It allows the spinal cord to connect to the brain. Two bumps called occipital *condyles* are on either side of the foramen magnum. They sit on top of the first vertebra. When you nod your head, your occipital condyles are rocking back and forth on the first vertebra of the spinal column.
- Two *temporal bones* form the lower sides of the skull.
- A canal called the *external auditory meatus* (commonly called the ear canal) runs through each temporal bone. A large bump called the *mastoid process* is located on each temporal bone just behind each ear. Major neck muscles attach to your skull at the mastoid processes.
- A *sphenoid bone* forms part of the floor of the cranium. It is shaped like a butterfly. In the center is a deep depression called the *sella turcica*. The pituitary gland sits in this deep depression.

TABLE 24-1	**Differences Between the Male and Female Skeletons**
Part	**Differences**
Skull	Male skull is larger and heavier, with more conspicuous muscular attachments. Male forehead is shorter, facial area is less round, jaw is larger, and mastoid processes are more prominent than those of a female.
Pelvis	Male pelvic bones are heavier, thicker, and have more obvious muscular attachments. The obturator foramina and the acetabula are larger and closer together than those of a female.
Pelvic cavity	Male pelvic cavity is narrower in all diameters, and is longer, less roomy, and more funnel-shaped. The distances between the ischial spines and between the ischial tuberosities are less than in a female.
Sacrum	Male sacrum is narrower, sacral promontory projects forward to a greater degree, and sacral curvature is bent less sharply posteriorly than in a female.
Coccyx	Male coccyx is less movable than that of a female.

TABLE 24-2 Terms Used to Describe Skeletal Structures

Term	Definition	Examples
Condyle	A rounded process that usually articulates with another bone.	Medial and lateral condyles of the femur (see Figure 24-4a)
Crest	A narrow, ridge-like projection.	Iliac crest of the ilium (see Figure 24-11)
Epicondyle	A projection situated above a condyle.	Medial epicondyle of the femur (see Figure 24-4a)
Foramen	An opening through a bone that is usually a passageway for blood vessels, nerves, or ligaments.	Mental foramen of the mandible (see Figure 24-7)
Fossa	A relatively deep pit or depression.	Olecrannon fossa of the humerus (see Figure 24-10d)
Head	An enlargement on the end of a bone.	Head of the femur (see Figure 24-4a)
Process	A prominent projection on a bone.	Mastoid process of the temporal bone (see Figure 24-6)
Suture	An interlocking line of union between bones.	Lambdoidal suture between the occipital and parietal bones (see Figure 24-6)
Trochanter	A relatively large process.	Greater trochanter of the femur (see Figure 24-4a)
Tubercle	A small, knoblike process.	Greater tubercle of the humerus (see Figure 24-10b)
Tuberosity	A knoblike process usually larger than a tubercle.	Tibial tuberosity of the tibia (see Figure 24-4b)

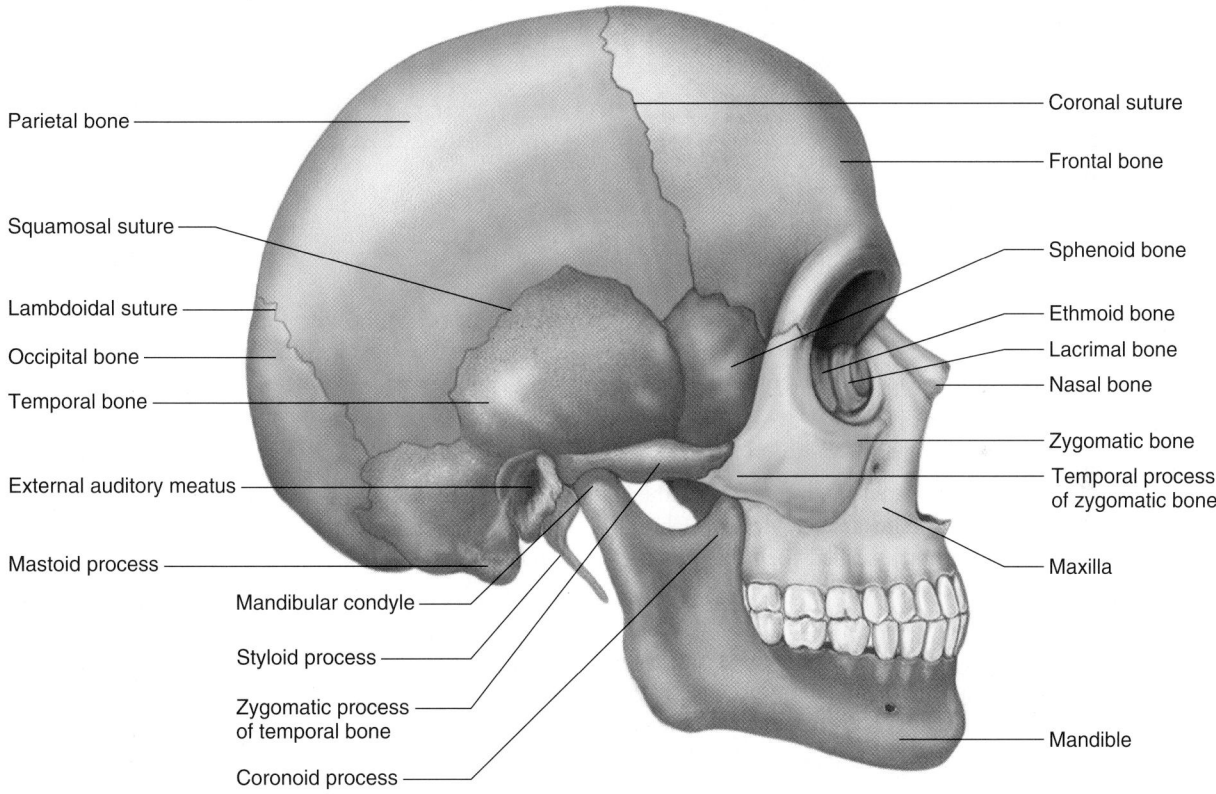

FIGURE 24-6 Lateral view of the skull.

- *Ethmoid bones* are between the sphenoid bone and the nasal bones. They also form part of the floor of the cranium.
- *Ear ossicles* are the body's smallest bones. They are the malleus, incus, and stapes and are in the middle ear cavities of the temporal bones.

The following are major facial bones:

- The *mandible* is the lower jaw bone and is the only movable bone in the skull. It attaches to the temporal bone in front of the external auditory meatus in an area known as the **temporal mandibular joint (TMJ).** The mandible anchors the lower teeth and forms the chin.
- The *maxillae* form the upper jaw bone of the facial skeleton, to which the upper teeth anchor.
- The *zygomatic bones* are the cheekbones. Several thin nasal bones fuse together to form the bridge of the nose.
- *Palatine bones* form the hard palate, which is the roof of the mouth.
- The *vomer* is a thin bone that divides the nasal cavity.

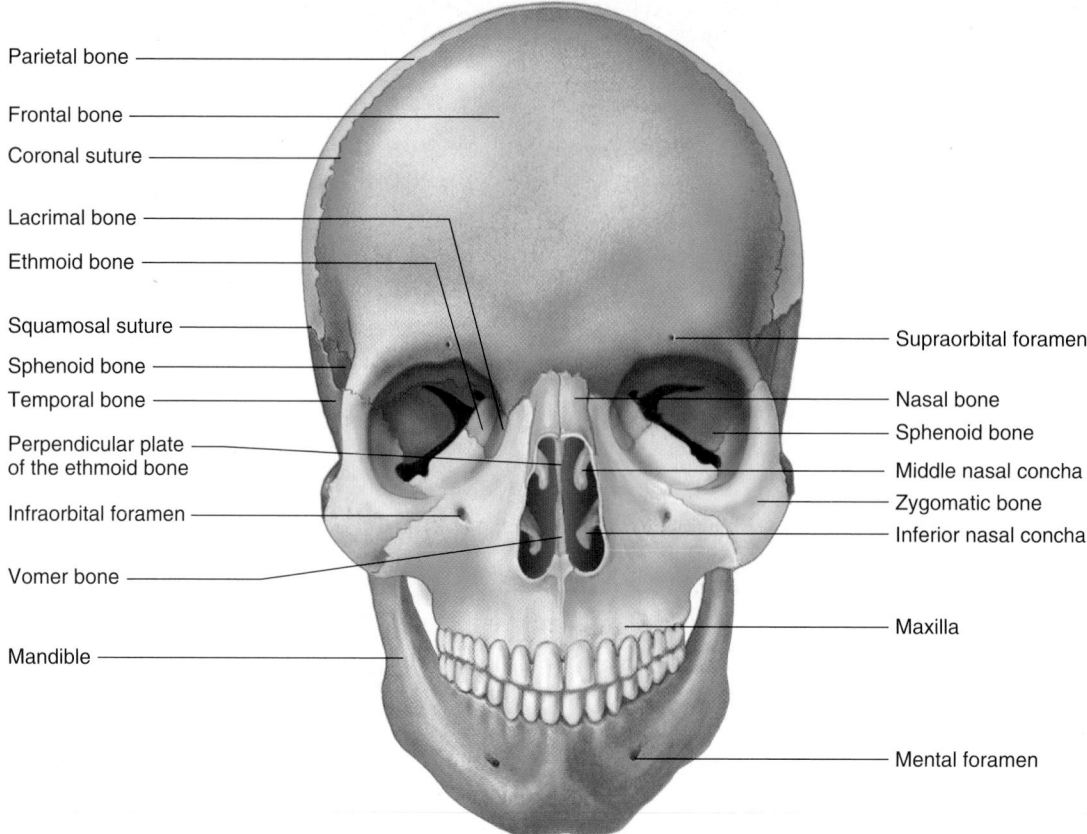

Labels on image:
Parietal bone
Frontal bone
Coronal suture
Lacrimal bone
Ethmoid bone
Squamosal suture
Sphenoid bone
Temporal bone
Perpendicular plate of the ethmoid bone
Infraorbital foramen
Vomer bone
Mandible

Supraorbital foramen
Nasal bone
Sphenoid bone
Middle nasal concha
Zygomatic bone
Inferior nasal concha
Maxilla
Mental foramen

FIGURE 24-7 Anterior view of the skull.

The Spinal Column

LO 24.6

The spinal column consists of 7 cervical vertebrae, 12 thoracic vertebrae, 5 lumbar vertebrae, a sacrum, and a coccyx (see Figure 24-8), all of which are further described below:

- *Cervical vertebrae,* which are located in the neck, are the smallest and lightest vertebrae. The first cervical vertebra is called the *atlas* and the second is called the *axis.* When you turn your head from side to side, your atlas is pivoting around your axis.
- *Thoracic vertebrae* are the posterior attachment for the 12 pairs of ribs. They have long, sharp, spinous processes that you can feel when you run your finger down someone's spine.
- *Lumbar vertebrae* are very sturdy structures. They form the small of the back and bear the most weight of all the vertebrae.
- The *sacrum* is a triangular-shaped bone that consists of five fused vertebrae.
- The *coccyx* (commonly called the tailbone) is a small, triangular-shaped bone made up of three to five fused vertebrae; it is considered nonessential in humans.

The Rib Cage

LO 24.7

The rib cage is made of 12 pairs of ribs and the **sternum** (see Figure 24-9). The sternum—often called the breastplate—forms the front middle portion of the rib cage. The cartilaginous tip of the sternum is known as the *xiphoid process.* The sternum joins with the clavicles and most ribs. All 12 pairs of ribs are attached posteriorly to thoracic vertebrae. The ribs themselves are classified in three groups based on their anterior attachment:

- True. The first seven pairs of ribs are *true ribs.* They attach directly to the sternum through pieces of cartilage called *costal cartilage.*
- False. Rib pairs 8, 9, and 10 are called *false ribs.* They do not attach directly to the sternum by individual cartilage, but instead attach to the costal cartilage of rib pair number 7.
- Floating. Rib pairs 11 and 12 are called *floating ribs* because they do not attach anteriorly to the sternum or to any other structure.

Bones of the Shoulders, Arms, and Hands

LO 24.8

The bones of the shoulders make up the pectoral girdle and include the clavicles and the scapulae (see Figure 24-10). They attach the arms to the axial skeleton.

- The **clavicles,** or collar bones, are slender in shape. Each joins with the sternum and a scapula.
- **Scapulae** (or shoulder blades) are thin, triangular-shaped flat bones located on the dorsal surface of the rib cage. Each scapula joins with the head of a humerus and a clavicle.

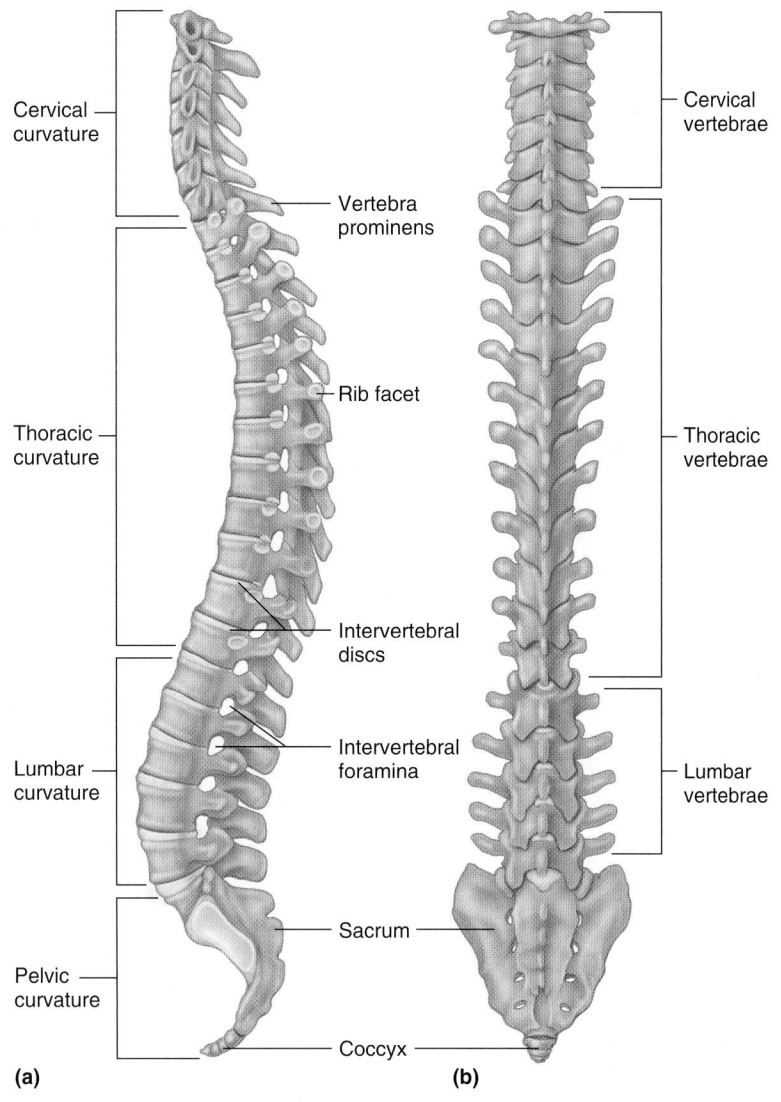

FIGURE 24-8 Vertebral column: (a) lateral view and (b) posterior view.

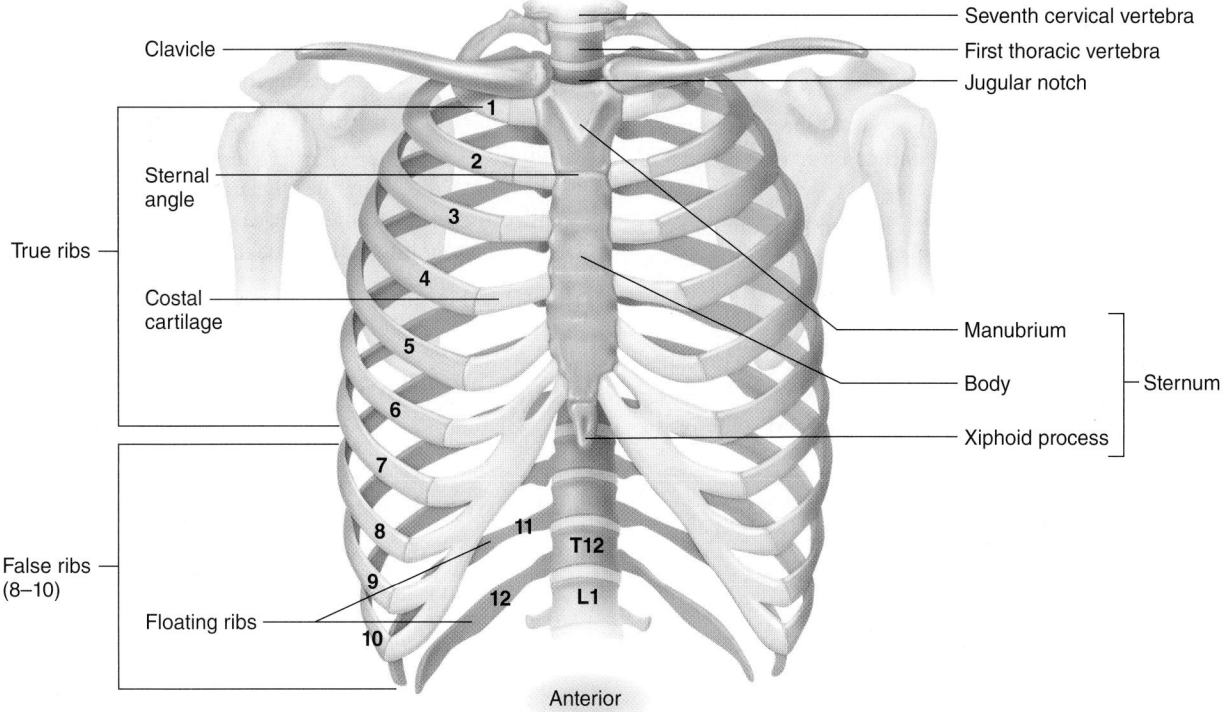

FIGURE 24-9 Thoracic rib cage showing pectoral girdle attachment of upper extremities.

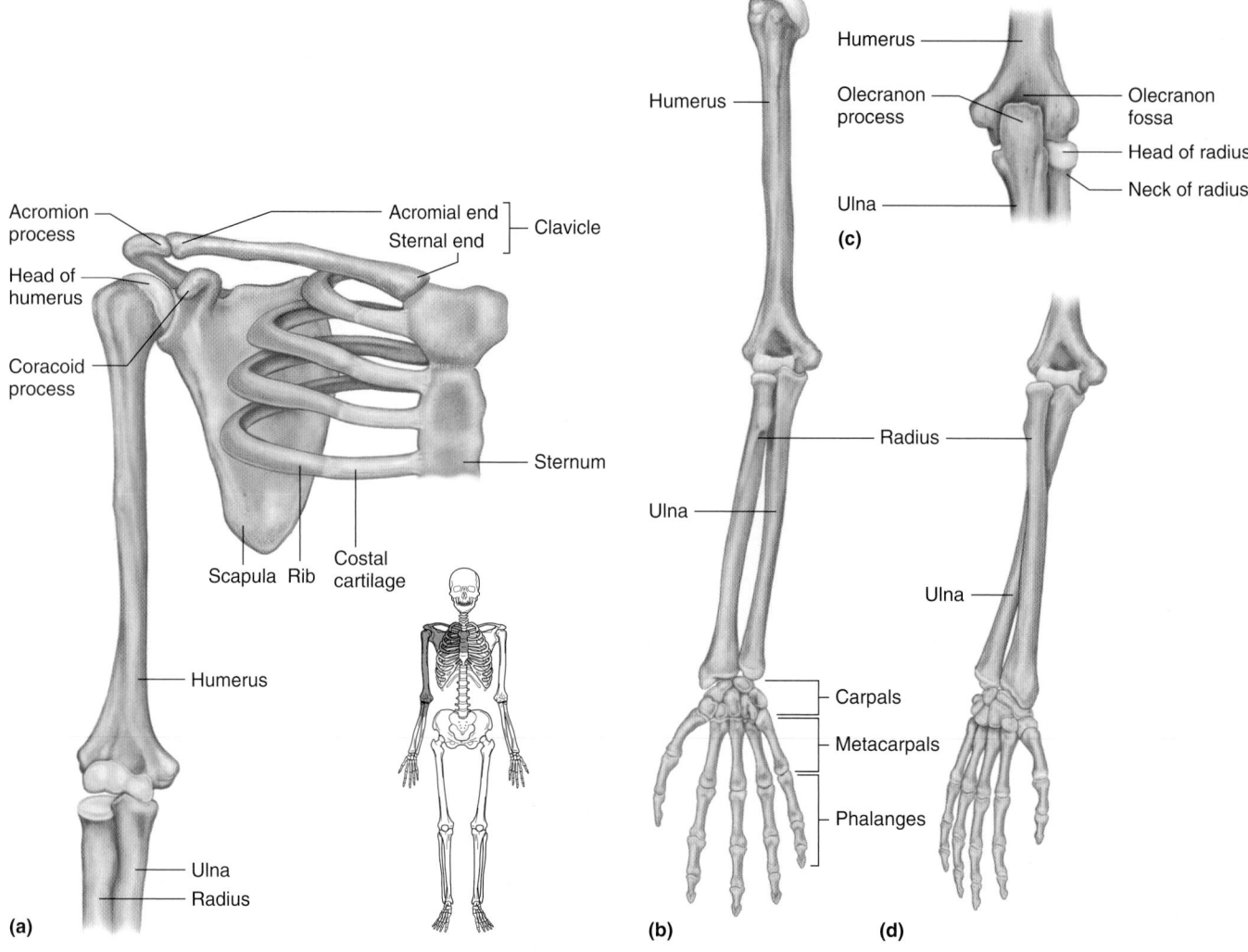

FIGURE 24-10 (a) The pectoral girdle with upper limb attached. (b) Frontal view of upper limb (palm anterior). (c) Frontal view of upper limb (palm posterior). (d) Posterior view of right elbow.

The upper limb, or arm, bones include the humerus, radius, and ulna:

- The *humerus* is located in the upper part of the arm. Its proximal end joins with the scapula, and its distal end attaches at the radius and the ulna.

- The **radius** is the lateral bone of the forearm. It is on the same side of the arm as your thumb. Proximally, it joins with the humerus and the ulna, and distally with the carpal (wrist) bones.

- The **ulna** is the medial bone of the lower arm. The proximal end of the ulna joins with the humerus to form the elbow joint. Distally, it also joins with the radius and some of the carpal bones of the wrist.

The bones of the hand include carpals, metacarpals, and phalanges:

- *Carpals* are wrist bones. Each wrist contains eight marble-sized carpal bones.

- **Metacarpals** form the palms of the hands. Each hand has five metacarpals.

- *Phalanges* are the bones of the fingers. There are 14 phalanges in each hand—three for each finger and two per thumb.

- The joints between the phalangeal bones are the proximal and distal *interphalangeal* (PIP and DIP) joints.

- The joints that join the phalanges to the metacarpals are called the *metacarpophalangeal* (MCP) joints. You probably know these joints as the knuckles.

Refer to Figure 24-10 for the bones of the shoulders, arms, and hands.

▶ Bones of the Hips, Legs, and Feet LO 24.9

The hip bones, also called *coxal* bones, attach the legs to the axial skeleton. They also protect pelvic organs. Each coxal bone has three parts: the ilium, the ischium, and the pubis.

- The *ilium* is the most superior part of a coxal bone. When you put your hands on your hips, you are touching the part of the ilium called the *iliac crest*.

- The *ischium* forms the lower part of a coxal bone and the pubis forms the front.

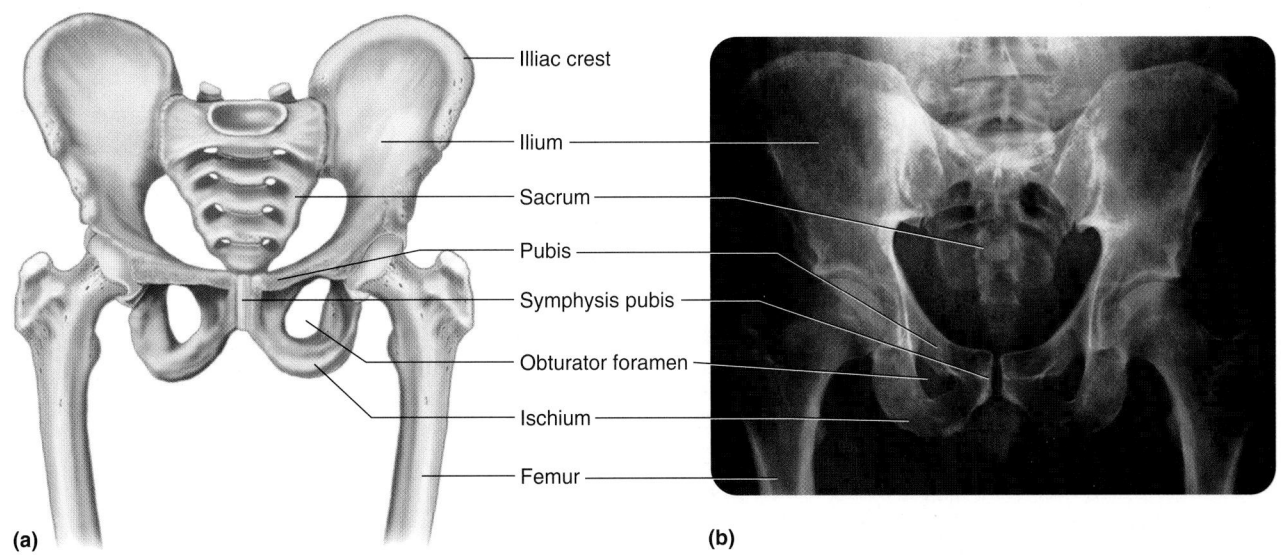

FIGURE 24-11 (a) Pelvic girdle. (b) Radiograph of the pelvic girdle.

- The *pubis* bones of each coxal bone join together to form the *pubic symphysis*, which is also referred to as the *pelvic girdle* (see Figure 24-11).

The bones of the lower limb, or leg, include the femur, the patella, the tibia, and the fibula.

- The femur is the thigh bone and the largest bone in the body. Its proximal end joins with the hip bone at the *acetabulum* (or hip socket). Ligaments and muscles hold it in place.
- The distal end of the femur attaches to the *tibia* and the **patella** (kneecap). The patella is a sesamoid bone—a small, rounded bone in front of the knee joint.
- The *tibia* (or shinbone) is the medial bone of the lower leg. Its proximal end joins with the femur and fibula, and distally to the ankle bones.
- The **fibula** is the lateral bone of the lower leg. It is much thinner than the tibia. It joins with the ankle bones at its distal end. Figure 24-12 illustrates the bones of the lower extremity.

The bones of the foot include the tarsals, the metatarsals, and the phalanges.

- The *tarsal* bones form the back of the foot. The *calcaneus,* or heel bone, is the largest tarsal bone. There are seven tarsal bones per foot.
- **Metatarsals** are bones that form the front of the foot. There are five metatarsals per foot.
- The bones of the toes are called *phalanges*. Each foot contains 14—two for each big toe and three in all the other toes. The joints between these lower phalanges are interphalangeal joints, just like those of the fingers.
- The joints that join the toes to the foot are called *metatarsophalangeal* (MTP) joints.

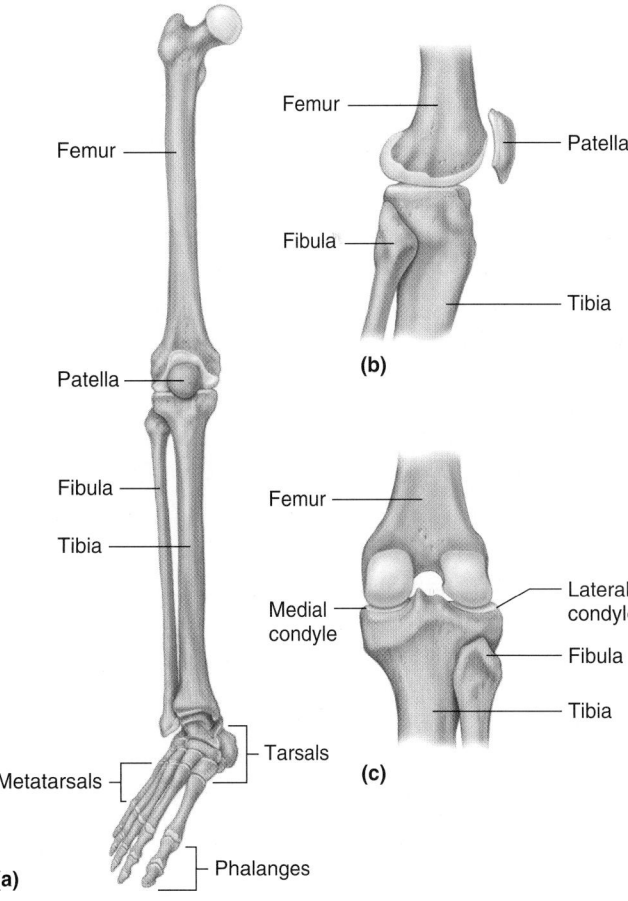

FIGURE 24-12 (a) Anterior view of the right lower limb. (b) Lateral view of the right knee. (c) Posterior view of the right knee.

▶ Joints

Joints are the junctions between bones. Based on their structure, joints can be classified as fibrous, cartilaginous, or synovial.

- The bones of *fibrous joints* are connected together with short fibers. So, the bones of this type of joint do not normally move against each other. Most fibrous joints are found between cranial bones and facial bones. Fibrous joints in the skull are called **sutures.**

- The bones of *cartilaginous joints* are connected together with a disc of cartilage. This type of joint is slightly movable. The joints between vertebrae are cartilaginous joints.

- The bones of *synovial joints* are covered with hyaline cartilage and are held together by a fibrous joint capsule (see Figure 24-13). The joint capsule is lined with a synovial membrane, which secretes a slippery fluid called *synovial fluid.* This fluid allows the bones to move easily against each other. Bones are also held together through tough, cord-like structures called *ligaments.* Synovial joints are freely movable. Examples of synovial joints are the elbows, knees, shoulders, and knuckles.

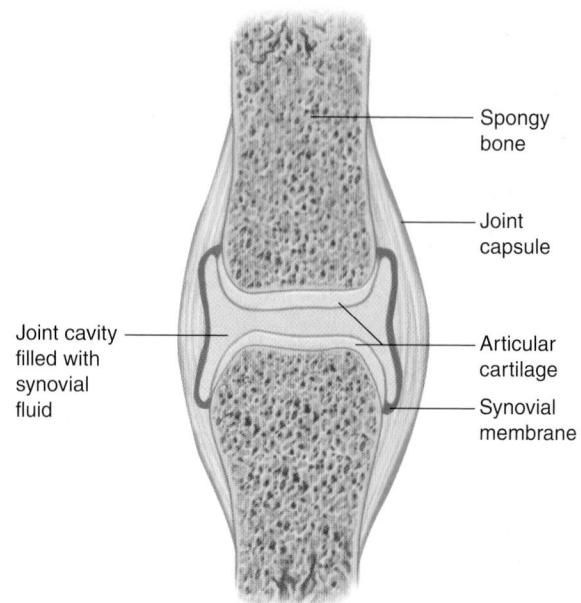

Spongy bone

Joint capsule

Joint cavity filled with synovial fluid

Articular cartilage

Synovial membrane

FIGURE 24-13 Structure of a synovial joint.

PATHOPHYSIOLOGY

Common Diseases and Disorders of the Skeletal System

Arthritis is a general term meaning "joint inflammation." Although there are more than 100 types of arthritis, we will discuss the two most common types: osteoarthritis and rheumatoid arthritis.

OSTEOARTHRITIS, also known as *degenerative joint disease (DJD),* is the most common type of joint disorder, affecting nearly everyone to some degree by the age of 70. DJD primarily affects the weight-bearing joints of the hips and knees, and the cartilage between the bones and the bones themselves begin to break down.

Causes. Research points to inflammatory processes or metabolic disorders as the etiology of DJD.

Signs and Symptoms. These include joint stiffness, aching, and pain, especially with weather changes. There is often fluid around the joint and grating noises with joint movement.

Treatment. Anti-inflammatory drugs, including aspirin and NSAIDS (nonsteroidal anti-inflammatory drugs) like naproxen and Feldene®, may be used. Intra-articular steroid injections may be tried for severe cases. In some cases, a series of injections of hyaluronic acid-containing medications are used when other treatments do not work. These injections serve as joint fluid replacement. Some success has been found with transplanting harvested cartilage cells from the patient's healthy knee cartilage, which are then grown in the lab and reinjected into the patient's diseased joint. Surgical scraping of the joint may also be done to remove deteriorated bone fragments. As a last resort, joint replacement may be recommended.

RHEUMATOID ARTHRITIS (RA) is the second most common form of arthritis. RA is a chronic systemic inflammatory disease that attacks the smaller joints, typically of the hands and feet, as well as the surrounding tissues of those joints. There may be flares or attacks of pain and inflammation followed by periods of remission. RA is three times more common in women than in men.

Causes. RA is believed to be an autoimmune disease, triggering joint inflammation.

Signs and Symptoms. In this disease, the body's immune system attacks the synovial membrane, causing edema (swelling) and congestion. Tissue becomes granular and thick, eventually destroying the joint capsule and bone. Scar tissue forms, bones atrophy, and visible deformities become apparent due to the bone malalignment and immobility. Patients also have moderate to severe pain in the affected joints.

Treatment. Treatment includes anti-inflammatory drugs, exercise, heat or cold treatments, and cortisone injections. Researchers are working with genetic techniques to block the immune system reaction. Low-impact aerobic exercise may be helpful, and some patients find warm water exercises beneficial, too.

Go to CONNECT to see an animation about *Osteoarthritis vs. Rheumatoid Arthritis.*

BURSITIS is inflammation of a bursa, which is a fluid-filled sac that cushions tendons. It occurs most commonly in the elbow, knee, shoulder, and hip.

Causes. Overuse of and trauma to joints are the most common causes of this condition. Bacterial infections can also cause bursitis.

Signs and Symptoms. These include joint pain and swelling, and tenderness in the structures surrounding the joint.

Treatment. The most common treatments are bed rest, pain medications, steroid injections, aspiration of excess fluid from the bursa, and antibiotics.

EWING SARCOMA FAMILY OF TUMORS (ESFT) is a group of tumors that affect different tissue types. However, the tumors primarily affect bone.

Causes. Causes of ESFT are not clear, but it mostly affects Caucasians between the ages of 10 and 20. The tumors are usually located in the lower extremities but may also occur in the pelvis, chest wall, upper extremities, spine, and skull.

Signs and Symptoms. Fever, pain in the tumor location, fractures, and bruises in the tumor location are the primary symptoms.

Treatment. Treatment options include surgery, chemotherapy, radiation therapy, a bone marrow transplant, or a stem cell transplant.

GOUT, also known as *gouty arthritis*, is a type of arthritis that usually occurs more frequently with age.

Causes. Gout is caused by deposits of uric acid crystals in the joints. People with gout cannot properly break down uric acid and remove it from their bloodstream.

Signs and Symptoms. Symptoms include sudden or chronic joint pain, commonly in the great toe, joint swelling and stiffness, and fever.

Treatment. The most common treatments are pain medications and changes to the patient's diet. Patients should eliminate from their diet certain foods that cause the formation of uric acid (meats, fish, beer, or wine). There are medications available that increase uric acid elimination by the kidneys (uricosuric agents) or decrease uric acid production (xanthine oxidase inhibitors).

KYPHOSIS is an abnormal curvature of the spine, most often at the thoracic (chest) level. This condition is often referred to as humpback.

Causes. Adolescent kyphosis may result from growth retardation or improper development of the epiphyses as a result of rapid growth. Poor posture may exacerbate or worsen this condition. The adult form of kyphosis is frequently the result of aging and degenerative disc disease of the intervertebral discs and vertebral fracture from underlying osteoporosis.

Signs and Symptoms. In adolescent kyphosis, there may be no symptoms other than visible back curvature. There may be mild pain, tiredness, tenderness, or stiffness of the thoracic spine. In adult kyphosis, the upper back is rounded and there may be pain, back weakness, and fatigue.

Treatment. Childhood kyphosis can be treated with exercise, a firm mattress, and a back brace if needed until growth is completed to keep the spine in alignment. Spinal fusion or grafting may be needed in rare cases of neurological damage

or disabling pain. Harrington rods may also be used to keep the vertebrae aligned.

LORDOSIS is an exaggerated inward (convex) curvature of the lumbar spine. Sometimes this condition is called swayback.

Cause. Wearing high heels is a frequent cause. The positioning of the feet with the elevated heel height causes an inward positioning of the back as a counter-balancing measure.

Signs and Symptoms. The main sign is visual inward curvature of the lower back. There may be mild pain with this exaggerated curvature.

Treatment. Avoiding excessive heel height is the best prevention. Once the condition begins, exercise and appropriate footwear will at least keep the condition stable.

OSTEOGENESIS IMPERFECTA (OI) is more commonly called *brittle-bone disease*. People with this disease have decreased amounts of collagen in their bones, which leads to very fragile bones. There are eight types of this disease:

- Type I—the mildest form of OI, which occurs more often than any of the other types.
- Type II—the most severe form of OI, normally fatal within a few weeks of birth.
- Type III—also a severe type of OI, however, infants usually live longer than those with Type II.
- Type IV—a moderate form of OI that is usually diagnosed later in childhood.
- Type V—similar to Type IV except that large callouses form around bone fractures. This type accounts for only 5% of OI cases.
- Type VI—an extremely rare, moderate form of OI characterized by a defect in mineralization of the bone.
- Type VII—a moderate form caused by inheritance of a recessive gene mutation. Similar to Type IV. Moderately abnormal bone growth occurs in this type of OI.
- Type VIII—similar to OI Types II and III, and growth deficiency is severe; however, sclera are white in Type VIII.

Cause. The disorder is hereditary and often runs in families.

Signs and Symptoms. These include fractures (all types); blue sclera (types 1, 2, 3, and 4); dental problems (types 3 and 4); hearing loss (type 1); a triangular face (type 3); abnormal spinal curves (types 1, 3, 4, 5, and 6); very small stature (types 2, 3, 4, 7, and 8); a small chest (types 2 and 3); fractures at birth (types 2 and 3); loose joints (type 4); muscle weakness (types 1, 3, and 4); and respiratory difficulties (types 1, 2, 3, and 8).

Treatment. Because this disease has many symptoms, the list of treatments is extensive and includes fracture repair, surgery to strengthen bones by inserting metal rods into them, dental procedures, physical therapy, braces to prevent bone deformities, wheelchairs and other supportive aids, medications, and counseling. Other surgeries may be required to treat lung and heart problems that sometimes occur with this disease.

OSTEOPOROSIS is a condition in which bones become thin (more porous) over time. It is a very common disorder in the United States and affects women more than men and Caucasians more than any other race. This condition occurs because of hypocalcemia in which bone is broken down to release calcium and is not replaced in sufficient amounts, thus bone density decreases.

Causes. These include hormone deficiencies (estrogen in women and testosterone in men), a sedentary lifestyle, a lack of calcium and vitamin D in the diet, bone cancers, corticosteroid excess (usually as a result of endocrine diseases), smoking, excess alcohol consumption, and steroid use.

Signs and Symptoms. There are usually no symptoms in the early stages of this disease. Patients at high risk, especially those with a family history of osteoporosis, should request bone densitometry studies to catch the disease before symptoms begin. Patients in later stages of the disease may experience fractures (usually of the spine, wrists, or hips), back and neck pain, a loss of height over time, and an abnormal curving of the spine (kyphosis).

Treatment. The most common treatments include: medications to prevent bone loss and relieve bone pain; hormone replacement therapy; lifestyle changes to prevent bone loss (including regular exercise and diets or supplements that include calcium, phosphorus, and vitamin D); moderation in use of alcohol; and stopping smoking.

Go to CONNECT to see an animation about *Osteoporosis.*

OSTEOSARCOMA is a type of bone cancer usually affecting the leg bones that originates from osteoblasts, the cells that make bony tissue. It occurs most often in children, teens, and young adults and more often in males than females.

Causes. The etiology of this type of cancer is unclear.

Signs and Symptoms. Primary symptoms include pain in affected bones (usually the legs), swelling around affected bones, and an increase in pain with movement of the affected bones.

Treatment. Treatments include surgery, chemotherapy, and radiation therapy. Amputation of the affected limb, followed by a prosthesis fitting, may be needed in some cases to prevent metastasis.

PAGET'S DISEASE causes bones to enlarge and become deformed and weak. It usually affects people over the age of 40.

Causes. This disease may be caused by a virus or various hereditary factors.

Signs and Symptoms. Bone pain, deformed bones, and fractures are common symptoms. Patients may experience headaches and hearing loss if the disease affects skull bones.

Treatment. Treatments include surgery to remodel bones, hip replacements, medications to prevent bone weakening, and physical therapy.

SCOLIOSIS is an abnormal, S-shaped, lateral curvature of the thoracic or lumbar spine.

Causes. This disorder can develop prenatally when vertebrae do not fuse together. It can also result from diseases that cause weakness of the muscles that hold vertebrae together. Other causes of scoliosis are unknown, but they may be genetic.

Signs and Symptoms. A patient with scoliosis usually has a spine that looks bent to one side, with one shoulder or hip appearing to be higher than the other. Patients often experience back pain.

Treatment. Treatment includes different types of back braces, surgery to correct spinal curves, and physical therapy to strengthen the muscles of the back and abdomen.

SUMMARY OF LEARNING OUTCOMES

LEARNING OUTCOMES	KEY POINTS
24.1 Describe the structure of bone tissue.	Bones consist of the following substances: osteons or Haversian systems, bone matrix between osteocytes (bone cells), collagen fibers and proteins, the lamella, and canaliculi. Long bones include the femur and humerus; short bones include the carpals and tarsals; flat bones include the ribs and the frontal bone; irregular bones include the vertebrae and bones of the pelvic girdle. The diaphysis is the shaft of the long bone. The epiphysis is an end of a long bone. Articular cartilage covers the end of the long bones. The endosteum lines the medullary cavity. The periosteum is the membrane surrounding the diaphysis.
24.2 Explain the functions of bones.	Bone functions include giving shape to body parts, protecting soft structures of the body, and assisting in movement. The red bone marrow is responsible for hematopoiesis. Bones also store calcium.

LEARNING OUTCOMES	KEY POINTS
24.3 Explain intramembranous and endochondral ossification.	Bones grow through the two types of ossification: intramembranous ossification and endochondral ossification. The cartilage plate between the diaphysis and the epiphysis allows for growth of the long bone.
24.4 Describe the skeletal structures and one location of each structure.	Skeletal structures include the following: condyles, crests, epicondyles, foramina, fossae, heads, processes, sutures, trochanters, tubercles, and tuberosities.
24.5 Locate the bones of the skull.	The major bones of the skull are the frontal, parietal, temporal, and occipital bones. The fontanels are the membranous structures that connect the incompletely developed cranial bones. Within the skull are the mastoid processes, sphenoid, ethmoid, and ear ossicles. The facial bones include the mandible, maxillae, zygomatics, nasal and palatine bones, and the vomer. Locations shown in Figures 24-6 and 24-7.
24.6 Locate the bones of the spinal column.	The spinal column includes cervical, thoracic, and lumbar vertebrae; the sacrum; and the coccyx. Locations shown in Figure 24-8.
24.7 Locate the bones of the rib cage.	There are 12 pairs of ribs, a sternum, and the xiphoid process. Locations shown in Figure 24-8.
24.8 Locate the bones of the shoulders, arms, and hands.	Each upper extremity includes the clavicle, scapula, humerus, radius, ulna, carpals, metacarpals, and phalanges. Locations shown in Figure 24-10.
24.9 Locate the bones of the hips, legs, and feet.	The bones of the hip, leg, and foot include the coxal bones, the femur, patella, tibia, fibula, metatarsals, tarsals, and phalanges. Locations shown in Figures 24-11 and 24-12.
24.10 Categorize the three major types of joints and give examples of each.	The three joint types are fibrous joints (for example, sutures of the skull), cartilaginous joints (for example, the joints between vertebrae), and synovial joints (for example, the elbow). A synovial joint consists of hyaline-covered bones held together by a fibrous joint capsule, which is lined by a synovial membrane that secretes synovial fluid. Ligaments hold the bones of these joints together.
24.11 Describe the common diseases and disorders of the skeletal system.	There are many common diseases and disorders of the bones and the skeletal system with varied signs, symptoms, and treatments. Examples include arthritis, bursitis, EFT, gout, kyphosis, lordosis, and scoliosis, as well as osteoporosis and osteosarcoma.

CASE STUDY CRITICAL THINKING

Recall John Miller from the beginning of the chapter. Now that you have completed the chapter, answer the following questions regarding his case.

1. Explain to John what bursitis is and what causes it.
2. What treatment might the doctor prescribe for John's bursitis?

1. (LO 24.1) The tiny canals of cancellous bone that allow for the spread of nutrients are called
   a. Lamella
   b. Lacunae
   c. Osteons
   d. Canaliculi
   e. Osteoblasts

2. (LO 24.3) Which substance is necessary for bone to absorb calcium?
   a. Vitamin C
   b. Phosporus
   c. Vitamin D
   d. Protein
   e. Carbohydrates

3. (LO 24.4) Articulation is another name for a
   a. Fossa
   b. Joint
   c. Foramen
   d. Suture
   e. Tubercle

4. (LO 24.5) Neck muscles attach to the skull via the _____ process.
   a. Mastoid
   b. Xiphoid
   c. Styloid
   d. Zygomatic
   e. Coracoid

5. (LO 24.9) The acetabulum is the
   a. Hip bone
   b. Knee joint
   c. Hip socket
   d. Shoulder bone
   e. Shoulder socket

6. (LO 24.11) A lateral curvature of the spine is known as
   a. Lordosis
   b. Kyphosis
   c. Osteoporosis
   d. Scoliosis
   e. Sarcoma

7. (LO 24.11) The medical term for brittle-bone disease is
   a. Ewing sarcoma family of tumors
   b. Osteogenesis imperfecta
   c. Rheumatoid arthritis
   d. Osteoporosis
   e. Paget's disease

8. (LO 24.1) Which of the following is the term for the shaft of a long bone?
   a. Spine
   b. Epiphysis
   c. Crest
   d. Periosteum
   e. Diaphysis

9. (LO 24.1) The bones of the rib cage are
   a. Long bones
   b. Flat bones
   c. Irregular bones
   d. Short bones
   e. Sesamoid bones

10. (LO 24.4) Which of the following is the term meaning an interlocking line of union between bones?
    a. Suture
    b. Condyle
    c. Process
    d. Articulation
    e. Fossa

Analyze the following medical terms, presented throughout the chapter. Using a medical dictionary (or Appendix I) place a / mark between each word part. Define each word part and then define the whole word.

EXAMPLE: mast/oid = mast means "breast" + oid means "resembling"
Mastoid means "resembling a breast." (A mastoid process resembles a breast.)

1. arthritis
2. bursitis
3. scoliosis
4. costal
5. coxal
6. metacarpophalangeal
7. metatarsophalangeal
8. osteoblast
9. osteoclast
10. osteocyte
11. osteoporosis
12. osteosarcoma
13. hematopoiesis
14. interphalangeal
15. intramembranous
16. synovial
17. tarsal
18. temporal

The Muscular System

PATIENT INFORMATION

Patient Name	Gender	DOB
Ken Washington	Male	12/1/19XX

Attending	MRN	Allergies
Paul F. Buckwalter, MD	891-12-743	Sulfa

Ken F. Washington, a 52-year-old male patient, has arrived for a follow-up visit from a recent hospitalization for a stroke. Until this hospitalization, he had no major health issues. However, he now has weakness in his left arm and his speech is difficult to understand. The physician has ordered a physical therapy evaluation and treatment as needed. The patient has been placed on an exercise regimen for his left-arm weakness.

Keep Ken in mind as you study this chapter. There will be questions at the end of the chapter based on the case study. The information in the chapter will help you answer these questions.

LEARNING OUTCOMES

After completing Chapter 25, you will be able to:

25.1 Describe the functions of muscle.
25.2 Compare the three types of muscle tissue including their locations and characteristics.
25.3 Explain how muscle tissue generates energy.
25.4 Describe the structure of a skeletal muscle.
25.5 Recognize the terms *origin* and *insertion*.
25.6 Identify the major skeletal muscles of the body, giving the action of each.
25.7 Summarize the changes that occur to the muscular system as a person ages.
25.8 Describe the causes, signs and symptoms, and treatments of various diseases and disorders of the muscular system.

KEY TERMS

acetylcholine
acetylcholinesterase
agonist
antagonist
aponeurosis
creatine phosphate
fascicle
insertion
lactic acid
multi-unit smooth muscle

myofibrils
origin
prime mover
sarcolemma
sarcoplasm
sarcoplasmic reticulum
sphincter
striations
synergist
visceral smooth muscle

Introduction

Your bones and joints do not produce movement all by themselves. Instead, your muscles—by alternating between contraction and relaxation—cause your bones and supported structures to move. The human body has more than 600 individual muscles. Although each muscle is a distinct structure, muscles act in groups to perform particular movements. In this chapter, you will explore the differences among three muscle tissue types, the structure of skeletal muscles, muscle actions, and the names of skeletal muscles.

Functions of Muscle   LO 25.1

Muscle tissue is unique because it has the ability to contract. This contraction allows muscles to perform various functions. In addition to allowing the human body to move, muscles provide stability, control body openings and passages, and warm the body.

Movement

Skeletal muscles are attached to bones by tendons. Because skeletal muscles cross joints, when these muscles contract, the bones they attach to move. This allows for various body motions, like walking or waving your hand. Facial muscles are attached to the skin of the face; when they contract, different facial expressions are produced, such as smiling or frowning. Smooth muscle is found in the walls of various organs, like the stomach, intestines, and uterus. The contraction of smooth muscle in these organs produces the movement of their contents, such as the movement of food material through the intestine or the birth of a child being pushed from the mother's uterus. Cardiac muscle of the heart produces the atrial and ventricular contractions that pump blood into the blood vessels.

Go to CONNECT to see an animation about *Muscle Contraction.*

Stability

You rarely think about it, but muscles are holding your bones tightly together so your joints remain stable. There are also very small muscles holding your vertebrae together to stabilize your spinal column.

Heat Production

When muscles contract, heat is released, which helps the body maintain a normal temperature. This is why moving your body—say, jogging in place for a few seconds—can make you warmer if you are cold.

Control of Body Openings and Passages

In addition to providing important structural support for your bones and joints, muscles also form valve-like structures called **sphincters** around various body openings and passages. These sphincters control the movement of substances into and out of these passages. For example, a urethral sphincter prevents urination until you relax it to permit urination.

Types of Muscle Tissue   LO 25.2

There are three types of muscle tissue: skeletal, smooth, and cardiac. Study Table 25-1 to review their locations and features.

Muscle cells or myocytes are called muscle fibers because of their long lengths. The cell membrane of a muscle fiber is called a **sarcolemma.** The cytoplasm of this cell type is called **sarcoplasm,** and the endoplasmic reticulum is called **sarcoplasmic reticulum.** Most of the sarcoplasm is filled with long structures called **myofibrils.** The arrangement of filaments in myofibrils produce the **striations**—stripes—observed in skeletal and cardiac muscle cells. Motor neurons, which release neurotransmitters onto the fibers, control muscle fibers. See Figure 25-1 for an illustration of the structure of a skeletal muscle.

TABLE 25-1	Types of Muscle Tissue					
Muscle Group	**Major Location**	**Major Function**	**Striated (Yes/No)**	**Mode of Control**	**Rate of Contraction**	**Intercalated Discs**
Skeletal muscle	Attached to bones and the skin of the face	Produces body movements and facial expressions	Yes	Voluntary	Fast to contract and relax	No
Smooth muscle	Walls of hollow organs, blood vessels, and iris	Moves contents through organs; vasoconstriction	No	Involuntary	Slow to contract and relax	No
Cardiac muscle	Wall of the heart	Pumps blood through heart	Yes	Involuntary	Groups of muscle fibers contract as a unit	Yes

Skeletal Muscle

Skeletal muscle fibers respond only to the neurotransmitter **acetylcholine,** which causes skeletal muscle to contract. Once contraction has occurred, skeletal muscles release an enzyme called **acetylcholinesterase,** which breaks down acetylcholine. This allows the muscle to relax.

Smooth Muscle

There are two types of smooth muscle: multi-unit and visceral. **Multi-unit smooth muscle** is found in the iris of the eye and the walls of blood vessels. This muscle type contracts in response to neurotransmitters and hormones. **Visceral smooth muscle** contains sheets of muscle cells that closely contact each other. It is found in the walls of hollow organs like the stomach, intestines, bladder, and uterus. Muscle fibers in visceral smooth muscle respond to neurotransmitters, but they also stimulate each other to contract; so, the muscle fibers tend to contract and relax together. This type of muscle produces an action called peristalsis. *Peristalsis* is a rhythmic contraction that pushes substances through tubes of the body, such as in the lower two-thirds of the esophagus, where peristalsis moves the food bolus, or in the Fallopian tubes, where these muscle movements propel the ovum or egg through the tubes to the uterus.

Two neurotransmitters are involved in smooth muscle contraction—acetylcholine and norepinephrine. Depending on the smooth muscle type, these neurotransmitters cause or inhibit contractions.

Cardiac Muscle

Groups of cardiac muscle are connected to each other through *intercalated discs*—discs with tunnels that physically connect the cardiac muscle cells. These discs allow the fibers in each

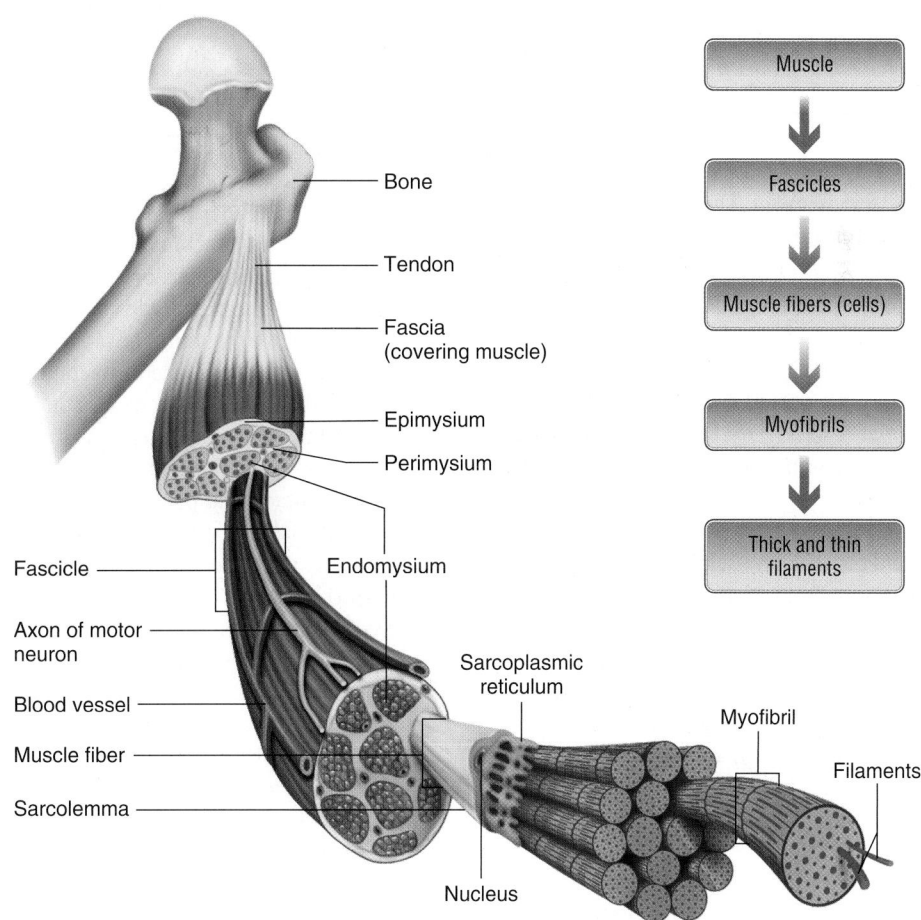

FIGURE 25-1   Structure of a skeletal muscle.

group to contract and relax together—a design that allows the heart to work as a pump. First, the atria (holding chambers) contract and relax together, then the ventricles (pumping chambers) contract to send blood to the lungs and body, after which they relax and the cycle starts again. Cardiac muscle is also self-exciting, which means that it does not need nerve stimulation to contract. Nerves only speed up or slow down the contraction of the heart. Like smooth muscle, cardiac muscle responds to two neurotransmitters—acetylcholine and norepinephrine. Acetylcholine slows the heart rate, and norepinephrine speeds it up.

Production of Energy for Muscle   LO 25.3

Because a lot of ATP (adenosine triphosphate)—a type of chemical energy—is needed for sustained or repeated muscle contractions, a muscle cell must have multiple ways to store or make this substance. So, muscle cells make this energy in three ways:

* **Creatine phosphate** production. Creatine phosphate production is a rapid way for a muscle to produce energy. When ATP is used during muscle contraction, it loses a phosphate and, therefore, energy. Imagine a desk toy that has five ball bearings suspended by strings. You create potential energy by lifting one of the ball bearings away from the others. When you release the ball bearing—breaking the bond between your fingers and the ball—the potential energy is released and the ball bearing hits the others, causing them to swing back and forth for several minutes. As with the ball bearing, energy stored in the phosphate bond is released when the bond is broken. Creatine phosphate "donates" a phosphate group, restoring energy potential.

* *Aerobic respiration*—an energy-forming biochemical process that requires oxygen—uses the body's store of glucose to make ATP. A cell breaks down glucose into pyruvic acid using oxygen (hence the term *aerobic*). The pyruvic acid is further converted into acetyl coenzyme A, which begins a series of reactions known as the *Krebs cycle* or the citric acid cycle. The oxygen needed for this method is stored in the muscle pigment called *myoglobin*, which also gives muscle its pinkish color.

* **Lactic acid** production occurs when a cell is low in oxygen and must convert pyruvic acid to lactic acid. This conversion produces a small amount of ATP for the cell, but because lactic acid is a waste product, it must then be released from the cell.

Oxygen Debt

Oxygen debt occurs when skeletal muscle is used strenuously for several minutes. When pyruvic acid is converted to lactic acid for energy production, the lactic acid builds up and causes muscle fatigue. The lactic acid is brought to the liver via the bloodstream to be converted back into glucose, which requires more energy. The amount of oxygen the liver cells need to make enough ATP for this conversion results in the oxygen debt. This process explains why your body still burns energy even after you are done exercising.

Muscle Fatigue

Muscle fatigue is a condition in which a muscle has lost its ability to contract. It usually develops because of an accumulation of lactic acid. It can also occur if the blood supply to a muscle is interrupted or if a motor neuron loses its ability to release acetylcholine onto muscle fibers. Cramps—painful, involuntary contractions of muscles—can accompany muscle fatigue. For this reason, if you have just finished an intense workout, it is important to replenish your electrolytes by drinking fluids and eating foods that are good sources of sodium, potassium, and calcium.

Structure of Skeletal Muscles   LO 25.4

Skeletal muscles are the major organs that make up the muscular system. A skeletal muscle consists of connective tissues, skeletal muscle tissue, blood vessels, and nerves. When you see marbling in a steak, you are actually viewing connective tissues. The red portion of the steak is the muscle tissue.

The following connective tissue coverings are associated with skeletal muscles (see Figure 25-1):

* *Fascia*. This structure covers entire skeletal muscles and separates them from each other.
* *Tendon*. This tough, cord-like structure is made of fibrous connective tissue that connects muscles to bones.
* **Aponeurosis.** This tough, sheet-like structure is made of fibrous connective tissue. It typically attaches muscles to other muscles.
* *Epimysium*. This tissue is a thin covering that is just deep to the fascia of a muscle. It surrounds the entire muscle.
* *Perimysium*. This connective tissue divides a muscle into sections called **fascicles.**
* *Endomysium*. This covering of connective tissue surrounds individual muscle cells.

Attachments and Actions of Skeletal Muscles   LO 25.5

The two types of attachments for skeletal muscles are known as origins and insertions. An **origin** is an attachment site for the less movable bone during muscle contraction. An **insertion** is an attachment site for the more movable bone during muscle contraction. For example, the biceps brachii (the muscle on the anterior upper arm) attaches to two places on the scapula and to one site on the radius. When the biceps brachii contracts, the radius moves and the arm bends at the elbow. So, the origin of the biceps brachii is where it attaches to the scapula. The insertion site of the biceps brachii is its attachment site on the radius (see Figure 25-2).

Most of the time, body movement is not produced by only one muscle, but by a group of muscles. However, one muscle is responsible for most of the movement; this muscle is called the **prime mover** or **agonist.** Other muscles help the prime mover by stabilizing joints; these muscles are called **synergists.** An **antagonist** is a muscle that produces a movement opposite to the prime mover. When the prime mover contracts, the antagonist must relax in order to produce a smooth body movement. For example, when you bend your arm at the elbow, the prime mover (agonist) is the biceps brachii. The synergist muscles are the brachialis and brachioradialis. The antagonist is the triceps brachii because its action is to extend the arm at the elbow. While the prime mover and synergists contract, the agonist relaxes; when the antagonist contracts, the prime mover and synergists relax.

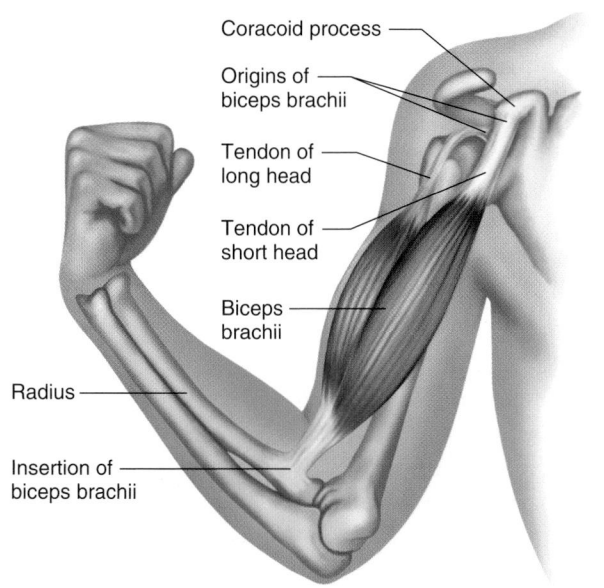

FIGURE 25-2   Origins and insertion of biceps brachii.

The body movements produced by skeletal muscles include the following:

- *Flexion*—bending a body part or decreasing the angle of a joint
- *Extension*—straightening a body part or increasing the angle of a joint
- *Hyperextension*—extending a body part past the normal anatomical position

- *Dorsiflexion*—pointing the toes up
- *Plantar flexion*—pointing the toes down
- *Abduction*—moving a body part away from the midline of the body
- *Adduction*—moving a body part toward the midline of the body
- *Rotation*—twisting a body part—for example, turning your head from side to side
- *Circumduction*—moving a body part in a circle—for example, moving your arm in a circular motion
- *Pronation*—turning the palm of the hand down or lying face down
- *Supination*—turning the palm of the hand up or lying face up
- *Inversion*—turning the sole of the foot medially
- *Eversion*—turning the sole of the foot laterally
- *Retraction*—moving a body part posteriorly
- *Protraction*—moving a body part anteriorly
- *Elevation*—lifting a body part—for example, elevating your shoulders as in a shrugging gesture
- *Depression*—lowering a body part—for example, lowering your shoulders

See Figures 25-3, 25-4, and 25-5 for illustrations of these types of movements. As a medical assistant, it is important to understand these movements so you can assist with judging and measuring your patients' ability to perform range of motion (ROM) exercises when assessing injuries and illnesses.

FIGURE 25-3   Adduction, abduction, dorsiflexion, plantar flexion, hyperextension, extension, and flexion.

FIGURE 25-4   Rotation, circumduction, supination, and pronation.

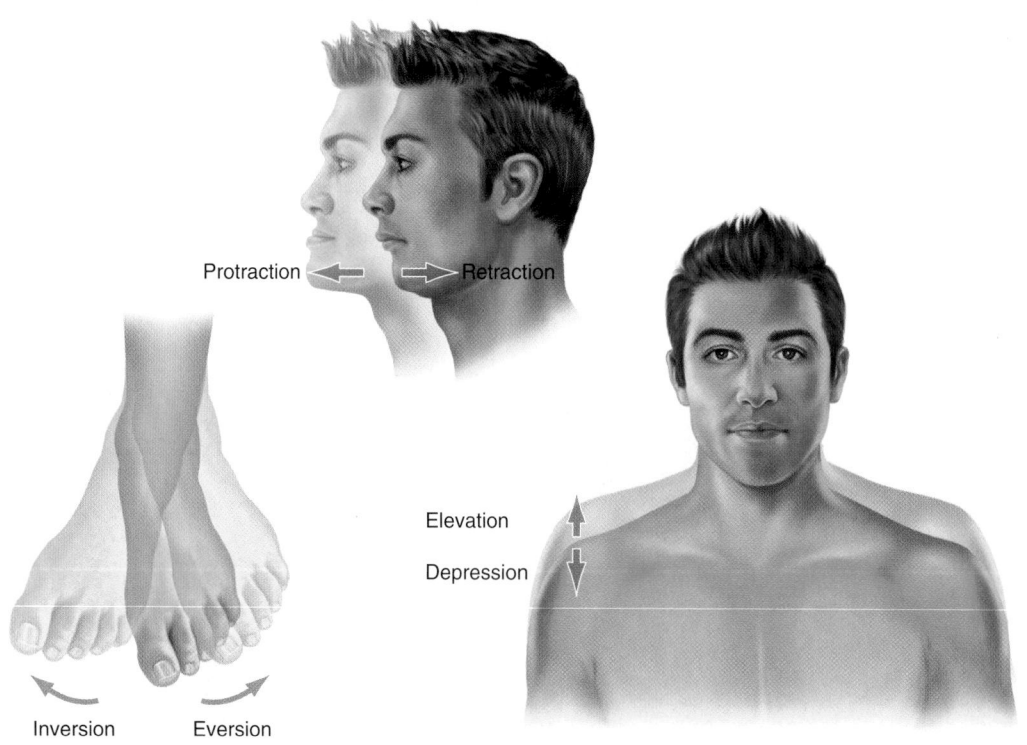

FIGURE 25-5   Eversion, inversion, protraction, retraction, elevation, and depression.

▶ Major Skeletal Muscles

LO 25.6

The name of a skeletal muscle often describes it in some way. Usually, the name indicates the location, size, action, shape, or number of attachments of the muscle. For example, the pectoralis major is named for its large size (major) and its location (pectoral, or chest, region). The sternocleidomastoid is named for its attachment sites—*sterno* (sternum), *cleido* (clavicle), and *mastoid* (the mastoid process of the temporal bone, located behind the ear). As you study muscles, you will find it easier to remember them if you think about what the name describes.

Muscles of the Head

The muscles of the head include those that move the head, provide facial expression, and move the jaw. See Figures 25-6 and 25-7 for illustrations of the various muscles. Muscles that move the head include the following, and hints to assist you with remembering the locations for some of these muscles are provided in parentheses:

- Sternocleidomastoid. This muscle pulls the head to one side and also pulls the head to the chest. (sterno = sternum, cleido = clavicle, mastoid = mastoid)

- Splenius capitis. This muscle rotates the head and allows it to bend to the side. (capit = head)

Muscles of facial expression include the following:

- Frontalis. This muscle raises the eyebrows. (frontal = pertaining to the front)

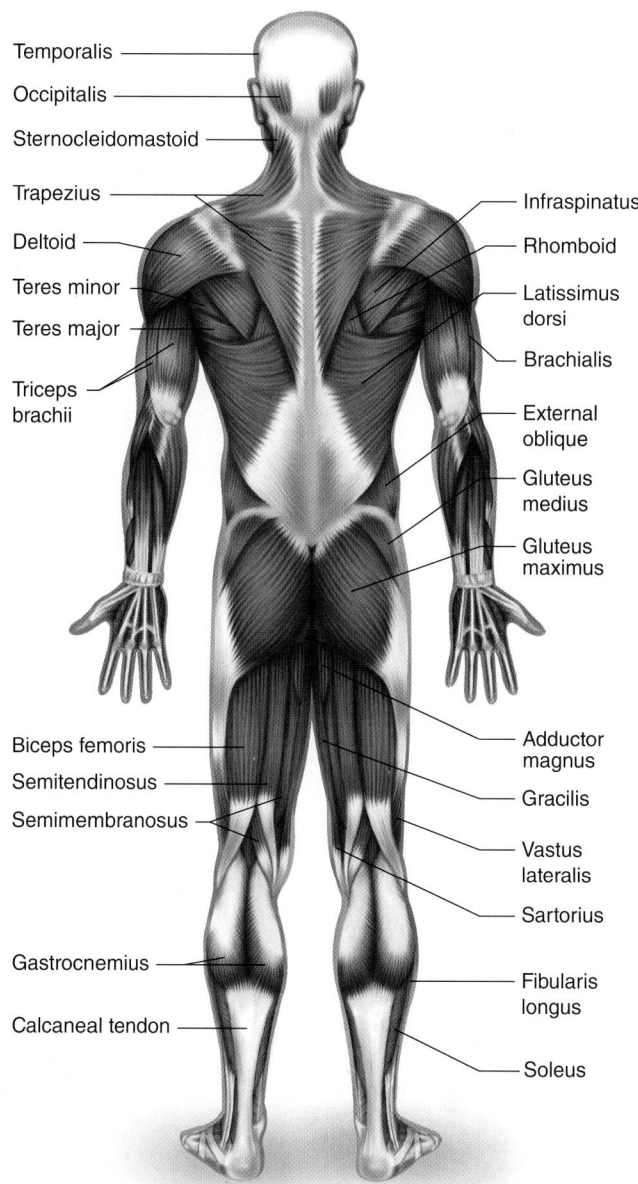

FIGURE 25-7 Posterior view of superficial skeletal muscles.

- Orbicularis oris. This muscle allows the lips to pucker. (oris = oro or mouth)
- Orbicularis oculi. This muscle allows the eyes to close. (oculi = eye)
- Zygomaticus. This muscle pulls the corners of the mouth up. (zygomat = cheekbone)
- Platysma. This muscle pulls the corners of the mouth down.

The muscles of the jaw allow for mastication (chewing) and include the following:

- Masseter and temporalis. These muscles close the jaw. (masseter as in mastication or chewing; temporo = temple)
- Internal and external pterygoids. These muscles help position the jaw.
- Sternohyomastoid. This muscle opens the jaw. (hyo = hyoid bone)

FIGURE 25-6 Anterior view of superficial skeletal muscles.

(a)

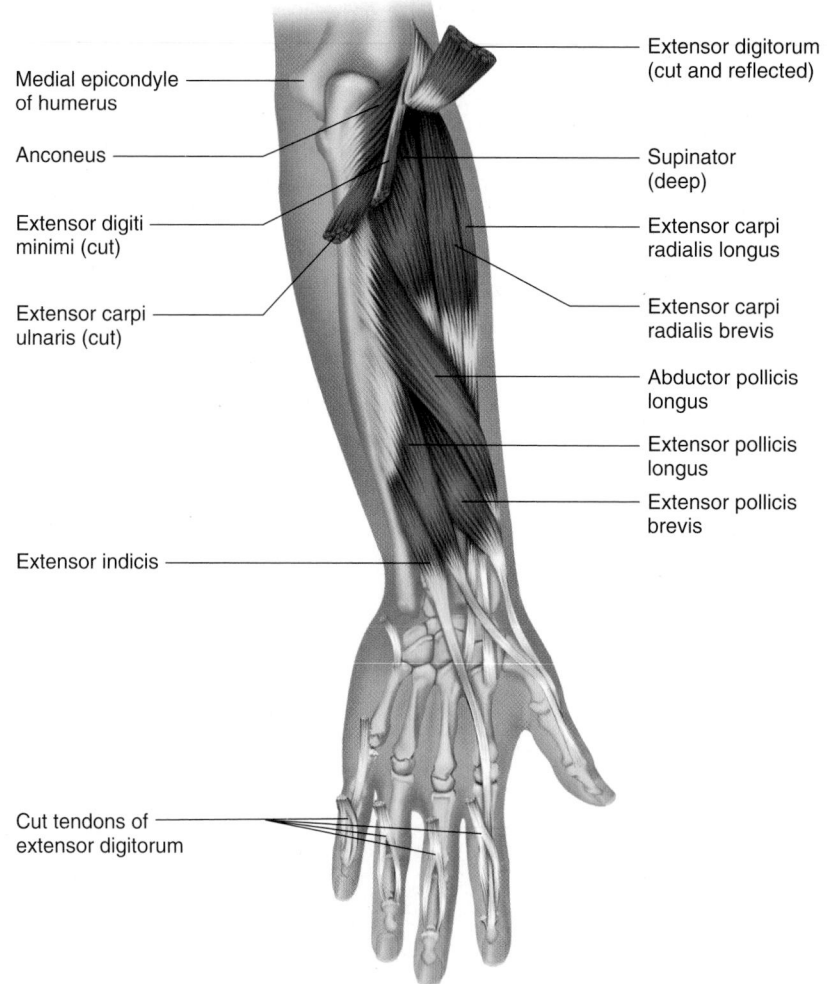

(b)

FIGURE 25-8   Muscles of the (a) anterior and (b) posterior forearm.

Arm Muscles

Muscles that move the arm include muscles of the arm and forearm (see Figures 25-6, 25-7, and 25-8). These muscles include:

- Pectoralis major. This muscle pulls the arm across the chest; it also rotates and adducts the arms. (pectoro = chest)
- Latissimus dorsi. This muscle acts to extend, adduct, and rotate the arm inwardly. (latissimus = butterfly, dorsi = back)
- Deltoid. This muscle acts to abduct and extend the arm at the shoulder.
- Subscapularis. This muscle rotates the arm medially. (sub = below, scapulo = shoulder blade)
- Infraspinatus. This muscle rotates the arm laterally. (infra = below, spinat = spine)

Muscles that move the forearm include the following:

- Biceps brachii. This muscle flexes the arm at the elbow and rotates the hand laterally. (bi = two, ceps = insertion, brachii = arm)
- Brachialis. This muscle flexes the arm at the elbow. (brachii = arm)
- Brachioradialis. This muscle flexes the forearm at the elbow. (brachii = arm, radio = radius)
- Triceps brachii. This muscle extends the arm at the elbow. (tri = three, ceps = insertion, brachii = arm)
- Supinator. This muscle rotates the forearm laterally (supination). (supine = palm up)
- Pronator teres. This muscle rotates the forearm medially (pronation). (prone = palm down)

Muscles of the Wrist, Hand, and Fingers

Muscles that move the wrist, hand, and fingers can be seen in Figures 25-6, 25-7, and 25-8. These muscles include the following:

- Flexor carpi radialis and flexor carpi ulnaris. These muscles flex and abduct the wrist. (radio = radius, ulna = ulna)
- Palmaris longus. This muscle flexes the wrist.
- Flexor digitorum profundus. This muscle flexes the distal joints of the fingers but not the thumb. (digits = fingers)
- Extensor carpi radialis longus and brevis. These muscles extend the wrist and abduct the hand. (carpo = wrist, radio = radius, long = long, brev = brief or short)
- Extensor carpi ulnaris. This muscle extends the wrist. (carpo = wrist, ulna = ulna)
- Extensor digitorum. This muscle extends the fingers but not the thumb. (digit = finger)

Respiratory Muscles

The muscles of respiration—breathing—include the following:

- Diaphragm. This muscle separates the thoracic cavity from the abdominal cavity; its contraction causes inspiration—breathing in.

- External and internal intercostals. The contractions of these muscles expands and then lowers the ribs during breathing. See Figure 25-9 on the next page for an illustration of the internal intercostal muscle. (inter = between, costo = rib)

Abdominal Muscles

The muscles of the abdominal wall include the following:

- External and internal obliques. These muscles compress the abdominal wall. (oblique = diagonal)
- Transverse abdominis. This muscle also compresses the abdominal wall. (transverse = across)
- Rectus abdominis. This muscle acts to flex the vertebral column and compress the abdominal wall. (rectus = erect)

See Figures 25-6, 25-7, and 25-9 for illustrations of these muscles.

Muscles of the Pectoral Girdle

The muscles that move the pectoral girdle (shoulder) include the following:

- Trapezius. This muscle raises the arms and pulls the shoulders downward. (trapezius = trapezoid)
- Pectoralis minor. This muscle pulls the scapula downward and raises the ribs. (pectoro = chest, minor = smaller)

See Figures 25-6, 25-7, and 25-9 for illustrations of these muscles.

Leg Muscles

The leg muscles include muscles of the thigh and lower leg (see Figures 25-6 and 25-7). Muscles that move the thigh include the following:

- Iliopsoas major. This muscle flexes the thigh.
- Gluteus maximus. This muscle extends the thigh.
- Gluteus medius and minimus. These muscles abduct the thighs and rotate them medially.
- Adductor longus and magnus. These muscles adduct the thighs and rotate them laterally. (adduct = toward the midline)
- Biceps femoris, semitendinosus, and semimembranosus. These three muscles are known as the *hamstring group*. They act to flex the leg at the knee and extend the leg at the thigh.
- Rectus femoris, vastus lateralis, vastus medialis, and vastus intermedius. These four muscles are known as the *quadriceps group;* they act to extend the leg at the knee.
- Sartorius. This muscle flexes the leg at the knee and thigh. It also abducts the thigh, rotating the thigh laterally but rotating the lower leg medially; it carries out the act of sitting cross-legged.

Muscles of the Ankle, Foot, and Toes

Muscles that move the ankle, foot, and toes include the following:

- Tibialis anterior. This muscle inverts the foot and points the foot up (dorsiflexion).
- Extensor digitorum longus. This muscle extends the toes and points the foot up.

FIGURE 25-9 Muscles of the anterior chest and abdominal wall.

CAUTION: HANDLE WITH CARE

Muscle Strains and Sprains

Strains are injuries that excessively stretch muscles or tendons. Sprains are more serious injuries that consist of tears to tendons, ligaments, and/or the cartilage of joints. You can teach patients to prevent these types of injuries by doing the following:

- Warm up. Warming up muscles for just a few minutes before an intense activity raises muscle temperature. This increase in temperature prevents injuries by making muscle tissue more pliable.

- Stretch. Stretching improves muscle performance and should always be done after the warm-up or after exercising. A person should never stretch further than he can hold for 10 seconds.

- Cool down. Slowing down the exercise before completely stopping prevents dizziness and fainting. If a person suddenly stops exercising, blood can pool in the legs and is prevented from reaching the brain. Cooling down also helps to remove lactic acid from muscles.

If sprains or strains do occur, immediate RICE treatment is recommended:

- R is for rest. Resting minimizes bleeding, further injury, and swelling. Sometimes a splint, sling, or crutches may be needed.

- I is for ice. Ice minimizes swelling and pain. A bag filled with crushed ice conforms better to a body part than one filled with ice cubes. A bag full of frozen peas or other small vegetables can also be used. The ice should be applied for 10 minutes and then removed for 10 minutes. This should be kept up for about an hour and repeated several times during a 48-hour period.

- C is for compression, which minimizes swelling. A bandage should be loosely wrapped around the injured area and the bag of ice. Compression should be applied and removed along with the ice.

- E is for elevation. The injured muscle should be elevated, which minimizes swelling, and elevation should be continued as long as swelling is present.

If the patient does not think his or her symptoms have improved in several days to a week, a physician should be contacted to rule out a more serious injury, such as a torn ligament or muscle, or even a bone fracture.

- Gastrocnemius. This muscle flexes the foot and flexes the leg at the knee. It is more commonly referred to as the calf muscle.
- Soleus. This muscle also flexes the foot.
- Flexor digitorum longus. This muscle flexes the foot and toes.

See Figures 25-6 and 25-7 for illustrations of these muscles.

▶ Aging and the Musculoskeletal System

LO 25.7

Although the aging of the skeletal system causes more obvious difficulties for patients with diseases and conditions like arthritis, fractures, and osteoporosis, muscular decline often goes hand-in-hand with these changes. Aging causes a decline in the speed and strength of muscle contractions even though the actual endurance of muscle fibers changes very little. Elderly patients often have increasing difficulty with dexterity and gripping ability. Mobility may decrease related to the combined decline of the musculoskeletal system. The patient's diet and exercise history, as well as family history, also have a direct impact on the patient's mobility and activity level as he or she ages.

Assistive devices like railings, tub and shower seats, and gripping devices can assist patients who are experiencing difficulties. Exercise routines, particularly pool exercises like swimming and physical therapy, are often helpful in maintaining strength and mobility.

PATHOPHYSIOLOGY

LO 25.8

Common Diseases and Disorders of the Muscular System

BOTULISM is usually thought of as a disease that affects the gastrointestinal tract, but it can also affect various muscle groups. This disease most commonly affects infants. Although a person can survive this disease, its effects may be long-lasting.

Causes. This disease is a rare but serious disorder caused by the bacterium *Clostridium botulinum*, which normally lives in soil and water. If this bacterium gets on food, it produces a toxin that can lead to a type of food poisoning. The foods most likely to contain *Clostridium botulinum* are canned vegetables, cured pork, raw fish, honey, and corn syrup. A person can also acquire this bacterium through improperly cleaned open wounds.

Signs and Symptoms. This disease causes many symptoms, including dysphagia (difficulty swallowing), paralysis, muscle weakness, nausea and vomiting, abdominal cramps, double vision, dyspnea (difficulty breathing), poor feeding and suckling in infants, the inability to urinate, the absence of reflexes, and constipation. The signs and symptoms usually appear 8 to 40 hours after the toxin is ingested. The diagnosis is usually made by either a blood test to identify the toxin or an analysis of the suspected food.

Treatment. Treatment includes emergency hospitalization, intubation—inserting a tube into the upper airway to open airways—mechanical ventilation if respiratory muscles are impaired, intravenous fluids or nasogastric (through nose to stomach) feeding if swallowing is impaired, and the administration of an antitoxin.

Prevention Tips. You can instruct patients to prevent botulism by observing the following guidelines:

- Never give honey or corn syrup to infants.
- Sterilize home-canned food containers properly (250°F for 35 minutes).
- Do not use foods from bent or bulging cans.
- Never eat foods that smell as if they may have spoiled.
- Cook and store foods properly.

FIBROMYALGIA is a fairly common condition that results in chronic pain primarily in joints, muscles, and tendons. It most ordinarily affects women between the ages of 20 and 50.

Causes. The causes of this disorder are poorly understood. Fibromyalgia may be caused or exacerbated by sleep disturbance, emotional distress, decreased blood flow to muscles, a virus, or any combination of these factors.

Signs and Symptoms Symptoms include fatigue, tenderness in different areas of the body, sleep disturbances, and chronic facial pain. The diagnosis is usually made by ruling out other possible diseases. It is not normally diagnosed unless a person has muscle and joint pain for at least 3 months in certain body areas.

Treatment. Treatment is varied and includes antidepressants, anti-inflammatory medications, physical therapy, lifestyle changes to reduce stress, counseling to improve coping skills, reduction or elimination of caffeine to improve sleeping, and diet supplements to improve nutrition.

MUSCULAR DYSTROPHY (MD) is a group of inherited disorders characterized by muscle weakness and a loss of muscle tissue. There are at least seven types of muscular dystrophy, and they are distinguished from each other by types of symptoms, the age at when symptoms appeared, and the cause.

Causes. The causes of this disorder are primarily hereditary. Genetic fetal testing is available.

Signs and Symptoms. The signs and symptoms vary widely and depend on the type of muscular dystrophy. The symptoms of Duchenne muscular dystrophy—the most common and widely known type—progress steadily and are eventually fatal. Other types cause mild symptoms, and patients usually have normal life expectancies. Specific signs and symptoms include: muscle weakness in various muscle groups, depending on the type of dystrophy; difficulty walking; drooling; a delayed development of motor skills; frequent falls; mental retardation in some types; a curved spine; the formation of a claw hand or clubfoot; a loss of muscle mass; the accumulation of fat or fibrous connective tissue in muscles; and arrhythmias (irregular heart rhythms) in some types. The progression of the muscular weakness may also include eventual paralysis of the affected muscle groups. The diagnosis is primarily made through a muscle biopsy. Other tests include deoxyribonucleic acid (DNA) testing; an EMG (electromyography) test, which tests muscle weakness; or an ECG (electrocardiogram), which tests cardiac function.

Treatment. Treatment includes physical therapy to maintain muscle function, the use of braces and wheelchairs, various medications based on the type of MD, and spinal surgery.

MYASTHENIA GRAVIS is a condition in which affected people experience muscle weakness. In this autoimmune condition, a person produces antibodies that prevent muscles from receiving neurotransmitters from neurons. It most commonly affects young women and older men, especially if they have other autoimmune disorders.

Causes. This disease is usually considered an autoimmune disorder.

Signs and Symptoms. The signs and symptoms usually get better with rest and worsen with activity. They include double vision; muscle weakness; dysphagia (difficulty swallowing); difficulty talking, chewing, lifting, or walking; fatigue; drooling; and difficulty breathing. The diagnosis may be difficult, but a single-fiber EMG test is often useful. This test measures the response of a muscle fiber to nervous stimulation. Other tests include acetylcholine receptor antibody tests and the Tensilon® test. In a positive Tensilon test, muscle activity increases after medication is given that blocks the breakdown of acetylcholine.

Treatment. Treatments include lifestyle changes to avoid excessive stress, getting adequate rest and heat, the use of an eye patch to treat double vision, medications to improve communication between nerves and muscles, medications to suppress the immune system, plasma-pheresis to remove harmful antibodies from blood, and removal of the thymus.

RHABDOMYOLYSIS is a condition in which the kidneys have been damaged in relation to serious muscle injuries.

Causes. Kidneys become damaged because of toxins released from muscle cells. When muscles are damaged, excessive amounts of the pigment myoglobin are released, which is then broken down into harmful chemicals. Muscles are most often damaged through trauma; excessive use (for example, marathon running); overdoses of cocaine, heroin, and other drugs; alcoholism; and a blockage of the blood supply to the muscles.

Signs and Symptoms. Symptoms include dark urine, muscle tenderness, muscle weakness, muscle stiffness, seizures, joint pain, and fatigue. The diagnosis includes urinalysis for the presence of myoglobin, creatine phosphokinase (CPK), and creatinine; blood is also tested for the presence of myoglobin, CPK, or high levels of potassium. CPK is an enzyme released into the blood when muscles are damaged. Creatinine is a protein released by the breakdown of muscle tissue.

Treatment. Treatment includes hydration to rapidly eliminate toxins from the kidneys, diuretics to help flush toxins from the body, medications to flush excess potassium from the body, and therapy for kidney failure.

TENDONITIS is described as the painful inflammation of a tendon as well as of the tendon-muscle attachment to a bone. The most common locations for tendonitis are the shoulder, hip, heel, and hamstrings. Tendonitis may also be associated with bursitis, the inflammation of the bursa located in synovial joints like the shoulder, elbow, and knee.

Causes. Tendonitis usually occurs after a sports-related activity that results in injury to the muscle tendon or tendon-to-bone attachment. Other musculoskeletal disorders may also cause or exacerbate this condition.

Signs and Symptoms. These include pain at the joint or muscle attachment that results in limited range of motion (ROM) of the affected area.

Treatment. For the initial injury, using ice for the first 12 to 24 hours will minimize inflammation. After this initial time period, applying heat will help with joint and muscle pain. If calcium deposits are found in the tendon, which can be confirmed by X-ray, heat will aggravate the condition, whereas continued use of ice packs will help to relieve the discomfort. Resting the affected area and taking oral analgesics will also help control pain.

TETANUS is commonly called lockjaw. This disease has a high mortality rate, especially in infants. Immediate treatment is necessary to prevent death or long-lasting effects. However, tetanus is completely preventable through regular vaccinations.

Causes. A toxin produced by the bacterium *Clostridium tetani*, which lives naturally in soil and water, causes this disease. People most commonly acquire this bacterium through open wounds caused by objects contaminated with soil.

Signs and Symptoms. Symptoms usually appear between 5 and 10 days after infection. Muscle spasms in the jaw, neck, and facial muscles are usually the first signs. Other signs and symptoms include worsening of the muscle spasms that spread to other body locations and may cause bone fractures, dyspnea (breathing difficulties), irritability, fever, profuse sweating, and drooling. The diagnosis is usually based on the type of wound and the characteristic signs and symptoms of the disease. Tetanus antibody tests can also be used in diagnosis, but cultures of the wound site often produce false-negative findings.

Treatment. Administering antitoxin and antibiotics is a key treatment. Others include wound cleaning, muscle relaxants, sedation, and bed rest. The insertion of an endotracheal tube and mechanical ventilation may be needed for patients with severe breathing difficulties.

TORTICOLLIS is also known as wry neck. This disease is a cervical deformity in which the head bends toward the affected side while the chin rotates to the opposite side.

Causes. Torticollis may be acquired or congenital. It is caused by spasm or shortening of the sternocleidomastoid muscle. Breech or other difficult birth is often the cause of the congenital form as a result of the previously noted malpositioning, or from injury or scar tissue from ruptured muscle fibers before or during the birth process. The acquired form is the result of underlying disease, cervical spine injury, or chronic muscle spasms.

Signs and Symptoms. There is obvious malpositioning of the head and neck in an affected individual.

Treatment. For the congenital form, passive exercises to stretch the muscles as well as corrected head positioning during sleep (to maintain the straightening accomplished through the exercises) may be helpful. The treatment for acquired torticollis should consist of treating the underlying disease if possible. Otherwise, heat, cervical traction, a neck brace, exercise, massage, and psychotherapy to help the patient deal with the psychological and emotional effects related to the deformity are all treatment options.

TRICHINOSIS is an infection caused by parasites (worms).

Causes. This disease is caused by worms that are usually ingested by eating undercooked meat. Once ingested, the worms can leave the digestive tract and infect skeletal muscles, the heart, the lungs, and the brain. This disease is preventable by not eating wild animal meat. Proper cooking will also prevent trichinosis. There is no cure for this disease once the worms leave the digestive tract and infect other tissues.

Signs and Symptoms. Common symptoms include abdominal pain, diarrhea, muscle pain, fever, and pneumonia. In more serious cases, arrhythmias, heart failure, and encephalitis (swelling of the brain) can result. The diagnosis is usually based on the symptoms, a blood test to determine if there is an increase in eosinophils (white blood cells) in blood, or a muscle biopsy that reveals the presence of the worms.

Treatment. Patients with this disease are treated with medications to kill worms in the digestive tract and with anti-inflammatory drugs to reduce muscle pain and swelling.

SUMMARY OF LEARNING OUTCOMES

LEARNING OUTCOMES	KEY POINTS
25.1 Describe the functions of muscle.	The functions of muscles include movement, stability, control of body openings and passages, and the production of heat. Valve-like muscular structures called sphincters control passage of substances into and out of organs like the stomach and bladder.
25.2 Compare the three types of muscle tissue including their locations and characteristics.	The three types of muscle tissue are striated, voluntary skeletal muscle; smooth, involuntary visceral muscle; and specialized striated and involuntary cardiac muscle.
25.3 Explain how muscle tissue generates energy.	There are three ways muscles create energy. Creatine phosphate is a rapid method for muscles to create energy; aerobic respiration uses stored glucose to produce ATP in the Krebs cycle; and lactic acid production occurs when a cell is low in oxygen and converts pyruvic acid to lactic acid.
25.4 Describe the structure of a skeletal muscle.	Skeletal muscle is composed of connective tissues, skeletal muscle tissue, blood vessels, and nerves. The coverings of skeletal muscles include fascia, tendon, aponeurosis, epimysium, perimysium, and endomysium.
25.5 Recognize the terms *origin* and *insertion*.	The origin of a muscle is the attachment site of the muscle to the less movable bone during muscle contraction. The insertion of a muscle is the attachment site for the muscle to the more movable bone during muscle contraction.

25.6 Identify the major skeletal muscles of the body, giving the action of each.	The major muscles of the head are sternocleidomastoid, splenius capitis, frontalis, orbicularis oris and oculi, zygomaticus, platysma, masseter, and temporalis. The upper extremity muscles include pectoralis major, latissimus dorsi, deltoid, subscapularis, infraspinatus, biceps brachii, brachialis, brachioradialis, triceps brachii, supinator, pronator teres, flexor carpi radialis and ulnaris, plamaris longus, flexor digitorum profundus, extensor carpi radialis longus and brevis, extensor carpi ulnaris, and extensor digitorum. The major respiratory muscles are the diaphragm and the external and internal intercostals. The abdominal muscles include external and internal obliques, transverse abdominis, and rectus abdominis. The pectoral girdle muscles include trapezius and pectoralis minor. The muscles of the lower extremity include iliopsoas major; gluteus maximus, medius, and minimus; adductor longus and magnus; biceps femoris; semitendinosus and semimembranosus; rectus femoris; vastus lateralis, medialis, and intermedius; sartorius; tibialis anterior; extensor digitorum longus; gastrocnemius; soleus; and flexor digitorum longus.
25.7 Summarize the changes that occur to the muscular system as a person ages.	The common diseases of aging include arthritis, fractures, osteoporosis, and muscular decline. Aging causes a decline in strength and speed of muscle contractions. Dexterity and gripping abilities lessen and mobility often decreases related to skeletal and muscular decline.
25.8 Describe the causes, signs and symptoms, and treatments of various diseases and disorders of the muscular system.	There are many common diseases and disorders of the muscular system with varied signs, symptoms, and treatments. Some of these include: botulism, fibromyalgia, muscular dystrophy, myasthenia gravis, rhabdomyolysis, tendonitis, tetanus, torticollis, and trichinosis.

CASE STUDY CRITICAL THINKING

Recall Ken Washington from the beginning of the chapter. Now that you have completed the chapter, answer the following questions regarding his case.

1. Relate the benefits of exercise to the musculoskeletal system.
2. Identify the arm muscles Ken will need to strengthen.

1. (LO 25.2) Groups of cardiac muscle are connected by
   a. Striations
   b. Multiunits
   c. Intercalated discs
   d. Fascia
   e. myofibrils.

2. (LO 25.2) Skeletal muscle responds to which of the following neurotransmitters?
   a. Epinephrine
   b. Acetylcholine
   c. Norepinephrine
   d. Dopamine
   e. Glucagon

3. (LO 25.5) Increasing the angle of a joint produces which of the following body movements?
   a. Extension
   b. Plantar flexion
   c. Flexion
   d. Hyperextension
   e. Elevation

4. (LO 25.6) Which muscle acts to abduct and extend the arm at the shoulder?
   a. Biceps brachii
   b. Gluteus maximus
   c. Triceps brachii
   d. Deltoid
   e. Brachioradialis

5. (LO 25.6) Which muscle separates the thoracic and abdominal cavities and assists in respiration?
   a. Internal/external obliques
   b. Internal/external intercostals
   c. Diaphragm
   d. Pectoralis major
   e. Serratus anterior

6. (LO 25.6) Which of the following muscles assist with mastication?
   a. Masseter
   b. Frontalis
   c. Platysma
   d. Zygomaticus
   e. Orbicularis oculi

7. (LO 25.8) The medical term for a condition known as wry neck is
   a. Tetanus
   b. Fibromyalgia
   c. Rhabdomyolysis
   d. Tendonitis
   e. Torticollis

8. (LO 25.8) Trichinosis is caused by a/an
   a. Autoimmune disorder
   b. Parasitic worm
   c. Cervical deformity
   d. Soil bacteria
   e. Genetic mutation

9. (LO 25.5) The attachment site for the more movable bone during muscle contraction is the
   a. Origin
   b. Agonist
   c. Synergist
   d. Insertion
   e. Antagonist

10. (LO 25.5) Pointing the toes downward is known as
    a. Plantar flexion
    b. Abduction
    c. Inversion
    d. Dorsiflexion
    e. pronation.

Analyze the following medical terms, presented throughout the chapter. Using a medical dictionary (or Appendix I) place a / mark between each word part. Define each word part and then define the whole word.

EXAMPLE: myo / globin = myo means "muscle" + globin means "protein"
Myoglobin means "muscle protein"

1. abduction
2. adduction
3. circumduction
4. dorsiflexion

5. eversion
6. fibromyalgia
7. hyperextension
8. inversion

9. tendonitis
10. myocytes
11. triceps
12. rhabdomyolysis

The Cardiovascular System

CASE STUDY

Patient Name	Gender	DOB
John Miller	M	12/5/19XX

Attending	MRN	Allergies
Paul F. Buckwalter, MD	082-09-981	Bee stings

John Miller, a 65-year-old patient, was referred to the cardiologist's office for an evaluation. The patient had recently started an exercise program for weight loss. For the last 3 weeks, following exercise, he had noticed radiating chest pain (angina pectoris) that stopped after rest. This condition had worsened in the last week. The cardiologist ordered a stress echocardiogram (a test that visualizes the heart during increasing stress). The stress echocardiogram results suggested that the patient had coronary artery disease (CAD). The patient was scheduled for a cardiac catheterization the next morning. It was noted in the patient's chart that he smoked two packs of cigarettes per day.

Keep John in mind as you study this chapter. There will be questions at the end of the chapter based on the case study. The information in the chapter will help you answer these questions.

ACTIVSim™

LEARNING OUTCOMES

After completing Chapter 26, you will be able to:

26.1 Describe the structures of the heart and the function of each.
26.2 Explain the cardiac cycle, including the cardiac conduction system.
26.3 Compare pulmonary and systemic circulation.
26.4 Differentiate among the different types of blood vessels and their functions.
26.5 Explain blood pressure and tell how it is controlled.
26.6 Describe the causes, signs and symptoms, and treatments of various diseases and disorders of the cardiovascular system.

KEY TERMS

atrioventricular node
bundle of His
cardiac output
chordae tendineae
coronary sinus
diastolic pressure
embolus
endocardium
epicardium
hepatic portal system

myocardium
pericardium
pulmonary circulation
Purkinje fibers
sinoatrial node
systemic circulation
systolic pressure
vasoconstriction
vasodilation

I. C (7)   Analyze pathology as it relates to the interaction of body systems

I. C (9)   Describe implications for treatment related to pathology

I. C (12)   Describe the relationship between anatomy and physiology of all body systems and medications used for treatment in each

IV. C (11)   Define both medical terms and abbreviations related to all body systems

2. **Anatomy & Physiology**
   Graduates:
   b. Identify and apply the knowledge of all body systems, their structure and functions, and their common diseases, symptoms, and etiologies
   c. Assist the physician with the regimen of diagnostic and treatment modalities as they relate to each body system.

3. **Medical Terminology**
   Graduates:
   b. Build and dissect medical terms from roots/suffixes to understand the word element combinations that create medical terminology
   c. Understand the various medical terminology for each specialty
   d. Recognize and identify acceptable medical abbreviations

▶ Introduction

The cardiovascular system consists of the heart and blood vessels. It is responsible for sending blood to the lungs to pick up oxygen and to the digestive system to pick up nutrients in order to deliver oxygen and nutrients to all the organ systems in the body. This system also circulates waste products to certain organ systems so these wastes can be removed from the blood.

▶ The Heart   LO 26.1

The heart is a cone-shaped organ about the size of a loose fist. It is located within the mediastinum (central part of the chest) and extends from the level of the second rib to about the level of the sixth rib. Although many people think the heart is found in the left side of the chest, it is located only slightly left of the midline of the body. The heart is bordered laterally by the lungs, posteriorly by the vertebral column, and anteriorly by the sternum. Inferiorly, the heart rests on the diaphragm.

Cardiac Membranes

A membrane called the **pericardium** covers the heart and the large blood vessels attached to it (see Figure 26-1). The pericardium consists of an outer fibrous layer that covers two inner layers. The innermost layer is called the *visceral pericardium*, and it forms the outer layer of the heart wall. The layer on top of the visceral pericardium is called the *parietal pericardium*. The *fibrous pericardium* and the parietal pericardium form the pericardial sac. The space between the parietal pericardium and visceral pericardium is called the *pericardial cavity*. The pericardial cavity contains pericardial fluid, a slippery, serous fluid that reduces friction between the membranes when the heart contracts.

The Heart Wall

The wall of the heart (see Figure 26-2) is composed of the following three layers:

- **Epicardium.** This outermost layer is the visceral pericardium. It contains fat, which helps to cushion the heart.
- **Myocardium.** This middle layer is the thickest layer of the wall and is made primarily of cardiac muscle.
- **Endocardium.** This innermost layer is thin and very smooth, and stretches as the heart pumps blood. This layer contains part of the cardiac electrical conduction system, which is discussed later in this chapter.

Heart Chambers and Valves

The heart contains four hollow chambers, two on the left and two on the right (see Figure 26-3). The upper chambers of the heart are called *atria* (the singular form is *atrium*). They have thin walls and receive blood returning to the heart from the lungs and the body. The atria are separated from each other by a walled membrane known as the *interatrial septum*. The bottom chambers of the heart are the *ventricles*. The septum separating the ventricles is the *interventricular septum*. The ventricles function to pump blood into the arteries, which send the blood to the lungs and the body. The *atrioventricular septum* is the wall that separates the atria from the ventricles.

The four valves within the heart that keep blood flowing in one direction are the tricuspid and the bicuspid (mitral) valves located between the atria and ventricles, and the pulmonary semilunar and aortic semilunar valves, which are located between the ventricles and their arteries.

Right lung   Left lung

Superior
vena cava

Aorta

Pulmonary trunk
Left auricle
Fibrous pericardium
Cut edge of
parietal pericardium

Right auricle
Right atrium

Heart (covered
by visceral
pericardium)

Right ventricle

Left ventricle

Diaphragm

Pericardial cavity

FIGURE 26-1   Location and membranes of the heart.

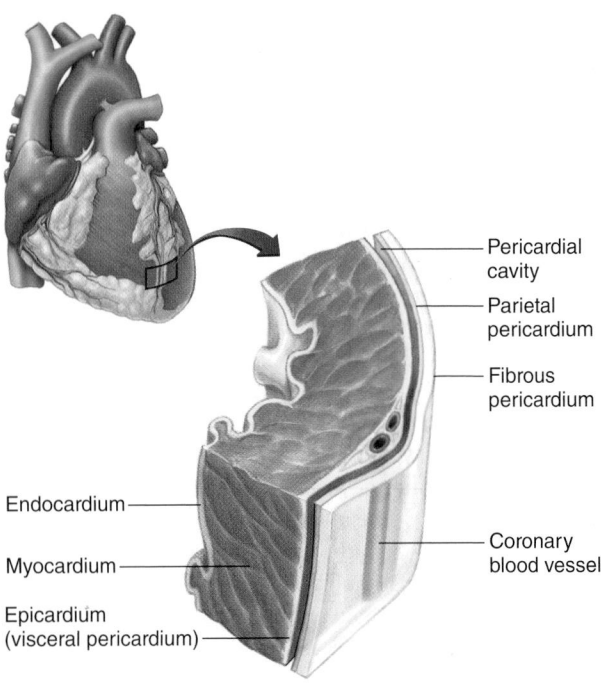

Pericardial
cavity

Parietal
pericardium

Fibrous
pericardium

Endocardium

Coronary
blood vessel

Myocardium

Epicardium
(visceral pericardium)

FIGURE 26-2   Layers of the wall of the heart.

Tricuspid Valve The *tricuspid valve* has three cusps and is situated between the right atrium and the right ventricle. It prevents blood from flowing back into the right atrium when the right ventricle contracts. This valve is also called the *right atrioventricular (AV) valve*. The cusps of this valve are anchored by cordlike structures called **chordae tendineae** to bumps of cardiac muscle called *papillary muscles*. These muscles contract when the ventricles contract to close the valve.

Bicuspid Valve The *bicuspid valve* has two cusps and is located between the left atrium and the left ventricle. It prevents blood from flowing back into the left atrium when the left ventricle contracts. This valve is also known as the *mitral valve* and the *left AV valve*. Like the tricuspid valve, the bicuspid valve also has chordae tendineae attached to papillary muscles.

Pulmonary Semilunar Valve The *pulmonary semilunar valve* is situated between the right ventricle and the trunk of the pulmonary arteries. It prevents blood from flowing back into the right ventricle. Because its cusps

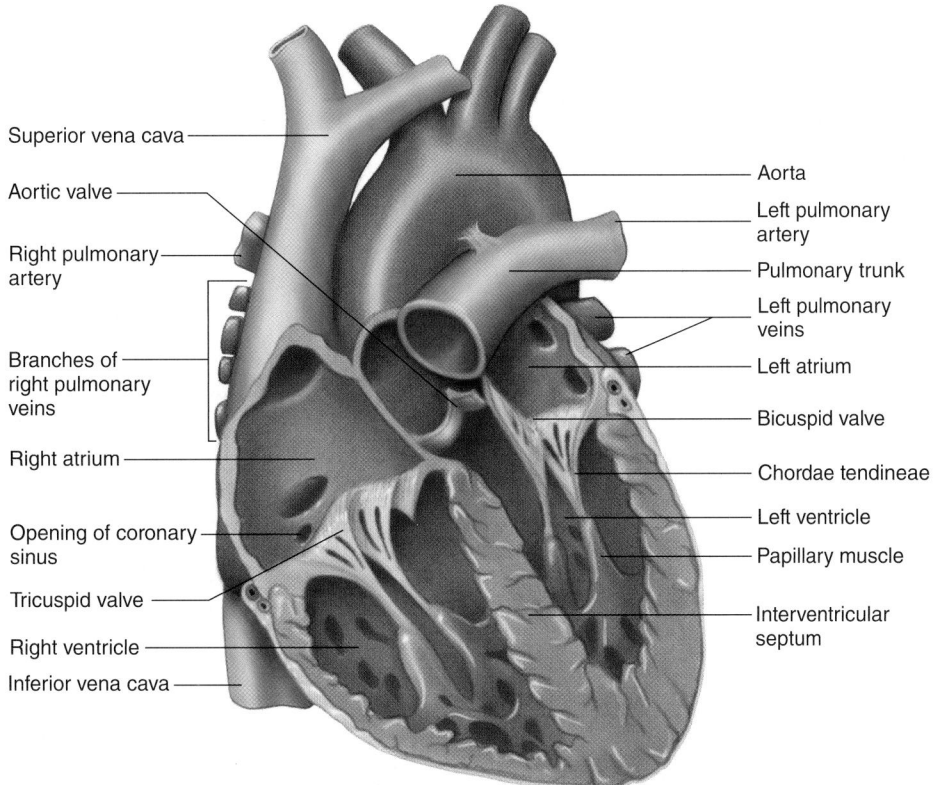

FIGURE 26-3 The chambers and valves of the heart are visible in this coronal section.

Labels (clockwise):
- Superior vena cava
- Aortic valve
- Right pulmonary artery
- Branches of right pulmonary veins
- Right atrium
- Opening of coronary sinus
- Tricuspid valve
- Right ventricle
- Inferior vena cava
- Aorta
- Left pulmonary artery
- Pulmonary trunk
- Left pulmonary veins
- Left atrium
- Bicuspid valve
- Chordae tendineae
- Left ventricle
- Papillary muscle
- Interventricular septum

are shaped like a half moon, this valve is called a *semilunar valve*.

Aortic Semilunar Valve The *aortic semilunar valve* is situated between the left ventricle and the aorta. It prevents blood from flowing back into the left ventricle and is also known as a semilunar valve because of the shape of its cusps.

▶ Cardiac Cycle   LO 26.2

One heartbeat makes up one cardiac cycle. In one cardiac cycle, the top chambers (atria) of the heart contract and relax together and then the bottom chambers (ventricles) of the heart contract and relax together. In other words, a cardiac cycle consists of one complete cardiac contraction and one complete cardiac relaxation. Here are the actions that occur:

- Right atrium contracts → tricuspid valve opens → blood flows into the right ventricle.
- Left atrium contracts → bicuspid valve opens → blood flows into the left ventricle.
- Right ventricle contracts → tricuspid valve closes, pulmonary semilunar valve opens → blood is pushed into the trunk of the pulmonary artery.
- Left ventricle contracts → bicuspid valve closes, aortic semilunar valve opens → blood is pushed into the aorta.

The following factors influence the cardiac cycle:

- Exercise. Strenuous exercise increases the heart rate because skeletal muscles need more oxygen.
- Parasympathetic nerves. The parasympathetic nerve to the heart is the vagus nerve, and it generally keeps the heart rate relatively low.
- Sympathetic nerves. The sympathetic nerves increase the heart rate during times of stress. Parasympathetic and sympathetic nerves are discussed in more detail in *The Nervous System* chapter.
- Cardiac control center. This center is located in the medulla oblongata. When blood pressure rises, this control center sends impulses to decrease the heart rate. When blood pressure falls, it sends impulses to increase the heart rate.
- Body temperature. An increase in body temperature usually increases the heart rate. This explains the high heart rate when a person runs a fever.
- Potassium ions. A low concentration of potassium ions in the blood decreases the heart rate, but a high concentration causes an arrhythmia (abnormal heart rate).
- Calcium ions. A low concentration of calcium ions in the blood depresses heart actions, but a high concentration causes heart contractions called *titanic contractions*, which are longer than normal heart contractions.

Go to CONNECT to see an animation on *Cardiac Cycle.*

Heart Sounds

During one cardiac cycle, you can hear two heart sounds. The sounds are called *lubb* and *dubb*. These sounds are generated when valves in the heart snap shut. Lubb is the first heart sound and occurs when the ventricles contract and the tricuspid and bicuspid valves snap shut. Dubb is the second heart sound and occurs when the atria contract and the pulmonary and aortic semilunar valves snap shut.

Physicians listen to heart sounds to diagnose certain conditions. For example, if an AV valve (tricuspid or bicuspid) is damaged, it will not close completely. This allows blood to leak back into the atria when the ventricles contract and produces an abnormal heart sound called a *murmur*. Murmurs may indicate serious heart conditions, although many heart murmurs are harmless.

Cardiac Conduction System

The cardiac conduction system consists of a group of structures that send electrical impulses through the heart. When cardiac muscle receives an electrical impulse, it contracts (see Figure 26-4). The components of the cardiac conduction system are the sinoatrial node, atrioventricular node, bundle of His, and Purkinje fibers.

- **Sinoatrial node (SA node).** This node is located in the wall of the right atrium and generates an impulse that flows to the atrioventricular node. The SA node is also known as the natural pacemaker of the heart because it generates the heart's rhythmic contractions.

- **Atrioventricular node (AV node).** This node is located between the atria, just above the ventricles. After the impulse reaches the AV node, the atria contract and the impulse is sent to the bundle of His.

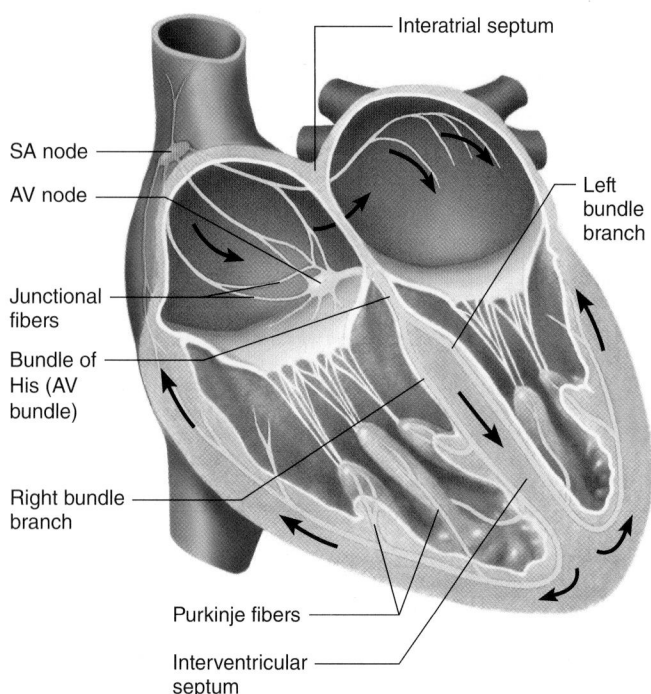

FIGURE 26-4 Cardiac conduction system.

(a)

(b)

FIGURE 26-5 Electrocardiogram: (a) a normal ECG and (b) waves of a normal ECG pattern.

- **Bundle of His.** This structure, also known as the *atrioventricular* or *AV bundle*, is located between the ventricles and splits into two branches, forming the left and right *bundle branches*, before sending the electrical impulse to the Purkinje fibers.

- **Purkinje fibers.** These fibers are located in the lateral walls of the ventricles. After the impulse flows through the Purkinje fibers, the ventricles contract and the SA node starts the flow of a new impulse.

Physicians use a test called an electrocardiogram (ECG or EKG) to tell if the cardiac conduction system is working properly. In a normal ECG, the waves shown in Figure 26-5 are produced. The first wave (P wave) indicates that an electrical impulse was sent through the atria, causing them to contract (depolarization). The Q, R, and S waves occur together and make up the QRS complex. This complex indicates that an electrical impulse was sent through the ventricles, causing them to contract (depolarization). Finally, the T wave indicates electrical changes that occur in the ventricles as they relax (repolarization). You will learn more about the electrical conduction system of the heart and ECGs, including how to perform them, in the *Cardiovascular and Respiratory Testing* chapter.

▶ Circulation

LO 26.3

Blood flows through the body through two main circuits. The *pulmonary circuit* provides oxygen, and the *systemic circuit* distributes the oxygen to the entire body.

Pulmonary Circuit

The pulmonary circuit, or **pulmonary circulation,** is the route blood takes from the heart to the lungs and back to the heart again. The function of this circuit is to oxygenate blood. It also allows carbon dioxide to leave blood and enter the lungs (see Figure 26-6). Blood low in oxygen (deoxygenated) and rich in carbon dioxide enters the right atrium of the heart through large veins called the inferior and superior *venae cavae*. From the right atrium, the blood flows through the tricuspid valve into the right ventricle. When the right ventricle contracts, blood is pushed through the pulmonary semilunar valve into a larger artery called the *pulmonary trunk*. The pulmonary trunk branches into the left and right pulmonary arteries, which carry blood to the lungs.

In the lungs, blood picks up oxygen and gets rid of carbon dioxide. Blood rich in oxygen and low in carbon dioxide then returns to the heart through the four pulmonary veins. The pulmonary veins empty the oxygenated blood into the left atrium.

Systemic Circuit

The systemic circuit, or **systemic circulation,** is the route blood takes from the heart through the body and back to the heart. The function of this circuit is to deliver oxygen and nutrients to body cells. It also picks up carbon dioxide and waste products from body cells (see Figure 26-6).

From the left atrium, blood flows through the bicuspid (mitral) valve into the left ventricle. When the left ventricle contracts, blood is pushed through the aortic semilunar valve into the aorta. The aorta distributes blood into its branches and throughout the body.

In the body, the blood gives oxygen to cells and picks up carbon dioxide. Veins of the body pick up the oxygen-poor blood and empty it into the venae cavae, and the whole system starts all over again with pulmonary circulation.

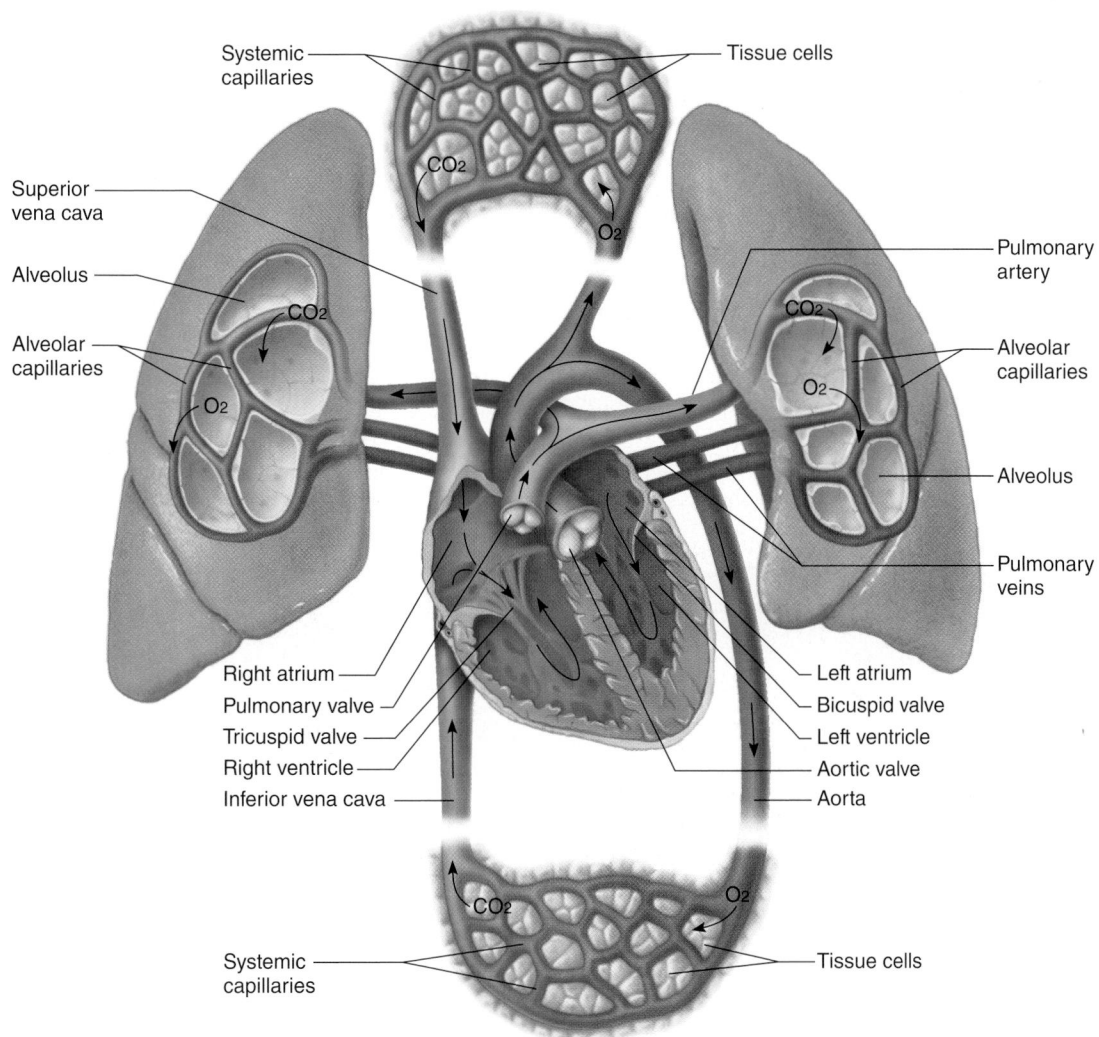

FIGURE 26-6 Pathway of blood through the heart and lungs and on to other body parts. The right side of the heart delivers blood to the lungs, and the left side delivers blood to all other body parts.

▶ Blood Vessels

LO 26.4

Blood circulation takes place in blood vessels that form a closed pathway to carry blood from the heart to cells and back again. These vessels include arteries, arterioles, veins, venules, and capillaries.

Arteries and Arterioles

Arteries are the strongest of the blood vessels. The muscular layer of arteries contains smooth muscle and is thicker than the muscular layer of other types of blood vessels (see Figure 26-7). Arteries, the largest of which is the aorta, carry blood away from the heart and are under high pressure, which is the main reason they need thick walls. The muscular wall of an artery can constrict to increase blood pressure, or it can dilate to decrease blood pressure. Small branches of arteries are called *arterioles*.

Coronary Arteries The tissues of the heart receive their blood supply through coronary arteries. Branches of the coronary arteries eventually give rise to very small blood vessels called *capillaries*. The capillaries of the heart are in the myocardium and allow oxygen to diffuse into the cardiac muscle cells. Blockage of one or more of the coronary arteries may cause chest pain, or angina, and if this is not corrected may lead to myocardial infarction (MI). See Educating the Patient: Chest Pain for more information about types of chest pain. Blood leaving the capillaries in the heart goes to the cardiac veins. Cardiac veins eventually deliver the oxygen-poor blood to a large vein called the **coronary sinus.** The coronary sinus empties the blood into the right atrium.

Other Major Arteries As stated earlier, arteries carry blood away from the heart. Most of them carry oxygen-rich blood, although the pulmonary arteries carry oxygen-poor blood from the heart to the lungs. The aorta comes directly off the left ventricle and is the largest artery in the body. It has many branches that supply blood to various

TABLE 26-1	Major Arteries of the Body
Artery	**Anatomic Location or Organ Supplied**
Lingual	Tongue
Facial	Face
Occipital	Back of scalp and neck
Maxillary	Teeth, jaw, and eyelids
Ophthalmic	Eye
Axillary	Armpit area
Brachial	Upper arm
Ulnar	Forearm and hand
Radial	Forearm and hand
Intercostals	Rib area
Lumbar	Posterior abdominal wall
External iliac	Anterior abdominal wall
Common iliac	Legs, gluteal area, and pelvic organs
Femoral	Thigh
Popliteal	Posterior knee
Tibial	Lower leg and foot

parts of the body. Many other arteries in the body are paired, meaning there is a left and a right artery of the same name. Major arteries are summarized in Table 26-1. Also see Figure 26-8.

Veins and Venules

Veins are blood vessels that carry blood toward the heart. Blood is under no pressure in the veins and does not move very easily. Therefore, the movement of blood through veins requires skeletal muscle contractions and valves. When skeletal muscles contract, they squeeze the veins and blood is pushed through them, much like the way toothpaste is pushed out of a tube. The valves in veins prevent blood from flowing backward (see

(a)   (b)

FIGURE 26-7 Arteries have much thicker walls than other blood vessels. (a) Cross-section of an artery. (b) Cross-section of a vein.

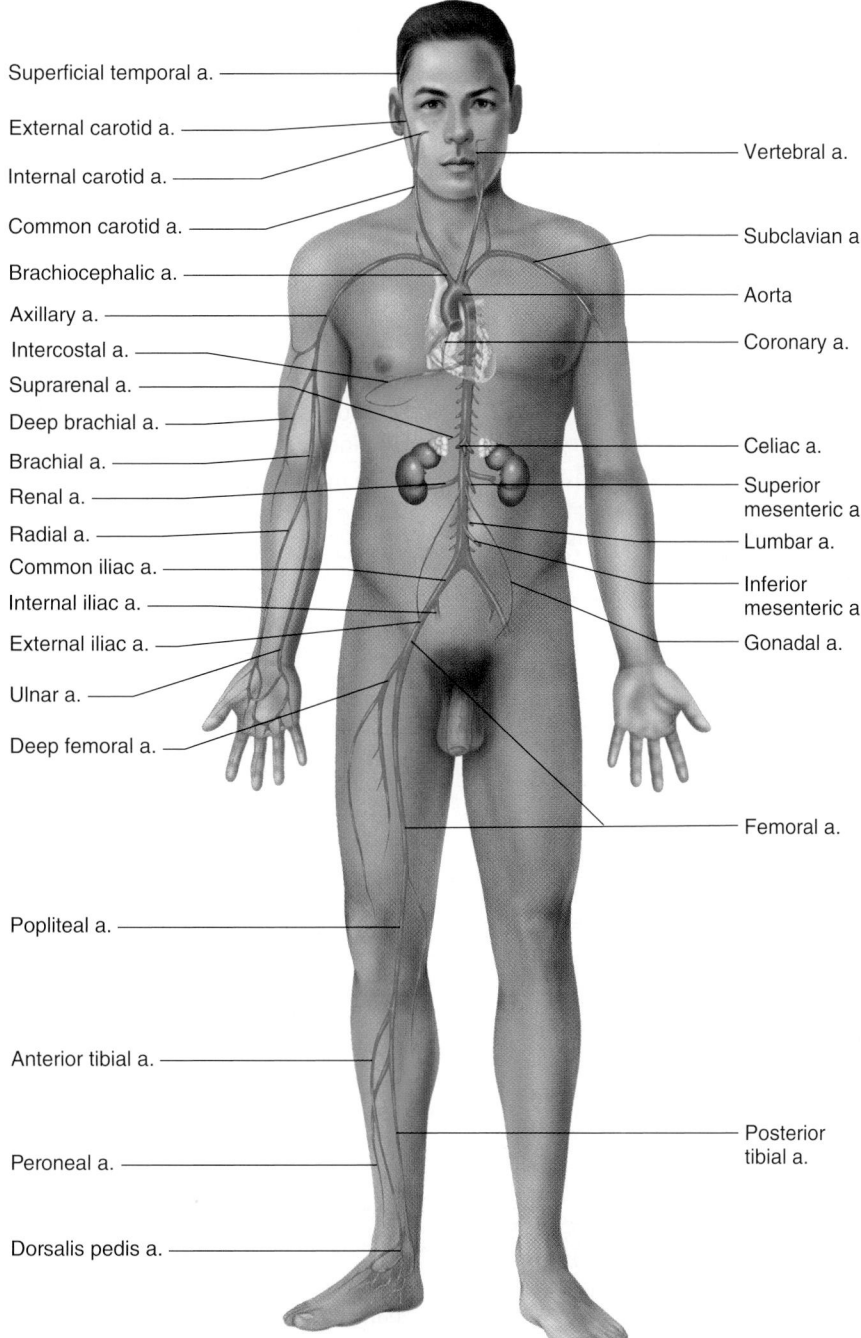

Superficial temporal a.
External carotid a.
Internal carotid a.
Common carotid a.
Brachiocephalic a.
Axillary a.
Intercostal a.
Suprarenal a.
Deep brachial a.
Brachial a.
Renal a.
Radial a.
Common iliac a.
Internal iliac a.
External iliac a.
Ulnar a.
Deep femoral a.
Popliteal a.
Anterior tibial a.
Peroneal a.
Dorsalis pedis a.

Vertebral a.
Subclavian a.
Aorta
Coronary a.
Celiac a.
Superior mesenteric a.
Lumbar a.
Inferior mesenteric a.
Gonadal a.
Femoral a.
Posterior tibial a.

FIGURE 26-8   Major arteries of the body (a. stands for *artery*).

Figure 26-9). *Varicose veins* occur when valves are destroyed and blood pools in the veins, causing them to become dilated or expanded.

The sympathetic nervous system also influences the flow of blood through veins. The sympathetic nervous system causes vein walls to constrict, which forces blood through the veins. This happens only if blood pressure gets abnormally low in the arteries.

Venules are very small blood vessels that are formed when capillaries merge together (see Figure 26-10). Venules merge together to make veins, the largest of which are the superior and inferior venae cavae. Veins carry blood toward the heart. The muscular layer in the walls of veins is thinner than the layer found in arteries.

Most veins in the body carry oxygen-poor blood. The exceptions are the pulmonary veins, which carry oxygenated blood from the lungs to the heart. Large veins often have the same names as the arteries they run next to. However, there are exceptions. For example, the veins next to carotid arteries are the jugular veins.

Chest Pain

Chest pain is a common reason people go to the emergency room every year. Although all chest pains should be taken seriously, they do not always indicate life-threatening heart conditions. There are two primary causes of chest pain: cardiac and noncardiac. Use the information in this box to teach patients about the conditions that cause chest pain.

Cardiac Causes

The cardiac causes of chest pain include the following:

- Myocardial infarction (MI). Commonly called *heart attacks,* myocardial infarctions are caused by the complete blockage of coronary arteries and are life-threatening conditions. The pain associated with a heart attack is often described as pressure or fullness in the chest. Sometimes pain also occurs in the back, neck, face (especially jaw), shoulder, or arms (the left arm more than the right). Other signs and symptoms include shortness of breath, sweating, nausea, and dizziness. Women have fewer of the "classic signs" of MI, such as chest pain, and should be educated about this.

- Angina. Angina is caused by a narrowing of coronary arteries and is not immediately life-threatening. However, it is an indication that the heart muscle is not receiving enough oxygen. The pain of angina is usually described as a tight feeling in the chest and is often brought about by stress or physical activity. This type of chest pain usually goes away after the stress or physical activity stops. A doctor should monitor patients with angina regularly. Most patients with angina carry sublingual nitroglycerin with them to help alleviate their chest pain.

- Pericarditis. This condition is characterized by inflammation of the sac surrounding the heart. It usually produces a sharp and localized pain in the chest. It is not immediately life-threatening but should be treated. This condition often produces a fever.

- Coronary spasms. In this condition, coronary arteries temporarily spasm and limit blood flow to cardiac muscle tissue. The pain accompanied by coronary spasms is similar to that of angina. It should be treated as soon as possible.

Noncardiac Causes

The noncardiac causes of chest pain include the following:

- Heartburn. Heartburn occurs when acids from the stomach are pushed into the esophagus; it is known as gastroesophageal reflux disease or GERD. Heartburn pain is described as a burning sensation. This pain usually follows a meal and gets worse if a patient bends forward or tries to lie on his or her back.

- Panic attacks. During times of intense stress or fear, chest pains can occur and are often accompanied by increased heart and breathing rates, as well as excessive sweating.

- Pleurisy. This condition occurs when the membranes surrounding the lungs become inflamed. Pleurisy produces a sharp chest pain that usually feels worse when a patient coughs or inhales.

- Costochondritis. This condition occurs when the cartilage attached to ribs becomes inflamed. The chest pain associated with this condition feels much like the pain of a heart attack but generally occurs only when someone pushes on the patient's chest.

- Pulmonary embolism. This condition occurs when a blood clot blocks an artery in the lungs. The pain associated with it is severe and sharp, and it increases when a patient inhales deeply or coughs. A pulmonary embolism also can produce shortness of breath, an increased heart rate, and dizziness. This condition is life-threatening.

- Sore muscles. Chest pain from sore muscles usually occurs only during body movements such as raising the arms.

- Broken ribs. Fractures of the ribs tend to produce sharp and localized chest pains.

- Inflammation of the gallbladder (cholecystitis) or pancreas (pancreatitis). Pain associated with these conditions usually begins in the abdomen and spreads to the chest.

Determining the Cause

Tests used to determine the cause of chest pain include the following:

- Electrocardiogram (ECG/EKG) is useful in determining if an MI is occurring or has already occurred.

- Stress tests are ECGs performed while a patient is exercising or has been given drugs to increase her heart rate. Stress tests are useful for determining the health of coronary blood vessels while under stress.

- Blood tests are useful in determining if a heart attack has occurred. When heart tissue is damaged, certain enzyme levels such as CPK and LDH are found to be elevated in the blood.

- Chest X-rays show the size and shape of the lungs and heart and can therefore indicate any serious conditions.

- Nuclear scans follow radioactive substances through the blood vessels of the heart and lungs. They can reveal narrow or obstructed arteries.

- Electron beam computerized tomography (EBCT), a procedure much like a CT scan of the arteries, is useful for finding narrowed arteries.

- Cardiac catheterization uses a contrast medium that is followed through coronary arteries. It also can show narrowing of the arteries. According to the American Heart Association, from 1979 to 2005 the number of cardiac catheterizations performed in this country increased 342%, a staggering statistic.

- Echocardiogram is a procedure that uses sound waves (ultrasound) to visualize the shape of the heart.

- Endoscopy involves inserting a tube with a tiny camera down the throat and into the stomach. It helps to diagnose disorders of the stomach or esophagus that might produce chest pains.

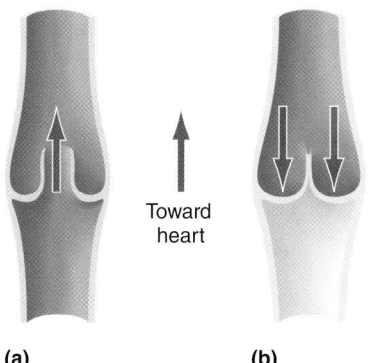

FIGURE 26-9 Venous valve: (a) valve opens when blood is flowing toward the heart and (b) valve closes to prevent blood from flowing away from the heart.

Toward heart

(a)   (b)

TABLE 26-2	Major Veins of the Body
Vein	**Anatomic Location or Organ Drained**
Jugular	Head and neck
Brachiocephalic	Head and neck
Axillary	Armpit area
Brachial	Upper arm
Ulnar	Lower arm and hand
Radial	Lower arm and hand
Intercostal	Rib area
Azygos	Thorax and abdomen
Iliac	Pelvic organs, legs, and gluteal areas
Femoral	Thighs
Popliteal	Knees
Saphenous	Legs
Hepatic	Liver to the inferior vena cava
Hepatic Portal System	
Gastric	Stomach to the liver
Splenic	Spleen, pancreas, and stomach to the liver
Mesenteric	Intestines to the liver
Hepatic portal	Gastric, splenic, and mesenteric veins to the liver

Arteriole

Capillary

Venule

FIGURE 26-10 This light micrograph of a capillary network shows the capillaries merging to become venules.

Large veins empty blood into venae cavae. The superior vena cava generally collects blood from veins above the heart, and the inferior vena cava collects blood from veins below the heart. The major veins of the body are summarized in Table 26-2. Also see Figure 26-11.

Veins of digestive organs carry blood from the digestive tract to the liver. The liver then processes nutrients in the blood and returns it to general circulation through the hepatic veins. The collection of veins carrying blood to the liver is called the **hepatic portal system.**

Capillaries

Capillaries are branches of arterioles; they are the smallest type of blood vessel. They connect arterioles to venules and have very thin walls that are only about one cell layer thick. These thin walls allow substances to pass into and out of capillaries (see

Figure 26-12). For example, oxygen and nutrients can pass out of a capillary into a body cell, and carbon dioxide and other waste products can pass out of a body cell into a capillary. In fact, capillaries are often referred to as *exchange vessels* because they are the only type of blood vessels that allow substances to move in and out of the blood.

Tissues that require a lot of oxygen, such as muscle and nervous tissues, have a lot of capillaries. Capillary openings have *precapillary sphincters* that control the amount of blood that flows into them. When the sphincter relaxes, more blood flows into the capillary.

The substances that move through the capillary wall (oxygen, carbon dioxide, nutrients, water, and metabolic wastes) do so through diffusion, filtration, and osmosis. When blood first enters a capillary, it has high concentrations of oxygen and nutrients. The body cells surrounding the capillary usually have low concentrations of oxygen and nutrients but high concentrations of carbon dioxide and other waste products. Substances naturally diffuse from an area of high concentration to an area of low concentration. Therefore, oxygen and nutrients diffuse out of the capillary and into body cells. At the same time, carbon dioxide and waste products diffuse out of the body cells and into the capillary.

Because blood is under pressure as it enters the capillary, water is forced through the capillary wall via filtration. This allows water to enter a body cell. By the time blood leaves a capillary, it has a high solid concentration and a low water concentration; water therefore moves back into the capillary through osmosis. Water always moves toward the greater concentration

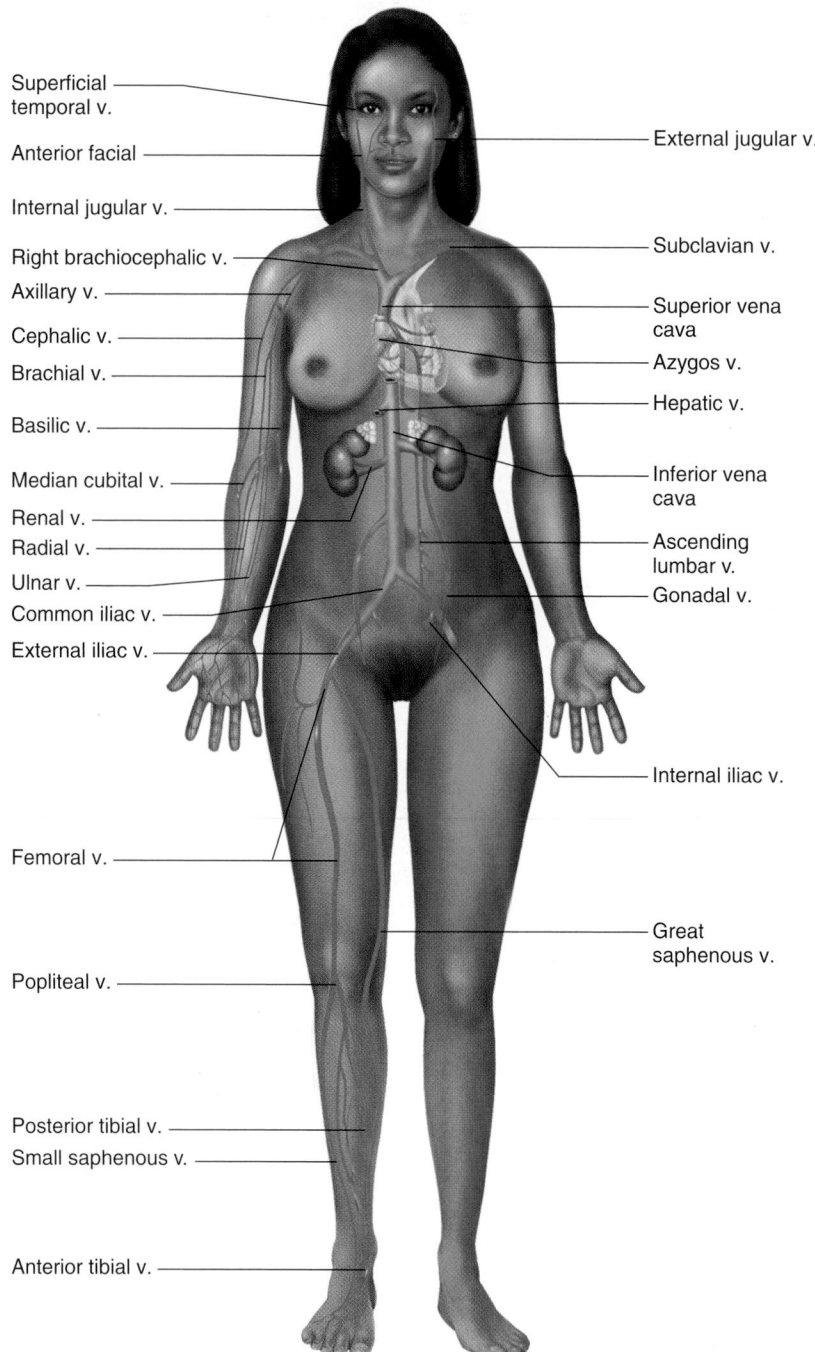

FIGURE 26-11 Major veins of the body (v. stands for *vein*).

Labels (left side, top to bottom):
Superficial temporal v.
Anterior facial
Internal jugular v.
Right brachiocephalic v.
Axillary v.
Cephalic v.
Brachial v.
Basilic v.
Median cubital v.
Renal v.
Radial v.
Ulnar v.
Common iliac v.
External iliac v.
Femoral v.
Popliteal v.
Posterior tibial v.
Small saphenous v.
Anterior tibial v.

Labels (right side, top to bottom):
External jugular v.
Subclavian v.
Superior vena cava
Azygos v.
Hepatic v.
Inferior vena cava
Ascending lumbar v.
Gonadal v.
Internal iliac v.
Great saphenous v.

of solids, if possible. The *Organization of the Body* chapter provides more detailed explanations about diffusion, filtration, and osmosis.

▶ Blood Pressure

LO 26.5

Blood pressure is defined as the force that blood exerts on the inner walls of blood vessels. Blood pressure is highest in arteries and lowest in veins. In the clinical setting, blood pressure refers to the pressure in arteries.

Arterial blood pressure rises and falls as the ventricles of the heart contract and relax. When the ventricles contract, blood pressure is greatest in the arteries. This pressure is called the **systolic pressure** or systole. When the ventricles relax, blood pressure in arteries is at its lowest. This pressure is called the **diastolic pressure** or diastole. Blood pressure is usually reported as the systolic number over the diastolic number. For example, in the blood pressure reading 120/80, 120 denotes the systolic pressure and 80 refers to the diastolic pressure.

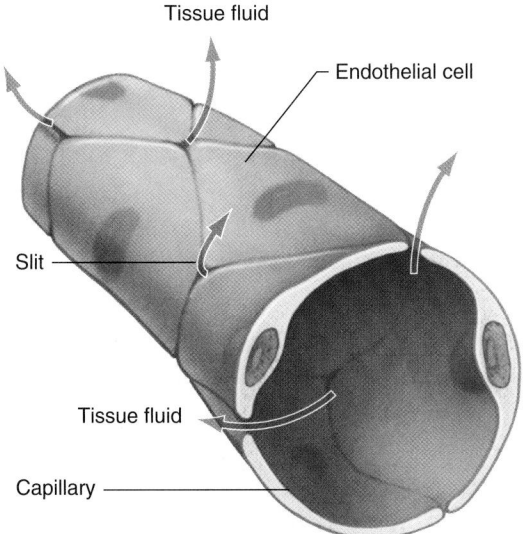

FIGURE 26-12 Structure of a capillary wall.

You can feel the surge of blood through arteries when you take a pulse. The pulse is created as the artery expands when pressure increases and then subsequently relaxes as blood pressure decreases. Common places to feel a pulse are the carotid and radial arteries.

Many factors affect blood pressure. The most common factors include cardiac output, blood volume, vasoconstriction, and blood viscosity (thickness). **Cardiac output** is the total amount of blood pumped out of the heart in one minute. As cardiac output increases and decreases, blood pressure increases and decreases. When a person loses a large amount of blood, his blood pressure significantly decreases. If blood pressure falls too low, **vasoconstriction,** which is the tightening of blood vessel walls, helps to raise blood pressure. In contrast, if blood pressure is too high, **vasodilation,** which is the widening of blood vessels, decreases the blood pressure. Under certain circumstances, such as dehydration, blood becomes more viscous, or thicker, than normal. This also decreases blood pressure.

Blood pressure is controlled to a large extent by the amount of blood pumped out of the heart. The amount of blood entering the heart should be equal to the amount of blood pumped out of the heart. The heart has a way to ensure that this happens. When blood enters the left ventricle, the wall of the ventricle is stretched. The more the wall is stretched, the harder it will contract and the more blood it will pump out. This is referred to as *Starling's law of the heart*. If only a small amount of blood enters the left ventricle, it will not be stretched very much and therefore will not contract very forcefully. In this case, not much blood is pumped out of the heart.

Baroreceptors also help regulate blood pressure. Baroreceptors measure blood pressure and are located in the aorta and carotid arteries. If pressure increases in these blood vessels, this information is sent to the cardiac center in the medulla oblongata. The cardiac center then knows to decrease the heart rate, which lowers blood pressure. If pressure gets too low in the aorta, baroreceptors pick up this information and relay it to the cardiac center. The cardiac center then increases the heart rate to raise blood pressure.

PATHOPHYSIOLOGY

Common Diseases and Disorders of the Cardiovascular System

An **ANEURYSM** is a ballooned, weakened arterial wall. The most common locations of aneurysms are the aorta and arteries in the brain, legs, intestines, and spleen. An aortic aneurysm is a bulge in the wall of the aorta. Most aortic aneurysms occur in the abdominal aorta (abdominal aortic aneurysm), but some occur in the thoracic aorta (see Figure 26-13). Most aortic aneurysms do not rupture; however, when they do, the resulting hemorrhage is a serious life-threatening emergency.

Causes. Most causes are unknown. One identified risk to developing an aneurysm is atherosclerosis, which is a hardening of the fatty plaque deposits within the arteries that is usually associated with a high-cholesterol diet. Smoking and obesity also increase the risk of atherosclerosis. Congenital conditions may cause an aneurysm—some individuals are born with weak aortic walls. A traumatic injury to the chest also may be a risk factor. The risk of developing an aneurysm can be reduced by not smoking, by losing excess weight, and by having low-fat, low-cholesterol diet. Periodic screening is an option for patients with a family history of aortic aneurysms.

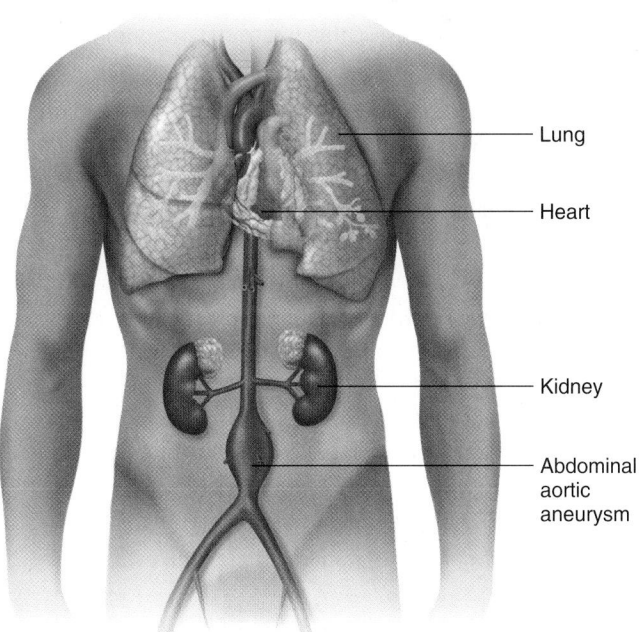

FIGURE 26-13 Abdominal aneurysms can occur without symptoms, but if they rupture they are frequently life threatening.

Signs and Symptoms. There are usually no signs or symptoms of an aneurysm, although hypertension can be a sign. When symptoms do exist, the most common are a pulsation in the abdomen and back pain. A sudden pain in the abdomen or back, dizziness, a fast pulse, or a loss of consciousness are signs that an aneurysm has ruptured.

Treatment. The primary treatment is surgery to repair the aneurysm.

ARRHYTHMIAS are abnormal heart rhythms in which the heart beats too quickly (tachycardia) or too slowly (bradycardia). The most common type of heart arrhythmia is atrial fibrillation, which is a sporadic and rapid beating of the atria. The most serious type of heart arrhythmia is ventricular fibrillation, which produces ineffective contractions of the ventricles. Most sudden cardiac deaths are caused by ventricular fibrillation.

Causes. These abnormal rhythms usually result when electrical impulses of the cardiac conduction system do not flow correctly through the heart. The long list of risk factors and causes includes electrical shock, certain drugs, herbal supplements containing ephedra (although most have been removed from the market because of the high risk of arrhythmias), high blood pressure, previous heart attack, decreased blood flow to the heart, coronary artery disease, heart valve disorders, weakening of the heart muscle (cardiomyopathy), some genetic diseases such as Wolff-Parkinson-White syndrome, thyroid conditions, diabetes mellitus, sleep apnea, electrolyte imbalances (including potassium, sodium, and calcium), excess alcohol consumption, smoking, caffeine consumption, and drugs such as amphetamines or cocaine.

Signs and Symptoms. Symptoms include shortness of breath, dizziness or fainting, an uncharacteristically rapid or slow heart rate, a fluttering feeling in the chest, and chest pain.

Treatment. The first management of arrhythmias should be to treat the underlying cause. Other treatment options include the following:

- Vagal maneuvers to slow the heart rate, such as holding the breath, straining (bearing down as if the patient is having a bowel movement), or putting one's face in cool water.
- Various medications such as beta blockers and anti-arrhythmics.
- Pacemakers.
- Radiofrequency catheter ablation, a procedure that destroys a small amount of heart tissue to change the flow of the electrical current through the heart.
- *Maze* procedure, which is an operation to form scars in the atria. These scars correct the electrical flow through the heart.
- Implantation of an ICD (implantable cardioverter defibrillator), a device that regulates heart rhythms.
- Cardiopulmonary resuscitation if there is no evidence of blood flow.
- Electrical shock (defibrillation) to reset heart rhythms.
- Surgery to correct heart defects such as narrow coronary arteries.

ENDOCARDITIS is an inflammation of the innermost lining of the heart, including the heart valves.

Causes. Bacterial infections are the most common cause of endocarditis. Patients are more susceptible to this condition if they have abnormal heart valves.

Signs and Symptoms. Common signs and symptoms include weakness, fever, excessive sweating, general body aches, difficulty breathing, and blood in the urine.

Treatment. The treatment for this condition is intravenous antibiotics followed by oral antibiotics for up to 6 weeks.

MYOCARDITIS is an inflammation of the muscular layer of the heart. It is relatively uncommon but very serious because it leads to weakening of the heart wall.

Causes. The most common cause of myocarditis is a viral infection, but it also may be caused by exposure to certain chemicals, allergens, and bacteria.

Signs and Symptoms. Signs and symptoms include fever as well as chest pains that feel like a heart attack. Difficulty breathing, decreased urine output, fatigue, and fainting also may accompany myocarditis.

Treatment. Treatment normally includes steroids to reduce inflammation, bed rest, and a low-sodium diet.

PERICARDITIS is inflammation of the pericardium, which is the group of membranes that surround the heart.

Causes. This condition is most commonly caused by complications of viral or bacterial infections. However, heart attacks and chest injuries also can lead to pericarditis.

Signs and Symptoms. Symptoms include sharp, stabbing chest pains, especially during deep breaths. Fever, fatigue, and difficulty breathing while lying down are also common symptoms.

Treatment. The treatment usually includes painkillers. Diuretics are used to remove excess fluids around the heart. If bacteria caused the pericarditis, antibiotics are used. In chronic cases, surgery may be required to remove part of the membranes surrounding the heart.

CONGESTIVE HEART FAILURE is a slowly developing condition in which the heart weakens over time. Eventually, the heart is no longer able to pump enough blood to meet the body's needs.

Causes. There are many risk factors for this condition, including smoking, being overweight, a diet high in cholesterol, a lack of exercise, atherosclerosis, history of MI, high blood pressure, a damaged heart valve, excessive alcohol consumption, and diabetes mellitus. Congenital heart defects (those present at birth) and drugs that weaken the heart (especially cocaine, heroin, and some antineoplastic drugs for cancer) also may contribute to the development of this disorder. This condition may be prevented by controlling high blood pressure and high cholesterol, not smoking, maintaining a healthy diet, engaging in regular exercise, and treating any existing atherosclerosis or diabetes.

Signs and Symptoms. Signs and symptoms include shortness of breath; constant wheezing; prominent neck veins; fluid retention

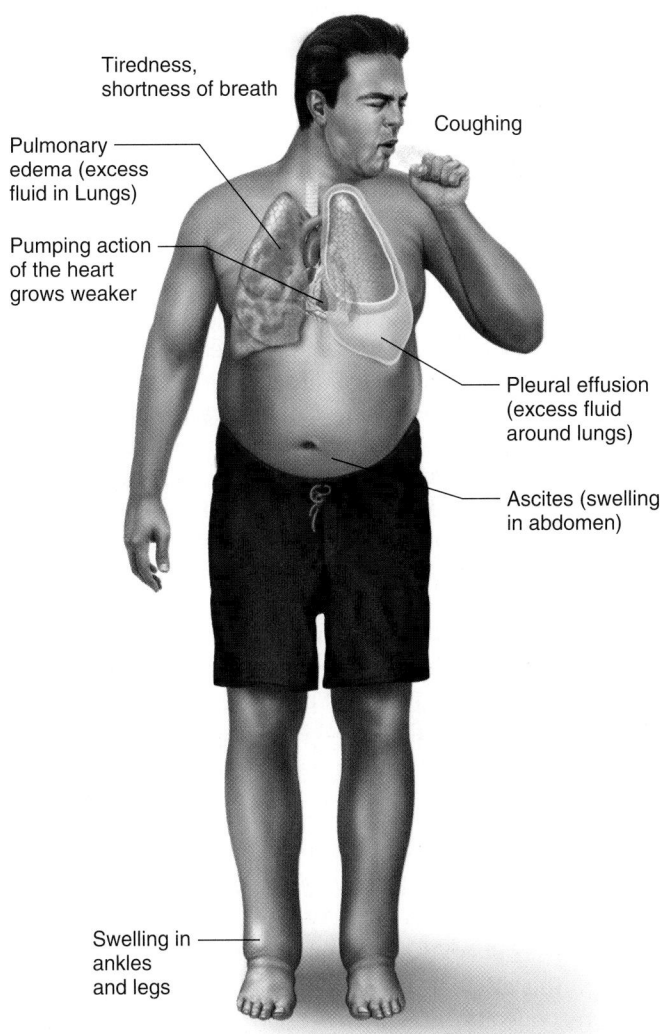

Tiredness, shortness of breath

Coughing

Pulmonary edema (excess fluid in Lungs)

Pumping action of the heart grows weaker

Pleural effusion (excess fluid around lungs)

Ascites (swelling in abdomen)

Swelling in ankles and legs

FIGURE 26-14 When the heart muscle is damaged and weak, a patient will suffer symptoms of heart failure.

that causes swelling in the legs, feet, or abdomen; nausea; dizziness; and an irregular or rapid heartbeat. (See Figure 26-14.)

Treatment. Common treatment options include medications to slow a rapid heartbeat, diuretics to decrease edema and fluid accumulation in the lungs, and medications to reduce blood pressure. In more serious cases, surgery to repair defective heart valves or other heart defects, implantation of a cardiac pacemaker, or a heart transplant may be needed.

Go to CONNECT to see animations about *Heart Failure Overview, Left-Side Heart Failure,* and *Right-Side Heart Failure.*

CORONARY ARTERY DISEASE (CAD) is also known as *atherosclerosis.* It affects more Americans than any other type of heart disease. The American Heart Association estimates that one in three American adults has one or more types of coronary artery disease.

Causes. This condition is characterized by the narrowing of coronary arteries. Usually the narrowing is produced by the buildup of fat, cholesterol, and calcium in the arteries. The risk factors for developing this condition include high levels of LDL (low density lipoprotein) cholesterol in the blood, a diet high in fat and cholesterol, smoking, high blood pressure, obesity, a lack of exercise, and diabetes mellitus. As with congestive heart failure, this condition may be prevented by controlling high blood pressure and high cholesterol, not smoking, having a healthy diet, engaging in regular exercise, and treating any existing diabetes and/or atherosclerosis.

Signs and Symptoms. There are often no signs or symptoms until a heart attack occurs. The most common symptoms include angina (a type of chest pain caused by a decreased blood flow to the heart), shortness of breath, tightness in the chest, fatigue, and swelling in the legs or feet (edema).

Treatment. Treatment includes lipid-lowering agents such as Mevacor® or Lipitor®, in addition to a low-fat diet and exercise, aspirin therapy, and medications to slow a rapid heartbeat. Surgery such as coronary angioplasty or, in severe cases or those not responding to angioplasty, CABG (coronary artery bypass grafting) to repair, widen, or detour around narrowed coronary arteries may be needed.

Go to CONNECT to see an animation about *Coronary Artery Disease (CAD).*

HYPERTENSION, commonly known as high blood pressure, is defined as a consistent resting blood pressure measured at 140/90 mm Hg or higher. This condition is commonly known as the "silent killer" because it increases a person's risk of heart attack, stroke, heart failure, and kidney failure, often while presenting no symptoms to the patient. The American Heart Association estimates that 73,000,000 American adults have hypertension, with African Americans having a higher incidence than Caucasians.

Causes. Many of the causes are unknown. Known causes and risk factors include narrowing of the arteries, various medications such as oral contraceptives and cold medicines, kidney disease, endocrine disorders, pregnancy, drug use (especially cocaine and amphetamines), sleep apnea, obesity, smoking, a high-sodium diet, excessive alcohol consumption, stress, and diabetes.

Signs and Symptoms. There are usually no symptoms with hypertension. When symptoms are present, they include excessive sweating, muscle cramps, fatigue, frequent urination, headaches, dizziness, and an irregular heart rate.

Treatment. The first management tool of hypertension control should be to treat the underlying cause if known. Other common treatments include a low-sodium, low-cholesterol diet, regular exercise, various medications to slow the heart rate and dilate blood vessels, diuretics to reduce blood volume, and lifestyle changes such as managing stress and stopping smoking. Patient compliance is the key to the successful management of hypertension, which usually cannot be cured, only controlled. Because hypertension itself often has no symptoms and medications often have side effects, patients frequently stop their anti-hypertensive regimes because "I felt better off the medication." Be sure they understand that medication compliance is crucial to their treatment and long-term health. They must tell the physician when a medication is not working for them because there are often many other options available for treatment.

Go to CONNECT to see an animation about *Hypertension*.

MITRAL VALVE PROLAPSE (MVP) is a condition in which the mitral valve falls into the left atrium during systole. This prevents the valve from sealing properly. In severe cases, blood may flow back into the atrium. Although most cases are mild, MVP can become worse over time. It also increases the risk of heart valve infections and endocarditis.

Causes. The cause of MVP is unknown in most cases. However, it may be hereditary, and it has been linked to autonomic nervous system disorders.

Signs and Symptoms. In mild cases, symptoms may not develop. In more severe cases, palpitations, shortness of breath, and chest pain may occur.

Treatment. No treatment is needed for mild cases. Medications are used to treat symptoms and to help prevent complications such as infection. In very severe cases, surgery may be required to repair the valve.

MURMURS are simply abnormal heart sounds. Normally, heart sounds are clear, strong, and smooth as valves close completely, and blood flows over the lining of the heart with no resistance. Not all murmurs indicate a heart disorder. Murmurs are graded from 1 to 6; 1 is barely audible and the least serious.

Causes. Not all the causes of heart murmurs are known. In children, the failure of the foramen ovale or ductus arteriosis to close completely after birth can cause murmurs. Other causes include stress and defective heart valves that do not close completely.

Signs and Symptoms. The signs and symptoms vary considerably depending on the cause and severity of the heart murmur. Severe symptoms include weakness, pallor, edema (fluid retention), and other signs commonly associated with heart failure.

Treatment. In many cases, no treatment is required. Surgery to correct valvular defects or other heart defects may be needed in more serious cases.

A **MYOCARDIAL INFARCTION,** commonly called a *heart attack*, is characterized by damage to cardiac muscle because of a lack of blood supply. Historically, heart attacks have been fatal, and they often still are, but with new treatments, more and more people survive MIs. However, they can be left with permanent damage because cardiac muscle does not grow back once it is lost.

Causes. The causes and contributing factors include blockage of coronary arteries as a result of atherosclerosis or a blood clot. Drugs such as cocaine also can cause coronary arteries to spasm. Preventing an MI includes treating or reducing the risk of atherosclerosis, including the use of lipid-lowering agents to lower cholesterol. This condition may be further prevented by controlling high blood pressure, not smoking, having a healthy diet, engaging in regular physical exercise, and avoiding the use of drugs such as cocaine.

Signs and Symptoms. Common symptoms include recurring, squeezing chest pain; pain in the shoulder, arm, back, teeth, or jaw; chronic pain in the upper abdomen; shortness of breath, especially on exertion; sweating (diaphoresis); dizziness or fainting; and nausea or vomiting.

Treatment. The first treatment, if possible, is chewing an aspirin at the onset of symptoms. In an unconscious patient without a pulse or respiration, CPR (cardiopulmonary resuscitation) should be administered. Other treatment options include the use of a defibrillator (if available) and thrombolytic drugs to destroy the blood clots that block a coronary artery. It should be noted these drugs are only effective if begun within 3 hours of the first symptom, so time is crucial. Anticoagulant medications, such as heparin and warfarin, should be administered to thin the blood. Medications that slow the heart rate, such as atenalol, may also be administered. Surgery to replace or repair blocked coronary arteries (angioplasty or CABG) may be necessary. According to the American Heart Association, in 2005 there were 469,000 cardiac bypasses in the United States and 1,265,000 percutaneous catheterization transluminal angioplasties, and the numbers are rising.

Stenosis of the heart valves is a condition in which the valves do not open fully.

AORTIC STENOSIS is a narrowing of the aortic valve, and **MITRAL STENOSIS** is narrowing of the mitral valve. In both, the valve does not fully open, so blood flow from the heart decreases, and pressure inside the left ventricle increases.

Causes. This disorder can be congenital or can occur later in life. Non-congenital cases often occur in patients who have had rheumatic fever.

Signs and Symptoms. Common signs and symptoms include shortness of breath, angina, palpitations, dizziness, weakness and fatigue.

Treatment. Mild cases may not be treated. Medications are used to treat heart failure or arrhythmias, if they occur. For people who have had rheumatic fever, antibiotics may also be given. Surgery or valvuloplasty is performed in severe cases.

THROMBOPHLEBITIS is a condition in which a blood clot and inflammation develop in a vein. It most commonly occurs in the leg veins. The danger of this disorder is that the blood clot may break loose, becoming an *embolus*. Once it reaches the heart, it is pumped to the lungs. If it blocks a blood vessel, it will cause a pulmonary embolism (an obstruction in the lungs). If the blood clot reaches the aorta and is pumped into arterial circulation, it can block a coronary artery, causing an MI (heart attack), or it can block a cerebral artery in the brain, causing a CVA (stroke).

Causes. The causes and risk factors include prolonged inactivity, oral contraceptives, post-menopausal hormone replacement therapy (HRT), certain types of cancer, paralysis in the arms or legs, the presence of a venous catheter, a family history of this condition, varicose veins, and trauma to veins.

Signs and Symptoms. The most common symptoms are tenderness and pain in the affected area; redness, swelling, and tenseness of the affected areas; fever; and a positive Homan's sign which is pain behind the knee, caused by a blood clot, when the foot is forceably dorsiflexed.

Treatment. This disorder is most often treated by the application of heat to the affected area, elevation of the legs, anti-inflammatory drugs, anticoagulant medications, wearing support stockings, and the removal of varicose veins. Surgery to remove the clot may be needed in some cases.

VARICOSE VEINS are twisted, dilated veins usually seen in the legs. They affect women more often than men. When varicose veins occur in the rectum, they are called *hemorrhoids.*

Causes. Varicose veins may be caused by prolonged sitting or standing, damage to valves in the veins, a loss of elasticity in the veins, obesity, pregnancy, oral contraceptives, or hormone replacement therapy. Family history also seems to play a part in the development of varicose veins. In some cases, varicose veins may be prevented or at least minimized through exercise and elevation of the legs.

Signs and Symptoms. Signs and symptoms include discomfort in the legs, discolorations around the ankles, clusters of veins, and enlarged, dark veins seen through skin.

Treatment. The treatment of varicose veins includes the following:

- Sclerotherapy, a procedure that prevents blood from flowing through varicose veins.
- Laser surgery to prevent blood from flowing through affected veins.
- Vein stripping, which involves removing affected veins.
- Insertion of a catheter in the affected veins in order to destroy them.
- Endoscopic vein surgery to close off affected veins.

SUMMARY OF LEARNING OUTCOMES

LEARNING OUTCOMES	KEY POINTS
26.1 Describe the structures of the heart and the function of each.	The structures of the heart include the pericardium, epicardium, myocardium, and endocardium. The chambers of the heart consist of the upper atria and the lower ventricles. The septa are the interatrial, interventricular, and atrioventricular. The four valves within the heart are the tricuspid, the bicuspid, the pulmonary semilunar, and the aortic semilunar valves.
26.2 Explain the cardiac cycle, including the cardiac conduction system.	One cardiac cycle consists of one complete heartbeat. The atria contract and relax together, and the ventricles contract and relax together. As each chamber contracts, associated valves open and close to control the flow of blood through the heart. Contractions are initiated by the cardiac conduction system, which consists of the sinoatrial node, the atrioventricular node, the bundle of His, and Purkinje fibers.
26.3 Compare pulmonary and systemic circulation.	Pulmonary circulation: Right atrium → tricuspid valve → right ventricle → pulmonary semilunar valve → pulmonary trunk → pulmonary arteries → lungs → pulmonary veins → left atrium. Systemic circulation: Left atrium → bicuspid valve → left ventricle → aortic semilunar valve → aorta → arteries → arterioles → capillaries → venules → veins → venae cavae → right atrium.
26.4 Differentiate among the different types of blood vessels their functions.	Types of blood vessels include arteries and arterioles, which bring blood from the heart to the body; veins and venules, which carry blood back from the body to the heart; and capillaries, which act as the connectors between the arterioles and venules. The largest artery in the body is the aorta. Other major arteries include lingual, facial, occipital, maxillary, ophthalmic, axillary, brachial, ulnar, radial, intercostals, lumbar, external iliac, common iliac, femoral, popliteal, and tibial. The largest veins in the body are the superior and inferior venae cavae. Other major veins are jugular, brachiocephalic, axillary, brachial, ulnar, radial, intercostals, azygos, iliac, femoral, popliteal, saphenous, hepatic, gastic, splenic, mesenteric, and hepatic portal.

LEARNING OUTCOMES	KEY POINTS
26.5 **Explain blood pressure and tell how it is controlled.**	Blood pressure is the force exerted on the inner wall of blood vessels by blood as it flows through vessels. It is highest in arteries and lowest in veins. Clinically, blood pressure refers to the force of blood within the arteries. Blood pressure is largely controlled by the amount of blood pumped out of the heart, but various other events also may raise and lower blood pressure.
26.6 **Describe the causes, signs and symptoms, and treatments of various diseases and disorders of the cardiovascular system.**	Many different types of cardiac and blood diseases are described within this chapter. The signs, symptoms, and treatments are as varied as the diseases themselves. The last section of this chapter outlines the most common of these diseases, their signs and symptoms, as well as their treatments.

CASE STUDY CRITICAL THINKING

Recall John Miller from the beginning of this chapter. Now that you have completed this chapter, answer the following questions regarding his case.

1. What symptoms suggest that this patient is suffering from coronary artery disease and not some other disorder?

2. Why is it important to test the heart under stress rather than obtaining a resting echocardiogram?

3. Why is a cardiac catheterization needed in addition to the stress echocardiogram?

4. What lifestyle changes should this patient make to prevent future heart attacks?

EXAM PREPARATION QUESTIONS

1. (LO 26.1) Which heart valve is between the left atrium and left ventricle?
  a. Tricuspid
  b. Bicuspid
  c. Pulmonary semilunar
  d. Aortic semilunar
  e. Right atrioventricular

2. (LO 26.2) Which part of the cardiac conduction system receives electrical impulses from the bundle branches?
  a. AV node
  b. SA node
  c. Bundle of His
  d. Purkinje fibers
  e. Chordae tendineae

3. (LO 26.4) Which vessels are also known as the "exchange vessels"?
  a. Arteries
  b. Arterioles
  c. Veins
  d. Venules
  e. Capillaries

4. (LO 26.3) Which chamber of the heart receives oxygenated blood from the lungs?
  a. Left atrium
  b. Right atrium
  c. Pulmonary trunk
  d. Left ventricle
  e. Right ventricle

5. (LO 26.6) Which of the following causes of chest pain is *not* cardiac in nature?
  a. Angina
  b. Pericarditis
  c. Costochondritis
  d. Myocardial infarction
  e. Coronary spasms

6. (LO 26.5) The amount of pressure in the arteries when the ventricles contract is called
  a. Cardiac output
  b. Vasodilation
  c. Vasoconstriction
  d. Diastole
  e. Systole

7. (LO 26.1) The layer of the heart wall that is made mostly of cardiac muscle that allows the heart to contract and relax is the
   a. Pericardial space
   b. Myocardium
   c. Epicardium
   d. Visceral pericardium
   e. Endocardium

8. (LO 26.6) A condition in which a blood clot and inflammation develop in a vein is
   a. Mitral stenosis
   b. Varicose veins
   c. Thrombophlebitis
   d. Myocardial infarction
   e. Pericarditis

9. (LO 26.4) The largest veins in the body are the
   a. Hepatic portal veins
   b. Jugular veins
   c. Venae cavae
   d. Pulmonary veins
   e. Femoral veins

10. (LO 26.5) The total amount of blood pumped out of the heart in one minute is known as the
    a. Cardiac output
    b. Systolic pressure
    c. Systemic circulation
    d. Coronary sinus
    e. Diastolic pressure

M E D I C A L   T E R M I N O L O G Y   P R A C T I C E

Analyze the following medical terms, presented throughout the chapter. Using a medical dictionary (or Appendix I) place a / mark between each word part. Define each word part and then define the whole word.

EXAMPLE: vaso / spasm = vaso means "vessel" + spasm means "cramp or twitching"
   Vasospasm means "twitching or cramping of a vessel"

1. atherosclerosis
2. atrioventricular
3. baroreceptor
4. echocardiogram
5. electrocardiogram
6. intercostal
7. myocardium
8. pericarditis
9. stenosis
10. thrombophlebitis
11. vasoconstriction
12. ventricular

PATIENT INFORMATION

Patient Name	Gender	DOB
Cindy Chen	F	7/15/19XX

Attending	MRN	Allergies
Alexis N. Whalen, MD	324-86-542	NKA

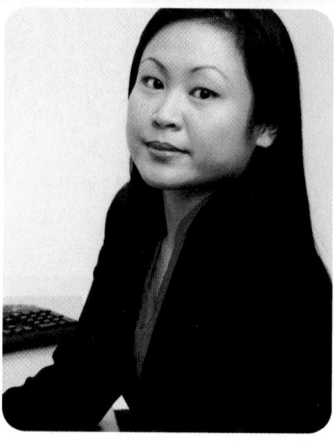

Cindy Chen is a 28-year-old Asian female complaining of inability to sleep and nervousness. She tested positive for HIV in 2005, although she has been asymptomatic on antiviral drugs. She currently lives with her aunt and is going to school for phlebotomy. When looking at her chart, you notice that she has lost 20 pounds since her last visit. Dr. Whalen has ordered a series of blood tests including helper T cell tests and CBC with platelet count.

Keep Cindy in mind as you study the chapter. There will be questions at the end of the chapter based on the case study. The information in the chapter will help you answer these questions.

ACTIV**Sim**™

L E A R N I N G   O U T C O M E S

After completing Chapter 27, you will be able to:

27.1 Describe the components of blood, giving the function of each component listed.

27.2 Explain how bleeding is controlled.

27.3 Explain the differences among blood types A, B, AB, and O; including in the discussion which blood types are compatible.

27.4 Explain the difference between Rh-positive blood and Rh-negative blood.

27.5 Describe the causes, signs and symptoms, and treatments of various diseases and disorders of the blood.

K E Y   T E R M S

agglutination
agranulocyte
basophil
coagulation
eosinophil
erythrocyte
erythropoietin
fibrinogen
globulins
granulocyte

hematocrit
hemostasis
leukocyte
lymphocyte
monocyte
neutrophil
platelets
serum
thrombocytes
thrombus

I. C (7) Analyze pathology as it relates to the interaction of body systems

I. C (8) Discuss implications for disease and disability when homeostasis is not maintained

I. C (9) Describe implications for treatment related to pathology

I. C (10) Compare body structure and function of the human body across the life span

I. C (12) Describe the relationship between anatomy and physiology of all body systems and medications used for treatment in each

IV. C (11) Define both medical terms and abbreviations related to all body systems

2. Anatomy & Physiology
Graduates:

b. Identify and apply the knowledge of all body systems, their structure and functions; and their common diseases, symptoms, and etiologies

c. Assist the physician with the regimen of diagnostic and treatment modalities as they relate to each body system

3. Medical Terminology
Graduates:

b. Build and dissect medical terms from roots/suffixes to understand the word element combinations that create medical terminology

c. Understand the various medical terminology for each specialty

d. Recognize and identify acceptable medical abbreviations

▶ Introduction

Your blood is a type of connective tissue that is made up of multiple parts, including red and white blood cells, cell fragments called platelets, and plasma (the fluid part of the blood). The average-sized adult body contains approximately 4 to 6 liters of blood, or approximately 8% of the total body weight. Blood volume varies from person to person depending on the person's size, the amount of adipose tissue in the body, and the concentrations of certain ions in the blood. In general, partly because of their smaller size, females generally have less blood volume than males. Blood can be considered the fluid of life because of the many essential functions it performs. It carries oxygen and nutrients to tissues, and carbon dioxide and wastes away from tissues. It also acts as the transport mechanism for hormones and aids in regulating body temperature.

▶ Components of Blood   LO 27.1

Red Blood Cells

Red blood cells (RBCs), also called **erythrocytes,** are biconcave-shaped cells, similar to a doughnut with a depression where the hole should be, that are small enough to pass through capillaries (see Figure 27-1).

The percentage of red blood cells in a sample of blood is called the **hematocrit.** A healthy person normally has a hematocrit level of about 45%. Most of the "formed elements" or cells found in blood are red blood cells, with only about 1% being white blood cells and platelets. The rest of blood (approximately 55%) is plasma (see Figure 27-2).

Mature RBCs do not contain nuclei. They lose their nuclei in order to make room for a pigment called *hemoglobin.* The function of hemoglobin is to carry oxygen from the lungs to

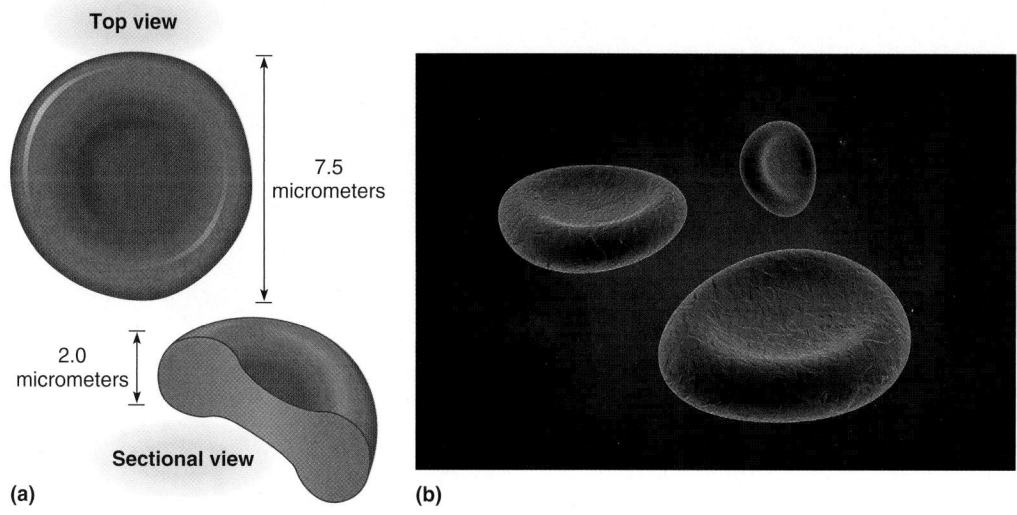

FIGURE 27-1 Red blood cells: (a) bioconcave shape of red blood cells and (b) scanning electron micrograph of red blood cells.

Centrifuged Blood Sample

Liquid
(plasma)

"Buffy coat" (white blood cells and platelets)

Red blood cells

Peripheral Blood Smear

White blood
cells

Red blood cells

Platelets

FIGURE 27-2 Centrifuged blood sample and peripheral blood smear slide seen through a microscope showing blood components.

the body tissues, and to carry carbon dioxide from the tissues to the lungs for release from the body. Hemoglobin that carries oxygen is called *oxyhemoglobin* and is bright red; hemoglobin that is not carrying oxygen is called *deoxyhemoglobin* and is a darker red. Often, because the deoxyhemoglobin is now carrying carbon dioxide, it is referred to as *carboxyhemoglobin*. Through blood testing, the amount of oxygen and carbon dioxide in the blood can be measured.

An RBC count consists of the number of red blood cells in 1 cubic millimeter (roughly 20 drops) of blood. A normal RBC count is between 4 million and 6.5 million RBC/milliliter. Because the function of an RBC is to transport oxygen throughout the body, a low count reflects a decreased ability to carry oxygen, causing a condition known as *anemia*. Likewise, if the RBC count is adequate but the amount of hemoglobin within the red blood cells is decreased, thus impairing the ability to carry adequate oxygen, anemia may also be diagnosed.

During fetal development, RBCs are made in the yolk sac, the liver, and the spleen. However, once a baby is born, most blood cells are produced in red bone marrow by cells called *hemocytoblasts*. The average life span of an RBC is only about 120 days, so red bone marrow is constantly making new cells. The hormone **erythropoietin,** produced by the kidneys, stimulates the red bone marrow and is responsible for regulating the production of RBCs. The kidneys release erythropoietin when oxygen concentrations in the blood get low.

Iron is necessary to make hemoglobin. In addition to iron, vitamin B_{12} and folic acid (vitamin B_9) are two dietary factors that affect RBC production. These vitamins are necessary for DNA synthesis, so red bone marrow, like all actively dividing tissue, is affected when DNA cannot be produced. As stated earlier, too few RBCs or too little hemoglobin can result in anemia, a common condition of many types, which will be discussed in more detail in the Pathophysiology: Common Diseases and Disorders for the Blood System section of this chapter.

As RBCs age, macrophages in the liver and spleen destroy them. When an RBC is destroyed, a pigment called *biliverdin* is released from the cell. The liver usually converts biliverdin into an orange-colored pigment called *bilirubin*. Bilirubin is used to make bile, which is needed for the digestion of fats. However, when there is too much bilirubin, it builds up in the bloodstream. This causes the individual's skin and the sclera of the eyes to appear yellow-orange in color, a condition known as *jaundice* (or icterus).

White Blood Cells

White blood cells (WBCs), commonly called **leukocytes,** are divided into two categories: granulocytes and agranulocytes. **Granulocytes** have granules (small particles) in their cytoplasm and include neutrophils, eosinophils, and basophils. **Agranulocytes** do not have granules in their cytoplasm and include monocytes and lymphocytes.

Neutrophils account for about 55% of all WBCs (see Figure 27-3). As phagocytes, they are important for destroying bacteria, viruses, and toxins in the blood. **Eosinophils** account for about 3% of all WBCs and are effective in getting rid of viruses and parasitic infections like worms (see Figure 27-4). Eosinophils also help control inflammation and allergic reactions. **Basophils** account for less than 1% of all WBCs. They release substances like histamine, which promotes inflammation, and heparin, which is an anticoagulant (see Figure 27-5).

Monocytes account for about 8% of all WBCs and are important for destroying bacteria, viruses, and toxins in the blood (see Figure 27-6). **Lymphocytes** account for about 33% of all WBCs

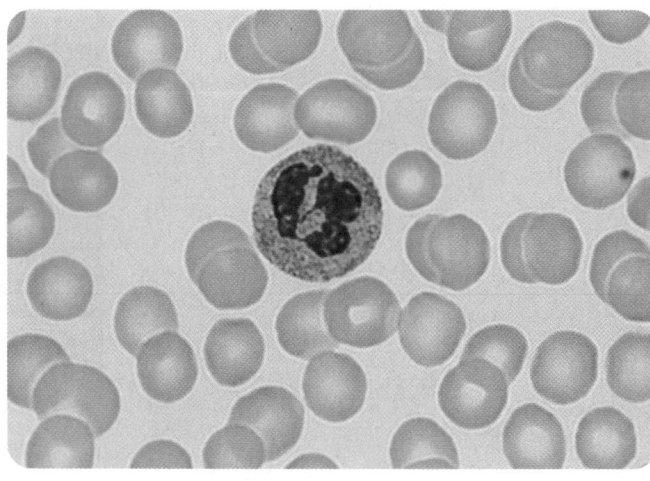

FIGURE 27-3 Neutrophils have distinct nuclei with many lobes.

FIGURE 27-4 Eosinophils have cytoplasmic granules that stain red.

FIGURE 27-5 Basophils have cytoplasmic granules that stain deep blue.

FIGURE 27-6 Monocytes have large kidney-shaped nuclei. They do not have cytoplasmic granules.

FIGURE 27-7 Lymphocytes have large round nuclei.

and provide immunity for the body (see Figure 27-7). Lymphocytes and their specific function in the immune system will be discussed further in *The Lymphatic and Immune Systems* chapter.

A WBC count is the number of WBCs in 1 cubic millimeter of blood. This count is normally between 5,000 and 10,000 cells. A WBC count above normal is called *leukocytosis.* This condition often results from bacterial infections. A WBC count below normal is called *leukopenia* and is caused by some viral infections and various other conditions.

A differential WBC count lists the percentages of the different types of leukocytes in a sample of blood. This is a useful test because certain diseases and conditions change the usual balance among the different types of WBCs. For example, neutrophil numbers increase at the beginning of a bacterial or viral infection, but monocyte numbers do not increase until about 2 weeks after a bacterial infection. Eosinophil numbers increase during viral or worm infections as well as with allergic reactions. In AIDS, lymphocyte numbers fall, particularly lymphocytes known as T-lymphocytes or T cells. You will gain more in-depth knowledge about T cells in *The Lymphatic and Immune Systems* chapter.

Some WBCs stay in the bloodstream to fight infections, whereas others leave the bloodstream by squeezing through blood vessel walls to reach other tissues. This squeezing of a cell through a blood vessel wall, which is called *diapedesis,* is shown in Figure 27-8.

FIGURE 27-8 Diapedesis of white blood cells into surrounding tissue.

Blood Platelets

Platelets are fragments of cells that are found in the blood-stream (refer back to Figure 27-2). Platelets are also called **thrombocytes** (thrombo = clot; cyte = cell) and are important in the blood-clotting process. Platelets come from cells called *megakaryocytes* found in red bone marrow. A normal platelet count is between 150,000 and 450,000 platelets per microliter of blood.

Blood Plasma

Plasma is the liquid portion of blood. It is mostly water but also contains a mixture of proteins, nutrients, gases, electrolytes, and waste products. The three major types of proteins in plasma are albumins, globulins, and fibrinogen. *Albumins* are the smallest of the plasma proteins and are important for pulling water into the bloodstream to help maintain blood pressure. **Globulins** transport lipids and some fat-soluble vitamins in plasma. Some globulins become antibodies. **Fibrinogen** is important in the blood-clotting process. The term **serum** refers to the fluid that is left when all clotting factors are removed from plasma. You will learn more about serum in the *Processing and Testing Blood Specimens* chapter.

Nutrients in plasma include amino acids, glucose, nucleotides, and lipids that have all been absorbed from the digestive tract. Because lipids are not water soluble and because plasma is mostly water, lipids must combine with molecules called *lipoproteins* to be transported. The different types of lipoproteins are chylomicrons, very low-density lipoproteins (VLDL), low-density lipoproteins (LDL), and high-density lipoproteins (HDL). You will learn more about lipids and their effect on the body in the *Nutrition and Health* chapter.

The gases dissolved in plasma include oxygen, carbon dioxide, and nitrogen. Many electrolytes are also dissolved in plasma. They include sodium, potassium, calcium, magnesium, chloride, bicarbonate, phosphate, and sulfate. Molecules that contain nitrogen but are not proteins make up a group called *nonprotein nitrogenous substances.* They include amino acids, urea, and uric acid. Urea and uric acid are waste products produced by cells.

▶ Bleeding Control
LO 27.2

Hemostasis refers to the control of bleeding. Three basic processes occur during hemostasis:

1. Blood vessel spasm
2. Platelet plug formation
3. Blood coagulation

When a blood vessel is broken, the smooth muscle of its wall responds to the damage by contracting, which in turn, causes the blood vessel to spasm. This spasm begins to reduce the amount of blood lost through the vessel. Platelets begin to flood the area, sticking to the injured vessel and to each other to form a platelet plug. The platelet plug slows or controls the bleeding temporarily (see Figure 27-9).

A blood clot eventually replaces the platelet plug. The formation of a blood clot is called blood **coagulation.** In this process, the plasma protein fibrinogen is converted to fibrin. Once fibrin forms, it sticks to the damaged area of the blood vessel, creating a meshwork that entraps blood cells and platelets. The resulting mass—the blood clot—stops bleeding until the vessel has repaired itself (see Figure 27-10).

When a blood vessel is injured, it is normal for a blood clot to form. However, sometimes blood clots form on the side of a blood vessel with no known injury; this abnormal blood clot is called a **thrombus.** A thrombus is dangerous because a portion of it can break off and start moving through the bloodstream. The moving portion of the thrombus is called an *embolus.* An embolus is dangerous because, as discussed in the *Cardiovascular System* chapter, it can eventually block a small artery in the lungs, heart, or brain causing pulmonary embolism, myocardial infarction, or CVA (stroke), respectively. All of these are serious and possibly fatal conditions if not treated, or if treatment cannot be initiated quickly enough to stop the condition from progressing.

(a)   (b)   (c)

FIGURE 27-9 Vasoconstriction and platelet plug formation leading to blood clot.

FIGURE 27-10 Scanning electron micrograph of a blood clot. Yellow fibrin threads are covering red blood cells.

▶ ABO Blood Types

LO 27.3

The ABO blood group consists of four different blood types: A, B, AB, and O. They are distinguished from each other in part by their antigens and antibodies.

Agglutination is the clumping of RBCs following a blood transfusion. This clumping is not desirable because it leads to severe anemia. Agglutination occurs because proteins called *antigens* on the surface of RBCs bind to antibodies in plasma (see Figure 27-11). To prevent agglutination, antigens should not be mixed with antibodies that will bind to them. Fortunately, most antibodies do not bind to antigens on blood cells; only very specific ones bind to them. There are four different blood types.

Type A Blood

People with type A blood have antigen A on the surface of their RBCs. They also have antibody B in their plasma. Antibody B will only bind to antigen B.

Type B Blood

People with type B blood have antigen B on the surface of their RBCs. They also have antibody A in their plasma. Antibody A will only bind to antigen A.

If a person with type A blood is given type B blood, then the antibody B in the recipient's blood will bind with the RBCs of the donor blood because those cells have antigen B on their surfaces. As a result, agglutination occurs, and the donated RBCs are destroyed. This is why a person with type A blood should not be given type B blood (and vice versa).

(a)

(b)

(c)

(d)

FIGURE 27-11 Agglutination: (a) red blood cells with antigen A are added to blood that contains antibody anti-A; (b) antibody anti-A reacts with antigen A, causing the agglutination of blood; (c) normal blood; and (d) agglutinated blood.

Type AB Blood

People with type AB blood have both antigen A and antigen B on the surface of their RBCs. They have neither antibody A nor antibody B in their plasma. People with type AB blood are called *universal recipients* because most of them can receive all ABO blood types. They can receive these blood types because they lack antibody A and antibody B in their plasma, so there is no reaction with antigens A and B of the donor blood.

Type O Blood

People with type O blood have neither antigen A nor antigen B on the surface of their RBCs. However, they do have both antibody A and antibody B in their plasma. People with type O blood are called *universal donors* because their blood can be given to most people, regardless of the recipient's blood type. Type O blood will not agglutinate when given to other people because it does not have the antigens to bind to antibody A or antibody B. Table 27-1 summarizes the ABO blood group. Also see Figure 27-12 for a pictorial representation of each blood type.

TABLE 27-1 ABO Blood Type Overview

Blood Type	Antigen Present	Antibody Present	Blood Type That Can Be Received
A	A	B	A and O
B	B	A	B and O
AB	A and B	None	All blood types
O	None	A and B	O only

▶ The Rh Factor   LO 27.4

The *Rh antigen* is a protein first discovered on RBCs of the rhesus monkey, hence the name Rh. People who are Rh-positive have RBCs that contain the Rh antigen. People who are Rh-negative have RBCs that do not contain the Rh antigen. If a person who is Rh-negative is given Rh-positive blood, then the Rh-negative person's blood will make antibodies that bind to the Rh antigens. If the Rh-negative person is given Rh-positive blood a second time, the antibodies will bind to the donor cells and agglutination will occur.

Clinically, it is very important for a female to know her Rh type if she is pregnant or wishes to become pregnant. If an Rh-negative female mates with an Rh-positive male, there is a 50% chance her fetus will be Rh-positive. When the blood of an Rh-positive fetus mixes with the blood of a mother who is Rh-negative, the mother develops antibodies against the fetus's RBCs. Typically, the first Rh-positive fetus (infant) does not suffer any effects from these antibodies because it takes so long for the mother's body to generate them. However, if the mother conceives a second Rh-positive fetus, her antibodies will attack this fetus's blood right away. The second fetus then develops a condition called *erythroblastosis fetalis,* and the baby is born severely anemic, often needing multiple blood transfusions at birth and often several times as a neonate (see Figure 27-13). Erythroblastosis fetalis is prevented by giving an Rh-negative woman the drug RhoGAM. RhoGAM prevents an Rh-negative mother from making antibodies against the Rh antigen.

Type A blood

Type B blood

Type AB blood

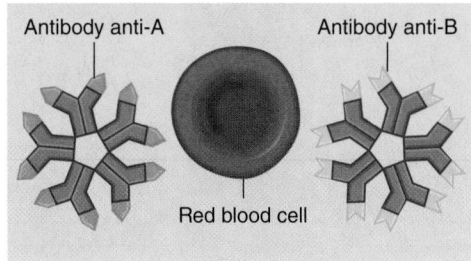

Type O blood

FIGURE 27-12 Blood Types A, B, AB, and O.

FIGURE 27-13 Development of antibodies in an Rh-negative woman in reaction to the blood of her Rh-positive fetus.

Common Diseases and Disorders of the Blood System

ANEMIA is a condition in which a person does not have enough RBCs or hemoglobin in the blood to carry an adequate amount of oxygen to the body's cells. It is the most common blood disorder in the United States and can be a sign of a more serious disorder. It generally affects more women than men. Many types of anemia can be prevented through a healthy diet high in iron, vitamin B_{12}, and folic acid. Other types of anemia require medical attention for more serious, underlying conditions.

Causes. The many causes of this condition include the following:

- Iron deficiency. This is the most common cause of anemia. Iron is needed to make hemoglobin, which is the pigment that carries most oxygen in the blood. Pregnant women and women with heavy menstrual cycles are most susceptible to this type of anemia.

- Chronic blood loss. Slow blood loss can occur in conditions such as ulcers, colon polyps, or colon cancer.

- Vitamin deficiency. Vitamin B_{12} and folic acid are needed to make enough RBCs.

- Inability to absorb vitamin B_{12}. This condition is called *pernicious anemia*. Some intestinal disorders prevent the absorption of vitamin B_{12}.

- Side effect of medication. Some oral contraceptives, seizure medications, and anti-neoplastic drugs used to treat cancer can cause anemia.

- Chronic illness. Chronic diseases like AIDS, cancer, rheumatoid arthritis, leukemia, and kidney failure can cause anemia.

- Bone marrow disorder. When the bone marrow fails to produce enough blood cells, aplastic anemia results. This is a life-threatening type of anemia. Toxins, chemotherapy, and radiation therapy can all destroy bone marrow.
- Destruction of RBCs. Some blood diseases, like sickle cell disease, cause RBCs to be destroyed faster than they can be made. These types of anemia are called *hemolytic anemias*.

Signs and Symptoms. Signs and symptoms of all forms of anemia include tiredness, weakness, pallor (paleness), tachycardia, numb or cold hands and feet, dizziness, headache, and jaundice.

Treatment. Injections of vitamin B$_{12}$ may be necessary. Treatment often begins with addressing the underlying causes, like an ulcer or colon polyps. Other treatment options include administering various medications, discontinuing the use of medications that can cause anemia, and blood transfusions or bone marrow transplants if defective or diseased bone marrow is the cause.

LEUKEMIA is a condition in which the bone marrow produces a large number of abnormal WBCs that prevent normal WBCs from carrying out their defensive functions. This disorder is sometimes referred to as cancer of the WBCs. There are several different kinds of leukemia: acute lymphocytic (lymphatic) leukemia, acute myelogenous leukemia, chronic lymphocytic (lymphatic) leukemia, and chronic myelogenous leukemia.

Causes. Causes include mutations (changes) in WBCs, chemotherapy for the treatment of other cancers, genetic factors (for example, the inheritance of abnormal genes), and exposure to environmental and chemical agents that cause changes in the WBCs.

Signs and Symptoms. The many signs and symptoms include fatigue, dyspnea on exertion (DOE), an enlarged liver (hepatomegaly) or spleen (splenomegaly), swollen (nontender) lymph nodes, abnormal bruising, cuts that heal slowly, frequent infections, nosebleeds, bleeding gums, chronic fever, unexplained weight loss, and excessive sweating.

Treatment. Treatment options include chemotherapy, radiation therapy, medications to strengthen the immune system, antibodies to destroy mutated WBCs, bone marrow transplant, and stem cell transplant.

SICKLE CELL ANEMIA is a condition in which abnormal hemoglobin causes RBCs to change to a sickle (crescent) shape. These sickle-shaped RBCs get stuck in capillaries. Sickle cell anemia affects about 1 in every 500 African Americans and 1 in every 1,400 Latino Americans born in the United States.

Causes. The primary cause is hereditary. As an autosomal recessive disorder, a person with this disease must inherit a sickle cell gene from both parents. If only one sickle cell gene is inherited, the person is said to have sickle cell trait and may have only mild symptoms of the disease. However, the person with sickle cell trait may pass on the trait or the disease to his or her children. This condition may be prevented through genetic screening of the parents.

Signs and Symptoms. The many signs and symptoms include anemia, periodic episodes of pain called *crises*, chest pain, numbness in the hands or legs, fainting, fatigue, swollen hands and feet, jaundice, frequent infections, sores on the skin, delayed growth, stroke, seizures, and breathing difficulties. Retina damage, which causes visual problems, and spleen, liver, or kidney and lung damage also may be seen.

Treatment. There is no cure for sickle cell disease, but treatment includes antibiotics to treat infections, blood transfusions, pain medications, bone marrow transplants, supplemental oxygen, and medications to promote the development of normal hemoglobin.

POLYCYTHEMIA VERA is a disease of the bone marrow that results in an abnormally high number of blood cells, especially red blood cells, causing the blood to thicken. It occurs more often in men than in women, and it usually occurs after the age of 40.

Causes. A genetic mutation causes polycythemia. However, the cause of the mutation is not known.

Signs and Symptoms. The signs and symptoms of polycythemia include difficulty breathing and shortness of breath, dizziness, excessive bleeding, enlarged spleen, and headache. Itching and a reddened skin color, especially in the face, may also be seen.

Treatment. Treatment involves reducing the thickness of the blood. Up to a pint of blood may be removed each week until the blood count becomes normal. Frequent blood counts are performed to monitor the blood, and further bloodletting, known as *therapeutic phlebotomy*, is performed when needed. Chemotherapy may also be used in some cases to reduce production of red blood cells, and aspirin may be prescribed to help prevent clots.

THALASSEMIA is an inherited form of anemia with a defective hemoglobin chain, causing microcytic (small), hypochromic (pale), and short-lived RBCs.

Causes. The primary cause is hereditary. Patients of Mediterranean descent are most likely to carry the defective autosomal recessive gene that causes this disease. Like sickle cell disease, thalassemia comes in two forms. *Thalassemia major* is the disease. Patients with *thalassemia minor* have only minimal symptoms, if any; this is considered to be a "carrier" form of the disease. Also like sickle cell, both parents must send the defective gene to the child in order for the child to be diagnosed with this disease. Inheriting only one gene results in the carrier status.

Signs and Symptoms. Thalassemia major is evident in infancy with anemia, fever, failure to thrive, and splenomegaly (enlarged spleen). It is confirmed by the characteristic changes in RBCs noted on microscopic examination. As the child matures, splenomegaly may interfere with breathing. In addition, skin becomes freckled or bronzed from the iron deposits created by the rapidly destroyed RBCs. Headache, nausea, and anorexia are common signs and symptoms.

Treatment. There is no cure for thalassemia. Frequent transfusions are necessary to treat the anemia caused by the destruction of the defective RBCs. A splenectomy may be recommended. Symptoms are otherwise treated as needed, including pain medication for the acute episodes known as crises, which are similar to those of sickle cell patients. Patients and their families may require counseling to help them deal with the day-to-day reality of living with this disease.

LEARNING OUTCOMES	KEY POINTS
27.1 **Describe the components of blood, giving the function of each component listed.**	The formed elements in blood include: red blood cells that are responsible for oxygen and carbon dioxide transport; white blood cells (granulocytes and agranulocytes) that are responsible for working with the immune system by fighting infection; and platelets, which assist in blood clotting. The liquid component of blood is called *plasma*; when all clotting factors and formed elements are spun out of plasma, the remaining liquid is called *serum*.
27.2 **Explain how bleeding is controlled.**	Hemostasis refers to the control of bleeding. Three basic processes occur during hemostasis: blood vessel spasm, platelet plug formation, and blood coagulation. Clot formation is coagulation. It involves fibrinogen converting to fibrin, which sticks to the damaged area of the blood vessel, creating a meshwork that entraps blood cells and platelets.
27.3 **Explain the differences among blood types A, B, AB, and O; including in the discussion which blood types are compatible.**	The four blood types are A, B, AB, and O. The antibodies attached to each type (except AB, which has no antibodies) require that each blood type receive only its specific antigen type during transfusions. So, A receives A or O; B receives B or O; AB as the universal receiver can receive any blood type; and O, although the universal donor, may receive only type O blood.
27.4 **Explain the difference between Rh-positive blood and Rh-negative blood.**	The Rh factor (named for the rhesus monkey) is an antigen that may be attached to any blood type. Its importance arises during transfusions (Rh-negative blood cannot receive Rh-positive blood) and also during pregnancy if the mother is Rh-negative but the fetus received the Rh-positive antigen from the father. The effect on the first fetus will be little; unless treated, however, any subsequent Rh-positive fetus will suffer effects of erythroblastosis fetalis because the mother's blood developed antibodies against the Rh-positive factor during the initial pregnancy.
27.5 **Describe the causes, signs and symptoms, and treatments of various diseases and disorders of the blood.**	There are many common diseases and disorders of the cardiovascular system with varied signs, symptoms, and treatments. Some of these include anemia, leukemia, sickle cell anemia, polycythemia vera, and thalassemia.

CASE STUDY CRITICAL THINKING

Recall Cindy Chen from the beginning of the chapter. Now that you have completed the chapter, answer the following questions regarding her case.

1. What information about Cindy's blood will be gained by the CBC and platelet count?

2. A helper T cell is a type of white blood cell (WBC). Why would information about Cindy's WBCs, particularly T cells, be of interest to her physician, considering her HIV status?

1. (LO 27.1) Which of the following is the hormone responsible for regulating the production of RBCs?
   a. Hemoglobin
   b. Erythropoietin
   c. Biliverdin
   d. Oxyhemoglobin
   e. Hematocrit

2. (LO 27.1) Which blood cell type does not contain a nucleus?
   a. RBCs
   b. Leukocytes
   c. Agranulocytes
   d. Granulocytes
   e. Serum

3. (LO 27.2) Which term refers to control of bleeding?
   a. Hemoglobin
   b. Hematocrit
   c. Platelets
   d. Agglutination
   e. Hemostasis

4. (LO 27.2) The other term for blood coagulation is
   a. Plug
   b. Fibrin
   c. Clot
   d. Granulation
   e. Agglutination

5. (LO 27.3) Which blood type is the universal donor?
   a. Blood type A
   b. Blood type B
   c. Blood type AB
   d. Blood type O
   e. Rh factor negative

6. (LO 27.3) Which process could indicate a transfusion reaction because of a blood typing mismatch?
   a. Coagulation
   b. Clotting
   c. Hemorrhage
   d. Bleeding
   e. Agglutination

7. (LO 27.4) Which combination could be a potential problem for an unborn fetus?
   a. Rh-negative Mom/Rh-positive Dad/first pregnancy
   b. Rh-positive Mom/Rh-negative Dad/first pregnancy
   c. Rh-negative Mom/Rh-positive Dad/second pregnancy
   d. Rh-positive Mom/Rh-negative Dad/second pregnancy
   e. Either a or c

8. (LO 27.4) RhoGAM is used to prevent
   a. Iron deficiency anemia
   b. Erythroblastosis fetalis
   c. Leukemia
   d. Transfusion reactions
   e. Hemophilia

9. (LO 27.5) Which of the following is a cause of anemia?
   a. Vitamin B_{12} deficiency
   b. Blood loss
   c. RBC destruction
   d. Bone marrow destruction
   e. All of the above are potential causes for anemia

10. (LO 27.5) Which blood disorder is hereditary?
    a. Sickle cell anemia
    b. Thalassemia
    c. Leukemia
    d. Both a and b
    e. Both b and c

MEDICAL TERMINOLOGY PRACTICE

Analyze the following medical terms, presented throughout the chapter. Using a medical dictionary (or Appendix I) place a / mark between each word part. Define each word part and then define the whole word.

EXAMPLE: hemo / rrhage = hemo means "blood" + rhagge means "excessive flow"
Hemorrhage means "excessive flow of blood"

1. erythrocytes
2. leukocytes
3. granulocytes
4. agranulocytes
5. anemia
6. thrombocytes
7. hemostasis
8. erythroblastosis fetalis
9. leukemia
10. hemolytic
11. hematoma
12. venogram

The Lymphatic and Immune Systems

CASE STUDY

Cindy Chen is a 28-year-old Asian female complaining of inability to sleep and nervousness. She tested positive for HIV in 2005, and is asymptomatic and on antiviral drugs. She currently lives with her aunt and is going to school to become a phlebotomist. When looking at her chart, you notice she has lost 20 pounds since her last visit. Dr. Whalen has ordered a series of blood tests, including helper T cell tests and CBC with platelet count.

Keep Cindy in mind as you study the chapter. There will be questions at the end of the chapter based on the case study. The information in the chapter will help you answer these questions.

LEARNING OUTCOMES

After completing Chapter 28, you will be able to:

28.1 Describe the pathways and organs of the lymphatic system.
28.2 Compare the nonspecific and specific body defense mechanisms.
28.3 Explain how antibodies fight infection.
28.4 Describe the four different types of acquired immunities.
28.5 Describe the causes, signs and symptoms, and treatments of major immune disorders.

KEY TERMS

- anaphylaxis
- antibodies
- antibody-mediated response
- antigens
- autoimmune disease
- cell-mediated response
- complements
- cytokines
- hapten
- immunoglobulins
- innate immunity
- interstitial fluid
- lymph
- lymphocytes
- lymphokines
- macrophages
- major histocompatibility complex (MHC)
- monokines
- natural killer (NK) cells
- phagocytosis

CAAHEP

I. C (4)   List major organs in each body system

I. C (5)   Describe the normal function of each body system

I. C (6)   Identify common pathology related to each body system

I. C (7)   Analyze pathology as it relates to the interaction of body systems

I. C (9)   Describe implications for treatment related to pathology

I. C (10)   Compare body structure and function of the human body across the life span

I. C (12)   Describe the relationship between anatomy and physiology of all body systems and medications used for treatment in each

IV. C (11)   Define both medical terms and abbreviations related to all body systems

ABHES

2. **Anatomy & Physiology**

Graduates:

b. Identify and apply the knowledge of all body systems; their structure and functions; and their common diseases, symptoms, and etiologies

c. Assist the physician with the regimen of diagnostic and treatment modalities as they relate to each body system

3. **Medical Terminology**

Graduates:

b. Build and dissect medical terms from roots/suffixes to understand the word element combinations that create medical terminology

c. Understand the various medical terminology for each specialty

d. Recognize and identify acceptable medical abbreviations

▶ Introduction

Your immune system works like a personal coat of armor, responsible for protecting your body against bacteria, viruses, fungi, toxins, parasites, and cancer. This important system, present in every human being, works with the organs of the lymphatic system—the thymus, spleen, and lymph nodes—to clear the body of various disease-causing agents.

▶ The Lymphatic System   LO 28.1

The lymphatic system is a network of connecting vessels that collects fluids between cells. These lymphatic vessels then return this fluid—lymph—to the bloodstream. The lymphatic system also picks up lipids from the digestive organs and transports them to the bloodstream. Finally, the lymphatic system defends the body against disease-causing agents called pathogens.

Lymphatic Pathways

Lymphatic pathways start with tiny vessels called lymphatic capillaries. The lymphatic capillaries merge to make lymphatic vessels. Lymphatic vessels eventually merge to make lymphatic trunks, and the trunks merge into lymphatic collecting ducts. Imagine a tree. The leaves represent the lymphatic capillaries, the limbs and gradually enlarging limbs and trunk represent the lymphatic vessels and trunk, and the roots are the lymphatic collecting ducts.

Lymphatic capillaries extend into the spaces between cells called interstitial spaces. Lymphatic capillaries have thin, permeable walls that are designed to pick up fluids in interstitial spaces. Once fluid enters the lymphatic capillaries, it is called **lymph.** Lymphatic capillaries deliver lymph to lymphatic vessels, and lymphatic vessels deliver the fluid to lymph nodes.

The cells inside the lymph nodes can remove pathogens from lymph or start an immune response against the pathogen.

Lymph fluid travels away from the lymph nodes through efferent lymphatic vessels. These efferent lymphatic vessels eventually deliver lymph to lymphatic trunks, and the trunks deliver the lymph to lymphatic collecting ducts (see Figures 28-1 and 28-2). There are two major lymphatic collecting ducts in the body: the thoracic duct and the right lymphatic duct. Both of these ducts empty lymph into the bloodstream, usually near the right and left subclavian veins in the thoracic cavity (see Figure 28-3).

The right lymphatic duct, which is much smaller than the thoracic duct, collects all the lymph from the right side of the head and neck, the right arm, and the right side of the chest. The thoracic duct collects lymph from the left side of the head and neck, the left arm, the left side of the thorax, the entire abdominopelvic area, and both legs (see Figure 28-3).

Go to CONNECT to see an animation about *Lymph and Lymph Node Circulation.*

Tissue Fluid and Lymph

Fluid, called **interstitial** (tissue) **fluid,** constantly leaks out of blood capillaries into the spaces between cells. Interstitial fluid is high in nutrients, oxygen, and small proteins. Most of this fluid is picked up by body cells. However, some of the fluid persists between cells and is destined to become lymph.

Once lymph enters the lymphatic vessels, the squeezing action of neighboring skeletal muscles pushes it through the vessels. Lymphatic vessels contain valves that prevent the backflow of lymph. Breathing movements also squeeze lymphatic vessels, which promotes lymph movement. If lymph is not pushed through a lymphatic vessel, it leaks back out of the

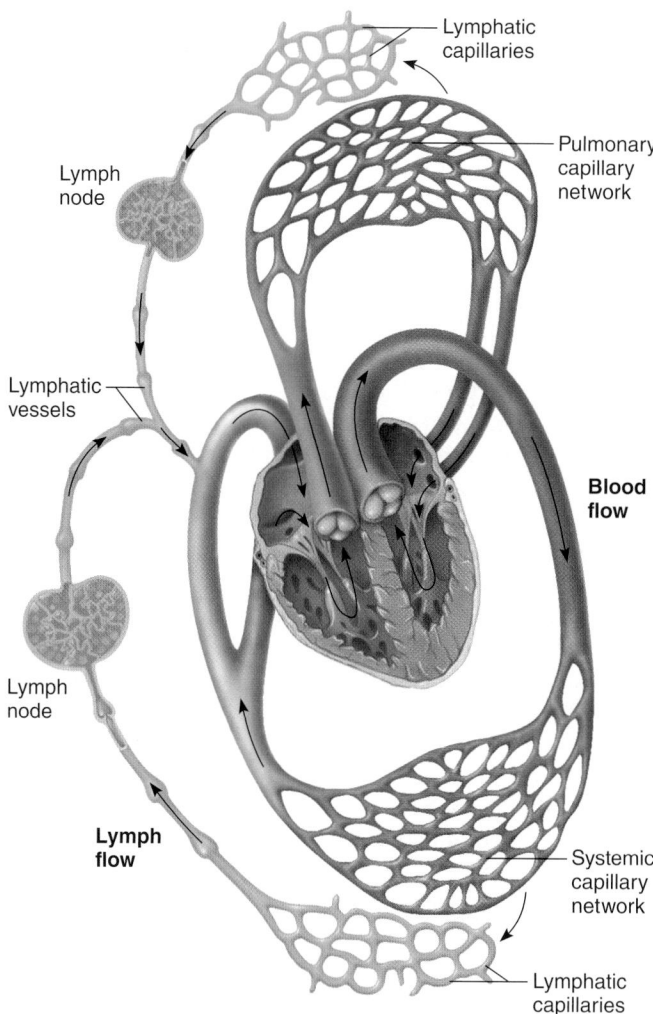

FIGURE 28-1 Schematic flow of lymph from the lymphatic capillaries to the bloodstream.

lymphatic capillaries. When this happens, the surrounding tissue swells, creating a condition called edema.

Lymph Nodes

Lymph nodes are very small, glandular structures that usually cannot be felt easily. They are located along the paths of larger lymphatic vessels and are spread throughout the body. One side of a lymph node, called the hilum, is indented. Nerves and blood vessels enter the node through the hilum.

Some lymphatic vessels—called afferent lymphatic vessels (afferent, meaning "to")—carry lymph to a lymph node on the side away from the hilum. Four or five afferent vessels are associated with each node. Lymphatic vessels that carry lymph out of a node are called efferent vessels (efferent, meaning "away from"). A lymph node usually has only one or two efferent vessels (see Figure 28-4). Because more lymph enters the node than can exit at one time, lymph tends to pool, or stay, in the node for some period of time.

Two important cell types are found inside lymph nodes: macrophages and lymphocytes. **Macrophages** digest pathogens in the lymph, and **lymphocytes** start an immune response

FIGURE 28-2 Lymphatic pathway.

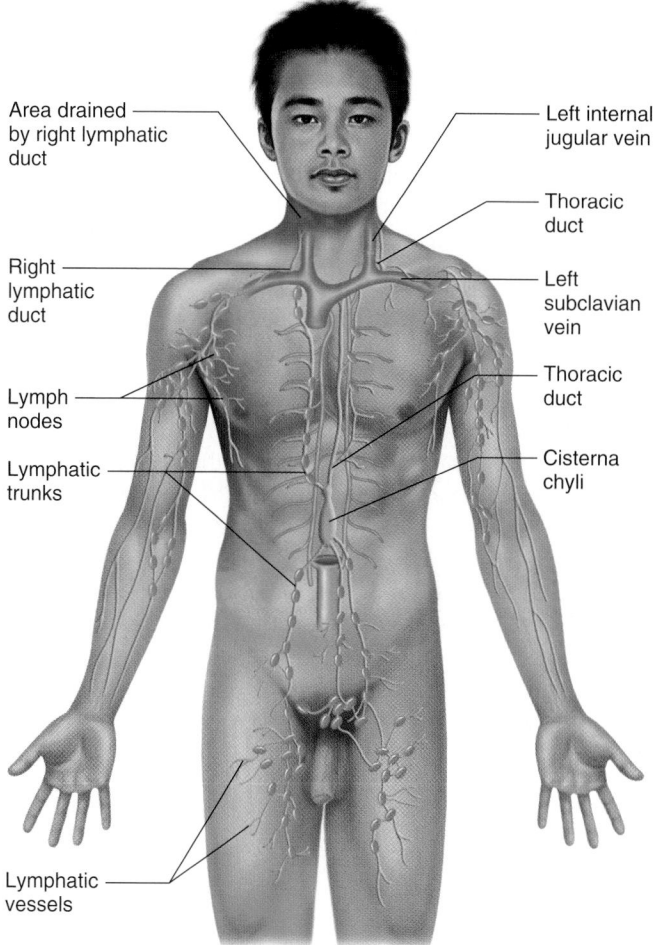

FIGURE 28-3 Areas drained by the right lymphatic duct (shaded) and thoracic duct (not shaded).

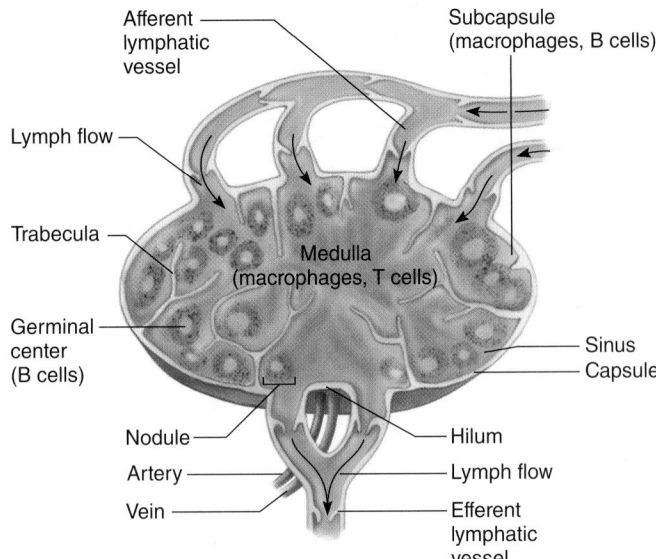

Afferent lymphatic vessel

Subcapsule (macrophages, B cells)

Lymph flow

Trabecula

Medulla (macrophages, T cells)

Germinal center (B cells)

Sinus

Capsule

Nodule

Hilum

Artery

Lymph flow

Vein

Efferent lymphatic vessel

FIGURE 28-4 Section of a lymph node.

against the pathogens. Lymph nodes are also responsible for the generation of some lymphocytes.

The Thymus and Spleen

The thymus is a soft, bilobed (meaning, it has two lobes) organ located just above the heart in the mediastinum. The thymus in an infant is large because it assists with the production of lymphocytes for the child's immature immune system. As a person ages, the thymus shrinks, becoming almost nonexistent as the immune system becomes fully functional. The thymus carries out the same functions as a lymph node, but it is also responsible for the production of lymphocytes and the hormone called thymosin. Thymosin stimulates the production of mature lymphocytes.

The spleen is the largest lymphatic organ. Located in the upper-left quadrant of the abdominal cavity, the spleen is filled with blood, macrophages, and lymphocytes. It filters blood in much the same way that lymph nodes filter lymph. The spleen also removes worn-out red blood cells from the bloodstream. If a person's spleen must be removed due to injury or disease, the patient's liver takes over most of the spleen's functions.

▶ Defenses Against Disease

LO 28.2

An infection is the presence of a pathogen—a disease-causing agent like a bacterium, virus, toxin, fungus, or protozoan—in or on the body. The body has mechanisms called nonspecific defenses or **innate immunity** to protect itself from pathogens in general. The body also has mechanisms to protect itself against specific pathogens; these mechanisms, called immunities, are considered specific defenses.

Nonspecific Defenses

The nonspecific mechanisms that protect the body against pathogens include species resistance, mechanical and chemical barriers, and phagocytosis. Fever and inflammation are also effective in protecting the body from invading organisms.

Species Resistance Species resistance means that a species typically gets only diseases unique to that species. For example, humans do not get diseases that affect plants. Humans also do not get most diseases that affect animals.

Mechanical Barriers The covering of the body (skin) and the linings of the tubes of the body (mucous membranes) provide mechanical barriers against pathogens. Intact skin is impermeable or resistant to most pathogens. Intact mucous membranes, although generally impermeable, do permit the entry of a few pathogens.

Chemical Barriers Chemicals and enzymes in body fluids provide chemical barriers that destroy pathogens. For example, acids in the stomach destroy pathogens that are swallowed. Lysozymes in tears destroy pathogens on the surface of the eye. Salt in sweat kills bacteria, and interferon in blood blocks viruses from infecting cells.

Phagocytosis Phagocytes are cells that surround and destroy pathogens and unwanted debris in the body. Neutrophils and monocytes are the most active phagocytes in blood. They can also leave the bloodstream to attack pathogens in other tissues. When a monocyte leaves the bloodstream, it becomes a macrophage, which is simply a larger phagocytic cell. The process of destroying pathogens by this method is called **phagocytosis.**

Fever An elevated body temperature is a fever. It causes the liver and spleen to take iron out of the bloodstream. Many pathogens need iron to survive in a body, so when their iron sources are gone, they die. Fever also activates phagocytic cells in the body to attack pathogens.

Inflammation When an area of the body becomes injured or infected with a pathogen, inflammation can result. In inflammation, blood vessels in the injured area dilate and become leaky. Because blood vessels dilate, more blood enters the area, bringing phagocytic white blood cells (WBC) to the area to attack the pathogen. The blood also brings proteins to replace injured tissues and clotting factors to stop any bleeding. The clotting factors also "wall off" the area so pathogens cannot spread. Because blood vessels become leaky, more fluid accumulates in the injured area, which leads to edema. The excess fluid often irritates pain receptors. The four cardinal signs of inflammation are redness, heat, swelling, and pain.

Specific Defenses

Specific defenses are called immunities. They protect the body against specific pathogens. For example, a person who has chickenpox develops a specific defense that prevents him or her from getting chickenpox again. However, this specific defense does not protect the person from any other disease. For example, a person may contract herpes zoster (shingles), which is caused by the same varicella virus as chickenpox. A person may not get chickenpox again, but the virus may resurface as herpes zoster.

Antigens are simply defined as foreign substances in the body. Pathogens have many antigens on their surfaces. The immune system is programmed to recognize antigens in the body. Foreign substances in the body that are too small to start an immune response by themselves are called **haptens**. Haptens often join to proteins in the blood, where they are then able to trigger an immune response. Penicillin is an example of a hapten.

Antibodies and complements are the major proteins involved in specific defenses. **Antibodies** are proteins the body produces in response to specific antigens, and **complements** are proteins in serum that work with antibodies to eliminate or destroy antigens.

Lymphocytes and macrophages are the major WBCs involved in specific defenses. The cells of the lymphatic system produce proteins known as **cytokines,** which assist in immune response regulation. Lymphocytes and macrophages produce cytokines known as **monokines**. Monokines assist in regulation of the immune response by increasing B cell production and stimulating red bone marrow to produce more WBCs.

B Cells and T Cells

Two major types of lymphocytes are B cells and T cells. Although both B cells and T cells circulate in the blood, most of the lymphocytes in blood are T cells. B cells and T cells are also found in lymph nodes, the spleen, the thymus, the lining of digestive organs, and bone marrow.

Both T cells and B cells recognize antigens in the body; however, they respond to antigens in different ways. T cells bind to antigens on cells and attack them directly. This type of response is called a **cell-mediated response.** T cells also respond to antigens by secreting cytokines called **lymphokines,** which increase T-cell production and directly kill cells that have antigens.

B cells, on the other hand, do not attack antigens directly. They respond to antigens by becoming plasma cells. The plasma cells then make antibodies against the specific antigen. The antibodies attach to antigens in the humors (fluids) of the body; this response is called a humoral or **antibody-mediated response.** B cells become activated when a specific antigen binds to receptors on their surfaces. Each group of B cells only recognizes one type of antigen. Once activated, B cells divide to make plasma cells and memory B cells. Plasma cells make antibodies, which travel through the fluids of the body and bind to the antigens that activated the B cells. Memory B cells trigger a faster and stronger immune response the next time the person is exposed to the same antigen because they already know to respond to the antigen—just as you know what to expect the second time you play a computer game and can thus play faster and better. (See Figures 28-5 and 28-6.)

As seen in Figure 28-5 before a T cell can respond to an antigen, it must be activated. T-cell activation begins when a macrophage ingests and digests a pathogen that has antigens on it. The macrophage then takes some of the antigens from the pathogen and puts them on its cell membrane next to a large protein complex called a **major histocompatibility complex**

(MHC). Every human being has a unique MHC (similar to an internal fingerprint), and it is present on every cell in the body. A T cell that has a receptor for the antigen recognizes and binds to the antigen and the MHC on the surface of the macrophage. The T cell is now activated and begins to divide to form other types of T cells and T memory cells. It is important to note that T cells cannot be activated without macrophages and MHC proteins.

Some activated T cells form cytotoxic T cells that are important in protecting the body against viruses and cancer cells. Other activated T cells become helper T cells that carry out many important roles in immunity. Helper T cells increase antibody formation, memory cell formation, B cell formation, and phagocytosis. Some activated T cells become memory T cells that "remember" the pathogen that activated the original T cell. When a person is later exposed to the same pathogen, memory cells trigger an immune response that is more effective than the first immune response. The production of memory cells prevents a person from suffering from the same disease twice.

Natural Killer Cells

Natural killer (NK) cells are another type of lymphocyte. They primarily target cancer cells but also protect the body against many types of pathogens. Like cytotoxic T cells, NK cells kill harmful cells on contact. They secrete chemicals that produce holes in the membranes of harmful cells, which cause the cells to burst. Unlike B cells and T cells, NK cells do not have to recognize a specific antigen to start destroying pathogens.

▶ Antibodies

LO 28.3

Antibodies are also called **immunoglobulins.** The following is a list of different types of immunoglobulins (Ig):

- IgA is an antibody found in secretions of the body like breast milk, sweat, tears, saliva, and mucus. It prevents pathogens from entering the body.
- IgD is an antibody found on the cell membranes of B cells. It is thought to control the activity of the B cells.
- IgE is an antibody found wherever IgA is located. It is involved in triggering allergic reactions.
- IgG is an antibody that primarily recognizes bacteria, viruses, and toxins. It can also activate complements.
- IgM is a large antibody that primarily binds to antigens on food, bacteria, or incompatible blood cells. It also activates complements.

When antibodies bind to antigens, they take one of the following actions:

- They allow phagocytes to recognize and destroy antigens.
- They make antigens clump together, causing them to be destroyed by macrophages. This is how incompatible blood cells are destroyed.
- They cover the toxic portions of antigens to make them harmless.

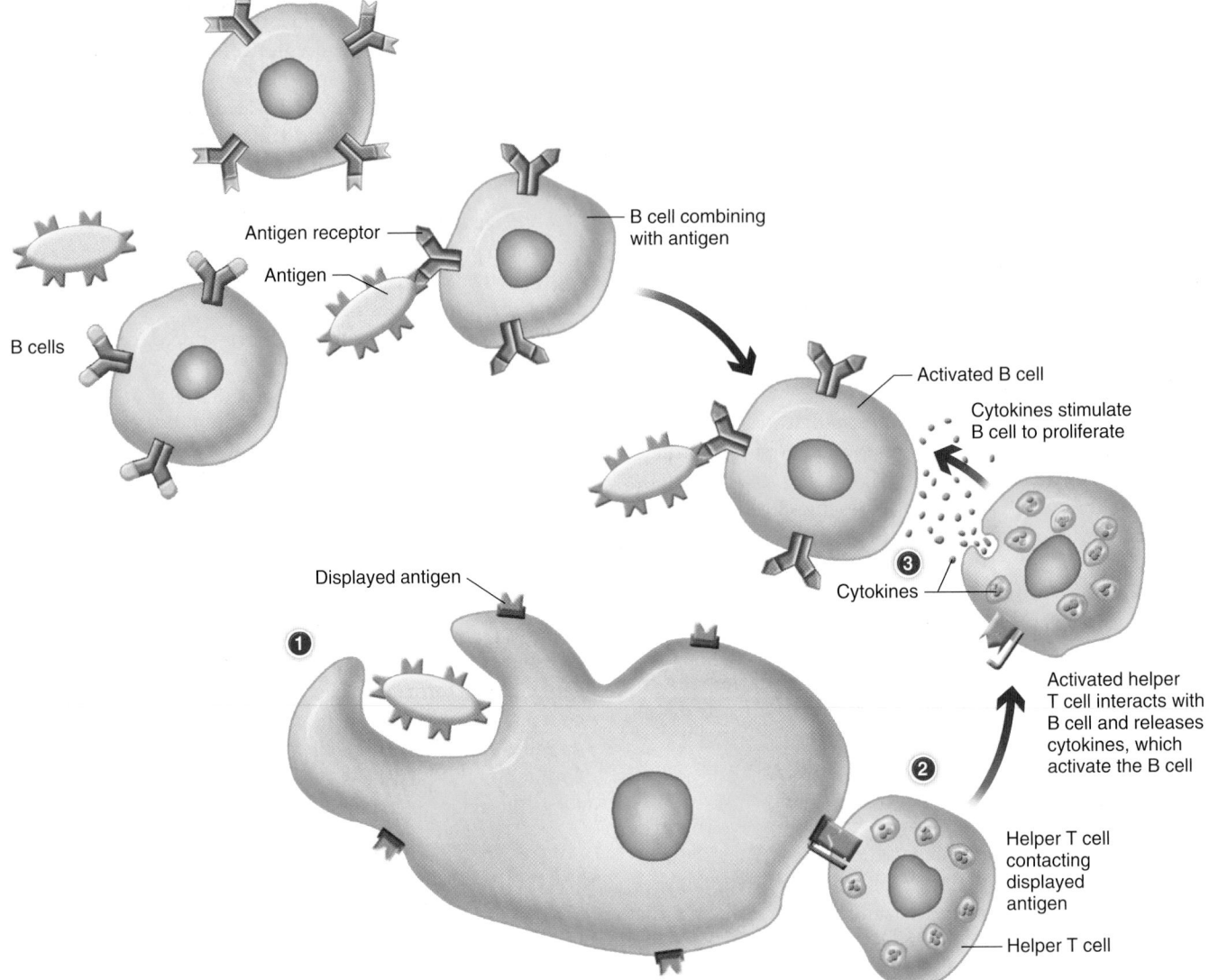

FIGURE 28-5 T cell and B cell activation. (1) A macrophage displays an antigen on its cell membrane. (2) A helper T cell binds to the antigen on the macrophage and becomes activated. (3) An activated helper T cell releases cytokines to help an activated B cell proliferate. Notice that the B cell must also bind to an antigen to become activated.

- They activate complements, which are proteins in serum that attack pathogens by forming holes in them. Complement proteins also attract macrophages to pathogens and can stimulate inflammation.

▶ Immune Responses and Acquired Immunities

LO 28.4

A primary immune response occurs the first time a person is exposed to an antigen. This response is slow and takes several weeks to occur. In this response, memory cells are made. A secondary immune response occurs the next time a person is exposed to the same antigen. This response is quick and usually prevents a person from developing a disease from the antigen. Memory cells carry out the secondary immune response.

A person is born with very few immunities but normally develops or acquires them as long as his immune system is healthy. The four types of immunities a person can acquire are (1) naturally acquired active immunity, (2) artificially acquired active immunity, (3) naturally acquired passive immunity, and (4) artificially acquired passive immunity.

Naturally Acquired Active Immunity

A person develops this immunity by being naturally exposed to an antigen and subsequently making antibodies and memory cells against the antigen. Having an infectious disease, caused by pathogens, leads to the development of this type of immunity, which is usually long-lasting.

Antigen

Antigen receptor

Receptor-antigen combination

Activated B cell

Cytokines from helper T cell

Proliferation

Clone of B cells

Proliferation and Differentiation

Proliferation and Differentiation

Released antibodies

Endoplasmic reticulum

Clone of B cells

Plasma cell (antibody-secreting cell)

Memory cell (dormant cell)

Plasma cell (antibody-secreting cell)

Memory cell (dormant cell)

FIGURE 28-6 An activated B cell multiplies to become memory cells and plasma cells. Plasma cells secrete antibodies.

Artificially Acquired Active Immunity

A person develops this immunity by being injected with a pathogen and subsequently making antibodies and memory cells against the pathogen. Immunizations and vaccines cause this type of immunity, which is also usually long-lasting.

Naturally Acquired Passive Immunity

A person receives this immunity from his mother. When a mother breast-feeds, she passes antibodies to her baby through breast milk. A mother also passes antibodies to her baby across the placenta, which is a short-lived immunity.

Artificially Acquired Passive Immunity

A person receives this immunity when she is injected with antibodies. For example, if a snake bites her, a physician will inject her with antibodies (antivenom) to neutralize the venom. This type of immunity is short-lived.

PATHOPHYSIOLOGY

LO 28.5

Common Diseases and Disorders of the Immune System

As science and medicine develop a better understanding of the immune system and its relationship to causing disease, multiple diseases and disorders involving many body systems are now thought to have an autoimmune component.

An **autoimmune disease** is one in which the body begins to attack its own antigens. Examples of autoimmune diseases include scleroderma (integumentary system), rheumatoid arthritis (skeletal system), multiple sclerosis (nervous system), glomerulonephritis (urinary system), Crohn's disease (digestive system), and insulin-dependent (type 1) diabetes mellitus (endocrine system). Although the reason is unknown, autoimmune disorders affect women almost 75% of the time, often during childbearing years.

A number of diseases and disorders can challenge the immune system. Among them, HIV infection, AIDS, cancer, and allergies are the most significant. HIV and AIDS are discussed in the *Microbiology and Disease* chapter. In this section, you will focus on specific immune system disorders. For other diseases with possible or probable autoimmune components, please refer to the appropriate body system in the Common Diseases and Disorders Appendix III at the back of the book.

Cancer. **CANCER** is defined as the uncontrolled growth of abnormal cells. Healthy cells normally know when to stop reproducing, but cancer cells have lost this ability. Occasionally, normal cells create growths, but these are benign, which means they are not cancerous. Cancer cells, however, often form growths called malignant tumors, which may become fatal. In many cases, these cancerous cells or tumors damage normal cells of tissues and organs, causing organ systems to fail.

At least 200 different types of cancers are known. In the United States, the three most common cancer types in men are prostate, lung, and colon cancer. The three most common types in women are breast, lung, and colon cancer. Lung cancer kills more people in the United States than any other type of cancer.

Causes. The causes of cancer are mostly unknown, but certain risk factors have been identified, including a suppressed immune system, radiation, tobacco, and some viruses. Many other factors are suspected. One of the best ways to prevent cancer is to avoid smoking and other known risk factors. A factor known to cause the formation of cancer is called a carcinogen.

Diagnosis. Most cancers are diagnosed with a biopsy, which is a removal of tissues for examination. CT scans are also used to help diagnose most cancer types. Other diagnostic tests include blood counts, an analysis of blood chemistry, and X-rays.

Signs and Symptoms. The symptoms of different types of cancer vary, but the following symptoms are usually observed in most types: fever, chills, unintended weight loss, fatigue, and a general sense of not feeling well.

Treatment. The treatment of cancer differs depending on the type and stage of cancer. The stage of cancer refers to how large a tumor is and how far cancer cells have spread throughout the body. Table 28-1 provides a summary of cancer staging.

TABLE 28-1	Cancer Staging
Stage	**Description**
Stage 0	Very early cancer. Cancer cells are localized in a few cell layers.
Stage I	Cancer cells have spread to deeper cell layers, or some may have spread to surrounding tissues.
Stage II	Cancer cells have spread to surrounding tissues but are considered contained in the primary cancer site.
Stage III	Cancer cells have spread beyond the primary cancer site to nearby areas.
Stage IV	Cancer cells have spread to other organs of the body.
Recurrent	Cancer cells have reappeared after treatment.

If tumors are localized and have not spread, the cancer can often be treated successfully by surgically removing the tumor. Other treatment options are chemotherapy, radiation therapy, newer immune therapies, and transplants, such as bone marrow transplant, which may be successful for curing certain types of cancer. Even if a cancer cannot be cured, its progression can sometimes be slowed, allowing the patient to live additional years.

ALLERGIES, cause an allergic reaction which is an immune response to a substance, like pollen, that is not normally harmful to the body. An allergy can also be an excessive immune response. Substances that trigger allergic responses are called *allergens*. Allergic reactions, involve IgE antibodies and mast cells. IgE antibodies increase and respond when exposed to an allergen (trigger). The IgE antibodies bind to these allergens and cause mast cells to release histamine and heparin. These chemicals trigger allergic reactions such as sneezing or wheezing, or worse.

To help prevent this reaction a patient receiving allergy shots is injected with tiny amounts of the allergen. This causes the body to produce IgG antibodies that will prevent IgE antibodies from binding to the allergen. IgG antibodies do not trigger immune responses because they do not activate mast cells.

Most allergies do not cause life-threatening conditions, but some do. One life-threatening condition that can result is **anaphylaxis**, when blood vessels dilate so quickly that blood pressure drops too fast for organs to adjust. Without treatment, patients may go into anaphylactic shock and die.

Signs and Symptoms. The signs and symptoms of allergies vary depending on what part of the body is exposed to allergens. Inhaled allergens often cause a runny nose, sneezing, coughing, or wheezing. Ingested allergens may cause nausea, diarrhea, or vomiting. Skin allergens cause rashes. Allergens in the blood, like penicillin, are often the most life-threatening for people who are allergic to them because the allergens can affect many organ systems.

Treatment. Many allergies are effectively treated with over-the-counter medications called antihistamines. Prescription-strength antihistamines are also available. Various types of nasal sprays and decongestants can also reduce allergy symptoms. When a person experiences anaphylaxis, an injection of epinephrine is usually an effective treatment. Epinephrine causes vaso-constriction, which increases blood pressure.

Go to CONNECT to see an animation about *Immune Response: Hypersensitivity.*

ACQUIRED IMMUNODEFICIENCY SYNDROME (AIDS) is the development of severe signs and symptoms caused by the human immunodeficiency virus (HIV) as it destroys lymphocytes—particularly T lymphocytes—which leaves the immune system weakened and susceptible to many other diseases. Because a person may be infected with HIV for years before developing symptoms, it is important for all high-risk individuals to be tested.

Causes. AIDS is caused by the human immunodeficiency virus (HIV).

Signs and Symptoms. Symptoms of AIDS include T-cell counts below 200 (normal is more than 400); fever; diaphoresis; weakness; weight loss; frequent infections, including herpetic ulcers of the mouth, skin, and genitals; TB; yeast infections of the mouth, esophagus, and vagina; meningitis; and encephalitis. Cytomegalovirus (CMV), a specific type of herpetic virus, may also affect the eyes and other internal organs. Kaposi's sarcoma is a skin cancer commonly seen in AIDS patients.

Treatment. Although there is no cure for AIDS, treatments are available in the United States that significantly delay the progression of the disease for many patients. These treatments include the use of various antiviral drugs, but many of these drugs have serious side effects. Antibiotics are also used to treat infections.

CHRONIC FATIGUE SYNDROME (CFS) is a condition in which a person feels severe tiredness that cannot be relieved by rest and is not related to other illness.

Causes. The causes are primarily unknown, although a unique virus known as the Epstein-Barr virus (EBV) is suspected as a possible cause. This condition may also be caused by an autoimmune response against the nervous system.

Signs and Symptoms. The most common symptom is severe fatigue. Other signs and symptoms include mild fever, sore throat, tender lymph nodes in the neck or armpit, general body aches, joint pain, sleep disturbances, and depression.

Treatment. Treatment includes antiviral drugs, medications to treat the depression associated with this condition, and pain medications.

LYMPHEDEMA is the blockage of the lymphatic vessels that drain excess fluids from various areas of the body.

Causes. This condition may be caused by parasitic infections, trauma to the vessels, tumors, radiation therapy, cellulitis (a skin infection), and surgeries such as mastectomies and biopsies in which lymph tissues have been removed.

Signs and Symptoms. The common symptom is tissue swelling that lasts longer than a few days or increases over time.

Treatment. Treatment options include compression stockings for swelling in the legs or arms, elevation of the affected limb, or surgery to remove abnormal lymphatic tissue. Physical therapy and massage therapy are also helpful in the early stages of lymphedema to spread the fluid into surrounding tissues for reabsorption.

MONONUCLEOSIS is also known as mono. Because it frequently affects teenagers and is a highly contagious viral infection spread through the saliva of the infected person, it has earned the nickname "the kissing disease." Mono is also spread through coughing and sneezing.

Causes. Mononucleosis can be caused by either the Epstein-Barr virus or CMV.

Signs and Symptoms. Unexplained fever, extreme fatigue, and sore throat are common. Other symptoms include weakness; headache; and swollen, tender lymph nodes.

Treatment. Rest, proper nutrition, and antibiotics to prevent secondary infections usually result in recovery from acute symptoms in a week or two, although complete recovery may take a month or longer.

SYSTEMIC LUPUS ERYTHEMATOSUS (SLE), commonly referred to as lupus, is an autoimmune disorder that affects a few or, sometimes, many organ systems of the body. In this condition, people produce antibodies that target their own cells and tissues. As with many autoimmune disorders, lupus affects women much more often than men.

Causes. This disorder may be caused by some drugs or by bacterial infections. Except for its autoimmune component, its actual cause is unknown.

Signs and Symptoms. The list of signs and symptoms is extensive and may include any or all of the following:

- Fatigue
- General body aches
- Fever
- Weight loss (anorexia)
- Hair loss
- Arthritis
- Numbness of the fingers and toes
- "Butterfly" rash on the face
- Sensitivity to sunlight (photophobia)
- Vision problems
- Nausea
- Nosebleeds (epistaxis)
- Headaches
- Mental disorders
- Seizures
- Abnormal blood clots
- Chest pains
- Inflammation of heart tissues (carditis)
- Anemia
- Shortness of breath
- Fluid accumulation around the lungs
- Renal failure
- Blood in the urine (hematuria)

Treatment. Treatment options include anti-inflammatory medications, including steroids, and protective clothing and creams to prevent damage from sunlight. Dialysis, immunosuppressive medications, and kidney transplants may be necessary for more serious cases.

LEARNING OUTCOMES	KEY POINTS
28.1 **Describe the pathways and organs of the lymphatic system.**	The lymph system is composed of pathways known as lymph vessels. In addition to the lymph vessels, the organs of the lymphatic system include lymph nodes, located throughout the body; the thymus, in the mediastinum; and the spleen, located in the upper-left quadrant of the abdominal cavity.
28.2 **Compare the nonspecific and specific body defense mechanisms.**	Nonspecific body defenses include species resistance, mechanical and chemical barriers, phagocytosis, fever, and inflammation. Specific defenses are immunities or defenses against specific antigens created by B cells, T cells, and natural killer (NK) cells.
28.3 **Explain how antibodies fight infection.**	Antibodies work in the following ways: phagocytosis, antigen clumping, covering (inactivating) toxic portions of antigens, and activating complements. Antibodies are also known as immunoglobulins. IgA prevents pathogens from entering the body; IgD controls B cell activity; IgE works with IgA in triggering allergic reactions; IgG recognizes bacteria, viruses, and toxins and activates complements; and IgM binds to antigens on food, bacteria, or incompatible blood cells. IgM also activates complements.
28.4 **Describe the four different types of acquired immunities.**	The four types of immune response are naturally acquired active immunity, such as when a person becomes ill and develops immunity; artificially acquired active immunity, as when an injection is given against a pathogen, preventing illness; naturally acquired passive immunity, which occurs when an infant has its mother's immunity for a short while after birth and through breast milk; and artificially acquired passive immunity, which occurs after injection of antibodies such as with an antivenom.
28.5 **Describe the causes, signs and symptoms, and treatments of major immune disorders.**	There are many common diseases and disorders of the immune system with varied signs, symptoms, and treatments. Some of these include cancer, allergies, AIDS and HIV infection, as well as other autoimmune diseases, in which the body attacks its own antigens.

CASE STUDY CRITICAL THINKING

Recall Cindy Chen from the beginning of the chapter. Now that you have completed the chapter, answer the following questions regarding her case.

1. Explain the function of the helper T cell within her immune system.

2. Why might Cindy be more susceptible to other diseases than the general population?

3. If Cindy is HIV positive, does that mean she has visible symptoms? Why or why not?

1. (LO 28.1) The fluid found between cells is called
   a. Lymph
   b. Interstitial fluid
   c. Plasma
   d. CSF
   e. Cellular fluid

2. (LO 28.1) The thoracic duct collects lymph from which of the following areas of the body?
   a. Right side of the head and neck
   b. Right side of the chest
   c. Right leg
   d. Right arm
   e. Left side of the head and neck

3. (LO 28.2) Innate immunity is the other name for which of the following types of body protection?
   a. Specific immunity
   b. Artificial immunity
   c. Humoral immunity
   d. Nonspecific immunity
   e. Temporal immunity

4. (LO 28.2) The types of white blood cells that are involved in specific defenses are lymphocytes and
   a. Macrophages
   b. Neutrophils
   c. Eosinophils
   d. Basophils
   e. Leukophils

5. (LO 28.3) Which of the following cells do not attack antigens directly?
   a. Lymphokines
   b. B cells
   c. T cells
   d. NK cells
   e. Alpha cells

6. (LO 28.3) Which antibody is involved in triggering allergic reactions?
   a. IgA
   b. IgD
   c. IgE
   d. IgM
   e. IgB

7. (LO 28.4) A patient who has been bitten by a rattlesnake is given antivenom. What type of acquired immunity does this provide?
   a. Naturally acquired active immunity
   b. Artificially acquired active immunity
   c. Naturally acquired passive immunity
   d. Artificially acquired passive immunity
   e. Humorally acquired active immunity

8. (LO 28.5) Which of the following is a known carcinogen?
   a. Family history
   b. Weight gain
   c. Sedentary lifestyle
   d. Smoking
   e. Black vegetables

9. (LO 28.5) Which of the following is a life-threatening condition that can be caused by allergies?
   a. Anaphylaxis
   b. AIDS
   c. Lymphedema
   d. Mononucleosis
   e. HIV

10. (LO 28.5) An example of an autoimmune disease is
    a. Chickenpox
    b. Rheumatoid arthritis
    c. Influenza
    d. Atherosclerosis
    e. Strep throat

MEDICAL TERMINOLOGY PRACTICE

Analyze the following medical terms, presented throughout the chapter. Using a medical dictionary (or Appendix I) place a / mark between each word part. Define each word part and then define the whole word.

EXAMPLE: **patho** / **logy** = patho means "disease" + logy means "study of"
   Pathology means "study of disease"

1. antihistamine
2. autoimmune
3. carcinogenic
4. cytotoxic
5. immunoglobulin
6. interstitial
7. leukocyte
8. lymphedema
9. lymphocyte
10. macrophage
11. mononucleosis
12. phagocytosis

The Respiratory System

PATIENT INFORMATION	Patient Name	Gender	DOB
	Mohammad Nassar	M	5/17/20XX
	Attending	**MRN**	**Allergies**
	Elizabeth H. Williams, MD	423-90-687	NKA

Mohammad Nassar is a 15-year-old male complaining of increased difficulty breathing over the last two days. From his chart, you see that Mohammad has a history of asthma and is on a maintenance dose of albuterol 4 mg extended-release tablets twice a day. Dr. Williams has ordered a peak expiratory flow test and has referred Mohammad for allergy testing.

Keep Mohammad in mind as you study the chapter. There will be questions at the end of the chapter based on the case study. The information in the chapter will help you answer these questionss.

After completing Chapter 29, you will be able to:

29.1 Describe the structure and function of each organ in the respiratory system.

29.2 Describe the events involved in the inspiration and expiration of air.

29.3 Explain how oxygen and carbon dioxide are transported in the blood.

29.4 Compare various respiratory volumes and tell how they are used to diagnose respiratory problems.

29.5 Describe the causes, signs and symptoms, and treatments of various diseases and disorders of the respiratory system.

alveoli
bronchi
bronchioles
dyspnea
epiglottis
expiration
glottis
inspiration
larynx
nares

nasal conchae
paranasal sinuses
pharynx
pleura
respiratory volume
surfactant
thoracocentesis
thoracostomy
thorax
trachea

I. C (4)   List major organs in each body system

I. C (5)   Describe the normal function of each body system

I. C (6)   Identify common pathology related to each body system

I. C (7)   Analyze pathology as it relates to the interaction of body systems

I. C (9)   Describe implications for treatment related to pathology

I. C (10)   Compare body structure and function of the human body across the life span

I. C (12)   Describe the relationship between anatomy and physiology of all body systems and medications used for treatment in each

2. **Anatomy & Physiology**
   Graduates:
   b. Identify and apply the knowledge of all body systems, their structure and functions, and their common diseases, symptoms, and etiologies
   c. Assist the physician with the regimen of diagnostic and treatment modalities as they relate to each body system

3. **Medical Terminology**
   Graduates:
   b. Build and dissect medical terms from roots/suffixes to understand the word element combinations that create medical terminology
   c. Understand the various medical terminology for each specialty
   d. Recognize and identify acceptable medical abbreviations

▶ Introduction

The function of the respiratory system is to move air in and out of the lungs. This process is called ventilation, respiration, or breathing. The respiration process delivers oxygen (O_2) to body cells via the bloodstream. It also removes a waste product—carbon dioxide (CO_2)—from the blood. The exchange of oxygen and carbon dioxide in the lungs is called *external respiration*. This same exchange within the hemoglobin of the red blood cells (RBCs) is known as *internal respiration*.

▶ Organs of the Respiratory System   LO 29.1

The organs of the respiratory system are the nose, pharynx, larynx, trachea, bronchial tree (including the bronchi and bronchioles), and the lungs (see Figure 29-1). The nose is made of bones and cartilage and the skin covering them. The openings of the nose are the nostrils, which in medicine are referred to as the **nares.** The hairs of the nostrils prevent large particles from entering the nose.

The Nasal Cavity and Paranasal Sinuses

The nasal cavity is simply the hollow space behind the nose. The nasal cavity is divided into a left and right portion by the nasal septum. Structures called **nasal conchae** extend from the lateral walls of the nasal cavity. Most of the nasal cavity is lined with a mucous membrane that warms and moistens air as it passes through the nasal cavity. The nasal conchae support this mucous membrane and increase the surface area of the nasal cavity.

The nasal cavity is also lined with cells that possess *cilia*, which are microscopic, hair-like projections from the mucous membrane. As mucus traps dust and other particles in the nasal cavity, the cilia push the mucus toward the pharynx, where it is swallowed. The enzymes of the stomach then destroy these foreign particles and pathogens, thus helping to protect the respiratory system from disease.

The **paranasal sinuses** are air-filled spaces within the skull bones that open into the nasal cavity. The paranasal sinuses reduce the weight of the skull and equalize pressure between the inside of the skull and the outside environment. The sinuses also give your voice its tone. When your paranasal sinuses are "stopped up" with mucus, they cause the tone of your voice to change. The bones of the skull that contain the sinuses include the frontal, sphenoid, ethmoid, and maxillae bones. When sinus membranes become inflamed due to allergies or infection (sinusitis), they swell, which results in a sinus headache.

The Pharynx

The **pharynx** is an organ of the respiratory system as well as the digestive system. During inspiration, air flows from the nasal or oral cavity into the pharynx. From the pharynx, air flows into the larynx.

The Larynx and Vocal Cords

The **larynx** is more commonly called the voice box. It sits superior to and is continuous with the trachea or windpipe. It moves air in and out of the trachea and produces the sounds of a person's voice. The larynx is mostly made of cartilage and muscle tissue. There are three cartilages in the larynx (see Figure 29-2). The largest cartilage is called the *thyroid cartilage*, and it forms the anterior wall of the larynx. During the puberty of a male, testosterone causes the thyroid cartilage to enlarge to produce the "Adam's apple." A smaller cartilage called the *epiglottic cartilage* forms the framework of the **epiglottis,** the flap-like structure that closes off the larynx during swallowing so food and liquids do not enter the respiratory system. The third cartilage

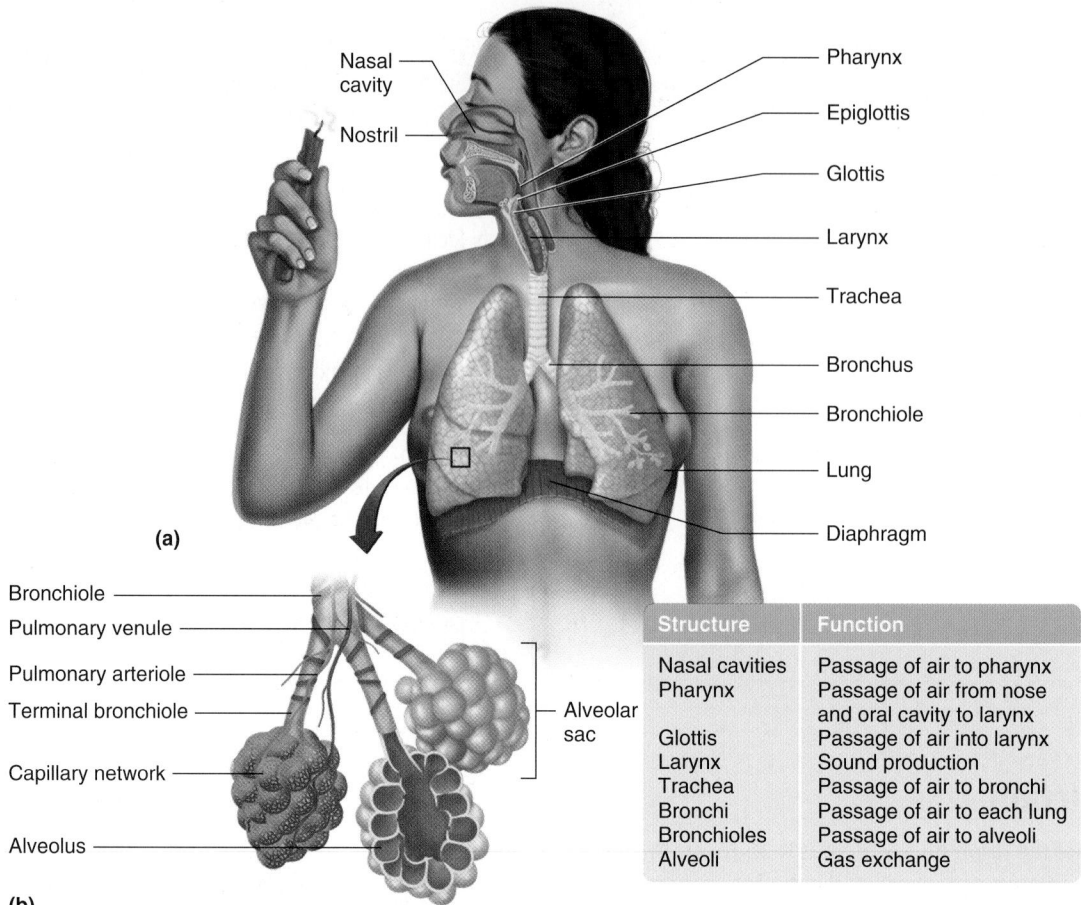

FIGURE 29-1 (a) Organs of the respiratory system and (b) a bronchiole with alveolar sac, covered by capillary network, whole, and in cross-section.

Structure	Function
Nasal cavities	Passage of air to pharynx
Pharynx	Passage of air from nose and oral cavity to larynx
Glottis	Passage of air into larynx
Larynx	Sound production
Trachea	Passage of air to bronchi
Bronchi	Passage of air to each lung
Bronchioles	Passage of air to alveoli
Alveoli	Gas exchange

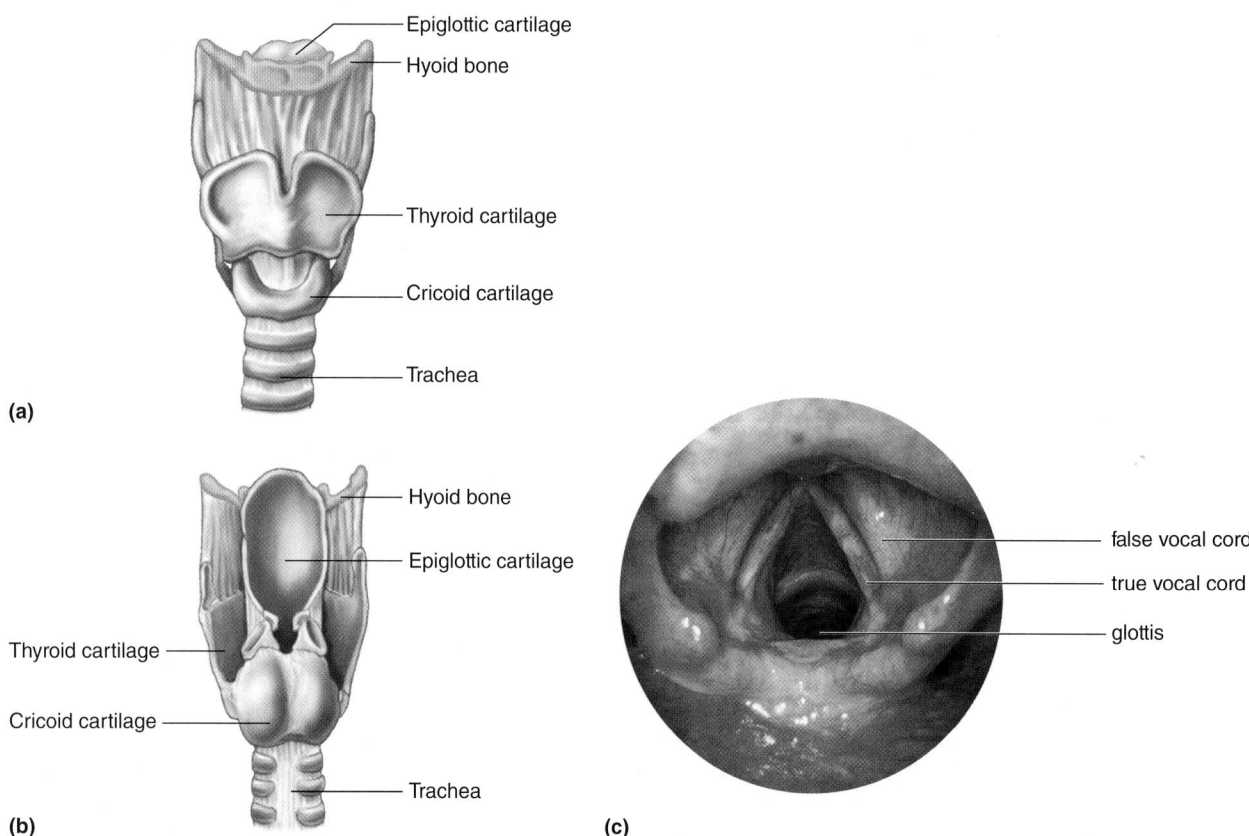

FIGURE 29-2 (a) Anterior view of larynx, (b) posterior view of larynx, and (c) photograph of the vocal cords and glottis.

of the larynx is called the *cricoid cartilage*. It forms most of the posterior wall of the larynx and a small part of the anterior wall.

The vocal cords stretch between the thyroid cartilage and the cricoid cartilage. The opening between the vocal cords is called the **glottis** (see Figure 29-2c). The upper vocal cords are referred to as *false vocal cords* because they do not produce sound. The lower vocal cords are called *true vocal cords* because muscles stretch and relax them to produce different types of sounds. When the true vocal cords are stretched, the voice becomes higher in pitch. When they are relaxed, the voice becomes lower in pitch. Men have thicker vocal cords, which is why their voices are deeper than female voices.

The Trachea, Bronchi, and Bronchioles

The **trachea** (windpipe) is a tubular organ made of rings of cartilage and smooth muscle. It extends from the larynx to the bronchi. The trachea is lined with cells that possess cilia that constantly move mucus up to the pharynx, where it is swallowed. Mucus traps bacteria, viruses, and other harmful substances a person inhales. The digestive juices of the stomach then destroy the harmful substances.

Smoking destroys cilia, so the only way a smoker can get mucus out of his trachea is to cough. Smokers often feel the urge to cough more frequently than nonsmokers in an effort to move mucus to the pharynx.

The distal end of the trachea branches and starts a series of tubes called the *bronchial tree*. The first branches off the trachea are called primary, or main stem, **bronchi.** The branches of the primary bronchi are called secondary bronchi. The secondary bronchi branch into tertiary bronchi. Tertiary bronchi then branch into **bronchioles.** At the ends of the bronchioles are air sacs called alveoli (see Figure 29-1b).

Alveoli are thin sacs made of only one layer of simple squamous epithelial cells and are surrounded by capillaries. They are considered the "working tissue" of the lung because it is in the alveoli that the exchange of oxygen and carbon dioxide takes place. Many physicians refer to the alveoli as the *pulmonary parenchyma* (*parenchyma* means "working tissue"). Through the process of diffusion, red blood cells in the capillaries release carbon dioxide into the alveoli. Conversely, the alveoli release oxygen into the blood through the thin walls of the capillaries. This exchange is known as *internal* or *cellular respiration*.

The Lungs

The lungs are cone-shaped organs that contain connective tissue, the bronchial tree, nerves, lymphatic vessels, and many blood vessels. The right lung is larger than the left because the heart is also located in the left **thorax,** or chest area. The right lung is divided into three lobes, known as the right upper, middle, and lower lobes. The left lung is divided into the left upper and lower lobes. The double-walled membrane that surrounds the lungs is called the **pleura.** The outer membrane is known as the parietal pleura, and the innermost membrane is the visceral pleura. The pleura produces a slippery, serous fluid called *pleural fluid* that helps decrease friction as the membranes move against each other during breathing.

The lungs themselves contain the bronchial tree and alveoli. Some alveolar cells secrete a fatty substance called **surfactant**

that helps maintain the inflation of the alveoli so they do not collapse in on themselves between inspirations. Premature infants often suffer from respiratory distress syndrome (RDS) (formerly known as hyaline membrane disease—see the Pathophysiology section) because their lungs do not yet create enough surfactant. This causes them to often have great difficulty maintaining adequate lung inflation.

▶ The Mechanisms of Breathing LO 29.2

Breathing, or pulmonary ventilation, consists of two events—**inspiration** and **expiration**. During inspiration, or inhalation, air, which is 21% oxygen, flows from the nasal or oropharynx through the sinuses into the larynx, trachea, and bronchial tree, eventually reaching the alveoli of the lungs. Air flows into the airways during inspiration because the thoracic cavity enlarges. When the thoracic cavity enlarges, pressure decreases in the cavity. The atmospheric pressure outside the body is greater than the pressure inside the cavity, and air passively flows from an area of high pressure to an area of low pressure. The following events enlarge the thoracic cavity and therefore lead to inspiration (see Figure 29-3a):

- The diaphragm contracts. As it does so, it flattens, which increases the amount of space in the thoracic cavity.
- The intercostal muscles raise the ribs, further enlarging the thoracic cavity.

During expiration, or exhalation, air rich with carbon dioxide flows out of the airways. Air flows out because the thoracic cavity becomes smaller, which increases the pressure inside the cavity. When the pressure inside the cavity becomes greater than the atmospheric pressure, air flows out. The following events lead to expiration (see Figure 29-3b):

- The diaphragm relaxes. As it does so, it domes up into the thoracic cavity, which decreases the space in the cavity.
- The intercostal muscles lower the ribs; this further decreases the size of the thoracic cavity.

Breathing is controlled by the respiratory center of the brain, which is located in the pons and medulla oblongata. The medulla oblongata controls both the rhythm and the depth of breathing. The pons controls the rate of breathing.

Other factors that affect breathing are the carbon dioxide levels in the blood and the pH of the blood. When carbon dioxide levels rise in the blood, the rate and depth of breathing increase. The rate and depth of breathing also increase when the blood pH drops. Fear and pain also increase the breathing rate. Breathing rapidly and deeply is called *hyperventilation,* which decreases the amount of carbon dioxide in the blood. However, it should be noted that in patients with chronic obstructive pulmonary disease (COPD), decreased oxygen levels stimulate respiratory rates. Therefore, giving a patient with COPD a high level of oxygen may actually decrease his or her breathing reflex.

Go to CONNECT to see animations about *Acid-Base Balance: Acidosis* and *Acid-Base Balance: Alkalosis.*

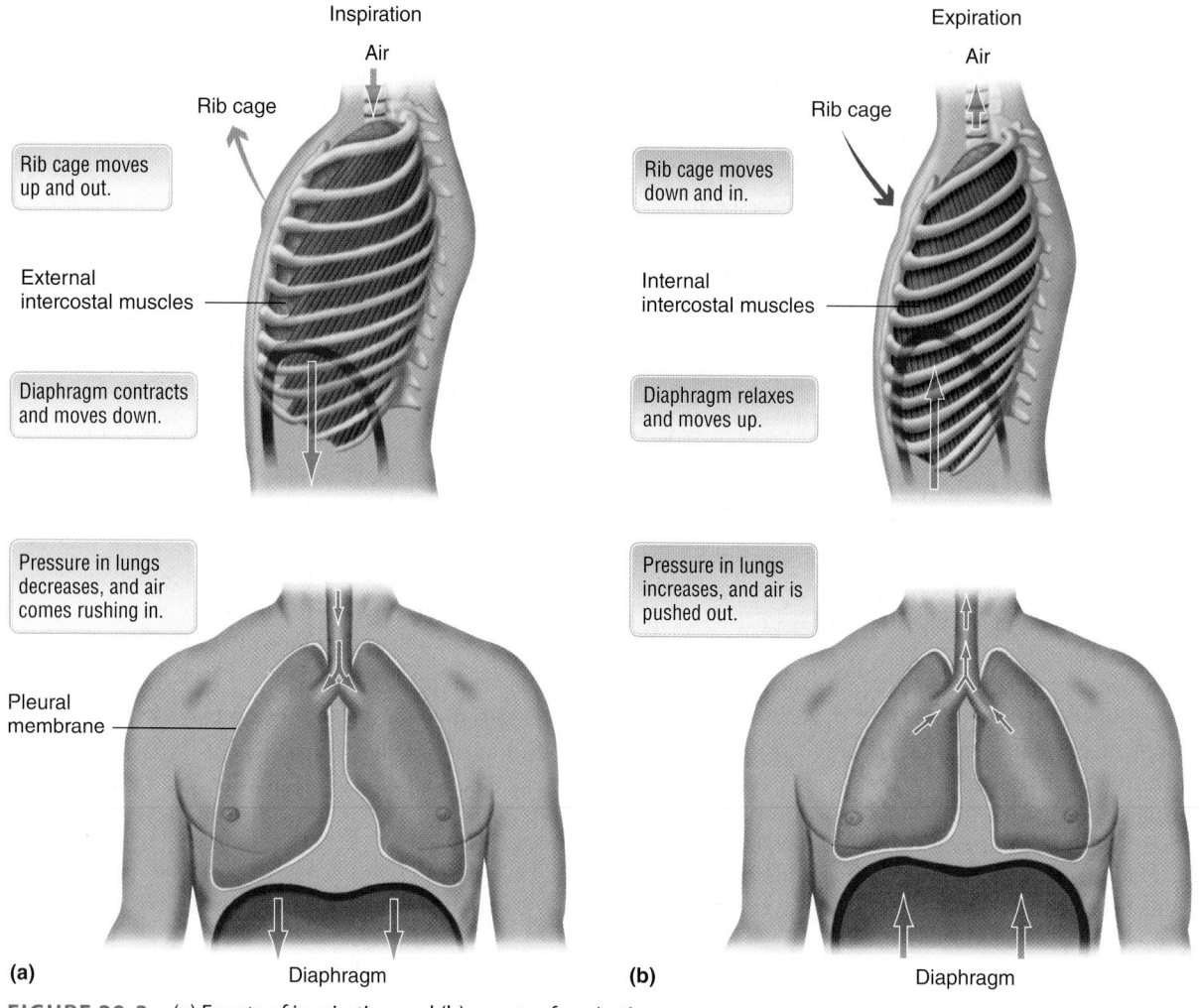

FIGURE 29-3 (a) Events of inspiration and (b) events of expiration.

The inflation reflex also helps to regulate the depth of breathing. Stretch receptors in pleural membranes are activated when the lungs are stretched past a certain point. This triggers a decrease in the depth of breathing to prevent overinflation of the lungs.

Normal, everyday situations also alter our breathing patterns. Consider these common occurrences:

- Coughing. A deep inspiration occurs and the glottis is closed. As the air forces the glottis open, a rush of air is forced up to clear the lower respiratory passages.
- Sneezing. The same process occurs as in coughing except that air is moved to the nasal passages by lowering the uvula. This causes a clearing of the upper respiratory passages.
- Laughing. A deep breath is expelled in short bursts, expressing happiness.
- Crying. The same respiratory process occurs as in laughing, but the expression is one of sadness.
- Hiccups. Also spelled hiccoughs; these are spasmodic contractions of the diaphragm against a closed glottis. Interestingly, the purpose for this is not known.
- Yawning. A deep inspiration that increases the amount of air brought to the alveoli, which aids in blood oxygenation.

- Speaking. Air is forced through the larynx, vibrating the vocal cords. Words are formed by the tongue, lips, and teeth, allowing for verbal communication.

▶ The Transport of Oxygen and Carbon Dioxide in the Blood
LO 29.3

Once oxygen gets into the bloodstream, most of it binds to the heme portion of hemoglobin in red blood cells. Hemoglobin bound to oxygen is called *oxyhemoglobin* and is bright red in color. Some oxygen stays dissolved in plasma and does not bind to hemoglobin, but this is generally a lesser amount than that which attaches to the RBCs. Carbon dioxide also binds to hemoglobin, but at the globin or protein portion of the hemoglobin, forming *carboxyhemoglobin*. However, unlike oxygen, much of the carbon dioxide enters the plasma for transport through the body, after being converted into carbonic acid by the RBCs. Carbonic acid can quickly be converted into the buffer bicarbonate as needed by the blood to maintain its narrow constant pH level of 7.35–7.45 (see *The Cardiovascular System* chapter).

Carbon monoxide is a colorless, odorless gas. Poisonous to humans, it is particularly dangerous because it binds to the same heme area of hemoglobin as does oxygen. In fact, it binds more tightly to this molecule than oxygen. When hemoglobin is exposed to carbon monoxide, the carbon monoxide "overrules" oxygen, leading to carbon monoxide poisoning.

BODY**ANIMAT3D**
POWERED BY
connect

Go to CONNECT to see an animation about *Oxygen Transport and Gas Exchange.*

▶ Respiratory Volumes
LO 29.4

During different intensities of breathing, different volumes of air move in and out of the lungs. These volumes, called **respiratory volumes,** can be measured to assess the healthiness of the respiratory system. Respiratory capacities can be calculated by adding certain respiratory volumes together. Several different measurements related to lung volume and capacity can be made (see Table 29-1). You will learn more about these respiratory volumes and the process of measuring them in the *Cardiovascular and Respiratory Testing* chapter.

TABLE 29-1 Respiratory Air Volumes and Capacities

Name	Volume*	Description
Tidal volume (TV)	500 mL	Volume moved in or out of the lungs during a respiratory cycle
Inspiratory reserve volume (IRV)	3,000 mL	Volume that can be inhaled during forced breathing in addition to resting tidal volume
Expiratory reserve volume (ERV)	1,100 mL	Volume that can be exhaled during forced breathing in addition to resting tidal volume
Residual volume (RV)	1,200 mL	Volume that remains in the lungs at all times
Inspiratory capacity (IC)	3,500 mL	Maximum volume of air that can be inhaled following exhalation of resting tidal volume: IC = TV + IRV
Functional residual capacity (FRC)	2,300 mL	Volume of air that remains in the lungs following exhalation of resting tidal volume: FRC = ERV + RV
Vital capacity	4,600 mL	Maximum volume of air that can be exhaled after taking the deepest breath possible: VC = TV + IRV + ERV
Total lung capacity (TLC)	5,800 mL	Total volume of air that the lungs can hold: TLC = VC + RV
Forced Vital Capacity (FVC)	Varies depending on gender, age, and height	Amount of air exhaled with force after inhaling as deeply as possible.
Peak Expiratory Flow (PEF)	Varies depending on gender, age, and height	Greatest rate of flow during forced exhalation.

* Values are typical for a tall, young adult.

EDUCATING THE PATIENT

Snoring

Snoring occurs when the muscles of the palate, tongue, and throat relax. Airflow then causes these soft tissues to vibrate. These vibrating tissues produce the harsh sounds characteristic of snoring.

Snoring causes daytime sleepiness and is sometimes associated with a condition known as obstructive sleep apnea (OSA). In OSA, the relaxed throat tissues cause airways to collapse, which prevents a person from breathing. Snoring affects approximately 50% of men and 25% of women older than age 40. The common causes of snoring include:

- Enlargement of the tonsils or adenoids
- Being overweight
- Alcohol consumption
- Nasal congestion
- A deviated (crooked) nasal septum

The severity of snoring varies among people. The Mayo Clinic's Sleep Disorders Center uses the following scale to determine the severity of snoring:

- Grade 1: Snoring can be heard from close proximity to the face of the snoring person.

- Grade 2: Snoring can be heard from anywhere in the bedroom.
- Grade 3: Snoring can be heard just outside the bedroom with the door open.
- Grade 4: Snoring can be heard outside the bedroom with the door closed.

You can educate patients about making lifestyle modifications and using aids to help reduce their snoring:

- Lose weight
- Change the sleeping position from the back to the side
- Avoid the use of alcohol and medications that cause sleepiness
- Use nasal strips to widen the nasal passageways
- Use dental devices to keep airways open

In addition, patients may benefit from a CPAP (continuous positive airway pressure) machine, which uses a mask attached to a pump that forces air into their passageways while they sleep. If these therapies are not effective, patients may need surgery such as a uvulotomy to trim excess tissues in the throat, or laser surgery to remove a portion of the soft palate.

Common Diseases and Disorders of the Respiratory System

ALLERGIC RHINITIS is a hypersensitivity reaction to various airborne allergens.

Causes. There are many causes, which may be seasonal, such as hay fever, or continual, such as those caused by dust, molds, colognes, cigarette smoke, animal dander, and mites.

Signs and Symptoms. There are numerous signs and symptoms, which may include sneezing; itchy, watery eyes; red, swollen eyelids; congested nasal mucous membranes; and nasal discharge.

Treatment. Treatment commonly includes the use of over-the-counter (OTC) antihistamines and decongestants. Severe cases may be treated with prescription medication such as Allegra® and OTC medication such as Zyrtec®. Patients should also avoid known allergens. Air filters and air conditioners assist in keeping allergen counts down. Seeking the assistance of an allergist for desensitization injections may be an option for long-term management.

ASTHMA is a condition in which the tubes of the bronchial tree become obstructed as a result of inflammation.

Causes. The causes include allergens (pollen, pets, dust mites, etc.), cigarette smoke, pollutants, perfumes, cleaning agents, cold temperatures, and exercise (in susceptible individuals).

Signs and Symptoms. Symptoms include difficulty breathing, a tight feeling in the chest, and wheezing, and coughing, all of which can cause a feeling of suffocation and increased anxiety.

Treatment. Treatment includes avoiding allergens, the use of steroidal and nonsteroidal inhalers such as Advair® and Flovent®, as well as oral medications such as Singulair® and other bronchodilators to reduce inflammation. See Figure 29-4. Patients should avoid smoky environments; those who smoke should stop. Strongly scented items such as perfumes, hair products, and cleaning agents should also be avoided.

BODYANIMAT3D
POWERED BY
connect

Go to CONNECT to see an animation about *Asthma*.

ATELECTASIS is more commonly called collapsed lung. It may occur after abdominal or thoracic surgery or because of pleural effusion, which may consist of blood, fluid, air, or pus in the pleural cavity. The medical names for these conditions are hemothorax (blood in the pleural cavity), hydrothorax (fluid), pneumothorax (air), and pyothorax (pus).

Causes. These include underlying cystic fibrosis and COPD in which patients may have a chronic form of atelectasis. Cancer patients and those with inflammatory conditions such as pleurisy (pleuritis—see below) may also be subject to chronic atelectasis. Acute atelectasis may occur after any injury to the ribs or trauma to the thorax. Post-surgical patients are also susceptible.

FIGURE 29-4 Individuals with asthma may use an inhaler with steroidal or nonsteroidal medication for treatment.

Signs and Symptoms. These include **dyspnea** (difficulty breathing), cyanosis (a blue coloration of skin and mucous membranes), diaphoresis (excessive perspiration), anxiety, tachycardia, and intercostal muscle retraction. Depending on the cause of the atelectasis, there may also be chest pain.

Treatment. In acute cases, thoracocentesis may be needed to drain the pleural cavity. For chronic atelectasis, treatment may include chest percussion, postural drainage, coughing, deep breathing exercises, and intermittent positive-pressure breathing (IPPB).

BRONCHITIS is inflammation of the bronchi and often follows a cold. Bronchitis that occurs frequently often indicates more serious underlying conditions, such as asthma or emphysema. Smokers are much more likely to develop bronchitis than are nonsmokers. Repeated episodes of bronchitis increase a person's chance of eventually developing lung cancer.

Causes. This condition can be caused by viruses and gastroesophageal reflux disease (GERD), a condition in which acids move from the stomach into the esophagus. Exposure to cigarette smoke, pollutants, and household cleaner fumes can also contribute to the development of bronchitis.

Signs and Symptoms. The signs and symptoms include chills, fever, coughing up yellow-gray or green mucus, tightness in the chest, wheezing, and dyspnea.

Treatment. This condition can be treated with rest, fluids, nonprescription and prescription cough medicines, and the use of a humidifier. Antibiotics are usually prescribed only for smokers. Patients who also have asthma may need to use inhalers. They should also wear masks if they may be exposed to lung irritants.

CHRONIC OBSTRUCTIVE PULMONARY DISEASE (COPD)

is a group of lung disorders that limit airflow to the lungs and usually cause enlargement of the alveoli in the lungs. Emphysema and chronic bronchitis are the most common types of COPD.

Causes. The primary causes are smoking and air pollution.

Signs and Symptoms. Common signs and symptoms include dyspnea, hypoxia (inadequate oxygenation of the cells), fatigue, and frequent coughing.

Treatment. Treatment should first be focused on lifestyle changes, especially smoking cessation. Other treatment options include respiratory therapy and the use of inhalers. In more serious cases, a lung transplant may be necessary.

Go to CONNECT to see an animation about *COPD*.

EMPHYSEMA

EMPHYSEMA is a chronic condition that damages the alveoli of the lungs. It is heavily associated with smoking, which causes stretching of the spaces between the alveoli and paralyzes the cilia of the respiratory system.

Causes. The most common causes are cigarette smoking and exposure to cigarette smoke; pollutants; and the dust from grains, cotton, wood, or coal.

Signs and Symptoms. Symptoms include shortness of breath that progresses over time, chronic cough, unintended weight loss, and fatigue. Pulmonary function tests and arterial blood gases become increasingly more abnormal as the disease progresses. In advanced cases, patients develop the characteristic barrel chest caused by the muscular changes in the chest as the patient struggles to breathe.

Treatment. Stopping smoking and preventing exposure to cold environments and pollutants should be the first treatment measures. Vaccinations to prevent the flu and pneumonia as well as antibiotics to control the respiratory infections associated with emphysema may also be administered. In addition, patients can be treated with bronchodilators, supplemental oxygen, inhaled steroids, and respiratory therapy. The most serious cases may require either surgery to remove damaged lung tissue or a lung transplant, without which patients will develop respiratory and/or heart failure, resulting in death.

Go to CONNECT to see animations about *Respiratory Tract Infections* and *Respiratory Failure.*

INFLUENZA

INFLUENZA is more commonly called the flu. Babies, the elderly, people with suppressed immune systems, and those with chronic respiratory illnesses, such as COPD, are at the highest risk of developing influenza. The flu normally lasts between 5 and 10 days.

Causes. This disease is caused by a number of different viruses that attack the respiratory system. It can be prevented through a yearly flu vaccination. Note that each year there are multiple strains of influenza. Therefore, the vaccine available each year is for the known strains for that year. Explain this to patients so they understand they need a flu shot each year for that year's specific strains of the virus.

Signs and Symptoms. Common symptoms include a runny nose (rhinorrhea), sore throat (pharyngitis), sneezing, fever or chills, a dry cough, muscle pain, fatigue, anorexia (loss of appetite), and diarrhea.

Treatment. OTC analgesics and antipyretics can alleviate the aches and pains as well as the fever associated with the flu. Other treatment options include bed rest, fluids, and antiviral medications.

LARYNGITIS

LARYNGITIS is an acute inflammation of the larynx. Chronic laryngitis is associated with lung cancer.

Causes. The causes of this condition are varied and include the following: viruses; bacteria; polyp formation in the larynx; excessive talking, shouting, or singing; allergies; smoking; frequent heartburn; the frequent use of alcohol; damage to nerves that supply the larynx; and a stroke (CVA, or cerebrovascular accident) that paralyzes vocal cord muscles.

Signs and Symptoms. Signs and symptoms include a hoarse voice (dysphonia), sore throat (pharyngitis), a dry cough and throat, and tickling sensations in the throat.

Treatment. The most common treatment options are antibiotics, the management of heartburn, the avoidance of cigarettes and alcohol, and voice rest. The treatment of more serious cases includes removing laryngeal polyps and surgery to tighten the vocal cords.

LEGIONNAIRE'S DISEASE

LEGIONNAIRE'S DISEASE is an acute type of bacterial pneumonia. As with many respiratory diseases, smokers are much more susceptible to pneumonia than are nonsmokers.

Causes. This disease is caused by Legionnaire bacilli that usually grow in the standing water of air conditioning systems.

Signs and Symptoms. The symptoms include fever, which may spike as high as 105°F, fatigue, anorexia, dyspnea, frequent coughing, chest pain, muscle aches, and headache. Complications may include hypotension, arrhythmia, respiratory and renal failure, as well as shock, which is often fatal.

Treatment. Treatments include antibiotics, antipyretics, and respiratory therapy, including oxygen and ventilator support if needed. Supportive therapy, such as IV fluids, is also used.

LUNG CANCER

LUNG CANCER is closely associated with smoking and exposure to secondhand smoke, and kills more people in the United States than any other type of cancer. Smoking accounts for approximately 85% of all lung cancer cases. See Figure 29-5.

Causes. The primary causes are smoking and exposure to radon, asbestos, and industrial carcinogens.

Signs and Symptoms. The respiratory symptoms include a cough that worsens over time, hemoptysis (coughing up

(a) Healthy lung, mediastinal surface   **(b)** Smoker's lung with carcinoma

FIGURE 29-5   A healthy lung is pink, unlike a lung with cancer caused by smoking, as shown on the right.

blood), dyspnea, wheezing, shortness of breath, and recurrent bronchitis. Other symptoms are chest pain, dysphonia, unintended weight loss, and bone pain if the cancer has spread.

Classification. Lung cancer is classified as follows:

- *Small cell lung cancer.* This type occurs almost exclusively in smokers. It is the most aggressive type and spreads readily to other organs. Small cell lung cancer that spreads to other organs is termed *extensive*.
- *Squamous cell lung cancer.* This type of lung cancer arises from the epithelial cells that line the bronchi and bronchioles of the lungs. It occurs most commonly in men.
- *Adenocarcinoma.* This type arises from the mucus-producing cells of the lungs. It develops most commonly in women and nonsmokers.
- *Large cell carcinoma.* This type of lung cancer arises from the peripheral parts of the lungs.

Stages. Squamous cell lung cancer, adenocarcinoma, and large cell carcinoma are staged as follows:

- Stage 0: Cancer is found only in the lining of the bronchi and bronchioles of the lungs.
- Stage 1: Cancer has spread from the lining of the bronchi and bronchioles to lung tissues.
- Stage 2: Cancer has spread to the lymph nodes or the chest wall.
- Stage 3: Cancer has spread to the lymph nodes and to other organs within the chest.
- Stage 4: Cancer has spread to organs outside the chest.

Small cell lung carcinoma is staged as follows:

- Limited-Stage Small Cell Lung Cancer: Cancer is found in one lung, the tissues between the lungs and nearby lymph nodes only.
- Extensive-Stage Small Cell Lung Cancer: Cancer has spread outside of the lung in which it began or to other parts of the body.

Treatment. Treatment varies, depending on the type of cancer and the stage. Stopping smoking and avoiding exposure to secondhand smoke should be the first treatment considerations. Common treatment options include chemotherapy and radiation therapy. More serious cases may require the surgical removal of tumors (if they are confined), a lobectomy (the removal of a lung lobe or lobes), or a pneumonectomy (the removal of an entire lung).

PLEURAL EFFUSION is a buildup of fluid in the pleural cavity.

Causes. Effusions are caused by either an overproduction of pleural fluid or an inadequate absorption of the fluid. These often result from an underlying disease, such as congestive heart failure, cirrhosis, tuberculosis, cancer, lupus, or rheumatoid arthritis.

Signs and Symptoms. As the fluid builds in the pleural space, the lungs begin to compress, reducing the gaseous exchange of oxygen and carbon dioxide. Infective processes may result in a pus buildup, which is known as empyema.

Treatment. **Thoracocentesis** is done to remove the fluid and/or pus. **Thoracostomy,** which requires insertion of a tube to continually drain the fluid, may be required to maintain drainage of the acute phase of the illness. Oxygen may be administered to increase oxygen concentration in the lung. Antibiotics may also be required for any infective process.

PLEURITIS or *pleurisy* is a condition in which the pleura becomes inflamed. This often causes the membranes to stick together or can cause an excess amount of fluid to form between the membranes.

Causes. Causes include viruses, pneumonia, autoimmune diseases such as lupus or rheumatoid arthritis, tuberculosis, a pulmonary embolism, inflammation of the pancreas, and trauma to the chest.

Signs and Symptoms. Symptoms include fever or chills; a dry cough; shortness of breath; and a sharp, stabbing chest pain during respiration.

Treatment. Analgesics may be prescribed to relieve chest pain. Anti-inflammatory drugs, antibiotics, and the removal of fluid around the lungs by thoracocentesis are the primary treatment options.

PNEUMOCONIOSIS is the name given to lung diseases that result from years of exposure to different environmental or occupational types of dust. There are three basic types: *anthracosis, asbestosis*, and *silicosis*.

Causes. Anthracosis (black lung disease) results from exposure to coal dusts. Asbestosis results from lung exposure to asbestos. Silicosis arises from exposure to silica sand from sand blasting and ceramic manufacture.

Signs and Symptoms. These include tachypnea, nonproductive cough, progressive dyspnea on exertion, pulmonary hypertension, recurrent respiratory infections, and eventual right ventricular hypertrophy. In all cases, fibrous tissue takes over healthy lung tissue, which destroys the alveoli and takes over the air passageways.

Treatment. Treatment for all types includes avoiding respiratory infections, using bronchodilators, and using supplemental oxygen as needed. Respiratory therapy can also be useful in helping patients rid themselves of respiratory secretions.

PNEUMONIA, also known as *pneumonitis,* is characterized by an inflammation of the lungs caused by a bacterial, viral, or fungal infection. There are at least 50 different types of pneumonia, and they range from mild to serious. Double pneumonia refers to inflammation of both lungs.

Causes. Pneumonia can be caused by bacteria, viruses, fungi, and parasites. It can also be caused by foreign matter that enters the lungs (for example, stomach contents that enter the lungs after vomiting), known as aspiration pneumonia. This disorder may be prevented by not smoking and, for some types of pneumonia, by pneumococcal vaccinations.

Signs and Symptoms. Common signs and symptoms include fever or chills, headache, chest or muscle pain, fatigue, dyspnea, and sputum consisting of rust-colored, green, or yellowish mucus.

Treatment. Rest, fluids, OTC pain medications, and antibiotics are the most common treatments. In severe cases, oxygen and ventilator support may be required.

PNEUMOTHORAX is a collection of air in the chest around the lungs, which may cause atelectasis.

Causes. Some causes of this disorder are unknown. Various respiratory diseases and trauma to the chest, such as a stabbing wound, can also contribute to the development of pneumothorax.

Signs and Symptoms. The primary symptoms include tightness in the chest or a sharp chest pain, shortness of breath, and a rapid heart rate.

Treatment. The insertion of a chest tube (thoracostomy) to remove air from the chest and surgery to repair chest wounds are the primary treatments.

PULMONARY EDEMA is a condition in which fluids fill spaces within the lungs. This disorder makes it very difficult for the lungs to oxygenate the blood. It most commonly occurs when the heart cannot pump all the blood it receives from the lungs. Left heart failure occurs when blood then backs up in the lungs, causing fluids to seep into lung spaces.

Causes. The many causes of this condition include the following: congestive heart failure, myocardial infarction (heart attack), cardiomyopathy, heart valve disorders, lung infections, allergic reactions, smoke inhalation, drowning, various drugs such as narcotics and heroin, chest injuries, and high altitudes. This disorder may be prevented by avoiding high altitudes and smoking. Preventing heart disease may also reduce the chance of developing this disorder.

Signs and Symptoms. The symptoms of pulmonary edema are shortness of breath; difficulty breathing, especially when lying down (a condition known as *orthopnea*); a feeling of suffocating; wheezing; a productive cough that produces pink mucus; rapid weight gain; pallor; and profuse sweating, which is known as diaphoresis.

Treatment. Treatment includes oxygen therapy, diuretics to eliminate excess fluids, and morphine to reduce anxiety and shortness of breath.

A **PULMONARY EMBOLISM** is a blocked artery in the lungs. Usually the artery is blocked by a blood clot that has traveled from a vein in the legs. If an artery in the lungs is completely blocked, death can occur quickly from resultant respiratory failure.

Causes. People at the highest risk of developing this condition are those who have had previous heart attacks, cancer, a fractured hip, or chronic lung diseases. Women who use birth control pills and individuals who have a pacemaker may be at risk for developing a pulmonary embolism. In addition, long periods of inactivity, increased levels of clotting factors in the blood (usually caused by certain cancers), injury to veins, or a stroke that causes paralysis of the arms or legs may cause this condition. A sedentary lifestyle as well as auto or airplane travel—or any activity that requires prolonged sitting or standing—are also major risk factors for developing a pulmonary embolism. A half-dose aspirin (formerly known as a baby aspirin) taken daily, as well as plenty of fluids and frequent movement of the arms and legs, may help prevent the development of a pulmonary embolism.

Signs and Symptoms. Symptoms include fainting, a sudden shortness of breath, hemoptysis (coughing up blood), wheezing, tachycardia (a rapid heartbeat), diaphoresis (profuse sweating), and chest pain that may spread to a shoulder, arm, or the face.

Treatment. Support stockings can be used to promote circulation. The patient should rest until the blood clot has dissolved and may be prescribed thrombolytic (clot-dissolving) medications, such as TPA. Anticoagulants, typically warfarin (Coumadin), may be used to prevent new blood clots from forming in the deep veins of the body. Finally, a filter may be surgically implanted in the vena cava to prevent blood clots from reaching the lungs.

RESPIRATORY DISTRESS SYNDROME (RDS), which was formerly known as hyaline membrane disease, kills apparently healthy infants. At highest risk are newborns to infants 8 months of age, especially "preemies."

Causes. The etiology is unknown. The underlying problem is known to be a lack of surfactant in the lungs. Surfactant helps prevent the alveoli from totally collapsing on expiration. Without it, the alveoli collapse, resulting in poor oxygenation due to difficulty with reinflation of the alveoli.

Signs and Symptoms. RDS is usually diagnosed soon after birth, when the infant's breathing becomes rapid and shallow. The infant's nares flare, and the accessory muscles are used to aid in respiration. The infant will also exhibit "grunting" noises in an attempt to breathe.

Treatment. Treatment must be immediate, preferably in a neonatal intensive care unit (NICU). Oxygen therapy, an endotracheal tube, ventilator support, and artificial surfactant are all used in an attempt to keep the alveoli inflated. Infants who survive RDS may be at higher risk for respiratory infections later, but this threat lessens as their lungs continue to mature.

SEVERE ACUTE RESPIRATORY SYNDROME (SARS) is a respiratory disease that is very contagious and sometimes fatal. It was first identified in 2003.

Causes. SARS is caused by viruses associated with the common cold as well as by unknown viruses. It can be prevented by thoroughly washing the hands, wearing a mask, and avoiding exposure to individuals with this disease.

Signs and Symptoms. Signs and symptoms include fever or chills, headache, a dry cough, and muscle aches.

Treatment. Rest and antiviral drugs are the primary treatments.

SINUSITIS is an inflammation of the membranes lining the sinuses of the skull.

Causes. Bacteria, excess mucus production in the sinuses (often from the "common cold"), the blockage of sinus openings, and the destruction of cilia that move mucus out of sinuses can cause this disorder.

Signs and Symptoms. Fever, cough, headache, pharyngitis, facial pain, and nasal congestion are the common signs and symptoms.

Treatment. Treatment options include the use of nasal decongestants, nasal steroid sprays, a humidifier, applications of heat to the face, and antibiotics. Surgery to clear the sinuses or unblock sinus openings may be required.

SUDDEN INFANT DEATH SYNDROME (SIDS) claims the life of more than 7,000 babies a year in the United States. There are no characteristic signs or symptoms. Usually a baby with this disorder simply goes to sleep and never wakes up.

Causes. The causes of SIDS are unknown, but certain risk factors have been identified:

- Male babies are more likely to die of SIDS.
- Babies are most susceptible between the ages of 2 weeks and 6 months.
- Premature or low birth weight babies are more likely to have SIDS.
- A baby with a sibling who died of SIDS is more likely to also die of this disorder.
- African American or Native American babies are more likely to die of SIDS.
- Babies who were prenatally exposed to alcohol, cocaine, heroin, or nicotine are at a higher risk of developing SIDS.
- Babies who sleep on their stomachs are approximately three times more likely to die of SIDS.

Treatment. Proper sleep positioning on the baby's back is best for all infants, especially those known to be at risk, those with previous apneic episodes, and those who have lost a sibling to SIDS. At-risk infants may also be sent home with an apnea monitor that will sound an alarm if breathing ceases. Research into this disease is ongoing. Support groups are available and are suggested for families who have experienced the tragedy of losing a child to SIDS.

TUBERCULOSIS (TB) kills more than 2 million people worldwide each year. Although it primarily affects the lungs, it can spread to other parts of the body.

Causes. This disease is caused by various strains of the bacterium *Mycobacterium tuberculosis*. Widespread tuberculosis may be complicated by the following factors:

- HIV infection. HIV infection makes a person more vulnerable to TB.
- Crowded living conditions. This factor allows TB to spread easily; TB, therefore, is found in some prisons and homeless shelters.
- Poverty. Poverty prevents some patients with TB from seeking or completing therapy.
- Drug-resistant bacterium. Drug-resistant strains of the bacterium that causes TB have increased.
- Long-term therapy. Current treatments require antibiotic therapy for many months, which some patients with TB do not complete.

Signs and Symptoms. The symptoms include a cough that lasts more than 3 weeks, unintended weight loss, fever or chills, fatigue, night sweats, pain when breathing or difficulty breathing, and pain in other affected areas.

Treatment. The first step should be TB testing to detect carriers of this disease, who should then be treated. Therapy for TB normally lasts 6 months to a year, but drug-resistant cases of TB may require years of drug therapy. Isolating the patient during the contagious phase of the disease (usually 2 to 4 weeks after treatment begins) is required. Also, during the initial stages of treatment, the patient should be encouraged to receive adequate bed rest and maintain an adequate, nutritious diet.

UPPER RESPIRATORY (TRACT) INFECTION (URI) is the term often used for *coryza,* or the common cold.

Causes. URIs are caused by a family of viruses known as *rhinovirus*. The viruses are airborne and also transmitted by contact with contaminated surfaces and on the hands. Children are frequent sources of transmission.

Signs and Symptoms. This is a generally self-limiting condition of approximately 1 week's duration, which follows an initial incubation period of 2 to 5 days. Symptoms include pharyngitis, nasal congestion, rhinitis, headache, fever, and general malaise. There may be a nonproductive cough, especially at night.

Treatment. Care is usually symptomatic and includes antipyretics, analgesics, decongestants, and cough suppressants. Adequate rest and plenty of fluids to flush the system are also helpful. Antibiotics are ordinarily only prescribed for patients with an underlying illness or complication.

SUMMARY OF LEARNING OUTCOMES

LEARNING OUTCOMES	KEY POINTS
29.1 Describe the structure and function of each organ in the respiratory system.	The function of the respiratory system is to move air in and out of the lungs in a process known as ventilation, respiration, or breathing. The larynx contains the vocal cords, which stretch between the thyroid and cricoid cartilages. The lungs contain connective tissue, the bronchial tree, nerves, lymphatic vessels, and blood vessels. The bronchial tree consists of the primary, secondary, and tertiary branches of the bronchi, the bronchioles, and the alveoli.
29.2 Describe the events involved in the inspiration and expiration of air.	During inspiration, the diaphragm contracts and the intercostal muscles raise the ribs, increasing the space in the thoracic cavity. This decreases the pressure within the cavity so that the air outside the body passively flows into the thoracic cavity. During expiration, the diaphragm relaxes, pushing up into the thoracic cavity, and the intercostal muscles lower the ribs, forcing the air to flow out of the body. Breathing is controlled by the respiratory center of the brain, located in the pons and medulla oblongata.
29.3 Explain how oxygen and carbon dioxide are transported in the blood.	Most of the oxygen in the bloodstream binds to the hemoglobin within red blood cells, resulting in oxyhemoglobin, although a small amount does not bind to hemoglobin and remains dissolved in the plasma. Carbon dioxide binds to hemoglobin, resulting in carboxyhemoglobin. Most of the carbon dioxide that enters the blood reacts with water in plasma and cerebrospinal fluid to form carbonic acid. As carbonic acid ionizes, it releases hydrogen and bicarbonate ions, which attach to hemoglobin making its way back to the lungs to be exhaled.
29.4 Compare various respiratory volumes and tell how they are used to diagnose respiratory problems.	Respiratory volumes are measured to check the health of the respiratory system. The volumes are: tidal volume, inspiratory and expiratory reserve volumes, residual volume, inspiratory capacity, functional residual capacity, vital capacity, and total lung capacity. The normal capacities are found in the chapter.
29.5 Describe the causes, signs and symptoms, and treatments of various diseases and disorders of the respiratory system.	There are many common diseases and disorders of the respiratory system with varied signs, symptoms, and treatments. Some of these include allergic rhinitis, asthma, atelectasis, bronchitis, chronic obstructive pulmonary disease (COPD), emphysema, influenza, laryngitis, Legionnaire's disease, lung cancer, pleural effusion, pleuritis, pneumoconiosis, pneumonia, pneumothorax, pulmonary edema, pulmonary embolism, respiratory distress syndrome (RDS), severe acute respiratory syndrome (SARS), sinusitis, sudden infant death syndrome (SIDS), tuberculosis (TB), and upper respiratory (tract) infection (URI).

Recall Mohammad from the beginning of the chapter. Now that you have completed the chapter, answer the following questions regarding his case.

1. Why is asthma considered a life-threatening condition?

2. Why did the doctor refer Mohammad for allergy testing?

3. In addition to the prescribed medication, what can Mohammad do to help reduce his symptoms?

1. (LO 29.1) Which of the following is/are known as the pulmonary parenchyma?
   a. Nares
   b. Bronchi
   c. Bronchioles
   d. Alveoli
   e. Larynx

2. (LO 29.2) What is responsible for raising and lowering the rib cage during respiration?
   a. Diaphragm
   b. Lungs
   c. Intercostal muscles
   d. Respiratory center
   e. Spinal cord

3. (LO 29.5) Lack of surfactant is responsible for which of the following in premature infants?
   a. SARS
   b. RDS
   c. COPD
   d. Pneumonia
   e. Asthma

4. (LO 29.1) Which structure covers the larynx during swallowing?
   a. Epiglottis
   b. Glottis
   c. Conchae
   d. Hyoid
   e. Uvula

5. (LO 29.5) Which condition is commonly known as a collapsed lung?
   a. Bronchitis
   b. Pleuritis
   c. Coryza
   d. Pneumonia
   e. Atelectasis

6. (LO 29.3) Most of the carbon dioxide in the blood remains in the plasma in which of the following forms?
   a. Carboxyhemoglobin
   b. Carbon monoxide
   c. Bicarbonate
   d. Carbonic acid
   e. Oxyhemoglobin

7. (LO 29.4) Which term refers to the total amount of air the lungs can hold?
   a. Total lung capacity
   b. Vital capacity
   c. Tidal volume
   d. Expiratory reserve volume
   e. Inspiratory reserve volume

8. (LO 29.2) Which of the following everyday occurrences alters our breathing patterns?
   a. Blinking
   b. Swallowing
   c. Yawning
   d. Watching TV
   e. Studying

9. (LO 29.5) The most common types of COPD are emphysema and which other disorder?
   a. Pleuritis
   b. Chronic bronchitis
   c. Asthma
   d. Pleural effusion
   e. Legionnaire's disease

10. (LO 29.2) Which of the following occurs during expiration?
    a. Air flows into the lungs
    b. The diaphragm contracts
    c. The diaphragm flattens
    d. The thoracic cavity enlarges
    e. The intercostal muscles lower the ribs

Analyze the following medical terms, presented throughout the chapter. Using a medical dictionary (or Appendix I) place a / mark between each word part. Define each word part and then define the whole word.

EXAMPLE: **pharyng** /**itis** = pharyng means "throat" + itis means "inflammation"
Pharyngitis means "inflammation of the throat"

1. anthracosis
2. bronchitis
3. epiglottis
4. lobectomy

5. pneumothorax
6. pulmonary
7. pyothorax
8. rhinitis

9. thoracostomy
10. uvulotomy
11. costochrondritis
12. dyspnea

The Nervous System

PATIENT INFORMATION

Patient Name	Gender	DOB
Nancy Evans	F	1/29/19XX

Attending	MRN	Allergies
Elizabeth H. Williams, MD	654-88-099	Amoxicillin

During the patient interview, you ask the patient her name and date of birth. She states, "I am Nancy Evans, I am Welsh, I was born in January but I don't remember what year." You look at the chart and note that her name is Nancy Evans and she was born on January 29, 1945. Her husband is in the waiting room; after obtaining Nancy's permission, you ask him to come to the interview area. He confirms Nancy's complete name and date of birth and then states, "She seems to forget everything these days."

Keep Nancy in mind as you study the chapter. There will be questions at the end of the chapter based on the case study. The information in the chapter will help you answer these questions.

L E A R N I N G   O U T C O M E S

After completing Chapter 30, you will be able to:

30.1 Describe the general functions of the nervous system.

30.2 Summarize the structure of a neuron.

30.3 Explain the function of nerve impulses and the role of synapses in their transmission.

30.4 Describe the structures and functions of the central nervous system.

30.5 Compare the structures and functions of the somatic and autonomic nervous systems in the peripheral nervous system.

30.6 Recognize common tests that are performed to determine neurologic disorders.

30.7 Describe the causes, signs and symptoms, and treatments of various diseases and disorders of the nervous system.

K E Y   T E R M S

afferent nerves

autonomic nervous system (ANS)

axon

cell body

central nervous system (CNS)

cerebrospinal fluid (CSF)

dendrite

dermatome

efferent nerves

ganglia

interneurons

meninges

neuroglia

neurotransmitter

parasympathetic division

paresthesias

peripheral nervous system (PNS)

plexus

somatic nervous system (SNS)

sympathetic division

I. C (5) Describe the normal function of each body system

I. C (6) Identify common pathology related to each body system

I. C (7) Analyze pathology as it relates to the interaction of body systems

I. C (8) Discuss implications for disease and disability when homeostasis is not maintained

I. C (9) Describe implications for treatment related to pathology

I. C (10) Compare body structure and function of the human body across the life span

I. C (12) Describe the relationship between anatomy and physiology of all body systems and medications used for treatment in each

IV. C (11) Define both medical terms and abbreviations related to all body systems

2. Anatomy & Physiology
Graduates:

b. Identify and apply the knowledge of all body systems, their structure and functions, and their common diseases, symptoms, and etiologies

c. Assist the physician with the regimen of diagnostic and treatment modalities as they relate to each body system

3. Medical Terminology
Graduates:

b. Build and dissect medical terms from roots/suffice to understand the word element combinations that create medical terminology

c. Understand the various medical terminology for each specialty

d. Recognize and identify acceptable medical abbreviations

Introduction

The nervous system is highly complex. It controls all other organ systems and is important for maintaining balance within those systems. Disorders of the nervous system are numerous and often difficult to diagnose and treat because of this system's complexity.

General Functions of the Nervous System

LO 30.1

The nervous system is divided into two major parts—the **central nervous system (CNS)** and the **peripheral nervous system (PNS)**. The CNS consists of the brain and the spinal cord; the peripheral nervous system consists of peripheral nerves, which are located throughout the rest of the body.

The peripheral nervous system is split into two separate sections: the **somatic nervous system (SNS),** which governs your body's skeletal or voluntary muscles, and the **autonomic nervous system (ANS),** which is in charge of your body's automatic functions, such as the respiratory and gastrointestinal systems.

In addition, there are three different types of nerve cells or neurons that carry out the actual functions of the nervous system: (1) The sensory or **afferent nerves** are responsible for detecting sensory information from the environment or from inside the body and bringing it to the CNS for interpretation. (2) The motor or **efferent nerves** bring information or impulses from the central nervous system to the PNS to control the movement or action of a muscle or gland. (3) Within the CNS (brain or spinal cord) are the interpretive neurons known as **interneurons** that lie between the sensory and motor nerves.

These neurons act as go-betweens or interpreters between the afferent and efferent nerves.

An example of this process would be noting a red light while driving. The sensory neurons in your eyes note the color and send the information to the brain's cerebral cortex where the interpretation takes place. The interneurons pick up the signal, interpret it, and send the information to the motor neurons that you are supposed to stop your vehicle, which in turn sends the instructions to your right foot to step on the brake pedal of your vehicle. This entire transaction, of course, takes place in milliseconds, allowing you to stop in time.

Neuron Structure

LO 30.2

Neurons are the functional cells of the nervous system. They transmit electrochemical messages called *nerve impulses* to other neurons and *effectors* (muscles or glands). An important characteristic of neurons is that they lose their ability to divide. Therefore, when neurons are destroyed by disease, they cannot be replaced.

The *neuroglial cells* or **neuroglia,** which do not transmit impulses, function as support cells for neurons. (See Figure 30-1.) Neuroglial cells never lose their ability to divide. The three types of neuroglia are:

- *Astrocytes*—star-shaped cells that anchor blood vessels to the nerve cells

- *Microglia*—small cells that act as phagocytes, watching for and engulfing invaders

- *Oligodendrocytes*—specialized neuroglial cells that assist in the production of the myelin sheath, which will be discussed in further detail later

FIGURE 30-1 A typical neuron surrounded by neuroglial cells.

All neurons have a **cell body** and processes called *nerve fibers* that extend from the cell body.

The cell body is the portion of the neuron that contains the nucleus and the typical organelles of any cell. (Refer to the *Organization of the Body* chapter.) It is responsible for generating the large amount of proteins and energy the neuron needs to carry out its important functions.

Extending from the cell body are two types of nerve fibers: **axons** and **dendrites.** A neuron may have one or more dendrites but typically has only one axon. Dendrites are usually short and branch profusely near the cell body. Their function is to receive information for the neuron. Axons are typically long and branch profusely after they have extended far away from the cell body. Their function is to send information (nerve impulses) away from the cell body.

In the peripheral nervous system, neuroglial cells called *Schwann cells* wrap themselves around some axons. The axons are coated by the cell membranes of the Schwann cells. The cell membranes contain large amounts of *myelin*, which is a fatty substance that insulates the axons and allows them to send nerve impulses quickly. The axons thus coated are referred to as *white matter.* Those not insulated by the myelin sheath are known as *gray matter.*

▶ Nerve Impulse and Synapse LO 30.3

Neuron cell membranes have a *cell membrane potential.* This means the membrane is *polarized.* Just like a battery is polarized—one end is negative and the other end is positive—neuron cell membranes are polarized because the inside is negatively charged and the outside is positively charged. This is true in most other types of body cells as well. The outside of cell membranes is positively charged because more positive ions are on the outside. The inside of cell membranes is negatively charged because more negative ions are on the inside. This membrane potential is very important for the function of neurons (see Figure 30-2).

BODY**ANIMAT3D**
POWERED BY
connect

Go to CONNECT to see an animation about *Nerve Impulse.*

(a)

Region of depolarization

(b)

Region of repolarization

(c)

FIGURE 30-2 Nerve impulse: (a) At rest, or in its polarized state, more Na⁺ is on the outside of the membrane, which makes the outside positive and the inside relatively negative (less positive). (b) When Na⁺ moves into the cell, the membrane depolarizes, and the inside becomes more positive. (c) The membrane repolarizes when K⁺ and later Na⁺ move to the outside of the cell membrane.

Potassium and sodium ions are both positively charged and play important roles in generating nerve impulses. When a neuron is at rest or without stimulation, the outside of its membrane is positively charged and the inside is negatively charged because the number of sodium and potassium ions is greater outside the membrane. As long as the neuron is at rest, it remains in this polarized state.

However, a neuron responds to stimuli such as heat, pressure, and chemicals by changing the amount of polarization across its membrane to make the outside of the membrane less positive. When this happens, the neuron has *depolarized,* or become less polar. To make the outside of the membrane less positive, some of the sodium ions flow to the inside of the cell membrane. If the membrane of an axon becomes depolarized enough, an action potential (a nerve impulse) is created. This *action potential* or nerve impulse is the flow of electric current along the axon membrane. Eventually, the axon membrane becomes polarized again by the return of positively charged ions to the outside of the cell membrane. The return to the original polarized (resting) state is called *repolarization*.

An unmyelinated axon does not conduct a nerve impulse as quickly as a myelinated axon does. Also, the speed of the nerve impulse is related to the diameter of the axon. The larger the diameter, the faster the nerve impulse travels to the end of the axon.

When traveling down an axon, a nerve impulse eventually reaches the *synaptic knob* at the end of the axon branches. Synaptic knobs contain small sacs called *vesicles*, which produce chemicals called **neurotransmitters.** Neurotransmitters are released by the synaptic knob to allow impulse transmission to continue to the postsynaptic structures, which consist of the dendrites, cell bodies, and axons of other neurons (see Figure 30-3). This space between the axon of one neuron and the dendrite of the next is sometimes referred to as the synaptic space.

There are about 50 different neurotransmitters. Most neurons release only one type of neurotransmitter, but some release more than one type. Their functions include causing muscles to contract or relax, causing glands to secrete products, activating neurons to send nerve impulses, or inhibiting neurons from sending nerve impulses.

▶ Central Nervous System   LO 30.4

The CNS includes the spinal cord and brain (see Figure 30-4). The tissues of the CNS are so delicate that a *blood-brain barrier* and layers of membranes protect them. Tight capillaries form the blood-brain barrier, which prevents certain substances from entering the tissues of the CNS. For example, various waste products and drugs do not cross the blood-brain barrier well. Inflammation, however, can make this barrier more permeable.

Meninges are membranes that protect the brain and spinal cord. The three layers of meninges are dura mater, arachnoid mater, and pia mater. *Dura mater* is the toughest and outermost layer of the meninges. The space above the dura mater is called the *epidural space*; below the dura mater is the *subdural space*. The middle layer, named for its spider web–like appearance, is the *arachnoid mater*. *Pia mater* is the innermost and most delicate layer. It sits directly on top of the brain and spinal cord and holds blood vessels onto the surface of these structures. Between the arachnoid mater and pia mater is an area

FIGURE 30-3 Synapse. When a nerve impulse reaches a synaptic knob, it releases a neurotransmitter onto the postsynaptic structure.

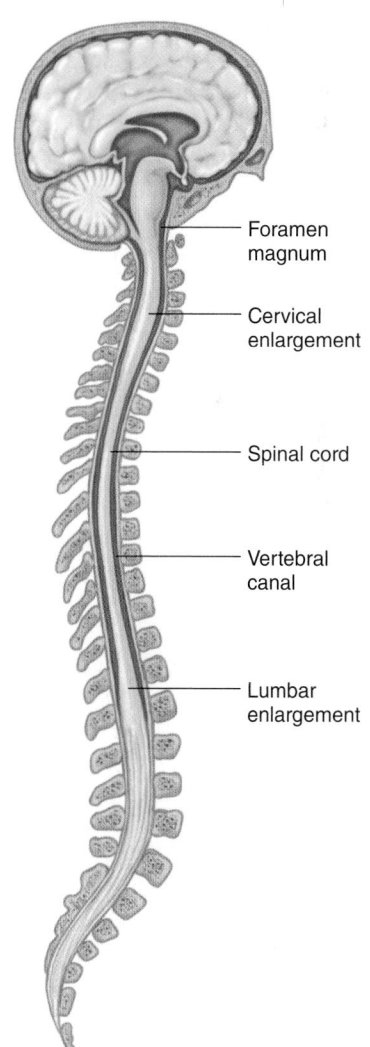

FIGURE 30-4 The central nervous system (CNS) consists of the brain and spinal cord. The spinal cord ends at the level of the third lumbar vertebra.

called the *subarachnoid space*. It contains **cerebrospinal fluid (CSF),** which cushions the CNS.

Spinal Cord

The spinal cord is a slender structure that is continuous with the brain. The spinal cord descends into the vertebral canal and ends around the level of the first or second lumbar vertebra. The spinal cord is divided into 31 spinal segments: 8 cervical segments, 12 thoracic segments, 5 lumbar segments, 5 sacral segments, and 1 coccygeal segment. The thickening of the spinal cord in the neck region is called the *cervical enlargement* and contains the motor neurons that control the arm muscles. Another thickening of the spinal cord occurs in the lumbar region. Called the *lumbar enlargement,* this thickening contains the motor neurons that control the leg muscles (see Figure 30-4).

Gray Matter and White Matter When you view a cross-section of the spinal cord, you observe two differently colored areas. The inner tissue is termed *gray matter* because it is darker than the outer tissue, which is termed *white matter.* The white matter contains the myelinated axons of neurons and is divided into columns (funiculi). The columns contain groups of axons called *nerve tracts.* The gray matter contains the neuron cell bodies and their dendrites and has bulges or sections called *horns.* A canal called the *central canal* contains CSF and runs through the center of the gray matter down the entire length of the spinal cord.

Ascending and Descending Tracts One function of the spinal cord is to carry sensory information up to the brain. The tracts that carry sensory information up to the brain are called *ascending tracts.* Another function of the spinal cord is to carry motor information down from the brain to muscles and glands in tracts called *descending tracts.*

Reflexes Another important function of the spinal cord is to participate in reflexes. A *reflex* is a predictable, automatic response to a stimulus. (See Figure 30-5). For example, if you touch something hot, the predictable response is that you will pull your finger away from the hot surface in a withdrawal reflex. The information that flows through a typical reflex moves in the following order: from receptors, to sensory neurons, to interneurons, to motor neurons, to effectors. In this example of the withdrawal reflex, the receptors are in the skin at the fingertips. These receptors send their information to sensory neurons that relay the information to interneurons in the spinal cord. The interneurons immediately relay the information to motor neurons that activate the muscles (effectors) in the arm. The arm muscles coordinate the movement of pulling your finger away from the painful stimulus. A person can consciously inhibit a reflex because the information also goes to the cerebral cortex—the part of the brain that handles conscious decisions.

Interneuron

Sensory neuron

Extensor relaxes

Extensor contracts

Motor neurons

Flexor relaxes

Motor neurons

Flexor contracts

⊕ = Stimulation

⊖ = Inhibition

FIGURE 30-5   The cross-section of the spinal cord and a spinal nerve illustrates a reflex arc.

Brain

The brain is divided into four major areas: the cerebrum, the diencephalon, the brainstem, and the cerebellum (see Figure 30-6).

Cerebrum   The cerebrum is the largest part of the brain. It is divided into two halves called cerebral hemispheres. A thick bundle of nerve fibers called the *corpus callosum* connects the two hemispheres. The grooves on the surface of the cerebrum are called *sulci*. The "bumps" of brain matter between the sulci are called *gyri*, or convolutions. A deep groove called the longitudinal fissure runs between the two longitudinal hemispheres.

Lobes   Each cerebral hemisphere is divided into *lobes*— frontal, parietal, temporal, and occipital. The frontal lobes contain motor areas that allow a person to consciously decide to produce a body movement such as walking or tapping a pencil. Somatosensory areas are located in the parietal lobes. These areas interpret sensations felt on or within the body. For example, if you feel a light touch on your right hand, the somatosensory area interprets the sensation and where it is occurring. The temporal lobes contain auditory areas that interpret sounds. Visual areas are located in the occipital lobes, and they interpret what a person sees.

Cortex   The outermost layer of the cerebrum is called the *cerebral cortex*. It is composed of gray matter and therefore contains neuron cell bodies and dendrites. This layer contains nearly 75% of all neurons in the entire nervous system. Beneath the cerebral cortex is white matter. Besides

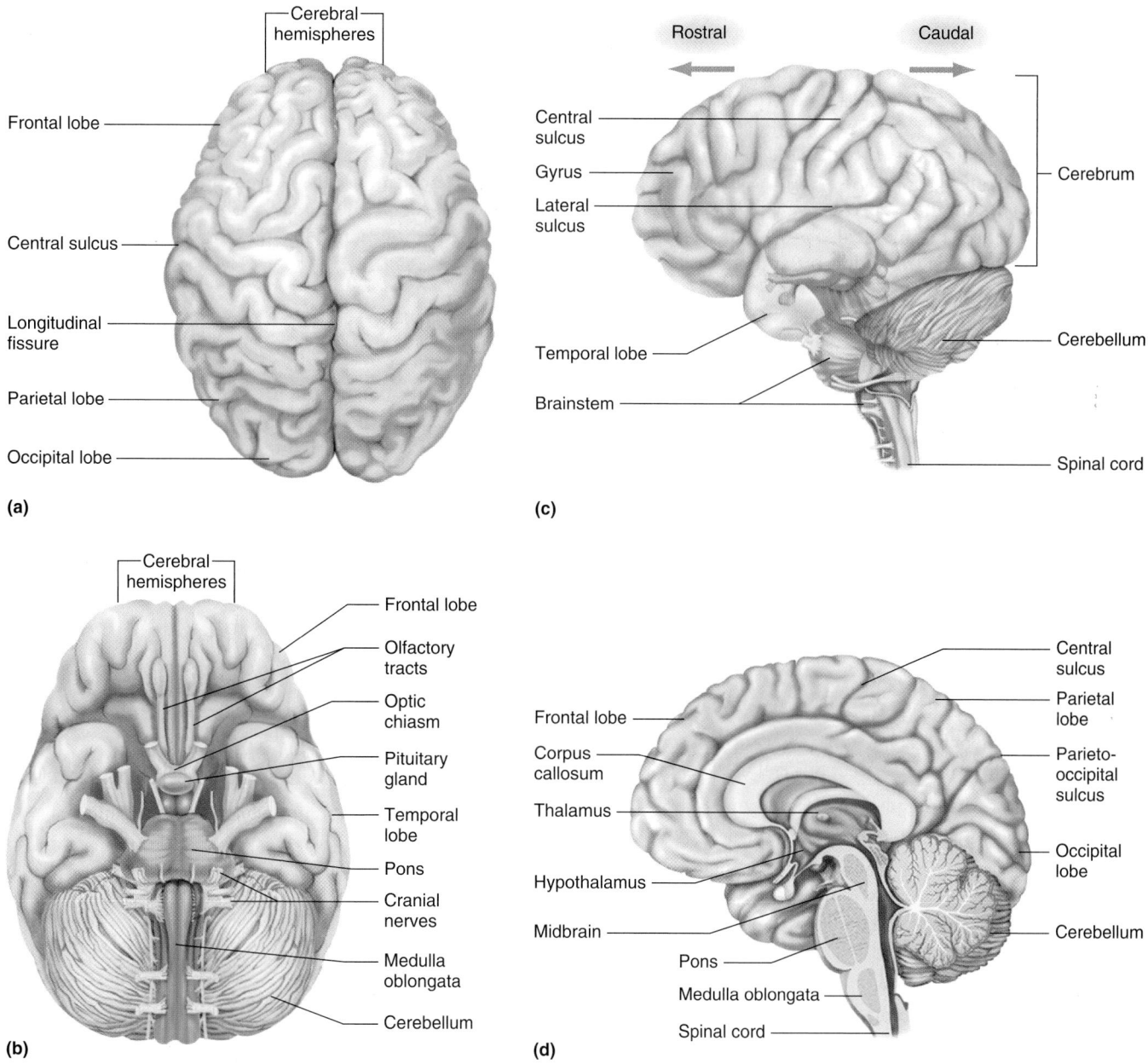

FIGURE 30-6   Four views of the brain: (a) superior, (b) inferior, (c) left lateral, and (d) sagittal section.

interpreting sensory information and initiating body movements, the cortex also stores memories and creates emotions.

Ventricles *Ventricles* are interconnected cavities within the brain. They are filled with CSF. Recall that this fluid is also found in the subarachnoid space of the meninges and the central canal of the spinal cord. Therefore, CSF is located within the brain and spinal cord and also around the brain and spinal cord. This fluid protects and cushions the CNS.

Diencephalon The *diencephalon* is located between the cerebral hemispheres and is superior to the brainstem. The diencephalon includes the thalamus and hypothalamus. The *thalamus* serves as a relay station for sensory information that heads to the cerebral cortex for interpretation. If sensory information does not pass through the thalamus before it reaches the cerebral cortex, it cannot be interpreted correctly. For example, say you are feeling pain in your left forearm. This information goes up the spinal cord and through the thalamus, and then to the cerebral cortex for interpretation. If the information did not go through the thalamus, the cerebral cortex might interpret that you are feeling cold instead of pain in your left forearm. The *hypothalamus* maintains homeostasis by regulating hunger, thirst, and body temperature. It also provides a link between the nervous system and the endocrine system.

Brainstem The *brainstem* is a structure that connects the cerebrum to the spinal cord. The three parts of the brainstem are the midbrain, the pons, and the medulla oblongata. The *midbrain* lies just beneath the diencephalon. It controls both visual and auditory reflexes. Seeing something in your peripheral vision and automatically turning your head to view it more clearly is an example of a visual reflex.

The *pons* is a rounded bulge on the underside of the brainstem situated between the midbrain and the medulla oblongata. It contains nerve tracts to connect the cerebrum to the cerebellum. The pons also regulates respiration.

The *medulla oblongata* is the most inferior portion of the brainstem and is directly connected to the spinal cord. It controls many vital activities such as heart rate, blood pressure, and respiration. It also controls reflexes associated with coughing, sneezing, and vomiting.

Cerebellum The cerebellum is inferior to the occipital lobes of the cerebrum and posterior to the pons and medulla oblongata. It coordinates complex skeletal muscle contractions needed for body movements. For example, when you walk, many muscles have to contract and relax at appropriate times. Your cerebellum coordinates these activities. The cerebellum also coordinates fine movements such as threading a needle, playing an instrument, and writing.

EDUCATING THE PATIENT
Preventing Brain and Spinal Cord Injuries

In the United States alone, almost half a million people a year suffer brain and spinal cord injuries. The most common causes of these injuries are motor vehicle accidents, sports and recreational accidents—especially diving—and violence. People at the highest risk for spinal cord injuries are children and teens. However, most brain and spinal cord injuries can be prevented. Use the following tips to educate patients on preventing these types of injuries.

Prevention Tips

- Know the depth of water into which you are diving. More than 90% of diving injuries occur in 5 feet of water or less.

- Explore diving areas before diving. For example, know where rocks are located before you dive.

- Do not drive or do any recreational activity while under the influence of alcohol or drugs. Both affect good judgment and control. Alcohol-related traffic crashes are the leading cause of disabling brain and spinal cord injuries.

- Always wear a helmet when riding a bike or motorcycle, or doing any sporting activity in which you might fall such as horse riding or skateboarding. Your risk of brain injury is 85% greater during a biking accident if you are not wearing

a helmet. Make sure your helmet fits properly. Make sure to replace your helmet if you have hit your head while wearing it; the helmet may be compromised from the fall and thus unsafe.

- Always wear appropriate protective gear while playing any sport.

- Avoid surfing headfirst.

- Always wear your safety belt in the car.

- Make sure children use car seats appropriate for their age and weight.

- Be familiar with ways to get help quickly in emergencies.

- Follow traffic rules and signs while walking, biking, or driving.

- Follow safety rules on playgrounds.

- Store firearms and ammunition in separate and locked places.

- Teach children the safety rules to follow if they find a gun.

Go to CONNECT to see an animation about *Spinal Cord Injury*.

▶ Peripheral Nervous System

LO 30.5

The peripheral nervous system (PNS) consists of nerves that branch off the CNS. These *peripheral nerves* are classified into two types: cranial nerves and spinal nerves.

Cranial Nerves

Cranial nerves are peripheral nerves that originate from the brain. Roman numerals and names designate the twelve cranial nerves (see Figure 30-7):

I.   *Olfactory nerves* carry smell information to the brain for interpretation.

II. *Optic nerves* carry visual information to the brain for interpretation.

III. *Oculomotor nerves* are found in the muscles that move the eyeball, eyelid, and iris.

IV. *Trochlear nerves* act in the muscles that move the eyeball.

V.   *Trigeminal nerves* carry sensory information from the surface of the eye, the scalp, facial skin, the lining of the gums, and the palate to the brain for interpretation. They also are found in the muscles needed for chewing.

VI. *Abducens nerves* act in the muscles that move the eyeball.

VII. *Facial nerves* are found in the muscles of facial expression as well as in the salivary and tear glands. These nerves also carry sensory information from the tongue.

VIII. *Vestibulocochlear nerves* carry hearing and equilibrium information from the inner ear to the brain for interpretation.

IX. *Glossopharyngeal nerves* carry sensory information from the throat and tongue to the brain for interpretation. They also act in the muscles of the throat.

X.   *Vagus nerves* carry sensory information from the thoracic and abdominal organs to the brain for interpretation. These nerves are also found in the muscles in the throat, stomach, intestines, and heart.

Cranial nerves

- Olfactory bulb, termination of olfactory nerve (CN I)
- Olfactory tract
- Optic chiasm
- Optic nerve (CN II)
- Infundibulum
- Optic tract
- Oculomotor nerve (CN III)
- Trochlear nerve (CN IV)
- Trigeminal nerve (CN V)
- Abducens nerve (CN VI)
- Facial nerve (CN VII)
- Vestibulocochlear nerve (CN VIII)
- Glossopharyngeal nerve (CN IX)
- Vagus nerve (CN X)
- Hypoglossal nerve (CN XII)
- Accessory nerve (CN XI)
- Spinal cord

Pons

Medulla oblongata

FIGURE 30-7 The cranial nerves. A view of the inferior surface of the brain shows the 12 pairs of cranial nerves.

XI. *Accessory nerves* are found in the muscles of the throat, neck, back, and voice box.

XII. *Hypoglossal nerves* are found in the muscles of the tongue.

Spinal Nerves

Spinal nerves are peripheral nerves that originate from the spinal cord (see Figure 30-8). There are 31 pairs of spinal nerves: 8 pairs of cervical nerves (numbered C1 through C8), 12 pairs of thoracic nerves (numbered T1 through T12), 5 pairs of lumbar nerves (numbered L1 through L5), 5 pairs of sacral nerves (numbered S1 through S5), and 1 pair of coccygeal nerves (Cx). Except for C1, each spinal nerve innervates a skin segment known as a **dermatome.** A map of the dermatomes with the spinal nerve responsible for the skin area is shown in Figure 30-9.

Two roots, a *ventral root* and a *dorsal root*, form each spinal nerve. The ventral root contains axons of motor neurons only,

and the dorsal root contains axons of sensory neurons only. The dorsal root also contains a dorsal root ganglion, which contains the cell bodies of sensory neurons.

Except in the thoracic region, the main portions of spinal nerves fuse together to form nerve **plexuses.** The major nerve plexuses are the cervical, brachial, and lumbosacral plexuses. Nerves coming off the cervical plexus supply the skin and the muscles of the neck. The phrenic nerve also originates from the cervical plexus. This nerve controls the diaphragm, which is a muscle needed for breathing.

The brachial plexus includes nerves that control muscles in the arms. The lumbosacral plexus supplies the lower abdominal wall, external genitalia, buttocks, thighs, legs, and feet. The largest nerve of the body, the sciatic nerve, originates from this plexus. This nerve controls the leg muscles. The coccygeal plexus is the source of the anococcygeal nerve, which innervates the anus and the back of the thighs.

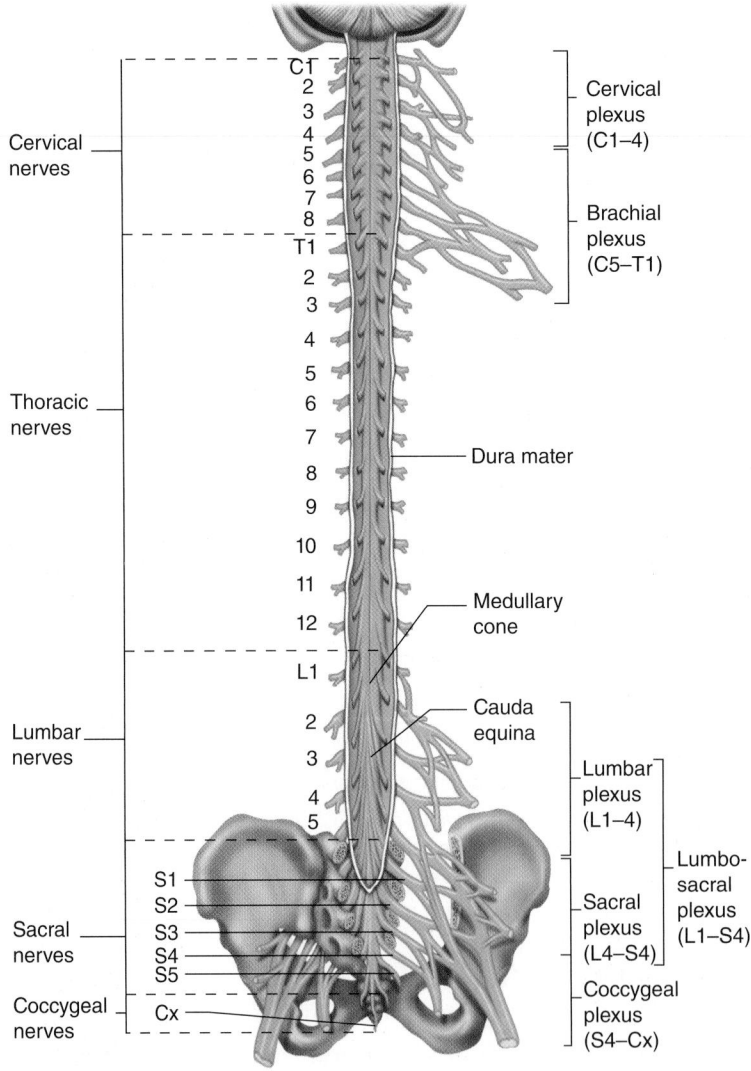

FIGURE 30-8 Spinal cord, spinal nerves, and plexuses.

FIGURE 30-9 Dermatome maps. A dermatome is an area of skin supplied by a single spinal nerve. These diagrams only approximate the dermatomal distribution.

Somatic and Autonomic Nervous Systems

The PNS is divided into a somatic nervous system (SNS) and an autonomic nervous system (ANS). The SNS consists of nerves that connect the CNS to skin and skeletal muscle. The SNS is often called the "voluntary" nervous system because it controls skeletal muscles, which are under voluntary control. The ANS consists of nerves that connect the CNS to organs and other structures such as the heart, stomach, intestines, glands, blood vessels, and bladder (among others). The ANS controls organs not under voluntary control, so it is often referred to as the "involuntary" nervous system.

In the ANS, motor neurons from the brain and spinal cord communicate to other motor neurons located in ganglia. **Ganglia** are collections of neuron cell bodies outside the CNS. The motor neurons of ganglia then communicate to various organs and blood vessels.

The two divisions of the ANS are the sympathetic and the parasympathetic (see Figures 30-10 and 30-11). The **sympathetic division** prepares organs for "fight-or-flight" stressful or emergency situations. For example, the sympathetic division prepares the heart for a stressful or frightening situation by increasing the heart rate. The **parasympathetic division** prepares the body for resting and digesting by, for example, keeping the heart rate

relatively low. Notice that sympathetic and parasympathetic actions are antagonistic, meaning they function in opposite ways. Most of the body's organs are under parasympathetic control.

Many neurons of the sympathetic division are located in the thoracic and lumbar regions of the spinal cord. For this reason, this division is also called the thoracolumbar division. The sympathetic neurons usually release the neurotransmitter norepinephrine into organs and glands. Norepinephrine increases the heart and breathing rates, slows down the activity of the digestive glands, slows down the muscles of the stomach and the intestines, and dilates the pupils. Sympathetic nerves also control the constriction of blood vessels. When blood vessels constrict, blood pressure increases, which is a needed response during an emergency situation.

Many neurons of the parasympathetic division are located in the brainstem and the sacral regions of the spinal cord. For this reason, this division is also referred to as the craniosacral division. All parasympathetic neurons release acetylcholine to organs and glands. Acetylcholine is a neurotransmitter that slows the heart and breathing rates, constricts the pupils, activates digestive glands, and activates the muscles of the stomach and intestines. Most blood vessels in the body do not receive communication from parasympathetic nerves.

FIGURE 30-10 Divisions of the ANS. Most parasympathetic fibers release acetylcholine onto visceral effectors. Most sympathetic fibers release norepinephrine onto visceral effectors.

▶ Neurologic Testing

LO 30.6

Patients with nervous system disorders may have a wide variety of signs and symptoms, but the most common are headache, muscle weakness, and **paresthesias** (loss of feeling). A typical neurologic examination can determine the following:

- State of consciousness. This state can vary from normal to a state of coma. A patient in a coma cannot respond to stimuli and cannot be awakened. Other terms used to describe states of consciousness include stupor (difficulty being awakened), delirium (being confused or having hallucinations), vegetative (having no cortical function), and asleep (can be aroused with normal stimulation).
- Reflex activity. Reflex tests primarily determine the health of the PNS.
- Speech patterns. Abnormal speech patterns include a loss of the ability to form words correctly or to form sentences that make sense.
- Motor patterns. Abnormal motor patterns include the loss of balance, abnormal posture, or inappropriate, involuntary movements of the body. For example, chorea is an exaggerated and sudden jerking of a body part.

Diagnostic Procedures

Common diagnostic procedures to determine neurologic disorders include the following tests:

- Lumbar puncture. When a physician needs to examine CSF, a lumbar puncture is performed. A needle is used to remove CSF from the subarachnoid space, usually below the third lumbar vertebra of the spinal column. Analysis of this fluid provides a great deal of information about the patient's health. For example, cancer cells in CSF often indicate a brain tumor or spinal cord tumor. White blood cells in this fluid indicate infections such as meningitis. Red blood cells indicate abnormal bleeding.
- Magnetic resonance imaging (MRI). This procedure allows the brain and spinal cord to be visualized from many angles. It uses powerful magnets to generate images and is useful in detecting tumors, bleeding, or other abnormalities.
- Positron emission tomography (PET) scan. This procedure uses radioactive chemicals that collect in specific areas of the brain. These chemicals allow images of those specific areas to be generated. This test is useful in detecting blood flow to areas of the brain, brain tumors, and the diagnosis of such diseases as Parkinson's and Alzheimer's.
- Cerebral angiography. This procedure uses contrast material that can be visualized in the blood vessels of the brain. It is useful in detecting aneurysms (abnormal, blood-filled bulges in blood vessels).
- Computerized tomography (CT) scan. This common procedure produces images that provide more information than a standard X-ray. It is useful in detecting tumors and other abnormal structures.

FIGURE 30-11 Comparison of the parasympathetic and sympathetic divisions. The parasympathetic and sympathetic divisions of the ANS have the same basic components, but they differ in origin and in the locations of preganglionic cell bodies, axon lengths, and amount of branching.

- Electroencephalogram (EEG). This test detects electrical activity in the brain. It is useful in diagnosing various states of consciousness.
- X-ray. This procedure is useful in detecting skull or vertebral fractures.

Cranial Nerve Tests

Disorders of the cranial nerves can be determined using the following tests:

- The olfactory nerves (I) are tested by asking a patient to smell various substances.
- Cranial nerves III, IV, and VI are tested by asking a patient to track the movement of the physician's finger. If a patient cannot move her eyeballs properly, there may be damage to one of these nerves. Recall that these nerves control the muscles that move the eyeballs.
- Cranial nerve V controls the muscles needed for chewing. To assess this nerve, a patient is asked to clench his teeth. The physician then feels the jaw muscles. If the muscles feel limp or weak, this nerve may be damaged.

- If a person can no longer make facial expressions, then cranial nerve VII may be damaged. This nerve controls the muscles needed to make facial expressions.
- If a patient cannot extend his tongue and move it from side to side, cranial nerve XII may be damaged. This nerve controls tongue movement.

Reflex Testing

Testing a patient's reflexes allows a physician to evaluate the components of a reflex as well as the overall health of the individual's nervous system. The absence of a reflex is called areflexia. Hyporeflexia is a decreased reflex, and hyperreflexia is a stronger than normal reflex. The following are common reflex tests:

- Biceps reflex. The absence of this reflex may indicate spinal cord damage in the cervical region.
- Knee reflex. The absence of this reflex may indicate damage to lumbar or femoral nerves.
- Abdominal reflexes. These reflexes are tested to evaluate damage to thoracic spinal nerves.

Common Diseases and Disorders of the Nervous System

ALZHEIMER'S DISEASE is a progressive, degenerative disease that occurs in the brain.

Causes. Fiber tangles within neurons, degenerating nerve fibers, and a decreased production of neurotransmitters cause the symptoms of this disorder. Alzheimer's is associated with advanced age, family history, certain genes, and possibly some environmental factors. Many causes have not yet been determined.

Signs and Symptoms. Common symptoms include memory loss, confusion, personality changes, language deterioration, impaired judgment, and restlessness.

Treatment. There is no cure, but with medications such as Aricept®, Cognex®, Razadyne®, and Namenda, as well as proper nutrition, physical exercise, social activity, and calm environments, the disease progress may be slowed and managed.

AMYOTROPHIC LATERAL SCLEROSIS (ALS), commonly known as Lou Gehrig's disease, is a fatal disorder characterized by the degeneration of neurons in the spinal cord and brain.

Causes. Most causes are unknown, but they are likely to involve hereditary and environmental factors.

Signs and Symptoms. Early symptoms include cramping of hand and feet muscles, persistent tripping and falling, chronic fatigue, and slurred speech. Signs and symptoms that appear in later stages include breathing difficulty and muscle paralysis.

Treatment. There is no cure for this disorder; however, physical, speech, and respiratory therapies help to manage the symptoms. Some medications relieve muscle cramping, but currently only the drug riluzole is approved by the U.S. Food and Drug Administration (FDA) specifically for ALS.

BELL'S PALSY is a disorder in which facial muscles are very weak or totally paralyzed.

Causes. This condition can result from damage to cranial nerve VII (the facial nerve), but many times the cause is unknown. It is more common in people with diabetes, the flu, or a cold.

Signs and Symptoms. The most common signs and symptoms are a loss of feeling in the face, the inability to produce facial expressions, headache, and excessive tearing or drooling.

Treatment. Treatments include the use of eyedrops, anti-inflammatory medications, and pain relievers. Symptoms usually diminish or go away within 5 to 10 days.

BRAIN TUMORS and **CANCERS** are abnormal growths in the brain. A brain tumor with cancer cells is termed malignant. Malignant tumors that start in any tissue of the brain are called primary brain cancers. Those that start in other body parts and spread to the brain are classified as secondary brain cancers. The most common primary brain tumors are gliomas that arise from neuroglial cells.

Causes. Like most cancers, the causes are gene mutations. Factors associated with gene mutations include exposure to toxins, an impaired immune system, and hereditary factors.

Signs and Symptoms. The signs and symptoms depend on the size and location of the tumor. Common symptoms include headache, seizures, nausea, weakness in the arms or legs, fatigue, changes in speech patterns, and a loss of memory.

Treatment. Treatment often includes surgery, radiation therapy, chemotherapy, and gene therapy. The success of the treatment depends on the type of tumor, the location and extent of the tumor, the tumor's response to treatment, and the patient's overall health.

EPILEPSY and **SEIZURES** occur when parts of the brain receive a burst of electrical signals that disrupt normal brain functioning. Seizures may be either petit mal (partial) or grand mal (generalized). Petit mal seizures may appear as loss of awareness of the present, whereas grand mal seizures result in the classic tonic-clonic seizure. Epilepsy is the condition of having repeated, long-term seizures.

Causes. Causes vary but may include birth trauma, high fevers, alcohol and drug withdrawal, head trauma, infections, brain tumors, and certain medications. Many causes are unknown.

Signs and Symptoms. The signs and symptoms may include visual disturbances, nausea, generalized abnormal feelings, a loss of consciousness, and uncontrolled muscle contractions and tremors.

Treatment. The primary treatment is medication to prevent seizures. Surgery is sometimes an option in patients with partial seizures.

GUILLAIN-BARRÉ SYNDROME is a disorder in which the body's immune system attacks part of the PNS. It usually has a sudden and unexpected onset.

Causes. The destruction of myelin by the body's immune system produces the signs and symptoms. Viral infections, immunizations, and pregnancy sometimes trigger the disease.

Signs and Symptoms. Symptoms may include weakness or tingling sensations in the legs or arms that can progress to paralysis. Difficulty breathing and an abnormal heart rate are more dangerous signs and symptoms. The disease normally runs its course, and with proper medical treatment, it is not fatal.

Treatment. Various supportive therapies, such as the use of respirators and heart machines, are necessary until the disease subsides. Physical therapy is used to keep muscles strong.

HEADACHES affect almost everyone at some point in life. A wide variety of factors produce headaches. Most headaches do not require medical attention, but a physician should evaluate repetitive and severe headaches. Headache types commonly include tension headaches, migraines, and cluster headaches.

Tension headaches are classified as either episodic (random) or chronic (frequent).

Episodic tension headaches are the most common type of tension headache.

Causes. This type of headache is often the result of temporary stress or anger.

Signs and Symptoms. Symptoms include pain or soreness in the temples and the contraction of head and neck muscles.

Treatment. Most of these headaches can be managed by taking an over-the-counter (OTC) medicine, and relief usually occurs in 1 or 2 hours.

CHRONIC TENSION HEADACHES occur almost daily and persist for weeks or months.

Causes. This type of headache may be the result of stress or fatigue, but it may also be associated with physical problems, psychological issues, or depression.

Signs and Symptoms. As with episodic tension headaches, the symptoms include pain or soreness in the temples and the contraction of head and neck muscles.

Treatment. People who suffer from chronic headaches should seek medical treatment.

MIGRAINES are the most severe type of headache. They are responsible for more "sick days" than any other headache type. Almost 30 million people in the United States suffer from migraines.

Causes. Hormones may influence migraines, which may explain why women experience migraines at least three times more often than men do. Migraines are considered vascular headaches because they are associated with the distension of the arteries of the brain.

Signs and Symptoms. Migraines often begin as dull pains that develop into throbbing pains accompanied by nausea and sensitivity to light and noise. There are many types of migraines, but the two most common classifications are migraine with aura and migraine without aura. Auras may include the appearance of jagged lines or flashing lights, tunnel vision, hallucinations, or the detection of strange odors. The auras may last up to an hour and usually go away as the headache begins. Most migraine headaches last about 4 hours, but some can last up to a week.

Treatment. When treating migraines, a physician may prescribe a drug to relieve the pain but also try to identify the factors that trigger it. Many medicines, both OTC and prescription, are available to treat migraines.

CLUSTER HEADACHES are so named because the attacks come in groups. They are the most severe type of migraines. More men than women experience these types of headaches.

Causes. Some research indicates that alcohol consumption can bring on attacks of cluster headaches.

Signs and Symptoms. Common symptoms include a runny nose, watery eyes, and swelling below the eyes. Cluster headaches normally last about 45 minutes to an hour, although they can last longer. It is common for a patient with this disorder to experience 1 to 4 headaches a day during a cluster time span. Cluster time spans can last weeks or months.

Treatment. Various drugs are available for the treatment of these headaches.

MENINGITIS is an inflammation of the meninges.

Causes. Causes may include bacterial, viral, and fungal infections. Some types of meningitis can be prevented with vaccines.

Signs and Symptoms. Fever, headache, vomiting, stiffness in the neck, sensitivity to light, drowsiness, and joint pain usually accompany this disorder.

Treatment. The treatment varies depending on the type of meningitis. Intravenous antibiotics are used for bacterial meningitis, supportive therapy for viral meningitis, and antifungal drugs for fungal meningitis. Bacterial meningitis can be fatal.

MULTIPLE SCLEROSIS (MS) is a chronic disease of the CNS in which myelin is destroyed.

Causes. The causes are mostly unknown, but some known causes are viruses, genetic factors, and immune system abnormalities.

Signs and Symptoms. Depending on the type of MS, symptoms can range from mild to severe. In severe cases, a person loses the ability to walk or speak.

Treatment. There is no cure for MS, but supportive treatments may lessen the symptoms. Some medications, including interferon, Copaxone®, prednisone, and Solu-Medrol, are available to treat and slow the progression of symptoms.

NEURALGIAS are a group of disorders commonly referred to as nerve pain. They most frequently occur in the nerves of the face.

Causes. There are many causes of neuralgia, including trauma, chemical irritation of the nerves, bacterial infections, and diabetes. Many times the causes are unknown.

Signs and Symptoms. Sudden and severe skin pain is the most common symptom. The pain occurs repeatedly in the same body area. Numbness of skin areas is also common.

Treatment. Many times the disorder goes away spontaneously, and treatment, other than pain medication, is not needed. Other treatments include injections of anesthetics or surgery to remove the affected nerves.

PARKINSON'S DISEASE is a motor system disorder. It is slowly progressive and degenerative.

Causes. Most causes are undetermined, although it is known that patients with this disease lack certain chemicals (neurotransmitters) in the brain. Brain tumors, certain drugs, carbon monoxide, or repeated head trauma may produce Parkinson's disease.

Signs and Symptoms. The most common signs and symptoms include tremor and stiffness of the arms and legs as well as a lack of coordination and balance. A mask face, where the patient shows little or no facial emotion, is also common, as is stooped posture with a shuffling gait.

Treatment. There is no cure, but medications such as dopamine, selegiline, and Symmetrel alleviate some symptoms and slow the progression of this disease. Surgery is useful in some cases of Parkinson's.

SCIATICA occurs when the sciatic nerve is damaged.

Causes. The sciatic nerve is commonly damaged by excessive pressure on the nerve from prolonged sitting or lying down. It is also easily damaged from trauma to the pelvis, buttocks, or thighs.

Signs and Symptoms. The most usual symptoms include numbness, pain, or tingling sensations on the back of a leg or foot. Weakness of leg and foot muscles can also develop.

Treatment. This disorder is usually treated with pain and anti-inflammatory medication or steroids. Physical therapy is also needed following trauma to the nerve.

STROKE occurs when brain cells die because of an inadequate blood flow. Stroke is sometimes referred to as a "brain attack."

The medical term is *cerebrovascular accident* (CVA). It is not uncommon for a stroke to be preceded by *transient ischemic attacks* (TIAs) or *"mini strokes,"* which are caused by brief interruptions of blood supply to the brain.

Causes. Most strokes are caused by the blockage of an artery in the neck or brain. They may also be caused by aneurysms that burst.

Signs and Symptoms. Signs and symptoms may include paralysis, speech problems, memory and reasoning deficits, coma, and possibly death. Symptoms vary depending on the location of the stroke within the brain.

Treatment. Because neurons in the brain cannot be replaced, the effects of a stroke can be permanent. However, physical, occupational, and speech therapy are often very useful in lessening the effects of a stroke.

Go to CONNECT to see an animation about *Stroke*.

SUMMARY OF LEARNING OUTCOMES

LEARNING OUTCOMES	KEY POINTS
30.1 Describe the general functions of the nervous system.	The central nervous system (CNS) is composed of the brain and spinal cord. The peripheral nervous system (PNS) consists of the peripheral nerves located throughout the body. Three types of neurons carry out the functions of the nervous system: the afferent (sensory) nerves detect sensation or other stimuli from the body or environment and bring it to the CNS for interpretation, the efferent (motor) nerves produce movement or other functions at the direction of the CNS, and the interpretive interneurons act as "interpreters" between the afferent and efferent nerves.
30.2 Summarize the structure of a neuron.	All neurons are composed of a cell body, the shorter and more numerous dendrites that receive information for the cell body, and the longer axons that function to bring impulses from the cell body to the dendrite of the next neuron.
30.3 Explain the function of nerve impulses and the role of synapses in their transmission.	Nerve impulses send information either from the CNS to the PNS or vice versa. A synapse is the space between the axon of one neuron and the dendrite of the next. At the end of each axon is the synaptic knob, which contains vesicles that produce neurotransmitters. These are released by the synaptic bulb to allow impulse transmission to continue to the next neuron.
30.4 Describe the structures and functions of the central nervous system.	The brain consists of the cerebrum, diencephalon, brainstem, and cerebellum. The blood-brain barrier is a layer of tightly woven capillaries that protects the delicate tissues of the CNS. The meninges are a triple-layered membrane protecting the brain and spinal cord. The spinal cord is continuous with the brain and consists of 31 spinal segments. The basic function of the spinal cord is to carry sensory information from the body to the brain and motor information from the brain to the muscles and glands of the body. Cerebrospinal fluid (CSF) is located within the subarachnoid space of the brain and within the central canal of the spinal cord. It cushions the brain and spinal cord.

LEARNING OUTCOMES	KEY POINTS
30.5 **Compare the structures and functions of the somatic and autonomic nervous systems in the peripheral nervous system.**	The somatic nervous system (SNS) connects the CNS to the skin and skeletal muscle (voluntary functions). The autonomic nervous system (ANS) connects the CNS to the internal organs (involuntary functions). The ANS is divided into the sympathetic system, which prepares the body for "fight or flight" (stressful) situations, and the parasympathetic system, which is the body's everyday "resting" system for normal situations.
30.6 **Recognize common tests that are performed to determine neurologic disorders.**	Tests commonly used to determine neurologic disorders include tests of the reflexes and cranial nerves, as well as diagnostic procedures such as lumbar puncture, MRI, PET, cerebral angiography, CT scan, EEG, and X-ray.
30.7 **Describe the causes, signs and symptoms, and treatments of various diseases and disorders of the nervous system.**	There are many common diseases and disorders of the nervous system with varied signs, symptoms, and treatments. Some of these include Alzheimer's disease, Amyotrophic lateral sclerosis (ALS), Bell's palsy, brain tumors, cancer, epilepsy, seizures, Guillain-Barré syndrome, headaches, chronic tension headaches, migraines, cluster headaches, meningitis, multiple sclerosis (MS), neuralgias, Parkinson's disease, sciatica, and stroke.

CASE STUDY CRITICAL THINKING

Recall Nancy Evans from the beginning of the chapter. Now that you have completed the chapter, answer the following questions regarding her case.

1. Forgetfulness is a common sign of what type of neurological disorder?

2. What are some of the possible causes for this disease?

3. Is there a definitive cure for this disease? What are the treatment options?

EXAM PREPARATION QUESTIONS

1. (LO 30.6) Which of the following is NOT a common symptom of patients with neurological disorders?
   a. Headache
   b. Paresthesia
   c. Fever
   d. Muscle weakness
   e. Numbness

2. (LO 30.6) Which of the following diagnostic procedures is done to detect blood flow within the brain for diagnosing brain tumors, Parkinson's, and Alzheimer's diseases?

   a. MRI
   b. PET scan
   c. CT scan
   d. Cerebral angiography
   e. X-ray

3. (LO 30.4) The _____ are interconnecting cavities of the brain filled with CSF.
   a. Ventricles
   b. Lobes
   c. Convolutions
   d. Gyri
   e. Sulci

4. (LO 30.1) What kind of neurons connect the neurons that carry messages to the CNS with those that carry messages from the CNS to the muscles and glands?
   a. Efferent neurons
   b. Sensory neurons
   c. Afferent neurons
   d. Motor neurons
   e. Interneurons

5. (LO 30.2) Which type of neuroglial cells anchor blood vessels to the nerve cells?
   a. Microglia
   b. Oligodendrocytes
   c. Astrocytes
   d. Schwann cells
   e. Satellite cells

6. (LO 30.4) What is the name of the tough, outer layer of the meninges?
   a. Dura mater
   b. Epidural space
   c. Arachnoid mater
   d. Subdural space
   e. Pia mater

7. (LO 30.3) Which two ions are responsible for cell membrane depolarization and repolarization?
   a. Na^+ and Ca^{++}
   b. Na^+ and Cl^-
   c. Ca^{++} and Cl^-
   d. K^+ and Na^+
   e. K^+ and SO_4-

8. (LO 30.5) Collections of neuron cell bodies outside the CNS that communicate with organs and blood vessels are called
   a. Ganglia
   b. Plexuses
   c. Dermatomes
   d. Ventral roots
   e. Dorsal roots

9. (LO 30.5) Which of the following cranial nerves are found in the muscles of the tongue?
   a. Olfactory nerves (I)
   b. Oculomotor nerves (III)
   c. Trigeminal nerves (V)
   d. Facial nerves (VII)
   e. Hypoglossal nerves (XII)

10. (LO 30.7) In which nervous system disorder are the facial muscles paralyzed?
   a. Amyotrophic lateral sclerosis
   b. Epilepsy
   c. Bell's palsy
   d. Guillain Barré syndrome
   e. Meningitis

MEDICAL TERMINOLOGY PRACTICE

Analyze the following medical terms, presented throughout the chapter. Using a medical dictionary (or Appendix I) place a / mark between each word part. Define each word part and then define the whole word.

EXAMPLE: **crani/otomy** = crani means "skull" + otomy means "incision"
Craniotomy means "incision into the skull"

1. angiography
2. areflexia
3. astrocyte
4. cerebral

5. electroencephalogram
6. hyperreflexia
7. hypothalamus
8. interneuron

9. neuralgia
10. neurotransmitter
11. meningitis
12. anesthesia

CASE STUDY

Peter Smith is a 73-year-old male with mild type II diabetes. He states that he has needed to urinate more frequently during the last two weeks, and he feels a burning sensation when he urinates. He has also been very tired lately. The physician ordered a fasting blood glucose and a urinalysis.

Keep Peter in mind as you study the chapter. There will be questions at the end of the chapter based on the case study. The information in the chapter will help you answer these questions.

LEARNING OUTCOMES

After completing Chapter 31, you will be able to:

31.1 Describe the structure, location, and functions of the kidney.

31.2 Explain how nephrons filter blood and form urine.

31.3 Compare the locations, structures, and functions of the ureters, bladder, and urethra.

31.4 Describe the causes, signs and symptoms, and treatments of various diseases and disorders of the urinary system.

KEY TERMS

Bowman's capsule
detrusor muscle
distal convoluted tubule
glomerulus
hilum
lithotripsy
loop of Henle
micturition
nephrons
proximal convoluted
  tubule

renal column
renal corpuscle
renal cortex
renal medulla
renal pelvis
renal pyramids
renal sinus
renal tubule
trigone
ureters
urethra

I. C (4) List major organs in each body system

I. C (5) Describe the normal function of each body system

I. C (6) Identify common pathology related to each body system

I. C (7) Analyze pathology as it relates to the interaction of body systems

I. C (8) Discuss implications for disease and disability when homeostasis is not maintained

I. C (9) Describe implications for treatment related to pathology

I. C (10) Compare body structure and function of the human body across the life span

I. C (12) Describe the relationship between anatomy and physiology of all body systems and medications used for treatment in each

IV. C (11) Define both medical terms and abbreviations related to all body systems

2. Anatomy & Physiology
Graduates:

b. Identify and apply the knowledge of all body systems, their structure and functions, and their common diseases, symptoms, and etiologies

c. Assist the physician with the regimen of diagnostic and treatment modalities as they relate to each body system

3. Medical Terminology
Graduates:

b. Build and dissect medical terms from roots/suffice to understand the word element combinations that create medical terminology

c. Understand the various medical terminology for each specialty

▶ Introduction

The organs of the urinary system are the kidneys, ureters, urinary bladder, and urethra (see Figure 31-1). This system removes waste products from the bloodstream. These waste products are excreted from the body in the form of urine. **Nephrons** are microscopic structures within the kidneys that filter blood, remove waste products, and form urine.

▶ The Kidneys

LO 31.1

The kidneys remove metabolic waste products from the blood. These metabolic wastes are combined with water and ions to form urine, which is excreted from the body. The kidneys also

FIGURE 31-1 Organs of the urinary system.

secrete the hormone *erythropoietin,* which stimulates the red bone marrow to produce red blood cells, and the hormone *renin,* which helps to regulate blood pressure. All three of these functions are important in maintaining the body's internal environment or homeostasis, which is a balanced, stable state within the body.

The kidneys are reddish-brown, bean-shaped organs. Tough, fibrous capsules cover them. The kidneys are *retroperitoneal* in position, which means they lie behind the peritoneal cavity. They lie on either side of the vertebral column at about the level of the lumbar vertebrae; the left kidney is slightly higher than the right, which is displaced by the liver.

The surface area of the concave depression of the kidney is called the **renal sinus.** The renal artery, renal vein, and ureter enter the kidney here in the area known as the **hilum.** The ureter is the tube that drains urine from the kidney, carrying it to the bladder. Inside the kidney, this same area is called the **renal pelvis,** formed by the expansion of the ureter inside the kidney. The renal pelvis itself further divides into small tubes known as *calyces* (calyx is the singular).

The outermost layer of the kidney is the **renal cortex,** and the middle portion is the **renal medulla.** The renal medulla is divided into triangular-shaped areas called **renal pyramids.** The renal cortex covers the pyramids and also dips down between them. The portion of the cortex between pyramids is called a **renal column** (see Figure 31-2).

Blood enters the kidney through the renal artery and goes through the filtration process explained in the next section. It then exits the kidney via the renal vein.

Nephrons

Nephrons remove waste products from the blood. Each kidney contains about one million nephrons, which are located in the renal medulla. Nephrons are made of a **renal corpuscle**

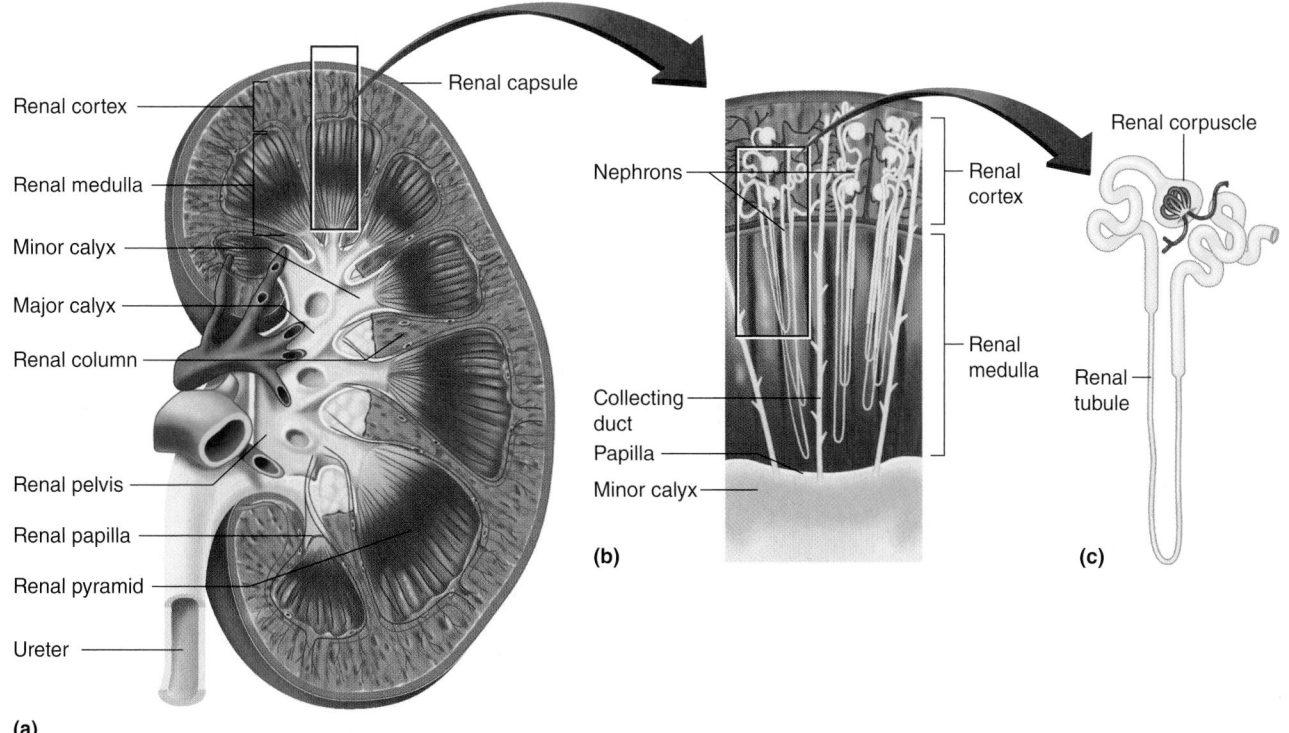

FIGURE 31-2   (a) Longitudinal section of a kidney, (b) the location of nephrons, and (c) a single nephron.

and a **renal tubule** (see Figure 31-2). A renal corpuscle is composed of a mass of capillaries called a **glomerulus;** the capsule that surrounds the glomerulus is called the **Bowman's capsule,** or *glomerular capsule.* Blood filtration occurs in the renal corpuscle.

Renal tubules extend from the Bowman's capsule of a nephron. The three parts of a renal tubule are the **proximal convoluted tubule,** the **loop of Henle** (*nephron loop*), and the **distal convoluted tubule.** The proximal convoluted tubule is directly attached to the Bowman's capsule and eventually straightens out to become the loop of Henle. The loop of Henle curves back toward the renal corpuscle and starts to twist again, becoming the distal convoluted tubule. Distal convoluted tubules from several nephrons merge to form collecting ducts. These ducts collect urine and deliver it to the renal pelvis, which in turn empties urine into the ureters (see Figures 31-2 and 31-3).

Afferent arterioles bring blood to the tightly packed, increasingly narrow capillaries of the glomeruli. This narrowing causes the filtration of the blood. The blood is forced through the capillary walls, similar to what occurs when water drips through a coffee filter in a drip coffee-maker. *Efferent arterioles* deliver blood to *peritubular capillaries,* which are wrapped around the renal tubules of the nephron. Blood leaves the peritubular capillaries through the veins of the kidneys. By the time the blood leaves the peritubular capillaries, it has been cleansed of waste products. Blood flows through a nephron in the following pathway:

afferent arteriole → glomerulus → efferent arteriole → peritubular capillaries → veins of the kidney

▶ Urine Formation

LO 31.2

The three processes of urine formation are glomerular filtration, tubular reabsorption, and tubular secretion.

Glomerular Filtration

Glomerular filtration takes place in the renal corpuscles of nephrons. In this process, the fluid part of blood is forced from the glomerulus (the capillaries) into Bowman's capsule (see Figure 31-4). The fluid in Bowman's capsule is called the *glomerular filtrate.*

Glomerular filtration depends on filtration pressure, which is the amount of pressure that forces substances (filtrate) out of the glomerulus into Bowman's capsule. Filtration pressure is largely determined by blood pressure. If a person's blood pressure is too low, glomerular filtrate will not form. If the blood pressure increases, filtration pressure also increases, causing the rate of filtration and the amount of glomerular filtrate to increase as well.

The sympathetic nervous system (SNS) largely controls the rate of filtration. If blood pressure or blood volume drops, the SNS causes the afferent arterioles in the kidneys to constrict. When this constriction occurs, glomerular filtration pressure decreases and less glomerular filtrate is formed. When less glomerular filtrate is formed, less urine is ultimately formed. This allows the body to retain fluids that are needed to raise blood pressure and blood volume.

Tubular Reabsorption

Tubular reabsorption is the second process in urine formation. In this process, the glomerular filtrate flows into the proximal

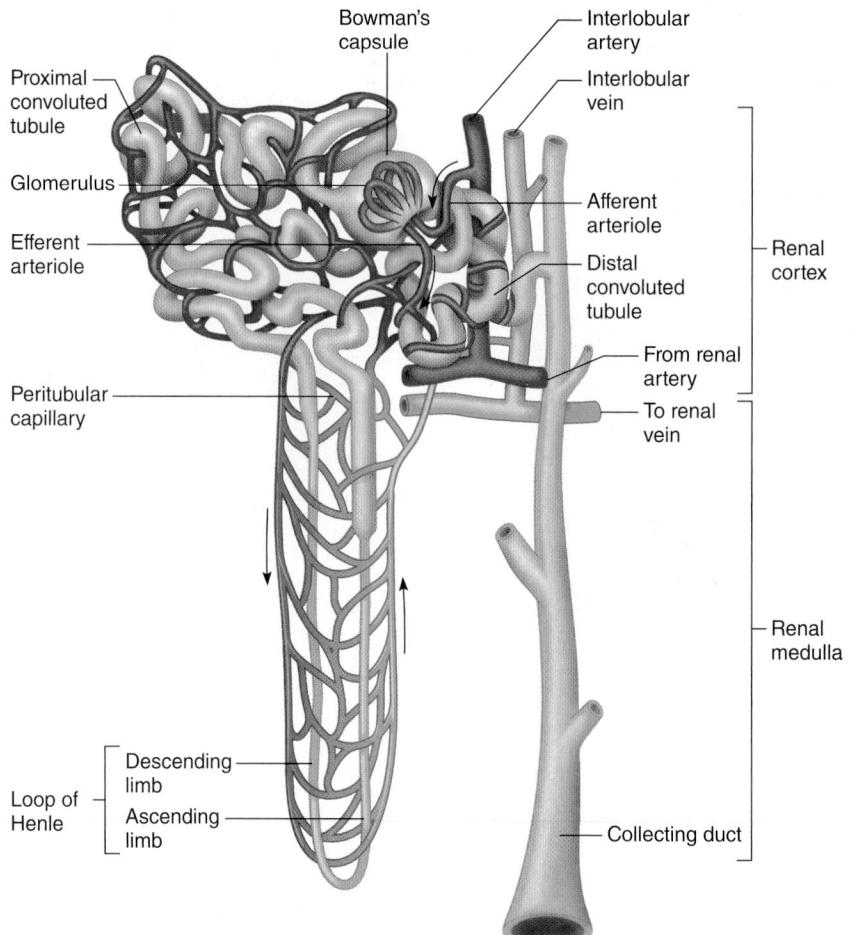

FIGURE 31-3 Structure of a nephron and its associated blood vessels.

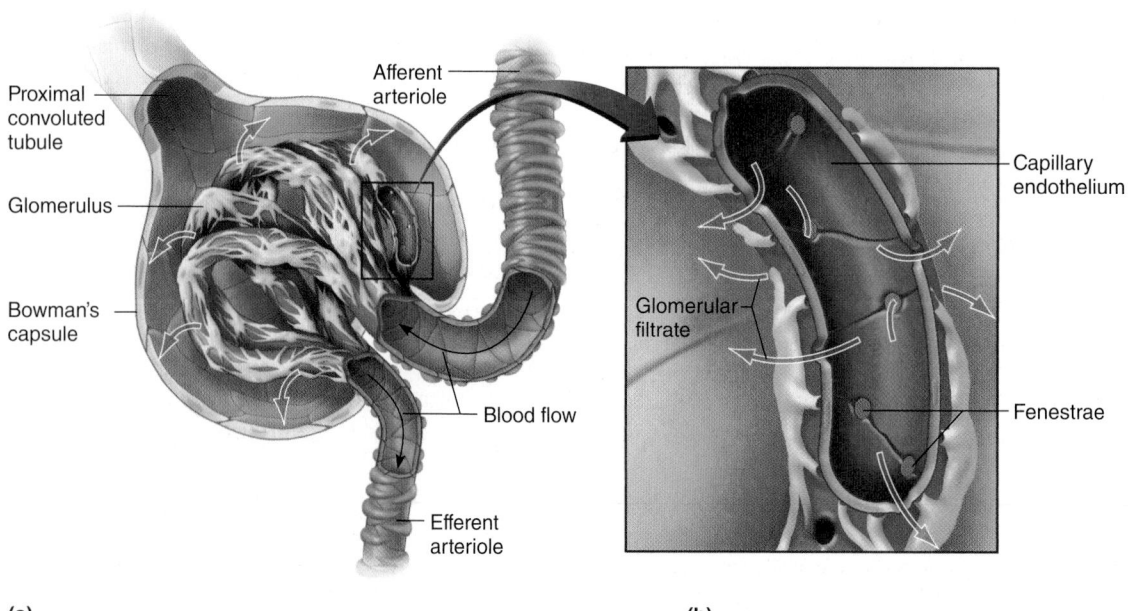

(a)

(b)

FIGURE 31-4 Glomerular filtration. (a) Substances move out of glomerular capillaries and into Bowman's capsule. (b) Glomerular capillaries have large holes called *fenestrae* that allow substances to move out of them and into Bowman's capsule.

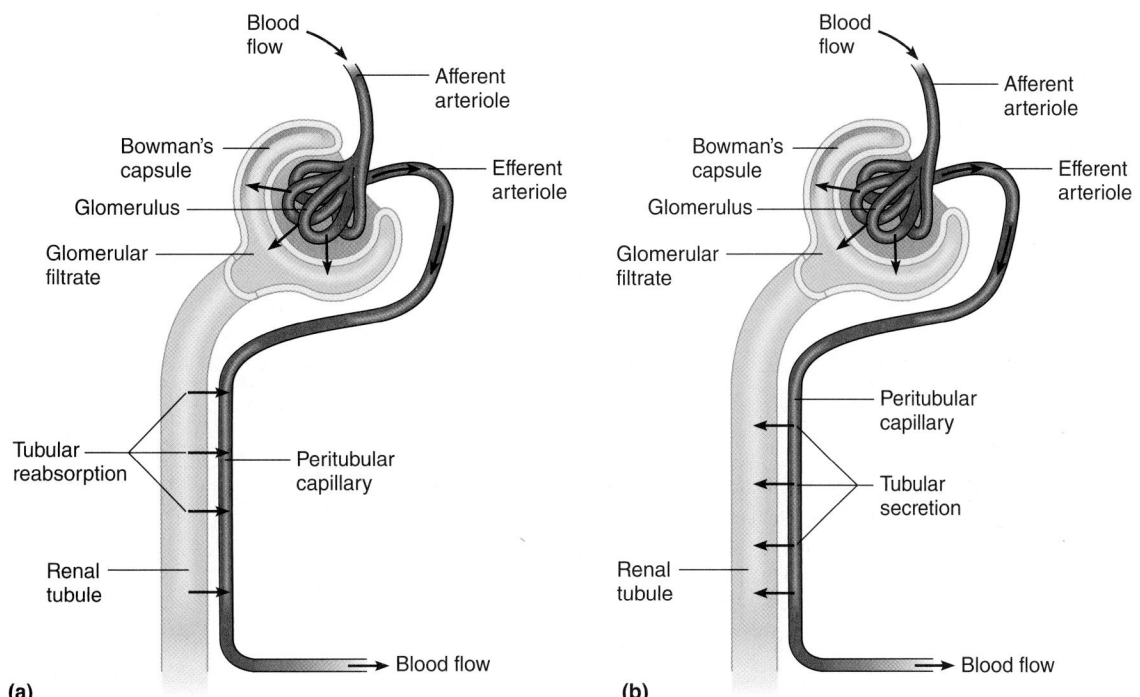

FIGURE 31-5 (a) Tubular reabsorption. Substances move from the glomerular filtrate into the blood of peritubular capillaries. (b) Tubular secretion. Substances move out of the blood of the peritubular capillaries into the renal tubule.

convoluted tubule (see Figure 31-5a). The body needs to keep many of the substances (nutrients, water, and ions) that are found in glomerular filtrate. In tubular reabsorption, all the substances to be kept pass through the wall of the renal tubule into the blood of the peritubular capillaries.

Water reabsorption varies depending on the presence of two hormones: antidiuretic hormone (ADH) and aldosterone. Both of these hormones increase water reabsorption, which decreases urine production. This fluid retention and the resultant increase in blood pressure is one of the reasons why diuretics, which rid the body of excess fluid, are successful in treating some forms of hypertension.

Tubular Secretion

Tubular secretion is the third process of urine formation. In tubular secretion, substances move out of the blood in the peritubular capillaries and into the renal tubules (see Figure 31-5b). Substances that are secreted include drugs, hydrogen ions, and waste products, all of which will be excreted in the urine.

Urine Composition

The final solution that reaches the collecting ducts of the kidneys is urine. Urine is mostly made of water but also normally contains urea, uric acid, trace amounts of amino acids, and various ions. *Urea* and *uric acid* are waste products formed by the breakdown of proteins and nucleic acids. The secretion of these waste materials helps maintain the body's acid-base balance.

Go to CONNECT to see an animation about *Renal Function.*

The Ureters, Urinary Bladder, and Urethra
LO 31.3

The remaining organs in the urinary system transport and store urine after it is formed in the kidneys.

The Ureters

The **ureters** are long, muscular tubes that carry urine from the kidneys to the urinary bladder. They propel urine toward the bladder through rhythmic muscular contractions of the ureters called *peristalsis.*

The Urinary Bladder

The urinary bladder is a distensible (expandable) organ that is located in the pelvic cavity. Its function is to store urine (up to 600 mL on average) until it is eliminated from the body. The internal floor of the bladder contains three openings—one for the urethra and two for the ureters. These three openings form a triangle called the **trigone** of the bladder. The wall of the bladder contains smooth muscle, called the **detrusor muscle.** This muscle contracts to push urine from the bladder into the urethra (see Figure 31-6).

The process of urination is called **micturition.** The stretching of the bladder triggers this process—usually when the bladder contains approximately 150 mL of urine. The major events of micturition are the following:

1. The urinary bladder distends as it fills with urine.
2. The distension stimulates stretch receptors in the bladder wall, signaling the micturition center in the spinal cord.

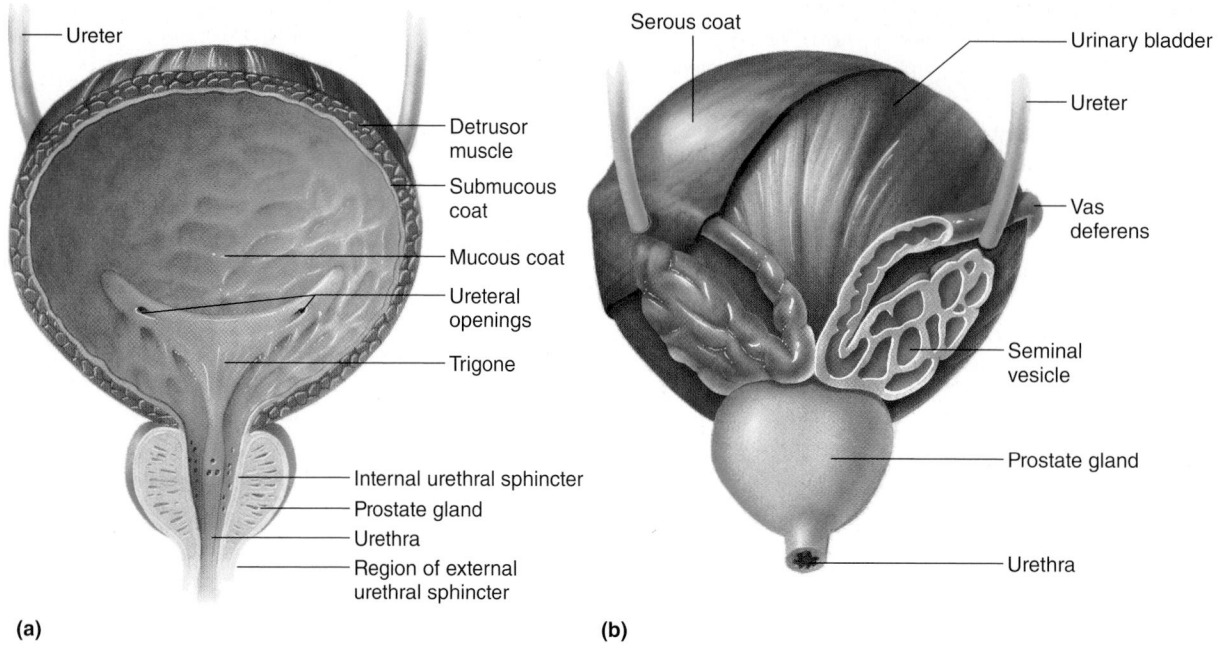

(a)   **(b)**

FIGURE 31-6   Male urinary bladder: (a) anterior view and (b) posterior view.

3. Parasympathetic nerves stimulate the detrusor muscle, which begins rhythmic contractions that trigger the sense of the need to urinate.

4. The brain stem and cerebral cortex send impulses to voluntarily contract the external urethral sphincter and to inhibit the micturition impulse.

5. Upon the decision to urinate, the external urethral sphincter is relaxed and impulses from the pons and hypothalamus start the micturition reflex.

6. Contraction of the detrusor muscle occurs and urine is expelled through the urethra.

The Urethra

The **urethra** is a tube that moves urine from the bladder to the outside world. In females, the urethra is much shorter than in males. This anatomic difference, combined with the fact that the anus, vagina, and urethra are in close proximity in females, makes females much more susceptible to urinary tract infections (UTIs).

EDUCATING THE PATIENT
Preventing Urinary Cystitis in Women

In females, the openings for the digestive, urinary, and reproductive systems are all within close proximity to each other in a highly functional design. However, when you combine this design with the female's shorter urethra (relative to men), women are much more likely than men to suffer from urinary tract infections (UTIs) and cystitis, more commonly known as bladder infections. As a medical assistant, if you understand why this is so, you will be able to assist your female patients when they have a UTI, with its pain (dysuria), urgency, and frequency, and give them helpful tips to prevent these painful episodes. Educate your female patients to take these steps:

1. *Urinate when the urge occurs.* When you "hold it," urine stays in the bladder and the upper urethra, allowing bacteria to grow and cause infection.

2. *Drink lots of clear fluids.* This is known as "pushing fluids." The more clear liquids you drink, the more urine is created and the system is flushed on a regular basis. Cranberry juice is highly recommended as a preventive fluid, as well as part of the treatment if infection does occur.

3. *Wipe front to back.* Teach your female patients they should wipe "front to back" after a bowel movement. Doing so prevents contamination of both the vagina and urethra by gastrointestinal (GI) bacteria such as *E. coli*. Maintaining excellent hygiene in the perineal area is an important component of UTI and cystitis prevention.

4. *Urinate after sexual intercourse.* Explain to your sexually active patients that urinating immediately after sexual intercourse will also help prevent episodes of cystitis. The urine will flush out contamination that could enter the bladder causing an infection.

If cystitis or UTI does strike despite preventive methods, reassure your patient that antibiotics and lots of fluids should take care of the problem. If the patient suffers from more than three infections during a year, a urologic workup may be advisable to look for underlying anatomical anomalies.

Common Diseases and Disorders of the Urinary System

ACUTE KIDNEY (RENAL) FAILURE is a sudden loss of kidney function.

Causes. There are many causes and risk factors of kidney failure, including burns, dehydration, low blood pressure, hemorrhaging, allergic reactions, obstruction of the renal artery, various poisons, alcohol abuse, trauma to the kidneys and skeletal muscles, blood disorders, blood transfusion reactions, kidney stones, urinary tract infections, enlarged prostate, childbirth, immune system disorders, and food poisoning involving the bacteria *E. coli.*

Signs and Symptoms. The signs and symptoms include decreased or no urine production, excessive urination, swelling of the extremities, bloating, mental confusion, coma, seizures, hand tremors, nosebleeds, easy bruising, pain in the back or abdomen, hypertension, abnormal heart or lung sounds, abnormal urinalysis, and an increase in potassium levels.

Treatment. The first treatment measure is modifying the diet to decrease the amount of protein consumed. Controlling fluid intake and potassium levels is also recommended. Antibiotics and dialysis may also be needed. If the underlying cause can be treated, acute renal failure may be reversed and kidney function returned to normal.

CHRONIC KIDNEY (RENAL) FAILURE is a condition in which the kidneys slowly lose their ability to function. The patient may be asymptomatic until the kidneys have lost about 90% of their function.

Causes. This disorder results from diabetes, hypertension, glomerulonephritis, polycystic kidney disease, kidney stones, obstruction of the ureters, and acute kidney failure.

Signs and Symptoms. The list of signs and symptoms is extensive and includes headache, mental confusion, coma, seizures, fatigue, frequent hiccups, itching, easy bruising, abnormal bleeding, anemia, excessive thirst, fluid retention, nausea, hypertension, abnormal heart or lung sounds, weight loss, white spots on the skin or increased pigmentation, high potassium levels, an increased or decreased urine output, urinary tract infections, and abnormal urinalysis results.

Treatment. This disorder can be treated with antibiotics; blood transfusions; medications to control anemia; restriction of fluids, electrolytes, and protein; control of high blood pressure; and dialysis. The most serious cases may require surgery to repair a ureteral obstruction or a kidney (renal) transplant.

CYSTITIS is a urinary bladder infection. Women are much more likely to develop this disorder than men because of the short length of their urethras. The urethral opening in women is also close to the anal opening, allowing bacteria from this area to be more easily introduced into the urinary tract.

Causes. This infection is caused by various types of bacteria (especially those found in the rectum) and may be caused by the placement of a catheter in the bladder. Good hygiene, urinating promptly when the urge occurs, and, for females, wiping from front to back can help to prevent this infection.

Signs and Symptoms. Common symptoms include fatigue, chills, fever, and a painful, frequent need to urinate, often with only small amounts of urine produced. Urine is often cloudy and blood may be present in the urine.

Treatment. This infection is treated with antibiotics and, when needed, pain medication. The patient should also be urged to drink lots of clear liquids.

GLOMERULONEPHRITIS is an inflammation of the glomeruli of the kidney. Chronic glomerulonephritis is one of the causes of chronic renal disease.

Causes. This disorder is caused by renal diseases, immune disorders, and bacterial infections.

Signs and Symptoms. The signs and symptoms are hiccups, drowsiness, coma, seizures, nausea, anemia, high blood pressure, increased skin pigmentation, abnormal heart sounds, abnormal urinalysis results, blood in the urine, and a decreased or increased urine output.

Treatment. Treatment begins with a low-sodium, low-protein diet. Medications to control high blood pressure, corticosteroids to reduce inflammation, and dialysis are other treatment options.

INCONTINENCE is a temporary or long-lasting condition in which a person (other than a child) cannot control urination. Women are more likely to develop incontinence than men are.

Causes. This condition can be caused by various medications, excessive coughing (for example, in smokers), UTIs, nervous system disorders, and bladder cancer. In men, prostate problems can lead to the development of this disorder. Weakness of the urinary sphincters from surgery, trauma, or pregnancy can also cause incontinence. It may be prevented by avoiding urinary bladder irritants such as coffee, cigarettes, diuretics, and various medications.

Signs and Symptoms. The primary symptom is the involuntary leakage of urine.

Treatment. Treatment includes various medications, incontinence pads, removal of the prostate, Kegel exercises to increase the control of urinary sphincters, and surgery to repair damaged bladders or urethral sphincters.

POLYCYSTIC KIDNEY DISEASE is a disorder in which the kidneys enlarge because they are filled with cysts. The disease develops relatively slowly, with symptoms worsening over time.

Causes. The causes are hereditary (via an inherited dominant gene from a parent).

Signs and Symptoms. Fatigue, hypertension, anemia, pain in the back or abdomen, joint pain, heart murmurs, the formation of kidney stones, kidney failure, blood in the urine, and liver disease are the symptoms of this disorder.

Treatment. Treatment includes medications to control anemia and high blood pressure, blood transfusions, draining of the cysts, dialysis, and surgery to remove one or both kidneys.

PYELONEPHRITIS is a complicated UTI. It begins as a bladder infection and spreads to one or both kidneys. This condition can develop suddenly, or it may be chronic.

Causes. This disorder is caused by bacteria, a bladder infection, kidney stones, or an obstruction of the urinary system ducts.

Signs and Symptoms. Signs and symptoms include fatigue, mental confusion, fever, nausea, pain in the back or abdomen, enlarged kidneys, painful urination, and cloudy or bloody urine.

Treatment. Treatment includes intravenous fluids, pain medication, and antibiotics.

RENAL CALCULI are commonly called kidney stones. They can become lodged in the ducts within the kidneys or ureters.

Causes. This condition is caused by gouty arthritis, defects of the ureters, overly concentrated urine, and UTIs.

Signs and Symptoms. The signs and symptoms include fever, nausea, severe back or abdominal pain, a frequent urge to urinate, blood in the urine, and abnormal urinalysis results.

Treatment. Treatment includes pain medication, intravenous fluids, medications to decrease stone formation, surgery to remove kidney stones, and **lithotripsy** (a procedure that uses shock waves to break up stones).

S U M M A R Y   O F   L E A R N I N G   O U T C O M E S

LEARNING OUTCOMES	KEY POINTS
31.1 Describe the structure, location, and functions of the kidney.	The retroperitoneal kidneys are composed of the outer renal cortex and inner renal medulla. Their function is to remove metabolic wastes from the body.
31.2 Explain how nephrons filter blood and form urine.	A nephron is a single kidney cell. It is composed of a renal corpuscle composed of the glomerulus and the Bowman's capsule and the three sections of the renal tubule: the proximal convoluted tubule, the loop of Henle, and the distal convoluted tubule. The nephrons filter blood and form urine through three processes: glomerular filtration, tubular reabsorption, and tubular secretion.
31.3 Compare the locations, structures, and functions of the ureters, bladder, and urethra.	The ureters are long tubes extending from each renal pelvis that bring urine to the bladder for storage. The urethra is the muscular tube extending from the bladder that allows urine to be expelled from the body.
31.4 Describe the causes, signs and symptoms, and treatments of various diseases and disorders of the urinary system.	There are many common diseases and disorders of the urinary system with varied signs, symptoms, and treatments. Some of these include acute kidney (renal) failure, chronic kidney (renal) failure, cystitis, glomerulonephritis, incontinence, polycystic kidney disease, pyelonephritis, and renal calculi.

C A S E   S T U D Y   C R I T I C A L   T H I N K I N G

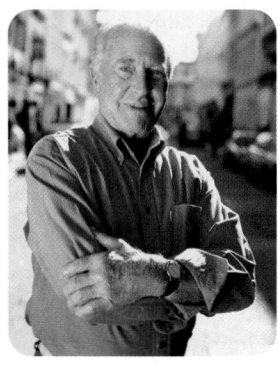

Recall Peter Smith from the beginning of the chapter. Now that you have completed the chapter, answer the following questions regarding his case.

1. What is the likely diagnosis for Mr. Smith?

2. Why did the physician order both a urinalysis and a blood glucose test?

3. Based on the laboratory test results, the physician prescribed an antibiotic for Mr. Smith. What can you advise Mr. Smith to do in addition to taking the antibiotic as prescribed?

1. (LO 31.4) _____ is a complicated UTI that begins as a bladder infection and spreads to one or both kidneys.
   a. Cystitis
   b. Glomerulonephritis
   c. Pyelonephritis
   d. Polycystic kidney disease
   e. Chronic renal failure

2. (LO 31.2) In which of the following processes do substances move into the renal tubules?
   a. Glomerular filtration
   b. Tubular secretion
   c. Tubular reabsorption
   d. Micturition
   e. Urination

3. (LO 31.2) Distal convoluted tubules from several nephrons merge together to form the
   a. Bowman's capsule
   b. Glomerulus
   c. Loop of Henle
   d. Collecting ducts
   e. Renal pyramids

4. (LO 31.2) Water reabsorption amounts vary depending on which two hormones?
   a. ADH and aldosterone
   b. ADH and erythropoietin
   c. Aldosterone and renin
   d. Aldosterone and ADH
   e. Erythropoietin and renin

5. (LO 31.1) _____ is the hormone from the kidneys that stimulates the bone marrow to produce RBCs.
   a. Renin
   b. ADH
   c. Aldosterone
   d. Hematopoietin
   e. Erythropoietin

6. (LO 31.1) The outermost layer of the kidney is the renal
   a. Cortex
   b. Pelvis
   c. Medulla
   d. Tubule
   e. Sinus

7. (LO 31.1) The _____ is the structure that surrounds the glomerulus.
   a. Loop of Henle
   b. Proximal convoluted tubule
   c. Distal convoluted tubule
   d. Bowman's capsule
   e. Renal pyramid

8. (LO 31.2) The rate of glomerular filtration is controlled mainly by the
   a. Blood pressure
   b. Sympathetic nervous system
   c. Somatic nervous system
   d. Parasympathetic nervous system
   e. Central nervous system

9. (LO 31.2) Which of the following is *not* a normal component of urine?
   a. Water
   b. Ions
   c. Glucose
   d. Uric acid
   e. Urea

10. (LO 31.3) The _____ is a triangular area formed by the urethral and ureteral openings into the bladder.
    a. Detrusor muscle
    b. Renal pyramid
    c. Ttrigone
    d. Hilum
    e. Calyx

Analyze the following medical terms, presented throughout the chapter. Using a medical dictionary (or Appendix I) place a / mark between each word part. Define each word part and then define the whole word.

EXAMPLE: **nephro / logy** = nephro means "kidney" + logy means "study of"
Nephrology means "study of the kidney"

1. antidiuretic
2. cystitis
3. dysuria
4. erythropoietin

5. glomerulonephritis
6. lithotripsy
7. nephritis
8. peristalsis

9. peritubular
10. pyelonephritis
11. retroperitoneal
12. uric

The Reproductive Systems

L E A R N I N G   O U T C O M E S

After completing Chapter 32, you will be able to:

32.1 Summarize the organs of the male reproductive system including the locations, structures, and functions of each.

32.2 Describe the causes, signs and symptoms, and treatment of various disorders of the male reproductive system.

32.3 Summarize the organs of the female reproductive system including the locations, structures, and functions of each.

32.4 Describe the causes, signs and symptoms, and treatment of various disorders of the female reproductive system.

32.5 Explain the process of pregnancy, including fertilization, the prenatal period, and fetal circulation.

32.6 Describe the birth process, including the postnatal period.

32.7 Compare several birth control methods and their effectiveness.

32.8 Explain the causes of and treatments for infertility.

32.9 Describe the causes, signs and symptoms, and treatments of the most common sexually transmitted infections.

K E Y   T E R M S

amnion
Bartholin's glands
blastocyst
Cowper's glands
ductus arteriosus
ductus venosus
embryo
fetus
foramen ovale
infundibulum

menarche
menopause
oogenesis
ovulation
placenta
primary germ layer
seminiferous tubules
spermatogenesis
testes
zygote

I.C (4) List major organs in each body system

I.C (5) Describe the normal function of each body system

I.C (6) Identify common pathology related to each body system

I. C (7) Analyze pathology as it relates to the interaction of body systems

I.C (9) Describe implications for treatment related to pathology

I. C (12) Describe the relationship between anatomy and physiology of all body systems and medications used for treatment in each

IV.C (11) Define both medical terms and abbreviations related to all body systems

2. Anatomy & Physiology

Graduates:

b. Identify and apply the knowledge of all body systems, their structure and functions, and their common diseases, symptoms, and etiologies

c. Assist the physician with the regimen of diagnostic and treatment modalities as they relate to each body system

3. Medical Terminology

Graduates:

b. Build and dissect medical terms from roots/suffixes to understand the word element combinations that create medical terminology

c. Understand the various medical terminology for each specialty

d. Recognize and identify acceptable medical abbreviations

▶ Introduction

The male and female reproductive systems function together to produce offspring. The female reproductive system nurtures a developing offspring. If a female breast-feeds, her breasts, considered accessory organs of both her reproductive and integumentary systems, are also used to nurture the newborn baby. The male and female reproductive systems also produce a number of important hormones before and during the reproductive years.

▶ The Male Reproductive System   LO 32.1

The male reproductive system is responsible for developing sperm. Accessory organs also produce substances that provide an environment for the sperm that allows it to reach the female ova (eggs).

Testes

Testes are considered the primary organs of the male reproductive system because they produce the male sex cells (sperm) (see Figure 32-1). They also produce the male hormone *testosterone*. Most males have two testes that are held just below the pelvic cavity in the *scrotum*. During the fetal stage, the testes develop in the abdominopelvic cavity of the fetus. Shortly before or soon after birth, the testes descend into the scrotal sac located just below the pelvic cavity. A fibrous capsule encloses each testis and invades the testis to divide it into lobules. Each lobule is filled with **seminiferous tubules,** which are filled with *spermatogenic cells.* These cells give rise to sperm cells. Between the seminiferous tubules are the *interstitial cells,* which produce testosterone.

Sperm Cell Formation Spermatogenic cells of the seminiferous tubules begin the process of making sperm cells, but the sperm cells do not mature until they travel to the *epididymis.* **Spermatogenesis** is the process of sperm cell formation. At the beginning of spermatogenesis, the cells are called *spermatogonia.* Spermatogonia contain 46 chromosomes. These cells undergo mitosis as shown in Figure 22-1 in the *Organization of the Body* chapter, and the resulting cells are called *primary spermatocytes.* Primary spermatocytes also contain 46 chromosomes. At about the time of puberty, primary spermatocytes undergo a process called *meiosis* (see Figures 32-2 and 32-3a). In meiosis, each primary spermatocyte divides to make two secondary spermatocytes. Each secondary spermatocyte divides to make two *spermatids.* Therefore, from one primary spermatocyte, four spermatids are formed. Spermatids develop flagella to become mature sperm cells. They contain only 23 chromosomes.

Go to CONNECT to see an animation about *Meiosis vs. Mitosis.*

Structure of Sperm Cells A mature sperm (see Figure 32-3b) has the following three parts: the head, the midpiece, and the tail.

The Head The head is oval in structure and holds a nucleus with 23 chromosomes. The head is covered with an enzyme-filled sac called an *acrosome,* which helps the sperm penetrate an ovum at the time of fertilization.

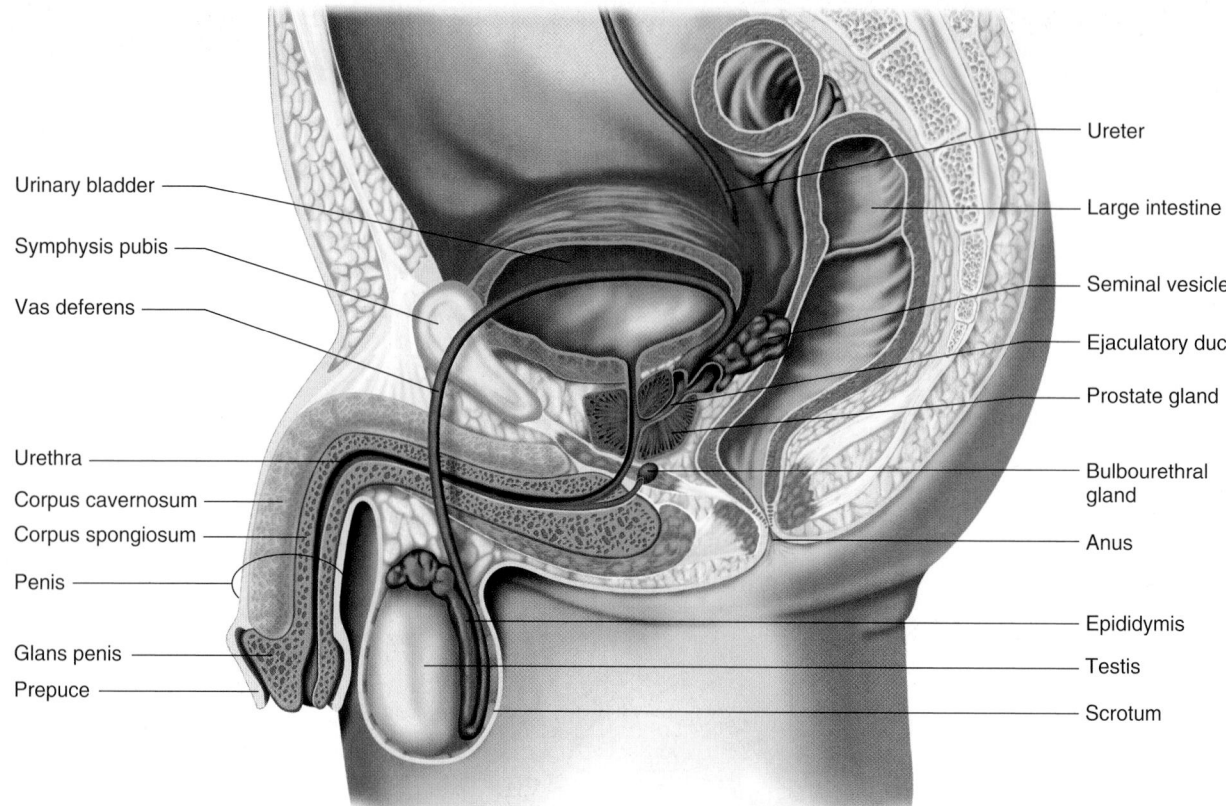

FIGURE 32-1 Sagittal view of male reproductive organs. The male reproductive system produces sperm and delivers them in a form that keeps them viable long enough to fertilize an ovum.

The Midpiece This portion of the sperm is between the head and tail. It is filled with mitochondria that generate the energy the cell needs to move.

The Tail The tail is a flagellum that propels the sperm forward in the female reproductive tract.

Internal Accessory Organs of the Male Reproductive System

The internal accessory organs of the male reproductive system are the epididymis, vas deferens, seminal vesicles, prostate gland, and bulbourethral or Cowper's glands.

Epididymis An epididymis sits on top of each testis. It is a highly coiled tube that receives spermatids from seminiferous tubules as these cells are formed. Inside the epididymis, spermatids mature to become sperm cells.

Vas Deferens A tube called a *vas deferens* is connected to each epididymis. These tubes carry sperm cells from the epididymis to the urethra in the male pelvic cavity. When a male has a vasectomy, these tubes are cut and tied, or *fulgurated,* to prevent sperm from reaching the ovum.

Seminal Vesicles Seminal vesicles are sac-like organs that secrete an alkaline *seminal fluid* that is rich in sugars and *prostaglandins.* Sperm cells use the sugars to make energy, and the prostaglandins stimulate muscular contractions in the female reproductive system. These muscular contractions, known as *peristalsis,* help to propel sperm forward in the female reproductive tract. Seminal vesicles release their product into the vas deferens just before ejaculation. Seminal fluid makes up approximately 60% of semen volume.

Prostate Gland The muscular prostate gland surrounds the proximal portion of the urethra. It produces a milky, alkaline fluid and secretes this fluid into the urethra just before ejaculation. The alkaline nature of this fluid helps to protect the sperm when they enter the acidic environment of the female vagina. Prostatic fluid makes up approximately 40% of semen volume. During ejaculation, the muscular contractions of the prostate help expel semen.

Bulbourethral Glands Bulbourethral glands, or **Cowper's glands,** are inferior to the prostate gland. They produce a mucus-like fluid that is secreted into the urethra before ejaculation. This fluid lubricates the end of the penis in preparation for sexual intercourse.

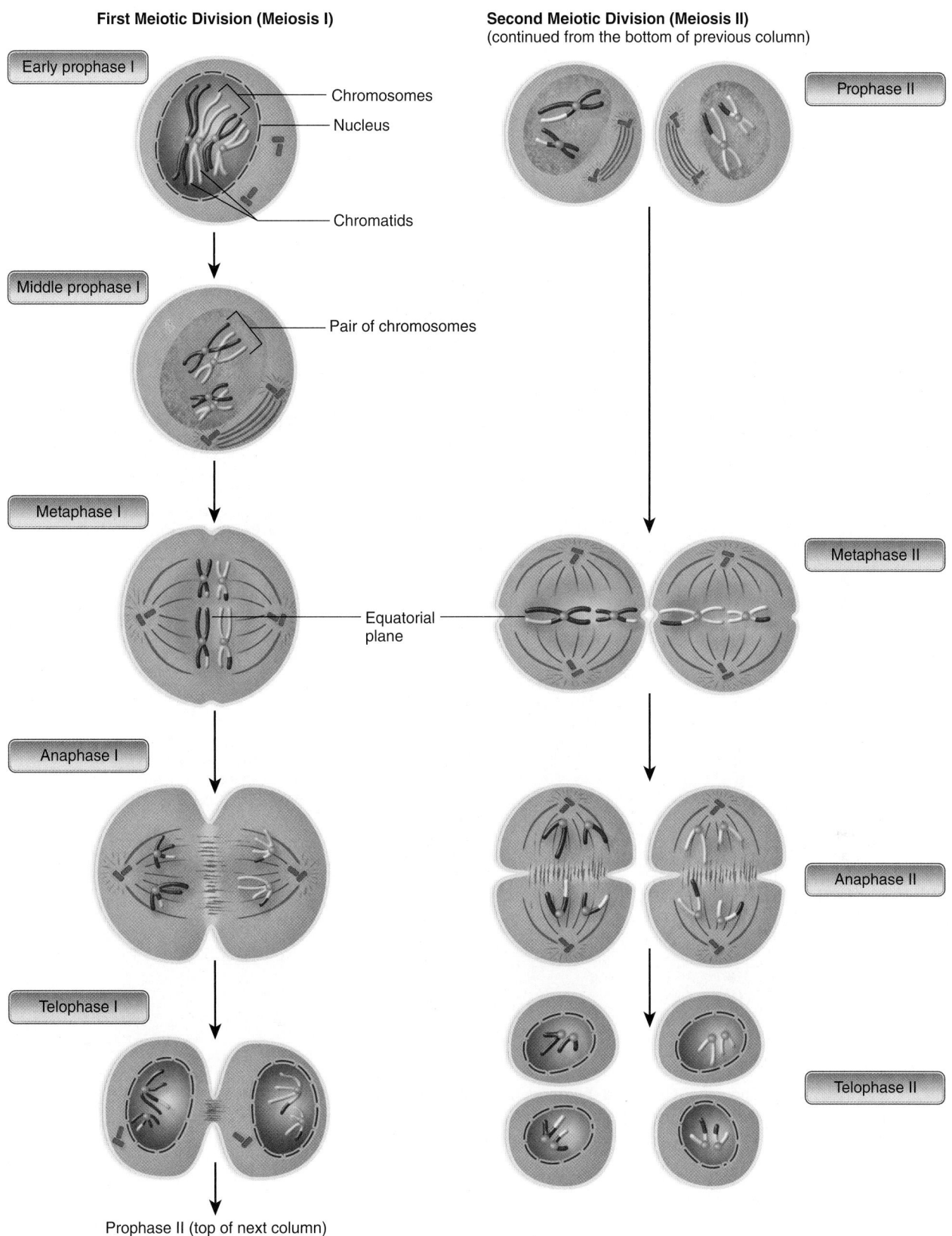

First Meiotic Division (Meiosis I)

Early prophase I

Chromosomes
Nucleus

Chromatids

Middle prophase I

Pair of chromosomes

Metaphase I

Equatorial plane

Anaphase I

Telophase I

Prophase II (top of next column)

Second Meiotic Division (Meiosis II)
(continued from the bottom of previous column)

Prophase II

Metaphase II

Anaphase II

Telophase II

FIGURE 32-2 The process of meiosis, including prophase, metaphase, anaphase, and telophase.

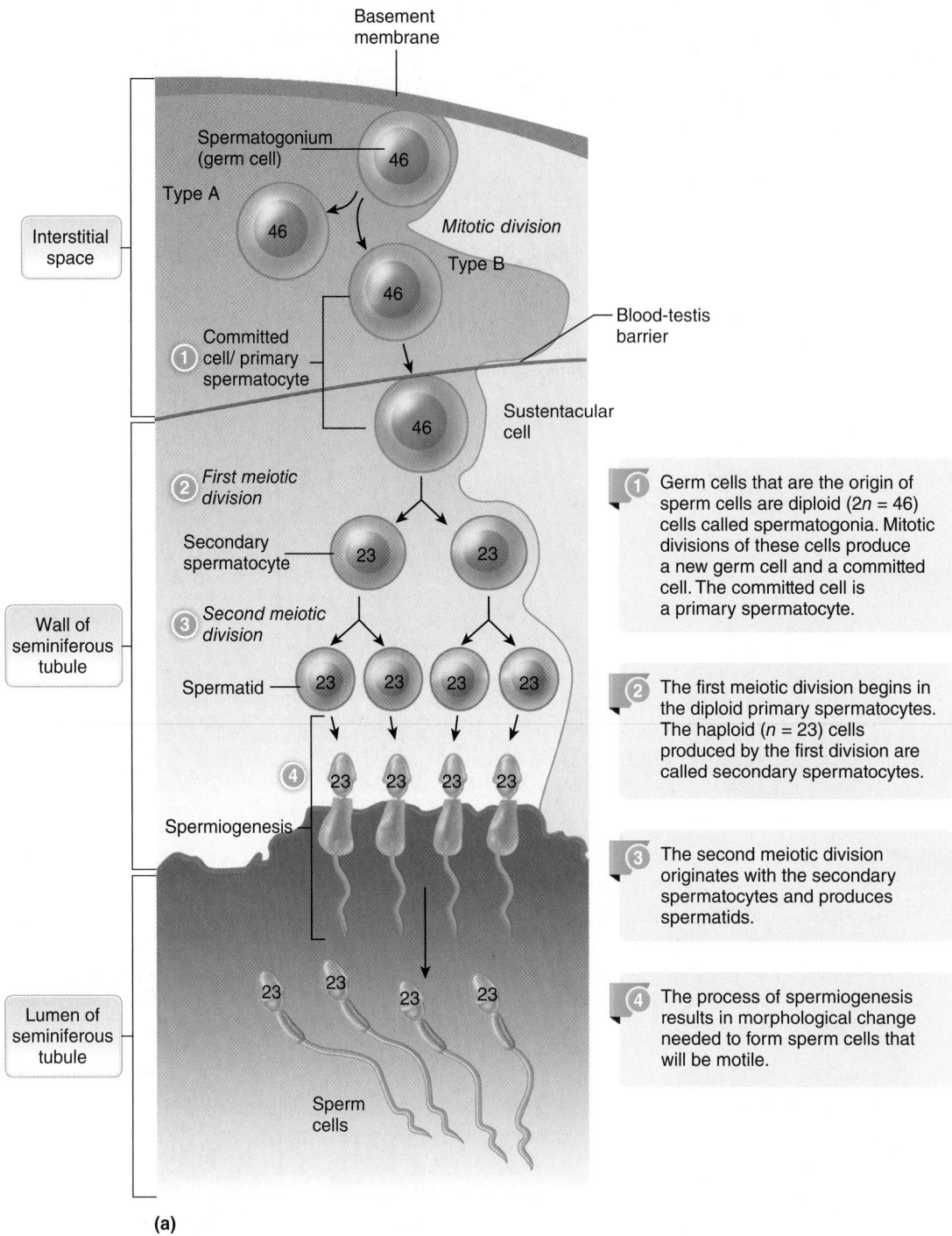

Basement membrane

Spermatogonium (germ cell)

Type A

Interstitial space

Mitotic division

Type B

Committed cell/ primary spermatocyte

Blood-testis barrier

Sustentacular cell

First meiotic division

Secondary spermatocyte

Second meiotic division

Wall of seminiferous tubule

Spermatid

Spermiogenesis

Lumen of seminiferous tubule

Sperm cells

(1) Germ cells that are the origin of sperm cells are diploid ($2n = 46$) cells called spermatogonia. Mitotic divisions of these cells produce a new germ cell and a committed cell. The committed cell is a primary spermatocyte.

(2) The first meiotic division begins in the diploid primary spermatocytes. The haploid ($n = 23$) cells produced by the first division are called secondary spermatocytes.

(3) The second meiotic division originates with the secondary spermatocytes and produces spermatids.

(4) The process of spermiogenesis results in morphological change needed to form sperm cells that will be motile.

(a)

FIGURE 32-3   Spermatogenesis and spermiogenesis: (a) The processes of spermatogenesis and spermiogenesis take place in the wall of the seminiferous tubule. (b) Structural changes occur during spermiogenesis as a sperm cell forms from a spermatid.

Semen   Semen is a mixture of sperm cells and fluids from the seminal vesicles, prostate gland, and bulbo-urethral glands. This alkaline mixture contains nutrients and prostaglandins. Total semen volume is between 1.5 and 5.0 mL per ejaculate, with a sperm count between 40 and 250 million/mL. A normal sperm count is more than 80 million.

External Organs of the Male Reproductive System

The two male external reproductive organs are the scrotum and the penis (see Figure 32-1).

Scrotum   The scrotum is a pouch of skin that holds the testes. It is lined with a serous membrane that secretes fluid to ensure that the testes move freely within it. The

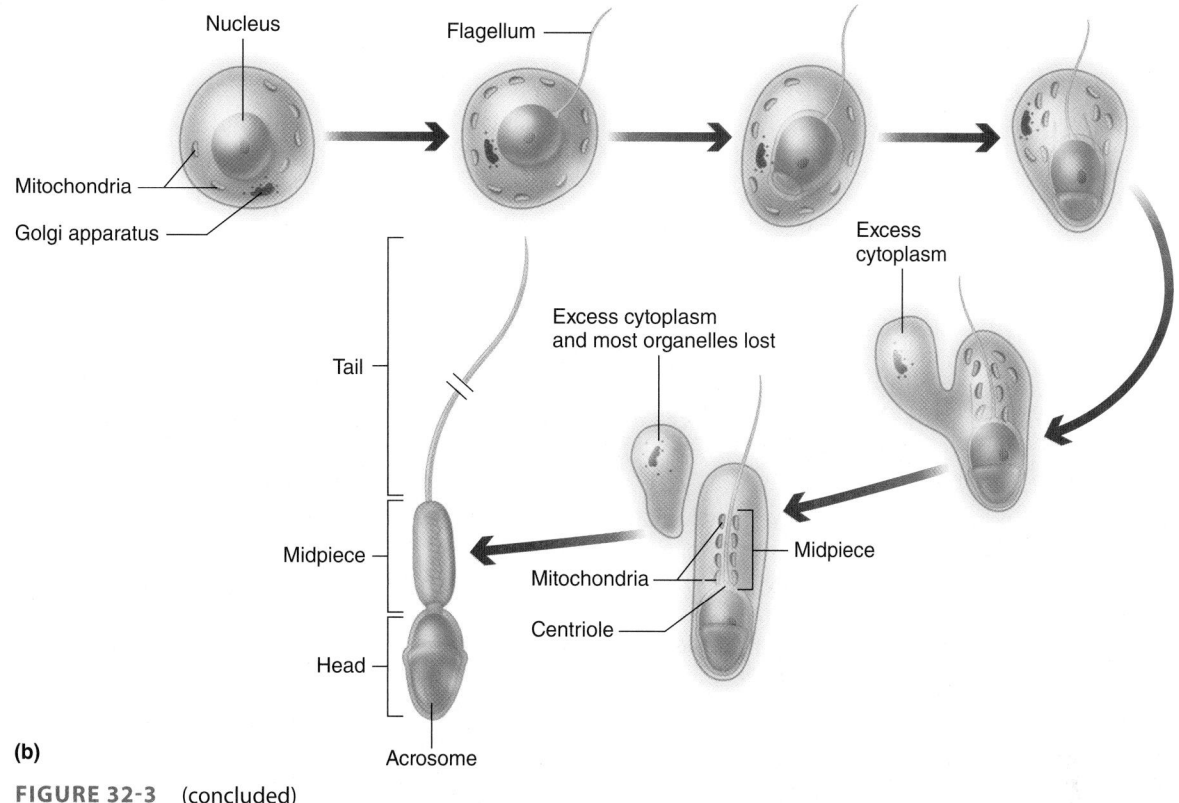

(b)

FIGURE 32-3 (concluded)

scrotum holds the testes away from the rest of the body, keeping their temperature about one degree lower than the rest of the body, which is necessary for the viability of the sperm.

Penis The penis is a cylindrical organ that moves urine and semen out of the body. The shaft, or body, of the penis contains specialized *erectile tissue* that surrounds the urethra, which runs the length of the penis. The end of the penis is enlarged into a cone-shaped structure called the *glans penis*. If a male has not been circumcised, a piece of skin, called the *prepuce,* covers the glans penis. The function of the penis is to deliver sperm to the female reproductive tract. The penis also functions in urination because it contains the urethra, which drains urine from the bladder.

Erection, Orgasm, and Ejaculation

During sexual arousal, the parasympathetic nervous system causes erectile tissue of the penis to become engorged with blood, which produces erection of the penis. During orgasm, sperm cells are propelled out of the testes toward the urethra. The secretions of the prostate, seminal vesicles, and bulbourethral glands are also released into the urethra. The movement of the sperm and secretions into the urethra is called *emission.* The process of *ejaculation* occurs when semen is forced out of the urethra. After ejaculation, sympathetic nerve fibers cause

the erectile tissue to release blood, and the penis gradually returns to a flaccid or nonerect state.

Male Reproductive Hormones

The hypothalamus, the anterior pituitary gland, and the testes secrete hormones that regulate male reproductive functions. At the onset of puberty and throughout life, the hypothalamus releases a hormone called *gonadotropin releasing hormone (GnRH).* GnRH stimulates the anterior pituitary gland to release *follicle-stimulating hormone (FSH)* and *luteinizing hormone (LH).* FSH causes spermatogenesis to begin, and LH stimulates interstitial cells to produce *testosterone.*

Testosterone is responsible for the development of male secondary sex characteristics that are typically unique to males. Examples of these characteristics include chest hair, thick facial hair, a thickening and strengthening of muscles and bones, and the thickening of vocal cords that produces a deeper voice. Testosterone also stimulates the maturation of male reproductive organs.

Testosterone levels are regulated by negative feedback in the following cycle: Blood testosterone levels increase to above normal levels, which causes the hypothalamus to release GnRH. In response, the anterior pituitary ceases the secretion of LH and FSH, in turn causing the testosterone level to fall. When the testosterone level falls below normal, GnRH is again secreted by the hypothalamus, triggering the release of LH and FSH by the anterior pituitary, and the cycle begins again.

Common Diseases and Disorders of the Male Reproductive System

BENIGN PROSTATIC HYPERTROPHY or **BPH** is the nonmalignant enlargement of the prostate gland. This condition is common in older men.

Causes. BPH is related to the hormonal changes that occur as part of the aging process.

Signs and Symptoms. Men with BPH often complain of frequent urination, especially at night, as well as painful urination and difficulty starting or stopping the urinary stream, including "dribbling" at the end of urination.

Treatment. Diagnosis is often confirmed by digital rectal exam (DRE), in which the physician inserts a gloved finger into the rectum and palpates the prostate. Blood tests (PSA) and a biopsy may be done to rule out cancer. Once cancer is ruled out, medications such as Avodart or Flomax may manage the problem, or *transurethral resection of the prostate (TURP)* may be performed to remove the enlarged tissue.

EPIDIDYMITIS is inflammation of an epididymis. Most cases start out as an infection of the urinary tract that spreads to an epididymis.

Causes. The causes include the use of certain medications, placement of a catheter in the urethra, and bacteria—especially those that cause gonorrhea and chlamydia.

Signs and Symptoms. Signs and symptoms include fever, pain in the testes, a lump in the testes, swelling of the scrotum, painful ejaculation, blood in the semen, pain during urination, discharge from the urethra, and enlarged lymph nodes in the pelvic area.

Treatment. Treatment includes pain medication, antibiotics for both the patient and his sexual partner, elevation of the scrotum, and ice packs applied to the scrotum.

IMPOTENCE or **ERECTILE DYSFUNCTION (ED)** is a disorder in which a male cannot achieve or maintain an erect penis to complete sexual intercourse. It is estimated that half of all men between the ages of 40 and 70 years have some degree of impotence. Most causes are physical and not psychological.

Causes. Psychological causes include anxiety, stress, and depression. Common physical causes include diabetes; high blood pressure; anemia; coronary artery disease (CAD); peripheral vascular disease (PVD); low testosterone production; various medications; smoking; excessive alcohol consumption; and drugs such as cocaine, marijuana, and heroin.

Signs and Symptoms. Signs and symptoms are an inability to achieve an erection or an inability to maintain an erection long enough to complete sexual intercourse.

Treatment. The first treatment step should be lifestyle changes to quit smoking and stop using alcohol and/or drugs. Counseling to reduce anxiety and depression may also be helpful. Other treatment options include oral medications such as Viagra or Cialis, penile injections of medications, and penile implants if oral medications do not work.

PROSTATE CANCER is one of the most common cancers in men older than age 40, and the risk of developing prostate cancer increases with age. Awareness about this malignancy is growing, and access to screenings such as digital rectal exam (DRE) is becoming widely available. Therefore, many cases in the United States are being diagnosed before symptoms even occur.

Causes. The causes are mostly unknown, although decreased testosterone production may contribute to the development of this disease, explaining why risk increases with age.

Signs and Symptoms. Common symptoms include anemia, weight loss, incontinence, difficulty starting or stopping urination, painful urination, pain in the lower back or abdomen, pain during bowel movements, high levels of prostate-specific antigen (PSA) in the blood, blood in the urine, and bone pain in advanced cases when cancer cells have spread (metastasized) to the bone.

Treatment. Treatments include hormone therapy, chemotherapy, radiation therapy to shrink or destroy the tumor, as well as surgery to remove the prostate, known as *prostatectomy.*

Go to CONNECT to see an animation about *Prostate Cancer.*

PROSTATITIS is an inflammation of the prostate gland. If it develops suddenly, it is called *acute prostatitis.* The slow development of this condition is termed *chronic prostatitis.*

Causes. This condition can be caused by excessive alcohol consumption, bacterial infection, a catheterization, trauma to the urethra or urinary bladder, and scarring of the urethra or prostate because of frequent infections. Urinating frequently can help to prevent this infection.

Signs and Symptoms. Signs and symptoms include fever; pain in the scrotum, pelvic area, or abdomen; difficult, frequent, and/or painful urination; blood in the urine; painful ejaculation; blood in the semen; discharge from the urethra; a low sperm count; and white blood cells in urine or semen.

Treatment. This condition is treated with antibiotics. Surgery may also be required to repair any damage to the urethra.

TESTICULAR CANCER is a malignant growth of one or both testicles. Unlike prostate cancer, which tends to occur in older males, testicular cancer occurs in males ages 15 to 30 and is a much more aggressive malignancy.

Causes. Predisposing factors include cryptorchidism (undescended testicles during infancy). Family history may also be a factor.

Signs and Symptoms. A hard, painless lump in one testicle is a common early symptom. Patients may complain of groin or abdominal pain as the disease progresses.

Treatment. Orchiectomy or removal of the involved testis is usually performed, followed by radiation therapy and chemotherapy. Caught in the early stages, testicular cancer has up to a 95% success rate, verifying the need for males to perform testicular self-exams on a monthly basis. You will learn how to instruct patients in this important exam technique in the *Assisting in Reproductive and Urinary Specialties* chapter.

▶ The Female Reproductive System LO 32.3

Ovaries and Ovum Formation

The ovaries are considered the primary female sex organs because they produce the female sex cells, called *ova* (see Figures 32-4 and 32-5). They also produce *estrogen* and *progesterone,* the female hormones. Most females have two ovaries. They are oval in shape and are located in the pelvic cavity. Each ovary is divided into an inner area called the *medulla* and an outer area called the *cortex.* The medulla contains nerves, lymphatic vessels, and many blood vessels. The cortex contains small masses of cells called *ovarian follicles.* Epithelial tissue and dense connective tissue cover each ovary.

Before a female child is born, *primordial follicles* develop in her ovarian cortex. Each primordial follicle contains a large cell called a *primary oocyte* (immature ovum) and smaller cells called *follicular cells.* Unlike males, who make sperm cells throughout their entire life, a female is born with the maximum number of primary oocytes she will ever produce.

Oogenesis is the process of ovum formation. At the onset of puberty, some primary oocytes are stimulated to continue meiosis (see Figure 32-2). When a primary oocyte divides, it produces one *polar body* (a nonfunctional cell) and a *secondary oocyte.* The secondary oocyte is released from an ovary each month during a process called **ovulation.** When the secondary oocyte is fertilized, it divides to form a mature, fertilized ovum. Therefore, the process of meiosis begins before a female is born and is completed only if a secondary oocyte is fertilized. The mature ovum contains 23 chromosomes; when it combines with a sperm cell, the resulting cell contains 46 chromosomes.

Internal Accessory Organs of the Female Reproductive System

The female reproductive internal accessory organs are the fallopian tubes, uterus, and vagina.

Fallopian Tubes A fallopian tube, or *oviduct,* opens near each ovary, and the other end connects to the uterus. The

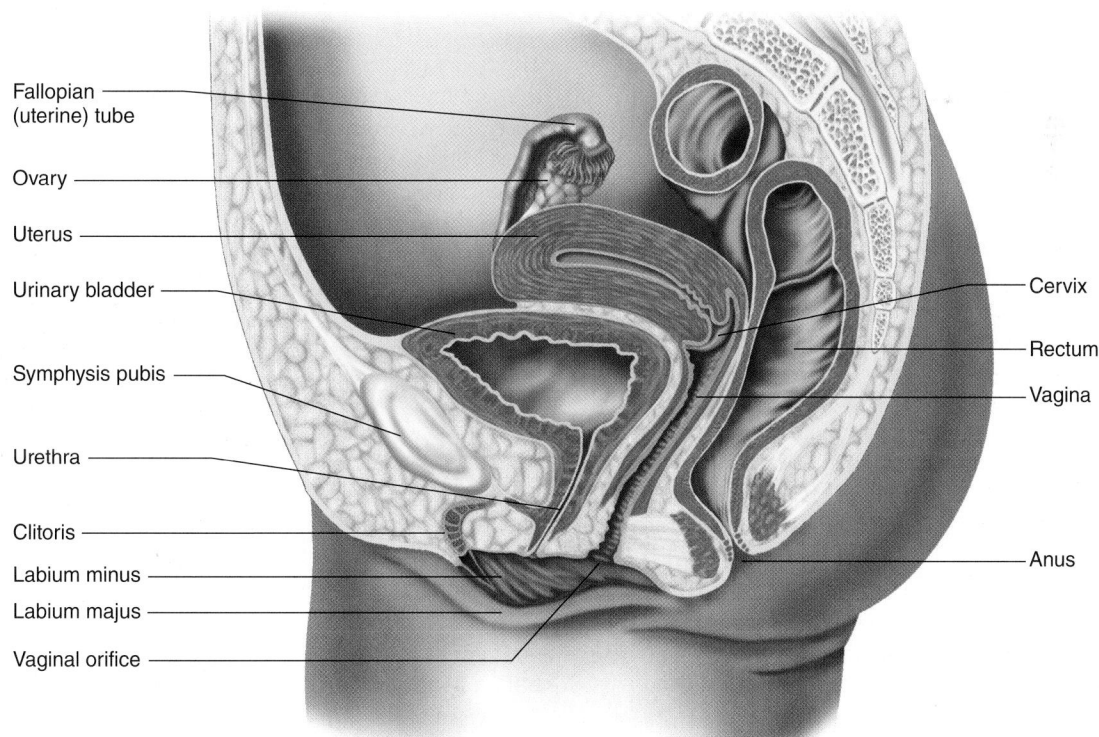

Fallopian (uterine) tube
Ovary
Uterus
Urinary bladder
Symphysis pubis
Urethra
Clitoris
Labium minus
Labium majus
Vaginal orifice
Cervix
Rectum
Vagina
Anus

FIGURE 32-4 Sagittal view of female reproductive organs. The female reproductive system produces ova for fertilization and provides the place and means for a fertilized ovum to develop.

FIGURE 32-5   Anterior view of internal female reproductive organs. Ovulation of an oocyte is also demonstrated.

fringed, expanded end of a fallopian tube near an ovary is called an **infundibulum.** The infundibulum ends in *fimbriae,* or finger-like projections. The infundibulum and its fimbriae "catch" an ovum as it leaves an ovary. Fallopian tubes are muscular tubes that are lined with mucous membrane and cilia. This construction allows the tube to propel the ovum toward the uterus using peristalsis and the sweeping motions of cilia.

Uterus   The uterus is a hollow, muscular organ that receives a developing embryo and sustains its development. The upper domed portion of the uterus is called the *fundus,* the main portion is called the *body,* and the narrow, lower portion that extends into the vagina is called the *cervix.* The opening of the cervix is called the *cervical orifice.*

The wall of the uterus has three layers: the endometrium, myometrium, and perimetrium. The *endometrium* is the innermost lining of the uterus. It is vascular with a rich blood supply and also contains numerous tubular glands that secrete mucus. The *myometrium* is the middle, thick, muscular layer. The *perimetrium* is a thin layer that covers the myometrium. It secretes serous fluid that coats and protects the uterus.

Vagina   The vagina is a tubular, muscular organ that extends from the uterus to the outside of the body. The muscular folds of the vagina, called *rugae,* allow it to expand to receive an erect penis during sexual intercourse, and to provide a passageway for delivery of offspring as well as for uterine secretions. The opening of the vagina is posterior to the urinary opening and anterior to the anal opening. The wall of the vagina has three layers: an innermost mucosal layer that secretes mucus, a middle muscular layer, and an outermost fibrous layer. The opening of the vagina to the outside is known as the *vaginal os,* the *vaginal orifice,* or the *vaginal introitus.*

External Accessory Organs of the Female Reproductive System

Mammary glands are accessory organs of the female reproductive and integumentary systems (see Figure 32-6). Their reproductive function is the secretion of milk for newborn offspring.

Mammary glands are located beneath the skin in the breast area. A nipple is located near the center of each breast. The pigmented area that surrounds the nipple is called the *areola.* Each gland is made of 15 to 20 lobes and contains *alveolar glands* that make milk under the influence of the hormone *prolactin.* The hormone *oxytocin (OT)* induces *lactiferous ducts* to deliver milk through openings in the nipples. If a woman wants to breast-feed, she must produce adequate amounts of prolactin and oxytocin.

External Genitalia of the Female Reproductive System

The female external genitalia, collectively known as the vulva, include the following structures: mons pubis, labia majora, labia minora, clitoris, urethral meatus, vaginal orifice, Bartholin's glands, and perineum.

Labia Majora   The labia majora are rounded folds of adipose tissue and skin that protect the other external female reproductive organs. At their anterior ends, the labia majora form the *mons pubis,* which is a fatty area that overlies the pubic symphysis. The labia majora and mons pubis are typically covered in pubic hair in post-pubescent females.

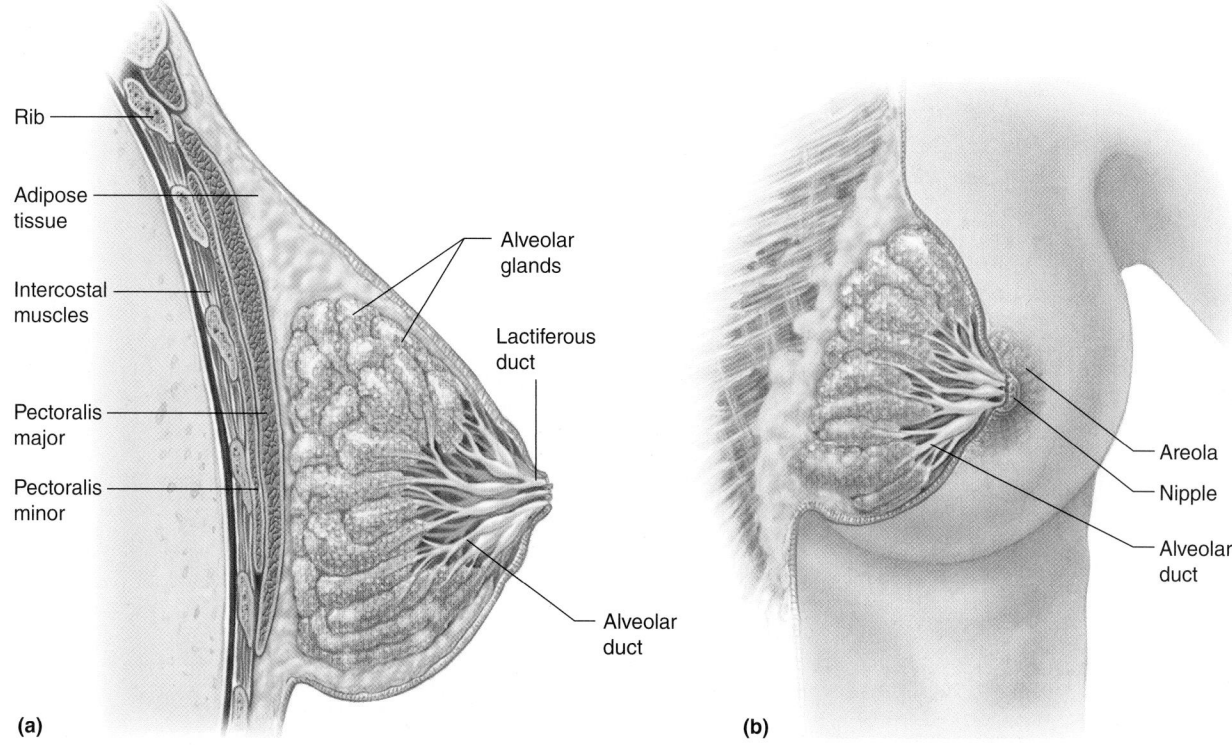

FIGURE 32-6   Mammary glands: (a) sagittal view and (b) anterior view.

Labia Minora The labia minora are folds of skin between the labia majora. They are pinkish in color because of their high degree of vascularity. They merge together anteriorly to form a hood over the clitoris.

The space enclosed by the labia minora is called the *vestibule.* The **Bartholin's glands,** sometimes referred to as the *vestibular glands,* secrete mucus into this area during sexual arousal. This mucus eases insertion of the penis into the vagina.

Clitoris The clitoris is anterior to the urethral meatus. It contains the female erectile tissue and is rich in sensory nerves.

Perineum The perineum is the area between the vagina and the anus. This is the area that is sometimes "clipped" during the birth process, in a procedure known as an *episiotomy.*

Erection, Lubrication, and Orgasm
During sexual arousal, nervous stimulation causes the clitoris to become erect and the Bartholin's glands to become active. At the same time, the vagina elongates. If the clitoris is sufficiently stimulated, an orgasm occurs. During orgasm, the walls of the uterus and fallopian tubes contract to help propel sperm toward the upper ends of the fallopian tubes.

Female Reproductive Hormones
Beginning at puberty, the hypothalamus secretes increasing amounts of GnRH. This causes the anterior pituitary gland to release FSH and LH, which stimulate the ovary to produce estrogen and progesterone, and also to mature the ovarian follicles. The estrogen and progesterone are responsible for the female secondary sex characteristics: breast development, increased vascularization of the skin; and increased fat deposits in the breasts, thighs, and hips.

Female Reproductive Cycle
The female reproductive cycle is also called the *menstrual cycle.* See Figure 32-7. It consists of regular changes in the uterine lining that leads to a monthly "period," or shedding of the uterine lining, along with bleeding. The first menstrual period is known as **menarche. Menopause** is the termination of the menstrual cycle because of normal aging of the ovaries. The following steps are the major hormonal changes that occur during one reproductive cycle:

1. The anterior pituitary gland releases FSH, which stimulates an ovarian follicle to mature.
2. The maturing follicle secretes estrogen. Estrogen causes the uterine lining to thicken.
3. The anterior pituitary gland releases a sudden surge of LH, which triggers ovulation.
4. Following ovulation, follicular cells of the follicle become a *corpus luteum.*
5. The corpus luteum secretes progesterone, which causes the uterine lining to become more vascular and glandular.
6. If the released oocyte is not fertilized, the corpus luteum degenerates, causing estrogen and progesterone levels to fall.
7. The decline in estrogen and progesterone levels causes the uterine lining to break down, and menses (elimination of the uterine lining, with bleeding) starts.
8. When the anterior pituitary releases FSH, the reproductive cycle begins again.

FIGURE 32-7 A typical 28-day menstrual cycle.

Menstruation
↓ estrogen and progesterone cause uterine lining to shed.

Follicular Phase
FSH causes growth of follicles on the ovary. Growing follicle causes the uterine lining to become more vascular.

Ovulation
LH triggers ovulation and egg is released.

Luteal Phase
Corpus luteum secretes progesterone causing uterine lining to grow. Ovum (egg) dies if not fertilized. Corpus luteum degenerates causing estrogen and progesterone levels to fall.

PATHO PHYSIOLOGY

LO 32.4

Common Diseases and Disorders of the Female Reproductive System

According to the American Cancer Society, **BREAST CANCER** is the second leading cause of cancer deaths in women after lung cancer. Depending on tumor size and how far cancer cells have spread, breast cancer is classified in stages from 0 to 4, with stage 4 cancer being the most serious. Early diagnosis through regular mammograms and breast self-exams greatly increases the success of treatment. Teaching female patients about breast self-exam and its importance in the early detection of breast cancer is an important aspect of being a medical assistant. You will learn how to teach women this technique in the *Assisting in Reproductive and Urinary Specialties* chapter.

Causes. The causes are largely unknown, although breast cancer may be related to hormonal changes or the presence of certain genes.

Signs and Symptoms. Signs and symptoms include a lump in the breast that is usually painless and firm, a lump in the armpit, discharge from the nipples, dimpled skin on the breast or nipple, and breast pain. Swelling of the breast into the adjacent arm and bone pain may be present in advanced cases. Inflammatory breast cancer may present only as a painless rash of the affected breast with none of the other typical symptoms.

Treatment. Nonsurgical treatment methods include hormone therapy, radiation therapy, and chemotherapy. Surgical options include surgery to remove affected lymph nodes, lumpectomy (surgery to remove a lump), and mastectomy (surgery to remove a breast).

Go to CONNECT to see an animation about *Breast Cancer.*

CERVICAL CANCER generally develops slowly, although adenocarcinoma of the cervix, which tends to be a more rapidly spreading cancer, is the exception to this rule. With early detection by a yearly Pap smear (a test looking for abnormal cervical cells), treatment is often successful. Note that the new recommendation for Pap smear screenings is now every other year if a woman's previous screenings have been negative for 5 years and if the woman is in a monogamous relationship and not on birth control pills.

Causes. A weak immune system may be a factor in the development of this cancer. Risk factors also include sexual intercourse early in life, multiple sexual partners, and infection with the human papilloma virus (HPV).

Signs and Symptoms. Primary symptoms include frequent vaginal discharge, sporadic vaginal bleeding, vaginal bleeding after sexual intercourse, and abnormal cells in the cervix. Patients who are in later stages of this disease may experience pain in the pelvic area or legs, or bone fractures.

Treatment. Radiation therapy, chemotherapy, the removal or destruction of diseased tissue with cryosurgery or laser surgery, and the removal of the uterus (hysterectomy) are the treatments for this disease.

CERVICITIS is an inflammation of the cervix, which is usually caused by an infection.

Causes. Causes include bacterial or viral infections and allergic reactions to spermicidal creams and latex condoms.

Signs and Symptoms. Frequent vaginal discharge, pain during intercourse, and vaginal bleeding after intercourse are common signs and symptoms.

Treatment. This condition is treated with antibiotics and by changing the contraception method.

DYSMENORRHEA is the condition of experiencing severe menstrual cramps that limit normal daily activities.

Causes. Causes include anxiety, endometriosis, pelvic inflammatory disease (PID), fibroid tumors in the uterus, ovarian cysts, abnormally high levels of prostaglandins, and multiple sexual partners.

Signs and Symptoms. Common symptoms are abdominal pain, including sharp or dull pain in the pelvic area just prior to and during the menstrual period.

Treatment. Nonsurgical treatments include pain medication, anti-inflammatory drugs, medications that inhibit prostaglandin formation, oral contraceptives, and antibiotics in the case of PID. Surgical treatments include hysterectomy and surgery to remove cysts or fibroids.

ENDOMETRIOSIS is a condition in which tissues that make up the lining of the uterus grow outside the uterus.

Causes. The cause of this disorder is unknown; it may be inherited.

Signs and Symptoms. Signs and symptoms include infertility, heavy bleeding from the uterus, pain in the abdomen or pelvis, painful periods, spotting between periods, and pain during sexual intercourse.

Treatment. Oral contraceptives, pain medications, and various hormone therapies may be prescribed. Surgical treatments include laser surgery to remove endometrial tissue outside the uterus and hysterectomy.

FIBROCYSTIC BREAST DISEASE is the presence of abnormal cystic tissues in the breasts. The cysts vary in size related to the menstrual cycle. It is a common disorder and occurs in more than 60% of women in the United States between age 30 and 50. It is rare in women who have gone through menopause because it is related to hormonal changes occurring during the menstrual cycle. It is important to note that fibrocystic breast disease is not considered to put a woman at higher risk of breast cancer.

Causes. This disorder is caused by hormonal changes associated with the menstrual cycle and ingestion of various dietary substances, including caffeine, nicotine, and sugar. Birth control pills may also aggravate this condition.

Signs and Symptoms. Common symptoms include breasts that feel "lumpy," breast tenderness or pain, itchy nipples, and dense tissues as seen in a mammogr.

Treatment. Treatments include changing one's diet, and taking vitamin supplements such as vitamin E, B complex, and magnesium. Wearing support bras may help with pain control.

FIBROIDS are benign (noncancerous) tumors that grow in the uterine wall. They are known to affect one out of four women in their thirties and forties and appear to be more common in women of African descent.

Causes. The causes are mostly unknown, although it has been found that the tumors enlarge as estrogen levels increase. Heredity appears to play a role.

Signs and Symptoms. The signs and symptoms are pressure in the abdomen, severe menstrual cramps, abdominal gas, heavy menstrual bleeding, and intermenstrual bleeding. Back and leg pain may also occur.

Treatment. Treatment includes pain medications, hormone treatments to shrink tumors, surgery to remove tumors, hysterectomy, and surgery to decrease the blood supply to the uterus.

OVARIAN CANCER is considered more deadly than other types of cancer because its signs and symptoms are usually mild or indistinct until the disease has spread to other organs, making early detection difficult. Current statistics suggest that about 1 woman in 67 will develop ovarian cancer. Women with a family history of ovarian cancer may be counseled to consider prophylactic *oophorosalpingectomy* (removal of the ovaries and fallopian tubes) prior to actually developing ovarian cancer.

Causes. The causes are unknown, although the presence of certain genes has been indicated as a risk factor. Some oral contraceptives may lower the risk of developing this disease.

Signs and Symptoms. Abdominal and pelvic discomfort, unusual menstrual cycles, indigestion, bloating, nausea, and excessive hair growth are signs and symptoms. Diagnosis is made after ultrasound, a CA 125 blood test, and an ovarian biopsy.

Treatment. Treatment options include radiation therapy, chemotherapy, and surgery to remove the ovaries and reproductive organs.

PREMENSTRUAL SYNDROME (PMS) is a collection of symptoms that occur just before a menstrual period.

Causes. The causes are mostly unknown, although hormone fluctuations during the menstrual cycle are implicated.

Signs and Symptoms. The signs and symptoms include anxiety, depression, irritability, acne, fatigue, food cravings, bloating, aches in the head or back, abdominal pain, breast tenderness, muscle spasms, diarrhea, weight gain, and loss of sex drive.

Treatment. PMS is commonly treated with pain medications, diuretics, medications to treat depression or anxiety, and oral contraceptives. Many women have also found changes in diet to be helpful, including limiting caffeine, sugar, and sodium. The addition of B complex vitamins may also be helpful.

UTERINE (ENDOMETRIAL) CANCER is most common in postmenopausal women. In the United States, it accounts for approximately 6% of cancer deaths in women.

Causes. The causes are mostly unknown, although it may be related to increased levels of estrogen.

Signs and Symptoms. Signs and symptoms include abdominal pain; abnormal bleeding from the uterus; pelvic pain; and a thin, white vaginal discharge in postmenopausal women.

Treatment. Treatment includes radiation therapy, chemotherapy, and surgery to remove the uterus, fallopian tubes, and ovaries.

VAGINITIS (inflammation of the vagina) and **VULVOVAGINITIS** (inflammation of the vulva and vagina) are usually associated with an abnormal vaginal discharge. Some vaginal discharge is normal for all women, and it varies throughout the menstrual cycle. Normal vaginal discharge is clear, whitish, or yellowish in color.

Causes. This condition can be caused by yeast infections, tampon use, poor hygiene, bacteria, antibiotics, and sexually transmitted infections (STIs). Vaginitis may be prevented through good hygiene and safe sex practices.

Signs and Symptoms. Common symptoms include fever, vulvar and vaginal itching and swelling, an abnormal increase or decrease in the amount of vaginal discharge, an abnormal color of vaginal discharge (brown, green, or pinkish), a change in the consistency of vaginal discharge (frothy or cheese-like), and vaginal discharge that has an abnormal odor.

Treatment. The patient may be given medications for fungal or bacterial infections, or the patient and her sexual partner may be treated for STIs.

▶ Pregnancy

LO 32.5

Pregnancy is defined as the condition of having a developing off-spring in the uterus. Pregnancy results when a sperm cell unites with an ovum in a process called fertilization (see Figure 32-8).

Fertilization

Prior to fertilization, an ovum is released from an ovary and travels through a fallopian tube. During sexual intercourse, the male deposits semen into the vagina. Sperm cells must travel up through the uterus to the fallopian tubes to fertilize the ovum.

Prostaglandins in semen stimulate the flagella of sperm cells to undulate, causing the swimming action of sperm. Prostaglandins also stimulate muscles in the uterus and fallopian tubes to contract. These contractions (peristalsis) help the sperm reach the ovum. Normally about 10 to 14 days after

ovulation, high estrogen levels stimulate the uterus and cervix to secrete a thin watery fluid that also promotes the movement of sperm toward the ovum.

Although many sperm cells normally reach an ovum, only one sperm cell unites with the ovum, penetrating the follicular cells and a layer called the *zona pellucida*, which surrounds the cell membrane of the ovum. The acrosome of this sperm releases enzymes to help the sperm penetrate the membrane of the ovum. Once a sperm unites with an ovum, the ovum releases enzymes to prevent other sperm from invading it. The enzymes cause the zona pellucida to become hard and therefore impenetrable to other sperm.

The nucleus of the ovum (with 23 chromosomes) and the nucleus of the sperm (with 23 chromosomes) fuse together to make one nucleus that contains 46 chromosomes. The cell that is formed by this union is called a **zygote.**

FIGURE 32-8 Stages of early embryo development.

The Prenatal Period

The prenatal period is the time before the offspring is born. It is divided into an *embryonic period* (weeks 2 through 8 of pregnancy) and a *fetal period* (week 9 to the delivery of the offspring). It is further divided into three periods known as trimesters, which consist of three calendar months each. See Points on Practice: The Pregnant Patient.

About one day after the zygote forms, it begins to undergo mitosis at a relatively rapid rate. This rapid cell division is called *cleavage,* and the resulting ball of cells is called a *morula.* The morula travels down the fallopian tube to the uterus. Fluid then invades the morula, and this organism is called a **blastocyst.** The blastocyst implants in the endometrial wall of the uterus. The process of moving from zygote formation to implantation of the blastocyst takes about one week. Once the blastocyst implants, a group of cells in the blastocyst, called the *inner cell mass,* gives rise to an **embryo.** Other cells in the blastocyst, along with cells of the uterus, eventually form the **placenta.**

The Embryonic Period The embryonic period extends from the second week of pregnancy to the end of the eighth week of development. During this stage, the placenta, *amnion, umbilical cord,* and *yolk sac* form, along with most of the internal organs and external structures of the embryo (see Figure 32-9). The cells of the inner cell mass organize into layers called **primary germ layers.** All organs are formed from the primary germ layers, which include the ectoderm, mesoderm, and endoderm.

- The *ectoderm* gives rise to nervous tissue and some epithelial tissue.
- The *mesoderm,* the middle layer, gives rise to connective tissues and some epithelial tissue.
- The *endoderm* gives rise to epithelial tissues only.

The placenta allows nutrients and oxygen from maternal blood to pass to embryonic blood. It also allows waste products from the fetal blood to pass into maternal blood. The **amnion** is a protective, fluid-filled sac that surrounds the embryo. The *umbilical cord* contains three blood vessels—one umbilical vein that carries oxygenated blood from the placenta to the embryo, and two umbilical arteries that carry deoxygenated blood from the embryo back to the placenta.

The yolk sac makes new blood cells for the fetus, as well as cells that eventually become the sex cells of the baby. By the end of the embryonic stage, the baby closely resembles a human because all external structures (arms, hands, legs, feet, etc.) have formed.

The Fetal Period The fetal period begins at the end of the eighth week of development and ends at birth. During this period, the growth of the offspring, which is now called a **fetus,** is rapid. By the twelfth week, bones have begun to harden and the external reproductive organs are distinguishable as male or female.

The growth rate of the fetus slows down in the fifth month but skeletal muscles become active. In the sixth month, the fetus starts to gain substantial weight. In the seventh month, the eyelids open. In the last 3 months of pregnancy, fetal brain cells divide rapidly and organs continue to grow. The testes of the male descend into the scrotum. The last organ systems to completely develop are the digestive and respiratory systems. By the end of the ninth month, the fetus is usually positioned upside down in the uterus in preparation for delivery.

Fetal Circulation

Throughout prenatal development, the placenta and umbilical blood vessels carry out the exchange of nutrients, oxygen, and waste products between maternal and fetal blood. Therefore, the fetus does not need to send blood to the lungs to pick up oxygen, nor does it need to send blood to the liver to process nutrients.

Fetal circulation has some important differences from normal circulation, which are illustrated in Figure 32-10. In the adult heart, blood flows from the right atrium into the right ventricle so it can be pumped to the lungs. In the fetal heart, a

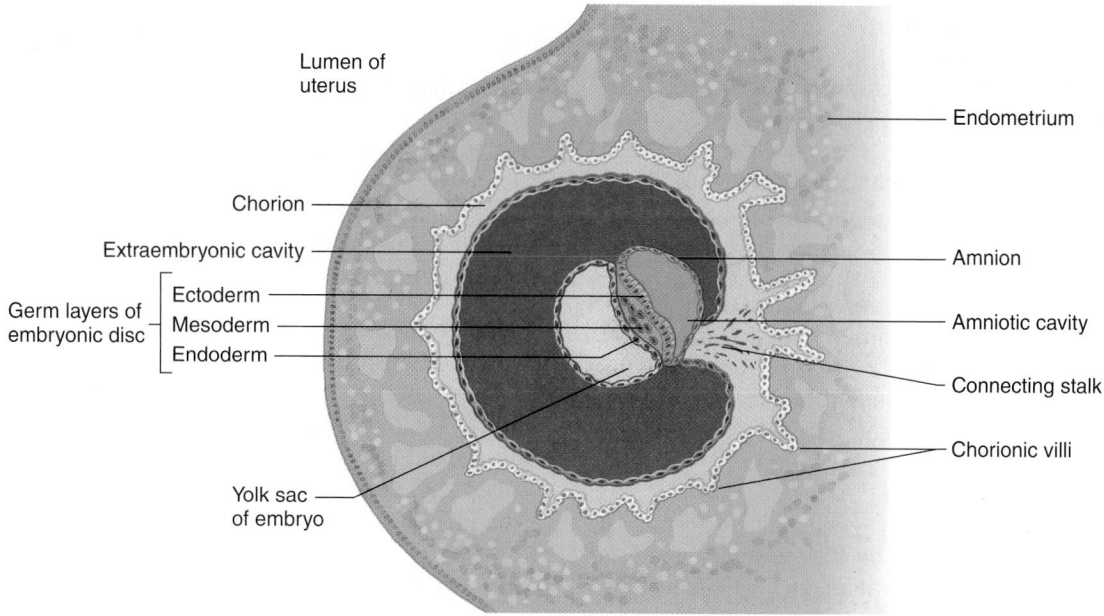

FIGURE 32-9 Primary germ layers and membranes associated with an embryo.

Aortic arch

Superior vena cava

Foramen ovale
(becomes fossa ovalis)

Inferior vena cava

Ductus venosus
(becomes ligamentum
venosum)

Hepatic portal vein

Umbilical vein
(becomes ligamentum
teres)

Placenta

Ductus arteriosus
(becomes ligamentum
arteriosum)

Pulmonary artery

Pulmonary veins

Pulmonary trunk

Left atrium

Left ventricle

Abdominal aorta

Left renal artery

Common iliac artery

Umbilical arteries
(become medial
umbilical ligaments)

Internal iliac artery

Umbilical vein

Umbilical arteries

Decreasing
blood
oxygen
level

FIGURE 32-10   Fetal circulation.

POINTS ON PRACTICE

The Pregnant Patient

The pregnant patient goes through three distinct stages known as *trimesters.* Each trimester has specific events associated with it.

First Trimester

The first trimester is from week 1 to week 12. During weeks 1 to 8 the product of conception is an embryo; after week 8 it is a fetus. Week 12 marks the end of the first trimester, or one-third of the pregnancy. It is usually during the first trimester that women confirm they are pregnant. "Morning sickness" commonly occurs during this stage.

Second Trimester

Fine, soft hair (lanugo) appears on the shoulders, back, and head of the fetus during the fourth month. By the 20th week,

fetal movement may be felt, and the pregnant woman begins to show fullness in the abdomen. Identifiable periods of fetal sleep and wakefulness occur as the second trimester ends at the completion of the sixth month.

Third Trimester

The last trimester encompasses the most noticeable period of growth, both in the fetus and in the mother. By the end of 30 weeks, the fetus most likely has assumed a head-down position and has a 50% chance of survival if it is born at this time. The fetus is said to have come full term after it is approximately 9 months (40 weeks) old.

More information about caring for a pregnant patient is found in the *Assisting with Reproductive and Urinary Specialties* chapter.

hole called the **foramen ovale** is located between the right and left atria. This hole allows most of the fetal blood to flow from the right atrium into the left atrium. However, some fetal blood does flow from the right atrium into the right ventricle, and the right ventricle then delivers the blood to the pulmonary trunk.

In the fetus, there is also a connection between the pulmonary trunk and the aorta called the **ductus arteriosus.** This connection allows blood to flow from the pulmonary trunk into the aorta. In the adult, this connection closes and blood flows from the pulmonary trunk to the lungs. The fetus also contains a blood vessel called the **ductus venosus** that allows most of the blood to bypass the liver. After a baby is born, the foramen ovale, ductus arteriosus, and ductus venosus normally close.

Hemoglobin within the fetus has a much higher affinity for oxygen than does the normal hemoglobin that is found after birth and during growth. Therefore, the fetus's blood is adapted to carry more oxygen.

Hormonal Changes during Pregnancy

Many hormonal changes take place when a woman is pregnant. Following implantation of the embryo, the embryo cells begin to secrete *human chorionic gonadotropin (HCG)*. HCG maintains the corpus luteum in the ovary so it will continue to secrete estrogen and progesterone. The placenta also secretes large amounts of progesterone and estrogen.

Progesterone and estrogen stimulate the uterine lining to thicken and inhibit the anterior pituitary gland from secreting FSH and LH to prevent ovulation during pregnancy. Estrogen and progesterone also stimulate the development of the mammary glands, inhibit uterine contractions, and stimulate the enlargement of female reproductive organs.

A hormone called *relaxin,* which comes from the corpus luteum, inhibits uterine contractions and relaxes the ligaments of the pelvis in preparation for childbirth. The placenta also secretes *lactogen,* a hormone that stimulates the enlargement of mammary glands. *Aldosterone,* which is secreted from the adrenal gland, increases sodium and water retention. The secretion of *parathyroid hormone (PTH)* increases, helping to maintain high calcium levels in the blood.

▶ The Birth Process
LO 32.6

The birth process ends pregnancy. This process begins when progesterone levels fall. When this happens, uterine contractions are no longer inhibited and the uterus secretes prostaglandins that stimulate uterine contractions, which cause the posterior pituitary gland to release oxytocin. Oxytocin stimulates strong uterine contractions until the birth process ends. The birth process itself occurs in three stages after the fetus settles into position in the mother's pelvis (see Figure 32-11a).

(a)

(b)

(c)

(d)

FIGURE 32-11 Stages of the birth process: (a) the fetal position before birth, (b) dilation of the cervix, (c) delivery of the fetus, and (d) delivery of the placenta.

1. *Dilation* (see Figure 32-11b). The cervix thins and softens, known as *effacement,* dilating to approximately 10 cm. Regular contractions occur at this stage and the amniotic sac ruptures. If rupture does not occur, the sac may be surgically punctured. This stage normally lasts 8 to 24 hours.

2. *Expulsion* (see Figure 32-11c). Also known as *parturition,* this is the actual childbirth stage. Forceful contractions and abdominal compressions force the fetus from the uterus into the vagina. This stage may take 30 minutes or only a few minutes.

3. *Placental stage* (see Figure 32-11d). This stage is also referred to as the *afterbirth.* Approximately 10 to 15 minutes after the birth, the placenta separates from the uterine wall and is expelled. Uterine contractions continue during this stage and the blood vessels constrict to prevent hemorrhage. Normal blood loss is less than 350 mL (12 oz).

If the fetus is not in the usual head-down position, the child is said to be *breech,* in which the buttocks or feet present first. If the fetus cannot be turned manually, forceps may be used to assist in the birth. Alternately, a *cesarean section* (C-section) may be performed to deliver the infant through the abdominal wall.

The Postnatal Period

The *postnatal period* is the 6-week period following birth. The first 4 weeks of the postnatal period are called the *neonatal period* and the offspring is called a *neonate.* The neonatal period is marked by adjustment to life outside the uterus. The lungs of the neonate must expand, which is why the baby's first breath is forceful. The newborn's liver is immature, so the baby must obtain most of its glucose from fat stores in the skin. The newborn urinates a lot because the kidneys are too immature to concentrate urine well. In addition, body temperature tends to be unstable. The newborn's umbilical vessels constrict, and the foramen ovale, ductus arteriosus, and ductus venosus close.

Milk Production and Secretion

During pregnancy, hormones stimulate the breasts to enlarge. After childbirth, prolactin causes the mammary glands to produce milk. The hormone oxytocin stimulates the ejection of milk from mammary gland ducts. As long as milk is removed from the mammary glands, milk production continues. Once a female stops breast-feeding, the hypothalamus inhibits the release of prolactin and oxytocin and milk production stops.

▶ Contraception

LO 32.7

Birth control methods, also referred to as *contraception,* reduce the risk of pregnancy (see Figure 32-12). Although many birth control methods are available, some are more reliable than others. The following are the most commonly used birth control methods:

- Coitus interruptus. Also known as withdrawal, the penis is withdrawn from the vagina before ejaculation. This method is not reliable because small amounts of semen may enter the vagina before ejaculation.

FIGURE 32-12 Couples use various forms of contraception. To provide adequate patient teaching, you should be knowledgeable of these methods.

- Rhythm method. Also known as periodic abstinence, this method requires abstinence from sexual intercourse around the time a female is ovulating. However, predicting ovulation can be difficult; therefore, this type of contraception can be unreliable.

- Mechanical barriers. Mechanical barriers prevent sperm from entering the female reproductive tract. They include condoms, diaphragms, and cervical caps. Spermicides are often used in conjunction with barrier methods, particularly condoms and diaphragms.

- Chemical barriers. Chemical barriers destroy sperm in the female reproductive tract. They primarily include spermicides.

- Oral contraceptives. Birth control pills are oral contraceptives. They normally include low doses of estrogen or progesterone that prevent the LH surge necessary for ovulation. These pills therefore prevent ovulation. Newer oral contraceptives are being developed in which the woman takes the pill daily for 3 months and then is off for 1 week, so that a period only occurs four times a year.

- Injectable contraceptives. Depo-Provera is one brand of injectable contraceptive. It prevents ovulation and alters the lining of the uterus so that implantation of a blastocyst is not likely.

- Insertable contraceptives. NuvaRing is one of the newest forms of contraception. The woman inserts the ring vaginally and leaves it in for 3 weeks. She removes the ring at the beginning of the fourth week to allow for menstruation on the same schedule she would experience using most oral contraceptives.

- Contraceptive implants. Contraceptive implants are small rods of progesterone that are implanted beneath the skin. They also prevent ovulation.

- Transdermal contraceptives. Commonly called "the Patch," transdermal contraceptives are applied to the skin once a week and removed on the seventh day for a 3-week cycle. No patch is applied during the fourth week to allow for the menstrual period.

- Intrauterine devices. An intrauterine device (IUD) is a small, solid device that a physician places in the uterus. It prevents the implantation of a blastocyst.

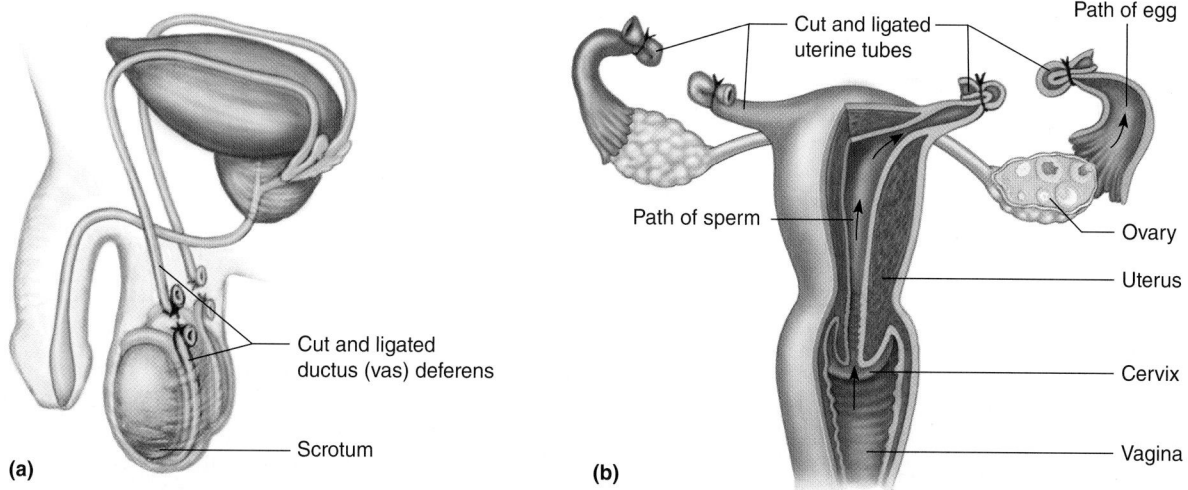

FIGURE 32-13 (a) Vasectomy involves cutting and ligating the vas deferens. (b)Tubal ligation involves cutting and ligating each fallopian tube.

- Surgical methods. *Tubal ligation* is a surgical method used in females to prevent pregnancy. In this process, each fallopian tube is cut and tied or fulgurated to prevent sperm from reaching the oocyte. *Vasectomy* is a surgical method used in males to prevent pregnancy. In this process, each vas deferens is cut and tied or fulgurated to prevent sperm from being ejaculated. Figure 32-13 illustrates these birth control methods.

Infertility

LO 32.8

Infertility is the inability to conceive a child. A couple that has never been pregnant and has tried for 12 months to achieve pregnancy is said to have *primary infertility*. If a couple has had at least one pregnancy but has not been able to get pregnant again after 1 year, they are said to have *secondary infertility*.

In the United States, about 15% of infertility causes are unknown, about 35% are the result of problems in the male, and about 50% are because of problems in the female. Common causes of infertility as a result of male factors include the following:

- Impotence
- Retrograde ejaculation
- Low or absent sperm count
- Use of various medications or drugs
- Decreased testosterone production
- Scarring of the male reproductive tract from STIs
- Previous mumps infection that infected the testes
- Inflammation of the epididymis or testes

Infertility because of female factors includes these common causes:

- Scarring of fallopian tubes from sexually transmitted infections (STIs)
- Pelvic inflammatory disease (PID)
- Inadequate diet
- Lack of ovulation

- Lack of menstrual cycles
- Endometriosis
- Abnormal shape of the uterus or cervix
- Hormone imbalances
- Cysts in ovaries
- Being older than age 40

Women are most likely to get pregnant in their early twenties. By the time a woman reaches age 40, her chance of conceiving a child is less than 10% each month. In general, infertility in men is not age related.

Infertility Tests

A number of tests are used to diagnose infertility. They include the following:

- Semen analysis. This test determines the semen thickness and the number and motility of sperm cells in a sample.
- Monitoring morning body temperature. If a woman's body temperature does not rise slightly once a month, which is best determined by taking her temperature first thing in the morning, she may not be ovulating.
- Blood hormone measurements. In females, various hormone levels can be monitored to predict ovulation and the general health of the ovaries. In males, testosterone levels are measured.
- Endometrial biopsy. This test determines the health of the uterine lining.
- Urinary analysis for luteinizing hormone. The absence of this hormone in urine may indicate a lack of ovulation.
- Hysterosalpingogram. This type of X-ray uses contrast media to visualize the shape of the uterus and the fallopian tubes. If a woman has excess scar tissue in her fallopian tubes, the contrast cannot run through them.
- Laparoscopy. Laparoscopy is a procedure used to visualize pelvic organs.

Treatment of Infertility

Many treatments are available for infertility, but often there is no cure for this condition. Common treatments include surgery to repair abnormal or scarred fallopian tubes, fertility drugs to increase ovulation, and hormone therapies. When infertility cannot be cured, procedures such as artificial insemination, in vitro fertilization, or the use of a surrogate may help a couple to have a child.

PATHOPHYSIOLOGY

Sexually Transmitted Infections Occurring in Both Sexes

AIDS (ACQUIRED IMMUNODEFICIENCY SYNDROME) is covered in detail in the *Microbiology and Disease* chapter.

Causes. The human immunodeficiency virus (HIV) causes AIDS.

Signs and Symptoms. These are numerous and include decreased T-cell count; flu-like symptoms; and a host of opportunistic infections, including *Pneumocystis carinii* pneumonia (PCP), Kaposi's sarcoma (KS), and cytomegalovirus (CMV).

Treatment. Antiviral medications have been successful in decreasing the viral load and maintaining T-cell counts in some patients, but there are many side effects to these drugs, and they require a strict medicine regime. Other medications include drugs to support the immune system and to treat opportunistic infections as they arise.

CHLAMYDIA is the most commonly reported STI in the United States. Chlamydia may be grossly underreported because, for women, there are often no symptoms until the disease has spread.

Causes. Chlamydia is caused by the bacterium *Chlamydia trachomatis*.

Signs and Symptoms. For females, there may be no symptoms. If they do occur, it will be 2 to 3 weeks after exposure. Symptoms may include abnormal vaginal discharge and burning on urination. As the disease progresses to other reproductive organs, pelvic inflammatory disease (PID) occurs and can cause abdominal pain, pain during intercourse, and intermenstrual bleeding. Men may have a penile discharge and pain on urination. In women, PID is a common cause of infertility; men seldom have serious complications related to chlamydia.

Treatment. Both partners must be treated to avoid reinfection. Effective antibiotics against chlamydia include azithromycin and doxycycline. Patients must complete the medication cycle and avoid sexual contact until both partners are cured. Because of the high rate of reinfection, women should be retested 3 to 4 months after treatment.

GENITAL WARTS, also known as *Condyloma acuminata*, are one of the most common STIs in the world affecting both men and women. It is important to note that not everyone infected with human papillomavirus (HPV) has symptoms. HPV has been implicated in an increased risk of cervical cancer in women.

Causes. HPV is the cause of genital warts.

Signs and Symptoms. Genital warts appear weeks or months after infection in the vulva, vagina, and cervix in women. In men, warts appear on the scrotum and penis. They have also been known to appear around the anus and on the thighs and groin. It is important to note that HPV can be spread even if the patient has no outward signs of the disease.

Treatment. Imiquimod cream, 20% podophyllin anti-miotic solutions, and TCA (trichloroacetic acid) may be used to remove warts. Cryosurgery, cautery, and laser surgery may also be used; however, the virus remains in the patient's body. Currently, there is no treatment to rid the body of the virus. Vaccines to prevent infection with HPV are being developed and tested.

GONORRHEA is a bacterial STI that is common in the United States. The Centers for Disease Control and Prevention (CDC) estimates 700,000 new infections per year.

Causes. Gonorrhea is caused by *Neisseria gonorrhoea,* a bacteria that thrives in the warm, moist areas of the reproductive tract, urethral tract, mouth, throat, eyes, and anus.

Signs and Symptoms. Men often have no symptoms. If they do appear, it will be 2 to 3 days after exposure, when the patient will experience burning on urination and/or white, yellow, or greenish penile discharge. Women may also be asymptomatic, but common symptoms include dysuria, increased vaginal discharge, and intermenstrual bleeding. Gonorrheal infections, like chlamydia, may lead to PID in women. In men, it may lead to epididymitis.

Treatment. Antibiotics are effective against gonorrhea, and both partners must be treated. However, drug-resistant strains of gonorrhea are developing, making successful treatment more difficult. It is not unusual for a patient with gonorrhea to also be diagnosed with chlamydia or other STIs, which also need to be tested for and treated if found to be present. In addition, gonorrhea lives well and actively in the throat, even if there is not an active genitourinary infection, which can lead to additional co-infection.

HERPES SIMPLEX infections include those caused by both herpes simplex 1 and herpes simplex 2.

Causes. Herpes viruses cause both infections. In most cases, herpes simplex 1 causes oral blisters known as cold sores, and herpes simplex 2 causes what is commonly known as genital herpes, although herpes simplex 1 has also been known to cause the genital type of infection. The herpes infection may also be passed from an infected mother to her child during pregnancy and birth with potentially fatal outcomes.

Signs and Symptoms. Many infected persons, both male and female, have minimal or no symptoms. Typical symptoms of genital herpes include blisters on or around the genitals or rectum. These blisters break, leaving tender ulcers in their wake for 2 to 4 weeks. The number and severity of outbreaks tend to decrease over a period of years.

Treatment. There is no treatment to rid the patient of the herpes virus; however, antiviral medications such as Acyclovir may shorten outbreaks when they occur. Daily suppressive therapies with medications like Valtrexmay reduce the risk of transmission. Pregnant women with active outbreaks should deliver the child via a C-section.

PUBIC LICE are known commonly as crabs and medically known as *Pediculosis pubis.*

Causes. These can be caused by a parasitic infestation in the genital area, most commonly spread through sexual contact.

Signs and Symptoms. Symptoms include itching in the genital area with visible evidence of eggs known as nits, as well as crawling lice. Lice only live while on a human body. If they fall off the body, they will die in 24 to 48 hours.

Treatment. Patients should use a lice-killing shampoo of 1% permethrin or pyrethrin. All laundry and clothing must be washed in hot water and dried using the hot dryer cycle for at least 30 minutes. Nits remaining in hair may be removed by hand. All partners should be treated and sexual contact should be avoided until treatment is completed.

SYPHILIS is the one bacterial STI whose incidence in women is decreasing, according to the CDC. However, it is increasing in males, especially in those who have sex with other males.

Causes. Syphilis is caused by the bacterium *Treponema pallidum.*

Signs and Symptoms. Primary-stage syphilis usually involves the appearance of a painless sore known as a *chancre,* which appears 10 to 90 days after exposure. It remains for 3 to 6 weeks, disappearing even without treatment. If untreated, the disease lies dormant, progressing to the second stage, which is characterized by a nonpruritic rash and lesions in the mucous membranes. The rash may be associated with flu-like symptoms. Again, all symptoms disappear without treatment. After a long latent period without symptoms, often years later, the third stage becomes apparent, with damage to the brain, eyes, heart, blood vessels, liver, and bones. This damage may lead to muscular incoordination, paralysis, numbness, blindness, dementia, and, finally, death.

Treatment. The cure for syphilis in its early stage is a single dose of intramuscular penicillin. Additional doses are needed for disease present longer than a year. Other antibiotics are also effective for patients allergic to penicillin. The patient must avoid sexual contact until treatment is completed to avoid further spread of the disease.

TRICHOMONIASIS (also known as trichomonas infection or the abbreviation "trich") is a common, curable STI.

Causes. Trichomonas infection is caused by the protozoan parasite *Trichomonas vaginalis.*

Signs and Symptoms. The vagina is the most common site of infection for females; the urethra is the most common site for males. Male patients may have penile irritation, dysuria, or a mild penile discharge, but more often than not, men have no symptoms. Females often have a frothy yellow-green vaginal discharge with a strong "fishy" odor to it. Itching and irritation of the vulva are also common.

Treatment. Oral metronidazole (Flagyl) is the treatment of choice. Both partners, even those who are asymptomatic, must be treated to avoid reinfection. Sexual contact should be avoided until after treatment is completed.

SUMMARY OF LEARNING OUTCOMES

LEARNING OUTCOMES	KEY POINTS
32.1 **Summarize the organs of the male reproductive system including the locations, structures, and functions of each.**	The organs of the male reproductive system include the testes, responsible for sperm and hormone production; the accessory organs of vas deferens, seminal vesicles, prostate gland, and bulbourethral glands; scrotum; and penis.
32.2 **Describe the causes, signs and symptoms, and treatment of various disorders of the male reproductive system.**	The diseases of the male reproductive system vary widely between simple inflammation and cancers, with varied signs, symptoms, and treatments. Some of these include benign prostatic hypertrophy, epididymitis, impotence (also called erectile dysfunction, or ED), prostate cancer, prostatitis, and testicular cancer.
32.3 **Summarize the organs of the female reproductive system including the locations, structures, and functions of each.**	The organs of the female reproductive system include the ovaries, fallopian tubes, uterus, and vagina. The external accessory organs include the mons pubis, labia majora and labia minora, clitoris, urethral meatus, vaginal orifice, Bartholin's glands, perineum, and mammary glands.

LEARNING OUTCOMES	KEY POINTS
32.4 **Describe the causes, signs and symptoms, and treatment of various disorders of the female reproductive system.**	The diseases of the female reproductive system vary widely between simple inflammation and cancers, with varied signs, symptoms, and treatments. Some of these include breast cancer, cervical cancer, cervicitis, dysmenorrhea, endometriosis, fibrocystic breast disease, ovarian cancer, premenstrual syndrome (PMS), uterine (endometrial) cancer, vaginitis, and vulvovaginitis.
32.5 **Explain the process of pregnancy, including fertilization, the prenatal period, and fetal circulation.**	Fertilization occurs with the union of a sperm cell and an ovum, usually within the fallopian tubes, but it may occur anywhere in the female reproductive tract. The fertilized ovum, now a blastocyst, implants in the endometrial wall of the uterus. The embryonic period occurs from week 2 through week 8 of the pregnancy; the fetal period is from week 9 through delivery.
32.6 **Describe the birth process, including the postnatal period.**	The birth process ends pregnancy and occurs in three stages: Dilation (effacement), in which the cervix thins and softens and dilates up to 10 cm; expulsion (parturition), in which the baby is expelled from the vagina; and placental stage (afterbirth), in which the placenta is expelled through the vagina.
32.7 **Compare several birth control methods and their effectiveness.**	Some of the contraceptive methods include coitus interruptus; the rhythm method; mechanical barriers; chemical barriers; oral contraceptives; injectable, implantable, and insertable contraceptives; transdermal contraceptives; and surgical methods.
32.8 **Explain the causes of and treatments for infertility.**	The causes of infertility are varied, with about 15% of infertility from unknown causes. There are a number of infertility tests and treatments; the treatment plan depends on the reason for the infertility.
32.9 **Describe the causes, signs and symptoms, and treatments of the most common sexually transmitted infections.**	There are many sexually transmitted infections occurring in both sexes, all passed between sexual partners (both heterosexual and same-sex partners), with varied signs, symptoms, and treatments. Some of these include AIDS (acquired immunodeficiency syndrome), chlamydia, genital warts, gonorrhea, pubic lice, syphilis, and trichomoniasis.

C A S E   S T U D Y   C R I T I C A L   T H I N K I N G

Recall Raja Lautu from the beginning of the chapter. Now that you have completed the chapter, answer the following questions regarding her case.

1. From Raja's symptoms, which STI might you suspect she is experiencing?

2. What causes this STI, and how is it treated?

3. Why is it important for her sexual partner to be treated?

1. (LO 32.1) Testosterone is produced in the _____ of the testes.
   a. Seminiferous tubules
   b. Epididymis
   c. Vas deferens
   d. Interstitial cells
   e. Bulbourethral gland

2. (LO 32.3) The innermost layer of the uterus is the
   a. Endometrium
   b. Myometrium
   c. Perimetrium
   d. Infundibulum
   e. cervical orifice.

3. (LO 32.4) In _____, the normal uterine lining is found outside of the uterus.
   a. PID
   b. Endometriosis
   c. PMS
   d. Dysmenorrhea
   e. Trichomoniasis

4. (LO 32.6) A newborn is described as a neonate until it reaches the age of
   a. 4 weeks
   c. 2 months
   b. 6 weeks
   d. 6 months
   e. 1 year

5. (LO 32.7) "The Patch" is a _____ method of contraception.
   a. Barrier
   b. Mechanical
   c. Transdermal
   d. Chemical
   e. Surgical

6. (LO 32.2) An enlargement of the prostate gland due normal hormonal changes as a man ages is known as
   a. Epididymitis
   b. Erectile dysfunction
   c. Prostatitis
   d. Testicular cancer
   e. Benign prostatic hypertrophy

7. (LO 32.3) The union of the nucleus of an ovum and a the nucleus of a sperm to create one nucleus containing 46 chromosomes results in a(n)
   a. Blastocyst
   b. Embryo
   c. Zygote
   d. Inner cell mass
   e. Morula

8. (LO 32.8) Which of the following is *not* a test performed to diagnose infertility?
   a. Semen analysis
   b. Endometrial biopsy
   c. Hysterosalpingogram
   d. Amniocentesis
   e. Blood hormone measurements

9. (LO 32.9) The most commonly reported STI in the United States is
   a. Gonorrhea
   b. Chlamydia
   c. Syphilis
   d. AIDS
   e. Trichomoniasis

10. (LO 32.5) The structure in a fetus that allows most of the blood to bypass the liver is the
    a. Ductus venosus
    b. Foramen ovale
    c. Ductus arteriosus
    d. Fossa ovalis
    e. Ligamentum arteriosum

Analyze the following medical terms, presented throughout the chapter. Using a medical dictionary (or Appendix I) place a / mark between each word part. Define each word part and then define the whole word.

EXAMPLE: spermato/cyte = spermato means "sperm" + cyte means "cell"
Spermatocyte means "sperm cell"

1. blastocyst
2. ectoderm
3. endometrium
4. episiotomy
5. hysterectomy
6. lactiferous
7. neonate
8. oogenesis
9. oviduct
10. vasectomy
11. vaginosis
12. oophorectomy

33

The Digestive System

L E A R N I N G   O U T C O M E S

After completing Chapter 33, you will be able to:

33.1 Describe the organs of the alimentary canal and their functions.

33.2 Explain the functions of the digestive system's accessory organs.

33.3 Identify the nutrients absorbed by the digestive system and where they are absorbed.

33.4 Describe the causes, signs and symptoms, and treatments of various common diseases and disorders of the digestive system.

K E Y   T E R M S

alimentary canal
bile
bolus
cardiac sphincter
chemical digestion
cholesterol
chyme
diverticula
esophageal hiatus
feces

glycogen
lipid
mechanical digestion
nutrient
palate
peritoneum
sphincter
triglycerides
uvula

CAAHEP

I.C (4)   List major organs in each body system

I. C (5)   Describe the normal function of each body system

I. C (6)   Identify common pathology related to each body system

I. C (7)   Analyze pathology as it relates to the interaction of body systems

I. C (9)   Describe implications for treatment related to pathology

I. C (10)   Compare body structure and function of the human body across the life span

I. C (12)   Describe the relationship between anatomy and physiology of all body systems and medications used for treatment in each

IV. C (11)   Define both medical terms and abbreviations related to all body systems

ABHES

2. Anatomy & Physiology

Graduates:

b. Identify and apply the knowledge of all body systems; their structure and functions; and their common diseases, symptoms, and etiologies

c. Assist the physician with the regimen of diagnostic and treatment modalities as they relate to each body system

3. Medical Terminology

Graduates:

b. Build and dissect medical terms from roots/suffixes to understand the word element combinations that create medical terminology

c. Understand the various medical terminology for each specialty

d. Recognize and identify acceptable medical abbreviations

Introduction

Digestion is the mechanical and chemical breakdown of foods into forms that your body cells can absorb. The digestive system's organs carry out digestion and can be divided into two categories: organs of the alimentary canal and accessory organs. Organs of the **alimentary canal** form a tube or pathway that extends from the mouth to the anus. They are the mouth, pharynx, esophagus, stomach, small intestine, large intestine, and anal canal. The accessory organs include the teeth, tongue, salivary glands, liver, gallbladder, and pancreas (Figure 33-1). You may find it helpful to review the "Organization of the Body" chapter to revisit the abdominal regions and quadrants while studying the organs described in this chapter.

Characteristics of the Alimentary Canal   LO 33.1

The wall of the alimentary canal, also known as the digestive tract, consists of four layers:

- *Mucosa.* The mucosa is the innermost layer of the wall and is made mostly of epithelial tissue that secretes enzymes and mucus into the lumen, or passageway, of the canal. This layer also is active in absorbing nutrients.

- *Submucosa.* The submucosa is the layer just outside the mucosa. It contains loose connective tissue, blood vessels, glands, and nerves. The blood vessels in this layer carry absorbed nutrients throughout the body.

- *Muscular layer.* This layer lies between the submucosa and the canal's outermost layer. It is made of layers of smooth muscle tissue and contracts to move materials through the canal.

- *Serosa.* The serosa is the double-walled outermost layer of the canal and is also known as the **peritoneum**. The innermost wall of the serosa is known as the *visceral peritoneum*. It secretes serous fluid to keep the outside of the canal moist, preventing it from sticking to other organs or to its outer layer, the *parietal peritoneum*, also called the abdominal lining.

Smooth muscle in the canal's wall can contract to produce two basic types of movements: churning and peristalsis. Churning mixes substances in the canal. Peristalsis propels substances through the tract (Figure 33-2).

The Mouth

The mouth, also known as the *buccal cavity*, takes in food and reduces its size through chewing—a process known as **mechanical digestion.** The mouth also starts the process of **chemical digestion** of food because saliva (spit) contains the enzyme amylase, which breaks down carbohydrates.

The cheeks consist of skin, adipose tissue, skeletal muscles, and an inner lining of moist, stratified squamous epithelium. The cheeks hold food in the mouth. The lips contain sensory nerve fibers that can judge the temperature of food before it enters the mouth. The tongue is made mostly of skeletal muscles and is covered by a mucous membrane. The body of the tongue is held to the floor of the oral cavity by a flap of mucous membrane called the *lingual frenulum.* The tongue mixes food in the mouth and holds it between the teeth. It also contains taste buds. The back of the tongue contains two lumps of lymphatic tissue called *lingual tonsils* that destroy bacteria and viruses on the back of the tongue.

The **palate** is the roof of the mouth. It separates the oral cavity from the nasal cavity. The front of the palate—the hard palate—is rigid because it has bony plates in it. The back of the palate, or soft palate, lacks bony material so it is not rigid. The back of the soft palate hangs down into the throat. This portion

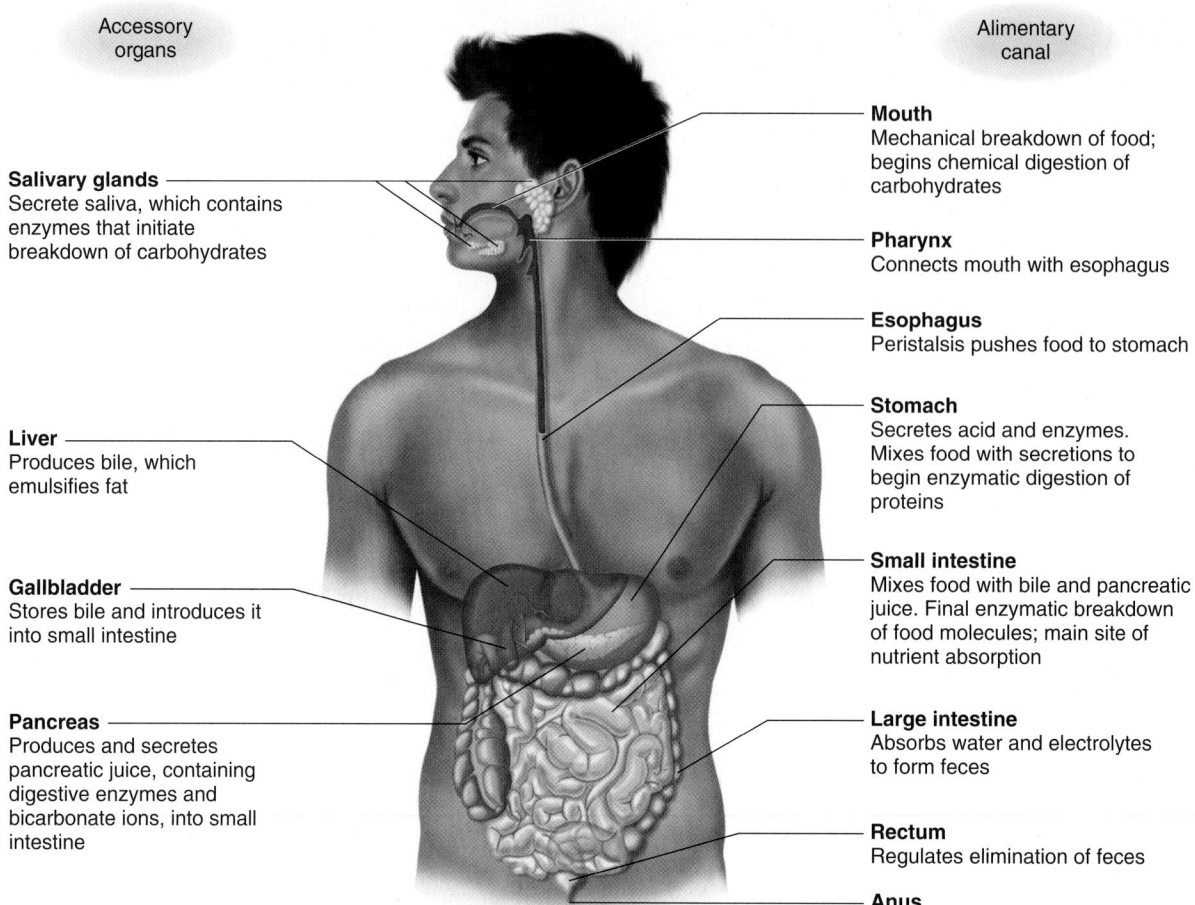

Accessory organs

Salivary glands
Secrete saliva, which contains enzymes that initiate breakdown of carbohydrates

Liver
Produces bile, which emulsifies fat

Gallbladder
Stores bile and introduces it into small intestine

Pancreas
Produces and secretes pancreatic juice, containing digestive enzymes and bicarbonate ions, into small intestine

Alimentary canal

Mouth
Mechanical breakdown of food; begins chemical digestion of carbohydrates

Pharynx
Connects mouth with esophagus

Esophagus
Peristalsis pushes food to stomach

Stomach
Secretes acid and enzymes. Mixes food with secretions to begin enzymatic digestion of proteins

Small intestine
Mixes food with bile and pancreatic juice. Final enzymatic breakdown of food molecules; main site of nutrient absorption

Large intestine
Absorbs water and electrolytes to form feces

Rectum
Regulates elimination of feces

Anus

FIGURE 33-1 Major organs of the digestive system.

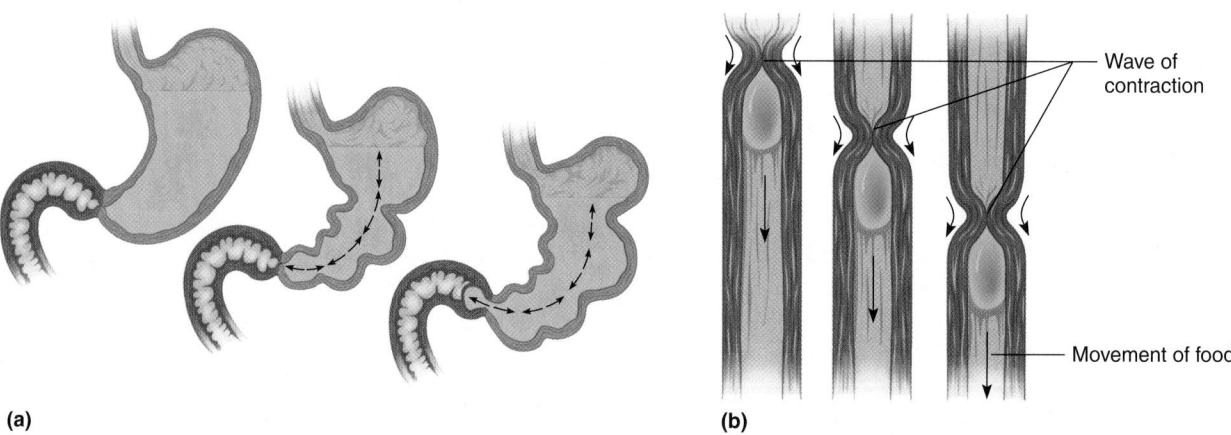

Wave of contraction

Movement of food

(a)   (b)

FIGURE 33-2 Movements through the alimentary canal: (a) Churning movements move substances back and forth to mix them. (b) Peristalsis moves contents along the canal.

of the soft palate is called the **uvula**. It prevents food and liquids from entering the nose during swallowing (Figure 33-3).

At the back of the mouth, where the oral cavity joins the pharynx in the area known as the *oropharynx*, are two masses of lymphatic tissue called *palatine tonsils*. Just above the palatine tonsils, in the area known as the *nasopharynx* (the nasal cavity joins the pharynx here), are two more masses of lymphatic tissue called the *pharyngeal tonsils*, or *adenoids*. These

masses of lymphatic tissue protect the area from bacteria and viruses.

Humans have 32 teeth—16 on the upper jaw and 16 on the lower jaw—which work to decrease the size of food particles. Different types of teeth are adapted to handle food in different ways. The most medial teeth, called *incisors*, act as chisels to bite off food pieces. Teeth called *cuspids*, also known as the canines, are the sharpest teeth and designed to tear tough food (Figure 33-4).

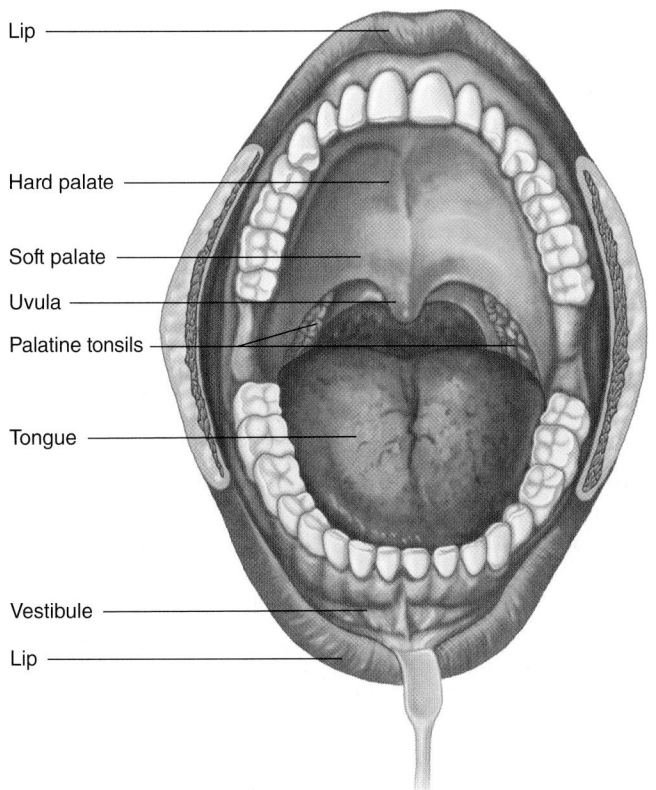

FIGURE 33-3 Structures of the mouth.

Labels for Figure 33-3:
Lip
Hard palate
Soft palate
Uvula
Palatine tonsils
Tongue
Vestibule
Lip

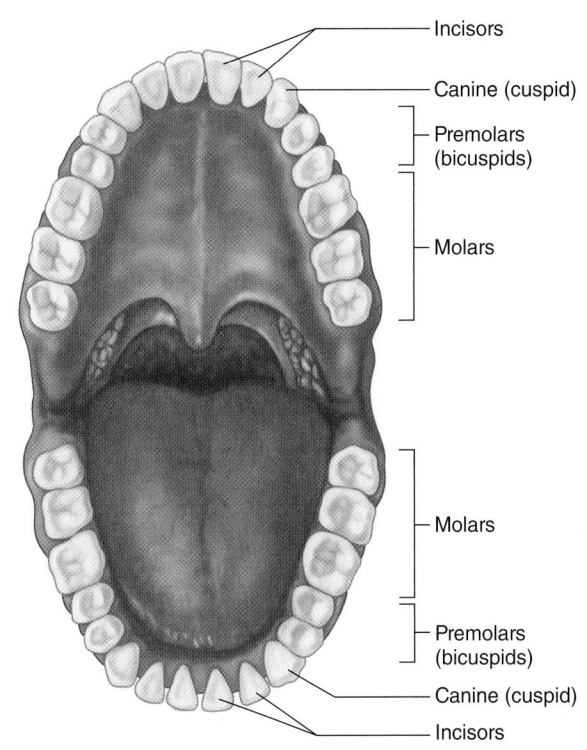

FIGURE 33-5 Types of teeth.

Labels for Figure 33-5:
Incisors
Canine (cuspid)
Premolars (bicuspids)
Molars
Molars
Premolars (bicuspids)
Canine (cuspid)
Incisors

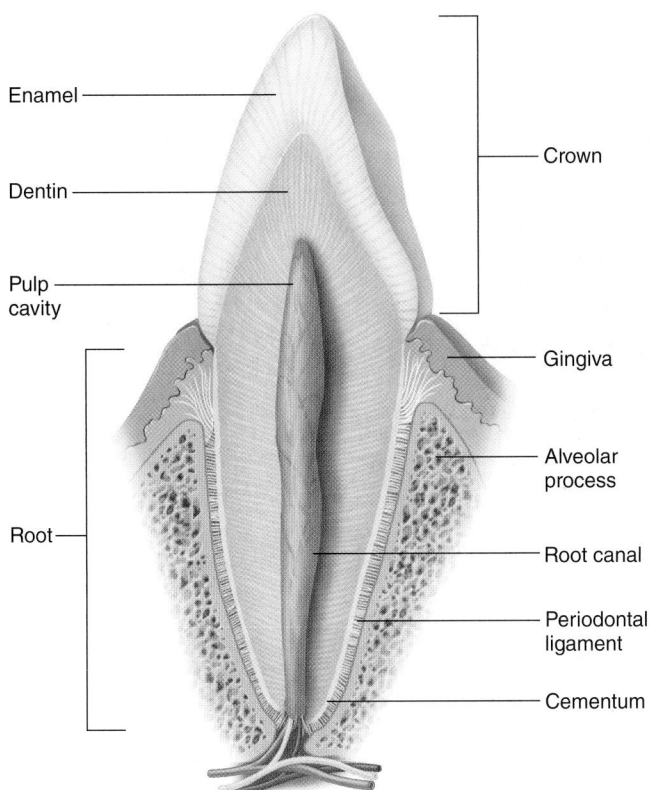

FIGURE 33-4 Structure of a cuspid tooth.

Labels for Figure 33-4:
Enamel
Dentin
Pulp cavity
Root
Crown
Gingiva
Alveolar process
Root canal
Periodontal ligament
Cementum

The back teeth, called *bicuspids* and *molars*, are flat and designed to grind food (Figure 33-5).

Salivary glands secrete saliva—a mixture of water, enzymes, and mucus—and are made of two types of cells: serous cells and mucous cells. Serous cells secrete a fluid made mostly of water, and they also secrete amylase. Mucous cells secrete mucus. The mass created by food mixed with the saliva and mucous mixture is called a **bolus.**

All major salivary glands are paired (Figure 33-6):

- *Parotid glands* are the largest of the salivary glands, located beneath the skin just in front of the ears.
- *Submandibular glands* are located in the floor of the mouth just inside the surface of the mandibles (jaws).
- *Sublingual glands* are the smallest of the salivary glands, located in the floor of the mouth beneath the tongue.

The Pharynx

The pharynx, commonly called the throat, is a long, muscular structure that extends from the area behind the nose to the esophagus. It connects the nasal cavity with the oral cavity for breathing through the nose. It also pushes food into the esophagus (Figure 33-7).

The divisions of the pharynx are:

- *Nasopharynx:* the portion behind the nasal cavity.
- *Oropharynx:* the portion behind the oral cavity.
- *Laryngopharynx:* the portion behind the larynx. The laryngopharynx continues as the esophagus.

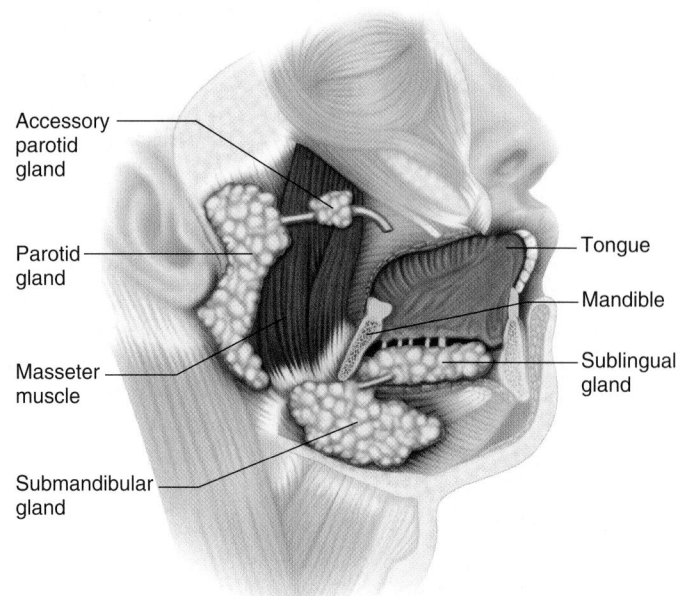

Accessory parotid gland

Parotid gland

Masseter muscle

Submandibular gland

Tongue

Mandible

Sublingual gland

FIGURE 33-6 Major salivary glands.

Swallowing is largely a reflex. In other words, it is an automatic response that does not require much thought. The following events occur during swallowing:

1. The soft palate rises, causing the uvula to cover the opening between the nasal cavity and the oral cavity.
2. The epiglottis covers the opening of the larynx so food does not enter it (see Figure 33-7).
3. The tongue presses against the roof of the mouth, forcing food into the oropharynx.
4. The muscles in the pharynx contract, forcing food toward the esophagus.
5. The esophagus opens.
6. The muscles of the pharynx push food into the cardiac sphincter.

The Esophagus

The esophagus is a muscular tube that connects the pharynx to the stomach (Figures 33-7 and 33-8). It descends through the thoracic cavity, through the diaphragm, and into the abdominal cavity, where it joins the stomach. The hole in the diaphragm that the esophagus goes through is called the **esophageal hiatus.** This hiatus is a place where hernias commonly occur. A hernia develops when an organ pushes through a wall that contains it.

Frontal sinus

Nasal cavity

Hard palate

Vestibule

Tongue

Tooth

Lip

Hyoid bone

Sphenoidal sinus

Pharyngeal tonsils

Opening of auditory tube

Soft palate

Nasopharynx

Oral cavity

Uvula

Palatine tonsils

Oropharynx

Lingual tonsil

Epiglottis

Laryngopharynx

Esophagus

Trachea

FIGURE 33-7 Sagittal section of the mouth, nasal cavity, and pharynx.

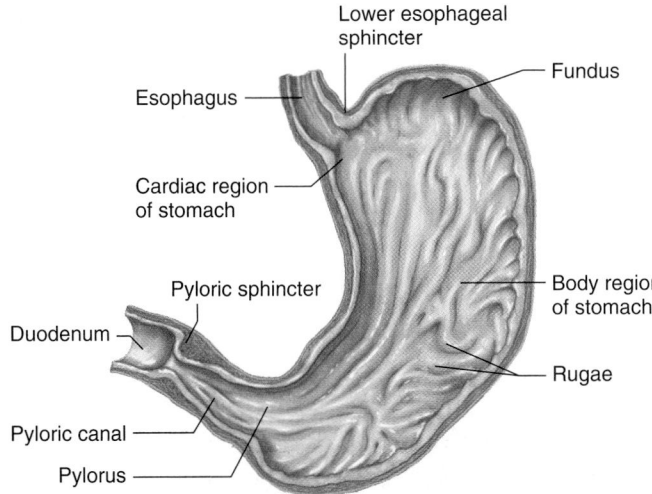

FIGURE 33-8 Regions of the stomach.

A hiatal hernia occurs when the stomach gets pushed up into the thoracic cavity through the esophageal hiatus.

The **cardiac sphincter**, also known as the *esophageal sphincter*, controls the movement of food into the stomach. **Sphincters** are circular bands of muscle located at the openings of many tubes in the body. They open and close to allow or prevent the movement of substances out of a tube.

The Stomach

The stomach lies below the diaphragm in the left upper quadrant of the abdominal cavity. The folds of the inner lining of the stomach are called *rugae*. The stomach receives the food bolus from the esophagus, mixes food with gastric juice (secretions of the stomach lining), starts protein digestion, and moves food into the small intestine. The mixture of food and gastric juices is called **chyme.** Once chyme is well mixed, stomach contractions push it into the small intestine a little at a time. It takes 4 to 8 hours for the stomach to empty following a meal. The stomach does not absorb many substances, but it can absorb alcohol, water, and some fat-soluble drugs.

The beginning portion of the stomach that is attached to the esophagus is called the *cardiac region*. The portion of the stomach that balloons over the cardiac region is the *fundus*. The main part of the stomach is called the *body*, and the narrow portion connected to the small intestine is the *pylorus*. The *pyloric sphincter* controls the movement of substances from the pylorus of the stomach into the small intestine (Figure 33-8).

The lining of the stomach contains gastric glands, which are made of the following cell types:

- *Mucous cells:* Secrete mucus to protect the lining of the stomach.
- *Chief cells:* Secrete pepsinogen, which becomes *pepsin* in the presence of acid. Pepsin digests proteins.
- *Parietal cells:* Secrete hydrochloric acid, which is necessary to convert pepsinogen to pepsin. They also secrete *intrinsic factor*, which is necessary for vitamin B_{12} absorption.

When a person smells, tastes, or sees appetizing food, the parasympathetic nervous system stimulates the gastric glands to secrete their products. A hormone called *gastrin*, made by the stomach, also stimulates the gastric glands to become active. A hormone called *cholecystokinin (CCK)*, made by the small intestine, inhibits gastric glands.

If a patient is unable to swallow for any reason, a gastrostomy tube or G tube may be inserted into the patient's stomach so he can be fed liquid meals, like Ensure, through this tube.

The Small Intestine

The small intestine is a coiled, tubular organ that extends from the stomach to the large intestine. It fills most of the abdominal cavity. The small intestine carries out most of the digestion in the body and is responsible for absorbing most of the nutrients into the bloodstream.

The beginning of the small intestine is called the *duodenum*. It is C-shaped and relatively short. The middle portion of the small intestine is called the *jejunum*. It is coiled and forms the majority of the small intestine. If a patient's stomach is diseased or removed, a jejunostomy or J tube may be inserted into the jejunum to allow her to receive nutrition.

The last portion of the small intestine is called the *ileum*, and it is directly attached to the large intestine. The jejunum and ileum are held in the abdominal cavity by a fan-like tissue called the *mesentery* that attaches to the posterior wall of the abdomen (Figure 33-9).

The lining of the small intestine contains cells that have *microvilli*. Microvilli greatly increase the surface area of the small intestine so it can absorb nutrients more efficiently. The lining of the small intestine also contains glands that secrete various substances. The secretions of the small intestine include mucus and water. Water aids in digestion, but some toxins cause the secretion of too much water, and this leads to diarrhea—which in turn aids the body in eliminating the toxins. Mucus protects the lining of the small intestine. The following are the major enzymes the small intestine secretes:

- *Peptidases.* These enzymes digest proteins.
- *Sucrase, maltase, and lactase.* These enzymes digest sugars. A person who cannot produce lactase will not be able to digest

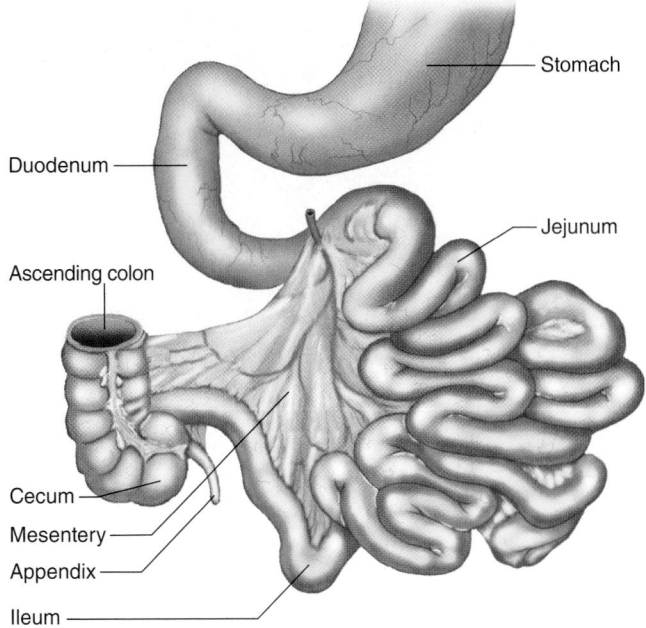

FIGURE 33-9 Parts of the small intestine.

lactose, which is the sugar in dairy products. This causes a condition called *lactose intolerance.*

- *Intestinal lipase.* This enzyme digests fats.

The parasympathetic nervous system and stretching of the wall of the small intestine are the primary factors that trigger the small intestine to secrete its products. The small intestine absorbs almost all nutrients (water, glucose, amino acids, fatty acids, glycerol, and electrolytes). The wall of the small intestine contracts to mix chyme and to propel it toward the large intestine. If chyme moves too quickly through the small intestine, nutrients are not absorbed and diarrhea results. The *ileocecal sphincter* controls the movement of chyme from the ileum to the *cecum*, which is the beginning of the large intestine.

The Large Intestine

The large intestine extends from the ileum of the small intestine to where it opens to the outside of the body as the anus. The beginning of the large intestine is the cecum. Projecting off the cecum is the *vermiform appendix,* which is made mostly of lymphoid tissue. It was once thought to have no function, but it is now thought to have a role in immunity. The cecum eventually gives rise to the ascending colon, which is the portion of the large intestine that runs up the right side of the abdominal cavity. If you remember that the appendix is in the right lower quadrant (RLQ), it will be easy to remember that the ascending colon also goes up the right side of the abdomen. The ascending colon becomes the transverse colon as it crosses the abdominal cavity; from there, it becomes the descending colon as it descends the left side of the abdominal cavity. In the pelvic cavity, the descending colon then forms the S-shaped tube called the *sigmoid colon.*

The Rectum and Anal Canal

Eventually, the sigmoid colon straightens out to become the *rectum.* The last few centimeters of the rectum are known as the *anal canal*, and the opening of the anal canal to the outside of the body is called the *anus* (Figure 33-10).

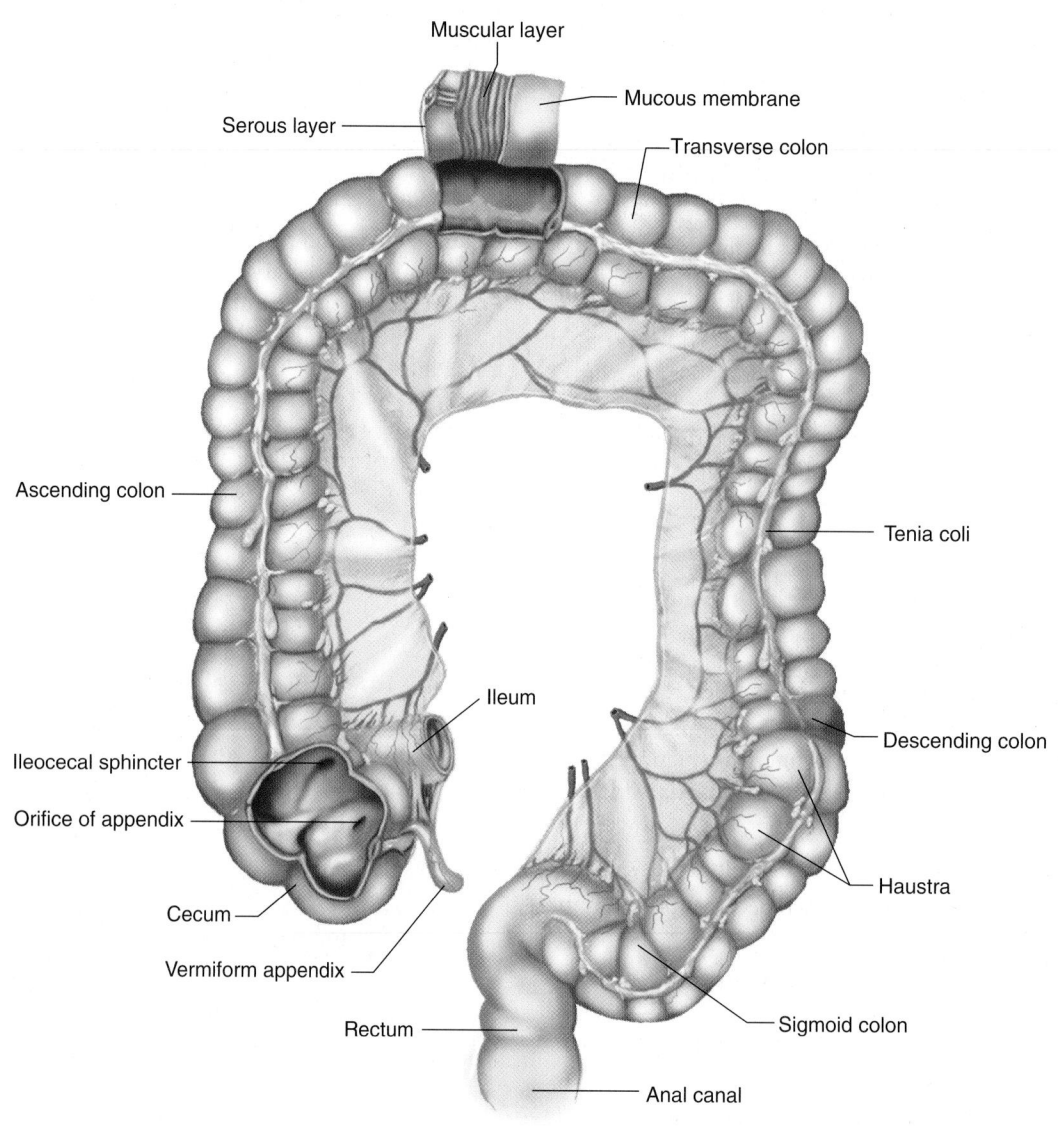

FIGURE 33-10 Parts of the large intestine.

The lining of the large intestine secretes mucus to aid in the movement of substances. As chyme leaves the small intestine and enters the large intestine, the proximal portion of the large intestine absorbs water and a few electrolytes from it. The left-over chyme is then called **feces,** which are made of undigested solid materials, a little water, ions, mucus, cells of the intestinal lining, and bacteria.

The contractions of the large intestine propel feces forward, but these contractions normally occur periodically and as mass movements. Mass movements trigger the *defecation reflex,* which allows the anal sphincters to relax and feces to move through the anus in the process of elimination. The squeezing actions of the abdominal wall muscles also aid in the emptying of the large intestine.

▶ Characteristics of the Digestive Accessory Organs

LO 33.2

Although they do not form part of the alimentary canal, the digestive system's accessory organs play important roles in digestion. They deliver enzymes and other substances to the alimentary canal to assist with the digestive process.

The Liver

The liver is quite large and fills most of the upper-right abdominal quadrant. Part of its function is to store vitamins and iron. It is reddish-brown in color and enclosed by a tough capsule that divides the liver into a large right lobe and a small left lobe (Figure 33-11). Each lobe is separated into smaller divisions called *hepatic lobules*. Branches of the *hepatic portal vein* carry blood from the digestive organs to the hepatic lobules. The hepatic lobules contain macrophages that destroy bacteria and viruses in the blood. Each lobule contains many cells called *hepatocytes*. Hepatocytes process the nutrients in blood and make **bile,** which is used in the digestion of fats. Bile leaves the liver through the hepatic duct. The *hepatic duct* merges with the *cystic duct* (the duct from the gallbladder) to form the *common bile duct*. This duct delivers bile to the duodenum.

The Gallbladder

The gallbladder is a small, sac-like structure located beneath the liver (Figures 33-11 and 33-12). Its only function is to store bile, which leaves the gallbladder through the cystic duct. The hormone cholecystokinin causes the gallbladder to release bile. The salts in bile break large fat globules into smaller ones so the digestive enzymes can more quickly digest them. Bile salts also increase the absorption of fatty acids, cholesterol, and fat-soluble vitamins into the bloodstream.

The Pancreas

The pancreas is located behind the stomach. Pancreatic *acinar cells* produce pancreatic juice, which ultimately flows through the pancreatic duct to the duodenum (Figure 33-12). Pancreatic juice contains the following enzymes:

- *Pancreatic amylase*, which digests carbohydrates
- *Pancreatic lipase*, which digests lipids
- *Nucleases,* which digest nucleic acids
- *Trypsin, chymotrypsin, and carboxypeptidase,* which digest proteins

The pancreas also secretes bicarbonate ions into the duodenum that neutralize the acidic chyme arriving from the stomach. The parasympathetic nervous system stimulates the pancreas to release its enzymes. The hormones secretin and cholecystokinin also stimulate the pancreas to release digestive enzymes. Secretin and cholecystokinin come from the small intestine.

Go to CONNECT to see an animation about *Food Absorption.*

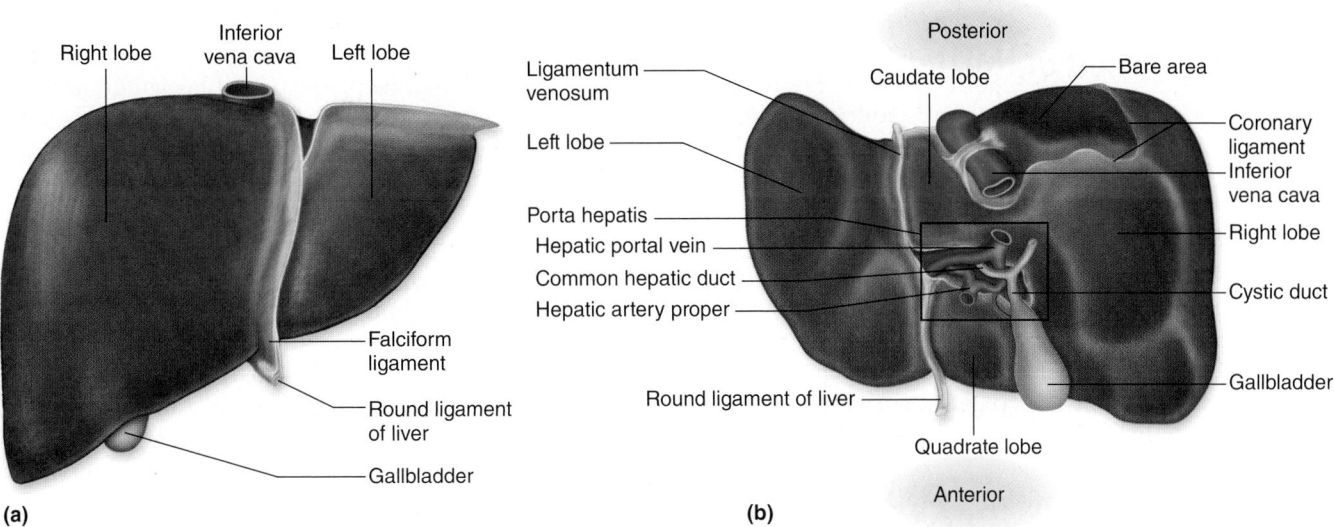

(a)

Right lobe | Inferior vena cava | Left lobe

Falciform ligament

Round ligament of liver

Gallbladder

(b)

Posterior

Ligamentum venosum

Caudate lobe

Bare area

Left lobe

Coronary ligament

Inferior vena cava

Porta hepatis

Hepatic portal vein

Common hepatic duct

Hepatic artery proper

Right lobe

Cystic duct

Round ligament of liver

Gallbladder

Quadrate lobe

Anterior

FIGURE 33-11 The liver is located in the right upper quadrant of the abdomen. (a) Anterior and (b) posteroinferior views show the four lobes of the liver, the gallbladder, inferior vena cava, hepatic portal vein, and hepatic artery (together known as the porta hepatis).

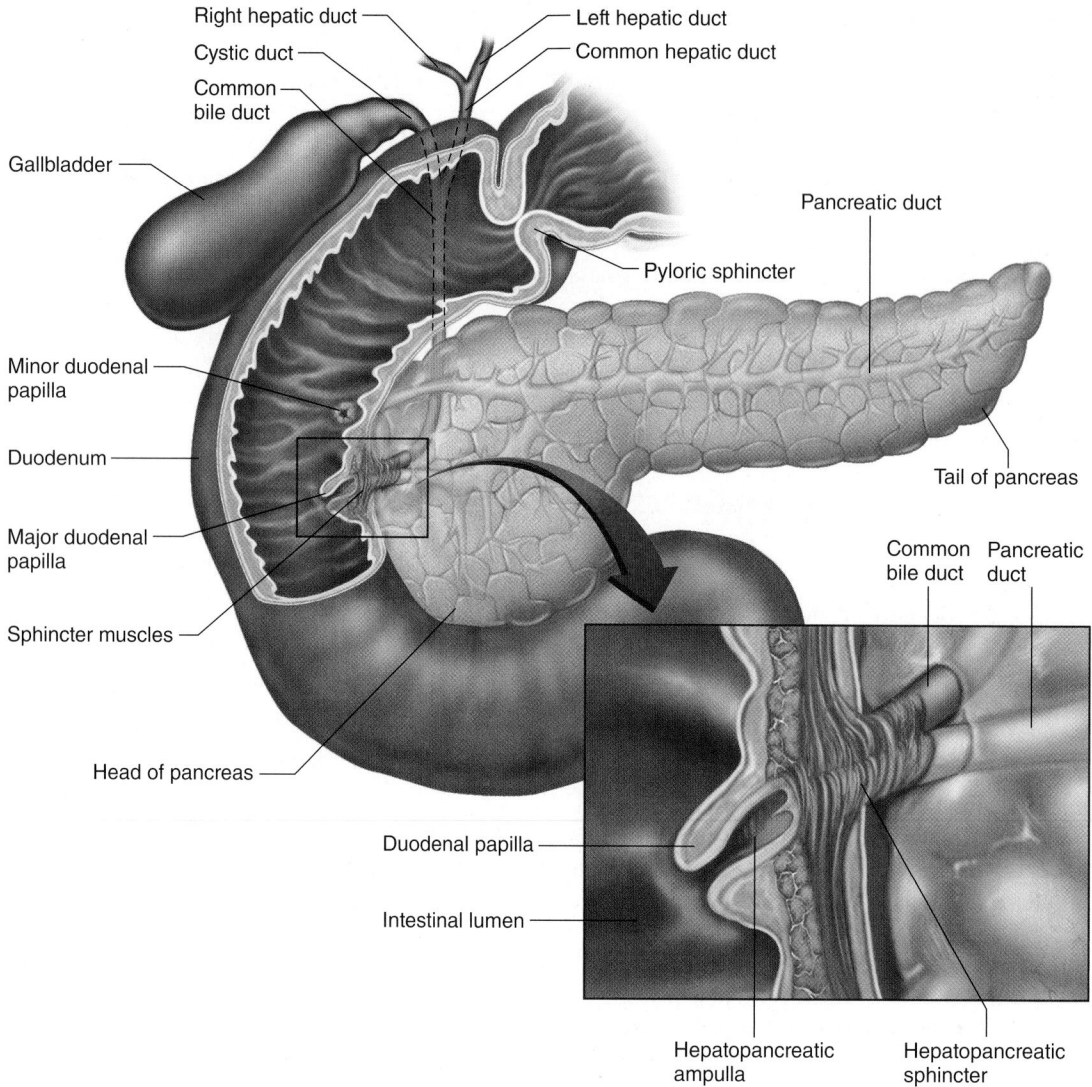

Right hepatic duct — — Left hepatic duct
Cystic duct — — Common hepatic duct
Common
bile duct
Gallblader

Pancreatic duct

— Pyloric sphincter

Minor duodenal
papilla

Duodenum

Major duodenal
papilla

Tail of pancreas

Sphincter muscles

Common Pancreatic
bile duct duct

Head of pancreas

Duodenal papilla

Intestinal lumen

Hepatopancreatic   Hepatopancreatic
ampulla   sphincter

FIGURE 33-12   Pancreas and its connections to the gallbladder and duodenum.

▶ The Absorption of Nutrients   LO 33.3

Necessary food substances are known as **nutrients.** They include carbohydrates, proteins, lipids, vitamins, minerals, and water.

Three types of carbohydrates that humans ingest are starches (polysaccharides), simple sugars (monosaccharides and disaccharides), and cellulose. Starches come from foods such as pasta, potatoes, rice, and breads. Monosaccharides and disaccharides are obtained from sweet foods and fruits. *Cellulose* is a type of carbohydrate found in many vegetables that humans cannot digest. So, cellulose provides fiber or bulk for the large intestine, which helps the large intestine to empty more regularly.

Harvard Medical International states a connection has been made between higher-fiber diets and a decrease in colon diseases, including cancer. This may be because fiber increases

water absorption and bulk, causing more rapid emptying of the colon and decreasing the production of benign growths like adenomas or polyps, which increase the risk of cancer. Fiber may also neutralize toxins produced by GI (gastrointestinal) tract bacteria.

Most body cells use the monosaccharide glucose to make ATP. ATP (adenosine triphosphate) is a type of chemical energy needed by the body. When a person has an excess of glucose, it can be stored in the liver and skeletal muscle cells as **glycogen. Lipids** (fats) are obtained through various foods. The most abundant dietary lipids are **triglycerides.** They are found in meats, eggs, milk, and butter. **Cholesterol** is another common dietary lipid and is found in eggs, whole milk, butter, and cheeses. Lipids are used by the body primarily to make energy when glucose levels are low. Excess triglycerides are stored in adipose tissue. Cholesterol is essential to cell growth and function; cells use it to make cell membranes

Aging and the Digestive System

As a person gets older, natural effects of aging cause changes in the digestive system, which can have important effects on both nutrition and medication dosages. As a medical assistant, you should be aware of these changes and their consequences for elderly patients.

In general, as a person ages, the mucus lining thins and the blood supply and number of smooth muscle cells within the alimentary canal decrease, which lead to decreased motility. The decreasing motility often causes gastroesophageal reflux disease (GERD) and constipation. The decreasing blood supply also affects the patient's ability to absorb medications and nutrients. Gastric secretions from the stomach, liver, and pancreas decrease, and the liver's ability to detoxify the blood also lessens. This makes adjusting medication dosages more difficult until it is clear (through lab tests or patient response) how rapidly and how much medication the patient's body

is absorbing. If the patient drinks alcohol, he may notice a difference in the way alcohol affects him. Advancing age also leaves the patient more likely to develop ulcerations and cancers of the GI system, including colorectal cancer, which is the second-leading cause of cancer deaths in the United States, according to the American Cancer Society.

Many elderly people state that their sense of taste is altered and that food loses some of its enjoyment. If the patient is lonely or feels isolated as a result of her social situation, and/or if depression is a component, her diet will likely change because "it is no fun or too much work to cook just for myself."

The medical assistant should be aware of these possibilities, looking for clues like weight loss, depression, or patient comments, and should relate information to the healthcare provider with a goal of securing social service assistance for the patient if needed.

and some hormones. People should have the essential fatty acid linoleic acid in their diet because the body cannot make it. This fatty acid is found in corn and sunflower oils. People also need a certain amount of fat to absorb fat-soluble vitamins.

The fat-soluble vitamins are vitamins A, D, E, and K; the water-soluble vitamins are all the B vitamins and vitamin C. The many functions of vitamins are summarized in Table 33-1.

Minerals—primarily found in bones and teeth—make up about 4% of total body weight. Cells use minerals to make enzymes, cell membranes, and various proteins like hemoglobin. The most important minerals to the human body are calcium, phosphorus, sulfur, sodium, chlorine, and magnesium. The body needs trace elements, including iron, manganese, copper, iodine, and zinc, in very small amounts.

Foods rich in protein include meats, eggs, milk, cheese, fish, chicken, turkey, nuts, seeds, and beans. Protein requirements vary from individual to individual, but all people must take in proteins that contain certain amino acids (called *essential amino acids*) because the body cannot make them. The body uses proteins for growth and tissue repair.

TABLE 33-1	Common Vitamins and Their Importance in the Body
Vitamin	**Function**
Vitamin A	Needed for the production of visual receptors, mucus, the normal growth of bones and teeth, and the repair of epithelial tissues.
Vitamin B$_1$ (thiamine)	Needed for carbohydrate metabolism.
Vitamin B$_2$ (riboflavin)	Needed for carbohydrate and fat metabolism and for the growth of cells.
Vitamin B$_6$	Needed for protein, antibody, and nucleic acid synthesis.
Vitamin B$_{12}$ (cyanocobalamin)	Needed for myelin production and carbohydrate and nucleic acid metabolism.
Biotin	Needed for protein, fat, and nucleic acid metabolism.
Folic acid	Needed for the production of amino acids, DNA, and red blood cells.
Pantothenic acid	Needed for carbohydrate and fat metabolism.
Niacin	Needed for carbohydrate, protein, fat, and nucleic acid metabolism.
Vitamin C (ascorbic acid)	Needed for the production of collagen, amino acids, and hormones and for iron absorption.
Vitamin D	Needed for calcium absorption.
Vitamin E	Antioxidant that prevents the breakdown of certain tissues.
Vitamin K	Needed for blood clotting.

PATHOPHYSIOLOGY

LO 33.4

Common Diseases and Disorders of the Digestive System

APPENDICITIS is an inflammation of the appendix. If not treated promptly, it can be life-threatening.

Causes. This disorder may be caused by an appendix blocked by feces or a tumor, infection, or other *idiopathic* (unknown) cause.

Signs and Symptoms. The signs and symptoms include lack of appetite, pain in the RLQ that may radiate throughout the abdomen and even down the right leg, nausea, slight fever, and an increased white blood cell (WBC) count.

Treatment. The primary treatments are antibiotics to prevent infection and an *appendectomy* to remove the appendix.

CIRRHOSIS is a chronic liver disease in which normal liver tissue is replaced with nonfunctional scar tissue.

Causes. This disease is often an autoimmune disease. It may also be caused by some medications and alcohol consumption. Hepatitis B and C infections can also contribute to the development of cirrhosis.

Signs and Symptoms. This disease has many symptoms, including anemia, fatigue, mental confusion, fever, vomiting, blood in the vomit, an enlarged liver, jaundice, unintended weight loss, swelling of the legs or abdomen, abdominal pain, decreased urine output, and pale feces.

Treatment. Alcohol consumption should be discontinued. A patient with cirrhosis may be given various medications, including antibiotics and diuretics. A liver transplant may be needed for the most seriously ill patients.

Go to CONNECT to see an animation about *Liver Failure*.

CHOLELITHIASIS, or gallstones, are hard deposits that usually consist of either cholesterol or bilirubin. They are more common in women than in men.

Causes. Gallstones can be caused by a variety of factors, including diabetes, cirrhosis, and other medical conditions; rapid weight loss; failure of the gallbladder to empty completely, which may occur during pregnancy; and organ transplant.

Signs and Symptoms. Some people who have gallstones do not have symptoms. If symptoms do occur, they may include pain in the right upper quadrant (RUQ) of the abdomen, fever, jaundice, nausea and vomiting, and clay-colored feces.

Treatment. Surgery to remove the stones is the most common treatment for people who have symptoms associated with gallstones. The most commonly used procedure is *laparoscopic cholecystectomy*. Another procedure, *lithotripsy*, is also a treatment option. It uses electrohydraulic shock waves to dissolve or break up the stones without the need for surgery. Medications are also used in some cases, but they take a long time to work.

COLITIS is inflammation of the large intestine. This condition can be chronic or short lived, depending on the cause.

Causes. Colitis can be caused by a viral or bacterial infection or the use of antibiotics. Ulcers in the large intestine, Crohn's disease, various other diseases, and stress may also contribute to the development of this disorder.

Signs and Symptoms. The primary symptoms are abdominal pain, bloating, and diarrhea.

Treatment. The first goal of therapy is to treat the underlying causes. Changing antibiotics, treating existing ulcers, and drinking plenty of fluids are treatment options. In advanced cases, surgery to remove the affected area of the colon, known as a *colectomy*, may be recommended. If too much of the colon is affected, a *colostomy* may be performed. In this procedure, the majority of the colon is removed and the opening to the outside of the body is moved to the abdomen where an appliance known as an ostomy, usually with a collecting device commonly called a bag, collects fecal material.

COLORECTAL CANCER usually comes from the lining of the rectum or colon. This type of cancer is curable if treated early.

Causes. The causes are mostly unknown, although research is putting some blame on high-fat/low-fiber diets. Polyps in the colon or rectum can become cancerous, leading to this disease. Colorectal cancer may be prevented through regular screenings for polyps, which is done with a procedure known as a colonoscopy.

Signs and Symptoms. Anemia, unintended weight loss, abdominal pain, blood in the feces, narrow feces, or changes in bowel habits are all common symptoms.

Treatment. Chemotherapy is the first line of treatment. Surgery to remove a cancerous tumor or the affected portions of the colon or rectum (colectomy or colostomy) may be needed in more advanced cases.

CONSTIPATION is the condition of difficult defecation, which is the elimination of feces.

Causes. The primary causes are lack of physical activity, lack of fiber and adequate water in the diet, the use of certain medications, and thyroid and colon disorders.

Signs and Symptoms. Common signs and symptoms include infrequent bowel movements (for example, no bowel movement for 3 days), bloating, abdominal pain and pain during bowel movements, hard feces, and blood on the surface of feces.

Treatment. Treatment includes an increase in dietary fiber; adequate fluid intake; regular exercise; and the use of stool softeners, laxatives, and enemas (for extreme cases only).

CROHN'S DISEASE is a common disorder called *inflammatory bowel disease*. It typically affects the end of the small intestine.

Causes. This is an autoimmune disorder.

Signs and Symptoms. The signs and symptoms of Crohn's disease include fever, tender gums, joint pain, GI ulcers, abdominal pain and gas, constipation or diarrhea, abnormal abdominal sounds, weight loss, intestinal bleeding, and blood in the feces.

Treatment. The first treatment is to change the patient's diet. Other treatments include medications to reduce inflammation, including steroids, as well as antibiotics and bowel "rest" in which IV (intravenous) feedings are given so the patient's digestive system is not used. For the most serious cases, surgery to remove the affected part of the intestine may be needed. This procedure is known as an *enterectomy*.

DIARRHEA is the condition of watery and frequent feces. Many cases of diarrhea do not require treatment because they usually stop within a day or two.

Causes. The causes of diarrhea include bacterial, viral, or parasitic infections of the digestive system. It may also be caused by the ingestion of toxins; food allergies, including lactose intolerance; ulcers; Crohn's disease; laxative use; antibiotics; chemotherapy; and radiation therapy. Diarrhea related to infections may be prevented by washing hands thoroughly and cooking food properly.

Signs and Symptoms. The symptoms include abdominal cramps, watery feces, and the frequent passage of feces.

Treatment. Patients should drink fluids to prevent dehydration. The underlying causes, if known, should be treated. Medications and dietary changes are the primary treatment options. In severe cases, antidiarrheal medications such as Lomotil may be prescribed.

DIVERTICULITIS is inflammation of diverticula in the intestine. **Diverticula** are abnormal dilations or pouches in the intestinal wall. When the diverticula are not inflamed, the condition is known as **DIVERTICULOSIS.**

Causes. The causes are mostly unknown. Lack of fiber in the diet and a bacterial infection of the diverticula can cause this disorder. Patients have found that certain foods, like peanuts and seeds, aggravate this disorder.

Signs and Symptoms. Signs and symptoms include fever, nausea, abdominal pain, constipation or diarrhea, blood in the feces, and a high WBC.

Treatment. Treatments include a high-fiber diet, antibiotics, and keeping a food diary to track foods that cause flare-ups. A *colectomy* (surgery to remove the affected portion of the intestine) may be necessary in severe cases.

GASTRITIS is an inflammation of the stomach lining. It is often referred to as an "upset stomach."

Causes. Gastritis can be caused by bacteria or viruses, some medications, alcohol use, spicy foods, excessive eating, poisons, and stress. Cooking food properly to kill harmful bacteria and viruses can help to prevent this condition.

Signs and Symptoms. Symptoms include nausea, lack of appetite, heartburn, vomiting, and abdominal cramps. An upper endoscopy may be done to confirm the diagnosis and rule out more serious conditions, such as an ulcer or cancer.

Treatment. Lifestyle changes should be implemented to avoid foods or medications that irritate the stomach lining. Treatment with various medications to reduce the production of stomach acids, such as Pepcid and Nexium, can provide relief from the symptoms of this disorder.

HEARTBURN is also called **GASTROESOPHAGEAL REFLUX DISEASE (GERD)**. It occurs when stomach acids are pushed into the esophagus.

Causes. Alcohol, some foods, a defective cardiac sphincter, pregnancy, obesity, a hiatal hernia, and repeated vomiting can contribute to the development of this disease.

Signs and Symptoms. Common symptoms include frequent burping, difficulty swallowing, a sore throat, a burning sensation in the chest following meals and nausea when lying down, and blood in the vomit.

Treatment. Treatment includes weight loss, making dietary changes, reducing alcohol consumption, taking medications such as Pepcid and Nexium, and elevating the head, neck, and chest when lying down.

HEMORRHOIDS are varicose veins of the rectum or anus.

Causes. Hemorrhoids are caused by constipation, excessive straining during bowel movements, liver disease, pregnancy, and obesity.

Signs and Symptoms. Signs and symptoms include itching in the anal area, painful bowel movements, bright red blood on feces, and veins that protrude from the anus.

Treatment. Constipation can be avoided or lessened by eating a high-fiber diet. Other treatments include stool softeners, medications to reduce hemorrhoid inflammation, and the surgical removal of hemorrhoids (*hemorrhoidectomy*).

HEPATITIS is inflammation of the liver. There are many different types of hepatitis.

Causes. Causes include bacteria, viruses, parasites, immune disorders, alcohol and drug use, and an overdose of acetaminophen. Preventive measures include getting hepatitis B (HBV) vaccinations, practicing safer sex, avoiding undercooked food (especially seafood), and using prescription or over-the-counter drugs (especially those containing acetaminophen) at their recommended dosages or as prescribed by a physician.

Signs and Symptoms. Symptoms include mild fever, bloating, lack of appetite, nausea, vomiting, abdominal pain, weakness, jaundice, itching in various body parts, an enlarged liver, dark urine, and breast development in males.

Treatment. Patients should avoid using alcohol and drugs. Various medications may be prescribed.

A **HIATAL HERNIA** occurs when a portion of the stomach protrudes into the chest through an opening in the diaphragm.

Causes. The causes are mostly unknown, although obesity and smoking are considered risk factors. Eating small meals can be an effective preventive measure.

Signs and Symptoms. Signs and symptoms include excessive burping, difficulty swallowing, chest pain, and heartburn.

Treatment. Treatments are weight reduction, medications to reduce stomach acid production, and surgical repair of the hernia.

INGUINAL HERNIAS occur when a portion of the large intestine protrudes into the inguinal canal, which is located where the thigh and the body trunk meet. In males, the hernia can also protrude into the scrotum.

Causes. The causes are mostly unknown, although these hernias may be caused by weak muscles in the abdominal walls.

Signs and Symptoms. A lump in the groin or scrotum or pain in the groin that gets worse when bending or straining are the common symptoms.

Treatment. Pain medications may be prescribed. Surgery to repair the hernia is needed, in which the large intestine is pushed back into the abdominal cavity.

ORAL CANCER usually involves the lips or tongue but can occur anywhere in the mouth. This type of cancer tends to spread rapidly to other organs.

Causes. The causes are mostly unknown, although the use of tobacco products and alcohol are known risk factors. Poor oral hygiene and ulcers in the mouth can also cause oral cancer.

Signs and Symptoms. Signs and symptoms include difficulty tasting; problems swallowing; and ulcers on the tongue, lip, or other mouth structures. Leukoplakia or hardened white patches in the mucous membrane of the mouth are considered precancerous lesions. A healthcare professional should examine them and biopsy them if they look suspicious.

Treatment. Radiation therapy, chemotherapy, and surgical removal of the malignant area are the treatment options.

PANCREATIC CANCER is the fourth leading cause of cancer deaths in the United States.

Causes. The causes are mostly unknown, although smoking and alcohol consumption are considered risk factors.

Signs and Symptoms. Common signs and symptoms include depression, fatigue, lack of appetite, nausea or vomiting, abdominal pain, constipation or diarrhea, jaundice, and unintended weight loss.

Treatment. Treatment includes radiation therapy, chemotherapy, and surgical removal of the tumor.

STOMACH CANCER most commonly occurs in the uppermost or cardiac portion of the stomach. It appears to occur more frequently in Japan, Chile, and Iceland than in the United States.

Causes. The causes are mostly unknown, although stomach ulcers may contribute to the development of stomach cancer.

Signs and Symptoms. Signs and symptoms include frequent bloating, lack of appetite, feeling full after eating small amounts, nausea, vomiting (with or without blood), abdominal cramps, excessive gas, and blood in the feces.

Treatment. Treatment includes radiation therapy, chemotherapy, and surgical removal of the tumor.

STOMACH ULCERS occur when the lining of the stomach breaks down.

Causes. Bacteria (particularly *Helicobacter pylori*), smoking, alcohol, excessive aspirin use, and hypersecretion of stomach acid can all cause stomach ulcers. They may be prevented by stopping smoking and avoiding aspirin, certain foods, and alcohol.

Signs and Symptoms. Symptoms include nausea, abdominal pain, vomiting (with or without blood), and weight loss. Diagnosis can be confirmed by an upper endoscopy.

Treatment. Treatment options include antibiotics, medications to reduce stomach acid production, *partial gastrectomy* (surgery to remove the affected portion of the stomach), and *vagotomy* (cutting the vagus nerve) to reduce the production of stomach acid.

SUMMARY OF LEARNING OUTCOMES

LEARNING OUTCOMES	KEY POINTS
33.1 Describe the organs of the alimentary canal and their functions.	The pathway of food through the alimentary canal starts with the mouth and continues through the pharynx, esophagus, stomach, small intestine, large intestine, and anal canal. The mouth takes in food and the teeth assist in reducing its size through chewing. The tongue mixes food and holds it between the teeth. The salivary glands produce saliva to moisten and break down food. The pharynx is a long muscular tube connecting the oral and nasal cavities. It pushes food into the esophagus. The esophagus is a muscular tube that pushes food toward the stomach through muscular contractions. The stomach receives the food, mixes it with gastric juices to start protein digestion, and moves it into the small intestine. The small intestine carries out most of the nutrient absorption. The large intestine's primary job is to rid the body of solid waste by defecation.
33.2 Explain the functions of the digestive system's accessory organs.	The accessory organs to the digestive system include the liver, gallbladder, and pancreas. The liver stores vitamins and iron and produces macrophages to fight infection. It also secretes bile for fat digestion. The gallbladder stores the bile produced by the liver. The pancreas produces pancreatic juices that assist in carbohydrate, lipid, and protein digestion.

LEARNING OUTCOMES	KEY POINTS
33.3 **Identify the nutrients absorbed by the digestive system and where they are absorbed.**	Nutrients absorbed by the body include carbohydrates, proteins, lipids, vitamins, minerals, and water. Most of the absorption takes place in the small intestine.
33.4 **Describe the causes, signs and symptoms, and treatments of various common diseases and disorders of the digestive system.**	There are many common diseases and disorders of the digestive system with varied signs, symptoms, and treatments. Some of these include appendicitis, cirrhosis, cholelithiasis, colitis, colorectal cancer, constipation, Crohn's disease, diarrhea, diverticulitis, diverticulosis, gastritis, heartburn (also called gastroesophageal reflux disease, or GERD), hemorrhoids, hepatitis, hiatal hernia, inguinal hernia, oral cancer, pancreatic cancer, stomach cancer, and stomach ulcers.

CASE STUDY CRITICAL THINKING

Recall Sylvia Gonzales from the beginning of this chapter. Now that you have completed the chapter, answer the following questions regarding her case.

1. What is the function of the gallbladder?

2. If Sylvia did not want to have surgery, what other treatment options are available?

3. Will Sylvia need to change her diet once her gallbladder is removed?

EXAM PREPARATION QUESTIONS

1. (LO 33.1) Which layer of the digestive tract is the most active in absorbing nutrients?
 a. Mucosa
 b. Submucosa
 c. Muscular
 d. Serosa
 e. Visceral

2. (LO 33.2) Which of the following organs is an accessory organ of the digestive process?
 a. Stomach
 b. Small intestine
 c. Liver
 d. Esophagus
 e. Pharynx

3. (LO 33.1) Although it hangs from the soft palate, the _____ is not one of the tonsils.
 a. Lingual
 b. Uvula
 c. Palatine
 d. Pharyngeal
 e. Adenoid

4. (LO 33.1) When an organ pushes through the wall that contains it, a(n) _____ develops.
 a. Sphincter
 b. Aneurysm
 c. Ulcer
 d. Hernia
 e. Bolus

5. (LO 33.4) Also known as inflammatory bowel disease, _____ often affects the end of the small intestine.
 a. Diverticulitis
 b. Crohn's disease
 c. GERD
 d. Colitis
 e. Cholelithiasis

6. (LO 33.2) Which of the following is made by the liver?
 a. Amylase
 b. Trypsin
 c. Secretin
 d. Bilirubin
 e. Bile

7. (LO 33.3) Which of the following is *not* a type of carbohydrate?
   a. Monosaccharides
   b. Polysaccharides
   c. Cellulose
   d. Disaccharides
   e. Triglycerides

8. (LO 33.3) Why do people need to include fiber in their diet?
   a. To help the large intestine empty more regularly
   b. To make energy when glucose levels are low
   c. To make cell membranes and hormones
   d. To help the body absorb fat-soluble vitamins
   e. To help synthesize antibodies and nucleic acids

9. (LO 33.4) Which of the following terms is used to describe difficult defecation?
   a. Cirrhosis
   b. Constipation
   c. Cholelithiasis
   d. Diarrhea
   e. Crohn's disease

10. (LO 33.4) Which disorder is commonly referred to as an "upset stomach"?
    a. GERD
    b. Diverticulitis
    c. Gastritis
    d. Hiatal hernia
    e. Crohn's disease

M E D I C A L   T E R M I N O L O G Y   P R A C T I C E

Analyze the following medical terms, presented throughout the chapter. Using a medical dictionary (or Appendix I) place a / mark between each word part. Define each word part and then define the whole word.

EXAMPLE: gastr/oid = gastr means "stomach" + oid means "resembling"
Gastroid means "resembling the stomach"

1. bicuspid
2. carboxypeptidase
3. diverticulosis
4. hepatocyte

5. idiopathic
6. laryngopharynx
7. nuclease
8. polysaccharide

9. pyloric
10. sublingual
11. hematemesis
12. gastroenteritis

The Endocrine System

LEARNING OUTCOMES

After completing Chapter 34, you will be able to:

34.1 Describe the general functions of hormones and the endocrine system.

34.2 Identify the hormones released by the pituitary gland, thyroid gland, parathyroid glands, adrenal glands, pancreas, and other hormone-producing organs, and give the functions of each.

34.3 Explain the effect of stressors on the body.

34.4 Describe the causes, signs and symptoms, and treatments of various endocrine disorders.

KEY TERMS

endocrine gland
exocrine gland
feedback loop
gonads
G-protein
hormone
islets of Langerhans
nonsteroidal hormone

parathyroid glands
pineal body
prostaglandins
steroidal hormone
stressor
thymus gland
thyroid gland

I. C (4)	List major organs in each body system	
I. C (5)	Describe the normal function of each body system	
I. C (6)	Identify common pathology related to each body system	
I. C (7)	Analyze pathology as it relates to the interaction of body systems	
I. C (8)	Discuss implications for disease and disability when homeostasis is not maintained	
I. C (9)	Describe implications for treatment related to pathology	
I. C (10)	Compare body structure and function of the human body across the life span	
I. C (12)	Describe the relationship between anatomy and physiology of all body systems and medications used for treatment in each	
IV. C (11)	Define both medical terms and abbreviations related to all body systems	

2. Anatomy & Physiology
Graduates:
b. Identify and apply the knowledge of all body systems, their structure and functions, and their common diseases, symptoms, and etiologies
c. Assist the physician with the regimen of diagnostic and treatment modalities as they relate to each body system

3. Medical Terminology
Graduates:
b. Build and dissect medical terms from roots/suffixes to understand the word element combinations that create medical terminology
c. Understand the various medical terminology for each specialty
d. Recognize and identify acceptable medical abbreviations

▶ Introduction

The endocrine (*endo-*, meaning "within," and *-crine*, meaning "to secrete") system includes the organs of the body that secrete hormones directly into body fluids such as blood. Hormones help to regulate the chemical reactions within cells. They therefore control the functions of the organs, tissues, and other cells. In this chapter, you will learn about the processes and organs of the endocrine system. Figure 34-1 shows the organs of the endocrine system, as well as the heart and kidney, both of which secrete a hormone, although hormone secretion is not the primary function of either of them. As shown, the gastrointestinal (GI) tract also secretes hormones, but again hormone secretion is not its primary function.

▶ Hormones   LO 34.1

Endocrine glands are ductless glands. This means they release their hormones directly into the tissues where they act or to the bloodstream, which carries them to their target cells. As you study each gland discussed in this chapter, refer to Figure 34-1 for its location.

Hormones are chemicals secreted by a cell that affect the functions of other cells. Once released, most hormones enter the bloodstream, which transports them to their target cells. A hormone's target cells are those that contain the receptors for the hormone. A hormone cannot affect a cell unless the cell has receptors for it, in much the same way that a locked door needs the key specifically cut to open its lock. Table 34-1 outlines the endocrine glands, the hormone(s) secreted by each, and the action resulting from each hormone.

Types of Hormones

Many hormones in the body are derived from steroids. Steroids are soluble in lipids and can therefore cross cell membranes easily. Once a **steroidal hormone** is inside a cell, it binds to its receptor, which is commonly in the cell's nucleus. The hormone-receptor complex turns a gene on or off. When new genes are turned on or off, the cell begins to carry out new functions, and this is ultimately how steroidal hormones affect their target cells. Examples of steroidal hormones are estrogen, progesterone, testosterone, and cortisol.

Nonsteroidal hormones are made of amino acids or proteins. Proteins cannot easily cross the cell membrane. Therefore, these hormones bind to receptors on the cell's surface. The hormone-receptor complex in the membrane usually activates a G-protein. The **G-protein** causes enzymes inside the cell to be turned on. Different chemical reactions then begin inside the cell, and the cell takes on new functions.

Prostaglandins are local hormones, also known as *tissue hormones*. They are derived from lipid molecules and typically do not travel in the bloodstream to find their target cells. Instead, their target cells are located close by. They have the same effects as other hormones and are produced by many body organs, including the kidneys, stomach, uterus, heart, and brain.

Negative and Positive Feedback Loops

Hormone levels are controlled by a mechanism known as a **feedback loop,** which can be negative or positive (see Figure 34-2). In a negative feedback loop, a stimulus such as eating raises blood sugar levels. This increase is detected by the

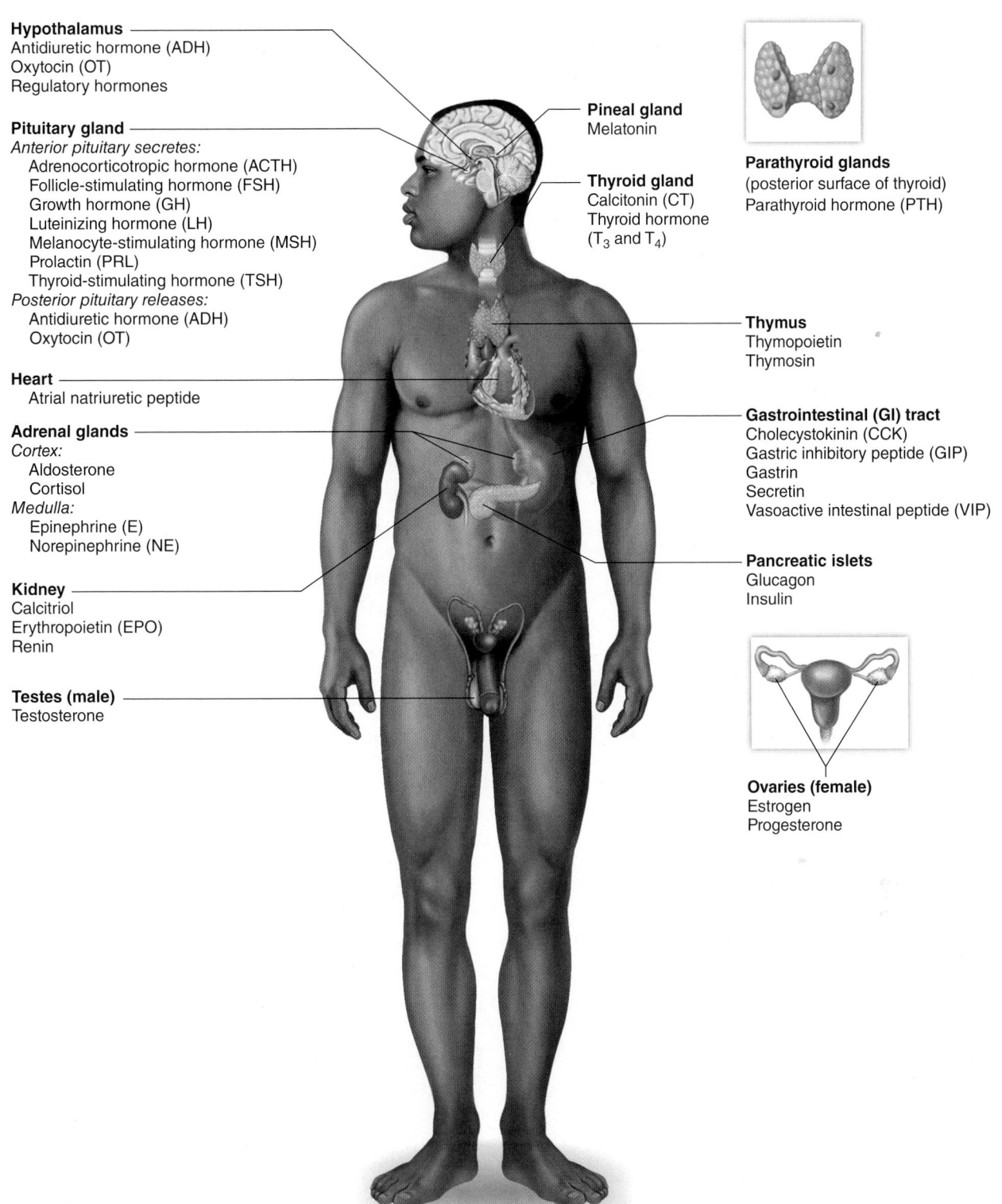

Hypothalamus
Antidiuretic hormone (ADH)
Oxytocin (OT)
Regulatory hormones

Pituitary gland
Anterior pituitary secretes:
 Adrenocorticotropic hormone (ACTH)
 Follicle-stimulating hormone (FSH)
 Growth hormone (GH)
 Luteinizing hormone (LH)
 Melanocyte-stimulating hormone (MSH)
 Prolactin (PRL)
 Thyroid-stimulating hormone (TSH)
Posterior pituitary releases:
 Antidiuretic hormone (ADH)
 Oxytocin (OT)

Heart
 Atrial natriuretic peptide

Adrenal glands
Cortex:
 Aldosterone
 Cortisol
Medulla:
 Epinephrine (E)
 Norepinephrine (NE)

Kidney
Calcitriol
Erythropoietin (EPO)
Renin

Testes (male)
Testosterone

Pineal gland
Melatonin

Thyroid gland
Calcitonin (CT)
Thyroid hormone
(T$_3$ and T$_4$)

Parathyroid glands
(posterior surface of thyroid)
Parathyroid hormone (PTH)

Thymus
Thymopoietin
Thymosin

Gastrointestinal (GI) tract
Cholecystokinin (CCK)
Gastric inhibitory peptide (GIP)
Gastrin
Secretin
Vasoactive intestinal peptide (VIP)

Pancreatic islets
Glucagon
Insulin

Ovaries (female)
Estrogen
Progesterone

FIGURE 34-1 Endocrine system—endocrine glands and other organs that secrete hormones are found throughout the body. They produce various types of hormones.

pancreas, which secretes the hormone insulin in response. As cells of the liver take up glucose to store it as glycogen and the body cells take up glucose for energy, the blood glucose levels decline and the insulin release stops as blood glucose levels normalize.

In a positive feedback loop, a stimulus also begins the process, as when a nursing infant suckles at the mother's breast. The suckling sends an impulse to the hypothalamus, which in turn signals the posterior pituitary to release oxytocin. The oxytocin stimulates milk production and ejection

TABLE 34-1 Endocrine Glands: Their Hormones and Actions

Gland	Hormone	Action Produced
Hypothalamus (produces)	Antidiuretic hormone (ADH)	Stored and released by posterior pituitary
	Oxytocin (OT)	Stored and released by posterior pituitary
Anterior pituitary	Growth hormone (GH)	Promotes growth and tissue maintenance
	Melanocyte-stimulating hormone (MSH)	Stimulates pigment regulation in epidermis
	Adrenocorticotropic hormone (ACTH)	Stimulates adrenal cortex to produce its hormones
	Thyroid-stimulating hormone (TSH)	Stimulates the thyroid to produce its hormones
	Follicle-stimulating hormone (FSH)	(F) Stimulates ovaries to produce ova and estrogen (M) Stimulates testes to produce testosterone
	Luteinizing hormone (LH)	(F) Stimulates ovaries for ovulation and estrogen production (M) Stimulates testes to produce testosterone
	Prolactin (PRL)	(F) Stimulates breasts to produce milk (M) Works with and complements LH
Posterior pituitary (releases)	Antidiuretic hormone (ADH)	Stimulates kidneys to retain water
	Oxytocin (OT)	Stimulates uterine contractions for labor and delivery
Pineal body	Melatonin	Regulates biological clock; linked to onset of puberty
Thyroid	T_3 and T_4	Protein synthesis and increased energy production for all cells
	Calcitonin	Increases bone calcium and decreases blood calcium
Parathyroid	Parathyroid hormone (PTH)	Agonist to calcitonin; decreases bone calcium and increases blood calcium
Thymus	Thymosin and Thymopoietin	Both hormones stimulate the production of T lymphocytes
Adrenal cortex	Aldosterone	Stimulates body to retain sodium and water
	Cortisol	Decreases protein synthesis; decreases inflammation
Adrenal medulla	Epinephrine and Norepinephrine	Prepare the body for stress; increase heart rate, respiration, and blood pressure
Pancreas (islets of Langerhans)	Alpha cells—Glucagon	Increases blood sugar; decreases protein synthesis
	Beta cells—Insulin	Decreases blood sugar; increases protein synthesis
Gonads: Ovaries (Female)	Estrogen and Progesterone	Secondary sex characteristics; female reproductive hormones
Testes (Male)	Testosterone	Secondary sex characteristics; male reproductive hormone

from the mammary glands. Milk continues to be released as long as the infant continues to nurse.

▶ Hormone Production   LO 34.2

Hormones are produced in various organs and glands throughout the body. For example, the brain has several sites of hormone production, including the hypothalamus, pituitary gland, and pineal body. The pancreas, kidneys, stomach, and reproductive organs also produce important hormones.

The Hypothalamus

The hypothalamus is located in the diencephalon of the brain (see *The Nervous System* chapter) and produces the hormones *oxytocin* and *antidiuretic hormone (ADH)*. These hormones are transported to the posterior pituitary, where they are stored and released as directed by the hypothalamus.

The Pituitary Gland

The pituitary gland, also known as the *hypophysis*, is located at the base of the brain and controlled by the hypothalamus. This gland is well protected by a bony structure called the sella turcica. The pituitary is divided into two lobes: the anterior lobe and the posterior lobe (see Figures 34-1 and 34-3).

Anterior Lobe of the Pituitary Gland The anterior lobe of the pituitary gland, also known as the *adenohypophysis*, secretes the following hormones:

* *Growth hormone (GH).* As its name suggests, this hormone stimulates an increase in the size of the body's muscles and bones. It is important in childhood for growth. It also stimulates tissue repair. Growth hormone is also known as *somatotropin.*

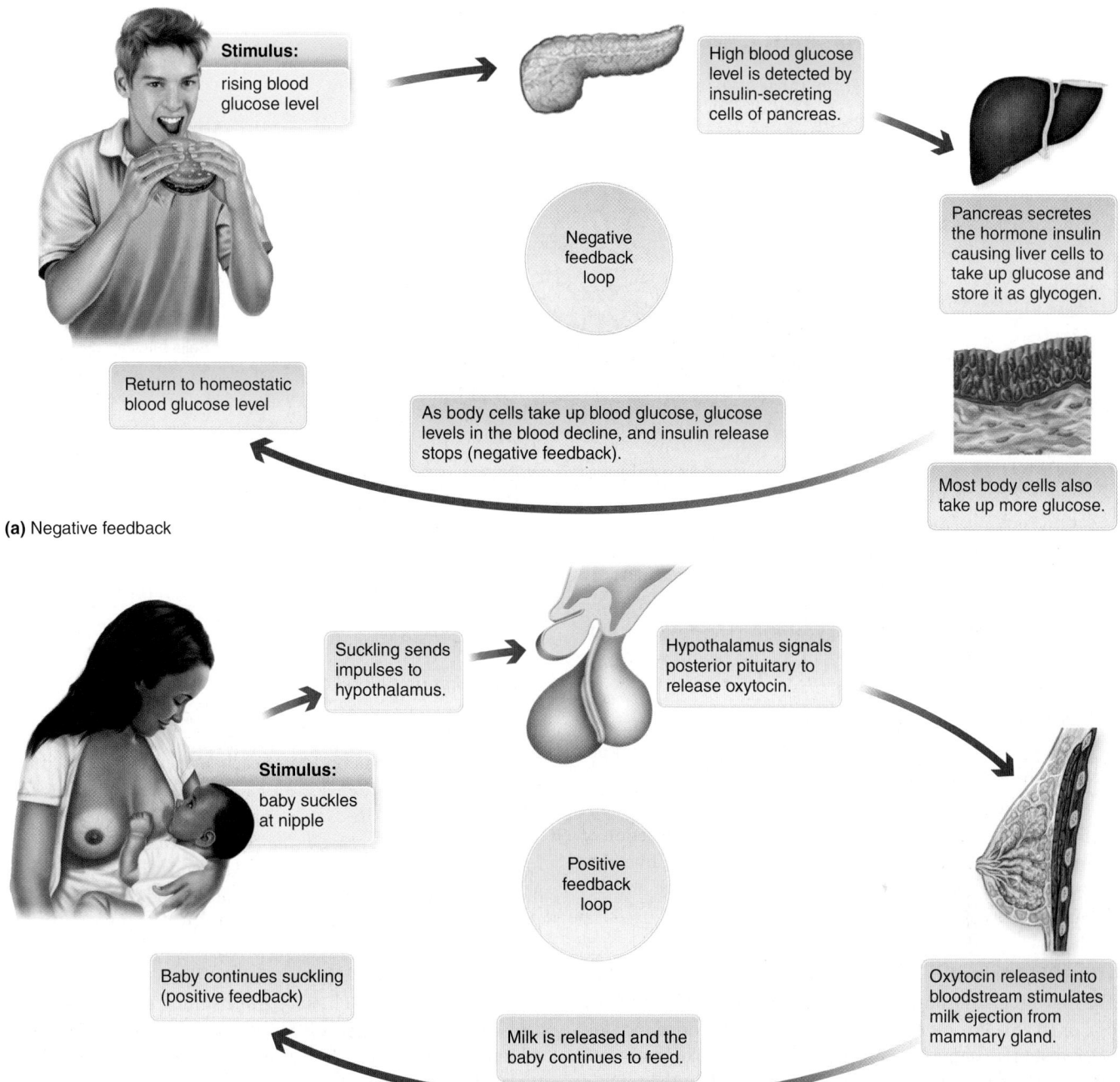

(a) Negative feedback

(b) Positive feedback

FIGURE 34-2 Positive and negative feedback loops in the endocrine system—the initial step in any feedback pathway is the stimulus. (a) A negative feedback loop occurs when the end product of a pathway turns off or slows down the pathway, whereas (b) a positive feedback loops is involved when the end product of a pathway stimulates further pathway activity.

- *Melanocyte-stimulating hormone (MSH).* This hormone stimulates synthesis of melanin and its disbursement to the skin cells of the epidermis.
- *Adrenocorticotropic hormone (ACTH).* This hormone stimulates the adrenal cortex to release its hormones.
- *Thyroid-stimulating hormone (TSH).* This hormone stimulates the thyroid gland to release its hormones.
- *Follicle-stimulating hormone (FSH).* In females, this hormone stimulates the production of estrogen by the ovaries. More significantly, FSH stimulates maturation of the

ova (eggs) before ovulation. In males, it stimulates sperm production.
- *Luteinizing hormone (LH).* In females, this hormone stimulates ovulation (the release of an egg from the ovaries) and the production of estrogen. In males, it stimulates the production of testosterone.
- *Prolactin (PRL).* In females, this hormone stimulates milk production by the mammary glands. Because of this function, it is sometimes called the lactogenic hormone. In males, prolactin is known to enhance the functioning of LH.

FIGURE 34-3 Location of the pituitary gland.

Posterior Lobe of the Pituitary Gland The posterior lobe of the pituitary gland, also known as the *neurohypophysis*, secretes the following hormones:

- *Antidiuretic hormone (ADH).* This hormone stimulates the kidneys to conserve water. It therefore decreases urine output and helps to maintain blood pressure.
- *Oxytocin (OT).* In females, this hormone causes contractions of the uterus during childbirth. It also causes the ejection of milk from mammary glands during breast-feeding. In males, oxytocin stimulates the contraction of the prostate and vas deferens during sexual arousal.

The Thyroid Gland and Parathyroid Glands

The **thyroid gland** consists of two lobes and sits below the voice box or larynx. It is covered by a capsule and is divided into follicles that store some of the hormones the thyroid gland produces. Two major types of hormones produced by the thyroid gland are *thyroid hormones* and *calcitonin*. There are two main thyroid hormones: *triiodothyronine (T_3)* and *thyroxine (T_4)*. The T stands for thyroid, and the numeral refers to the number of iodine atoms that are needed for each of these hormones to work properly.

Thyroid hormones increase cells' energy production, stimulate protein synthesis, and speed up the repair of damaged tissues. In children, they are important for normal growth and the development of the nervous system. Calcitonin lowers blood calcium levels by activating osteoblasts, which use excess blood calcium to build new bone tissue.

Most people have four **parathyroid glands.** They are small glands embedded into the posterior surface of the thyroid gland. The only hormone secreted by the parathyroid glands is called *parathormone* or *parathyroid hormone (PTH).* This hormone acts as an agonist to calcitonin by raising blood calcium levels through the activation of osteoclasts. Osteoclasts are bone-dissolving cells. When they dissolve bone, calcium levels in bone decrease as calcium is released into the bloodstream. This action raises blood calcium levels.

The Adrenal Glands

An adrenal gland sits on top of each kidney. It is divided into two portions: the adrenal medulla and the adrenal cortex. The adrenal medulla is the central portion of the gland and secretes *epinephrine* and *norepinephrine.* These hormones produce the same effects that the sympathetic nervous system produces. They increase heart rate, breathing rate, blood pressure, and all the other actions that prepare the body for stressful situations.

The adrenal cortex is the outermost portion of the adrenal gland. It secretes many hormones, but the two major ones are aldosterone and cortisol. *Aldosterone* stimulates the body to retain sodium, which helps it to retain water. It is important for maintaining blood pressure. *Cortisol* is released when a person is stressed. It decreases protein synthesis, so it slows down the repair of tissues. Its advantage is that it also decreases inflammation, which decreases pain.

The Pancreas

The pancreas is located behind the stomach. It is an endocrine gland as well as an exocrine gland. It is considered an **exocrine gland** because it secretes digestive enzymes into a duct that leads to the small intestine. It is considered an endocrine gland because it contains structures known as **islets of Langerhans** that secrete hormones into the bloodstream. The islets of Langerhans consist of two types of cells: alpha cells, which secrete glucagon, and beta cells, which secrete insulin.

Insulin promotes the cells' uptake of glucose. It therefore reduces glucose concentrations in the bloodstream. It also promotes the transport of amino acids into cells and increases protein synthesis. *Glucagon* increases glucose concentrations in the bloodstream and slows down protein synthesis.

Other Hormone-Producing Organs

The **pineal body** is a small gland located between the cerebral hemispheres. It secretes a hormone called *melatonin*. Melatonin helps to regulate your circadian rhythms, which are more commonly known as your biological clock. Your biological clock helps you decide when you should be awake or asleep. Melatonin is also thought to play a role in the onset of puberty.

The **thymus gland** lies between the lungs. It secretes a hormone called *thymosin*, which promotes the production of certain lymphocytes known as T lymphocytes. Refer to *The Cardiovascular System* chapter for further information about thymosin and the function of T cells.

Sometimes referred to as the **gonads**, the ovaries and testes are reproductive organs that secrete hormones. The ovaries release estrogen and progesterone, and the testes produce testosterone. The functions of these hormones are discussed in *The Reproductive Systems* chapter.

The stomach and small intestines also secrete hormones. The stomach produces gastrin, and the small intestine releases *secretin* and *cholecystokinin*. These hormones are discussed in *The Digestive System* chapter.

The heart secretes a hormone called *atrial natriuretic peptide*, which regulates blood pressure. The kidneys secrete a hormone called *erythropoietin*, which stimulates blood cell production.

▶ The Stress Response LO 34.3

Any stimulus that produces stress is termed a **stressor.** Stressors include physical factors such as extreme heat or cold, infections, injuries, heavy exercise, and loud sounds. Stressors also include psychological factors such as personal loss, grief, anxiety, depression, and guilt. Even positive stimuli such as sexual arousal, joy, and happiness can be stressors.

The body's physiologic response to stress consists of a group of reactions called the *general stress syndrome*, which is primarily caused by the release of hormones. This syndrome results in an increase in the heart rate, breathing rate, and blood pressure. Glucose and fatty acid concentrations also increase in the blood, which leads to weight loss. Prolonged stress causes the release of cortisol. Cortisol slows down body repair because it prevents protein synthesis and inhibits immune responses, which is why a person under stress becomes more susceptible to illness.

PATHOPHYSIOLOGY LO 34.4

Common Diseases and Disorders of the Endocrine System

Refer to Table 34-2 for a quick reference to diseases and disorders of the endocrine system. The table lists hormones according to the hyposecretion or hypersecretion of individual hormones. They are listed in "head-to-toe" order according to the organ that makes the hormone.

ACROMEGALY is a disorder in which too much growth hormone is produced in adults (see Figure 34-4).

Causes. This disorder is caused by an increased production of growth hormone or by a tumor of the pituitary gland.

Signs and Symptoms. The primary signs and symptoms include enlargement of the bones in the entire skull as well as in the hands and feet, and thickening of the skin. Other symptoms include

TABLE 34-2	Endocrine System Diseases/Conditions: Quick Reference Guide	
Hormone	**Hypo- or Hypersecretion**	**Disease or Condition**
GH (Somatotropin)	Hyposecretion (children)	Dwarfism
	Hypersecretion (children)	Gigantism
	Hypersecretion (adults)	Acromegaly
ACTH	Hyposecretion (adrenal cortex—cortisol)	Addison's disease
	Hypersecretion (adrenal cortex—cortisol)	Cushing's syndrome
ADH	Hyposecretion	Diabetes insipidus (dehydration)
	Hypersecretion	Edema, hypertension
T_3/T_4	Hyposecretion (congenital/children)	Cretinism
	Hyposecretion (adults)—*severe cases*	Hypothyroidism and *Myxedema*
	Hypersecretion (adults or children)	Graves' disease (hyperthyroidism)
Glucagon	Hyposecretion	Hypoglycemia
	Hypersecretion	Hyperglycemia
Insulin	Hyposecretion	Hyperglycemia (Diabetes mellitus)
	Hypersecretion	Hypoglycemia (hyperinsulinism)

Age 9   Age 16   Age 33   Age 52

FIGURE 34-4 Acromegaly is caused by the secretion of excessive growth hormone (GH) in adulthood. The face and hands are most notably affected, as seen in this individual at ages 9, 16, 33, and 52.

headache, fatigue, profuse sweating, pain (especially in the arms and legs), gaps between the teeth, weight gain, excessive hair production, cardiovascular diseases, arthritis, and vision problems.

Treatment. Treatment includes medications to lower the production of growth hormone, radiation therapy to reduce the size of a pituitary tumor, or surgery to remove a pituitary tumor.

ADDISON'S DISEASE is a condition in which the adrenal glands fail to produce enough corticosteroids. It affects about 1 in every 25,000 people (see Figure 34-5).

Causes. The cause of this disease is most often unknown. It may be caused by an autoimmune dysfunction. It can be caused by cancer and other serious diseases that damage the adrenal glands.

Signs and Symptoms. The signs and symptoms may begin long before a diagnosis is made. They include weakness, fatigue, and dizziness after rising from a sitting or reclining position. Other symptoms include weight loss, muscle pain, lack of appetite, nausea, vomiting, diarrhea, and dehydration.

Treatment. Because this disease can be life-threatening, the first treatment is to administer corticosteroids. Medications or other hormones may be prescribed to help balance the levels of sodium and potassium.

CUSHING'S SYNDROME is also known as *hypercortisolism*. In this condition, a person produces too much cortisol (see Figure 34-6).

Causes. This syndrome is caused by an excessive production of ACTH (a hormone that increases the production of cortisol), a tumor of the adrenal gland (the source of cortisol), a tumor of

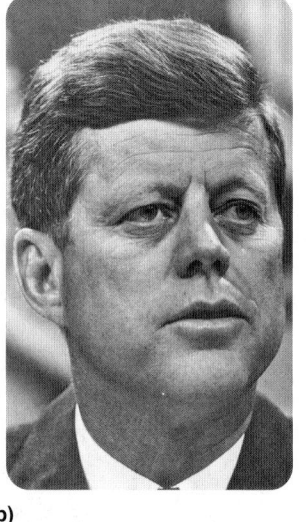

(a)   (b)

FIGURE 34-5 Addison's disease. (a) John F. Kennedy prior to being treated for Addison's disease. (b) In 1960, Kennedy's face shows the facial swelling that was one of the effects of cortisone treatment for Addison's disease.

(a)   (b)

FIGURE 34-6 Cushing's syndrome. (a) Photo prior to the onset of Cushing's syndrome. (b) The same person after the onset of Cushing's syndrome. Notice the rounding or fullness of the face.

the pituitary gland (the source of ACTH), or the long-term use of steroidal hormones.

Signs and Symptoms. Common symptoms include a round or full face ("moon face"), a hump of fat between the shoulders ("buffalo hump"), thin arms and legs with a large abdomen, fatigue, thin skin, acne, frequent thirst, frequent urination, mental disabilities, a loss of menstrual cycle in females, high blood pressure, high blood glucose levels, and body aches in the muscles, back, or head.

Treatment. The first treatment includes lifestyle changes, especially stopping the use of steroidal hormones. Radiation therapy or surgery may be needed to treat any tumors.

DIABETES INSIPIDUS is a condition in which the kidneys fail to reabsorb water, causing excessive urination.

Causes. The primary cause is the hyposecretion of ADH.

Signs and Symptoms. These include excessive thirst, even with a more-than-adequate fluid intake. Other signs and symptoms include excessive urination and, in severe cases, muscle cramps and cardiac arrhythmias related to electrolyte imbalances caused by the excessive fluid loss.

Treatment. The primary treatment is increased fluid intake. Other treatments include surgery for any tumor of the pituitary that may cause the inadequate secretion of ADH. Changes in diet and medication help increase water retention.

DIABETES MELLITUS is a chronic disease characterized by high glucose levels in the blood. There are at least three different types of diabetes mellitus. Type 1 is referred to as *early onset diabetes* or *insulin-dependent diabetes mellitus*, and it usually develops during childhood. Type 2 is the most common type and is often called *late-onset diabetes* or *noninsulin-dependent diabetes mellitus* because, historically, it is primarily diagnosed in adults. Of concern in recent years is a national surge in the number of adolescents and teens being diagnosed with type 2 diabetes. This is being directly linked to a lack of exercise and excessive weight gain in this age group. Gestational diabetes occurs only in pregnant women and is usually temporary, although a history of gestational diabetes has been found to put the patient at higher risk of developing type 2 diabetes later in life. Women with gestational diabetes should be monitored closely for type 2 diabetes. African Americans, Hispanics, and Native Americans are more likely to develop diabetes than any other ethnic groups.

Causes. This disease is caused by the production of too little or no insulin by the pancreas. Other causes include body cells having too few insulin receptors, obesity, high blood pressure, pregnancy, and high cholesterol levels in the blood.

Signs and Symptoms. There are many signs and symptoms of this disease. They include high levels of glucose in the blood, excessive thirst, frequent urination, fatigue, increased appetite, unexplained weight loss, blurry vision, impotence in men, nausea, skin wounds that heal slowly, high glucose and ketone levels in the urine, and lower extremity problems (due to poor circulation).

Treatment. Treatment includes daily injections of insulin, oral medications to increase insulin production, oral medications to increase the body's sensitivity to insulin, frequent monitoring of glucose levels in the blood, and frequent monitoring of ketone levels in the urine. Lifestyle changes are important and should include reducing weight (especially if obese), changing eating habits, and getting regular exercise. Lifestyle changes to prevent injury to legs and feet may also be needed. More information on diet and treatment for diabetic patients may be found in the *Nutrition and Health* chapter.

Complications. Left untreated, diabetes can result in long-term and life-threatening complications. Blood vessels become thickened, which can damage vital organs including the kidneys, eyes, heart, and brain. Long-term damage can result in kidney disease, blindness, and atherosclerosis (the buildup of fatty deposits in blood vessels). Circulation worsens, which not only affects organs but also may result in slower overall healing and ulcers that develop in the lower extremities, particularly the feet. Because of the body's decreased ability to heal, these ulcers may require amputation of the affected foot and possibly part of the leg (below-knee amputation, or BKA). Further information on diabetic emergencies, including insulin shock and diabetic coma, may be found in the *Emergency Preparedness* chapter.

Go to CONNECT to see animations about *Type 1 Diabetes* and *Type 2 Diabetes*.

DWARFISM is a condition in which too little growth hormone (somatotropin) is produced in childhood (see Figure 34-7).

Causes. This condition can be caused by an under-production of the growth hormone during childhood, trauma to the pituitary gland, or by a pituitary tumor.

Signs and Symptoms. Signs and symptoms include short height, abnormal facial features, cleft lip or palate, delayed puberty, headaches, frequent urination, and excessive thirst.

Treatment. Treatment is the administration of supplemental growth hormone.

GIGANTISM is a condition in which too much growth hormone is produced during childhood (see Figure 34-8).

Causes. This condition is caused by overproduction of growth hormone during childhood. It can also be caused by a tumor in the pituitary gland.

Signs and Symptoms. Very tall height, delayed sexual maturity, thick facial bones, thick skin, weakness, and vision problems are common symptoms.

Treatment. Treatment includes medications to reduce growth hormone levels, radiation therapy, and surgery to remove the tumor.

GOITER is an enlargement of the thyroid gland causing (sometimes disfiguring) swelling of the neck (see Figure 34-9).

Causes. Typically, a simple goiter is caused by a deficiency of iodine in the diet. Iodine is needed for the thyroid to produce thyroid hormones.

FIGURE 34-7 Pituitary dwarfism is caused by hyposecretion of growth hormone.

FIGURE 34-8 Gigantism results from hypersecretion of growth hormone.

FIGURE 34-9 An iodine deficiency causes simple (endemic) goiter and results in high levels of TSH.

Signs and Symptoms. These include overgrowth of the follicles of the thyroid gland, which causes enlargement of the gland and of the neck, and abnormal thyroid function tests (TFTs).

Treatment. The most common treatment is iodine supplementation in the diet. In the United States, salt contains iodine, so goiters are seldom seen. Because a goiter may not shrink even after adequate iodine is introduced into the diet, surgery may be required to remove some or most of the enlarged gland.

GRAVES' DISEASE is a disorder in which a person develops antibodies that attack the thyroid gland (see Figure 34-10). This attack causes the thyroid to produce too many thyroid hormones. Graves' disease is the most common type of hyperthyroidism in the United States.

Causes. This disease is caused by an overproduction of thyroid hormones. It is also considered an autoimmune disorder.

Signs and Symptoms. The most common signs and symptoms include exophthalmos (protrusion of the eyes) and goiter (thyroid enlargement). Other symptoms include insomnia, unexplained weight loss, anxiety, muscle weakness, increased appetite, excessive sweating, vision problems, and an increased heart rate.

FIGURE 34-10   Signs of Graves' disease, a form of hyperthyroidism, include protruding eyes and goiter.

Treatment.   Treatment includes medications to reduce heart rate, sweating, and nervousness; radiation to destroy the thyroid gland; surgery to remove the thyroid gland (thyroidectomy); and supplemental thyroid hormones if the gland is destroyed or removed.

BODYANIMAT3D
POWERED BY
connect

Go to CONNECT to see an animation about *Hyperthyroidism.*

CRETINISM is an extreme form of hypothyroidism that is present prior to or soon after birth (see Figure 34-11).

Causes.   The cause is hypothyroidism at birth related to the absence or malformation of the thyroid gland, abnormal formation of thyroid hormones, or pituitary failure that results in a lack of thyroid stimulation.

Signs and Symptoms.   Stunted growth, abnormal bone formation, mental retardation, low body temperature, and overall sluggishness are the primary signs and symptoms.

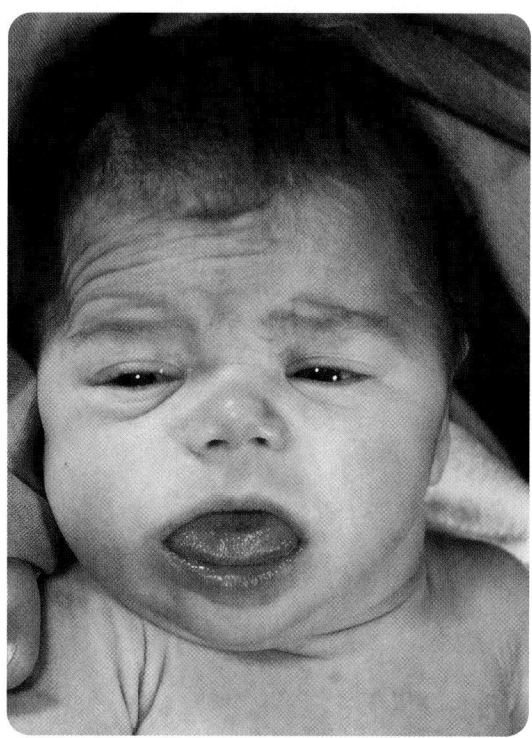

FIGURE 34-11   Cretinism is the result of an underactive thyroid gland during infancy and childhood.

Treatment.   The treatment is thyroid hormone replacement.

MYXEDEMA is a disorder in which the thyroid gland does not produce adequate amounts of thyroid hormone. It is a severe type of hypothyroidism that is most common in females over age 50.

Causes.   Causes include the removal of the thyroid, radiation treatments to the neck area, and obesity. This disorder may be congenital.

Signs and Symptoms.   Signs and symptoms include weakness, fatigue, weight gain, depression, general body aches, dry skin and hair, hair loss, puffy hands or feet, a decreased ability to taste food, abnormal menstrual periods, pale or yellow skin, a slow heart rate, low blood pressure, anemia, an enlarged heart, high cholesterol levels, or coma.

Treatment.   Treatment consists of giving supplemental thyroid hormones intravenously or orally and closely monitoring the levels of thyroid hormones.

SUMMARY OF LEARNING OUTCOMES

LEARNING OUTCOMES	KEY POINTS
34.1 **Describe the general functions of hormones and the endocrine system.**	Endocrine glands are ductless glands, releasing hormones directly into the bloodstream and tissues. The organs of the endocrine system produce hormones that regulate the chemical reactions within cells, controlling the functions of organs, tissues, and other cells. Hormone levels are controlled by positive and negative feedback loops.

LEARNING OUTCOMES	KEY POINTS
34.2 **Identify the hormones released by the pituitary gland, thyroid gland, parathyroid glands, adrenal glands, pancreas, and other hormone-producing organs, and give the functions of each.**	The pituitary gland releases the following hormones: GH, MSH, ACTH, TSH, FSH, LH, PRL, ADH, and OT. The thyroid gland releases calcitonin, T_3, and T_4, which are important in growth and protein synthesis. The parathyroid gland releases PTH, which balances the action of calcitonin. The adrenal medulla secretes epinephrine and norepinephrine, which work with the sympathetic nervous system. The adrenal cortex produces many hormones, but the two major ones are aldosterone and cortisol. The two types of hormone-releasing of cells in the pancreas are alpha cells, which release glucagon, and beta cells, which release insulin. The pineal body releases melatonin; the thymus releases thymosin and thymopoietin; ovaries release estrogen and progesterone (females); and the testes (males) release testosterone. The kidneys produce erythropoietin, and the heart produces atrial natriuretic peptide. Each hormone's specific function may be found in Table 34-1.
34.3 **Explain the effect of stressors on the body.**	Stressors are stimuli that produce a stress response, a physiologic response to the stimulus that changes the body's functioning in some way.
34.4 **Describe the causes, signs and symptoms, and treatments of various endocrine disorders.**	The diseases and disorders of the endocrine system are as varied as the organs and hormone dysfunctions that cause them. An overview of these conditions is found in Table 34-2.

CASE STUDY CRITICAL THINKING

Recall Ken Washington from the beginning of the chapter. Now that you have completed this chapter, answer the following questions regarding his case:

1. What gland is likely to be causing Ken's problems?

2. What is Ken's likely diagnosis?

3. What treatment options are available?

4. What other condition is often caused by treating this condition, and how is it managed?

EXAM PREPARATION QUESTIONS

1. (LO 34.1) Which of following hormone types is also known as a tissue hormone?
   a. Steroidal hormones
   b. Nonsteroidal hormones
   c. G-proteins
   d. Prostaglandins
   e. Thyroid hormones

2. (LO 34.2) Which endocrine organ listed below also has a digestive function?
   a. Adrenal medulla
   b. Adrenal cortex
   c. Pancreas
   d. Pineal body
   e. Thymus

3. (LO 34.2) Which hormone assists the kidneys in retaining fluid?
   a. ACTH
   b. ADH
   c. PTH
   d. FSH
   e. MSH

4. (LO 34.2) The numeral in "T_3" and "T_4" stands for the number of _____ atoms needed for the hormones to work properly.
   a. Chloride
   b. Potassium
   c. Calcium
   d. Iodine
   e. Sodium

5. (LO 34.4) From which endocrine disease did President John F. Kennedy suffer?
   a. Cushing's syndrome
   b. Addison's disease
   c. Acromegaly
   d. Hypothyroidism
   e. Graves' disease

6. (LO 34.3) Which hormone is released when a person is under prolonged stress?
   a. Glucagon
   b. Aldosterone
   c. Melatonin
   d. Oxytocin
   e. Cortisol

7. (LO 34.2) Which of the following hormones is not produced by the anterior pituitary?
   a. Growth hormone
   b. Follicle-stimulating hormone
   c. Oxytocin
   d. Luteinizing hormone
   e. Prolactin

8. (LO 34.1) Nonsteroidal hormones require which of the following to turn on enzymes inside target cells?
   a. Amino acids
   b. Prostaglandins
   c. Calcitonin
   d. G-protein
   e. Prolactin

9. (LO 34.4) A condition in which the body produces too much cortisol is
   a. Cushing's syndrome
   b. Graves' disease
   c. Myxedema
   d. Gigantism
   e. Diabetes insipidus

10. (LO 34.4) When too much growth hormone is produced in adults, the result is
   a. Dwarfism
   b. Gigantism
   c. Cretinism
   d. Myxedema
   e. Acromegaly

MEDICAL TERMINOLOGY PRACTICE

Analyze the following medical terms, presented throughout the chapter. Using a medical dictionary (or Appendix I) place a / mark between each word part. Define each word part and then define the whole word.

EXAMPLE: aden/oma = aden means "gland" + oma means "tumor"
Adenoma means "tumor of a gland"

1. acromegaly
2. adrenocorticotropic
3. antidiuretic
4. exocrine
5. hypothalamus
6. melanocyte
7. natriuretic
8. nonsteroidal
9. parathyroid
10. thymopoietin
11. hyperparathyroidism
12. exocrine

CASE STUDY

Patient Name	Gender	DOB
Valarie Ramirez	Female	8/4/19XX

Attending	MRN	Allergies
Paul F. Buckwalter, MD	829-78-462	Penicillin

Valarie Ramirez, a 33-year-old female, arrives at the office with something in her eye. While riding her motorcycle yesterday, something flew up under her helmet visor. She has been using Visine® eyedrops, but when she woke up this morning, her eye felt worse. You notice her right eye is red and swollen. You prepare Valarie for the physician to examine her eye.

Keep Valarie in mind as you study this chapter. There will be questions at the end of the chapter based on the case study. The information in the chapter will help you answer these questions.

LEARNING OUTCOMES

After completing Chapter 35, you will be able to:

35.1 Describe the anatomy of the nose and the function of each part.

35.2 Describe the anatomy of the tongue and the function of each part.

35.3 Describe the anatomy of the eye and the function of each part, including the accessory structures and their functions.

35.4 Explain the visual pathway through the eye and to the brain for interpretation.

35.5 Describe the causes, signs and symptoms, and treatments of various disorders of the eyes.

35.6 Describe the anatomy of the ear and the function of each part, and explain the role of the ear in maintaining equilibrium.

35.7 Explain how sounds travel through the ear and are interpreted in the brain.

35.8 Describe the causes, signs and symptoms, and treatments of various disorders of the ears.

KEY TERMS

auricle	organ of Corti
cerumen	ossicles
choroid	oval window
cochlea	papillae
conjunctiva	refraction
cornea	retina
eustachian tube	semicircular canals
external auditory canal	sensory adaptation
labyrinth	tympanic membrane
lacrimal apparatus	vestibule

I. C (1) Describe structural organization of the human body

I. C (2) Identify body systems

I. C (4) List major organs in each body system

I. C (5) Describe the normal function of each body system

I. C (6) Identify common pathology related to each body system

I. C (7) Analyze pathology as it relates to the interaction of body systems

I. C (8) Discuss implications for disease and disability when homeostasis is not maintained

I. C (9) Describe implications for treatment related to pathology

I. C (10) Compare body structure and function of the human body across the life span

I. C (12) Describe the relationship between anatomy and physiology of all body systems and medications used for treatment in each

IV. C (11) Define both medical terms and abbreviations related to all body systems

2. Anatomy & Physiology
Graduates:

b. Identify and apply the knowledge of all body systems; their structure and functions; and their common diseases, symptoms, and etiologies

c. Assist the physician with the regimen of diagnostic and treatment modalities as they relate to each body system

3. Medical Terminology
Graduates:

b. Build and dissect medical terms from roots/suffixes to understand the word element combinations that create medical terminology

c. Understand the various medical terminology for each specialty

▸ Introduction

The special senses are smell, taste, vision, hearing, and equilibrium. They are called special senses because their sensory receptors are located within relatively large sensory organs in the head—the nose, tongue, eyes, and ears. Although the skin is also considered a sense organ (in fact, it is the largest sense organ), touch is not considered a special sense but rather a generalized one (refer to *The Integumentary System* chapter). As you read this chapter, keep in mind that no matter how a stimulus starts, it is sent, via the nervous system, to the brain for interpretation (and then reaction, if necessary). This chapter introduces the structure and function of the special sense organs.

As a medical assistant, you will likely be asked to assist with or perform examinations and treatments for common disorders of the eyes and ears. So, you will need to understand how these important sense organs function.

▸ The Nose and the Sense of Smell   LO 35.1

Smell receptors, also called *olfactory receptors*, are chemoreceptors. This means that they respond to changes in chemical concentrations. Chemicals that activate smell receptors must be dissolved in the mucus of the nose. This explains why a person with either a "dry nose" or excessive mucus related to an upper respiratory tract infection or allergies has trouble smelling.

Smell receptors are located in the olfactory organ, found in the upper part of the nasal cavity. Humans have a relatively poor sense of smell compared to animals because chemicals must diffuse all the way up the nasal cavity to activate smell

receptors. There are also fewer smell receptors in the human nose compared to most animal noses.

Once smell receptors are activated, they send their information to the olfactory nerves. The olfactory nerves send the information along olfactory bulbs and tracts to different areas of the cerebrum. The cerebrum interprets the information as a particular type of smell (see Figure 35-1). An interesting fact about our sense of smell is that it undergoes **sensory adaptation,** which means that the same chemical can stimulate smell

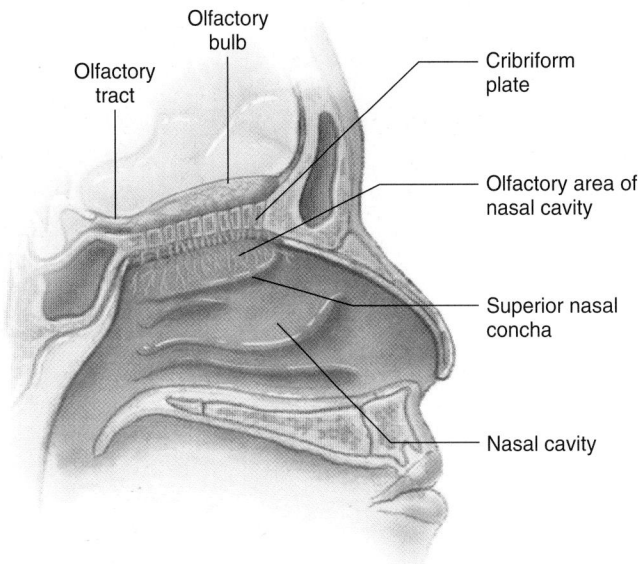

FIGURE 35-1   The olfactory area (organ) is located in the superior part of the nasal cavity.

receptors for only a limited amount of time. In a relatively short period of time, the smell receptors fatigue and no longer respond to the same (odor) chemical, and it can no longer be smelled. Sensory adaptation explains why you smell perfume when you first encounter it, but after a few minutes, you cannot smell it or may be less aware of it.

The Tongue and the Sense of Taste

LO 35.2

Taste or gustatory receptors are located on taste buds. Taste buds are microscopic structures found on the **papillae** (bumps) of the tongue. They cannot be seen with the naked eye. Some taste buds are also scattered on the roof of the mouth and in the walls of the throat.

Each taste bud is made of taste cells and supporting cells. The taste cells function as taste receptors, and the supporting cells simply fill in the spaces between the taste cells. Like the olfactory cells of smell, taste cells are types of chemoreceptors. They are activated by chemicals found in food and drink that must be dissolved in saliva as part of the digestive process (see Figure 35-2).

There are four types of taste cells, and each type is activated by a particular group of chemicals to produce the following four primary taste sensations:

- Sweet. Taste cells that respond to "sweet" chemicals are concentrated at the tip of the tongue.
- Sour. Taste cells that respond to "sour" chemicals are concentrated on the sides of the tongue.
- Salty. Taste cells that respond to "salty" chemicals are concentrated on the tip and sides of the tongue.

- Bitter. Taste cells that respond to "bitter" chemicals are concentrated at the back of the tongue.

In addition to these four well-known taste sensations, in the 1980s, science recognized a taste known as *umami*. In 1908, a Japanese scientist discovered that glutamic acid found in kelp produced a savory, meaty taste that he named umami. This unique taste is found most notably in tomatoes and also in meats, fish, and dairy products, including breast milk. Although discovered and named in the early 1900s, it was not until the 1980s that studies found that glutamate, the substance responsible for this unique taste, created a fifth basic taste that has become universally recognized.

When taste cells are activated, they send their information to several cranial nerves. This information eventually reaches the gustatory cortex in the cerebrum's parietal lobe. The gustatory cortex interprets the information as a particular taste. For example, although it is not an actual taste sensation, eating spicy foods activates pain receptors on the tongue that the brain then interprets as "spicy."

The Eye and the Sense of Sight

LO 35.3

The sense of sight comes from the eyes and is also supported by visual accessory organs.

Vision

Your visual system consists of the eyes; the optic nerve, which connects the eye to the vision center of the brain; and several accessory structures. If these parts of the system are healthy and normal, you are able to see normally.

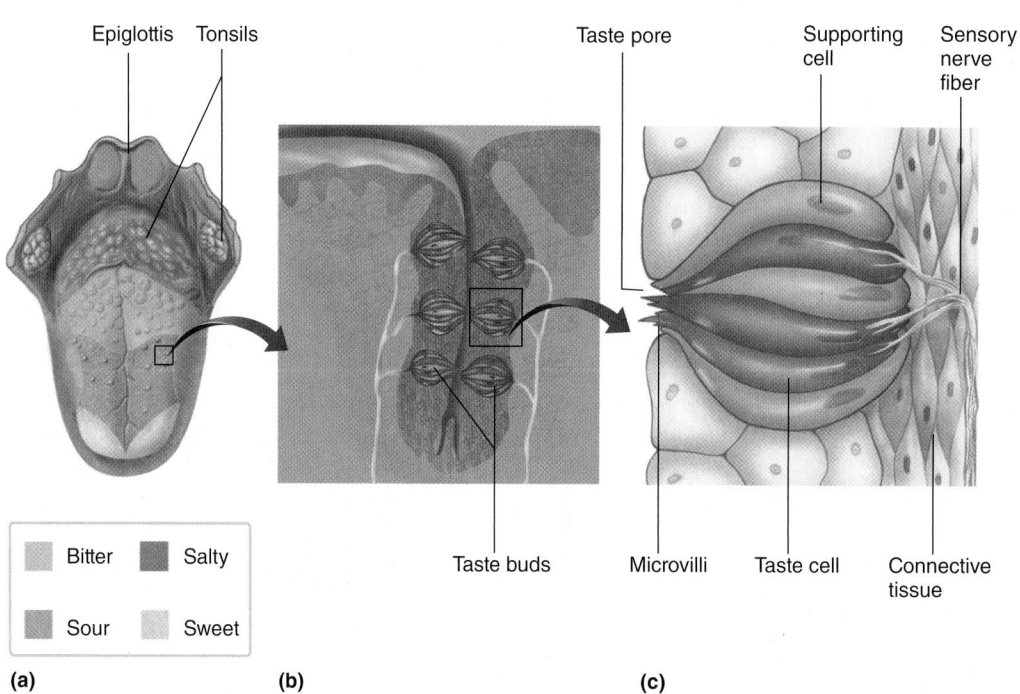

FIGURE 35-2 Tongue and taste buds. (a) Areas of the tongue are sensitive to different tastes, as indicated. (b) Taste buds are located on and in papillae. (c) Taste buds are composed of taste cells and supporting cells.

The Eye

The eye is a complex organ that processes light to produce images. It is made up of three main layers, two chambers, and a number of specialized parts, as shown in Figure 35-3.

The Outer Layer The white of the eye—the *sclera*—is the tough, outermost layer of the eye. This layer, through which light cannot pass, covers all except the front of the eye. Here, the sclera gives way to the cornea in an area known as the corneal-scleral junction or *limbus*. The **cornea** is a transparent area on the front of the eye that acts as a window to let light into the eye. Although there are no blood vessels in the sclera, numerous sense receptors exist to detect even the smallest particles on the eyeball's surface.

The Middle Layer The **choroid** is the middle layer of the eye, which contains most of the eye's blood vessels. In the anterior part of the choroid are the iris and the ciliary body. The iris is the colored part of the eye. It is made of muscular tissue. As this tissue contracts and relaxes, an opening at

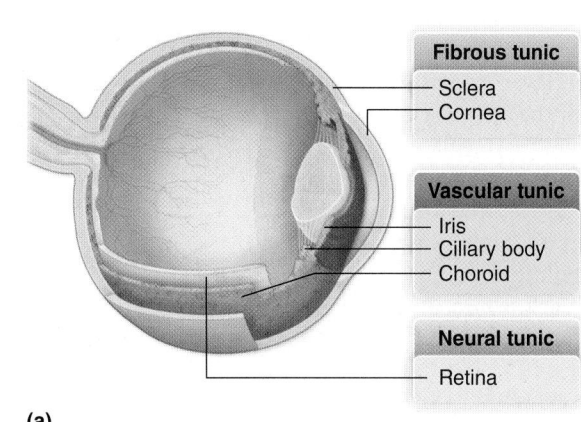

(a)

(b)

FIGURE 35-3 Anatomy of the internal eye—sagittal views depict (a) the three layers of the eye and (b) internal eye structures.

its center (the pupil) grows larger or smaller. The size of the pupil regulates the amount of light that enters the eye. In bright light, the pupil becomes constricted (smaller). In dim light, it becomes dilated (larger).

The ciliary body is a wedge-shaped thickening in the eyeball's middle layer. Muscles in the ciliary body control the shape of the lens—making the lens more or less curved for viewing either near or distant objects. The lens is a clear, circular disk located just posterior to the iris. Because the lens can change shape, it helps the eye focus images of near or faraway objects. This process is called *accommodation*. Clouding and hardening of the lens, which often occur with aging, lead to visual changes in a condition known as *cataracts*. This condition will be discussed in more detail later in the *Assisting with Eye and Ear Care* chapter.

The Inner Layer The eye's inner layer consists of the **retina.** Nerve cells at the posterior of the retina sense light. The area where the optic nerve enters the retina is known as the optic disc. This area contains no sensory nerves itself and is referred to as the *blind spot*. There are two types of nerve cells, each named for its shape. *Rods* are highly sensitive to light. They function in dim light but do not provide a sharp image or detect color, only black, white, and shades of gray. They give you your limited "night vision" as well as peripheral vision. *Cones* function best in bright light. They are sensitive to color and provide sharper images. They are responsible for the ability to differentiate tones and hues of color. Deficiencies in the number or types of cones are responsible for the various types of color blindness, which is generally an inherited condition.

The Chambers of the Eye Each eyeball is divided into two chambers: the anterior and the posterior.

The Anterior Chamber The anterior chamber is in front of the lens and is filled with a watery fluid called *aqueous humor*. Aqueous humor provides nutrients to and bathes the structures in the anterior chamber of the eyeball. When there is an accumulation of aqueous humor, a person develops a visual condition known as *glaucoma*. This disorder will be discussed in more detail in the *Assisting with Eye and Ear Care* chapter.

The Posterior Chamber The posterior chamber of the eyeball is behind the lens and is filled with a thick, jelly-like fluid called *vitreous humor*. Vitreous humor keeps the retina flat and helps to maintain the eye's shape.

Visual Accessory Organs
Visual accessory organs assist and protect the eyeball. They include the orbits, eyebrows, eyelids and eyelashes, conjunctivas, the lacrimal apparatus, and extrinsic eye muscles.

Eye Orbits The eye sockets, or *orbits,* form a protective shell around the eyes. Eyebrows protect the eyes by reducing the chances that sweat and direct sunlight will enter them.

FIGURE 35-4   Lacrimal apparatus.

Eyelids Each eyelid is composed of skin, muscle, and dense connective tissue. The muscle in the eyelid is called the *orbicularis oculi* and is responsible for blinking and squinting. Blinking the eyelids prevents the mucous membrane surface of the eyeball from drying. A moist eyeball surface is much less likely to grow bacteria than a dry one is. Blinking also protects the eyes, keeping foreign material from entering them with the assistance of the eyelashes, which catch foreign substances, including perspiration and dust.

Conjunctivas **Conjunctivas** are mucous membranes that line the inner surfaces of the eyelids and cover the anterior surface of each eyeball. They are called mucous membranes because they produce mucus that keeps the surface of the eyeballs moist.

The Lacrimal Apparatus The **lacrimal apparatus** consists of lacrimal glands and nasolacrimal ducts (see Figure 35-4). *Lacrimal glands,* located on the lateral edge of each eyeball, produce tears. Tears are mostly water, but they also contain enzymes (lysozymes) that can destroy bacteria and viruses as part of the body's system to protect itself. Tears also have an outer oily layer that prevents them from evaporating. *Nasolacrimal ducts,* located on the medial aspect of each eyeball, drain tears into the nose. When a person cries, the abundance of tears entering the nose produces the "runny nose" associated with crying.

Extrinsic Eye Muscles Extrinsic eye muscles are skeletal muscles that move the eyeball. Each eyeball has six extrinsic eye muscles attached to it that move the eyeball superiorly, inferiorly, laterally, or medially. (See Figure 35-5.)

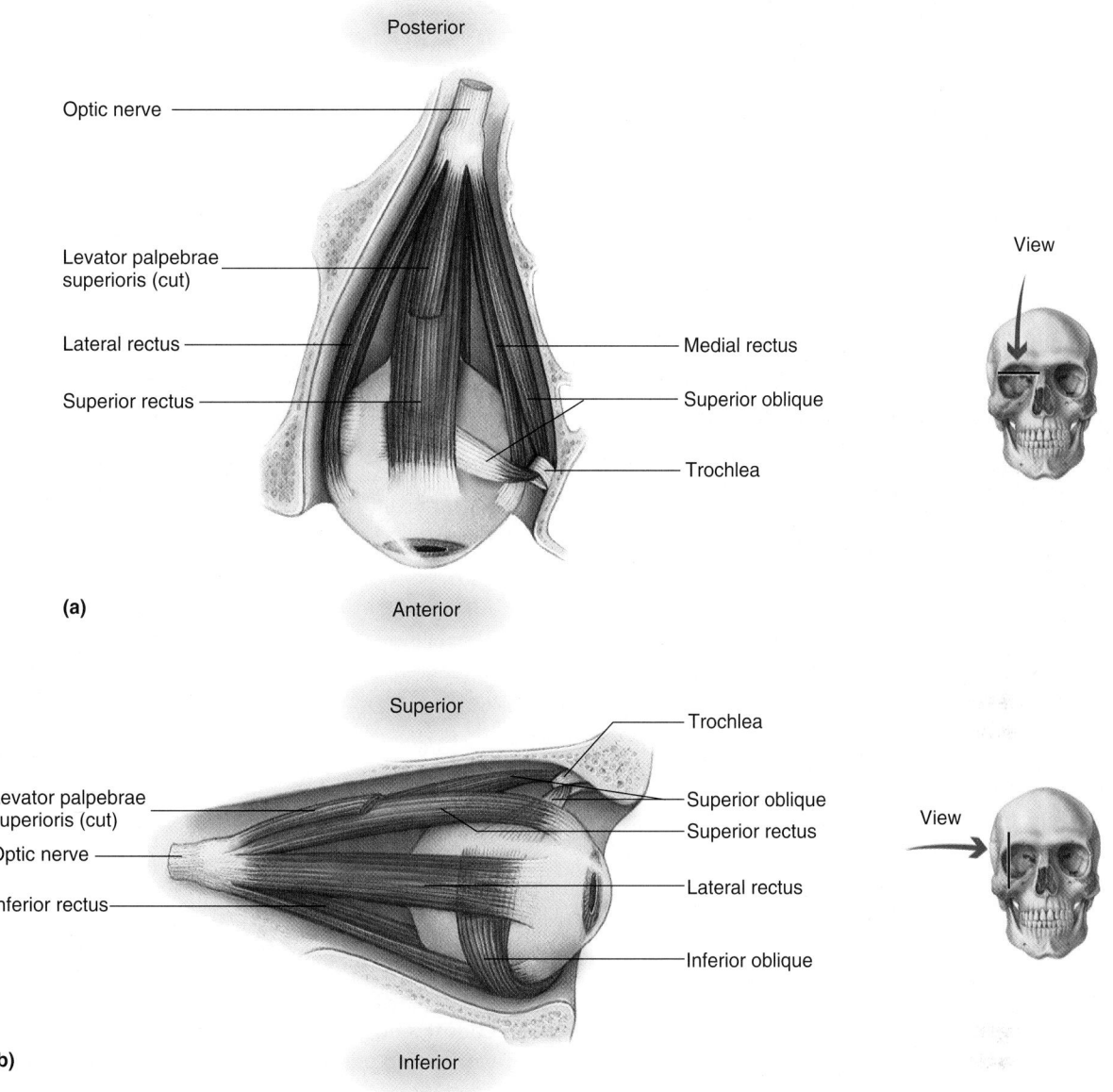

Posterior

Optic nerve

Levator palpebrae
superioris (cut)

Lateral rectus

Superior rectus

Medial rectus

Superior oblique

Trochlea

(a)

Anterior

View

Superior

Trochlea

Levator palpebrae
superioris (cut)

Optic nerve

Inferior rectus

Superior oblique

Superior rectus

Lateral rectus

Inferior oblique

View

(b)

Inferior

FIGURE 35-5 The six extrinsic eye muscles move the eyeball superiorly, inferiorly, laterally, or medially.

▶ Visual Pathways

LO 35.4

The eye works much like a camera. Light reflected from an object, or produced by one, enters the eye from the outside and passes through the cornea, pupil, lens, and fluids in the eye. The cornea, lens, and fluids help focus the light onto the retina by bending it in a process known as **refraction.** As in a camera, light patterns carry an image of an object. The image is projected upside-down—on film in a camera and on the retina in an eye. The retina converts the light into nerve impulses. These impulses are transmitted along the optic nerve to the brain. This nerve, which consists of about a million fibers, serves as a flexible cable connecting the eyeball to the brain.

Parts of the optic nerve fuse together then cross at a structure called the optic chiasm—an x-shaped structure, located at the base of the brain. The visual area in the occipital lobes of the cerebrum is responsible for interpreting vision. Because visual information crosses in the optic chiasm, about half of the visual information detected in each eye is interpreted on the opposite side of the brain. So, half of what a person sees in the right eye is interpreted in the left side of the brain and vice versa, where it is brought together as one image. The brain interprets these impulses, turns the image right-side up, and "develops" a picture of the object from which the light originally came. See Table 35-1 for a summary of the parts of the eye and their functions.

TABLE 35-1   The Functions of the Parts of the Eye

Structure	Function
Aqueous humor	Nourishes and bathes structures in the anterior eye cavity
Vitreous humor	Holds the retina in place; maintains the shape of the eyeball
Sclera	Protects the eye
Cornea	Allows light to enter the eye; bends light as it enters the eye (refraction)
Choroid	Supplies nutrients and provides a blood supply to the eye
Ciliary body	Holds the lens; controls the shape of the lens for focusing
Iris	Controls the amount of light entering the eye
Lens	Focuses light onto the retina (accommodation)
Retina	Contains visual receptors
Rods	Allow vision in dim light; detect black, white, and gray images; detect broad outlines of images
Cones	Allow vision in bright light; detect colors; detect details
Optic nerve	Carries visual information (stimuli) from rods and cones toward the brain

The Aging Eye

With age, a number of changes occur in the structure and function of the eye, including the following.

- The amount of fat tissue diminishes; this loss may cause the eyelids to droop.
- The quality and quantity of tears decrease.
- The conjunctiva becomes thinner and may be drier because of a decrease in tear production.
- The cornea begins to appear yellow, and a ring of fat deposits may appear around it.
- The sclera may develop brown spots.
- Changes in the iris cause the pupil to become smaller, limiting the amount of light entering the eye.
- The lens becomes denser and more rigid; this trend reduces the amount of light that reaches the retina and makes focusing more difficult.
- Yellowing of the lens causes problems in distinguishing colors.
- Changes in the retina may make vision fuzzy.
- The ability of the eye to adapt to changes in light intensities may be reduced; glare can become painful as this ability diminishes.

EDUCATING THE PATIENT

Eye Safety and Protection

Almost 90% of all eye injuries could be prevented by eye safety practices or proper protective eyewear. You can educate patients about preventing eye injuries in the home, at work, and during recreational activities.

Eye Safety in the Home

Patients should follow these suggestions to protect their eyes in the home:

- Pad or cushion the sharp corners and edges of furniture and home fixtures.
- Make sure adequate lighting and handrails are available on stairs.
- Keep personal use items (like cosmetics and toiletries), kitchen utensils, and desk supplies out of the reach of children.
- Keep toys with sharp edges out of the reach of children. Also, make sure toys intended for older children are kept away from younger children.
- Remove dangerous debris from the lawn before mowing it.
- Wear safely goggles when operating any type of power equipment.
- Keep dangerous solvents, paints, cleaners, fertilizers, and other chemicals out of the reach of children.
- Never mix cleaning agents.

Eye Safety at Work

Approximately 15% of eye injuries in the workplace lead to temporary or permanent vision loss. Eye injuries at work can be diminished if patients take the following precautions:

- Choose safety eyewear according to the type of work being performed and the type of eye protection needed.
- Wear safety eyewear whenever there is a chance of flying objects from machines.
- Wear safety eyewear whenever there is possible exposure—splash or splatter—to harmful chemicals, body fluids, or radiation.

Eye Safety During Sports and Recreational Activities

Eye injuries that commonly occur while playing a sport include scratched corneas, inflamed irises and retinas, bleeding in the anterior chamber of the eye, traumatic cataracts, and fractures of the eye socket. Wearing sports eye guards or goggles can prevent most sports eye injuries. These guards are recommended for baseball, basketball, soccer, football, rugby, and hockey. Protective goggles are recommended for mountain biking, motocross, and snow skiing. Virtually any type of contact sport requires appropriate eye protection.

- Night vision may be impaired.
- Peripheral vision is reduced, limiting the area a person can see and reducing depth perception.
- The vitreous humor breaks down, producing tiny clumps of gel or cellular material that cause floaters—dark spots or lines—that appear in a person's field of vision.

- Rubbing of the vitreous humor on the retina produces flashes of light or "sparks."

Because of changes that impair vision—such as reductions in the field of vision, in depth perception, and in visual clarity—elderly people may fall more often than younger people.

PATHOPHYSIOLOGY

LO 35.5

Common Diseases and Disorders of the Eyes

As with all the body's organs, the sense organs are also susceptible to various diseases and disorders. The following common diseases and disorders are specific to the eyes.

ASTIGMATISM occurs when the lens has an abnormal shape or the cornea is unevenly curved. This abnormality causes blurred images during near or distant vision. Astigmatism may cause vertical or horizontal lines to appear out of focus.

Causes. This condition is normally considered to be congenital.

Signs and Symptoms. There are no symptoms with this condition other than blurred vision. However, it can be diagnosed during an ophthalmic (eye) exam.

Treatment. Treatment includes corrective lenses or surgery, such as photorefractive keratectomy (PRK) or, more commonly now, laser-assisted in situ keratomileusis (LASIK) to reshape the cornea (see Figure 35-6). This procedure—done on an outpatient basis under local anesthesia—involves reshaping the cornea with a special laser. After LASIK surgery, 70% of patients have normal vision. A very small percentage of patients have postsurgical complications that cause their vision to worsen.

DRY EYE SYNDROME is one of the most common eye problems physicians treat. This syndrome results from a decreased production of the oil within tears, which normally occurs with age.

Causes. Dry eye can be caused by cigarette smoke; air conditioning; eye strain created by long hours at a computer monitor; some medications; contact lenses; hormonal changes associated with menopause; and hot, dry, or windy climates.

Signs and Symptoms. The common eye symptoms include burning, irritation, redness, itching, and excessive tearing.

Treatment. Artificial tears may provide relief to many patients, and drugs like Restasis® have helped patients with this condition make more of their own tears. People with this condition should drink 8 to 10 glasses of water a day and make a conscious effort to blink more frequently and avoid rubbing their eyes. In addition, punctual plugs can be inserted to trap tears on the eyes, which prevents the tears from entering the nasolacrimal duct and being drained.

ECTROPION is characterized by eversion (turning inside-out) of the lower eyelid.

Causes. Aging and skin relaxation or scar tissue may cause this condition.

Cornea is sliced with a sharp knife. Flap of cornea is reflected, and deeper corneal layers are exposed.

A laser removes microscopic portions of the deeper corneal layers, thereby changing the shape of the cornea.

Corneal flap is put back in place, and the edges of the flap start to fuse within 72 hours.

FIGURE 35-6 LASIK laser vision correction procedure.

Signs and Symptoms. Common signs and symptoms include redness, irritation, and drying of the conjunctiva. Poor tear drainage through the nasolacrimal system may also be present.

Treatment. Surgery to repair the defect may be needed if the condition is bothersome to the patient.

ENTROPION is characterized by an inversion (turning outside-in) of the lower eyelid.

Causes. Aging and scar tissue may cause this condition.

Signs and Symptoms. Signs include irritation of the sclera as the lashes brush against it, which may lead to corneal ulceration or scarring.

Treatment. Surgery is the only treatment option to correct this problem.

NYSTAGMUS is rapid, involuntary eye movements.

Causes. Alcohol and some drug use may cause nystagmus. Inner ear disturbances may also result in involuntary eye movements. Brain lesions and injury (including those that may occur during birth), and cerebrovascular accidents (CVA) or strokes, may also cause nystagmus.

Signs and Symptoms. Rapid, irregular eye movements that may be horizontal, vertical, or rotary, depending on the underlying cause of the nystagmus.

Treatment. Treatment focuses on the underlying cause of the disorder.

RETINAL DETACHMENT occurs when the layers of the retina separate. It is considered a medical emergency and if not treated right away, leads to permanent vision loss.

Causes. Retinal detachment is rare; however, it is more common as people age. This disorder is sometimes caused by fluids that seep between layers of the retina; this occurs most commonly in nearsighted people. In diabetics, vitreous body or scar tissue pulls the retina loose. Other causes include eye trauma that causes fluid to collect underneath the layers of the retina.

Signs and Symptoms. Signs and symptoms include light flashes, wavy vision, a sudden loss of vision (particularly of peripheral vision), and a larger amount of floaters.

Treatment. When detected early, a hole in the retina can be "sealed" so that the retina does not completely detach. Sealing the hole is usually accomplished through the use of lasers or a procedure called cryopexy—surgical fixation with cold.

If the retina has already detached, some vison can often be restored with the following procedures.

- Pneumatic retinopexy, which involves injecting a gas bubble into the posterior segment of the eye. The pressure from the gas bubble flattens the retina, and the retina is later fixed in place with a laser.
- Scleral buckle, which involves using a silicone band to hold the retina in place.
- Replacing the vitreous body with silicone oil to reattach the retina.

▶ The Ear and the Senses of Hearing and Equilibrium

LO 35.6

The organ of hearing is the ear. In addition to providing the sense of hearing, the ear aids the body in maintaining balance, or equilibrium. To assist with ear exams and procedures, you need to understand ear anatomy and the hearing process.

Structure of the Ear

The ear is divided into three parts: the external ear, middle ear, and inner ear (see Figure 35-7).

External Ear The external ear is composed of the **auricle** or **pinna** and the **external auditory canal.** The auricle is the flap of skin and cartilage that hangs off the side of the head. It collects sound waves. The external auditory canal is more commonly called the ear canal and is lined with skin that contains hairs and glands that produce **cerumen,** a wax-like substance commonly known as earwax. Cerumen lubricates the ear and protects it by trapping dirt, dust, and other microbes. This canal carries sound waves to the **tympanic membrane** or eardrum. The tympanic membrane is a fibrous partition located at the inner end of the external auditory canal. It separates the external ear from the middle ear.

Middle Ear The middle ear begins with the tympanic membrane, which is relatively thin and vibrates when sound waves hit it. On the other side of the tympanic membrane are three tiny bones called ear **ossicles**—the *malleus* (hammer), *incus* (anvil), and *stapes* (stirrup). When the tympanic membrane vibrates, it causes the ossicles to vibrate and hit a membrane called the **oval window.** The oval window ends the middle ear and marks the beginning of the inner ear.

The middle ear is connected to the throat by a tube called the **eustachian** (auditory) **tube.** This tube helps maintain equal pressure on both sides of the eardrum, which is important for normal hearing. Because the middle ear is connected to the throat by this tube, any throat infection can easily spread to the ear and vice versa.

Inner Ear The inner ear is a complex system of communicating chambers and tubes known as the **labyrinth.** It is divided into three portions: **semicircular canals,** a **vestibule,** and a **cochlea** (see Figure 35-8). Each ear has three semicircular canals that detect the body's balance. The cochlea is

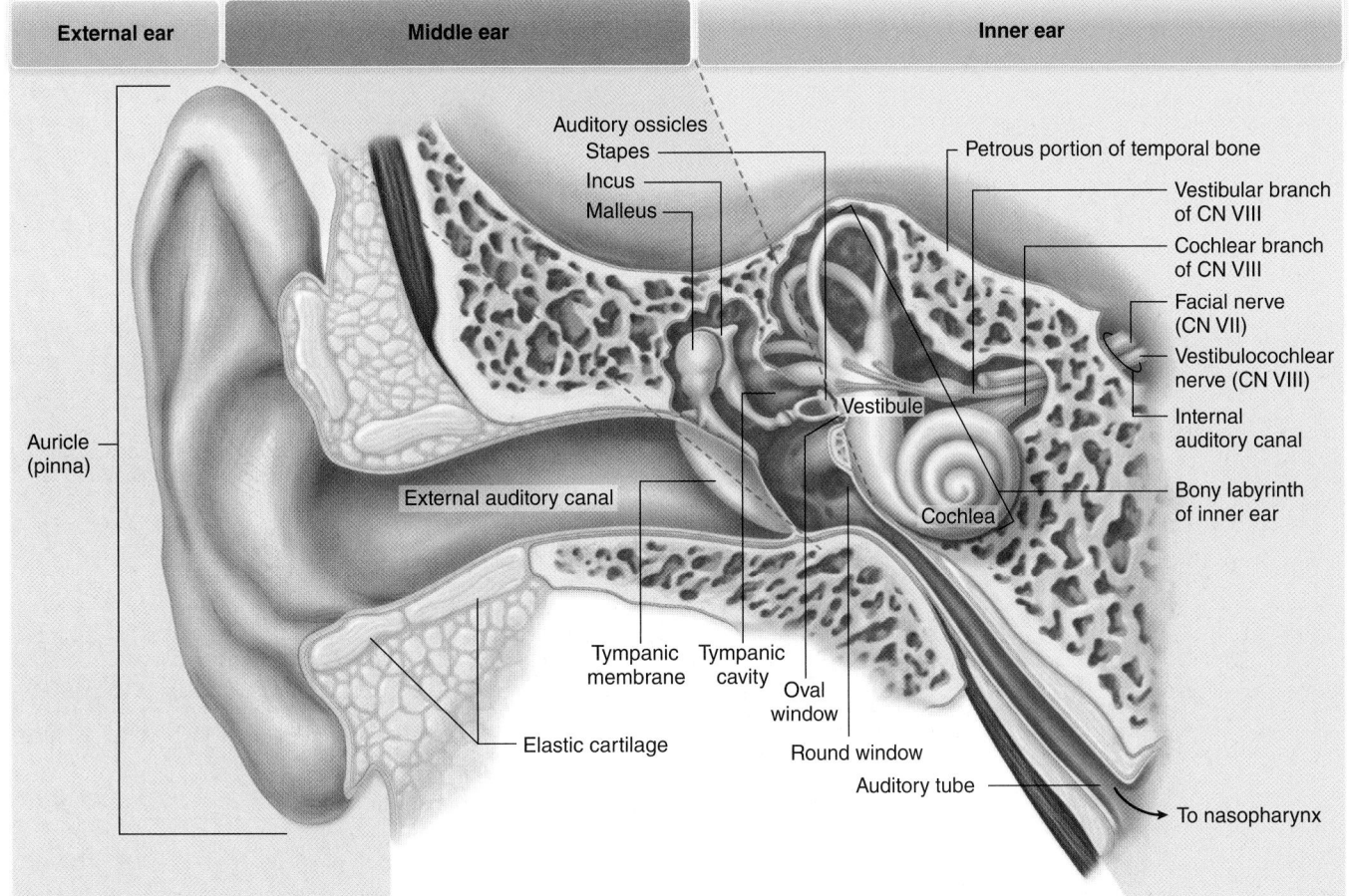

| External ear | Middle ear | Inner ear |

Auditory ossicles
Stapes
Incus
Malleus

Petrous portion of temporal bone

Vestibular branch of CN VIII

Cochlear branch of CN VIII

Facial nerve (CN VII)

Vestibulocochlear nerve (CN VIII)

Internal auditory canal

Bony labyrinth of inner ear

Auricle (pinna)

Vestibule

Cochlea

External auditory canal

Elastic cartilage

Tympanic membrane

Tympanic cavity

Oval window

Round window

Auditory tube

To nasopharynx

FIGURE 35-7   Anatomic regions of the right ear—the ear is divided into external, middle, and inner regions.

shaped like a snail's shell and contains hearing receptors, including the **organ of Corti,** which is known as the organ of hearing. The vestibule is the area between the semicircular canals and the cochlea. Like the semicircular canals, it functions in equilibrium. When the head moves, the *perilymph* and *endolymph* fluids in the semicircular canals and vestibule move. This activates both equilibrium and hearing receptors. The equilibrium receptors send the information along vestibular nerves to the cerebrum for interpretation. The cerebrum can then advise the body if it needs to make any adjustments to prevent a fall.

When sound waves of different volumes and frequencies activate the hearing receptors in the cochlea, they send their information to auditory nerves. Auditory nerves (vestibulocochlear nerves) deliver the information to the auditory cortex in the cerebrum's temporal lobe. The auditory cortex interprets the information as sounds.

▶ The Hearing Process   LO 35.7

A sound consists of waves of different frequencies that move through the air. The external ear initiates sound conduction when it collects these waves and channels them to the tympanic membrane. Here, the waves make the tympanic membrane

vibrate. The vibrations, in turn, are amplified by the middle ear's ossicles. The amplified waves enter the inner ear and the cochlea. These waves cause tiny hairs that line the cochlea to bend. Movements of the hairs trigger nerve impulses. The auditory nerve transmits these impulses to the brain, where they are perceived as sound.

Sound waves are also conducted through the bones of the skull directly to the inner ear—a process called bone conduction. This alternative pathway for sound bypasses the external and middle ears. When you hear your own voice, the sound has reached your inner ear mainly through bone conduction. By comparing a person's ability to sense sounds by bone conduction and through the entire ear, doctors can often identify what part of the ear is causing a hearing problem. For example, if bone conduction is normal, a hearing problem likely involves the middle or external ear rather than the inner ear.

The Aging Ear
As a person grows older, a number of changes occur in the ear. The external ear appears larger because of continued cartilage growth and the loss of skin elasticity. The earlobe gets longer and may have a wrinkled appearance. The glands that produce cerumen become less efficient, producing earwax that is

FIGURE 35-8   Right inner ear—the inner ear is composed of a bony labyrinth cavity that houses a fluid-filled membranous labyrinth. Within the bony labyrinth are the vestibular organs for equilibrium and balance, and the cochlea for hearing.

much drier and prone to impaction. The ear canal also becomes narrower.

In the middle ear, changes in the eardrum cause it to shrink and appear dull and gray. The joints between the bones of the middle ear degenerate, so they do not move as freely. In the inner ear, the semicircular canals become less sensitive to changes in position, and this reduced sensitivity affects balance.

Problems with equilibrium make the elderly prone to falls. Some ear disorders, like hearing loss and Mèniére's disease, are also more common in older individuals.

BODYANIMAT3D
POWERED BY
connect

Go to CONNECT to see an animation about *Hearing Loss: Sensorineural.*

How to Recognize Hearing Problems in Infants

Hearing problems in infants are not easy to recognize. The following general guidelines can be used to teach parents how to identify normal hearing in infants. Any deviations from these guidelines may indicate a hearing loss.

Infants up to 4 months old:

- They should be startled by loud noises (barking dog, hand clap, etc.).

- When sleeping in a quiet room, they should wake up at the sound of voices.

- Around the fourth month of age, they should turn their head or move their eyes to follow a sound.

- They should recognize the mother's or primary caregiver's voice better than other voices.

Infants 4 to 8 months of age:

- They should regularly turn their heads or move their eyes to follow sounds.

- Their facial expressions should change at the sound of familiar voices or loud noises.

- They should begin to enjoy certain sounds such as rattles or ringing bells.

- They should begin to babble at people who talk to them.

Babies 8 to 12 months of age:

- They should turn quickly to the sound of their name.

- They should begin to vary the pitch of the sounds they produce in their babbling.

- They should begin to respond to music.

- They should respond to the instruction "no."

Common Diseases and Disorders of the Ears

The following common diseases and disorders are specific to the ears.

ACOUSTIC NEUROMA is a benign tumor of the cranial nerve involved in hearing and balance.

Causes. A malfunction in a gene responsible for controlling the growth of Schwann cells—a type of neuroglial cell. (See *The Nervous System* chapter for more information.) This gene is found on chromosome 22.

Signs and Symptoms. Gradual hearing loss in one ear is the most common symptom. Patients may also experience balance problems and tinnitus—ringing in the ears.

Treatment. Since acoustic neuromas often grow slowly, the physician may monitor the tumor if the patient is not experiencing severe symptoms. Large tumors or those causing severe symptoms may be treated with radiation therapy or surgical removal.

CERUMEN IMPACTION is a condition that consists of the buildup of earwax within the external auditory canal.

Causes. Cerumen impaction may be caused by improper cleaning of cerumen from the ear canal—using cotton-tipped applicators—or by over-active ceruminous glands producing more than the normal amount of cerumen.

Signs and Symptoms. The most common sign is some degree of hearing loss because of the blockage of sound waves. Some patients may also complain of ear pain, ringing in the ear, or a feeling that the ear is stopped up.

Treatment. Treatment includes ear irrigation to remove the blockage. Severely hardened cerumen may require an earwax softener such as Debrox to soften and loosen the cerumen before the impaction can be removed.

HEARING LOSS, also known as deafness, is the loss of the ability to hear sounds at normal levels.

Causes. The two types of hearing loss are conductive and sensorineural. Conductive hearing loss is caused by a blockage of sound waves caused by cerumen impaction, a foreign body, otosclerosis (hardening of the stapes), or a tumor. Sensorineural hearing loss involves damage to the auditory nerve. Causes may include infection, medications, head trauma, and vascular disorders. In some cases, both types of hearing loss may be evident.

Signs and Symptoms. Patients may report gradual or sudden difficulty hearing voices, television, and other sounds within their environment. People around them may notice the need for increased volume when listening to television or the radio, or notice that the patient is speaking in a louder voice than necessary. Sudden hearing loss requires immediate medical attention.

Treatment. The treatment depends on the type of hearing loss involved. Any obstruction should be removed by irrigation or surgery if necessary. If hearing loss is a medication side effect, medication changes may be necessary. Hearing aids may be the

answer for many patients. Cochlear implants may be an option for those not assisted adequately with hearing aids, as long as the auditory nerve remains intact.

OTITIS is inflammation of the ear. All three areas of the ear may be inflamed. **OTITIS EXTERNA** is infection of the outer ear also known as swimmer's ear. The infection can be localized, as with a boil or abscess, or the entire ear canal lining can be affected. **OTITIS MEDIA** is a middle ear infection, and **OTITIS INTERNA** (labyrinthitis) is an inner ear infection.

Causes. Bacterial infections are often to blame for otitis externa. Otitis media often results from the spread of an upper respiratory infection from the throat that enters the eustachian tube and infects the middle ear. Labyrinthitis, especially the purulent or infective type, occurs from a spread of otitis media to the inner ear.

Signs and Symptoms. Pain in the ear with associated hearing loss is the primary symptom. Patients with otitis externa may include itching and pus in the ear. Labyrinthitis also often causes vertigo and nausea. Purulent (pus-containing) drainage may also occur in some forms of otitis media.

Treatment. Antibiotics or antifungals are given to treat the causative agent. Anti-inflammatory or pain medication and fever reducers may also be given to make the patient more comfortable. Antihistamines and anti-nausea medications may also be used to treat otitis interna.

OTOSCLEROSIS is the immobilization of the stapes within the inner ear, which is a common cause of conductive hearing loss.

Causes. Genetics seems to play a role. This disease occurs more frequently in females than in males.

Signs and Symptoms. These include a slow and progressive hearing loss that may be accompanied by tinnitus.

Treatment. Surgical removal of the stapes (stapedectomy) with insertion of a prosthetic stapes may result in at least a partial hearing restoration.

PRESBYCUSIS is hearing loss because of the aging process.

Causes. Factors like prolonged exposure to loud noise, infection, injury, certain medications, and some diseases are thought to be causes of presbycusis. For example, as part of the natural aging process, the auditory system deteriorates, resulting in a loss of hair cells (sensory receptors) in the organ of Corti. Changes in the blood supply to the ear or reduced function of the tympanic membrane or ossicles are also contributing factors.

Signs and Symptoms. Signs and symptoms include gradual, progressive hearing loss, usually of high-frequency sounds first. Typically both ears are affected and the patient has difficulty hearing high-pitched tones as well as normal conversation. Tinnitus may accompany this loss and the patient may become depressed and frustrated at his developing inability to communicate well as a result of the hearing loss.

Treatment. In most cases, hearing aids are prescribed to alleviate some of the hearing loss, although the condition itself is irreversible.

LEARNING OUTCOMES	KEY POINTS
35.1 Describe the anatomy of the nose and the function of each part.	Olfactory receptors—the sense receptors for the sense of smell—are found in the olfactory organ located in the upper part of the nasal cavity.
35.2 Describe the anatomy of the tongue and the function of each part.	Gustatory receptors are found on the taste buds, which are located on the papillae (bumps) of the tongue.
35.3 Describe the anatomy of the eye and the function of each part, including the accessory structures and their functions.	The eye is composed of three layers. The sclera is the outer protective layer and includes the cornea. The middle vascular layer is the choroid consisting of the iris, pupil, ciliary body, and lens, and is the area of light regulation and focusing. The innermost layer is the retina containing the rods and cones, the optic nerve, and the optic disc. This is where the nerve impulse is picked up and brought to the brain for interpretation. The accessory organs are the orbits, eyelids, conjunctivas, lacrimal apparatus, and extrinsic eye muscles, all of which are protective for the eye.
35.4 Explain the visual pathway through the eye and to the brain for interpretation.	The cornea, lens, and fluids focus light on the retina. The retina converts the image into nerve impulses that the optic nerve transmits to the brain for interpretation.
35.5 Describe the causes, signs and symptoms, and treatments of various disorders of the eyes.	There are many common diseases and disorders of the eyes with varied signs, symptoms, and treatments. Some of these include astigmatism, dry eye syndrome, ectropion, entropion, nystagmus, and retinal detachment.
35.6 Describe the anatomy of the ear and the function of each part, and explain the role of the ear in maintaining equilibrium.	There are three parts to the ear. The external ear includes the auricle or pinna and the external auditory canal to the tympanic membrane. The middle ear begins at the tympanic membrane and ends at the oval window and includes the ear ossicles. The inner ear is composed of the labyrinth and contains the organ of Corti as well as perilymph and endolymph—the fluids of hearing. The semicircular canals and vestibule in the inner ear function in the body's equilibrium and balance, sending impulses to the vestibular nerves, which bring information to the cerebrum for interpretation.
35.7 Explain how sounds travel through the ear and are interpreted in the brain.	The outer ear collects sound waves and channels them to the tympanic membrane, which vibrates. The vibrations are amplified by the ear ossicles and enter the inner ear and cochlea. The movements of the hairs in the cochlea trigger nerve impulses that the auditory nerve transmits to the brain.
35.8 Describe the causes, signs and symptoms, and treatments of various disorders of the ears.	There are many common diseases and disorders of the ears with varied signs, symptoms, and treatments. Some of these include acoustic neuroma, cerumen impaction, hearing loss, otitis, otitis externa, otitis media, otitis interna, otosclerosis, and presbycusis.

Recall Valarie Ramirez from the beginning of the chapter. Now that you have completed the chapter, answer the following questions regarding her case.

1. Describe the structures of the eye that might be affected by Valarie's motorcycle injury.

2. What can you tell Valarie about protecting her eyes when she rides her motorcycle again?

1. (LO 35.1 and LO 35.2) Which of the special senses utilize chemoreceptors?
   a. Smell and hearing
   b. Taste and vision
   c. Smell and taste
   d. Vision and hearing
   e. Smell and vision

2. (LO 35.3) Which of the following is the other name for the corneal-scleral junction?
   a. Optic chiasm
   b. Limbus
   c. Blind spot
   d. Orbicularis oculi
   e. Ciliary body

3. (LO 35.3) The changing of the lens shape is called
   a. Astigmatism
   b. Accommodation
   c. Refraction
   d. Focusing
   e. Ectropion

4. (LO 35.3) The fluid in the anterior eye chamber is
   a. Aqueous humor
   b. Lacrimal humor
   c. Vitreous humor
   d. Orbital humor
   e. Vestibular humor

5. (LO 35.2) Taste buds are found on the
   a. Supporting cells
   b. Papillae
   c. Chemoreceptors
   d. Esophagus
   e. Gingiva

6. (LO 35.3) The mucous membranes that line each eye are known as
   a. Lacrimal glands
   b. Cornea
   c. Conjunctivas
   d. Aqueous tissues
   e. Chonchae

7. (LO 35.6) Which of the following marks the beginning of the inner ear?
   a. Tympanic membrane
   b. Eustachian tube
   c. Stapes
   d. Auditory canal
   e. Oval window

8. (LO 35.6) Another name for the auricle of the ear is the
   a. Exteral auditory canal
   b. Pinna
   c. Malleus
   d. Eustachian tube
   e. Earlobe

9. (LO 35.7) The process by which sound waves bypass the external and middle ear is known as
   a. Bone conduction
   b. Tympanic conduction
   c. Sensorineural conduction
   d. Air conduction
   e. Ossicular pathway

10. (LO 35.6) Which of the following structures is involved with equilibrium?
    a. Limbus
    b. Ossicles
    c. Eustachian tube
    d. Organ of Corti
    e. Semicircular canals

Analyze the following medical terms, presented throughout the chapter. Using a medical dictionary (or Appendix I) place a / mark between each word part. Define each word part and then define the whole word.

EXAMPLE: **ophthalo/scope** = ophthalo means "eye" + scope means "instrument used to examine"
Ophthaloscope means "instrument used to examine the eye"

1. amblyopia
2. auditory
3. conjunctivitis
4. ectropion
5. endolymph

6. entropion
7. glaucoma
8. ophthalmologist
9. optician
10. optometrist

11. otosclerosis
12. perilymph
13. semicircular
14. sensorineural
15. tympanic

Patient Interview and History

CASE STUDY

Patient Name	Gender	DOB
Peter Smith	Male	3/28/19XX

Attending	MRN	Allergies
Paul F. Buckwalter, MD	428-69-544	NKA

Peter Smith, a 73-year-old male with mild type II diabetes, calls to schedule an appointment. He states that he is feeling very anxious and fatigued and is having difficulty eating and sleeping. He arrives at the clinic with his wife and needs to check in.

During the patient interview, he states that he wakes up in the middle of the night almost nightly. He also has many nights when he cannot even fall asleep. In addition, he has lost about 8 pounds in the last month. His symptoms started when his son died 6 months ago.

Keep Mr. Smith in mind as you study this chapter. There will be questions at the end of the chapter based on the case study. The information in the chapter will help you answer these questions.

McGraw Hill ACTIVSim™

LEARNING OUTCOMES

After completing Chapter 36, you will be able to:

36.1 Identify the skills necessary to conduct a patient interview.

36.2 Recognize the signs of anxiety; depression; and physical, mental, or substance abuse.

36.3 Use the six Cs for writing an accurate patient history.

36.4 Carry out a patient history using critical thinking skills.

KEY TERMS

addiction
chief complaint
clarification
mirroring
objective data

reflection
restatement
subjective data
substance abuse
verbalizing

I. P (6)	Perform patient screening using established protocols
I. A (1)	Apply critical thinking skills in performing patient assessment and care
I. A (2)	Use language/verbal skills that enable patients' understanding
IV. C (2)	Identify nonverbal communication
IV. C (4)	Identify techniques for overcoming communication barriers
IV. C (6)	Differentiate between subjective and objective information
IV. C (7)	Identify resources and adaptations that are required based on individual needs, i.e., culture and environment, developmental life stage, language, and physical threats to communication
IV. C (12)	Organize technical information and summaries
IV. P (1)	Use reflection, restatement and clarification techniques to obtain a patient history
IV. P (2)	Report relevant information to others succinctly and accurately
IV. P (3)	Use medical terminology, pronouncing medical terms correctly, to communicate information, patient history, data and observations
IV. P (11)	Respond to nonverbal communication
IV. A (2)	Apply active listening skills
IV. A (3)	Use appropriate body language and other nonverbal skills in communicating with patients, family and staff
IV. A (5)	Demonstrate sensitivity appropriate to the message being delivered
IX. P (2)	Perform within scope of practice
IX. P (3)	Apply HIPAA rules in regard to privacy/release of information
IX. P (5)	Incorporate the Patient's Bill of Rights into personal practice and medical office policies and procedures
IX. P (7)	Document accurately in the patient record
IX. A (1)	Demonstrate sensitivity to patient rights

3. **Medical Terminology**

Graduates:

d. Recognize and identify acceptable medical abbreviations

4. **Medical Law and Ethics**

Graduates:

a. Document accurately

b. Institute federal and state guidelines when releasing medical records or information

f. Comply with federal, state, and local health laws and regulations

5. **Psychology of Human Relations**

Graduates:

a. Define and understand abnormal behavior patterns

b. Identify and respond appropriately when working/caring for patients with special needs

e. Advocate on behalf of family/patients, having ability to deal and communicate with family

9. **Medical Office Clinical Procedures**

Graduates:

a. Obtain chief complaint, recording patient history

11. **Career Development**

Graduates:

b. Demonstrate professionalism by:

(3) Maintaining confidentiality at all times

(4) Being cognizant of ethical boundaries

(8) Being courteous and diplomatic

(9) Conducting work within scope of education, training, and ability

▷ Introduction

As a medical assistant, it is your job to prepare the patient and the patient's chart before the physician enters the exam room to examine the patient. You are the first contact with the patient in the exam room. How you conduct yourself during those first few moments can make a major difference in the patient's attitude and perception of the medical office. The patient must cooperate fully to provide the information the physician needs for an accurate diagnosis and successful treatment. Conducting the patient interview and recording the necessary medical history are essential to the practitioner's exam process.

▷ The Patient Interview and History

LO 36.1

The first step in the exam process is the patient interview. A well-conducted initial interview in the exam room helps establish a beneficial relationship between you and the new patient while providing a detailed exchange of pertinent information. Subsequent interviews with established patients may take less time; however, all patient interviews require good communication skills.

When you interview a patient, you will ask the patient (or an attending family member) for specific information about the reason for his or her visit. If the visit is for a medical problem, you will ask about his or her symptoms and determine the patient's chief complaint. The **chief complaint** is a subjective statement made by the patient describing the patient's most significant symptoms or signs of illness. Medicare and most insurers require this information. When a patient makes an office visit for a routine checkup, you will ask the patient about general health and lifestyle and about any changes in health status since the last visit.

A patient's medical and health history is the basis for all treatment rendered by the practitioner. The history also provides information for research, reportable diseases, and insurance claims. The information contained on the chart becomes a legal record of the treatment rendered to the patient. It must be complete and accurate to be a good defense in case of legal action. Document all information regarding the patient precisely and accurately.

www.mhhe.com/BoothMA5e

Recording a Chief Complaint

Patient Rights, Responsibilities, and Privacy

It is important to remember that all the data you obtain are subject to legal and ethical considerations. Most states have adopted a version of the American Hospital Association's (AHA) Patient's Bill of Rights, written in 1973 and revised in 1992. Although AHA has replaced this bill of rights with "The Patient Care Partnership: Understanding Expectations, Rights, and Responsibilities," each state encourages healthcare workers to be aware of and provide for the patient's rights. Familiarize yourself with the information about patient rights contained in the following bullets. All patients have the right to

- Receive considerate and respectful care.
- Receive complete and current information concerning his or her diagnosis, treatment, and prognosis.
- Know the identity of physicians, nurses, and others involved with his or her care as well as know when those involved are students, residents, or trainees.
- Know the immediate and long-term costs of treatment choices.
- Receive information necessary to give informed consent prior to the start of any procedure or treatment.
- Have an advance directive concerning treatment or be able to choose a representative to make decisions.
- Refuse treatment to the extent permitted by law.
- Receive every consideration of his or her privacy.
- Be assured of confidentiality.
- Obtain reasonable responses to requests for services.
- Obtain information about his or her healthcare and be allowed to review his or her medical record and to have any information explained or interpreted.
- Know whether treatment is experimental and be able to consent or decline to participate in proposed research studies or human experimentation.
- Expect reasonable continuity of care.

- Ask about and be informed of the existence of business relationships between the hospital and others that may influence the patient's treatment and care.
- Know which hospital policies and practices relate to patient care, treatment, and responsibilities.
- Be informed of available resources for resolving disputes, grievances, and conflicts, such as ethics committees or patient representatives.
- Examine his or her bill and have it explained, and be informed of available payment methods.

Medical assistants also should know that patients have certain responsibilities when they seek medical care. Patients are responsible for

- Providing information about past illnesses, hospitalizations, medications, and other matters related to their health status. If an incorrect diagnosis is made because a patient fails to give the physician the proper information, the physician is not liable.
- Participating in decision making by asking for additional information about their health status or treatment when they do not fully understand information and instructions.
- Providing healthcare agencies with a copy of their written advance directive if they have one.
- Informing physicians and other caregivers if they anticipate problems in following a prescribed treatment.
- Following the physician's orders for treatment. If a patient willfully or negligently fails to follow the physician's instructions, that patient has little legal recourse.
- Providing healthcare agencies with necessary information for insurance claims and working with the healthcare facility to make arrangements to pay fees when necessary.

Additionally, in April 2003, enforcement of the Health Insurance Portability and Accountability Act (HIPAA) began. If this act is not followed, individual healthcare workers can be subject to fines up to $250,000 and 10 years in jail. The privacy standards of this act ensure the following:

- Healthcare facilities must provide patients with a written notice of their practices regarding the use and disclosure of all individually identifiable health information.
- Healthcare facilities may not use or disclose protected health information for any purpose that is not in the privacy notice.
- Patient consent is required when protected information is used or disclosed for purposes of treatment, payment, or health operations.
- Written authorization is required for other types of disclosures.
- Hospitals must make the privacy notice available either prior to, or at the time of, the delivery of care.
- A privacy notice must be posted in a clear and prominent location within the hospital facility.

Communicating with Professionalism

Remember, the first impression you make with patients in the exam room can be everlasting, as it can affect the way patients view the entire office's practice, including the physicians. As a medical assistant, communicating with professionalism is key. In addition to your awareness of patient rights, responsibilities, and privacy, your overall professionalism and poise can be a direct result of your verbal communication skills. If you use improper language skills, like poor grammar or slang, or appear to have sloppy body language, you may give the patient the perception that you are not educated or intelligent. Your communication skills will have a direct impact on your career. Take care and pride in what you know and how you communicate. Think before you speak or react and you will learn to avoid communication pitfalls.

Interviewing Skills

To conduct a successful patient interview and obtain history and health information, you will need to apply a variety of skills, including the following:

- Using effective listening.
- Being aware of nonverbal clues and body language.
- Using a broad knowledge base.
- Summarizing to form a general picture.

Using Effective Listening Listening attentively is one of the most important skills you will need for a successful interview. When you listen to what the patient is saying, you not only listen for details but also try to get an overall view of the patient's situation. As you become more experienced in conducting patient interviews, these skills will improve. One way to be a good listener is to hear, think about, and respond to what the patient has said. This technique is called *active listening*. Passive listeners simply sit back and hear. When you are an active listener, you look at the patient, pay attention, and provide feedback. For example, you may use the technique of **restatement**. Simply repeat what the patient says, in your own words, back to the patient. This helps to ensure that you have understood the meaning of the patient's words.

Being Aware of Nonverbal Clues and Body Language
Verbal communication is the asking and answering of questions. To conduct a successful interview, you also must be aware of nonverbal communication. The patient's tone of voice, facial expression, and body language are examples of nonverbal communication. These signs often communicate more than words could ever say. For example, a patient who has difficulty making eye contact may be embarrassed by some symptoms and may need your extra patience and encouragement to report symptoms fully. A child or adolescent may deny or exaggerate pain. Pay attention to the patient's facial expression and how much the patient guards the area in question.

Using a Broad Knowledge Base To conduct a successful interview, you must have a broad knowledge base so that you can ask questions that will elicit the most meaningful information about the patient. You must take every opportunity to expand your knowledge base by learning more about medical terminology, anatomy and physiology, symptoms, and diseases.

Summarizing to Form a General Picture You will gather a variety of subjective and objective data as you conduct a patient interview. You must consider the relative importance of each piece of information so that you can summarize the data to formulate a general picture of the patient. It is always a good idea to repeat back a summary of information to the patient. This will ensure that all important data are recorded. Patients will sometimes forget to add something, and repeating the summary may jog their memory.

Interviewing Successfully

One of the main goals of the patient interview is to give the patient an opportunity to fully explain, in her own words, the reason for the current office visit. These eight steps will help you conduct a successful interview.

1. Do your research before the patient interview.
2. Plan the interview.
3. Approach the patient and request the interview.
4. Make the patient feel at ease.
5. Conduct the interview in private without interruptions.
6. Deal with sensitive topics with respect.
7. Do not diagnose or give a diagnostic opinion.
8. Formulate the general picture.

Doing Research Before the Patient Interview Before the interview, review the patient's medical record for history, medications, and chronic problems (for example, diabetes or high blood pressure). Note whether the patient has family problems that might have an impact on health issues. Make sure that all currently ordered diagnostic testing, laboratory work, and consultation results are in the chart. If you discover that you are missing a result, you have some time to retrieve it from the facility while the patient is in the office.

Planning the Interview Develop an interview plan by having a general idea of the questions you will ask. For example, if a patient is being treated for high blood pressure, you might ask about headaches or tinnitus (ringing in the ears), which are common signs of high blood pressure. Planning the interview helps you maintain your focus and ensures that you will obtain all the necessary information.

It is important to be organized before the interview takes place. Follow the office policies when gathering patient information. For example, you may record the patient's height, weight, and vital signs before you begin the interview. Make sure that you follow office policy on the types of information you will need to ask the patient during the interview. For example, some physicians prefer that you record the patient's medication list before the exam, whereas others prefer to record the medication list themselves. Planning for the types of information that you need to collect will save time for the visit itself.

Approaching the Patient and Requesting the Interview Ask the patient for permission before conducting the interview. You may need to explain that questions about the reason for the visit and the patient's current health situation are necessary to plan the most effective care. It is more courteous to seek permission to ask questions than to say that you "need to take a history." Asking permission helps the patient feel more comfortable and emphasizes the importance of the interview process. It also makes the patient feel more like a participant in the medical care being provided.

Making the Patient Feel at Ease Using certain words or phrases known as icebreakers can help set the stage for the interview. Icebreakers put the patient at ease and create a relaxed atmosphere. Examples of icebreakers include acknowledging the patient's reason for the visit, introducing yourself, or commenting about the weather. Icebreakers that also convey a sincere and sensitive interest in the patient are asking the patient how she prefers to be addressed or clarifying the pronunciation of a difficult name.

Another way to convey an image of a professional who is sensitive to the patient's needs is to sit with the patient and appear relaxed. By appearing relaxed, you help the patient relax and encourage a more open and comfortable interview. Eye contact is important when interviewing a patient. Sometimes patients will feel intimidated if they are forced to look up at you. If the patient sits in a chair, then it is best that you sit; if the patient sits on the examining table, then it is appropriate to stand while recording the visit. Remember, if you are entering data into an electronic record, there is a patient in the room with you. If you pay more attention to inputting information into the computer than looking at and speaking with your patient, she may feel as if she is just another patient and not an individual being cared for by you.

Conducting the Interview in Private without Interruptions After setting the stage for the interview, ensure privacy by showing the patient to a private room or area or by closing the door if the patient is already in a private room. You can then begin to ask relevant questions. Some approaches are more effective than others, as shown in Table 36-1. Listening carefully to the patient's responses may lead you to ask questions other than those in your interview plan.

TABLE 36-1	**Methods of Collecting Patient Data**
Effective Methods	**Characteristics**
Asking open-ended questions	Requires more than a yes or no answer; allows the patient to more fully explain the situation, resulting in more relevant data. Instead of asking, "Do you have a cough?" ask, "Can you tell me about your symptoms?"
Asking hypothetical questions	Allows you to determine the patient's knowledge of the situation and whether it is accurate. For example, ask a patient who has been prescribed nitroglycerin for chest pain, "What would you do if you have chest pain?"
Mirroring patient's responses and verbalizing the implied	Allows nonthreatening ways for the patient to discuss the situation further and to provide underlying meaning. **Mirroring** means restating what the patient says in your own words. **Verbalizing** means stating what you believe the patient is suggesting by his response. You might say, "So the pain started about 3 days ago and has been getting worse each day, and today it has not let up at all."
Focusing on patient	Shows the patient that you are really listening to what he is saying. You maintain eye contact (as culturally appropriate), assume a relaxed and open body posture, and use the proper responses.
Encouraging patient to take the lead	Motivates the patient to discuss or describe the situation in his own way. Ask a question such as, "Where would you like to begin?"
Encouraging patient to provide additional information	Conveys sincere interest in the patient by continuing to explore topics in more detail when appropriate. You might ask the patient if he has experienced a symptom before or if he associates it with a change in routine. This provides for **clarification** or increased understanding of the problem.
Encouraging patient to evaluate his situation	Provides an idea of the patient's point of view about the situation; allows you to determine the patient's knowledge of the situation and possible fears. Ask the patient, "What do you think is going on here?" This will allow you and the patient to use **reflection**. Reflection is when a thought, idea, or opinion is formed as a result of deeper thought, in this case stimulated by a question.
Ineffective Methods	**Characteristics**
Asking closed-ended questions	Provides little information because closed-ended questions offer the patient little freedom to explain his answers. Closed-ended questions require only yes or no answers.
Asking leading questions	Leading questions suggest a desired response instead of the patient's true response. The patient tends to agree with such statements instead of elaborating on them. An example of a leading question is, "You seem to be making progress, don't you agree?" This type of question limits the patient's response.
Challenging patient	The patient may feel you are disagreeing with what he is saying if you ask an emotional or challenging question or use a certain tone of voice. The patient may become defensive, which might block further communication. An example of challenging the patient is, "You are not having that much pain from this small wound, are you?"
Probing	Continuing to question a patient after he appears to have finished giving information can make him feel that you are invading his privacy. The patient may become defensive and withhold information.
Agreeing or disagreeing with patient	When you agree or disagree with a patient, it implies that the patient is either "right" or "wrong." This action can block further communication.

Developing a rapport with the patient is essential. Keep the atmosphere relaxed, do not rush, maintain eye contact, and use the patient's name in conversation. Avoid interruptions, like taking phone calls and letting people walk in and out of the room. Make sure that you do not use "pet names" for your patients, such as "honey" or "sweetie." Doing so can offend some patients and can be misinterpreted as being insincere.

Dealing with Sensitive Topics with Respect Sometimes you will have to ask patients questions about sensitive topics. Such topics may be related to sexuality, lifestyle, or behaviors that put a person at risk for diseases. You must approach these topics gently so that the patient does not feel threatened by the questioning. You can show respect for the patient's rights and privacy by knowing when to stop. Both verbal and nonverbal clues can guide you in this area. It is also important to be conscious of your body language when dealing with sensitive subjects. You may find yourself exposed to situations that you do not have any prior experience with and "shock" may register on your face.

Avoiding Making a Diagnosis or Giving a Diagnostic Opinion Only the physician can make a diagnosis, based on the patient's symptoms and complaints. If the patient asks for your opinion about a diagnosis, explain that the physician should be asked about diagnoses. If pressed, you may need to say you are not able to give opinions about a diagnosis and the physician will answer any questions he or she may have. Never go beyond your scope of practice or job description.

Formulating the General Picture Summarize the key points of the interview. Ask the patient whether he or she has questions or other information to add. You will be most successful with the interview process if you remain alert and organized but flexible. Procedure 36-1, at the end of the chapter, demonstrates the proper approach to an interview.

Go to CONNECT to see a video about *Using Critical Thinking Skills During an Interview.*

▶ Your Role as an Observer LO 36.2

During the pre-exam stage of the office visit, you will gather most of your information through verbal and nonverbal communication. The nonverbal communication that occurs during the interview and history taking, however, sometimes reveals more about a patient than the patient's words. Listening attentively and observing the patient closely may help you detect a problem that might otherwise go unnoted.

Anxiety

Anxiety is a common emotional response in patients. Some patients respond with anxiety to a specific fear, such as fear of pain. Others simply feel anxious when they are in an unfamiliar situation. For example, many patients have what is called "white coat syndrome," which is anxiety related to seeing a physician.

To recognize anxiety, you must understand that it varies from mild to severe. A patient with mild anxiety may have a heightened ability to observe and to make connections. A patient with severe anxiety has difficulty focusing on details, feels panicky, and is virtually helpless. A heightened focus or a lack of focus in a patient can hinder your ability to get the information and cooperation you need. When you observe signs of anxiety in a patient, make every effort to help her relax and release or reduce the anxious feelings. You may be able to help by allowing the patient to describe her feelings. If a patient becomes agitated while discussing a physical complaint, you may need to postpone talking about the matter until the patient is calmer. In either situation, give support in nonverbal ways by trying to make the patient as comfortable as possible. Give the patient time to respond and then wait quietly, provide privacy, make eye contact, and communicate at the patient's level of understanding.

Depression

Depression can be difficult to recognize, as some of its symptoms are the same as those of many common illnesses. For example, fatigue and sleep disturbances are symptoms of both depression and hypothyroidism. To complicate matters, many patients with major depression develop great skill in hiding depression or are unaware they are suffering from it. Consequently, many patients—especially the elderly—have undiagnosed depression.

To recognize depression, you must be aware of common symptoms associated with the condition. Classic symptoms of depression are profound sadness and fatigue. In addition, a depressed person may have difficulty falling asleep at night or getting up in the morning. The depressed patient may suffer from loss of appetite, loss of energy, or both.

Depression seems to occur most frequently during late adolescence, in middle age, and after retirement. In late adolescence, depression can be difficult to distinguish from addiction and substance abuse. Depression in middle age is often triggered by life events like financial troubles or death of a family member. It is sometimes confused with midlife crises. And in the elderly, depression is common but often mistaken for senility. If you observe any signs of depression, indicate them in the patient's chart and alert the physician.

As mentioned in the previous paragraph, depression, addiction, and substance abuse in adolescents can be difficult to distinguish, as the signs of substance abuse or addiction can be mistaken for those of depression. The reverse is also true. And sometimes all three conditions exist simultaneously. If you have any clues that point to one of these conditions in an adolescent patient, notify the physician immediately. For symptoms that may be signs of these disorders, see the Caution: Handle with Care section.

Physical and Psychological Abuse

Abuse can involve people from all walks of life and of all ages. Abuse can be physical, psychological, or both. As a medical

CAUTION: HANDLE WITH CARE

Signs of Depression, Substance Abuse, and Addiction in Adolescents

Signs of depression, substance abuse, and addiction are often hard to distinguish in adolescents. Part of the difficulty is that adolescents are particularly skilled at hiding signs of all three disorders.

Various signs may indicate depression in an adolescent. One teenager may lose interest in or be unable to enjoy everyday activities. Another may sleep for long periods and have difficulty getting up in the morning, whereas yet another may sleep very little. Chronic fatigue or aches and pains may signal depression, as may trouble with concentration or school absenteeism. These signs also may indicate substance abuse or addiction.

It is important to know the difference between substance abuse and addiction. **Substance abuse** refers to the use of a substance, even an over-the-counter drug, in a way that is not medically approved. Inappropriate use includes such practices as using diet pills to stay awake or consuming large quantities of cough syrup that contains codeine. It also includes taking larger-than-prescribed doses of a medication. Substance abusers are not necessarily addicts, however.

Addiction refers to a physical or psychological dependence on a substance. Addiction usually involves a pattern of behavior that includes an obsessive or compulsive preoccupation with a substance and the security of its supply, as well as a high rate of relapse after withdrawal.

As a medical assistant, you should not try to make a diagnosis. Quite likely, an adolescent with one or more of these disorders will be uncooperative and refuse to answer relevant questions. You must be aware, however, of physical signs or behaviors that may be associated with depression, substance abuse, or addiction in an adolescent patient. The following signs or behaviors are important clues that you should report immediately to the doctor.

- The patient complains of altered eating habits or disturbed sleep patterns (either too much or too little sleep).
- The patient's weight has changed drastically (either up or down) since the previous office visit.
- The patient appears lethargic or sullen, or exhibits radical mood changes.
- The patient has slurred speech.
- The patient appears to have illogical thought patterns.
- The patient appears to have needle tracks (anywhere on the body, especially on the arms or legs).
- The patient has pinpoint (highly constricted) pupils.

---

assistant, you are in a unique position to detect abuse in the patients you see.

Although you must not make hasty judgments, you may suspect abuse when a patient speaks in a guarded way. An unlikely explanation for an injury also may be a sign of abuse. There may be no history of the injury, or the history may be suspicious. In either case, the following injuries may be signs of physical abuse:

- Head injuries and skull fractures.
- Burns (especially those that appear to be deliberate, such as from a cigarette or an iron).
- Broken bones.
- Bruises (especially multiple bruises, those that are clearly in the shape of an object, and those in various stages of healing).

Although a patient can recover physically from abuse, the emotional and psychological scars may last a lifetime. Other signs of physical abuse (including sexual abuse and neglect) and signs of psychological abuse include the following:

- A child's failure to thrive.
- Severe dehydration or being underweight.
- Delayed medical attention.
- Hair loss.
- Drug use.
- Genital injuries.

Women, children, and elderly patients are more likely to be abused. Pay extra attention to these patients when performing the interview. If you suspect abuse, report it to your supervisor or physician. Prepare a list of local abuse hotline numbers for potential abuse victims.

The Interview and Abuse

Again, because women, children, and the elderly are more likely to be victims of abuse, it is crucial to pay extra attention to them during the interview.

Women According to the Domestic Violence Resource Center, 85% of victims of domestic violence are women and those ages 20 to 24 are at the greatest risk. Victims stay in abusive relationships for a variety of reasons, including fear of the abuser, threats of suicide by the abuser, financial dependence, lack of housing options, low self-esteem, and isolation. Women who are abused often feel shame. They may make excuses for their abuser or simply will not talk about it. It is important that you not be embarrassed to approach the subject of abuse with the patient. As with any other sensitive topic, you should not worry about embarrassing or insulting the patient by asking sensitive questions. Be kind, supportive, and nonjudgmental while interviewing a woman you suspect may be a victim of abuse. Careful listening and encouragement will build rapport with the patient, making the interview easier for the patient and more productive for you.

TABLE 36-2 Symptoms Associated with Commonly Abused Drugs

Drug Names/Type	Trade or Other Name	Symptoms, Effects
Amphetamines/stimulants	Benzedrine, Dexedrine, methamphetamine, black beauty, speed, uppers	Altered mental status, from confusion to paranoia; hyperactivity, then exhaustion; insomnia; loss of appetite
Anabolic steroids	Anadrol, Depo-testosterone, roids, juice	Irritability, aggression, nervousness, male-pattern baldness
Barbiturates/sedatives	Amobarbital, phenobarbital, Butisol, secobarbital, yellow jackets, red birds	Slowed thinking, slowed reflexes, slowed respiration, loss of anxiety
Benzodiazepines/sedatives	Ativan, diazepam, Librium, Valium, downers, candy	Poor coordination, drowsiness, increased self-confidence
Cocaine/stimulant	Coke, snow, crack	Alternating euphoria and apprehension, intense craving for more of the drug
Ecstasy/psychoactive	Adam, XTC, MDMA	Confusion, depression, anxiety, paranoia, increased heart rate and blood pressure
GHB/depressants	G, liquid ecstasy, Georgia homeboy	Slow pulse and breathing, lowered blood pressure, drowsiness, poor concentration
Heroin	Big H, Black Tar, Dope, Smack	Track marks, slowed or slurred speech, vomiting
Inhalants	Solvents: paint thinner Gases: aerosol, butane, or propane	Stimulation, intoxication, hearing loss, arm or leg spasms
LSD (lysergic acid diethylamine)/hallucinogen	Acid, microdot	Heightened sense of awareness, grandiose hallucinations, mystical experiences, flashbacks
Marijuana/cannabinoids/hashish	Pot, grass, joints, reefer, weed, chronic, Mary Jane, hash, boom	Altered thought processes, distorted sense of time and self, impaired short-term memory
Opium, morphine, codeine/opiate narcotics	Monkey, white stuff	Decreased level of consciousness, detachment, drowsiness, impaired judgment
PCP (phencyclidine)/hallucinogen	Angel dust, hog, rocket fuel, DOA, peace pill	Decreased awareness of surroundings, hallucinations, poor perception of time and distance, possible overdose and death

Children Children pose a unique situation during the patient interview. For infants and younger children, you will be asking the parent or other caregiver about the child's condition. However, no matter what the age of the child, you should consider the child first. Communicate with the child, observe for nonverbal signs of pain or other problems, and ask questions whenever possible.

Remember, children are often the targets of violence, much of which occurs in the home. In addition to being physically, emotionally, or sexually abused, children can be abused by being neglected. In addition to watching for physical signs of abuse during the interview, watch for any problems in the relationship between the child and caregiver. If you suspect a problem, report it to the physician.

The Elderly Physical and mental disabilities can make elderly people dependent on a caregiver. So, elderly patients may or may not be able to communicate with you verbally during the patient interview. You may need to communicate verbally with their caregiver. However, always observe elderly patients for nonverbal signs of problems, such as grimacing, foul odors, or bruising, even if they cannot speak to you verbally. The caregiver may perceive the patient as a burden and abuse can occur. Disabilities may make the elderly person defenseless against abuse. If you suspect a problem, report it to the physician.

Drug and Alcohol Abuse

Substance abuse and addiction to drugs or alcohol are serious social problems. Symptoms of substance abuse or addiction differ from drug to drug, as indicated in Table 36-2. Addiction, however, typically causes a gradual decline in the quality of someone's work or relationships. The patient may behave erratically, have frequent mood changes, suffer from loss of appetite, and be constantly tired.

Someone who is abusing alcohol may have no apparent signs or symptoms at first. As time goes on, however, that person may suffer from blackouts (failure to remember what happened while drinking) or may become secretive and guilty about drinking and deny that there is a problem. She may suffer from bruises, trembling hands, or chronic stomach problems. Even though the patient may feel she does not have a substance abuse or addiction problem, healthcare team members may recognize a problem. When this occurs, their job is to try to persuade the patient to seek help.

▶ Documenting Patient Information

LO 36.3

Whenever you interview a patient, keep in mind that the patient chart is a legal document. The chart can be used as evidence in a court of law. So, you must meet certain guidelines when recording data.

The Six Cs of Charting

To help ensure that you record patient data accurately, you must follow the six Cs of charting. These guidelines are as follows:

1. *Client's words* must be recorded exactly. The doctor may uncover clues to use in diagnosing the patient's condition. Place quotation marks to indicate what the patient said.

2. *Clarity* is essential when you describe the patient's condition. You must use medical terminology and precise descriptions.

3. *Completeness* is required on all the forms used in the patient record.

4. *Conciseness* can save time and space when you are recording information.

5. *Chronological order* and dates on all entries in patient records are critical in the documentation of patient care. This information also can be used for legal questions regarding medical services. Most charts are arranged with the most recent information on top. This type of charting is known as *reverse chronological order*.

6. *Confidentiality* is essential to protect the patient's privacy. You cannot discuss a patient's records, forward them to another office, fax them, or show them to anyone except the doctor unless the patient gives you written permission to do so. The only exception is when the records must be sent to ensure continuity of care of the patient and the patient is unable to grant permission.

Contents of Patient Charts

In most medical offices, patient records are electronic. Whether they are electronic or paper, all records must contain the following standard information:

- The patient registration form carries the date of the patient's current visit and generally lists the patient's age, address, medical insurance, occupation, education, racial or ethnic background, marital status, number of children, and nearest relative. There is a section that allows the patient to indicate his or her preference about telephone contact, such as leaving messages, or relaying information to designated family members or friends. Some medical offices also use e-mail to communicate with patients. Make sure the patient understands the privacy information section and chooses the appropriate action.

- Patient medical history usually includes the chief complaint, history of the present illness, past medical history (including medical treatment, surgeries, known allergies, and current medications), family history, and social and occupational history (including diet, exercise, smoking, and use of alcohol or drugs). This section also may be used to record the results of a general physical exam. See Figure 36-1 for one example.

- Test results include those performed in the office and those received from other physicians, hospitals, or independent laboratories. Physicians may have tests run on a patient's blood, urine, or tissue samples to aid in their diagnoses. Figure 36-2a and b shows examples of laboratory reports of a panel of chemical tests on blood performed by an outside laboratory.

Well-woman template (excerpt)

GYN History: No concerns DELETE
Gravida 0 Past Pregnancies Post-Menopausal
Average interval between menses: DEL 28-31 days MenstrInt irregular P1
Length of menses: DEL DurDay P1
Flow: DEL MenstrFlo normal heavy light P1
Dysmenorrhea: DEL yes no controlled with NSAIDs controlled with OCPs H8
Post-coital bleeding: DEL yes no R7
Intermenstrual bleeding: DEL yes no R7
Pelvic pain: DEL yes no R7
Dyspareunia: DEL yes no R7
Vaginal discharge: DEL yes no VAG D/C DETAILS R7
GYN surgery: DEL GYNSURG none P1
Contraception: DEL Contracep P3 I

Menopausal Symptoms: none N/A DELETE
Hot flashes: DEL yes no tolerable intolerable R1
Night sweats: DEL yes no R1
Sleep disturbances: DEL yes no R11
Vaginal dryness: DEL yes no R7
Mood/cognitive disturbances: DEL yes no R11

FIGURE 36-1 Medical history form in an electronic health record.

- Records from other physicians or hospitals are accompanied by a copy of the patient's written authorization to release the records.

- The physician's diagnosis and treatment plan are specific and detailed.

- Operative reports include a record of all procedures, surgeries, follow-up care, and additional notes the physician makes regarding the patient's case. Continuation forms can be used for additional information. Some medical offices also keep a separate log of telephone calls to and from the patient.

- Informed consent forms verify that the patient has understood the treatment offered and the possible outcomes or side effects of it. The patient signs the consent form but may withdraw consent if she decides to change or discontinue treatment.

- A discharge summary form is used when a patient is hospitalized. This form includes information that summarizes the reason the patient entered the hospital; tests, procedures, or operations performed in the hospital; medications administered; and the disposition, or outcome, of the case.

- Correspondence with or about the patient is marked or stamped with the date the physician's office received the document.

When recording information in the patient chart, be sure to date and initial every entry. This documentation makes it easy to tell which items you entered into the chart and which items others entered. The physician usually initials reports before they are filed to prove that she saw them.

Building a Patient Past Medical History and Family Health History

Methods of Charting

Various methods of charting are used on the medical record. Most methods are based on a series of steps to document the information. These steps are referred to as the SOAP method of documentation (Figure 36-3). Understanding the parts of SOAP will help you document information in a logical manner.

1. *Subjective data.* You obtain **subjective data** from conversation with the patient or an attending family member.

Main Info | Extra Info

ID	TEST001
Date of the Analysis	5/4/2014
Patient Name	Smith, Peter
Date requested	5/3/2014

Test type	COMPLETE BLOOD COUNT
Pathologist	Henderson, John
Physician	Buckwalter, Paul F.

Lab Test Criteria

W	E	Analyte	Result	Lower Limit	Upper Limit	Units	Remarks
☐	☐	RBC	5.3	4.7	6.1	(males) million cells/mcL	
☐	☐	Hb	15.2	13.8	17.2	(males)gm/dL	
☐	☐	HCT	45.6	40.7	50.3	(males)%	
☐	☐	MCV	82	80	95	femtoliter	
☐	☐	MCH	29	27	31	pg/cell	
☐	☐	MCHC	33	32	36	gm/dL	
☐	☐	Platelets	289,000	150,000	400,000	Platelets/mcL	
☐	☐	WBC	9600	4,500	10,000	cells/mcL	
☐	☐	Neutrophils	57	40	60	%	
☐	☐	Lymphocytes	32	20	40	%	
☐	☐	Monocytes	7	2	8	%	
☐	☐	Eosinophils	3	1	4	%	
☐	☐	Basophils	1	0.5	1	%	

Lab Report

Waiting request:0 received-0 sent   lab@BWWassociates

(a)

FIGURE 36-2 Laboratory reports provide physicians with valuable information about patients' health. Test results are accompanied by normal ranges appropriate for the laboratory's testing procedures. (a) Electronic health record report. (b) Paper report.

Subjective data include thoughts, feelings, and perceptions, including the chief complaint. An example of subjective information is the patient's statement about his or her chief complaint: "I have an itchy red rash on my left hand that I noticed 3 days ago." The chief complaint should always be recorded in the patient's own words.

2. *Objective data.* **Objective data** are readily apparent and measurable, such as vital signs or test results and the physician's exam. An example of objective data is the examination of the rash by the physician.

3. *Assessment.* Assessment is the physician's diagnosis or impression of the patient's problem.

4. *Plan of action.* Options for treatment, the type of treatment chosen, medications, tests, consultations, patient education, and follow-up are included in a plan of action. The plan of action may include an order for injection or other treatment that you as the medical assistant will need to perform.

Three common methods for maintaining notes on a patient chart include

1. Conventional or source-oriented medical records (SOMR). Information is arranged according to who supplied those data—the patient, the doctor, a specialist, or someone else. The medical form may have a space for patient remarks followed by a section for the doctor's comment.

2. Problem-oriented medical records (POMR). This method is used more extensively by large clinics or practices that may have more than one physician who may see the same patient. POMR includes a problem list that is dated and numbers are assigned to each patient condition or problem. At the patient's initial visit, conditions or problems are identified by a number throughout the record until the problem is resolved. The POMR has four components:

   • *Database.* This includes the patient's medical history, diagnostic and laboratory results, and physical exam

Morris A. Turner, MD

C.L.I.A #21.1862

266 Line Road
Montelair, Delaware 00956
800-555-1567

Med**LAB**

John Miller	09/12/12	09/12/12	09/13/12
Patient Name	Date Drawn	Date Received	Date of Report

Sex **M** Age **65**	Alexis N. Whalen, MD BWW Medical Associates, PC 305 Main Street, Port Snead YZ 12345-9876	23341	67294
		ID Number	Account Number
166241809			897211
Patient ID, Soc. Sec. Number			Specimen Number

Test name	Result		Units	Reference range
	Abnormal	Normal		
Chem-screen panel				
Glucose		76.0	MG/DL	65.0–115
Sodium		139.0	MMOL/L	134–143
Potassium		4.00	MMOL/L	3.60–5.10
Chloride		107.0	MMOL/L	96.0–107
BUN		17.0	MG/DL	6.00–19.0
BUN/creatinine ratio		14.2		
Uric acid		4.30	MG/DL	2.20–6.20
Phosphate		2.40	MG/DL	2.40–4.50
Calcium		9.50	MG/DL	6.60–10.0
Magnesium		1.75	MEG/L	1.40–2.00
Cholesterol	237.0		MG/DL	130–200
Chol. percentile	90.0		PERCENTILE	1.00–75.0
HDL cholesterol	41.0		MG/DL	48.0–89.0
Chol./HDL ratio		5.80		
LDL Chol, calculated	175.0		MG/DL	65.5–130
Triglycerides		104.0	MG/DL	00.0–200
Total protein		6.60	GM/DL	6.40–8.00
Albumin		4.10	GM/DL	3.70–4.80
Globulin		2.50	GM/DL	2.20–3.60
Alb/glob ratio		1.64		1.10–2.10
Total bilirubin		0.60	MG/DL	0.20–1.30
Direct bilirubin		0.15	MG/DL	0.00–0.20
Alk. phosphatase		44.0	UNITS/L	25.0–125
G-glutamyl transpep		8.00	UNITS/L	1.00–63.0
AST (SGOT)		21.0	IU/L	1.00–40.0
ALT (SGPT)		14.0	IU/L	1.00–50.0
LD		134.0	IU/L	90.0–250
Iron		130.0	MCG/DL	35.0–180

(b)

FIGURE 36-2 (concluded)

reports. This is the foundation of the problem-oriented medical record.

- *Problem list.* Each patient condition or problem is listed individually, assigned a number, and dated.
- *Diagnostic and treatment plan.* Laboratory and other diagnostic tests are completed and the physician's treatment plan for the condition is documented.
- *Progress notes.* The physician enters notes on every condition or problem recorded on the problem list. Progress notes are entered chronologically and include the chief complaint, problems, conditions, treatments, and responses to treatment.

3. Computerized medical records. This method uses a combination of SOMR and POMR but provides accessibility by the physician or other healthcare workers at any time from a computer terminal. This accessibility enhances the patient's continuity of care between departments and specialty physicians in other practices because everyone is looking at the same record.

OUTLINE FORMAT PROGRESS NOTES

Patient Name _Chen_ _Cindy_ _M._ Date of Birth _07 / 15 / XX_ Chart # _H234_
               Last   First   Middle

Prob. No. or Letter	Date	Subjective	Objective	Assess	Plans
	6/16/XX	Patient complaining of pain in lower right quadrant. Has been running fever of between 100.5° F and 101.3° F since Sunday morning. Has queasy feeling in stomach and has been unable to eat since yesterday morning.			
			BP 125/75. Temperature 101.2° F. Abdominal exam revealed rebound tenderness and distension in lower right quadrant.		
				Appendicitis	
					1. Admit to hospital
					2. Surgically remove appendix.

Signature _Paul F. Buckwalter, MD_

Start each Progress Note (Subjective, Objective, Assessment, and Plans) at the appropriate shaded column to create an outline form. Write through the intervening columns to the right margin of the page.

© 1976 BIBBERO SYSTEMS, INC., PETALUMA, CA   TO REORDER CALL TOLL FREE: (800)BIBBERO (800 242-2376)
FORM # 26-7215-01

PROGRESS NOTES

FIGURE 36-3 When you use the SOAP approach to documenting patient information, start each progress note at the appropriate shaded column to create an outline form. Write through the intervening columns to the right margin of the page.

Common Chart Terminology and Abbreviations

Most of the information that you collect verbally from a patient will be documented in the patient's medical record. Table 36-3 lists some of the most common abbreviations used in the medical chart. Abbreviations used must be accepted by the facility where you are employed as well as The Joint Commission (TJC).

To help reduce medical errors, The Joint Commission, previously the Joint Commission on Accreditation of Healthcare Organizations (JCAHO), issued a list of abbreviations, acronyms, and symbols that should not be used. All medication orders, progress notes, consultation reports, operative reports, and clinical orders are subject to this "do not use" list. Table 36-4 provides a list of "do not use" and other abbreviations, acronyms, and symbols that you should avoid when charting.

▶ Recording the Patient's Medical History

LO 36.4

A patient's medical history includes pertinent information about the patient and the patient's family. Age, previous illnesses, surgical history, allergies, medication history, and family medical history are key items.

TABLE 36-3	Common Medical Abbreviations		
Abortion	Ab	Headache	HA
Abnormal	Abnl	History of	H/O
Antibiotics	Abx	History and physical	H & P
Against medical advice	AMA	Left	L
As much as possible	AMAP	Right	R
Awake and oriented	A&O	Low back pain	LBP
Both	B	Low birth weight	LBW
Biopsy	BX	Last menstrual period	LMP
Childhood diseases	CHD	No known allergies	NKA
Complains of	C/O	Packs per day	PPD
Cause of death	COD	Rule out	R/O
Chest X-ray	CXR	Range of motion	ROM
Date of birth	DOB	Shortness of breath	SOB
Date of conception	DOC	Sudden unexplained/ unexpected death	SUD
Digital rectal exam	DRE		
Estimated delivery date	EDD	Seizure	Sz
Follow-up	F/U	Tonsillectomy and adenoidectomy	T & A
Fracture	FX	Years old	Y/O
Growth and development	G & D	Within normal limits	WNL

TABLE 36-4 TJC "Do Not Use" Abbreviations, Acronyms, and Symbols

Abbreviation	Potential Problem	Preferred Term
U (for unit)	Mistaken as zero, four, or cc.	Write "unit"
IU (for international unit)	Mistaken as IV (intravenous) or 10 (ten).	Write "international unit"
Q.D., QD, qd, q.d., Q.O.D., QOD, q.o.d, qod (Latin abbreviation for once daily and every other day)	Mistaken for each other. The period after the Q can be mistaken for an "I" and the "O" can be mistaken for "I."	Write "daily" and "every other day"
Trailing zero (X.0 mg), lack of leading zero (.X mg)	Decimal point is missed.	Never write a zero by itself after a decimal point (X mg), and always use a zero before a decimal point (0.X mg).
MS MSO$_4$ MgSO$_4$	Confused for one another. Can mean morphine sulfate or magnesium sulfate.	Write "morphine sulfate" or "magnesium sulfate"

Other Abbreviations, Acronyms, and Symbols to Avoid

Abbreviation	Potential Problem	Preferred Term
μg (for microgram)	Mistaken for mg (milligrams), resulting in one-thousand-fold dosing overdose.	Write "mcg"
c.c. (for cubic centimeter)	Mistaken for U (units) when poorly written.	Write "mL" for milliliters
> (greater than) < (less than)	Misinterpreted as the number "7" or the letter "L"; confused for one another.	Write "greater than" and "less than"
Abbreviations for drug names	Misinterpreted due to similar abbreviations for multiple drugs.	Write drug names in full
Apothecary units	Unfamiliar to many practitioners. Confused with metric units.	Use metric units
@	Mistaken for the number "2" (two).	Write "at"
H.S. (for half-strength or Latin abbreviation for bedtime)	Mistaken for either half-strength or hour of sleep (at bedtime). qH.S. mistaken for every hour. All can result in a dosing error.	Write out "half-strength" or "at bedtime"
T.I.W. (for three times a week)	Mistaken for three times a day or twice weekly, resulting in an overdose.	Write "3 times weekly" or "three times weekly"
S.C. or S.Q. (for subcutaneous)	Mistaken as SL for sublingual, or "5 every"	Write "Sub-Q," "subQ," or "subcutaneously"
D/C (for discharge)	Interpreted as discontinue whatever medications follow (typically discharge meds).	Write "discharge"
A.S., A.D., A.U. (Latin abbreviation for left, right, or both ears) O.S., O.D., O.U. (Latin abbreviation for left, right, or both eyes)	Mistaken for each other (e.g., AS for OS, AD for OD, AU for OU, etc.).	Write "left ear," "right ear," or "both ears"; "left eye," "right eye," or "both eyes"

When recording a patient history, you must do more than just fill out the form (Figure 36-4). You must review the pieces of information, organize them, determine their importance, and document the facts. When you write your first histories, you may find it to be a lengthy process. When you become more experienced, however, you will be able to write histories more quickly. Whenever you write information on the chart, you must consider its completeness and accuracy. First determine the chief complaint or the main reason for the patient visit. For example, the patient may have a rash or pain. Then ask more questions. A good interview technique is the "PQRST" interview technique. It will help you remember the types of questions that are appropriate for the condition. Each letter stands for a word that will remind you to ask more specific questions about the chief complaint or problem the patient is having.

P: Provoke or Palliative

Q: Quality or Quantity

R: Region or Radiation

S: Severity Scale

T: Timing

See Table 36-5 for questions and charting examples using the PQRST interview technique.

You will need to chart other information prior to the physician visit. Figure 36-5b shows a form used by the medical assistant and the licensed practitioner when seeing a patient. When keying information in an electronic record, it is just as important to correctly type the information into the record. Pay special attention to spelling when entering data into the chart or electronic record. If you do not know how to spell a word, look it up. Use only TJC-approved and office-recognized abbreviations (see Tables 36-3 and 36-4). Many facilities have a document identifying these abbreviations. Electronic health records often use drop-down-type boxes or menus with common medical information provided. Take care to click the correct box when using drop-down menus. Remember, the chart is a legal document, so special attention to detail is required when charting.

The Progress Note

Many offices use a variation of the progress note for established patients who are seen for routine visits or follow-ups like

HEALTH HISTORY
(Confidential)

Name _____
Age _____ Birthdate _____ Date of last physical examination _____ Today's Date _____
What is your reason for visit? _____

SYMPTOMS Check (✓) symptoms you currently have or have had in the past year.

GENERAL
- ☐ Chills
- ☐ Depression
- ☐ Dizziness
- ☐ Fainting
- ☐ Fever
- ☐ Forgetfulness
- ☐ Headache
- ☐ Loss of sleep
- ☐ Loss of weight
- ☐ Nervousness
- ☐ Numbness
- ☐ Sweats

MUSCLE/JOINT/BONE
Pain, weakness, numbness in:
- ☐ Arms ☐ Hips
- ☐ Back ☐ Legs
- ☐ Feet ☐ Neck
- ☐ Hands ☐ Shoulders

GENITO-URINARY
- ☐ Blood in urine
- ☐ Frequent urination
- ☐ Lack of bladder control
- ☐ Painful urination

GASTROINTESTINAL
- ☐ Appetite poor
- ☐ Bloating
- ☐ Bowel changes
- ☐ Constipation
- ☐ Diarrhea
- ☐ Excessive hunger
- ☐ Excessive thirst
- ☐ Gas
- ☐ Hemorrhoids
- ☐ Indigestion
- ☐ Nausea
- ☐ Rectal bleeding
- ☐ Stomach pain
- ☐ Vomiting
- ☐ Vomiting blood

CARDIOVASCULAR
- ☐ Chest pain
- ☐ High blood pressure
- ☐ Irregular heart beat
- ☐ Low blood pressure
- ☐ Poor circulation
- ☐ Rapid heart beat
- ☐ Swelling of ankles
- ☐ Varicose veins

EYE, EAR, NOSE, THROAT
- ☐ Bleeding gums
- ☐ Blurred vision
- ☐ Crossed eyes
- ☐ Difficulty swallowing
- ☐ Double vision
- ☐ Earache
- ☐ Ear discharge
- ☐ Hay fever
- ☐ Hoarseness
- ☐ Loss of hearing
- ☐ Nosebleeds
- ☐ Persistent cough
- ☐ Ringing in ears
- ☐ Sinus problems
- ☐ Vision – Flashes
- ☐ Vision – Halos

SKIN
- ☐ Bruise easily
- ☐ Hives
- ☐ Itching
- ☐ Change in moles
- ☐ Rash
- ☐ Scars
- ☐ Sore that won't heal

MEN only
- ☐ Breast lump
- ☐ Erection difficulties
- ☐ Lump in testicles
- ☐ Penis discharge
- ☐ Sore on penis
- ☐ Other

WOMEN only
- ☐ Abnormal Pap smear
- ☐ Bleeding between periods
- ☐ Breast lump
- ☐ Extreme menstrual pain
- ☐ Hot flashes
- ☐ Nipple discharge
- ☐ Painful intercourse
- ☐ Vaginal discharge
- ☐ Other

Date of last
menstrual period _____
Date of last
Pap smear _____
Have you had
a mammogram? _____
Are you pregnant? _____
Number of children _____

CONDITIONS Check (✓) conditions you have or have had in the past.
- ☐ AIDS
- ☐ Alcoholism
- ☐ Anemia
- ☐ Anorexia
- ☐ Appendicitis
- ☐ Arthritis
- ☐ Asthma
- ☐ Bleeding Disorders
- ☐ Breast Lump
- ☐ Bronchitis
- ☐ Bulimia
- ☐ Cancer
- ☐ Cataracts

- ☐ Chemical Dependency
- ☐ Chickenpox
- ☐ Diabetes
- ☐ Emphysema
- ☐ Epilepsy
- ☐ Glaucoma
- ☐ Goiter
- ☐ Gonorrhea
- ☐ Gout
- ☐ Heart Disease
- ☐ Hepatitis
- ☐ Hernia
- ☐ Herpes

- ☐ High Cholesterol
- ☐ HIV Positive
- ☐ Kidney Disease
- ☐ Liver Disease
- ☐ Measles
- ☐ Migraine Headaches
- ☐ Miscarriage
- ☐ Mononucleosis
- ☐ Multiple Sclerosis
- ☐ Mumps
- ☐ Pacemaker
- ☐ Pneumonia
- ☐ Polio

- ☐ Prostate Problem
- ☐ Psychiatric Care
- ☐ Rheumatic Fever
- ☐ Scarlet Fever
- ☐ Stroke
- ☐ Suicide Attempt
- ☐ Thyroid Problems
- ☐ Tonsillitis
- ☐ Tuberculosis
- ☐ Typhoid Fever
- ☐ Ulcers
- ☐ Vaginal Infections
- ☐ Venereal Disease

MEDICATIONS List medications you are currently taking

ALLERGIES To medications or substances

Pharmacy Name _____ Phone _____

(All information is strictly confidential)

FAMILY HISTORY Fill in health information about your family.

Relation	Age	State of Health	Age at Death	Cause of Death
Father				
Mother				
Brothers				
Sisters				

Check (✓) if your blood relatives had any of the following:

Disease	Relationship to you
Arthritis, Gout	
Asthma, Hay Fever	
Cancer	
Chemical Dependency	
Diabetes	
Heart Disease, Strokes	
High Blood Pressure	
Kidney Disease	
Tuberculosis	
Other	

PREGNANCY HISTORY

Year of Birth	Sex of Birth	Complications if any

HOSPITALIZATIONS

Year	Hospital	Reason for Hospitalization and Outcome

Have you ever had a blood transfusion? ☐ Yes ☐ No
If yes, please give approximate dates.

SERIOUS ILLNESS/INJURIES

	DATE	OUTCOME

HEALTH HABITS Check (✓) which substances you use and describe how much you use.
- Caffeine
- Tobacco
- Drugs
- Other

OCCUPATIONAL CONCERNS Check (✓) if your work exposes you to the following:
- Stress
- Hazardous Substances
- Heavy Lifting
- Other

Your occupation: _____

I certify that the above information is correct to the best of my knowledge. I will not hold my doctor or any members of his/her staff responsible for any errors or omissions that I may have made in the completion of this form.

Signature _____ Date _____
Reviewed By _____ Date _____

FIGURE 36-4   The health history form must be complete and accurate. The patient should start the form and the medical assistant should check and complete it.

TABLE 36-5 Example Questions When Using the PQRST Interview Technique

PQRST Interview Technique	Chief Complaint: *Itching/Rash under Arms*	Chief Complaint: *Pain in the Left Shoulder*
P: Provoke or Palliative	• What causes the itching to occur? • Does anything make the itching go away?	• When did you first notice the pain? • Is there anything you do that reduces the pain?
Q: Quality or Quantity	• How severe is the rash/itching? • How often does the itching occur?	• Can you describe the pain: dull, aching, burning, or sharp? • When does the pain occur?
R: Region or Radiation	• Where is the itching/rash?	• Where do you feel the pain? • Does the pain move from one location to another?
S: Severity Scale	• Is the rash/itching interfering with your daily life?	• Is the area red or tender to the touch? • Is there any swelling? • Rate the pain on a scale of 1 to 10, with 10 being the worst. (See Figure 36-6.)
T: Timing	• When did you first notice the rash/itching?	• How long have you had the pain? • Is the pain intermittent or continuous? • How long does the pain last?

hypertension arthritis, or flu (see Figures 36-3 and 36-5). The medical history form is primarily used for new patients the physician is seeing for the first time. Some important guidelines to consider when using a progress note include

- It must be arranged in reverse chronological order.
- Every entry must be initialed and signed by the person making the entry. Typically, the first initial, last name, and credentials are used. For example, K. Haddix, RMA (AMT).
- Entries most commonly made on progress notes include documentation for prescription refills, follow-up visits, telephone conversations with patients, appointment cancellations or no shows, and referrals and consultation efforts made by the office for the patient.
- The patient name must be recorded on every progress note along with any other identifying information such as birth date or chart number.
- All entries must be dated. All entries typically include the time and must always include the date.

Procedure 36-2, at the end of this chapter, will guide you in how to use a progress note.

Polypharmacy

Many patients will take a variety of different medications to treat several conditions, such as hypertension, elevated cholesterol, and diabetes. Some patients take several medications for the same condition, with each one treating a different aspect of the condition. The chapters *Principles of Pharmacology* and *Medication Administration* provide detailed information regarding various medications. During the patient interview, it is important to document medications the patient is currently taking. The patient will often see several physicians or specialists, and it is important for your office to be up to date about the treatments

a patient is currently receiving. This reduces the likelihood of polypharmacy or unnecessarily repeating medical tests.

Some offices may use a medication flowsheet for the physicians to record patient medication histories. In some cases, the medical assistant gathers the information for the current medication flowsheet (see Figure 36-7). A helpful hint for organizing this task is to develop a form or card for the patient to use (if the office does not already have a form) and gather the initial medication history. Then instruct the patient to use the list and to have it updated by the other physicians that he or she sees. A drug reference guide or the Internet will assist you with the spelling of medications.

The Health History Form

The medical office usually has a standard medical history form that is used for all patients. The specific arrangement and wording of items on this form, however, may vary from office to office. The following sections contain brief descriptions of each of the parts of this form. Procedure 36-3, at the end of this chapter, will assist in your practice of obtaining medical histories.

Go to CONNECT to see a video about *Obtaining a Medical History*.

Personal Data This information is obtained from the administrative sheet and includes the patient's name, birth date, and other basic data.

Chief Complaint Abbreviated as CC, the chief complaint is the reason the patient came to visit the practitioner. It should be short and specific and should cover subjective and/or objective data stated by the patient.

BWW

BWW Medical Associates, PC
305 Main Street, Port Snead YZ 12345-9876
Tel: 555-654-3210, Fax: 555-987-6543
Web: BWWAssociates.com

Paul F. Buckwalter, MD
Alexis N. Whalen, MD
Elizabeth H. Williams, MD

PROGRESS NOTES

Name ___Cindy Chen___   Chart # ___01769___

DATE	
10/12/XX	Patient c/o headache and cough X 3 days. HA is dull ache, pain scale 7/10
	cough — non-productive. ———————— Kaylyn Haddix RMA (AMT)

(a)

Name ___Cindy Chen___   DOB ___07/15/XX___   Date ___08/28/XX___
ALLERGIES ___NKA___

Review of Systems

Systems	NL	Note	Systems	NL	Note
Constitutional			Musculoskeletal		
Eyes			Skin/breasts		
ENT/mouth			Neurologic		
Cardiovascular			Psychiatric		
Respiratory			Endocrine		
GI			Hem/lymph		
GU			Allergy/immun		

Current Medicines	Date	Current Diagnosis
ClaritinD PRN		
MVI †qd		
Ortho Novum 7/7/7 †qd		

Note

H: _5'7"_ W: _140_ T: _97.8_ P: _88_ R: _20_
B/P Sitting _122/78_ or Standing _____ Supine _____

Last Tetanus _06/12/XX_
L.M.P. _08/20/XX_

O2 Sat: _98%_
Pain Scale: _6/10_

Social Habits	Yes	No
Tobacco		✓
Alcohol	✓	
Rec. Drugs		✓

CC: (L) shoulder pain X 3 days due to fall.
"Sharp pain that hurts when I move"

HPI:

(b)

FIGURE 36-5 These forms are completed by the medical assistant prior to the physician visit. All information must be complete and accurate. (a) Progress note. (b) Medical visit form.

History of Present Illness This history includes detailed information about the chief complaint, including when the problem started and what the patient has done to treat the problem (including any medications taken). For example, a chief complaint might be "sore throat" and the history of the present illness would include when the sore throat started (e.g., 3 days ago), how severe the pain is on a scale of 1 to 10 (e.g., pain scale rating of 6 out of 10), and what treatments have been used (e.g., throat lozenges and four to six aspirin daily).

Past Medical History The past medical history includes any and all health problems both present and past, including major illnesses and surgery. The past medical history also includes important information about medications and allergies. It should list any medications taken by the patient, including their dosages and the reasons for taking them. Over-the-counter and herbal medications should be listed as well. Known or suspected allergies to medications or other substances should be listed and clearly visible. Some facilities use a red sticker or other means on charts

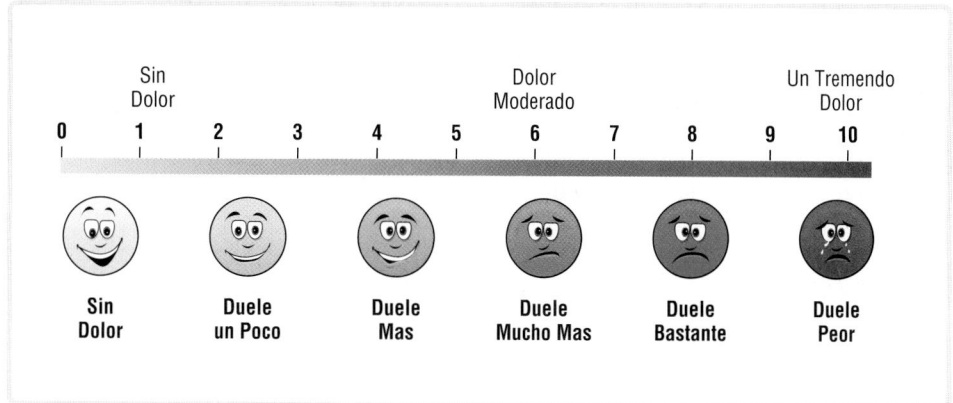

FIGURE 36-6 Assessing a patient's pain, considered the fifth vital sign, is part of the interview and history-taking process. A chart similar to this is used to make the process easier for the patient and the medical assistant.

BWW

BWW Medical Associates, PC
305 Main Street, Port Snead YZ 12345-9876
Tel: 555-654-3210, Fax: 555-987-6543
Web: BWWAssociates.com

Paul F. Buckwalter, MD
Alexis N. Whalen, MD
Elizabeth H. Williams, MD

MEDICATION FLOWSHEET

Patient Name		Allergies	

DATE		MEDICATION	REFILLS
Start	Stop	Dosage/Direction/Amount	Date/Amount/Initials

FIGURE 36-7 Medication flowsheet.

to identify allergies immediately. Most electronic health record programs automatically run drug allergy and drug-drug interaction checks. If you are entering medication data into an EHR program that does not have this feature, make sure you flag patient drug allergies according to office policy.

Family History This section includes information about the health of the patient's family members. Many times, the family history can help lead a practitioner to the cause of a current medical problem. Obtain specific information about family members' current ages and medical conditions or, if deceased, their age at death and the cause. Ask open-ended questions about the siblings, parents, and grandparents. Because the death of a parent or sibling or the limited knowledge of an adopted child can be difficult to discuss, use great care and sensitivity when asking these questions.

Social and Occupational History Information like marital status, sexual behaviors and orientation, occupations, hobbies, and the use of chemical substances help determine a patient's risk for disease. Patients should be asked about their use of alcohol, tobacco, recreational drugs, or other chemical substances. Be aware that patients may feel uncomfortable or may refuse to provide certain information. Depending on the circumstances, you may ask the question later in the interview. For example, an adolescent child may not want to answer questions about his sexual behaviors in front of his parents. Occupational information regarding the patient's level of stress, exposure to hazardous substances, and heavy lifting also may be included here.

Review of Systems Some of this information may be started by the patient but is completed by the practitioner. This systematic review of each of the body systems includes questions and an exam by the practitioner. The information is obtained in an orderly fashion but may vary depending on the physician or practitioner.

PROCEDURE 36-1 Using Critical Thinking Skills During an Interview

Procedure Goal: To be able to use verbal and nonverbal clues and critical thinking skills to optimize the process of obtaining data for the patient's chart.

OSHA Guidelines: This procedure does not involve exposure to blood, body fluids, or tissues.

Materials: Patient chart or electronic health record, pen (if using a paper record).

Method: Procedure steps.

Example 1: Getting at an Underlying Meaning

1. You are interviewing a female patient with type 2 diabetes who has recently started insulin injections. She is in the office for a follow-up visit.

2. Use open-ended questions such as, "How are you managing your diabetes?"
   RATIONALE: Open-ended questioning allows the patient to explain the situation in her own words and often provides more information than closed-ended questioning.

3. The patient states that she "just can't get used to the whole idea of injections."

4. To encourage her to verbalize her concerns more clearly, you can mirror her response or restate her comments in your own words. For example, you might say, "You seem to be having some difficulty giving yourself injections."

RATIONALE: This response should encourage her to verbalize the specific area in which she is having problems such as loading the syringe, injecting herself, finding the time for the injections, and so on.

5. Verbalize the implied, which means that you state what you think the patient is suggesting by her response.
   RATIONALE: Restating her response ensures you have understood.

6. After you determine the specific problem, you will be able to address it in the interview or note it in the patient's chart for the doctor's attention.

Example 2: Dealing with a Potentially Violent Patient

1. You are interviewing a 60-year-old male patient who is new to the office. He appears agitated. You ask his reason for seeing the doctor today.

2. The patient explains that he does not want to talk to "some assistant" about his problem. He just wants to see the doctor.

3. You say that you respect his wish not to discuss his symptoms but explain that you need to ask him a few questions so that the doctor can provide the proper medical care.
   RATIONALE: The patient has the right to refuse to answer a question, even if it is a reasonable one.

4. The patient begins to yell at you, saying he wants to see the doctor and does not "want to answer stupid questions."

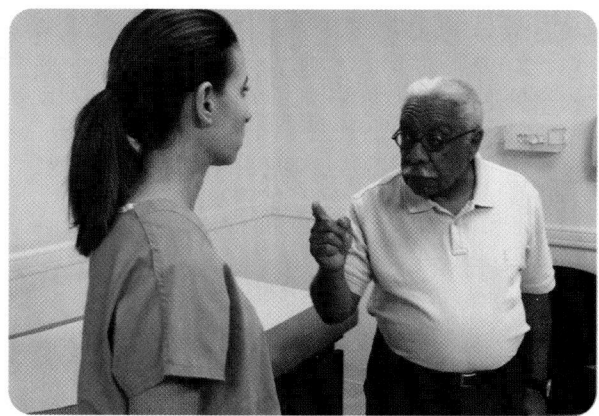

FIGURE Procedure 36-1 Example 2 Step 4 Do not try to handle by yourself a patient who may become violent. Ask for help from other staff members.

5. The fact that the patient appears agitated and begins to raise his voice in anger should be a warning to you that he may become violent. It would be best not to handle this patient by yourself.

6. If you are alone with the patient, leave the room and request assistance from another staff member.

Example 3: Gathering Symptom Information About a Child

1. A parent brings a 5-year-old boy to the office because the child is complaining about stomach pain.

2. To gather the pertinent symptom information, ask the child various types of questions.
   RATIONALE: Talking to the child first allows him to feel that his view of the problem is important.

   a. Can he tell you about the pain?
   RATIONALE: Open-ended questioning allows him to tell you about his problem in his own words.

   b. Can he tell you exactly where it hurts?

FIGURE Procedure 36-1 Example 3 Step 2 Gather any symptom information you can from the child. Then ask the parent or caregiver similar questions.

   c. Is there anything else that hurts?

3. To confirm the child's answers, ask the parent to answer similar questions.

4. You should then ask the parent additional questions. Begin with an open-ended question, as above. Follow up with specific questions such as these:

   a. How long has he had the pain?

   b. Is the pain related to any specific event (like going to school)?

5. Ask the child to confirm the parent's answers. He may be able to provide additional information at this time.

PROCEDURE 36-2 Using a Progress Note

Procedure Goal: To accurately record a chief complaint on a progress note.

OSHA Guidelines: This procedure does not involve exposure to blood, body fluids, or tissues.

Materials: Progress note, patient chart or electronic health record, pen (if using a paper record).

Method: Procedure steps.

1. Wash your hands.

2. Review the patient's chart notes from the patient's previous office visit. Verify that all results for any previously ordered laboratory work or diagnostics are in the chart.
   RATIONALE: Ensures that all reports have been reviewed by the physician.

3. Greet the patient and escort her to a private exam room.

4. Introduce yourself and ask the patient her name.

5. Using open-ended questions, find out why the patient is seeking medical care today.

   RATIONALE: Asking open-ended questions like "What is the reason for your visit today?" and "How long have you been feeling this way?" will encourage the patient to provide more details.

6. Accurately document the chief complaint on the progress note. Document vital signs. Initial or sign the chart entry according to office policy.

> Patient here for recurrent sore throat and nasal stuffiness. VS - T 99.7°F P 84 R 22 BP 118/74 Ht 65 inches, Wt 153 lbs., Throat culture, blood for CBC. Return 1 wk. _____ *G. Drake CMA(AAMA)*

7. File the progress note in chronological order within the patient's chart if the record is a paper record.
   RATIONALE: This ensures that the most current patient information is reviewed by the physician and the medical staff.

8. Thank the patient and offer to answer any questions she may have. Explain that the physician will come in soon to examine her.

9. Wash your hands.

PROCEDURE 36-3 Obtaining a Medical History

Procedure Goal: To obtain a complete medical history with accuracy and professionalism.

OSHA Guidelines: This procedure does not involve exposure to blood, body fluids, or tissues.

Materials: Medical history form, patient chart, pen or electronic medical record.

Method: Procedure steps.

1. Wash your hands.
2. Assemble the necessary materials. Review the medical history form and plan your interview.
   RATIONALE: This saves time and improves the effectiveness of the visit, plus it will assist in determining the appropriate questions to ask.
3. Invite the patient to a private exam room and correctly identify the patient by introducing yourself and asking his or her name and date of birth.
4. Explain the medical history form while maintaining eye contact. Make the patient feel at ease.
5. Using language that the patient can understand, ask appropriate, open-ended questions related to the medical history form. Listen actively to the patient's response.
6. Accurately document the patient's responses.
7. Thank the patient for his or her participation in the interview. Offer to answer any questions.
8. Sign or initial the medical history form and file it in the patient's chart.
9. Inform the physician that you are finished with the medical history according to the physician's office policy.
10. Wash your hands.

SUMMARY OF LEARNING OUTCOMES

LEARNING OUTCOMES	KEY POINTS
36.1 Identify the skills necessary to conduct a patient interview.	The skills necessary to conduct an interview include effective listening, awareness of nonverbal cues, use of a broad knowledge base, and the ability to summarize a general picture.
36.2 Recognize the signs of anxiety; depression; and physical, mental, or substance abuse.	Anxiety can range from a heightened ability to observe to a difficulty in being able to focus. Depression can be demonstrated through severe fatigue, sadness, difficulty sleeping, and lost of appetite. Abuse can be physical (like an injury) or psychological (like neglect).
36.3 Use the six Cs for writing an accurate patient history.	The six Cs for writing an accurate patient history include client's words, clarity, completeness, conciseness, chronological order, and confidentiality.
36.4 Carry out a patient history using critical thinking skills.	When obtaining a patient history, you can use open-ended questions, active listening, clarification, restatement, reflection, and the PQRST interview technique; review the information obtained, determine the importance, and then document the facts accurately.

CASE STUDY CRITICAL THINKING

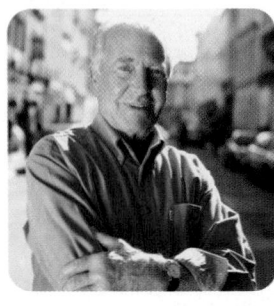

Recall Peter Smith from the beginning of the chapter. Now that you have completed the chapter, answer the following questions regarding his case.

1. What is the most likely diagnosis for this patient?
2. What specific symptoms make you suspect this condition?

1. (LO 36.3) Which item below represents objective data?
   a. Headache
   b. Pain
   c. Itching
   d. Rash
   e. Nausea

2. (LO 36.1) Which of the following is an open-ended question?
   a. How long have you had the rash under your arm?
   b. So, have you had a headache for three days on the left side of your head?
   c. Can you tell me more about your symptoms?
   d. How long does your pain last?
   e. Does your left arm hurt?

3. (LO 36.1) Which of the following is the most effective question to use during a patient interview?
   a. Do you agree that you are getting better when you use the medicine?
   b. Have you had a headache every day this week?
   c. Do you agree you should not have taken so much medication?
   d. What do you think is going on here?
   e. You haven't been taking your medicine, have you?

4. (LO 36.2) Which type of patient is the least likely victim of abuse?
   a. A 2-year-old child
   b. A 48-year-old male
   c. A 78-year-old male
   d. A 35-year-old female
   e. An 85-year-old female

5. (LO 36.3) Which of the following is an accepted abbreviation?
   a. HA
   b. OU
   c. HS
   d. ASA
   e. AU

6. (LO 36.4) In the PQRST interview technique, the "P" stands for
   a. Prescription
   b. Problem
   c. Provoke
   d. Plan
   e. Prevent

7. (LO 36.2) The intentional use of a medication or other substance in a way that is not medically approved is known as
   a. Medication error
   b. Substance abuse
   c. Polypharmacy
   d. Addiction
   e. Palliation

8. (LO 36.3) Which of the following is considered subjective data?
   a. Rash
   b. Fever
   c. Increased pulse rate
   d. Headache
   e. Hypertension

9. (LO 36.1) "You seem to be having trouble taking your medication, don't you agree?" is an example of
   a. Asking a leading question
   b. Asking an open-ended question
   c. Asking a hypothetical question
   d. Focusing on the patient
   e. Mirroring the patient's response

10. (LO 36.4) Asking a patient if his pain moves from one location to another is an example of which part of the PQRST interview technique?
    a. P
    b. Q
    c. R
    d. S
    e. T

Go to CONNECT to see activities about *Building the Medical Face Sheet* and *Printing the Face Sheet*.

Access the OLC to practice in a live EHR program. Refer to the EHR Appendix IV at the end of the book for more information and directions.

37

Vital Signs and Measurements

C A S E   S T U D Y

PATIENT INFORMATION		
Patient Name Shenya Jones	**Gender** Female	**DOB** 11/3/19XX
Attending Elizabeth H. Williams, MD	**MRN** 124-86-564	**Allergies** cinnamon, peanuts

Shenya Jones, a 34-year-old female, arrives at the office with a swelling and a red pustule on her face. She states the problem started two days ago as a small pimple near her nose. It became irritated then extremely swollen and painful overnight. Now this morning, she noted yellow drainage at the lesion site and the swelling has increased. The area of drainage is approximately 1 cm in diameter. The upper lip, side of the face, and nose are all swollen. You have taken her vital signs but must ask her about her level of pain and measure the area of drainage.

Keep Shenya in mind as you study this chapter. There will be questions at the end of the chapter based on the case study. The information in the chapter will help you answer these questions.

LEARNING OUTCOMES

After completing Chapter 37, you will be able to:

37.1 Describe the five vital signs.
37.2 Identify various methods of taking a patient's temperature.
37.3 Describe the process of obtaining pulse and respirations.
37.4 Carry out blood pressure measurements.
37.5 Summarize orthostatic or postural vital signs.
37.6 Illustrate various body measurements.

KEY TERMS

afebrile
apnea
auscultated blood
  pressure
bradycardia
calibrate
febrile
hyperpnea
hyperpyrexia
hypertension
hypotension

orthostatic hypotension
palpatory method
positive tilt test
postural hypotension
rales
sphygmomanometer
stethoscope
tachycardia
tachypnea
thermometer

CAAHEP

I. P (1) Obtain vital signs

II. C (7) Analyze charts, graphs and/or tables in the interpretation of healthcare results

II. P (3) Maintain growth charts

IV. P (2) Report relevant information to others succinctly and accurately

IX. P (7) Document accurately in the patient record

ABHES

2. **Anatomy and Physiology**
   Graduates:
   c. Assist the physician with the regimen of diagnostic and treatment modalities as they relate to each body system

4. **Medical Law and Ethics**
   Graduates:
   f. Comply with federal, state, and local health laws and regulations

8. **Medical Office Business Procedures Management**
   Graduates:
   y. Perform routine maintenance of administrative and clinical equipment
   kk. Adapt to individualized needs
   ll. Apply electronic technology

9. **Medical Office Clinical Procedures**
   Graduates:
   b. Apply principles of aseptic techniques and infection control
   c. Take vital signs

▶ Introduction

Vital signs are one of the most important assessments you can make when preparing the patient to be examined by the practitioner. Temperature, pulse, respirations, blood pressure, and pain assessment give information about how a patient will adjust to changes within the body and in the environment. Changes in the vital signs can indicate an abnormality.

Measurements like height, weight, and head circumference can indicate physical growth and development, especially in infants and children. These measurements also are used to evaluate health problems, like obesity, and other measurements are completed to evaluate a patient's condition. For example, you may need to measure the size of a wound or bruise or the diameter of an arm or leg. In all cases, you must be accurate when performing and recording vital signs and body measurements. The practitioner uses your results when making a diagnosis.

▶ Vital Signs   LO 37.1

As a medical assistant, you will usually take the vital signs before the doctor examines the patient. Vital signs include temperature, pulse, respirations, blood pressure, and pain; these measurements provide the doctor with information about the patient's overall condition.

In some offices, pre-exam procedures such as vital signs are performed in a general area outside the patient exam room. In other offices and in most pediatric offices, these measurements are taken in the exam room. In either case, you typically take the measurements before the patient disrobes. Follow the standard procedure used in your office and be sure to follow the HIPAA regulations and provide for the privacy of your results. Assessment of pain, which was discussed in the *Patient Interview and History* chapter, is considered the fifth vital sign. It is typically evaluated during the patient interview and recorded with the other vital signs.

Vital signs are usually measured at every office visit. There is a standard range of values for each measurement, as shown in Table 37-1, and each patient has an individual baseline value that is normal for that patient. The difference between a patient's current values and normal values can help the physician in making a diagnosis. You must follow closely the guidelines from the Department of Labor's Occupational Safety and Health Administration (OSHA) for taking measurements of vital signs (Table 37-2). These guidelines are intended to prevent transmission of disease to or from the patient. They help protect the patient and you, and keep the workplace safe.

▶ Temperature   LO 37.2

When you take a patient's temperature, you will determine whether the patient is **febrile** (has a body temperature above the patient's normal range) or **afebrile** (has a body temperature at about the patient's normal range). A fever is usually a sign of inflammation or infection. An exceptionally high fever is known as **hyperpyrexia**. Body temperature is the

TABLE 37-1 Normal Ranges for Vital Signs*

Vital Sign	Age					
	0–1 year	1–2 years	2–5 years	6–12 years	Greater than 12 years	Adult
Temperature						
Oral (°F)	—	—	—	95.9–99.5	97.6–99.6	97.8–99.1
Rectal (°F)	99–100	97.9–100.4	97.9–100.4	97.9–100.4	98.6–100.6	98.8–100.1
Pulse (beats per minute)	100–160	90–150	80–140	70–120	60–100	60–100
Respirations (per minute)	30–60	24–40	22–34	18–30	12–16	12–18
Blood Pressure (mmHg)**†						
Systolic	80–114	84–117	85–123	91–135	104–147	Less than 120
Diastolic	34–67	39–72	44–82	53–91	60–97	Less than 80

*Normal vital signs vary. Always compare your results with previous results obtained on the patient.

**Classifications for adult blood pressure are shown in Table 37-4.

†Pediatric blood pressure ranges vary greatly based on height percentiles and gender. Always consult the physician regarding specific ranges for each patient.

TABLE 37-2 OSHA Guidelines for Taking Measurements of Vital Signs

Situation	OSHA Guidelines
Before and after all patient contact	• Examination area cleaned according to OSHA standards • Aseptic hand washing
• Temperature by oral or rectal route • Contact with patient with lesions • Contact with patient suspected of having infectious disease	• Gloves always worn for rectal route • Gloves worn for oral route if contact precautions exist • Biohazard bags used for disposal of used thermometer sheaths, otoscope tips, alcohol swabs, dressings, and bandages
In presence of patient suspected of having an airborne infectious disease (particularly sneezing)	• Mask worn • Patient weighed, measured, and examined in room away from staff and other patients • Protective clothing (laboratory coat, gown, or apron) worn • Biohazard bags used as above

balance between heat produced by metabolic processes and heat lost from the body; it varies based upon numerous factors. These factors include the time of day (usually higher at night due to exercise and food intake), age, gender, physical exercise, emotion, pregnancy, drugs, food, environmental changes, and the metabolism (a slow metabolism, as seen in hypothyroidism, would cause a lower temperature). The location where the temperature is measured also can affect the result.

You can take a temperature in one of five locations: mouth (oral), ear (tympanic), rectum (rectal), armpit or axilla (axillary), and temporal artery (temporal). Temperature can be measured in degrees Fahrenheit (°F) or degrees Celsius (centigrade; °C). Table 37-3 gives equivalent values for these two temperature scales. Normal adult oral temperature is considered to be about 98.6°F or 37.0°C. See the Points on Practice box to review formulas and example conversions.

Temperature is measured with either an electronic or disposable **thermometer**.

Electronic Digital Thermometers
Electronic digital thermometers are used frequently in medical offices. These thermometers provide a digital readout of the

TABLE 37-3 Fahrenheit and Celsius Equivalents for Temperature

°F	°C	°F	°C	°F	°C	°F	°C
95.0	35.0	98.4	36.9	101.8	38.8	105.2	40.7
95.2	35.1	98.6	37.0	102.0	38.9	105.4	40.8
95.4	35.2	98.8	37.1	102.2	39.0	105.6	40.9
95.6	35.3	99.0	37.2	102.4	39.1	105.8	41.0
95.8	35.4	99.2	37.3	102.6	39.2	106.0	41.1
96.0	35.6	99.4	37.4	102.8	39.3	106.2	41.2
96.2	35.7	99.6	37.6	103.0	39.4	106.4	41.3
96.4	35.8	99.8	37.7	103.2	39.6	106.6	41.4
96.6	35.9	100.0	37.8	103.4	39.7	106.8	41.6
96.8	36.0	100.2	37.9	103.6	39.8	107.0	41.7
97.0	36.1	100.4	38.0	103.8	39.9	107.2	41.8
97.2	36.2	100.6	38.1	104.0	40.0	107.4	41.9
97.4	36.3	100.8	38.2	104.2	40.1	107.6	42.0
97.6	36.4	101.0	38.3	104.4	40.2	107.8	42.1
97.8	36.6	101.2	38.4	104.6	40.3	108.0	42.2
98.0	36.7	101.4	38.6	104.8	40.4		
98.2	36.8	101.6	38.7	105.0	40.6		

Math for Measurements

When performing vital signs and measurements, certain basic math conversions may be required. You may need to convert a temperature from Fahrenheit (°F) to Celsius (°C) or weight from pounds (lb) to kilograms (kg). Review the following formulas and examples in preparation for practice.

To convert °C to °F, use this formula:
°F = (°C × 9/5) + 32

Example: Convert 37.6 °C to °F:

°F = (37.6 × 9/5) + 32

°F = (338.4/5) + 32

°F = 67.68 + 32

°F = 99.68, rounded to the nearest tenth equals 99.7

To convert °F to °C, use this formula:
°C = (°F − 32) × 5/9

Example: Convert 99.6 °F to °C:

°C = (99.6 − 32) × 5/9

°C = 67.6 × 5/9

°C = 338/9

°C = 37.55, rounded to the nearest tenth equals 37.6

To convert kgs to lbs, use this formula:
lbs = kgs × 2.205

Example: Convert 52.4 kg to lbs:

lbs = 52.4 × 2.205

lbs = 115.542, rounded to the nearest tenth equals 115.5

To convert lbs to kgs, use this formula:
kgs = lbs × 0.454

Example: Convert 134 lbs to kg:

kgs = 134 × 0.454

kgs = 60.836, rounded to the nearest tenth equals 60.8

FIGURE 37-1 The electronic digital thermometer provides a digital readout of the patient's temperature.

FIGURE 37-2 The tympanic thermometer measures infared energy emitted from the tympanic membrane. The result, converted to body temperature, is displayed within seconds of insertion of the shielded tip into the ear.

patient's temperature (Figure 37-1). They are accurate, fast, easy to read, and comfortable for the patient. Separate probes and tips are available for oral and rectal use. Most units have an audible indicator, like a beep, to let you know when the temperature has registered and is displayed.

Another type of electronic thermometer is the tympanic thermometer, which is designed for use in the ear. See Figure 37-2. This thermometer measures infrared energy emitted from the tympanic membrane (eardrum). This energy is converted into a temperature reading. The tip is covered with a disposable sheath to prevent cross-contamination.

A third type of electronic thermometer is a temporal scanner (Figure 37-3). This thermometer measures the infrared heat of the temporal artery and the ambient temperature (the temperature around the area) at the site where the temperature is taken. These two readings are synthesized and the body temperature is displayed on the screen.

FIGURE 37-3 This temporal scanner is passed across the forehead to measure the temperature of the blood in the temporal artery.

Disposable Thermometers

Disposable, single-use thermometers are usually made of thin strips of plastic with specially treated dot or strip indicators (Figure 37-4). The indicators change color according to the temperature. This type of thermometer is used for oral and axillary or skin temperature measurements, particularly in children. Although not as accurate, disposable thermometers are useful for patients in their homes.

Taking Temperatures

Using the proper instrument and technique provides the most accurate temperature readings and prevents the spread of infection. All temperature measurements should be recorded to the nearest one-tenth of a degree. The procedure for taking temperatures is described in Procedure 37-1 at the end of this chapter.

Measuring Oral Temperatures To take an oral temperature, make sure the patient is able to hold the thermometer in the mouth. The patient also must be able to breathe through the nose. Place the thermometer under the tongue in either pocket just off-center in the lower jaw (Figure 37-5). The patient should hold the thermometer with lips closed. Wait at least 15 minutes after a patient has been eating, drinking, or smoking before taking an oral temerature; otherwise, you may obtain an inaccurate result.

Measuring Tympanic Temperatures Proper technique must be used when measuring a tympanic temperature. These thermometers are easy to use, but you must follow manufacturers' instructions precisely. First, remove the thermometer from its recharging cradle and then wait for the indicator light to show that the unit is ready. Attach a disposable sheath and place the thermometer in the opening

FIGURE 37-5 When taking an oral temperature, place the thermometer under the tongue to the side of the mouth as shown here.

of the ear so that the fit is snug. To make sure you have a tight fit and the thermometer is pointing at the eardrum, pull the ear up and back for adults and down and back for children. Press the button and the result will be displayed within seconds. Be certain to press the correct button to read the temperature. Another button on the thermometer releases the sheath. You do not want to release the sheath into the patient's ear. See the Caution: Handle with Care box for potential problems that can occur with tympanic thermometers.

Measuring Rectal Temperatures Rectal temperatures are usually 1°F higher than oral temperatures and are considered the most accurate measurement of body temperature. Temperatures are sometimes measured rectally in infants and in adults in whom an oral temperature cannot be taken. Gloves are always worn and the patient is placed on his or her side. The left side is the preferred position because the rectum is angled in this direction. This position promotes comfort and prevents accidental puncture of the rectal wall. The tip of the thermometer should be inserted slowly and gently until it is covered or until you feel resistance, at approximately 1 inch for adults and ½ inch for infants and small children. For safety, always hold the thermometer in place while taking the temperature.

FIGURE 37-4 A disposable thermometer like this one is a convenient method for taking temperature. Thermometer reading after taking a normal temperature (a) and an elevated temperature (b).

Tympanic Thermometers: What You Need to Know

Tympanic thermometers are popular and are useful with uncooperative patients and with patients who have been eating, drinking, or smoking. Tympanic temperatures are fast and accurate when performed properly. To prevent inaccurate readings, here is a summary of what you need to know.

Why the Eardrum?

The eardrum is an ideal place to measure temperature because it shares the same blood supply with the hypothalamus, the organ that controls body temperature.

How Do Tympanic Thermometers Work?

Tympanic thermometers convert the infrared energy, a type of heat energy emitted from the eardrum, into a temperature reading, usually within seconds. Most tympanic thermometers run on a rechargeable battery that must be recharged between uses.

Where Problems Can Occur

The technique for taking a tympanic temperature may vary slightly, depending on which brand of thermometer you use. Most units have an indicator to let you know when the thermometer is ready for use. Some units require taking the temperature within a certain period after removing the thermometer from its charging base. Read the manufacturer's instructions for specific information.

There can be problems if the outer opening of the ear is not sealed completely when the probe is placed at the ear canal or the thermometer is not aimed at the eardrum. You may need to tug gently on the ear to position the thermometer properly and aim it at the eardrum.

If the thermometer has been charging for several hours before use, the initial reading may be inaccurately high. So, some experts believe you should take two measurements on the first patient after charging the unit and record only the second reading.

Even with good technique, problems can sometimes occur. For example, excessive or impacted cerumen (earwax) or otitis media (ear infection) may prevent an accurate reading. If you obtain a reading that does not appear to match the patient's general condition, repeat the temperature measurement to be sure. It also may be necessary to use a different method. Additionally, if a patient has otitis media, the tympanic temperature reading may be higher than the actual body temperature.

Measuring Axillary Temperatures To take an axillary temperature, first have the patient sit or lie down. Place the tip of the thermometer in the middle of the axilla (armpit), with the shaft facing forward. The patient's upper arm should be pressed against his side and his lower arm should be crossed over the stomach to hold the thermometer in place. Make sure the tip of the thermometer touches skin on all sides of the probe.

Measuring Temporal Temperatures The temporal scanner is a quick, noninvasive procedure for taking temperatures. You gently stroke the thermometer across the forehead, crossing over the temporal artery (on the side of the forehead at the temple). An infared scanner measures the difference in the temperature of the forehead and that of the temporal artery and then electronically calculates the patient's body temperature. As with all electronic devices, check the manufacturer's instructions before using.

Go to CONNECT to see a video about *Measuring and Recording Temperature.*

▶ Pulse and Respiration   LO 37.3

Pulse and respiration are related because the circulatory and respiratory systems work together. Pulse is measured as the number of times the heart beats in 1 minute. Respiration is the number of times a patient breathes in 1 minute. One breath, or respiration, equals one inhalation and one exhalation. Usually, if either the pulse or respiration rate is high or low, the other is also. The usual ratio of the pulse rate to the respiration rate is about 4:1 (for example, a pulse of 80 and a respiration of 20). In general, the younger the patient, the higher the normal pulse and respiration rate. Additionally, adult female rates tend to be faster than those for males. You should be familiar with these rates and how to perform the procedure. See Table 37-1 and Procedure 37-2, at the end of this chapter.

Pulse

A pulse rate gives information about the patient's cardiovascular system. It is an indirect measurement of the patient's cardiac output or the amount of blood the heart is able to pump in one minute. If the pulse is abnormally fast—**tachycardia**, or slow—**bradycardia**, or weak, or irregular, the patient may have a medical problem.

Measure the pulse of adults at the radial artery, where it can be felt in the groove on the thumb side of the inner wrist. Press lightly on this pulse point with your fingers and not your thumb (a pulse is located in your thumb, and you may feel it instead of the patient's pulse). Count the number of beats you feel in 1 minute and note the rhythm and volume. The rhythm can be regular or irregular. The volume can be weak, strong, or bounding. A bounding pulse feels like it is leaping out and then quickly disappearing with each pulse beat and sometimes can be seen at the pulse site. You may be asked to document the pulse volume on a numerical scale from 0 to 4+. The characteristics of this scale are

- 0 = no palpable pulse
- 1+ = weak
- 2+ = faint pulse
- 3+ = normal pulse
- 4+ = bounding pulse

Office policy may direct that you count the pulse for 30 seconds and multiply the results by 2 to obtain the beats per minute. If you measure a pulse for less than 1 minute and notice that the rhythm is irregular or the pulse is weak or bounding, you must count for 1 full minute and document the irregularities.

Pulse sites other than the radial pulse may be used for various reasons. For example, in young children, the radial artery may be hard to feel. You may instead take the pulse at the brachial artery, which is in the bend of the elbow (the antecubital space) or on the inner side of the upper arm. If you cannot feel the brachial pulse, then take the pulse over the apex (the left lower corner) of the heart, where the strongest heart sounds can be heard. Count the apical pulse (the heartbeat at the apex of the heart) while you listen with a **stethoscope**, an instrument that amplifies body sounds. The apex is located in the fifth intercostal space between the ribs on the left side of the chest, directly below the center of the clavicle. Though the condition is rare, you may encounter a patient with *dextrocardia*—a congenital condition where the heart is pointed toward the right side of the chest. In this case, you will find the apical pulse

on the right side of the chest, directly below the clavicle in the fifth intercostal space. Consult Figure 37-6 for placement of the stethoscope. You also may use other locations to take a pulse. Figure 37-7 shows the location of common pulse points.

Electronic Pulse The pulse may be measured electronically using a device attached to the finger or sometimes the nose or earlobe. Figure 37-8 shows one type of device used as part of an electronic blood pressure machine. A pulse

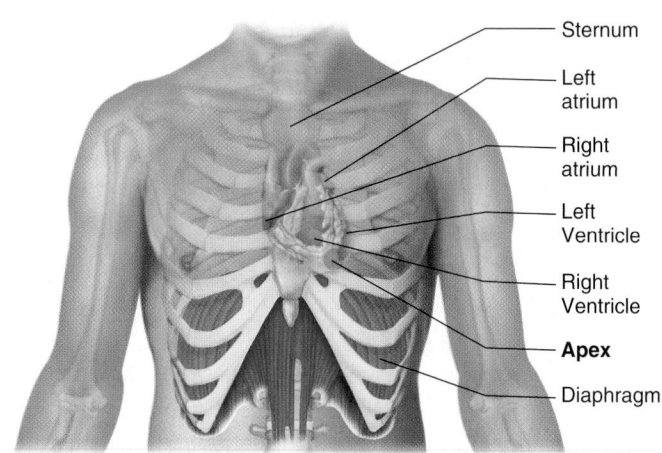

FIGURE 37-6 A stethoscope is used over the apex of the heart to listen for the heart sounds and measure the heart rate in patients in whom pulse is not otherwise detectable.

FIGURE 37-7 There are many locations on the body where major arteries are close enough to the surface to allow a pulse to be felt and counted.

FIGURE 37-8 Pulse, blood pressure, and oxygen saturation can all be measured with this electronic blood pressure device.

FIGURE 37-9 A pulse oximeter measures the pulse and oxygen saturation of the blood.

FIGURE 37-10 Attach the clip firmly to the finger.

FIGURE 37-11 Make sure there is good skin contact when using a nose bridge pulse oximeter.

oximeter machine, which measures the oxygen level of the blood, also can be used (Figure 37-9).

When using these devices, be certain to attach the clip firmly to the finger or lobe. See Figure 37-10. When using a nose bridge pulse oximeter, make sure there is good skin contact. The nose bridge pulse oximeter should only be used with patients who have good peripheral circulation. See Figure 37-11. The finger clip uses an infrared light to measure the pulse and oxygen levels, so it works best when no nail polish is present on the patient's finger. The pulse reading and the oxygen saturation of the blood will display on the screen. If the pulse is outside the normal range (see Table 37-1), it should be taken again or performed manually. If the oxygen level is less than 92%, the patient should be asked to take deep breaths during the procedure to increase her oxygen level. An oxygen level below 92% that does not improve with deep breaths should be reported.

Respiration

Respiration rate indicates how well a patient's body is providing oxygen to tissues. The best way to check respiration is by watching, listening, or feeling the movement at the patient's chest, stomach, back, or shoulders. If you cannot see the chest movement, then place your hand over the patient's chest, shoulder, or abdomen and listen and feel for the movement of air.

Respirations also may be counted with a stethoscope. Place the stethoscope on one side of the spine in the middle of the back to count respirations. You need to count respirations subtly because once the patient is aware that respiration is being measured, he may unintentionally alter his breathing. If using a stethoscope, tell the patient that you want to listen to his lungs. When you are not using a stethoscope, count the respirations while you have your hand on the pulse site.

Respirations are counted for one full minute in order to determine the rate, rhythm, and effort (quality). Counting for less than a minute may cause you to miss certain breathing abnormalities. The rhythm should be regular. The quality of effort should be normal, shallow, or deep. Irregularities such as hyperventilation (excessive rate and depth of breathing usually due to hysteria), dyspnea (difficult or painful breathing), tachypnea (rapid breathing), or **hyperpnea** (abnormally rapid, deep, or labored breathing) are indications of possible disease and should be noted. Rales and rhonchi are types of noisy breathing that can indicate an abnormality. **Rales**—crackling sounds—indicate fluid in the lung and can be heard in patients with pneumonia, atelectasis, pulmonary edema, or other conditions. Rhonchi—deep snoring or rattling sounds—are associated with asthma, acute bronchitis, or any condition involving partial obstruction of the lung's airway. They may be noted in pneumonia, bronchitis, asthma, or other pulmonary diseases. Cheyne-Stokes respirations are characterized by periods of increasing and decreasing depth of respiration between periods of **apnea** (the absence of respiration). This pattern of breathing may be seen in patients with strokes, head injuries, brain tumors, and congestive heart failure.

Go to CONNECT to see a video about *Measuring and Recording Pulse and Respirations.*

▶ Blood Pressure

LO 37.4

Blood pressure (also known as arterial blood pressure) is the force at which blood is pumped against the walls of the arteries. The standard unit for measuring blood pressure is millimeters of mercury (mm Hg). The pressure measured when the left ventricle of the heart contracts is known as the systolic pressure. The pressure measured when the heart relaxes is known as the diastolic pressure. The diastolic pressure indicates the minimum amount of pressure exerted against the vessel walls at all times.

According to the Joint National Committee of Prevention, Detection, Evaluation, and Treatment of High Blood Pressure, expected adult systolic readings are less than 120 mm Hg and adult diastolic readings are less than 80 mm Hg. These values may increase with advancing age. A systolic reading between 120 and 139 mm Hg and a diastolic reading between 80 and 90 mm Hg is considered prehypertension. A reading between 140 mm Hg and 159 mm Hg systolic and between 90 mm Hg and 99 mm Hg diastolic is considered Stage 1 hypertension. A systolic reading above 160 mm Hg and above 100 mm Hg diastolic is considered Stage 2 hypertension. Table 37-4 outlines blood pressure classifications.

Factors Affecting Blood Pressure

High blood pressure, known as **hypertension**, is a common health problem. If the blood pressure reading is consistently elevated after 2 or more visits to the physician, the patient may be diagnosed with hypertension. According to the American Heart Association, more the 76 million Americans over the age of 20 have high blood pressure. Hypertension may be categorized as essential or secondary. There is no identifiable cause for essential hypertension. According to the Joint National Committee, 95% of all hypertension is essential. Secondary hypertension occurs as a result of some other condition like kidney or heart disease. There are many factors that affect the blood pressure. Internal factors such as cardiac output (amount of blood pumped by the heart), blood volume (amount of blood in the body), vasoconstriction (peripheral resistance), and blood viscosity (thickness) regulate the blood pressure within the body.

Malignant hypertension is high blood pressure with other conditions such as renal or heart failure or *papilledema* (swelling of the optic nerve). Patients with elevated blood pressure are frequently checked more than once during an office visit and also may be monitoring their blood pressure at home.

Go to CONNECT to see an animation about *Hypertension.*

Hypotension, or low blood pressure, is not generally a chronic health problem. Slightly low blood pressure may be normal for some patients and does not usually require treatment. Severe hypotension may be present with shock, heart failure, severe burns, and excessive bleeding.

Blood Pressure Measuring Equipment

Blood pressure is measured with an instrument called a **sphygmomanometer**. A sphygmomanometer consists of an inflatable cuff, a pressure bulb or automatic device for inflating the cuff, and a manometer to read the pressure. The three basic types of sphygmomanometers differ in how the pressure is displayed.

Aneroid Sphygmomanometers Aneroid sphygmomanometers have a circular gauge that registers pressure. The needle on the gauge rotates as pressure rises. This type of sphygmomanometer is very accurate as long as calibration is done on a regular basis. Each measurement line indicates 2 mm Hg (Figure 37-12).

FIGURE 37-12 Each line on the aneroid gauge indicates 2 mm Hg. To prevent inaccuracies, look directly at this gauge when performing a blood pressure test.

TABLE 37-4	Blood Pressure Classifications	
Classification	**Systolic (mm Hg)**	**Diastolic (mm Hg)**
Normal	Less than 120	and less than 80
Prehypertension	120–139	or 80–89
Stage 1 Hypertension	140–159	or 90–99
Stage 2 Hypertension	Greater than 160	or greater than 100

FIGURE 37-13 This electronic sphygmomanometer displays the patient's blood pressure, pulse, and oxygen saturation. If you question any of the results, repeat the test using a manual method.

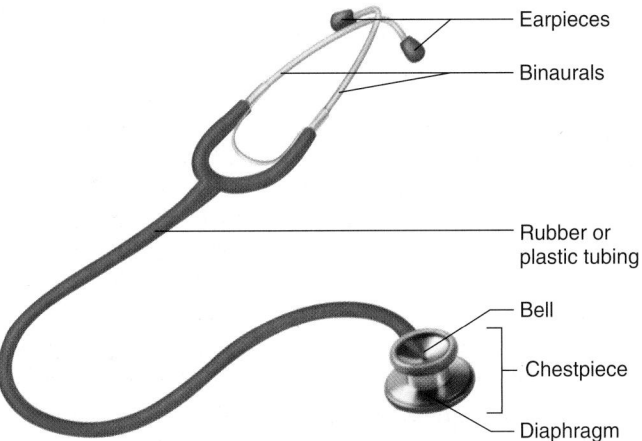

FIGURE 37-14 The stethoscope amplifies body sounds.

Electronic Sphygmomanometers Electronic sphygmomanometers provide a digital readout of blood pressure (Figure 37-13). Unlike aneroid sphygmomanometers, these devices do not require use of a stethoscope to determine blood pressure. They are easy to use but can be costly. Accuracy can sometimes be an issue, so maintain the equipment according to the manufacturer's instructions. If you question the results of an electronic blood pressure measurement, take it again with an aneroid cuff.

Mercury Sphygmomanometers Mercury sphygmomanometers contain a column of mercury that rises with an increase in pressure as the cuff is inflated.

Mercury instruments are gradually being replaced because the government has restricted the use of mercury due to its effects on the environment. Additionally, in 2007, the World Health Organization in conjunction with Healthcare Without Harm began an initiative to eliminate the use of mercury thermometers and sphygmomanometers by the year 2017. Consequently, no new mercury sphygmomanometers are being manufactured in the United States.

Calibrating the Sphygmomanometer

To ensure that sphygmomanometers are working properly, you or a medical supply dealer must calibrate them regularly. To **calibrate** means to standardize a measuring instrument. Follow the manufacturer's instructions for an electronic sphygmomanometer.

Do not use a sphygmomanometer unless you are certain it is calibrated because inaccurate readings can result. To calibrate an aneroid sphygmomanometer, follow these steps:

1. Check that the recording needle on the dial rests within the small square at the bottom of the dial.
2. To calibrate the dial, use a Y connector to attach the dial to a pressure bulb and a calibrated manometer.

3. Use the pressure bulb to elevate both manometer readings to 250 mm Hg. As you let the pressure fall, record both readings at four different points.
4. The difference between paired readings should not exceed 3 mm Hg.
5. If the sphygmomanometer does not calibrate properly, check the manufacturer's instructions and send the sphygmomanometer for repair if needed. Do not use a sphygmomanometer that is not properly calibrated.

The Stethoscope

A stethoscope amplifies body sounds, making them louder. It consists of earpieces, binaurals, rubber or plastic tubing, and a chestpiece (Figure 37-14). For best results, the earpieces should fit snugly and comfortably in your ears. When placing them in your ears, face the angle of the earpiece up and forward for the best fit.

The chestpiece consists of two parts: the diaphragm and the bell. The diaphragm is the larger, flat side of the chestpiece, which is covered by a thin, plastic disk. The diaphragm—best at amplifying high-pitched sounds, like bowel and lung sounds—must be placed firmly against the skin for proper amplification of sound.

The bell is the cone-shaped side of the stethoscope chestpiece. It must be held lightly against the skin to amplify sound. The bell is best at amplifying low-pitched sounds, like vascular and heart sounds. With practice, you may find you prefer to use one side rather than the other for various purposes.

Measuring Blood Pressure

To measure blood pressure, wrap the cuff of the sphygmomanometer around the patient's upper arm, just above the brachial artery's pulse point (Figure 37-15). This pulse point is located in the bend of the elbow, or the antecubital space. When measuring blood pressure, you should first determine the palpatory pressure that represents the target peak inflation. With the cuff placed just above the the brachial artery pulse, palpate the radial pulse. This **palpatory method** provides an approximation of the systolic blood pressure to ensure an adequate level of inflation when the actual measurement is made. Inflate the cuff until you can no longer feel the radial pulse and note the pressure at that point. Allow the arm to rest for 30 to 60 seconds or remove the

FIGURE 37-15 The blood pressure cuff should be one inch above the elbow with the center of the bladder directly above the brachial pulse.

cuff and replace. To determine the **auscultated blood pressure,** meaning it is determined by listening with a stethoscope, inflate the cuff to 30 mm Hg above the palpatory result, or approximately 180 to 200 mm Hg. Then, while you release the air in the cuff, listen with the stethoscope placed over the brachial pulse point. You will hear vascular sounds that will change. These sounds are called Korotkoff sounds and they have 5 phases:

- Phase 1—The first tapping sound you hear represents the systolic pressure.
- Phase 2—A strong heartbeat changes to a softer, swishing sound.
- Phase 3—The resumption of a crisp, tapping sound.
- Phase 4—Sounds become muffled.
- Phase 5—The point at which the sound disappears; this represents the diastolic pressure.

As the pressure in the cuff decreases, a strong heartbeat changes to a softer, swishing sound (phase 2). Sometimes the sound will vanish temporarily. This happens when the blood vessels beneath the cuff become congested and is often a sign of hypertension. When the congestion clears, the sound resumes. The period when the sound either changes or vanishes is called the *auscultatory gap.* Blood pressure is usually recorded with the systolic and diastolic sounds separated by a slash—for example, 116/76. If there is a pressure difference greater than 10 mm Hg between the muffled sound and its disappearance, the blood pressure may be recorded with all three sounds, noted as 120/80/60. The process of taking blood pressure is described in Procedure 37-3, at the end of this chapter.

Special Considerations in Adults Blood pressure is elevated during and just after exercise. If a patient has engaged in strenuous activity before the exam, you should wait 15 minutes before taking blood pressure measurements. This waiting period also applies to patients with ambulatory disabilities, to those who are obese, and to those who have a known blood pressure problem. If you ensure that patients have relaxed for 15 minutes before you measure their blood pressure, you should get an accurate reading.

Blood pressure also may be elevated when a patient is anxious or under stress. The patient may be aware that a blood pressure reading is high or low and upset about the reading. If the patient

seems stressed or upset, allow him to rest for about 5 minutes before measuring his blood pressure. To help the patient relax, try to engage the person in conversation rather than calling attention to the fact that you are waiting to take his blood pressure. If the patient still appears anxious or under stress, take his blood pressure anyway and make a notation for the physician (who may want to repeat the measurement later in the visit).

However, there are certain instances when you should not take a blood pressure measurement on a particular arm. Blood pressure should not be taken on an arm that is on the same side as a mastectomy (breast removal) or on an arm that has an injury, a blocked artery, or a device under the skin (implant) at the site. In such cases, use the other arm or the upper leg, placing the stethoscope over the popliteal artery behind the knee. Note the measurements and their locations in the patient's chart.

Be sure you use the proper size cuff when taking blood pressure. The bladder inside the cuff should encircle 80% to 100% the distance around the arm or leg. Although the standard adult cuff can be used for most adults, some may require the larger size. Using an improper size may result in an inaccurate reading.

Go to CONNECT to see a video about *Taking the Blood Pressure of Adults and Older Children.*

▶ Orthostatic or Postural Vital Signs
LO 37.5

Orthostatic vital signs usually consist of taking the blood pressure and pulse. The vital signs are taken in different positions to assess for **orthostatic** or **postural hypotension.** This means that as the patient moves from a lying to standing position, the blood pressure becomes low and, as a result, the pulse increases. This usually indicates some sort of fluid loss or malfunctioning of the cardiovascular system, which may be the result of vomiting, diarrhea, or prolonged bed rest.

Orthostatic vital signs are taken in three different positions. BP and pulse are taken with the patient lying down, then sitting up, and then standing. It is recommended to wait 2 to 5 minutes before taking the vital signs after repositioning to allow the body's systems to adjust. Do not allow the patient's arm to hang down while taking the blood pressure as this could cause a false blood pressure increase. Instead, rest the patient's arm on the bed or table. Watch the patient carefully since there is an increased chance of passing out during these position changes. If there is an increase in the pulse rate of more than 10 bpm and the blood pressure drops more than 20 points, then the patient is considered to have orthostatic hypotension. This is sometimes documented as a **positive tilt test.** A positive tilt test may be due to dehydration, heart disease, diabetes, medications, or a nervous system disorder.

▶ Body Measurements
LO 37.6

Certain measurements are obtained prior to the patient's being seen by the practitioner. These include height and weight for adults and older children, and weight, length, and head circumference for infants. Usually, these measurements are taken before or after the vital signs, depending on the office policy. Depending on the patient, you may choose to take the patient's vital signs first. For example, if a patient may become upset about her weight, you should take her vital signs first so that the patient's vital signs will not be affected by the weight results. Anxiety can cause a patient's pulse, respirations, and blood pressure to increase. Follow the policy at your facility.

Measurements provide baseline values for a patient's current condition. Any extreme or abnormal changes may indicate a disease or disorder and should be noted for the practitioner. For children and adolescents, these measurements should be taken at each office visit, which allows the physician to follow growth and development.

Measurements are also important in determining the extent of an injury or illness and certain treatment regimens. For example, dosages of certain medications are based on patient weight, or a wound or bruise may be measured to determine how well it is healing. These measurements also may be necessary for correct interpretation of certain diagnostic tests, like electrocardiography.

Metric conversions for weight and height measurements are given in Tables 37-5 and 37-6. To complete these conversions yourself, review the Points on Practice feature, Math for Measurements.

Measuring the Weight of Adults

An adult's and child's weight is taken at each office visit. Weight should be listed in the patient's chart to the nearest quarter of a pound. In some cases it will need to be converted to metric units. See Table 37-5. The steps for weighing an adult or child are described in Procedure 37-4.

Measuring the Height of Adults

The height of an adult should be measured at the patient's initial visit and whenever a complete physical exam is performed

TABLE 37-6		Metric Conversions for Height			
in	cm	in	cm	in	cm
20	51	42	107	62	157
22	56	44	112	64	163
24	61	46	117	66	168
26	66	48	122	68	173
28	71	50	127	70	178
30	76	52	132	72	183
32	81	54	137	74	188
34	86	56	142	76	193
36	91	58	147	78	198
38	97	60	152	80	203
40	102				

Note: cm = in × 2.54; in = cm × 0.394. Conversions are rounded to the nearest whole number.

or at least yearly. Height for children is typically measured at each visit. Height should be measured to the nearest quarter of an inch. In some cases it will need to be converted to metric units. See Table 37-6. Measure the patient's height after weighing the patient. Most office scales have a height bar located in the center of the scale. This bar is calibrated in inches and quarter inches. The steps for measuring the height of an adult are described in Procedure 37-4.

Go to CONNECT to see a video about *Measuring Adults and Children.*

Body Mass Index

A reliable indicator of healthy weight is body mass index (BMI), which is calculated based on height and weight. You may be asked to calculate a patient's BMI. Use the CDC's BMI chart to calculate the patient's BMI (Figure 37-16). There are also handheld BMI calculators available. See the chapter on *Nutrition and Health* for more information on healthy weight management.

TABLE 37-5		Metric Conversions for Weight			
lb	kg	lb	kg	lb	kg
10	4.5	95	43.1	180	81.7
15	6.8	100	45.4	185	84.0
20	9.1	105	47.7	190	86.3
25	11.4	110	49.9	195	88.5
30	13.6	115	52.2	200	90.8
35	15.9	120	54.5	205	93.1
40	18.2	125	56.8	210	95.3
45	20.4	130	59.0	215	97.6
50	22.7	135	61.3	220	99.9
55	25.0	140	63.6	225	102.2
60	27.2	145	65.8	230	104.4
65	29.5	150	68.1	235	106.7
70	31.8	155	70.4	240	109.0
75	34.1	160	72.6	245	111.2
80	36.3	165	74.9	250	113.5
85	38.6	170	77.2		
90	40.9	175	79.5		

Note: kg = lbs × 0.454; lb = kg × 2.205. Conversions are rounded to nearest tenth.

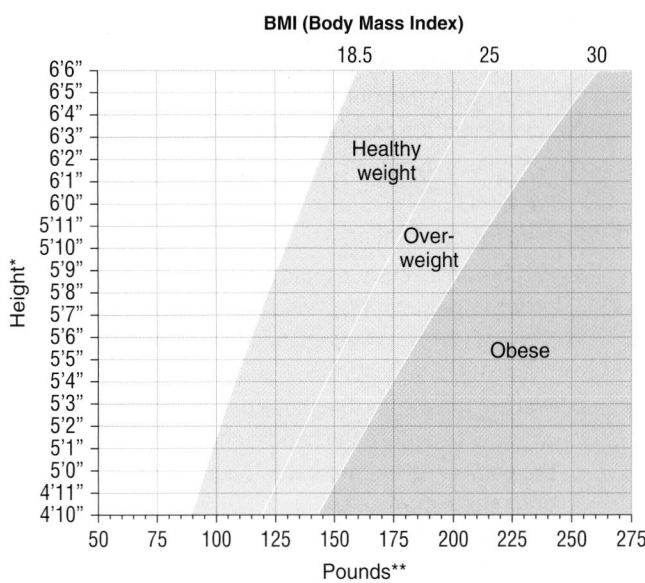

FIGURE 37-16 Use a BMI chart to calculate a patient's body mass index.

Other Body Measurements

In some facilities, you may be asked to obtain other body measurements. For example, if a patient has edema (swelling) of an arm or leg, you might be asked to measure the diameter. You should measure both arms or legs to determine the difference in size. If a patient has a wound, bruise, or other injury, you may need to measure its length and width to evaluate the healing process. Additionally, sometimes an infant will need his chest circumference measured, or an adult may require a measurement around his abdomen, which is known as *abdominal girth*.

Recording Vital Signs

PROCEDURE 37-1 Measuring and Recording Temperature

Procedure Goal: To accurately measure the temperature of patients while preventing the spread of infection.

OSHA Guidelines:

Materials: Thermometer, probe cover if required by thermometer, lubricant for rectal temperature, gloves, trash receptacle, patient's chart, and a black pen if recording in a paper record.

Method: Procedure steps.

1. Gather the equipment and make sure the thermometer is in working order.

2. Identify the patient and introduce yourself.

3. Wash your hands and explain the procedure to the patient.

4. Prepare the patient for the temperature.
   a. *Oral*. If the patient has had anything to eat or drink, or has been smoking, wait at least 15 minutes before measuring the temperature orally.
   RATIONALE: Inaccurate reading could result.
   b. *Rectal*. Have the patient remove the appropriate clothing; assist as needed. Have the patient lie on his or her left side and drape for comfort.
   RATIONALE: Proper positioning is necessary for the patient's safety and comfort.
   c. *Axillary*. Assist the patient to expose the axilla. Provide for privacy and comfort. Pat dry the axilla.
   RATIONALE: Perspiration or heavy deodorant prevents the thermometer from coming in direct contact with the skin.
   d. *Temporal or tympanic*. Remove the patient's hat if necessary.

5. Prepare the equipment.
   a. Prepare an electronic thermometer by inserting the probe into the probe cover if necessary.
   RATIONALE: Probe covers are needed to prevent contamination of the probe.
   b. Prepare the disposable thermometer by removing the wrapper to expose the handle end. Avoid touching the part of the thermometer that goes in the mouth or on the skin.
   RATIONALE: Touching the thermometer could interfere with an accurate reading.
   c. Prepare the temporal scanner by removing the protective cap and making sure the lens is clean.

RATIONALE: This will ensure an accurate reading.

6. Measure the temperature.
   a. *Oral*. Place the thermometer under the tongue in the back of the mouth on one side. Have the patient hold it in place with his or her lips and tongue. Wait for the electronic thermometer to beep or indicate completion. For a disposable thermometer, wait the required time, usually 60 seconds.
   b. *Rectal*. Put on gloves. Lubricate the thermometer tip. Raise the buttock to expose the anus with one hand and insert the thermometer into the anal canal, 1½ inches for adults and ½ to 1 inch for infants and children. Hold the thermometer securely in place until the indicator beeps or blinks.
   RATIONALE: Injury could occur if the thermometer is inserted too far or if the patient moves during the procedure.
   c. *Axillary*. Place the thermometer into the axilla, making sure the tip is in direct contact with the top of the axilla and is touching skin on all sides. Hold the arm firmly against the body until the indicator light blinks or beeps or the proper amount of time has passed.
   RATIONALE: Ensures accuracy.
   d. *Tympanic*. Hold the outer edge of the ear (pinna) with your free hand. Gently pull the pinna up for adults and down for children (see figure). Insert the probe into the ear canal directed to the eardrum and sealing the ear canal. Press the scan button.
   RATIONALE: Ensures accuracy.

(a)

FIGURE Procedure 37-1 Step 6d When placing an aural thermometer, seal the ear canal by holding the pinna (outer ear) upward and outward for an adult (a) and downward and backward for a child (b).

(b)

FIGURE Procedure 37-1 Step 6d

e. *Temporal.* Position the probe flat on the center of the exposed forehead. Press and hold the SCAN button and then slide the thermometer straight across the forehead until it beeps and the red light blinks.

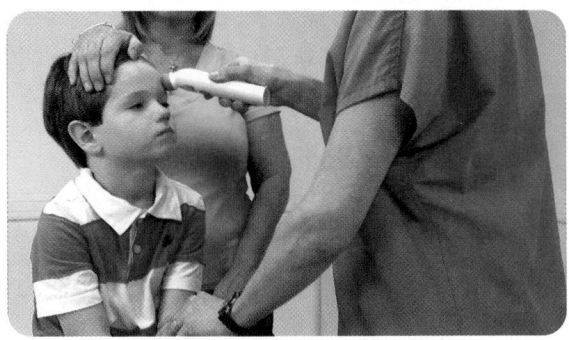

FIGURE Procedure 37-1 Step 6e   A temporal scanner is a safe, fast, and noninvasive method for taking temperature.

7. Remove and read the measurement in the display or on the thermometer. Discard the disposable thermometer. Eject and discard the probe cover for an electronic thermometer. Replace the cap and/or place the thermometer into the charging base.
   RATIONALE: Contaminated items should be removed and the thermometer should be protected and charged until the next use.

8. Record the results. Chart by including the date and location where the temperature was taken.
   - Oral: 98.6
   - Rectal: 99.6 R
   - Axillary: 97.6 Ax
   - Temporal: 97.6 Temp or TA
   - Tympanic: 97.6 Tymp

   RATIONALE: The temperature varies depending upon the location; this location should be charted to ensure an accurate diagnosis.

9. Help the patient to replace clothing as necessary. Clear the area and provide for safety and comfort for the patient.

10. Wash your hands.

PROCEDURE 37-2 Measuring and Recording Pulse and Respirations

Procedure Goal: To accurately measure the pulse and respirations of a patient while keeping the patient unaware the respirations are being counted.

OSHA Guidelines:

Materials: Watch with a second hand, patient's chart, and black pen if recording in a paper chart.

Method: Procedure steps.

1. Gather the equipment and wash your hands.
2. Introduce yourself and identify the patient.
3. Explain the procedure saying, "I am going to take your vital signs. We'll start with your pulse first." Do not tell him you are counting the respirations.
   RATIONALE: If the patient is aware you are counting respirations, he may unconsciously change his breathing rate.

4. Ask the patient to sit or lie in a comfortable position. Have the patient rest his arm on a table. The palm should be facing downward.

5. Position yourself so you can observe and/or feel the chest wall movements. You may want to lay the patient's arm over the chest to feel the respiratory chest movements.

6. Place two to three fingers on the radial pulse site. Find the radial bone on the thumb side of the wrist, then slide your fingers into the groove on the inside of the wrist to locate the pulse.

7. Count the pulse for 15 to 30 seconds if regular. Note the rhythm and volume. If irregular, count for a full minute. Remember or note the number if necessary.
   RATIONALE: An irregular pulse is counted for a full minute to ensure accuracy and to note abnormalities.

8. Without letting go of the wrist, observe and feel the respirations, counting for one full minute. Observe for rhythm, volume, and effort.

9. Once you are certain of both numbers, release the wrist and record them. If the pulse was taken for less than one

minute, obtain the number of beats per minute. Multiply the number of beats counted in 30 seconds by 2 or the number of beats counted in 15 seconds by 4.

10. Document results with the date and time. (Example: 6/18/12 P 88 regular and strong R 16 regular.)

11. Report any findings that are a significant change from a previous result or outside the normal values, as shown in Table 37-1.

PROCEDURE 37-3 Taking the Blood Pressure of Adults and Older Children

Procedure Goal: To accurately measure blood pressure in adults and older children.

OSHA Guidelines:

Materials: Aneroid or mercury sphygmomanometer, stethoscope, alcohol gauze squares, patient's chart, and black pen if recording in a paper chart.

Method: Procedure steps.

1. Gather the equipment and make sure the sphygmomanometer is in working order and is correctly calibrated.
   RATIONALE: Calibration helps ensure an accurate result.

2. Identify the patient and introduce yourself.

3. Wash your hands and explain the procedure to the patient.

4. Have the patient sit in a quiet area. If she is wearing long-sleeved clothing, have her loosely roll up one sleeve. If she cannot, have her change into a gown.

5. Have the patient rest her bared arm on a flat surface so that the midpoint of the upper arm is at the same level as the heart.
   RATIONALE: Doing so ensures an accurate reading.

6. Select a cuff that is the appropriate size for the patient. The bladder inside the cuff should encircle 80% of the arm in adults and 100% of the arm in children younger than the age of 13. If you are not sure about the size, use a larger cuff.
   RATIONALE: The proper cuff size ensures an accurate reading.

7. Locate the brachial artery in the antecubital space.

8. Position the cuff so that the midline of the bladder is above the arterial pulsation. Then wrap and secure the cuff snugly around the patient's bare upper arm. The lower edge of the cuff should be 1 inch above the antecubital space, where the head of the stethoscope is to be placed.
   RATIONALE: If the blood pressure cuff touches the stethoscope, it could interfere with your ability to hear.

9. Place the manometer so that the center of the aneroid dial is at eye level and easily visible and so that the tubing from the cuff is unobstructed.

10. Close the valve of the pressure bulb until it is finger-tight.

11. Inflate the cuff rapidly to 70 mm Hg with one hand and increase this pressure by 10 mm Hg increments while palpating the radial pulse with your other hand. Note the level of pressure at which the pulse disappears and subsequently reappears during deflation. This procedure is the palpatory method.

12. Open the valve to release the pressure, deflate the cuff completely, and wait 30 seconds or remove and replace the cuff.
    RATIONALE: If you do not deflate the cuff completely and wait, blood may pool in the artery and give a falsely high reading.

13. Place the earpieces of the stethoscope in your ear canals and adjust them to fit snugly and comfortably. When placed in the ears, they should point up or toward the nose. Switch the stethoscope head to the diaphragm position. Confirm the setting by listening as you tap the stethoscope head gently.

14. Place the head of the stethoscope over the brachial artery pulsation, just above and medial to the antecubital space but below the lower edge of the cuff. Hold the stethoscope firmly in place between the index and middle fingers, making sure the head is in contact with the skin around its entire circumference.
    RATIONALE: Do not hold the stethoscope with the thumb because the pulse of your thumb can interfere with the reading.

15. Inflate the bladder rapidly and steadily to a pressure 20 to 30 mm Hg above the level previously determined by palpation. Then partially open (unscrew) the valve and deflate the bladder at approximately 2 mm per second while you listen for the appearance of the Korotkoff sounds.

16. As the pressure in the bladder falls, note the level of pressure on the manometer at the first appearance of repetitive sounds. This reading is the systolic pressure.

17. Continue to deflate the cuff gradually, noting the point at which the sound changes from strong to muffled.

18. Continue to deflate the cuff, and note when the sound disappears. This reading is the diastolic pressure.

19. Continue to listen for an additional 10 mm Hg, listening carefully for a return of the repetitive sounds.
    RATIONALE: To ensure there is no auscultatory gap.

20. Deflate the cuff completely and remove it from the patient's arm.

21. Record the numbers, separated by slashes, in the patient's chart. Chart the date and time of the measurement, the arm on which the measurement was made, the subject's position, and the cuff size when a nonstandard size is used.
RATIONALE: The value recorded is an exact measurement of the auscultated blood pressure.

22. Fold the cuff and replace it in the holder.

23. Inform the patient that you have completed the procedure.

24. Disinfect the earpieces and diaphragm of the stethoscope with gauze squares moistened with alcohol.

25. Properly dispose of the used gauze squares and wash your hands.

PROCEDURE 37-4 Measuring Adults and Children

Procedure Goal: To accurately measure weight and height of adults and children.

OSHA Guidelines:

Materials: For an adult or older child, adult scale with height bar, disposable towel; for toddler, adult scale with height bar or height chart, disposable towel.

Method: Procedure steps.

Adult or Older Child: Weight

1. Identify the patient and introduce yourself.

2. Wash your hands and explain the procedure to the patient.

3. Check to see whether the scale is in balance by moving all the weights to the left side. The indicator should be level with the middle mark. If not, check the manufacturer's directions and adjust it to ensure a zero balance. If you are using a scale equipped to measure either kilograms or pounds, check to see that it is set on the desired units and that the upper and lower weights show the same units.
RATIONALE: Proper functioning of the scale ensures an accurate result.

4. Place a disposable towel on the scale or have the patient leave her socks on.
RATIONALE: Prevents cross-contamination of the scale from various patients' feet.

5. Ask the patient to remove her shoes, if that is the standard office policy.
RATIONALE: Follow the policy and use the same procedure for all visits for consistency of results.

6. Ask the patient to step on the center of the scale, facing forward. Assist as necessary.

7. Place the lower weight at the highest number that does not cause the balance indicator to drop to the bottom.
RATIONALE: To ensure accuracy.

8. Move the upper weight slowly to the right until the balance bar is centered at the middle mark, adjusting as necessary.
RATIONALE: To ensure accuracy.

9. Add the two weights together to get the patient's weight.

10. Record the patient's weight in the chart to the nearest quarter of a pound or tenth of a kilogram.

11. Return the weights to their starting positions on the left side.

Adult or Older Child: Height

12. With the patient off the scale, raise the height bar well above the patient's head and swing out the extension.
RATIONALE: Doing so prevents hitting the patient with the extension bar.

13. Ask the patient to step on the center of the scale and to stand up straight and look forward.
RATIONALE: Standing straight is necessary for accuracy.

14. Gently lower the height bar until the extension rests on the patient's head.

FIGURE Procedure 37-4 Step 14   The medical assistant adjusts the height bar to meet the top of the patient's head.

15. Have the patient step off the scale while you hold the height bar before reading the measurement.
RATIONALE: To better visualize the height measurement.

16. If the patient is fewer than 50 inches tall, read the height on the bottom part of the ruler; if the patient is more than 50 inches tall, read the height on the top movable part of the ruler at the point at which it meets the bottom part of the ruler. Note that the numbers increase

on the bottom part of the bar and decrease on the top, moveable part of the bar. Read the height in the right direction.

17. Record the patient's height.
18. Have the patient put her shoes back on, if necessary.
19. Properly dispose of the used towel and wash your hands.

Toddler: Weight

1. Identify the patient and obtain permission from the parent to weigh the toddler.
2. Wash your hands and explain the procedure to the parent.
3. Check to see whether the scale is in balance and place a disposable towel on the scale or have the patient wear shoes or socks, depending upon the facility's policy.
4. Ask the parent to hold the patient and to step on the scale. Follow the procedure for obtaining the weight of an adult.
5. Have the parent put the child down or hand the child to another staff member.

RATIONALE: This is done to find the difference between the two weights.

6. Obtain the parent's weight.
7. Subtract the parent's weight from the combined weight to determine the child's weight.
8. Record the patient's weight in the chart to the nearest quarter of a pound or tenth of a kilogram.

Toddler: Height

9. Measure the child's height in the same manner as you measure adult height, or have the child stand with his back against the height chart. Measure height at the crown of the head.
10. Record the height in the patient's chart.
11. Properly dispose of the towel (if used) and wash your hands.
    RATIONALE: Doing so prevents infection.

SUMMARY OF LEARNING OUTCOMES

LEARNING OUTCOMES	KEY POINTS
37.1 Describe the five vital signs.	Vital signs include temperature, pulse, respirations, blood pressure, and assessment of pain.
37.2 Identify various methods of taking a patient's temperature.	Using either an electronic digital or disposable thermometer, a patient's temperature may be measured by the oral, tympanic, rectal, axillary, or temporal method.
37.3 Describe the process of obtaining pulse and respirations.	Pressing lightly at the radial artery using your fingers, count the number of beats you feel in 1 minute to get the pulse. While still keeping fingers on the patient's pulse site, observe and feel the patient's respirations, and count the respirations for one full minute. See Procedure 37-2.
37.4 Carry out blood pressure measurements.	To obtain a blood pressure, have the patient sit in a quiet area, rest his or her bared arm on a flat surface at heart level, locate the brachial artery, snugly secure the cuff above the brachial artery, use the palpatory method to determine the approximate systolic pressure, use a stethoscope to auscultate the systolic and diastolic blood pressure.
37.5 Summarize orthostatic or postural vital signs.	Orthostatic or postural vital signs consist of taking the blood pressure and pulse in different positions, from lying to sitting to standing, waiting 2 to 5 minutes between repositioning to allow the body's sytems to adjust to the change.
37.6 Illustrate various body measurements.	For adults and older children the measurements obtained are the height and weight; for infants they are the weight, length, and head circumference. See Procedure 37-4. BMI, extremities and wounds are also measured.

Recall Shenya from the beginning of the chapter. Now that you have completed the chapter, answer the following questions regarding her case.

1. What is the best technique for determining the fifth vital sign, "pain"?

2. The physician is going to give Shenya an antibiotic injection and needs to know her weight in kilograms. You measured her weight as 136 pounds. Convert this weight to kilograms.

E X A M   P R E P A R A T I O N   Q U E S T I O N S

1. (LO 37.4) If a patient's blood pressure is 138/82, it is considered
   a. Normal
   b. Abnormal
   c. Prehypertension
   d. Tachycardia
   e. Stage 1

2. (LO 37.1) When taking a patient's oral temperature, you should wear gloves if
   a. The patient is in for a routine physical exam
   b. There are contact precautions for the patient
   c. The patient is less than 5 years old
   d. You suspect the patient has a fever
   e. The patient cannot hold the thermometer in her mouth

3. (LO 37.2) Using the formula to convert degrees Fahrenheit to degrees Celsius, determine which of the following is equal to 99.8°F (round to the nearest tenth).
   a. 37.7°C
   b. 37.7°F
   c. 37.6°C
   d. 35.8°C
   e. 36.7°C

4. (LO 37.2) How would you abbreviate a rectal temperature of 99.7 degrees Fahrenheit?
   a. T 97.9 R
   b. P 99.7 R
   c. T 99.7 Ax
   d. T 99.7 R
   e. T 99.7

5. (LO 37.3) The average ratio of the pulse rate to the respiration rate is
   a. 1:4
   b. 1:2
   c. 3:1
   d. 4:1
   e. 5:2

6. (LO 37.3) Abnormally rapid, deep, or labored breathing is known as
   a. Hyperpyrexia
   b. Hyperpnea
   c. Tachypnea
   d. Hypertension
   e. Bradypnea

7. (LO 37.3) Which of the following are crackling noises heard when the patient breathes?
   a. Rhonchi
   b. Apnea
   c. Cheyne-Stokes
   d. Asthma
   e. Rales

8. (LO 37.4) Low blood pressure is known as
   a. Papilledema
   b. Hypertension
   c. Tachycardia
   d. Hypotension
   e. Bradycardia

9. (LO 37.6) When measuring a patient's weight in pounds, it is important to round to the nearest
   a. ¼ pound
   b. Pound
   c. ½ pound
   d. Ounce
   e. ⅛ pound

10. (LO 37.5) Taking a patient's blood pressure in different positions is used to assess for
   a. Heart failure
   b. Hypertension
   c. Postural hypotension
   d. Vasoconstriction
   e. Kidney disease

Go to CONNECT to see activities about *Taking the Vitals Only, Vitals as Part of an Office Visit, Recording Vitals for Children,* and *Viewing the Vitals.*

Access the OLC to practice recording vital signs in a live EHR program. Refer to the EHR Appendix IV at the back of the book for more information and directions.

PATIENT INFORMATION		
Patient Name	**Gender**	**DOB**
Valarie Ramirez	F	8/4/XX
Attending	**MRN**	**Allergies**
Paul F. Buckwalter, MD	829-78-462	Penicillin

Valarie Ramirez, a 33-year-old female, is at the office for a pre-employment general physical exam. Her vital signs are BP 122/80, T 98.6 P 84 R 20, Height 62 inches, and Weight 140 pounds. While you are interviewing her, she shows you a wart on her right hand and says it is very painful and would like it taken off.

Keep Valarie Ramirez in mind as you study this chapter. There will be questions at the end of the chapter based on the case study. The information in the chapter will help you answer these questions.

Mc
Graw
Hill **ACTIVSim**™

LEARNING OUTCOMES

After completing Chapter 38, you will be able to:

38.1 Identify the purpose of a general physical exam.

38.2 Describe the role of the medical assistant in a general physical exam.

38.3 Explain safety precautions used during a general physical exam.

38.4 Carry out the steps necessary to prepare the patient for an exam.

38.5 Carry out positioning and draping a patient in each of the nine common exam positions.

38.6 Apply techniques to assist patients from different cultures and patients with physical disabilities.

38.7 Identify the six examination methods used in a general physical exam.

38.8 List the components of a general physical exam.

38.9 Describe follow-up steps after a general physical exam.

KEY TERMS

auscultation
clinical diagnosis
culture
differential diagnosis
digital examination
fenestrated drape
hyperventilation
inspection
kyphosis
manipulation
mensuration
nasal mucosa
palpation
percussion
prognosis
quadrant
respiratory hygiene/
  cough etiquette
scoliosis
sign
symmetry
symptom

I. P (10) Assist physician with patient care

I. A (2) Use language/verbal skills that enable patients' understanding

III. P (3) Select appropriate barrier/personal protective equipment (PPE) for potentially infectious situations

IV. P (6) Prepare a patient for procedures and/or treatments

IX. P (7) Document accurately in the patient record

X. A (3) Demonstrate awareness of diversity in providing patient care

2. Anatomy and Physiology

Graduates:

c. Assist the physician with the regimen of diagnostic and treatment modalities as they relate to each body system

4. Medical Law and Ethics

Graduates:

f. Comply with federal, state, and local health laws and regulations

5. Psychology of Human Relations

Graduates:

b. Identify and respond appropriately when working/caring for patients with special needs

e. Advocate on behalf of family/patients, having ability to deal and communicate with family

8. Medical Office Business Procedures Management

Graduates:

c. Schedule and manage appointments

cc. Communicate on the recipient's level of comprehension

dd. Serve as liaison between physician and others

kk. Adapt to individualized needs

9. Medical Office Clinical Procedures

Graduates:

b. Apply principles of aseptic techniques and infection control

d. Recognize and understand various treatment protocols

l. Prepare patient for examinations and treatments

m. Assist physician with routine and specialty examinations and treatments

p. Advise patients of office policies and procedures

q. Instruct patients with special needs

r. Teach patients methods of health promotion and disease prevention

▶ Introduction

Whether a patient comes for a regular checkup or to have a problem diagnosed and treated, the physical exam is the first step in the process for the physician or other licensed practitioner. As the medical assistant, your role during the physical exam is to make the patient comfortable and assist the physician as necessary. A skilled medical assistant who is sensitive to patient needs and proficient in performing these skills can create an atmosphere that results in a positive outcome for the patient during the exam.

▶ The Purpose of a General Physical Exam

LO 38.1

Physicians perform general physical exams for two general purposes. The first is to examine a healthy patient to confirm an overall state of health and to provide baseline values for vital signs and measurements. The second is to examine a patient to diagnose a medical problem.

To confirm a patient's health status, physicians usually perform exams on a routine basis, such as once a year. Some exams are done to fulfill a requirement before an individual starts school, begins a new job, or starts an exercise program.

To diagnose medical problems, physicians usually focus on a particular organ system, as indicated by the patient's chief complaint. Because organ systems are so interdependent, however, physicians generally perform an overall physical exam even when a specific medical problem exists.

During a general physical exam, physicians check all the major organs and body systems. They can determine much about a patient's general condition of health from the exam. If appropriate, they also try to make an initial or **clinical diagnosis**—a diagnosis based on the signs and symptoms of a disease. A **sign** is objective information that can be detected by a person other than the affected person. Some examples of signs are blood in the stool or a bloody nose. A **symptom** is subjective information supplied by the patient. Anxiety, back pain, abdominal pain, and fatigue are examples of symptoms. Only the patient can perceive these sensations, which are typically part of the chief complaint.

After forming an initial diagnosis of a patient's problem, physicians may order laboratory or other diagnostic tests. These tests are done to confirm a clinical diagnosis or to rule out other possible disorders, and are necessary when a patient has symptoms that may indicate more than one condition. Determining the correct diagnosis when two or more diagnoses are possible is called making a **differential diagnosis**.

Laboratory and diagnostic tests also may aid physicians in developing a **prognosis**, or a forecast of the probable course and outcome of the disorder and the prospects of recovery. In addition, such tests help physicians formulate a treatment plan or appropriate drug therapy. Physicians may ask to have these tests repeated as part of the follow-up evaluation of a patient's progress.

The Role of the Medical Assistant   LO 38.2

Your job as a medical assistant is to assist both the licensed practitioner and the patient during the general physical exam. Your presence enables the licensed practitioner to perform the exam as efficiently and professionally as possible. Patients benefit from the positive and caring attention, and you contribute to their confidence in the care they receive.

Your role starts before the actual exam. First, you interview the patient, document an accurate history, determine vital signs, and measure weight and height.

Generally, your responsibilities during the exam include ensuring all instruments and supplies are readily available to the licensed practitioner. You also ensure that patients are physically and emotionally comfortable during the exam by helping them into position and keeping them aware of what is going to happen. It is important to observe the patient for signs that indicate distress or the need for assistance. Providing comfort and safety to the patient and competent assistance to the physician are key during a general physical exam.

Safety Precautions   LO 38.3

As you prepare for and assist with a general physical exam, you will practice safety measures. Some of these are outlined by the Department of Labor's Occupational Safety and Health Administration (OSHA) and the Department of Health and Human Services' Centers for Disease Control and Prevention (CDC). Recall that OSHA standards and guidelines are designed to protect employees and make the workplace safe. The CDC establishes the guidelines intended to protect both patients and healthcare professionals in the medical office and the hospital setting. Taken together, these safety measures help protect you, the physician, and the patient from disease transmission.

Safety measures that you must take before, during, and after a general physical exam include the following:

- Perform a thorough aseptic handwashing before and after contact with each patient and before and after each procedure. Waterless, alcohol-based hand cleanser may be used between patients if no gross contamination or visible soilage is on your hands.

- Wear gloves whenever there is a possibility that you may come in contact with blood, body fluids, nonintact skin, or moist surfaces, both during the patient exam and when handling specimens.

- Instruct symptomatic patients to maintain **respiratory hygiene/cough etiquette** by covering their mouth and nose when coughing; using tissues and disposing of them in a no-touch receptacle; observing hand hygiene; and wearing a surgical mask or maintaining a distance of greater than three feet if possible.

- Wear a mask in the presence of a patient suspected of having an infectious disease that is transmitted by airborne droplets, such as tuberculosis (TB) or meningitis.

- Patients with highly contagious infectious diseases, like diphtheria or chickenpox, must be examined under isolation precautions, such as in a private room. Wear personal protective equipment during contact. Review Points on Practice: Selecting Personal Protective Equipment for more information about the appropriate equipment to wear when coming in contact with patients with infectious diseases.

- Discard in biohazardous waste containers all disposable equipment and supplies that come in contact with a patient's blood or body fluids.

- Clean and disinfect the exam room following each patient's exam.

- Sanitize, disinfect, and sterilize equipment, as appropriate, after each patient's exam.

Preparing the Patient for an Exam   LO 38.4

As a medical assistant, you will need to prepare the patient both emotionally and physically.

Selecting Personal Protective Equipment (PPE)

You must always ensure that you create an environment that protects people from disease-causing microorganisms. The Occupational Safety and Health Administration guidelines include the types of precautions needed and patients requiring these precautions. In addition to applying Standard Precautions, there are some infections that require the use of additional PPE.

Table 38-1 identifies the condition, the precaution type, and the appropriate PPE to wear.

All PPE, once contaminated, must be removed properly to avoid cross contamination from the patient to your skin or mucous membranes. You must guard against touching the outside surface of your contaminated gloves, gown, or mask.

TABLE 38-1   PPE for Infection and Precaution Type

Infection	Precaution Type	Appropriate PPE
Abscess	Contact	Gloves and gown.
AIDS	Standard	Use appropriate PPE when exposed to blood or body fluids.
Anthrax	Standard	Use appropriate PPE when exposed to blood or body fluids.
Chickenpox (Varicella)	Airborne/Contact	Respirator (or mask and goggles) and gloves.
Diphtheria	Contact Droplet	Gloves and gown.
• Cutaneous		Mask and goggles when working within 3 feet of patient.
• Pharyngeal		
Gastroenteritis	Standard/Contact	Use appropriate PPE when exposed to blood or body fluids; avoid contact with fecal material by donning gloves and gown.
Hepatitis		
• A	Contact	Gloves and gown.
• B	Standard	Use appropriate PPE when exposed to blood or body fluids.
• C	Standard	Use appropriate PPE when exposed to blood or body fluids.
• E	Standard	Use appropriate PPE when exposed to blood or body fluids.
Herpes Zoster (Shingles)	Contact	Gloves and gown. *Note:* Individuals who have not had chickenpox should avoid contact with patients with shingles.
Influenza	Droplet	Mask and goggles when working within 3 feet of patient.
Measles	Airborne	Mask and goggles or respirator.
Meningitis	Standard/Droplet	Use appropriate PPE when exposed to blood or body fluids; use mask and goggles when working within 3 feet of patient.
Mumps	Droplet	Mask and goggles when working within 3 feet of patient.
Pertussis	Droplet	Mask and goggles when working within 3 feet of patient.
Poliomyelitis	Standard	Use appropriate PPE when exposed to blood or body fluids.
Rotavirus	Contact	Gloves and gown.
Rubella	Droplet	Mask and goggles when working within 3 feet of patient.
Scabies	Contact	Gloves and gown.
Staphylococcal disease	Contact	Gloves and gown.
Streptococcal disease	Contact/Droplet	Gloves, gown, mask, and goggles.
Tuberculosis	Airborne	Mask and goggles or respirator.

Emotional Preparation

To prepare patients, begin by explaining exactly what will occur during the exam. Use simple, direct language that patients can understand. Describe what patients can expect to feel and how their cooperation can contribute to the procedure's success. As discussed in the *Assisting in Pediatrics* chapter, emotional preparedness is particularly important when dealing with children, who deserve to have the same sort of information and reassurance as adults. Mature adults may require special attention to communication during emotional preparation, as discussed in the *Assisting in Geriatrics* chapter.

If you are a male medical assistant, a female physician may ask you to remain in the room when she examines a male patient. Likewise, if you are a female medical assistant, a male physician may ask you to remain in the room when he examines a woman. These measures are for the protection of both the patient and the physician. Such policies depend on the standard procedures in each medical practice or facility.

Physical Preparation

To ensure the patient is physically prepared before the physician enters the exam room, give the patient an opportunity to empty his bladder and/or bowels in order to be more comfortable during the exam. Collect a urine specimen at this time, if needed.

Ensure the room temperature is comfortable and when the patient is ready, ask him to disrobe and put on an exam gown or cover himself with a drape. The extent of disrobing depends on the type of exam and the physician's preference. If the physician requests a gown for the patient, show the patient how to put on the gown. Include specific instructions on whether the gown should open in the back or front and whether it should be left open or tied. Leave the exam room while the patient disrobes to give him privacy, unless he needs and requests assistance.

Be aware of the patient's modesty and comfort at all times. Imagine what it feels like to visit a physician and as you disrobe and put on the gown, you notice that it is too small and it's beginning to tear. In order to ensure patient comfort, make sure a variety of sizes are available for patient use. Use your critical thinking skills when selecting a patient gown. Your patient will remember this gesture and appreciate your consideration.

▶ Positioning and Draping   LO 38.5

During the exam, the patient may need to assume a variety of positions, which facilitate the physician's exam of certain areas of the body. The physician will indicate which positions are needed for specific exams. You will help the patient assume these positions. To protect yourself from injury when positioning a patient, always follow the basic rules of good body mechanics. These include lifting with your strongest muscles, including your legs and arms, rather than your back; keeping your feet apart; and bending from the hip and knees.

Some positions are embarrassing or physically uncomfortable for patients. If you perceive embarrassment, explain the need for the position and help the patient assume the position when necessary. Consider cultural differences and be understanding to each individual's needs. Most important, help minimize the time a patient spends in any embarrassing or uncomfortable position.

If a patient is physically uncomfortable in a position, you may be able to ease the discomfort by using a small pillow to support part of the body. You may have to help the patient maintain a position during the exam. Always try to make the patient as comfortable as possible.

When you need to make changes in the patient's position, do so gradually. If your office is equipped with an examining table that can be adjusted automatically, learn to use the controls efficiently to maximize patient comfort. Always tell the patient what movement to expect.

When patients have assumed the correct position, cover them with an appropriate drape. Drapes vary in size. Make sure you choose one that will help keep the patient warm and maintain privacy. You will position drapes differently depending on the exam position and the parts of the patient's body that the physician examines.

Exam Positions

The positions commonly used during a medical exam include (see Figure 38-1)

- Sitting
- Supine (Recumbent)
- Dorsal Recumbent
- Lithotomy
- Fowler's
- Prone
- Sims'
- Knee-Chest or Knee-Elbow
- Proctologic

Sitting In the sitting position, the patient sits at the edge of the examining table without back support (see Figure 38-1a). The physician examines the patient's head, neck, chest, heart, back, and arms. While the patient is in the sitting position, the physician evaluates the patient's ability to fully expand the lungs. She then checks the upper body parts for **symmetry**, the degree to which one side is the same as the other. In the sitting position, the drape is placed across the patient's lap for men or across the patient's chest and lap for women.

If a patient is too weak to sit unsupported, another position is necessary, such as the supine position.

Supine (Recumbent) In the supine, or recumbent, position, the patient lies flat on the back with the hands to the side (Figure 38-1b) or on the abdomen. (*Supine* means "lying down face-up"; *recumbent* means "lying down." Both terms are used to describe this position.) This is the most relaxed position for many patients. A physician can examine the head, neck, chest, heart, abdomen, arms, and legs when a patient is in this position. The patient is normally draped from the neck or underarms down to the feet.

The supine position may not be comfortable for patients who become short of breath easily or for a pregnant patient late in her pregnancy. Also, patients with a back injury or lower back pain may find it uncomfortable. You can make these patients more comfortable by placing a pillow under their heads and under their knees. Some patients, however, may need to be placed in the dorsal recumbent position.

Dorsal Recumbent In the dorsal recumbent position, the patient lies face-up, with his back supporting all his weight. (The term *dorsal* refers to the back.) This position is the

FIGURE 38-1 These positions may be used during the general physical examination.

(a) Sitting position

(b) Supine position

(c) Dorsal recumbent position

(d) Lithotomy position

(e) Fowler's position

(f) Prone position

(g) Sims' position

(h) Knee-elbow position

(i) Proctologic position

same as the supine position, except the patient's knees are drawn up and the feet are flat on the table, as shown in Figure 38-1c. Again, the hands can be at the patient's side or on the abdomen. The physician may examine the head, neck, chest, and heart while a patient is in this position. The patient is normally draped from the neck or underarms down to the feet.

Patients who have leg disabilities may find the dorsal recumbent position uncomfortable or even impossible. On the other hand, patients who are elderly or have painful disorders like arthritis or back pain may find the dorsal recumbent position more comfortable than the supine position because the knees are bent. This position is sometimes used as an alternative to the lithotomy position when patients have severe arthritis or joint deformities.

Lithotomy The lithotomy position is used during examination of the female genitalia. In this position, the patient lies on her back with her knees bent and her feet in stirrups attached to the end of the examining table. You may need to help the patient place her feet in the stirrups. She should then slide forward to position her buttocks near the edge of the table, as shown in Figure 38-1d.

Many women are embarrassed and physically uncomfortable in this position, so you should not ask a patient to remain in this position any longer than necessary. Use a large drape that covers the patient from the breasts to the ankles. Placing the drape with one point or corner between the legs will make the exam easier in this position.

A patient with severe arthritis or joint deformities in the hips or knees may have difficulty assuming the lithotomy position. She may be able to place only one leg in the stirrup, or she may need your assistance in separating her thighs. An alternative position for such a patient is the dorsal recumbent position. Other patients who may have difficulty with the lithotomy position are those who are obese or in the late stages of pregnancy.

Fowler's In Fowler's position, the patient lies back on an examining table on which the head is elevated at a 45-degree angle, as shown in Figure 38-1e. The physician may examine the head, neck, and chest areas while the patient is in this position. The patient is usually draped from the neck or underarms down to the feet.

Fowler's position is one of the best positions for examining patients who are experiencing shortness of breath or individuals with a lower back injury.

Prone In the prone position, the patient is lying flat on the table, face-down. The patient's head is turned to one side, and his arms are placed at his sides or bent at the elbows, as shown in Figure 38-1f. The patient is normally draped from the upper back to the feet.

With the patient in this position, the physician can examine the back, feet, or musculoskeletal system. The prone position is unsuitable for women in advanced stages of pregnancy, obese patients, patients with respiratory difficulties, or the elderly.

Sims' In the Sims' position, the patient lies on the left side. The patient's left leg is slightly bent, and the left arm is placed behind the back so the patient's weight is resting primarily on the chest. The right knee is bent and raised toward the chest, and the right arm is bent toward the head for support, as shown in Figure 38-1g. The patient is draped from the upper back to the feet.

Sims' position is used during anal or rectal exams and may also be used for perineal and certain pelvic exams. Patients with joint deformities of the hips and knees may have difficulty assuming this position.

Knee-Chest or Knee-Elbow In the knee-chest position, the patient is lying on the table face-down, supporting the body with the knees and chest. The patient's thighs should be at a 90-degree angle to the table and slightly separated. The head is turned to one side, and the arms are placed to the side or above the head. The patient may need your assistance to assume this position correctly and to maintain it during the exam.

The knee-chest position is used during exams of the anal and perineal areas and during certain proctologic procedures. Some patients—those who are pregnant, obese, or elderly—may have difficulty assuming this position. An alternative that puts less strain on the patient and is easier to maintain is the knee-elbow position, shown in Figure 38-1h. This position is the same as the knee-chest position except that the patient supports body weight with the knees and elbows rather than the knees and chest. In either of these two positions, the patient is commonly covered with a **fenestrated drape**, in which a special opening provides access to the area to be examined.

Proctologic The proctologic, or jackknife, position may be used as an alternative to the Sims' or knee-chest position. In the proctologic position, the patient is bent at the hips at a 90-degree angle. The patient can assume this position by standing next to the examining table and bending at the waist until the chest rests on the table. If an adjustable examining table is available, the patient can assume the position

by lying prone on the table, which is then raised in the middle with both ends pointing down. This places the patient at the correct 90-degree angle, as shown in Figure 38-1i. In either variation of this position, the patient is draped with a fenestrated drape, as in the knee-chest position.

The steps for placing patients into these positions are described in Procedure 38-1, Positioning a Patient for an Exam, at the end of this chapter.

Go to CONNECT to see a video about *Positioning a Patient for an Exam.*

▶ Special Patient Considerations   LO 38.6

Patients from other cultures and patients with disabilities may require special considerations during a general physical exam.

Patients from Different Cultures

You can expect to assist with a general physical exam for patients from other cultures. A **culture** is defined as a pattern of assumptions, beliefs, and practices that shape the way people think and act. Avoid the temptation to stereotype an individual or group on the basis of a single patient's behavior. Stereotyping can lead to incorrect judgments, which may influence the care you provide to patients. Avoid making judgments about patients or cultural groups on the basis of your experience with other patients or with your own family and friends. Remember, if their culture is different than yours, then your culture also seems different to them.

Patients from different cultures may not be familiar with the medical exam and may not know what to expect. These patients may be more modest than other patients and may have a greater need for privacy. They may not want the physician to examine certain areas of their bodies. Procedure 38-2, Communicating Effectively with Patients from Other Cultures and Meeting Their Needs for Privacy, at the end of this chapter describes techniques you can use to help ensure effective communication with patients from other cultures while meeting their privacy needs.

Go to CONNECT to see a video about *Communicating Effectively with Patients from Other Cultures and Meeting Their Needs for Privacy.*

Patients with Physical Disabilities

Patients with physical disabilities have different strengths and weaknesses and vary in their ability to ambulate (move from place to place). Many patients with physical disabilities require the use of wheelchairs, canes, walkers, or other special equipment that permits or enhances mobility.

Depending on the extent of their disability, these patients may require extra assistance in preparing for a general physical exam. You may need to help them disrobe, move from a mobility device to the examining table, and assume certain positions on or off the examining table. At all times, you should ask another staff member for assistance if you are not sure whether you can safely move or lift a patient on your own. Procedure 38-3,

Transferring a Patient in a Wheelchair for an Exam, at the end of this chapter outlines the steps you would take to transfer a patient from a wheelchair to the examining table.

Go to CONNECT to see a video about *Transferring a Patient in a Wheelchair for an Exam.*

▶ Exam Methods

LO 38.7

The six methods for examining a patient during a general physical exam enable the practitioner to gather important information about the patient's condition. Although practitioners may have their own preference, the methods are normally performed in the following sequence:

1. Inspection
2. Auscultation
3. Palpation
4. Percussion
5. Mensuration
6. Manipulation

Inspection

Inspection is the visual exam of the patient's entire body and overall appearance. During inspection, the physician assesses posture, mannerisms, and hygiene. The physician also inspects parts of the body for size, shape, color, position, symmetry, and the presence of abnormalities like rashes or growths. You can help the physician perform the inspection by making sure good lighting is available and that the patient's body parts are properly exposed.

Auscultation

Auscultation is the process of listening to body sounds. Physicians use auscultation to detect the flow of blood through an artery and perform auscultation extensively in the general exam to assess sounds from the heart, lungs, and abdominal organs. They use a stethoscope to hear most of these sounds (see Figure 38-2).

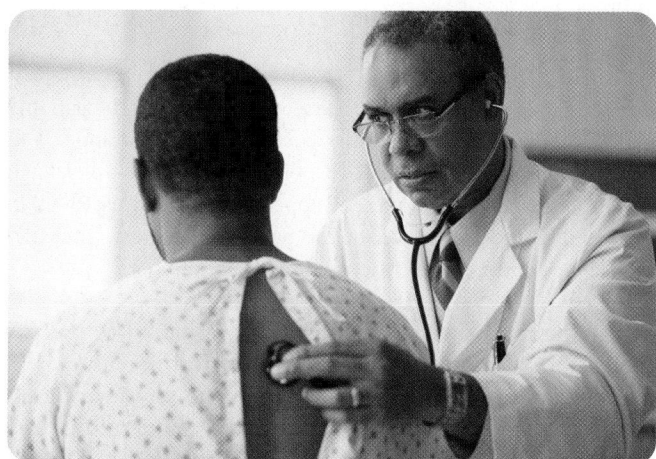

FIGURE 38-2 Auscultation, or listening to body sounds, can be done using a stethoscope.

Palpation

The physician uses **palpation** (touch) extensively in the general physical exam to assess characteristics such as texture, temperature, shape, and the presence of vibrations or movements. The physician may palpate superficially (on the skin surface), or she may palpate with additional pressure. She uses extra pressure when assessing characteristics of underlying tissues and organs. Depending on the characteristic the physician is measuring, she may perform palpation using the fingertips, one hand, two hands (bimanual), or the palm of the hand.

Percussion

Percussion involves tapping or striking the body to hear sounds or feel vibrations. Physicians use percussion to determine the location, size, or density of a body structure or organ under the skin. For example, physicians use percussion to determine whether the lungs contain air or fluid.

The physician may perform percussion by striking the body directly with one or two fingers. More commonly, however, he performs indirect percussion by placing one finger of one hand on the area and striking it with a finger from the other hand.

Mensuration

Mensuration is the process of measuring. In addition to the measurements you take before the exam—weight and height—you may need to take other measurements during the exam. For example, measurements may be done to monitor the growth of the uterus during pregnancy or to note the length and diameter of an extremity or wound. You will usually use a tape measure or small ruler to take measurements.

Manipulation

Manipulation is the systematic moving of a patient's body parts. Physicians may palpate an area of the body while manipulating it to check for abnormalities that affect movement. Physicians often use manipulation to determine a joint's range of motion (ROM).

▶ Components of a General Physical Exam

LO 38.8

Each physician performs the general physical exam in a certain order. Most physicians begin by assessing the patient's overall appearance and the condition of the patient's skin, nails, and hair. They usually then proceed with the exam in the following order, using the exam methods described in the previous section:

1. Head
2. Neck
3. Eyes
4. Ears
5. Nose and sinuses
6. Mouth and throat
7. Chest and lungs
8. Heart

9. Breasts

10. Abdomen

11. Genitalia

12. Rectum

13. Musculoskeletal system

14. Neurological system

Learn the standard order that licensed practitioners in your facility follow when performing the general exam. You also should be familiar with the components of the exam and the instruments and supplies needed for each component (see Table 38-2 and Figure 38-3).

The following are basic items needed for a general physical exam:

- Penlight
- Otoscope/ophthalmoscope
- Vision chart
- Color vision chart
- Audiometer
- Nasal speculum
- Gloves
- Tongue depressor
- Stethoscope
- Vaginal speculum (for female internal exam only)
- Lubricant (for rectal exam)
- Tape measure

FIGURE 38-3   Some common instruments and supplies for the general physical examination are (A) color vision chart, (B) ophthalmoscope, (C) otoscope, (D) tongue blades (depressors), (E) near vision chart, (F) penlight, (G) vaginal speculum, (H) gloves, (I) lubricant, and (J) stethoscope.

TABLE 38-2	**Components and Materials for a General Physical Exam**
Component	**Materials Required***
General appearance (skin, nails, hair)	No special materials needed
Head	No special materials needed
Neck	No special materials needed
Eyes and vision	Penlight, ophthalmoscope, vision and color vision charts
Ears and hearing	Otoscope and audiometer
Nose and sinuses	Penlight and nasal speculum
Mouth and throat	Gloves and tongue depressor
Chest and lungs	Stethoscope
Heart	Stethoscope
Breasts	No special materials needed
Abdomen	Stethoscope
Genitalia (women)	Gloves, vaginal speculum, and lubricant
Genitalia (men)	Gloves
Rectum	Gloves and lubricant
Musculoskeletal system	Tape measure
Neurological system	Reflex hammer and penlight

*Gloves should always be worn if your hands will come in contact with the patient's nonintact skin, blood, body fluids, or moist surfaces. Additional appropriate PPE should be worn when patients have a suspected or actual infectious disease.

Certain parts of the exam may be your responsibility and you should know how to perform them. You also should understand the physician's responsibilities. Part of the medical assistant's role in the general exam is to ensure the patient is as comfortable as possible. You can do this by helping to protect the patient's modesty as much as you can. For example, when the physician removes a drape or gown to expose an area for inspection, watch the patient for signs of embarrassment. If you notice any such signs, do your best to keep the patient covered without hindering the physician's exam. The steps for assisting the physician with a general physical exam are outlined in Procedure 38-4, Assisting with a General Physical Exam, at the end of this chapter.

Go to CONNECT to see a video about *Assisting with a General Physical Exam.*

General Appearance

The physician usually begins the exam by reviewing the patient's general appearance and noting whether the patient appears to be in good health and of an acceptable weight. The physician also notes whether the patient appears to be distressed or in pain and assesses the level of the patient's alertness. Then the physician examines the patient's skin, nails, and hair.

Skin   The physician may prefer to examine all of the patient's skin at one time or to look at certain areas of skin while examining specific body parts. The physician notes the skin's color, texture, moisture level, temperature, and elasticity. The condition of the skin is a good indicator of overall health. If the physician notices any lesions, he wears gloves to prevent possible transmission of microorganisms.

The physician also may request that a specimen be taken from a lesion or wound for later examination to determine the infecting microorganism.

Nails When the physician examines the patient's nails, he looks at both the nails and the nail beds. The condition of the nails may indicate poor nutrition, disease, infection, or injury. If needed, remind the patient to remove nail cosmetics prior to the appointment.

Hair The physician notes the patient's pattern of hair growth and the texture of the hair on the patient's scalp and on the rest of the body. Sudden hair loss or changes in hair growth may be indicators of an underlying disease.

Head

After reviewing the patient's general appearance, the physician examines the patient's head. He looks for any abnormal condition of the scalp or skin, puffiness around the eyes or lips or in other areas of the face, or any abnormal growths.

Neck

To check the neck, the physician palpates the patient's lymph nodes, thyroid gland, and major blood vessels. Enlarged lymph nodes may be a sign of infection or a blood cancer. An enlarged thyroid gland may indicate thyroid disease. The physician also checks the neck for symmetry and range of motion.

Eyes

The physician examines the patient's eyes—particularly the eyelids and conjunctiva—for the presence of disease or abnormalities. He checks eye muscles by observing the patient's ability to follow the movement of a finger. He checks the pupils for their response to light (the pupils should contract—become smaller—when a penlight is directed toward them). Then he uses an ophthalmoscope to examine the patient's retinas and other internal structures of the eyes. You may be required to perform various vision tests either before or after the general physical exam.

Ears

The physician checks the patient's outer ears for size, symmetry, and the presence of lesions, redness, or swelling. Using an otoscope, he then examines the inner structures of the patient's ears. The physician may ask you to assist in keeping the patient's head still during the otoscopic exam, particularly when the patient is a young child. Although this procedure is usually painless, patients with an ear infection may find it uncomfortable or painful.

The physician checks the patient's ear canals for redness, drainage, lesions, foreign objects, or the presence of excessive cerumen (a waxy secretion from the ear, also known as earwax). During the most important part of the ear exam, the physician assesses the color, shape, and reflectiveness of the eardrums. If an eardrum bulges outward or reflects light abnormally, the middle ear could be infected. One of your responsibilities may be to perform various hearing tests either before or after the general physical exam.

Nose and Sinuses

When examining the nose, the physician checks for the presence of infection or allergy. She uses a penlight to view the color of the **nasal mucosa** (lining of the nose) and notes any discharge, lesions, obstructions, swelling, or inflammation. Mucosa that is red or swollen and is accompanied by a yellowish discharge usually indicates an infection. A pale, swollen mucosa accompanied by a clear discharge indicates an allergy. When examining adults, the physician uses the nasal speculum to view the structures of the nose.

The physician may use palpation to check for tenderness in a patient's sinuses. Tenderness is an indication of inflammation or swelling.

Mouth and Throat

The condition of the patient's mouth provides a general impression of overall health and hygiene. Using a tongue depressor to draw back the patient's cheeks, the physician examines the lining of the cheeks, the underside of the tongue, and the floor of the mouth. Changes in color or any lesions in these areas may indicate possible infection or oral cancer. The physician also assesses the condition of the teeth and gums. When examining children, he counts the number of teeth. Most physicians leave this part of the exam of infants and toddlers until last because children of this age tend to resist opening their mouths.

The physician also examines the patient's throat carefully, as it is a common site of infection. He uses a tongue depressor to press the patient's tongue down and out of the way while asking the patient to say "ah." This procedure allows the physician to view the throat and tonsils more clearly while checking them for redness or swelling, which can indicate the presence of infection.

Chest and Lungs

The physician usually assesses the patient's chest and lungs while the patient sits at the end of the examining table. The physician may remove the patient's gown or lower the drape from the waist up. Then he asks the patient to breathe normally or to take deep breaths. A patient who becomes dizzy during deep breathing may be hyperventilating. **Hyperventilation** is overly deep breathing that leads to a loss of carbon dioxide in the blood. You can help by having the patient breathe into a paper bag. If no bag is available, the patient can breathe into cupped hands.

The physician inspects the patient's chest from the back, side, and front. He checks its shape, symmetry, and postural position and looks for the presence of any type of deformity. For example, **kyphosis**, better known as humpback, is commonly seen in the elderly.

The physician then uses a stethoscope to auscultate the chest from the back, side, and front. He listens to the lung sounds during both normal and deep breathing. The stethoscope allows him to hear abnormal breathing that may result from disorders such as bronchitis, asthma, or pneumonia. The physician also palpates the chest and performs percussion to check for the presence of fluid or a foreign mass in the lungs.

Heart

The physician usually examines the patient's heart and vascular system at the same time as, or immediately after, the lung exam. He may palpate the area first to locate the correct anatomical landmarks for placing the stethoscope. He may use percussion to check the heart's size. The patient should not speak while the physician auscultates the heart sounds with the stethoscope. The physician notes the heart's rate, rhythm, intensity, and pitch.

Breasts

During a general physical exam, every woman should have a complete breast exam to check for signs of cancer. The physician begins the exam with the patient in a sitting position. The physician asks the patient to hold her arms at her sides while he inspects the breasts for symmetry, contour, masses, and retracted areas. He then asks the patient to raise her arms above her head while he palpates the lymph nodes under her arms.

Next, the physician asks the patient to lie down and place her hand under her head on the first side to be examined. (The physician may ask you to place a small pillow or folded towel under the patient's shoulder blade on the same side.) This procedure allows the breast tissue to flatten evenly against the chest wall, permitting easier palpation. The physician then palpates the breast in a circular, systematic manner to check for lumps, examines the areola and nipple, and then repeats the procedure on the other side.

The breasts of men are also checked. When examining male patients, the physician palpates the patient's breasts and lymph nodes in the same manner that he does with his female patients. He also checks the breasts for lesions or swelling.

Abdomen

The physician examines the patient's abdomen while the patient is in a supine position with arms down at the sides. The abdominal muscles should be completely relaxed for this part of the exam. The physician may ask you to place a small pillow under the patient's head or knees (or both) to help keep the abdomen relaxed. If the patient is wearing a gown, it is raised to just under the breasts. If the patient is draped, the drape must be lowered to just above the genitalia to allow a complete view of the area. A separate drape should be placed to cover a female patient's breasts.

The order of exam methods for the abdomen should be followed correctly. The physician begins with inspection and auscultation, followed by percussion and palpation. Following this order allows the physician to listen to bowel sounds before palpating the abdominal organs. Palpation of the abdominal area can change bowel sounds in such a way that the physician could misdiagnose a patient's condition.

The physician begins with an inspection of the abdominal skin's color and surface and follows with an inspection of the abdomen's shape and symmetry. He then uses auscultation to check bowel and vascular sounds and uses percussion to note the size and position of the organs. Lastly, he uses palpation to check muscle tone and to determine the presence of any tenderness or masses.

The physician describes observations based on a system of landmarks that map out the abdominal region. The abdomen is typically divided into four equal sections, or **quadrants**. Some physicians divide the abdomen into nine sections, similar to a tic-tac-toe board. For example, if a patient has had her appendix removed, the physician might note that the patient has an abdominal scar on the right lower quadrant.

Female Genitalia

Female patients may feel self-conscious or anxious in the lithotomy position—most commonly used during examination of the genitalia. The medical assistant may help the patient relax during this procedure to assist the patient in maintaining the position. This type of exam may be performed by a specialist or by a primary care physician. The procedure for a gynecologic exam is described in detail in the *Assisting in Reproductive and Urinary Specialties* chapter.

Male Genitalia

During the genitalia exam, men may be just as embarrassed or uncomfortable as women. If the physician performing the assessment is female, a male medical assistant, if available, should be in the room to protect both the patient and the physician from potential lawsuits.

The procedure begins with the patient in the supine position. The physician puts on gloves and visually inspects the patient's penis for signs of infection or structural abnormalities, palpating any lesions. The physician then examines the scrotum in the same manner, palpating the testicles for lumps. The patient is asked to stand while the physician checks for any bulges in the groin that may indicate a hernia. At the same time, the physician palpates the local lymph nodes to check for any abnormality.

Rectum

The physician usually examines the rectum after examining the genitalia. You may need to assist an adult patient into a dorsal recumbent or Sims' position. Female patients may already be in the lithotomy position for this exam. The physician normally examines a child when the child is in the prone position and inspects only the external areas of the rectum.

In adults, the physician uses a **digital examination** to palpate the rectum for lesions or irregularities. Physicians recommend that patients older than age 40 have a yearly digital examination for early detection of colorectal cancer. For this exam, the physician puts on a clean pair of gloves. You may assist by applying lubricant to the physician's gloved index finger before the exam begins.

After performing the procedure, the physician may request that any stool found on the glove be tested for the presence of occult blood using a guaiac-based fecal occult blood test. The presence of occult blood in the stool is a possible indication of colorectal cancer or gastrointestinal bleeding. This test—often called by its brand name, Hemoccult or Seracult test—involves placing a sample of stool on a special cardboard slide. You assist by presenting the slide to the physician. To produce an accurate test, three consecutive bowel movements are tested;

this sample is usually the first. After the exam, you may be responsible for instructing the patient on how to collect the additional two samples. The procedure is outlined on the package of the occult blood-testing kit and in the *Processing and Testing Urine and Stool Specimens* chapter.

After the rectal exam, offer the patient the opportunity to clean the anal area before you adjust the drape. Dispose of gloves and soiled materials in a biohazardous waste container.

Musculoskeletal System

If the physician did not examine the patient's back during the chest exam, he does so during the musculoskeletal assessment. The physician checks for good posture from the back and side. He may ask the patient to walk so he can assess her gait. The physician always asks a child to bend at the waist so he can check for the presence of **scoliosis,** a lateral curvature of the spine.

During the musculoskeletal assessment, the physician determines range of motion, the strength of various muscle groups, and body measurements. The physician also examines the arms, hands, legs, and feet for any lesions, deformities, or circulatory problems.

The physician checks a patient's range of motion to detect joint deformities and to learn whether the patient has any limitations in movement caused by an injury or other conditions, like arthritis. Checking a patient's range of motion also allows the physician to follow a patient's progress during recovery from an injury or surgery.

Neurological System

The physician's neurologic assessment includes an evaluation of the patient's reflexes, mental and emotional status (including intelligence, speech, and behavior), and sensory and motor functions. The physician often performs the neurologic assessment at the same time as the musculoskeletal assessment because both systems are involved in movement and coordination.

The physician may incorporate certain aspects of the neurologic assessment into other parts of the exam. For example, testing how a patient's pupils react to light is part of an eye exam, but because this test also examines the patient's light reflex, the test includes a neurological assessment as well. To check reflexes, the physician uses a reflex hammer to tap tendons in different areas of the patient's body.

Most exams of children also include an intellectual assessment, in which the physician asks the child general questions appropriate to the child's age. Physicians may also test the mental status and memory of older adults to detect disorders like senility and Alzheimer's disease in patients who show signs of confusion or complain of memory loss.

▶ After the Exam
LO 38.9

After the physician completes the exam, you should assist in making the patient comfortable. Help her into a sitting position, then allow her to perform any necessary self-hygiene. Additional, tests and procedures may be ordered. Depending upon what is ordered, you will either complete them before the patient dresses or after she is dressed. In addition, you may be responsible

for patient education as well as follow-up care needed for the patient based on the physician's recommendations.

Additional Tests and Procedures

Post-exam procedures may include taking body fat measurements, obtaining blood samples, or preparing the patient for a diagnostic or therapeutic procedure, such as an X-ray or physical therapy session. Other procedures medical assistants may perform before the patient dresses include cold or heat therapy, applying a bandage, collecting specimens, or administering certain medications.

If the physician has not ordered any additional procedures—or if wearing clothing does not interfere with the procedures ordered—the patient may dress. Help the patient get off the examining table and allow her to dress in privacy. Make sure she knows you are available to assist if she needs help dressing. Tests and procedures that can be done after the patient has dressed include urinalysis, pulmonary function tests, administration of oral medications, and eye or ear irrigation or medication administration.

Patient Education

The general physical exam provides you with the opportunity to assess the patient's educational needs. Based on the findings of the patient's interview, history, and exam, you may identify areas in which the patient will benefit from additional education.

Pay special attention to educating patients about risk factors for disease. For example, women are often instructed about the risk factors for breast cancer, and men are instructed about the risk factors for prostate cancer. The physician also may request that you teach patients how to administer certain medications or how to perform self-help or diagnostic techniques. These procedures may involve collecting samples for occult blood testing or urine testing, applying cold or hot packs, or instilling eye drops. It is important to teach the patient the correct way to perform a diagnostic test. If a specimen is incorrectly obtained, the test results will be inaccurate.

Regardless of the type of instruction, be sure to address patients at a language level they can understand without talking down to them. To ensure they understand fully, ask patients to repeat each instruction and to perform each demonstration. Give patients written instructions they can refer to at home.

Follow-Up

After the exam, you must help the patient follow up on all of the physician's recommendations. Follow-up may include these actions:

- Scheduling the patient for future visits at the office.
- Making outside appointments for certain diagnostic tests, like mammograms or other radiologic procedures, or for therapeutic procedures, such as physical therapy.
- Helping the patient and the patient's family plan for home nursing care after an illness or surgical procedure.
- Helping the patient obtain help from community or social service organizations, such as adult day care, counseling, or meal programs.

Follow-up appointments can vary depending on the outcome of the patient visit. Patient follow-up can be scheduled to review diagnostic testing or laboratory results and to discuss possible treatment methods for any abnormal test results. Another type of follow-up visit is to monitor previous treatments for diagnosed conditions, like hypertension or diabetes.

During the follow-up exam, it is important to make sure patient preparation is appropriate for the type of exam scheduled. For example, it is not necessary for a patient to disrobe for a follow-up exam for hypertension. Use your critical thinking skills and follow office procedures to prepare patients correctly for the various types of patient visits.

PROCEDURE 38-1 Positioning a Patient for an Exam

Procedure Goal: To effectively assist a patient in assuming the various positions used in a general physical exam.

OSHA Guidelines:

Materials: Adjustable examining table or gynecologic table, stepstool, exam gown, and drape.

Method: Procedure steps.

1. Identify the patient and introduce yourself.
2. Wash your hands.
3. Explain the procedure to the patient.
4. Provide a gown or drape, if the physician has requested one, and instruct the patient in the proper way to wear it after disrobing. Allow the patient privacy while disrobing and assist only if the patient requests help.
   RATIONALE: Taking an extra minute to explain to the patient how to wear the gown will make the visit more efficient and the patient more comfortable.
5. Explain to the patient the necessary exam and the position required.
6. Ask the patient to step on the stool or the pullout step of the examining table. If necessary, assist the patient onto the examining table.
7. Assist the patient into the required position:
   a. *Sitting.* Do not use this position for patients who cannot sit unsupported.
   b. *Supine (Recumbent).* Do not use this position for patients with back injuries, low back pain, or difficulty breathing. Place a pillow or other support under the head and knees for comfort, if needed.
   c. *Dorsal Recumbent.* This position may be difficult for someone with leg disabilities. It may be used for patients when lithotomy is difficult.
   d. *Lithotomy.* This position is used to examine the female genitalia, with the patient's feet placed in stirrups. Assist as necessary. The patient's buttocks should be near the edge of the table. Drape the client with a large drape to help prevent embarrassment.
   e. *Fowler's.* Adjust the head of the table to the desired angle. Help the patient move toward the head of the table until the patient's buttocks meet the point at which the head of the table begins to incline upward.

   f. *Prone.* In this position, the patient lies face down. It is not used for later stages of pregnancy, obese patients, patients with respiratory difficulty, or certain elderly patients.
   g. *Sims'.* In this position, the patient lies on her left side with her left leg slightly bent and her left arm behind her back. Her right knee is bent and raised toward her chest and her right arm is bent toward her head. This position may be difficult for patients with joint deformities.
   h. *Knee-Chest.* This position is difficult for patients to assume. The patient is face-down, supporting his weight on his knees and chest, or in an alternative knee-elbow position. These positions are used for rectal and perineal exams. Keep the patient in this position for the shortest amount of time possible.

FIGURE Procedure 38-1 Step 7h Patient in the knee-chest position on examining table.

   i. *Proctologic.* This position also is used for rectal and perineal exams. In this position, the patient bends over the examining table with his chest resting on the table.

FIGURE Procedure 38-1 Step 7i Patient in the proctologic position.

8. Drape the client to prevent exposure and avoid embarrassment. Place pillows for comfort as needed.
   RATIONALE: The patient's comfort and safety are mandatory.

9. Adjust the drapes during the exam.

10. On completion of the exam, assist the patient out of the position as necessary and provide privacy as the patient dresses.

PROCEDURE 38-2 Communicating Effectively with Patients from Other Cultures and Meeting Their Needs for Privacy

Procedure Goal: To ensure effective communication with patients from other cultures while meeting their privacy needs.

OSHA Guidelines: This procedure does not involve exposure to blood, body fluids, or tissue.

Materials: Exam gown and drapes.

Method: Procedure steps.

Effective Communication

1. When it is necessary to use a translator, direct conversation or instruction to the translator.
   RATIONALE: Translators will reduce the risk of litigation and improve patient outcomes.

FIGURE Procedure 38-2 Step 1   Medical assistant using a translator for effective communication with patient.

2. Direct conversation and demonstrations of what to do, such as putting on an exam gown, to the patient.

3. Confirm with the translator that the patient has understood the instruction or demonstration.

4. Allow the translator to be present during the exam if the patient prefers.

5. If the patient understands some English, speak slowly, use simple language, and demonstrate instructions whenever possible.

Meeting the Need for Privacy

6. Before the procedure, thoroughly explain to the patient or translator the reason for disrobing. Indicate that you will allow the patient privacy and ample time to undress.

7. If the patient is reluctant, reassure him that the physician respects the need for privacy and will look at only what is necessary for the exam.
   RATIONALE: Some patients from certain cultures are embarrassed when exposed.

FIGURE Procedure 38-2 Step 7   Medical assistant providing a gown to the patient.

8. Provide extra drapes if you think doing so will make the patient feel more comfortable.

9. If the patient is still reluctant, discuss the problem with the physician; the physician may be able to negotiate a compromise with the patient.

10. During the procedure, ensure the patient is undraped only as much as necessary.

11. Whenever possible, minimize the amount of time the patient remains undraped.

PROCEDURE 38-3 Transferring a Patient in a Wheelchair for an Exam

Procedure Goal: To assist a patient in transferring from a wheelchair to the examining table safely and efficiently.

OSHA Guidelines:

Materials: Adjustable examining table or gynecologic table, stepstool (optional), exam gown, and drape.

Method: Procedure steps. *Caution:* Never risk injuring yourself; call for assistance when in doubt. As a rule, you should not attempt to lift more than 35% of your body weight.

Preparation for Transfer

1. Identify the patient and introduce yourself.
2. Wash your hands.
3. Explain the procedure in detail.
4. Position the wheelchair at a right angle to the end of the examining table. This position reduces the distance between the wheelchair and the end of the examining table across which the patient must move.
5. Lock the wheels of the wheelchair.
   RATIONALE: To prevent the wheelchair from moving during the transfer.

FIGURE Procedure 38-3 Step 5 Lock the wheels on the wheelchair before a transfer.

6. Lift the patient's feet and fold back the foot and leg supports of the wheelchair.
7. Place the patient's feet on the floor. The patient should have shoes or slippers with nonskid soles. Place your feet in front of the patient's feet.
   RATIONALE: These actions prevent the patient from slipping.
8. If needed, place a stepstool in front of the table and place the patient's feet flat on the stool.

Transferring the Patient by Yourself

9. Face the patient, spread your feet apart, align your knees with the patient's knees, and bend your knees slightly.
   RATIONALE: If you lift while bending at the waist instead of bending your knees, you can cause serious injury to your back.
10. Have the patient hold onto your shoulders.
11. Place your arms around the patient, under the patient's arms.
12. Tell the patient you will lift on the count of 3, and ask the patient to support as much of her own weight as possible (if she is able).
13. At the count of 3, lift the patient.

FIGURE Procedure 38-3 Step 13 Medical assistant transferring the patient by herself from wheelchair to exam table.

14. Pivot the patient to bring the back of the patient's knees against the table.
15. Gently lower the patient into a sitting position on the table. If the patient cannot sit unassisted, help her move into a supine position.
16. Move the wheelchair out of the way.
17. Assist the patient with disrobing as necessary, providing a gown and drape.

Transferring the Patient with Assistance

18. Working with your partner, both of you face the patient, spread your feet apart, position yourselves so that one of each of your knees is aligned with the patient's knees, and bend your knees slightly.
    RATIONALE: If you lift while bending at your waist instead of bending your knees, you can cause serious injury to your back.
19. Have the patient place one hand on each of your shoulders and hold on.
20. Each of you places your outermost arm around the patient, one under each of the patient's arms. Then interlock your wrists.

FIGURE Procedure 38-3 Step 20 Interlock your wrists to lift the patient when transferring the patient with assistance.

21. Tell the patient you will lift on the count of 3, and ask the patient to support as much of her own weight as possible (if she is able).

22. At the count of 3, you should lift the patient together.

23. The stronger of the two of you should pivot the patient to bring the back of the patient's knees against the table.

24. Working together, gently lower the patient into a sitting position on the table. If the patient cannot sit unassisted, help her move into a supine position.

25. Move the wheelchair out of the way.

26. Assist the patient with disrobing as necessary, providing a gown and drape.

PROCEDURE 38-4 Assisting with a General Physical Exam

Procedure Goal: To effectively assist the physician with a general physical exam.

OSHA Guidelines:

Materials: Supplies and equipment will vary depending on the type and purpose of the exam and the physician's practice preferences. Supplies may include the following: gown, drape, adjustable examining table, gloves, laryngeal mirror, lubricant, nasal speculum, otoscope and ophthalmoscope, pillow, reflex hammer, tuning fork, sphygmomanometer, stethoscope, tape measure, tongue depressors, and a penlight.

Method: Procedure steps.

1. Wash your hands and adhere to Standard Precautions throughout the procedure.
   RATIONALE: Safe, aseptic technique greatly reduces the transmission of an infectious disease.

2. Gather and assemble the equipment and supplies.

3. Arrange the instruments and equipment in a logical sequence for the physician's use.

6. Obtain vital statistics according to the physician's preference.

7. Obtain the patient's weight and height (with shoes removed).

8. Obtain a urine specimen before the patient undresses for the exam.

9. Explain the procedure and exam to the patient.
   RATIONALE: This builds the patient's confidence with the office and prepares the patient physically and emotionally.

10. Obtain blood specimens or other laboratory tests according to the chart or verbal order.

11. Provide the patient with an appropriate gown and drape, and explain where the opening for the gown is placed.

12. Obtain the ECG if ordered by the physician.

13. Assist patient to a sitting position at the end of the table with the drape placed across her legs.

14. Inform the physician the patient is ready and remain in the room to assist the physician.

15. You may be asked to shut off the light in the exam room to allow the patient's pupils to dilate sufficiently for a retinal exam.

16. Hand the instruments to the physician as requested.

FIGURE Procedure 38-4 Step 3 Assemble and arrange equipment for general physical exam.

4. Greet and properly identify the patient using at least two patient identifiers.
   RATIONALE: To prevent treatment errors.

5. Review the patient's medical history with the patient if office policy requires it.

FIGURE Procedure 38-4 Step 16 Hand the instruments to the physician as needed.

17. Assist the patient to a supine position and drape her for an exam of the front of the body.

18. If a gynecological exam is needed, assist and drape the patient in the lithotomy position.

19. If a rectal exam is needed, assist and drape the patient in the Sims' position.

20. Assist the patient to a prone position for a posterior body exam.

21. When the exam is complete, assist the patient to a sitting position and ask the patient to sit for a brief period of time.

    RATIONALE: Some patients experience dizziness when they first sit up.

22. Ask the patient if he or she needs assistance in dressing.

23. After the patient has left, dispose of contaminated materials in an appropriate container.

24. Remove the table paper and pillow covering and dispose of them in the proper container.

25. Disinfect and clean the counters and the examining table.

26. Sanitize and sterilize the instruments, if needed.

27. Prepare the room for the next patient by replacing the table paper, pillowcase, equipment, and supplies.

28. Document the procedure.

    Example Documentation:

> Patient here for yearly exam VS 98.8-88-24 BP 110/68 Ht 5'6" Wt 168, UA and blood for CBC and chem12 to lab, 12-lead ECG completed and placed on chart _____ *Kaylyn Haddix RMA (AMT)*

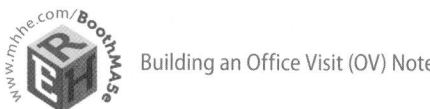 Building an Office Visit (OV) Note

SUMMARY OF LEARNING OUTCOMES

LEARNING OUTCOMES	KEY POINTS
38.1 Identify the purpose of a general physical exam.	A general physical exam is done either to confirm an overall state of health or to examine a patient to diagnose a medical problem.
38.2 Describe the role of the medical assistant in a general physical exam.	The medical assistant assists the patient and the physician during an exam. Making the patient physically and emotionally comfortable, as well as providing materials and assistance to the physician, are essential to a successful exam.
38.3 Explain safety precautions used during a general physical exam.	During an exam, the medical assistant should perform hand hygiene, wear gloves and other personal protective equipment, ensure respiratory hygiene/cough etiquette, use isolation precautions, dispose of biohazardous waste, and clean and disinfect the exam room as necessary to provide for safety.
38.4 Carry out the steps necessary to prepare the patient for an exam.	The medical assistant should prepare the patient for an exam emotionally, by using simple direct language, and physically, by providing for the patient's comfort and privacy when positioning him or her according to the type of exam or procedure and by modifying techniques to meet the needs of special patients.
38.5 Carry out positioning and draping a patient in each of the nine common exam positions.	The nine common exam positions include sitting, supine, dorsal recumbent, lithotomy, Fowler's, prone, Sims', knee-chest/knee-elbow, and proctologic.
38.6 Apply techniques to assist patients from different cultures and patients with physical disabilities.	When assisting with the physical exam, avoid judging and stereotyping patients from different cultures and obtain a translator for proper communication if necessary. Assist patients who have physical disabilities with transfers and other tasks they cannot accomplish themselves.
38.7 Identify the six examination methods used in a general physical exam.	The six examination methods used in a general physical exam include inspection, auscultation, palpation, percussion, mensuration, and manipulation.

LEARNING OUTCOMES	KEY POINTS
38.8 **List the components of a general physical exam.**	A general physical exam typically includes an evaluation of the general appearance, head, neck, eyes, ears, nose and sinuses, mouth and throat, chest and lungs, heart, breasts, abdomen, genitalia, rectum, musculoskeletal system, and neurological system.
38.9 **Describe follow-up steps after a general physical exam.**	In order to assist the patient with follow-up after the exam, you may schedule future visits, schedule visits outside of the office, help plan for home care, and, if within your scope of practice, provide education related to the patient's condition.

CASE STUDY CRITICAL THINKING

Recall Valarie Ramirez from the beginning of the chapter. Now that you have completed the chapter, answer the following questions regarding her case.

1. What would you chart as her chief complaint?

2. What things will you do during her exam to make her more comfortable?

3. What are the most likely position(s) she will be put in during her examination and why would these positions be used?

4. If you were unable to communicate with Valarie successfully, what measures should you take to improve communication and meet her privacy needs?

EXAM PREPARATION QUESTIONS

1. (LO 38.7) When the physician uses a stethoscope to listen to body sounds, he is performing
   a. Auscultation
   b. Percussion
   c. Inspection
   d. Palpation
   e. Mensuration

2. (LO 38.3) Which safety measure should the medical assistant perform with every patient?
   a. Wear gloves
   b. Use isolation precautions
   c. Perform hand hygiene
   d. Transfer the patient to the exam table
   e. Place all waste in a biohazardous container

3. (LO 38.5) Which of the following positions would be used to examine the female genitalia?
   a. Prone
   b. Sims'
   c. Fowler's

   d. Proctologic
   e. Lithotomy

4. (LO 38.1) The patient is complaining of pain in her left foot. This would be considered a
   a. Sign
   b. Symptom
   c. Prognosis
   d. Clinical diagnosis
   e. Differential diagnosis

5. (LO 38.2) You are asked to do all of the following during a general physical exam. Which one is outside of your scope of practice?
   a. Prepare the instruments and supplies
   b. Give the patient a pillow while the physician conducts the exam
   c. Determine the vital signs, height, and weight
   d. Provide the patient with emotional support
   e. Check the patient's abdomen when he complains of pain

6. (LO 38.4) What would be your best response to a nervous, young female patient who is going to have a general physical exam by a male physician when she asks, "Will this hurt?"
   a. An exam is not painful; you don't need to worry.
   b. No, you just have to lie still. I will be here with you the whole time.
   c. Yes, you can expect a lot of pain, but I will be here with you the whole time.
   d. You won't have any discomfort. Dr. Buckwalter is very gentle.
   e. The exam may be uncomfortable at times, but I will be here to help keep you comfortable.

7. (LO 38.6) When assisting with a patient from another culture during an exam, which of the following would *least* likely be necessary?
   a. Extra drapes
   b. Translator
   c. Wheelchair
   d. Direct demonstrations
   e. Thorough explanations

8. (LO 38.8) What is the purpose of a digital examination?
   a. To check for blood in the urine
   b. To determine if a female patient has breast cancer
   c. To check for rectal lesions or irregularities
   d. To locate a landmark on the abdomen
   e. To listen to the patient's breathing

9. (LO 38.9) Which of the following would *not* be one of your duties after the physician has completed a general physical exam?
   a. Schedule a future visit to check the blood pressure
   b. Administer a medication
   c. Provide patient education
   d. Document a chief complaint
   e. Help the family plan for in-home care

10. (LO 38.3) A patient is suspected of having TB. What PPE should you wear?
    a. Mask only
    b. Mask and goggles when working within 3 feet of patient
    c. Gown and gloves
    d. Gloves, gown, mask, and goggles
    e. Mask and goggles or respirator

 Access the OLC to practice in a live EHR program. Refer to the EHR Appendix IV at the back of the book for more information and directions.

Go to CONNECT to see EHR activities about *Documenting a Physical Exam* and *Documenting a Procedure.*

Assisting in Reproductive and Urinary Specialties

C A S E   S T U D Y

PATIENT INFORMATION

Patient Name	Gender	DOB
Raja Lautu	F	2/23/19XX

Attending	MRN	Allergies
Elizabeth H. Williams, MD	224-86-564	Benzalkonium Chloride

Raja Lautu, a 42-year-old woman, has arrived at the office for her annual gynecological physical. After her physical exam, she is scheduled for her annual digital mammogram. The digital mammogram results reveal a small, abnormal density close to the chest wall on the right breast. Dr. Williams speaks to Ms. Lautu and then schedules an ultrasound to determine if the density is fluid-filled or solid. The right breast ultrasound reveals a solid mass close to the chest wall. Since the mass is solid, the physician orders a right stereotactic fine-needle breast biopsy, which reveals a grade II infiltrating ductal carcinoma (IDC).

Keep Raja Lautu in mind as you study the chapter. There will be questions at the end of the chapter based on the case study. The information in the chapter will help you answer these questions.

L E A R N I N G   O U T C O M E S

After completing Chapter 39, you will be able to:

39.1 Carry out the role of the medical assistant in the medical specialty of gynecology.

39.2 Carry out the role of the medical assistant in the medical specialty of obstetrics.

39.3 Identify diagnostic and therapeutic procedures performed in obstetrics and gynecology.

39.4 Relate the role of medical assisting to the medical specialty of urology.

39.5 Identify diagnostic tests and procedures performed in urology.

39.6 Recognize diseases and disorders of the reproductive and urinary systems.

K E Y   T E R M S

amenorrhea
dysmenorrhea
induction
infertility
last menstrual period (LMP)
loop electrosurgical excision procedure (LEEP)

menarche
menopause
menorrhagia
menstruation
metrorrhagia
postcoital
speculum
vasectomy

I. C (6)   Identify common pathology related to each body system

I. C (7)   Analyze pathology as it relates to the interaction of body systems

I. C (9)   Describe implications for treatment related to pathology

I. C (10) Compare body structure and function of the human body across the life span

I. C (12) Describe the relationship between anatomy and physiology of all body systems and medications used for treatment in each

I. P (10) Assist physician with patient care

IV. P (6) Prepare a patient for procedures and/or treatments

IV. P (8) Document patient care

IX. P (7) Document accurately in the patient record

2. **Anatomy and Physiology**

   Graduates:

   b. Identify and apply the knowledge of all body systems; their structure and functions; and their common diseases, symptoms, and etiologies

   c. Assist the physician with the regimen of diagnostic and treatment modalities as they relate to each body system

3. **Medical Terminology**

   Graduates:

   c. Understand the various medical terminology for each specialty

4. **Medical Law and Ethics**

   Graduates:

   a. Document accurately

   f. Comply with federal, state, and local health laws and regulations

5. **Psychology of Human Relations**

   Graduates:

   b. Identify and respond appropriately when working/caring for patients with special needs

9. **Medical Office Clinical Procedures**

   Graduates:

   d. Recognize and understand various treatment protocols

   e. Recognize emergencies and treatments and minor office surgical procedures

   f. Screen and follow up patient test results

   l. Prepare patient for examinations and treatments

   m. Assist physician with routine and specialty examinations and treatments

   p. Advise patients of office policies and procedures

   q. Instruct patients with special needs

   r. Teach patients methods of health promotion and disease prevention

10. **Medical Laboratory Procedures**

    Graduates:

    b. Perform selected CLIA-waived tests that assist with diagnosis and treatment
       6. Kit testing
          a. Pregnancy

▶ Introduction

Obstetrics (OB) involves the study of pregnancy, labor, delivery, and the period following labor, called postpartum. This field is often combined with gynecology (GYN), which is care of the female reproductive system. An OB/GYN practices both specialties. A urologist diagnoses and treats disorders and diseases of both the female and male urinary systems, as well as the male reproductive system. For this reason, the specialty fields of OB/GYN and urology are discussed together in this chapter. Excellent knowledge of the reproductive and urinary systems (both male and female) is a must to work in these specialties. As a medical assistant, you will need to recall diseases and disorders, examinations, diagnostic tests, and treatments for each of these systems. Most importantly, you must be able to assist the physician, physician assistant, nurse practitioner, or midwife, or other licensed practitioner during exams, treatments, and procedures, and provide patient education unique to these specialties.

Assisting with the Gynecologic Patient

LO 39.1

Gynecologic patients are females and as females mature, they experience many physical changes throughout their bodies. These changes, including menstruation and menopause and the hormones that cause them, are common reasons for women to visit their OB/GYN licensed practitioner.

Menstruation

Menstruation is a woman's normal cycle of preparation for conception (the union of egg and sperm that initiates pregnancy). The normal age range of **menarche**—the beginning of menstruation—is 10 to 15 years of age. Each month (averaging every 28 days), the endometrium, which lines the uterus, is shed in vaginal bleeding. If the woman becomes pregnant, this shedding does not occur and the woman misses her menstrual period.

A period lasts an average of 5 days, with durations of 3 to 7 days considered normal. Menstrual cycles are prompted by changes in hormonal (estrogen and progesterone) levels.

Menopause

Menopause, like menstruation, is a natural occurrence. It is the cessation (the end) of the menstrual cycle. Menopause usually occurs between ages 45 and 55. Several stages surround menopause. Premenopause is the time period before menopause, during which the menstrual periods may be irregular. The time just before and after menopause is called perimenopause. During perimenopause, a woman may experience irregular periods, hot flashes, and vaginal dryness, all caused by changing levels of estrogen. Because hormonal change is occurring, the woman may experience mood swings or other psychological changes. Menopause can also be brought on by the surgical removal of the uterus and ovaries, known as a hysterectomy, and discussed later in this chapter. The symptoms and treatment for menopause are the same for both surgical and naturally occurring menopause.

The Gynecologic Exam

The gynecologic exam is intended to provide an overview of a woman's health and to offer the opportunity for important cancer-screening exams and tests. The American College of Obstetricians and Gynecologists (ACOG) has specific recommendations regarding when a woman should have a gynecologic exam and tests related to the female reproductive system. These recommendations are outlined in Table 39-1.

During the exam, a female medical assistant should be in the exam room to assist a male licensed practitioner. In this case, the medical assistant could act as a witness to provide legal protection. Your role during the exam is similar to that for the general physical exam. In this role, you will complete the following:

TABLE 39-1 ACOG Examination and Screening Recommendations

Age	Exam(s) Needed	Frequency
< 21	Cervical cytology	Three years after onset of sexual activity, then annually
	Pelvic exam	As medical history dictates
21–29	Pelvic exam and cervical cytology	Annually
< 25 Adolescents	Chlamydia screening	When sexually active
	Gonorrhea screening	When sexually active (can use urine-based screening)
19–64	HIV screening	When sexually active
30–64	Pelvic exam and cervical cytology	Annual; under certain conditions, decreased to every 2 to 3 years after 3 normal tests
> 65	Pelvic exam	Annual
	Cervical cytology	Discontinued after 3 normal tests under certain conditions

- Ask the patient to empty her bladder; if a urine specimen is needed, it should be collected at this time.
- Provide the patient with a gown before the exam and give her privacy while she changes.
- During the interview, discuss her gynecologic and general health and inquire about any changes in appetite, weight, or emotional status.
- Observe for signs of problems such as substance abuse, sexually transmitted diseases, or domestic violence. It is crucial that you bring to the licensed practitioner's attention any clues you notice during your interview. See the Caution: Handle with Care feature Detecting Domestic Violence.
- Determine the first day of her **last menstrual period** (**LMP**).
- Then have her sit on the examining table while you check her vital signs.

The Licensed Practitioner's Interview

The gynecologic physical exam is more than an internal pelvic exam. It is an evaluation of the patient's total health and a review of factors that could be an indication of possible cancer or sexually transmitted infections (STIs). STIs, previously known as STDs (sexually transmitted diseases), are discussed later in this chapter. The licensed practitioner asks questions about the patient's menstrual cycle and about any abnormal discharge or discomfort during sexual intercourse. These questions help the licensed practitioner determine what tests need to be ordered. The licensed practitioner also examines the breasts and listens to the patient's heart and lungs before beginning the gynecologic exam.

Breast Exam

While reviewing the patient's chart, the licensed practitioner checks to see when the last mammogram was performed. He will also ask the patient about any other concerns or changes

Detecting Domestic Violence

Licensed practitioners and medical assistants are in a position to detect signs of domestic violence. These signs can be seen in unusual bruising or injuries that the patient may try to hide or excuse. You may hear signs in a patient's tone of voice or choice of words during a conversation in the office or over the telephone. Many times patients who are abused blame themselves. When the patient's injuries do not match his or her story, this may indicate the likelihood of abuse. Observe the male or female who constantly answers questions for his or her partner. You play an important role in noticing these signs, and you must inform the licensed practitioner of any signs that you detect.

You must also create a supportive office environment where the patient can seek help. Encourage the licensed practitioner to join the American Medical Association's National Coalition of Physicians Against Family Violence if she is not already a member. This organization provides posters—which often help patients feel encouraged to discuss domestic violence—in addition to pamphlets and other information. Reporting suspected domestic violence is mandatory in some states. You should have a folder that contains lists of the phone numbers for domestic violence hotlines, women's shelters, and other helpful resources. You can offer the following general guidelines to women.

- Ignoring the problem never works—silence does not help anyone.
- Understand that abusive family members may not be able to help themselves.
- Call for help if a physical threat exists.

in her breasts. Since the breast self-exam is now an optional screening tool for breast cancer, the physician may or may not ask whether she knows how to perform a breast self-exam (BSE) and how often she is performing this exam. The licensed practitioner will then perform a clinical breast exam (CBE) by examining the patient's breasts and underarm areas to check for abnormal lumps that could be cancerous.

Patients must understand the need for regular breast exams including mammograms (discussed later in this chapter), clinical breast exams, optional breast self-exams, and additional tests if needed. When interviewing the patient and after the exam, you should take a moment to emphasize the following breast cancer detection guidelines of the American Cancer Society and National Cancer Institute:

- Yearly mammograms are recommended starting at age 40 and continuing for as long as a woman is in good health.

- A clinical breast exam is recommended about every 3 years for women in their 20s and 30s and every year for women 40 and over.
- Women should know how their breasts normally look and feel and report any breast change promptly to their health-care provider. A breast self-exam is an option for women starting in their 20s.
- Women with a family history, a genetic tendency, or certain other factors should be screened with an MRI (discussed later in the chapter) in addition to mammograms. The number of women who fall into this category is less than 2% of all the women in the United States.

In some cases, you may be asked to instruct the patient in performing the BSE. Review the Educating the Patient feature How to Perform a Breast Self-Exam.

How to Perform a Breast Self-Exam

The breast self-exam, although now considered an optional screening method for breast cancer, is still an important part of breast cancer prevention. As a medical assistant, you may be responsible for reinforcing patient education about the monthly breast self-exam. Check the office policy to see which of several methods it recommends for teaching BSE.

Consider the following when teaching the BSE:

1. Explain the purpose of the BSE. Make sure the patient knows that she should perform the BSE around the same date of each month after her period ends, if she is still menstruating. (At this time, the breasts are most normal and least swollen and lumpy.) Have the patient mark her calendar as a monthly reminder.

2. Emphasize that the BSE is not a substitute for mammograms or regular breast exams by a licensed practitioner.

3. Demonstrate the breast self-exam according to the method used at your facility. For example, the National Cancer Institute has established one method and the instructions are provided on their Internet site.

4. Observe the patient's self-exam technique. (If the patient is reluctant to examine herself in front of you, have her repeat the highlights of the procedure or use the synthetic model.)

5. Review and reinforce teaching as needed. Provide patient educational materials that explain how to perform the BSE.

Pelvic Exam

During the pelvic exam, the licensed practitioner checks the external genitalia, cervix, vaginal wall, internal reproductive organs, and rectum. Exam methods include palpation and inspection with a **speculum,** an instrument that expands the vaginal opening to permit viewing of the vagina and cervix (see Figure 39-1). The licensed practitioner wears gloves and may use a lubricant for patient comfort.

Your role is to assist the patient into position, with her feet in the stirrups of the examining table and her buttocks at the end of the table. Drape her so that only the area between the thighs is exposed. Assist the licensed practitioner by having gloves and instruments ready for use and by applying lubricant, if indicated, to the licensed practitioner's gloved fingers.

You also may warm the speculum for the patient's comfort. Be prepared to provide reassurance and explanation to a patient who appears to be uncomfortable or nervous. Encourage her to breathe deeply to help relax the pelvic muscles and reduce discomfort. After checking the vagina and cervix and

while the speculum is still in place, the licensed practitioner will most likely take a Papanicolaou (Pap) smear.

The licensed practitioner also may take a sample for testing with potassium hydroxide (KOH) or saline solution. KOH is added to a cervical smear on a glass slide. The KOH helps dissolve epithelial cells and mucus, thus improving visualization of any fungus that might be present. A saline solution is used to create a wet mount specimen. A wet mount specimen is used to view bacteria, yeast, and trichomoniasis. Trichomoniasis, commonly call "trich," is a vaginal infection that is caused by a microscopic organism and is transferred during sexual intercourse.

The licensed practitioner then removes the speculum and begins the bimanual phase of the exam. Bimanual means she is using two hands rather than the speculum. She may ask for your assistance in removing the examining gloves, putting on new gloves, and lubricating two fingers. Placing those fingers in the vagina and using the other hand to palpate the abdomen, the licensed practitioner assesses the position of the uterus. She may then place a lubricated finger in the rectum and palpate for abnormal growths with the other hand by pressing on the lower abdomen.

When the licensed practitioner completes the exam, she usually asks the patient if she has any questions or concerns. After the licensed practitioner leaves the exam room, be sure to ask the patient whether she has additional questions. You may need to provide written information in addition to answering the patient's questions orally. Materials are available from a variety of sources, including the AMA, government agencies, and pharmaceutical companies. The website of the National Women's Health Information Center is one excellent resource. See Procedure 39-1, at the end of this chapter, on how to assist with a gynecological exam. The Caution: Handle with Care feature Guidelines for Cervical Specimen Collection and Submission provides information about how to ensure an adequate specimen for optimal screening.

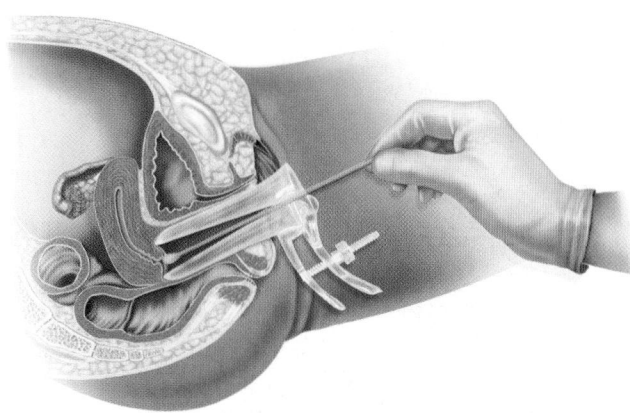

FIGURE 39-1 A speculum is used to expand the vaginal opening to help view the vagina and cervix and obtain specimens.

Go to CONNECT to see a video about *Assisting with a Gynecological Exam.*

CAUTION: HANDLE WITH CARE

Guidelines for Cervical Specimen Collection and Submission

In order to ensure that the cervical specimen collected is adequate for optimal screening, the American Society of Cytopathology has certain clinical guidelines for collecting patient information. As a medical assistant, you will be responsible for helping the licensed practitioner implement these guidelines, which include

- Scheduling a patient appointment about 2 weeks after the patient's last menstrual period.
- Instructing patients not to douche; use tampons, foams, or jellies; or have sexual intercourse 48 hours prior to the test.
- Completing a lab requisition form, which includes the following information:
  - Patient name (note any recent name changes)
  - Date of birth

- Menstrual status (last menstrual period, hysterectomy, etc.)
- Any patient risk factors
- Specimen source
- Completing a specimen label, which includes the following materials and information:
  - Liquid samples
    - Complete all requested information on the label and affix it to the vial.
  - Glass slide
    - Label the frosted end of the slide with the patient's first and last name.
    - Include an additional patient identifier, such as the patient record number.

▶ Assisting with the Obstetrical Patient

LO 39.2

When a woman discovers she is pregnant, one of the first things she wants to know is the baby's due date. One simple method to estimate the delivery date for a pregnant woman is called Nägele's rule. Begin with the first day of the patient's last menstrual period, subtract 3 months, and add 7 days plus 1 year. For example, if the first day of the last menstrual period was June 30, 2012, subtracting 3 months would give you March 30, 2011. After the addition of 7 days plus 1 year, April 6, 2013, would be the estimated delivery date.

Prenatal Care

Pregnant women should be attentive to nutrition, exercise, medical monitoring, and childbirth classes. They should avoid using tobacco, alcohol, and drugs. Normal changes occur during pregnancy, such as morning sickness (usually in the first trimester), weight gain, urinary frequency, fatigue, depression, constipation, and swollen hands and feet. Review Figure 39-2 and Table 39-2 regarding the trimesters of pregnancy and what changes may be expected.

You may perform or assist with routine tests for pregnant women, or you may send them to an outside laboratory. These tests may include the complete blood count (CBC), Rh-antibody determination, blood typing, Pap smear, urinalysis, and hematocrit. Other tests may include tests for syphilis (rapid plasma reagin, or RPR), hepatitis B antibodies, HIV, and chlamydia.

Encouraging the obstetric patient to have regular checkups and to take proper care of herself may be part of your job. Prenatal visits become more frequent as the pregnancy

1 month (first trimester)

1st trimester (from conception to 12 weeks): Mother finds out she is pregnant and experiences morning sickness.

4 months (second trimester)

2nd trimester (from 12 weeks to 24 weeks): Abdomen becomes full and fetal movement is noticed.

7 months (third trimester)

3rd trimester (from 24 weeks to 40 weeks): Noticeable growth occurs in fetus, enlarging the abdomen.

Placenta

Umbilical cord

Mucus plug in cervical canal

Rectum

Vagina

Urinary bladder

Symphysis pubis

Urethra

9 months

FIGURE 39-2   The fetus develops over the course of three trimesters.

TABLE 39-2 Changes during Pregnancy

Stage of Pregnancy	Normal Changes	Example Complications
1st trimester (weeks 1 to 12)	Missed period, fatigue, morning sickness, frequent urination, moodiness, heartburn, constipation, swollen and tender breasts	Ectopic pregnancy—severe dizziness with vaginal bleeding and abdominal pain
2nd trimester (weeks 12 to 24)	Weight gain up to 4 pounds a month; fetal movement around 16 weeks; stretched, enlarging breasts; back, pelvis, and hip pain; mild contractions known as Braxton Hicks or "false labor"	Deep vein thrombosis—blood clot in a leg vein causing pain and swelling Preterm labor—painful uterine contractions that have a regular pattern and don't go away with movement
3rd trimester (weeks 24 to 40)	Unable to sleep on back; leg cramps; frequent urination; strange dreams; nasal congestion; heartburn; constipation; hemorrhoids; varicose veins; puffiness, especially the feet	Pregnancy-induced hypertension—extreme swelling of the hands and face, headache, and blurred vision

progresses. Unless complications occur, a typical schedule for prenatal visits includes

- Initial prenatal visit.
- Monthly visits during the 2nd trimester.
- Visits every other week during the 3rd trimester up to 36 weeks' gestation.
- Once-a-week visits from 36 weeks until delivery.

In addition to assisting with prenatal examinations, you may also help teach and support both parents throughout the pregnancy. You must document all information given to or taken from the patient. Providing information on the effects of using drugs or alcohol during pregnancy is particularly important. See the Caution: Handle with Care feature Alcohol and Drugs during Pregnancy.

The following are your responsibilities when assisting with routine prenatal patient visits:

- Ask the patient about any problems and record any symptoms she reports.
- Ask the patient to empty her bladder and obtain a urine specimen in the cup you provide.
- Weigh the patient and note her weight in the chart.
- Perform the reagent urine test (chemical analysis) and note the results in her chart.
- Give the patient a drape and ask her to undress from the waist down if the licensed practitioner will be performing an internal exam.

- Assist the patient to the examining table. Some positions (such as the prone—on the stomach—and lithotomy—on the back with the feet up—positions) are not recommended for a pregnant patient, especially during late stages of pregnancy. Other positions may be difficult or impossible for a pregnant woman to achieve.
- Take her vital signs. Record them in her chart.
- Assist the licensed practitioner as needed with the exam. Provide the flexible centimeter tape measure and Doppler, an instrument used to listen to the fetal heartbeat.
- Assist the patient from the examining table after the exam.

Procedure 39-2, at the end of this chapter, outlines steps to take that ensure that a pregnant woman's needs are addressed during an exam.

Prenatal Care by the Licensed Practitioner

The licensed practitioner carefully monitors the progress of a pregnancy. She watches blood pressure, weight changes, and urinalysis results for possible signs of preeclampsia. Increased blood pressure (hypertension), unusual weight gain because of edema, and protein in the urine are signs of this serious complication of pregnancy. The licensed practitioner examines urine specimens for possible urinary tract infections (UTIs) and occasionally asks for other laboratory tests, such as a CBC. She may prescribe special vitamins and iron as dietary supplements.

During the prenatal period, the licensed practitioner will monitor for many conditions, including placenta previa,

CAUTION: HANDLE WITH CARE

Alcohol and Drugs during Pregnancy

Everything a pregnant woman eats, drinks, or smokes will affect her developing baby. Alcohol, for example, crosses the placental barrier and directly affects fetal development. Drinking alcohol during pregnancy can cause fetal alcohol syndrome (FAS). This syndrome may include fetal growth deficiencies, mental retardation or learning disabilities, heart defects, cleft palate, a small head, a small brain, and deformed limbs. Preventing FAS by teaching all pregnant patients about

the potential effects of alcohol on their unborn babies is crucial. If a pregnant patient who is an alcoholic expresses a desire to stop drinking, inform the licensed practitioner, who may wish to discuss with her admission to an alcoholic rehabilitation program. You may also refer the patient to Alcoholics Anonymous or a similar community group for assistance. Drug use during pregnancy poses similar problems for a woman's developing fetus.

abruptio placenta, and gestational diabetes. Placenta previa is indicated by bright red vaginal bleeding that is painless. Abruptio placenta is a more serious condition that includes vaginal bleeding and back and abdominal pain. Gestational diabetes is indicated by an increase in glucose in the blood or urine.

Labor

When working in an OB/GYN office, you will need to know the signs of labor and when to tell the patient to go to the hospital. Most practices provide patient instructions regarding when to seek medical care and procedures to follow if they believe they are in labor. For example, most patients will be told to go to the hospital if they are having regular contractions—6 or more per hour for at least two hours. Also, a sudden surge of fluid from the uterus indicates that the "water broke," which signals impending labor and requires the patient to go to the delivering healthcare facility.

Delivery

Delivery of an infant is typically through the vagina. After the labor process and delivery, the licensed practitioner clamps, ties, and cuts the umbilical cord and presents the baby to the mother. Women either go into labor spontaneously or may need to have their labor induced. **Induction** of labor means that the patient is admitted to the delivering healthcare facility, then given medication to start uterine contractions. If labor is spontaneous, most women go to the delivering facility as directed by their licensed practitioner. However, the medical assistant may need to schedule inductions at the delivering healthcare facility.

If the pregnant woman cannot deliver the baby vaginally, the licensed practitioner may deliver the baby by performing an operation known as a cesarean section, or C-section. Several conditions may require a cesarean section, such as a large baby or a breech position. Again, the medical assistant may need to schedule C-sections with the delivering healthcare facility.

Deliveries can be an emergency. Although not a common occurrence or a typical job responsibility for a medical assistant, if you are working in a busy obstetrical practice, knowing the steps of emergency childbirth may be appropriate. You could be called upon to assist a physician during an in-office emergency delivery.

Breastfeeding

Human milk is the preferred form of nutrition for an infant. Colostrum, the first milk the mother produces after delivery, is rich in antibodies that provide passive natural immunity to the baby. Breastfeeding is economical and convenient. There is no need to buy or make formula or wash bottles and nipples. Breast milk is always available to the baby at the correct temperature.

A woman's success at breastfeeding depends largely on her desire to breastfeed, her satisfaction with it, and her available support systems. You can support patients who choose to breastfeed by providing them with pamphlets and other written materials. Emphasize how essential the mother's nutritional intake is and explain that she needs to follow a high-protein, high-calorie diet. Patients who need help may be referred to lactation consultants or support groups such as the La Leche League.

Bottle Feeding

Bottle feeding is an acceptable alternative for women who choose not to breastfeed or for one reason or another are unable to breastfeed. There are several acceptable formulas available including milk-based, soy-based, and special formulas for low-birth-weight infants. The type of formula is recommended by the licensed practitioner. If an infant is to be bottle-fed, parents must be given instruction about the type of formula and how to prepare it correctly. Regular, full-fat cow's milk should not be given to a child until after his or her first birthday.

Postpartum

Postpartum is a period after the delivery of an infant. During this time women experience many changes and challenges as their body is trying to get back to normal. These include

- Shrinking of the uterus back to its prepregnancy size, which typically takes about six weeks.
- Sharp abdominal pains, known as afterpains, that occur while the uterus is shrinking. These usually subside about the third day.
- Sore muscles of the arms, neck, or jaw for women who have labored and/or delivered vaginally.
- Difficulty with urination and bowel movements.
- Postpartum bleeding (lochia), which may last up to 4 weeks and can come and go up to 2 months.
- Recovery from a vaginal tear, episiotomy (surgical incision for a vaginal delivery), or abdominal incision for C-section.
- Pain that may occur from pelvic bone separation during vaginal delivery.
- Emotional stress related to coping with the physical changes and the needs of the new family.

The postpartum patient returns to the licensed practitioner at least once after the delivery of her baby to be evaluated. As a medical assistant you will need to ask questions regarding her recovery and document any complaints or concerns. You also may need to assist with a physical exam or provide information about birth control if asked to do so by the physician. Recall methods of birth control from *The Reproductive Systems* chapter.

▶ OB/GYN Diagnostic and Therapeutic Tests and Procedures LO 39.3

Many OB/GYN offices have their own small laboratories for immediate results, especially for pregnancy-related tests. Other diagnostic tests and procedures are sent to outside laboratories or performed at outpatient surgery centers or hospitals.

Pregnancy Test

Pregnancy tests are done on a specimen of blood or urine (the patient's first urine of the morning). These tests detect whether or not the hormone human chorionic gonadotropin (HCG)—produced during pregnancy—is present. A variety of testing kits are available, including over-the-counter urine self-test kits that the patient can use at home. These tests are not foolproof; false positives and false negatives do occur. For example, an abnormal pregnancy can result in a lower level of HCG that is not detectable by the tests. Urine specimens that contain blood, protein, or drugs also can give a false-positive result. False negatives may result from testing too early after getting pregnant or from a urine specimen that is too dilute. Dilute urine occurs when the woman has consumed too much fluid and the urine does not have enough HCG to cause the test to react as a positive. The tests are also subject to human error. The licensed practitioner confirms pregnancy after taking the patient's history, performing an exam, and ordering a pregnancy test. You can review and practice this procedure, presented in the *Processing and Testing Urine and Stool Specimens* chapter.

Tests for Sexually Transmitted Infections

The licensed practitioner diagnoses and treats sexually transmitted infections (STIs) by taking bacterial and tissue cultures, examining lesions, ordering blood tests, and discussing the patient's history, as appropriate for the specific disease. Some facilities do not permit the release of these results, even to the parents of a minor, without the patient's written consent. Be sure you are familiar with your state's regulations regarding the reporting of STIs to the state epidemiology department.

Radiologic Tests

Several radiologic tests are used in obstetrics and gynecology. The gynecologist uses X-ray, ultrasonography, CT scan, and MRI. X-rays are avoided when a patient is pregnant. If it is crucial for a pregnant woman to have an X-ray, a lead apron must cover her abdomen, and she must be made aware that the X-ray could possibly cause an abnormality in the fetus. As a medical assistant, you will usually schedule the appointment for radiologic tests. Tell the patient when and where to go for the test and answer her questions about the procedure. Medical assistants need further training to assist with X-ray procedures.

Hysterosalpingography Hysterosalpingography is an X-ray exam of the fallopian or uterine tubes and the uterus that uses a contrast medium, such as dye or air. Because the procedure is quite uncomfortable, the licensed practitioner may prescribe a sedative.

Mammogram A mammogram is a picture of the breast on film or digital media. Digital mammograms are more easily stored and transported and require less radiation. Mammography can detect cancer about 2 years before it can be palpated with a BSE. The first, or baseline, mammogram is taken for later comparison. The procedure involves compressing the breast to obtain a clear X-ray (Figure 39-3). Recall our patient Raja Lautu, whose routine mammogram revealed an abnormality that was later found to be cancerous. Detailed information

FIGURE 39-3 Mammography consists of two views of each breast and is achieved by compressing the breast between the radiography plates.

may need to be discussed with the patient before she has a mammogram. Review the Educating the Patient feature Checking for Breast Cancer to help you prepare the patient for a mammogram.

Go to CONNECT to see an animation about *Breast Cancer*.

Fetal Screening

Tests for determining the health of an unborn child are performed on many women. Some, like an ultrasound, may be performed routinely. Other tests are used only for women whose unborn babies are at high risk of having birth defects. This includes women over 35, couples with a family history of genetic defects, and couples who have had a previous child with a birth defect. Fetal screening tests can indicate the presence of several types of birth defects, including Down syndrome and spina bifida. The licensed practitioner will consider the patient's age and medical history and the age of the unborn baby when ordering fetal screening tests.

Alpha Fetoprotein Alpha fetoprotein (AFP) is a protein produced by the unborn child that normally passes into the mother's blood. A blood test determines whether the AFP level in the blood is normal. Too little or too much AFP in the blood can indicate a fetal abnormality known as a neural

Checking for Breast Cancer

A mammogram may be ordered if a licensed practitioner detects a suspicious lump in a patient's breast or as part of the yearly screening. In either case, you should remain calm when preparing the patient for her first mammogram.

Preparing the Patient for a Mammogram

To alleviate some of the patient's fears, explain exactly what a mammogram is. Provide the patient with the following information:

1. A mammogram is a special type of X-ray of the breast that is used to detect cancer and other breast abnormalities.

2. A technician specially trained in performing mammography will position the patient's breast along a flat, plastic plate. A second plate will be brought into position and pressure will be applied for about 20 to 30 seconds to flatten the breast (to obtain a clearer X-ray) while the X-ray is taken. This will be done in two directions (planes) for each breast.

3. Mammography is generally not a painful procedure, but some women may find it uncomfortable. Many professionals suggest that patients avoid scheduling a mammogram during the week prior to a menstrual period to reduce potential discomfort.

4. The mammography appointment normally takes half an hour to an hour. The actual mammography takes only about 15 minutes.

5. Because the patient will have to undress from the waist up, she should wear a separate top and slacks or a skirt rather than a dress.

6. The patient should have no creams, powders, or deodorants on her breasts or underarms when the mammography is performed because chemicals in these preparations can produce misleading images in the mammogram.

7. If the patient has films from previous mammograms, it is important for the radiologist to see the films for a comparison study. If you schedule a mammogram, make sure you instruct the patient to obtain previous mammogram films prior to the screening if the films are located in a facility other than the one scheduled.

In addition, it is important in your role as a medical assistant during this procedure to answer any questions the patient has and to provide patient education materials related to mammography and breast disease. If your office refers patients to a particular facility that you are familiar with, give the patient an idea of how long she can expect to wait for the results. Ensure her that she will be notified as soon as the licensed practitioner receives the report. You may want to schedule a follow-up visit at this time, based on when results are expected. Tell the patient that if she has any questions at all, she should call the licensed practitioner.

---

tube defect. A neural tube defect is a developmental abnormality of the brain or spinal cord. AFP is also measured in amniotic fluid collected by amniocentesis. The licensed practitioner may order a blood test known as a triple screen or triple test. In addition to AFP, maternal levels of human chorionic gonadotropin and estriol are tested. These substances, like AFP, are only present during pregnancy. The triple test is used to detect neural tube defects and is a better indicator of Down syndrome than AFP alone. This test is generally done between the 15th and 22nd weeks of pregnancy.

Ultrasound Ultrasound translates the echoes of sound waves into a picture of an internal part of the body. The picture or image is called a sonogram, and it can help identify and diagnose cysts and tumors in the abdominal cavity or obstructions of the urinary tract. Ultrasound is painless and safe to use on pregnant women to determine fetal size and position. It is also used to guide a licensed practitioner in performing amniocentesis as well as chorionic villus sampling (CVS) for chromosomal abnormalities and other inherited disorders. A patient who is going to have an ultrasound exam during early pregnancy should be instructed not to urinate before the test because a full bladder allows a better view of the uterus. The patient is asked to lie on an examining table and a gel or lotion is applied to the surface

of her skin on the abdomen. This gel or lotion helps enhance sound wave conduction and reduce friction of the transducer on the skin (Figure 39-4).

Invasive Procedures

Many surgical OB/GYN procedures require the use of needles or other instruments to obtain tissue or amniotic fluid samples. Some procedures are used for obstetric reasons only; others may be used gynecologically and obstetrically.

Pap Smear A Pap smear is used to determine the presence of abnormal or precancerous cells. As discussed earlier, during a pelvic exam, cells from the cervix, endocervix, and vagina are smeared on a special, properly labeled slide. They are then sprayed with a fixative and sent to a laboratory for microscopic analysis. Obtaining accurate Pap smear results is an important tool in the successful treatment of cervical cancer. See Points on Practice: Pap Smear Technologies. The Pap test results are classified according to level of abnormality. The Bethesda system is used for interpreting the results. Review Table 39-3 to better understand Pap smear results.

Amniocentesis Amniocentesis is a procedure performed when a genetic or metabolic defect is suspected in a fetus. The test involves removing from the uterus a small amount

(a)

(b)

FIGURE 39-4 (a) An ultrasound technician lightly rubs the transducer over a pregnant woman's abdomen to reveal the anatomy of her fetus. (b) Routine ultrasounds are usually two-dimensional, as shown here; however, three-dimensional ultrasounds may be done.

POINTS ON PRACTICE

Pap Smear Technologies

During a Pap smear, a false-negative test occurs when abnormal cells are not detected. This can occur as a result of the following:

- Too many cells left on the sampling device (brush, broom, or spatula).
- Too many cells piled on top of one another on the slide.
- Epithelial cells hidden by extraneous material (blood, mucus, etc.).

A false-negative result could cause a delay in treatment of a year or more, depending on the timing of the next Pap smear. In an effort to reduce false-negative Pap smear readings, advances in the processing methods of cytologic specimens have been developed. The thin-layer preparation of cells is a liquid-based sampling technique. The licensed practitioner collects cervical cells in much the same way as for traditional Pap smears, using a brush or broom-like device. Once collected, the cells are suspended in a liquid preserving medium rather than being smeared directly onto a glass slide. The cells are then sent to an outside laboratory, where they are filtered or centrifuged and placed on a slide in a thin layer. This method has been shown

to produce samples that are more accurately interpreted by cytotechnologists. A cytotechnologist is a healthcare professional who uses a microscope to examine cells for changes that might indicate the presence of cancer. The advantages of thin-layer preparation over conventional specimen preparation include the following:

- Artifacts caused by air-drying are reduced because cells are placed in a fixative solution immediately.
- The possibility of hidden cells is reduced because cells are placed on the slide in a single layer.
- Blood and cellular debris are removed from the field of view because they are washed away or filtered out.
- The fluid left over after the thin-layer slide preparation may be used for additional testing (e.g., DNA testing for human papillomavirus).

If your office uses a thin-layer cell preparation system, make sure you read and follow all instructions for handling specimens. These instructions can be found in the package inserts for the individual tests.

TABLE 39-3   Understanding Pap Smear Results*

Classification	What It Means	Tests and Treatments That May Be Indicated
Unsatisfactory	Inadequate sampling or other interfering substance.	The test must be repeated.
Negative	Cells appear normal and no identifiable infection is evident.	Continue routine Pap smears.
Benign	Noncancerous cells, but smear shows infection, irritation, or normal cell repair.	Continue routine Pap smears.
A typical cells of uncertain significance: either ASC-US or ASC-H	Abnormal cells are present but it is uncertain what these cells may indicate.	Repeat the Pap smear; sometimes changes can go away without treatment. Estrogen cream for women who are at or near menopause. Follow-up test of cells for presence of high-risk HPV (human papillomavirus). If HPV is present, a colposcopy is performed.
Low-grade changes (mild dysplasia)	Cells have changes that are not cancer but have the potential to be cancer. Cell changes may be caused by HPV infection.	HPV testing; repeat Pap test; colposcopy, and if abnormal tissue is found, then endocervical curettage or biopsy.
High-grade changes (moderate to severe dysplasia or carcinoma in situ, depending upon amount and location of cells)	Cells have more evident changes and look very different than normal cells.	Colposcopy and biopsy; LEEP procedure, cryotherapy, laser therapy, or conization.
Squamous cell carcinoma	Cells invade deep into the cervix and other tissues or organs.	Immediate treatment including surgical removal. Rare finding in well-screened populations such as the United States.

*Based on the Bethesda System for Classification of Papanicolaou Smear.

of amniotic fluid, which surrounds the fetus. The licensed practitioner inserts a needle, which is guided with ultrasonography, through the anesthetized lower abdominal wall. Fetal skin cells obtained from the fluid are then grown in a culture and examined for chromosomal abnormalities. The level of AFP also may be measured in amniotic fluid.

Chorionic Villus Sampling Chorionic villus sampling (CVS) is a test done on patients over 35 or those with a history of genetic disorders to determine problems with the fetus. A sample of the chorionic villi (finger-shaped projections) of the placenta is collected either through amniocentesis or directly through the vagina. Collection through the vagina and cervix is done by using a small flexible tube with a long thin needle. As in amniocentesis, an ultrasound is used as a guide to locate the correct spot for sampling. Unlike amniocentesis, which is usually done between 15 and 20 weeks, a sampling can be taken through the vagina as early as 10 to 12 weeks. This provides parents the results earlier in the pregnancy so a decision can be made whether to continue or end the pregnancy.

Biopsy Biopsy is the surgical removal of tissue for later microscopic exam. It is the most accurate and, in some cases, the only way to diagnose breast and other cancers. Biopsy of the endometrium, which is the mucous membrane lining the uterus, may help the licensed practitioner diagnose uterine cancer and show whether ovulation is occurring. It also may indicate whether infection, polyps, or abnormal cells are present. If a patient's Pap smear indicates abnormal cells, a cervical or endocervical biopsy may be performed to rule out or diagnose cervical cancer. Procedure 39-3, at the end of this chapter, explains how to assist with a cervical biopsy.

To assist with these biopsies, you must have knowledge of the female anatomy, the order of the procedure, and the instruments

used. You also will need to instruct patients about having an escort, appropriate clothing, and any special dietary restrictions. A careful medical history must be obtained to screen for problems like possible allergic reactions. The day before the biopsy, you might call the patient to confirm the appointment and address any concerns. A biopsy is considered minor surgery and consequently requires observance of Standard Precautions and sterile technique. Depending on the extent and site of the biopsy, the patient may receive sedation or local anesthesia. During the procedure, you may be responsible for clipping excess material from sutures (stitches) and any other special assistance the licensed practitioner requests. You must place the biopsy specimen in a sterile, solution-filled container provided by the laboratory. You also may assist with or perform the cleaning and bandaging of the site after the procedure.

Colposcopy Colposcopy is the exam of the vagina and cervix with an instrument called a colposcope. See Figure 39-5. The licensed practitioner first cleanses the cervix with saline solution. She then cleanses the cervix with acetic acid, which makes abnormal tissue appear white. The licensed practitioner inserts the colposcope into the vagina and uses the attached magnifying lens to identify abnormal cells, such as cancerous or precancerous cells. The abnormal cells may not be cancerous but may be caused by infection or medication.

This procedure is often performed prior to a biopsy or LEEP procedure after results of a Pap smear show the presence of abnormal cells. LEEP procedures are described later in this chapter.

Dilation and Curettage (D&C) A D&C consists of widening the opening of the cervix (dilation) and scraping the uterine lining (curettage). Reasons for the D&C procedure include assessing the size and shape of the uterus, removing polyps and fibroids from the endometrium, obtaining endometrial specimens for biopsy, performing an abortion, and

FIGURE 39-5 A colposcope is used to examine the vagina and cervix for abnormal cells.

completing an incomplete miscarriage. Other diagnoses for which a D&C may be performed include abnormal uterine bleeding, abnormal menstrual bleeding, **postcoital** bleeding, spotting between periods, postmenopausal bleeding, and an imbedded intrauterine device (IUD).

The procedure is usually performed in a hospital or outpatient surgical facility. You must inform the patient that she will need to have someone take her to and from the facility and that she will have anesthesia before the licensed practitioner performs a routine pelvic exam. For the D&C procedure, the licensed practitioner swabs the vagina with an antiseptic and inserts a speculum. After dilating the cervix, the licensed practitioner uses a curette to remove a portion of the endometrium to assess the texture. Both cervical and endometrial tissue may be sent to a laboratory for examination. Exploration of the uterine cavity and removal of any abnormal growths complete the procedure. Instruct the patient not to have intercourse, take tub baths, or use tampons for 1 week after the procedure. She should also avoid strenuous activity.

Stereotactic Core Biopsy/Fine-Needle Aspiration In a fine-needle aspiration, the licensed practitioner uses a fine needle to remove by vacuum a sample of tissue from a cyst, lump, or tumor of the breast. The term *stereotactic* means that the licensed practitioner finds the target to aspirate using three-dimensional coordinates from a radiographic mammogram, computed tomography, or MRI. This procedure may be used instead of mammography to diagnose breast disorders in pregnant patients, thus avoiding the use of radiation. Patients with fibrocystic breast disease (involving multiple cystic lumps within the breast tissue) may have needle aspiration of a cyst followed by replacement of the cystic fluid with a steroid to prevent recurrence.

Hysterectomy A hysterectomy is the surgical removal of the uterus. If surgery includes removal of one or both fallopian tubes, it is called a hysterosalpingectomy. Surgical removal of the uterus, the fallopian tubes, and the ovaries is called a hysterosalpingo-oophorectomy. A hysterectomy or a related surgery may be performed for the following reasons: cervical or endometrial cancer; severe endometriosis; unusual bleeding; a leiomyoma, or fibroid; defects of pelvic supports; pregnancy-related problems; and pelvic adhesions or other causes of uterine pain not controllable by other methods.

Inform the patient that an abdominal hysterectomy is major surgery that requires hospitalization. It also requires preadmission urine and blood tests, cleansing enemas, and shaving of the pelvic area. Normal activities, including sexual intercourse, can usually be resumed within a few weeks. Premenopausal women who have hysterectomies or hysterosalpingectomies may begin menopause sooner than they otherwise would have. Premenopausal women who have hysterosalpingo-oophorectomies will experience menopause immediately after the surgery.

Laparoscopy A laparoscope is a long, tubular instrument. It contains fiber-optic threads that illuminate the organs and a lens that resembles a small telescope. A licensed practitioner can use the laparoscope to view the internal female organs. Laparoscopy is used to help determine the cause of **infertility** (the inability to conceive), to obtain tissue samples, to remove abnormal growths, and to surgically sterilize a patient. It is also used in the treatment of ectopic pregnancies, endometriosis, and laparoscopy-assisted hysterectomy.

In a laparoscopy, the patient is anesthetized before a tube is inserted into a small incision in or near the navel. Carbon dioxide or another gas is pumped into the abdomen to spread the organs apart, making them easier to see. The patient's body is then tilted with her head lower than her hips to allow the intestines to move away from the lower abdomen. This positioning permits a clearer view of the ovaries, uterus, and fallopian tubes.

Loop Electrosurgical Excision Procedure (LEEP) A **loop electrosurgical excision procedure (LEEP)** is when the physician uses a thin wire loop electrode attached to the speculum to cut away abnormal cervical tissue that was discovered during a Pap smear. The tissue is then sent to a lab for further testing. This procedure may last about 20 to 30 minutes and may be done as part of a colposcopy. A small amount of smoke may be seen during this procedure.

Cryosurgery Cryosurgery is using extremely cold temperatures to freeze and destroy abnormal tissues such as venereal warts, treat precancerous tumors, and control bleeding. The procedure is done through the vagina using a vaginal speculum and a special probe. Compressed gases flow through the probe making it as low as −50 degrees Celsius. The extreme cold freezes and kills the tissues. A second treatment might be done after three minutes. Patients may experience slight cramping during the procedure. After the procedure, sexual intercourse and douching should be avoided and discharge may be seen.

▶ Assisting in Urology   LO 39.4

The urologist focuses on the male and female urinary systems as well as the male reproductive system. Urologists perform surgical procedures such as hernia repairs and vasectomies. In a urologist's office, you would assist with general exams; collect and process

Testicular Self-Exam

Although testicular cancer is rare, it is currently the most common cancer in American males between the ages of 15 and 34. The American Cancer Society recommends that all men perform a monthly testicular self-exam from age 15 onward to increase the chances of early detection. Although testicular cancer is one of the most curable cancers, early detection is vital to its treatment.

A TSE should be performed in the following manner after a warm shower or bath, when scrotal skin is relaxed.

1. The man first observes the testes for changes in appearance, such as swelling. He then manually examines each testicle, gently rolling it between the fingers and thumbs of both hands to feel for hard lumps (see Figure 39-6).
2. After examining each testicle, the man should locate the area of the epididymis and spermatic cord. This area can be felt as a cordlike structure originating at the top back of each testicle.

A man who perceives an abnormality during a TSE should be examined by a physician right away. Warning signs of testicular cancer include a heavy or dragging feeling in the groin, enlargement of one testicle, and a dull ache in the groin.

FIGURE 39-6   Males from age 15 onward should perform a monthly testicular self-exam.

urine, blood, and other specimens; obtain cultures; and participate in patient education about conditions and about presurgical and postsurgical care. So, you need to understand the urinary system and the diseases and disorders you are likely to encounter.

You must be thorough when you take a patient's history for a urologist. Much information about urinary problems is obtained by questioning the patient about changes in frequency or urgency of urination, difficulty or pain with urination (dysuria), and incontinence. The physical exam usually includes palpation of the kidneys and bladder and visual inspection of the external genitalia. Women are examined in the lithotomy position, and men are usually seated when the exam begins. During examination of the male reproductive system, the urologist inspects and palpates the patient's penis and scrotum. The genitalia are usually examined with the patient standing and the chest and abdomen draped. The physician usually examines the inguinal region for a hernia and, in men over 40, checks the prostate gland. This gland is examined by digital insertion into the rectum. The physician instructs the patient as needed in performing a regular testicular self-exam (TSE). This instruction, discussed in the Educating the Patient feature Testicular Self-Exam, may also be your responsibility.

BODYANIMAT3D
POWERED BY
connect

Go to CONNECT to see an animation about *Prostate Cancer*.

▸ Urological Diagnostic Tests and Procedures

LO 39.5

Urologists sometimes use imaging techniques such as CT scans and MRIs. Pyelography is an X-ray of the kidney area with an iodine-based contrast agent. It is used to diagnose renal

(kidney-related) disorders. Urologists also use several other diagnostic techniques.

Urine and Blood Tests

Urinalysis is the most commonly ordered test in a urology practice. Urine can be tested for the presence of bacteria, blood, and other substances. Blood testing is also done for a variety of reasons, including monitoring for dysfunctions of the prostate gland and for certain sexually transmitted infections (STIs).

Semen Analysis and Smears

Semen samples may be obtained to determine fertility or to evaluate the success of a **vasectomy** (surgical sterilization by cutting of the vas deferens in a male patient). The patient usually collects these samples at home, but you may be required to provide the patient with a container, written instructions, and laboratory paperwork. Smears are used in diagnosing infections.

Cystometry

Cystometry is used to measure urinary bladder capacity and pressure. Using a catheter passed through the urethra, the physician fills the bladder with carbon dioxide gas. The test results are examined to diagnose bladder function disorders.

Cystoscopy

In cystoscopy, the physician examines the walls of the bladder and urethra by visualization and inspection. A special viewing instrument, called a cystoscope, is used for this procedure. The cystoscope is inserted into the bladder through the urethra.

Testicular Biopsy

Testicular biopsy, an invasive procedure, involves obtaining a tissue sample of a mass for laboratory examination. The patient will need your emotional support because he will most likely be very anxious about the nature of the lump.

▶ Diseases and Disorders of the Reproductive and Urinary Systems
LO 39.6

Many of the diseases and disorders encountered in OB/GYN and urology practices have been mentioned in the context of the procedures in this chapter. Tables 39-4 and 39-5 outline

TABLE 39-4	Common Obstetric and Gynecologic Diseases and Disorders	
Condition	**Description**	**Treatment**
Cancer	Common occurrence in cervix, endometrium (uterus), and ovaries; cells divide uncontrollably, eventually forming a tumor or other growth of abnormal tissue; most often seen in women between the ages of 50 and 60; symptoms differ for each type of cancer.	Surgery (hysterectomy), radiation, chemotherapy, hormones; for ovarian cancer, surgical removal of all reproductive organs, affected lymph nodes, appendix, and some muscle tissue, followed by chemotherapy (to extend survival time).
Ectopic pregnancy	Fertilized egg unable to move out of fallopian tube into uterus for implantation; patient experiences pain within a few weeks of conception; can be fatal.	Surgery to remove the embryo from the fallopian tube before the tube ruptures.
Endometriosis	Endometrial tissue present outside uterus, usually in pelvic area; not life-threatening but may cause sterility; symptoms include abnormal menstruation and pain (sometimes severe) in lower abdominal area and back.	Hormone therapy, hysterectomy for severe cases, endometrial ablation (1-day surgery, alternative to hysterectomy), leuprolide acetate injection.
Fibrocystic breast disease	Benign, fluid-filled cysts or nodules in breast; sometimes confused with malignant growths in breast until complete diagnostic tests are performed; symptoms include pain and tenderness.	Depending on severity, vitamin E supplements, hormones, compresses, analgesics, aspiration, biopsy; restricted caffeine intake.
Fibroids, or leiomyomas	Common, benign, smooth tumors of muscle cells (not fibrous tissue) grouped in uterus; symptoms include excessive menstruation and bloating; diagnosis by bimanual examination and ultrasound	Surgery for severe cases
Menstrual disturbances	May be (1) **amenorrhea** (absence of menstruation), (2) **dysmenorrhea** (painful menstruation), (3) **menorrhagia** (excessive amount of menstrual flow or prolonged period of menstruation), or (4) **metrorrhagia** (bleeding between menstrual periods).	Treatment according to symptoms; analgesics; possibly D&C or cryosurgery; for severe cases, hysterectomy.
Ovarian cysts	Sacs of fluid or semisolid material, usually benign and without symptoms; occur anytime between puberty and menopause; extensive ovarian cysts may cause pelvic discomfort, lower back pain, and abnormal bleeding.	Analgesics and bed rest if severe pain; hormone therapy; surgery is usually reserved for cysts that rupture or are large enough to put pressure on surrounding organs.
Pelvic inflammatory disease (PID)	Acute, chronic infection of reproductive tract; causes include untreated STIs, such as gonorrhea and chlamydia, and organisms such as staphylococci and streptococci; symptoms include vaginal discharge, fever, and general discomfort.	Antibiotics
Pelvic support problems (uterine prolapse, rectocele, cystocele)	Abnormal weakening of vaginal tissue, unusual increase in abdominal pressure, congenital weakening (weakness since birth); symptoms include urine leakage, pelvic heaviness ("bottom falling out"), pain or discomfort in pelvic area, pulling or aching feeling in lower back, abdomen, or groin.	Kegel or perineal exercises to strengthen muscles, insertion of pessary (device to hold pelvic organs in place), surgery to repair muscles.
Polyps	Red, soft, and fragile growths, with slender stem attachment, sometimes found on mucous membranes of cervix or endometrium; may cause pain.	Depending on size and shape, may be removed in office or hospital.
Premenstrual dysphoric disorder (PMDD)	A severe form of premenstrual syndrome that affects 5% of women; symptoms have a very disrupting effect on the patient's life; screening tests and physician evaluation are necessary for diagnosis.	Medications, including antidepressants, anti-anxiety drugs, analgesics, hormones, and diuretics; exercise, relaxation, diet modification, vitamins, minerals, and herbal preparations are also useful.
Premenstrual syndrome (PMS)	Symptoms include swelling, bloating, weight gain, breast tenderness, headaches, and mood shifts 1 week to 10 days before menstruation.	Vitamins, diuretics, hormones, oral contraceptives, tranquilizers, other medications; stress-reduction methods as needed; restricted intake of dietary sodium, alcohol, and caffeine.
Sexual function disorders	Interruption or lack of sexual response cycle (excitement, plateau, orgasm, and resolution); unhealthy view of one's feelings about oneself as a woman and feelings toward sex; sometimes caused by painful intercourse, abusive partner, unrealistic demands on oneself, or menopause.	Counseling (for both woman and partner) to teach relaxation, effective communication, and identification of cycle stages and natural responses.
Vaginitis	Inflammation of vagina caused by bacteria, viruses, yeasts, or chemicals in sprays, douches, or tampons; symptoms include itching, redness, pain, swelling.	Treatment prescribed according to cause; avoiding douches, tampons, tight pants, wiping from back to front; sometimes avoiding sex during treatment.

TABLE 39-5   Common Urologic Diseases and Disorders

Condition	Description	Treatment
Epididymitis	Bacterial infection of the epididymis; causes pain, swelling, and sometimes fever.	Rest and antibiotic medications.
Hydrocele	Excess fluid in the scrotum; usually caused by infection of the epididymis or testes; can also result from a congenital defect or occurs after injury.	Aspiration of fluid to relieve discomfort.
Impotence	Inability either to achieve or to maintain an erection; the cause may be physical, as when it results from cardiovascular or endocrine disease, or it may be a side effect of a medication such as certain diuretics and chemotherapy agents; the cause may also be psychological or emotional.	Treatment depends on the cause or causes and may include medication, counseling, or surgical procedures.
Incontinence	Loss of bladder control, which results in anything from mild urine leaking to uncontrollable wetting; most bladder-control problems happen when muscles are too weak or too active. Stress incontinence occurs when the muscles that keep the bladder closed are too weak and urine leaks during a sneeze, when laughing, or when lifting a heavy object.	Treatment depends on the cause and severity of the problem. It may include simple exercises, medicines, special devices or procedures prescribed by a licensed practitioner, or surgery.
Kidney Stones	Chemical substances in the urine form crystals in the kidney, ureter, or bladder; if kidney stones cannot pass through the ureter, they can cause excruciating pain.	Some stones pass; however, large stones often must be removed surgically or broken up by means of sound waves (lithotripsy) or laser techniques.
Prostate cancer	The most common type of cancer among men; often no symptoms are evident, but sometimes a nodule may be felt on palpation of the prostate; if the growth is large enough, problems with urination may occur. A blood test known as a prostate specific antigen (PSA) is used for screening in men over 50 years of age; an abnormal elevation of the PSA could indicate prostate cancer.	Treatment options include radiation therapy and removal of the prostate.
Prostatic hypertrophy	Enlargement of the prostate gland; occurs most commonly in men over 50; may constrict the urethra, causing difficulty in urinating and repeated urinary infections.	Medications to reduce the hypertrophy and surgery are common treatments.
Prostatitis	Inflammation of the prostate, usually bacterial; symptoms are pain on urination and, often, fever; patients are instructed to avoid sitting for long periods.	Antibiotic medications and sitz baths.
Sexually transmitted infections (STIs)	Numerous diseases are acquired through sexual contact and affect both reproductive and urinary systems.	Treatment includes prevention through education as well as specific treatments depending upon the disease.
Urethritis	Inflammation of the urethra. Like cystitis, it is usually caused by bacterial infection.	Antibiotics.

common obstetric, gynecologic, and urologic diseases and disorders.

Sexually Transmitted Infections (Diseases)

Sexually transmitted diseases (STDs)—diseases acquired through sexual contact with an infected person—are now frequently called sexually transmitted infections. You may have asked yourself why the term *sexually transmitted infection* is preferred instead of the term *sexually transmitted disease*. The term *infection* more accurately describes conditions in which sexual partners may not have symptoms and may not be aware that they have an infection. Many of these infections are actually curable. Also the term *infection* carries less of a social stigma than the term *disease*. STI is now used by many leading sexual health organizations. Urologists and gynecologists are both involved in the diagnosis and treatment of STIs.

Your role as an educator is vital in dealing with patients who have STIs. Some patients may be hesitant to ask for information. Providing educational materials in the exam room will help answer their questions and put them at ease. These materials deal with sensitive or embarrassing topics, and the patient's privacy must be maintained. Patient education about prevention and treatment of STIs is needed. See the Educating the Patient feature Teaching Patients About Sexually Transmitted Infections for more information on this topic.

When assisting the licensed practitioner in treating a patient who has an STI, you will emphasize to the patient the importance of completing the course of therapy and avoiding sexual contact while the infection is still active. Sexual partners also must be treated to avoid reinfection. Several types of STIs are fairly common. Other types are very serious. Review the *Reproductive Systems* chapter and the *Microbiology and Disease* chapter to become familiar with these infections.

Teaching Patients About Sexually Transmitted Infections

You must provide complete and detailed information with a nonjudgmental and supportive attitude when you teach patients about STIs. Begin with the principle that all STIs are preventable. The key to prevention is avoiding sexual activities in which blood, semen, or vaginal secretions pass from one person to another. Although there are various levels of protection in connection with STIs, the only absolute methods of "safe sex" are abstinence (no sex) and masturbation (self-stimulation). The next level is mutual monogamy, in which partners have sex only with each other. Emphasize that monogamy provides protection from STIs only if neither partner has an STI when the relationship begins. A final level of prevention applies to people who do not practice abstinence or mutual monogamy but wish to protect themselves and others from STIs. The following measures provide some protection:

- Use a latex condom and spermicide for every act of intercourse. (Use a latex condom during vaginal, oral, or anal sex.)
- Use only water-based lubricants with latex condoms. (Oil- and petroleum-based lubricants can break down latex, causing the condom to tear or break.)
- Know all your sexual partners, and discuss STI prevention with them.
- Have a physician regularly screen you for STIs because many people, especially men, have no signs when they are infected.

- Consult a physician if any signs of STIs develop, such as a blister, sore, discharge, rash, or abdominal pain.

Encourage patients to ask questions and discuss any concerns they have. Explain the need to make follow-up appointments with a physician if appropriate. Teaching a patient who has been diagnosed with an STI how to treat or manage the disease is especially important. Make sure the patient understands all directions and the necessity for treatment. Bacterial infections such as chlamydia, gonorrhea, and syphilis can be cured with antibiotics as long as the patient takes all the medication in the prescribed manner. Viral infections such as AIDS, genital herpes, and genital warts cannot be cured, although they can be treated and managed to differing degrees.

Emphasize to patients with an STI that they should avoid all sexual contact until the infection has been treated completely. Many STIs can be spread through any type of genital contact, including vaginal intercourse, anal sex, and oral sex. Herpes can be spread through kissing if there are herpes sores in the mouth. Encourage patients to inform each person with whom they had sexual contact that they have contracted an STI. Explain that unless all sexual partners are treated successfully, the disease will pass back and forth indefinitely.

You can reinforce your education efforts by providing patients with materials on the prevention and treatment of STIs. Keep a variety of pamphlets, books, and other resources in your office to help patients cope with and manage STIs.

PROCEDURE 39-1 Assisting with a Gynecological Exam

Procedure Goal: To assist the licensed practitioner and maintain the client's comfort and privacy during a gynecological exam.

OSHA Guidelines:

Materials: Gown and drape; vaginal speculum; specimen collection equipment, including cervical brush, cervical broom, and/or scraper; cotton-tipped applicator; potassium hydroxide solution (KOH); exam gloves; tissues; laboratory requisition; water-soluble lubricant; examining table with stirrups; exam light; microscopic slide(s); thin-layer collection vial (or slides if used); tissues; spray fixative; pen; and pencil.

Method: Procedure steps.

1. Gather equipment and make sure all items are in working order. Correctly label the slide and/or the collection vials.
   RATIONALE: Slides or vials should be properly labeled to avoid confusing one patient's sample with another's.

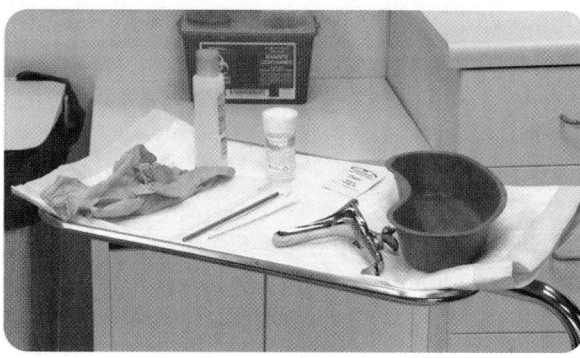

FIGURE Procedure 39-1 Step 1 Gather the necessary equipment.

FIGURE Procedure 39-1 Step 1   Label the vial and/or slide for the specimen that will be obtained.

2. Identify the patient and explain the procedure. The patient should remove all clothing, including underwear, and put the gown on with the opening in the front.

FIGURE Procedure 39-1 Step 2   Have the patient remove all clothing and put on the gown with the opening in the front.

3. Ask the patient to sit on the edge of the examining table with the drape until the licensed practitioner arrives.

4. When the licensed practitioner is ready, have the patient place her feet into the stirrups and move her buttocks to the edge of the table. This is the lithotomy position.
RATIONALE: Putting the patient in the lithotomy position too early can cause the patient to experience back and leg cramps.

5. Provide the licensed practitioner with gloves and an exam lamp as she examines the genitalia by inspection and palpation. Put on gloves per standard precautions guidelines.

6. Pass the speculum to the licensed practitioner. To increase patient comfort, you may place it in warm water before handing it to the licensed practitioner. Lubricant is not typically recommended prior to the Pap smear because it may interfere with the test results.

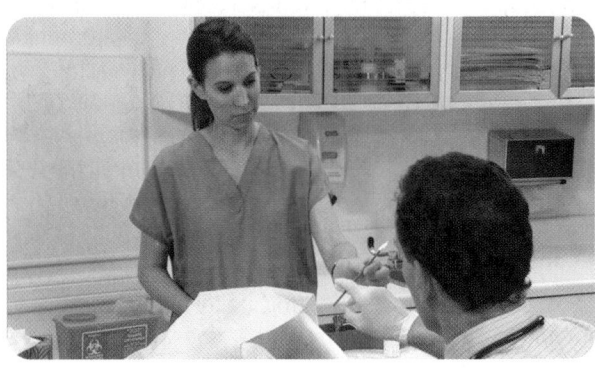

(a)

FIGURE Procedure 39-1 Step 6   Hand the speculum to the practitioner when needed.

(b)

FIGURE Procedure 39-1 Step 6   A speculum is used to view the internal structures during a gynecological exam.

7. For the Pap (Papanicolaou) smear, be prepared to pass a cotton-tipped applicator and cervical brush, broom, or scraper for the collection of the specimens. Have the labeled slide or vial available for the licensed practitioner to place the specimen on the slide. Depending on the licensed practitioner, the specimen collected, the method of collection, and the method of preparation, two or more slides or collection vials may be necessary. They may be labeled based on where the specimen was collected: endocervical (E), vaginal (V), and cervical (C).

8. Once the specimen is on the slide, a cytology fixative must be applied immediately. A spray fixative is common and should be held 6 inches from the slide and sprayed lightly with a back and forth motion. Allow the slide to dry completely.

RATIONALE: The fixative holds the cells in place until a microscopic exam is performed.

Cells collected for thin-layer preparation should be washed into the collection vial and transported to an outside lab for processing and analysis.

9. After the licensed practitioner removes the speculum, a digital exam is performed to check the position of the internal organs. Provide the licensed practitioner with additional lubricant as needed.

10. Upon completion of the exam, help the patient switch from the lithotomy position to a supine or sitting position.

11. Provide tissues or moist wipes for the patient to remove the lubricant and ask the patient to get dressed. Assist as necessary or provide for privacy. Explain the procedure for communicating the laboratory results.

12. After the patient has left, don gloves and clean the exam room and equipment. Dispose of the disposable speculum, specimen collection devices, and other contaminated waste in a biohazardous waste container.

13. Store the supplies, straighten the room, and discard the used exam paper on the table.

14. Prepare the requisition slip and place the specimen and requisition slip in the proper place for transport to an outside laboratory.

15. Remove your gloves and wash your hands.

16. Document the specimen and complete the laboratory log if needed.

Example Documentation:

> PAP smear specimen labeled and sent to MedLAB lab. _____
>
> _____ *K Haddix RMA (AMT)*

PROCEDURE 39-2 Assisting during the Exam of a Pregnant Patient

Procedure Goal: To assist the licensed practitioner and meet the special needs of the pregnant woman during the general physical exam.

OSHA Guidelines:

Materials: Patient education materials, examining table, exam gown, drape.

Method: Procedure steps.

Providing Patient Information

1. Identify the patient and introduce yourself.

2. Assess the patient's need for education by asking appropriate questions and having the patient describe what she already knows about the information you are providing.

3. Provide any appropriate instructions or materials.

4. Ask the patient whether she has any special concerns or questions about her pregnancy that she might want to discuss with the licensed practitioner.

5. Communicate the patient's concerns or questions to the licensed practitioner; include all pertinent background information on the patient.
   RATIONALE: Maintains your scope of practice and ensures that the patient receives correct information.

Ensuring Comfort during the Exam

6. Identify the patient and introduce yourself.

7. Wash your hands.

8. Explain the procedure to the patient.

9. Provide a gown or drape and instruct the patient in the proper way to wear it after disrobing. (Allow the patient privacy while disrobing and assist only if she requests help.)

10. Assist the patient onto the examining table. Ask the patient to step on either the stool or the pullout step of the examining table.
    RATIONALE: Pregnant women may need assistance during the later stages of pregnancy.

11. Help the patient into the position requested by the licensed practitioner, observing the patient for any difficulties she may have in achieving the requested position.

12. Provide and adjust additional drapes as needed.

13. Minimize the time the patient must spend in uncomfortable positions by making sure that the licensed practitioner has all supplies and equipment for the exam before it begins.

14. If the patient appears to be uncomfortable during the procedure, ask whether she would like to reposition herself or take a break; assist as necessary.

15. To prevent pelvic pooling of blood and subsequent dizziness or hyperventilation, allow the patient time to adjust to sitting before standing after she has been lying on the examining table. Assist the patient off the exam table if needed.

PROCEDURE 39-3 Assisting with a Cervical Biopsy

Procedure Goal: To assist the physician in obtaining a sample of cervical tissue for analysis.

OSHA Guidelines:

Materials: Gown and drape, tray or Mayo stand, disposable cervical biopsy kit (disposable forceps, curette, and spatula in a sterile pack), transfer forceps, vaginal speculum, biopsy specimen container, clean basin, sterile cotton balls, sterile gauze squares, sanitary napkin.

Method: Procedure steps.

1. Identify the patient and introduce yourself.

2. Look at the patient's chart and ask the patient to confirm information or explain any changes. Specific patient information you need to ask about and note in the chart includes the following:
   - Date of birth and Social Security number (verify that you have the correct chart for the correct patient).
   - Date of last menstrual period.
   - Method of contraception, if any.
   - Previous gynecologic surgery.
   - Use of hormone replacement therapy or other steroids.

3. If within your scope of practice, describe the biopsy procedure to the patient, noting that a piece of tissue will be removed to diagnose the cause of her problem. Explain that it may be painful but only for the brief moment during which tissue is taken.

4. Give the patient a gown, if needed, and a drape. Direct her to undress from the waist down and to wrap the drape around herself. Tell her to sit at the end of the examining table.

5. Wash your hands and put on exam gloves.

6. Using sterile method, open the sterile pack to create a sterile field on the tray or Mayo stand and arrange the instruments with transfer forceps. Add the vaginal speculum and sterile supplies to the sterile field.
   RATIONALE: The instruments and supplies must stay sterile because this is an invasive procedure.

7. When the physician arrives in the exam room, ask the patient to lie back, place her heels in the stirrups of the table, and move her buttocks to the edge of the table.
   RATIONALE: Placing the patient in the lithotomy position too early can cause the patient's back and legs to cramp.

8. Assist the physician by arranging the drape so that only the genitalia are exposed, and place the light so that the genitalia are illuminated.

9. Use transfer forceps to hand instruments and supplies to the physician as he requests them. You may don sterile gloves and hand the physician supplies and instruments directly.

10. When the licensed practitioner is ready to obtain the biopsy, tell the patient that it may hurt. If she seems particularly fearful, instruct her to take a deep breath and let it out slowly.

11. When the physician hands you the instrument with the tissue specimen, place the specimen in the specimen container and discard the instrument in the appropriate container.

12. Label the specimen container with the patient's name, the date and time, cervical or endocervical (as indicated by the physician), the physician's name, and your initials.

13. Place the container and the cytology laboratory requisition form in the envelope or bag provided by the laboratory.

14. When the physician has completed the procedure and removed the speculum, properly clean instruments as needed and dispose of used supplies and disposable instruments. Metal speculums, if used, should be placed in a clean basin for later sanitization, disinfection, and sterilization.

15. Remove the gloves and wash your hands.

16. Tell the patient that she may get dressed. Inform her that she may have some vaginal bleeding for a couple of days, and provide her with a sanitary napkin. Instruct her not to take tub baths or have intercourse and not to use tampons for 2 days. Encourage her to call the office if she experiences problems or has questions.

17. Document the procedure as appropriate.
    Example documentation:

Cervical specimen labeled and sent to MedLAB lab. _____
_____ *Kaylyn R. Haddix RMA (AMT)*

LEARNING OUTCOMES	KEY POINTS
39.1 **Carry out the role of the medical assistant in the medical specialty of gynecology.**	Medical assistants assist with gynecological exams, provide patient teaching for OB/GYN and breast health issues, and must handle cervical and other specimens correctly.
39.2 **Carry out the role of the medical assistant in the medical specialty of obstetrics.**	Medical assistants assist with examinations for pregnant females, providing for their needs, and provide education for the pregnant patient and new mother.
39.3 **Identify diagnostic and therapeutic procedures performed in obstetrics and gynecology.**	Diagnostic and therapeutic procedures performed in OB/GYN include pregnancy tests, tests for STIs, radiologic tests such as mammograms, fetal screening, Pap smears, D&C, and fine-needle aspiration.
39.4 **Relate the role of medical assisting to the medical specialty of urology.**	Medical assistants assist with urological exams and diagnostic tests. Patient education for urologic patients regarding TSE and other information is also the duty of a medical assistant working in urology.
39.5 **Identify diagnostic tests and procedures performed in urology.**	Various urologic diagnostic tests and procedures are performed, including semen analysis, cystometry, cystoscopy, and testicular biopsy.
39.6 **Recognize diseases and disorders of the reproductive and urinary systems.**	Diseases and disorders of the reproductive and urinary systems are listed for review in Table 39-4, Common Obstetric and Gynecologic Diseases and Disorders, and Table 39-5, Common Urologic Diseases and Disorders.

C A S E   S T U D Y   C R I T I C A L   T H I N K I N G

Recall Raja from the beginning of the chapter. Now that you have read the chapter, answer the following questions regarding her case.

1. How often should Raja have a pelvic exam, cervical cytology, HIV screen, and mammogram?

2. What should have been discussed with Raja before she had the mammogram?

3. How is stereotactic fine-needle biopsy performed?

1. (LO 39.2) A pregnant patient, Molly Holiday, has started feeling the movement of her baby. What is her current stage of pregnancy?
   a. 1st trimester
   b. Menarche
   c. 3rd trimester
   d. 2nd trimester
   e. 4th trimester

2. (LO 39.4) A TSE is
   a. Surgery that involves bypassing a blockage in the heart
   b. An imaging procedure that uses magnets and radio waves
   c. An examination of the testicles by the patient
   d. Scanning of the blood flow and metabolic activity in the brain
   e. An examination of the testicles by the physician

3. (LO 39.2) A pregnant patient is monitoring her blood glucose level with a glucometer. She most likely has
   a. Type II diabetes
   b. Type I diabetes
   c. Gestational diabetes
   d. Hyperthyroidism
   e. Diabetes mellitus

4. (LO 39.1) Which of the following indicates the LMP?
   a. The last day of the last menstrual period
   b. The first day of the last menstrual period
   c. A late menstrual period
   d. A likely menopausal pregnancy
   e. The heaviest flow day of the last menstrual period

5. (LO 39.1) A speculum is used to
   a. Evaluate for a DVT
   b. Evaluate the LMP
   c. Perform a basic physical exam
   d. Perform a vaginal exam
   e. Examine the breasts

6. (LO 39.3) Which of the following patients would most likely have an alpha fetoprotein test?
   a. 28-year-old male patient with urinary frequency and urgency
   b. 36-year-old female in her third trimester of pregnancy
   c. 27-year-old female with vaginal discharge
   d. 54-year-old female with urinary incontinence
   e. 35-year-old female in her 2nd trimester of pregnancy

7. (LO 39.5) Which of the following diagnostic tests would *least* likely be performed on a male urologic patient?
   a. Colposcopy
   b. Testicular biopsy
   c. Semen analysis
   d. Urinalysis
   e. Cystoscopy

8. (LO 39.1) At what age should most women start having yearly mammograms, according to the American Cancer Society and National Cancer Institute?
   a. 20
   b. 30
   c. 40
   d. 50
   e. 65

9. (LO 39.6) Your 27-year-old female patient has a menstrual disturbance. Which of the following does she *least* likely have?
   a. Amenorrhea
   b. Menorrhea
   c. Dysmenorrhea
   d. Metrorrhagia
   e. Menorrhagia

10. (LO 39.6) Your male patient has an infection that is not an STI. Which of the following is most likely the problem?
    a. Hydrocele
    b. Vaginitis
    c. Epididymitis
    d. Gonorrhea
    e. Prostatic hypertrophy

Assisting in Pediatrics

PATIENT INFORMATION

Patient Name	Gender	DOB
Chris Matthews	M	11/19/20XX

Attending	MRN	Allergies
Alexis N. Whalen, MD	324-95-786	NKA

Chris Matthews is an 8-year-old male patient whose mother states he has had diarrhea for 3 days. He kept her up all night last night going to the bathroom at least three times. He says his stomach hurts but has not vomited although is eating very little. While you are preparing to weigh the patient, he initially does not want to get on the scale and begins to cry. After his mother has persuaded him to get on the scale and you have obtained all the measurements and vital signs, you check his immunization record. While doing so, you see a note on Chris's chart indicating he is home-schooled and his parents are against immunizations.

Keep Chris in mind as you study this chapter. There will be questions at the end of the chapter based on the case study. The information in the chapter will help you answer these questions.

McGraw Hill ACTIVSim™

L E A R N I N G   O U T C O M E S

After completing Chapter 40, you will be able to:

40.1 Relate growth and development to pediatric patient care.

40.2 Identify the role of the medical assistant during pediatric examinations.

40.3 Discuss pediatric immunizations and the role of the medical assistant.

40.4 Explain variations of pediatric screening procedures and diagnostic tests.

40.5 Describe common pediatric diseases and disorders and their treatment.

40.6 Recognize special health concerns of pediatric patients.

K E Y   T E R M S

addiction	immunizations
bilirubin	jaundice
contraindications	menarche
enuresis	puberty
fontanels	substance abuse

I. C (9)   Describe implications for treatment related to pathology

I. C (10) Compare body structure and function of the human body across the life span

I. P (1)   Obtain vital signs

I. P (6)   Perform patient screening using established protocols

I. P (10) Assist physician with patient care

I. A (1)   Apply critical thinking skills in performing patient assessment and care

I. A (2)   Use language/verbal skills that enable patients' understanding

II. P (3) Maintain growth charts

IV. P (6) Prepare a patient for procedures and/or treatments

IV. P (8) Document patient care

IV. A (10) Demonstrate respect for individual diversity, incorporating awareness of one's own biases in areas including gender, race, religion, age, and economic status

IX. P (7) Document accurately in the patient record

2. **Anatomy and Physiology**
   Graduates:
   b. Identify and apply the knowledge of all body systems, their structure and functions, and their common diseases, symptoms, and etiologies
   c. Assist the physician with the regimen of diagnostic and treatment modalities as they relate to each body system

3. **Medical Terminology**
   Graduates:
   c. Understand the various medical terminology for each specialty

4. **Medical Law and Ethics**
   Graduates:
   a. Document accurately
   f. Comply with federal, state, and local health laws and regulations

5. **Psychology of Human Relations**
   Graduates:
   a. Define and understand abnormal behavior patterns
   b. Identify and respond appropriately when working/caring for patients with special needs
   e. Advocate on behalf of family/patients, having ability to deal and communicate with family
   f. Identify and discuss developmental stages of life
   g. Analyze the effect of hereditary, cultural, and environmental influences

8. **Medical Office Business Procedures/Management**
   Graduates:
   cc. Communicate on the recipient's level of comprehension
   ii. Recognize and respond to verbal and non-verbal communication
   kk. Adapt to individualized needs

9. **Medical Office Clinical Procedures**
   Graduates:
   c. Take vital signs
   d. Recognize and understand various treatment protocols
   g. Maintain medication and immunization records
   j. Prepare and administer oral and parenteral medications as directed by physician
   l. Prepare patient for examinations and treatments
   m. Assist physician with routine and specialty examinations and treatments
   p. Advise patients of office policies and procedures
   q. Instruct patients with special needs

Introduction

Pediatrics is a specialty area of medicine that involves the care of children up to the age of 18, and in some cases 21. To be a good pediatric medical assistant, you must first like children of all ages. If you do, you will be better able to relate to them and to communicate with them effectively. The pediatrician specializes in the healthcare of children, monitoring their development and diagnosing and treating their illnesses. Just as with other specialty fields, there are subspecialties of pediatrics, such as surgery and oncology.

As a medical assistant working in pediatrics, your primary areas of responsibility include parent or caregiver education, adherence to immunization schedules, and recognition of special health concerns. You also will assist with the pediatric patient's physical exam and treatment. Relating to the child, as well as being a liaison between the parent or caregiver and the physician, is essential to your job.

Developmental Stages and Care   LO 40.1

Different periods of childhood present different changes and challenges. This chapter focuses on the life stages from birth through the teenage years. Understanding the child's stages of growth and development will improve your skills as a medical assistant. During each stage of growth, the following developmental milestones occur:

- Physical development is the actual bodily changes that occur.
- Intellectual-cognitive development refers to the thinking skills the child is developing.
- Psycho-emotional development refers to the changes in feelings experienced during a particular period.
- Social development is the way a person relates to others.

The stages of growth and development for pediatric patients include neonate, infant, toddler, preschooler, elementary school child, middle school child, and adolescent. As you explore each stage, you will also review the related aspects of care to help you provide the necessary care and patient education.

Neonate

An infant is called a *neonate* from birth to one month of age. Many changes take place in this short time.

Physical Development The full-term infant usually weighs between 7 and 9 pounds and is 18 to 22 inches in length. The newborn infant's head seems large in comparison to the rest of her body. No wonder—the head is usually one-fourth of the infant's entire length! An adult head is usually only about one-ninth of the body length. An infant's head has two soft spots, or **fontanels**, which are tough cartilage (Figure 40-1). The anterior, or front, fontanel is diamond-shaped. The baby's pulse can sometimes be seen here. The infant can move her head from side to side. However, because the neck muscles are not strong enough to hold the head up, the person holding the infant must provide support.

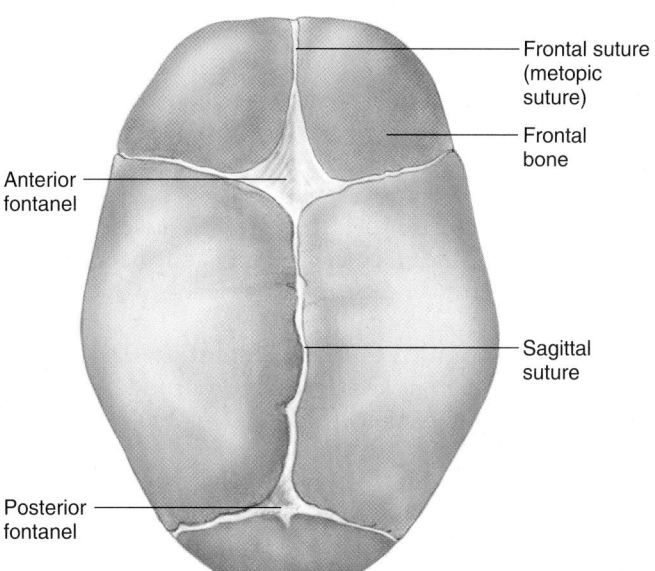

FIGURE 40-1   Be aware of the newborn's fontanels or "soft spots." These areas are open at birth so that the brain can grow. They close as the infant ages.

The newborn baby's skin is usually loose, wrinkled, and somewhat red in appearance. During the first week of life, this skin may start to peel. This is not harmful, and nothing needs to be done about it. The part of the umbilical cord still attached to the baby's body is a "stump" about 1 to 1½ inches in length. At birth it has a white, waxy appearance, then turns darker and usually falls off around the tenth day of life (Figure 40-2).

Sometimes infants develop neonatal **jaundice**—a yellowish color of the skin—in the first few days of life. This is caused by an accumulation of **bilirubin**, the waste product from the normal breakdown of the red blood cells. Babies have large numbers of red blood cells at birth. Their immature liver is unable to handle the breakdown of these cells. The waste product accumulates, giving the skin a yellowish tint. The whites of the

FIGURE 40-2   The umbilical cord usually falls off when the baby is about 10 days old.

eyes also may appear yellow, and the urine and feces may have a dark yellow color.

Certain reflexes can be observed in the newborn. Some are protective. For example, blinking is a reflex that protects the eyes. Everyone, including newborns, has this reflex. Other reflexes are due to the infant's immature nervous system. The physician will check reflexes as part of an examination. Infants can see objects within eight inches of their eyes. They probably detect brightness rather than color. Their eyes tend to turn outward or may even cross. Infants seem to prefer high-pitched tones.

Intellectual-Cognitive Development Newborns will become calm when picked up and held firmly. They tune out disturbing stimulation by sleeping.

Social Development Early on, infants respond to stimulation and establish an individual activity pattern. Generally, an infant responds to a soft, gentle voice and tries to focus on the voice and face. Newborns can show excitement and distress.

Aspects of Care: Neonate Consider the following when caring for neonates or providing parent or caregiver education.

- Sponge baths with tepid water and limited amounts of mild infant cleansing soap are given until the cord has fallen off. The infant's face should be washed with tepid water. No oil should be rubbed on the baby. Lotions and powders also should be avoided.

- If an infant is to be breast-fed, parents are given instruction about frequency of feedings, duration of feedings, and care of the mother and her breasts while breast-feeding. If an infant is to be bottle-fed, parents must be given instruction about the type of formula and how to prepare it correctly. Parents also should be taught about bowel movements and spitting up.

- The treatment for jaundice in the newborn is keeping the infant well hydrated with breast milk or formula. If necessary, the infant is placed under ultraviolet light, making sure that the infant's eyes are protected. Some neonates may need to use a bili-blanket, which is a special type of phototherapy device that helps the infant eliminate the bilirubin, thus improving the jaundice (Figure 40-3). Blood tests will be performed fairly often to ensure that the bilirubin level does not become dangerously high.

The Infant: One Month to One Year

Many changes occur in an infant during the first year. Parents cherish the wonder of their growing, developing child during this period.

Physical Development Growth is rapid during the first year of life. Infants triple their birth weight by their first birthday. They develop in a cephalocaudal fashion with the earliest development starting at the head and moving down. Infants first gain control of the head, neck, and shoulders,

FIGURE 40-3   A newborn with excessive bilirubin may be sent home with an ultraviolet light bili-blanket to help reduce the jaundice.

and then the arms, torso, and legs. This is why an infant finds and uses his hands before he finds and uses his feet. Larger groups of muscles develop before the smaller groups of muscles develop. The nervous system develops rapidly. Changes are seen in reflexes and in the development of coordinated movement and eye-hand coordination. The following is a brief look at some specific types of physical development in infants.

- By about three weeks of age, infants can focus on objects.

- By about four weeks, infants can follow an object with their eyes and make eye-to-eye contact. The infant can lift his head when lying on his abdomen.

- At two months, infants can follow objects with their eyes from one side to the other, listen to sounds, bat at objects, and respond to sounds. At this age, the infant may string together vowel sounds.

- By three months, an infant may raise the head and shoulders while on the abdomen and may hold up the head (Figure 40-4). When the infant is pulled to a sitting position, the head remains in line with the backbone.

- By four months, the infant may roll from stomach to back and may begin to play with a rattle placed in the hand. Teething may begin at this time.

- By five months, the infant may transfer a rattle from one hand to the other.

- At six months, the infant rolls from back to stomach, may be able to sit up briefly, and can reach to retrieve a dropped object. The two bottom front teeth have probably erupted, or emerged, from the gums.

- At nine months, the infant is able to sit and to creep on hands and knees. The infant is beginning to use the pincer grasp. The infant can put consonants with vowels and make repetitive sounds such as "mama" and "dada."

- At 12 months, the child can hold onto a piece of furniture and move around it, perhaps taking a step or two. With tooth development and the pincer grasp, the infant can pick up and eat small pieces of food.

FIGURE 40-4 A three-month-old infant should be able to hold up her head when lying on her stomach.

Intellectual-Cognitive Development At one month of age, an infant can make contact. This progresses to recognition of familiar faces and then to "making faces" at four to five months. At around six months of age, the child is making babbling sounds and by nine months is able to play games like peek-a-boo. The infant begins to understand cause and effect. If the infant drops a toy and someone retrieves it, the infant will drop it again. This becomes a game. At 12 months, an infant can follow simple directions.

Psycho-emotional Development By the time a child is one month old, he or she can smile at another smiling face. By three months, the infant smiles spontaneously and displays pleasure in making sounds. At four months, the infant can vocalize a mood. At six months, there may be abrupt mood changes. At nine months, the infant displays pleasure in playing simple games, and by one year has learned to express many emotions. For infants to develop physically and emotionally, it is important that their physical needs be addressed quickly and calmly. Physical contact and cuddling are ways to help infants develop a sense of security and trust.

Social Development Infants become social beings very quickly. By one month of age, infants are able to smile. At three months, the infant responds to voices. This can be seen when the infant pays attention and coos along with a person speaking in a quiet and gentle manner. At six months, the baby "babbles" and is interested in his or her own voice. Imitative play becomes an important part of the infant's interaction with others. At nine months, the first development of words can be observed. This leads to increased interaction with family and others.

Aspects of Care: One Month to One Year Consider the following when caring for infants or providing parent or caregiver education.

- Regular health checkups and immunizations should be followed. Immunizations will be discussed later in this chapter.

- Infants need tactile stimulation for growth and development. Physical contact and cuddling, as well as prompt attention to their needs, help infants develop a sense of security and trust, which is necessary for them to thrive.

- In the first six months, the mother's breast milk or infant formula meets the growing infant's needs. The physician, with your assistance, will provide guidance about the introduction of solid foods to the diet.

- Ensure infant safety. See the Educating the Patient feature Keeping Infants and Toddlers Safe.

The Toddler: One to Three Years

Children from the age of one to three years need constant attention from parents and others. Although they grow less rapidly during this period, their growth is still fast, and their communication skills begin to take shape in their use of language.

Physical Development Weight gain slows between one and two years. The arms and legs grow more than the trunk and head, and now seem to be in proportion to the child's overall size. Girls usually reach half of their adult height between 1½ and 2 years of age; boys reach half of their expected adult height between 2 and 2½ years. Growth charts, as shown in Figure 40-5, are used to determine a child's growth in relation to average rates. Procedure 40-2, Maintaining Growth Charts, at the end of this chapter provides more information about how to record height, weight, and head circumference on a growth chart.

Most toddlers will walk independently by 15 months of age. At 18 months, a toddler can squat to reach for a toy, kneel and remain upright, and precisely perform the pincer grasp. The toddler may use a spoon for self-feeding. By two years of age, the child can run, throw a ball, and scribble with a pencil. The child may want to feed herself or himself. At three years, the child is very active. Children of this age can dress themselves, ride a tricycle, throw a ball, draw simple shapes, and use a pair of child's scissors. Many children are toilet-trained between two and three years of age.

Intellectual-Cognitive Development During the toddler years, the child begins to learn about the world through play. Children enjoy imitating sweeping, raking, and making things they have seen adults make. A major task for the toddler is to develop independence. Toddlers are curious about their world and their play may involve experimenting.

The toddler progresses with speech in the following ways:

- Speaks a few single words at 12 to 15 months.
- Makes sentences containing 6 to 20 words at two years.
- Repeats nursery rhymes at three years.

At 15 months, the child enjoys looking at books. Between two and three years of age, the toddler seems to be constantly asking, "Why?" By three years of age, the child may participate

FIGURE 40-5 The curved lines on these growth charts are used to chart the growth for boys from birth to age 36 months. The child's length, height, and head circumference are measured and recorded, then plotted on this graph to show progress.

in the retelling of familiar stories and can draw and recognize simple shapes. During the toddler years, the child also enjoys playing with blocks.

Psycho-emotional Development At one year of age, children are able to express many emotions. As children move from one year to three years, they gain some control over ways of expressing their feelings. Temper tantrums may become a problem between 18 months and 2 to 2½ years of age. A child of 15 months may respond to "No," but by the time the toddler approaches 18 to 21 months, he or she is resisting authority and is the one who is saying "No!" Children of this age need consistent limits. If the child learns that a certain behavior will gain nothing, the behavior will stop fairly soon. As toddlers approach three years of age, they become sensitive to the feelings of others and may be characterized as affectionate.

Social Development Between one and two years, the toddler is unlikely to be able to truly play with another child. Play may involve taking toys from another child rather than

sharing. Between two and three years, children become able to share and play with others. Adult guidance is necessary for the toddler to develop an awareness of what is appropriate when playing with other children.

Aspects of Care: One to Three Years Consider the following when caring for toddlers or providing parent or caregiver education. Safety is of utmost importance. During the toddler years, it is very important to allow a child to increase independence in a safe environment.

- Toddlers need opportunities to work on their fine-motor skills, such as those used in writing with crayons.

- Toddlers are developing their language skills, so simple explanations provide a positive environment for development.

- Setting limits helps the child to develop boundaries in relationships and behavior. At the same time, the environment should not be one in which the child is constantly told, "No."

- Safety is of utmost importance with a toddler. See the Educating the Patient feature Keeping Infants and Toddlers Safe.

Keeping Infants and Toddlers Safe

Teaching the parents or caregivers of infants and children about safety may be the responsibility of the medical assistant. Use the following points when teaching parents or caregivers:

- Keep emergency phone numbers close to the phone for family and sitter.
- Make sure the crib meets federal safety standards.
- Never hold the infant or toddler on your lap in a car. Use an approved car seat placed in the back of the vehicle. Use the current recommendations for forward-facing or rear-facing infant car seats. (See Figure 40-6.)
- Never leave the child unattended in the car.
- Do not put pillows, comforters, or plush toys in the infant's crib.
- Prevent falls. Place the baby on a low surface and use correctly installed gates across stairs.
- Prevent choking. Check toys for small objects that might come loose. Be sure that clothing does not have cords around the neck.
- Do not leave hanging toys over the crib once the child begins to reach, pull, and roll over.
- Keep all cords on window blinds, lamps, and electrical equipment out of reach.
- Never leave a child unattended around, near, or in any kind of water, including the water in toilets, mop buckets, or pools.

FIGURE 40-6   Infants and toddlers should be in approved car seats. Check the Internet site of the American Academy of Pediatrics for proper type and size.

- Set the water temperature of the household hot water tank at 120°F. Turn pot handles inward, away from the edge of the stove, while cooking. Cover electrical outlets.
- Keep medicines and chemicals, including household cleaners, out of reach or in locked cabinets. Post the local poison control center's phone number in an accessible location.

The Preschooler: Three to Five Years

The child of three to five years is preparing to go out into the world.

Physical Development Individual differences, such as heredity, account for differences in height and weight among children between the ages of three and five years. During this time, it is best not to compare the preschooler's size to that of another preschooler. Each child's growth should be monitored and compared to the size documented on his or her on-going growth chart. Girls progress more rapidly toward their adult height and weight than do boys. The respiratory rate and the heart rate begin to slow down, coming closer to the adult range. Bones begin to ossify, or harden, between the ages of two and seven. During these years, it is important for children to be active in their play. They also need adequate calcium intake for the development of strong bones. Most children will have achieved nighttime bowel and bladder control by the time they are three or four years of age. If lack of bowel and/or bladder control persists beyond four or five years, this should be brought to the physician's attention.

During the three-to-five-year period, many skills are achieved, including going up and down stairs using an alternating step approach, riding a tricycle, skipping, hopping on one foot, and throwing a ball. Girls are usually about a year ahead of boys in small muscle coordination and fine-motor skills. A child of three can draw simple shapes and use a pencil to imitate the way an adult writes. At four, the child can draw a simple human figure and can cut with blunt scissors, though not well at this age. A child of five can reproduce some shapes, letters, and numbers. By the age of five, some children also may have learned how to tie their shoes.

Intellectual-Cognitive Development Language grows by leaps and bounds during these years. The imaginative child of three years has a vocabulary of about 900 words, forms simple sentences, and can tell simple stories that may be very "I"-oriented. At four years of age, the child's vocabulary is about 1600 words, sentences are complete, and the favorite question is "Why?" Parents need to give very simple answers such as, "Because it will keep you safe right now." The child's vocabulary at age five exceeds 2000 words, and the stories the child tells involve more detail. At this age, the child has learned the difference between telling stories and lying.

Psycho-emotional Development The three-year-old child is very easy and pleasant. Children of this age usually enjoy music. A child at this age has an increasing sense of self, but imagination may lead the child to have unfounded worries and fears, especially at night. At four years of age, negativity may increase. Parents hear more of the "Nos" that they heard when the child was two years old. The four-year-old child is testing limits and needs guided opportunities for freedom. Once a child reaches five years, life settles down a little. The child is more self-assured, well-adjusted, and home-centered. At this age, the child likes to follow the rules, may want to "play by the rules," and is capable of accepting some responsibility.

Social Development Three-year-old children know what gender they are. The child knows how to take turns and may enjoy brief activities in a group with other children. A three-year-old child likes to "help." Four-year-old children are very social and enjoy playing simple group games, like tag and hide-and-seek. At five years, the child continues to be very social, enjoys playing with other children, and likes games in which the "rules" are observed.

Aspects of Care: Three to Five Years Consider the following when caring for children from 3 to 5 years or providing parent or caregiver education.

- The child of five years should receive a complete preschool developmental assessment and physical that includes an evaluation of hearing and vision.
- Immunizations, discussed later, must be up to date when the child enters kindergarten.
- Children of about three years may have night terrors. Parents should discuss these with the pediatrician if they are severe or persistent.
- Children may use delaying tactics at bedtime and may need to be shown repeatedly that there is nothing in the closet or under the bed. A nightlight is useful.
- Nighttime routines are important in helping a child feel secure.

The Elementary School Child: Six to Ten Years

The following describes the stages of development of the six- to ten-year-old child.

Physical Development During childhood, girls may be taller and heavier than boys. Bones continue to ossify. Permanent teeth replace "baby teeth." Muscles continue to develop. Regular exercise is needed to encourage strength and coordination. At nine and ten years of age, the reproductive system also will be developing.

Intellectual-Cognitive Development Knowledge explosion happens once a child enters school. On entering school, the six-year-old child has a brief attention span. By ten years old, she or he is able to focus for longer periods of time. Most children of this age like to talk. As children move from five or six years of age toward nine and ten years, they are better able to separate fantasy from reality. They develop a sense of what is right and wrong, of honesty and fairness.

Psycho-emotional Development When children approach ten years of age, they may be more influenced by their peers than by their parents. During these years, children are beginning to develop a sense of self and also learn gender-related roles. Children of six to eight years of age may have trouble thinking about disasters that they hear about. As children approach ten years of age, they are better able to grasp concepts of time and distance. A nine- to ten-year-old child may want to do something to help others. School-age children may be very sensitive to criticism and to what they see as failure.

Social Development School is central to the life of a child between six and ten years of age. Although team sports and activities become important, parents need to avoid allowing the child to become overwhelmed with too many organized activities at this time. Children also need time to be quiet and alone. Outdoor activities help to use up some of the child's energy. Appropriate social behaviors are learned during this stage.

Aspects of Care: Six to Ten Years Consider the following when caring for six- to ten-year-olds or providing parent or caregiver education.

- Structure and a schedule help to maintain order and discipline.
- Monitor physical activities to prevent injury. The American Academy of Pediatrics advises against elementary-school-age children participating in contact sports.
- Consistency in daily activities and in discipline helps the child to develop intellectually, emotionally, and socially.
- Regular health and dental care and maintenance of immunizations are required.
- Communicable diseases are common.

The Middle School Child: 11 to 13 Years

The following sections will give you some insight into the stages of development of the 11- to 13-year-old child.

Physical Development In the United States and most Western cultures, the onset of puberty occurs in females at around 12 or 13 years of age, but some may experience changes as early as nine. **Puberty** refers to the physiological changes that make a person capable of sexual reproduction. By the time a girl reaches middle school, a significant occurrence may be the onset of menstruation. It is important for everyone to remember that even though her body may be maturing, she is still only between 9 and 12 years old. Males tend to go through the changes of puberty later than females (Figure 40-7). The average age for males to experience these changes is around 14 years. Hormonal changes may contribute to development of skin problems and acne.

Intellectual-Cognitive Development Grades may slip during this time. So much physical growth is taking place and so many physiological changes are occurring that less energy is available to concentrate on academics. Preadolescents may tend to exaggerate and "bend the truth."

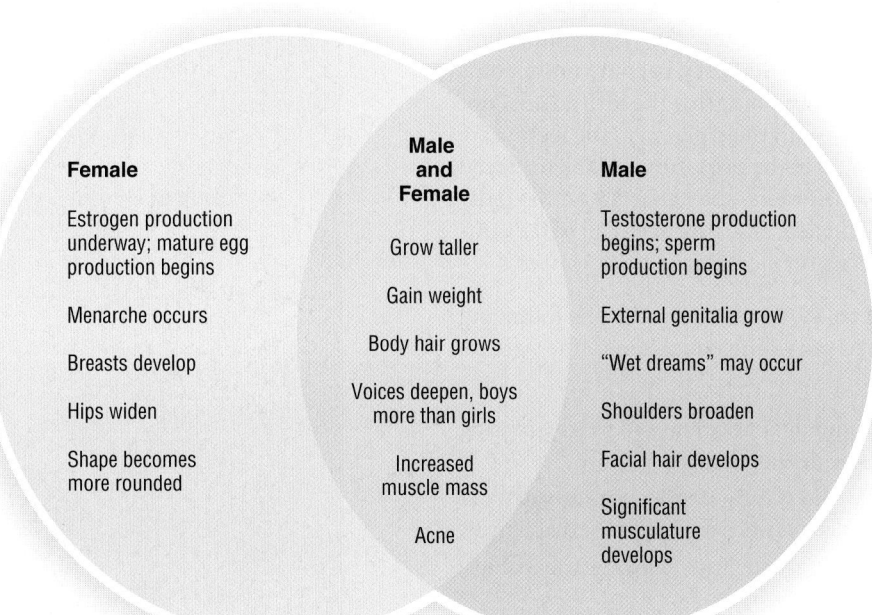

Female

Estrogen production underway; mature egg production begins

Menarche occurs

Breasts develop

Hips widen

Shape becomes more rounded

Male and Female

Grow taller

Gain weight

Body hair grows

Voices deepen, boys more than girls

Increased muscle mass

Acne

Male

Testosterone production begins; sperm production begins

External genitalia grow

"Wet dreams" may occur

Shoulders broaden

Facial hair develops

Significant musculature develops

FIGURE 40-7 Some changes during puberty are the same for males and females. Others are unique to one sex.

Psycho-emotional Development Although preadolescents crave independence, they are also very unsure of themselves. They are experiencing a wide range of physical changes and, at the same time, are learning the roles of sexuality. It is very important for preadolescents to receive accurate information about their changing bodies and feelings from appropriate and reliable sources. Middle-school-age students may not be comfortable asking parents questions about sexuality. Conflict may arise at this time. Parents may find that the preadolescent is easily annoyed and may be temperamental. Frequently, the preadolescent child will take on the behaviors of his or her peer group.

Social Development During the middle school years, children are learning about their own sexual identity and may not be comfortable in heterosexual relationships. Girls express an earlier interest in male-female relationships than do boys. Children of this age need to be able to turn to an adult with whom they are comfortable, so they can ask personal and intimate questions.

Aspects of Care: 11 to 13 Years Consider the following when caring for preadolescents or providing parent or caregiver education.

- A preadolescent needs to be assured that he or she is valued and loved.
- Consistency in discipline is very important.
- Parents should not be hypercritical or make too many demands.
- Friendships and associations should be monitored.
- Overscheduling of the child's time should be avoided.

The Adolescent: 14 to 19 Years

The teen years can be full of excitement for teenagers and their family and friends. They also can be difficult years. Tremendous physiological changes during this time may cause internal conflicts that can turn into external clashes. Parents may feel anxious about their child's quest for independence and about the child's upcoming departure from the home. The process of developing independence, a personal identity, and future plans is important during this stage.

Physical Development During the later teen years, females attain their adult height and weight. Males may continue to grow in height until 25 years of age. Physical growth and development in the teenage years are centered on normal sexual change. Girls usually have reached **menarche**, the onset of menstruation. Boys may have nocturnal emissions of seminal fluid (also called wet dreams). Weight control can be a concern. Some health problems of adulthood can be traced back to lifelong habits of poor dietary choices and lack of exercise begun in adolescence.

Intellectual-Cognitive Development During the early adolescent years, the child may have taken the word of an adult or a peer without question. Now, the teen asks questions and needs to work out answers that fit into his or her values. Adolescents often do not see the connection between behavior and consequences. This may lead to experimentation with drugs, alcohol, or sex.

Psycho-emotional Development An adolescent knows the socially acceptable and appropriate ways to express feelings, but the pressures felt by adolescents may result in angry outbursts. Anger that is directed inward can be harmful. Anxiety and sometimes depression are part of adolescence.

Social Development Friendships are very important to adolescents. As teens get older, they become more comfortable with their parents and outgrow the attitude of "not wanting to be seen dead" with their parents. The teen years are wonderful and difficult at the same time. Problems faced by teens include eating disorders, substance abuse, sexually transmitted infection, suicide, and violence. You will examine these special concerns further later in this chapter.

Aspects of Care: 14 to 19 Years Consider the following when caring for teens or providing education to the parents or caregiver.

- Teens need adequate amounts of calcium and weight-bearing exercise for strong bone development.
- Teens should know the risks of early, unplanned pregnancy and sexually transmitted infections when engaging in sexual activity.
- The adolescent needs to spend time enjoying friendships, sporting events, and social events.
- People who are caring for teens should
  - Listen.
  - Give them the facts.
  - Trust them.
  - Provide them with firm and friendly discipline.
  - Be consistent.
  - Educate them with their independence in mind.
  - Set limits and stick to them.
  - Set examples of good behavior and good taste.
  - Remember how it feels to be an adolescent.

▶ Pediatric Examinations

LO 40.2

Many of the exam procedures for a pediatric patient are the same as those for an adult. While you prepare the child or adolescent for the exam, you may discuss with the parent, caregiver, or child topics such as eating habits, sleep patterns, daily activities, immunization schedules, and toilet training. Discussions should be appropriate for the child's developmental stage. This discussion will provide important clues to possible abnormal physical, cognitive-intellectual, psycho-emotional, and social development. Additional discussion topics such as sexually transmitted infections, drugs, and alcohol may be appropriate for an adolescent. Point out potential problems to the doctor.

You can help relieve a child's fear by calmly explaining procedures before they occur, giving the reason for each procedure, and being cheerful and mindful of a child's feelings. Allowing a child to examine some of the blunt instruments may also lessen fear (Figure 40-8). If a patient is physically resistant to the exam, you may need to call for assistance from the doctor or caregiver, or the child may need to be restrained.

Try to speak in terms aimed at the child's age level and kneel if necessary to make eye contact with the child. Treat the child with respect and provide positive reinforcement when a child is cooperative. Avoid making light of crying or pain. Make a game out of some aspect of a procedure and provide a small token reward at the end of a visit. For infants, a gentle approach, such as talking quietly and holding them comfortably, is helpful.

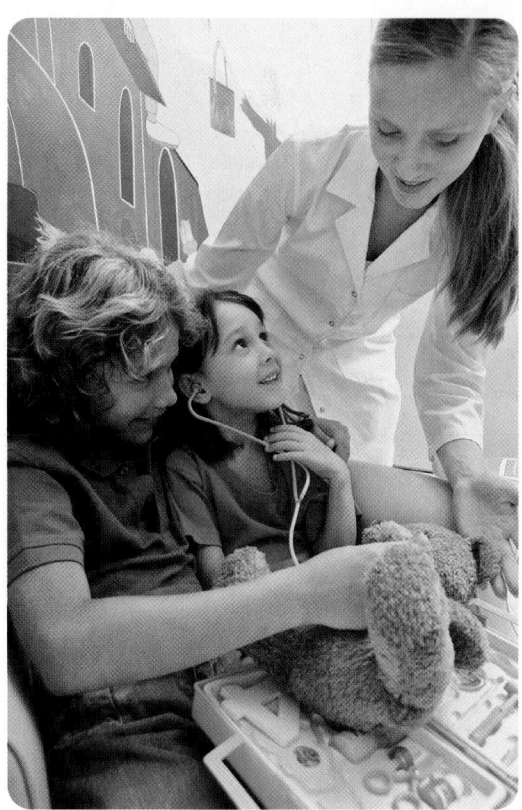

FIGURE 40-8 Providing a pediatric patient with a diversion may help lessen the child's fear.

Be mindful of adolescents' sensitivity toward rapid growth and physical, sexual, and social development when you prepare them for examination. Adolescents and preadolescents often feel awkward and self-conscious about being examined. They also may prefer to dress alone and to be alone with the doctor. Some children are afraid of going to the doctor's office.

Well-Child Examination

Parents should bring their infants and children to the pediatrician for regular checkups and growth monitoring. The American Academy of Pediatrics (AAP) recommends the following frequency:

- Infants need seven well-baby exams during their first year, at these intervals: 3 to 5 days, 1 month, 2 months, 4 months, 6 months, 9 months, and 1 year.
- Children in the second and third years of life should have checkups at 15, 18, 24, and 30 months.
- From the age of 3, children should have checkups every year.

The AAP has developed recommendations for these examinations. See Table 40-1 for a summary of the components of the well-child examination based on the age of the child.

Follow Standard Precautions and prepare for the physical exam the same way you would for an adult, except for draping and positioning. Ask the parent of an infant or toddler to remove all the child's clothing except the diaper. Then keep the child covered until the physician enters the exam room. An infant or toddler may be crying during the exam. To assist the physician in hearing chest sounds with a stethoscope, ask the parent to allow the infant to suck on a pacifier, if used, to quiet

POINTS ON PRACTICE

Assisting with an Exam for an Infant or Child

When assisting with an exam for an infant or child, you will need to take some special considerations. The techniques you use to prepare an infant or child emotionally and physically should be modified based on the patient's age and ability.

Emotional

Speak to infants and children calmly during the procedure and praise them when they are cooperative. Infants and toddlers are likely to be afraid of you because you are a stranger. Approach these children slowly, smile, and use a gentle voice. Children of preschool age are sometimes uncooperative and challenging. Remain calm, perform the procedures quickly, and restrain the child (with assistance from the parent) when appropriate. To prevent children from getting injured, watch them at all times.

Physical

Base your choice of an exam position for children on each child's age and ability to cooperate. Although young infants are usually examined on an examining table, older infants and toddlers may need to be examined while held on a parent's lap. Some toddlers may cooperate while standing on the examining table with a parent nearby. Preschool children can usually be placed on the examining table if a parent is nearby. Regardless of their position, watch children at all times to prevent injury. When examining young children, doctors typically perform percussion (tapping on the surface to hear the underlying structures) and auscultation (listening) first because children are more likely to be calm and quiet at the outset. Doctors always examine painful areas last. Doctors may examine older children's genitalia last because after a certain age, children tend to find such an exam embarrassing.

TABLE 40-1	Recommendations for Preventive Pediatric Healthcare*
Developmental Stage	**Components of the Examination**
Infancy (birth to 12 months)	History and physical
	Length/height and weight
	Head circumference
	Weight for length
	Immunizations
	Newborn metabolic/hemoglobin screening
	Developmental/behavioral assessments
Early Childhood (12 months to 4 years)	History and physical
	Length/height and weight
	Head circumference up to 24 months
	Body mass index starting at 24 months
	Weight for length up to 18 months
	Blood pressure and vision screening starting at 3 years
	Hearing starting at 4 years
	Immunizations
	Developmental/behavioral assessments
Middle Childhood (5 years to 10 years)	History and physical
	Length/height and weight
	Body mass index
	Blood pressure
	Vision and hearing screening
	Oral health at 6 years
	Immunizations
Adolescence (12 years to 21 years)	History and physical
	Length/height and weight
	Body mass index
	Blood pressure
	Vision and hearing screening
	Ages 18–21 dyslipidemia screening

*Adapted from the American Academy of Pediatrics, *Recommendations for Preventive Pediatric Health Care*, copyright 2008.

the crying. Feeding the child during the exam is not encouraged because stomach sounds interfere with clear auscultation (listening to body sounds with a stethoscope). Distracting infants and toddlers with mobiles, shiny surfaces, or toys may help the exam go more smoothly. Review the Points on Practice feature Assisting with an Exam for an Infant or Child for additional information about the pediatric exam.

▶ Pediatric Immunizations   LO 40.3

As discussed in the *Basic Safety and Infection Control* chapter, you should know that one of the necessary elements in the cycle of infection is the transmission of the pathogen to a susceptible host. To reduce the susceptibility of the host to infection, **immunizations** are given. An immunization is the administration of a vaccine or a toxoid (a weakened toxin) to protect susceptible individuals from infectious diseases. When a healthy patient is vaccinated with a weakened strain of a virus, the patient's lymphocytes manufacture antibodies against that virus. These antibodies remain in the body, making it immune to that virus in the future. Killed-virus vaccines, which are used to immunize against influenza, do not provide protection for as long a period as live-virus vaccines. Toxoids are used to produce active immunity against diseases such as tetanus and diphtheria.

Immunizations are usually given during regular check-ups (Figure 40-9). Immunizing children against diseases such as hepatitis B, diphtheria, tetanus, pertussis (whooping cough), poliomyelitis, measles, mumps, rubella (German measles), chickenpox, and *Haemophilus influenzae* type B (Hib) is recommended. Many vaccines have largely eliminated the threat of these once-prevalent, life-threatening diseases. The first vaccine, for hepatitis B, is given to a newborn the day after birth. Some vaccines require a series of doses to give immunity. Booster doses may be required for a particular vaccine at a later age. The Centers for Disease Control and Prevention (CDC) recommends that physicians take every reasonable opportunity to vaccinate a child, to ensure that the child receives the protection he needs.

FIGURE 40-9 Immunizations are part of routine well-child visits in a pediatric practice.

As a medical assistant, you will play a vital role in the immunization process. Your duties may include

- Scheduling appointments and follow-up visits at the appropriate time based on the immunization schedule.
- Educating parents about the benefits and risks of vaccines and obtaining informed consent.

- Administering the vaccine correctly.
- Keeping careful immunization records, including the vaccine type, the date of vaccination, and the vaccine lot number.
- Ensuring proper vaccine storage and handling, including checking the temperature of the refrigerator and freezer daily.

Immunization Recommendations

The Advisory Committee on Immunization Practices, the American Academy of Pediatrics, and the American Academy of Family Physicians jointly publish immunization schedules for children. When working in a pediatrician's office, you should be familiar with the current guidelines regarding these vaccination schedules because immunization guidelines change occasionally. New guidelines, methods, and vaccines are constantly being developed. See Figure 40-10 for the birth to age 6 and the ages 7–18 immunization schedules.

Informed Consent

The physician may ask you to explain the benefits and risks of an immunization to the parents. You will need to explain that the side effects of immunizations are usually mild, such as a slight fever or soreness, and of short duration. Review with the parent the vaccine information statement for the specific

| Recommended Immunization Schedule for Persons Aged 0 Through 6 Years—United States - 2011 | | | | | | | | | | | |
| For those who fall behind or start late, see the catch-up schedule | | | | | | | | | | | |
Vaccine / Age ▶	**Birth**	**1 month**	**2 months**	**4 months**	**6 months**	**12 months**	**15 months**	**18 months**	**19–23 months**	**2–3 years**	**4–6 years**
Hepatitis B[1]	HepB	HepB				HepB					
Rotavirus[2]			RV	RV	RV[2]						
Diphtheria, Tetanus, Pertussis[3]			DTaP	DTaP	DTaP	see footnote[3]	DTaP				DTaP
Haemophilus influenzae type b[4]			Hib	Hib	Hib[4]	Hib					
Pneumococcal[5]			PCV	PCV	PCV	PCV				PPSV	
Inactivated Poliovirus[6]			IPV	IPV		IPV					IPV
Influenza[7]						Influenza (Yearly)					
Measles, Mumps, Rubella[8]						MMR		see footnote[8]			MMR
Varicella[9]						Varicella		see footnote[9]			Varicella
Hepatitis A[10]						HepA (2 doses)				HepA Series	
Meningococcal[11]										MCV4	

(a)

| Recommended Immunization Schedule for Persons Aged 7 Through 18 Years—United States - 2011 | | | |
| For those who fall behind or start late, see the schedule below and catch-up schedule | | | |
Vaccine / Age ▶	**7–10 years**	**11–12 years**	**13–18 years**
Tetanus, Diphtheria, Pertussis[1]		Tdap	Tdap
Human Papillomavirus[2]	see footnote[2]	HPV (3 doses) (females)	HPV Series
Meningococcal[3]	MCV4	MCV4	MCV4
Influenza[4]		Influenza (Yearly)	
Pneumococcal[5]		Pneumococcal	
Hepatitis A[6]		HepA Series	
Hepatitis B[7]		HepB Series	
Inactivated Poliovirus[8]		IPV Series	
Measles, Mumps, Rubella[9]		MMR Series	
Varicella[10]		Varicella Series	

(b)

▢ Range of recommended ages for all children   ▢ Range of recommended ages for catch-up immunization   ▢ Range of recommended ages for certain high-risk groups

FIGURE 40-10 Recommended immunization schedules for (a) birth to age 6 and (b) ages 7 to 18. For more information, an updated schedule, or the catch-up schedule, check the Centers for Disease Control website at www.cdc.gov/vaccines.

DIPHTHERIA TETANUS & PERTUSSIS **VACCINES**

WHAT YOU NEED TO KNOW

Many Vaccine Information Statements are available in Spanish and other languages. See www.immunize.org/vis.

1. Why get vaccinated?

Diphtheria, tetanus, and pertussis are serious diseases caused by bacteria. Diphtheria and pertussis are spread from person to person. Tetanus enters the body through cuts or wounds.

DIPHTHERIA causes a thick covering in the back of the throat.
- It can lead to breathing problems, paralysis, heart failure, and even death.

TETANUS (Lockjaw) causes painful tightening of the muscles, usually all over the body.
- It can lead to "locking" of the jaw so the victim cannot open his mouth or swallow. Tetanus leads to death in up to 2 out of 10 cases.

PERTUSSIS (Whooping Cough) causes coughing spells so bad that it is hard for infants to eat, drink, or breathe. These spells can last for weeks.
- It can lead to pneumonia, seizures (jerking and staring spells), brain damage, and death.

Diphtheria, tetanus, and pertussis vaccine (DTaP) can help prevent these diseases. Most children who are vaccinated with DTaP will be protected throughout childhood. Many more children would get these diseases if we stopped vaccinating.

DTaP is a safer version of an older vaccine called DTP. DTP is no longer used in the United States.

2. Who should get DTaP vaccine and when?

Children should get 5 doses of DTaP vaccine, one dose at each of the following ages:
- 2 months
- 4 months
- 6 months
- 15–18 months
- 4–6 years

DTaP may be given at the same time as other vaccines.

3. Some children should not get DTaP vaccine or should wait

- Children with minor illnesses, such as a cold, may be vaccinated. But children who are moderately or severely ill should usually wait until they recover before getting DTaP vaccine.

- Any child who had a life-threatening allergic reaction after a dose of DTaP should not get another dose.

- Any child who suffered a brain or nervous system disease within 7 days after a dose of DTaP should not get another dose.

- Talk with your doctor if your child:
  - had a seizure or collapsed after a dose of DTaP,
  - cried non-stop for 3 hours or more after a dose of DTaP,
  - had a fever over 105°F after a dose of DTaP.

Ask your health care provider for more information. Some of these children should not get another dose of pertussis vaccine, but may get a vaccine without pertussis, called **DT**.

4. Older children and adults

DTaP is not licensed for adolescents, adults, or children 7 years of age and older.

But older people still need protection. A vaccine called **Tdap** is similar to DTaP. A single dose of Tdap is recommended for people 11 through 64 years of age. Another vaccine, called **Td**, protects against tetanus and diphtheria, but not pertussis. It is recommended every 10 years. There are separate Vaccine Information Statements for these vaccines.

| Diphtheria/Tetanus/Pertussis | 5/17/2007 |

FIGURE 40-11 Review the vaccine information sheet with the parent and obtain a signature before administering a vaccine.

immunization you will be administering (Figure 40-11). Advise parents that the benefits of immunity greatly outweigh the risks. Then obtain informed consent for the child's immunization. Provide a copy of the vaccine information statement and then have the parent sign so the immunization can be given. Remember that religious or other personal beliefs may prohibit parents from consenting to immunizations for their child. Some parents may want to delay or slow down the number of immunizations given at one time. Give immunizations as ordered and record all appropriate information in the patient's chart.

Administering Immunizations

In many states, medical assistants may administer immunizations. Most immunizations are given as injections. You might be required to give more than two vaccinations in a single visit. Careful site selection is important when giving multiple injections. Refer to the *Medication Administration* chapter for information about administering various types of injections and selecting an appropriate injection site. Some vaccines, such as live polio, are given orally. Most vaccinations may be administered even if the child has a mild illness. The physician will make the decision to vaccinate a child who is ill based on the disease and the severity of the symptoms. For the most part, if a child has a fever, the physician may postpone the immunization until the fever has subsided. However, do not postpone the visit if the child has an upper respiratory infection without a fever. Remember that the child does not need to restart a series of immunizations. He can simply receive the next scheduled immunization as soon as possible.

Before administering a childhood immunization, check for any contraindications to its use. A **contraindication** is known risk or reason not to give the immunization. For example, pertussis vaccine must not be given to a child with a progressive neurological disorder. It also must not be administered to a child who developed seizures, persistent crying, or a high fever after receiving a previous pertussis vaccine. In such a situation, the doctor would direct you to administer diphtheria and tetanus toxoids instead of the diphtheria and tetanus toxoid and pertussis vaccine (DTP).

Immunization Records

Under the National Childhood Vaccine Injury Act of 1988, you must record certain information about immunizations in a child's permanent medical record. Required information includes

- The vaccine's type, manufacturer, and lot number.
- The date of administration.

- The name, address, and title of the healthcare professional who administered the vaccine.

You also must document

- The administration site and route.
- The vaccine's expiration date.

Parents should maintain an accurate, up-to-date immunization record for each child. They should be encouraged to bring this record with them to each healthcare visit. Each state and/or the CDC issues an immunization record form, which may be available in languages other than English. Complete a form after each child's first immunization. Instruct the parents to keep the form and bring it with the child for each subsequent immunization so that you can update the record. Chris's immunization record is shown in Figure 40-12. Advise parents that this record is important to keep because it acts as proof of immunization,

(a)

Vaccine (circle specific type given)		Date Given	Doctor or Clinic
1	Hep B	2/25/XX	BWW Assoc.
2	Hep B	3/21/XX	BWW Assoc.
3	Hep B	8/12/XX	BWW Assoc.
1	Hep A	5/12/XX	BWW Assoc.
2	Hep A		
Other			
Other			
Other			
Other			

Please fold on dotted line

1	*Flu (TIV/LAIV)		
2	*Flu (TIV/LAIV)		
Yearly	*Flu (TIV/LAIV)		
Yearly	*Flu (TIV/LAIV)		
Other			
Other			
Other			

All children ages 6 months through 8 years who receive seasonal influenza vaccine for the first time should be given 2 doses. Children who receive only one dose in the first year of vaccination should receive two doses in their second year of vaccination.

*Seasonal   Please fold on dotted line

Immunization Record

Name _____ Matthews, Chris _____
(Last, First, MI)

Date of Birth _____ 11/19/XX _____

Physician or Clinic _____ BWW Associates _____
Alexis M. Whalen MD

Notice to Parents: Please take this card with you when you visit your doctor or clinic and have them fill in the information.

(b)

Vaccine (circle specific type given)		Date Given	Doctor or Clinic
1	DtaP/DT/Td	4/08/XX	BWW Assoc.
2	DtaP/DT/Td	6/10/XX	BWW Assoc.
3	DtaP/DT/Td	8/12/XX	BWW Assoc.
4	DtaP/DT/Td		
5	DtaP/DT/Td		
1	Tdap/Td		
1	Hib	4/08/XX	BWW Assoc.
2	Hib	6/10/XX	BWW Assoc.
3	Hib	8/12/XX	BWW Assoc.
4	Hib		
1	IPV	4/08/XX	BWW Assoc.
2	IPV	6/10/XX	BWW Assoc.
3	IPV	5/12/XX	BWW Assoc.
4	IPV		
5	IPV		
1	MMR/MMRV	5/12/XX	BWW Assoc.
2	MMR/MMRV		
1	Varicella	5/12/XX	BWW Assoc.
2	Varicella		
1	Rotavirus	4/08/XX	BWW Assoc.
2	Rotavirus	6/10/XX	BWW Assoc.
3	Rotavirus	8/12/XX	BWW Assoc.
1	PCV	4/08/XX	BWW Assoc.
2	PCV	6/10/XX	BWW Assoc.
3	PCV	8/12/XX	BWW Assoc.
4	PCV	5/12/XX	BWW Assoc.
1	MCV		
1	HPV		
2	HPV		
3	HPV		
other			

DH 686, 8/09 Stock Number 5740-000-0686-5

FIGURE 40-12 Example immunization record of Chris Matthews. (a) Front. (b) Back.

required by daycare centers, schools, the military, and other organizations. This record also may be helpful when parents consult another doctor, in case of emergency, or when moving to a new location.

Vaccine Storage and Handling

Vaccines must be stored properly. As a medical assistant, in order to ensure vaccine safety and effectiveness, you are responsible for proper storage and handling from the time a vaccine arrives at your facility until it is administered to the patient. Follow these general guidelines.

- Store vaccines at the recommended temperatures immediately upon arrival at your facility. Check and record temperatures of refrigerators and freezers daily.
  - Store refrigerated vaccines between 35°F and 46°F (2°C and 8°C).
  - Store frozen vaccines between –58°F and +5°F (–50°C and –15°C).
- Rotate your supply of vaccines so those with the shortest expiration date are used first. Place the vaccine with the longest expiration date behind the vaccine that will expire the soonest. Remove expired vaccines from usable stock immediately.
- Prepare vaccines just prior to administration to the patient.
- Follow infection control guidelines when preparing and administering vaccines.

▶ Pediatric Screening and Diagnostic Tests

LO 40.4

Pediatricians look for any sign of growth abnormality during routine well-child visits. Physicians compare a child's physical, cognitive-intellectual, psycho-emotional, and social signs to charts showing national averages. In general, physicians look for signs that the child is in the appropriate stage of growth for her age. Similar to the medical assistant's role in adult patient exams, during the pediatric exam, the medical assistant may assist with or perform many tasks, including taking vital signs and body measurements, performing vision and hearing tests, collecting specimens, and administering medications and immunizations.

Vital Signs

Some variations in technique and results should be considered when performing vital signs on pediatric patients. In addition to the normal vital signs range variations (review Table 37-1 from the *Vital Signs and Measurements* chapter), some other things should be taken into account. Taking a child's or an infant's temperature can be a challenge. If the infant or child is likely to cry or become agitated, take the temperature last. Measure pulse, respiration, and blood pressure (if ordered) before you take the temperature to avoid having these measurements elevated because of the child's agitation. Oral thermometers are not appropriate for children younger than 5 years of age because these children are too young to safely hold the thermometer in their mouths. Instead, take axillary, rectal, tympanic, or

temporal temperatures. If you use a rectal thermometer, hold it in place until the temperature registers to prevent the thermometer from being expelled or injuring the patient. Tympanic and temporal thermometers are especially useful in pediatric offices because of their speed and safety.

Blood pressure in children or infants is not routinely measured at each visit. Instead, the measurement is taken as per the doctor's orders. The procedure is the same as that for taking blood pressure in adults, except for these modifications:

1. Ideally, take the patient's blood pressure before performing other tests or procedures that may cause anxiety. In this way, you can avoid a falsely high result.
2. Be sure to use the correct cuff size for the child or infant. The bladder width should not exceed two-thirds the length of the upper or lower arm. The bladder should cover three-fourths of the extremity's circumference.
3. Do not attempt to estimate an infant's blood pressure using the palpatory method (discussed in the *Vital Signs and Measurements* chapter). It is typically not used.
4. Inflate the pressure cuff to 20 mm Hg above the point at which the radial pulse disappears.
5. Deflate the cuff at a rate of 2 mm Hg per second.
6. You may continue to hear a heartbeat on a child or infant until the pressure reaches zero, so note when the strong heartbeat becomes muffled.

Body Measurements

Children and infants are weighed and measured at each office visit. Children who can stand may be weighed on an adult scale. If toddlers cannot remain still on an adult scale, weight may be determined by weighing an adult holding the toddler, then subtracting the adult's weight. Infants are weighed on infant scales, which typically measure pounds and ounces. Infant scales are sometimes built into a pediatric examining table.

The height of children and the length of infants are measured at each office visit. Measure children in the same manner as you measure an adult. Some offices are equipped with height bars or wall charts that are separate from a scale. Use these devices in the same way as those attached to a scale. Measure infants while they are lying down; in this instance, you are measuring length instead of height. Some pediatric examining tables have a built-in bar for measuring length. You also can use a tape measure or yardstick.

The circumference of an infant's head is an important measure of growth and development and is used to evaluate diseases such as hydrocephalus or excessive cerebrospinal fluid in the cranial cavity, which causes enlargement of the head. You may be asked to perform or assist with this measurement (Figure 40-13) when you measure the infant's length. Measurement of head circumference may be performed at the same time as weight and length, or it may be part of the general physical exam. The steps for measuring

Go to CONNECT to see a video about *Measuring Infants.*

FIGURE 40-13 The medical assistant uses a flexible tape to measure the circumference of an infant's head.

infants are described in Procedure 40-1 at the end of this chapter. Review the *Vital Signs and Measurements* chapter and the procedures for weighing and measuring children.

General Eye and Vision Exam

As part of the general exam, the pediatrician examines the interior of the child's eyes with a special instrument called an *ophthalmoscope*. You will probably perform the visual acuity test (Figure 40-14). Make a game of covering the child's eye if

FIGURE 40-14 Making a game out of the visual acuity test helps put a child at ease.

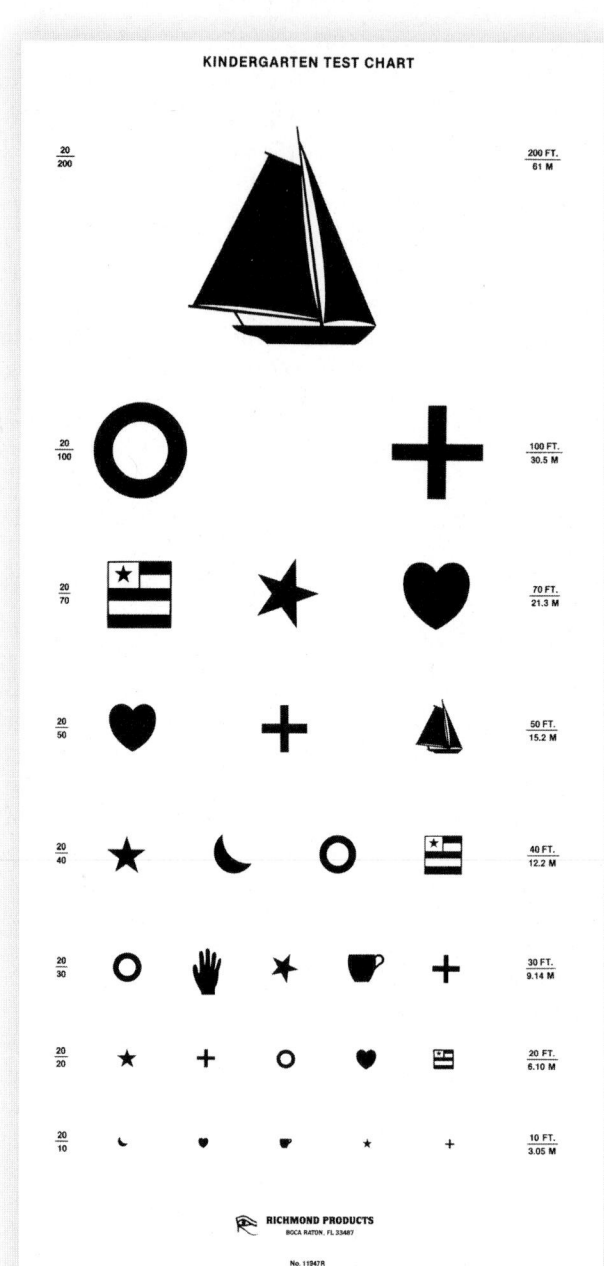

FIGURE 40-15 A kindergarten test chart is used to check the vision of a child who cannot read.

the child resists this part of the procedure. Use a pediatric vision chart as shown in Figure 40-15 for patients who cannot read. If the caregiver brought the child in specifically for a vision test, record in the child's chart whatever symptoms the caregiver mentions. Follow the procedure in the *Assisting with Eye and Ear Care* chapter and use these modifications when performing vision screening on a pediatric patient:

- Watch for signs of visual difficulty during the test, such as tilting the head in a certain direction, blinking, squinting, or frowning.

- Use a pointer to select one symbol at a time in random order to prevent patients from memorizing the order.

- It is common to start with children at the 40- or 30-foot line or larger if low vision is suspected and then proceed to the 20-foot line.
- Note the smallest line on which they can identify three out of four or four out of six symbols correctly.

General Ear and Hearing Exam

A pediatric ear exam is important because so many children have ear infections or upper respiratory infections involving the ear. Because children's eustachian tubes are more horizontal than those of adults, fluid collects more easily in the tubes and can promote bacterial growth. The tubes are also short and connected to the throat, making it easy for any upper respiratory infections to travel to the ear.

You may be asked to perform a hearing test on a pediatric patient. For children use the procedure found in the *Assisting with Eye and Ear Care* chapter. When performing a hearing test on an infant or toddler, follow these steps:

1. In a quiet location have the patient sit, lie down, or be held by the parent.
2. Instruct the parent to be silent during the procedure.
3. Position yourself so your hands are behind the child's right ear and out of sight.
4. Clap your hands loudly. You also may use a special device, such as a rattle or clicker, to generate sounds of varying loudness. Observe the child's response. (Never clap or create noise directly in front of the ear because this can damage the eardrum.)
5. Record the child's response as positive or negative for loud noise.
6. Position one hand behind the child's right ear, as before.
7. Snap your fingers or make a softer noise using a special device. Observe the child's response.
8. Record the response as positive or negative for moderate noise.
9. Repeat the above steps for the left ear and record all results.

Diagnostic Testing

Diagnostic procedures on adults, such as x-rays, blood and urine tests, and throat cultures, are also used for children. The pediatrician basically uses the same laboratory tests and radiologic tests. He performs some diagnostic tests in the office and needs the same types of specimens. Throat cultures, urine, and blood specimens are collected with a few extra considerations, explained in the following paragraphs.

Throat Culture Because streptococcal infection can be especially serious in a child, some pediatricians perform a rapid test for the presence of streptococcal bacteria so they can immediately start the appropriate medical treatment. If the test is positive, the physician begins treatment with antibiotics specifically for this type of bacteria. To confirm a negative test result, physicians may also do a throat culture. A throat culture can determine which of the streptococcal bacteria are present or whether other organisms are causing the symptoms. The results can indicate a possible change in medication. Review the method for obtaining a throat culture in the Obtaining a Throat Culture procedure in the chapter *Microbiology and Disease*. Having a small child lie down rather than sit may make the process easier. If the child refuses to open the mouth, gently squeeze the nostrils shut. The child will eventually open the mouth to breathe. Enlist the parent's help to restrain the child's hands if necessary.

Pediatric Urine Specimen When you collect a urine specimen from a pediatric patient, involve the child (if age-appropriate) and the parents or guardians. Explain the procedure thoroughly and ask specific questions, including the following:

- If the child is in diapers, ask whether there is a problem of persistent diaper rash. (Rash may indicate a change in urine composition because of renal dysfunction.)
- Is the child excessively thirsty? (In this case, the patient may not be taking in enough fluids for the amount of urine being excreted. Excessive thirst, combined with increased urinary frequency and volume, is symptomatic of diabetes.)
- Has the child experienced any difficulty urinating or a urine stream change? (These signs may suggest an obstruction in the urinary tract.)
- Does the child cry when urinating? (If so, the child may have pain or burning on urination, which can indicate a urinary tract infection.)
- If the child is in diapers, ask how many diapers are wet each day. Has the number changed recently? (Responses to these questions can rule out or confirm a urine volume change. For example, a child with a fever and increased perspiration might experience decreased urine volume.)
- Has the child experienced deterioration in bladder control, such as bed-wetting (**enuresis**)? (The child may be under stress or may have a small bladder capacity or a urinary tract infection.)
- If the child is having problems with toilet training and is older than 4 years old, ask whether the child learned to sit, stand, and talk at the age-appropriate times. (If so, the child may have a urinary system dysfunction.)

When you collect a urine specimen from a child who is toilet-trained, follow the same procedures as for an adult. If the child is an infant or not toilet-trained, however, follow the steps outlined in Procedure 40-3, at the end of this chapter, and shown in Figure 40-16. The *Processing and Testing Urine and Stool Specimens* chapter provides additional information.

Blood Drawing Procedures and Children Collecting blood may be part of your responsibility in a pediatric office. The *Collecting, Processing, and Testing Blood Specimens* chapter will provide detailed information about this task. Note that when working with children, it is a challenge to explain blood-drawing procedures to them, and that many children become visibly upset by the situation. If possible, it

Male   Female

FIGURE 40-16 When you apply a pediatric urine bag, make sure there are no leaks. Follow the steps in Procedure 40-3 at the end of this chapter.

is best to talk with the parents or caregivers before working with the child. The adults can provide the best insight into how their child handles stressful situations.

Your primary concern when working with infants is to complete tests accurately. Because an infant's veins are often too small for adequate blood collection, the best site for drawing blood is usually the heel, using a dermal puncture.

When working with children, address them directly. Speak clearly in a calm, soothing voice and explain the procedure briefly in terms they can understand. If they ask whether the process will hurt, be honest. A parent, guardian, or coworker should hold a very young child during a venipuncture or dermal puncture to prevent the child from moving. If a child is extremely distressed, it may be best to go on to another patient while the child calms down.

After you have begun the procedure, give the child status reports such as, "We're almost finished!" and make comments like, "You've been very brave." This also helps to calm nervous parents or caregivers. When the procedure is complete, offer a compliment on some aspect of the child's behavior. Gather your supplies and samples as quickly as possible to avoid alarming the child with the sight of blood-collection tubes. If parents or caregivers have questions, encourage them to discuss the tests with the child's physician.

▶ Pediatric Diseases and Disorders   LO 40.5

Many common disorders found in children are not specific diseases. Upper respiratory infections, including colds and viral influenza, occur frequently among children. Do not make assumptions regarding diagnosis or treatment. When reported symptoms include fever, sore throat, runny nose, and earache, any number of conditions could be the cause. Encourage the parent to bring the child to the office. You should, however, tell the doctor as soon as possible when a child has an extremely high fever. The doctor may want the child to go to an emergency room. Do not recommend aspirin for fever in children, as aspirin use in children has been associated with Reye syndrome, a potentially fatal disease of the central nervous system (CNS) and liver. Acetaminophen (Tylenol) or ibuprofen (Motrin) is preferred for treating fever in children. However,

you should check with the doctor before recommending any fever-reducing medication such as Tylenol or Motrin.

Common Diseases and Disorders

When you work in a pediatric office, you should know the signs and symptoms of childhood diseases. These include infectious diseases such as chickenpox, influenza, croup, measles, mumps, pertussis, rubella, scarlet fever, and tetanus, which are discussed in the *Microbiology and Disease* chapter. In addition to infectious diseases, there are several other common diseases of childhood, which are outlined in Table 40-2.

Less Common Diseases and Disorders

Some less common diseases and disorders also can be found in children. You need to be aware of the basic symptoms and the treatments for these disorders.

AIDS Most childhood cases of human immunodeficiency virus (HIV) infection are transmitted from a mother to her infant. The transmission of HIV from an HIV-positive mother to her child during pregnancy, labor, delivery, or breast-feeding is called mother-to-child transmission. In the absence of any interventions, transmission rates range from 15–45%. This rate can be reduced to levels below 5% with effective interventions. All babies born to HIV-positive mothers have HIV antibodies that are detectable through testing at birth. The antibodies persist for a period of 15 to 18 months, but not all of these babies remain permanently infected. AIDS has no cure, but treating the pregnant woman and newborn child with antiviral agents has been shown to lower the rate of HIV infection in the child.

Juvenile Rheumatoid Arthritis Juvenile rheumatoid arthritis (JRA) is an autoimmune disease of the joints that occurs in children aged 16 or younger. The symptoms of JRA include swelling, pain, and stiffness of the joints. The knees, hands, and feet are most commonly affected. The severity of the disease ranges from mild to severe and may affect the eyes and internal organs. A child with JRA will have periods of remission (a lessening of symptoms) and flare-up (a worsening of symptoms). JRA is diagnosed based on the severity of symptoms, specific laboratory tests, and X-rays. Treatment of this disease includes nonsteroidal anti-inflammatory drugs (NSAIDs), disease-modifying anti-rheumatic drugs (DMARDs), corticosteroids, biologic agents, and physical therapy.

As a medical assistant, your role in caring for children with JRA includes emphasizing the value of exercise and physical therapy, stressing the importance of taking medications as directed, and offering assistance by providing patient education brochures and information regarding local support groups and organizations.

Attention Deficit Hyperactivity Disorder and Learning Disabilities Attention deficit hyperactivity disorder (ADHD) and learning disabilities (LD) are found in children, adolescents, and adults. These disorders can cause

TABLE 40-2　Common Pediatric Diseases and Disorders

Condition	Description	Treatment
Head lice	Small insects easily spread among children by head-to-head contact and by sharing objects such as combs and hairbrushes. Lice live on the scalp and lay eggs strongly attached to hair shafts; symptoms include itchy scalp. Identify this condition by locating crawling lice or nits (eggs) attached to hair; examine parted hair carefully at the scalp and bottom of hair strands.	Anti-lice shampoo or 1% permethrin cream rinse; removal of eggs with fine-tooth comb; disinfection of clothing, bedding, and washable toys by machine washing and drying in hot cycles or by dry cleaning; tight bagging for 30 days of items that cannot be washed; disinfection of combs and brushes (used for hair) by washing in anti-lice shampoo.
Herpes simplex virus (HSV)	In children, this virus causes cold sore blisters on or near the mouth; diagnosis made by inspecting lesions. The first stage (2–12 days before appearance of blister) involves tingling and itching sensations; later, the blister ruptures and forms a yellow crust. An outbreak takes about 3 weeks to heal completely.	Application of ice cube to blister, which may promote faster healing; ointments to alleviate cracking and discomfort; avoidance of sun exposure because it may trigger an outbreak.
Impetigo	Highly contagious dermatologic disease caused by staphylococcal, or sometimes streptococcal, bacteria; transmitted by direct contact. Causes inflammation and pustules, which are small lymph-filled bumps that rupture and become encrusted before healing; frequently seen around the mouth and nostrils.	Avoidance of scratching lesions and sharing utensils, towels, bed linens, or bath or pool water that could cause further transmission; careful washing of affected areas two to three times per day to keep lesions clean and dry; topical antibacterial cream.
Infectious conjunctivitis ("pink eye")	Highly contagious streptococcal or staphylococcal bacterial infection of the conjunctiva of the eye; transmitted by direct contact. Causes redness, pain, swelling, and discharge; usually begins in one eye and spreads to other.	Avoidance of scratching eyes and sharing utensils, towels, or bed linens that could cause further transmission; warm compresses to relieve discomfort; antibiotic drops or ointment.
Pinworms	Parasites transmitted by swallowing worm eggs, by touching something that the infected person has touched, or by putting infested sand or dirt into mouth. When the eggs hatch in the body, worms attach to intestinal lining; mature females travel to areas just outside the rectum to lay eggs, which causes itching.	Medication is usually given to the whole family to treat and prevent further infestation.
Ringworm	Contagious fungal infection involving the scalp, groin, feet, or other areas of body, causing flat, dry, and scaly or moist and crusty lesions; lesions develop into a clear center with an outer ring. When the scalp is affected, may cause bald patches.	Oral and topical antifungal medication; isolation to prevent spreading; frequent changing of towels and bedding, with no sharing with others in family; caution that the child should not use others' combs or brushes.
Streptococcal sore throat ("strep throat")	Contagious disease caused by streptococcal bacteria and spread by droplet. Symptoms include headache, high fever, vomiting, and extremely painful, swollen, and red or white sore throat; causes difficulty swallowing. Complications include progression to rheumatic fever (with arthritis, nephritis, and inflammation of endocardium, or inner lining of heart).	Streptococci-specific antibiotics given as soon as possible; because of potential complications, therapy based on the practitioner's experience is sometimes given without confirmed diagnosis from throat culture; antibiotics are adjusted with confirmation of infecting organism; possible hospitalization in acute cases.

gross motor disability, inability to read or write, hyperactivity, distractibility, impulsiveness, and generally disruptive behavior. ADHD encompasses all conditions formerly identified as hyperactivity, or hyperkinesis, and attention deficit. LD encompasses a wide range of conditions that interfere with learning, including dyslexia (reading problems), dysgraphia (writing problems), and dyscalculia (math problems).

ADHD is misunderstood, misdiagnosed, and overdiagnosed in children. Some physicians fail to recognize ADHD as a cause of academic, social, and emotional problems. Others are quick to attribute too many such problems to ADHD. When ADHD is the correct diagnosis, methylphenidate hydrochloride (Ritalin) and other drugs may alleviate the symptoms, but not without risk of adverse effects, such as insomnia, increased heart rate and blood pressure, and interference with growth rate. Successful treatment usually requires a combination of drug and behavioral therapies and educational, psychological, and emotional support tailored to the child.

Cerebral Palsy　Cerebral palsy, a birth-related disorder of the nerves and muscles, is the most frequent crippling disease in children. It is caused by brain damage that occurs before, during, or shortly after birth or in early childhood. Signs of spastic cerebral palsy (the most common form) include hyperactive tendon reflexes, rapid alteration between muscular contraction and relaxation, permanent muscle shortening, and underdevelopment of extremities. Among people who have this disease, 40% are mentally retarded, 25% have seizures, and 80% have impaired speech. There is no known cure, but the effects of the disorder can be alleviated with physical therapy, speech therapy, orthopedic surgery, splints, skeletal muscle relaxants, and anticonvulsant medication.

Congenital Heart Disease Congenital heart disease is caused by a cardiovascular malformation in the fetus before birth. If the fetus survives, the newborn is usually small. The defect may be so small, however, that it may not be recognized until days, months, or even years later. Some patients have such a mild case of the disease that no treatment is necessary. Others require only low-risk surgery. In still others, major high-risk surgery is necessary. Many patients diagnosed with the problem are treated with antibiotics to avoid secondary infections.

A cardiovascular defect can be caused by genetic mutations (changes in the genes), maternal infections (such as rubella or cytomegalovirus), maternal alcoholism, or maternal insulin-dependent diabetes. Blue lips and fingernails—signs of cyanosis in a newborn—are obvious indications of a cardiac defect.

Down Syndrome Down syndrome is a genetic disorder resulting from one extra chromosome in each of the millions of cells formed during development of the fetus. It is the most common chromosomal abnormality in humans, and it is not caused by any parental behavior, such as diet or activity. The estimated risk for a Down syndrome birth increases, however, as maternal age increases. Down syndrome is characterized by low muscle tone, which can be alleviated with physical therapy. Characteristic facial features are also evident (Figure 40-17). These include broad face, flattened nasal bridge, narrow nasal passages (increasing the risk of congestion), slanting eyes (vision problems are common), and small teeth and ears. Mild to severe impaired intellectual disability is also a characteristic of Down syndrome.

Hepatitis B Infection with the hepatitis B virus (HBV) can lead to a serious and chronic liver infection. A child can carry the virus for years and only later develop liver failure or liver cancer. The virus can be transmitted across the placenta or during birth if the mother is infected. The disease also may be transmitted sexually, by blood transfusion, or by direct contact. It is frequently seen among drug abusers who share needles. Immunization is available, and children should be immunized starting the day after birth. Children who have not been immunized should begin to receive the series of immunizations for protection from infection.

Respiratory Syncytial Virus The respiratory syncytial virus (RSV) is a major cause of lower respiratory disease in infants and young children. RSV is most often seen in the winter and spring as outbreaks of pneumonia, bronchiolitis, and tracheobronchitis. It is highly contagious, and reinfection is common. Treatment is difficult because the infection is viral rather than bacterial. Antibiotics are thus effective for treating only the possible secondary infections that develop during or after contracting RSV. You may be asked to obtain nasal smears to assist in the diagnosis of RSV. More information about collecting specimens is found in the *Microbiology and Disease* chapter.

Sudden Infant Death Syndrome Sudden infant death syndrome (SIDS) is the sudden death of an infant, which occurs during sleep, that remains unexplained after all possible causes have been carefully ruled out. Most SIDS cases occur between 2 and 4 months of age. Victims appear to be healthy and are more likely to be male than female. When necessary, recommend and refer families to support groups that are helpful to the parents of a SIDS infant. The American SIDS Institute provides this advice as well as family support for victims of SIDS. Counseling and information are also available through local health organizations. Placing the infant on his back to sleep is highly recommended to help prevent SIDS. Other things that can be done to reduce the risk of SIDS include

- Obtain good prenatal care.
- Do not smoke, drink, or take drugs when pregnant.
- Avoid pregnancy during the teenage years.
- Wait at least one year between pregnancies.
- Use a firm mattress and avoid covers, toys, pillows, and bumper pads.
- Keep the baby's crib in the parent's room until the baby is 6 months old, or use a monitor.
- Do not let babies sleep in adult beds.
- Do not overheat the infant with covers or clothing while sleeping.
- Avoid exposing the baby to smoke.
- Breast-feed whenever possible.
- Avoid exposure to people with respiratory infections; wash hands and clean anything that comes in contact with the baby.
- Offer the baby a pacifier.

Spina Bifida Spina bifida is a defect of spinal development that results when tissues fail to close properly around the spinal cord during the first trimester of pregnancy. Neurologic symptoms are common because the spinal cord is not fully

FIGURE 40-17 A child with Down syndrome usually has distinct facial features.

FIGURE 40-18 Spina bifida occurs when the tissue around the spinal cord does not develop completely. It can be mild, with no symptoms, or severe, causing neurologic symptoms such as paralysis of the lower extremities.

protected by the spine's bony and connective tissues. These symptoms may vary with the defect's severity, ranging from foot weakness and bladder or bowel problems to paralysis of the lower extremities and mental retardation. In less severe cases the skin over the spinal cord often has a depression, tuft of hair, or port wine stain. In more severe cases, the newborn has a sac sticking out of the mid to lower back (Figure 40-18).

The treatment and outcome of spina bifida are based on the extent of damage. Surgical closure or implants are sometimes required. Unfortunately, the neurologic conditions cannot be reversed. However, some research has indicated that taking folic acid while trying to get pregnant and during the first trimester of pregnancy may reduce the risk of spina bifida.

Viral Gastroenteritis Gastroenteritis is an inflammation of the stomach and intestines. Gastroenteritis caused by a virus may be called the flu, traveler's diarrhea, or food poisoning. Viral gastroenteritis usually subsides within 1 to 2 days. It can be serious in young children, however, because it can cause extreme fluid loss that results in dehydration and electrolyte imbalances.

Symptoms include fever, nausea, abdominal cramping, diarrhea, and vomiting. Gastroenteritis is treated with bed rest, increased fluid intake, dietary modifications (usually only clear liquids), and medication for vomiting and diarrhea if necessary. Antibiotics may be prescribed if evidence of bacterial involvement is present.

▶ Pediatric Patient Special Concerns LO 40.6

In addition to well-child exams, immunizations, and the diseases discussed in the previous sections, there are some special concerns for pediatric patients. Medical assistants should be aware of problems such as child abuse or neglect; eating disorders; depression, substance abuse, and addiction; violence; suicide; and sexually transmitted infections, and unwanted pregnancies.

Detecting Child Abuse or Neglect

Child abuse is an all-too-common and potentially fatal problem. It frequently goes unnoticed. Whenever a child comes to the office, you should watch for any signs of serious problems in the relationship between the parent or caregiver and the child. Also notice any signs of physical injury, such as unexplained bruises or burns. Any suspicious lesion on a child's genitalia also should prompt an investigation of sexual abuse. Possible signs of neglect include a dirty or neglected appearance, hunger, extreme sadness or fear, and an inability to communicate. Note any suspicions in the chart and report them to the doctor before he sees the patient. The doctor will respond to your information by examining the child for clues to indicate the following:

- Internal injuries: tenderness when palpated or auscultated.
- Malnutrition: tooth discoloration, unhealthy gums or skin color.
- Lack of cognitive ability: dulled neurologic responses.

Studies show that certain risk factors are usually present in parents who abuse their children. Risk factors for child abuse or neglect include stress, single parenthood, inadequate knowledge of normal developmental expectations, lack of family support, family hostility, financial problems, and mental health problems. Other risk factors include prolonged separation of parent and child, ambivalent feelings toward the child, and a mother younger than 16 years. Additional risk factors include an unhealthy or unsafe home environment, inappropriate supervision, substance abuse, a parental crime record, a negative attitude toward pregnancy, and a history of parents having been abused.

Intervention, such as home visits by healthcare professionals, can significantly lower the rate of child abuse. These professionals provide information on normal child growth and development and routine health needs, serve as informational support persons, and refer families to appropriate services when they require assistance. Keep in mind that according to the law, suspected child abuse and neglect must be reported. If you suspect that a child is being abused or neglected while you are working as a medical assistant, you must inform your supervising licensed practitioner and contact the child protection agency in your community. Keep the child protection agency telephone number posted in your office.

Eating Disorders

Adolescents feel pressured to look good. Whether this pressure comes from modern media—be it magazines, television, movies, or the Internet—or from an adolescent's peer group, it's often focused on being slim and beautiful, which may include watching the scale and dieting, wearing stylish clothing, and having a certain hairstyle. This pressure may lead adolescents to develop abnormal eating behaviors such as anorexia nervosa. Although not limited to adolescents, patients with anorexia basically starve themselves by not eating. Males and females may suffer from anorexia, but it is more common in females.

Signs of Depression, Substance Abuse, and Addiction in Adolescents

Signs of depression, substance abuse, and addiction are often hard to distinguish in adolescents, partly because adolescents are particularly skilled at hiding the signs of all three disorders. However, various signs may indicate depression in an adolescent. One teenager may lose interest in or be unable to enjoy everyday activities. Another may sleep for long periods and have difficulty getting up in the morning, whereas yet another may sleep very little. Chronic fatigue or aches and pains may signal depression, as may trouble with concentration or school absenteeism. These signs also may indicate substance abuse or addiction.

It is important to know the difference between substance abuse and addiction. **Substance abuse** refers to the use of a substance, even an over-the counter drug, in a way that is not medically approved. Inappropriate use includes practices such as using diet pills to stay awake or consuming large quantities of cough syrup that contains codeine. It also includes taking larger-than-prescribed doses of a medication. Substance abusers are not necessarily addicts, however.

Addiction refers to a physical or psychological dependence on a substance. Addiction usually involves a pattern of behavior that includes an obsessive or compulsive preoccupation with a substance and the security of its supply, as well as a high rate of relapse after withdrawal.

As a medical assistant, you should not try to make a diagnosis. Quite probably an adolescent with one or more of these disorders will be uncooperative and refuse to answer relevant questions. You must be aware, however, of physical signs or behaviors that may be associated with depression, substance abuse, or addiction in an adolescent patient. The following signs or behaviors are important clues that you should report immediately to the doctor:

- The patient complains of altered eating habits or disturbed sleep patterns (either too much or too little sleep).
- The patient's weight has changed drastically (either up or down) since the previous office visit.
- The patient appears lethargic or sullen or exhibits radical mood changes.
- The patient has slurred speech.
- The patient appears to have illogical thought patterns.
- The patient appears to have needle tracks (anywhere on the body, especially on the arms or legs).
- The patient has pinpoint (highly constricted) pupils.

Another eating disorder is bulimia nervosa—a pattern of binge eating and purging. Purging is done by vomiting, taking excessive doses of laxatives, abusing diuretics such as Diurex water pills, or exercising excessively. However, a teen suffering from bulimia may still be of normal weight. Additional information about eating disorders is found in the *Nutrition and Health* chapter.

Depression, Substance Abuse, and Addiction

Signs of depression, addiction, and substance abuse in adolescents can be difficult to distinguish. Signs of substance abuse or addiction can be mistaken for depression. The reverse is also true. Sometimes all three conditions exist simultaneously. The use of alcohol, tobacco, club drugs, marijuana, cocaine, and heroin is an important concern with adolescents. Club drug examples include GHB, a central nervous system (CNS) depressant; ecstasy, a mental stimulant that increases physical energy; and Rohypnol, a sedative-hypnotic similar to Xanax. The abuse of controlled prescription drugs, such as Ritalin or OxyContin, is equally dangerous. Family members should be aware and willing to discuss signs of adolescent depression, substance abuse, and addiction with the doctor. Although these signs are difficult to evaluate in a short office visit, as the medical assistant, you should also be alert to them. If the doctor determines that a teen has a substance abuse problem, medical and health counseling services should be provided. Review the Caution: Handle with Care feature Signs of Depression, Substance Abuse, and Addiction in Adolescents for more information about this pediatric special concern.

Violence

Violence takes many forms. Teens of many cultures are exposed to violence in movies, television, video games, and music. Excessive exposure leads to insensitivity toward violence. Teens also may be victims of physical, emotional, psychological, or sexual violence at home. Bullying, browbeating, or abusing is recognized as a cause of violence at school. Many youths who have carried out homicidal acts of violence were deeply disturbed by repeated bullying experiences such as being teased, taunted, and rejected by peers. Most students are able to tolerate moderate amounts of teasing, but students who are depressed and harbor resentment and anger for a long time may explode in a violent way. In other cases, the teen may turn inward and commit suicide, which is discussed later. The medical assistant should be aware of the following warning signs of potential violence, including

- Frequent physical fighting.
- Increased or serious use of drugs or alcohol.
- Increase in risk-taking behavior.
- Gang membership or strong desire to be in a gang.
- Trouble controlling feelings such as anger.
- Withdrawal from friends and usual activities.
- Feeling rejected or alone.
- Having been a victim of bullying.
- Feeling constantly disrespected.
- Failing to acknowledge the feelings or rights of others.

Suicide

According to the Centers for Disease Control, suicide is the third leading cause of death for people aged 15 to 24. Unintentional or accidental injury and homicide are the first and second causes, respectively. The suicide rate among young people is greater for males than for females. Females are more likely to attempt suicide than males, but males are more likely to be successful in their first attempt at suicide. Be alert for warning signs, which include

- Depression.
- Anger that is directed inward, toward the self.
- Alcohol and/or other substance abuse.
- Changes in habit—carelessness, sloppiness, and a lack of interest in personal appearance.
- Giving away personal possessions.
- Giving verbal hints about committing suicide.

If you notice these signs or if you hear someone talking about committing suicide, you should listen and take the person seriously. Never assume that it's "just talk." Discuss your concerns with the licensed practitioner immediately.

Sexually Transmitted Infections and Pregnancy Prevention

Sexually transmitted infections (STIs) threaten long-term health and well-being. They are spread by bloodborne pathogens and require public education for teens as well as adults. Since teens may engage in sex, they should be aware of STIs and their effects. Teens also should know about pregnancy prevention. Information and education are available through schools, local and state departments of health, television ad campaigns, the Internet, and the Centers for Disease Control and Prevention. Further information about STIs is found in the chapter titled *The Reproductive Systems*. Additional information about birth control is found in the chapter *Assisting in Reproductive and Urinary Specialties*.

PROCEDURE 40-1 Measuring Infants

Procedure Goal: To accurately measure weight and length of infants and infant head circumference.

OSHA Guidelines:

Materials: Pediatric examining table or infant scale, cardboard, pencil, yardstick, tape measure, disposable towel.

Method: Procedure steps.

Weight

1. Identify the patient and obtain permission from the parent to weigh the infant.
2. Wash your hands and explain the procedure to the parent.
3. Ask the parent to undress the infant.
   RATIONALE: The infant's clothing and diaper can affect the results.

FIGURE Procedure 40-1 Step 3   Mother undressing her infant.

4. Check to see whether the infant scale is in balance, and place a disposable towel on it.
   RATIONALE: Balancing the scale ensures accuracy.
5. Have the parent place the child face-up on the scale (or on the examining table if the scale is built into it). Keep one hand over the infant at all times, and hold a diaper over a male patient's penis to catch any urine the infant might void.
   RATIONALE: Keeping one hand over the infant can prevent a fall, and holding a diaper over a male patient's penis prevents contamination of yourself and the weighing area with urine.
6. Place the lower weight at the highest number that does not cause the balance indicator to drop to the bottom.
   RATIONALE: Doing so ensures accuracy.

FIGURE Procedure 40-1 Step 6   Move the lower weight first.

7. Move the upper weight slowly to the right until the balance bar is centered at the middle mark, adjusting as necessary.
   RATIONALE: Doing so ensures accuracy.

FIGURE Procedure 40-1 Step 7   Center the balance bar at the middle mark.

8. Add the two weights together to get the infant's weight.
9. Record the infant's weight in the chart or on the growth chart in pounds and ounces or to the nearest tenth of a kilogram.
10. Return the weights to their starting positions on the left side.

Length: Scale with Length (Height) Bar

11. If the scale has a height bar, move the infant toward the head of the scale or examining table until her head touches the bar.

FIGURE Procedure 40-1 Step 11   Moving the infant toward the head of the scale to measure height.

12. Have the parent hold the infant by the shoulders in this position.
13. Holding the infant's ankles, gently extend the legs and slide the bottom bar to touch the soles of the feet.
    RATIONALE: The legs are held to ensure that the correct length will be measured.
14. Note the length and release the infant's ankles.
15. Record the length in the patient's chart or on the growth chart.

Length: Scale or Examining Table without Length (Height) Bar

16. If neither the scale nor the examining table has a height bar, have the parent position the infant close to the

head of the examining table and hold the infant by the shoulders in this position.

17. Place a stiff piece of cardboard against the crown of the infant's head and mark a line on the paper.
18. Holding the infant's ankles, gently extend the legs and draw a line on the paper to mark the heel, or note the measure on the yardstick.
    RATIONALE: The legs are held to ensure that the correct length will be measured.

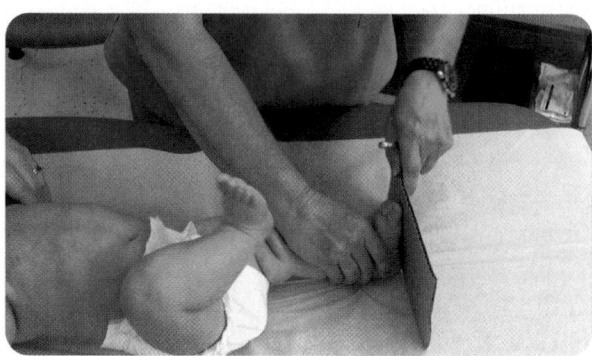

FIGURE Procedure 40-1 Step 18   Holding the infant's ankle to extend the leg and measure for correct length at the heel.

19. Release the infant's ankles and measure the distance between the two markings on the towel or paper using the yardstick or a tape measure.
20. Record the length in the patient's chart or on the growth chart.

Head Circumference

21. With the infant in a sitting or the supine position, place the tape measure around the infant's head at the forehead.

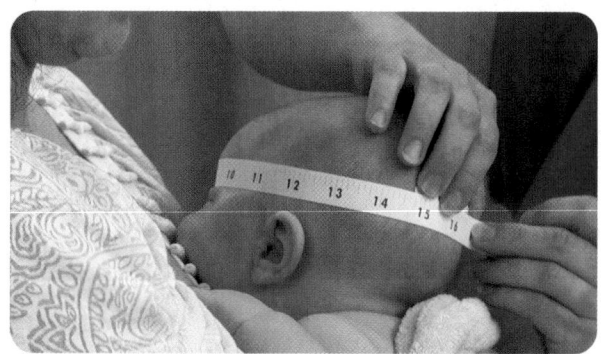

FIGURE Procedure 40-1 Step 21   Wrapping the tape measure around the infant's head at the forehead.

22. Adjust the tape so that it surrounds the infant's head at its largest circumference.
23. Overlap the ends of the tape and read the measure at the point of overlap.
24. Remove the tape and record the circumference in the patient's chart or on the growth chart.
25. Properly dispose of the used towel and wash your hands.

PROCEDURE 40-2 Maintaining Growth Charts

Procedure Goal: To accurately document the height, weight, and head circumference of a pediatric patient on a growth chart.

OSHA Guidelines: This procedures does not require exposure to blood or body fluids.

Materials: Appropriate growth chart, calculator or BMI calculator, pencil and pen.

Method: Procedure steps.

1. Obtain accurate measurements: Weight and stature (height) are measured for children 2 to 20 years who are able to stand. Weight, length, and head circumference are measured for children fewer than 36 months or 3 years who are measured while lying down.

2. Select the growth chart to use based on the age and gender of the child being weighed and measured. For boys and girls less than 36 months whom you will be measuring while lying down, use length-for-age, weight-for-age, head circumference-for-age, and weight-for-length. When measuring height in a standing position of boys and girls age 2 to 20 years, use weight-for-age, stature-for-age, and BMI-for-age. Charts are available in the workbook that accompanies this textbook or on the website of the Centers for Disease Control and Prevention.
   RATIONALE: The correct growth chart must be used because growth charts are used as a comparison to other patients in the same age category.

3. Record the patient's name and record number at the top of the form.

4. Record the mother's and father's stature (height) and the gestational age (pregnancy week) at which the infant was born.

5. Record the date of birth, birth weight, length, and head circumference, and add notable comments, for example, breast-feeding. *Note:* These data are not included for growth charts for children aged 2 to 20 years.

6. Determine the age based upon the date of birth. For infants determine the age to the nearest month by subtracting the birthdate from the date of the measurement as follows: To subtract, it will be necessary to convert months to days and years to months if either the month or day in the birth data is larger than in the date of measurements. When converting one month to days, subtract 1 from the number of months in the date of measurement, then add 28, 30, or 31, as appropriate, to the number of days.

   a. Example A: Patient was born on March 26, 2011, and today is January 13, 2013.

	Year	Month	Day
Date of measurement	2013	1	13
Convert one month to days	2013	(−1)	(+31)
		0	44
Convert one year to months	(−1)	(+12)	
	2012	12	44
Birthday	2011	3	26
Child's Age	1	9	18

Round day to months: 0–15 days = 0 months and 16 to 31 days = 1 month.

When charting for example A patient, you would use 1 year 10 months.

   b. Example B: Child was born on November 27, 2007, and today is May 15, 2014.

	Year	Month	Day
Date of measurement	2014	5	15
Convert one month to days	2014	(−1)	(+30)
		4	45
Convert one year to months	(−1)	(+12)	
	2013	16	45
Date of birth	2007	11	27
Child's Age	6	5	18

Round 5 months and 18 days to 6 months, making the patient 6 years and 6 months. Since the age is over 2 years, round months to nearest ¼ year:

   0–1 month = 0 year
   2–4 months = ¼ year
   5–7 months = ½ year
   8–10 months = ¾ year
   11–12 months = 1 year

When charting for example B patient, you would use 6 ½ years.

7. Record the date, age, weight, height (stature), and head circumference. Add comments as appropriate such as "patient uncooperative."

8. Calculate the body mass index (BMI) if using the BMI-for-Age chart. First, convert weight and stature measurements to the correct decimal value using the table below.

Fraction	Ounces	Decimal
⅛	2	0.125
¼	4	0.25
⅜	6	0.375
½	8	0.5
⅝	10	0.625
¾	12	0.75
⅞	14	0.875

Use a calculator and one of the following formulas to determine the BMI:

- BMI = Weight (kg) ÷ Stature (cm) ÷ Stature (cm) × 10,000

  Example A: Weight = 3.6 kg; Stature = 98 cm

  BMI = 3.6 ÷ 98 ÷ 98 × 10,000

  BMI = 3.7

- BMI = Weight (lb) ÷ Stature (in) ÷ Stature (in) × 703

  Example B: Weight = 36 lbs; Stature = 44½ in

  BMI = 36 ÷ 44.5 ÷ 44.5 × 703

  BMI = 12.8 (rounded from 12.78)

Note: You can also calculate the BMI using an online calculator such as the one found on the National Lung and Blood Institute's website.

9. Plot the measurement on the graph using the data you entered on the chart from the current visit.

- Find the child's age on the horizontal axis. When plotting weight-for-length, find the length on the horizontal axis. Use a straight edge or right-angle ruler to draw a vertical line up from that point.
- Find the appropriate measurement (weight, length, stature, head circumference, or BMI) on the vertical axis. Use a straight edge or right-angle ruler to draw a horizontal line across from that point until it intersects the vertical line.
- Make a small dot where the two lines intersect.

To ensure accuracy, you may want to use a pencil first to mark the small dot, then mark over with pen or a fine tip marker to make the document part of the legal healthcare record.

PROCEDURE 40-3 Collecting a Urine Specimen from a Pediatric Patient

Procedure Goal: To collect a urine specimen from an infant or a child who is not toilet-trained.

OSHA Guidelines:

Materials: Urine specimen bottle or container, label, sterile cotton balls, soapy water, sterile water, plastic disposable urine collection bag.

Method: Procedure steps.

1. Confirm the patient's identity and be sure all forms are correctly completed.
2. Explain the procedure to the child (if age-appropriate) and to the parents or guardians.
3. Wash your hands and put on exam gloves.
4. Have the parent(s) pull the child's pants down and take off the diaper.
5. Position the child with the genitalia exposed.
6. Clean the genitalia. For a male patient, wipe the tip of the penis with a soapy cotton ball and then rinse it with a cotton ball saturated with sterile water. Allow to air-dry. For a female patient, use soapy cotton balls to clean the labia majora from front to back, using one cotton ball for each wipe. Again, use cotton balls saturated in sterile water to rinse the area and allow it to air-dry.

   RATIONALE: The area must be thoroughly cleaned so that microorganisms from the head of the penis or vulva do not contaminate the specimen.

7. Remove the paper backing from the plastic urine collection bag and apply the sticky, adhesive surface over the penis and scrotum (in a male patient) or vulva (in a female patient). Seal tightly to avoid leaks. Do not include the child's rectum within the collection bag or cover it with the adhesive surface.
8. Diaper the child.
9. Remove the gloves and wash your hands.
10. Check the collection bag every half-hour for urine. You must open the diaper to check; do not just feel the diaper.

    RATIONALE: The diaper should not be wet, and feeling the diaper without looking could dislodge the bag.
11. If the child has voided, wash your hands and put on exam gloves.
12. Remove the diaper, take off the urine collection bag very carefully so that you do not irritate the child's skin, wash off the adhesive residue, rinse, and pat dry.
13. Diaper the child.
14. Place the specimen in the specimen container and cover it.
15. Label the urine specimen container with the patient's name, ID number, and date of birth; the physician's name; the date and time of collection; and your initials.
16. Remove the gloves and wash your hands.
17. Complete the laboratory request form.
18. Record the collection in the patient's chart.

    Example Documentation:

> Urine specimen collected per pediatric urine bag. Sent to MEDLab with requisition slip for complete UA _____ *Kaylyn Haddix RMA (AMT)*

LEARNING OUTCOMES	KEY POINTS
40.1 Relate growth and development to pediatric patient care.	Growth and development occur in stages throughout life, including neonate, infant, toddler, preschooler, elementary school child, middle school child, and adolescent. Each stage of development occurs through physical, cognitive-intellectual, psycho-emotional, and social milestones.
40.2 Identify the role of the medical assistant during pediatric examinations.	The medical assistant must be able to communicate with pediatric patients of all stages, gather and provide educational information to the parent or caregiver, assist with diagnostic and screening procedures, and serve as a liaison between the patient and the physician.
40.3 Discuss pediatric immunizations and the role of the medical assistant.	Immunizations provide patients with protection from infectious diseases. Throughout life, especially during childhood, immunizations are recommended. The medical assistant may schedule appointments, provide education, obtain informed consent, administer the medication, maintain the immunization record, and properly handle and store the immunizations.
40.4 Explain variations of pediatric screening procedures and diagnostic tests.	Screening procedures and diagnostic tests for pediatric patients vary depending upon the age and size of the child. When performing vital signs, body measurements, vision and hearing tests, specimen collection, or administration of immunizations and medications, follow the specific guidelines for the procedure and child.
40.5 Describe common pediatric diseases and disorders and their treatment.	Some childhood diseases include chickenpox, influenza, measles, mumps, rubella, scarlet fever, and tetanus. Other diseases are outlined in Table 40-2.
40.6 Recognize special health concerns of pediatric patients.	The medical assistant should be alert to signs of special health concerns of pediatric patients, including child abuse and neglect; eating disorders; depression, substance abuse, and addiction; violence; suicide; and sexually transmitted infections and birth control.

CASE STUDY CRITICAL THINKING

Now that you have completed this chapter, review the case study at the beginning of the chapter and answer the following questions.

1. Considering Chris Matthews's age, what special aspects of care should you be aware of while caring for him?

2. What information (chief complaint) should you chart regarding Chris?

3. According to his immunization record (see Figure 40-12), what immunizations are missing?

4. What screening and diagnostic tests would you perform or assist the physician in performing?

1. (LO 40.1) When Chris was a neonate, he had a high level of bilirubin in his blood. As a medical assistant, you know that he had _____ and needed _____.
   a. Jaundice; hospitalization
   b. Jaundice; medication
   c. Hypobilirubinemia; a bili-blanket
   d. Jaundice; a bili-blanket
   e. Hyperbilirubinemia; hospitalization

2. (LO 40.1) Which of the following statements indicates that the parents of a 12-month-old, named Ian, understand the importance of safety for their child?
   a. "Ian loves to sit on my lap when we drive to the grocery store. It keeps him quiet and happy."
   b. "Ian got some new toys from his cousin. It says they are for 3-year-olds or older but he plays with them all the time."
   c. "Ian learned how to turn on the water in the bathtub so I had my husband set the water temperature on the hot water tank to 140 degrees."
   d. "We put locks on all the cabinets to keep Ian from opening them."
   e. "Ian never puts anything in his mouth. He is such a good boy, we let him play with whatever he wants."

3. (LO 40.2) Which of the following would be the most important information to point out to a physician about a pediatric patient?
   a. A 3-year-old boy is not potty trained yet
   b. An 18-month-old girl just started having temper tantrums
   c. An adolescent patient wants his parents not to be in the room during his examination
   d. A 5-year-old girl doesn't want to go to bed at night
   e. A 7-year-old does not have any friends at school

4. (LO 40.2) If an infant is crying while the physician is listening to breath sounds, which of the following would be the best course of action?
   a. Have the physician wait until the infant stops crying to continue
   b. Provide the infant with a pacifier if he uses one
   c. Have the parent leave the room
   d. Blow in the infant's face
   e. Hold the infant more tightly in your arms

5. (LO 40.3) Immunizations are
   a. Vaccines or toxoids that protect susceptible individuals from infectious diseases
   b. Never given to a child who has minor cold symptoms
   c. Kept at room temperature
   d. Administered even if contraindications are present
   e. Recorded in the patient's chart only

6. (LO 40.4) Which method of temperature should *not* be used on a 2-year-old patient?
   a. Temporal
   b. Axillary
   c. Oral
   d. Rectal
   e. Tympanic

7. (LO 40.4) Which of the following vital signs would be taken last for an infant?
   a. Temperature
   b. Blood pressure
   c. Pulse
   d. Respiration
   e. Pain assessment

8. (LO 40.4) You are to collect a urine specimen on an infant in diapers. Which of the following questions would you *least* likely ask the infant's parent(s)?
   a. Has your baby experienced enuresis?
   b. How many diapers are wet each day?
   c. Does the baby have a persistent diaper rash?
   d. Does your baby cry when she wets her diaper?
   e. Has your baby had a fever?

9. (LO 40.5) A parent calls in stating that her 5-year-old son has a fever of 102 degrees and will not eat. What should you do?
   a. Suggest that the parent take the child to the emergency room
   b. Tell the parent to the give the child either Tylenol or Motrin right away
   c. Schedule the child for the first available appointment that day
   d. Tell the parent to give the child a cool bath to lower the child's temperature
   e. Have the parent call back if the child's fever goes over 102

10. (LO 40.6) Which of the following is an incorrect or untrue statement regarding child abuse and/or neglect?
    a. Report only cases of child abuse and/or neglect that you are sure occurred
    b. Unexplained bruises may be a sign
    c. Risk factors include young parent, single parent, financial problems, and family stress
    d. Intervention can lower the rate of child abuse
    e. Signs of abuse and neglect are not just physical

Assisting in Geriatrics

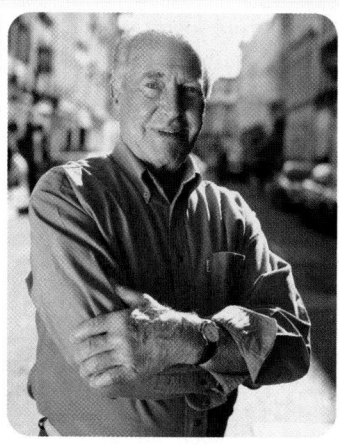

a few months ago. He arrives at the clinic with his nephew and needs to check in.

Keep Peter Smith in mind as you study this chapter. There will be questions at the end of the chapter based on the case study. The information in the chapter will help you answer these questions.

Peter Smith, a 73-year-old male with mild type II diabetes, calls to schedule an appointment. He states that he is feeling very anxious and fatigued and is having difficulty eating and sleeping since his wife passed away

LEARNING OUTCOMES

After completing Chapter 41, you will be able to:

41.1 Relate developmental changes in geriatric patients to medical assisting practice.

41.2 Describe common geriatric diseases and disorders and their treatment.

41.3 Identify variations of care for geriatric patients during examinations, screening procedures, diagnostic tests, and treatments.

41.4 Explain special health concerns of geriatric patients.

KEY TERMS

elderly
geriatrician
incontinence
kyphosis
lentigos
nocturia

osteoarthritis
osteoporosis
patient compliance
polypharmacy
preventive medicine
prolapse

I. C (6)	Identify common pathology related to each body system
I. C (7)	Analyze pathology as it relates to the interaction of body systems
I. C (9)	Describe implications for treatment related to pathology
I. C (10)	Compare body structure and function of the human body across the life span
I. C (12)	Describe the relationship between anatomy and physiology of all body systems and medications used for treatment in each
I. P (10)	Assist physician with patient care
I. A (1)	Apply critical thinking skills in performing patient assessment and care
IV. C (7)	Identify resources and adaptations that are required based on individual needs, i.e., culture and environment, developmental life stage, language, and physical threats to communication
IV. P (5)	Instruct patients according to their needs to promote health maintenance and disease prevention
IV. P (6)	Prepare a patient for procedures and/or treatments
IV. P (9)	Document patent education
IV. A (10)	Demonstrate respect for individual diversity, incorporating awareness of one's own biases in areas including gender, race, religion, age and economic status
IX. P (7)	Document accurately in the patient record

2. **Anatomy and Physiology**

Graduates:

b. Identify and apply the knowledge of all body systems, their structure and functions, and their common diseases, symptoms, and etiologies

c. Assist the physician with the regimen of diagnostic and treatment modalities as they relate to each body system

3. **Medical Terminology**

Graduates:

c. Understand the various medical terminology for each specialty

4. **Medical Law and Ethics**

Graduates:

a. Document accurately

5. **Psychology of Human Relations**

Graduates:

a. Define and understand abnormal behavior patterns

b. Identify and respond appropriately when working/caring for patients with special needs

e. Advocate on behalf of family/patients, having ability to deal and communicate with family

f. Identify and discuss developmental stages of life

9. **Medical Office Clinical Procedures**

Graduates:

d. Recognize and understand various treatment protocols

g. Maintain medication and immunization records

m. Assist physician with routine and specialty examinations and treatments

p. Advise patients of office policies and procedures

q. Instruct patients with special needs

r. Teach patients methods of health promotion and disease prevention

11. **Career Development**

b. Demonstrate professionalism by:
   (8) Being courteous and diplomatic

▶ Introduction

Geriatrics is the field of medicine concerned with the problems of aging. It is a subspecialty of internal medicine and family medicine. This field is growing because of increases in life span. Growing numbers of individuals are living longer, healthier lives. In fact, it is not uncommon now for individuals to live well into and beyond their 90s. Although there is no specific age at which a patient is prescribed geriatric treatment, in general, **elderly** patients (those over 65) will be cared for by a specialist in geriatrics. These specialists are called **geriatricians**.

According to the U.S. Census Bureau, by the year 2030, more than 20% of the population will be 65 years of age or older. Given that older people typically have more health concerns, you will find that as a medical assistant, at least 50% of your time will be spent caring for older patients. Keep in mind that just like children are not simply tiny adults, the elderly are not simply older versions of young adults. Geriatric patients have unique needs and concerns that will be discussed in this chapter. Knowledge of the geriatric patient's needs will prepare you to work as a medical assistant in a geriatric practice, as well as in a general medical practice.

▶ The Geriatric Patient   LO 41.1

As individuals age, they experience changes unique to aging. As a medical assistant, you should be aware of the physical changes that make the geriatric patient more prone to diseases and disorders. In addition, geriatric patients experience cognitive-intellectual, psycho-social, and emotional changes. Some aspects of geriatric patient care are age-specific.

Physical Changes of Aging

As the body ages, all body systems begin to show signs of aging. It is important to note that not all people experience all changes and that these changes occur at different rates. Let's explore the characteristic signs of aging for the body systems, outlined in the following paragraphs. These include the integumentary, nervous, musculoskeletal, cardiovascular, respiratory, immune, digestive, genitourinary, and endocrine systems.

Integumentary System Signs of aging in the integumentary system include

- Thinning and wrinkling skin due to decreased amounts of collagen and elastin in the dermis.
- Atrophy, or degeneration, of the subcutaneous layer of skin due to a decrease in adipose tissue.
- Decreased number of cells that produce pigment, or melanocytes, which protect against ultraviolet light. Melanocytes that are still present gather in common locations, causing the brown spots known as **lentigos** or "liver spots" (Figure 41-1).
- Graying, thinning hair.
- Brittle nails.
- Decreasing inflammatory response, resulting in slower healing.

Nervous System Signs of aging in the nervous system include

- Slower reaction time and thought processing.
- Decreased blood flow to the brain due to arteriosclerosis, a group of disorders that causes thickening of the artery walls.
- Shortened attention span and difficulty handling several tasks at one time, caused by decreased frontal lobe size.
- Shrinkage of temporal lobes, leading to weaker signals to the brain for processing.
- Impairment of fine motor activities like writing, caused by shrinkage of the substantia nigra, a layer of gray matter in the brain.
- Memory loss caused by changes in the part of the brain called the *hippocampus* and a lack of acetylcholine—a chemical that transmits messages between nerve cells or between nerve cells and muscle cells.

Special Senses Signs of aging in the special senses include

- Impaired vision and hearing.
- Altered or decreased taste sensations, which contribute to undereating and possible malnutrition.

Musculoskeletal System Signs of aging in the musculoskeletal system include

- **Osteoporosis** or decreased bone density, leading to increased incidence of fracture, particularly fractures of the hip.
- **Osteoarthritis** (OA) or degenerative joint disease (DJD) (Figure 41-2).
- Decreased numbers of musculoskeletal fibers.

Cardiovascular System Signs of aging in the cardiovascular system include

- Decreased cardiac output, especially during exercise.
- Arteriosclerosis.
- Postural hypotension or loss of blood pressure when standing or sitting up abruptly.
- Increased risk of heart disease.

FIGURE 41-1 Fair-skinned individuals are more likely to have lentigos, also called liver spots only because they are the color of the liver.

FIGURE 41-2 Also known as degenerative arthritis or degenerative joint disease, osteoarthritis occurs mostly in individuals over the age of 45 years and causes pain, stiffness, and swelling.

FIGURE 41-3 Kyphosis, a type of curvature of the spine also known as "humpback," occurs with age due to degeneration of the spine from osteoporosis.

Respiratory System Signs of aging in the respiratory system include

- Some loss of elasticity of the lungs.
- Calcification of the intercostal cartilage (located between the ribs) and the development of **kyphosis** (curvature of the spine), making it difficult for the lungs to expand properly (Figure 41-3).
- Increased shortness of breath, caused by the physical changes listed above.

Immune System Signs of aging in the immune system include

- Susceptibility to infectious diseases.
- Susceptibility to autoimmune diseases such as cancer and rheumatoid arthritis.

Digestive System Signs of aging in the digestive system include

- Constipation, caused by lack of exercise and poor diet.
- Fecal incontinence, caused by lack of muscle tone.

Genitourinary System Signs of aging in the genitourinary system include

- Decreased number of nephrons, which are the functional units of the kidney.

- Reduced tolerance for stress, so the kidneys may respond to disease in other parts of the body.
- Loss of voluntary control of urination.

Endocrine System Signs of aging in the endocrine system include

- Decreased thyroid function.
- Loss of estrogen production in postmenopausal females.
- Decreasing levels of aldosterone, a hormone that has a role in regulating blood pressure.
- Increase in the time it takes for levels of the hormone cortisol to return to normal after stressful events.
- Deficiencies in response to insulin by various organs.

Cognitive-Intellectual Development

In addition to the age-related physical changes to the body systems, developmental changes in the cognitive-intellectual, psycho-emotional, and social areas also occur among geriatric patients. Mature adults may take longer to process information. However, they can and do continue to learn. Long-term memory seems to remain intact. Short-term memory may be less acute. If they do not have a disease like Alzheimer's, they can continue to perform the same functions as they always have. Their accumulated wealth of information and life experiences makes mature adults great teachers.

Psycho-Emotional Development

Many changes may occur in the life of the mature adult. In Western cultures, people retire when they are about 65 to 70 years of age. Retirement is a major change that may have benefits or may cause difficulties. For example, people who no longer have a career may feel a sense of loss and grief. Those who have developed interests outside of their careers may make a smoother transition to retirement. In addition, many times older adults keep working because of financial need.

The deaths of a spouse and of friends are more common life events as a person ages and with which the mature adult must deal. In addition, mature adults face the reality of their own eventual death. Sometimes, physical ailments and the inability to physically and mentally do what they used to do can lead to increasing dependence on other family members—frequently, middle-aged children.

Social Development

Mature adults may experience an increased spirituality. Individuals who are financially and physically able may prefer to remain in their own home and familiar neighborhood. Others choose to move to their "dream" retirement home or community. Most mature adults in the United States live independently, contributing numerous volunteer hours to their communities. Frequently, relationships with grandchildren are a source of great pleasure.

Aspects of Care

Although all patient needs vary, as a medical assistant working with mature adults, you should consider the following points when caring for and providing patient education to geriatric patients:

- Encourage regular weight-bearing and aerobic exercises to reduce and prevent bone loss.
- Provide patient education regarding a balanced nutritional plan. Specifics of a nutritional plan may need to be discussed with a nutritionist or other licensed healthcare practitioner, particularly if there are complicating medical conditions, such as cardiovascular disease or diabetes.
- Question mature adults about their sleeping patterns. As adults reach the age of maturity, their periods of extended sleep may decrease, but short periods of rest during the day may help to offset that loss. Adequate rest helps an individual to be alert and better able to perform the tasks of the day. Disturbances in sleep or excessive fatigue should be reported to a healthcare practitioner.
- Encourage socialization. Social contact persists throughout adult life and should be encouraged. As an adult matures, retires from the world of work, and maybe even loses a spouse, opportunities for socialization may decrease. It is essential that an individual join with other community members to maintain contact. Frequently, this may be accomplished through volunteer activities.
- Encourage the patient to continue to get regular healthcare checkups, dental care checkups, and breast and prostate exams.
- Remember that the old adage "Use it or lose it!" applies. Keeping the brain active is necessary to prevent loss of function. Studies have shown that individuals who maintain active interests in the world around them maintain mental function better than those individuals who do not.

▶ Diseases and Disorders of Geriatric Patients

LO 41.2

Aging-associated diseases, or diseases that increase in frequency as individuals age, include cardiovascular disease, hypertension, cancer, arthritis, cataracts, diabetes mellitus, and Alzheimer's disease. Other disorders, such as constipation, diarrhea, and osteoporosis—while not serious for young and middle-aged adults—can be major problems for the elderly. Diseases and disorders that commonly affect mature adults, as well as their treatments, are summarized in Table 41-1.

BODYANIMAT3D
POWERED BY
connect

Go to CONNECT to see an animation about *Alzheimer's Disease.*

▶ Assisting with Geriatric Care

LO 41.3

Usually, examination, screening, diagnostic procedures, and treatments for geriatric patients are similar to those for younger adults. However, as a medical assistant, you should be aware of variations in the care and treatment of elderly patients. Notice the vast differences in the capabilities of people of this age group and do not stereotype all elderly patients as frail or confused

(most are not). Each patient deserves to be treated according to her own individual abilities. Always treat geriatric patients with respect. Regardless of their physical or mental state, elderly patients are adults. Do not talk down to them. Good communication is necessary. For more information about communication with geriatric patients, see Points on Practice: Talking with the Geriatric Patient.

Patient Education

Patient education for elderly patients is especially valuable because it can help them prevent or manage health problems and remain independent. You may need to educate some older patients about the importance of taking measures to protect their health. You may work with elderly patients who have hearing or vision problems or physical limitations that restrict their ability to perform certain tasks. Practice good communication in addition to keeping the following suggestions in mind when educating elderly patients.

- Speak in clear, low-pitched tones. High-pitched voices are more difficult for people with hearing impairments to understand. When asking questions, give the patient time to answer and confirm the response to prevent misunderstandings. Avoid both overly simple "yes" or "no" questions that the patient might answer without thinking and overly complex questions that might confuse the patient.
- Treat each patient as an individual. Some older people have trouble understanding directions. Try to communicate with them at the highest level they can understand. Remember, never talk down to patients.
- Put instructions in writing. Because some elderly patients have problems with memory, detailed written instructions are an essential aspect of patient care. Patients can refer to the instructions as necessary or ask a relative to do so.
- Adjust procedures as needed. When demonstrating a procedure to elderly patients, keep in mind any physical limitations they may have and adjust the procedure accordingly. Make sure patients understand the instructions by asking them to perform the procedure for you.

Denial or Confusion

Sometimes elderly patients, just like many other adult patients, deny that they are ill. A patient's perception of how he feels may be quite different from his actual state of health. The reverse situation also can occur. Elderly patients may overreact to a problem and consider themselves sicker than they really are. They may become dependent, passive, or anxious.

Elderly patients also may over- or underestimate their ability to perform certain tasks or to deal with certain limitations. Elderly patients may be confused if they have some impairment in memory, judgment, or other mental abilities. Signs of confusion can occur with Alzheimer's disease, senility, depression, head injury, or misuse of medications or alcohol. Elderly patients may or may not be aware of their condition. They may have difficulty understanding instructions.

TABLE 41-1 Diseases of the Elderly

Disease	Description	Treatment
Alzheimer's disease	Severely debilitating brain disorder. Warning signs include changes in personality, mood, or behavior; recent memory loss and increased forgetfulness; decreased ability to perform familiar tasks; difficulty with use of language and abstract thinking; decreased powers of judgment; and disorientation to time or place.	Because there is no cure, the primary role of caregivers is to provide comfort and safety to the patient. Medications like Aricept are available that can slow the symptoms of the disease.
Arthritis	Chronic inflammatory disease of joint tissues; symptoms include pain, swelling, and stiffness in joints.	Anti-inflammatory medication for inflammation and pain; surgery, including joint replacement in severe cases.
Cancer	Abnormal growth of cells that are able to invade other tissues.	Surgery, chemotherapy, or radiation therapy. Under-diagnosis and treatment as well as side effects of treatment are concerns for geriatric patients.
Cardiovascular diseases	Arrhythmias: abnormal heart rates.	Medication or surgery to control the heart rate.
	Coronary artery disease: blockages of the arteries surrounding the heart.	Stop smoking, improve cholesterol with medication or diet and exercise, angioplasty and/or placement of stents, or coronary artery bypass surgery.
	Valvular diseases: abnormalities of the heart valves.	Most frequently require a surgical repair of the affected valve.
	Congestive heart failure.	Medication to reduce fluid around the heart (diuretics) and to improve the beating of the heart (digoxin, beta blockers).
Cataracts	Lens of the eye becomes cloudy and opaque, causing decreased vision.	Sunglasses, improved lighting, and changing of glasses are helpful. Cataract surgery to replace the lens.
Constipation-diarrhea cycle	The cycle of constipation followed by diarrhea occurs when people's diets lack the fiber and liquids to maintain healthy bowel function and they use harsh laxatives to treat their constipation. The patient then complains of diarrhea and asks for antidiarrheal medication, which in turn causes constipation again.	Encourage elderly patients to eat more high-fiber foods, such as cereals, fruits, and vegetables, and to increase their fluid intake, as well as increase their activity level if possible.
Diabetes mellitus Type II	High levels of sugar (glucose) in the blood. Symptoms include fatigue, hunger, increased thirst, increased urination, and even blurred vision.	Diet, exercise, and weight control. Monitoring of blood sugar. Oral medications like Glucophage (metformin), or insulin injections.
Hypertension	An elevation of blood pressure over 140 systolic and 90 diastolic. There are often no symptoms or symptoms are mild.	Medications to reduce blood pressure. Diet restrictions to reduce fat and sodium and lose weight. Increase exercise to lose weight and strengthen heart.
Hyperlipidemia	A condition in which lipid (fat) levels are above normal. These include cholesterol and triglycerides. Although not just a disease of the elderly, it tends to be more common and serious with age. High cholesterol levels can lead to atherosclerosis, the accumulation of fatty deposits along the inner walls of arteries (Figure 41-4). These deposits, along with other substances in the blood, can form an atherosclerotic plaque. This plaque can narrow the opening in an artery to the point of obstructing blood flow. Atherosclerosis is a primary cause of cardiovascular disease and stroke.	Teach patients about eating foods with lower amounts of cholesterol and increasing exercise. Provide patients with printed materials about hyperlipidemia and cholesterol. The doctor may prescribe medication to lower cholesterol (statins) in patients when diet modification and exercise are not effective.
Osteoporosis	An endocrine and metabolic disorder of the musculoskeletal system. Thinning of bone tissue and loss of bone density occur over time, leading to fractures. More common in women than men, this disorder may be caused by inadequate calcium consumption, estrogen deficiency, or alcoholism.	Prevention methods include regular weight-bearing and strength exercises and a diet high in calcium (perhaps including supplemental calcium). Prescription medications, such as Fosamax or Actonel, and hormone replacement therapy also are used.

The Importance of Touch

Therapeutic touch is based on an ancient therapy called the laying on of hands. It was reconceived in the early 1970s by a registered nurse (RN). Essentially, the hands are used to direct human energies to help or heal someone who is ill. Although little scientific evidence exists about the effectiveness of this therapy, it is known that touch can improve health and well-being.

Because they often live alone, many elderly patients experience a lack of physical touch. Using touch—offering to hold a patient's hand or placing an arm around his shoulder—communicates that you care about the patient and may improve his health and well-being (Figure 41-5).

Incontinence

Elderly patients may suffer from urinary **incontinence** or involuntary leakage of urine. Many people are too embarrassed to ask for help or are unaware of possible solutions. In general, if a patient has urinary incontinence that interferes

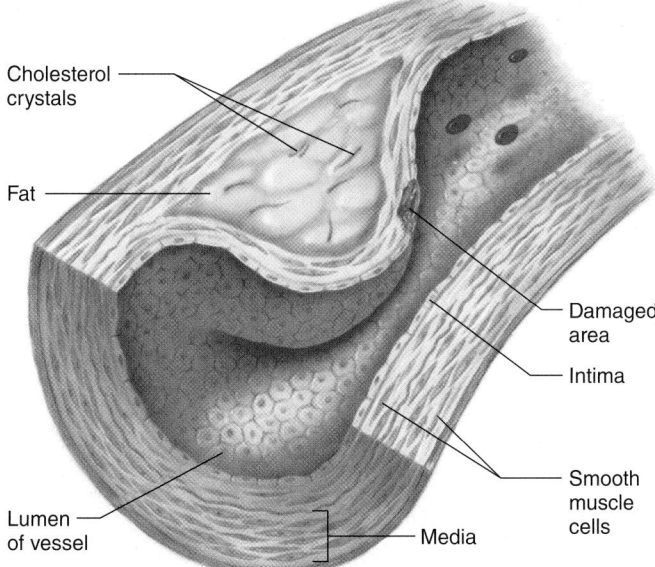

FIGURE 41-4 High cholesterol can lead to atherosclerosis. Help patients reduce their cholesterol through proper diet and exercise, along with medication, if prescribed.

FIGURE 41-5 The importance of touch: Elderly patients may appreciate your touch as a sign of caring. Consider offering to hold their hand or placing an arm around their shoulder.

POINTS ON PRACTICE

Talking with the Geriatric Patient

Communication is key to successful practice as a medical assistant. The following tips will help you and the patient communicate with each other more effectively.

- Make sure you select a private setting for the patient interview.

- Many older patients are hard of hearing but not deaf. Speak slightly more slowly than you normally would. Speak clearly and loudly (but do not shout—shouting will insult and anger an older patient who does hear well). Enunciate well and use a lower tone of voice (elderly people lose the ability to hear high-frequency sounds first). If the patient asks you to repeat a question, rephrase it instead of repeating it verbatim.

- Look at the patient directly so that she knows you care about what she has to say and so that you can make sure she understands what you tell or ask her.

- You can show respect for the patient's age by addressing the patient with Mr., Mrs., Ms., or Miss, unless the patient asks to be called by his or her first name.

- Be patient. Some older patients live alone or in relative isolation and may be out of practice with the two-way communication skills that make a conversation or interview go smoothly. The simple act of being interviewed, even for what may seem to you a straightforward medical history, may unsettle the older patient. For example, he may need to stop and think of a word here and there. Do not supply the word. Wait and let the patient think of it on his own. Also, do not rush through your questions. Rushing will only make the patient feel anxious and incompetent if he feels he cannot keep up with you.

- Practice active listening skills. Pay attention to the patient's verbal and nonverbal cues. Do not interrupt the patient. After the patient finishes giving each answer, repeat it to give her a chance to correct you if you misheard or misunderstood.

- If you are interviewing the patient to obtain a medical history, explain before you begin the type of questions you will ask and how the information will be used.

- If you need to use medical terminology, try also to express the same information in lay terms. For example, you might ask, "Do you use a diuretic or pill to help you eliminate fluids?"

- Be cheerful and friendly but not sugary-sweet. Do not talk down to older patients; they are not stupid.

- Avoid sounding surprised or excited by any answer to a question or to any information the patient gives.

- Under no circumstances use endearments such as dear, honey, or sweetie.

- Look for ways to make a connection so that the patient feels relaxed and comfortable. For example, in the course of taking a patient's history, you might find out that he enjoys swimming. Ask him to tell you about it.

- Show an interest in the patient as a person. Ask about something she is interested in. For example, a patient might be wearing a piece of handmade jewelry. Ask where it came from. She might have a wonderful story to tell.

Go to CONNECT to see a video on *Obtaining Information from a Geriatric Patient.*

with day-to-day life, the physician should be notified of the problem. Incontinence will sometimes cause a patient to drink less, making her prone to urinary tract infections and other problems.

Preventive Medicine

Many elderly patients are either not aware of or do not practice the concept of **preventive medicine** (measures taken to prevent illness). Many come from environments in which people went to a doctor only when they were very ill. So, they do not realize the importance of preventive measures such as regular check-ups, digital rectal exams, immunizations, and colonoscopy. Also, older women often do not recognize the need for regular mammograms and Pap smears to detect cancers of the breast and cervix.

As a medical assistant, you should use any educational tools available to you to make elderly patients more aware of the importance of preventive measures. If you reinforce the doctor's recommendations with education, you increase the chance that patients will heed the advice they are given.

Lack of Compliance When Taking Medications

Often, geriatric patients need several medications, and many of them find it difficult to keep track and take the right medication at the right time. Sometimes patients have difficulty swallowing or simply decide not to take a medication because they feel they do not need it. In your role as a medical assistant, you can help by telling geriatric patients about available medication reminder boxes, timers, or medication organizers. These devices can help ensure **patient compliance** (obedience in following the physician's orders). Patient compliance helps patients remain healthier and get well faster.

Collecting Urine Specimens

Consider the following when you are collecting urine from a geriatric patient: Bladder muscles weaken with age, often leading to incomplete bladder emptying and chronic urine retention, which can cause urinary tract infection, **nocturia** (excessive nighttime urination), and incontinence. Incontinence can interfere with collecting a 24-hour urine specimen.

Weakening of the supports of the uterus may cause it to **prolapse** (work its way down the vaginal canal). The uterus pulls with it the vaginal walls, bladder, and rectum. This weakening—often the result of several childbirths—may not occur until a woman is postmenopausal. Symptoms include pressure, incontinence, and urinary retention. Normal activities, such as walking up the stairs, can aggravate the problem. This condition can interfere with collecting a 24-hour specimen.

Find out whether the patient ever loses bladder control. If so, ask whether it occurs suddenly or whether a feeling of intense pressure precedes it. These symptoms can be a sign of weakening of the bladder muscles, which can also interfere with collecting a 24-hour specimen.

Keep in mind that some elderly patients need assistance in providing a urine specimen. For example, you may have to accompany the patient to the bathroom and hold the specimen container. (Wash your hands before and after doing so, and wear gloves while providing this help.)

If necessary, offer repeated explanations or reminders about the procedure or the specimens that need to be provided.

Blood-Drawing Procedures

The challenges presented by elderly patients may test your technical skills as well as your interpersonal skills. Physically, some older adults are frail and may not withstand blood-drawing procedures as easily as younger patients. Changes in skin condition often make elderly patients more prone to bruising and other injuries. Decreased circulation may make it difficult to collect enough blood for an adequate sampling. Be aware of these issues and take extra precautions when drawing blood on an elderly patient.

Hot and Cold Therapy

Elderly patients are usually more sensitive than others to cold and heat. As you may have noticed with elderly friends and relatives, there is a reduced ability to tolerate temperature changes. Sudoriferous (sweat-producing) glands of the skin decrease in number and, with less perspiration, high temperatures are more difficult to adjust to. At the same time, the loss of adipose tissue and decreased circulation result in a lessened ability to retain heat, which increases sensitivity to cold.

Along with possible poor circulation, geriatric patients also may have arthritis; impaired sensation; kidney, heart, or lung disease; or atherosclerosis. They also may have impaired skin integrity—thinning of the skin, resulting in increased risk of skin tearing, bruising, and burning. When administering cryotherapy (cold therapy) or thermotherapy (heat therapy), stay with an elderly patient during its application to check the patient's skin frequently for excessive paleness or redness.

Nutritional Guidelines

Universal nutritional guidelines for aging patients have not been developed. It is known, however, that energy and metabolic requirements usually decline with age, which calls for some dietary modification. The Food and Nutrition Board of the National Academy of Science recommends a 10% decrease in caloric intake for people over age 50 compared with that of young adults. Men and women older than age 75 should decrease their intake another 10% to 15%. The exact adjustment, however, depends on the individual patient's condition and needs.

Because protein requirements do not change, elderly patients should select foods that provide ample protein in a smaller quantity of food. To achieve daily nutritional goals, patients may require supplements for iron, calcium, and other minerals, such as phosphorus and magnesium.

Aging is often accompanied by decreased gastrointestinal muscle tone, so elderly patients should increase their intake of high-fiber foods and drink plenty of water. Of course, all people need to have an adequate amount of daily water. However, elderly patients sometimes restrict their fluid intake because they may need to urinate frequently, do not remember, or do not understand the importance of keeping the body well hydrated by consuming enough fluid. See Procedure 41-1, Educating Adult Patients About Daily Water Requirements, at the end of this chapter. Poor fluid intake also can quickly lead to urinary tract infections in mature adults.

Although all people need a certain amount of fat in their diet to help the body absorb vitamins, too much may lead to atherosclerosis. Elderly individuals should keep fat intake to 20% of their total calories.

Certain factors can impair or impede eating in this age group and may even lead to malnutrition. If you recognize any of these factors, discuss them with the patient's doctor:

- Physical factors, such as chewing difficulty caused by tooth loss or poorly fitting dentures, swallowing difficulty, and lack of appetite caused by altered taste, smell, or sight.
- Medications, which may adversely affect food intake or nutrient use.
- Social factors, including apathy toward food caused by depression, grief, or loneliness.
- Economic factors, including homelessness or lack of money for food or transportation.

Immunizations

Influenza and influenza-related pneumonia represent a serious health risk for patients older than age 65. Although elderly patients can be immunized against influenza each year and influenza-related pneumonia one time, they may have misconceptions about vaccinations. Another recommended vaccine for individuals over 65 is the shingles vaccine. No matter the vaccine, geriatric patients may worry about the expense, getting the disease from the vaccine, or the need for a vaccination when they do not feel ill.

Explain to patients who are concerned about the cost of vaccinations that if they are not enrolled in one of the many insurance plans that cover immunization, Medicare Part B covers the cost. For those worried about the potential side effects of immunization, describe the mild symptoms they may encounter and emphasize that the symptoms are short-lived. You also might mention that compared to the potential dangers of contracting a serious infection, the symptoms are quite mild.

Because older patients are much more likely than younger patients to develop side effects as a result of immunizations, instruct older patients so that they recognize and immediately report any adverse effects. That way, the physician can treat elderly patients before their illness becomes severe.

▶ Geriatric Patient Special Concerns LO 41.4

As you can see, geriatric patients require a lot of special consideration. Four additional special concerns when working with the elderly include falls, depression, elder abuse, and polypharmacy.

Preventing Falls in the Elderly

Falls can occur at any age, but in the elderly, they can have especially serious consequences. Bones become brittle with age due to osteoporosis, and falls can cause breaks in major bones, such as the hip and wrist. Complications from falls and bone fractures can lead to death in individuals in this age group.

The elderly are prone to falling because of vision problems, possible poor health, slowing reflexes, and changes in the ear that cause equilibrium problems. In addition, medications can increase the risk of falls because they may make the patient less alert.

As a medical assistant, you should discuss a safety checklist with elderly patients and their families. Point out that by taking the precautions listed, elderly patients can reduce the risk of falling. Make sure patients and their families understand the following instructions:

- Remove reading glasses before getting up and walking around.
- Make sure that potentially hazardous areas, such as stairs and doorway entrances, are well lit.
- Use night-lights in the bedroom and bathroom to help prevent night falls.
- When getting up from a reclining or recumbent position, sit at the edge of the bed for a few minutes before trying to stand to allow blood flow and blood pressure to adjust.
- Wear well-fitting shoes with low heels and slippers with non-slip soles.
- Use a cane or walker if you are unsteady on your feet.
- Secure rugs and floor coverings to the floor to prevent slippage.
- Attach all electrical cords to the walls or floor moldings.
- Place sturdy banisters along all stairs inside and outside the home.
- Install secure handrails near the bathtub and toilet.
- Use nonslip mats in the bathtub and shower.
- Minimize clutter in the home.
- Store frequently used items within easy reach.

Depression

Depression is common in the elderly, but many of the symptoms of depression mimic those of other conditions. As a medical assistant, you can help elderly patients—and their families—recognize the signs of depression. Recall Peter from our case study. What symptoms does he have? Do you think he has depression? Knowing what to look for may help patients seek help sooner than they otherwise would and receive prompt diagnosis and treatment. See the Caution: Handle with Care feature Helping Elderly Patients with Depression for a discussion of symptoms and treatment of depression in the elderly.

Elder Abuse

Even though you may need to communicate verbally with an elderly patient's caregiver, always observe the elderly patient for nonverbal signs of problems such as grimacing, foul odors, or bruising even if they cannot speak to you verbally. Disabilities may make the elderly person defenseless against abuse, and a medical assistant should be alert to signs of abuse.

CAUTION: HANDLE WITH CARE

Helping Elderly Patients with Depression

Studies published by the National Institutes of Health (NIH) indicate that at least 5% of elderly people attending primary care clinics suffer from depression. For elderly people in nursing homes, that percentage rises to between 15% and 25%. The NIH also indicates that only about 10% of elderly people who need treatment for depression ever receive it. Additionally, the NIH considers depression in people age 65 and older to be a major public health concern. In fact, suicide is more common among the elderly than any other age group. One reason for the low rate of treatment is that many older people—and their families—believe that depression is a normal consequence of growing old.

After all, older people may experience many difficult life changes, including enduring the deaths of a spouse and siblings, adjusting to retirement, being alone, dealing with a relocation, suffering economic hardship, and managing a variety of physical ailments. Because of these circumstances, doctors and family may miss the signs of depression.

Recognizing the Symptoms

There is, unfortunately, no specific diagnostic test for depression, so a diagnosis must be made on the basis of symptoms. The symptoms of depression in the elderly are similar to those in other age groups and include the following:

- Decreased ability to enjoy life or to show an interest in activities or people.
- Slow thinking, indecisiveness, or difficulty in concentrating.
- Increased or decreased appetite.
- Increased or decreased time spent sleeping.
- Recurrent feelings of worthlessness.
- Loss of energy and motivation.
- Exaggerated feelings of sadness, hopelessness, or anxiety.
- Recurrent thoughts of death or suicide.

The failure to realize that symptoms like these indicate an illness prevents many older people from seeking help. Yet there is evidence that treatment for depression in the elderly can be highly effective.

Treatment for Depression

Treatment for depression generally combines a course of antidepressant drugs with psychotherapy. Older patients generally respond to antidepressants more slowly than younger patients, so older patients may not experience relief until more than 6 weeks after starting treatment. For this and other reasons, compliance in taking medications for depression is a problem with the elderly. Many elderly patients do not understand depression and the importance of taking medications as prescribed. They also may be frightened by the idea of taking medication for a mental problem. Psychotherapy aims to help older patients talk through their anxieties, develop coping skills, and improve the quality of their lives. Again, compliance is a problem. Many older adults are unwilling to admit that they have a mental health problem and refuse to follow up on referrals to mental health professionals.

Benefits of Treatment

Elderly patients who follow a course of treatment for depression benefit in several of ways. They gain

- Relief from many of the symptoms associated with depression.
- Relief from some of the pain and suffering associated with physical ailments.
- Improved physical, mental, and social well-being.

Healthcare providers, including you as the medical assistant, can play a significant role in recognizing symptoms of depression in elderly patients and in encouraging them to get the treatment they need.

It is difficult to detect elder abuse. There is no uniform and comprehensive definition of this type of abuse, and bruises from falls and other accidents can be mistaken for abuse. Also, the signs of neglect can be similar to the signs of some chronic medical conditions. There are three basic categories of elder abuse: domestic elder abuse, institutional elder abuse, and self-neglect, or self-abuse. Elders can be abused physically, sexually, or psychologically. Elders may also be neglected, abandoned, or exploited materially or financially. Elders may even choose to neglect or abuse themselves. More than one type of abuse can occur simultaneously. Elder abuse occurs in all racial, socioeconomic, and religious groups. However, most victims are older women with chronic illness or disabilities. Risk factors or situations that increase the possibility of elder abuse include

- History of alcoholism, drug abuse, or violence in the family.
- History of mental illness in the abuser or victim.

- Isolation of the victim from family members and friends other than the abuser.
- Recent stressful events affecting the abuser or victim.

Signs of neglect include the following:

- Foul odor from the patient's body.
- Poor skin color.
- Inappropriate clothing for the season.
- Soiled clothing.
- Extreme concern about money.

You can assist the doctor by taking a careful history. Ask the patient about living arrangements, social contact, and emotional stress. Note the interaction between the caregiver and the patient. If you suspect abuse, inform the doctor. He will then be able to direct the physical exam toward possible internal injuries, malnutrition, or lack of cognitive ability. Most states require doctors who suspect elder abuse or neglect to report their concerns to a designated office. Early intervention usually results in better living arrangements for both the patient and the caregiver.

Polypharmacy

Age-related changes in the body can affect drug absorption, metabolism, distribution, and excretion. These normal changes can be exaggerated by various diseases or disorders. So, as people age, they have an increased risk of drug toxicity, adverse effects, or lack of therapeutic effects. Because of this risk, be especially alert when assessing an elderly patient who is on drug therapy.

Many elderly patients have complex, chronic diseases with unusual symptoms. This situation can make it difficult to tell whether a problem is caused by a drug. Listen closely to elderly patients and their family members; they are more likely to notice subtle changes than you are.

Patient and family education are important with elderly patients, particularly if they engage in **polypharmacy** (take several medications concurrently). Polypharmacy is common in elderly patients and possible drug-drug interactions can be severe. See the Caution: Handle with Care feature Preventing Unsafe Polypharmacy.

If an elderly patient is forgetful or confused, talk to the doctor about simplifying the medication schedule to reduce the risk of drug administration errors or omissions. If the patient has vision problems, provide drug instruction sheets in large type. To do this, type instructions on a word processor in a large type size, enlarge the instructions on a photocopier, or clearly handwrite the instructions in large block letters. You also might contact a local association for the blind or visually impaired for devices and tips.

CAUTION: HANDLE WITH CARE

Preventing Unsafe Polypharmacy

Before administering any drug by any route, you must know every drug, both prescription and nonprescription, that the patient is taking. Many patients, especially elderly ones, visit several doctors. It is entirely possible that each doctor may prescribe one or more drugs without being aware of other drugs the patient is taking. This practice can result in polypharmacy, which means taking several drugs at once. Polypharmacy can be safe, but if the doctor is unaware of the total drug profile, serious drug interactions can result.

When asking patients to identify *all* other drugs they are taking, including OTC drugs, keep in mind that patients may forget to mention all their medicines, OTC drugs, supplements, or herbal remedies to the doctor. Drugs that patients often forget to mention include antacids (such as Tums or Rolaids), supplements that are part of a food or drink (such as flavored drinks with glucosamine-chondroitin), or medicines that are used only as needed, such as medicine for migraine headaches, vitamins, and herbal remedies such as gingko biloba or omega 3.

To help prompt patients about drugs they may have forgotten, ask patients who have seen an orthopedist or cardiologist whether pain medication has been prescribed. Ask women who have seen a gynecologist if they are using a patch or other form of hormone replacement therapy. Ask all patients if they take any other dietary supplement, OTC medication, and/or herbal remedy. If a patient has been referred to any other doctor for any reason, ask whether that doctor prescribed medication. After determining the total drug profile, you should

- Update the patient's record (this should be done with every visit to your facility).
- Consider possible drug interactions, consulting online drug interaction checkers or other drug references, such as the *PDR*, if needed.
- Inform the doctor of your findings.

PROCEDURE 41-1 Educating Adult Patients About Daily Water Requirements

Procedure Goal: To teach patients how much water their bodies need to maintain health.

OSHA Guidelines: This procedure does not involve exposure to blood, body fluids, or tissues.

Materials: Patient education literature, patient's chart, and device to document education.

Method: Procedure steps.

1. Explain the importance of water to the body. Point out the water content of the body and the many functions of water in the body, including maintaining the body's fluid balance, lubricating the body's moving parts, and transporting nutrients and secretions.

2. Add any comments applicable to an individual patient's health status, such as issues related to medication use, physical activity, fluid limitation, or increased fluid needs. For example, geriatric patients have decreased gastrointestinal motility and require water to avoid constipation.
   RATIONALE: Some elderly patients purposely limit their fluid intake because of incontinence or physical limitations that make getting to a bathroom difficult, so it is necessary to provide specific comments about their exact fluid needs.

3. Explain that people obtain water by drinking water and other fluids and by eating foods that contain water. On average, an adult should drink six to eight glasses of water a day to maintain a healthy water balance in which intake equals excretion. People's daily need for water varies with size and age, the temperatures to which they are exposed, the degree of physical exertion, and the water content of foods eaten. Make sure you reinforce the physician's or dietitian's recommendations for a particular patient's water needs.

4. Caution patients that soft drinks, coffee, and tea are not good substitutes for water and that it would be wise to filter out any harmful chemicals contained in the local tap water or to drink bottled water, if possible. A good rule of thumb is that for every soft drink, coffee, or tea, the patient should drink the same amount of water to ensure hydration.

5. Provide patients with tips about reminders to drink the requisite amount of water. Some patients may benefit from using a water bottle of a particular size, so they know they have to drink, say, three full bottles of water each day. Another helpful tip is to make a habit of drinking a glass of water at certain points in the daily routine, such as first thing in the morning and after lunch or right before bedtime if it does not interrupt your sleep.

FIGURE Procedure 41-1 Step 5 Using a water bottle can help patients remember to drink a certain amount of water each day.

6. Provide patients with printed materials documenting the amount of water to drink and methods to ensure that their fluid intake is adequate.

7. Remind patients that you and the physician are available to discuss any problems or questions.

8. Document any formal patient education sessions or significant exchanges with a patient in the patient's chart, noting whether the patient understood the information presented.
   RATIONALE: Many insurance companies require evidence of preventative health counseling, and documentation is an important aspect of patient insurance coverage.

> **Example Documentation:**
> Water needs explained to patient including the body's use of water, the need to increase water, and tips for increasing water in diet. Patient stated she understood the need to increase water and would implement a plan to increase her intake of water. No questions asked. _____
> _____ _K. Booth RMA (AMT)_

LEARNING OUTCOMES	KEY POINTS
41.1 Relate developmental changes in geriatric patients to medical assisting practice.	Geriatrics is a subspecialty of internal medicine or family practice. Geriatricians typically care for patients over the age of 65. These patients have multiple physical changes as well as psycho-emotional, cognitive-intellectual, and social development variations to consider when working as a medical assistant.
41.2 Describe common geriatric diseases and disorders and their treatment.	Common aging-associated diseases and disorders include cardiovascular disease, hypertension, cancer, arthritis, cataracts, diabetes mellitus, Alzheimer's disease, constipation, diarrhea, and osteoporosis. Understanding these will help you prepare to care for geriatric patients.
41.3 Identify variations of care for geriatric patients during examinations, screening procedures, diagnostic tests, and treatments.	When working with geriatric patients, you must treat them with respect and dignity. Be aware of their physical and mental changes so that you can adapt your care to meet their needs.
41.4 Explain special health concerns of geriatric patients.	Each of the following special concerns should be handled appropriately when caring for the elderly: falls, elder abuse, depression, and polypharmacy.

CASE STUDY CRITICAL THINKING

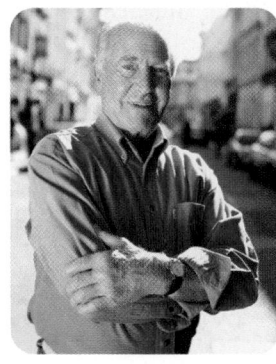

Recall Peter Smith from the beginning of the chapter. Now that you have completed this chapter, answer the following questions regarding his case.

1. Considering Mr. Smith's age, what special aspects of care should you be aware of while caring for him?

2. Why would Mr. Smith be prone to falls and what can you do to help prevent them?

3. You need to collect a urine specimen from Mr. Smith. What special considerations should you take?

4. What symptoms does Mr. Smith have and why is it important for you to recognize them?

EXAM PREPARATION QUESTIONS

1. (LO 41.1) Which of the following is the *least* likely to occur with a geriatric patient?
   a. Incontinence
   b. Kyphosis
   c. Hyperbilirubinemia
   c. Polypharmacy
   e. Lentigos

2. (LO 41.1) Your 68-year-old patient suffers from pain and swelling of his left knee. He also has poor vision and hearing. He needs education about how to care for his knee. Which of the following would be the best technique?
   a. Looking at your patient education sheet, give him simple directions at his level

b. Perform patient education in an open area of the clinic to prevent him from being uncomfortable

c. Have him go to a small class to teach him about his care

d. Speak in clear high-pitched tones so he can hear you

e. Look directly at the patient, speaking slightly slower in low-pitch tones

3. (LO 41.2) Which of the following patients is most likely to suffer from urinary incontinence?

a. A 78-year-old female patient with a prolapsed uterus

b. A 65-year-old male patient with nocturia due to an enlarged prostate

c. A 76-year-old female patient taking 12 different prescription medications and two over-the-counter supplements

d. A 68-year-old male patient with a history of alcoholism

e. An 82-year-old patient who uses a walker for ambulation

4. (LO 41.2) Your 68-year-old patient suffers from disorientation to time and place. Which of the following is the most likely problem?

a. Cataracts

b. Valvular disease

c. Polypharmacy

d. Alzheimer's disease

e. Osteoporosis

5. (LO 41.3) When speaking to Peter Smith, which of the following is the best way to address him?

a. Hi, Pete, how are you doing today?

b. Mr. Smith, how are you feeling today?

c. Sir, I would like to take your vital signs.

d. What is your chief complaint today, mister?

e. Hi there, honey, will you sit down right here so we can start the interview?

6. (LO 41.3) Your elderly patient refuses an immunization. Which of the following is the *least* likely reason?

a. He is worried about the expense

b. He had a severe reaction to a previous immunization

c. He does not feel bad and does not want to feel bad

d. He does not want to be stuck by a needle

e. He is afraid he will get the disease from the vaccine

7. (LO 41.3) When providing nutritional education for an elderly patient, which of the following statements is *most* accurate?

a. You will need to decrease the amount of protein in your diet.

b. As you age, you will require more calories in your diet.

c. High-fiber food and plenty of water should be included in your diet.

d. Your daily intake of fat should be at least 30% or more.

e. The medications you take will not affect your dietary intake.

8. (LO 41.2) Which medication would most likely be given to an elderly patient with congestive heart failure?

a. Statin

b. Glucophage

c. Actonel

d. Aricept

e. Digoxin

9. (LO 41.4) Which of following is *not* a practice of preventive medicine?

a. Biopsy

b. Colonoscopy

c. Mammogram

d. Immunization

e. Pap smear

10. (LO 41.4) Which of the following patients is engaging in polypharmacy?

a. A 78-year-old female patient with a prolapsed uterus

b. A 65-year-old male patient with nocturia due to an enlarged prostate

c. A 76-year-old female patient taking 12 different prescription medications and two over-the-counter supplements

d. A 68-year-old male patient with a history of alcoholism

e. An 82-year-old patient who uses a walker for ambulation

Assisting in Other Medical Specialties

CASE STUDY

Valarie Ramirez, a 33-year-old female, arrives at the clinic for a follow-up check for the removal of a painful wart on her right hand. During the patient interview, she states she is not having trouble with her hand; however, she has noticed in the mirror that she has a lump on the front of her neck at the bottom. She denies any other symptoms but thought she should tell the doctor. Her vital signs are BP 122/78 T 98.8 P 88 R 20 Ht. 5' 2" Wt. 135 lbs.

Keep Valarie in mind as you study this chapter. There will be questions at the end of the chapter based on the case study. The information in the chapter will help you answer these questions.

LEARNING OUTCOMES

After completing Chapter 42, you will be able to:

42.1 Describe the medical specialties of allergy, cardiology, dermatology, endocrinology, gastroenterology, neurology, oncology, and orthopedics.

42.2 Identify common diseases and disorders related to cardiology, dermatology, endocrinology, gastroenterology, neurology, oncology, and orthopedics.

42.3 Relate the role of the medical assistant in examinations and procedures performed in the medical specialties of allergy, cardiology, dermatology, endocrinology, gastroenterology, neurology, oncology, and orthopedics.

KEY TERMS

angiography

arthroscopy

balloon angioplasty

benign

cardiac catheterization

colonoscopy

computed tomography

coronary artery bypass graft (CABG)

echocardiography

electroencephalography (EEG)

electromyography

intradermal test

magnetic resonance imaging (MRI)

malignant

patch test

positron emission tomography (PET)

scratch test

sigmoidoscopy

stent

Wood's light examination

I. C (6)	Identify common pathology related to each body system
I. C (7)	Analyze pathology as it relates to the interaction of body systems
I. C (9)	Describe implications for treatment related to pathology
I. C (12)	Describe the relationship between anatomy and physiology of all body systems and medications used for treatment in each
I. P (10)	Assist physician with patient care
IV. P (6)	Prepare a patient for procedures and/or treatments
IV. A (10)	Demonstrate respect for individual diversity, incorporating awareness of one's own biases in areas including gender, race, religion, age and economic status
IX. P (7)	Document accurately in the patient record

2. **Anatomy and Physiology**
   Graduates:
   b. Identify and apply the knowledge of all body systems, their structure and functions, and their common diseases, symptoms, and etiologies
   c. Assist the physician with the regimen of diagnostic and treatment modalities as they relate to each body system

3. **Medical Terminology**
   Graduates:
   c. Understand the various medical terminology for each specialty

4. **Medical Law and Ethics**
   Graduates:
   a. Document accurately

5. **Psychology of Human Relations**
   Graduates:
   b. Identify and respond appropriately when working/caring for patients with special needs

9. **Medical Office Clinical Procedures**
   Graduates:
   l. Prepare a patient for examinations and treatments
   m. Assist physician with routine and specialty examinations and treatments
   p. Advise patients of office policies and procedures
   q. Instruct patients with special needs

▶ Introduction

As a medical assistant, you may choose employment in a medical specialty. This chapter introduces you to many of the specialties, their diseases and disorders, the types of exams involved, and how the medical assistant can assist with diagnostic testing. Certain specialized tests and the correct methods to administer them also are included in this chapter. As with any other practice, when working in a medical specialty, keep in mind that you also perform basic administrative and clinical skills and will have the responsibility of communicating with and educating patients. Certain concerns and questions are common to patients within a specialty area. Being prepared to address these concerns and questions will allow you to help patients effectively and fulfill a vital role on the healthcare team.

▶ Working in Other Medical Specialties

LO 42.1

Physicians working in medical specialties focus on one body system (such as the skin) or a single type of disease (such as cancer). The medical specialties discussed here include allergy, cardiology, dermatology, endocrinology, gastroenterology, neurology, oncology, and orthopedics.

Allergy

An allergist specializes in diagnosing and treating allergies. Allergies involve inappropriate immune system responses, or allergic reactions, to normally harmless substances called *allergens*. During an allergic reaction, inflammation and tissue damage occur. Common allergens include certain foods (like eggs and nuts), pollens, medications, insect venom, and animal saliva or dander.

Allergic reactions may show themselves locally—with a skin rash or nasal congestion—or may manifest themselves throughout the body. The most severe kind of allergic reaction is anaphylaxis, or anaphylactic shock, which is life threatening. When anaphylaxis occurs, immediate medical intervention is needed to save the patient's life. You should know emergency medical intervention for anaphylaxis when preparing to work in an allergist's office. You may need to teach patients who have severe allergies how to use an epinephrine autoinjector. See the Educating the Patient feature.

EDUCATING THE PATIENT

Using an Epinephrine Autoinjector

When working in a medical office that treats people with allergies, you must be familiar with epinephrine so you can teach patients how to self-administer it. Epinephrine is a drug used to treat allergies so severe that exposure to the allergen may be life threatening. The following reactions indicate the possibility of anaphylaxis, or anaphylactic shock:

- Flushing
- Sharp drop in blood pressure
- Hives
- Difficulty breathing
- Difficulty swallowing
- Convulsions
- Vomiting
- Diarrhea and abdominal cramps

If a patient with a severe allergy experiences any or all of these symptoms, the reaction can be fatal unless emergency treatment is given immediately. So, patients who cannot always control their exposure to an allergen—for example, bee or wasp venom—must have access to an epinephrine autoinjector for emergency intramuscular use. These prepackaged injectors (Figure 42-1) deliver either 0.3 mg of epinephrine—a single dose for an adult—or 0.15 mg of epinephrine—a single dose for a child. A patient who is exposed to the allergen should use the injector if the allergy is confirmed or if the allergy is suspected and signs of anaphylaxis appear. Teach the patient to follow these steps when using an autoinjector:

1. Remove the autoinjector from the packaging (box and/or plastic tube).
2. Pull back the gray cap.
3. Place the black tip of the injector on the outside of the upper thigh. (If needed, the injector can go through clothing.)
4. Press firmly into the thigh and hold for 10 seconds.
5. Remove the autoinjector and massage the injection site for a few minutes.
6. Call your physician or go to a nearby hospital emergency room.

An autoinjector is designed as emergency supportive therapy only. It is not a replacement or substitute for immediate medical or hospital care. Make sure the patient is thoroughly familiar with the parts of the autoinjector, how to activate it, how to use it, and what to do next. Ask the patient to explain the use of the autoinjector to you. If the patient is very young or otherwise unable to use the autoinjector reliably, teach a family member or companion how to use it.

FIGURE 42-1 Epinephrine autoinjectors come prepackaged, containing the correct amount of the drug for an adult or a child.

Cardiology

A *cardiologist* is a physician who specializes in heart diseases and disorders. To assist a cardiologist, you must be familiar with the structure of the cardiovascular system and the typical exams and measurements associated with it. You also need to know about common heart diseases and their treatments. Many diagnostic tests are performed in this specialty, including electrocardiography and stress testing. Imaging techniques, like X-rays and **echocardiography** (see Figure 42-2), also may be employed. You will assist with or perform some of these tests. Because managing a heart condition often involves many lifestyle changes, educating the patient about topics like diet and exercise will be especially important in this specialty. You also will provide emotional support to patients with serious illnesses.

Dermatology

Dermatologists diagnose and treat skin diseases and disorders such as acne, eczema, and skin cancer. Some skin conditions

FIGURE 42-2 An echocardiograph shows the structures and function of the heart.

involve only the skin itself; others are a sign of disease elsewhere in the body. To assist in a dermatologist's office, you must understand the basic elements of dermatologic exams and procedures. In addition to developing familiarity with skin disorders and their treatments, you also need to understand the terminology used to describe skin lesions, as outlined in *The Integumentary System* chapter. Assisting with positioning and draping during a skin examination and taking skin scrapings or wound cultures might be among your duties in a dermatologist's office. You might perform procedures such as administering sunlamp treatments and applying topical medications. You also will instruct patients about caring for a skin condition or wound site at home.

Endocrinology

Endocrinologists treat diseases and disorders of the endocrine system, which includes glands that regulate and coordinate the body's systems. Hormonal imbalances can affect the basic processes of growth, metabolism, and reproduction. Patients with thyroid imbalances, diabetes, or menopause frequently go to endocrinologists. In the endocrinologist's office, you will assist with exams and collect specimens for analysis.

Gastroenterology

Gastroenterologists diagnose and treat disorders of the entire gastrointestinal (GI) tract, from the mouth to the anus, as well as the liver and pancreas. (Proctologists treat disorders of the rectum and anus only.) A patient who sees a GI specialist has usually been referred by a family doctor, internist, or pediatrician who suspects a GI problem requiring additional expertise. You will need to understand the basic elements of GI exams and procedures to assist in a gastroenterologist's office. You also must be familiar with common GI disorders, their treatments, and the terminology used to describe them. In a gastroenterologist's office, you will tell patients how to prepare for exams like a **colonoscopy**, whether in the office, a radiology facility, or a hospital. Colonoscopy is discussed later in this chapter.

Neurology

Neurologists diagnose and treat diseases and disorders of the central nervous system (CNS) and associated systems. Nervous system injuries or diseases can result in loss of sensation, loss or impairment of voluntary movement, seizures, or mental confusion. Your duties in a neurologist's office include assisting with exams by readying equipment for use, positioning the patient, and handing the doctor tools and other items. You may be asked to perform parts of these exams. You also may assist with certain diagnostic tests, like **electroencephalography (EEG)** (see Figure 42-3). Your responsibilities may include instructing and educating patients and their families about procedures, disorders, and treatments.

Oncology

An oncologist specializes in the detection and treatment of tumors and cancerous growths. The term *cancer* refers to a

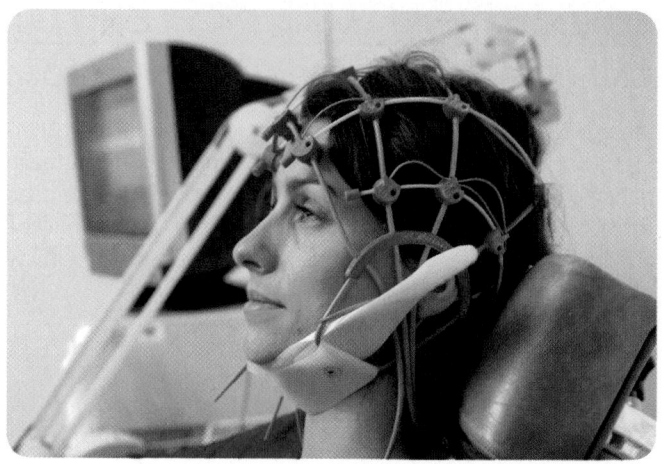

FIGURE 42-3 Electroencephalography (EEG) is performed by placing electrodes on the patient's forehead and scalp.

number of oncologic diseases that affect different body systems. All cancers are characterized by the uncontrolled growth and spread of abnormal cells. A tumor is a lump of abnormal cells. Tumors are classified as **benign** or **malignant**. Benign tumors contain abnormal cells, but the cells do not invade and actively destroy surrounding tissue. Malignant tumors contain cells that grow uncontrollably, invading and actively destroying the tissue around them. Malignant, or cancerous, growths are capable of *metastasis*—the transfer of abnormal cells to body sites far removed from the original tumor. When cells become malignant, the process is called *carcinogenesis*. You will encounter patients with a variety of medical conditions in an oncologist's office, so you must be aware of the common types of cancer, what their symptoms are, and how they are treated (Table 42-1). Part of your job may involve preparing patients for the side effects of cancer treatment and helping patients deal with them. Patient and family education and support are essential.

Orthopedics

Orthopedics is the medical specialty focusing on disorders, injuries, and diseases of the muscular and skeletal systems. The two systems are so interdependent they are sometimes referred to as the musculoskeletal system, especially by orthopedists. In an orthopedist's office, you will be asked to assist with general exams. Other responsibilities may include assisting with X-rays, helping with casting, applying hot or cold treatments, and educating patients about therapy regimens.

▶ Diseases and Disorders of Medical Specialties

LO 42.2

The medical assistant working in medical specialties should have a basic knowledge of the diseases and disorders related to these specialties. Understanding the conditions that commonly

TABLE 42-1	Common Cancers by System		
System	Cancer Type	Symptoms	Treatment
Reproductive (female)	Breast	Lump or thickening in breast, changed appearance, discharge	Surgery (lumpectomy or mastectomy), radiation, chemotherapy
	Endometrial	Postmenopausal bleeding	Surgery, radiation, chemotherapy
	Cervical	Usually none; possible painless vaginal bleeding and an abnormal Pap smear (Papanicolaou smear)	Surgery, radiation, chemotherapy
	Ovarian	Usually none; possible abdominal pain and bloating	Surgery, radiation, chemotherapy
Reproductive (male)	Prostate	Often none; possible difficult, frequent, or painful urination	Surgery, radiation, chemotherapy
	Testicular	Lump in testicle	Surgery, radiation, chemotherapy
Respiratory	Lung (including bronchus)	Often no early symptoms; later, new cough or cold that lingers; chest, shoulder, and/or back pain; wheezing and shortness of breath; hoarseness; coughing up blood; swelling in the face and neck; difficulty in swallowing; weight loss and anorexia; increased fatigue; recurrent respiratory infections	Surgery, radiation, chemotherapy
Digestive	Colorectal	Changes in bowel habits, blood in stools, rectal or abdominal pain	Surgery combined with radiation or chemotherapy
	Liver	Abdominal pain, fatigue, jaundice	Surgery, liver transplant
	Esophageal	Often no early symptoms; later, difficulty swallowing and/or regurgitation of food	Surgery, radiation, chemotherapy
	Oral cancer (mouth and throat)	May begin with painless sore or mass; later, difficulty chewing or swallowing	Surgery, radiation, chemotherapy
	Stomach	Indigestion, weight loss, nausea	Surgery, chemotherapy
Circulatory	Leukemia (all types)	Fatigue, paleness, repeated infections	Chemotherapy, bone marrow transplants
	Non-Hodgkin lymphoma	Enlarged lymph nodes, itching, fever, weight loss	Chemotherapy, radiation
Urinary	Kidney (renal cell) cancer	Blood in urine, pain in side that does not go away; lump or mass in side or abdomen; weight loss for no known reason; fever; feeling very tired	Surgery, targeted therapy, radiation therapy
	Bladder	Blood in urine; urgent need to empty bladder; urinary frequency; feeling the need to empty the bladder without results; feeling pain when emptying the bladder	Surgery, chemotherapy, biological therapy, radiation therapy
Endocrine	Thyroid	A lump in the front of the neck; hoarseness or voice changes; swollen lymph nodes in the neck; trouble swallowing or breathing; pain in the throat or neck that does not go away	Surgery, thyroid hormone therapy, radioactive iodine therapy, external radiation therapy, chemotherapy
	Pancreatic	Dark urine, pale stools, and yellow skin and eyes from jaundice; pain in the upper part of the abdomen; pain in the middle part of the back that does not go away when shifting position; nausea and vomiting; stools that float in the toilet	Surgery, chemotherapy, targeted therapy, radiation therapy
Nervous	Malignant tumors of brain and brainstem	Headaches, nausea, and vomiting; changes in speech, vision, or hearing; problems balancing or walking; changes in mood, personality, or ability to concentrate; problems with memory; muscle jerking or twitching; numbness or tingling in the arms or legs	Surgery, radiation, chemotherapy
Skeletal	Osteosarcoma (most often in knee and upper arm) Chondrosarcomas: malignant tumors of cartilage (most often in hip, femur, humerus)	Persistent unusual pain or swelling in or near a bone.	Surgery, chemotherapy, radiation therapy, immunotherapy, cryosurgery, vaccine therapy

Source: Adapted from American Cancer Society (cancer.org) and National Cancer Institute (www.cancer.gov).

occur in certain medical specialties will improve your ability to assist the physician and patients in specialty practices.

Cardiology Diseases and Disorders

Cardiology is a common specialty practice because of the prevalence of cardiovascular diseases and disorders. Every year since 1918, the number one cause of death in the United States has been cardiovascular disease, or a disease of the heart and blood vessels. Approximately 2500 Americans die every day from coronary artery disease (CAD)—narrowing of the blood vessels surrounding the heart that causes a reduction of blood flow to the heart. Cardiovascular disease claims more lives than the next four leading causes of death altogether. Unbelievably, one out of every three American adults has some form of CAD. You may know someone who has hypertension (high blood pressure) or other heart conditions. Maybe someone you know has had an MI (myocardial infarction, or heart attack). Several factors put patients at risk for heart disease, including inactivity, obesity, high blood pressure, cigarette smoking, high cholesterol, and diabetes. As a medical assistant working in a cardiology office, you should be able to teach patients about ways to reduce or prevent heart disease, stroke, or heart attack (see Table 42-2). Many of the diseases or disorders seen in a cardiology office are outlined in Table 42-3. Treatment for cardiovascular disease frequently includes medications, discussed in the *Principles of Pharmacology* chapter.

Dermatologic Conditions and Disorders

The condition of the skin plays a large part in a person's appearance. Patients with skin disorders, therefore, may worry about their attractiveness to and acceptance by others. Allow patients to express their anxieties; in return, provide encouragement about the course and outcome of their treatment. Table 42-4 discusses some of the most common dermatologic conditions and disorders. These and other diseases and disorders of the skin and accessory organs are discussed in *The Integumentary System* chapter.

Endocrine Diseases and Disorders

The most common diseases and disorders seen in an endocrinologist's office are ones related to the pancreas, thyroid, and reproductive organs. However, an endocrinologist would treat any disorder related to the endocrine system. Diabetes occurs when the pancreas does not secrete enough insulin or the body is

TABLE 42-2	Ways to Reduce or Prevent Heart Disease, Stroke, or Heart Attack

The American Heart Association now recommends that you watch your ABCs:

A. Avoid tobacco.
 1. Stop smoking. A smoker's risk is twice that of a nonsmoker. Even exposure to environmental tobacco smoke (secondhand smoke, passive smoking) may increase heart disease risk.
 2. Decrease stress.
 3. Maintain healthy blood pressure. Find ways to lower blood pressure and to keep the numbers down. The goal is a blood pressure of less than 120/80 mmHg.
 4. Maintain healthy blood cholesterol. Cholesterol will cause fat to lodge in your arteries, sooner or later causing a heart attack or stroke. Keep the total cholesterol less than 200 mg/dL.

B. Be more active.
 1. Increase physical activity. The goal is to increase physical activities on most days of the week to 30 to 60 minutes of physical activity. Increasing activity will decrease
 a. Stress
 b. High blood pressure
 c. High blood cholesterol
 d. Obesity

C. Choose good nutrition. Maintain a well-balanced diet, which helps to decrease the following:
 1. Alcohol consumption
 2. Stress
 3. High blood cholesterol
 4. Diabetes
 5. Obesity

Source: Adapted from The American Heart Association's guidelines.

TABLE 42-3	Cardiovascular Diseases	
Category of Disease/Disorder	**Common Conditions***	**Treatment**
Arterial/vascular disorders	Aneurysm	Medication, surgery
	Arteriosclerosis	Medication, lifestyle and diet management, surgery
	Atherosclerosis	Medication, lifestyle and diet management, surgery
	Hypertension	Medication, lifestyle and diet management, stress management
	Varicose veins	Wearing elastic stockings, weight loss, elevation of legs, surgery
Coronary artery disease	Angina pectoris	Medication, rest, lifestyle management
	Myocardial infarction	Medication, oxygen administration, rest, lifestyle management
Dysrhythmias	Atrial fibrillation	Medication, cardioversion (electric shock to the heart)
	Conduction delays or blocks (problems with electrical transmission within the heart)	Medication, pacemaker
	Tachycardia	Medication, diet management
Heart failure	Congestive heart failure	Medication, diet management, rest
	Cardiomyopathy (weakening of the heart muscle)	Medication, heart transplant
Inflammation of the heart tissue	Endocarditis (inflammation of heart lining and valves)	Medication, valve surgery
	Myocarditis	Specific treatment for underlying cause, medication, rest
	Pericarditis	Medication, rest
Valvular diseases	Aortic stenosis	Surgical replacement of valve
	Mitral stenosis	Medication, rest, valve surgery
	Mitral valve prolapse	Medication (usually antibiotic prophylaxis to prevent subacute bacterial endocarditis)

*Cardiovascular diseases and disorders are described in more detail in *The Cardiovascular System* chapter.

TABLE 42-4 Common Dermatologic Conditions and Disorders

Condition	Description/Symptoms	Treatment/Prevention
Acne vulgaris (acne)	Inflammation of the follicles of the skin's sebaceous (oil) glands causing skin eruptions. Pimples, blackheads, and cysts are seen on the face, back, and other areas.	Antibiotics, contraceptives, and retinoid are used to manage the outbreaks. Retinoid can damage a fetus, so it is not taken if a woman is pregnant or could get pregnant.
Basal cell carcinoma	Risk factors: overexposure to the sun, X-rays, irritants, various chemical carcinogens, presence of premalignant lesions. Most common are malignant basal cell carcinomas on areas exposed to the sun, like the face and neck. Higher-than-average risk of developing skin cancer: those who have had severe, blistering sunburns in their teens or 20s; those who have fair skin and hair and light-colored eyes; and those who work outdoors.	Treatments for skin cancer vary with the type of cancer and its extent. Treatments include surgery, electrosurgery, cryosurgery, radiation therapy, and chemotherapy.
Contact dermatitis	Caused by irritants such as rough fabrics, cosmetics, pollen, or plants like poison ivy or poison oak. Symptoms include redness, itching, edema, and lesions.	Treatment depends on the cause and type of lesions. Anti-inflammatory or antihistamines; oral corticosteroids are prescribed for severe inflammation.
Eczema	Skin inflammation that may be an allergic response to allergens, like chemicals or foods.	Combination of therapy and lifestyle changes to control flare-ups; oral or topical (applied to the skin) medication and phototherapy (light therapy).
Malignant melanoma	Originates in cells that produce the pigment melanin; this is the most dangerous type of skin cancer. Malignant cells may spread through the bloodstream or lymphatic system to the liver, lungs, and other parts of the body. A sudden or continuous change in the appearance of a mole may signal melanoma.	Treatments for skin cancer vary with the type of cancer and its extent. Treatments include surgery, electrosurgery, cryosurgery, radiation therapy, and chemotherapy.
Moles	Raised or unraised brown, black, or tan spot less than 6 mm in diameter. Has even coloring and a round or oval shape and clear borders. Monitor for bleeding, itching, or changes in color, size, shape, or texture.	May be surgically removed.
Psoriasis	Patches of red, thickened skin with silver scales mostly found on the knees, elbows, scalp, face, palms, and soles of the feet. More common in adults than in children. Diagnose through microscopic exam of skin scrapings.	Topical creams and ointments, light therapy, and systemic and combination therapies.

(Continued)

TABLE 42-4 (Concluded)

Condition	Description/Symptoms	Treatment/Prevention
Ringworm	Most often affects the feet (athlete's foot, or tinea pedis), groin (jock itch, or tinea cruris), and scalp (tinea capitis). Flat lesions are dry and scaly or moist and crusty, and develop a clear center with an outer ring. Creates scaly bald patches on scalp.	Topical antifungal medications; oral medications if severe. Contagious, so patient should not share bedding, combs, towels, or other personal items.
Squamous cell carcinoma	Appear on sun-exposed areas and look ulcerated or have a crust. They invade deeper into the skin and have a greater tendency to spread to other body areas.	Treatments for skin cancer vary with the type of cancer and its extent. Treatments include surgery, electrosurgery, cryosurgery, radiation therapy, and chemotherapy.
Warts (verrucae)	Benign skin tumors that result from a viral skin infection. If a wart is scratched open, the virus may spread by contact to another part of the body or to another person. Several kinds: • Common warts are raised, rounded, flesh-colored lesions that usually occur on the hands and fingers. • Plantar warts appear on the soles of the feet. • Venereal warts appear on the genitalia and anus and are transmitted through sexual contact.	Treatment depends on the type of wart. Some warts go away without treatment. Removed by burning or freezing the wart tissue. Instruct the patient to keep the wart removal site clean and dry until a scab forms or the wart falls off.

resistant to insulin. A deficiency of insulin or a resistance to it interferes with the metabolism of carbohydrates, proteins, and fats, raising the glucose level in the blood. This condition is known as *hyperglycemia*. The symptoms of diabetes are often subtle and include frequent urination, excessive thirst, extreme hunger, unexplained weight loss, fatigue, and blurry vision. Common types of diabetes include Type I, Type II, and gestational diabetes, discussed in *The Endocrine System* chapter. No matter the type of diabetes, the goal is basically the same: Keep blood sugar levels within a normal range, eat a healthy diet, exercise regularly, and see a healthcare provider routinely (see Figure 42-4).

Disorders related to the thyroid gland include hypothyroidism and hyperthyroidism. Hypothyroidism is characterized by decreased activity of the thyroid gland and underproduction of the hormone thyroxine. This shortage can cause cretinism in children, with resulting mental and physical retardation. Underproduction of thyroxine in adults results in myxedema. Patients with this condition have fatigue, low blood pressure, dry skin and hair, facial puffiness, and goiter or an enlarged thyroid gland. Treatment for hypothyroidism consists of thyroid hormone supplements.

Hyperthyroidism, also called Graves' disease, is characterized by increased thyroid gland activity. The patient has anxiety, irritability, elevated heart rate and blood pressure, tremors, and weight loss despite an increased appetite. Treatment includes the administration of radioactive iodine, antithyroid drugs, or surgery to remove part or all of the thyroid gland. Many patients require supplemental thyroid hormones following treatment for a hyperactive thyroid.

Gastrointestinal Diseases and Disorders

The level of discomfort from GI disorders can be misleading in relation to severity. There may be severe pain with intestinal gas, which is not serious, whereas there is virtually no pain in the initial stage of appendicitis, which is potentially life threatening. Be sure your notes are accurate and complete when a patient reports GI symptoms. Note the level of the patient's pain and whether over-the-counter (OTC) drugs have been administered. Common diseases and disorders treated by a GI specialist are outlined in Table 42-5 and discussed in *The Digestive System*.

Neurologic Diseases and Disorders

Common diseases of the neurologic system are described in Table 42-6. Trauma can also cause damage to the nervous system; such injuries can result in loss of sensation and voluntary

FIGURE 42-4 Patients with diabetes can use a glucometer to monitor their own blood glucose levels.

TABLE 42-5 Common Gastrointestinal Diseases and Disorders

Condition*	Description	Treatment
Anal fissure	Ulcer in anal wall; may develop into fistula (an abnormal duct to the rectum).	Depends on extent; may require surgery to repair
Cholecystitis	Inflammation of the gallbladder caused by fatty foods, gallstones, or infection. Symptoms: Pain, nausea, diarrhea.	Avoidance of fatty foods if intolerant; lithotripsy to break up stones; antibiotic for bacterial infection
Cholelithiasis	Gallstones.	Lithotripsy, antibiotics to prevent secondary infection
Colitis	Inflammation of the colon caused by bacteria, food intolerance, anxiety, or emotional disorder.	Diet modification (clear liquid for acute phase), medication, psychotherapy, fluid replacement, colostomy for severe cases
Constipation	Hard feces or stools.	Diet modification, stool-softener medication, enema, surgery if necessary for impaction
Diarrhea	Abnormally frequent, watery bowel movements.	Diet modification, antibiotics for bacterial infection, medication to prevent dehydration
Diverticulitis	Inflammation of diverticulum.	Diet modification, surgery for severe cases
Gastritis	Inflammation of stomach lining.	Diet modification, drug therapy
Gastroesophageal reflux (GERD)	Gastric acid rising from stomach into esophagus.	Diet modification, small meals, antacids, upright eating, remaining upright for several hours after eating, surgery (rarely)
Hemorrhoids	Enlargement of rectal or anal veins.	Diet modification, surgery
Hernia	Organ pushes through a muscle or wall containing it. Common abdominal hernias include hiatal hernia and inguinal hernia.	Surgery to repair muscle
Stomatitis (canker sores)	Sore gums or other oral areas caused by herpes virus or acidic body chemistry; exacerbated by emotional distress, acidic foods. Symptoms: ulcerations (canker sores) with burning, sometimes swelling.	Bland diet, avoidance of stress, medicated mouth rinses, topical anesthetic

*Gastrointestinal diseases and disorders are described in more detail in *The Digestive System* chapter.

TABLE 42-6 Common Diseases of the Neurological System

Condition*	Description	Treatment
Alzheimer's disease	Disabling disease that involves dementia and deterioration of physical function	Frequent stimulation to possibly help slow deterioration, and medications that may slow progression of some symptoms
Bell's palsy	Disease that causes sudden weakness or paralysis on one side of the face because of damage to the facial nerve	Usually resolves without treatment in 1 to 8 weeks
Encephalitis	Inflammation of brain tissue usually caused by viral infection; symptoms: fever, headache, vomiting, stiff neck, drowsiness	Medication, rest
Epilepsy	Disease caused by misfiring of nerve groups in the brain, resulting in seizures	Medication
Herpes zoster	Disease caused by the virus that causes chickenpox; symptoms: painful blisters that form along path of one or more nerves	Medication to relieve pain
Meningitis	Inflammation of the meninges	Medication like antibiotics and drugs to reduce swelling
Migraine headaches	Severe headaches caused by vascular disturbance	Medication
Multiple sclerosis	Degenerative disease of the central nervous system	Anti-inflammatory medications
Neuritis	Inflammation of one or more nerves; symptoms: severe pain and discomfort or paralysis of the affected area	Medication and rest
Parkinson's disease	Progressive neurological disease	Medication to relieve symptoms
Sciatica	Inflammation of the sciatic nerve	Medication to relieve pain, rest, heat applications

*Neurological diseases and disorders are described in more detail in *The Nervous System* chapter.

motion. Paralysis on one side of the body, as a result of damage to the opposite side of the brain, is called hemiplegia. Paraplegia involves motor or sensory loss in the lower extremities. Paralysis of the arms, legs, and muscles below the place where the spinal cord is damaged is called quadriplegia.

Encephalopathy is a term for a disease of the brain that alters brain function or structure. Encephalopathy may be caused by an infectious agent, metabolic dysfunction, brain tumor, increased pressure in the skull, prolonged exposure to toxic elements, chronic progressive trauma, poor nutrition, or

TABLE 42-7   Common Diseases and Disorders of the Musculoskeletal System

Condition*	Description	Treatment
Arthritis	Inflammation of joints	Anti-inflammatory medications, heat, rest, exercise, occupational and physical therapy, surgery (arthroplasty)
Bursitis	Inflammation of one or more bursae (sacs surrounding joints)	Anti-inflammatory medications
Carpal tunnel syndrome	Compression of the median nerve, causing wrist pain and numbness	Rest and occupational adjustments, splinting of wrists, injection of corticosteroids, surgical decompression of nerve
Dislocation	Displacement of bones at joint so that parts that are supposed to make contact no longer come together; occurs most often to fingers, shoulder, knee, and hip	Relocation, or shifting bones back into place; anti-inflammatory medications
Herniated intervertebral disk (HID)	Protruding contents of disk compress nerve roots, causing severe pain	Rest, traction, physical therapy, muscle relaxants, surgery
Osteomyelitis	Infection of bone; principal symptom is pain	Antibiotics and analgesics, surgery
Osteoporosis	Decreased bone mass, resulting in brittle, easily fractured bones	Exercise, dietary supplements, hormone therapy, drug therapy
Paget's disease	Chronic condition that causes bone deformities	Exercise, dietary supplements, hormone therapy, drug therapy
Scoliosis	Abnormal curving of spine	Back brace, surgery
Sprain	Injury to ligament caused by joint overextension	Rest, support, application of cold, anti-inflammatory medications
Tendonitis	Inflammation of tendon	Rest, support, anti-inflammatory medications

* Musculoskeletal diseases and disorders are described in more detail in *The Skeletal System* and *The Muscular System* chapters.

lack of oxygen or blood flow to the brain. The most prevalent sign of encephalopathy is an altered mental state. Common neurological symptoms of encephalopathy are progressive loss of memory and cognitive ability, slight personality changes, inability to concentrate, lethargy, and progressive loss of consciousness.

Orthopedic Diseases and Disorders

Table 42-7 lists many of the diseases and disorders you will encounter in an orthopedic specialty. For example, back pain—especially lower back pain—is a common disorder. It can have many causes, including muscle strain, osteoarthritis, or the presence of a tumor. Treatments include the application of heat, administration of analgesics or muscle relaxants, exercise therapy, special braces, traction, and surgery.

Another condition commonly encountered in the orthopedist's office is a fracture, or break in a bone. Fractures and their treatment are discussed in detail in the *Emergency Preparedness* chapter.

▶ Exams and Procedures in Medical Specialties

LO 42.3

As a medical assistant, understanding the anatomy and physiology of various body systems and the specific exam and procedural steps for each specialty area is key. Most specialists' offices have a procedure manual for you to use as a reference when learning new procedures. You will assist with exams and procedures and perform certain procedures on your own. This section will introduce you to basic exams and procedures performed in medical specialties.

Allergy Exams and Testing

An allergy exam involves a medical history and, usually, several diagnostic tests. You may assist with these tests or perform them yourself under a physician's supervision. Skin tests, for example, involve introducing solutions containing suspected allergens onto or just below the skin. Any reaction is observed and assessed.

Allergy treatments include allergen avoidance, medications, and desensitization to a substance by means of

EDUCATING THE PATIENT
Creating a Dust-Free Environment

Patients with household dust allergies will need to reduce their dust exposure as much as possible. One way they can do this is to keep their environment, especially their bedroom, as clean as possible. Share these guidelines from The National Institute of Allergy and Infectious Diseases with your patients.

- Prepare the room by removing all contents, cleaning and scrubbing all woodwork, removing carpeting and drapery (if possible), and closing doors and windows. Maintain the room by cleaning it thoroughly once a week. This includes floors, the tops of doors, and windowsill and frames. Use a special vacuum filter and wash any curtains often.

- Keep the bed and bedding as dust free as possible by encasing box springs and mattress in a dustproof cover and washing all pajamas in 130°F water.

- Keep furniture in the room to a minimum, use furnace air filters (high-efficiency particulate absorption (HEPA) filters are best), avoid stuffed animals, and keep pets out of the bedroom.

injections. Part of your job will be to encourage patients to make necessary lifestyle changes to avoid allergens. See Educating the Patient: Creating a Dust-Free Environment. You also will help patients adhere to regimens of injections or medication.

Three tests are commonly performed in the allergist's office: the **scratch test**, the **intradermal test**, and the **patch test**. The *radioallergosorbent (RAST)* test is performed in a laboratory. Prior to the scratch, patch, or intradermal test patients are asked to stop taking antihistamines and steroids. These medications could interfere with the test results. The RAST test has the advantage of allowing the patients to continue to take antihistamines to control their allergies while being tested.

Scratch Test A scratch test tests the patient for specific allergies. Extracts of suspected allergens are applied to the patient's skin, usually on the arms or back. One site is always a negative control—a solution like the one used to carry the allergens but containing no allergen is applied. Then the skin is scratched to allow the extracts to penetrate. A scratch test may be performed using sterile needles or lancets. Some allergists prefer to use applicators that allow the tester to apply allergens to and puncture the skin in several places at once, as shown in Figure 42-5. Be sure to let the patient know the procedure may cause some discomfort and that itching afterward can be relieved with cold packs. See Procedure 42-1, Assisting with a Scratch Test Examination, at the end of this chapter. The doctor interprets the test results. Because a delayed reaction is possible, the doctor may wish to recheck the scratch sites in 24 hours. When the results of the scratch test are inconclusive, another test, like an intradermal test, may be ordered.

Intradermal Test This test introduces dilute solutions of allergens into the skin of the inner forearm or upper back with a fine-gauge needle. The intradermal test is more sensitive than the scratch test. A small blister, also known as a wheal, which is filled with the introduced fluid, appears on the skin over the injection site. The allergic reaction time is about 15 to 30 minutes, although some substances may cause delayed reactions. If no reaction appears, the test can be repeated with a more concentrated solution to confirm the result. If a severe reaction occurs, the doctor will order epinephrine to be administered.

The tuberculin test, or purified protein derivative (PPD) test, is a type of intradermal skin test. An extract from the tubercle bacillus is injected into the skin. The results are read in 48 to 72 hours. Raising and hardening of the skin around the area (induration), rather than redness alone, indicate a positive reaction. The procedure for administering an intradermal injection is found in the *Medication Administration* chapter.

Patch Test You perform a patch test by placing a linen or paper patch on uninvolved skin and then using a dropper to soak the patch with the suspected allergen (Figure 42-6). Cellophane or another occlusive material, usually covered with an adhesive patch, is then applied over the linen or paper patch. Among other things this test is used to discover the cause of contact dermatitis.

Radioallergosorbent Test (RAST) The RAST measures blood levels of antibodies to specific allergens. You obtain a blood sample from the patient and send it to a laboratory.

FIGURE 42-5 A multiple applicator allows the medical assistant to apply several allergens at one time.

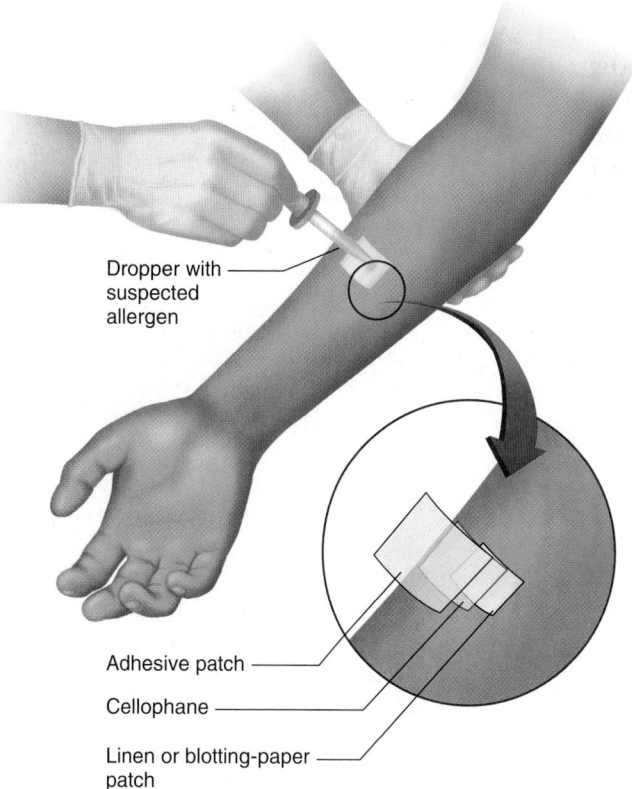

Dropper with suspected allergen

Adhesive patch

Cellophane

Linen or blotting-paper patch

FIGURE 42-6 A patch test is usually done on the arm and is read in 48 hours.

There, the blood serum is exposed to suspected allergens and the levels of antibodies are measured. This test usually provides more information than skin testing but is more expensive.

Cardiology Exams

A general cardiovascular exam usually begins with cardiac auscultation to obtain a blood pressure reading and an evaluation of overall cardiac health. The cardiologist also palpates the heart and chest wall and the vessels in the extremities to detect abnormal vibrations, pulses, swelling, or temperature. In addition, an electrocardiogram may be obtained.

Electrocardiogram An electrocardiogram (ECG or EKG) provides a measurement of the heart's electrical activity. Electrocardiography—a routine part of a cardiovascular exam—is a painless and safe diagnostic test. Electrodes are placed on the skin in particular areas of the chest and limbs. The heart's electrical activity is shown as a tracing on a strip of graph paper. Review the full procedure for performing an ECG in the *Cardiovascular and Respiratory Testing* chapter.

Stress Test A stress test involves recording an ECG while the patient is exercising on a stationary bicycle, treadmill, or stair-stepping ergometer (see Figure 42-7). This test measures the patient's response to a constant or increasing workload. Part of your job may involve keeping the equipment properly maintained and calibrated. You also may be responsible for administering the test itself, but a doctor should always

be present, however, because of the risk of cardiac crisis. Before the test, the patient has a screening appointment with the doctor, during which you take a careful medical history and explain pretest requirements. On the day of the test, be sure the patient has followed pretest directions, like abstaining from smoking or consuming alcohol, and has signed the proper consent form. The patient is prepared as for an ECG by having electrodes attached to the skin. Show the patient how to use the exercise device. Review additional information regarding exercise electrocardiography (stress testing) in the *Cardiovascular and Respiratory Testing* chapter.

A type of stress test called the stress thallium ECG is performed by injecting the radioisotope thallium (201 Tl) into the patient's veins at the time of peak stress. The patient is checked several minutes later to find out how much thallium has been taken up by the heart. Damaged areas do not take up the thallium as rapidly as healthy areas do. In addition, when a patient cannot perform the physical exercise needed for a stress test, a chemical stress test is done. The patient is given a medication that will cause the heart to act like it would if the patient was exercising.

Holter Monitor This is an ECG device that includes a digital or cassette recorder, allowing readings to be taken over a specific period of time. Electrodes are attached to the patient's chest wall in the physician's office. The patient wears a recording device on a belt or sling (Figure 42-8). The patient returns home, and the device monitors heart activity for 24 or more hours. Review additional information regarding ambulatory electrocardiography (Holter monitoring) in the *Cardiovascular and Respiratory Testing* chapter.

Radiography and Imaging Techniques

Various radiography techniques are used in cardiology. Chest X-rays can reveal conditions like cardiac enlargement. In radionuclide studies, the patient ingests or is injected with a radioactive contrast medium, often referred to as a dye. X-rays are then taken. For example, fluoroscopy studies are X-ray exams

FIGURE 42-7 A stress test measures the electrical activity of the heart under a constant or increasing amount of exertion.

FIGURE 42-8 A Holter monitor allows the physician to assess heart function during periods of normal activity.

in which a contrast medium is injected and pictures of the heart in motion are projected onto a closed-circuit television screen. A venogram allows evaluation of the deep veins of the legs. **Angiography** is an X-ray examination of a blood vessel after the injection of a contrast medium. The test, performed in a hospital, evaluates the function and structure of one or more arteries.

Ultrasound, a noninvasive diagnostic method, is also used in cardiology. Doppler ultrasonography tests the body's main blood vessels for conditions such as weaknesses in vessel walls or blocked arteries. With the use of a handheld probe, sound waves are transmitted through the skin and are reflected by the blood cells moving through the blood vessels.

Echocardiography tests the structure and function of the heart through the use of reflected sound waves, or echoes. Sound waves of an extremely high frequency are projected through the chest wall into the heart and are reflected back through a mechanical device. The echoes, recorded on paper or video, can indicate conditions like structural defects and fluid accumulation.

Heart magnetic resonance imaging (MRI) is a diagnostic procedure that uses strong magnets and radio waves to produce images of the heart. This procedure is noninvasive and does not use ionizing radiation, so it is safer than other imaging techniques. Detailed pictures of the heart and heart vessels can be obtained using heart MRI.

Cardiac catheterization is an invasive diagnostic method in which a catheter (a slender, hollow tube) is inserted into a vein or artery in the right or left arm or leg and passed through the blood vessels into the heart. The cardiologist can use this method to take blood samples for analysis, measure the pressure in the heart's chambers, and view the heart's motions with the aid of fluoroscopy. During cardiac catheterization, the physician may choose to perform a **balloon angioplasty** to open partially blocked coronary arteries. This procedure involves passing a slender, hollow tube through the artery at the blockage site. The balloon at the end of the tube is then inflated, compressing the blockage and widening the artery. A metal mesh tube known as a **stent** may be placed in the artery in order to keep it open. These stents are usually coated with medications that prevent the reclosure of the blood vessel.

If the blockage is extensive, the patient may need surgery known as **coronary artery bypass graft (CABG)**, which involves bypassing the blockage with a vessel taken from another area. All of these procedures are performed in the hospital.

Dermatology Exams

During a whole-body skin examination, the dermatologist examines the visible top layer of the entire surface of the skin, including the scalp, the genital area, and the areas between the toes. The physician uses a magnifying lens and a bright light to look for lesions, especially suspicious moles or precancerous growths. Your role in this exam includes preparing patients and helping them into the proper position before examining each skin area. During the exam, drape patients to protect their privacy as much as possible while exposing the area to be examined. The physician also may ask you to take photographs or make sketches of lesions to aid in detecting future changes.

Another type of dermatologic exam is the **Wood's light examination**, in which the physician inspects the patient's skin under an ultraviolet lamp in a darkened room. This examination highlights certain abnormal skin characteristics and aids in diagnosis. The dermatologist also may perform more limited, focused exams to evaluate specific skin conditions or disorders.

Endocrine Exams and Tests

Before an exam, you will take a thorough medical history. The physician will assess the patient's skin condition, weight, and cardiac functioning for clues about illness. An endocrinologist will perform a complete physical exam, including palpation of glands. Most of the endocrine glands are located deep within the body; only the thyroid, the testes, and, to some extent, the ovaries can be examined with palpation or auscultation. Therefore, you may need to collect essential diagnostic urine and blood tests.

Other diagnostic tools used in endocrinology include radiologic tests like X-rays and iodine scans. In a thyroid scan, the patient receives an oral or intravenous (IV) dose of radioactive iodine, and the thyroid is X-rayed as the material is absorbed. Ultrasound also can be employed to view glands or detect tumors. Urine and blood may be tested for the presence of glucose or hormones.

Gastrointestinal Exams

The gastroenterologist's examination of the patient's GI tract covers the mouth (lips, oral cavity, and tongue), the abdomen and lower thorax, the lower sigmoid colon, the rectum, and the anus. Depending on the patient's symptoms, the physician may perform an invasive exam procedure during the patient's first visit. Formerly, such procedures were performed only in hospitals or special medical facilities. Now, many GI specialists' offices are equipped for these procedures and the management of possible resulting emergencies.

You must prepare the patient and provide reassurance during exams and help patients be as comfortable as possible. Your duties during the procedures will vary according to your state's scope of practice and the physician for whom you work. Instruct patients in advance to arrange for someone to drive them to and from the exam. After a procedure in which patients have had a local anesthetic at the back of the throat, caution them to avoid eating until the drug has been eliminated from the body. Otherwise, they could choke or aspirate food particles into the trachea.

Endoscopy *Endoscopy* generally refers to any procedure in which a scope is used to visually inspect a canal or cavity within the body. Most endoscopic exams are performed with a flexible fiber-optic tube that has a lighted instrument on the end. These exams provide direct visualization of a body cavity and a means for collecting tissue biopsies and removing polyps, as in the colon. Endoscopy helps diagnose tumors, ulcers, structural abnormalities, and other problems. It is particularly useful in performing procedures that formerly would have required an incision, like removing stones from the bile duct.

FIGURE 42-9 To perform a peroral endoscopy, the physician inserts a scope through the patient's mouth.

Peroral Endoscopy Peroral endoscopy involves inserting the scope by way of the mouth (Figure 42-9). The patient is sedated and the gag reflex is inhibited with a local anesthetic. The peroral endoscopic procedures include esophagoscopy (esophagus only), gastroscopy (stomach only), duodenoscopy (duodenum only), and panendoscopy (esophagus, stomach, and duodenum) also referred to as an EGD (esophagogastroduodenoscopy).

Colonoscopy Colonoscopy—performed by inserting a colonoscope through the anus—can provide direct visualization of the large intestine. The gastroenterologist uses this procedure to determine the cause of diarrhea, constipation, bleeding, or lower abdominal pain. A colonoscopy also is performed on patients over 50 to screen for abnormal growths called polyps that can lead to colon cancer.

Patient preparation is designed to clear the colon of fecal material so the colon can be seen clearly. The type of preparation varies depending upon the practice where you are working. For example, one regimen requires the patient to follow a liquid diet for 24 to 48 hours before the procedure, then take a cathartic on the two evenings prior to the colonoscopy. Patients may also need to use one or more prepackaged enema preparations the night before and the day of the procedure. Teach the patient the colon cleansing regimen and then tell him to expect diarrhea and possibly mild cramps.

Immediately before the procedure, instruct patients to empty the bladder. Patients should be given a sedative or an analgesic before undergoing the procedure. Patients lie in the Sims' position as the scope is guided through the large intestine. The doctor may manipulate the abdomen to facilitate passage of the scope.

Proctoscopy Proctoscopy is an examination of the lower rectum and anal canal. After an initial digital exam, the proctoscopy is performed with a 3-inch instrument called a proctoscope. This exam can detect hemorrhoids, polyps, fissures, fistulas, and abscesses.

Sigmoidoscopy Sigmoidoscopy is similar to colonoscopy, except that only the sigmoid area of the large intestine (the S-shaped segment between the descending colon and the rectum) is examined. Sigmoidoscopy also aids in diagnosing colon cancer, ulcerations, polyps, tumors, bleeding, and other lower intestinal problems. Patient preparation involves using one or two prepackaged enemas either the night before or the morning of the procedure, depending on the physician's instructions. The method for assisting the physician during a sigmoidoscopy is described in Procedure 42-2, at the end of this chapter.

Diagnostic and Laboratory Testing A GI specialist may order laboratory analysis of stomach contents (obtained by gastric lavage) to determine the presence of bacteria or gastric bleeding. Another important test for GI specialists is the occult blood test, in which the feces are analyzed for occult, or hidden, bleeding from the intestinal tract. This is discussed in the *Testing and Processing Urine and Stool Specimens* chapter.

Gastroenterologists sometimes use imaging techniques, such as X-rays, ultrasound, radionuclide imaging, computed tomography (CT), and magnetic resonance imaging. Most GI radiologic exams are not performed in an office, but you should know enough about them to answer patients' questions. Generally, these exams are performed in a hospital X-ray laboratory or an outpatient facility. You may be responsible for scheduling tests at such facilities for patients. You also may help prepare the patient for these exams. However, in some cases, the patient should discuss specific preparation with personnel from the other facility.

Cholecystography Cholecystography is a gallbladder function test performed by X-ray with a contrast agent. The patient swallows tablets of the contrast agent the night before the test. X-rays taken 12 to 14 hours later should show the contrast agent in the gallbladder. The patient then swallows a substance high in fat, which should make the gallbladder contract and empty the contrast agent into the duodenum. If the contrast agent is not taken up by the gallbladder or if the gallbladder does not contract properly, the physician can determine whether there is bile duct obstruction or gallstones. See the *Diagnostic Imaging* chapter for further information about cholecystography.

Ultrasound Ultrasound is used commonly for diagnosing problems in the gallbladder, pancreas, spleen, and liver. The patient should have nothing to eat or drink after midnight of the night before and on the morning of the exam. Some gastroenterologists may perform ultrasound exams in the office.

Barium Swallow The barium swallow (also called an upper GI series) is used to detect abnormalities in the esophagus, stomach, and small intestine. The patient swallows a liquid containing barium—an insoluble contrast agent. This material is viewed using fluoroscopy (moving X-ray images) as

FIGURE 42-10 During a barium enema, the barium is tracked on X-rays.

the liquid is swallowed and passes into the stomach. X-ray films are taken at frequent intervals to record the diagnostic images. The patient is asked to move into various positions while the barium is tracked through the small intestine. To prepare for this test, the patient should have nothing to eat or drink after midnight the night before and on the morning of the procedure. Refer to the *Diagnostic Imaging* chapter for more information.

Barium Enema A barium enema (also called a lower GI series) is used to detect abnormalities in the large intestine. Barium is given as an enema in this test. A balloon-like tube is inflated in the rectum during the X-ray and the patient is asked to move into various positions to ensure that the barium is distributed completely (Figure 40-10). Patients must eat no meats or vegetables for 1 to 3 days before the test to avoid incorrect indications on the X-ray. For 24 hours before the test, they must also follow a liquid diet, which includes drinking special liquid laxative preparations and more than a quart of water. Specific steps vary depending on the facility, but the intent is to cleanse the colon completely. See the *Diagnostic Imaging* chapter for more information.

Radionuclide Imaging Radiology subspecialists trained in nuclear medicine perform nuclear medicine studies with radionuclide imaging. The patient is first injected with a radioactive substance, then waits a prescribed length of time for the radioactive substance to be taken up by the body part being imaged. The patient is scanned or photographed with a special gamma camera, which can read the radioactive areas to determine abnormalities in their composition. This technique is commonly used for liver, spleen, thyroid, and bone scans.

Neurologic Exams and Diagnostic Testing

The neurologist evaluates five categories of neurologic function in a complete exam:

- Cognitive function (mental status)
- Cranial nerves
- Motor system
- Reflexes
- Sensory system

Cognitive function can be assessed by observing general appearance and grooming as well as by asking patients specific questions. The neurologist also determines the status of the cranial nerves, which affect smell and taste, eye movements, hearing, voice quality, facial expression, and facial mobility. The physician may, for example, ask patients to close their eyes and then identify familiar smells. The neurologist observes patients' faces for symmetry of movement and tests visual and auditory acuity. The physician assesses motor ability by testing coordination, observing gait, and determining muscle strength. Finally, the neurologist tests patients' reflexes and examines the function of the sensory system in areas of tactile sensation, pain and temperature sensitivity, and awareness of vibration. You are likely to assist the physician in completing these exams, and you may perform certain components yourself.

Common diagnostic tests in neurology include electroencephalography and various radiologic tests. You may assist in performing these tests. Invasive tests may not be done at the physician's office. In such cases, you will need to schedule the procedures, instruct patients about pretest preparations, and educate them about the procedure and what to expect.

Electroencephalography Electroencephalography records the electrical activity of the brain on a strip of graph paper. The tracing is an electroencephalogram (EEG). Electrodes are attached to the patient's scalp and readings are taken while the patient is at rest and engaged in specific activities. An EEG can be used to detect or examine conditions such as tumors, seizure disorders, or brain injury. You may assist with electrode placement or, after training, obtain the EEG on your own.

Imaging Procedures Several imaging techniques are used as neurological diagnostic tools. Types of procedures include angiograms, brain scans, CT, MRI, myelography, and skull X-rays.

Cerebral Angiography Cerebral angiography (or angiogram) is a radiologic study of the cerebral blood vessels. After a contrast medium is injected into an artery, X-rays are taken to visualize the cerebral blood vessels.

Brain Scan A brain scan is performed by injecting the patient with radioisotopes and, after a period of time, using a scanner to detect the material. The radioisotopes tend to gather in areas of abnormality, such as tumors or abscesses.

FIGURE 42-11 Magnetic resonance imaging is used to diagnose disorders in many specialties.

Computed Tomography **Computed tomography**, often called a CT scan, is a radiographic exam that produces a three-dimensional, cross-sectional view of the brain. Often one scan is done without a contrast medium. Then a contrast medium is injected for greater clarity. CT scans can help diagnose a wide range of conditions, including tumors, blood clots, and brain swelling.

Magnetic Resonance Imaging **Magnetic resonance imaging (MRI)** is a viewing technique that enables physicians to see areas inside the body without exposing the patient to X-rays or surgery. The procedure, which takes 30 to 60 minutes, requires the patient to lie still on a padded table that is moved into a tunnel-like structure (Figure 42-11). A powerful magnetic field produces an image of internal body structures. Newer MRI scanners are open for patients who are unable to tolerate being inside a tunnel-like structure.

Positron Emission Tomography **Positron emission tomography**, often called a **PET** scan, studies the blood flow and metabolic activity in the brain to help physicians identify certain neurological and CNS disorders. These disorders include Parkinson's disease, multiple sclerosis, Alzheimer's disease, transient ischemic attack (TIA), amyotrophic lateral sclerosis (ALS), Huntington's disease, epilepsy, stroke, cancer, and schizophrenia.

Myelography Myelography is an X-ray visualization of the spinal cord after the injection of a radioactive contrast medium or air into the spinal subarachnoid space (between the second and innermost of three membranes covering the spinal cord). This test can reveal tumors, cysts, spinal stenosis, or herniated disks.

Skull X-Ray Skull X-rays may be used to detect breaks in the skull and to locate tumors.

Other Tests Other diagnostic tests—including lumbar puncture and electromyography—do not involve imaging techniques. A lumbar puncture, or spinal tap, involves collecting a sample of cerebrospinal fluid (CSF) to diagnose infection, to measure CSF pressure, and to check for blood cells and proteins in the fluid. A needle is inserted between two lumbar vertebrae and into the subarachnoid space. The collected fluid is sent to a laboratory for analysis. **Electromyography** is used to detect neuromuscular disorders or nerve damage. Needle electrodes are inserted into some of the patient's skeletal muscles. When the muscles contract, a monitor records the nerve impulses and measures conduction time.

Oncology Exams and Diagnostic Testing

An exam in an oncologist's office focuses on the area of the body where a problem is suspected. The oncologist's goal is to detect, diagnose, and treat cancer. Cancer is detected and diagnosed through a variety of procedures. You will schedule some of these tests and provide pretest instructions and explanations to patients.

A biopsy is a common procedure an oncologist may perform, and you may assist with the procedure. There are several types of biopsies. A physician performs an incisional, or open, biopsy by making an incision and removing a piece of tissue. A needle biopsy is performed by removing tissue with a needle inserted through the skin into the growth or area. Needle aspiration is performed by removing fluid from a lump or cyst with a needle. Procedure 42-3, at the end of this chapter, describes the steps in assisting with a needle biopsy. During a biopsy, Standard Precautions and sterile technique must be maintained. Always place the specimen in a prepared, labeled container provided by the laboratory. Transport it according to laboratory instructions, attaching the proper accompanying forms. After the biopsy, you might assist with or perform the cleaning and bandaging of the site.

In addition to a biopsy, you may obtain blood specimens for some tests and assist in other diagnostic procedures, including

- X-rays
- CT scan
- MRI
- Blood tests, especially those to detect tumor markers, such as carcinoembryonic antigen (CEA) (increased levels of CEA indicate a variety of cancers), CA125, and CA15-3
- Ultrasonography

Cancer Treatment

Cancer treatments fall into three general categories: surgery, radiation therapy, and chemotherapy. Often, a combination of these treatment methods is used. All methods damage healthy as well as cancerous cells. The success of treatment depends on many factors, and recovery varies greatly from patient to patient.

Surgery Surgical removal of the tumor and some surrounding tissue is one method of cancer treatment. It is most

TABLE 42-8	Chemotherapy Drugs	
Category	**Mechanism of Action**	**Examples**
Alkylating agents	Hinder cell division	Chlorambucil, cyclophosphamide
Antimetabolites	Interfere with folic acid and nucleic acid synthesis	Methotrexate, fluorouracil
Antibiotics	Break DNA strands	Actinomycin, bleomycin
Antimitotic agents	Affect cell division	Vinblastine, paclitaxel

effective when the tumor appears to be contained within a particular organ or is localized in an area of the skin. Surgery is often followed, however, by either radiation therapy or chemotherapy.

Radiation Therapy Radiation therapy uses radiation to kill and stop the growth of tumor cells. It is often used in conjunction with surgery or chemotherapy. Radiation therapy is effective because although radiation affects all living cells, it has the most damaging effect on cells that are undergoing rapid division, like cancer cells.

Chemotherapy Chemotherapy is also used in conjunction with other therapies. Chemotherapy is the use of strong anticancer drugs to kill malignant cells. As with radiation therapy, rapidly dividing cells like cancer cells are most strongly affected by these medications. A variety of chemotherapy drugs are available, each with slightly different mechanisms of action. Table 42-8 describes common classes of chemotherapy drugs and outlines their major categories, their mechanism of action, and some examples in each category. These drugs can be used alone or in combination, depending on the type of cancer being treated. Although it is unlikely you will prepare or administer anticancer drugs, you need to be aware that they are highly toxic. General protective guidelines including using PPE must be followed whenever there is risk of contact with the drugs or patients' body fluids.

Orthopedic Exams and Procedures

An orthopedist uses inspection, palpation, and a variety of diagnostic tests to assess the structure and function of the musculoskeletal system. The patient is asked to stand, walk, and perform several range-of-motion exercises. The physician notes the degree of mobility the patient has, in some cases using a device called a *goniometer*. A complete exam takes some time, and you may need to help drape, position, or physically support the patient, especially if the patient is elderly or incapacitated. You also may be responsible for instructing the patient about care for a musculoskeletal condition, including how to perform therapeutic exercises.

Orthopedists use a variety of diagnostic tests. Bone and muscle biopsies may be performed to detect disorders like bone infection and muscle atrophy. Electromyography is another diagnostic tool used in this specialty. An orthopedist also may order urine and blood tests to detect levels of substances like calcium or phosphorus.

As in most other specialties, X-rays play a vital role in diagnosis and may be performed right in the orthopedist's office. X-rays are especially useful in determining the nature and extent of a bone injury. Other common radiographic exams in the orthopedic specialty include

- CT scan
- MRI
- Angiography (for affected vascular structures)
- Myelography (for spinal disorders)
- Diskography (for intervertebral disk disorders)
- Arthrography (for joint disorders)
- Bone scans

These procedures are discussed in more detail in the *Diagnostic Imaging* chapter.

Arthroscopy enables the orthopedist to see inside a joint—usually the knee, shoulder, or hip—with an arthroscope. This tubular instrument includes an optical system; when the tube is inserted into the joint, it can be visualized (Figure 42-12). Arthroscopy is used to give the physician a closer look at conditions such as injuries and degenerative joint diseases and to guide surgical procedures.

Joint replacement surgery is often used to treat knee and hip joints severely damaged by arthritis, disease, or injury. Hip replacement may be indicated in cases of severe arthritis pain, femoral neck fractures, or hip joint tumors. Knee pain that does not respond to medications or physical therapy or a knee damaged by severe arthritis may indicate the need for knee replacement. Both surgeries require that the damaged joint be removed and an artificial joint inserted in its place. Physical therapy is usually started soon after surgery. Most patients fully recover in 3 to 12 months.

FIGURE 42-12 Arthroscopy can be used for diagnosis as well as biopsy and surgical repair.

PROCEDURE 42-1 Assisting with a Scratch Test Examination

Procedure Goal: To assist a licensed practitioner in determining substances to which a patient has an allergic reaction.

OSHA Guidelines:

Materials: Disposable sterile needles or lancets, allergen extracts, control solution, cotton balls, alcohol, timer, adhesive tape, ruler, cold packs or an ice bag.

Method: Procedure steps.

1. Wash your hands and assemble the necessary materials.
2. Identify the patient and introduce yourself.
3. Show the patient into the treatment area. Explain the procedure and discuss any concerns. Confirm whether the patient followed pretesting procedures such as discontinuing medications.
   RATIONALE: Antihistamines and steroids may interfere with the test.
4. Assist the patient into a comfortable position and don exam gloves.
5. Swab the test site, usually the upper arm or back, with an alcohol prep pad.
6. Identify the sites with tape labels.
   RATIONALE: The sites must be easily identified so you can record reactions to individual antigens.

7. Apply small drops of the allergen extracts and control solution onto the test site at evenly spaced intervals, about 1½ to 2 inches apart.
8. Open the package containing the first needle or lancet, making sure you do not contaminate the instrument.
9. Assist the physician with the scratch procedure or perform the procedure if it is within your scope of practice. Using a new sterile needle or lancet for each site, scratch the skin beneath each drop of allergen, no more than ⅛-inch deep.
10. Start the timer for the 20-minute reaction period.
11. After the reaction time has passed, cleanse each site with an alcohol prep pad. (Do not remove identifying labels until the physician has checked the patient.)
12. Assist the physician or examine and measure the sites.

Negative   +1   +2   +3   +4
           5 mm   10 mm   15 mm   20 mm

FIGURE Procedure 42-1 Step 12   Physicians classify skin reactions as either negative (no greater than the reaction to the control) or positive. Positive reactions are rated on a scale of +1 to +4, depending on the size of the wheal.

13. Apply cold packs or an ice bag to sites as needed to relieve itching.
14. Properly dispose of used materials and instruments.
15. Clean and disinfect the area according to OSHA guidelines.
16. Remove the gloves and wash your hands.
17. Document the test results in the patient's chart, if required, and initial your entries.

    Example Documentation:

    > Scratch test to back results. Pollen +2, Fragrance mix 0, Benzalkonium chloride +4, Animal dander +3 _____ *Kaylyn R. Haddix RMA (AMT)*

FIGURE Procedure 42-1 Step 6   Label each site with the name of the allergen or an accepted abbreviation.

PROCEDURE 42-2 Assisting with a Sigmoidoscopy

Procedure Goal: To assist the physician during the examination of the rectum, anus, and sigmoid colon using a sigmoidoscope.

OSHA Guidelines:

Materials: Sigmoidoscope, suction pump, lubricating jelly, drape, patient gown, and tissues.

Method: Procedure steps.

1. Wash your hands and assemble and position materials and equipment according to the physician's preference.
2. Test the suction pump.
3. Identify the patient and introduce yourself.
4. Show the patient into the treatment room. Explain the procedure and discuss any concerns the patient may have.
5. Instruct the patient to empty the bladder, take off all clothing from the waist down, and put on the gown with the opening in the back.
6. Don exam gloves and assist the patient into the knee-chest or Sims' position. Immediately cover the patient with a drape.
7. Use warm water to bring the sigmoidoscope to slightly above body temperature; lubricate the tip.
   RATIONALE: To ensure patient comfort.
8. Assist as needed, including handing the doctor the necessary instruments and equipment.
9. Monitor the patient's reactions during the procedure and relay any signs of pain to the doctor.
10. Clean the anal area with tissues after the exam.
11. Properly dispose of used materials and disposable instruments.
12. Remove the gloves and wash your hands.
13. Help the patient gradually assume a comfortable position.
    RATIONALE: The patient should sit up slowly so he does not become faint.
14. Instruct the patient to dress.
15. Don clean gloves.
16. Sanitize reusable instruments and prepare them for disinfection and/or sterilization, as necessary.
17. Clean and disinfect the equipment and the room according to OSHA guidelines.
18. Remove the gloves and wash your hands.

PROCEDURE 42-3 Assisting with a Needle Biopsy

Procedure Goal: To assist the licensed practitioner with removing tissue from a patient's body so it can be examined in a laboratory.

OSHA Guidelines:

Materials: Sterile drapes; tray or Mayo stand; antiseptic solution; cotton balls; local anesthetic; disposable sterile biopsy needle or disposable sterile syringe and needle; sterile sponges; specimen bottle with fixative solution; laboratory packaging; and sterile wound-dressing materials.

Method: Procedure steps.

1. Identify the patient and introduce yourself.
2. Instruct the patient as needed and discuss any concerns the patient may have.
3. Wash your hands and assemble the necessary materials.
4. Prepare the sterile field and instruments.
5. Don exam gloves.
6. Position and drape the patient.
7. Cleanse the biopsy site. Prepare the patient's skin.
   RATIONALE: To reduce the possibility of infection.
8. Remove the gloves, wash your hands, and don clean exam gloves.
9. Assist the doctor as needed when she injects anesthetic.
10. Perform a surgical scrub and don sterile gloves if you will be handing the physician's sterile instruments.
11. Place the sample in a properly labeled specimen bottle, complete the laboratory requisition form, and package the specimen for immediate laboratory transport.
    RATIONALE: The specimen must be properly labeled and accompanied by a completed laboratory requisition form to ensure the specimen is not lost and the appropriate tests are completed in the lab.
12. Apply a dressing to the patient's wound site.
13. Properly dispose of used supplies and instruments.
14. Clean and disinfect the room according to OSHA guidelines.
15. Remove the gloves and wash your hands.
16. Document as needed.
    Example Documentation:

> Needle biopsy performed by Dr. Buckwalter. Specimen labeled and sent to MEDLab. _____ *Kaylyn R. Haddix RMA (AMT)*

LEARNING OUTCOMES	KEY POINTS
42.1 **Describe the medical specialties of allergy, cardiology, dermatology, endocrinology, gastroenterology, neurology, oncology, and orthopedics.**	The medical specialties discussed in this chapter include allergy, which is diagnosing and treating allergies (inappropriate immune system responses); cardiology, which is the study and treatment of heart diseases and disorders; dermatology, or the diagnosis and treatment of skin diseases and disorders such as acne, eczema, and skin cancer; endocrinology, or the treatment of diseases and disorders of the endocrine system, which includes glands that regulate and coordinate the body systems; gastroenterology, or the diagnosis and treatment of disorders of the entire gastrointestinal (GI) tract, from the mouth to the anus, as well as the liver and pancreas; neurology, or the diagnosis and treatment of diseases and disorders of the central nervous system (CNS) and associated systems; oncology, which is a medical specialty that is concerned with the detection and treatment of tumors and cancerous growths; and orthopedics, which is the medical specialty focusing on disorders, injuries, and diseases of the muscular and skeletal systems.
42.2 **Identify common diseases and disorders related to cardiology, dermatology, endocrinology, gastroenterology, neurology, oncology, and orthopedics.**	Many common diseases and disorders are identified in the specialty practices. You should have an understanding of the implications of these diseases on the patient and the necessary treatments.
42.3 **Relate the role of the medical assistant in examinations and procedures performed in the medical specialties of allergy, cardiology, dermatology, endocrinology, gastroenterology, neurology, oncology, and orthopedics.**	Exams and diagnostic tests performed in allergy, cardiology, dermatology, endocrinology, gastroenterology, neurology, oncology, and orthopedics specialties are numerous. During most of these exams and tests, your role may include patient safety and comfort, educating the patient about the necessary preparation and the procedure, and assisting the physician.

CASE STUDY CRITICAL THINKING

Recall Valarie Ramirez from the beginning of the chapter. Now that you have completed the chapter, answer the following questions regarding her case.

1. How would you chart Valarie's chief complaint?

2. The physician thinks Valarie has a thyroid nodule that may be cancer. Which two types of specialists may she need to visit?

3. The physician wants to evaluate the thyroid nodule by performing a needle biopsy. What will be your responsibilities during this procedure?

1. (LO 42.1) In which medical specialty practice would you most likely be working if you are assisting with a scratch test?
   a. Dermatology
   b. Cardiology
   c. Oncology
   d. Allergy
   e. Endocrinology

2. (LO 42.3) You just finished patient education for a patient who is to have a colonoscopy tomorrow. At which of the following specialty practices do you most likely work?
   a. Cardiology
   b. Gastroenterology
   c. Surgery
   d. Urology
   e. Oncology

3. (LO 42.3) A patient has a growth on his arm and the physician removes some of the tissue of the growth. He most likely had a
   a. Needle aspiration
   b. Wood's light examination
   c. Needle biopsy
   d. CABG
   e. RAST test

4. (LO 42.1) Which specialist would do a whole-body skin examination?
   a. Dermatologist
   b. Cardiologist
   c. Oncologist
   d. Allergist
   e. Endocrinologist

5. (LO 42.1) If a patient is suffering from diabetes Type I, what specialist would he most likely visit?
   a. Dermatologist
   b. Cardiologist
   c. Oncologist
   d. Allergist
   e. Endocrinologist

6. (LO 42.2) The patient has been diagnosed with the most dangerous type of skin cancer. What type of cancer does he have?
   a. Basal cell
   b. Melanoma
   c. Squamous cell
   d. Diabetic
   e. Arthritic

7. (LO 42.2) The patient has been diagnosed with Alzheimer's disease and will most likely see a specialist in
   a. Neurology
   b. Cardiology
   c. Endocrinology
   d. Oncology
   e. Dermatology

8. (LO 42.2) The type of medication used to treat cancer is
   a. Antibiotic
   b. Radiation
   c. Retinoid
   d. Contraceptives
   e. Chemotherapy

9. (LO 42.3) The patient has been instructed to sit up slowly after a sigmoidoscopy. What is the most likely reason?
   a. To prevent bleeding
   b. To maintain asepsis
   c. To prevent the patient from getting faint
   d. To check for a reaction
   e. To ensure the test is done accurately

10. (LO 42.3) After a scratch test, you charted +4 pollen. What does this most likely mean?
    a. The test was negative
    b. The test was mildly positive
    c. The test was +4 on a scale of 1 to 10
    d. The test was positive with a wheal of 10 mm
    e. The test was positive with a wheal of 20 mm

C A S E   S T U D Y

PATIENT INFORMATION

Patient Name	Gender	DOB
Valarie Ramirez	Female	8/4/19XX

Attending	MRN	Allergies
Paul F. Buckwalter, MD	829-78-462	Penicillin

eye and determined that there is a small amount of debris in the eye. The physician has asked you to assist with eye irrigation.

Keep Valarie in mind as you study this chapter. There will be questions at the end of the chapter based on the case study. The information in the chapter will help you answer these questions.

Valarie Ramirez, a 33-year-old female, has been examined by the physician after complaining that something flew into her eye while she was riding her motorcycle yesterday. The physician has examined the

L E A R N I N G   O U T C O M E S

After completing Chapter 43, you will be able to:

43.1 Describe the medical assistant's role in eye exams and procedures performed in a medical office.

43.2 Discuss various eye disorders encountered in a medical office.

43.3 Identify ophthalmic exams performed in the physician's office.

43.4 Summarize ophthalmologic procedures and treatments.

43.5 Describe the medical assistant's role in otology.

43.6 Describe disorders of the ear encountered in the medical office.

43.7 Recall various hearing and other diagnostic ear tests.

43.8 Summarize ear procedures and treatments.

K E Y   T E R M S

astigmatism
audiologist
audiometer
cochlear implant
conductive hearing loss
decibels
frequency
hyperopia
myopia

ophthalmoscope
otologist
presbyopia
refraction examination
sensorineural hearing loss
slit lamp
tinnitus
tonometer

I. C (6) Identify common pathology related to each body system

I. C (7) Analyze pathology as it relates to the interaction of body systems

I. C (9) Describe implications for treatment related to pathology

I. C (12) Describe the relationship between anatomy and physiology of all body systems and medications used for treatment in each

I. P (10) Assist physician with patient care

I. A (1) Apply critical thinking skills in performing patient assessment and care

I. A (2) Use language/verbal skills that enable patients' understanding

IV. C (7) Identify resources and adaptations that are required based on individual needs, i.e., culture and environment, developmental life stage, language, and physical threats to communication

IV. P (6) Prepare a patient for procedures and/or treatments

IV. P (8) Document patient care

IX. P (7) Document accurately in the patient record

2. **Anatomy and Physiology**
   Graduates:
   b. Identify and apply the knowledge of all body systems, their structure and functions, and their common diseases, symptoms and etiologies
   c. Assist the physician with the regimen of diagnostic and treatment modalities as they relate to each body system

3. **Medical Terminology**
   Graduates:
   c. Understand the various medical terminology for each specialty

4. **Medical Law and Ethics**
   Graduates:
   a. Document accurately

5. **Psychology of Human Relations**
   Graduates:
   b. Identify and respond appropriately when working/caring for patients with special needs

9. **Medical Office Clinical Procedures**
   Graduates:
   m. Assist physician with routine and specialty examinations and treatments
   p. Advise patients of office policies and procedures
   q. Instruct patients with special needs

Introduction

Think about how often you use your eyes and ears. You use your eyes to *read* the words on this page and watch the rise and fall of a patient's chest while counting their respirations. Both your eyes and ears are needed when watching the dial on a sphygmomanometer while listening for the first Korotkoff sound while taking a blood pressure. These are daily activities for a medical assistant. Good eye and ear care is critical for you and for your patients. In this chapter, you will explore the role of ophthalmology and otology in patient care, various eye and ear disorders, and exams and procedures related to the eye and ear, including vision and hearing tests.

Ophthalmology

LO 43.1

Ophthalmology is a branch of medicine specializing in the anatomy, function, and diseases of the eye. An ophthalmologist specializes in medical and surgical eye problems, treating the eyes and related tissues. The most common eye disorders that an ophthalmologist treats are visual defects, which are often correctable with eyeglasses or contact lenses. Ophthalmologists also treat eye injuries and remove foreign bodies from the eye. More serious

disorders, like cataracts and glaucoma, require medication or surgery. In an ophthalmologist's office, you may perform some of the procedures that involve measuring various aspects and functions of the eye, such as visual acuity, color vision, and intraocular pressure. You also may perform some of these exams in a general practice office or an optometrist's office. Optometrists diagnose and treat visual defects only with glasses or contacts. Review eye anatomy and pathophysiology in the *Special Senses* chapter.

Eye Diseases and Disorders

LO 43.2

You may encounter a wide range of eye diseases and disorders in an ophthalmologist's or general practitioner's office. Some, such as a sty or conjunctivitis, do not greatly affect vision and may be treated by a general practitioner. Others affect the eye's internal workings and require a specialist's attention.

Disorders of External Eye Structures

Some disorders affect external eye structures, such as the eyelid and the eyelashes.

Blepharitis Blepharitis is a chronic inflammation of the eyelid's edges, more common in older individuals than in younger people. It can be caused by infection or by the same skin condition that causes dandruff. Symptoms include red, swollen eyelids with scaling or crusting of skin at the edges. The patient's eyes may be irritated and itchy. Proper eye care and hygiene often clear up the condition successfully. Antibiotic creams may be necessary in severe cases.

Ptosis Ptosis is a drooping of the upper eyelid in which the lid partially or completely covers the eye. It is caused by weakness of or damage to the muscle that raises the eyelid or by problems with the nerve that controls the muscle. Often no treatment is required, although surgery may be performed if the condition interferes with vision or if the patient is concerned about appearance.

Sty A sty (external hordeolum) is the result of an eyelash follicle infection. The microorganism most often responsible for the infection is *Staphylococcus aureus*. A red, painful swelling appears on the eye's edge and typically forms a white head of pus. The head bursts and drains before it heals in about a week. Applying warm, moist compresses to the sty may help it drain sooner.

Disorders of Structures at the Front of the Eye

Another group of disorders affects structures at the front of the eye, which include the conjunctiva and the cornea.

Conjunctivitis Conjunctivitis, or pinkeye, is an inflammation of the conjunctiva caused by an allergy, irritant, or infection. It is a common disorder that is annoying but normally not serious.

Allergic conjunctivitis occurs when a person has an allergic reaction to pollen, makeup, or other substance. The symptoms are itchy, red eyes. The doctor may prescribe medication to relieve troublesome symptoms and suggest avoidance of the trigger whenever possible. Irritants like dust, smoke, wind, pollutants, and excessive glare also may cause conjunctivitis.

Infectious conjunctivitis can be caused by either a bacterial or a viral infection. Both forms are easily spread and have symptoms including redness and a gritty feeling in the eye. Bacterial infections typically produce pus, which may form a crust on the eye during sleep. Viral infections usually produce a watery discharge. Although eye irrigation or saline drops may be used to soothe eyes affected by either type of infection, only bacterial infections are treated with antibiotic drops or ointment.

Because you may not know the cause of a patient's conjunctivitis (allergies, irritants, bacteria, viruses), take precautions to avoid spreading infection. As with any potentially infectious disease, use Standard Precautions in medical settings. Wear appropriate personal protective equipment when dealing with any patient who has conjunctivitis.

Corneal Ulcers and Abrasions Ulcers (lesions) on the cornea may be the result of injury, infection, or both. An injury like an abrasion (scratch) on the cornea can become infected with bacteria, viruses, or fungi. The symptoms of a corneal ulcer include pain or discomfort and unclear vision.

Treatment consists of antibiotic eyedrops or ointments and drops that temporarily paralyze the eye's ciliary muscles—those that control the shape of the lens—to help control pain. Patching the eye is no longer recommended because doing so creates a warm, moist environment that supports further growth of microorganisms.

Disorders Involving Internal Eye Structures

Another group of disorders affects structures inside the eye. Cataracts, for example, affect the lens, while glaucoma can damage several internal eye structures.

Cataracts Cataracts are cloudy or opaque areas in the normally clear lens of the eye. Cataracts develop gradually, blocking the passage of light through the eye. The result is a progressive loss of vision in one or both eyes. In severe cases, you can actually see the cloudy lens through the eye's pupil (Figure 43-1).

Cataracts are more common in the elderly than in younger people because the lens deteriorates with aging. Cataracts also can be caused by iritis, injury, ultraviolet radiation, or diabetes. Some cataracts are congenital. Treatment includes surgically removing the lens and using an artificial lens in its place. The artificial lens may be in the form of special eyeglasses, special contact lenses, or an intraocular lens inserted at the time of cataract surgery.

Glaucoma Glaucoma is a condition in which fluid pressure builds up inside the eye. This pressure damages the eye's internal structures and gradually destroys vision. Glaucoma is the second leading cause of blindness in the United States and the first cause among African Americans. According to Prevent Blindness America, 2.3 million Americans over age 40 have glaucoma.

Capillaries in the ciliary body produce aqueous humor—a sticky, watery fluid that circulates between the lens and the cornea. In a patient with healthy eyes, this fluid drains out of this

FIGURE 43-1 The lens of an eye with a cataract has a clouded appearance.

area through the angle formed by the iris and the cornea. The aqueous humor then diffuses into a vascular channel (Schlemm's canal) that encircles the cornea where it meets the sclera—the white of the eye (see the *Special Senses* chapter). The aqueous humor then returns to the systemic circulation (the circulation of the blood to body tissues). However, in a patient with glaucoma, the fluid drains out of the eye too slowly or fails to drain at all. The result is a buildup of intraocular pressure. Retinal nerve fibers are damaged and blood vessels are destroyed, leading to loss of vision and possible blindness.

Glaucoma is treated with medication that reduces pressure in the eye. Drops, pills, or both may be prescribed to reduce the production of aqueous humor. Sometimes, an iridotomy—a type of laser surgery procedure in which a small hole is created in the iris that allows excess fluid to drain—is performed. If the surgery is not effective, an iridectomy (partial removal of the iris) is done to create a larger opening in the iris to allow drainage.

Iritis Iritis, also known as anterior uveitis, is an inflammation of the iris and sometimes the ciliary body. There are nearly 37,000 cases of uveitis per year in the United States; 90% of these are anterior uveitis—iritis. The cause is often unknown but may be associated with eye trauma, infection, and some autoimmune diseases. White blood cells from the inflamed area and protein that leaks from small blood vessels float in the aqueous humor. The symptoms of iritis are pain or discomfort in one or both eyes; pain may be worse in bright light. The eye is red and loss of vision may occur. Left untreated, iritis can lead to other complications, like glaucoma and cataracts. Iritis is treated with anti-inflammatory drops or ointment.

Disorders of the Retina

Several serious disorders affect the retina—the internal layer of the back of the eye. These disorders include retinal detachment, diabetic retinopathy, and macular degeneration.

Retinal Detachment Retinal detachment occurs when the retina separates from the underlying choroid layer—the middle, vascular layer of the eye. When this separation occurs, vision is damaged.

Early symptoms of detachment include flashes of light or floating black shapes, both of which can occur as the hole in the retina forms. Patients occasionally describe their field of vision as being like a window shade that has been pulled down. Peripheral vision is lost as the retina detaches. Vision becomes progressively blurred as detachment continues.

A hole in the retina can be fixed with cryopexy—surgical fixation with cold. During the procedure, the physician places a freezing probe on the outside of the eye over the area of the retinal tear, freezing the area and creating a thin scar that seals the hole. If the retina has already detached, some vision can often be restored with new surgical and laser treatments.

Diabetic Retinopathy Diabetic retinopathy is a complication of diabetes. People who have had diabetes for a long time or who do not keep their condition under control experience damage to small blood vessels that supply the retina. The vessels initially leak fluid, which distorts vision. As the disease progresses, fragile new blood vessels grow on the retina and bleed into the vitreous humor—the thick, jelly-like fluid that fills the posterior eye chamber. Scar tissue also may form on the retina. The result is loss of vision. The damage usually cannot be repaired, but the disorder can be controlled to prevent further loss of vision.

Macular Degeneration The macula is the area of the retina responsible for the central area of a person's visual field. For unknown reasons, the macula begins to deteriorate as some individuals age. Macular degeneration causes loss of vision in the center of an image; peripheral vision remains intact. Macular degeneration is the leading cause of blindness among the elderly in the United States. According to the National Eye Institute, 1.75 million Americans have age-related macular degeneration.

When an individual develops macular degeneration, the loss of sharp vision occurs very gradually and without pain. One of the first signs is difficulty in reading. The loss of vision often appears as a dark spot in the center of the field of vision. If macular degeneration is detected early, laser surgery may restore some vision or prevent further loss.

Disorders Involving Eye Movement

Normally, both eyes move together when people look at objects. However, a deviation of one eye is called strabismus. In young children, misaligned or unbalanced eye muscles cause strabismus. This misalignment makes it appear as though the child is looking in two different directions. A condition called amblyopia may occur as the misaligned eye becomes "lazy." The brain tends to ignore what the lazy eye sees; if the condition is not treated, vision will be affected in this eye. Treatment involves putting a patch over the fully working eye to force the child to use the other eye. Eyeglasses may be used along with the patch. In some cases, surgery on the eye muscle is required.

Strabismus in adults usually results from problems with the nerves connecting the brain and the eye muscles or with the muscles themselves. Conditions that can cause such problems include diabetes, high blood pressure, brain injury, muscular dystrophy, and inflammation of certain cerebral arteries. Treatment depends on the cause of the condition.

Refractive Disorders

Refraction refers to the way light from objects is focused through the eye to form an image on the retina. The normal eye focuses light exactly at the retina, producing a clear image (Figure 43-2). In some people, the eye focuses light either in front of or behind the retina, so the image is not clear. The problem may be the result of an abnormal shape of the eye or due to abnormal focusing of the light by the cornea and lens. The most common refractive disorders are nearsightedness, farsightedness, presbyopia, and astigmatism.

(a)   Lens shape for distant vision   Lens shape for near vision (accommodation)

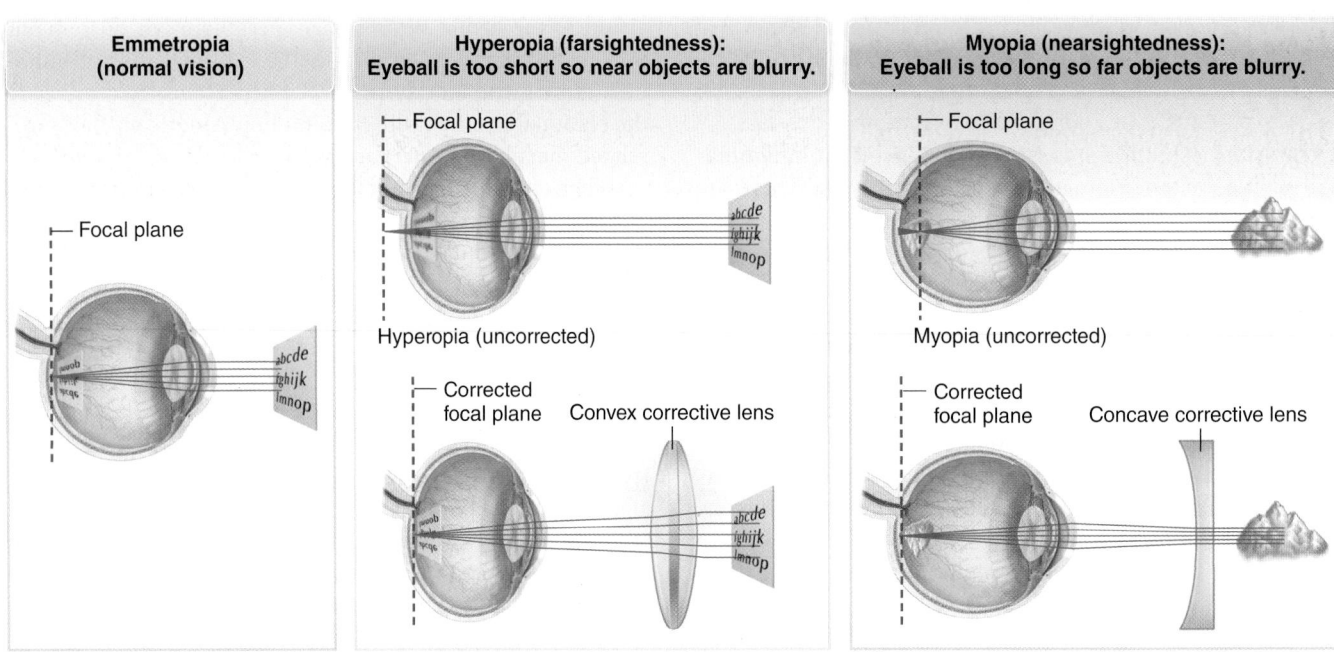

(b) Vision correction using (*center*) convex and (*right*) concave lenses.

FIGURE 43-2   (a) Lens shape for distant vision and lens shape for near vision (accommodation). (b) Emmetropia, hyperopia, and myopia.

Myopia (Nearsightedness) **Myopia** is the condition in which images of distant objects come into focus in front of the retina and are blurred (Figure 43-2). This condition occurs if the eye is too long or if the cornea and lens bend light rays more than normally. Nearby objects are usually seen clearly, but objects far away are unclear.

Nearsightedness is corrected with eyeglasses or contact lenses that have inwardly curving (concave) lenses. The lenses correct the bending of light rays so that they focus on the retina. Surgical and laser techniques are also used to correct myopia by changing the shape of the cornea.

Hyperopia (Farsightedness) and Presbyopia **Hyperopia**, or hypermetropia, causes images to come into focus behind the retina (Figure 43-2). The eyeball may be too short, or the cornea and lens may bend light rays less than

normally. Faraway objects are usually seen clearly, but nearby objects are unclear. If the hyperopia is mild, young eyes can compensate for the problem by a process known as accommodation. The ciliary muscles contract during accommodation, thickening the lens and increasing its convexity. These changes allow the image to come into focus on the retina.

Patients with mild farsightedness may have no symptoms or may have blurred vision. They may have symptoms of eyestrain (an aching in the eye) because the ciliary muscles are overworked. Farsightedness is corrected with eyeglasses or contact lenses that have outwardly turning (convex) lenses. Aging usually causes the ciliary muscles to weaken, so a person may need stronger eyeglasses over time.

Presbyopia is a condition that most commonly affects people starting in their mid-40s. Older eyes tend to lose the ability to accommodate because the lens becomes more rigid. As a result, images come into focus behind the retina, as they do with farsightedness. Individuals find they must hold reading materials farther away to see them clearly. Corrective lenses are used to treat this condition.

Astigmatism Sometimes vision is distorted because the cornea is unevenly curved or the lens has an abnormal shape. This condition is called **astigmatism**. Astigmatism is treated with lenses that correct the unevenness of the cornea or laser vision correction surgery known as LASIK. After surgery, patients may still need to wear glasses to correct presbyopia.

▶ Ophthalmic Exams   LO 43.3

An ophthalmologist performs an eye exam by inspecting the interior of the patient's eyes, including the retina, optic nerve, and blood vessels. The instrument used for this exam is an **ophthalmoscope,** a handheld instrument with a light, to view the inner eye structures. You will maintain and prepare this instrument for the physician's use, as described in Procedure 43-1, at the end of this chapter.

During the eye exam, the physician tests the patient's visual fields. The visual field is the entire area visible to the eye when the patient looks at an object straight ahead. Visual fields are assessed by the confrontation method. The doctor stands or sits about 2 feet in front of the patient. The patient covers one eye, and the doctor closes her own opposite eye. (This makes the visual fields of the two individuals roughly the same.) Then the doctor moves a pencil or other object into the patient's horizontal or vertical visual field, asking the patient to say, "Now" when the object comes into view. Defects in the field of vision are noted. The doctor then tests the convergence of the eyes (or how the eyes come together) by bringing the handheld object to the patient's nose as the eyes focus on it.

The ophthalmologist also routinely tests for glaucoma with the aid of a **tonometer** (Figure 43-3). The tonometer measures intraocular pressure, shown by the eyeball's resistance to indentation by either direct pressure or pneumatic pressure. Your role is to explain the procedure to the patient, instill anesthetizing eyedrops into the patient's eyes when required, assist the patient into position, and hand the doctor the instruments.

Another instrument the ophthalmologist may use during the exam is the **slit lamp** (Figure 43-4). This instrument consists of a magnifying lens combined with a light source. It is used to examine the eye's anterior structures including the eyelids, iris, lens, and cornea. Patients rest their chin on the device's chin rest and stare straight ahead while the doctor shines a narrow beam (slit) of light into the eye and looks at the eye through the instrument's lens. A special dye—fluorescein—may be used to help visualize foreign bodies or problems with the cornea.

The eye exam also may include a **refraction exam** to verify the need for corrective lenses. Normally, the lens and other parts of the eye work together to focus images on the retina. When errors of refraction exist, images are focused incorrectly, causing conditions like farsightedness and nearsightedness.

(a)

(b)

FIGURE 43-3 Two types of tonometers are (a) the applanation tonometer, which actually touches the eyeball during assessment, and (b) the noncontact, or airpuff, tonometer, which directs a puff of air at the cornea.

FIGURE 43-4 A slit lamp is used to examine the anterior structures of the eye.

FIGURE 43-5 The Phoroptor helps the ophthalmologist assess errors of refraction.

A refraction exam is performed with a retinoscope or a Phoroptor, the trademark name for a device that contains many different lenses. The doctor has the patient look through a succession of lens combinations to find out which one creates the clearest image (Figure 43-5).

Types of Vision Screening Tests

Screening tests are used to detect a number of common visual problems, including those involving the ability to see clearly, known as hyperopia, presbyopia, and myopia. Others may involve the ability to distinguish shades of gray or colors. When you record the results of vision tests, be sure to document for which eye you are recording the results and note if the test was done with corrective lenses (glasses or contacts). If vision is tested with glasses or contacts, you will note this with the abbreviation $\overline{cc}$ (with correction).

Screening for Visual Acuity Visual acuity screenings are a common procedure that medical assistants perform in physician offices either before or after the exam. The Snellen chart is the most common screening for distance visual acuity. The Jaeger chart is the most common screening for near vision. And the Ishihara book is the most common for color vision screening. Learning more about the anatomy of the eye and visual impairments will help you understand these screening procedures. In addition to performing the visual screening procedures, the medical assistant must observe for any actions by the patient to indicate visual difficulties, like squinting or leaning forward, and slow responses during the screening. Refer to Procedure 43-2, at the end of this chapter, for the correct methods to perform vision screening tests.

Certain patients may need special attention when having vision tests. For example, children may be anxious, uncooperative, or unable to follow directions. A patient with dementia or Alzheimer's disease also may require special attention during a vision test. Before the test, encourage a family member to stay with the patient so he is more comfortable. During the test, use simple language to explain the procedure and demonstrate whenever possible. Proceed through the exam slowly, one step at a time. Because the patient's memory and language skills may be impaired, you may need to repeat directions many times and help him name a particular object. If he appears to have trouble with one part of the exam, proceed to another part and return later to the part that was difficult for him.

Near Vision Refractive error in close vision is called hyperopia. In hyperopia, the eyeball is shorter than normal, resulting in objects being focused posterior to the retina (see Figure 43-2b). To test for near vision, special handheld charts are used. These cards contain letters, numbers, or paragraphs in various print sizes. They may be held and read at a normal reading distance or mounted in a plastic and metal frame and read through optical lenses. Presbyopia is visual impairment that results from aging and is caused by the loss of lens elasticity, which makes it difficult to see items close to you. The combination of myopia and presbyopia occurring together is the reason that many people require bifocal lenses as they age.

Contrast Sensitivity To test for the ability to distinguish shades of gray (contrast sensitivity), the Pelli-Robson contrast sensitivity chart, the Vistech Consultants vision contrast test system, or another testing system is used. Newer systems use special equipment to provide contrast variations in a projected image. These tests can detect cataracts or problems of the retina even before the sharpness of the patient's vision is impaired.

Color Vision To test color vision, illustrations like those of the Ishihara color system or the Richmond pseudoisochromatic color test are used. These illustrations contain numbers or symbols made up of colored dots that appear among other colored dots. The patient is asked to identify what he sees. A patient who is color-blind will not be able to report seeing the numbers or symbols. Color blindness may be inherited; it occurs more commonly in males. Changes in one's ability to see colors, however, may indicate a disease of the retina or optic nerve. Details on how to perform color vision and other vision tests can be found in Procedure 43-2, at the end of this chapter.

Go to CONNECT to see a video about *Performing Vision Screening Tests.*

▶ Ophthalmologic Procedures and Treatments   LO 43.4

The eye is an extremely delicate organ. Even what seems to be a minor injury or infection can have lasting consequences. You must use the greatest caution as well as proper technique—including sterile technique—when treating a patient's eyes. You also should provide patients with information on how to routinely care for their eyes. See the Educating the Patient feature for specific guidelines to follow when presenting eye care information.

Preventive Eye Care Tips

You can help patients take care of their eyes and protect their vision by providing them with guidelines to follow. Go over each item slowly and carefully. Ask whether the patient has questions before moving on to the next item. Answer all the patient's questions and make sure the patient understands the answers. Eye care tips include the following:

1. Get regular health checkups. Patients may not appreciate the connection between their general health and their eyes. Point out that high blood pressure and diabetes can cause eye problems.

2. Get regular eye examinations. Most people need eye examinations every 1 to 2 years. Patients with diabetes should see their eye care specialists more frequently.

3. Be alert for eye disease warning signs. Tell patients to call their eye care specialist immediately if they experience any of these signs:

   - Eye pain
   - Loss of vision
   - Double or blurred vision
   - Headache with blurred vision
   - Redness of the eye or eyelid
   - A gritty or sticky feeling around the eye
   - Excessive tearing
   - Difficulty seeing in the dark
   - Flashes of light
   - Halos around lights
   - Sensitivity to light
   - Loss of color perception

4. Wear sunglasses with ultraviolet protection to shield the eyes from bright sunlight, even in the winter. Recommend that patients ask to have ultraviolet protection added when purchasing new distance prescription glasses. Explain to patients that the cornea can get sunburned, which can be painful and damaging. Also tell patients that excessive exposure to the sun is a contributing factor in the development of cataracts and malignant melanoma of the eye—a dangerous type of skin cancer that may spread through the bloodstream or lymphatic system.

5. Wear protective eye equipment to prevent eye injury. Indicate to patients that they should wear protective eyewear every time they participate in sports, work with chemicals, or encounter a situation in which they may be exposed to flying debris.

6. Use nonprescription eye medications properly. Show patients how to use eyedrops, emphasizing that the tip of the dropper should never touch the eye. Explain that medications should be used only as indicated on the label and discarded after the condition has cleared up.

7. Never share eye makeup because bacterial infections can be passed via the applicators. To minimize contamination of the applicators, patients should take care of the applicators by storing them in a clean container and changing the applicator often. Patients should never place applicators on a dirty countertop.

Administering Medications to the Eye

Doctors commonly administer eye medications or perform eye irrigations to assist patients in eye tests, reduce pressure in the eyes, relieve eye pain, and treat eye infections and inflammation. Your responsibility as a medical assistant may include dispensing medications and explaining their use. Some medications are used to diagnose conditions; others are used to treat conditions. Only medications for ophthalmic use should be used in the eye. If you administer eye medications as part of your job, avoid touching a dropper or ointment tube tip to the eye. Doing so can injure the eye, cause infection, and contaminate the medication. Teach patients how to check medication labels carefully before administering them at home. For example, optic medications for eye use could easily be confused for otic medications for the ear. Medications other than optic medications may be too concentrated or may contain substances that will injure sensitive eye tissue.

Although most eye medications are administered for local effect, some contain drugs that are absorbed systemically (affecting the whole body). To prevent systemic absorption, the doctor may request that you apply pressure with one finger just below the inner corner of each eye after instilling medications. Continue applying pressure for 2 to 3 minutes, as directed. Procedure 43-3, at the end of this chapter, provides information on administering eye medications.

Eye Irrigation

When foreign materials like dust, sand, or chemicals enter the eye, they must be flushed out. Flushing—irrigation—should be done whenever possible, with a sterile solution especially formulated for this purpose. Someone's eye also may need to be irrigated to relieve discomfort from irritating substances, like smog, pollen, chemicals, or chlorinated water. Procedure 43-4, at the end of this chapter, will provide you with details about irrigating an eye. See the *Basic Safety and Infection Control* chapter for more information on using an eye wash station.

▶ Otology
LO 43.5

An **otologist** treats diseases and disorders of the ears. Procedures common to this specialty are sometimes performed by other physicians as well, especially general practitioners, internists, and allergists. In your role as a medical assistant, you also may assist with or perform auditory screening, administer ear medications, perform ear irrigations, and help with diagnostic tests like tympanometry. Otology specialists whose practices include problems affecting the nose and throat are called otorhinolaryngologists.

▶ Ear Diseases and Disorders   LO 43.6

When assisting physicians in administering various tests, treatments, and procedures, you may encounter a wide range of ear diseases and disorders in the medical office. Some—like cerumen impaction and otitis externa—do not have lasting effects on hearing and may be treated by a general practitioner. Others affect the ear's middle or inner parts and may require a specialist's attention.

Common Disorders of the Outer Ear

Several disorders affect the ear's external parts. These include cerumen impaction, otitis externa, and pruritus.

Cerumen Impaction A condition called cerumen impaction occurs when the ear canal becomes blocked by a buildup of cerumen (earwax). The wax can be softened with special eardrops, and irrigation can be performed to remove the wax. Refer to Procedure 43-7, at the end of this chapter, for more information about ear irrigation.

Otitis Externa Otitis externa is an infection of the outer ear, usually caused by bacteria or fungi. Also known as swimmer's ear, fungal infections are common in swimmers due to persistent moisture in the ear canal. This infection is treated with a combination of antibiotic or antifungal eardrops and an anti-inflammatory medication.

Pruritus A common problem in the elderly is pruritus—or itching—of the ear canal. Because the sebaceous glands produce less wax with aging, the ear becomes dry and itchy. Dryness can be overcome by a regular routine of lubricating the ear canal with a few drops of mineral oil.

Common Disorders of the Middle Ear

Middle ear disorders involve the eardrum and the chamber behind it. They include otitis media, mastoiditis, otosclerosis, and ruptured eardrum.

Otitis Media Otitis media is an inflammation of the middle ear characterized by fluid buildup, most commonly referred to as an ear infection. For detailed information on otitis media, see the Points on Practice feature Otitis Media: The Common Ear Infection.

Mastoiditis The mastoid bone is located just behind the ear. It is connected to the middle ear by air cells, or sinuses, in the bone. Sometimes, if left untreated, an infection in the middle ear can spread to the mastoid bone through these air cells. Although mastoiditis is fairly rare, it may be serious because the mastoid air cells are close to the organs of hearing,

important nerves, the covering of the brain, and the jugular vein. Severe cases of mastoiditis may require removal of the affected bone.

Otosclerosis Otosclerosis occurs when bone tissue grows abnormally around the stapes, or stirrup (the innermost of the three tiny bones that connect the eardrum and the inner ear). This overgrowth of tissue prevents the stapes from transmitting sound vibrations to the inner ear. The result is hearing loss in one or both ears. The condition is often hereditary.

Symptoms of otosclerosis include gradual loss of hearing and **tinnitus**—ringing in the ears. Surgery to replace the stapes—ossicular replacement prosthesis surgery—can restore or improve hearing in almost 90% of patients with otosclerosis. Alternatively, a hearing aid may improve hearing for some patients.

Ruptured Eardrum The eardrum may become ruptured in several ways: by a sharp object, an explosion, a blow to the ear, or a severe middle ear infection. Sometimes the eardrum is ruptured by a sudden change in air pressure, as might occur when flying in an airplane or diving. Symptoms include pain, partial hearing loss, and a slight discharge or bleeding. The symptoms typically last only a few hours. A ruptured eardrum usually heals on its own in 1 to 2 weeks, but the doctor may use a temporary patch to help close the defect.

Common Disorders of the Inner Ear

Disorders of the inner ear, or labyrinth, affect the cochlea and the semicircular canals. They include labyrinthitis, Ménière's disease, presbycusis, and tinnitus.

Labyrinthitis Labyrinthitis is an infection of the labyrinth, most commonly caused by a virus. Because the labyrinth includes the semicircular canals, which are involved in balance, this infection causes symptoms of dizziness or vertigo. The room may appear to spin and any movement exacerbates (worsens) the sensation, sometimes to the point of nausea and vomiting. Although disturbing, labyrinthitis disappears on its own within 1 to 3 weeks. The patient may need to rest in bed for a few days and medication can be given for symptoms.

Ménière's Disease Ménière's disease is caused by increased fluid in the labyrinth. The pressure of the fluid disturbs the sense of balance and may even rupture the labyrinth wall or damage the cochlea with its hearing receptors. One or both ears may be affected. Symptoms of this disorder include vertigo, nausea, vomiting, distorted hearing, and tinnitus. Some people may suffer hearing loss ranging from mild to severe. Medications may be used to combat vertigo, nausea, and vomiting. Other treatments that help some people include using diuretics and following a low-sodium diet.

Presbycusis Presbycusis is a type of sensorineural hearing loss. It is the most common form of hearing loss in older adults, affecting about 25% of people by the age of 60 or 70.

Otitis Media: The Common Ear Infection

Otitis media, commonly referred to as an ear infection, affects almost all children by age 6. This inflammation of the middle ear accounts for 22 million doctor visits each year—second only to routine well-child health exams.

Ear infections typically start when fluid becomes trapped in the middle ear. The lining of the middle ear and eustachian tube contains fluid similar to the mucus within the nasal passages. The normal flow of this fluid from the ear into the back of the nose where it joins the pharynx helps keep the middle ear and the eustachian tube free of bacteria. When a child gets a cold or flu, the lining of the eustachian tube and middle ear can become inflamed and can trap the fluid, which becomes infected.

There are four distinct types of otitis media to be aware of. One or both (bilateral) ears may be affected.

1. Acute otitis media typically refers to a bacterial infection of the middle ear that comes on suddenly. This type is common in children and typically follows an upper respiratory tract infection. The symptoms include pain, a feeling of fullness in the ear, some loss of hearing, and possible fever. In severe cases, the eardrum may rupture because of the fluid pressure. Acute infections are not usually treated with oral antibiotics at first. Most infections will resolve on their own without treatment so physicians will usually wait 48–72 hours before prescribing antibiotic treatment for a patient with acute otitis media.

2. Recurrent otitis media is diagnosed when a child contracts acute otitis repeatedly, perhaps once or twice every month.

3. Otitis media with effusion, also known as OME, involves an accumulation of fluid in the middle ear. Children with OME do not exhibit any symptoms, and they may not experience any discomfort.

4. Chronic otitis media is diagnosed when fluid is present in the ear and fails to clear up after 3 months or more. Infection may or may not be present. Without treatment, the undrained fluid thickens, resulting in possible changes in the shape of the eardrum, erosion of the ossicles—tiny bones of hearing, and mastoiditis. Chronic otitis media left untreated for a sufficient amount of time could result in facial paralysis, brain infections, and balance problems. These changes may cause temporary or permanent hearing loss if not treated. Antibiotics and reconstructive surgery may be used to treat this condition.

If a child suffers from recurrent or chronic otitis media, myringotomy—surgical incision of the eardrum with insertion of tubes—may be recommended to keep the fluid draining continuously. This procedure usually removes enough fluid

FIGURE 43-6   A pressure-equalizing tube inserted in the eardrum helps keep fluid from building up behind the eardrum.

so the infection clears up. Depending on the type of tube, it falls out on its own within 3 to 18 months of insertion. See Figure 43-6.

Ear infections may be difficult to identify, especially in a young child who cannot talk. The following symptoms may be indications of a possible ear infection, particularly if more than one is present:

- Tugging or rubbing the ear.
- Fever ranging from 100°F to 104°F.
- Difficulty balancing.
- Excessive crankiness.
- Difficulty hearing or speaking.
- An unwillingness to lie down. (The pain may become more severe in a reclining position because of increased pressure against the eardrum.)

Preventing ear infections is the best course of action. Several measures may be taken to reduce the likelihood of ear infections, including

- Preventing colds by teaching children to wash their hands often and not share cups and other eating utensils.
- Limiting a child's exposure to second-hand smoke.
- Breastfeeding for at least 6 months.
- Bottle feeding in an upright position—*never* put a baby to bed with a bottle.
- Keeping immunizations like flu shots and pneumococcal vaccines up to date.

Men are affected more often than women. Hearing loss can be treated effectively, however, with a hearing aid.

Tinnitus Tinnitus is more commonly called a ringing in the ears. This "ringing" can take several forms, including a buzzing, whistling, or hissing sound. The most common causes of tinnitus are damage to the hearing receptors from noise or toxins, age-related changes in the ear's organs, and aspirin use. Tinnitus can affect people at any age but is more common as people get older. If tinnitus becomes chronic, the patient may find relief by listening to quiet, soothing music or other distracting sounds or by using a device similar to a hearing aid that masks the noise with more pleasant sounds.

Hearing Loss

Hearing loss is actually a symptom of a disease, not a disease in itself. Contrary to what most people believe, hearing loss is not a normal part of the aging process and should always be evaluated for proper treatment. There are two types of hearing loss: conductive and sensorineural. The two types differ in the point at which the hearing process is interrupted.

A **conductive hearing loss** is caused by an interruption in the transmission of sound waves to the inner ear. Conditions that can cause conductive hearing loss include obstruction of the ear canal (as with cerumen impaction or tumor), infection of the middle ear, and otosclerosis or reduced movement of the ossicles (bones of hearing).

A **sensorineural hearing loss** occurs when there is damage to the inner ear, to the nerve that leads from the ear to the brain, or to the brain itself. In this kind of loss, sound waves reach the inner ear, but the brain does not perceive them as sound. This type of hearing loss can be hereditary, can be caused by repeated exposure to loud noises or viral infections, or can occur as a side effect of medications like aspirin and some antibiotics. Tinnitus suggests damage to the auditory nerve.

Sensorineural hearing loss can be differentiated from conductive hearing loss by hearing tests. It is also possible for both types of hearing loss to occur together.

Noise Pollution Prolonged exposure to loud noises is a common cause of hearing loss because of damage to the sensitive cells in the cochlea. People who work around noisy equipment—like construction workers, aircraft personnel, and machine operators—are likely to suffer from this type of hearing loss unless they protect their ears (Figure 43-7). Repeatedly listening to loud music from a personal stereo or car radio set at too high a volume also can damage the ears.

Go to CONNECT to see an animation about *Hearing Loss: Sensorineural.*

Working with Patients with a Hearing Impairment

You may come in contact with patients of all ages who have hearing impairments. Many patients wear hearing aids to amplify normal speech. Some patients, however, may not admit they have a problem—out of fear, vanity, or misinformation. It

FIGURE 43-7 Loud noises, like those produced by power tools, can damage hearing unless appropriate ear protectors are worn.

is estimated that one-third of patients between the ages of 65 and 74 and one-half of those between the ages of 75 and 79 suffer from some loss of hearing.

To improve communication with a patient whose hearing is impaired, you can do the following:

- Speak at a reasonable volume. Do not shout. Shouting can actually make your words harder to understand. A hearing aid filters out loud sounds, so the patient may not hear everything you say if you shout.

- Speak in clear, low-pitched tones. Elderly patients lose the ability to hear high-pitched sounds first.

- Avoid speaking directly into the patient's ear. Stand 3 to 6 feet away and face the patient so she can see your lip movements and facial expressions. Avoid covering your mouth with your hands. Speak at a normal rate.

- Avoid overemphasizing your lip movements, which makes lip reading difficult.

- Avoid hand gestures unless they are appropriate.

- If the patient does not understand what you say, restate the message in short, simple sentences. Have the patient repeat the message to verify that your words were understood.

- Treat patients who have a hearing impairment with patience and respect.

Go to CONNECT to see a video about *Obtaining Information from a Patient with a Hearing Aid.*

▶ Hearing and Other Diagnostic Ear Tests   LO 43.7

Various tests are performed to find out whether a person hears normally. If the tests reveal a problem, follow-up tests are conducted to determine the cause of the problem. You may assist with the testing or educate the patient about caring for her ears. See the Educating the Patient feature Preventive Ear Care Tips for more information.

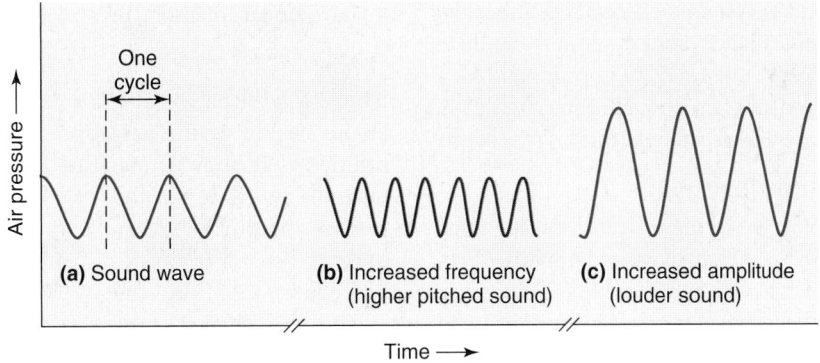

FIGURE 43-8 Sound frequency is determined by the number of waves per second that pass a specified point.

Hearing Tests

As part of a general examination, physicians may perform a simple hearing test with one or more tuning forks. Physicians use the tuning forks to determine whether there is a hearing loss. Tuning forks also can be helpful in differentiating conductive from sensorineural hearing loss.

If you have the necessary training, you may help perform a test that uses an audiometer. An **audiometer** is an electronic device that measures hearing acuity by producing sounds in specific frequencies and intensities. A **frequency** is the number of complete fluctuations—waves—of energy that pass a specific point in one second (Figure 43-8). Frequency is best described as the pitch of sound. High frequency is high-pitched and low frequency is low-pitched. The audiometer allows a physician or other health practitioner to test a person's hearing and to determine the nature and extent of a person's hearing loss.

Many types of audiometers are available. Some machines automatically generate the various tones at different **decibels** (units for measuring the relative intensity—loudness—of sounds on a scale from 0 to 130) and print out the patient's responses. Others must be manually adjusted and the results charted by hand. During the test, the patient wears a headset to hear the sounds produced by the audiometer. Depending on the particular unit, the patient indicates hearing a sound by raising a finger or pushing a button. In the former case, the person administering the test records the response. In the latter case, the response may be recorded automatically or by the test giver. Procedure 43-5, at the end of this chapter, provides additional information about measuring auditory acuity.

Adults and children who can understand directions and respond appropriately can be screened in this manner. If you work in a pediatrician's office, you also may help to check an infant's response to sounds. These tests require special techniques, as infants cannot understand directions. The general steps involved in performing hearing tests on infants are outlined in the "Assisting in Pediatrics" chapter.

Go to CONNECT to see a video about *Measuring Auditory Acuity.*

Tympanometry

A diagnostic test called tympanometry measures the eardrum's ability to move and thus gauges pressure in the middle ear. Tympanometry is used to detect diseases and abnormalities of the middle ear or ear canal including

* Cerumen impaction
* Middle ear fluid
* Middle ear tumor
* Ossicular detachment
* Tympanic membrane perforation
* Tympanic membrane scars

To perform the test, a small, soft-rubber cuff is placed over the external ear canal, producing an airtight seal. The tympanometer then automatically measures air pressure against the tympanic membrane and prints a graph of the results. Let the patient know that they will hear sounds during the test that may seem loud, but they need to remain as still as possible.

▶ Ear Treatments and Procedures   LO 43.8

Some common ear problems that you may encounter in the physician's office include cerumen impaction (a buildup of earwax in the ear canal), rupture of the eardrum, otitis media (inflammation of the middle ear), and otitis externa (inflammation of the outer ear). Physicians use various approaches and techniques with each problem to restore the health of a patient's ears. Physicians also employ special techniques and devices to improve patients' hearing and maintain their ear health. As a medical assistant, you can provide patients with information on preventive ear care techniques, as described in the Educating the Patient feature Preventive Ear Care Tips.

You also may administer ear medications, perform ear irrigations, and assist the physician in earwax removal.

Administering Medications to the Ear

Doctors often administer eardrops or perform ear irrigations to treat patients' ear infections or inflammation, relieve ear pain, or loosen earwax. Like eye medications, eardrops are ordered primarily for their local effects. They are not usually absorbed systemically, nor do they cause systemic effects. It is important that you warm the eardrops slightly before administration to avoid making the patient dizzy. Holding them in your hand for a minute or two will usually warm them enough. Procedure 43-6, at the end of this chapter, provides instructions for this procedure.

Earwax and Foreign Body Removal

Earwax—cerumen—may build up in the ear canal causing a full feeling in the ear, ear pain, partial hearing loss, and tinnitus. Cerumen normally protects the ear, but if a person produces too much, it can harden and block the ear canal. Also, cleaning your ear with cotton-tipped swabs can push the cerumen down into the ear canal. There are several treatments for removing earwax. In some cases, if the wax is close enough to reach, the physician may be able to remove the wax with an ear curette—a small instrument with a scoop or loop on one end. Home remedies include over-the-counter wax softening drops, mineral oil, and glycerin. These may work if the impaction is not too severe. But if the wax is extremely hard or is stuck to the ear canal, irrigation may be the best treatment.

Ear Irrigation Irrigating the ear may relieve inflammation or irritation of the ear canal and may help loosen and remove impacted cerumen (earwax) or a foreign body. This procedure is performed in the physician's office. Irrigation is contraindicated in (or inadvisable for) patients who

- currently have or have had a ruptured eardrum,
- have pressure equalizing tubes in their eardrum,
- have an ear infection, or
- have had ear surgery including mastoidectomy.

Always ask the patient about ear surgeries and other conditions before beginning the irrigation and make sure the irrigation solution is at body temperature before starting. This helps reduce the possibility of the patient becoming dizzy during the procedure. Procedure 43-7, at the end of this chapter, provides instructions for ear irrigation.

Go to CONNECT to see a video about *Performing Ear Irrigation.*

Microscopic Earwax and Foreign Body Removal

Occasionally, irrigation does not work to remove the cerumen impaction. With the help of a special microscope, an otologist can use suction or special instruments to remove the wax. Foreign bodies in the ear also are removed with the aid of a microscope. During the procedure, the physician looks through the microscope into the patient's ear canal. This gives her a better view of the ear, allowing her to get deeper into the ear canal without damaging the delicate structures within the ear. The patient must remain extremely still during this procedure. Your role as a medical assistant is to help keep the patient at ease and comfortable and to make sure the physician has the necessary instruments.

EDUCATING THE PATIENT

Preventive Ear Care Tips

You can help patients protect their ears and take care of their hearing by providing them with guidelines to follow. As with any patient education, go over items slowly, ask patients whether they have questions before moving on, and answer questions completely. Ear care tips include the following:

1. Get routine hearing exams. Screening for hearing problems is often part of a comprehensive physical exam. Encourage patients who have not had their hearing screened or who suspect they have hearing problems to arrange for testing by their doctor. Older patients, who may not admit they have a problem, may need special encouragement.

2. Avoid injury when cleaning the ears. Instruct patients in proper ear care. Point out that they should not put objects in the ear that might injure the eardrum or ear canal, which includes vigorous probing with cotton-tipped swabs.

3. Avoid injury from nonprescription ear care products. Tell patients to check with a doctor before using nonprescription products for softening earwax.

4. Use proper ear protection. Urge patients to wear ear protectors around loud work equipment and to avoid listening to loud music. It is especially important to keep the volume at a reasonable level when listening through earphones and through ear buds that fit directly into the external auditory canal.

5. Use all medications properly. Show patients how to use eardrops; emphasize that they must follow instructions precisely. Explain to patients that following instructions applies to all medications because many, including aspirin and some antibiotics, may cause hearing loss if used improperly.

6. Be alert for warning signs. Tell patients to call their doctor immediately if they experience any of these signs of ear problems:
   - Ear pain
   - Stuffiness
   - Discharge from the ear
   - Vertigo (dizziness)

Also have patients notify the doctor if they have any of these signs of hearing problems:
- Tinnitus (ringing).
- Hearing others' speech as mumbled sounds.
- Speaking in a very loud voice without being aware of it.

Hearing Aids

Hearing aids may be worn inside or outside the ear. If worn outside, they may be located behind the ear, mounted on eyeglasses, or worn on the body. Hearing aids consist of the following parts:

- A tiny microphone to pick up sounds;
- An amplifier to increase the volume of sounds; and
- A tiny speaker to transmit sounds to the ear.

You may need to teach patients how to obtain a hearing aid. You also can pass along tips to patients to help them take proper care of their hearing aids and to troubleshoot problems.

Obtaining a Hearing Aid A patient with signs of hearing loss should be referred to an otologist, a medical doctor specializing in the health of the ear, or an **audiologist,** a specialist who focuses on evaluating and correcting hearing problems. Audiologists are not medical doctors and do not treat diseases of the ear. Instead, they evaluate the patient's hearing, fit hearing aids, give instruction in the use of hearing aids, and provide service for hearing aids if necessary. It is important for hearing aids to fit properly. If they do not, sounds may not be transmitted well into the ear.

Care and Use of Hearing Aids Hearing aids run on batteries that typically last about 2 weeks. So, the patient must keep a fresh supply of batteries on hand. The hearing aid itself must be routinely cleaned or the microphone, switches, or dials may not work properly. Moisture can damage the aid, so it must not get wet. Hair sprays can clog hearing aid openings or interfere with the operation of moving parts. For these reasons, spray should be applied before a hearing aid is inserted. Cerumen often builds up behind hearing aids that are worn in the ear, reducing sound transmission. If buildup does occur, the cerumen plug should be removed by ear irrigation.

Other Devices and Strategies

People whose hearing cannot be substantially improved by hearing aids may need to use other devices or strategies to overcome the problem. These devices include appliances that light up as well as ring—like telephones, doorbells, smoke detectors, alarm clocks, and burglar alarms. Patients can purchase amplifiers for the telephone, television set, and radio. Many closed-captioned television programs are also available. To benefit from closed captioning, the patient must have a television set with a decoder that translates the captioning and displays the captions on the screen.

Cochlear Implants

A person who is profoundly deaf and cannot benefit from using a hearing aid may be a candidate for a **cochlear implant**, an electronic device that stimulates the auditory nerve. A cochlear implant has an external and an internal component. The external portion sits just behind the ear and the internal portion has an array of electrodes that are implanted directly in the cochlea. Cochlear implants do not amplify sound like a hearing aid but send signals through the auditory nerve to the brain. This gives patients the ability to detect warning signals like smoke alarms and recognize speech patterns so that they may be better understood. Hearing with a cochlear implant is not the same as normal hearing; patients have to learn to recognize sounds. Adults with cochlear implants can often learn to understand speech without using visual cues—like lip reading. Children can learn to speak with extensive speech therapy. More than 42,000 adults and 28,000 children in the United States have cochlear implants.

PROCEDURE 43-1   Preparing the Ophthalmoscope for Use

Procedure Goal: To ensure that the ophthalmoscope is ready for use during an eye exam.

OSHA Guidelines: This procedure does not involve exposure to blood, body fluids, or tissues.

Materials: Ophthalmoscope, lens, spare bulb, spare battery.

Method: Procedure steps.

1. Wash your hands.
2. Take the ophthalmoscope out of its battery charger. In a darkened room, turn on the ophthalmoscope light.
3. Shine the large beam of white light on the back of your hand to check that the instrument's tiny lightbulb is providing strong enough light.
4. Replace the bulb or battery if necessary. (The battery is located in the ophthalmoscope's handle.)
5. Make sure the instrument's lens is screwed into the handle. If it is not, attach the lens.

FIGURE Procedure 43-1 Step 3 Shine the ophthalmoscope light on your hand to check the strength of the beam.

PROCEDURE 43-2 Performing Vision Screening Tests

Procedure Goal: To screen a patient's ability to see distant or close objects, to determine contrast sensitivity, or to detect color blindness.

OSHA Guidelines:

Materials: Occluder or card; alcohol; gauze squares; appropriate vision charts to test for distance vision, near vision, and color blindness.

Method: Procedure steps.

Distance Vision

1. Wash your hands, clean the occluder with a gauze square dampened in alcohol, identify the patient, introduce yourself, and explain the procedure.

2. Mount one of the following eye charts at eye level: Snellen letter or similar chart (for patients who can read); Snellen E, Landolt C, pictorial, or similar chart (for patients who cannot read).

   If using the Snellen letter chart, verify that the patient knows the letters of the alphabet. With children or nonreading adults, use demonstration cards to verify that they can identify the pictures or direction of the letters. **RATIONALE:** If the patient does not understand the instructions, the results will not be accurate.

(b)

FIGURE Procedure 43-2 Step 2 (b) The Snellen E chart is used to test the vision of children and nonreading adults. (Reprinted with permission of Richmond Products, Inc.)

(a)

FIGURE Procedure 43-2 Step 2 (a) The Snellen letter chart is used to test the vision of people who can read.

3. Make a mark on the floor 20 feet away from the chart.

4. Have the patient stand with his or her heels at the 20-foot mark, or sit with the back of the chair at the mark.

5. Instruct the patient to keep both eyes open and not to squint or lean forward during the test.
   RATIONALE: Closing one eye, squinting, or leaning will lead to inaccurate results.

6. Test both eyes first, then the right eye, and then the left eye. (Different offices may test in a different order. Follow your office policy.)
   RATIONALE: Following a specific testing order based on office policy leads to consistency in the results of all medical records.

7. Have the patient read the lines on the chart (or identify the picture/direction), beginning with the 20-foot line. If the patient cannot read this line, begin with the smallest line the patient can read. (Some offices use a pointer to select one symbol at a time in random order to prevent patients from memorizing the order.)

8. Note the smallest line the patient can read or identify with no more than two errors. (Some offices only allow 1 error per line. Follow office policy when performing this test.)

9. Record the results as a fraction (for example, each eye 20/40 −1 if the patient misses one letter on a line or each eye 20/40 −2 if the patient misses two letters on a line).

10. Show the patient how to cover the left eye with the occluder or card. Again, instruct the patient to keep both eyes open and not to squint or lean forward during the test.

11. Have the patient read the lines on the chart.

12. Record the results of the right eye (for example, Right Eye 20/30).

13. Have the patient cover the right eye and read the lines on the chart.

14. Record the results of the left eye (for example, Left Eye 20/20).

15. If the patient wears corrective lenses, record the results using $\overline{cc}$ (if your office uses this abbreviation for "with correction") in front of the abbreviation (for example, $\overline{cc}$ both eyes 20/20).

    RATIONALE: For charting accuracy, vision correction must be noted using your office format.

16. Note and record any observations of squinting, head tilting, excessive blinking, or tearing.

17. Ask the patient to keep both eyes open and to identify the two colored bars, and record the results in the patient's chart.

18. Clean the occluder with a gauze square dampened with alcohol.

19. Properly dispose of the gauze square and wash your hands.

    RATIONALE: Maintain principles of aseptic technique at all times.

Near Vision

20. Wash your hands, identify the patient, introduce yourself, and explain the procedure.

21. Have the patient hold one of the following at normal reading distance (approximately 14 to 16 inches): Jaeger, Richmond pocket, or similar chart or card.

(a)

FIGURE Procedure 43-2 Step 21   (a) Have the patient hold the card at a comfortable reading distance.

V = .50 D.

The fourteenth of August was the day fixed upon for the sailing of the brig Pilgrim, on her voyage from Boston round Cape Horn, to the western coast of North America. As she was to get under way early in the after-noon, I made my appearance on board at twelve o'clock in full sea-rig, and with my chest, containing an outfit for a two or three years voyage, | which I had undertaken from a determination to cure, if possible, by an entire change of life, and by a long absence from books and study, a weak-ness of the eyes which had obliged me to give up my pursuits, and which no medical aid seemed likely to cure. The change from the tight dress coat, silk cap and kid gloves of an undergraduate at Cambridge, to the

V = .75 D.

loose duck trousers, checked shirt and tarpaulin hat of a sailor, though somewhat of a transfor-mation, was soon made, and I supposed that I should pass very well for a Jack tar. But it is impossible to deceive the practiced eye in these matters; and while I supposed myself to be looking as salt as Neptune himself, I was, no doubt, known for a landsman by every one on board, as soon as I hove in sight. A sailor has a peculiar cut to his clothes, and a way of wear-

V = 1.   D.

ing them which a green hand can never get. The trousers, tight around the hips, and thence hanging long and loose around the feet, a superabundance of checked shirt, a low-crowned, well-varnished black hat, worn on the back of the head, with half a fathom of black ribbon hanging over the left eye, and a peculiar tie to the black silk necker-chief, with sundry other *details*, are signs of which betray the beginner at once.

V = 1.25 D.

Beside the points in my dress which were out of the way, doubtless my complexion and hands would distinguish me from the regular *salt*, who, with a sun-browned cheek, wide step and rolling gait, swings his bronzed and toughened hands athwart-ships half open, as though just to ready to grasp a rope. "With all my imperfections

V = 1.50 D.

on my head," I joined the crew, and we hauled out into the stream and came to anchor for the night. The next day we were employed in prep-aration for sea, reeving and studding-sail gear, crossing royal yards, putting on chafing gear, and taking on board our powder. On the

V = 1.75 D.

following night I stood my first watch. I remained awake nearly all the first part of the night, from fear that I might not hear when I was called; and when I went on deck, so great were my ideas of the importance of my trust, that I

V = 2.   D.

walked regularly fore and aft the whole length of the vessel, looking out over the bows and taffrail at each turn, and was not a little surprised at the uncon-cerned manner in which the billows turned up their

Your glasses are of value to you only as they accurately inter-pret your prescription and this only as they are fitted and serviced in accordance with these needs. They are a therapeutic device.

 RICHMOND PRODUCTS
BOCA RATON, FL 33487

No. 11974 R

(b)

FIGURE Procedure 43-2 Step 21   (b) This near vision chart is used to test the ability to see objects at a normal reading distance. (Reprinted with permission of Richmond Products, Inc.)

22. Ask the patient to keep both eyes open and to read or identify the letters, symbols, or paragraphs.

    RATIONALE: If both eyes are not open, results may not be accurate.

23. Record the smallest line read without error.

24. If the card is laminated, clean it with a gauze square dampened with alcohol.

25. Properly dispose of the gauze square and wash your hands.

    RATIONALE: Maintain principles of aseptic technique at all times.

FOR TESTING AT 40 CM (16 INCHES)

				POINT	JAEGER	DISTANCE EQUIVALENT
62		‖				$\frac{20}{800}$
958				N60	J17	$\frac{20}{400}$
3 6 2 5				N30	J15	$\frac{20}{200}$
8 3 9	**Ɔ C O**	**T V H**		N14	J12	$\frac{20}{100}$
5 6 2 8	**C O O Ɔ**	**V H O T**		N12	J10	$\frac{20}{80}$
6 8 3 2 9	**O C Ɔ O O**	**O T H V T**		N10	J7	$\frac{20}{63}$
2 5 9 3 8	**C O O C O**	**H O T H V**		N8	J6	$\frac{20}{50}$
3 2 8 6 5	**Ɔ C O Ɔ O**	**T H O V H**		N6	J4	$\frac{20}{40}$
9 5 3 8 2	**C O O O O**	**H V T O V**		N5	J3	$\frac{20}{32}$
6 3 8 2 5	**O O O C O**	**O T V H T**		N4	J2	$\frac{20}{25}$
● ● ● ● ●	**O O O O O**	**H O T V O**		N3	J1	$\frac{20}{20}$

PUPIL GAUGE (mm.)

2 3 4 5 6 7 8 9

(c)

FIGURE Procedure 43-2 Step 21   (c) The Richmond pocket vision screener is also used to test near vision. (Reprinted with permission of Richmond Products, Inc.)

(a)

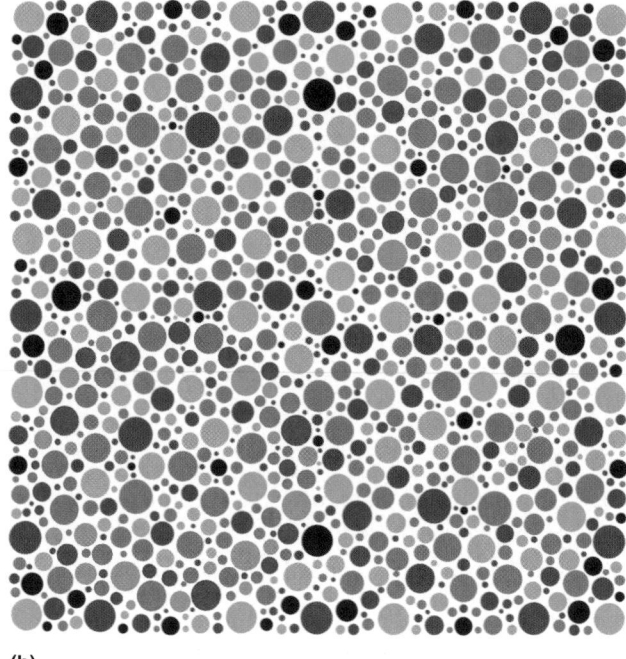

(b)

FIGURE Procedure 43-2 Step 27   (a) Have the patient hold the chart at a comfortable reading distance. (b) The Richmond pseudoisochromatic color chart is used to test a person's ability to see colors. (Reprinted with permission of Richmond Products, Inc.)

Color Vision

26. Wash your hands, identify the patient, introduce yourself, and explain the procedure.

27. Hold one of the following color charts or books at the patient's normal reading distance (approximately 14 to 16 inches): Ishihara, Richmond pseudoisochromatic, or similar color-testing system.

28. Ask the patient to tell you the number or symbol within the colored dots on each chart or page.

29. Proceed through all the charts or pages, usually totaling 24.

30. Record the number correctly identified and failed with a slash between them (for example, 23 passed/1 failed).

31. If the charts are laminated, clean them with a gauze square dampened with alcohol.

32. Properly dispose of the gauze square and wash your hands.

    RATIONALE: Maintain principles of aseptic technique at all times.

    Document the following information after you have completed the procedure:

    > Vision screening performed: Distance L 20/20 −1 R 20/20 −1 Both 20/20, Near L 20/50 R 20/40 −2, Color vision passed all color plates. _____
    > _____ _K. Booth RMA (AMT)_

PROCEDURE 43-3 Administering Eye Medications

Procedure Goal: To instill (introduce) medication into the eye for treatment of certain eye disorders.

OSHA Guidelines:

Materials: Medication (drops, cream, or ointment), tissues, eye patch (if applicable).

Method: Procedure steps.

1. Identify the patient, introduce yourself, and explain the procedure.
2. Review the doctor's medication order. This should include the patient's name, drug name, concentration, number of drops (if a liquid), into which eye(s) the medication is to be administered, and the frequency of administration.
   RATIONALE: The physician's order must be followed exactly.
3. Compare the drug with the medication order three times, checking the rights of medication administration.
   RATIONALE: To ensure necessary accuracy.
4. Ask whether the patient has any known allergies to substances contained in the medication.
5. Wash your hands and put on gloves.
6. Assemble the supplies.
7. Ask the patient to lie down or to sit back in a chair with the head tilted back.
8. Give the patient a tissue to blot excess medication as needed.
9. Remove an eye patch, if present.
10. Instruct the patient to look at the ceiling and to keep both eyes open during the procedure.
11. With a tissue, gently pull the lower eyelid down by pressing downward on the patient's cheekbone just below the eyelid with your nondominant hand. This pressure will open a pocket of space between the eyelid and the eye.

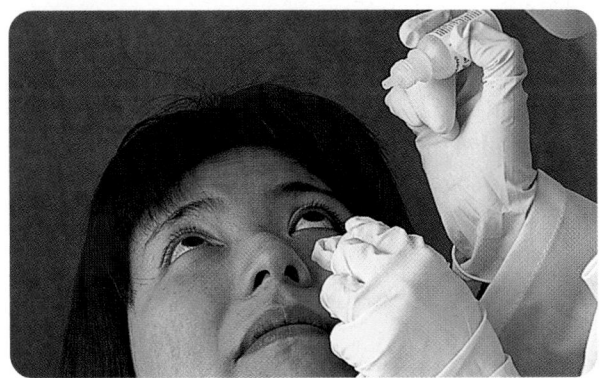

FIGURE Procedure 43-3 Step 11 Use a tissue to press down on the patient's cheekbone just below the eyelid, opening up a pocket of space between the eyelid and the eye.

Eyedrops

12. Resting your dominant hand on the patient's forehead, hold the filled eyedropper or bottle approximately ½ inch from the conjunctiva.
    RATIONALE: Touching the patient's skin with the dropper or bottle tip will cause contamination.

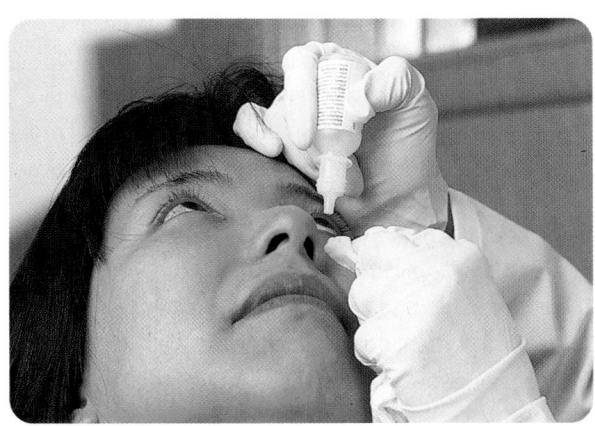

FIGURE Procedure 43-3 Step 12 The medication container should be approximately ½ inch from the conjunctiva as you prepare to instill drops in the patient's eye.

13. Drop the prescribed number of drops into the pocket. If any drops land outside the eye, repeat instilling the drops that missed the eye.

Creams or Ointments

14. Rest your dominant hand on the patient's forehead and hold the tube or applicator above the conjunctiva.
15. Without touching the eyelid or conjunctiva with the applicator, evenly apply a thin ribbon of cream or

FIGURE Procedure 43-3 Step 15 Apply a thin ribbon of cream or ointment along the inside of the lower eyelid on the conjunctiva.

ointment along the inside edge of the lower eyelid on the conjunctiva, working from the medial (inner) to the lateral (outer) side.

RATIONALE: Touching the patient's skin with the applicator will cause contamination.

All Medications

16. Release the lower lid and instruct the patient to gently close the eyes.
17. Repeat the procedure for the other eye as necessary.
18. Remove any excess medication by wiping each eyelid gently with a fresh tissue from the medial to the lateral side.
19. Apply a clean eye patch to cover the entire eye, if ordered.
20. Ask whether the patient felt any discomfort and observe for any adverse reactions. Notify the doctor as necessary.
21. Instruct the patient on self-administration of medication and patch application, if ordered.
22. Ask the patient to repeat the instructions.
23. Provide written instructions.
24. Properly dispose of used disposable materials.

FIGURE Procedure 43-3 Step 18   Use a tissue to remove excess medication from the eyelid.

25. Remove gloves and wash your hands.
26. Document administration in the patient's chart. Include the drug, concentration, the number of drops or amount, the time of administration, and the eye(s) that received the medication.

PROCEDURE 43-4 Performing Eye Irrigation

Procedure Goal: To flush the eye to remove foreign particles or relieve eye irritation.

OSHA Guidelines:

Materials: Sterile irrigating solution, sterile basin, sterile irrigating syringe and kidney-shaped basin, tissues.

Method: Procedure steps.

1. Identify the patient, introduce yourself, and explain the procedure.
2. Review the physician's order. This should include the patient's name, the irrigating solution, the volume of solution, and for which eye(s) the irrigation is to be performed.
3. Compare the solution with the instructions three times, checking the rights of medication administration.
   RATIONALE: To ensure necessary accuracy.
4. Wash your hands and put on gloves, a gown, and a face shield.
   RATIONALE: Splashing is possible when a syringe is used.
5. Assemble supplies.
6. Ask the patient to lie down or to sit with the head tilted back and to the side that is being irrigated. The solution should not spill over into the other eye.

   RATIONALE: Cross-contamination between the eyes must be avoided.
7. Place a towel or a disposable waterproof underpad over the patient's shoulder. Have the patient hold the kidney-shaped basin at the side of the head next to the eye to be irrigated.
8. Pour the solution into the sterile basin.
9. Fill the irrigating syringe with solution (approximately 50 mL).
10. Hold a tissue on the patient's cheekbone below the lower eyelid with your nondominant hand and press downward to expose the eye socket.
11. Holding the tip of the syringe ½ inch away from the eye, direct the solution onto the lower conjunctiva from the inner to the outer aspect of the eye. (Avoid directing the solution against the cornea because it is sensitive; do not use excessive force.)
    RATIONALE: To avoid contamination, do not let the tip touch the eye or skin. Excessive force could damage the cornea.
12. Refill the syringe and continue irrigation until the prescribed volume of solution is used.
13. Dry the area around the eye with tissues or gauze squares.
14. Properly dispose of used disposable materials.
15. Remove your gloves, gown, and face shield, and wash your hands.
16. Record the following in the patient's chart: procedure, type of solution, amount of solution used, time of administration, and eye(s) irrigated.
17. Put on gloves and clean the equipment and room according to OSHA guidelines.

PROCEDURE 43-5 Measuring Auditory Acuity

Procedure Goal: To determine how well a patient hears.

OSHA Guidelines:

Materials: Audiometer, headset, graph pad (if applicable), alcohol, gauze squares.

Method: Procedure steps.

Infants and Toddlers

1. Identify the patient and introduce yourself.
2. Wash your hands.
3. Pick a quiet location.
4. The patient can be sitting, lying down, or held by the parent.
5. Instruct the parent to be silent during the procedure.
6. Position yourself so your hands are behind the child's right ear and out of sight.
   RATIONALE: You want the child to respond to sound, not to sight.
7. Clap your hands loudly. Observe the child's response. (Never clap directly in front of the ear because this can damage the eardrum. As an alternative to clapping, use special devices, like rattles or clickers (which may be available in the office) to generate sounds of varying loudness.
8. Record the child's response as positive or negative for loud noise.
9. Position one hand behind the child's right ear, as before.
10. Snap your fingers. Observe the child's response.
11. Record the response as positive or negative for moderate noise.
12. Repeat steps 6 through 11 for the left ear.
    Document the following information after you have completed the procedure:

> Hearing test completed with patient on mother's lap. Patient responded to moderate noise in both ears. _____ P. Braithwaite CMA (AAMA)

Adults and Children

1. Wash your hands, identify the patient, introduce yourself, and explain the procedure.

2. Clean the earpieces of the headset with a sanitizing wipe according to manufacturer's instructions.
   RATIONALE: Maintain aseptic technique at all times.
3. Have the patient sit with his back to you.
   RATIONALE: To prevent the patient from using visual clues to pass the hearing test.
4. Assist the patient in putting on the headset and adjust it until it is comfortable.
5. Tell the patient he will hear tones in the right ear.
6. Tell the patient to raise his finger or press the indicator button when he hears a tone.
7. Set the audiometer for the right ear.
8. Set the audiometer for the lowest range of frequencies and the first degree of loudness (usually 15 decibels). (When using automated audiometers, follow the instructions printed in the user's manual.)
9. Press the tone button or switch and observe the patient.
10. If the patient does not hear the first degree of loudness, raise it two or three times to greater degrees, up to 50 or 60 decibels.
11. If the patient indicates that he has heard the tone, record the setting on the graph.
12. Change the setting to the next frequency. Repeat steps 9, 10, and 11.
13. Proceed to the midrange frequencies. Repeat steps 9, 10, and 11.
14. Proceed to the high-range frequencies. Repeat steps 9, 10, and 11.
15. Set the audiometer for the left ear.
16. Tell the patient that he will hear tones in the left ear and ask him to raise his finger or press the indicator button when he hears a tone.
17. Repeat steps 8 through 14.
18. Have the patient remove the headset.
19. Clean the earpieces with a sanitizing wipe.
20. Properly dispose of the used sanitizing wipe and wash your hands.
    RATIONALE: Maintain aseptic technique at all times.

PROCEDURE 43-6 Administering Eardrops

Procedure Goal: To instill medication into the ear to treat certain ear disorders.

OSHA Guidelines:

Materials: Liquid medication, cotton balls.

Method: Procedure steps.

1. Identify the patient, introduce yourself, and explain the procedure.
2. Check the physician's medication order. It should include the patient's name, drug name, concentration, the number of drops, into which ear(s) the medication

is to be administered, and the frequency of administration.

3. Compare the drug with the instructions three times, checking the rights of medication administration.
   RATIONALE: To ensure necessary accuracy.

4. Ask whether the patient has any allergies to ear medications.

5. Wash your hands and put on gloves.

6. Assemble supplies.

7. Warm the medication with your hands or by placing the bottle in a pan of warm water.
   RATIONALE: Internal ear structures are very sensitive to extreme heat or cold. Administering cold medications can result in severe vertigo (dizziness) or nausea.

8. Have the patient lie on his or her side with the ear to be treated facing up.

9. Straighten the ear canal by pulling the auricle upward and outward for adults, down and back for infants and children.

(a)

(b)

FIGURE Procedure 43-6 Step 9 (a) Straighten an adult's ear canal by pulling the auricle upward and outward. (b) Straighten an infant's or child's ear canal by pulling the auricle downward and back.

RATIONALE: Straightening the ear canal assures the medication reaches its destination.

10. Hold the dropper ½ inch above the ear canal.
    RATIONALE: The dropper must not be contaminated by touching the patient's skin or any other surface.

11. Gently squeeze the bottle or dropper bulb to administer the correct number of drops.

FIGURE Procedure 43-6 Step 11 Apply slow gentle pressure to the dropper bulb so you can count the drops and administer the prescribed number.

12. Have the patient remain in this position for 10 minutes.

13. If ordered, loosely place a small wad of cotton in the outermost part of the ear canal.

14. Note any adverse reaction, notifying the physician as necessary.

15. Repeat the procedure for the other ear, if ordered.

16. Instruct the patient on how to administer the drops at home.

17. Ask the patient to repeat the instructions.
    RATIONALE: For maximum effectiveness, it is important that the patient understands how to correctly continue treatment at home.

18. Provide written instructions.

19. Remove the cotton after 15 minutes.

20. Properly dispose of used disposable materials.

21. Remove gloves and wash your hands.

22. Record in the patient's chart the medication, the concentration, the number of drops, the time of administration, and which ear(s) received the medication.

PROCEDURE 43-7 Performing Ear Irrigation

Procedure Goal: To wash out the ear canal to remove impacted cerumen, relieve inflammation, or remove a foreign body.

OSHA Guidelines:

Materials: Fresh irrigating solution, clean basin, clean irrigating syringe, towel or absorbent pad, kidney-shaped basin, cotton balls.

Method: Procedure steps.

1. Identify the patient, introduce yourself, and explain the procedure.

2. Check the doctor's order. It should include the patient's name, the irrigating solution, the volume of solution, and for which ear(s) the irrigation is to be performed. If the doctor has not specified the volume of solution, use the amount needed to remove the wax.

3. Compare the solution with the instructions three times, checking the rights of medication administration.
   RATIONALE: To ensure necessary accuracy.

4. Wash your hands and put on gloves, a gown, and a face shield.
   RATIONALE: Splashing is possible when a syringe is used.

5. Look into the patient's ear to identify cerumen or a foreign body needing to be removed. You will know when you have completed the irrigation when the cerumen or foreign body is removed.
   RATIONALE: Identifying the cerumen or foreign body visually will help you assess when you have successfully completed the irrigation.

6. Assemble the supplies.

7. If the solution is cold, warm it to body temperature by placing the bottle in a pan of warm water.
   RATIONALE: Internal ear structures are very sensitive to extreme heat or cold. Administering cold liquids can result in severe vertigo or nausea.

8. Have the patient sit or lie on his or her back with the ear to be treated facing you.

9. Place a towel or disposable waterproof underpad over the patient's shoulder (or under the head and over the shoulder if the patient is lying down) and have the patient hold the kidney-shaped basin under the ear.

10. Pour the solution into the other basin.

FIGURE Procedure 43-7 Step 7   Warm the irrigation solution in a pan of warm water.

11. If necessary, gently clean the external ear with cotton moistened with the solution.

12. Fill the irrigating syringe with solution (approximately 50 mL).

13. Straighten the ear canal by pulling the auricle upward and outward for adults.
    RATIONALE: Straightening the ear canal allows the solution to reach its destination.

14. Holding the tip of the syringe ½ inch from the opening of the ear and tilted toward the top of the ear canal, slowly instill the solution into the ear. Allow the fluid to drain out during the process.
    RATIONALE: Do not contaminate the syringe by allowing it to touch the patient or by allowing the draining fluid to touch it.

15. Refill the syringe and continue irrigation until the canal is cleaned or the solution is used up.

16. Dry the external ear with a cotton ball and, if ordered, leave a clean cotton ball loosely in place for 5–10 minutes.

17. If the patient becomes dizzy or nauseated, allow him or her time to regain balance before standing up. Assist patient as needed.

18. Properly dispose of used disposable materials.

19. Remove your gloves, gown, and face shield, and wash your hands.

20. Record the following in the patient's chart: procedure and result, amount of solution used, time of administration, and ear(s) irrigated.

21. Put on gloves and clean the equipment and room according to OSHA guidelines.

LEARNING OUTCOMES	KEY POINTS
43.1 **Describe the medical assistant's role in eye exams and procedures performed in a medical office.**	The medical assistant may perform some of the procedures that involve measuring various aspects and functions of the eye, such as visual acuity, color vision, and intraocular pressure.
43.2 **Discuss various eye disorders encountered in a medical office.**	Disorders of the eye include those of the external eye structures, such as blepharitis, ptosis, and sty; disorders of the anterior eye structures, such as conjunctivitis and corneal abrasions; disorders involving internal eye structures, such as cataracts, glaucoma, iritis, and retinal disorders; and refractive disorders, such as myopia, hyperopia, astigmatism, and presbyopia.
43.3 **Identify ophthalmic exams performed in the physician's office.**	Ophthalmic exams performed in the physician's office include inspecting internal eye structures; testing visual fields; glaucoma testing; inspecting external eye structures; and refraction exams.
43.4 **Summarize ophthalmologic procedures and treatments.**	Ophthalmologic procedures and treatments include administering eye medications like eyedrops and ointments and performing eye irrigation.
43.5 **Describe the medical assistant's role in otology.**	Medical assistants in an otology office may assist with or perform auditory screening, administer ear medications, perform ear irrigations, and help with diagnostic tests such as tympanometry.
43.6 **Describe disorders of the ear.**	Ear diseases and disorders include those of the outer ear, such as cerumen impaction, otitis externa, and pruritus; middle ear disorders, such as otitis media, mastoiditis, otosclerosis, and ruptured ear drum; and those of the inner ear, such as labyrinthitis, Ménière's disease, presbycusis, tinnitus, and hearing loss.
43.7 **Recall various hearing and other diagnostic ear tests.**	Hearing and other diagnostic ear tests include audiometry and tympanometry.
43.8 **Summarize ear procedures and treatments.**	Ear treatments and procedures include administration of ear medications, ear irrigation, microscope-aided earwax or foreign body removal, hearing aid fitting, and cochlear implants.

CASE STUDY CRITICAL THINKING

Recall Valarie from the beginning of the chapter. Now that you have completed the chapter, answer the following questions regarding her case.

1. What is the medical assistant's role during the eye irrigation?

2. What are some of the reasons a physician might order an eye irrigation procedure?

1. (LO 43.2) Which of the following is the common name for an inflammation of the conjunctiva?
   a. Pruritus
   b. Pink eye
   c. Blepharitis
   d. Iritis
   e. Hordeolum

2. (LO 43.2) Drooping of the upper eyelid is known as
   a. Astigmatism
   b. Sty
   c. Ptosis
   d. Amblyopia
   e. Conjunctivitis

3. (LO 43.5) An otologist treats which of the following disorders?
   a. Glaucoma
   b. Refractive disorders
   c. Mastoiditis
   d. Cataracts
   e. All of the above

4. (LO 43.6) Ringing in the ears is known as
   a. Presbycusis
   b. Tinnitus
   c. Ménière's disease
   d. Labyrinthitis
   e. Otitis media

5. (LO 43.2) The buildup of which fluid causes glaucoma?
   a. Aqueous humor
   b. Lacrimal fluid
   c. Vitreous humor
   d. Cerumen
   e. Perilymph

6. (LO 43.2) Which of the following is not a visual disturbance?
   a. Presbyopia
   b. Astigmatism
   c. Refractive error
   d. Presbycusis
   e. Hyperopia

7. (LO 43.3) Which of the following would be determined by a refraction exam?
   a. Astigmatism
   b. Blepharitis
   c. Corneal ulcers
   d. Diabetic retinopathy
   e. Strabismus

8. (LO 43.6) Which of the following would improve communication with a hearing-impaired patient?
   a. Speak very loudly
   b. Speak in clear, low-pitched tones
   c. Speak directly into the patient's ear
   d. Overemphasize your lip movements so that the patient can read your lips
   e. Write everything down for the patient to read

9. (LO 43.7) The units for measuring the relative intensity of sounds on a scale from 0 to 130 are
   a. Frequencies
   b. Waves
   c. Audiometers
   d. Periods
   e. Decibels

10. (LO 43.6) Sensorineural hearing loss is caused by
    a. Damage to the inner ear
    b. Impacted cerumen
    c. Otitis media
    d. Tinnitus
    e. Otosclerosis

Assisting with Minor Surgery

CASE STUDY

Patient Name	Gender	DOB
Peter Smith	Male	3/28/19XX

Attending	MRN	Allergies
Paul F. Buckwalter, MD	428-69-544	NKA

PATIENT INFORMATION

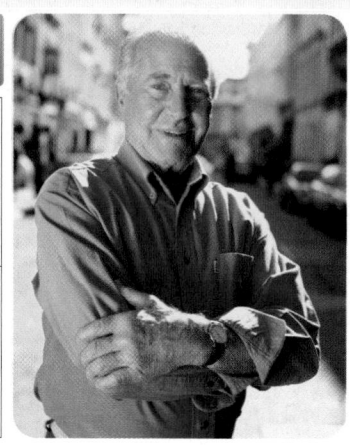

Peter Smith is a 73-year-old male with a history of mild depression. He arrives at the clinic holding a bloody towel over his left forearm. He is brought immediately back to the treatment area. He states that he cut himself with a large knife while cutting a pineapple. You take his vital signs while waiting for the physician. You

notice the blood is leaking through the towel. You need to control the bleeding.

You put on PPE, most importantly gloves, and apply a large dressing over the area, holding firm pressure. The physician arrives, examines the patient, and determines that the patient will need sutures.

Keep Mr. Smith in mind as you study this chapter. There will be questions at the end of the chapter based on the case study. The information in the chapter will help you answer these questions.

LEARNING OUTCOMES

After completing Chapter 44, you will be able to:

44.1 Define the medical assistant's role in minor surgical procedures.

44.2 Describe surgical procedures performed in an office setting.

44.3 Identify the instruments used in minor surgery and describe their functions.

44.4 Describe the procedures for medical and sterile asepsis in minor surgery.

44.5 Discuss the procedures used in a medical office to sterilize surgical instruments and equipment.

44.6 Summarize the medical assistant's duties in preoperative procedures.

44.7 Describe the medical assistant's duties during an operative procedure.

44.8 Implement the medical assistant's duties in the postoperative period.

KEY TERMS

anesthesia
anesthetic
approximate
cryosurgery
debridement
electrocauterization
formalin
incision
inflammatory phase
intraoperative

laceration
ligature
maturation phase
needle biopsy
postoperative
preoperative
proliferation phase
puncture wound
sterile field
suture

CAAHEP

I. P (10) Assist physician with patient care

III. C (8) Differentiate between medical and surgical asepsis used in ambulatory care settings, identifying when each is appropriate

III. P (2) Practice Standard Precautions

III. P (3) Select appropriate barrier/personal protective equipment (PPE) for potentially infectious situations

III. P (5) Prepare items for autoclaving

III. P (6) Perform sterilization procedures

III. A (3) Show awareness of patients' concerns regarding their perceptions related to the procedure being performed

IV. P (6) Prepare a patient for procedures and/or treatments

IV. P (8) Document patient care

IV. A (7) Demonstrate recognition of the patient's level of understanding in communications

IX. P (7) Document accurately in the patient record

ABHES

2. Anatomy and Physiology

   Graduates:

   c. Assist the physician with the regimen of diagnostic and treatment modalities as they relate to each body system

9. Medical Office Clinical Procedures

   Graduates:

   b. Apply principles of aseptic techniques and infection control

   e. Recognize emergencies and treatments and minor office surgical procedures

   h. Wrap items for autoclaving

   k. Prepare and maintain examination and treatment area

   i. Prepare patient for examinations and treatments

   n. Assist physician with minor office surgical procedures

   o. Perform:

      (4) Sterilization techniques

   p. Advise patients of office policies and procedures

10. Medical Laboratory Procedures

    Graduates:

    c. Dispose of biohazardous materials

Introduction

Minor surgical procedures are frequently performed in ambulatory care settings and office practices. Assisting with minor surgery requires a variety of duties and skills. As a medical assistant, you must be knowledgeable of the types of procedures performed where you are employed. You need to know how to prepare the patient for surgery, assist the practitioner during surgery, and care for the patient after surgery. Because all types of surgery require surgical asepsis, a working knowledge of this technique is mandatory.

The Medical Assistant's Role in Minor Surgery LO 44.1

Medical assistants play an important role in all aspects of minor surgical procedures. You will perform administrative tasks prior to the patient's surgery, including completing forms for insurance and obtaining signed informed consent from the patient. You will explain basic aspects of the surgical procedure and answer the patient's questions. Informing the doctor of all current prescription and over-the-counter (OTC) medications that the patient is currently taking is also an administrative task. Finally, you will make sure the patient knows how to follow the appropriate presurgical instructions.

In addition to presurgical administrative tasks, you also will perform many tasks directly related to the surgical procedure. You will make sure the surgical room is clean, neat, and properly lit. You will see that all the equipment, instruments, and supplies the doctor will use are clean, disinfected or sterilized, and properly arranged. You also may function as an unsterile assistant, ensuring the safety and comfort of the patient during the procedure and performing other duties. At other times, you may directly assist with the surgical procedure in a sterile capacity.

Following the surgical procedure, you will help dress the wound and perform other postoperative patient care, making sure the patient is not experiencing ill effects from the surgery or local anesthetic. You will educate the patient about wound care and proper procedures to follow after surgery and make sure the patient has safe transportation home. You also will clean the room and prepare it for the next patient.

Surgery in the Physician's Office LO 44.2

Minor surgical procedures are those that can be safely performed in the physician's office or clinic without general anesthesia. **Anesthesia** is a loss of sensation, particularly the feeling of pain. An **anesthetic** is a medication that causes anesthesia. A general anesthetic affects the entire body, whereas a local anesthetic affects only a particular area. Minor surgical procedures typically involve the use of a local anesthetic in the form of an injection or a cream applied to the skin.

Minor surgery is performed for many reasons, whether it be to diagnose an illness or repair an injury. Other procedures may be elective, or optional. Removal of a wart, skin tag (a small outgrowth of skin, occurring frequently on the neck as people get older), or other small growth for cosmetic reasons is an elective procedure. Some of the common minor surgical procedures you may assist the doctor with include the following:

- Repair of a laceration.
- Irrigation and cleaning of a puncture wound.
- Wound debridement.
- Removal of foreign bodies.
- Removal of small growths.
- Removal of a nail or part of a nail.
- Drainage of an abscess.
- Collection of a biopsy specimen.
- Cryosurgery.
- Laser surgery.
- Electrocauterization.

Common Surgical Procedures

Many surgical procedures are routinely performed in a doctor's office. You may perform some of these procedures on your own. For example, you may change dressings for surgical wounds, and under a doctor's orders, you may remove sutures (commonly called stitches) or staples after wounds have healed. Any procedure that requires an **incision** (a surgical wound made by cutting into body tissue) must be performed by a doctor.

Draining an Abscess An abscess is a collection of pus (white blood cells [WBCs], bacteria, and dead skin cells) that forms as a result of infection. A protective lining can form around an abscess and prevent it from healing. In such a case, the physician may make an incision in the lining of the abscess. This procedure is known as an incision and drainage (I&D). The physician may allow the abscess to drain on its own or insert a drainage tube.

Obtaining a Biopsy Specimen A biopsy specimen is a small amount of tissue removed from the body for examination under a microscope. Most biopsies involve cutting the tissue. For a **needle biopsy**, the doctor uses a needle and syringe to aspirate (withdraw by suction) fluid or tissue cells. (The procedure in the *Assisting in Other Medical Specialties* chapter describes how to assist with a needle biopsy.) All specimens must be placed in a preservative, most commonly a 10% **formalin** solution (a dilute solution of formaldehyde), to prevent changes in the tissue.

Mole Removal A mole, also called a *nevus*, is a small, discolored area of the skin. It may be raised or flat. Any mole that changes shape, size, or color should be evaluated for possible removal. Moles are typically removed by excision or by slicing flush with the skin. If the mole is excised, sutures are usually necessary. Moles that are removed by slicing flush with the skin do not require sutures but may need to be cauterized.

Caring for Wounds A wound is any break in the skin. The break may be accidental or intentional, as from a surgical procedure. There are several types of accidental wounds. A **laceration** is a jagged, open wound in the skin that can extend down into the underlying tissue. The jagged edges may have to be cut away before the wound is closed. A **puncture wound** is a deep wound caused by a sharp object. (See the *Emergency Preparedness* chapter for further information on types and care of accidental wounds.) Both surgical and accidental wounds require special care to prevent infection. Proper wound care that promotes healing without infection is discussed in the Caution: Handle with Care feature.

Cleaning a Wound The first step in preventing a nonsurgical wound from becoming infected is careful cleansing. The wound must be thoroughly cleaned with soap and water. Then, it must be irrigated with sterile saline solution or sterile water, applied with a syringe and needle.

A wound that has dead or sloughing tissue may require a special type of cleaning called **debridement**, the removal of debris or dead tissue from the wound. This procedure helps to expose healthy tissue and promote healing. The doctor may use one of a number of wound debridement methods:

- Surgical—cutting away tissue with scalpel and scissors.
- Chemical—using special compounds to dissolve tissue.
- Mechanical—applying a dressing that sticks to the wound, removing dead tissue when the dressing is removed, or irrigating the wound with sterile saline.
- Autolytic—applying a special dressing that helps the body's natural fluids dissolve dead tissue.

Wound Healing It is important to know how a wound heals so that you can care for it properly. A wound heals in three phases: inflammatory phase, proliferation phase, and maturation phase. The time it takes for a wound to heal depends on several factors, including the patient's age, nutritional status, and overall health. During the initial phase, or **inflammatory phase**, bleeding is reduced as blood vessels in the affected area constrict. Platelets, clotting factors, and WBCs play an important role in this phase. They seal the wound, clot the blood that has seeped into the area, and remove bacteria and debris from the wound. The wound contracts under the clot or scab that forms.

During the second phase, or **proliferation phase**, new tissue forms. Skin cells at the edges of the wound begin to move together to close off the wound. The scab that often forms over a wound actually slows down this movement of skin cells. The edges of the wound eventually come together and form a continuous layer, closing off the wound.

The proliferation phase speeds up if the edges of an incision or nonsurgical wound are **approximated** or brought together so the tissue surfaces are close. This intervention protects the area from further contamination and minimizes scab and scar formation. Small wounds can be held together with butterfly closures, sterile strips, or adhesive. Skin adhesive is a special type of glue used for closing small wounds. Larger wounds or those subject to strain may require suturing or stapling.

The **maturation phase** (the third phase) involves the formation of scar tissue. Scar tissue is important for closing large, gaping, or jagged wounds. The continuous layer of skin cells

CAUTION: HANDLE WITH CARE

Conditions That Interfere with Fast, Effective Wound Healing

The goals for treating both surgical and nonsurgical wounds are similar: to heal the wound without infection and to preserve normal skin function and appearance. Nonsurgical wounds often involve conditions that do not promote fast, effective healing. In these cases, the wounds require special attention to ensure good results.

Many types of nonsurgical wounds contain foreign material that can lead to infection. For example, a child may have a deep laceration from landing on a dirty, broken bottle when falling off a bicycle. These types of wounds always need vigorous cleaning. Some may need debridement.

Wounds heal better when the edges are brought closely together, or approximated. Jagged edges in a laceration make approximation harder. It is also difficult to approximate crushed tissue, as you would see with fingers closed in a car door. Crushing disrupts a tissue's blood supply by rupturing blood vessels throughout the affected area. A physician might debride this type of wound with a scalpel to remove severely damaged tissue and achieve a clean wound edge before suturing.

After a surgical or nonsurgical wound is closed and sutured, it is essential to keep the wound clean and dry to help prevent infection. Infection delays the healing process and can have other serious consequences.

A sutured wound heals more quickly and smoothly when no scab forms because the migrating skin cells encounter no barrier to their movement. Proper postoperative care, including daily cleaning with soap and water or a mild antiseptic, keeps a wound scab-free. Although skin cells migrate across the space of a wound more easily in a somewhat moist environment, a wet wound offers the ideal conditions for bacteria to grow and cause infection. Covering a wound with antiseptic ointment

and a clean, dry dressing keeps the wound slightly moist yet helps prevent infection.

Wound healing may be delayed in a number of instances not directly related to the surgery or injury. The presence of any of the following conditions can put a patient at risk for wound healing problems. Wounds in such patients may require extra attention and care.

- Poor circulation. This condition results in inadequate supplies of nutrients, blood cells, and oxygen to the wound, all of which delay the healing process.
- Aging. Physiologic changes that occur with age can decrease a person's resistance to infection.
- Diabetes. Patients with diabetes experience changes in their artery walls that result in poor circulation to peripheral tissues. These patients also may have a decreased resistance to infection.
- Poor nutrition. Patients who are undernourished, particularly those who are deficient in protein or vitamin C, do not have the physiologic resources for vigorous healing.
- High levels of stress. An increase in stress-related hormones can decrease resistance to infection.
- Weakened immune system. Patients who are on certain medications or who have certain chronic diseases may have weakened immune systems, putting them at increased risk of infection.
- Obesity. When someone is obese, the circulation directly under the skin is often poor, leading to slow healing.
- Smoking. Nicotine constricts the blood vessels in the skin, reducing circulation to the wound area and slowing healing.

---

formed during the second phase becomes thicker and pushes off the scab, leaving a scar. Scar tissue contains no nerves or blood vessels and lacks the resilience of skin.

BODYANIMAT3D
POWERED BY
connect

Go to CONNECT to see an animation about *Wound Healing*.

Closing a Wound Sutures are surgical stitches used to close a wound. Suture materials, or **ligature**, can be either absorbable or nonabsorbable. The body breaks down absorbable sutures, so they do not require removal after the wound has healed. They are typically made of gut (a sterile strand made of collagen fibers usually obtained from sheep or cow intestines). If a wound is particularly deep, the doctor may need to suture in layers, from inside to outside. In this case, absorbable sutures are used for the inner suturing. Removable (nonabsorbable) sutures are generally used for the outside layer. Nonabsorbable ligature must be removed after

wound healing is well under way. These sutures may be made of silk, nylon, or polyester. Suture materials come in thicknesses ranging from size 11-0 (smallest) to size 7 (largest). The needle is already attached to most prepackaged ligature.

Staples may be used to bring the edges of a wound together if there is considerable stress on the incision. For example, a long and deep surgical wound or a wound across the leg would have a strong tendency to gape open if not firmly secured. Surgical staples look somewhat like ordinary staples. They are inserted into the skin with a disposable staple unit.

Special Minor Surgical Procedures

Some types of minor surgical procedures require special surgical instruments. These procedures include laser surgery, cryosurgery, and electrocauterization. They all remove excess or abnormal tissue, as in the case of warts or skin lesions, and usually require surgical aseptic technique because they break the integrity of the skin.

Laser Surgery A laser emits an intense beam of light that is used to cut away tissue. Laser surgery is sometimes preferred over conventional surgery because it causes less damage to surrounding healthy tissue than does conventional surgery. Laser surgery also promotes quick healing and helps prevent infection.

When a laser is used in an office setting, close blinds and shades to keep out stray light. Remove any items—like the paper from wrapped sterile instruments or syringes—that could catch fire if they came in contact with the laser beam. Cover any shiny or reflective surfaces or use nonshiny instruments. Make sure that everyone in the room, including the patient, wears special safety goggles to protect the eyes. You should have a fire extinguisher in the room where it is out of the way but easily accesible. Post a standard laser warning placard in the room's entryway, per Occupational Safety and Health Administration (OSHA) regulations.

Position, drape, and prepare the patient as you would for conventional surgery. Place gauze around the surgical site and assist the physician with administration of a local anesthetic if requested. The physician uses the laser to vaporize the unwanted tissue; vaporized tissue is cleared away by the vacuum hose portion of the unit (see Figure 44-1). You may be asked to apply pressure to control any bleeding. Clean the wound with an antiseptic and apply a sterile dressing. Give the patient the normal instructions on wound care, including the recommendation to protect the site from sun exposure.

Cryosurgery The use of extreme cold to destroy unwanted tissue is called **cryosurgery**. Cryosurgery is often used to remove skin lesions and lesions on the cervix. Before cryosurgery, inform the patient that an initial sensation of cold will be followed by a burning sensation. Instruct the patient to remain as still as possible to prevent damage to nearby tissue.

The doctor may freeze the tissue by touching it with a cotton-tipped applicator dipped in liquid nitrogen or by spraying it with liquid nitrogen from a pressurized can. Sometimes, a special cryosurgical instrument is used, most often during surgery on the cervix.

Make the patient aware that more than one freezing cycle may be necessary. A local anesthetic is usually not required because the cold itself reduces sensation in the area. After the procedure, the area is cleaned with an antiseptic and a sterile dressing may be applied. An ice pack may be applied to reduce swelling and pain relievers may be given for pain.

Reassure the patient that some pain, swelling, or redness is normal after a cryosurgical procedure. Encourage the patient to use ice and pain relievers as necessary. Let the patient know that a large, painful, bloody blister may form. Left undisturbed, the blister usually ruptures in about 2 weeks. It should be left intact to promote healing and prevent infection. The patient should call the doctor if a blister becomes too painful. Be sure to provide the patient with complete wound care instructions.

Electrocauterization This is a technique whereby a needle, probe, or loop heated by electric current destroys the target tissue. A physician may use **electrocauterization** to remove growths like warts, to stop bleeding, and to control nosebleeds that either will not subside or continually recur.

Several types of electrocautery units are in use. Some are small, handheld units powered by battery or by ordinary household electric current. Other, larger units are designed for countertop placement or wall mounting. Some units use disposable probes and others employ reusable ones.

With certain units, a grounding pad or plate is placed on or under the patient's body during the procedure. This grounding completes the circuit and prevents electric shock to the patient, the physician, and staff members. Reassure the patient that grounding causes no discomfort.

A local anesthetic may be administered before the procedure. After electrocauterization, a scab or crust generally forms over the area. Healing may take 2 to 3 weeks. General wound care instructions are appropriate for this procedure, except that a dressing may be omitted to keep the area drier.

▶ Instruments Used in Minor Surgery
LO 44.3

The type of minor surgical procedure determines which surgical instruments are used. Surgical instruments have specific purposes and may be classified by function.

Cutting and Dissecting Instruments
Cutting and dissecting instruments have sharp edges and are used to cut (incise) skin and tissue. Figure 44-2 illustrates some of the basic cutting and dissecting instruments you will encounter. You must be careful when cleaning, sterilizing, and storing these instruments to avoid injuring yourself and to protect the instruments' sharp edges.

Scalpels A scalpel consists of a handle that holds a disposable blade. Scalpel handles are either reusable or disposable and vary in width and length. A scalpel's specific use

FIGURE 44-1 Suction eliminates vaporized tissue as a physician uses a laser to remove a wart from a patient's hand.

Surgical scissors

Sharp/ sharp   Sharp/ blunt   Blunt/ blunt   Blunt/ curved blunt   Curved sharp/ blunt

Lister bandage scissors   Spencer suture scissors   Scalpel handles with blades

DISPOSABLE SCALPEL

Various curettes

FIGURE 44-2 These are typical cutting and dissecting instruments used in minor surgical procedures.

determines the shape and size of its blade. General-purpose scalpels have wide blades and a straight cutting surface. A no. 15 blade is the most common one for performing minor procedures.

Scissors Surgical scissors come in various sizes. They may be straight or curved and have either blunt or pointed tips. Tissue scissors must be sharp enough to cut without damaging or ripping surrounding tissue. Suture scissors have blunt points and a curved lower blade. The lower blade is inserted under the suture material to cut it. Bandage scissors are used to remove dressings. They have a blunt lower blade to prevent injuring the skin next to the dressing. Clippers are scissor-like instruments used for cutting nails or thick materials.

Curettes The doctor uses a curette for scraping tissue. Curettes come in a variety of shapes and sizes and consist of a circular blade—actually a loop—attached to a rod-shaped handle. The blade is blunt on the outside and sharp on the inside. The inner part of the blade may also be serrated. Serrated blades may be used to take Pap (Papanicolaou) smears.

Blunt curettes, known as Buck ear curettes, are used to remove wax from the ear canal when a large amount of cerumen has accumulated.

Grasping and Clamping Instruments

Special instruments are used for grasping and clamping tissue. Grasping instruments are used to hold surgical materials or to remove foreign objects, like splinters, from the body. Clamping instruments are used to apply pressure and close off blood vessels. They also are used to hold tissue and other materials in position. Figure 44-3 shows some common grasping and clamping instruments.

Forceps Forceps are instruments that are commonly used to grasp or hold objects. Grasping types are usually shaped like tweezers and include thumb forceps and tissue forceps. Thumb forceps, also called smooth forceps, vary in shape and size. The blades of thumb forceps are tapered to a point and have small grooves at the tip. Tissue forceps (serrated forceps) have one or more fine teeth at the tips of the blades. When closed, these forceps hold tissue firmly. Holding forceps have handles with ratchets that lock the teeth in a closed position. Dressing, or sponge, forceps have ridges to hold a sponge or gauze when it is used to absorb body fluids.

Hemostats The most commonly used surgical instruments are hemostats. These surgical clamps vary in size and shape and are typically used to close off blood vessels. The serrated jaws of hemostats taper to a point. Like holding forceps, hemostats have handles that lock on ratchets, holding the jaws securely closed.

Towel Clamps Towel clamps are used to keep towels in place during a surgical procedure. This stability is important in maintaining a sterile field.

Retracting, Dilating, and Probing Instruments

Retracting instruments are used to hold back the sides of a wound or incision. Dilating and probing instruments may be used to enlarge, examine, or clear body openings, body cavities, or wounds. The shapes of these instruments vary with their functions. Some typical retracting, dilating, and probing instruments are shown in Figure 44-4.

Retractors The use of retractors allows greater access to and a better view of a surgical site. Some retractors must be held open by hand, while others have ratchets or locks to keep them open.

Dilators Dilators are slender, pointed instruments used to enlarge a body opening, like a tear duct.

Probes A surgical probe is a slender rod with a blunt, bulb-shaped tip. Probes are used to explore wounds or body cavities and to locate or clear blockages.

FIGURE 44-3 These are typical grasping and clamping instruments used in minor surgical procedures.

FIGURE 44-4 These are typical retracting, dilating, and probing instruments used in minor surgical procedures.

Suturing Instruments

Suturing instruments are used to introduce suture materials into and retrieve them from a wound. Some carry the suture material, whereas others manipulate the suture carriers. Examples of suturing instruments are shown in Figure 44-5.

Suture Needles Surgical suture needles carry suture material, or ligature, through the tissue being sutured. They are either pointed or blunt at one end and may have an eye at the other end to hold suture material. Ligature often comes prepackaged with the needle already connected. Prepackaged suture needles with attached ligature have no eye and produce less trauma to the tissue being sutured than do suture needles with eyes.

Suture needles may be straight, or they may be curved to allow deeper suture placement. Taper point needles (needles that taper into a sharp point) are used to suture tissues that are easily penetrated. They create only very small holes, thus minimizing tissue fluid leakage. Cutting needles (needles that have at least two sharpened edges) are used on tough tissues that are not easily penetrated, such as skin.

Several measurements are used to determine the size of a surgical needle. Needle length is the distance from the tip to the end, measuring along the body of the needle. Chord length is the straight-line distance from the tip to the end of the needle. (Chord length is not the same as needle length in curved needles.) The radius of a curved needle is determined by mentally continuing the curve of the needle into a full circle and finding the distance from the center of the circle to the needle body. The diameter is the thickness of the needle. Needle size generally corresponds to the size of suture material used. Smaller needles are used for delicate procedures, like eye surgery or repairing a facial laceration. Larger needles are used for suturing wounds of less delicate parts of the body, like the hands or legs.

Needle Holders Curved suture needles require special instruments to hold, insert, and retrieve them during suturing. Most needle holders look like hemostats with short, sturdy jaws.

Syringes and Needles

Sterile syringes and needles are used to inject anesthetic solutions, withdraw fluids, or obtain biopsy specimens. The size of the syringe and needle varies with the intended use. For example, a needle used to perform a biopsy is generally larger than needles used for most injections. (Syringes and needles used for injections are discussed and illustrated in the *Medication Administration* chapter.) Both syringes and needles are provided in individual sterile envelopes.

Instrument Trays and Packs

All the surgical instruments needed for a specific procedure are usually assembled beforehand. They are then sterilized together in a pack. Certain surgical supplies necessary for the procedure

FIGURE 44-5 These are typical suturing instruments.

FIGURE 44-6 This laceration tray contains scissors, several pairs of forceps, a needle holder, and sterile gauze. Suture material must be added for the procedure.

(like gauze) are included in the pack because they, too, must be sterile. Surgical trays can be quickly set up with these instrument packs. Individually wrapped items also may be added as needed.

These are the common types of instrument trays:

- Laceration repair tray (see Figure 44-6).
- Laceration repair with debridement tray.
- Incision and drainage tray.
- Foreign body or growth removal tray.
- Onychectomy (nail removal) tray.
- Vasectomy (male sterilization procedure) tray.
- Suture removal tray.
- Staple removal tray.

▶ Asepsis

LO 44.4

Maintaining asepsis during surgical procedures is always a priority. It is critical to the health and safety of both the patient and the healthcare professional. The two levels of aseptic technique are medical asepsis (clean technique) and surgical asepsis (sterile technique). Medical asepsis is discussed in detail in the *Basic Safety and Infection Control* chapter. You will use both levels of asepsis when assisting with minor surgery.

Personal Protective Equipment

Personal protective equipment, or PPE, includes all items used as a barrier between the wearer and potentially infectious or hazardous medical materials. PPE includes gloves, gowns, and masks and protective eyewear or face shields. OSHA regulations regarding PPE are discussed in detail in the *Basic Safety and Infection Control* chapter.

Gloves are of particular importance during surgical procedures. You should wear properly sized latex, nitrile, or vinyl gloves during any procedure that might expose you to potentially infectious or hazardous materials. (Gloves that are too big can catch on instruments or equipment and cause accidents.) When you wear gloves, you also protect the patient from any infectious organisms on your hands.

Vinyl, nitrile, and latex gloves can all prevent contamination of the hands with bacteria. Although latex gloves were the preference of healthcare professionals for many years, the incidence of latex allergy among healthcare professionals has grown. Allergic reactions to latex can range from a skin rash to shock and even death. Many healthcare institutions are switching to less allergenic low-powder or powderless nonlatex gloves. The powder in latex gloves, which makes them easier to put on, is one of the primary sources of latex allergy. The latex protein that causes the allergy mixes with the powder. When the gloves are removed, the powder containing the latex protein becomes airborne and is inhaled.

If you work in a facility that uses latex gloves, take these steps to prevent latex allergy:

- If possible use powder free gloves only.
- Thoroughly dry hands after washing.
- Frequently apply non-oil based lotion to the hands.
- Clean areas and equipment contaminated with latex-containing dust frequently.

If you notice latex allergy symptoms, consider consulting an allergist. You also should discuss your symptoms with your supervisor, who will recommend that you switch to hypoallergenic or vinyl gloves. If you have an allergy, the healthcare facility where you are employed is required to provide nonlatex gloves for your use.

Sharps and Biohazardous Waste Handling and Disposal

Sharp medical and surgical instruments have great potential for transmitting infection through cuts and puncture wounds. Used scalpels, needles, syringes, and other sharp objects should be disposed of in a puncture-resistant sharps container.

All items other than sharps that have come in contact with tissue, blood, or body fluids must be disposed of in a leakproof plastic bag or container. The container must either be red or be labeled with the orange-red biohazard symbol. The proper procedure for handling and disposing of sharps and biohazardous waste is discussed in detail in the *Basic Safety and Infection Control* chapter.

Surgical Asepsis

Unlike medical asepsis, surgical asepsis does not just reduce the quantity of microorganisms but completely eliminates them. The goal of surgical asepsis is to control microorganisms before they enter the body. To accomplish this, you will be responsible for sterilizing surgical instruments prior to their use during sterile procedures.

You will be expected to perform the following common procedures involving sterile technique:

- Creating a sterile field.
- Adding sterile items to the sterile field.
- Performing a surgical scrub.
- Putting on sterile gloves.
- Sanitizing, disinfecting, and sterilizing equipment.

Creating a Sterile Field A **sterile field** is an area free of microorganisms that is used as a work area during a surgical procedure. Always be aware that the sterile field is understood to become contaminated and must be redone in the following circumstances:

- An unsterile item touches the field.
- Someone reaches across the field.
- The field becomes wet.
- The field is left unattended and uncovered.
- You turn your back on the field.

The sterile field is often set up on a Mayo stand—a movable stainless steel instrument tray on a stand. Adjust the stand so the tray is above waist level. Remember, items placed below waist level are considered contaminated. Before beginning, disinfect the Mayo stand with 70% isopropyl alcohol and allow it to dry.

To create the sterile field, cover the stand with two layers of sterile material. This material can be sterile disposable drapes, separately sterilized muslin towels, or the muslin towels that the surgical instruments are wrapped in before autoclaving to produce office-sterilized sterile instrument packs. Commercially prepared sterile instrument packs, usually with disposable paper wrappings, are also used to create a sterile field. Procedure 44-1, at the end of this chapter, describes how to prepare a sterile field and how to open sterile packages.

When assembling the necessary supplies, place all unsterile items that may be used during the procedure outside the sterile field. Unsterile items include items that are sterile on the inside but not on the outside, such as a sterile gauze pack or a sterile liquid like alcohol, saline, or peroxide inside an unsterile bottle. Unsterile supplies should be arranged on a counter away from the sterile field. A typical arrangement of unsterile items used in surgery is shown in Figure 44-7. If you place an unsterile item within the sterile field, the field is no longer sterile and you must repeat the entire process.

Go to CONNECT to see a video about *Creating a Sterile Field.*

FIGURE 44-7 For each surgical procedure, unsterile surgical supplies must be gathered and arranged in an area separate from the sterile field.

Adding Sterile Items to the Sterile Field The outer 1 inch of the sterile field is considered contaminated. So, before you add sterile items to the sterile field, carefully plan where you will place the instruments so they are within the sterile field.

Instruments and Supplies If you have used sterile disposable drapes or separately sterilized muslin towels to create the sterile field, you will need to add the necessary instruments. Stand away from the sterile field and open the sterile instrument pack in the manner described in Procedure 44-1. Place the pack on a counter or hold it open in your hand. Transfer and arrange the instruments on the sterile field with sterile transfer forceps. Never reach across the sterile field.

Some instruments are sterilized individually in autoclave bags, and sterile supplies are often prepackaged. Stand away from the sterile field as you open an individual bag or package. You can pull the flaps of the packaging partway apart, then snap (remove from position by a sudden movement) the item onto the sterile field from a distance of 8 to 12 inches. Alternatively, you can use sterile forceps to grasp and place the items in the sterile field.

Pouring Sterile Solutions Sterile solutions are often required during the surgical procedure to rinse or wash the wound. These can be added to the sterile field after the sterile instruments. Several sterile solutions are commonly used during minor surgical procedures, including sterile water and physiological (normal) saline (0.9% sodium chloride).

Bottles of these sterile solutions come in a variety of sizes. Choose the smallest size that will meet the amount of solution needed during the procedure to help minimize cost, because unused solutions may be discarded.

When pouring a solution, cover the label on the bottle with the palm of your hand to keep the label dry. Pour a small amount of the liquid into a liquid waste receptacle to clean the lip of the bottle. As you pour the solution into a sterile bowl on the field, hold the bottle at an angle to avoid reaching over the sterile area. Hold the bottle fairly close to the bowl without touching it. Pour the contents slowly to avoid splashing the drape, which would contaminate the field.

When a sterile solution bottle is opened and may be used again during the procedure, do not let any unsterile object touch the inside of its cap. To accomplish this, place the cap on a clean location with the sterile inside of the cap facing up.

Performing a Surgical Scrub and Donning Sterile Gloves If you assist in a surgical procedure, you must perform a surgical scrub and wear sterile surgical gloves. Surgical scrub procedures are similar to those for aseptic handwashing, but there are several distinctions. Differences include the following:

- A sterile scrub brush is used instead of a nailbrush.
- Both hands and forearms are washed.

- The hands are kept above the elbows to prevent water from running from the arms onto washed areas.
- Sterile towels are used instead of paper towels.
- Sterile gloves are put on immediately after the hands are dried.

You may wonder why a surgical scrub is necessary if you are planning to wear sterile gloves. The answer is that there is always the possibility that a glove may be punctured. If the skin is as clean as possible, the risk of contamination from a punctured glove is minimized. Nevertheless, if a glove is damaged during a sterile procedure, you must consider anything touched by that glove after it is damaged to be contaminated. Contaminated items must be resterilized or replaced before you continue.

A surgical scrub removes microorganisms more effectively than does routine handwashing. Routine handwashing removes bacteria present on the skin's surface, whereas the surgical scrub removes bacteria in deeper layers of the skin—where the hair follicles and oil-producing glands exist. Procedure 44-2, at the end of this chapter, describes the process for performing a sterile scrub.

Sterile gloves are required for many procedures. You don sterile gloves after you perform the surgical scrub. The process for donning sterile gloves is described in Procedure 44-3, at the end of this chapter.

Remember, once you are wearing sterile gloves, you may touch only the items in the sterile field. So, you must remove any drape covering the sterile instrument tray before you glove. Sterile gloves provide a small margin of safety in preventing contamination; your movements must be controlled and precise to work within this margin to protect the sterile area.

Go to CONNECT to see videos about *Performing a Surgical Scrub* and *Donning Sterile Gloves.*

Sanitizing, Disinfecting, and Sterilizing Equipment

Many supplies used in a doctor's office are disposable. Many surgical instruments, however, are made of steel and are reusable. Preparing surgical instruments for reuse involves cleaning them with germicidal soap and water (a process called *sanitization*), then disinfecting and/or sterilizing them, depending on how the equipment will be used. These procedures are described more fully in the *Examination and Treatment Areas* chapter.

▶ Sterilization

LO 44.5

Sterilization is required for all instruments and supplies that will penetrate a patient's skin or come in contact with any other normally sterile areas of the body. Sterilization also is required for all instruments that will be used in a sterile field, even if they will not actually be used on a patient. An item is considered either sterile or unsterile. If you doubt the status of an item, consider it unsterile.

Before sterilizing an item, you must first sanitize it and, sometimes, disinfect it. Instruments and equipment that need to be sterilized include the following:

- Curettes (spoon-shaped instruments for removing material from a cavity wall or other surface).
- Instruments used during surgical procedures.
- Suture removal instruments.
- Vaginal specula (instruments used to enlarge the opening of the vagina and allow examination of the vagina and cervix).

Sterilize instruments and equipment by one of the following methods:

- Autoclaving.
- Chemical (cold) processes.

The Autoclave

The primary method for sterilizing instruments and equipment is the use of pressurized steam in an **autoclave** (Figure 44-8). This device forces the temperature of steam above the boiling point of water (212°F, or 100°C). Sterilization by autoclave is a widely accepted method of sterilization for two reasons:

1. Steam autoclaves can operate at a lower temperature than is required for dry heat sterilization. The moist heat from

FIGURE 44-8 Steam autoclaving is the most common method of sterilizing instruments and equipment. Understanding the gauges and timer is essential to proper operation of an autoclave.

FIGURE 44-9 Common wrapping products and sterilization indicators.

steam more quickly permeates the clean, porous wrappings in which all instruments are placed prior to loading them into the unit.

2. The moisture causes coagulation of proteins within microorganisms at a much lower temperature than is possible with dry heat. When cells containing coagulated protein cool, their cell walls burst; this kills the microorganisms.

General Autoclave Procedures In general, the autoclave process involves the following steps:

1. Prepare sanitized and disinfected instruments and equipment for loading into the autoclave by wrapping them in muslin, special porous paper, plastic bags, or envelopes and labeling each pack. (Include sterilization indicators.)

2. Check the water level in the autoclave; add distilled water if necessary.

3. Preheat the autoclave according to the manufacturer's guidelines. (Some models require putting instruments in before preheating.)

4. Perform any required quality control procedures (in addition to sterilization indicators in instrument packs).

5. Load the instruments and equipment into the autoclave. Allow adequate space around the items to ensure that steam reaches all areas.

6. Choose the correct setting based on the load type (unwrapped items, pouches, packs, liquids, etc.). If the autoclave is not automatic, set the autoclave for the correct time after the correct temperature and pressure have been reached.

7. Run the autoclave through the sterilization cycle, including drying time.

8. Remove the instruments and equipment from the autoclave.

9. Store the instruments and equipment properly for the next use. Rotate stored items so packages with the oldest date are used first. Do not use packages past their expiration date.

10. Clean the autoclave and the surrounding work area.

During each step of the process, assume the instruments and equipment are contaminated, and follow Standard Precautions:

- Wear gloves to avoid contamination by blood, body fluids, or tissues.
- Take measures to protect against needlesticks or cuts—for example, use forceps to handle sharps.
- Wash your hands thoroughly after all cleaning procedures.

Wrapping and Labeling All Items Wrap items in porous fabric, paper, or plastic before placing them in the autoclave. This material helps surround the items with the correct levels of moisture and heat. Instruments and equipment to be used immediately after autoclaving can be placed on trays with material above and below the items. Items that must be stored in a sterile state for later use are wrapped and sealed before autoclaving. Refer to Procedure 44-4, at the end of this chapter, for wrapping and labeling instructions.

A number of products are available for wrapping items for sterilization. Muslin (140 count) is the most commonly used wrapping fabric. Other products include permeable paper, disposable nonwoven fabric, and clear plastic envelopes with one side made of permeable material. Figure 44-9 shows several common wrapping products and sterilization indicators.

Instruments that will be used together should be wrapped together to form a sterile pack. Wrap the pack loosely so the steam can reach the instruments inside. After using a pack, consider all items (even those not used) unsterile and return them for sanitization, disinfection, and sterilization.

Clearly label each pack with a nontoxic marker to identify the item or items inside the wrapping and the person who completed the procedure. The label also must include the date to prevent use after expiring.

Go to CONNECT to see a video about *Wrapping and Labeling Instruments for Sterilization in the Autoclave.*

Preheating the Autoclave Check for solutions that may have boiled over and for deposits that may have formed on any of the inner surfaces. Make sure the water reservoir is filled to the proper level with distilled water. Also check the discharge lines and valves to make sure there are no obstructions. If lines or valves are blocked, air may remain trapped inside the chamber, rendering the load unsterile.

Following this inspection, preheat the unit according to the manufacturer's guidelines. Loading cold instruments into an overheated chamber can cause excess condensation, so be sure to understand and follow the preheating instructions.

Understanding Autoclave Settings Modern autoclaves are designed to operate as automatically as possible; however, manual autoclaves are still used. Because you are responsible for the sterility of the items processed by the autoclave, you must be able to identify the various gauges and interpret their readings correctly.

Manual autoclaves have three gauges and a timer. The jacket pressure gauge shows the outer chamber's steam pressure. The chamber pressure gauge shows the inner chamber's steam pressure. The temperature gauge shows the temperature inside the inner, or sterilization, chamber. The timer allows you to control the number of minutes the load is exposed to the high-temperature, pressurized steam.

Exact temperature and pressure requirements vary with the model and type of autoclave, and with the instruments and packaging in the load. In general, the temperature must reach 250°F to 270°F (121°F to 132°C) and the chamber pressure gauge must show 15 to 30 pounds of pressure. Follow the manufacturer's instructions precisely for each autoclave load. Procedure 44-5, at the end of this chapter, describes the general steps to follow for running a load through the preheated autoclave.

Sterilization Indicators and Quality Control It is important to monitor all sterilization procedures. This is accomplished through the use of various types of indicators and quality control measures.

Sterilization indicators are tags, inserts, tapes, tubes, or strips that confirm the items in the autoclave have been exposed to the correct volume of steam at the correct temperature for the correct length of time. Several types of indicators are available (Figure 44-10).

FIGURE 44-10 Sterilization indicators are manufactured in various types, sizes, and shapes.

For example, you place tags or inserts within the load, whereas you affix tapes to the outside of wrapped instrument packs. These types of indicators have designated areas or words that change color when the correct temperature has been reached. Some also show when the proper temperature, pressure, and duration have occurred. Although it is generally acceptable to rely on these indicators as a guarantee of sterility, they are, in reality, only indicators that the load has been exposed to conditions that usually result in sterile surfaces. They do not guarantee that the autoclave contents are actually sterile.

Biological indicators—containing bacterial spores—are used as a quality control method to confirm that sterilization has occurred. Bacterial spores come in various forms including strips, disks, and ampules. They are used because they are more resistant to common sterilization processes than non-spore-forming organisms. The general procedure for using biological indicators is as follows:

- Place a biological indicator in a load to be sterilized.
- Place another biological indicator outside the autoclave as a positive control.
- Run the load as usual.
- Interpret the biological indicator and positive control as directed by the manufacturer or send to an outside lab for processing.
- Incubate as recommended by the manufacturer.

In general, place indicators in a sufficient number of places in the load so you can be reasonably confident of the sterility of all items in the chamber. The following locations are suitable for indicator positioning:

- Within instrument packs.
- On the outside of wrapped instrument packs.
- Inside containers, especially those that cannot be positioned to allow steam to surround the item.
- Near the air exhaust valve.
- In any other areas into which steam might not be able to flow freely.

For more information regarding interpreting the results of a biological indicator, see the Caution: Handle With Care feature.

Preventing Incomplete Sterilization Although the autoclave is generally considered the simplest and most effective method for sterilizing instruments and equipment, certain pitfalls can cause incomplete sterilization. The four leading factors that cause incomplete sterilization are incorrect timing, insufficient temperature, overcrowding of packs, and inadequate steam levels. Once again, the manufacturer's guidelines provided with the autoclave unit are the best source of accurate information on how to operate it correctly.

Timing Guidelines After loading the autoclave, make sure the heating cycle lasts long enough to allow the steam to permeate all wrappings to reach the instruments and equipment inside. Timing for items to be sterilized should not be

Interpreting the Results of a Biological Indicator

If you do not send the biological indicator to an outside lab, you may be asked to interpret the results. If the indicator exposed to the sterilization cycle is positive for bacterial growth, then sterilization has not occurred. The load should be held, the chemical indicators checked, and the biological indicator test repeated. If the second test is positive, have the sterilizer serviced. Once the sterilizer has been serviced, retest with three consecutive tests in an empty chamber. If all three tests are negative, the sterilizer can be returned to service. If the indicator exposed to the cycle shows no bacterial growth, check the growth of the positive control. The positive control should show bacterial growth because it has not been exposed to the sterilization cycle. Note: If there is no growth on the positive control, you should repeat the quality control procedure with biological indicators from another manufactured lot number. Record the results of each biological indicator monitoring procedure in the sterilization log. Biological indicators should be used at the following times:

- If a new type of packaging material is used.
- If you have a new autoclave.
- After autoclave maintenance or repair.
- On a weekly basis as a general quality control measure.

started until the unit has reached the proper temperature. Automatic autoclaves have preset timing for each load type. You should keep up with the amount of time an automatic autoclave takes to complete a cycle, noting any differences between loads. Large differences in the amount of time it takes to complete a load cycle should alert you to a problem with the autoclave. Although following timing guidelines helps ensure sterilization, you also should use sterilization indicators.

If you have any doubt about the sterility of an instrument or piece of equipment, do not use it. Instead, put it aside for another cycle of sanitization, disinfection, and sterilization. The risks to patients and to you are too great to take chances.

Temperature Guidelines The length of the sterilization cycle is only one factor that has an impact on the final quality of autoclave operations. If the autoclave is manual, the unit must operate at the correct temperature. Unit thermometers and sterilization indicators help confirm correct temperatures have been reached.

Temperatures that are too high can cause problems as easily as those that are too low. If the temperature is too high inside the autoclave compartment, the steam does not have the correct level of moisture. The heat and moisture will not penetrate wrapped instrument packs, resulting in an unsterilized load.

If the temperature is too low, the steam contains too much moisture. Packs will be oversaturated and the drying cycle will be insufficient. Wet packs can easily pick up contaminants from surfaces they touch after you unload them from the autoclave. Common causes of low temperature are failing to preheat the autoclave chamber, loading cold instruments into an overheated chamber, opening the unit door too wide during drying, and overfilling the water reservoir. Always make sure you are familiar with the manufacturer's recommendations before running a load through an autoclave.

Overcrowding Packs or instruments placed in too close proximity in the autoclave chamber may not be sterilized because of the inability of the steam to penetrate or reach all surfaces.

Steam Level Guidelines If the correct level of steam is not present during the autoclave cycle, items will not be sterile at the end of the cycle. It is vital that the unit force all air out of the chamber at the beginning of the sterilization cycle. It is also essential that you place items in the chamber in positions that will not cause formation of air pockets.

To help ensure proper operation of the unit, check all release valves and discharge lines to make sure they are free from obstruction. Clogged valves and lines may prevent elimination of all air from the chamber.

To prevent the formation of air pockets, load items in the autoclave so that the steam can circulate freely around all sides of the items. Place containers on their sides to avoid trapping air. Besides allowing the free flow of steam, careful positioning helps ensure that all items dry thoroughly before you remove them from the autoclave.

Storing Sterilized Supplies After packs and instruments are sterilized in the autoclave, you must store them in a clean, dry location, where they will not be disturbed or shuffled around. This keeps the wrapping material from being torn or otherwise compromised.

The method you use to wrap an item for sterilization determines the item's sterile shelf life. As a general rule, double-layer fabric- or paper-wrapped packages are considered sterile for 30 days. The manufacturers of other wrapping products provide their own guidelines for sterile shelf life.

Return items for sanitization, disinfection, and sterilization after the sterile shelf life period has elapsed. Do not reuse any wrapping or labeling products. Instead, open the packs or wrappings and process each item as if it had never been cleaned.

Cleaning the Autoclave and Work Area Clean the autoclave after each use to prevent accumulation of deposits that might affect the unit's operation. You may use a nontoxic all-purpose cleaner, although specific cleaning products are available for autoclave use.

You are responsible for ensuring that routine cleaning is done correctly and thoroughly. When you clean the unit, also check for signs of cracking or wear in gaskets, drain valves, and tubing. Check the level of distilled water in the reservoir. Service representatives who specialize in the maintenance of your unit should periodically clean and check all seals and gauges.

The work area around the autoclave unit should be divided into two clearly marked areas: one for nonsterile, not-yet-autoclaved items and one for sterile equipment as it is removed from the unit. Do not use supplies from one area in the other. Be sure to move any sterile packs or equipment to the correct storage areas when cleaning the counters and other work surfaces. If anything is spilled on a sterile pack or instrument, return the item for sanitization, disinfection, and sterilization.

Chemical Sterilization

Chemical or cold sterilization involves the use of liquids to eliminate microorganisms on instruments and equipment that are sensitive to heat and steam. For example, in a gastroenterologist's office you may need to disinfect or sterilize an endoscope. Although each facility may perform this process differently, the process involves five steps after performing a leak test on the endoscope:

1. Clean: mechanically clean internal and external surfaces, including brushing internal channels and flushing each internal channel with water and a detergent or enzymatic cleaners.

2. Disinfect: immerse the endoscope in a high-level disinfectant or chemical sterilant and ensure contact of the germicide into all accessible channels, such as the suction/biopsy channel and air/water channel. Expose for the time recommended for specific products.

3. Rinse: rinse the endoscope and all channels with sterile water, filtered water or tap water (high-quality potable water that meets federal clean water standards at the point of use).

4. Dry: rinse the insertion tube and inner channels with alcohol, and dry with forced air after disinfection and before storage. Drying the endoscope is essential to greatly reduce the chance of recontamination of the endoscope by microorganisms that may be present in the rinse water.

5. Store: store the endoscope in a way that prevents recontamination and promotes drying, such as hanging it vertically.

▶ Preoperative Procedures LO 44.6

You must complete a number of steps before a surgical procedure, including performing various preliminary duties, preparing the surgical room, and physically preparing the patient for surgery.

Preliminary Duties

The first tasks you will perform before the surgery include providing **preoperative** (prior to surgery or "preop") instructions to the patient, completing various administrative tasks, and easing the patient's fears.

Preoperative Instructions When a patient is scheduled for a minor surgical procedure in the doctor's office, you must explain the preoperative instructions. Be prepared to answer the patient's questions about the procedure and possible risks. The patient may ask you, rather than the doctor, such questions or may need clarification of information provided by the doctor.

A patient may need to follow certain dietary and fluid restrictions before a minor surgical procedure. Not eating or drinking for a specific period of time is a common restriction. The patient's medications may also be restricted because of anesthetic administration during the procedure. Ask non-English-speaking patients to bring along a family member or other interpreter who can help them understand the forms they must sign and their instructions.

Instruct the patient to wear either comfortable, loose-fitting clothes that will not interfere with the procedure or clothing that can be removed easily. In most cases, patients also need to arrange for someone to drive them home and stay with them for 24 hours after the procedure.

Administrative and Legal Tasks You must ensure that all the necessary paperwork is completed before surgery. Routine administrative tasks include completing the required insurance forms and obtaining prior authorization from the patient's insurance company.

Make absolutely certain the patient reads, understands, and signs the surgical consent form. The patient needs a clear understanding of what to expect during and after the surgery to give informed consent as required by law. Sometimes surgery is performed on a child or a patient with limited understanding of legal documents. In such cases, the consent form must be signed by the patient's parent or legal guardian.

Failure to obtain the necessary paperwork prior to a surgical procedure can cause serious legal problems. The doctor and other staff members could be held legally liable if problems were to develop during or after the procedure.

It is common practice to call the patient the day before the surgery to confirm the appointment. This call also provides a chance to ensure that the patient follows the preoperative instructions. You may be responsible for making this call.

Easing the Patient's Fears Knowing what to expect during and after a surgical procedure will ease the patient's fears. This information allows him to plan daily activities and, if necessary, to arrange for help at home during the recovery period.

Some offices may have educational materials like brochures, fact sheets, or videotapes about the procedure the patient will undergo. You may assist in preparing or acquiring these materials if your office's policy includes such participation for medical assistants. This type of information may increase patient compliance with pre- and postoperative instructions.

Much of a patient's fear about a surgical procedure can be overcome if you spend sufficient time before the procedure explaining what to expect. Be prepared to answer the patient's questions honestly, calmly, and confidently. Your calm and knowledgeable manner will reassure the patient. If the answer to a question requires experience or knowledge beyond your own, pass the question on to the doctor.

Preparing the Surgical Room

Prior to surgery, the doctor should inform you of specific instructions concerning patient preparation. He also will tell you what special equipment or supplies are necessary for the procedure.

Because patients are likely to feel anxious before a procedure, it is best to have everything ready in the surgical room before you escort the patient into the room. Make sure the room is clean, neat, and free of waste from previous procedures. The examining table should have been cleaned and disinfected, and surface barriers (table paper and pillow covers) should have been changed.

Check to see that there is adequate lighting. Make sure that all equipment and supplies necessary for the procedure are available. Check the date and sterilization indicator on sterilized packs and supplies.

You will then wash your hands and prepare the sterile field as outlined in Procedure 44-1, at the end of this chapter. The sterile field and the instruments should be draped with a sterile towel.

Preparing the Patient

Just before the surgery, various concerns must be addressed and procedures completed in sequence. The initial tasks are followed by gowning and positioning the patient and preparing the patient's skin for surgery.

Initial Tasks Before leading the patient into the surgical room, find out whether he has followed the presurgical instructions. Restrictions on food and fluid intake are of particular concern. Also, ask what medications the patient is taking and whether he has taken that day's dosage.

Measure the patient's vital signs. Ask if there are any symptoms or problems the doctor should know about before the surgery. If any unusual signs or symptoms are present, notify the doctor. The doctor will want to examine the patient before proceeding.

Check the chart for medication orders, such as pain medication or a tranquilizer to calm the patient. Medications should be administered at this time so they can take effect before surgery.

Gowning and Positioning the Patient Some procedures require the patient to disrobe and put on a gown to expose the surgical site. If this is the case, you should offer to assist, if appropriate, or leave the room while the patient changes. You should then help the patient onto the table and into the position required for the procedure. You may use one or more small pillows to make the patient as comfortable as possible. Then adequately drape the patient to retain body heat and preserve personal dignity.

Sterile drapes are also used to create a sterile field on a patient's body around the surgical site. Drapes come in a variety of sizes and styles. A fenestrated drape has a round or slitlike opening cut out in the center to provide access to the surgical site.

Surgical Skin Preparation Proper preparation of the patient's skin before surgery reduces the number of microorganisms and the risk of surgical site infection (SSI). The prepared area should extend 2 inches beyond the surgical field—the area exposed in the center of the fenestrated drape. This extra margin allows for draping without contaminating the field.

Cleaning the Area Before proceeding with the surgical skin preparation, wash your hands and don exam gloves. Place a plastic-backed drape under the surgical site to absorb any liquids. Clean the site first with antiseptic soap and sterile water, using forceps and gauze sponges dipped in the solution. Begin at the center of the surgical site and work outward in a firm, circular motion (Figure 44-11). Discard the gauze sponge after each complete pass. Clean in concentric circles until you cover the full preparation area. Continue the process, repeating as necessary, for at least 2 minutes or the amount of time specified in the office's procedure manual. Cleaning takes more time if a wound is dirty or contains foreign materials. When procedures are performed on a hand or foot, clean the entire hand or foot. The skin and body openings, particularly the nose, mouth, and perineum, cannot be considered sterile. Nevertheless, the principles of aseptic technique require that you try to keep the area as contamination-free as possible.

Removing Hair from the Area Depending on office policy, you may be required to remove hair from the surgical site. Shaving often causes many small wounds on the skin, which

FIGURE 44-11 Clean the surgical site with antiseptic soap and sterile water. Begin at the center of the surgical site and work outward in a firm, circular motion. Clean in a circular, outward pattern 2 inches larger than the surgical field.

increases the risk of infection, and is not recommended. Some experts feel that hair should not be removed unless it is thick enough to interfere with surgery. If this is the case, hair may be trimmed with scissors or electric trimmers or smoothed out of the way. This should be done with care—to avoid damaging the skin—immediately before surgery.

Applying the Antiseptic Next, apply antiseptic solution to the area. Antiseptics are agents that are applied to the skin to limit the growth of microorganisms and to help prevent infection. Povidone iodine (Betadine) is most commonly used, but chlorhexidine gluconate (Hibiclens) or benzalkonium chloride (Zephiran Chloride) may also be used, particularly if the patient is allergic to iodine. Swab an area 2 inches larger than the surgical field with the antiseptic solution in a circular outward motion, starting at the surgical site. This is the same motion that is used for cleaning the surgical site. For surgery on a hand or foot, swab the entire hand or foot. Allow the antiseptic to air-dry; do not pat it dry—that would remove some of the solution's antiseptic properties.

When the area is dry, treat it as a sterile field. Instruct the patient not to touch the area. Cover the area with a sterile fenestrated drape, from front to back. Avoid reaching over the field. At this point, notify the physician that the patient is ready. Then prepare yourself to assist with the surgery.

▶ Intraoperative Procedures LO 44.7

Intraoperative procedures are procedures that take place during surgery. You may be asked to perform a wide variety of unsterile and sterile tasks during surgery, like preparing a local anesthetic for the doctor, monitoring the patient, processing specimens, and handing instruments to the doctor. The doctor also may ask you to explain to the patient step by step what will be done next during the procedure.

Administering a Local Anesthetic

Before beginning the surgical procedure, the physician will administer a local anesthetic. Some local anesthetics are injected. An injected anesthetic is packaged in a sterile vial (a small glass bottle with a self-sealing rubber stopper). Other local anesthetics come in a cream, gel, or spray form. These anesthetics are topical (applied directly to the skin) and affect only the area to which they are applied. The choice of administration method depends on how invasive or painful the procedure is likely to be.

Lidocaine (Xylocaine) is the most commonly used anesthetic, often used as a topical gel anesthetic. Tetracaine hydrochloride (Pontocaine), a long-acting anesthetic, is injected.

Topical Application A topical anesthetic is useful when the pain will be mild or when only the skin's upper layers are affected. It is common to use such agents to anesthetize the area of a small laceration prior to suturing. Sometimes an anesthetic cream is applied before a local anesthetic is injected to reduce or eliminate the pain caused by the injection. A topical anesthetic must usually remain on the skin for 10 to 15 minutes for the area to become sufficiently anesthetized.

Injections If a local anesthetic is to be injected, it is typically administered after the skin is prepared but before the patient is draped. In some cases, however, the anesthetic is injected prior to skin preparation to allow time for it to take effect. In either case, it is important to note the time of anesthetic administration in the patient's chart.

If the doctor is already wearing sterile gloves, you may be asked to assist in administering the anesthetic. Because administering an anesthetic is an unsterile task (the outside of the vial is unsterile), when performing it, follow proper procedure to protect the sterility of the doctor's gloves and the anesthetic solution.

First, check the label of the anesthetic vial two times to confirm that it is the correct solution. Then, clean the vial's rubber stopper with a 70% isopropyl alcohol solution and leave the alcohol pad on top of the stopper. Present the requested needle and syringe to the doctor by peeling half the outer wrapper away and allowing the doctor to remove them from the wrapper.

Remove the pad from the rubber stopper and hold the vial so the doctor can verify it is the proper medication. Turn the vial upside down and hold it securely around the base, without touching the sterile stopper. Be sure to hold the vial in front of you at shoulder height. Because significant force will be necessary to push the needle through the rubber stopper, brace the wrist of the hand holding the vial with your free hand. Hold the vial firmly so the doctor can withdraw the anesthetic from it (Figure 44-12). Check the vial a third time to confirm that it is the correct solution.

Potential Side Effects of the Anesthetic You should inform the patient of possible reactions to the anesthetic medication. Although rare, reactions may include dizziness, loss of consciousness, seizures, or cardiac arrest. Adverse reactions can occur if the anesthetic dose is too high or if it is absorbed too quickly. They also can occur if the patient is taking other medications that should not be mixed with the anesthetic. It is vital to document all medications (including OTC ones) that the patient is taking at the time of the surgery.

FIGURE 44-12 You must hold the anesthetic vial firmly to allow the physician to puncture the rubber stopper with the needle.

Use of Epinephrine Epinephrine is a sterile solution that is sometimes injected along with an anesthetic. It constricts the blood vessels, making them narrower, which reduces bleeding and prolongs the action of the local anesthetic. Epinephrine is used if the surgery site is an area with many small blood vessels that are expected to bleed profusely (like the head). Reducing bleeding makes it easier to see and to repair the wound.

Epinephrine should be used with caution, however, in patients with heart disease or respiratory disease. Epinephrine also prolongs the anesthesia because epinephrine slows the rate at which the anesthetic spreads into the tissue. This effect may or may not be desirable. There is some concern that epinephrine may increase wound infection rates. If the wound is highly contaminated, the physician may choose to use anesthetic without epinephrine.

Assisting the Physician during Surgery

Your role in surgical assisting depends on the type of surgery and the physician's preference. You may assist the physician in one of two capacities with different duties: as a floater—an unsterile assistant who is free to move about the room and attend to unsterile needs—or as a sterile scrub assistant—who assists in handling sterile equipment during the procedure.

The Floater If you are assisting as a floater (sometimes called a circulator), you will perform a routine hand wash and don exam gloves. Remember, you cannot touch sterile items in the sterile field because you have not performed a surgical scrub and are not wearing sterile gloves. Procedure 44-6, at the end of this chapter, outlines the tasks performed by a floater (unsterile assistant).

Monitoring and Recording One of a floater's most important duties is to monitor the patient during the procedure. You must measure vital signs regularly and observe the patient for reactions to the anesthetic. Record all observations in the patient's chart. Also, write down any information or notes the doctor requests. You must keep a record of time, including when the anesthetic is administered, when the procedure begins, and when the procedure is completed.

Processing Specimens When you serve as a floater during surgery, the doctor may ask you to receive and process specimens for laboratory examination. Most tissues are placed in a 10% formalin solution to preserve them before they are sent to the laboratory. If the container is not prefilled, half-fill the specimen container with the formalin solution ahead of time. Remove the lid of the specimen container without touching the rim. Hold the container out toward the doctor so she can place the tissue directly into it without contaminating the sample (Figure 44-13).

The container should be labeled with the following information:

- The patient's name and the doctor's name.
- The date and time of collection.
- The body site from which the specimen was obtained.
- Your initials.

FIGURE 44-13   Be sure to hold the specimen container so the doctor can place the tissue in it without touching the rim or outside of the container with the tissue.

If more than one specimen is obtained from a patient, place each specimen in a separate container. Label each container with the necessary information, along with a number to indicate the order in which the specimens are obtained (no. 1, no. 2, and so on). The physician will usually tell you the exact location of each specimen taken. You will also fill out a laboratory requisition slip to send along with the specimen(s). Specimen containers should be red or labeled with the biohazard symbol and placed in specially designed bags for transport.

Other Duties As a floater, you also may be asked to perform a number of other duties, including:

- Assisting with the injection of additional anesthetic.
- Adding additional sterile items to the sterile tray.
- Pouring sterile solutions.
- Keeping the surgical area clean and neat during the procedure.
- Repositioning the patient as necessary.
- Adjusting lighting.

The Sterile Scrub Assistant When you serve as a sterile scrub assistant, you perform a surgical scrub and wear sterile gloves. You may be asked to perform a variety of tasks under sterile conditions. Remember, do not touch unsterile items after putting on sterile gloves. Procedure 44-7, at the end of this chapter, outlines the tasks performed by a sterile scrub assistant.

Handling Instruments Your first duty as a sterile scrub assistant is, typically, to close the instruments on the sterile tray because they are left in the open position during sterilization. Your next duty is to rearrange the instruments on the tray in the order in which they will be used or according to the doctor's preference. Instruments are generally used in the following sequence:

- Cutting instruments.
- Grasping instruments.
- Retractors.

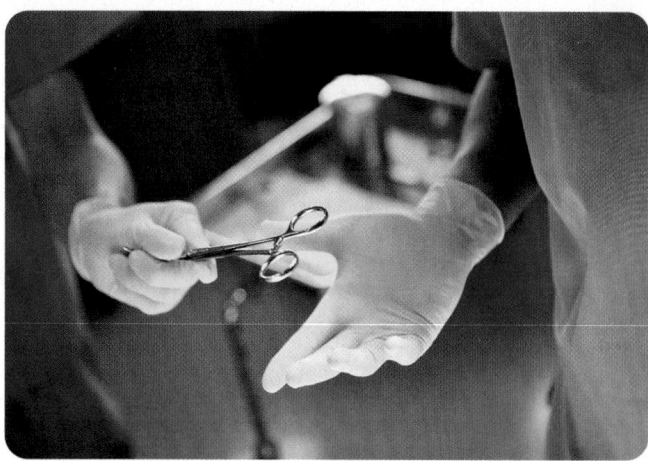

FIGURE 44-14 Holding the scissors by the hinge, slap the handles into the doctor's hand.

- Probes.
- Suture materials.
- Needle holders and scissors.

Prepare for swabbing by placing several sterile gauze squares in the dressing forceps, to be ready when needed. As the sterile scrub assistant, you will be asked to pass instruments to the doctor during the procedure. You must hold instruments so the doctor can grasp them safely and securely, without needing to reposition them in her hands. At the same time, the instruments must be handled properly to maintain their sterility.

When passing scissors and clamps, hold them by the hinge (Figure 44-14). You will have a clear view of the instrument's tip and the doctor will have full use of the handles. Firmly slap the instrument handles into the doctor's extended palm. The doctor's hand will close around the handles as a reflex action to the slapping. This technique reduces the risk of dropping an instrument. If the scissors or clamp is curved, the curve should follow the same curve as the doctor's hand.

When passing a scalpel, hold it above and just behind the cutting edge of the blade so the doctor can grasp the entire handle (Figure 44-15). Pass a needle holder with suture material so

FIGURE 44-15 Hold a scalpel above and just behind the cutting edge as you pass the handle into the palm of the doctor's hand.

the needle is pointing up, and hold the end of the suture material with your other hand to prevent the material from becoming tangled in the handles.

Other Duties As a sterile scrub assistant, you also may be asked to swab fluids from a wound or to retract the edges of a wound to help the doctor view the area. While the doctor is closing the wound, you may be required to cut the suture material after each stitch. The doctor may not verbalize every request to you. With practice and after experience with a particular doctor, you will learn how to respond to the doctor's actions.

When cutting suture materials, leave ⅛ inch of the material above the knot. This length prevents the suture from coming untied, but is short enough that it does not bother the patient.

▶ Postoperative Procedures   LO 44.8

You will be responsible for the patient's **postoperative** ("postop") follow-up after the surgical procedure. Your duties may include immediate care of the patient, proper cleaning of the surgical room, and follow-up care of the patient. Procedure 44-8, at the end of this chapter, outlines the tasks performed after a minor surgical procedure.

Immediate Patient Care

Patient care is your top priority as a medical assistant. Except for intravenous medications, you will administer postoperative medications the physician requests for the patient. You also will ensure that the patient remains lying down on the examining table for the prescribed length of time after the procedure. During this period, continue to monitor the patient's vital signs and watch for adverse reactions. Document your observations in the patient's chart.

Dressing the Wound You also may dress the wound during the monitoring period. Dressings are sterile materials used to cover an incision. They serve a number of functions. They protect the wound from further injury and keep the wound clean, thus preventing infection. Dressings also reduce bleeding, absorb fluid drainage, reduce discomfort to the patient, speed healing, and reduce the possibility of scarring. Gauze dressings are the most common type and come in a variety of sizes and shapes.

Before dressing the wound, don clean exam gloves. Place the sterile dressing over the site and secure it appropriately.

Bandaging the Wound It may be necessary to apply a bandage (a clean strip of gauze or elastic material) over the dressing to help hold it in place. Tube gauze may be needed for bandaging wounds on fingers or other extremities. Application of this type of gauze requires a special applicator. The applicator is a wire cage on which the gauze is loaded. Bandages also may be used to improve circulation, to provide support or reduce tension on a wound or suture and prevent it from reopening, or to prevent movement of that area of the body. Adhesive tape also may be used for these purposes. Some patients are allergic to the adhesive, but most tapes are now hypoallergenic. The patient is usually more comfortable after a bandage or adhesive tape has been applied.

Postoperative Instructions After the procedure, provide oral postoperative instructions to the patient. You may do this during the monitoring part of the postoperative period or afterward. These instructions include guidelines for pain management and instructions for wound care. Postoperative information also includes dietary or activity restrictions, if any, and when to come in for a follow-up appointment. It is a good idea to ask patients to repeat what you say so you know they understand the information.

Instructions should be provided in writing as part of a complete postoperative information packet. You may be asked to help prepare or update packet materials, especially if you routinely assist patients as they recover from minor surgery. A postoperative information packet might include the following information:

- Proper wound care instructions.
- Suggestions for pain relief and reduction of swelling, like medications and hot or cold packs.
- Dietary restrictions.
- Activity restrictions.
- Timing for a follow-up appointment or an appointment card.

Wound care instructions include details on changing the dressing, keeping the wound clean, recognizing signs of infection, and protecting the wound. The instructions may vary depending on the depth and size of the wound. In general, the bandage should be removed after the first 24 hours or if it becomes soaked with blood, wet, or dirty. A wet dressing allows bacteria and other contaminants to enter the wound. In most cases, the wound may be cleaned with soap and water after 24 to 48 hours. Once cleaned, gently dry the incision with a sterile gauze and cover with a clean, dry bandage.

You should teach the patient about the signs of infection. For more information, see Educating the Patient: When to Call the Doctor about a Wound. Encourage the patient to protect the incision from sun exposure for the first 6 months; doing so helps prevent the incision line from becoming darker than the surrounding skin.

The length of time it takes for a wound to heal varies with the site, the patient's age and health status, and the severity of the wound. So, each patient needs specific instructions on how long to continue with the dressings and when to return for suture or staple removal. He or she also may need specific information about limiting activities.

Patient Release Notify the doctor when the patient is stabilized and ready to leave. The doctor may want to further observe and instruct the patient. Be sure to offer assistance if the patient needs help getting dressed.

Then help the patient check out. Schedule the next appointment for the patient. Make sure the patient has the correct discharge packet. Confirm arrangements to transport the patient home. Finally, assist the patient to the car or other transport if this is part of office procedure.

EDUCATING THE PATIENT
When to Call the Doctor about a Wound

Whether a wound is post-surgical or from an accident, it is important for patients to know when they should call the doctor. Understanding when a wound needs medical attention can reduce the instances of scarring and infection. You can help by teaching them what to look for when they have a wound. Patients with any wounds should call the office if they have any of the following:

- Jagged or gaping edges.
- A face wound.
- Limited movement in the area of the wound.
- Tenderness or inflammation at the wound site.
- Purulent drainage.
- A fever greater than 100°F.
- Red streaks near the wound.
- A puncture wound.
- Bleeding that does not stop after 10 minutes of pressure.
- Sutures coming out on their own or too early.

If a patient insists on driving himself home, enter this information on the chart. Indicate the time and have the patient initial the entry. This documentation is important for legal reasons. It would clarify liability should an accident occur as a result of a reaction to the surgery or the anesthetic.

Go to CONNECT to see a video about *Assisting after Minor Surgical Procedures.*

Surgical Room Cleanup

If there is time during the monitoring period, begin to clean up the surgical area. If time is not available then, perform the cleanup routine after the patient has been released. Refer to the *Examination and Treatment Area* chapter sanitization and disinfection guidelines.

Follow-Up Care

During a follow-up appointment, the physician examines the patient's surgical wound. You may be asked to change the dressing or remove the wound closures. Typically, suture or staple removal takes place 5 to 10 days after minor surgery. The sutures or staples are ready for removal when a clean, unbroken suture line is observed. There should be no scabs, no seepage from the wound, and no visible opening. Any of these signs may indicate unhealed areas. Suture removal is described in Procedure 44-9, at the end of this chapter. Staple removal is similar, except that staple removal forceps, rather than thumb forceps and scissors, are used to remove the staples.

Go to CONNECT to see a video about *Suture Removal.*

PROCEDURE 44-1 Creating a Sterile Field

Procedure Goal: To create a sterile field for a minor surgical procedure.

OSHA Guidelines: This procedure does not involve exposure to blood, body fluids, or tissues.

Materials: Tray or Mayo stand, sterile instrument pack, sterile transfer forceps, cleaning solution, sterile drape, and additional packaged sterile items as required.

Method: Procedure steps.

1. Clean and disinfect the tray or Mayo stand.
2. Wash your hands and assemble the necessary materials.
3. Check the label on the instrument pack to make sure it is the correct pack for the procedure.
4. Check the date and sterilization indicator on the instrument pack to make sure the pack is still sterile.
   RATIONALE: Using an out-of-date pack puts the patient at risk for surgical site infection.
5. Place the sterile pack on the tray or stand and unfold the outermost fold away from yourself.
6. Unfold the sides of the pack outward, touching only the areas that will become the underside of the sterile field.
   RATIONALE: Touching the inside of the pack will contaminate the sterile field.
7. Open the final flap toward yourself, stepping back and away from the sterile field.

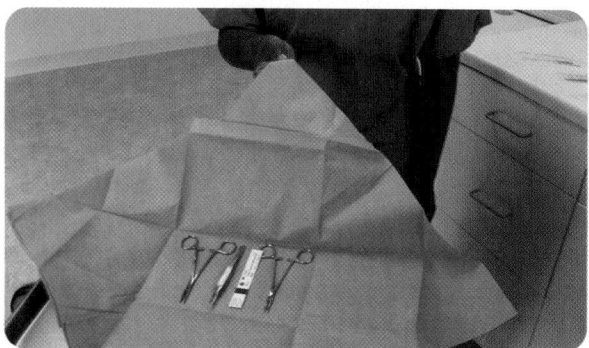

FIGURE Procedure 44-1 Step 7 Open the flap toward yourself last to avoid reaching over the sterile field.

8. Place additional packaged sterile items on the sterile field.
   - Ensure that you have the correct item or instrument and that the package is still sterile.
   - Stand away from the sterile field.
   - Grasp the package flaps and pull apart about halfway.

- Bring the corners of the wrapping beneath the package, paying attention not to contaminate the inner package or item.
- Hold the package over the sterile field with the opening down; with a quick movement, pull the flap completely open and snap the sterile item onto the field.

FIGURE Procedure 44-1 Step 8 Hold the package over the sterile field with the opening down. Pulling the flap open, snap the instrument onto the field.

9. Place basins and bowls near the edge of the sterile field so you can pour liquids without reaching over the field.
   RATIONALE: Reaching over the field may drop contaminants in the field.

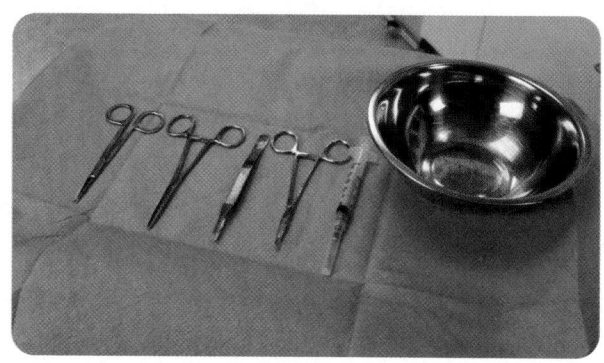

FIGURE Procedure 44-1 Step 9 Placing the bowl at the edge of the sterile field keeps you from reaching over the sterile field to pour liquids in the bowl.

10. Use sterile transfer forceps if necessary to add additional items to the sterile field.
11. If necessary, don sterile gloves after a sterile scrub to arrange items on the sterile field.

PROCEDURE 44-2 Performing a Surgical Scrub

Procedure Goal: To remove dirt and microorganisms from under the fingernails and from the surface of the skin, hair follicles, and oil glands of the hands and forearms.

OSHA Guidelines: This procedure does not involve exposure to blood, body fluids, or tissues.

Materials: Dispenser with surgical soap, sterile surgical scrub brush or sponge, and sterile towels.

Method: Procedure steps.

1. Remove all jewelry and roll up your sleeves to above the elbow.

2. Assemble the necessary materials.

3. Turn on the faucet using the foot or knee pedal.

4. Wet your hands from fingertips to elbows, keeping your hands higher than your elbows.
   RATIONALE: This prevents water from running down your arms and contaminating the washed area.

5. Under running water, use a sterile brush to clean under your fingernails.

6. Apply surgical soap and scrub your hands, fingers, areas between the fingers, wrists, and forearms with the scrub sponge, using a firm circular motion. Follow the manufacturer's recommendations to determine appropriate length of time (usually 2 to 6 minutes).
   RATIONALE: Scrubbing all surfaces dislodges microorganisms so they may be rinsed away.

FIGURE Procedure 44-2 Step 7 Keep your hands higher than your elbows when rinsing after a surgical scrub so water runs away from the fingertips.

8. Thoroughly dry your hands and forearms with sterile towels, working from the hands to the elbows.
   RATIONALE: Using sterile towels prevents recontaminating your hands.

FIGURE Procedure 44-2 Step 6 With a sterile scrub brush, use a circular motion to scrub every surface of your hands and forearms.

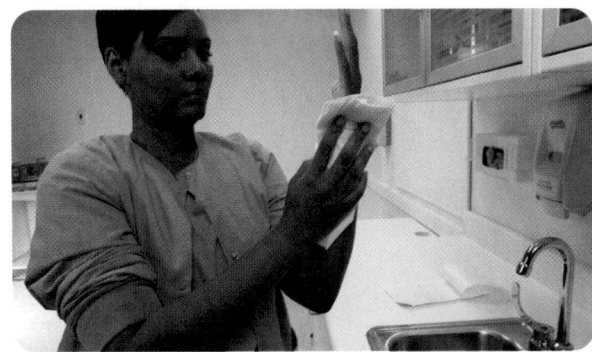

FIGURE Procedure 44-2 Step 8 Dry your hands with sterile towels, working from the hands to the elbows.

7. Rinse from fingers to elbows, always keeping your hands higher than your elbows.

9. Turn off the faucet with the foot or knee pedal. Use a sterile paper towel if a foot or knee pedal is not available.

PROCEDURE 44-3 Donning Sterile Gloves

Procedure Goal: To don sterile gloves without compromising the sterility of the gloves' outer surface.

OSHA Guidelines: This procedure does not involve exposure to blood, body fluids, or tissues.

Materials: Correctly sized, prepackaged, double-wrapped sterile gloves.

Method: Procedure steps.

1. Obtain the correct size gloves.

2. Check the package for tears and ensure that the expiration date has not passed.
   RATIONALE: A torn package should be considered unsterile.

3. Perform a surgical scrub.

4. Peel the outer wrap from gloves and place the inner wrapper on a clean surface above waist level.

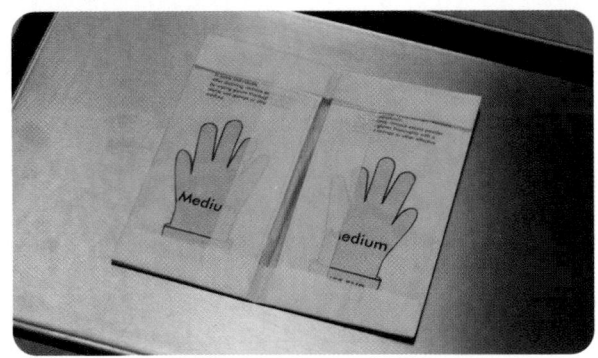

FIGURE Procedure 44-3 Step 4 Place the inner wrap on a clean surface, above waist level, with the cuff end closest to your body.

5. Position gloves so the cuff end is closest to your body.

6. Touch only the flaps as you open the package.

RATIONALE: Touching the inside of the package could contaminate the gloves.

7. Use instructions provided on the inner package, if available.

8. Do not reach over the sterile inside of the inner package.

9. Follow these steps if there are no instructions:

   a. Open the package so the first flap is opened away from you.

   b. Pinch the corner and pull to one side.

   c. Put your fingertips under the side flaps and gently pull until the package is completely open.

10. Use your nondominant hand to grasp the inside cuff of the opposite glove (the folded edge). Do not touch the outside of the glove. If you are right-handed, use your left hand to put on the right glove first, and vice versa.

    RATIONALE: Grabbing the inside of the glove allows you to put it on without contaminating its outside.

11. Holding the glove at arm's length and waist level, insert the dominant hand into the glove, palm facing up. Do not let the outside of the glove touch any other surface.

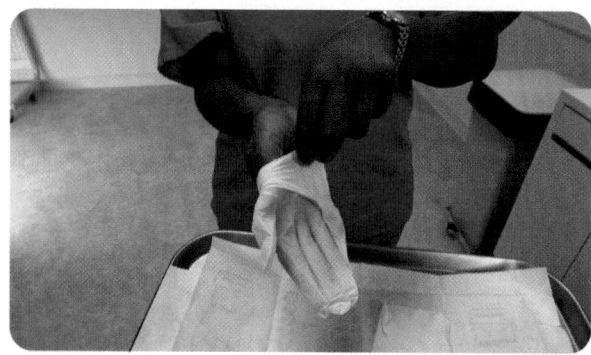

FIGURE Procedure 44-3 Step 11   When donning the glove, do not let the outside of the glove touch any other surface.

12. With your sterile gloved hand, slip the gloved fingers into the cuff of the other glove.

13. Pick up the other glove, touching only the outside. Do not touch any other surfaces.

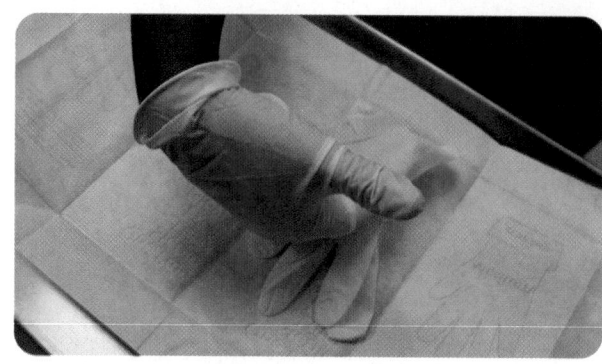

FIGURE Procedure 44-3 Step 13   Slip the fingers of your gloved hand into the other glove's cuff, touching only the outside.

14. Pull the glove up and onto your hand, ensuring that the sterile gloved hand does not touch your skin.

FIGURE Procedure 44-3 Step 14   Pull the glove up and onto your hand without touching the sterile gloved hand to your skin.

15. Adjust your fingers as necessary, touching only glove to glove.

16. Do not adjust the cuffs because your forearms may contaminate the gloves.

17. Keep your hands in front of you, between your shoulders and waist. If you move your hands out of this area, they are considered contaminated.

18. If contamination or the possibility of contamination occurs, change gloves.

19. Remove these gloves the same way you remove clean gloves, by touching only the inside.

    RATIONALE: Touching only the inside of the gloves reduces exposure to the patient's blood and body fluids.

PROCEDURE 44-4   Wrapping and Labeling Instruments for Sterilization in the Autoclave

Procedure Goal: To enclose instruments and equipment to be sterilized in appropriate wrapping materials to ensure sterilization and to protect supplies from contamination after sterilization.

OSHA Guidelines:

Materials: Dry, sanitized, and disinfected instruments and equipment; wrapping material (paper, muslin, gauze, bags, envelopes); sterilization indicators; autoclave tape; labels (if wrapping does not include space for labeling); and a waterproof pen.

Method: Procedure steps.

For Wrapping Instruments or Equipment in Pieces of Paper or Fabric

1. Wash your hands and don gloves before beginning to wrap the items to be sterilized.

2. Place a square of paper or muslin on the table with one point toward you. With muslin, use a double thickness. The paper or fabric must be large enough to allow all four points to cover the instruments or equipment you will be wrapping. It also must be large enough to provide an overlap, which will be used as a handling flap.

3. Place each item to be included in the pack in the center area of the paper or fabric "diamond." Items that will be used together should be wrapped together. Make sure, however, that surfaces of the items do not touch each other inside the pack so that steam can penetrate every surface of all instruments in the pack. Inspect each item to ensure it is operating correctly. Place hinged instruments in the pack in the open position. Wrap a small piece of paper, muslin, or gauze around delicate edges or points to protect against damage to other instruments or to the pack wrapping.

4. Place a sterilization indicator inside the pack with the instruments. Position the indicator correctly, following the manufacturer's guidelines (Figure a).
   RATIONALE: A sterilization indicator must always be placed inside the pack to ensure the contents have been sterilized properly.

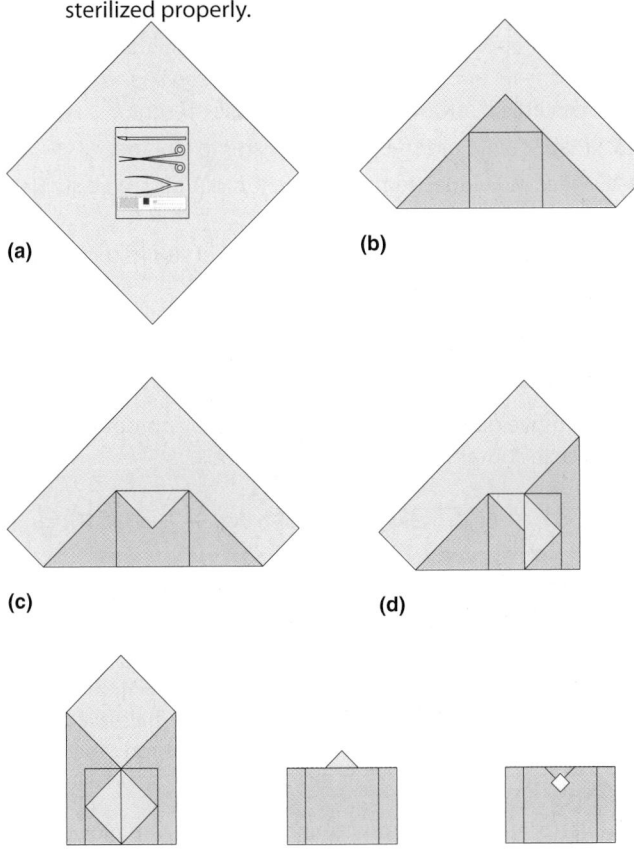

(a)   (b)

(c)   (d)

(e)   (f)   (g)

FIGURE Procedure 44-4 Step 4   Follow the sequence in this figure when you wrap instruments in a paper or fabric pack for sterilization in an autoclave.

5. Fold the bottom point of the diamond up and over the instruments in to the center (Figure b). Fold back a small portion of the point (Figure c).
   RATIONALE: This "handle" will be used later, when the sterile pack is opened.

6. Fold the right point of the diamond in to the center. Again, fold back a small portion of the point to be used as a handle (Figure d).

7. Fold the left point of the diamond in to the center, folding back a small portion to form a handle. The pack should now resemble an open envelope (Figure e).

8. Grasp the covered instruments (the bottom of the envelope) and fold this portion up, toward the top point (Figure f). Fold the top point down over the pack, making sure the pack is snug but not too tight.

9. Secure the pack with autoclave tape (Figure g). A "quick-opening tab" can be created by folding a small portion of the tape back onto itself. The pack must be snug enough to prevent instruments from slipping out of the wrapping or damaging each other inside the pack, but loose enough to allow adequate steam circulation through the pack.

10. Label the pack with your initials and the date. Then list the contents of the pack. If the pack contains syringes, be sure to identify the syringe size(s).
    RATIONALE: Dating helps you keep up with the date the pack expires. Items should be easily identified without opening the pack.

11. Place the pack aside for loading into the autoclave.

12. Remove gloves, dispose of them in the appropriate waste container, and wash your hands.

For Wrapping Instruments and Equipment in Bags or Envelopes

1. Wash your hands and put on gloves before beginning to wrap the items to be sterilized.

2. Insert the items into the bag or envelope as indicated by the manufacturer's directions. Hinged instruments should be opened before insertion into the package.
   RATIONALE: This allows steam to penetrate inside the hinge.

3. Close and seal the pack. Make sure the sterilization indicator is not damaged or already exposed.
   RATIONALE: If the sterilization indicator is damaged or already exposed, you have no way of knowing if the sterilization cycle was completed.

4. Label the pack with your initials and the date. Then list the contents of the pack. The pens or pencils used to label the pack must be waterproof; otherwise, the contents of the pack and date of sterilization will be obliterated.
   RATIONALE: Dating helps you keep up with the date the pack expires. Items should be easily identified without opening the pack.

5. Place the pack aside for loading into the autoclave.

6. Remove gloves, dispose of them in the appropriate waste container, and wash your hands.

PROCEDURE 44-5 Running a Load through the Autoclave

Procedure Goal: To run a load of instruments and equipment through an autoclave, ensuring sterilization of items by properly loading, drying, and unloading them.

OSHA Guidelines:

Materials: Dry, sanitized, and disinfected instruments and equipment, both individual pieces and wrapped packs; oven mitts; sterile transfer forceps; and storage containers for individual items.

Method: Procedure steps.

1. Wash your hands and don gloves before beginning to load items into the autoclave.

2. Rest packs on their edges and place jars and containers on their sides.

3. Place lids for jars and containers with their sterile sides down.

4. If the load includes plastic items, make sure no other item leans against them.
   RATIONALE: Pressure that results from the high temperatures can cause plastic items to bend or warp.

5. If your load is mixed—containing both wrapped packs and individual instruments—place the tray containing the instruments below the tray containing the wrapped packs.
   RATIONALE: This arrangement prevents any condensation that forms on the instruments from dripping onto the wrapped packs and saturating the wrapping.

6. Close the door and start the unit. For automatic autoclaves, choose the cycle based on the type of load you are running. Consult the manufacturer's recommendations before choosing the load type.

7. For manual autoclaves, start the timer when the indicators show the recommended temperature and pressure.

8. Right after the end of the steam cycle and just before the start of the drying cycle, open the door to the autoclave slightly (between ¼ and ½ inch).
   RATIONALE: Opening the door more than ½ inch causes cold air to enter the autoclave, possibly creating excessive condensation in the chamber. This condensation would cause incomplete drying. Consult the manufacturer's recommendations regarding opening the door. Some automatic autoclaves do not require opening the door during the drying cycle.

9. Dry according to the manufacturer's recommendations. Packs and large items may require up to 45 minutes for complete drying.

10. Unload the autoclave after the drying cycle is finished. Do not unload any packs or instruments with wet wrappings, or the objects inside will be considered unsterile and must be processed again.
    RATIONALE: Wet wrappings can transfer bacteria from your hands to the interior of the pack.

11. Unload each package carefully. Wear oven mitts to protect yourself from burns when removing wrapped packs. Use sterile transfer forceps to unload unwrapped individual objects.

12. Inspect each package or item, looking for moisture on the wrapping, underexposed sterilization indicators, and tears or breaks in the wrapping. Consider the pack unsterile if any of these conditions is present.

13. Place sterile packs aside for transfer to storage.

14. Place individual items that are not required to be sterile in clean containers.

15. Place items that must remain sterile in sterile containers; close container covers tightly.

16. As you unload items, avoid placing them in an overly cool location; the cool temperature could cause condensation on the instruments or packs.

17. Remove gloves, dispose of them in the appropriate waste container, and wash your hands.

PROCEDURE 44-6 Assisting as a Floater (Unsterile Assistant) during Minor Surgical Procedures

Procedure Goal: To provide assistance to the doctor during minor surgery while maintaining clean or sterile technique as appropriate.

OSHA Guidelines:

Materials: Sterile towel, tray or Mayo stand, appropriate instrument pack(s), needles and syringes, anesthetic, antiseptic, sterile water or normal saline, small sterile bowl, sterile gauze squares or cotton balls, specimen containers half-filled with preservative, suture materials, sterile dressings, and tape.

Method: Procedure steps.

1. Perform routine handwashing and don exam gloves.

2. Monitor the patient during the procedure; record the results in the patient's chart.

3. During the surgery, assist as needed.

4. Add sterile items to the tray as necessary.

5. Pour sterile solution into a sterile bowl as needed.

6. Assist in administering additional anesthetic.
   a. Check the medication vial two times.
   b. Clean the rubber stopper with an alcohol pad (write the date opened when using a new bottle); leave pad on top.
   c. Present the needle and syringe to the doctor.
   d. Remove the alcohol pad from the vial and show the label to the doctor.
   e. Hold the vial upside down and grasp the lower edge firmly; brace your wrist with your free hand.
   RATIONALE: This firmly supports the vial to sustain the force of the needle being inserted into the rubber stopper.

   f. Allow the doctor to fill the syringe.
   g. Check the medication vial a final time.
7. Receive specimens for laboratory examination.
   a. Uncap the specimen container; present it to the doctor for the specimen's introduction.
   b. Replace the cap and label the container.
   c. Treat all specimens as infectious.
   d. Place the specimen container in a transport bag or other container.
   e. Complete the requisition form to send the specimen to the laboratory.

PROCEDURE 44-7 Assisting as a Sterile Scrub Assistant during Minor Surgical Procedures

Procedure Goal: To provide assistance to the doctor during minor surgery while maintaining clean or sterile technique as appropriate.

OSHA Guidelines:

Materials: Sterile towel, tray or Mayo stand, appropriate instrument pack(s), needles and syringes, anesthetic, antiseptic, sterile water or normal saline, small sterile bowl, sterile gauze squares or cotton balls, specimen containers half-filled with preservative, suture materials, sterile dressings, and tape.

Method: Procedure steps.
1. Perform a surgical scrub and don sterile gloves. (Remember, remove the sterile towel covering the sterile field and instruments before gloving.)
   RATIONALE: You will be handling sterile instruments.
2. Close and arrange the surgical instruments on the tray.
   RATIONALE: They should be quickly and easily located.
3. Prepare for swabbing by inserting gauze squares into the sterile dressing forceps.
4. Pass the instruments as necessary.
5. Swab the wound as requested.
6. Retract the wound as requested.
7. Cut the sutures as requested.

PROCEDURE 44-8 Assisting after Minor Surgical Procedures

Procedure Goal: To provide assistance to the doctor during minor surgery while maintaining clean or sterile technique as appropriate.

OSHA Guidelines:

Materials: Examination gloves, antiseptic, tray or Mayo stand, sterile dressings, and tape.

Method: Procedure steps.
1. Monitor the patient.
2. Don clean exam gloves and clean the wound with antiseptic.

3. Dress the wound.
   RATIONALE: To protect the wound.
4. Remove the gloves and wash your hands.
5. Give the patient oral postoperative instructions in addition to the release packet.
   RATIONALE: The patient will need to understand wound care, medication use, and diet instructions for proper healing.
6. Discharge the patient.
7. Put on clean exam gloves.
8. Properly dispose of used materials and disposable instruments.
9. Sanitize reusable instruments and prepare them for disinfection and/or sterilization as needed.
10. Clean equipment and the exam room according to OSHA guidelines.
11. Remove the gloves and wash your hands.

PROCEDURE 44-9 Suture Removal

Procedure Goal: To remove sutures from a healing wound while maintaining sterile technique and protecting the integrity of the closed wound.

OSHA Guidelines:

Materials: Tray or Mayo stand, suture removal pack (suture scissors and thumb forceps or skin staple remover), sterile towel, antiseptic solution, hydrogen peroxide (3%), two small sterile bowls, sterile gauze squares, sterile strips or butterfly closures, sterile dressings, and tape.

Method: Procedure steps.

1. Clean and disinfect the tray or Mayo stand.

2. Wash your hands and assemble the necessary materials.

3. Check the date and sterilization indicator on the suture removal pack.
   RATIONALE: You must ensure that the pack has been subjected to a sterilization procedure and has not expired.

4. Unwrap the suture removal pack; place it on the tray or stand to create a sterile field.
   RATIONALE: You need to maintain a sterile field to avoid contaminating the wound.

5. Unwrap the sterile bowls; add them to the sterile field.
   RATIONALE: You need to maintain a sterile field to avoid contaminating the wound.

6. Pour a small amount of antiseptic solution into one bowl and a small amount of hydrogen peroxide into the other bowl.

7. Cover the tray with a sterile towel to protect the sterile field while you are out of the room.

8. Escort the patient to the exam room and explain the procedure.

9. Perform a routine hand wash, remove the towel from the tray, and don exam gloves.

10. Remove the old dressing.
    a. Lift the tape toward the middle of the dressing to avoid pulling on the wound.
    b. If the dressing adheres to the wound, cover the dressing with gauze squares soaked in hydrogen peroxide. Leave the wet gauze in place for several seconds to loosen the dressing.
    c. Save the old dressing for the doctor to inspect.

11. Inspect the wound for signs of infection.

12. Clean the wound with gauze pads soaked in antiseptic; pat it dry with clean gauze pads.

13. Remove the gloves and wash your hands.

14. Notify the doctor that the wound is ready for examination.
    RATIONALE: The doctor should determine if the sutures should be removed.

15. Once the doctor indicates the wound is sufficiently healed to proceed, don clean exam gloves.

16. Place a square of gauze next to the wound for collecting the sutures or staples as they are removed.

17. Sutures: Grasp the first suture knot with forceps.
    Staples: Slide the staple remover under the first staple.

18. Sutures: Gently lift the knot away from the skin to allow room for the suture scissors.

FIGURE Procedure 44-9 Step 18   Gently pulling each suture up and away from the skin creates room for the suture scissors.

Staples: Gently press down on the staple remover handle.

19. Sutures: Slide the suture scissors under the suture material and cut the suture where it enters the skin.
    RATIONALE: This minimizes the amount of exposed suture that travels beneath the skin during removal.
    Staples: Continue pressing down on the staple remover to straighten the staple so that it exits the skin.

20. Sutures: Gently lift the knot up and toward the wound to remove the suture without opening the wound.

FIGURE Procedure 44-9 Step 20   Lift the knot up and toward the wound to prevent opening the wound.

Staples: Observe the staple on each side to ensure it is completely out of the skin.

21. Place the suture or staple on the gauze pad; inspect to ensure the entire suture or staple is present.
    RATIONALE: Sutures inadvertently left in place may cause an infection.

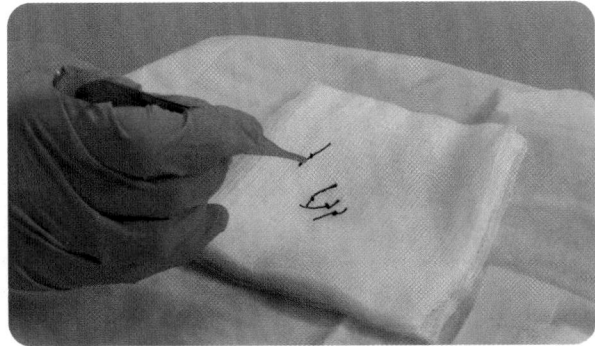

FIGURE Procedure 44-9 Step 21 Place sutures on a gauze square so you can count and inspect them.

22. Repeat the removal process until all sutures or staples have been removed.

23. Count the sutures or staples and compare the number with that indicated in the patient's record.

24. Clean the wound with antiseptic; allow it to air-dry.

25. Dress the wound as ordered, or notify the doctor if sterile strips or butterfly closures are to be applied.

26. Observe the patient for signs of distress, like wincing or grimacing.

27. Properly dispose of used materials and disposable instruments.

28. Remove the gloves and wash your hands.

29. Instruct the patient on wound care.

30. In the patient's chart, record pertinent information, like the condition of the wound and the type of closures used, if any.

31. Escort the patient to the checkout area.

32. Don clean gloves.

33. Sanitize reusable instruments; prepare them for disinfection and/or sterilization as needed.

34. Clean the equipment and exam room according to OSHA guidelines.

35. Remove the gloves and wash your hands.

SUMMARY OF LEARNING OUTCOMES

LEARNING OUTCOMES	KEY POINTS
44.1 **Define the medical assistant's role in minor surgical procedures.**	The medical assistant's role in minor surgery includes both administrative and clinical tasks. These include but are not limited to completing insurance forms, obtaining signed patient consent, preparing the surgical room, and assisting during a procedure.
44.2 **Describe surgical procedures performed in an office setting.**	Several special surgical procedures are performed in an office setting, including laser surgery, cryosurgery, and electrocauterization.
44.3 **Identify the instruments used in minor surgery and describe their functions.**	Various categories of instruments are used in minor surgery including instruments for cutting and dissecting, grasping and clamping, retracting, dilating and probing, suturing, and injecting, withdrawing fluids, and obtaining specimens.
44.4 **Describe the procedures for medical and sterile asepsis in minor surgery.**	Medical asepsis involves reducing the number of microorganisms to prevent the spread of disease. The goal of surgical asepsis is to eliminate all microorganisms.
44.5 **Discuss the procedures used in a medical office to sterilize surgical instruments and equipment.**	Instruments and equipment that must be sterilized before use should be sanitized to remove blood and gross tissue and then sterilized either in an autoclave or by chemical means.
44.6 **Summarize the medical assistant's duties in preoperative procedures.**	A medical assistant's preoperative duties include providing preoperative instructions to the patient, ensuring all necessary paperwork is completed, easing the patient's fears, and preparing the surgical room.

LEARNING OUTCOMES	KEY POINTS
44.7 **Describe the medical assistant's duties during an operative procedure.**	A medical assistant may serve in one of two capacities during a surgical procedure: either as an unsterile assistant known as a floater or as a sterile scrub assistant.
44.8 **Implement the medical assistant's duties in the postoperative period.**	A medical assistant's postoperative duties include giving immediate patient care, dressing and bandaging the wound, giving postoperative instructions, assisting with patient release, and cleaning the surgical room.

CASE STUDY CRITICAL THINKING

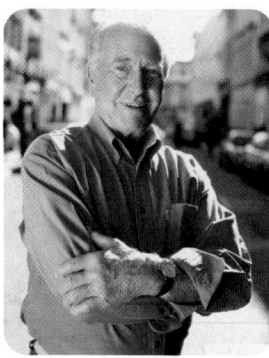

Recall Peter Smith from the beginning of the chapter. Now that you have completed the chapter, answer the following questions regarding his case.

1. What is the medical assistant's role during this minor surgical procedure?

2. Why is it important to document the number of sutures Dr. Buckwalter uses to close Peter's wound?

EXAM PREPARATION QUESTIONS

1. (LO 44.2) The removal of dead tissue from a wound is known as
  a. Incision
  b. Debridement
  c. Ligature
  d. Cauterization
  e. Approximation

2. (LO 44.3) An instrument used to clear a blockage is a
  a. Probe
  b. Scalpel
  c. Retractor
  d. Syringe
  e. Forceps

3. (LO 44.4) Why is it important to keep your hands higher than your elbows when performing a surgical scrub?
  a. To avoid touching the sink
  b. So the soap reaches the elbows
  c. To prevent water from contaminating the washed area
  d. It is not important to keep the hands higher than the elbows
  e. Your hands should be lower than your elbows

4. (LO 44.2) Another name for a mole is a
  a. Wart
  b. Hemangioma
  c. Ligature
  d. Birthmark
  e. Nevus

5. (LO 44.6) Which of the following is an antiseptic that may be used to clean a surgical site if the patient is allergic to iodine?
  a. Lidocaine
  b. Betadine
  c. Normal saline
  d. Zephiran chloride
  e. Hydrogen peroxide

6. (LO 44.2) A jagged, open wound of the skin is a/an
  a. Incision
  b. Avulsion
  c. Laceration
  d. Puncture
  e. Abrasion

7. (LO 44.4) When adding solutions to a sterile field, you should cover the label with your palm to keep it
   a. Sterile
   b. Dry
   c. From pouring too quickly
   d. From dripping
   e. Visible

8. (LO 44.5) After the steam autoclave finishes the steam cycle, the door should be opened
   a. ¼–½ inch
   b. 1–2 inches
   c. Completely
   d. Half-way
   e. Not at all

9. (LO 44.8) Sterile materials used to cover an incision are
   a. Bandages
   b. Sterile strips
   c. Sutures
   d. Drapes
   e. Dressings

10. (LO 44.3) What type of instrument is a curette?
   a. Probing and dilating
   b. Cutting and dissecting
   c. Grasping
   d. Retracting
   e. Clamping

PATIENT INFORMATION

Patient Name	Gender	DOB
Sylvia Gonzales	Female	9/1/19xx

Attending	MRN	Allergies
Alexis N. Whalen, MD	341-73-792	PCN

Sylvia Gonzales, a 51-year-old female, is at the office for a 3-month return check for her newly diagnosed Type II diabetes. She states that she has taken the medication she received for her "sugar" and she knows the doctor wants to a do a special "sugar test" this time. Her medication list includes Januvia 100 mg daily.

The physician has ordered a fasting blood sugar (FBS) and a hemoglobin A1C blood test. You will need to perform both of these waived tests in your office lab.

Keep Sylvia in mind as you study this chapter. There will be questions at the end of the chapter based on the case study. The information in the chapter will help you answer these questions.

LEARNING OUTCOMES

After completing Chapter 45, you will be able to:

45.1 Describe the purpose of the physician's office laboratory.

45.2 Identify the medical assistant's duties in the physician's office laboratory.

45.3 Identify important pieces of laboratory equipment.

45.4 Illustrate measures to prevent accidents.

45.5 Explain the goal of a quality assurance program in a physician's office laboratory.

45.6 Carry out communication with patients regarding test preparation and follow-up.

45.7 Carry out accurate documentation, including all logs related to quality control.

KEY TERMS

10x lens
artifact
centrifuge
Certificate of Waiver tests
compound microscope
control sample
objectives
ocular
oil-immersion objective
optical microscope
photometer

physician's office laboratory (POL)
proficiency testing program
qualitative test response
quality assurance program
quality control program
quantitative test result
reagent
reference laboratory
standard

I. P (11)	Perform quality control measures
III. C (9)	Discuss quality control issues related to handling microbiological specimens
III. C (10)	Identify disease processes that are indications for CLIA waived tests
III. C (11)	Describe Standard Precautions, including:
	a. Transmission based precautions
	b. Purpose
	c. Activities regulated
III. P (2)	Practice Standard Precautions
III. P (3)	Select appropriate barrier/personal protective equipment (PPE) for potentially infectious situations
III. A (1)	Display sensitivity to patient rights and feelings in collecting specimens
III. A (2)	Explain the rationale for performance of a procedure to the patient
III. A (3)	Show awareness of patients' concerns regarding their perceptions related to the procedure being performed
IV. A (3)	Use appropriate body language and other nonverbal skills in communicating with patients, family and staff
IX. C (14)	Describe the process to follow if an error is made in patient care
IX. P (6)	Complete an incident report

3. Medical Terminology

Graduates:

d. Recognize and identify acceptable medical abbreviations

4. Medical Law and Ethics

Graduates:

a. Document accurately

f. Comply with federal, state, and local health laws and regulations

9. Medical Office Clinical Procedures

Graduates:

b. Apply principles of aseptic techniques and infection control

f. Screen and follow up patient test results

i. Use standard precautions

10. Medical Laboratory Procedures

Graduates:

a. Practice quality control

c. Dispose of biohazardous materials

▶ Introduction

Laboratory testing of patients' specimens is an integral component of patient care. Medical assistants often perform a role in the clinical laboratory setting in the physician's office. This chapter will introduce you to the various types and uses of common laboratory equipment. You will learn about safety in the laboratory and steps to aid in preventing accidents. A discussion of the Clinical Laboratory Improvement Amendments of 1988 (CLIA '88) and this law's impact on the laboratory setting is included in this chapter to help you understand quality assurance, quality control procedures, and required recordkeeping.

▶ The Role of Laboratory Testing in Patient Care
LO 45.1

Laboratory analysis of blood, urine, or other body fluids and substances provides three kinds of information about a patient. First, regular monitoring through laboratory tests, like those that are part of an annual exam, can help a physician identify possible diseases or other problems. Second, specific tests can help confirm or contradict a physician's initial diagnosis. Third, laboratory testing can help a physician determine and monitor the proper dosage of a patient's medication.

Kinds of Laboratories

Some physicians prefer to have all laboratory tests performed by a **reference laboratory**, a laboratory owned and operated by an organization outside the practice. Other physicians choose to have some tests completed by the reference laboratory and some completed in the office in the **physician's office laboratory (POL)**.

Each method of managing laboratory analyses has advantages and disadvantages. Reference laboratories often have technological resources beyond those available in the POL. A reference laboratory offers a complete range of tests in all specialties and subspecialties: cytology, toxicology, immunology, blood banking, urinalysis, histology, serology, chemistry, microbiology, and hematology. Using a reference laboratory frees a physician's staff from testing duties and allows more time for patient care. Furthermore, some managed care companies have contracts with laboratory companies that require their subscribers to use a specific reference laboratory. On the other hand, processing tests in the POL produces quicker turnaround and eliminates the need for the patient to travel to other test locations.

The Purpose of the Physician's Office Laboratory

Office policy determines which tests, if any, will be performed at your location and which tests will be performed by a reference

FIGURE 45-1 A physician's office laboratory (POL) may be simple or elaborate, depending on the tests the office performs.

laboratory. A POL, like the one shown in Figure 45-1, is responsible for accurate and timely processing of routine tests and for reporting test results to the physician.

A POL usually processes chemical analyses, hematologic tests, microbiologic tests, and urinalyses. Chemical analyses are performed on blood and its components, urine, and other body fluids. Hematologic tests usually use samples of whole blood to identify problems with the count, size, or shape of blood cells that could indicate disease. Microbiologic tests include examining blood, urine, sputum, reproductive fluids, and fluids from wounds to identify the presence of pathogenic organisms like bacteria, viruses, fungi, protozoans, and parasites. Semen may be examined microscopically to determine sperm levels, appearance, and motility. Urinalysis includes chemical analysis of the urine sample, analysis of its physical characteristics, and microscopic examination of the sample to detect disease states.

▶ The Medical Assistant's Role   LO 45.2

As a medical assistant, you may be responsible for processing tests done in the POL, including preparing the patient for the test, collecting the sample, completing the test, reporting the results to the physician, and communicating information about the test from the physician to the patient. Your role in the POL requires you to integrate a great deal of information to serve both the physician and the patient effectively. You will need to master the following subjects:

- Use of laboratory equipment.
- Regulations governing laboratory practices and procedures.
- Precautions for accident prevention.
- Waste disposal requirements.
- Housekeeping and maintenance routines.
- Quality assurance and control procedures.
- Technical aspects of specimen collection and test processing, including expected results.
- Communication with patients.
- Reporting of test results to the physician.

- Recordkeeping of test specimens, procedures, and results.
- Inventory and ordering of equipment and supplies.
- Use of reference materials in the POL.
- Screening and follow-up of test results.

▶ Use of Laboratory Equipment   LO 45.3

As a medical assistant, you must be familiar with the operation of common laboratory equipment. Learning to use a specific piece of equipment may take the form of on-the-job training or attending training programs conducted by manufacturers' representatives. You may routinely use the following equipment:

- Autoclave.
- Centrifuge.
- Microscope.
- Electronic equipment and software.
- Equipment used for measurement.

Autoclave

A steam autoclave is used to sterilize, or eradicate, all organisms on the surfaces of instruments and equipment before they are used on a patient or in testing procedures. Use of the autoclave is discussed in the *Assisting with Minor Surgery* chapter.

Centrifuge

A **centrifuge** is a device for spinning a specimen at high speed until it separates into its component parts. The centrifuge in a POL is generally used to separate whole blood samples into blood components or to prepare urine samples for examination. Use of a centrifuge is described in greater detail in the *Processing and Testing Urine and Stool Specimens* chapter.

Microscope

The instrument used most often in a POL is the microscope, commonly used for the examination of blood smears and identification of microorganisms in body fluid samples. Although onsite blood smear evaluation is convenient and fast for both patient and physician, it is important to know which procedures are routinely covered. Only CLIA-approved microscopy procedures are eligible for payment by Medicare and Medicaid. Table 45-1 lists CLIA-approved provider-performed microscopy procedures.

TABLE 45-1	**CLIA-Approved Provider-Performed Microscopy Procedures**
Wet mounts—vaginal, cervical, or skin specimens	
Potassium hydroxide preparations	
Pinworm examinations	
Fern test (for the presence of amniotic fluid in vaginal secretions)	
Urinalysis by dipstick with microscopy	
Urinalysis; two or three glass test (for the presence of blood 1—at the beginning of the urine stream, 2—midstream, and/or 3—at the termination of urination)	
Fecal leukocyte examination	
Semen analysis (for presence or motility of sperm)	
Nasal smears for eosinophils	

FIGURE 45-2 The microscope is the most heavily used piece of equipment in a POL.

Labels (top to bottom):
Oculars (eyepieces)
Revolving nosepiece
Objectives
Stage
Slide clips
Condenser
Iris
Light source
Base
Arm
Focus controls — Fine, Coarse

The usual microscope in a POL is an **optical microscope** (Figure 45-2), which uses light, concentrated through a condenser and focused through the object being examined, to project an image. Most optical microscopes in POLs are **compound microscopes**, which use two lenses to magnify the image created by the condensed light.

You must be able to operate an optical microscope correctly. First, you need to become familiar with the component parts, described in the following paragraphs.

Oculars The **oculars** are the eyepieces through which you view the image. A microscope is either monocular, with a single eyepiece, or binocular, with two eyepieces. You can adjust the oculars on a binocular microscope to compensate for differences in visual acuity between your right and left eyes. You also can adjust the distance between oculars to match the distance between your eyes. The ocular contains a magnifying lens—called a **10x lens**—that usually magnifies an image 10 times.

Objectives Just below the ocular or oculars, the **objectives** are mounted on a swivel base called the *nose-piece*. An objective contains another magnifying lens. Generally, microscopes used in the POL have a three-piece objective system. An objective is moved into position directly under the ocular when needed.

Two of the objectives are dry objectives; this means there is air space between the specimen under examination and the objective. Condensed light passes through the specimen and the air space above the specimen as it travels toward the objective lens. These dry objectives are low- and high-power lenses,

usually 10x and 40x, respectively. When the low-power objective lens is combined with the ocular lenses, the total magnification factor is 100x (10 x times 10 x). The high-power lens and ocular lenses yield a magnification factor of 400x.

The third objective is an **oil-immersion objective**, which is used for specimens that need extreme magnification, like blood smears and bacteriological slides. It is designed to be lowered into a drop of immersion oil placed directly on the slide above the prepared specimen under examination. This design eliminates the air space between the microscope slide and the objective, where some of the light scatters beyond the objective. Placing the end of the objective in oil reduces the loss of light. A much sharper, brighter image results, allowing for greater magnification. An oil-immersion objective has a magnification factor of 100x. Combined with the ocular lenses, the total magnification factor is 1000x.

Arm and Focus Controls The ocular(s) and objectives, collectively referred to as the body tube, are attached to the base of the microscope by the arm. The microscope arm is also the location of the focus controls. The two focus controls—coarse and fine—move the body tube up and down to bring into focus the object being examined.

Stage and Substage The objectives and oculars are focused on a specimen placed on the microscope's stage. The stage is the platform on which the specimen slide rests, held in place by metal clips. Under the stage is the substage containing the condenser, which concentrates the light being directed through the sample, and the iris. The iris is a diaphragm that opens and closes like the shutter of a camera to increase or decrease the amount of light illuminating the specimen. The stage is controlled by the stage mechanisms, which control left-right and forward-backward movements of the stage, allowing you to examine different areas of the specimen without reseating the slide.

Light Source Under the stage and substage assemblies is the light source. Most POL microscopes use a built-in electric light source, and most of these are equipped with controls that allow you to adjust the light intensity. In place of a built-in light source, older microscopes use a mirror, which gathers and focuses light from a microscope lamp onto the specimen.

Specimen Slides and Coverslip Although the specimen slide is not technically part of the microscope assembly, it is necessary for using the microscope. All specimens must be placed on slides. Many specimens also require a coverslip, or cover glass. The slide and coverslip support and position the specimen. They also prevent contamination of the microscope by the specimen. Specimens that are to be stained or immersed in oil, like blood smears, do not require coverslips.

Using an Optical Microscope To use an optical microscope, you must be able to focus it using each of the three objectives. Procedure 45-1, at the end of this chapter, describes how to operate an optical microscope correctly.

CAUTION: HANDLE WITH CARE

Care and Maintenance of the Microscope

The microscope is the workhorse of the POL. For it to provide trouble-free service, however, it must be well cared for. Dust, oil, and other contaminants cause major problems with microscopes. Careless cleaning and haphazard storage will also eventually cause problems. These problems may include mechanical difficulties with the microscope or contamination of the specimen being examined. Foreign objects visible through a microscope, but unrelated to the specimen, are called **artifacts** and may be misinterpreted when the specimen is examined.

Clean the microscope after each use. Inspect the body tube, arm, and stage to make sure they are dust- and contaminant-free. Clean the ocular and objective lenses with lens paper, not tissue or other products. Tissue fibers are a common artifact. The eyepiece is an area in which skin oil, dust, and eye makeup

may collect, posing a risk of disease transmission and making images difficult to see. Use lens-cleaning products according to the manufacturer's guidelines. Excess amounts of these products may dissolve the cement holding the lenses in place, rendering the microscope useless.

When not in use, the microscope should be stored under its plastic cover. If there is a power cord, wrap it loosely around the base and secure it with a twist-tie or elastic band. Lower the low-power objective close to the stage and center the stage.

If the microscope must be moved, hold it by the arm and support it under the base. Never carry a microscope with one hand or by just the arm. Carry the cord so it does not dangle and pose a tripping hazard. Place the microscope on a sturdy table or bench, away from the edge.

You also will be responsible for the proper care and maintenance of the optical microscope in your office. Related concerns and techniques are described in the Caution: Handle with Care section.

Go to CONNECT to see a video about *Using a Microscope.*

Electronic Equipment and Software

Electronic equipment is used in the POL because it is safer, more accurate, and more efficient than manual methods; generally requires little maintenance; and does not require extensive training prior to its use. A wide variety of tasks, such as cell counting and complex chemical analyses, are performed with electronic equipment. A range of clinical laboratory software systems are available, which are used to create and maintain clinical data, making remote access and tracking between facilities easier. Manufacturers' instructions for operation and maintenance of these systems must be followed to ensure safety, efficiency, and reliable results.

A **photometer**, which measures light intensity, is a basic electronic component of many pieces of analytic laboratory equipment. A handheld glucometer (Figure 45-3), for example, contains a photometer that measures reflected light. Patients with diabetes and clinical personnel use a glucometer to monitor blood glucose levels.

Equipment Used for Measurement

Precise measurement is critical in the POL because it produces accurate test results. Much of this measurement is built into the electronic equipment or premeasured kits you will use. However, you will still need to perform various measurements manually when blood, semen, urine, and other body fluids are analyzed using manual tests. Some reagents also require measuring.

FIGURE 45-3 A handheld glucometer translates the amount of reflected light into the level of glucose in a blood sample.

Metric system units are commonly used in the POL. For information on metric system weight, height, and temperature measurements, see the *Vital Signs and Measurements* chapter. To learn how to convert between measurement systems, see the *Dosage Calculation* chapter.

A variety of equipment is used to provide accurate measurements. You must take these measurements carefully for them to be of value in the final test results. Other types of measuring equipment include:

- Pipettes (mechanical or manual)—used to measure small amounts of liquids.
- Volumetric or graduated flasks or beakers—used to measure the relatively large amounts of liquids necessary for reagents.
- A hemocytometer—a slide calibrated to the exact measurements needed to count blood cells and sperm under a microscope.
- Thermometers (generally in degrees centigrade)—used to provide legal documentation that refrigerators, bacterial incubators, and other appliances maintain the precise temperature range required for accurate laboratory work.

▶ Safety in the Laboratory

LO 45.4

Safety is a primary concern in any laboratory environment, and it is especially important in a physician's office laboratory because patients and laboratory workers may be at risk. For your own protection, as well as that of patients and coworkers, you must always be aware of and observe laboratory safety guidelines.

Use Standard Precautions when handling all body fluids, excretions, and secretions. If you have any doubt about whether you need to take precautions, take them. Even though some substances do not present a risk of transmitting bloodborne pathogens, they may present a high risk of transmitting other bacteria, viruses, or parasites. Follow these guidelines:

- Wear gloves when handling all body fluids, secretions, and excretions.
- Change gloves every time you move from patient to patient as you collect specimens for testing.
- Wash your hands immediately after removing used gloves.
- Wear other protective gear like eye protection and face masks during procedures in which there is a risk that droplets or spray may come in contact with your eyes, nose, or mouth.
- Take special care to avoid injury from sharp or pointed instruments or equipment. Although gloves protect you from surface exposure to potentially infected substances, they offer little protection against exposure from needlesticks or cuts. Never use needles or other sharp instruments unnecessarily.
- Use only recommended instruments and equipment. A once-common laboratory technique that has been discontinued is the use of a mouth pipette (a type of calibrated glass or plastic straw) to transfer specimens. Under no circumstances should you use a mouth pipette to transfer blood from one collection device to another; doing so puts you at risk for getting blood or or other hazardous fluids in your mouth.
- Take care to prevent spills and splashes when transporting specimens to the laboratory and when moving specimens in the laboratory.
- If a work surface becomes contaminated because of spilling or splashing, disinfect the area completely, using an approved solution such as 10% bleach, before beginning any other procedure.

- Dispose of waste products carefully and correctly.
- Be sure to remove protective gear before leaving the laboratory.

Biologic Safety

You will work with test specimens that may be contaminated with bloodborne or other pathogens. Treat every specimen as if it were contaminated. Additional information regarding OSHA's Bloodborne Pathogens Standard may be found in the *Basic Safety and Infection Contol* chapter. Follow Standard Precautions.

- If you have any cuts, lesions, or sores, do not expose yourself to potentially contaminated material. Consult your supervisor if you have any doubt about whether you can safely perform test procedures.
- Wash your hands before and after every procedure and whenever you come in contact with a potentially contaminated substance.
- Wear gloves at all times. Use other protective gear as appropriate to prevent exposing your eyes, nose, and mouth to potentially contaminated material.
- Mouth pipetting is prohibited at all times. Use specially made rubber suction bulbs to draw specimens mechanically.
- Work in a biologic safety cabinet (similar to a fume hood) when completing procedures that are likely to generate droplet sprays or splashes of potentially contaminated material.
- When transferring a blood specimen from a collection tube to another container, wear appropriate PPE (including a mask and goggles or a face shield) and cover the tube stopper with an absorbent pad or a commercial stopper remover to prevent spray or splatter from the tube. Do not rock the stopper back and forth because this could cause the tube to break. Always remove the stopper by opening it away from your face so the vapor pressure flows away from you. Place the stopper on a sterile gauze pad while you work with the collection tube. Do not allow the stopper to come in contact with other work surfaces. Keep the collection tube stoppered unless you are actively using it.
- Establish clean and dirty areas in the laboratory. Place all used instruments and equipment in the dirty area for sanitization, disinfection, and sterilization.
- Disinfect your work area at least once a day with a 10% bleach solution or a germ-killing solution approved by the Environmental Protection Agency (EPA). If a spill occurs, immediately disinfect the work area.
- Dispose of waste products immediately.
- Dispose of needles in the appropriate sharps container.
- If an instrument or piece of equipment must be serviced, be sure it has been decontaminated first.
- If you use a bleach solution for disinfection, change it daily.

Accident Reporting

Despite all precautions, laboratory accidents still occur. Armed with an understanding of the materials with which you are

MILLSTONE
INDUSTRIES

Central State Division
Incident Report

Name of Injured Employee _____

Department _____ Job Title _____

Supervisor _____

Date of Accident _____ Time _____

Nature of Injury _____

Was injured acting in a regular line of duty? _____

Was first aid given? _____ By whom? _____

Was designated emergency contact notified? _____

Did injured receive medical treatment? _____

Was injured tested for infection? _____ If no, why not? _____

Did injured go to ER? _____ Other? _____

Did injured leave work? _____ Date _____ Hour _____ A.M. P.M.

Did injured return to work? _____ Date _____ Hour _____ A.M. P.M.

Other Parties Involved _____

Names of Witnesses _____

Describe where and how accident occurred. _____

_____

What, in your opinion, caused the accident? _____

Has anything been done to prevent a similar accident? _____

Has the hazard causing the injury been reported by telephone or in writing? _____

_____   _____
Date   Employee's Signature

_____   _____
Date   Supervisor's Signature

**IF TREATMENT IS NEEDED, TAKE THE ORIGINAL AND DUPLICATE OF THIS FORM TO
THE EMERGENCY ROOM.**

This part for Employee Health Office use only

Was incident investigated? _____

Has injured had follow-up medical care? _____

Comments _____

Original copy to Employee Health Office   Duplicate copy to supervisor

FIGURE 45-4 In the event of an accident or exposure incident in the POL, OSHA regulations require completion of an incident report form.

working and basic first-aid procedures, you should be able to deal with most emergencies. Your office also should have written procedures to follow in the event of an accident. Familiarize yourself with the procedures beforehand so you will know what to do if an accident occurs.

If the accident involves exposure to blood or blood products, OSHA regulations require that several steps be followed:

1. Immediate cleaning of the area, including disinfection of contaminated surfaces and sterilization of contaminated instruments and equipment.

2. Notification of a designated emergency contact, as identified in your office's safety manual.

3. Documentation of the incident on a form similar to that shown in Figure 45-4, including the names of all parties

FIGURE 45-5 Certain substances require cleanup with specially formulated products such as these.

involved, the names of witnesses, a description of the incident, and a record of medical treatments given to those involved.

4. Medical evaluation and follow-up exam of the employees involved.

5. Written evaluation of the medical condition of the involved individuals and testing for infection, provided that such testing does not violate confidentiality regulations.

Housekeeping

There is a high risk of serious contamination in the laboratory, and housekeeping duties are designed to reduce this risk. Great care must be taken by following these guidelines to ensure good operating procedures and to reduce the risk of infection:

- Refer to your office's written policies and procedures to ensure you are performing housekeeping duties correctly and according to schedule.

- Immediately clean up spills or splashes of potentially contaminated material. Depending on the material, you may need to use special hazardous waste control products, like those shown in Figure 45-5. Be sure to dry the area if appropriate, or clearly indicate that the area is still wet.

- Clean laboratory equipment immediately after use. Contaminants often become hard to remove if they are left on for a long time.

- Dispose of waste products carefully and correctly.

- Use extreme caution when handling and disposing of sharps.

▶ Quality Assurance Programs   LO 45.5

The operation of a POL can have a significant impact on the health of the patients who depend on the medical practice for care. Accurate patient specimen testing is a primary concern. A **quality assurance program** is designed to monitor the quality of the patient care a medical laboratory provides. It also helps to ensure laboratory worker safety. An effective quality assurance program should be a written plan that includes both internal and external reviews of procedures. It serves to assess the quality of the tests performed in a clinical laboratory based on a set of written standards and procedures.

Clinical Laboratory Improvement Amendments

In response to public concern over the accuracy of laboratory tests, Congress enacted the Clinical Laboratory Improvement Amendments of 1988 (CLIA '88). This law placed all laboratory facilities that conduct tests for diagnosing, preventing, or treating human disease or for assessing human health under federal regulations administered by the Health Care Financing Administration (HCFA) and the CDC. State governments may implement their own standards, which must be at least as stringent as federal standards. If your state has its own standards, your office will operate under those standards. The state health department provides information about which standards to follow in a given locale.

CLIA '88 has had a major impact on office laboratories. Because of the complexity of the regulations and the expense required to meet them, many doctors have closed their laboratories or sharply reduced the number of tests they perform. Several attempts have been made to change the federal legislation, including an effort to exempt POLs from the regulations. As the healthcare debate continues, you may see changes in laboratory operations as a result of changes in CLIA '88 regulations.

As updated and implemented in 1992, CLIA '88 standards apply to four areas of laboratory operation: standards, fees, enforcement, and accreditation programs. Most of the regulations relate to laboratory standards. The specific standards that must be met depend on the test. Tests have been divided into these three categories, based on complexity: Certificate of Waiver tests, tests of moderate complexity, and tests of high complexity.

Certificate of Waiver Tests The **Certificate of Waiver tests**, as listed in Table 45-2, are laboratory tests defined as follows:

- The tests pose an insignificant risk to the patient if they are performed or interpreted incorrectly.

- The procedures involved are simple and accurate to such a degree that the risk of obtaining incorrect results is minimal.

- The tests have been approved by the Food and Drug Administration (FDA) for use by patients at home.

If laboratory management decides to perform these tests only, the office may apply for a Certificate of Waiver. When the certificate is granted, the laboratory is exempt from meeting various CLIA '88 standards that apply to the other two test

TABLE 45-2 Certificate of Waiver Tests

Urine tests	Urinalysis by dipstick (reagent strip) or tablet reagent (nonautomated) for bilirubin, glucose, hemoglobin, ketone, leukocytes, nitrite, pH, protein, specific gravity, and urobilinogen
	Ovulation (visual color comparison tests)
	Pregnancy (visual color comparison tests)
	Home-screening tests for drugs (opioids, cocaine, methamphetamines, cannabinoids, phencyclidine, methadone, bensodiaxepines, barbituates, oxycodone)
	Nicotine detection tests
	Urine chemistry analyzer for microalbumin and creatinine (semi-quantitative)
	Tumor-associated antigen for bladder cancer (using devices approved by the FDA for home use)
	Catalase
	Ascorbic acid
Blood tests	Erythrocyte sedimentation rate (ESR), nonautomated
	Hemoglobin by copper sulfate, nonautomated
	Spun microhematocrit
	Blood glucose (using devices approved by the FDA for home use)
	Hemoglobin by single analyte instruments, automated
	Prothrombin time
	Platelet aggregation
	Ketones in whole blood, over-the-counter test only
	Total cholesterol, high-density lipoprotein (HDL), low-density lipoprotein (LDL), and triglycerides
	Hemoglobin A1c
	Liver panel (alanine aminotransferase, alkaline phosphatase, amylase, gamma glutamyl transferase, aspartate aminotransferase, total bilirubin)
	Lactate in whole blood
	Chloride
	Carbon dioxide
	Calcium
	Sodium
	Potassium
	Urea
	Uric acid
	Creatinine
	Lead in whole blood
	Thyroid-stimulating hormone, rapid test
	Mononucleosis rapid test
	Helicobacter pylori rapid antibody test
	Lyme disease antibodies
	HIV antibody test
Fecal tests	Fecal occult blood
Saliva tests	Alcohol in saliva
Nasal smear tests	Influenza A and B antigens
	Respiratory syncytial virus
Vaginal smear tests	*Trichomonas vaginalis* antigens
	Vaginal pH
Throat swab tests	Strep A antigens
	Influenza A and B
Semen	Sperm concentration, home screening

CAUTION: HANDLE WITH CARE

Operating a Reliable Certificate of Waiver Laboratory

CLIA requires that Certificate of Waiver laboratories obtain a certificate of waiver, pay biennial certificate fees, and follow manufacturers' test instructions. They also require that Certificate of Waiver laboratories submit to random inspections and investigation if indicated. CLIA does not require laboratory personnel to have any specific qualifications or training, nor do they require quality control procedures or routine quality assessment, except as recommended by the manufacturer of each waived test. Although waived tests are simple to perform and interpret, they may have serious consequences if done incorrectly. Patient care decisions are often made based on the outcome of waived tests.

In order to help ensure quality testing procedures and reduce patient error, the Clinical Laboratory Improvement Advisory Committee (CLIAC) has made several recommendations for good practice in a Certificate of Waiver laboratory. These include laboratory management considerations and testing procedures before, during, and after the test. To ensure that you are operating a reliable laboratory, follow these recommendations:

Laboratory Management and Personnel

- Designate the person who will be responsible for laboratory supervision—usually a physician or someone with enough laboratory experience to make decisions about testing.
- Follow all applicable federal, state, and local regulations.
- Perform waived tests only.
- Follow manufacturer's instructions in the package insert.
- Do not make modifications to the instructions.
- Allow random inspections by authorized agencies like the Centers for Medicare and Medicaid Services (CMS).
- Establish a laboratory safety plan that follows OSHA guidelines.
- Have a designated area that has adequate space and conditions.
- Have enough personnel in the lab and train them appropriately.

- Have written documentation of each test performed.

Before the Test

- Confirm written test orders.
- Establish a procedure for patient identification.
- Give patients pretest instructions and determine whether they have followed them.
- Collect specimens according to package insert instructions.
- Label specimens appropriately.
- Never use expired reagents of test kits.

During the Test

- Perform quality control testing as indicated in the package insert.
- Correct any problem discovered during quality control testing before testing patient samples.
- Establish a policy for control testing frequency.
- Carefully follow all test-timing recommendations.
- Interpret test results using product inserts as a guide.
- Record test results according to your office policy.

After the Test

- Report test results to the physician in a timely manner.
- Follow package insert recommendations for follow-up or confirmatory testing.
- Follow OSHA regulations for disposing of biohazardous waste.
- Participate in quality assurance assessment programs:
  - Internal assessment—Perform routine, in-house testing to ensure a test's accuracy.
  - External assessment—Voluntary inspection of your facility by an outside agency.

categories. Such laboratories, however, are subject to the following: (1) random inspections to ensure that laboratories operating under a Certificate of Waiver are performing only those tests that qualify for the waiver and (2) investigation of the laboratory if there is any reason to believe the laboratory is not operating safely or if there have been complaints against the laboratory. See the Caution: Handle with Care feature Operating a Reliable Certificate of Waiver Laboratory for more information about good lab practice.

Tests of Moderate Complexity Tests of moderate complexity make up approximately 75% of all tests performed in

the laboratory. Among these tests are blood cell counts and cholesterol screening. Test procedures falling into this category include studies involving bacteriology, mycobacteriology, mycology, parasitology, virology, immunology, chemistry, hematology, and immunohematology.

A laboratory that performs moderate-complexity testing must be run by a pathologist who has an MD or PhD degree. Technicians performing the tests must have training beyond the high school level as defined by CLIA '88 regulations. All personnel must participate in a quality assurance program for laboratory procedures, and the laboratory is subject to periodic unannounced inspections and proficiency testing.

Tests of High Complexity Tests of high complexity include more complicated tests in the specialties and subspecialties, including tests in clinical cytogenics, histopathology, histocompatibility, and cytology, and any test not yet categorized by the CMS. Manufacturers' guidelines for testing products are often the best source for discovering a test's CMS determination. The CMS publishes a directory of all moderate- and high-complexity tests.

Like a laboratory that conducts moderate-complexity tests, a laboratory that conducts high-complexity tests is subject to inspection, proficiency testing, and participation in a quality assurance program, and it must be headed by a medical doctor or a scientist who has a PhD degree. Testing procedures can be performed only by qualified laboratory personnel whose training exceeds that provided by high schools and meets the requirements of CLIA '88 regulations. Medical assistants will need additional training and education to perform moderate- and high-complexity tests.

Components of Quality Assurance

Every quality assurance program must include the following components, in a measurable and structured system, to satisfy CLIA '88 requirements:

- Quality control.
- Instrument and equipment maintenance.
- Proficiency testing.
- Training and continuing education.
- Standard operating procedures documentation.

Quality Control and Maintenance

A **quality control program** is one component of a quality assurance program. The focus of the quality control program is to ensure accuracy in test results through careful monitoring of test procedures. To be in compliance with quality control standards, a laboratory must follow certain procedures.

Calibration Testing equipment must be calibrated regularly, in accordance with manufacturers' guidelines. Calibration ensures the equipment is operating correctly. Each calibration must be recorded in a quality control log like the one shown in Figure 45-6. Calibration routines are performed on a set of standards. A **standard** is a specimen, like the patient specimens you would normally process with the equipment, except that the value for each standard is already known. If the equipment does not yield the expected results during the calibration procedure, it must be adjusted until the expected results are obtained. Calibration routines are run on the standards alone, never with patient samples. They are used exclusively to ensure that the equipment is performing according to manufacturers' specifications. Check the manufacturer's instructions to determine how often the equipment should be calibrated. Calibration of some equipment must be performed by trained service personnel.

Control Samples Control samples are similar to standards in that they are specimens like those taken from a patient and have known values. Unlike standards, however, control samples are used before each patient sample is processed. Using a control sample serves as a check on the accuracy of the test. If the control tests do not fall within the manufacturer's prescribed ranges, patient samples are not analyzed, preventing erroneous results.

The control samples for certain laboratory procedures show both normal (negative) and abnormal (positive) results.

QUALITY CONTROL DAILY LOG

Name of Unit	Glucose Control Solution	Strip Lot No./ Exp. Date	Low Control Value 35–65 mg/dL	High Control Value 75–235 mg/dL	Analyzed By	Date	Remedial Action Taken If Control Values Abnormal	Retest After Remedial Action Taken
XYZ Glucometer	Check-strip control solution	Lot 851 10/15/XX	39 mg/dL	230 mg/dL	MSM	1/17/XX		
Mitchell Drugs Glucometer	Check-strip control solution	Lot 851 10/15/XX	50 mg/dL	267 mg/dL	MSM	1/17/XX	Machine cleaned	220 mg/dL high value
XYZ Glucometer	Check-strip control solution	Lot 851 10/15/XX	Unable to read	Unable to read	LMC	1/18/XX	Battery changed	38 mg/dL low 198 mg/dL high
Mitchell Drugs Glucometer	Check-strip control solution	Lot 851 10/15/XX	45 mg/dL	226 mg/dL	LMC	1/18/XX		

FIGURE 45-6 The quality control log shows the completion of every quality control check conducted on a piece of equipment.

Generally, positive and negative control samples are used with tests that yield a **qualitative test response** (the substance being tested for is either present or absent).

Other control samples—used for tests that yield **quantitative test results** (the concentration of a test substance in a specimen)—are formulated to show when results fall within a normal range. At least two control samples containing different concentrations of the test substance should be run for quantitative tests.

Reagent Control Control samples or standards are also run every time you open a new supply of testing products, such as staining materials, culture media, and reagents. **Reagents** are chemicals or chemically treated substances used in test procedures. A reagent is formulated to react in specific ways when exposed under specific conditions. One example of a reagent is the chemically coated strip used in blood glucose monitoring. A visual change on the reagent strip (also called a dipstick) occurs in the presence of glucose in a blood sample.

To ensure the quality of reagents, you should keep a reagent control log. If a defective reagent test is identified, it can be tracked to its source. A sample reagent control log is shown in Figure 45-7. Running controls on a routine basis gives you information about the equipment and the reagents used during the test. If a control consistently yields unexpected results (for example, a positive control yields a negative result), you should check the reagents first and then the equipment calibration.

Maintenance Testing instruments and equipment must be properly maintained and all maintenance procedures must be documented. Follow manufacturers' guidelines for performing instrument and equipment maintenance. A maintenance log provides a complete record of all work performed on an instrument or a piece of equipment (Figure 45-8).

Troubleshooting You may need to investigate the cause of a problem with a piece of equipment or a test. To do this, you should take a systematic approach to rule out the cause of the problem. For more information regarding investigating equipment and test malfunctions, see the Caution: Handle with Care feature Troubleshooting Problems in a Physician's Office Laboratory.

Documentation A quality control program depends first on careful adherence to procedures designed to identify problems with equipment calibration, errors in testing procedures, and defective testing supplies. The second component of a quality control program is the careful documentation of all procedures. Besides maintaining the quality control log, the reagent control log, and the equipment maintenance log, you also will complete the following records as part of a quality control program:

- Reference laboratory log, which lists specimens sent to another laboratory for testing.
- Daily workload log, which shows all procedures completed during the workday.

Proficiency Testing

All laboratories that perform moderate- and high-complexity tests as identified by CLIA '88 must participate in a proficiency testing program. **Proficiency testing programs** measure test

URINE REAGENT STRIP CONTROL LOG											Control Solution		Exp. Date		Lot #
Reagent Strip / Lot # & Exp. Date	Test	Specific Gravity	pH	Protein	Glucose	Ketone	Bilirubin	Blood	Nitrite	Urobi-linogen	Control Test Date	Remedial Action Taken If Reading Is Abnormal	Retest Date	Technician Initials
	Reagent Strip Expected Range													
	Test Results													
	Reagent Strip Expected Range													
	Test Results													

FIGURE 45-7 The reagent control log shows the quality testing performed on every batch or lot of reagent products.

ACME MEDICAL SUPPLIES
Equipment Maintenance Record

Practice	BWW Medical Associates		
Name of Equipment	Acme Microscope Model ABC-123		
Location	Lab	Purchase Date	12/1/20XX

Date	Cleaning	Maintenance/Repair	Technician Initials
6/5	Microscope	Cleaned	CJC
6/11	Microscope high objective	Cleaned	DWM
6/14	Microscope	Changed bulb	CJC
6/16	Microscope eyepiece	Lens cover replaced	CJC
6/17	Microscope high objective	Cleaned	CJC

FIGURE 45-8 A maintenance log must be kept for every piece of laboratory equipment. All work done on the equipment must be recorded in the log.

CAUTION: HANDLE WITH CARE

Troubleshooting Problems in a Physician's Office Laboratory

Working in a physician's office laboratory can be exciting and challenging. Part of your job as a medical assistant is to make sure the tests you perform are accurate. Occasionally, you will encounter a piece of equipment that is not working or test results and controls that are consistently too high or too low. You will need to troubleshoot these problems to determine their cause. Troubleshooting is a thorough and logical investigation for the cause of a problem. You must eliminate possible causes of the problem one at a time. The general steps to troubleshooting a piece of equipment or test kit are

- Follow a written procedure for troubleshooting tests and equipment.
- Recognize the problem (controls give clues to possible problems).
- Think about possible causes.
- Start by investigating the simplest cause first.
- Document your findings.
- Call your service company after you have checked everything you know to check.

When troubleshooting equipment, follow these steps:

- Check the power source at the machine, the wall outlet, the breaker box, or the battery.

- Check the equipment manual for troubleshooting information.
- Reboot the equipment by turning it off, waiting a few minutes, and then turning it back on.
- Check the service log for the date of the last maintenance.
- If you are able to repair the problem, run controls to verify the problem is fixed before testing patient samples.

When troubleshooting a test kit, follow these steps:

- Read the package insert to verify that you have performed the test correctly.
- Check to make sure you have used the correct reagents or test strips.
- Check the dates on the reagents or test strips to make sure they are not outdated.
- Make sure you are using the proper sample for the test.
- Repeat the test using control samples.
- If the controls are correct, repeat the test with the patient sample.

result accuracy and adherence to standard operating procedures. Generally, proficiency tests include two parts: (1) a control sample from the proficiency testing organization engaged by your laboratory and (2) forms that must be completed to record the steps in the testing procedure. The control sample is processed normally, under the same conditions as any patient sample. The results, the forms, and sometimes the control samples are returned to the proficiency testing organization, which then informs your office of whether it has passed or failed the test. A passing mark means that your laboratory can continue to perform that particular test. A failing mark can mean that your laboratory must discontinue that test and possibly other tests, too.

Training, Continuing Education, and Documentation

One of your employer's responsibilities is to provide opportunities for employee training and continuing education. Another is to provide written reference materials and documentation for all procedures conducted in the POL. Your responsibility is to consult reference materials and take part in available training to keep your skills sharpened and up to date.

It may seem unnecessary to refer to written instructions for procedures you perform many times a day. Changes can be made in a procedure for many reasons, however, and you must be aware of these changes. Here are some reference materials with which you should be familiar:

- Material Safety Data Sheets.
- Standard operating procedures.
- Safety manuals.
- Equipment manufacturers' user or reference guides.
- Clinical Laboratory Technical Procedure Manuals.
- Regulatory documentation (OSHA standards, CLIA '88 requirements).
- Maintenance and housekeeping schedules.

▶ Communicating with the Patient LO 45.6

In your job as a medical assistant, you will be involved with patients before they submit samples for laboratory testing, during the specimen collection procedure, and after the physician has interpreted the test results. It is your responsibility to ensure that patients understand what is expected of them every step of the way.

Before the Test

Certain tests require patients to prepare by fasting or restricting fluid intake. It is your duty to explain test preparations. Use simple, nontechnical language and check with patients to be sure they understand the information. In some cases, providing a written instruction sheet may be helpful.

Explaining the reason for the preparation can help ensure compliance or unearth potential problems. For example, if you explain to a patient that he is to refrain from drinking anything for a particular period, he might ask whether that includes the water he uses to take a certain medication. You can then make sure the patient receives the answers he will need for carrying out the physician's orders.

If you are the person who collects specimens, you need to determine whether patients have correctly completed the required test preparations. Test results are invalid in some cases if patients fail to follow test preparation guidelines. When preparations have not been completed correctly, discuss the situation with the physician or other appropriate staff member as required by your office to determine whether the specimen should still be collected. If the specimen is not collected, document the reason the test was not carried out as requested. Review the guidelines for specimen collection with the patient and schedule another appointment if appropriate.

During Specimen Collection

Before collecting a specimen, you must first be sure you have the right patient. Proper patient identification is an essential part of good laboratory practice. You do not want to collect a blood sample from someone who only needs a urinalysis. Patients do not always understand the tests they are having. It is up to you to make sure you have the right patient and are performing the test as it is ordered.

The instructions you deliver to patients during specimen collection vary with the nature of the specimen. Always deliver instructions clearly and in language patients can understand. Do not assume that patients do not need to hear the instructions, even if they have had the test before. Explain what you must do and what patients must do before moving to each new step in the process.

Patients are understandably nervous during many collection procedures. In addition to communicating technical information, you should provide any helpful advice that may make the test easier. Also provide reassurance as appropriate. For example, if a patient asks whether the blood-drawing procedure is painful, explain that a sharp stick or stinging sensation may be experienced when the needle is inserted but that no pain should be felt after that. Let the patient be your guide in determining how much information to provide. Some people want to know every detail, whereas others prefer to know as little as possible.

One important aspect of communicating with patients about testing procedures is your nonverbal communication skills. Even if you deliver accurate technical information and answer every question patients have, there can still be a breakdown in communication if your nonverbal signals do not support your verbal message. Follow these guidelines to ensure that your nonverbal actions are helping, not hindering, the communication process:

- Strike a balance between a strict, businesslike attitude and overly familiar friendliness. Your actions must impress on the patient that you are well informed about the procedure and that you care about the patient's understanding of it.
- Treat the patient with respect. Address the patient by name, using the appropriate courtesy title unless you have been invited to use the patient's first name or the patient is a child.

Provide privacy during specimen collection. Privacy needs may be met by using a separate room or contained area for drawing blood, for example; a private bathroom is best for collecting urine specimens.

- Recognize that the patient may be under stress because of the test procedure or the pending results. Some patients may be familiar with the test procedures, but others may not know what to expect. You may need to repeat instructions or explain what you are doing more than one time. Remain calm and patient. Never be abrupt or condescending.

- Direct your attention to the patient, particularly during a procedure that might be uncomfortable, like drawing blood. Unless an emergency develops, pay attention to nothing else at that time.

After Specimen Collection

If the patient must follow particular guidelines after you collect the specimen, explain them. Commonly, post-test instructions deal with care of venipuncture sites, signs and symptoms of infection, additional or continuing dietary restrictions, and the schedule for further testing if it is necessary.

When the Test Results Return

When you receive the test results, communicate them not to the patient but to the doctor. Only the doctor is qualified to interpret test results for the patient. Your role in reporting results comes after the doctor examines the test information and prepares a report. Sometimes, the doctor discusses the results with the patient. Other times, you will be asked to convey the test results to the patient along with instructions from the doctor. Answer only those patient questions that are within the range of your knowledge and experience. If the patient needs more information than you can provide, refer the patient to the doctor.

▶ Recordkeeping

LO 45.7

The importance of accurate and complete recordkeeping can be summed up in one statement: If it is not written down, it was not done. This motto applies to all your duties as a medical assistant. Besides recording information about quality control and equipment maintenance, you must keep track of every specimen that passes through your hands, or you may be called on to handle inventory control and record test results in patient records. You may need to use standard abbreviations for measures when recording test results. Table 45-3 provides a list of common abbreviations used in the laboratory.

Filling Out a Laboratory Requisition Form

As a medical assistant, it is your responsibility to ensure that the laboratory requisition form is properly completed. Missing information can lead to improper testing or lost results. The completed form should be included with the specimen collected or sent with the patient to the laboratory. Be sure to include the following information on all requisitions:

- Patient's full name, sex, date of birth, and address.
- Patient's insurance information.

TABLE 45-3	Abbreviations for Common Laboratory Measures
cm	centimeter
cm³	cubic centimeter
dL	deciliter
fl oz	fluid ounce
g	gram
L	liter
lb	pound
m	meter
mcg	microgram
mg	milligram
mL	milliliter
mm	millimeter
mm Hg	millimeters of mercury
oz	ounce
pt	pint
QNS	quantity not sufficient
QS	quantity sufficient
qt	quart
U	unit
wt	weight

- Physician's name, address, and phone number.
- Source of the specimen.
- Date and time of the specimen collection.
- Test(s) requested.
- Preliminary diagnosis.
- Any current treatment that might affect the results.

See Figure 45-9 for a sample laboratory requisition form.

Specimen Identification

All specimens must immediately be clearly identified with the patient's name, the patient's identification code (if your office uses one), the date and time the specimen was collected, the initials of the person who collected the specimen, the physician's name, and other information as required by the test procedure or your office. If you encounter an unidentified or incorrectly identified specimen, you must make an effort to track it to its source. The specimen will probably be discarded or destroyed, however, because there is no guarantee that it was identified correctly. Even if you do manage to identify it, it may have been compromised in some way.

Inventory Control

You will be responsible for taking inventory of equipment and supplies to ensure that the POL never runs out of them. To do so, you will keep a list of items that are used routinely and reordered systematically. Establish a regular schedule—perhaps weekly—for counting items in the POL. Then estimate when you will probably need to reorder an item and put the date on your calendar.

LAB USE ONLY

Acct #	
DATE	
TIME	

Laboratory Name & Address

Requesting Physician Information

Address

Phone Number

Patient Information

Patient Name (Last)	(First)		(MI)	Date of Birth / /
Address	City, State		Zip	Phone Number
Patient I.D. Number	Responsible Party (Last)	(First)	(Phone)	Male Female
Social Security Number	Physician			Date Time Specimen Collection

---

Bill: Check One
  Our account   Medicare
  Insurance Co./Patient

Complete the Following Information for Billing a Patient and/or a Third Party Agency

Policy Holder Name	Policy Holder Address: Policy Holder Phone Number:	Relation Self Spouse Child Other____
Insurance Co. Name	Address Insurance Co.	City , State, Zip
Employer		
Policy	Group #	
	PATIENT or GUARDIAN SIGNATURE:	DATE:

CHECK DESIRED TESTS   PLEASE PROVIDE ICD=9-CM#

√	ORGAN DISEASE PANELS, BLOOD	ICD-9	√	TEST, BLOOD	ICD-9	√	TEST, BLOOD	ICD-9	√	TEST, URINE	ICD-9
	ACUTE HEP. A,B,C			ESR			WBC with diff			U/A Routine	
	BASIC METABOLIC			EBV			PT				
	THYROID			FBS			PTT				
	ELECTROLYTES			Grp A β-hem strep			Bleeding time				
	HEPATIC FUNCTION			Hgb			PCO_2				
	LIPID PROFILE			Hct			PO_2				
	RENAL FUNCTION			HgbA1c			CO_2				
	TEST, BLOOD			HIV antibodies			HCO_3			**MICROBIOLOGY**	
	ACE			Insulin			Ca^{++}			AFB culture	
	ADH			Iron			Cl^-			C & S	
	ALT			Ketone bodies						Chlamydia screen	
	AFP			LD						Endocervical culture	
	Amylase			pH						GC screen	
	Acetone			Phenylalanine						Gram stain	
	AST			K^+ and Na^+			**TEST, URINE**			O & P	
	Bilirubin			Proteins, Albumin			Cys			Strep A culture	
	BUN			Proteins, Fibrinogen			CrCl			Throat culture	
	CEA			PSA			Glucose			Urine culture	
	Calcium, total			RBC			HCG			Viral culture	
	Carbon dioxide, total			Sickle cells			UBG			Wound culture	
	Cholesterol, total			TSH			UFC				
	Cholesterol, HDLs			T3			UK				
	Cholesterol, LDLs			T4			UNA				
	CK			Uric Acid			Uosm				
	CMV			WBC			UUN				

FIGURE 45-9 The laboratory requisition form must be accurately completed.

Patient Records

When recording test results, it may be your responsibility to identify unusual findings. Many offices require out-of-range test results to be circled or underlined in red. Follow the procedure established by your office. The physician usually initials or otherwise marks the records after examining them. Electronic health records automatically identify out-of-range tests when the results are entered.

PROCEDURE 45-1 Using a Microscope

Procedure Goal: To correctly focus the microscope using each of the three objectives for examination of a prepared specimen slide.

OSHA Guidelines:

Materials: Microscope, lens paper, lens cleaner, prepared specimen slide, immersion oil, and tissues.

Method: Procedure steps.

1. Wash your hands and don exam gloves.

2. Remove the protective cover from the microscope. Examine the microscope to make sure it is clean and that all parts are intact.

3. Plug in the microscope and make sure the light is working. If you need to replace the bulb, refer to the manufacturer's guidelines. (Be sure to note bulb replacements in the maintenance log for the microscope.) Turn the light off before cleaning the lenses.

4. Clean the lenses and oculars with lens paper. Avoid touching the lenses with anything except lens paper. Pay careful attention to the oculars, as they are easily dirtied by dust and eye makeup. If a lens is particularly dirty, use a small amount of lens cleaner. Oil-immersion lenses are prone to oil buildup if not cleaned properly. Too much lens cleaner, however, can loosen the cement that holds the lens in place.
   RATIONALE: The lenses must be clean to reduce artifacts.

5. Place the specimen slide on the stage. Slide the edges of the slide under the slide clips to secure the slide to the stage.

FIGURE Procedure 45-1 Step 5 Carefully secure the specimen slide on the stage of the microscope.

6. Adjust the distance between the oculars to a position of comfort.

7. Adjust the objectives so the low-power (10x) objective points directly at the specimen slide, as shown. Before swiveling the objective assembly, be sure you have sufficient space for the objective. Recheck the distance between the oculars, making sure the field you see through the eyepieces is a merged field, not separate left and right fields. Raise the body tube by using the coarse adjustment control and lower the stage as needed.
   RATIONALE: If the objective assembly is too close to the stage, you may hit the specimen slide and crack it. The specimen is then contaminated and cannot be used. The objective also may be damaged.

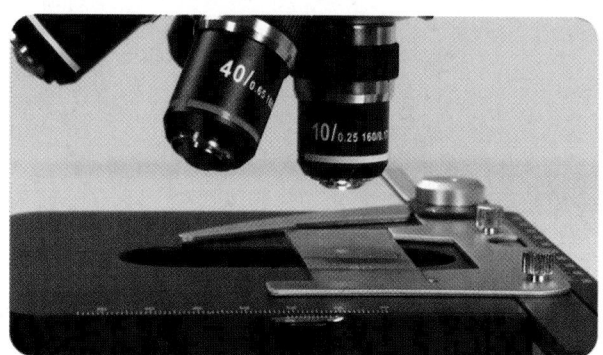

FIGURE Procedure 45-1 Step 7 Move the low-power objective into position above the specimen slide.

8. Turn on the light and, using the iris controls, adjust the amount of light illuminating the specimen so the light fills the field but does not wash out the image. (At this point, you are not examining the specimen image for focus but adjusting the overall light level.)

9. Observe the microscope from one side and slowly lower the body tube to move the objective closer to the stage and specimen slide. This adjustment is shown below. If you used the stage controls to lower the stage away from the objectives, you also may need to adjust those controls. Again, take care not to strike the stage with the objective. The objective should almost meet the specimen slide but not touch it.

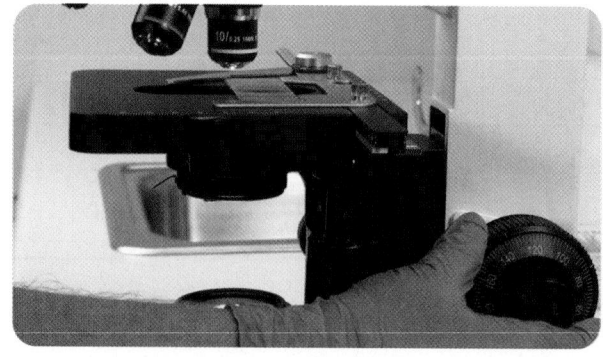

FIGURE Procedure 45-1 Step 9 When lowering the objective toward the stage and specimen slide, observe the microscope from the side to be sure you do not hit the stage with the objective and crack the slide.

10. Look through the oculars and use the coarse focus control to slowly adjust the image. If necessary, adjust the amount of light coming through the iris.

11. Continue using the fine focus control to adjust the image. When the image is correctly focused, the specimen will be clearly visible and the field illumination will be bright enough to show details but not so bright that it is uncomfortable to view or washed out.

12. Switch to the high-power (40x) objective. Use the fine focus controls to view the specimen clearly.
RATIONALE: Using the coarse adjustment could cause lens damage if the lens touches the slide.

13. Rotate the objective assembly so that no objective points directly at the stage and specimen slide. You will now have enough room to apply a drop of immersion oil to the slide. (Only dry slides, without coverslips, are used with the oil-immersion objective.)

14. Apply a small drop of immersion oil to the specimen slide, as shown below.

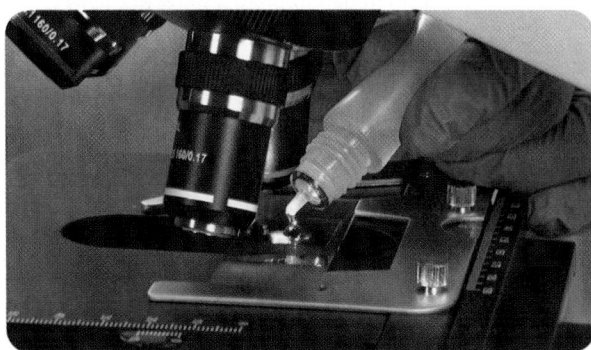

FIGURE Procedure 45-1 Step 14   Place a small drop of immersion oil directly on the dry specimen.

15. Gently swing the oil-immersion (100x) objective over the stage and specimen slide so it is surrounded by the immersion oil.

16. Examine the image and adjust the amount of light and focus as needed. Only use the fine focus adjustment with this objective. To eliminate air bubbles in the immersion oil, gently move the stage left and right.

17. After you have examined the specimen as required by the testing procedure, lower the stage and raise the objectives.

18. Remove the slide. Dispose of it or store it as required by the testing procedure. If you must dispose of the slide, be sure to use the appropriate biohazardous waste container. If you must store the slide, remove the immersion oil with a tissue.

19. Turn off the light. Unplug the microscope if that is your laboratory's standard operating procedure.

20. Clean the microscope stage, ocular lenses, and objectives. Be careful to remove all traces of immersion oil from the stage and oil-immersion objective. Clean the oil-immersion lens last.
RATIONALE: So that you do not get oil from the oil-immersion lens on the other lenses.

FIGURE Procedure 45-1 Step 20   Clean the oil-immersion lens last using a small amount of lens cleaner.

21. Rotate the objective assembly so the low-power objective points toward the stage. Lower the objective so it comes close to but does not rest on the stage.

22. Cover the microscope with its protective cover. Check the work area to be sure you have cleaned everything correctly and disposed of all waste material.

23. Remove the gloves and wash your hands.

SUMMARY OF LEARNING OUTCOMES	
LEARNING OUTCOMES	**KEY POINTS**
45.1 **Describe the purpose of the physician's office laboratory.**	The physician's office laboratory (POL) is responsible for accurate and timely processing of routine tests, usually involving blood or urine, and for reporting test results to the physician.
45.2 **Identify the medical assistant's duties in the physician's office laboratory.**	The medical assistant's duties in a physician's office laboratory include preparing the patient for the test, collecting the sample, completing the test, reporting the results to the physician, and communicating information about the test from the physician to the patient.

LEARNING OUTCOMES	KEY POINTS
45.3 **Identify important pieces of laboratory equipment.**	Common laboratory equipment includes autoclaves, centrifuges, microscopes, electronic equipment and software, and equipment used for measurement.
45.4 **Illustrate measures to prevent accidents.**	Preventing accidents in the physician's office laboratory begins by observing all safety guidelines including standard precautions, reporting all laboratory accidents in a timely manner, and maintaining appropriate housekeeping in the lab setting.
45.5 **Explain the goal of a quality assurance program in a physician's office laboratory.**	The goal of a quality assurance program in a physician's office laboratory is to monitor the quality of the patient care that a medical laboratory provides.
45.6 **Carry out communication with patients regarding test preparation and follow-up.**	It is the medical assistant's responsibility to ensure that patients understand what is expected of them before a test. Providing clear pretest instructions in both oral and written form is an essential part of the test procedure.
45.7 **Carry out accurate documentation, including all logs related to quality control.**	Accurate quality control documentation in a physician's office laboratory includes a reference laboratory log and a daily workload log.

CASE STUDY CRITICAL THINKING

Recall Sylvia Gonzales from the beginning of the chapter. Now that you have completed the chapter, answer the following questions regarding her case.

1. Identify equipment used by a medical assistant in an office laboratory.

2. You will be measuring Sylvia's fasting blood glucose using a glucometer. You know this is classified as a waived test. What does the classification of waived test mean?

3. The glucometer contains an instrument called a photometer. How is blood glucose measured using a photometer?

EXAM PREPARATION QUESTIONS

1. (LO 45.1) A laboratory owned by a company other than the physician's practice is a
   a. Physician's office laboratory
   b. Reference laboratory
   c. Pathology department
   d. Waived testing center
   e. High-complexity testing center

2. (LO 45.3) The eyepieces on a microscope are also called
   a. Objectives
   b. Condensers
   c. Oculars
   d. Irises
   e. Stages

3. (LO 45.3) An object visible through a microscope but unrelated to the specimen is a/an
   a. Iris
   b. Aperture
   c. Artifact
   d. Speck
   e. Inclusion

4. (LO 45.5) A test that poses little or no risk to the patient if it is performed or interpreted incorrectly is a
   a. Waived test
   b. Moderate-complexity test
   c. High-complexity test
   d. Quality assurance test
   e. Reference test

5. (LO 45.5) Which of the following is a test to determine the amount of a substance in a specimen?
   a. Qualitative
   b. Waived
   c. Complex
   d. Quantitative
   e. Assurance

6. (LO 45.3) A device for spinning a specimen at high speed until it separates into its component parts is a
   a. Refractometer
   b. Photometer
   c. Concentrator
   d. Condenser
   e. Centrifuge

7. (LO 45.4) The most common disinfectant used in a physician's office laboratory is
   a. Germicidal soap
   b. 10% bleach
   c. Hydrogen peroxide
   d. Betadine
   e. 70% alcohol

8. (LO 45.5) A laboratory that performs moderate-complexity testing must be run by a
   a. Pathologist
   b. Medical technologist
   c. Medical assistant
   d. Medical lab specialist
   e. CLIA-trained employee

9. (LO 45.5) Chemicals or chemically treated substances used in test procedures are known as
   a. Controls
   b. Standards
   c. Reagents
   d. Strips
   e. Negatives

10. (LO 45.3) An instrument in a medical laboratory that measures light intensity is a/an
    a. Photometer
    b. Microscope
    c. Condenser
    d. Analyte
    e. Reflector

Microbiology and Disease

PATIENT INFORMATION

Patient Name	Gender	DOB
Cindy Chen	F	07/15/19XX

Attending	MRN	Allergies
Alexis N. Whalen, MD	324-86-542	NKA

lives with her aunt and is going to school to become a phlebotomist. She has lost 20 pounds since her last visit to the clinic. The physician orders a series of blood tests, including the helper T cell test.

Keep Cindy in mind as you study the chapter. There will be questions at the end of the chapter based on the case study.

Cindy Chen, a 28-year-old Asian female complaining of the inability to sleep and nervousness, arrives at the office. She tested positive for HIV in 2005. Currently, she

The information in the chapter will help you answer these questions.

LEARNING OUTCOMES

After completing Chapter 46, you will be able to:

46.1 Explain the medical assistant's role in microbiology.

46.2 Summarize how microorganisms cause disease.

46.3 Describe how microorganisms are classified and named.

46.4 Discuss the role of viruses in human disease.

46.5 Review the symptoms of HIV/AIDS and hepatitis.

46.6 Discuss the role of bacteria in human disease.

46.7 Discuss the role of protozoa in human disease.

46.8 Discuss the role of fungi in human disease.

46.9 Discuss the role of multicellular parasites in human disease.

46.10 Describe the process involved in diagnosing an infection.

46.11 Identify general guidelines for obtaining specimens.

46.12 Carry out the procedure for transporting specimens to outside laboratories.

46.13 Compare two techniques used in the direct examination of culture specimens.

46.14 Carry out the procedure for preparing and examining stained specimens.

46.15 Carry out the procedure for culturing specimens in the medical office.

46.16 Describe how to perform an antimicrobial sensitivity determination.

KEY TERMS

acid-fast stain
aerobe
agar
anaerobe
bacillus
coccus
colony
culture
culture and sensitivity (C&S)
etiologic agent

facultative
Gram-negative
Gram-positive
Gram stain
KOH mount
mordant
spirillum
stain
vibrio
wet mount

M E D I C A L   A S S I S T I N G   C O M P E T E N C I E S

CAAHEP

I. C. (7)	Analyze pathology as it relates to the interaction of body systems
III. C (5)	List major types of infectious agents
III. C (9)	Discuss quality control issues related to handling microbiological specimens
III. P (2)	Practice Standard Precautions
III. P (7)	Obtain specimens for microbiological testing
III. P (8)	Perform CLIA waived microbiology testing

ABHES

3. **Medical Terminology**

 Graduates:

 c. Understand the various medical terminology for each specialty

4. **Medical Law and Ethics**

 Graduates:

 a. Document accurately

9. **Medical Office Clinical Procedures**

 Graduates:

 f. Screen and follow up patient test results.

 i. Use standard precautions

10. **Medical Laboratory Procedures**

 Graduates:

 a. Practice quality control

 b. Perform selected CLIA-waived tests that assist with diagnosis and treatment

    (5) Microbiology testing

    (6) b. Kit testing: Quick strep

 c. Dispose of biohazardous materials

 d. Collect, label, and process specimens

    (3) Perform wound collection procedures

    (4) Obtain throat specimens for microbiologic testing

▶ Introduction

Humans are surrounded by tiny living organisms invisible to the naked eye. For the most part, these microorganisms cause no problems; however, when they are pathogenic in nature or are displaced from their natural environment, they can cause infections and disease. This chapter addresses the different life forms of microorganisms and how they may be identified; it also teaches you the proper collection techniques for common types of specimens. You will learn about the processes involved in identifying microorganisms, the types of culture media used for these processes, how antimicrobial testing is done, and how quality control fits into ensuring reliable patient results.

▶ Microbiology and the Role of the Medical Assistant   LO 46.1

Microbiology is the study of *microorganisms*—simple forms of microscopic (visible only through a microscope) life found everywhere. Most microorganisms are made up of a single cell. Some microorganisms, called resident normal flora, which are normally found on the skin and within the human body, perform a number of important functions and typically do not cause disease. For example, microorganisms in the intestines

produce vitamins, help digest food, and help protect the body from infection.

Many microorganisms, however, do cause infections. These are referred to as *pathogens* (microorganisms capable of causing disease). Infections can be mild, like the common cold, or they can sometimes lead to serious conditions. Their proper diagnosis and treatment are essential to restoring good health.

You may assist the physician in performing a number of microbiologic procedures in the medical office that aid in diagnosing and treating infectious diseases, including obtaining specimens or assisting the physician in doing so, preparing specimens for direct examination by the physician, and preparing specimens for transportation to a microbiology laboratory for identification.

▶ How Microorganisms Cause Disease   LO 46.2

Microorganisms live all around us—in and on our bodies, in the air we breathe, in the water we drink, and on almost every surface we touch. The variety of pathogenic microorganisms is extensive. Successful pathogens have developed ways to evade the host defenses. Each classification of microorganism contains pathogens. Some examples of these appear in Table 46-1.

TABLE 46-1 Microbial Pathogens and Their Characteristics

Classification	Characteristics	Example	Disease
Prions*	• Infectious particle made of protein • Very small • No nucleic acid • Reproduction unknown	PrP^{sc}	• Creutzfeldt-Jakob Disease (CJD) • Bovine spongiform encephalopathy (BSE), or mad cow disease
Viruses	• DNA or RNA surrounded by a protein coat • Reproduced in living cells only • Very small • Acellular	Varicella-zoster virus	Chickenpox
Bacteria	• Single-celled • Reproduce quickly • Mostly asexual reproduction	Vibrio cholerae	Cholera
Protozoans	• Single celled • Reproduction mostly asexual	Entamoeba histolytica	Amebic dysentery
Fungi	• Multicellular • Reproduction is sexual & assexual	Candida albicans	Candidiasis
Helminths	• Multicellular • Parasitic • Contain specialized organs • Reproduction is sexual	Enterobius vermicularis	Pinworms

*Although evidence exists that prions are directly responsible for several diseases that cause progressive brain degeneration, like spongiform encephalopathies, some scientists believe prions merely aid another unknown infectious agent in causing disease. Prion research is ongoing.

Although everyone is surrounded by microorganisms, people are able to avoid infection most of the time for the following three reasons:

1. The majority of microorganisms are either beneficial or harmless. Pathogens comprise only a small portion of the total number of microorganisms that exist in a given environment.
2. The human body has a variety of defenses that allow it to resist infection.
3. Conditions must be favorable for a pathogen to grow and to be transmitted to a person who is susceptible (sensitive) to infection.

Microorganisms and Disease Mechanisms

Microorganisms can cause disease in a variety of ways. They may use up nutrients or other materials needed by the cells and tissues they invade, they may damage body cells directly by reproducing themselves within cells, or their very presence may make body cells the targets of the body's own defenses. Some microorganisms produce cell- and tissue-damaging toxins or poisons. Infecting microorganisms, or the toxins they produce, may remain localized or may travel throughout the body, damaging or killing cells and tissues. The resulting symptoms include local swelling, pain, warmth, and redness along with generalized symptoms of fever, tiredness, aches, and weakness. Infection by certain organisms also may cause skin reactions, gastrointestinal upset, or other symptoms. Recall from the *Safety and Infection Control* chapter the chain of infection and how pathogenic organisms are transmitted from one person to another.

▶ Classification and Naming of Microorganisms

LO 46.3

Scientists classify microorganisms on the basis of their structure. Common classifications include the following:

- Subcellular, which consist of hereditary material, either deoxyribonucleic acid (DNA) or ribonucleic acid (RNA), surrounded by a protein coat.
- Prokaryotic, which have a simple cell structure with no nucleus and no organelles in the cytoplasm.
- Eukaryotic, which have a complex cell structure containing a nucleus and specialized organelles in the cytoplasm.

Table 46-2 lists the characteristics that distinguish these classifications and the types of microorganisms found in each classification. Types of microorganisms include:

- Viruses.
- Bacteria.
- Protozoans.
- Fungi.
- Multicellular parasites.

TABLE 46-2	Classifications of Microorganisms	
Classification	**Characteristics**	**Examples**
Subcellular	Noncellular Nucleic acid surrounded by protein coat	Viruses
Prokaryotic	Simple structure Single chromosome No organelles	Bacteria
Eukaryotic	Highly structured Nucleus and cytoplasm Organelles	Protozoans, fungi, parasites

These types may be further divided into groups that share certain characteristics. For example, within the bacteria classification are the mycobacteria and rickettsiae groups.

Specific microorganisms are named in a standard way, using two words. The first word refers to the *genus* (a category of biologic classification between the *family* and the *species*) to which the microorganism belongs. The second word refers to the particular species of the organism. Each species represents a distinct kind of microorganism. For example, within the bacteria classification is the *Staphylococcus* genus. Then within that genus are various species like *Staphylococcus aureus* and *Staphylococcus epidermidis*. Although the two bacteria belong to the same genus, they differ greatly in their ability to cause disease. The first letter of the genus is always capitalized and the species name is always written in all lowercase letters.

▶ Viruses
LO 46.4

Viruses, which are among the smallest known infectious agents and cannot be seen with a regular microscope, are the cause of many common illnesses and conditions seen frequently in the medical office. Table 46-3 lists common viral pathogens. Because viruses are a simpler life form than the cell (see Figure 46-1), they can only live and grow within the living cells of other organisms.

▶ Significant Bloodborne Pathogens
LO 46.5

In the medical office, you will likely encounter patients who are living with HIV and hepatitis. As you learned in the *Basic Safety and Infection Control* chapter, proper technique when handling blood and body fluids is essential. You also must understand how HIV and hepatitis cause infection, risk factors for contracting these diseases, the progression of the infections, how they are treated, and special precautions you need to take with these patients.

AIDS/HIV Infection

HIV is a virus that infects and gradually destroys components of the immune system. AIDS is the condition that results from the advanced stages of this viral infection.

Over a period of time and in most cases, HIV infection develops into AIDS, which results in death. The pathogen gradually destroys helper T cells. *Helper T cells* are white blood cells that are a key component of the body's immune system, working in coordination with other white blood cells (B cells, macrophages, and so on) to combat infection.

The virus also attacks neurons, causing demyelination (destruction of the myelin sheath of a nerve), which results in neurological problems, including dementia. Unlike a person with a properly functioning immune system, most AIDS patients are prone to various opportunistic infections—infections caused by microorganisms that do not ordinarily cause disease in people with properly functioning immune systems. Virtually everyone is at risk for contracting HIV. Although its initial outbreak in the United States appeared in the male homosexual population, and currently homosexual and bisexual men comprise a large percentage of AIDS cases, the disease knows no limits.

Risk Factors The greatest risk factor for contracting HIV infection is unprotected sexual activity. The virus can be found in blood, semen, and vaginal secretions and can be transmitted to an uninfected person through mucous membranes in the vagina, rectum, or mouth, especially if there are

(a)

(b)

(c)

FIGURE 46-1 The three types of viral diseases often seen in medical offices are (a) influenza, (b) hepatitis, and (c) warts.

TABLE 46-3 Viral Pathogens

Disease	Causative Organism	Route of Transmission	Signs and Symptoms
Viral pharyngitis	Adenovirus	Direct person-to-person contact and respiratory droplet contact	Colds, pharyngitis, bronchitis, pneumonia, diarrhea, pink eye, fever, cystitis, gastroenteritis, and/or neurologic disease.
Infectious mononucleosis	Epstein-Barr virus	Direct contact with saliva from an infected person	Fever, sore throat, and swollen lymph glands.
Hepatitis	Hepatitis A virus	Fecal-oral	Fever, fatigue, loss of appetite, nausea, vomiting, abdominal pain, dark urine, clay-colored bowel movements, joint pain, and jaundice.
	Hepatitis B virus	Bloodborne, sexually transmitted infection (STI)	
	Hepatitis C virus	Bloodborne	
Cold sores	Herpes simplex virus, type 1	Direct contact with someone infected with Herpes simplex, type 1 (sharing eating utensils or drinking glasses, kissing)	Pain; tingling; small, painful, fluid-filled blisters on a raised, red area of the skin, typically around the mouth.
Genital herpes CMV	Herpes simplex virus, type 2 Cytomegalovirus	STI Direct contact, maternal-fetal transmission	Pain, itching, small red bumps, blisters, and ulcers. Healthy adults: usually asymptomatic but may have mild hepatitis and prolonged fever. Congenital: premature birth, liver problems, lung problems, spleen problems, small size at birth, small head size, seizures, hearing loss, vision loss, lack of coordination, and/or mental disability.
AIDS	HIV	Bloodborne, STI	Initial: flulike symptoms. Untreated or advanced: heart, kidney, and liver disease; cancer; and opportunistic infections.
Influenza	Influenza virus	Airborne, respiratory droplets	Fever, cough, sore throat, runny or stuffy nose, muscle or body aches, headaches, and fatigue.
Measles	Measles virus	Airborne, respiratory droplets	Blotchy rash, fever, cough, runny nose, conjunctivitis, malaise, and tiny white spots with bluish-white centers inside the mouth.
Mumps	Mumps virus	Airborne, respiratory droplets	Fever, headache, muscle aches, fatigue, loss of appetite, swollen and tender salivary (parotid) glands.
HPV infection	Human papillomavirus	STI	The majority of cases are asymptomatic. Some strains cause genital warts; others are associated with cervical cancer.
Upper respiratory infections, viral	Parainfluenza virus	Direct contact with respiratory secretions (droplets)	HPV1: croup. HPV3: bronchiolitis and pneumonia.
Polio	Poliovirus	Direct person-to-person contact	Fever, fatigue, nausea, headache, flulike symptoms, back and neck stiffness, limb pain, and/or paralysis.
Rabies	Rabies virus	Direct contact with saliva of rabid animal, usually through the bite of an infected animal	Initially: weakness, fever, headache. If untreated: cerebral dysfunction, anxiety, confusion, agitation, delirium, abnormal behavior, hallucinations, insomnia, and death.
Norovirus infection, acute gastroenteritis	Norovirus	Fecal-oral; foodborne (most common cause of foodborne illness in the United States)	Diarrhea, nausea, stomach pain, vomiting, fever, headache, and body aches.
Rotavirus infection	Rotavirus	Fecal-oral	Fever, diarrhea, abdominal pain, and vomiting.
Fifth disease	Parvovirus B19	Direct contact with respiratory secretions (droplets); can be spread through blood or blood products	Fever, runny nose, headache, rash on face (slapped cheek appearance) and body, and arthralgia.
RSV	Respiratory syncytial virus	Airborne, respiratory secretions (droplets)	Cough, sneezing, runny nose, fever, loss of appetite, wheezing, and dyspnea.
German measles (3-day measles)	Rubella virus	Airborne, respiratory secretions (droplets)	Fever, rash. If acquired during pregnancy, fetal symptoms may include deafness, cataracts, heart defects, mental retardation, and liver and spleen damage.
Chickenpox	Varicella-zoster virus	Direct contact with respiratory secretions (droplets); airborne, respiratory secretions (droplets)	High fever, fatigue, loss of appetite, headache, and itchy rash that becomes blistered then scabs over.

cuts or open sores in those areas. Some strains of the virus are more likely to infect the cells in the female reproductive tract (Langerhans cells). The HIV strain most common in the United States, however, targets the monocyte or lymphocyte white blood cells and is more prone to being passed along through anal sex and blood-to-blood contact.

The virus also can be spread by the sharing of needles used by intravenous drug users. The minute amount of blood left on a needle after injection provides an ample supply of the virus to transmit the infection to another host. Needles used in tattooing and piercing also can pose a risk. In all cases, needles should be new and sterile.

The virus can pass from mother to fetus during pregnancy, and to an infant during delivery or through breastfeeding. Approximately 25% of infants born to an untreated infected mother contract the disease, whereas only 2% of infants born to infected mothers who are treated contract HIV.

At one time, the virus also was being spread through the nation's blood supply via transfusion of HIV-contaminated blood products. This form of transmission has virtually stopped as a result of an aggressive screening program that began in 1985. All blood donations are tested for the virus and contaminated donations are destroyed.

Risk in the Medical Community
A small number of healthcare workers have contracted HIV as a direct result of occupational activities. There were 57 confirmed cases of healthcare-associated infection with HIV between 1981 and 2010. Investigations showed that infection in most of these cases occurred as a result of percutaneous exposure (exposure via puncture wound or needlestick). Mucocutaneous exposure (exposure through a mucous membrane) resulted in infection in a few cases.

Further analysis identified that in most cases, the infecting substance was HIV-infected blood. Concentrated virus cultures in the laboratory and visibly bloody body fluid caused a few of the cases.

Progress of the Infection
Current research has shown that development of AIDS occurs in three main stages:

1. Initial infection
2. Incubation period
3. Full-blown AIDS

Initial HIV infection can occur years before any symptoms appear. In some cases, the initial infection is marked by severe flulike symptoms. However, identification of the initial infection is almost always through hindsight.

The virus attacks helper T cells during this initial phase by first entering the cell. Then the host cell produces multiple copies of the virus. As a result, helper T cells die or are disabled. The body's immune system responds to the attack at this point, cleansing the blood supply of the virus, and the virus enters an inactive phase.

The incubation period begins when the virus incorporates its genetic material into the genetic material of the helper T cells. The virus is trapped within the lymph system and the host experiences few, if any, disease symptoms. Many doctors discover the infection in patients during this period when treating them for other illnesses. This incubation period, in which people are HIV-positive but do not have AIDS, generally lasts 8 to 15 years.

Sometime during the incubation period, HIV becomes active again and continues to attack and destroy helper T cells. As the number of helper T cells dwindles, the patient becomes more prone to opportunistic infections.

The threshold at which a patient is officially diagnosed with AIDS is the point at which there are 200 or fewer helper T cells per milliliter of blood. Once a person has full-blown AIDS—the third phase of infection—opportunistic infections take hold as the overall immune system deteriorates. Neurons are destroyed, resulting in neurological problems, including dementia.

Diagnosis
The initial diagnosis may be accomplished through the use of a rapid HIV test. Rapid tests are available for testing whole blood, blood plasma, urine, and oral fluids and the results are available within 20 minutes. These tests are used for initial testing only. To know for certain whether a person is infected with HIV, that person must have confirmatory blood tests specifically for HIV infection, which include

- Enzyme-linked immunosorbent assay (ELISA).
- Western blot test.
- Immunofluorescent antibody (IFA) test.

Positive results from two of the three HIV tests (ELISA plus one other) yield an accurate diagnosis in almost 100% of patients tested.

Home tests are available that involve an ELISA test followed by either a Western blot test or an IFA test if the ELISA results are positive. These tests are performed on a drop of the patient's blood, collected on a specially treated card. (Keep in mind that people who perform home tests may not report positive results to the proper authorities.) Patients should be made aware that:

- Only one home test, the Home Access HIV-1 Test System, is Food and Drug Administration (FDA)–approved, and even this test may give false results.
- If test results are positive, they will need medical care, including treatment and counseling.

In all cases involving HIV testing, you must follow measures to ensure protection of the patient's confidentiality. Knowledge about a patient's test results should be limited to those who will be treating the patient and appropriate authorities as required by law. The patient's decision on whether to reveal test results to family and friends should be respected at all times.

Symptoms
HIV infection can cause a variety of problems as it progresses to AIDS. Patients with AIDS may complain of any of the following symptoms:

- Systemic complaints, like weight loss, fatigue, fever, chills, and night sweats.
- Respiratory complaints, like sinus fullness, dry cough, shortness of breath, difficulty swallowing, and sinus drainage.

- Oral complaints, like gingivitis, oral lesions, and hairy leuko-plakia, which is a white lesion on the tongue.
- Gastrointestinal complaints, like diarrhea and bloody stool.
- Central nervous system (CNS) complaints, like depression, personality changes, concentration difficulties, and confusion or dementia.
- Peripheral nervous system complaints, like tingling, numbness, pain, and weakness in the extremities.
- Skin-related complaints, like rashes, dry skin, and changes in the nail bed.
- Kaposi's sarcoma, an unusual malignancy occurring in the skin and sometimes in the lymph nodes and organs, and manifested by reddish purple to dark blue patches or spots on the skin.

Because many other diseases can cause these symptoms, the occurrence of any one symptom is not necessarily indicative of AIDS. Be aware, however, that patients exhibiting a combination of symptoms should be tested. The two symptoms most indicative of AIDS are hairy leukoplakia and Kaposi's sarcoma.

Preventive Measures
The only way to prevent the spread of HIV infection is to avoid specific activities or to take safety precautions when engaging in these activities. Activities requiring preventive measures can be divided into three groups, based on the means of disease transmission:

- Sexual contact
- Sharing of intravenous needles
- Medical procedures

Prevention and Sexual Contact
The most effective method for preventing the spread of AIDS/HIV infection through sexual contact is to avoid high-risk sexual activity. Such high-risk activities or situations include:

- Having unprotected vaginal, oral, or anal sex, either homosexual or heterosexual, *unless* the individuals are involved in a long-term, monogamous relationship, they both have been tested and received negative results, and have not engaged in any unsafe sexual activity 6 months before the test or anytime after the test.
- Having multiple sexual partners, even when using protection against infection.
- Experiencing a concurrent infection with another sexually transmitted disease.

In addition, precautions must be taken when using a condom as a means of protection against infection. Proper condom use requires adherence to the following guidelines:

- A condom must be used every time the individual has sex and must never be reused.
- Only latex (not lambskin) condoms provide protection against HIV.
- If lubrication is required, the lubricant must be water-based, not petroleum-based (like petroleum jelly). Lubricants other than those specifically formulated for use with latex condoms

can damage the condom, rendering it permeable and eliminating its usefulness as a disease barrier.

- Condoms should be placed on the penis before any risk of leakage of seminal fluid occurs. Space should be left at the tip to act as a reservoir for ejaculated semen.
- The condom must remain in place from the beginning to the end of intercourse and should be held in place during withdrawal to prevent slippage. After withdrawal, the condom should be disposed of properly.

Prevention and Intravenous Drug Use
Intravenous drug users are at risk for infection when they share needles. The most effective means of preventing the spread of the pathogen among drug users is to avoid sharing or reusing needles.

Prevention and Medical Procedures
Preventing the spread of AIDS/HIV infection in the medical environment involves taking many precautions. You must take precautions to prevent the spread of infection between patients, between yourself and the patient, and when you are working with potentially contaminated equipment, supplies, or instruments.

Strict adherence to Standard Precautions when working with patients is the best method for preventing the spread of disease among patients and between the patient and you. (See the *Basic Safety and Infection Control* chapter for specific guidelines.)

Education as Prevention
As a medical assistant, you will encounter many opportunities to inform and educate patients about the dangers of HIV infection and AIDS, the ways in which the disease is spread, the ways in which it is not spread, and methods for preventing its spread. Use these opportunities to educate patients because one of the best preventive measures is providing accurate and thorough information to people.

Chronic Disorders of the AIDS Patient
The impaired immune system of the AIDS patient permits opportunistic infections, which further reduce the body's ability to fight off infection. These infections attack many different parts of the body.

One of the cornerstones of the care of patients who have AIDS is to prevent opportunistic infections and identify such infections as quickly as possible when they occur. Identifying malignancies, if they occur, is also of utmost importance. If you are familiar with the common disorders an AIDS patient faces, you will be better able to identify early signs of infection or malignancy and point them out to the doctor, in turn initiating early treatment, which is usually most effective. You can help patients who have been diagnosed with HIV to understand the risks they face and the measures best suited to preventing particular infections. Opportunistic infections include

- *Pneumocystis carinii* pneumonia
- Kaposi's sarcoma
- Non-Hodgkin's lymphoma
- Tuberculosis
- *Mycobacterium avium* complex (MAC) infection

- Meningitis
- Oral candidiasis
- Vaginal candidiasis
- Herpes simplex
- Herpes zoster

Drug Treatments A growing number of drugs are available for HIV/AIDS treatment, and billions of dollars are spent each year for research into such treatments and vaccines. Although there is no cure for either of these diseases, pharmaceutical companies are making great strides in creating new drugs that slow the virus's reproduction. Because more than 20 drugs are available for treatment, an individual with HIV or AIDS who has had no success with one regimen or treatment might find success with another. This is important for increasing life expectancy. Table 46-4 identifies different classifications of drugs currently approved by the FDA for the treatment of diseases associated with HIV infection and AIDS.

Treatment Goals The goals of drug treatment for HIV and AIDS include the following:

- Increasing the time between infection and symptomatic disease (AIDS).
- Improving the quality of life of those diagnosed with AIDS.
- Reducing transmission of HIV to uninfected persons.
- Reducing maternal-infant transmission.
- Reducing the number of HIV-related deaths.

Treatment Guidelines The Panel on Clinical Practices for Treatment of HIV Infection (the Panel) developed some basic guidelines for implementing HIV/AIDS treatment. These include initial and follow-up testing of viral load and CD4 T cell count (good indicators of the treatment's overall effectiveness) and drug resistance testing (especially useful for patients who have failed initial therapy). FDA-approved pharmaceutical agents used in HIV/AIDS treatment are divided into the six classes described in Table 46-4. Each of these drug classes has a different manner of working against the HIV virus. All of these classes, used in combination, are important weapons in the arsenal of treatments used to combat HIV/AIDS.

The Panel recommends a combination of drug treatment called *antiretroviral therapy (ART)*, which combines three or more HIV drugs. Taking three or more drugs has proven to be more effective than taking two or fewer because viral load decrease is only temporary in those taking one or two HIV drugs. Treatment during pregnancy is the only exception to this. Because many (but not all) HIV/AIDS drugs are contraindicated during pregnancy, pregnant patients are offered a single drug in order to limit passing HIV to their infants.

Initiating Therapy When therapy should begin is an important decision that must be made jointly by the patient and the physician. To help with this decision, the Panel has made several recommendations based on a combination of CD4 T cell count, viral load, and the presence or absence of symptoms. Starting therapy immediately is recommended if patients have severe symptoms (AIDS diagnosis) or if their CD4 T cell count is less than 200 cells/mm³. The physician should consider treatment if the CD4 T cell count is between 200 and 350 cells/mm³. In patients with a CD4 T cell count greater than 350 cells/mm³, no symptoms, and a viral load greater than 55,000 copies/mL, observation of the patient is recommended with a delay of treatment. The patient and physician should decide whether to take an aggressive or a conservative approach. If a conservative approach is taken, the patient should have routine CD4 T cell and viral load counts.

Delayed Treatment Delaying therapy has advantages and disadvantages. The benefits include postponing drug-related adverse effects, delaying the development of drug resistance, and preserving treatment options for the future. The risks of delaying treatment include irreversible immune system damage and an increased risk of the patient transmitting HIV to others.

TABLE 46-4 Antiretroviral Drugs Used in the Treatment of HIV/AIDS		
Classification	**Generic Name**	**Major Side Effects**
Fusion inhibitors—block viral entrance into the human cell	Enfuvirtide	Local injection site reactions (pain, erythema, induration, nodules and cysts, pruritus, and ecchymosis), increased incidence of bacterial pneumonia
Nonnucleoside reverse transcriptase inhibitors (NNRTIs)—block HIV's ability to make copies of itself	Efavirenz Atripla	Rash, neuropsychiatric symptoms, elevated liver enzymes, hyperlipidemia
Nucleoside reverse transcriptase inhibitors (NRTIs)—block HIV's ability to make copies of itself	Abacavir	Fever, rash, nausea, vomiting, diarrhea, abdominal pain, malaise or fatigue, sore throat, cough, or shortness of breath
Protease inhibitors (PIs)—block HIV's ability to make copies of itself	Atazanavir	Increased bilirubin levels, arrhythmias, hyperglycemia, and fat maldistribution
CCR5 antagonists—inhibit HIV attachment to human cells	Maraviroc	Abdominal pain, cough, dizziness, musculoskeletal symptoms, liver toxicity, fever, and upper respiratory tract infections
Integrase strand transfer inhibitors (INSTIs)—inhibit integration of viral DNA into the human chromosome, thus inhibiting replication	Raltegravir	Rash, nausea, headache, diarrhea, fever, and rhabdomyolysis

Early Treatment There are also advantages and disadvantages to beginning treatment early. Early treatment benefits include:

- Suppression of viral replication (the spread of the virus within the patient's system) to preserve immune function.
- Reduced risk of the patient transmitting HIV to others.
- Helping the patient live symptom-free longer.

The disadvantages of early treatment are:

- Development of drug toxicity.
- Drug resistance and the subsequent transmission of drug-resistant HIV strains to others.
- Adverse effects on the quality of life.
- Loss of treatment options in the future.

Each of these advantages and disadvantages must be carefully weighed by the patient and physician based on the patient's symptoms, lifestyle, and ability to comply with the treatment.

Go to CONNECT to see an animation about *HIV/AIDS*.

Hepatitis

Hepatitis is a viral infection of the liver that can lead to cirrhosis and death. Hepatitis virus variants differ in their means of transmission and in their presenting symptoms of infection. These variations include the following:

- Hepatitis A, caused by the hepatitis A virus (HAV). Hepatitis A is spread mainly through the fecal-oral route. People can be infected with HAV by drinking contaminated water, eating contaminated food, or having intimate contact with an infected person. HAV can spread in daycare settings when an attendant changes the diaper of an infected child, then helps another child with feeding before performing adequate handwashing. The disease is rarely fatal (the recovery rate is 99%) and there is a vaccine that prevents infection.
- Hepatitis B, the most common bloodborne hazard heathcare workers face. It is spread through contact with contaminated blood or body fluids and through sexual contact. Most patients recover fully from HBV infection, but some patients develop chronic infection or remain carriers of the pathogen for the rest of their lives. Adults and children with hepatitis B who develop lifelong infections may experience serious health problems, including cirrhosis (scarring of the liver), liver cancer, liver failure, and death. Preventing the spread of the infection is the most effective means of combating the disease. Following Standard Precautions and receiving HBV vaccination are the most effective ways to control the spread of the infection.
- Hepatitis C, which is also spread through contact with contaminated blood or body fluids and through sexual contact. There is no cure for this variant, which has resulted in more deaths than hepatitis A and hepatitis B combined. Many people become carriers of hepatitis C without knowing it because they do not experience any symptoms. If the infection causes immediate symptoms, they often resemble the flu. Although treatment exists to suppress the virus, nothing can prevent or stop the virus from replicating. Over time, it is likely to damage the liver, causing cirrhosis, liver failure, and cancer. As with hepatitis B, preventing the spread of the infection is the best way to combat the disease.

- Hepatitis D (delta agent hepatitis), which occurs only in people infected with HBV. Delta agent infection may make hepatitis B symptoms more severe, and it is associated with liver cancer. The HBV vaccine also prevents delta agent infection.
- Hepatitis E, caused by hepatitis E virus (HEV). Hepatitis E is transmitted by the fecal-oral route, usually through contaminated water. Chronic infection does not occur, but acute hepatitis E may be fatal in pregnant women.

Risk Factors Risk factors for HBV and HCV infection are the same. Although both infections can be spread through sexual contact—and high-risk sexual activity is a risk factor for hepatitis—the main risk factor is working in an occupation that requires exposure to human blood and body fluids. Other risk factors are listed below:

- Using intravenous drugs.
- Having hemophilia, a disorder characterized by a permanent tendency to bleed and requiring blood transfusions.
- Traveling internationally to areas with a high prevalence of hepatitis B.
- Having received blood transfusions before screening for HBV/HCV was in place.
- Receiving hemodialysis, a procedure in which toxic wastes are removed from a patient's blood.
- Living with a partner who has hepatitis B or hepatitis C.
- Having multiple sexual partners.

Risk in the Medical Community As described, the primary risk factor for HBV and HCV infection is occupational exposure to the virus. In fact, although exposure to HIV has received more publicity and causes the greatest fear, your risk of contracting hepatitis, particularly hepatitis B, is actually considerably greater if you have not had the Hepatitis B vaccine. Studies show that the risk of contracting HIV from a single needlestick exposure is approximately 0.5%, whereas the risk of contracting hepatitis B from a single needlestick exposure varies from 6% to as much as 33%. Several variables are responsible for the broad range of measured risk in HBV infection, including the recipient's immune status and the efficiency of the virus transmission.

Progress of the Infection Infection with hepatitis is a multistage process. The stages are as follows:

1. The prodromal stage, in which patients may experience general malaise, specific symptoms like nausea and vomiting, or no symptoms at all;
2. The icteric, or jaundice, stage, characterized by yellowness of the skin, eyes, mucous membranes, and excretions

FIGURE 46-2 Jaundice is caused by excess bilirubin, which is produced in the liver and deposited throughout the body and which results in the yellow appearance of the patient's eyes and skin.

(Figure 46-2), which usually appears 5 to 10 days after initial infection; and

3. The convalescent stage, which occurs after the two acute infection stages and can last from 2 to 3 weeks as symptoms gradually abate.

The acute illness lasts approximately 16 weeks for hepatitis B and hepatitis C. Although patients recover, they may remain infected with the virus for life.

Symptoms People infected with hepatitis may show no symptoms, may experience such mild or subtle symptoms that they do not realize they are seriously ill, or may experience severe symptoms. When you treat patients with hepatitis, any of these signs and symptoms may be present:

- Jaundice
- Diminished appetite
- Fatigue
- Nausea
- Vomiting
- Joint pain or tenderness
- Stomach pain
- General malaise

Diagnosis Diagnosis of hepatitis is made through an investigation of risk factors and exposure incidents as well as through several blood tests. Most of the blood tests indicate the presence of antigen-antibody systems that relate to infection by hepatitis. They also can be used to determine the stage of the disease.

Preventive Measures The best prevention against hepatitis is avoiding contact with contaminated substances. Follow Standard Precautions when working with all patients and be especially careful with patients who have unknown or hepatitis-positive status.

A vaccine is available to prevent HBV infection. In fact, OSHA has established guidelines that require your employer to offer you this vaccine at no charge. If you decline the offer, you must sign a waiver. Current standard medical practice recommends against declining the vaccine.

Vaccination against HBV does not protect you from other strains of hepatitis. There are currently no vaccines for HCV, for example.

In the past, HBV vaccination was recommended only for high-risk individuals, such as medical personnel, dialysis patients, homosexual men, and intravenous drug users. However, this program of vaccinating only selected individuals did not greatly reduce the incidence of infection. Today, the CDC recommends routine vaccination for everyone.

If you are exposed to hepatitis B and have not been vaccinated, you can receive a postexposure inoculation of hepatitis B immune globulin (HBIG). HBIG is given in large doses during the 7-day period after exposure. Shortly after beginning the treatment, you would also receive HBV vaccination. The HBIG inoculation is also used for infants born to HBV-infected mothers.

▶ Bacteria

LO 46.6

Bacteria are single-celled prokaryotic organisms that reproduce very quickly and are one of the major causes of disease. Under the right conditions—the right temperature, the right nutrients, and moisture—bacterial cells can double in number in 15 to 30 minutes. This rapid reproduction is one reason why untreated infections can be dangerous.

Classification and Identification

Bacteria can be classified according to their shape, their ability to retain certain dyes, their ability to grow with or without air, and certain biochemical reactions. Table 46-5 lists some representatives of the major groups of bacteria, with distinguishing characteristics and a few examples.

Shape The most common way to classify bacteria is according to their shape. The four common shape classifications are the coccus, bacillus, spirillum, and vibrio (see Figure 46-3).

A **coccus** (plural, cocci) is spherical, round, or ovoid. Cocci can be further divided into three types. *Staphylococci* are grapelike clusters of cocci commonly found on the skin. One species of this microorganism causes a variety of infections, including boils, acne, abscesses, food poisoning, and a type of pneumonia. *Diplococci* are pairs of cocci. The causative agents for gonorrhea and some forms of meningitis are diplococci. *Streptococci* are cocci that grow in chains. These microorganisms are responsible for infections like strep throat, certain types of pneumonia, and rheumatic fever.

A **bacillus** (plural, bacilli) is rod-shaped. Bacilli are responsible for a wide variety of infections, including gastroenteritis, tuberculosis, pneumonia, whooping cough, urinary tract infections (UTIs), botulism, and tetanus.

A **spirillum** (plural, spirilla) is spiral-shaped. Spirilla are responsible for infections like syphilis and Lyme disease.

A **vibrio** (plural, vibrios) is comma-shaped. Vibrios are responsible for diseases like cholera and some cases of food poisoning.

TABLE 46-5 Some Major Groups of Bacteria

	Gram-Positive Bacteria		
Genus	**Species**	**Shape**	**Characteristic**
Staphylococcus	aureus, epidermidis	Spherical, round, or ovoid	Clusters
Streptococcus	pyogenes, pneumoniae		Chains
Bacillus	subtilis	Straight rod	Aerobic
Clostridium	botullinum, tetani		Aanaerobic
	Gram-Negative Bacteria		
Genus	**Species**	**Shape**	**Characteristic**
Neisseria	meningitidis, gonorrhoeae	Spherical, round, or ovoid	Aerobic
Pseudomonas	aeruginosa	Straight rod	Aerobic
Haemophilus	influenzae		
Escherichia	coli		Facultative
Salmonella	typhi		
Shigella	dysenteriae		
Vibrio	cholerae	Comma	Facultative
Treponema	pallidum	Spiral	Move by undulating
	Other Groups		
Genus	**Species**	**Shape**	**Characteristic**
Mycobacterium	tuberculosis	Straight, curved, or branched rod	Acid-fast
Mycoplasma	pneumoniae	Variable	Have no rigid cell wall
Rickettsia	rickettsii		Intracellular parasites
Chlamydia	trachomatis	Spherical, round, or oval	Intracellular parasites

FIGURE 46-3 The four bacterial classifications by shape are (a) coccus, (b) bacillus, (c) spirillum, and (d) vibrio.

Ability to Retain Certain Dyes In addition to their shape, bacteria are commonly classified by how they react to certain stains. A **stain** is a solution of a dye or group of dyes that imparts a color to microorganisms. The most common staining procedure in use today is the **Gram stain,** a method of staining that differentiates bacteria according to the chemical composition of their cell walls. This procedure is often performed in the medical office. Another important stain is the **acid-fast stain,** a staining procedure for identifying bacteria with a waxy cell wall. The bacteria that cause tuberculosis can be stained with this procedure.

Ability to Grow in the Presence or Absence of Air Bacteria that grow best in the presence of oxygen are referred to as **aerobes.** Those that grow best in the absence of oxygen are referred to as **anaerobes.** Organisms that can grow in either environment are referred to as **facultative.** Although most common bacteria are aerobes, many of the bacteria that make up the body's resident normal flora are anaerobes. Not surprisingly, anaerobes are often responsible for infections within the body.

Biochemical Reactions Many closely related bacteria can be differentiated from one another only by certain biochemical reactions that occur within the bacterial cell. For example, one way to identify a particular bacterial strain is to look at what types of sugars the bacteria can grow on.

Special Groups of Bacteria

Several groups of bacteria have certain characteristics that set them apart from most other bacteria. These include the mycobacteria, rickettsiae, chlamydiae, and mycoplasmas.

Mycobacteria Mycobacteria are rod-shaped bacilli with a distinct cell wall that differs from that of most bacteria. Certain types of mycobacteria cause disease in humans. For example, *Mycobacterium tuberculosis* causes the respiratory disease tuberculosis and *Mycobacterium leprae* causes leprosy.

Rickettsiae Rickettsiae are very small bacteria that can live and grow only within other living cells. Rickettsiae are commonly found in insects like ticks and mites but may be transmitted to humans through bites. Rickettsiae are responsible for diseases such as Rocky Mountain spotted fever and typhus.

Chlamydiae Chlamydiae differ from other bacteria in the structure of their cell walls. Like rickettsiae, they can live and grow only within other living cells. In humans, chlamydiae can cause venereal disease, eye disease, certain types of pneumonia, and certain types of heart disease.

Mycoplasmas Mycoplasmas are small bacteria that completely lack the rigid cell wall of other bacteria. These bacteria cause a variety of human diseases, including venereal disease and a form of pneumonia.

Bacterial Pathogens

In spite of our efforts to erradicate disease-causing bacteria through the use of antibiotics, bacterial pathogens are still

with us. Table 46-6 lists some of these pathogens and the diseases they cause.

Drug-Resistant Microogranisms

Drug-resistant pathogens are the cause of many infections. Drug resistance has been linked to overuse of antibiotics. It is the responsibility of physicians, medical staff, and patients to use antibiotics wisely, as resistance to antimicrobial agents is a severe problem. Bacteria and other microorganisms that have developed resistance to antimicrobial drugs include the following:

- MRSA—methicillin/oxacillin-resistant *S. aureus*
- VRE—vancomycin-resistant enterococci
- VISA—vancomycin-intermediate *S. aureus*
- VRSA—vancomycin-resistant *S. aureus*
- ESBLs—extended-spectrum beta-lactamases, which are resistant to cephalosporins and monobactams
- PRSP—penicillin-resistant *Streptococcus pneumoniae*

MRSA and VRE are the most common multidrug-resistant organisms in patients who reside in nonhospital healthcare facilities (for example, nursing homes and other long-term-care facilities). People outside of healthcare facilities are increasingly at risk for MRSA, as community-associated MRSA, an infection found in otherwise healthy individuals, is on the rise in the United States. PRSP is more common in patients seeking care in physicians' offices and clinics, especially in pediatric settings. This is thought to be because penicillin is the most commonly prescribed antibiotic in outpatient settings.

Risk Factors

There are a number of risk factors for both the development of and infection with drug-resistant organisms. These risk factors include:

- Advanced age.
- Invasive procedures, which include dialysis, the presence of invasive devices, and urinary catheterization.
- Previous use of antimicrobial agents.
- Repeated contact with the healthcare system.
- Severity of the illness.
- Underlying diseases or conditions, especially chronic renal disease, insulin-dependent diabetes mellitus, peripheral vascular disease, and dermatitis or skin lesions.

Preventing Antibiotic Resistance in Healthcare Settings

In response to a growing concern over the emergence of antibiotic-resistant infections, the CDC began the Campaign to Prevent Antimicrobial Resistance in Healthcare Settings. This campaign has four strategies to reduce the incidence of antibiotic-resistant microorganisms:

- Prevent infection
- Diagnose and treat infection appropriately
- Use antibiotics carefully
- Prevent transmission of infections

TABLE 46-6	Bacterial Pathogens			
Disease	**Causative Organism**	**Characteristics**	**Route of Transmission**	**Signs and Symptoms**
Anthrax	*Bacillus anthracis*	Aerobic, Gram-positive, spore-forming bacillus	Contact with animals infected with or inhalation of *B. anthracis* spores, or consumption of raw or undercooked meat from infected animals	Cutaneous: raised, blistered skin lesion with development of black eschar (dead tissue). Inhalation: high fever, dyspnea, stridor, cyanosis, shock.
Whooping cough	*Bordetella pertussis*	Gram-negative bacterium	Airborne	Stage 1: runny nose, low-grade fever, and mild cough. Stage 2: bursts of rapid, uncontrollable coughs with characteristic "whoops" at the end of the cough; cyanosis; and exhaustion. Stage 3: recovery, less persistent cough.
Lyme disease	*Borrelia burgdorferi*	Spirochete that does not have typical Gram stain characteristics	Tick-borne (Ixodes tick)	Red, expanding, "bulls-eye" rash; fatigue; fever; chills; headache; muscle and joint aches; and swollen lymph nodes.
Campylobacteriosis	*Campylobacter jejuni*	Gram-negative, microaerophilic, spiral-shaped	Fecal-oral, foodborne	Diarrhea, sometimes bloody; abdominal cramps; and fever.
Chlamydia	*Chlamydia trachomatis*	Coccus; does not have typical Gram stain characteristics but is considered Gram-negative; obligate, intracellular bacteria (must live within an animal cell)	STI	Women: often "silent"; possible vaginal discharge and dysuria. Men: penile discharge and dysuria.
Botulism	*Clostridium botulinum*	Anaerobic, Gram-positive, spore-forming bacillus	Foodborne	Double vision, blurred vision, drooping eyelids, slurred speech, difficulty swallowing, dry mouth, and muscle weakness.
Pseudomembranous colitis	*Clostridium difficile*	Anaerobic, Gram-positive, spore-forming bacillus	Fecal-oral (healthcare-associated infection)	Watery diarrhea, fever, loss of appetite, nausea, and abdominal pain/tenderness.
Tetanus	*Clostridium tetani*	Anaerobic, Gram-positive bacillus (sometimes forms spores)	Direct contact through a deep cut	Early: lockjaw, neck, and abdomen stiffness, and difficulty swallowing. Late: severe muscle spasms and generalized tonic seizure–like activity.
Diphtheria	*Corynebacterium diphtheria*	Gram-positive bacillus	Direct person-to-person contact with respiratory droplets or cutaneous lesions	Sore throat; low-grade fever; presence of a pseudomembrane over the tonsils, throat, and nose.
E. coli diarrhea	*Escherichia coli*	Gram-negative bacillus	Foodborne (some strains do not cause disease)	Diarrhea, severe abdominal cramps, and vomiting.
Haemophilus influenzae Serotype b (Hib) disease (epiglottitis, pneumonia)	*Haemophilus influenzae*	Gram-negative coccobacillus	Direct contact with respiratory droplets	Epiglottitis: sore throat and difficulty breathing. Pneumonia: difficulty breathing and fever
Peptic ulcer	*Helicobacter pylori*	Microaerophilic, Gram-negative bacillus	Not well understood; may be fecal-oral or oral-oral	Peptic ulcer, gnawing or burning stomach pain.
Legionnaire's disease	*Legionella pneumophila*	Gram-negative bacillus	Water aerosol	High fever, chills, cough, chest pain, and pneumonia.
Leprosy	*Mycobacterium leprae*	Acid-fast bacillus	Airborne, respiratory droplets	Skin lesions, nodules, plaques, thickened dermis.
Tuberculosis	*Mycobacterium tuberculosis*	Acid-fast bacillus	Airborne, respiratory droplets	Bad cough lasting three weeks or longer, pain in the chest, coughing up blood or sputum, weakness or fatigue, weight loss, no appetite, chills, fever, and night sweats.
Mycoplasma pneumonia	*Mycoplasma pneumoniae*	Wall-less bacteria usually coccoid in shape with polar extensions	Direct contact with respiratory droplets	Fever, nonproductive cough, malaise, and headache.

TABLE 46-6 (concluded)

Disease	Causative Organism	Characteristics	Route of Transmission	Signs and Symptoms
Gonorrhea	Neisseria gonorrhoeae	Gram-negative diplococcus	STI	Women: most have no symptoms; some have dysuria and vaginal discharge. Men: dysuria and green, yellow, or white penile discharge. Left untreated can cause complications in both women and men.
Meningitis	Neisseria meningitidis	Gram-negative diplococcus	Direct contact with respiratory droplets	Stiff neck, fever, confusion, light sensitivity, nausea, and vomiting.
	Haemophilus influenzae	Gram-negative coccobacillus		
	Group B Streptococcus (Streptococcus agalactiae)	Gram-positive coccus		
	Listeria monocytogenes	Gram-positive, flagellated bacillus		
Pseudomonas infection (hot tub rash)	Pseudomonas aeruginosa	Gram-negative bacillus	Direct contact with water contaminated with P. aeruginosa	Itchy, red rash; pustules around hair follicles.
Rocky Mountain spotted fever	Rickettsia rickettsi	Gram-negative coccobacillus	Tick-borne (wood or dog tick)	Fever, rash (occurs 2–5 days after fever), headache, nausea, vomiting, abdominal pain, muscle pain, lack of appetite, and conjunctival inflammation.
Shigellosis	Shigella sonnei	Gram-negative bacillus	Fecal-oral	Diarrhea, fever, and stomach cramps.
Methicillin-resistant Staphylococcus aureus (MRSA) infections	Staphylococcus aureus	Gram-positive coccus	Direct contact	Red, swollen, painful pustules.
Bacterial pneumonia	Streptococcus pneumonia	Gram-positive diplococci	Direct person-to-person contact	Cough, chest pain, shortness of breath, malaise, and poor appetite.
Strep throat	Streptococcus pyogenes	Gram-positive coccus	Direct contact with respiratory droplets	Sore throat and fever.
Syphilis	Treponema pallidum	Gram-negative spirochete	STI	Primary stage: single sore (chancre) at site of the organism's entry into the body. Secondary stage: skin rash and mucous membrane lesions. Late stage: uncoordinated muscle movements, paralysis, numbness, gradual blindness, dementia.
Cholera	Vibrio cholerae	Gram-negative curved rod	Fecal-oral from contaminated water	Profuse watery diarrhea ("rice-water stools"), vomiting, rapid heart rate, loss of skin elasticity, dry mucous membranes, low blood pressure, thirst, muscle cramps, and restlessness or irritability.

▶ Protozoans

LO 46.7

Protozoans are single-celled eukaryotic organisms that are generally much larger than bacteria. Found in soil and water, most do not cause disease in people. Certain protozoans are pathogenic, however, and cause diseases like malaria, amebic dysentery (a type of diarrhea), and trichomoniasis vaginitis (a type of venereal disease; see Figure 46-4). Protozoal diseases are a leading cause of death in developing countries because the lack of proper sanitation in some areas promotes their spread. These diseases are also common in patients with depressed immune systems. Table 46-7 lists some of the parasitic protozoans and multicellular parasites that affect humans.

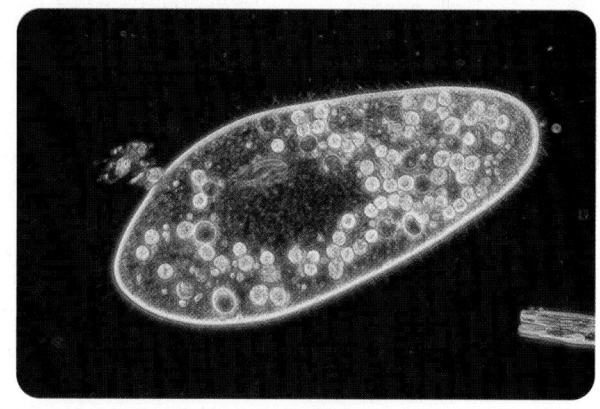

FIGURE 46-4 The protozoan *Trichomonas vaginalis* causes a common sexually transmitted infection in humans.

TABLE 46-7 Human Protozoal and Multicellular Parasites

Disease	Causative Organism	Notable Features	Route of Transmission	Signs and Symptoms
Intestinal				
Amebiasis	*Entamoeba histolytica*	Can become invasive and cause liver abscess	Fecal-oral	Loose stool, abdominal pain, abdominal cramping, bloody diarrhea, and fever.
Intestinal hookworm	*Necator americanus* and *Ancylostoma duodenale*	Larvae migrate to the intestinal tract	Larvae in soil contaminated with feces from an infected person penetrate bare feet and cause infection	Itching at the site of entry, abdominal pain, diarrhea, anorexia, and anemia due to loss of blood at the site of attachment in the intestine.
Round worm	*Ascaris lumbricoides*	Most common helminthic (worm) infection in the world	Contact with contaminated soil	Can be asymptomatic. Abdominal discomfort and intestinal blockage.
Cryptosporidiosis	*Cryptosporidium parvum* and *C. hominis*	Can be found in recreational water such as swimming pools and hot tubs contaminated with *Cryptosporidium*	Waterborne	Abdominal cramps and pain, dehydration, nausea, vomiting, fever, and weight loss.
Cyclosporiasis	*Cyclospora cayetanensis*	Outbreaks in the United States have been linked to imported fresh produce	Fecal-oral	Frequent, explosive, watery diarrhea; abdominal cramps; loss of appetite; weight loss; bloating; excessive gas; and fatigue.
Fish or broad tapeworm	*Diphyllobothrium latum*	Longest human tapeworm, reaching up to 30 feet in length	Foodborne from eating raw or undercooked fish infected with *D. latum*	Abdominal discomfort, diarrhea, vomiting, weight loss, and vitamin B_{12} deficiency.
Pinworm	*Enterobius vermicularis*	While the infected person is sleeping, female pinworms leave the intestine and lay their eggs on the skin surrounding the anus	Fecal-oral	Anal itching, nighttime restlessness due to anal itching.
Giardiasis	*Giardia intestinalis* (formerly *G. lamblia*)	Once outside the body, can live in soil or water for weeks or months	Fecal-oral	Greasy, floating stool; gas; diarrhea; abdominal pain and cramping; nausea; and dehydration.
Lung fluke (Paragonimiasis)	*Paragonimus kellicotti*	Linked to eating raw or undercooked crab or crayfish infected with *P. kellicotti*; ingested larvae migrate to the lungs	Foodborne	Initially diarrhea and abdominal pain, followed by fever, chest pain, fatigue, and cough.
Bloodborne/Vectorborne				
Chagas disease	*Trypanosome cruzi*	Found only in the Americas (mostly Latin America but also found in the United States)	Vector-borne (triatomine bugs)	Acute phase: fever, fatigue, body aches, headache, and diarrhea. Chronic phase: cardiomyopathy, heart failure, heart arrhythmia, enlarged esophagus, enlarged colon, and difficulty eating or passing stool.
Malaria	*Plasmodium falciparum, P. vivax, P. ovale, P. malariae*	Fifth most common cause of death worldwide from infectious disease	Vector-borne (mosquito)	Fever, chills, sweats, headache, nausea, body aches, and general malaise.
Skin				
Swimmer's itch (cercarial dermatitis)	*Austrobilharzia variglandis*	Ducks and geese are the most common host; however, the larvae will burrow into a human swimmer's skin	Contact with larvae in water	Tingling, burning, or itching of the skin; small reddish pimples and small blisters.
Head lice (pediculosis)	*Pediculus humanus capitis*	Can be transmitted by contact with clothing, combs, or brushes used by an infested individual	Direct contact with the hair of infested individual	Feeling that something is moving in your hair, itching, difficulty sleeping because of louse activity, and scalp sores.
Pubic lice (pthiriasis)	*Phthirus pubis*	Infestation has been linked to casual contact with personal items—like combs or hairbrushes—used by infested individuals.	Direct contact with an infested individual (usually sexual contact)	Genital itching, visible nits (eggs), or crawling adult lice.
Scabies	*Sarcoptes scabiei*	Symptoms are worse at night	Prolonged, direct contact with an infested individual	Intense itching and papular rash.
Bed bugs	*Cimex lectularius* and *C. hemipterus*	Bed bugs are not known to carry any disease and are not considered a public health threat	Exposure to bedding or furniture infested with *C. lectularius* or *C. hemipterus*	Bite marks on the head, neck, face, hands, or other body parts occurring at night while sleeping.
Muscle				
Trichinellosis	*Trichinella spiralis*	Currently uncommon in commercial pork; more cases in the United States are now associated with wild game	Foodborne from eating raw or undercooked pork or wild animals	Nausea, diarrhea, vomiting, fatigue, fever, abdominal pain, headache, chills, coughing, eye swelling, and joint pain.
Toxoplasmosis	*Toxoplasma gondii*	Forms cysts that may be found in skeletal muscle, myocardium, brain, and eyes	Foodborne, animal-to-human, mother-to-child (congenital)	Some have no or very mild symptoms; swollen lymph glands and muscle aches.
Vagina, Vulva, Urethra				
Trichomoniasis	*Trichomonas vaginalis*	Considered the most common and most curable STI	Sexual contact	Women: itching, burning, redness or soreness of the genitals, dysuria, and watery discharge with an unusual smell. Men: itching or irritation inside the penis, burning after urination or ejaculation, and some penile discharge.

Fungi

LO 46.8

A *fungus* (plural, fungi) is a eukaryotic organism that has a rigid cell wall at some stage in the life cycle. Fungi that grow mainly as single-celled organisms and reproduce by budding are referred to as *yeasts*, whereas fungi that grow into large, fuzzy, multicelled organisms that produce spores are called *molds*. Figure 46-5 shows the differences between these two types of fungi.

Most fungi do not cause disease in humans. Of those that do, the majority produce superficial infections like athlete's foot (tinea pedis), ringworm, thrush, and vaginal yeast infections. Fungi can produce serious, life-threatening illness, however, when they infect the internal tissues. This kind of infection can occur when patients have a depressed immune system, as in patients who are undergoing cancer treatment and patients with AIDS. Table 46-8 lists some of the most common fungal diseases and the organisms that cause them.

Multicellular Parasites

LO 46.9

A *parasite* is an organism that lives on or in another organism and uses that other organism for its own nourishment, or for some other advantage, to the detriment of the host organism. Viruses, rickettsiae, chlamydiae, and some protozoans are parasitic. Multicellular organisms also can be parasitic, and some of these organisms are microscopic during all or part of their lives. An infection caused by a parasite is called an *infestation*. Multicellular parasites that cause human disease include certain worms and insects, as illustrated in Figure 46-6 and listed in Table 46-7.

(a)

(b)

FIGURE 46-5 Because fungi lack the ability to make their own food, they depend on other life forms. (a) Single-celled fungi are called yeasts. (b) Multicelled fungi are called molds.

TABLE 46-8	**Pathogenic Fungi**		
Disease	**Causative Organism**	**Route of Transmission**	**Signs and Symptoms**
Aspergillosis	*Aspergillus fumigatus* and *A. flavus*	Airborne (inhalation of spores)	Wheezing, coughing, fever, chest pain, shortness of breath, and aspergilloma (fungus ball).
Blastomycosis	*Blastomyces dermatitidis*	Airborne (inhalation of spores)	Fever, chills, cough, muscle aches, joint pain, and chest pain.
Candidiasis • Oropharyngeal (thrush) • Vaginal • Invasive	*Candida albicans*	*C. albicans* is part of the body's resident normal flora; conditions that cause an imbalance in the resident normal flora cause an overgrowth of the fungus	• Oropharyngeal—white patches on the tongue and other oral mucous membranes, redness or soreness in the affected areas, difficulty swallowing, and cracking at the corners of the mouth. • Vaginal—genital itching, burning, thick white vaginal discharge. • Invasive—fever and chills.
Coccidioidomycosis (valley fever)	*Coccidioides*	Airborne (inhalation of spores)	Fever, cough, headache, rash on upper trunk or extremities, muscle aches, joint pain in the knees or ankles, skin lesions, chronic pneumonia, meningitis, bone or joint infection.
Ringworm	Dermatophytes (*Trichophyton rubrum* and *T. tonsurans*)	Direct contact with an infected person	Redness, scaling, cracking of the skin, or a ring-shaped rash; loss of hair at the site of infection.
Cryptococcosis	*Cryptococcus neoformans* and *C. gattii*	Airborne; *C. neoformans* is usually associated with large amounts of bird droppings	Shortness of breath, cough, fatigue, fever, headache, and meningitis.
Histoplasmosis	*Histoplasma capsulatum*	Airborne, usually associated with large amounts of bird or bat droppings	Fever, chest pains, and nonproductive cough.
Pneumocystis pneumonia (PCP)	*Pneumocystis jirovecii*	Airborne, inhalation of spores; most common opportunistic infection in people with HIV/AIDS	Fever, dry cough, shortness of breath, and fatigue.
Sporotrichosis	*Sporothrix schenckii*	Direct contact with spores	Small, painless nodule at contact site; lesion becomes larger over time and may ulcerate.

(a)

(c)

(d)

(e)

(b)

FIGURE 46-6 Parasitic worms, such as (a) tapeworms and (b) *Trichinella,* cause disease in humans when they are ingested. Parasitic insects, such as (c) mosquitoes, (d) deer ticks, and (e) mites, cause disease by biting or burrowing into the skin.

Parasitic Worms

People can be infested with a parasitic worm by ingesting its eggs or an immature form of the worm or by having the parasite penetrate the skin. As with the protozoans, infestation by these parasites is more common in developing nations with poor sanitation.

Worms that infect people include roundworms, flatworms, and tapeworms. Roundworms can occur in the intestines, as in the case of pinworms, a common infection in children. Other roundworms, like *Trichinella,* are found in muscle tissue. *Trichinella spiralis,* which causes the infection trichinosis, enters the human body in infected meat eaten raw or insufficiently cooked. People also may get flatworms and tapeworms by eating undercooked meats. A trained medical professional must inspect a patient's stool for the presence of the parasite or its eggs to diagnose an intestinal infection with a parasitic worm.

Parasitic Insects

Insects that can bite or burrow under the skin include mosquitoes, ticks, lice, and mites. These insects spread many viral, bacterial (including rickettsial), and protozoal diseases. The causative organisms can live in the insects' bodies and enter people's bodies when they are bitten by the insects. Such diseases include Lyme disease, malaria, Rocky Mountain spotted fever, and encephalitis. Lice are small insects that live on hair and skin and feed on blood. Scabies infestations are caused by mites that burrow under the skin.

How Infections Are Diagnosed   LO 46.10

To assist with the diagnosis and treatment of an infection, a medical assistant must work closely with other medical team members. The basic steps in diagnosis and treatment are summarized in Figure 46-7.

Step 1. Examine the Patient

When a patient comes into the office with signs or symptoms that suggest an infection, begin by taking the patient's vital signs and noting the patient's complaints. On the basis of these findings and the patient examination, the doctor can make a presumptive, or tentative, clinical diagnosis.

In many cases, signs and symptoms of a particular infection are so characteristic of the disease that the doctor need not

(a)

(b)

(c)

(d)

(e)

(f)

FIGURE 46-7 The steps in diagnosis and treatment of an infection: (a) Examine the patient. (b) Obtain one or more specimens. (c) Examine the specimen directly, by wet mount or smear. (d) Culture the specimen. (e) Determine the culture's antibiotic sensitivity. (f) Treat the patient as ordered by the physician.

perform additional tests to reach a diagnosis. An example might be a case of chickenpox or mumps. At other times, however, the doctor needs to gather additional information to confirm a diagnosis and determine the cause.

Step 2. Obtain One or More Specimens

To determine the cause of an infection, you may need to obtain specimens from one or more areas of the patient's body. Label each specimen properly and include with it the physician's presumptive diagnosis. If the sample is to be transported to an outside laboratory, ensure that it is transported in such a way that any pathogenic organisms remain alive (and safely contained) during transit.

Step 3. Examine the Specimen Directly

You must sometimes obtain more than one specimen from each site. The doctor or specially trained laboratory or microbiology personnel will then directly examine one specimen under the microscope. The specimen may be viewed in one of two ways:

- As a **wet mount,** a preparation of a specimen in a liquid that allows the organisms to remain alive and mobile while they are being identified.
- As a smear, in which a specimen is spread thinly and evenly across a slide.

If you make a smear, allow it to dry and then treat or stain it as ordered before it is examined microscopically. In some cases, direct examination allows the doctor to make a presumptive diagnosis of the microorganism.

Step 4. Culture the Specimen

If the physician still needs a more definitive identification of the microorganism, you may perform a **culture,** in which a sample of the specimen is placed in or on a substance that allows microorganisms to grow. A *culture medium* is a substance that contains all the nutrients a particular type of microorganism needs. Most media come in the form of a semisolid gel. After you inoculate (place a sample of the specimen in or on) the medium, place it in an incubator (a chamber that can be set to a specific temperature and humidity) to allow the microorganism to grow.

The culture is examined visually and microscopically after a specified time and a preliminary identification is made. The physician sets up additional tests to confirm the identification of the microorganism that has been isolated from the specimen. Most microbiology laboratories and some physicians' office laboratories are equipped to grow routine bacterial cultures and some fungal cultures. Physicians' office laboratories, in particular, may have to send other types of cultures, like virus cultures, to a specialized laboratory for identification.

Step 5. Determine the Culture's Antibiotic Sensitivity

In many cases of bacterial infection, a **culture and sensitivity (C&S)** is performed. This procedure involves culturing a specimen and then testing the isolated bacterium's susceptibility (sensitivity) to certain antibiotics. The results help the doctor determine which antibiotics might be most effective in treating the infection.

Step 6. Treat the Patient as Ordered by the Physician

On the basis of identification of the microorganism and antibiotic sensitivity, if determined, the physician can prescribe an *antimicrobial.* This agent, which kills microorganisms or suppresses their growth, should help clear up the patient's infection.

▶ Specimen Collection LO 46.11

Perhaps the most important step in isolating and identifying a microorganism as the cause of an infection is collecting the specimen. If this is done incorrectly, the organism may not grow in culture in a way that it can be identified, resulting in an untreated infection. Furthermore, if the specimen becomes contaminated during collection and the contaminant is mistakenly identified as the cause of the infection, the patient may receive incorrect or even harmful therapy.

In addition to vaginal specimens (discussed in detail in the *Assisting in Reproductive and Urinary Specialties* chapter), the most common types of culture specimens involve the following:

- Throat
- Urine
- Sputum
- Wound
- Stool

Specimen-Collection Devices

To help ensure optimal recovery of microorganisms, you must use the appropriate collection device and specimen container. Specimen-collection devices—usually provided by the lab—are available for the collection of sputum, urine, and stool specimens, as shown in Figure 46-8. These containers are designed

FIGURE 46-8 You may use specially designed collection containers to collect sputum, urine, and stool specimens.

FIGURE 46-9 Sterile swabs vary in size and material.

FIGURE 46-10 The CULTURETTE is used to obtain and transport microbiologic specimens to outside laboratories.
Source: Courtesy of Becton Dickson Microbiology Systems.

with large openings to allow specimen collection with minimal chance of contamination. They also have tight-fitting caps to prevent leakage and contamination.

Sterile Swabs The most common device for obtaining cultures is the sterile swab. Sterile swabs vary in the absorbent material at the tip and in the composition of the shaft (Figure 46-9).

Although cotton is absorbent, it is no longer used for culture swabs because natural chemicals in cotton inhibit the growth of certain microorganisms. Polyester, rayon, or calcium alginate fibers are preferred. Most swabs used to collect routine specimens have a wooden or plastic shaft for rigidity. Swabs with a small tip and a flexible wire shaft are made especially for culturing hard-to-reach areas and obtaining pediatric specimens. Some collection containers contain two swabs—one for a culture and one for a smear.

Collection and Transport Systems

Sterile, self-contained systems for obtaining and transporting specimens are commercially available from many suppliers. The CULTURETTE Collection and Transport System, manufactured by Becton Dickinson Microbiology Systems of Sparks, Maryland, is a well-known example. The unit, shown in Figure 46-10, contains a polyester swab and a small, thin-walled vial of transport medium in a plastic sleeve. If a specimen will not be tested within 30 minutes after it is obtained, the swab is replaced in the sleeve and the vial is crushed between the thumb and the index finger. The moisture and nutrients provided by the transport medium help keep the bacteria alive during transport to the laboratory.

Several collection systems are also available for culturing anaerobic organisms. These systems provide a means of generating an oxygen-free environment so the anaerobic organisms remain viable (alive and able to reproduce) during transport.

Specimen-Collection Guidelines

To collect specimens properly, you should follow a number of general guidelines.

- Obtain the specimen with great care to avoid causing the patient harm, discomfort, or undue embarrassment. If patients are to collect specimens on their own, give them clear, detailed instructions along with the proper container.
- Collect the material from a site where the organism is most likely to be found and where contamination is least likely to occur. For example, the best location to obtain a specimen for diagnosing strep throat is at the back of the throat in the area of the tonsils. A properly collected sputum specimen should contain mucus coughed up from the respiratory tract but should not contain saliva, which is a contaminant.
- Obtain the specimen at a time that allows optimal chance of recovery of the microorganism. Knowledge of the infectious disease process allows the doctor to determine the best time to collect a specimen. For example, certain viruses are more readily isolated during the early, symptomatic stage of an illness.
- Use appropriate collection devices, specimen containers, transport systems, and culture media to ensure optimal microorganism recovery. The purpose of such equipment and materials is to preserve the viability of any microorganisms so they will grow in culture. Special collection devices are available for certain body areas or suspected pathogens.
- Obtain a sufficient quantity of the specimen for performing the requested procedures. If, for example, both a culture and a direct examination of a swabbed specimen will be done, you must collect two specimens. Each procedure requires its own sample.
- Obtain the specimen before antimicrobial therapy begins. If the patient is already taking an antibiotic, note this fact on the laboratory request form or ask the doctor whether you should obtain the specimen.

After correctly collecting the specimen, you must label the container and include the appropriate requisition form. The label should contain the following information:

- Patient's name and identification number (if appropriate).
- Source (collection site) of the specimen.

- Date and time of collection.
- Doctor's name.
- Your initials (if you obtained the specimen).

The requisition form should include the following information:

- Patient's name, address, and identification number.
- Patient's age and gender.
- Patient's insurance billing information.
- Type and source of the microbiologic specimen (for example, discharge from wound, big toe).
- Date and time of microbiologic specimen collection.
- Test requested.
- Medications the patient is currently receiving.
- Doctor's presumptive diagnosis.
- Doctor's name, address, and phone number.
- Special instructions or orders.

Throat Culture Specimens

The doctor may request a throat culture on patients with signs or symptoms of an upper respiratory, throat, or sinus infection. In most cases, the doctor wants to determine whether the patient has strep throat, an infection caused by the bacterium *Streptococcus pyogenes,* a group A streptococcus. It is particularly important to diagnose and treat this infection because, left untreated, strep throat can lead to complications like rheumatic fever. Rheumatic fever is an inflammation of the heart tissue that occurs most frequently in school-age children.

When you obtain a throat culture specimen, avoid touching any structures inside the mouth as this will contaminate the specimen. The correct technique for obtaining a throat culture specimen is outlined in Procedure 46-1, at the end of this chapter.

Many doctors order rapid strep tests if strep is suspected. Antigen-antibody test kits for strep are available in a variety of brands and provide immediate indications of the strep antigen's presence on a throat swab, sparing the patient the expense and waiting period associated with having a culture done. The correct technique for performing a rapid strep test is outlined in Procedure 46-2, at the end of this chapter.

If your office does not culture microbiologic specimens, use a sterile collection system to obtain the specimen. If your office has the equipment to perform its own cultures, use a sterile swab and inoculate a culture plate directly with the swab. Specimens to be evaluated in the office should be cultured immediately after collection.

Go to CONNECT to see a video about *Obtaining a Throat Culture Specimen.*

Urine Specimens

To minimize contaminants in urine specimens, it is important to obtain a clean-catch midstream specimen. You must process urine specimens within an hour of collection or refrigerate them to prevent continued bacterial growth. (Collection of urine specimens for culturing is discussed in detail in the *Processing and Testing Urine and Stool Specimens* chapter.)

Sputum Specimens

To obtain sputum specimens, have the patient expectorate (cough up) mucus from the lungs into a wide-mouthed specimen container. Beforehand, instruct the patient to avoid contaminating the specimen with saliva. If sputum specimens are not cultured right away, they should be refrigerated.

Observe Standard Precautions whenever you handle sputum samples and wear a face shield or mask and goggles when collecting such specimens, especially if the patient is coughing. Even when tuberculosis is not suspected, the potential for its transmission always exists.

Wound Specimens

You usually obtain specimens from infected wounds and lesions by swabbing. The procedure is similar to that of a throat culture. Be sure you obtain representative material from a deep area and a surface area of the wound without contaminating the swab by touching areas outside the site.

▶ Transporting Specimens to an Outside Laboratory
LO 46.12

Many physicians' offices do not perform microbiologic testing onsite, choosing instead to send their culture specimens to an outside laboratory. This is particularly true for many specialized microbiologic procedures like virus cultures and bacteria cultures (including chlamydia) that require special techniques and equipment rarely found in a physician's office laboratory.

Your Main Objectives

When you collect and transport a microbiologic specimen to an outside laboratory, you have three main objectives:

1. To be sure you follow proper collection procedures and use the proper collection device. Most laboratories have specific directions for sample collection and packaging, and some laboratories may provide specific containers for these procedures. If you collect or package any specimens improperly, the laboratory may not accept them for testing, as they could be contaminated or no longer viable.

2. To maintain the samples in a state as close to their original as possible. You must take specific steps to prevent them from deteriorating.

3. To protect anyone who handles a specimen container from exposure to potentially infectious material. To do so, ensure that the specimen container has a tight-fitting lid. As extra protection against leakage, place the specimen container in a secondary container or zipper-type plastic bag (usually provided by the laboratory).

Methods of Transportation

Specimens to be tested by an outside laboratory may be transported in one of three ways:

- During regularly scheduled daily pickups by the laboratory.
- During an as-needed pickup by the laboratory.
- Through the mail.

FIGURE 46-11 When packaging and labeling a specimen for mail delivery, you must follow the procedures set by the CDC, based on US Public Health Service regulations.

Pickup by the laboratory is the most reliable and timely method of transporting microbiologic specimens. Although each laboratory has its own procedure, the general steps for preparing specimens for transport to a laboratory are outlined in Procedure 46-3, at the end of this chapter.

Sending Specimens by Mail

There may be times when you must send a specimen through the mail to a special reference laboratory for a test not normally done by a local laboratory. The US Postal Service accepts a package containing microbiologic specimens as long as the total volume of specimen material is less than 50 milliliters and it is packaged under strict regulations specified by the US Public Health Service.

When sending specimens through the mail, pack them securely with adequate cushioning material to prevent breakage and leakage. Leakage can contaminate the specimen, putting mail handlers at risk of contamination with infectious materials. The proper technique for packaging and labeling microbiologic specimens is outlined by the Centers for Disease Control and Prevention (CDC) and is shown in Figure 46-11.

Securely close the primary culture container and surround it with enough absorbent packing material to absorb the entire fluid contents if the container were to leak. Place these items together in a secondary container, commonly a metal container with a screw-top or snap-on lid. Then place the secondary container in an outer shipping carton made of cardboard or Styrofoam.

In addition to the address label, microbiologic specimens sent through the mail must have an Etiologic Agent label affixed to the package, as shown in Figure 46-11. This label uses the biohazard symbol to alert the mail carrier as to the nature of the contents. The term **etiologic agent** refers to a living microorganism or its toxin that may cause human disease.

▶ Direct Examination of Specimens LO 46.13

At times, the physician may directly examine the specimen under a microscope to detect the presence of microorganisms or to identify them. Two types of procedures that allow direct examination of microbiologic specimens are preparing wet mounts and preparing potassium hydroxide (KOH) mounts. You may be required to perform these procedures as part of your duties.

Wet Mounts

A wet mount permits quick identification of many microorganisms and is easy to prepare.

1. Wearing examination gloves, mix a small amount of the specimen with a drop of normal saline (0.9% sodium chloride [NaCl] solution) on a glass slide.

2. Apply a coverslip over the mixture.

3. Give the slide to the doctor for direct examination under the microscope.

If you obtain a specimen from a body site that is normally sterile, detection of microorganisms on a wet mount immediately tells the doctor whether there is infection. Wet mounts are also useful in determining whether a microorganism is motile (able to move), which helps in identifying the microorganisms.

Potassium Hydroxide (KOH) Mounts

A **KOH mount** is a type of wet mount used when a physician suspects that a patient has a fungal infection of the skin, nails, hair, or vagina. It is difficult to visualize a fungus directly in these types of specimens because the body produces a tough, hard protein called keratin that often masks any fungus present. The chemical potassium hydroxide (KOH) is added to the specimen to dissolve the keratin and allow visualization of any fungus.

To prepare a KOH mount, follow these steps:

1. Wearing examination gloves, suspend the specimen in a drop of 10% KOH on a glass slide.
2. Apply a coverslip.
3. Allow the specimen to sit at room temperature for 30 minutes to dissolve the keratin.
4. Provide the physician with the slide to examine for microscopic evidence of fungal structures.

▶ Preparation and Examination of Stained Specimens
LO 46.14

Although wet mounts are a useful tool for detecting microorganisms, microorganisms and their structures can be seen more clearly when you stain them with a dye or group of dyes. As with wet mounts and KOH mounts, the doctor can make a quick, tentative diagnosis with stained specimens. A stained specimen also enables the doctor to differentiate between types of infections, like bacterial and yeast infections, or between bacterial infections of one type and another. Stains also help doctors identify microorganisms that have grown on culture plates.

Preparation of Smears

The first step in staining a microbiologic specimen is to prepare a smear. To do so, simply apply a small amount of the specimen to a glass slide. Allow the sample to dry and then briefly heat the slide to "fix" the sample to the slide so it does not wash off during the staining process. The steps are described in detail in Procedure 46-4, at the end of this chapter.

Gram Stain

The Gram stain is the most frequently used stain for microscopic examination of bacteriologic specimens. This stain is a moderate-complexity test that you may perform in the medical office if you have additional training. The steps for performing a Gram stain are outlined in Procedure 46-5, at the end of this chapter.

A Gram stain involves performing a series of staining and washing steps on the heat-fixed smear. First, apply a purple stain called crystal violet (also known as gentian violet) to the smear. After washing the slide in water, apply iodine. The iodine acts as a **mordant,** a substance that can intensify or deepen the response of a specimen to a stain. Iodine helps bind the dye to the bacterial cell wall.

After washing the slide again in water, apply a decolorizing solution (alcohol or acetone-alcohol). Certain bacterial species retain the purple dye even after the decolorizer is added. These bacteria appear blue or violet and are **Gram-positive.**

Other bacteria lose their purple color when the decolorizer is added. To allow the physician to visualize these bacteria, apply a red counterstain (safranin) to the smear. Bacteria that lose the purple color and pick up the red color of the safranin are **Gram-negative**. Figure 46-12 illustrates Gram-positive and Gram-negative bacteria. It is important that you follow each step in the Gram stain process carefully to reduce the likelihood of misidentifying the microorganisms.

(a)

(b)

FIGURE 46-12   (a) Gram-positive organisms appear blue or violet after staining. (b) Gram-negative organisms appear red.

On the basis of a bacterium's staining characteristics and the shape and arrangement of cells, the physician can make a presumptive identification of an organism. For example, clusters of cocci that appear Gram-positive typically suggest an infection with staphylococci.

▶ Culturing Specimens in the Medical Office
LO 46.15

If your medical office is equipped with a laboratory and if you have had the necessary on-the-job training or additional courses, you may be required to culture certain specimens. It is, however, becoming more common for doctors' offices to send specimens to outside laboratories because of Clinical Laboratory Improvement Amendments of 1988 (CLIA '88) guidelines and the additional requirements concerning personnel and administrative work.

Culturing involves placing a sample of the specimen on or in a specialized culture medium, which contains nutrients that enable microorganisms like bacteria and fungi to grow. The medium is placed in an incubator set at 37°C (body temperature), the optimal temperature for growth. As the microorganism multiplies, a **colony**—a distinct group of the organisms—can be seen on the culture medium's surface. The microorganism is identified according to the colony appearance, its staining characteristics, and certain biochemical reactions. A microorganism's biochemical reactions are determined by their growth on specific types of culture media.

Culture Media

Culture media come in liquid, semisolid, and solid forms. In the medical office, you will most likely work with a semisolid. The medium contains **agar,** a gelatinlike substance derived from seaweed that gives the medium its consistency. This form of medium comes commercially prepared in culture plates—round, covered glass or plastic dishes called *petri dishes.*

Handle petri dishes on the outside only, so they do not become contaminated. You can avoid introducing contaminants by storing the petri dishes with the agar side up. Use the palm of your hand to pick up the agar-containing part of the dish when you are ready to inoculate it with a specimen.

Types of Media Many different types of semisolid media are commercially available. The type of medium used for culturing depends on the type of suspected organism and the site from which the specimen is obtained. Some types—called selective media—allow the growth of certain kinds of bacteria while inhibiting the growth of others. Selective media are commonly used for specimens that normally contain bacteria, like stool or vaginal samples.

Other types of media support the growth of most organisms and are referred to as nonselective media. The most common type of culture medium used in the laboratory is blood agar, a nonselective medium. Blood agar gets its red color from sheep's blood. Comparing the growth of a specimen on selective and nonselective media often provides important information about the microorganisms present.

You will typically use a blood agar plate when you culture a throat swab specimen. The organism that causes strep throat (*Streptococcus pyogenes*) can be identified when it grows on blood agar because it destroys the blood cells (hemolysis) in the agar, leaving a clear zone surrounding each colony.

Special Culture Units Small physicians' office laboratories often use commercial culture units with specific culturing purposes. Units for performing rapid urine culture, such as Uricult (manufactured by Orion Diagnostica, Somerset, New Jersey), are typical. Uricult consists of a small vial with a double-sided paddle attached to a screw-on top (Figure 46-13). Each side of the paddle contains a different type of medium on its surface. To culture a urine specimen, simply dip the media paddle into the clean-catch midstream urine specimen or catheterized specimen, coating both sides of the paddle. Then remove the paddle from the specimen, screw it into the vial, and place it upright in the incubator for 18 to 24 hours. If bacteria are present, they will grow on the surfaces of the media. Other units for culturing urine, throat specimens, vaginal specimens, and blood are also simple to use. These units usually enable you to obtain an estimate of the number of bacteria in the sample in addition to identifying the bacteria.

FIGURE 46-13 One common urine culture device consists of a lid and attached double-sided paddle that screws into a vial.

Inoculating a Culture Plate

Inoculating a culture plate involves transferring some or all of the specimen onto the plate. Before inoculating a plate, label it on the bottom (agar side) rather than the lid because the lid can be lost or switched. Label the plate with the patient's name, doctor's name, source of the sample, date and time of inoculation, and your initials. You can apply a label or write the information with a grease pencil or permanent marker.

In the case of a specimen swab, inoculate the plate by streaking the swab across the plate. Bacterial colonies can be identified by their appearance. This determination of the type of pathogen is referred to as a qualitative analysis of the specimen.

To perform a qualitative analysis of a specimen like urine, introduce only a small portion of the specimen onto the plate. A calibrated inoculating loop is used for this purpose. A loop is a small circle of wire or plastic attached to a long handle. When this loop is dipped into the specimen, a small specific amount of liquid can be transferred to the plate. Different sizes of calibrated loops deliver different volumes of fluid. For example, calibrated loops may allow you to pick up either 0.01 or 0.001 milliliter of liquid.

In addition, you may need to perform a separate determination—called a quantitative analysis—of the number of bacteria present in specimens such as urine. A quantitative analysis is important with a specimen like urine because a few bacteria may contaminate a urine sample during collection. A true infection is confirmed by the presence of a certain number of bacteria; any number beneath this level is typically considered contamination.

Inoculating for Qualitative Analysis To inoculate an agar plate for qualitative analysis, perform the first pass with a culture swab (as with a throat culture) or an inoculating loop (as with a urine culture). If you use a culture swab, roll and streak it back and forth across an area covering roughly one-third of the culture plate to deposit the microorganisms. When using an inoculating loop, spread the material by streaking the loop across one-third of the plate in the same

FIGURE 46-14 When inoculating a plate for qualitative analysis, roll and streak the culture swab or streak the inoculating loop of specimen material across one-third of the surface of the culture plate. Begin the next pass with a sterile loop.

Culture swab

Inoculating loop (sterile before pass begins)

Same loop (do not resterilize)

back-and-forth pattern. Figure 46-14 shows the correct pattern for inoculating a plate.

Because there may be several microorganisms in the specimen, you need to streak the inoculated (firstpass) area with a sterile loop to separate out individual colonies that can be identified on the remaining areas of the culture plate. Unless you use a sterile disposable loop, first sterilize the loop by heating it in a bacterial loop incinerator until it glows red. Allow the loop to cool and then pass it once across the inoculated area of the plate to pick up a small number of microorganisms. Then streak it in a back-and-forth pattern over the second one-third of the plate. Next, sterilize the loop again, pass it once across the second inoculated area of the plate, and then streak it back and forth over the last one-third of the plate. Each successive pass serves to reduce the microorganism concentration. This procedure allows isolated colonies, or colony-forming units, to be observed in the area of the last pass of the loop, as Figure 46-15 shows.

For throat cultures, the physician may simply want you to screen the sample for the presence of streptococcal organisms.

![Rahnella aquatilis culture plate]

FIGURE 46-15 You can see individual colony-forming units in the last third of an inoculated culture plate.

You may not need to use a loop to spread the microorganisms; the swab will be sufficient, as described in Procedure 46-1, at the end of this chapter, when preparing the specimen for screening.

Inoculating for Quantitative Analysis To perform a quantitative analysis of a urine specimen, use a calibrated loop to withdraw a portion of urine from the sample. Be sure the urine specimen is well mixed before taking the sample, as the microorganisms may settle to the bottom of the specimen cup. Sterilize, cool, and dip the calibrated loop into the sample. Transfer the entire volume to the surface of an agar plate by making a single streak down the center of the plate. Next, spread the specimen evenly across the plate at a right angle to the initial streak, using the same loop (without sterilizing it). Turn the plate and spread the material again, at a right angle to the last streak, over the entire surface. Figure 46-16 illustrates this technique.

After the microorganisms are allowed to grow for 24 hours, estimate the number of microorganisms by counting the number of colonies that appear on the surface of the plate. For example, if you use a 0.001 milliliter calibrated loop to streak the plate and 50 colonies grow, multiply the 50 colonies by 1000 to obtain the number of colonies per milliliter. In this case, you would estimate there are 50,000 colony-forming units per milliliter of urine. You must be especially careful that your counts and calculations are correct so the doctor has accurate information on which to base a diagnosis.

Incubating Culture Plates

After inoculating a plate, place it in an incubator set at 95°F to 98.6°F (human body temperature) to allow the bacteria to grow. Plates are always incubated with the agar side up, so any moisture that collects in the plate will fall on the inside of the lid and not on the microbes growing on the surface of the agar. How long plates are allowed to grow varies with the type of culture. Most bacteria grow sufficiently within 24 hours, but some require 48 hours. Fungi typically take longer to grow than bacteria and may grow at a slightly lower temperature (95°F to 96.8°F).

Interpreting Cultures

After incubation, cultures are assessed for growth and are interpreted. This process requires considerable skill and practice

FIGURE 46-16 When inoculating a plate for quantitative analysis, (a) streak the loop down the center of the plate. Next, (b) streak the loop at right angles to the first inoculation. Then, (c) turn the plate 90° and streak the entire surface once more.

because pathogens must often be differentiated from resident normal flora. This step may be performed by the physician, a microbiologist, or a technician who has been properly trained to do so through on-the-job training or additional coursework.

The process of interpreting a culture typically involves several determinations. The characteristics of the colonies growing on the agar are noted, along with their relative numbers. In addition, any changes in the media surrounding the colonies are noted because changes may reflect certain characteristics of the microorganism.

The physician decides at this point whether additional procedures are required. In the case of a throat culture, the presence of colonies of a characteristic shape, size, and color, surrounded by areas of hemolysis, suggests strep throat, as shown in Figure 46-17. A Gram stain and determination of bacterial shape may be all that is necessary for a confirmed diagnosis. Many cultures, however, require additional biochemical and, in some cases, serologic tests for definitive pathogen identification. Since this is an advanced skill, either the physician or an outside microbiology laboratory will make the final interpretation of the cultured microorganism.

▶ Determining Antimicrobial Sensitivity

LO 46.16

After a particular bacterial (or sometimes fungal) pathogen is identified, the organism's sensitivity (also called *susceptibility*) to several different antimicrobial agents must be determined. This information enables the doctor to choose an agent for treating the infection that is likely to be effective in curing it. If your office sends the specimens to a reference laboratory, the lab will report the results as sensitive (no growth), intermediate (little growth), or resistant (overgrown).

Performing an antimicrobial sensitivity test involves taking a sample of the isolated pathogen, suspending it in a small amount of liquid medium, and streaking it evenly on the surface of a culture plate. Small disks of filter paper containing various antimicrobial agents are placed on top of the inoculated agar plate. Although this step can be done manually using sterile forceps, a special dispenser is often used to place all the disks at once (Figure 46-18).

FIGURE 46-17 A positive strep throat culture contains distinctive colonies surrounded by areas of hemolysis.

FIGURE 46-18 Antimicrobial disk dispensers simplify placement of antimicrobial disks, help ensure that each disk contains a single antimicrobial agent, and reduce the probability of contaminating the culture.

The plate is then incubated at 98.6°F and the results are evaluated the following day. If a particular antimicrobial agent is effective against the microorganism, a clear zone will appear around the disk, indicating the growth was inhibited in the area of the agent, as seen in Figure 46-19. If there is growth right up to the disk, it means the agent is not effective against the organism. Each zone is measured in millimeters and compared to a standard chart to determine the degree of the antimicrobial agent's effectiveness. The doctor uses these results to choose an effective antimicrobial agent to treat the patient.

Many bacterial identification systems are now available as automated systems, which are used at most larger institutions and reference laboratories. They require special instrumentation with the capability of identifying the organism and determining the antibiotic susceptibility, a procedure known as MIC (minimum inhibitory concentration). This susceptibility testing is performed in special welled plates that test the organism against an antibiotic dilution to determine the minimum antibiotic concentration required to inhibit bacterial growth.

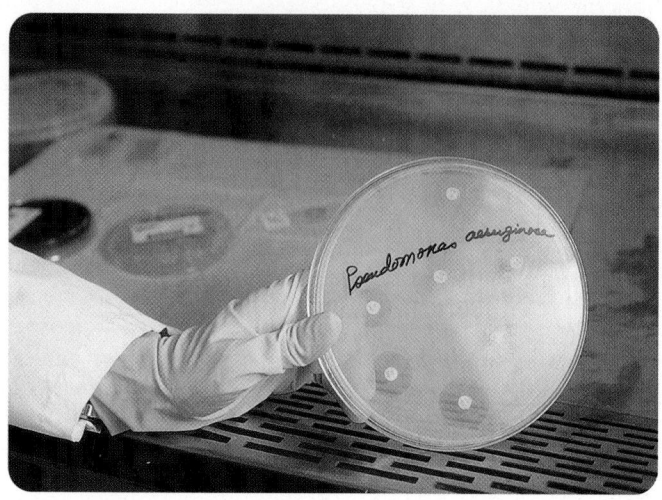

FIGURE 46-19 The effectiveness of different antimicrobial agents against an organism is apparent when an antimicrobial sensitivity test is performed.

PROCEDURE 46-1 Obtaining a Throat Culture Specimen

Procedure Goal: To isolate a pathogenic microorganism from the throat or to rule out strep throat.

OSHA Guidelines:

Materials: Tongue depressor, sterile collection system or sterile swab plus blood agar culture plate.

Method: Procedure steps.

1. Identify the patient, introduce yourself, and explain the procedure.
2. Assemble the necessary supplies; label the culture plate if used.
3. Wash your hands and don examination gloves, goggles, and a mask or face shield.
   RATIONALE: The patient may cough while you swab the throat.
4. Have the patient assume a sitting position. (Having a small child lie down rather than sit may make the process easier. If the child refuses to open the mouth, gently squeeze the nostrils shut. The child will eventually open the mouth to breathe. Enlist the help of the parent to restrain the child's hands if necessary.)
5. Open the collection system or sterile swab package by peeling the wrapper halfway down; remove the swab with your dominant hand.
6. Ask the patient to tilt back her head and open her mouth as wide as possible.
7. With your other hand, depress the patient's tongue with the tongue depressor.
8. Ask the patient to say "Ah."

9. Insert the swab and quickly swab the back of the throat in the area of the tonsils, twirling the swab over representative areas on both sides of the throat. Avoid touching the uvula (the soft tissue hanging from the roof of the mouth), the cheeks, or the tongue.

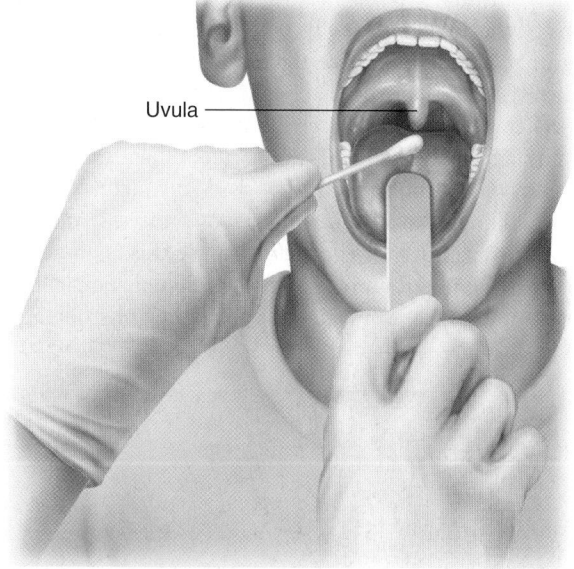

Uvula

FIGURE Procedure 46-1 Step 9 When obtaining a throat culture specimen, swab the back of the throat in the area of the tonsils on each side, taking care to avoid touching the uvula.

   RATIONALE: Touching these areas will contaminate the specimen.
10. Remove the swab and then the tongue depressor from the patient's mouth.
11. Discard the tongue depressor in a biohazardous waste container.

To Transport the Specimen to a Reference Laboratory

12. Immediately insert the swab back into the plastic sleeve, being careful not to touch the outside of the sleeve with the swab.

13. Crush the vial of transport medium to moisten the tip of the swab.

FIGURE Procedure 46-1 Step 13 The transport medium released from the crushed capsule keeps microorganisms alive while in transit to the laboratory for culturing.

RATIONALE: To keep the microorganisms alive during transport.

14. Label the collection system and arrange for transport to the laboratory.

To Prepare the Specimen for Evaluation in the Physician's Office Laboratory

12. Immediately inoculate the culture plate with the swab, using a back-and-forth motion.

13. Discard the swab in a biohazardous waste container.

14. Place the culture plate in the incubator.

When Finished with All Specimens

15. Remove the gloves and wash your hands.

16. Document the procedure in the patient's chart.

PROCEDURE 46-2 Performing a Quick Strep A Test on a Throat Swab Specimen

Procedure Goal: To determine the presence of Strep A antigen in a throat swab.

OSHA Guidelines:

Materials: Strep A testing kit, throat swab specimen, and a timer or watch.

Method: Procedure steps.

1. Review the laboratory requisition form and gather the supplies.

2. Confirm the patient's identity, introduce yourself, and explain the procedure.

3. Wash your hands and don gloves, goggles, and a mask or face shield.

4. Open the Strep A testing kit and check the expiration date on the kit.

5. Obtain a throat specimen with a sterile swab, being careful not to touch the tongue, teeth, or cheeks.
   RATIONALE: Swabbing only the throat reduces the likelihood of getting a false positive test result.

6. Complete the quality control tests provided with the testing kit.
   RATIONALE: To ensure the test is working correctly.

7. Put the required amount of the first reagent in the test tube or testing device provided in the kit.

8. Place the swab into the test tube or testing device. Following the manufacturer's instructions, swirl the swab and press it against the sides of the tube or device.

9. Add the second reagent as directed.

10. Read the results at the required time.

11. Dispose of testing supplies in the appropriate waste container according to OSHA requirements.

12. Remove your gloves and wash your hands.

13. Document the results in the patient's chart.

PROCEDURE 46-3 Preparing Microbiologic Specimens for Transport to an Outside Laboratory

Procedure Goal: To properly prepare a microbiologic specimen for transport to an outside laboratory.

OSHA Guidelines:

Materials: Specimen-collection device, requisition form, secondary container or a zipper-type plastic bag.

Method: Procedure steps.

1. Wash your hands and don examination gloves (and goggles and a mask or face shield if you are collecting a microbiologic throat culture specimen).

2. Obtain the microbiologic culture specimen.
   a. Use the collection system specified by the outside laboratory for the test requested.
   b. Label the microbiologic specimen-collection device at the time of collection.
   c. Collect the microbiologic specimen according to the guidelines provided by the laboratory and office procedure.
   RATIONALE: To ensure the specimen is correctly collected and handled.
3. Remove the gloves and wash your hands.
4. Complete the test requisition form.
5. Place the microbiologic specimen container in a secondary container or zipper-type plastic bag.
   RATIONALE: To prevent contaminating anyone who handles the specimen during transport.

6. Attach the test requisition form to the outside of the secondary container or bag, per laboratory policy.
7. Log the microbiologic specimen in the list of outgoing specimens.
   RATIONALE: So you can follow up on lab tests sent to outside laboratories.
8. Store the microbiologic specimen according to guidelines provided by the laboratory for that type of specimen (for example, refrigerated, frozen, or 37°C).
9. Call the laboratory for pickup of the microbiologic specimen, or hold it until the next scheduled pickup.
10. At the time of pickup, ensure the carrier takes all microbiologic specimens that are logged and scheduled to be picked up.
11. If you are ever unsure about collection or transportation details, call the laboratory.

PROCEDURE 46-4   Preparing a Microbiologic Specimen Smear

Procedure Goal: To prepare a smear of a microbiologic specimen for staining.

OSHA Guidelines:

Materials: Glass slide with frosted end, pencil, specimen swab, Bunsen burner, and forceps.

Method: Procedure steps.
1. Wash your hands and don exam gloves.
2. Assemble all the necessary items.
3. Use a pencil to label the frosted end of the slide with the patient's name.

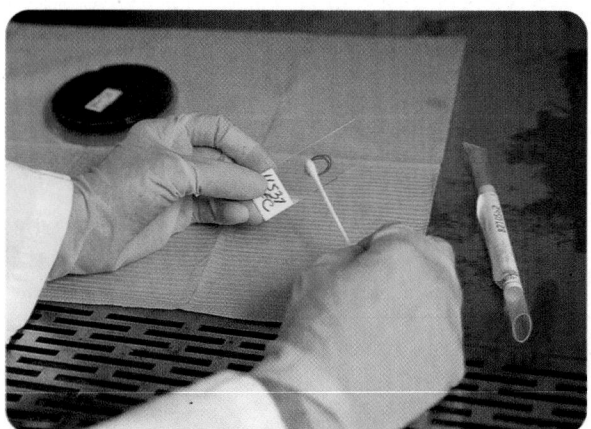

FIGURE Procedure 46-4 Step 4   Rolling the swab ensures that representative microorganisms collected on it are deposited on the slide.

4. Roll the specimen swab evenly over the smooth part of the slide, making sure all areas of the swab touch the slide.
   RATIONALE: To make sure a representative specimen is transferred to the slide.
5. Discard the swab in a biohazardous waste container. (Retain the microbiologic specimen for culture as necessary or according to office policy.)
6. Allow the smear to air-dry. Do not wave the slide to dry it.
   RATIONALE: Waving the slide may spread pathogens or contaminate the slide.
7. Heat-fix the slide by holding the frosted end with forceps and passing the clear part of the slide, with the smear side up, through the flame of a Bunsen burner three or four times. (Your office may use an alternate procedure for fixing the slide, such as flooding the smear with alcohol, allowing it to sit for a few minutes, and either pouring off the remaining liquid or allowing the smear to air-dry. Chlamydia slides come with their own fixative.)
   RATIONALE: The specimen must be fixed to the slide to prevent washing the microorganism off during staining or handling.
8. Allow the slide to cool before the smear is stained.
9. Return the materials to their proper location.
10. Remove the gloves and wash your hands.

PROCEDURE 46-5 Performing a Gram Stain

Procedure Goal: To make bacteria present in a specimen smear visible for microscopic identification.

OSHA Guidelines:

Materials: Heat-fixed smear, slide staining rack and tray, crystal violet dye, iodine solution, alcohol or acetone-alcohol decolorizer, safranin dye, wash bottle filled with water, forceps, and blotting paper or paper towels (optional).

Method: Procedure steps.

1. Assemble all the necessary supplies.
2. Wash your hands and don examination gloves.
3. Place the heat-fixed smear on a level staining rack and tray, smear side up.
4. Completely cover the specimen area of the slide with the crystal violet stain.

FIGURE Procedure 46-5 Step 4   Apply crystal violet. Wait 1 minute.

(Many commercially available Gram stain solutions have flip-up bottle caps that allow you to dispense stain by the drop. If the stain bottle you are using does not have an attached dropper cap, use an eyedropper.)

5. Allow the stain to sit for 1 minute; rinse the slide thoroughly with water from the wash bottle.

FIGURE Procedure 46-5 Step 5   Wash slide with water.

RATIONALE: Rinsing the slide after 1 minute stops the staining process and prevents overstaining specimen.

6. Use the forceps to hold the slide at the frosted end, tilting the slide to remove excess water.
7. Place the slide flat on the rack again and completely cover the specimen area with iodine solution.

FIGURE Procedure 46-5 Step 7   Apply iodine solution. Wait 1 minute.

8. Allow the iodine to remain for 1 minute; rinse the slide thoroughly with water.

FIGURE Procedure 46-5 Step 8   Rinse slide with water.

RATIONALE: The iodine helps increase cell staining.

9. Use the forceps or a gloved hand to hold and tilt the slide to remove excess water.
10. While still tilting the slide, apply the alcohol or decolorizer drop by drop until no more purple color washes off. (This step usually takes 10 seconds to 30 seconds.)
    RATIONALE: The decolorizing step is essential for differentiation between Gram-positive and Gram-negative bacteria.

FIGURE Procedure 46-5 Step 10   Apply decolorizing solution.

11. Rinse the slide thoroughly with water; use the forceps to hold and tip the slide to remove excess water.

FIGURE Procedure 46-5 Step 13   Rinse slide with water.

FIGURE Procedure 46-5 Step 11   Wash slide with water.

12. Completely cover the specimen with safranin dye.

FIGURE Procedure 46-5 Step 12   Apply safranin dye to slide. Wait 1 minute.

13. Allow the safranin to remain for 1 minute; rinse the slide thoroughly with water.

RATIONALE: To counterstain the specimen so Gram-negative organisms can be visualized.

14. Use the forceps to hold the stained smear by the frosted end and carefully wipe the back of the slide to remove excess stain.

15. Place the smear in a vertical position and allow it to airdry or blot it lightly between blotting paper to hasten drying. Take care not to rub the slide or the specimen may be damaged.

FIGURE Procedure 46-5 Step 15   Blot and allow slide to air-dry.

16. Sanitize and disinfect the work area.
17. Remove the gloves and wash your hands.

SUMMARY OF LEARNING OUTCOMES

LEARNING OUTCOMES	KEY POINTS
46.1 **Explain the medical assistant's role in microbiology.**	As an office medical assistant, you may assist the physician with several microbiologic procedures that aid in diagnosing and treating infectious diseases, including obtaining specimens or assisting the physician in doing so; preparing specimens for direct examination by the physician; and preparing specimens for transportation to a microbiology laboratory for identification.
46.2 **Summarize how microorganisms cause disease.**	Microorganisms can cause disease by using up nutrients or other materials needed by the cells and tissues they invade, damaging body cells, and producing toxins.

LEARNING OUTCOMES	KEY POINTS
46.3 Describe how microorganisms are classified and named.	Microorganisms are classified on the basis of their structure. Specific microorganisms are named in a standard way, using the genus (a category of biologic classification between the family and the species) to which the microorganism belongs and the particular species of the organism.
46.4 Discuss the role of viruses in human disease.	Viruses are among the smallest known infectious agents causing common diseases, including the common cold, influenza, chickenpox, croup, hepatitis, and warts.
46.5 Review the symptoms of HIV/AIDS and hepatitis.	The initial symptoms of AIDS are usually severe flulike symptoms followed later by systemic (weight loss, fatigue, night sweats), respiratory, oral, gastrointestinal, nervous system, and skin complaints. The general symptoms of hepatitis include jaundice, diminished appetite, fatigue, nausea, vomiting, joint pain or tenderness, stomach pain, and general malaise.
46.6 Discuss the role of bacteria in human disease.	Bacteria are single-celled prokaryotic organisms that reproduce very quickly and cause diseases like pneumonia, tuberculosis, meningitis, boils, urinary tract infections, Lyme disease, cholera, and tetanus.
46.7 Discuss the role of protozoa in human disease.	Protozoans are single-celled eukaryotic organisms found in soil and water. They can cause malaria, amebic dysentery, and trichomoniasis vaginitis.
46.8 Discuss the role of fungi in human disease.	Fungi are eukaryotic organisms including molds and yeasts. Diseases caused by fungi include athlete's foot, thrush, ringworm, and vaginal yeast infections.
46.9 Discuss the role of multicellular parasites in human disease.	Multicellular parasites include roundworms, tapeworms, flatworms, ticks, lice, and mites.
46.10 Describe the process involved in diagnosing an infection.	The steps involved in diagnosing an infection are to examine the patient, obtain one or more specimens, examine the specimen directly by either wet mount or smear, culture the specimen, and determine the culture's antibiotic sensitivity.
46.11 Identify general guidelines for obtaining specimens.	The general guidelines for obtaining specimens are to obtain the specimen with great care to avoid causing the patient harm, discomfort, or undue embarrassment; collect the material from a site; obtain the specimen at the proper time; use appropriate collection devices; obtain a sufficient quantity of the specimen; and obtain the specimen before antimicrobial therapy begins.
46.12 Carry out the procedure for transporting specimens to outside laboratories.	When transporting specimens to outside laboratories, the medical assistant should follow proper collection techniques using specific containers provided by the laboratory, maintain the samples in a state as close to their original as possible, and protect anyone who handles a specimen container from exposure to potentially infectious material.
46.13 Compare two techniques used in the direct examination of culture specimens.	Direct examination of culture specimens is accomplished in two ways: wet mounts and KOH mounts.
46.14 Carry out the procedure for preparing and examining stained specimens.	To prepare a stained specimen, the medical assistant must first prepare a smear, fix the sample to the slide so it does not wash off during the staining process, and follow a specific staining procedure. The sample is then observed under a microscope for certain characteristics.

LEARNING OUTCOMES	KEY POINTS
46.15 Carry out the procedure for culturing specimens in the medical office.	To culture a specimen, the medical assistant should place a sample of the specimen on or in a specialized culture medium and allow it to grow in an incubator for 24 to 48 hours.
46.16 Describe how to perform an antimicrobial sensitivity determination.	Performing an antimicrobial sensitivity test involves taking a sample of the isolated pathogen, suspending it in a small amount of liquid medium, and streaking it evenly on the surface of a culture plate. Small disks of filter paper containing various antimicrobial agents are placed on top of the inoculated agar plate. The plate is then incubated at 37°C and the results are evaluated the following day.

CASE STUDY CRITICAL THINKING

Recall Cindy Chen from the beginning of the chapter. Now that you have completed the chapter, answer the following questions regarding her case.

1. Why are Cindy's T-helper cells being tested?

2. What other tests might the physician order to confirm Cindy's diagnosis?

3. What special precautions should you take when drawing Cindy's blood?

EXAM PREPARATION QUESTIONS

1. (LO 46.1) Microorganisms normally found on the skin and other body tissues are known as
   a. Tissue pathogens
   b. Viruses
   c. Resident normal flora
   d. Colonies
   e. Infections

2. (LO 46.3) Which of the following is an example of a sub-cellular microorganism?
   a. Bacterium
   b. Virus
   c. Fungus
   d. Helminth
   e. Multicellular organism

3. (LO 46.10) A specimen that is spread thinly and evenly across a slide is a
   a. Smear
   b. Wet prep
   c. Culture
   d. Medium
   e. Streak

4. (LO 46.13) A KOH mount is used to detect which of the following?
   a. Gonococci
   b. Fungi
   c. Viruses
   d. Pinworms
   e. HIV

5. (LO 46.11) Which of the following is an appropriate guideline for collecting specimens?
   a. The specimen label includes the patient's name and number, source of specimen, date and time, doctor's name, and your initials.
   b. The best location to obtain a throat culture to diagnose strep throat is from the sides of the throat.
   c. When a patient is collecting a specimen on her own you should trust that she knows how to do it without an explanation.
   d. When a patient is taking an antibiotic you should never obtain a specimen.
   e. Allow the patient to use a container from home to collect a sputum specimen.

6. (LO 46.2) Organisms capable of causing disease are known as
   a. Commensals
   b. Flora
   c. Pathogens
   d. Facultative
   e. Aerobes

7. (LO 46.4) Infectious mononucleosis is caused by which of the following?
   a. Adenovirus
   b. Cytomegalovirus
   c. Norovirus
   d. Epstein-Barr virus
   e. Rotavirus

8. (LO 46.8) Athlete's foot, thrush, and ringworm are all caused by types of
   a. Prions
   b. Parasites
   c. Bacteria
   d. Viruses
   e. Fungi

9. (LO 46.14) A substance that can intensify or deepen a specimen's response to a stain is a/an
   a. Mordant
   b. Substrate
   c. Wash
   d. Dye
   e. Counterstain

10. (LO 46.9) An organism that lives on or in another organism and uses that other organism for its own nourishment is a/an
    a. Obligate
    b. Eukaryote
    c. Resident
    d. Parasite
    e. Prokaryote

47 Processing and Testing Urine and Stool Specimens

CASE STUDY

Ken Washington, a 61-year-old male patient, arrived today for a follow-up visit from a recent hospitalization for a stroke. Up until this hospitalization, he has had no major health issues. He now has weakness in his left arm and his speech is difficult to understand. His wife tells you that she has noticed some blood in the toilet after he urinates. She also tells you that he has had some pain when he urinates and often only urinates a small amount. Dr. Buckwalter would like for you to obtain a urine sample for a reagent test and also have Ken collect a 24-hour urine sample for analysis.

Keep Ken in mind as you study this chapter. There will be questions at the end of the chapter based on the case study. The information in the chapter will help you answer these questions.

LEARNING OUTCOMES

After completing Chapter 47, you will be able to:

47.1 Discuss the role of the medical assistant in collecting, processing, and testing urine and stool samples.

47.2 Carry out procedures for following guidelines when collecting urine specimens.

47.3 Describe the process of urinalysis and its purpose.

47.4 Carry out the proper procedure for collecting and processing a stool sample for fecal occult blood testing.

KEY TERMS

anuria
cast
catheterization
clean-catch midstream urine specimen
crystal
fecal occult blood test (FOBT)
first morning urine specimen
glycosuria
hematuria

O&P specimen
oliguria
phenylketonuria (PKU)
proteinuria
refractometer
supernatant
24-hour urine specimen
urinalysis
urinary pH
urine specific gravity
urobilinogen

I. P (14)	Perform CLIA waived urinalysis
I. P (16)	Screen test results
III. P (2)	Practice Standard Precautions
III. P (3)	Select appropriate barrier/personal protective equipment (PPE) for potentially infectious situations
III. P (7)	Obtain specimens for microbiological testing
III. P (8)	Perform CLIA waived microbiology testing
III. A (1)	Display sensitivity to patient rights and feelings in collecting specimens
III. A (2)	Explain the rationale for performance of a procedure to the patient
IX. P (7)	Document accurately in the patient record
IX. P (8)	Apply local, state and federal health care legislation and regulation appropriate to the medical assisting practice setting
IX. A (3)	Recognize the importance of local, state and federal legislation and regulations in the practice setting

3. Medical Terminology

Graduates:

d. Recognize and identify acceptable medical abbreviations

4. Medical Law and Ethics

Graduates:

f. Comply with federal, state, and local health laws and regulations

9. Medical Office Clinical Procedures

Graduates:

b. Apply principles of aseptic techniques and infection control

f. Screen and follow up patient test results

i. Use standard precautions

q. Instruct patients with special needs

r. Teach patients methods of health promotion and disease prevention

10. Medical Laboratory Procedures

Graduates:

a. Practice quality control

b. Perform selected CLIA-waived tests that assist with diagnosis and treatment

   (1) Urinalysis

   (6) Kit testing

      (a) Pregnancy

      (c) Dip sticks

c. Dispose of biohazardous materials

e. Instruct patients in the collection of a clean-catch mid-stream urine specimen

f. Instruct patients in the collection of a fecal specimen

▶ Introduction

Proper collection and testing of urine and fecal samples is a crucial step in the diagnostic process. The routine analysis of a urine specimen is a simple, noninvasive diagnostic test that provides a healthcare provider with a window to a patient's health. Many significant conditions may be noted with the assessment of the physical, chemical, and microscopic examinations of a patient's specimen. In this chapter, you will learn about various types of urine specimens and how to properly instruct or assist patients with their collection. Additionally, you will learn how to correctly process a specimen, including a random specimen and a chain of custody drug screen. You will learn to identify normal and abnormal constituents of urine samples and what may cause these abnormal elements to be present in a specimen. You also will learn about fecal samples, which are collected for a variety of reasons including detecting bacterial infections, detecting parasites, and screening for cancer. Teaching patients proper techniques for collecting stool samples is key to getting accurate test results.

▶ The Role of the Medical Assistant   LO 47.1

In your role as a medical assistant, you will help collect, process, and test urine and stool specimens. To perform your duties, you need to know about the anatomy and physiology of the kidneys, how urine is formed, and what its normal contents are. You also will need to understand the anatomy and physiology of the digestive system. This information will help you collect various specimen types, process them, and perform tests on them. Be sure to review the anatomy and physiology of the urinary system and the digestive system in *The Urinary System* and *The Digestive System* chapters (see Table 47-1 for a list of abbreviations commonly used in urine analysis and testing). Dealing

TABLE 47-1	Abbreviations Common to Urine Analysis and Testing		
ADH	antidiuretic hormone	RBCs	red blood cells
BIL; bili; BR	bilirubin	SPG; sp gr; sp.gr.	specific gravity
BJP	Bence Jones proteins	U/A	urinalysis
Ca	calcium	UBG	urobilinogen
CC	clean-catch (urine)	U/C	urine culture
CCMS	clean-catch, midstream (urine)	UC	urinary catheter
CL VOID	clean voided specimen (urine)	UC&S	urine culture and sensitivity
CrCl	creatinine clearance	UcaV	urinary calcium volume
CSU	catheter specimen (urine)	UCRE	urine creatinine
Cys	cysteine	UFC	urinary free cortisol
CYS	cystoscopy	UK	urine potassium
EMU	early morning urine(s)	Una	urinary sodium
HCG; hcg; hCG	human chorionic gonadotropin	Uosm	urine osmolarity
IVP	intravenous pyelogram	UTI	urinary tract infection
K	potassium	UUN	urinary urea nitrogen
pH	hydrogen ion concentration	UV	urinary volume
PKD	polycystic kidney disease	Vol	volume
PKU	phenylketonuria	WBCs	white blood cells

with a variety of patient groups who require special care, including elderly patients and pediatric patients, also will be an important part of your job.

Although you will not generally be dealing with bloodborne pathogens when obtaining and processing urine and stool specimens, you will deal with potentially infectious body waste. For this reason, you must take precautions to protect yourself, the patient, and others in the environment from transmitting disease-causing microorganisms. Most medical offices use Standard Precautions when dealing with urine. (See the *Basic Safety and Infection Control* chapter for detailed information on these precautions.) During all procedures, you must be sure to wear adequate personal protective equipment (PPE); handle and dispose of specimens properly; dispose of used supplies and equipment properly; and sanitize, disinfect, and/or sterilize all reusable equipment.

▶ Obtaining Urine Specimens   LO 47.2

It is essential to collect, store, and preserve urine specimens in ways that do not alter their physical, chemical, or microscopic properties. You must follow guidelines each time you obtain specimens and instruct patients in the proper guidelines to follow.

General Collection Guidelines

When you collect urine specimens from patients, follow these guidelines:

- Follow the procedure specified for the urine test that will be performed.

- Use the type of specimen container indicated by the laboratory. If a patient must bring in a specimen, be sure the container is provided by the physician's office or that it's appropriate for the testing protocol. If you provide the patient with a container that contains a preservative, make sure the appropriate warning labels are attached. You also should warn patients that the additive may contain acid and they should take care not to spill the acid on themselves.

- Label the specimen container before giving it to the patient or on receipt of a container the patient provides. Include the patient's name, the physician's name, the date and time of collection, and your initials. Label the side of the specimen container, not the lid, because lids may be lost or switched.

- If the patient is having an invasive test, such as catheterization, always explain the procedure to the patient completely, using simple, clear language.

- If you are assisting in the collection process, wash your hands before and after the procedure and wear gloves during the procedure.

- Complete all necessary paperwork, recording the collection in the patient's chart and making sure you use the correct laboratory request slip for the ordered test.

In many instances, patients need to collect a urine specimen at home. It is your responsibility to give patients instructions for obtaining the specific type of specimen. In addition, provide them with the following general instructions:

- Urinate into the container indicated by the laboratory. In most instances, urinate into a wide-mouthed, throw-away, spouted specimen container as instructed. Do not add anything to the container except the urine.

- If the collection container contains liquid or powdered preservative, do not pour it out.
- If any of the preservative spills on you, wash the area immediately and contact the physician's office.
- Always refrigerate the labeled collection container or keep it in a cooler or pail filled with ice.
- Be sure to keep the lid on the container.

Specimen Types

Many different tests are performed on urine. You may need to obtain different types of specimens for different tests, such as quantitative analysis or qualitative analysis. A quantitative analysis is a test that measures the amount of a specific substance in the urine. A qualitative analysis simply indicates the presence (or absence) of a substance in urine. Specimens vary in two ways: in the method used to collect them and in the time frame in which they are collected.

Quality assurance is essential in the physician's office laboratory. As discussed in the *Orientation to the Lab* chapter, control samples must be used every time you test patient specimens. These are the types of urine specimens:

- Random
- First morning
- Clean-catch midstream
- Timed
- 24-hour

Random Urine Specimen The random urine specimen is the most common type of sample. It is a single urine specimen taken at any time of the day and collected in a clean, dry container.

If a random urine specimen collection is to be done at the doctor's office, supply the patient with a urine specimen container. Show the patient to the bathroom and ask the patient to void a few ounces of urine into the specimen cup and to leave the cup on the sink. Retrieve the specimen when the patient leaves the bathroom and attach a properly completed label and requisition slip. Transport the specimen to the laboratory immediately. Urine specimens should be processed within 1 hour of collection. If this is not possible, refrigerate the specimen. Before processing refrigerated specimens, however, allow them to come to room temperature. If specimens will be shipped to an outside laboratory, chemical preservatives are added.

If patients are to collect a random urine specimen at home, have them use the container indicated by the laboratory. Either provide patients with a urine specimen container or instruct them to use a clean, wide-mouthed glass jar with a tight-fitting lid. Explain that a household dishwasher provides hot enough water to disinfect a jar adequately. Tell patients to refrigerate specimens until they bring them to the doctor's office and to keep them cool during transport.

First Morning Urine Specimen The **first morning urine specimen** is collected after a night's sleep. This type of specimen contains greater concentrations of substances that collect over time than do specimens taken during the day. A urine specimen container or clean, dry jar is used to collect the urine as per the laboratory's request.

Clean-Catch Midstream Urine Specimen The **clean-catch midstream urine specimen**, sometimes referred to as mid-void, may be collected and submitted for culturing to identify the number and the types of pathogens present. The presence of clinical symptoms or unexplained bacteria in a urinalysis specimen is an indication for urine culture. This method is not like other urine tests in which urine is simply voided into a specimen container. Instead, the clean-catch midstream method requires special cleansing of the external genitalia to avoid contamination by organisms residing near the urethral meatus (the external opening of the urethra). Voiding a small amount of urine into the toilet prior to collecting the midstream specimen flushes the normal flora out of the distal urethra to prevent possible contamination of the specimen. Procedure 47-1, at the end of this chapter, describes how to collect a clean-catch midstream urine specimen and how to instruct patients to perform this technique.

Go to CONNECT to see a video about *Collecting a Clean-Catch Midstream Urine Specimen.*

Timed Urine Specimen A physician may order a timed urine specimen to measure a patient's urinary output or to analyze substances. First, determine whether the required time period means that the patient must collect the specimen at home. If so, provide the patient with the proper collection container; written instructions on the process, including specimen preservation; and the following oral instructions:

- Discard the first specimen.
- Then collect *all* urine for the specified time (2 to 24 hours).
- Be sure the urine does not mix with stool or toilet paper.
- Keep the sample refrigerated until returning it to the physician's office or laboratory.

24-Hour Urine Specimen A **24-hour urine specimen** is collected over a 24-hour period and is used to complete a quantitative and qualitative analysis of one or more substances, such as sodium, chloride, and calcium. You need to instruct the patient in the proper collection process. If an outside laboratory will be testing the specimen, you will receive protocols for collection, preservation, and transport. Procedure 47-2, at the end of this chapter, outlines the steps in collecting a 24-hour urine specimen.

Catheterization

A urinary catheter is a sterile plastic tube inserted into the kidney, ureter, or bladder to provide urinary drainage. **Catheterization** is the procedure during which the catheter is inserted, and it is performed for various reasons, including to

- Relieve urinary retention.
- Obtain a sterile urine specimen from a patient.
- Measure the amount of residual urine in the bladder to determine how much urine remains after normal voiding (patient voids and is then catheterized; more than 50 milliliters is considered abnormal).
- Obtain a urine specimen if the patient cannot void naturally.
- Instill chemotherapy as a treatment for bladder cancer.
- Empty the bladder before and during surgery and before some diagnostic exams.

The two primary types of urinary catheters are:

- Drainage catheters, which are used to withdraw fluids and include an indwelling urethral (Foley) catheter placed in the bladder; a retention catheter in the renal pelvis; a ureteral catheter; a catheter for drainage through a wound that leads to the bladder (cystostomy tube); and a straight catheter to collect specimens or instill medications.
- Splinting catheters, which are inserted after plastic repair of the ureter and must remain in place for at least a week after surgery.

Catheterization is not routinely recommended because it can introduce infection. Some states do not permit medical assistants to perform catheterization, and in most healthcare institutions, only a physician or nurse can insert or withdraw a catheter. Check the protocol in your state. If you are not permitted to perform the procedure, you may be asked to assemble the necessary supplies and to assist the physician during the procedure.

Catheterization performed in a physician's office is usually done for diagnostic purposes using a specially prepared catheterization kit. This kit contains all necessary instruments and supplies, including a sterile instrument pack that is used to create a sterile field for the procedure.

If a patient is incontinent, the physician may use a bladder-drainage catheter to help drain the bladder and keep the patient dry. Another type of drainage catheter, the ureteral, is inserted into the ureter to help drain urine.

The indwelling urethral (Foley) catheter is designed to stay in place within the bladder (Figure 47-1). It consists of two tubes, one inside the other. The inside tube is connected to a balloon, which is filled with water or air to keep the catheter from slipping out of the bladder. Urine travels through the bladder and drains from the outside tube into a soft plastic container. The physician may order a leg bag to attach to the patient's thigh. The bag is anchored to the leg by two bands placed around the thigh. Make sure the bag is positioned so there is no tension on the catheter tube. To prevent back-flow into the patient's bladder, the container must always be lower than the bladder.

Special Considerations

When you obtain a urine specimen from a patient or take a history of a patient who may have a urinary problem, you need to consider the patient's sex, condition, and age. Some patients may require special care during collection procedures.

Special Considerations in Male and Female Patients Depending on the test, you may need to alter guidelines for collecting urine specimens from a male or female patient. Procedure 47-1 describes how to assist in collecting a clean-catch urine specimen from a female patient and from a male patient. In addition, when you take a medical history on a male or female patient, you will need to ask gender-specific questions as part of your assessment. For example, if a female patient leaks urine when laughing or coughing, she

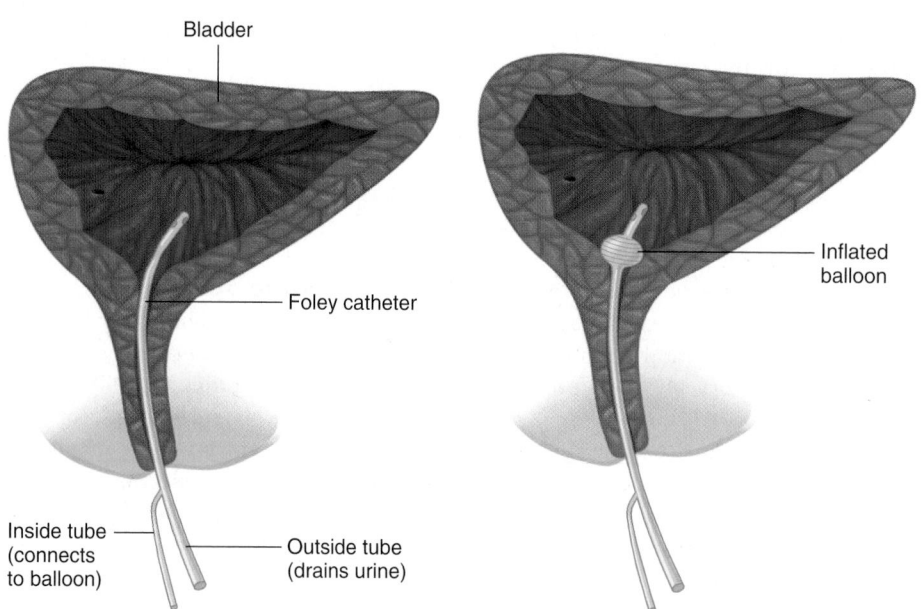

Bladder

Foley catheter

Inside tube (connects to balloon)

Outside tube (drains urine)

Inflated balloon

FIGURE 47-1 A Foley catheter stays in place within the bladder and has a collection container that is emptied periodically.

BWW Medical Associates, PC
305 Main Street, Port Snead YZ 12345-9876
Tel: 555-654-3210, Fax: 555-987-6543
Web: BWWAssociates.com

DRUG SCREEN CONSENT FORM

A urine drug test is required by _____ as part of your pre-employment screening. Please provide us with a list of all medications that you are presently taking.

_____

_____

_____

_____

I understand that my prospective or continued employment is contingent on a successful screening.

Date: _____ Signature: _____

Witness: _____

FIGURE 47-2   A consent form is a legal requirement when urine is collected for drug testing.

may have bladder dysfunction, which would affect the collection of a 24-hour urine specimen.

Special Considerations in Pregnant Patients

Pregnant women normally have increased urinary frequency. They also may be prone to urinary tract infections. At each prenatal visit, pregnant women must have their urine checked for abnormal levels of glucose (a screening test for diabetes) and abnormal levels of protein (a screening test for preeclampsia or renal problems).

Ask a pregnant patient whether she has any pain during urination or in the kidney area. A positive response may indicate a urinary tract infection or kidney stones. Also ask about urine leakage and whether she has previously been pregnant. Leakage may occur in a woman who has had multiple births because the pressure of the fetus on the bladder or delivery of the baby may have weakened the patient's bladder control. Additionally, ask whether any of the babies were delivered by forceps, which can injure urinary and genital structures.

Establishing Chain of Custody

Occasionally, you may need to obtain urine specimens for drug and alcohol analysis. When you do so, you must establish a proper chain of custody.

The specific steps to establish a chain of custody are described in Procedure 47-3, at the end of this chapter. Because of the medicolegal issues involved, it is important to follow the

procedure exactly to avoid breaking the chain. Also, because supplying a specimen for drug or alcohol testing could be self-incriminating, it is important to thoroughly explain the procedure to donors and have them sign a consent form (Figure 47-2). The consent form may be a part of the chain of custody form (CCF) (Figure 47-3), or it may be a separate form. The consent form states the purpose of the test and gives you permission to collect the specimen, prepare it for transport to the laboratory for analysis, and release the results to the agency requesting the test. Distribute copies of the CCF to the medical review officer, laboratory, patient, collector, and employer or other requesting party.

Inform the patient that medication (both prescription and nonprescription), drugs, and alcohol will show up in the test results. Encourage the patient to list on the consent form or CCF all substances consumed in the last 30 days, including what was taken and how much.

The CCF form indicates the source of the specimen. It verifies through signatures that the patient whose name is on the CCF and consent forms is the same person who provided the sealed specimen sent to the laboratory. Follow Procedure 47-3 at the end of this chapter when collecting a urine sample for drug or alcohol testing.

Preservation and Storage

Proper specimen preservation and storage are essential. Changes that can affect the physical, chemical, and

Morris A. Turner, MD

C.L.I.A #21.1862

266 Line Road
Montelair, Delaware 00956
800-555-1567

MedLAB

CHAIN OF CUSTODY FORM
SPECIMEN I.D.NO:

STEP 1—TO BE COMPLETED BY COLLECTOR OR EMPLOYER REPRESENTATIVE.

Employer Name, Address, and I.D. No.:   OR   Medical Review Officer Name and Address:

_____   _____
_____   _____
_____   _____

Donor Social Security No. or Employee I.D. No.: _____

Donor I.D. verified: ☐ Photo I.D.   ☐ Employer Representative _____
                                                                          Signature

Reason for test: (check one)   ☐ Preemployment ☐ Random   ☐ Postaccident
                                ☐ Periodic   ☐ Reasonable suspicion/cause
                                ☐ Return to duty ☐ Other (specify)

Test(s) to be performed: _____   Total tests ordered: ☐

Type of specimen obtained: ☐ Urine   ☐ Blood   ☐ Semen   ☐ Other (specify)
                        Submit only one specimen with each requisition.

STEP 2—TO BE COMPLETED BY COLLECTOR.

For urine specimens, read temperature within 4 minutes of collection.
Check here if specimen temperature is within range. ☐ Yes, 90°–100°F/32°–38°C
Or record actual temperature here: _____

STEP 3—TO BE COMPLETED BY COLLECTOR.

Collection site _____   Address _____
City _____   State _____   Zip _____   Phone _____
Collection date: _____   Time: _____   ☐ a.m.   ☐ p.m.

I certify that the specimen identified on this form is the specimen presented to me by the donor identified in step 1
above, and that it was collected, labeled, and sealed in the donor's presence.

Collector's name: _____ ·   Signature of collector _____

STEP 4—TO BE INITIATED BY DONOR AND COMPLETED AS NECESSARY THEREAFTER.

Purpose of change	Released by Signature	Received by Signature	Date
A. Provide specimen for testing			
B. Shipment to Laboratory			
C.			

Comments:

STEP 5—TO BE COMPLETED BY THE LABORATORY:

Specimen package seal(s) intact when received in lab?   ☐ Yes   ☐ No   If no, explain.
Laboratory receiver's initials _____

Copy 1 - Original - Must accompany specimen to laboratory.

FIGURE 47-3   The chain of custody form provides documentation that specific specimen collection safeguards have been followed.

microscopic properties of urine, and invalidate certain test results, occur in urine kept at room temperature for more than 1 hour.

Refrigeration is the most common method for storing and preserving urine. It prevents bacterial growth in a specimen for at least 24 hours. Refrigeration can cause other changes in the urine, however, that may affect the physical characteristics of sediment and specific gravity. Bringing the specimen back to room temperature before testing will correct these problems. You can also use chemical preservatives to preserve specimens, especially 24-hour specimens or those that must be sent a long distance to a laboratory.

Urinalysis

LO 47.3

Urinalysis is the evaluation of urine by various types of testing methods to obtain information about body health and disease. Urinalysis consists of three types of testing:

- Physical
- Chemical
- Microscopic

There are normal values for all tests done on urine. The normal value for a specific substance may be negative or none, "normal,"

or a range in concentration. Urine test results within normal ranges indicate health and normality. Table 47-2 identifies normal values for a variety of urine tests. Because a urine test is a screening test, all abnormal values must be followed up with a confirmatory test.

Urinalysis is done as part of a general physical exam to screen for certain substances or to diagnose various medical conditions (Table 47-3). For example, daily urine output provides a picture of renal function. With adequate fluid intake, the average adult daily urine output is 1250 milliliters, or approximately 5 cups per 24 hours. When total intake and output measurements are not approximately equal, urinary tract dysfunction may be the cause.

TABLE 47-2   Standard Urine Values

Physical Characteristics		Microscopic Examination	
Test	**Normal Values**	**Test**	**Normal Values**
Color	Pale yellow to yellow	***Epithelial cells***	
Clarity	Clear to slightly turbid	Renal	Negative
Reagent Strip Test		Squamous, adult females	Moderate
Bilirubin	Negative	Squamous, adult males	Few
Blood	Negative	Transitional	Rare
Glucose	Negative	Mucus	Rare–few
Ketone bodies (Acetone)	Negative	Protozoa	Negative
Leukocytes	Negative	Red blood cells	0–3/high-powered field
Nitrites	Negative	White blood cells	0–8/high-powered field
pH	4.5–8.0	Yeast	Few
Protein	Negative to trace	***24-Hour***	
Specific gravity	1.002–1.028	5-HIAA	2–8 mg
Urobilinogen	0.3–1.0 E.U.	Albumin (quantitative)	10–140 mg/L
Microscopic Examination		Ammonia	140–1500 mg
Bacteria	Negative	Calcium (quantitative)	100–300 mg
Casts		Catecholamines, total	<100 mcg
Epithelial cell	Negative	Chloride	110–120 mEq
Granular	Negative	Cortisol	10–100 mcg
Hyaline	Few	Creatine, nonpregnant women/men	<100 mg
Red blood cell	Negative	Creatine, pregnant women	≤12% of creatinine
Waxy	Negative	Creatinine, men	1.0–1.9 g
White blood cell	Negative	Creatinine, women	0.8–1.7 g
Crystals		Cystine and cysteine	< 38.1 mg
Amorphous phosphates	Normal	Glucose, quantitative	50–500 mg
Calcium carbonate	Normal	Phosphorus	0.4–1.3 g
Calcium oxalate	Normal	Potassium	25–120 mEq/L
Cholesterol	Negative	Protein (Bence Jones)	Negative
Cystine	Negative	Sodium	80–180 mEq
Leucine	Negative	Urea nitrogen	6–17 g
Sulfonamide	Negative	Uric acid	0.25–0.75 g
Triple phosphate	Normal	Urobilinogen, quantitative	1.0–4.0 mg
Tyrosine	Negative	Volume, adult females	600–1600 mL
Uric acid	Normal	Volume, adult males	800–1800 mL
		Volume, children	3–4 times adult rate/kg

Note: Individual laboratories may have slightly different reference values. Consult the reference values provided by the lab performing the test.

TABLE 47-3   Common Urine Tests According to Clinical Condition

Clinical Condition or Suspected Disease	Types of Urine Testing
Acidosis	Reagent stip* for pH Specific gravity
Alkalosis (metabolic, respiratory)	Reagent stip* for pH Specific gravity
Diabetes mellitus	Odor (fruity) Microscopic examination for fatty, waxy casts Reagent strip* for ketonuria and glycosuria Specific gravity
Drug abuse	Gas chromatography Mass spectrometry**
Genitourinary infections (prostatitis, urethritis, vaginitis)	Cultures for bacteria, yeasts, and parasites Microscopic examination for bacteria and RBCs
Human immunodeficiency virus (HIV)	Culture for virus (antibiotic added to kill bacteria) Other tests as indicated by specific symptoms
Hypercalcemia	Microscopic examination for calcium oxalate crystals Specific gravity
Hypertension	Microscopic examination for casts (hyaline, RBC) Specific gravity
Infectious diseases (bacteria) or other inflammatory diseases	Color and odor Cultures for bacteria, yeasts, and viruses Microscopic examination for bacteria and WBCs RBC casts (in severe cases) Reagent strip* for bacteria Turbidity
Metabolic disorders (except diabetes mellitus)	Color Microscopic examination for cystine crystals Reagent strip* for ketonuria, fructosuria, galactosuria, pentosuria, and pH
Nephron disorders (nephrotic syndrome, glomerulonephritis, nephrosis, nephrolithiasis, pyelonephritis)	Color Microscopic examination for casts (epithelial, fatty, waxy, RBC) and RBCs Reagent strip* for proteinuria Specific gravity Turbidity
Phenylketonuria	Color Reagent strip* for pH
Poisoning (arsenic, cadmium, lead, mercury)	Color Mass spectrometry**
Polycystic kidney disease	Proteinuria Urinary volume
Pregnancy	Reagent strip* for human chorionic gonadotropin (HCG)
Renal infections (acute glomerulonephritis, nephrotic syndrome, pyelonephritis, pyogenic infection)	Color Microscopic examination for epithelial cells (especially with tubular degeneration), numerous casts (granular, hyaline, WBC), RBCs, and WBCs Radioimmunoassay (RIA)** Reagent strip* for bacteria, albumin Specific gravity Turbidity Urinary volume

TABLE 47-3 *(concluded)*

Clinical Condition or Suspected Disease	Types of Urine Testing
Renal disease, renal failure, severe renal damage, acute renal failure, renal tubular degeneration	Microscopic examination for epithelial cells (especially with tubular degeneration) and numerous casts (hyaline, fatty, waxy, RBC) Reagent strip* for proteinuria (albumin), pH Specific gravity Turbidity Urinary volume
Sickle cell anemia	RBC casts
Starvation, dietary imbalance, extreme change in diet, dehydration	Color Odor (fruity) Reagent strip* for ketonuria Specific gravity
Urinary tract infection or mild inflammation (cystitis, pyelonephritis)	Color and odor Cultures for bacteria, yeasts, and viruses Microscopic examination for bacteria, WBC casts, RBCs, and WBCs Reagent strip* for bacteria, albumin, and pH Specific gravity Turbidity
Urinary obstruction (tumor, trauma, inflammation)	Color Microscopic examination for RBCs Specific gravity Urinary volume

*Federal listings of waived tests refer to these as *dipstick tests*.

**Drug screening and some other common urine tests must be performed by a forensic laboratory or other laboratory capable of performing gas chromatography, mass spectrometry, and radioimmunoassay.

The urinary system works with other body systems to help the body function normally. So, a disorder in another body system can affect urinary function. For example, the kidneys interact with the nervous system to help regulate blood pressure and control urination. Thus, a nervous system disorder can affect the circulatory and urinary systems. The cardiovascular system delivers blood to the kidneys for filtration, and the kidneys regulate fluid balance, which helps maintain circulation of blood and myocardial function. A cardiovascular system disorder can allow blood to be delivered to the kidneys at a pressure inadequate for filtration, which would affect urinary system function.

Physical Examination and Testing of Urine Specimens

After confirming that the specimen is properly labeled, the first step in urinalysis is the visual examination of physical characteristics. As part of quality assurance, examine it to make sure there is no visible contamination and that no more than 1 hour has passed since collection (or since the sample was refrigerated and brought back to room temperature). You will examine these physical characteristics:

- Color and turbidity
- Volume
- Odor
- Specific gravity

Color and Turbidity Normal urine ranges from pale yellow (straw-colored) to dark amber. The color, which comes from a yellow pigment called *urochrome*, depends on food and fluid intake, medications (including vitamin supplements), and waste products present in the urine. In general, a pale color indicates dilute urine and a dark color indicates concentrated urine.

Assess urine for turbidity, or cloudiness, by noting whether the urine is clear, slightly cloudy, cloudy, or very cloudy. Typically, urine is clear, although cloudy urine does not always indicate an abnormal condition.

The color of urine and any turbidity present can reveal medical conditions that require treatment. Table 47-4 provides more information on variations in urine color and turbidity and the possible causes or sources of these variations. Both pathologic (resulting from disease) and nonpathologic causes are noted.

Volume Normal urine volume, or output, varies according to the patient's age. Normal adult urine volume is 600 to 1800 milliliters per 24 hours (average of 1250 milliliters per 24 hours). Infants and children have smaller total urine volumes, although they produce more urine per unit of body weight. Urine volume is typically measured on a timed specimen (like a 24-hour urine specimen) rather than a random specimen.

Oliguria, insufficient production (or volume) of urine, occurs in conditions like dehydration, decreased fluid intake, shock, and renal disease. The absence of urine production is called **anuria.** Renal or urethral obstruction and renal failure can cause anuria.

TABLE 47-4 Urine Color and Turbidity: Possible Causes

Color and Turbidity	Pathologic Causes	Other Causes
Colorless or pale straw color (dilute)	Diabetes, anxiety, chronic renal disease	Diuretic therapy, excessive fluid intake (water, beer, and/or coffee)
Cloudy	Infection, inflammation, glomerular nephritis	Vegetarian diet
Milky white	Fats, pus	Amorphous phosphates, spermatozoa
Dark yellow, dark amber (concentrated)	Acute febrile disease, vomiting or diarrhea (fluid loss or dehydration)	Low fluid intake, excessive sweating
Yellow-brown	Excessive RBC destruction, bile duct obstruction, diminished liver cell function, bilirubin	Drugs (Primaquine)
Orange-yellow, orange-red, orange-brown	Excessive RBC destruction, diminished liver-cell function, bile, hepatitis, urobilinuria, obstructive jaundice, hematuria	Drugs (such as pyridium, rifampin), dyes
Salmon pink	No pathological cause	Amorphous urates
Cloudy red	RBCs, excessive destruction of skeletal or cardiac muscle	None
Bright yellow or red	RBCs (hemorrhage, myoglobin, hemoglobin), excessive destruction of skeletal or cardiac muscle, porphyria	Beets, drugs (such as phenazopyridine hydrochloride), dyes (such as food coloring and contrast media)
Dark red, red-brown	Porphyria, RBCs (menstrual contamination, hemorrhage, hemoglobin), blood from previous hemorrhage	Menstrual contamination
Green, blue-green	Biliverdin, *Pseudomonas* organisms, oxidation of bilirubin	Vitamin B, methylene blue, asparagus (for green)
Green-brown	Bile duct obstruction	Drugs (Cascara)
Brownish black	Methemoglobin, melanin	Drugs (levodopa)
Dark brown or black	Acute glomerulonephritis	Drugs (nitrofurantoin, chlorpromazine, iron preparations)

Odor Although urine odor is not typically recorded or considered a significant indicator of disease, it can provide clues about the body's condition. The odor of normal, freshly voided urine is distinct but not unpleasant and is sometimes characterized as aromatic. After urine has been standing for a while, bacteria in the specimen decompose the urea, which causes an odor similar to ammonia.

Diseases, the presence of bacteria, and particular foods (like asparagus and garlic) can cause changes in urine odor. For example, in the presence of urinary tract infections, urine is foul-smelling, and in patients with uncontrolled diabetes, the smell is characterized as fruity (because of the presence of ketones). Phenylketonuria, a congenital metabolic disease, produces a strange, "mousy" or "musty"odor in an infant's wet diaper.

Specific Gravity Urine specific gravity is a measure of the concentration or amount of substances dissolved in urine. Because the kidneys remove metabolic wastes and other substances from the blood, the specific gravity of the urine they produce is an indicator of kidney function. The physician's office laboratory uses one of these two methods to determine specific gravity:

1. Refractometer
2. Reagent strip (dipstick)

Specific gravity is a relative measure that is always compared to a standard. The standard for liquids is distilled water, which contains no dissolved substances.

$$\text{Specific gravity} = \frac{\text{Weight of sample}}{\text{Weight of distilled water}}$$

The specific gravity of distilled water is 1.000. You use special equipment to test for specific gravity (Figure 47-4).

The normal range of urine specific gravity is 1.002 to 1.028. Specific gravity fluctuates throughout the day in response to fluid intake. For example, a first morning urine specimen normally has a higher specific gravity than a specimen provided later in the day. An increase in urine specific gravity indicates that the kidneys cannot properly dilute the urine. The urine then becomes more concentrated, causing it to darken. Increased specific gravity may indicate conditions such as a urinary tract infection, dehydration (for example, from fever, vomiting, or diarrhea), adrenal insufficiency, hepatic disease, or congestive heart failure. A decrease in the specific gravity of urine causes a lighter than normal urine color, may indicate

FIGURE 47-4 Specific gravity is commonly determined using a refractometer or reagent strips.

that the kidneys cannot properly concentrate the urine, and may suggest conditions such as overhydration (excess fluid in the body), diabetes insipidus, chronic renal disease, or systemic lupus erythematosus.

Refractometer Measurement

A **refractometer** is an optical instrument that measures the refraction, or bending, of light as it passes through a liquid. The degree of refraction, or refractive index, is proportional to the amount of dissolved material in the liquid. You must calibrate a refractometer each day with distilled water by setting the instrument at 1.000 with the set screw. Two standard solutions (solutions of known specific gravity) also are used to ensure accuracy. Advantages of using a refractometer to measure urine specific gravity are that the process takes little time and requires little urine. Only a drop of urine is used for this determination. Procedure 47-4, at the end of this chapter, describes how to measure specific gravity with a refractometer.

Reagent Strip Measurement

You may use special reagent strips, or dipsticks, to test for specific gravity. Test pads along these plastic strips contain chemicals that react with substances in the urine and change color in precise ways. The reagent strip container includes a color chart for interpreting color changes on the test pads. When you evaluate urine specific gravity in this way, keep in mind that this type of test depends on precisely timed intervals identified by the manufacturer. Follow all directions exactly. Procedure 47-5, at the end of this chapter, describes how to perform a reagent strip test.

Go to CONNECT to see a video about *Performing a Reagent Strip Test.*

Chemical Testing of Urine Specimens

As a medical assistant, you may be asked to perform chemical tests on urine. Prior to performing chemical tests, always check for proper identification on the urine specimen to be tested. Chemical testing is usually done with reagent strips. It also can be performed with certain automated machines that use photometry.

The doctor orders chemical testing of urine to determine the status of body processes like carbohydrate metabolism, liver or kidney function, or acid-base balance. Other reasons for chemical testing include determining the presence of drugs, toxic environmental substances, or infections.

Testing with Reagent Strips As already described in the discussion of specific gravity, reagents (on plastic strips) are chemicals that react with a particular substance in urine and change color in precise ways. These changes indicate the presence of that substance and its amount or concentration in the urine specimen. For example, when a reagent strip is used to test for ketones, the reacted color on the strip will correspond either to a specific concentration of ketone bodies, like acetoacetic acid, or to the absence of ketones.

Reagent strips are used to test urine for a number of substances. In addition to ketones, these substances include nitrite, pH, blood, bilirubin, glucose, specific gravity, protein, and leukocytes.

There are numerous trade names for urine reagent strips (for example, Multistix and Chemstrip). Because not all reagents are reactive for the same chemicals, you must choose the appropriate strip according to the chemical test requested. All reagent strips are used once and discarded.

Follow the exact directions that come with the reagent strips to ensure accurate results. For quality assurance, take these basic precautions: Keep strips in tightly closed containers in a cool, dry area. Never remove them from the container until immediately before testing. Never touch the pads on the strip with your fingers or gloved hands. Examine strips for discoloration before use; discard discolored strips. Check the expiration date on the bottle; do not use strips that have expired. Use strips within 6 months of opening the container. Every time you open a new supply of reagents, run control samples to check for proper operation. Write the date opened on the bottle.

Although the process is essentially the same for all reagent strip tests, there are variations in time intervals before reading results. Some reagent strips are designed to test for several substances at once. The basic procedure for using reagent strips for chemical tests can be found in Procedure 47-5, at the end of this chapter.

Ketone Bodies Ketone bodies (or ketones) are intermediary products of fat and protein metabolism in the body. They include acetone, acetoacetic acid, and betahydroxybutyric acid. Only the first two substances can be determined by a reagent strip test. Normally, there are no ketones in urine. The presence of ketones in the urine may indicate that a patient is following a low-carbohydrate diet, or it may indicate that the patient has a condition such as starvation, excessive vomiting, or diabetes mellitus. Because ketones evaporate at room temperature, be sure to test urine immediately or cover the specimen tightly and refrigerate it until testing can be done.

pH Urinary pH is a measure of the urine's degree of acidity or alkalinity. Determination of pH can provide information about a patient's metabolic status, diet, medications being taken, and several conditions. The normal pH of freshly voided urine ranges from 4.5 to 8.0. The average urine pH is 6.0, which is slightly acidic. A pH of 7.0 is neutral, a lower pH is acidic, and a higher one is alkaline. Patients with alkaline urine may have conditions such as urinary tract infection or metabolic or respiratory alkalosis. Those with acidic urine may have conditions such as phenylketonuria or acidosis. Reagent strip tests on both urine and blood are used to measure pH in the body. (See the *Processing and Testing Blood Specimens* chapter for information on blood tests for pH.)

Blood A patient who has blood in the urine may be menstruating, have a urinary tract infection, or have trauma or bleeding in the kidneys. To test for blood in urine, use a reagent strip that reacts with hemoglobin. There are two indicators on the strip: one is for nonhemolyzed blood, the other for hemolyzed blood.

Colors on the strip range from orange through green to dark blue and may indicate **hematuria** (the presence of blood in the urine) caused by cystitis; kidney stones; menstruation; or ureteral, bladder, or urethral irritation. The presence of free hemoglobin in the urine is known as *hemoglobinuria*, a rare condition caused by transfusion reactions, malaria, drug reactions, snakebites, or severe burns. Injured or damaged muscle tissue—such as occurs in crushing injuries, myocardial infarction, muscular dystrophy, or contact sports injuries—can cause *myoglobinuria* (the presence of myoglobin in the urine). Reagent strip testing does not distinguish between these two conditions.

Bilirubin and Urobilinogen When hemoglobin breaks down, it converts into conjugated bilirubin in the liver and then to urobilinogen in the intestines. Presence of the bile pigment bilirubin in the urine (*bilirubinuria*) is one of the first signs of liver disease or conditions that involve the liver. When bilirubin is present, urine turns yellow-brown to greenish orange. You usually use a reagent strip to test for bilirubin. If the reagent strip test is positive, a confirmatory test called an Ictotest® is usually performed. The Ictotest® is a reagent tablet test that is more sensitive than the reagent strip test.

Although **urobilinogen** is present in the urine in small amounts, elevated levels of this colorless compound formed in the intestines may indicate increased red blood cell destruction or liver disease. Lack of urobilinogen in the urine may suggest total bile duct obstruction, as a result of which urobilinogen is not formed in the intestines or reabsorbed in the circulation. To test for urobilinogen, you use reagent strips.

Testing for either bilirubin or urobilinogen must be performed on a fresh urine specimen. Bilirubin decomposes rapidly in bright light to form biliverdin, which is not detected by the reagent strip test for bilirubin. Urobilinogen breaks down to urobilin on standing.

Glucose Glucose is present in patients with normal urine, but only in small quantities not detectable by the reagent strip test for glucose. **Glycosuria** (the presence of significant glucose in the urine) is common in patients with diabetes. Blood is more commonly tested for glucose than urine is because reagent strip tests may show false-negative results when used for testing urine.

Protein Although a small amount of protein is excreted in the urine every day, an excess of protein in the urine (**proteinuria**) usually indicates renal disease. Proteinuria is also common in pregnant patients or after heavy exercise.

Nitrite The presence of nitrite in the urine suggests a bacterial infection of the urinary tract. The test is not definitive, however, because some bacteria cannot convert nitrate to nitrite. Also, if an insufficient number of bacteria are present in the urine or if the urine has not incubated long enough in the bladder for a reaction to take place, a negative nitrite test

can occur. The best urine specimen to test for nitrites is the first morning specimen.

When testing for urinary nitrite, you must test the urine immediately or refrigerate the specimen. Bacteria can multiply in a specimen allowed to sit at room temperature, causing a false-positive test result. Bacteria also can further metabolize the nitrite already produced, causing a false-negative result.

Leukocytes Leukocytes appear in the urine in urinary tract or renal infections. Use strip tests for leukocyte esterase, a chemical seen when leukocytes are present, to test for leukocytes.

Other Types of Chemical Testing There are other types of chemical tests—like those that test for electrolytes and osmolality—that may be performed on urine specimens. Because these tests are performed in an outside laboratory rather than in a physician's office laboratory, you do not need to know the steps in each procedure.

Phenylketones The presence of phenylketones in a patient's urine indicates **phenylketonuria (PKU)**, a genetically inherited disorder in which the body cannot properly metabolize the nutrient phenylalanine. This disorder causes phenylketones to accumulate in the bloodstream, resulting in mental retardation. PKU can be treated successfully by limiting the dietary intake of phenylalanine, which makes up 5% of all natural protein, from early infancy. Although urine can be tested for the presence of phenylketones, blood testing is routine for newborns before discharge, at least 24 hours after birth.

Pregnancy Tests Pregnancy testing is based on detecting the hormone—called *human chorionic gonadotropin*, or *HCG*—secreted by the placenta. HCG levels vary throughout pregnancy: they usually peak at about 8 weeks, drop to lower levels in the second trimester, and then detectable levels recur in the last trimester. Many commercial pregnancy tests are manufactured for use both in the clinical setting and at home. These tests are sensitive, are easy to perform and interpret, and give quick results. Most tests are now designed as an enzyme immunoassay (EIA) test, which involves an antigen, an antibody specific for the antigen, and a second antibody conjugated to an enzyme. Newer technologies called *membrane EIAs* have been developed; in these tests, most of the reagents are incorporated into an absorbent membrane in a plastic case. Using either urine or serum, a sample is added through a chamber window, where it migrates through the membrane and combines with the reagents to produce a reaction. Although the technology used in the design of these tests is quite complex, the actual test itself is easy to set up and interpret (Procedure 47-6, at the end of this chapter). The tests are all designed with a control feature incorporated into the reagent pack for quality assurance of the test results.

Go to CONNECT to see a video about *Pregnancy Testing Using the EIA Method.*

Urine Tests for the Presence of STIs In response to increasing numbers of sexually transmitted infections, the CDC recommends that all sexually active females between the ages of 15 and 25 be screened annually for chlamydia. To accomplish this, several tests called *nucleic acid amplification tests (NAATs)* have recently been developed. These tests utilize urine samples to detect the presence of nucleic acid. Patients infected with either *Chlamydia trachomatis* or *Neisseria gonorrhoeae* will have nucleic acid in their urine. By amplifying nucleic acids specific to chlamydia and gonorrhea, the test can detect the presence of very small numbers of bacteria.

These tests have several advantages:

- Sample collection is noninvasive and the sample is easily collected.
- The tests are highly specific.
- The tests are highly sensitive. As little as one copy of bacterial nucleic acid can be detected in a urine specimen.
- Organisms do not have to be living to be detected.
- The tests are good screening tools for asymptomatic patients.

The tests also have some disadvantages:

- The tests are expensive.
- No living organisms remain for use in a follow-up culture. So, positive tests must be confirmed by culture from an endocervical or urethral swab.

Microscopic Examination of Urine Specimens

A microscopic examination of urine sediment may be performed to view elements only visible with a microscope. You will use a centrifuge to obtain sediment for analysis. A centrifuge spins test tubes containing fluid at speeds that cause heavier substances in the fluid to settle to the bottom of the tubes.

During microscopic examination, elements that are categorized and counted include the cells, casts, crystals, yeast, bacteria, and parasites that form sediment (precipitate) after urine is centrifuged. You may use the KOVA System®, manufactured by Hycor Biomedical, Irvine, California, to prepare urine sediment for microscopic examination. When you use the KOVA System®, the sediment is evenly distributed to four calibrated chambers before the microscopic elements are counted. Procedure 47-7, at the end of this chapter, describes how to process a urine specimen for microscopic examination of sediment.

Cells High-power magnification is used to classify and count cells. Three types of cells are found in urine (Figure 47-5):

- Epithelial cells
- White blood cells
- Red blood cells

Epithelial Cells Epithelial cells are classified as renal, transitional, or squamous. Renal epithelial cells can be round to oval and have a large, oval, and sometimes eccentric nucleus. Although a few of these cells appear normally in urine, several may indicate tubular damage in the kidneys. Damage in the renal tubules causes epithelial cells to die and slough off—shed. These shed cells can then be seen in a urine sample.

Transitional epithelial cells line the urinary tract from the renal pelvis (the beginning of the ureter) to the upper portion of

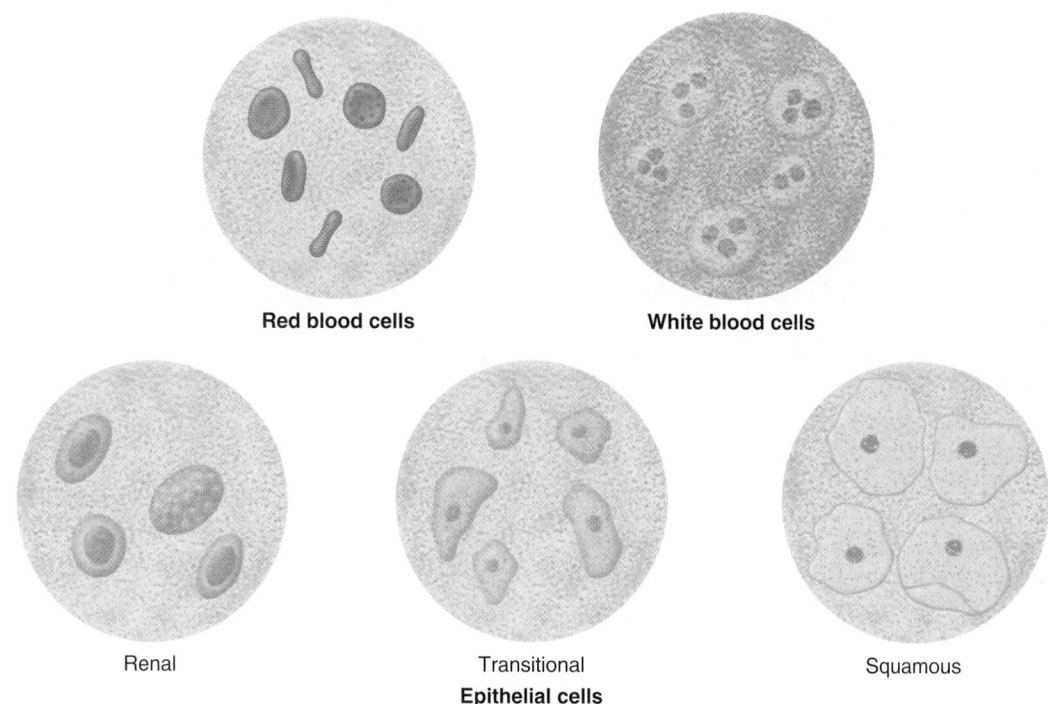

Red blood cells

White blood cells

Renal Transitional Squamous

Epithelial cells

FIGURE 47-5 The number and types of cells found in urine provide important diagnostic information about a patient's condition.

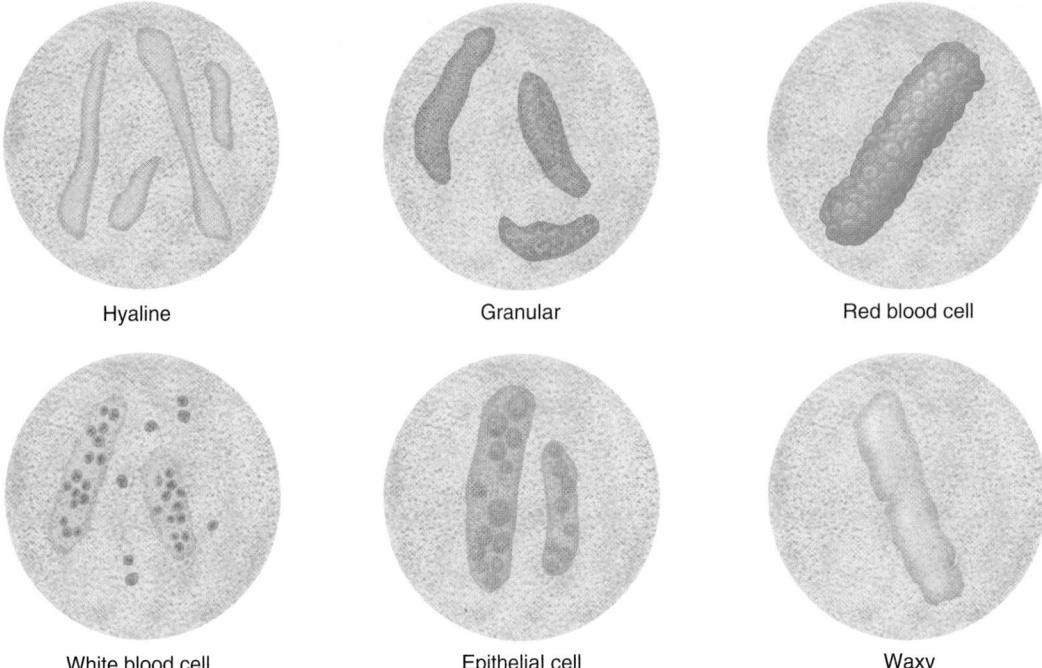

Hyaline

Granular

Red blood cell

White blood cell

Epithelial cell

Waxy

FIGURE 47-6 Casts, which are shaped like cylinders with flat or rounded ends, are formed when protein accumulates in the kidney tubules and is washed into the urine.

the urethra. They can be round to oval and may have a tail and, occasionally, two nuclei. Like the renal epithelial cell, a few appear normally in urine, but several may indicate tubular damage.

Squamous epithelial cells—large, flat, irregular cells with a small, round, centrally located nucleus—line the genitourinary tract's lower portion. They often occur in sheets or clumps and can be easily recognized under low-power magnification.

White Blood Cells White blood cells (WBCs) are larger than red blood cells, have a granular appearance, and usually contain a multilobed nucleus. They are typically found in large numbers in the urine (greater than the normal zero to 8 per high-power field) if inflammation is present or if the specimen was contaminated during collection.

Red Blood Cells Red blood cells (RBCs) are typically pale, round, nongranular, and flat or biconcave. They have no nucleus and enter the urinary tract during inflammation or injury. From zero to three RBCs per high-power field in urine are normal. However, numerous RBCs may indicate a variety of problems, including urinary infection, obstruction, inflammation, trauma, or tumor.

Casts Casts—cylinder-shaped elements with flat or rounded ends—form when protein from the breakdown of cells accumulates and precipitates in the kidney tubules and is washed into the urine. The protein then assumes the size and shape of the tubules. Think of a clogged drain in your bathroom sink. The drain may start out just slow at first but, after a while, very little water will pass through. If you remove the drain pipe, you will find the material plugging up the drain has taken on the shape of the pipe. It works the

same in the kidney tubules, but with different materials. Casts differ in composition and size (Figure 47-6). Classified according to their appearance and composition, casts can indicate renal pathologic conditions or can be caused by strenuous exercise. Types of casts include:

- Hyaline casts, which are pale, transparent, and cylinder-shaped with rounded ends and parallel sides. Composed of protein, they form because of diminished urine flow through individual nephrons. They are present in patients with kidney disease or in people who have exercised strenuously. A few hyaline casts observed in the urine is normal.

- Granular casts, which resemble hyaline casts and also can result from kidney disease or strenuous exercise. The granules are believed to come from degeneration of cellular inclusions.

- Red blood cell casts, which always indicate an abnormality and are hyaline casts with embedded red blood cells. Because of the RBCs, these casts sometimes appear brown.

- White blood cell casts, which are hyaline casts with leukocytes. These casts typically have a multilobed nucleus and may indicate pyelonephritis—an inflammation of the kidney and renal pelvis.

- Epithelial cell casts, which contain embedded renal tubular epithelial cells and indicate excessive kidney damage. Causes include shock, renal ischemia, heavy-metal poisoning, certain allergic reactions, and nephrotoxic drugs. These casts are often confused with white blood cell casts.

- Waxy casts, which are rare, yellow, glassy, brittle, smooth, and homogeneous structures with cracks or fissures and squared or broken ends. These casts occur with severe renal disease.

Crystals Crystals, naturally produced solids of definite form, are commonly seen in urine specimens, especially those permitted to cool. They usually do not indicate a significant disorder, except when found in large numbers in patients with kidney stones and in a few pathologic conditions (like hypercalcemia and some inborn errors of metabolism). Figure 47-7 shows common crystals found in urine specimens. Because different substances tend to crystallize in both acidic and alkaline (or basic) urine, it is important to determine the pH of a patient's urine before you try to identify any present crystals.

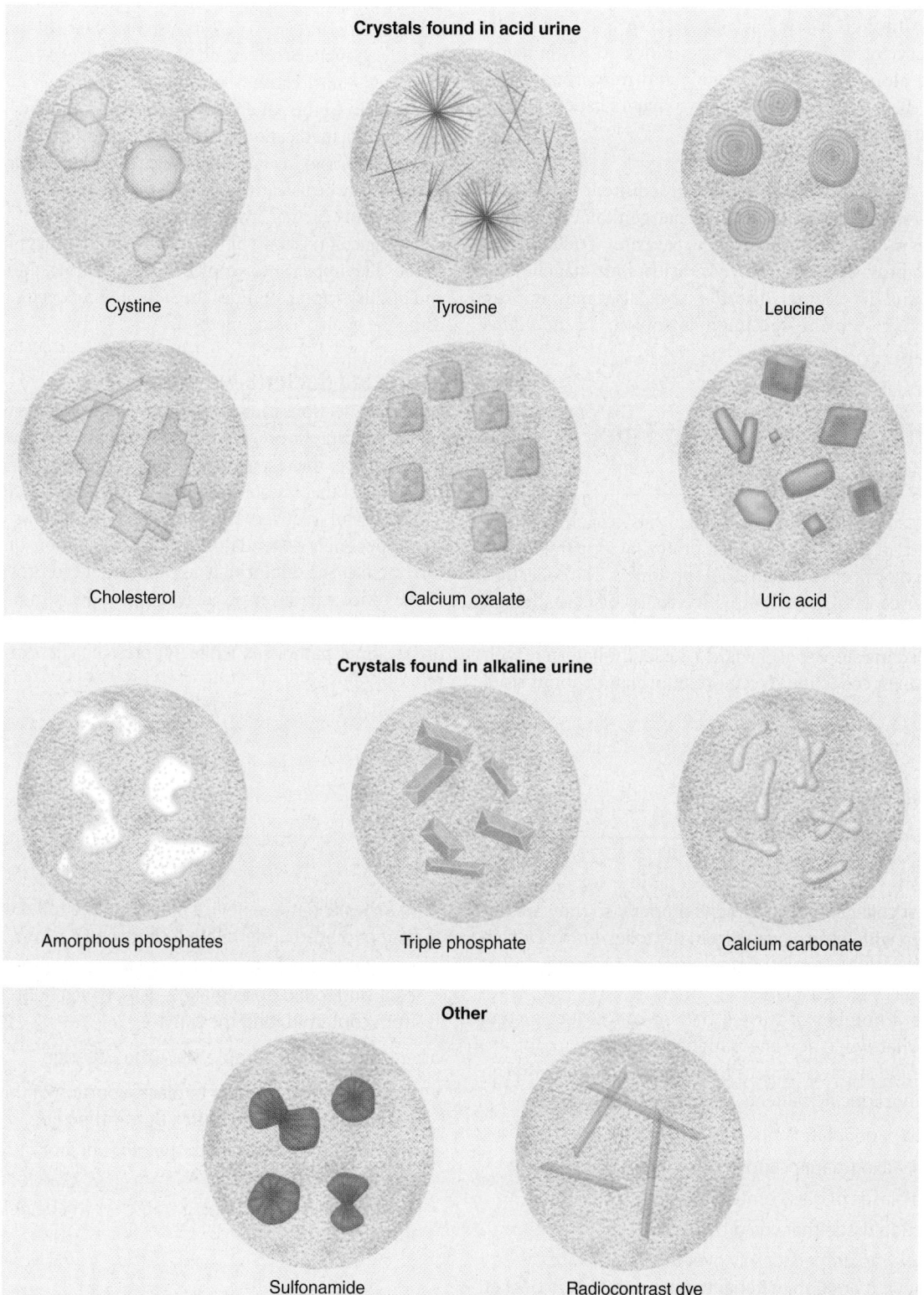

Crystals found in acid urine

Cystine   Tyrosine   Leucine

Cholesterol   Calcium oxalate   Uric acid

Crystals found in alkaline urine

Amorphous phosphates   Triple phosphate   Calcium carbonate

Other

Sulfonamide   Radiocontrast dye

FIGURE 47-7 You should be able to identify common crystals in urine and what they mean.

Yeast Cells Yeast cells, which are usually oval and may show budding, may be confused with RBCs. Yeast cells in urine sediment are associated with genitourinary tract infection, external genitalia contamination, vaginitis, urethritis, and prostatitis. These cells are also commonly seen in the urine of patients with diabetes.

Bacteria Although a few bacteria are normally found in urine, urinary tract infection may be indicated if the urine has bacteria along with a putrid odor and numerous white blood cells. Bacteria under high-power magnification appear rod- or cocci-shaped.

Parasites The presence of parasites in sediment may signal genitourinary tract infection or external genitalia contamination. The most common urinary parasite, *Trichomonas vaginalis* (a pear-shaped protozoan with four flagella), is typically found in vaginal disorders but also may appear in males. When a urine specimen is cooled, *Trichomonas* organisms die.

▸ Collecting and Processing Stool Specimens

LO 47.4

If the physician suspects that the patient has certain diseases, such as cancer or colitis, or bacterial, protozoal, or parasitic infections, you may need to obtain stool specimens. The collection technique varies with the suspected microorganism. Although both you and the patient may be embarrassed to discuss instructions for collecting stool specimens, do not let this interfere with proper specimen collection. For more information about stool sample collection, see the feature Educating the Patient: Collecting a Stool Sample.

Screening for Colorectal Cancer

The **fecal occult blood test (FOBT)** is a test for hidden (occult) blood in the stool. The presence of blood in the stool may indicate colorectal cancer, though other diseases and disorders like hemorrhoids and gastric ulcers also may cause blood in the stool. Some food—like broccoli and beets—and drugs—like aspirin and ibuprofen—may cause a false-positive test. It is important that you explain to the patient the importance of following all pretest dietary and medication instructions. The test is fast, easy, and inexpensive, making it a good choice for colorectal screening. The test also may be used to determine the cause of anemia. A positive test warrants further investigation for the cause of the bleeding, including colonoscopy, blood tests, and other diagnostic imaging studies like upper endoscopy or CT scan. Procedure 47-8, at the end of this chapter, outlines the steps in fecal occult blood testing using the guaiac testing method.

Suspected Bacterial Infection

Bacterial infections caused by species of the *Shigella* or *Salmonella* genus can cause loose, bloody, or mucus-tinged stools. A doctor who suspects that a patient has one of these types of infections may request that a stool specimen be obtained for culture.

Successful recovery of these pathogenic bacteria from a stool specimen depends on timely inoculation of special culture media. The doctor may ask the patient to provide a sample in the office whenever possible to avoid delay in processing the specimen. Several types of culture media promote the growth of intestinal pathogens while suppressing the growth of other microorganisms.

EDUCATING THE PATIENT
Collecting a Stool Sample

Patients must collect stool specimens properly so they are not contaminated with urine or water from the toilet, both of which can lead to inaccurate results. If the sample is contaminated, it will have to be collected again.

There are a number of ways a patient can collect a stool specimen. What works for one patient may not work for another. Obtaining stool specimens from young children also can be challenging. Educate patients to collect samples:

- On a clean paper plate;
- In a clean waxed-paper carton;
- In a clean plastic or glass container;
- On collection tissue that you provide;
- On plastic wrap draped loosely over the back half of the toilet seat with enough material to form a collection pocket in the middle;

- In a plastic hat-like device placed on the toilet under the seat or placed underneath a child; or
- In a child's diaper lined with plastic positioned toward the back and rolled up to make a dam, which helps keep urine from contaminating the sample.

After collecting the sample, have the patient:

- Use a tongue depressor to place a portion of the sample in a specimen container with a tight-fitting lid.
- Transport the specimen to the office or laboratory as soon as possible.
- Refrigerate the specimen if transport will be delayed.

Suspected Protozoal or Parasitic Infection

In cases of a suspected protozoal or parasitic infection, the physician may request an **O&P specimen**, short for *ova and parasites specimen*. This type of stool sample is examined for the presence of certain forms of protozoans or parasites, including their eggs (ova).

When a physician requests an O&P test, obtain both a fresh and a preserved stool specimen. A fresh specimen is examined both macroscopically and microscopically for the presence of microorganisms. A preserved specimen is also necessary because certain forms of these organisms are destroyed within a short time after leaving the body and may not be detected in the fresh specimen. You must always obtain a preserved specimen when stool samples are sent to an outside laboratory.

Special stool collection kits are available. They contain a specimen container for a fresh sample along with vials of two types of preservatives: formalin (a dilute solution of formaldehyde) and polyvinyl alcohol (PVA). Instruct the patient to place the stool sample in the specimen container and to mix portions of the specimen in each of the preservative vials. The laboratory will examine all specimens for the presence of microorganisms.

When a physician suspects that a patient has a protozoal or parasitic infection, he will request that a series of at least three stool specimens be examined. Three specimens are required because different diagnostic forms of the microorganism may be present in the stool at different times and some could be missed with only one sample. Because certain medications can interfere with detecting these microorganisms, the patient may be asked to refrain from using medications like antidiarrheal compounds, antacids, and mineral oil laxatives for at least a week before samples are obtained.

PROCEDURE 47-1 Collecting a Clean-Catch Midstream Urine Specimen

Procedure Goal: To collect a urine specimen that is free from contamination.

OSHA Guidelines:

Materials: Dry, sterile urine container with lid; label; written instructions (if the patient is to perform procedure independently); and antiseptic towelettes.

Method: Procedure steps.

1. Confirm the patient's identity and be sure all forms are correctly completed.
2. Label the sterile urine specimen container with the patient's name, ID number, date of birth, the physician's name, the date and time of collection, and the initials of the person collecting the specimen.

When the Patient Will Be Completing the Procedure Independently

3. Explain the procedure in detail. Provide the patient with written instructions, antiseptic towelettes, and the labeled sterile specimen container.
4. Confirm that the patient understands the instructions, especially not to touch the inside of the specimen container and to refrigerate the specimen until bringing it to the physician's office.
   RATIONALE: Touching the inside of the container will introduce microorganisms into the container and can interfere with the test results. The specimen should be refrigerated to keep bacteria from growing and causing a false-positive result.

When You Are Assisting a Patient

3. Explain the procedure and how you will be assisting in the collection.
4. Wash your hands and don exam gloves.

When You Are Assisting in the Collection for Female Patients

5. Remove the lid from the specimen container and place the lid upside down on a flat surface.
6. Use three antiseptic towelettes to clean the perineal area by spreading the labia and wiping from front to back. Wipe with the first towelette on one side and discard it. Wipe with the second towelette on the other side and discard it. Wipe with the third towelette down the middle and discard it. To remove soap residue that could cause a higher pH and affect chemical test results, rinse the area once from front to back with water.
   RATIONALE: The area must be thoroughly cleaned so microorganisms from the vulva do not contaminate the specimen.
7. Keeping the patient's labia spread to avoid contamination, tell her to urinate into the toilet. After she has expressed a small amount of urine, instruct her to stop the flow.
   RATIONALE: So microorganisms are washed away from the urethral opening.
8. Position the specimen container close to but not touching the patient.
9. Tell the patient to start urinating again. Collect the necessary amount of urine in the container. (If the patient cannot stop her urine flow, move the container into the urine flow and collect the specimen anyway.)
10. Allow the patient to finish urinating. Place the lid back on the collection container.

11. Remove the gloves and wash your hands.

12. Complete the test request slip and record the collection in the patient's chart.

When You Are Assisting in the Collection for Male Patients

5. Remove the lid from the specimen container and place the lid upside down on a flat surface.

6. If the patient is circumcised, use an antiseptic towelette to clean the head of the penis. Wipe with a second towelette directly across the urethral opening. If the patient is uncircumcised, retract the foreskin before cleaning the penis. To remove soap residue that could cause a higher pH and affect chemical test results, rinse the area once from front to back with water.
RATIONALE: The area must be thoroughly cleaned so microorganisms from the head of the penis do not contaminate the specimen.

7. Keeping an uncircumcised patient's foreskin retracted, tell the patient to urinate into the toilet. After he has expressed a small amount of urine, instruct him to stop the flow.
RATIONALE: So microorganisms are washed away from the urethral opening.

8. Position the specimen container close to but not touching the patient.

9. Tell the patient to start urinating again. Collect the necessary amount of urine in the container. (If the patient cannot stop his urine flow, move the container into the urine flow and collect the specimen anyway.)

10. Allow the patient to finish urinating. Place the lid back on the collection container.

11. Remove the gloves and wash your hands.

12. Complete the laboratory request form and record the collection in the patient's chart.

PROCEDURE 47-2   Collecting a 24-Hour Urine Specimen

Procedure Goal: To collect a urine specimen that is free from contaminants over a 24-hour period.

OSHA Guidelines:

Materials: Urine collection container (disposable urinal or collection hat), sterile urine storage containers, and written instructions.

Method: Procedure steps.

1. Review the laboratory requisition form and gather the supplies.

2. Confirm the patient's identity, introduce yourself, and check that all forms are completed correctly.

3. Label the sterile urine specimen storage containers with the patient's name, ID number, date of birth, and the physician's name.

4. Explain that the urine specimen storage container may have a preservative in it. Tell the patient what they should do if they get the preservative on their skin. (Usually flushing with cold water is sufficient; follow the manufacturer's provided instructions.)

5. Give the patient the following instructions:

   a. At the start of the observation period (usually early in the morning), void and discard the first urine specimen. This will start the collection period. Write the start date and time on the urine specimen storage containers.
   RATIONALE: So only the urine produced in a 24-hour period is collected.

   b. Do not discard the preservative in the urine specimen storage container.

   c. For the next 24 hours, each time the patient voids, collect the entire specimen in the provided specimen collection container.

   d. Carefully transfer the entire specimen in the urine storage container, being careful not to spill any urine. If the patient spills urine or accidently urinates in the toilet, have them call to reschedule the test.
   RATIONALE: All urine must be collected so an accurate measure of urine components may be obtained.

   e. Keep the specimen covered and in the refrigerator or in a cooler when not in use.

   f. 24 hours after you begin the test, void once more and transfer to the specimen storage container. Write the end date and time on the container.

   g. As quickly as possible, bring the specimen back to the office or deliver it to the laboratory if instructed to do so. Keep the specimen cool during transport.

6. When the patient returns the urine specimen, wash your hands, don gloves, and then be sure to do the following:

   a. Check that the container lid is secure.

   b. Clean the outside of the container with a tissue or gauze pad if necessary.

   c. Check that the start and end dates and times are recorded on the container.

   d. Note the volume of the collected specimen.

   e. Review the procedure with the patient to make sure the specimen was properly collected and stored during the collection period.

   f. Complete the necessary laboratory requisition forms.

   g. Notify the lab that the specimen is ready for transport.

   h. Keep the specimen cold until it is transported to the lab.

7. Remove the gloves and wash your hands.

8. Document the specimen collection including volume, dates and times, and lab tests requested.

PROCEDURE 47-3 Establishing Chain of Custody for a Urine Specimen

Procedure Goal: To collect a urine specimen for drug testing, maintaining a chain of custody.

OSHA Guidelines:

Materials: Dry, sterile urine container with lid; chain of custody form (CCF); and two additional specimen containers.

Method: Procedure steps.

1. Positively identify the patient. (Complete the top part of the CCF with the drug testing laboratory's name and address, the requesting company's name and address, and the patient's Social Security number. Make a note on the form if the patient refuses to give her Social Security number.) Ensure the number on the printed label matches the number at the top of the form.

2. Ensure the patient removes any outer clothing and empties her pockets, displaying all items.
   RATIONALE: So the patient does not bring anything into the room to adulterate the specimen, resulting in a false-negative result.

3. Instruct the patient to wash and dry her hands.

4. Instruct the patient that no water is to be running while the specimen is being collected. Tape the faucet handles in the *off* position and add bluing agent to the toilet.
   RATIONALE: So the patient cannot warm a specimen brought in from another source and has no water available to dilute the specimen.

5. Instruct the patient to provide the specimen as soon as it is collected so you may record the specimen's temperature.

6. Remain by the door of the restroom.

7. Measure and record the urine specimen's temperature within 4 minutes of collection. Make a note if its temperature is out of the acceptable range.
   RATIONALE: To determine that the patient voided the specimen and did not bring it from an outside source.

8. Examine the specimen for signs of adulteration (unusual color or odor).

9. *In the presence of the patient*, check the "single specimen" or "split specimen" box. The patient should witness you transferring the specimen into the transport specimen bottle(s), capping the bottle(s), and affixing the label on the bottle(s).
   RATIONALE: To maintain the chain of custody.

10. The patient should initial the specimen bottle label(s) *after* it is placed on the bottle(s).
    RATIONALE: To maintain the chain of custody.

11. Complete any additional information requested on the form, including the authorization for drug screening. This information will include
    - Patient's daytime telephone number
    - Patient's evening telephone number
    - Test requested
    - Patient's name
    - Patient's signature
    - Date

12. Sign the CCF; print your full name and note the date and time of the collection and the name of the courier service.

13. Give the patient a copy of the CCF.

14. Place the specimen in a leakproof bag with the appropriate copy of the form.

15. Release the specimen to the courier service.

16. Distribute additional copies as required.

PROCEDURE 47-4 Measuring Specific Gravity with a Refractometer

Procedure Goal: To measure the specific gravity of a urine specimen with a refractometer.

OSHA Guidelines:

Materials: Urine specimen, refractometer, dropper, and laboratory report form.

Method: Procedure steps.

1. Wash your hands and don exam gloves.

2. Check the specimen for proper labeling and examine it to make sure there is no visible contamination and that no more than 1 hour has passed since collection (or since the specimen has been removed from the refrigerator and brought back to room temperature).

3. Swirl the specimen.
   RATIONALE: To mix the specimen thoroughly.

4. Confirm that the refractometer has been calibrated that day. If not, you must calibrate it with distilled water. You also must use two standard solutions as controls to check the refractometer's accuracy. Follow Steps 6 through 11 using each of the three samples in place of the specimen. Clean the refractometer and the dropper after each use and record the calibration values in the quality control log.
   RATIONALE: To ensure the refractometer is standardized prior to testing the specimen.

5. Open the hinged lid of the refractometer.

6. Draw up a small amount of the specimen into the dropper.

7. Place one drop of the specimen under the cover.

8. Close the lid.

9. Turn on the light and look into the refractometer's eyepiece. As the light passes through the specimen, the refractometer measures the refraction of the light and displays the refractive index on a scale on the right with corresponding specific gravity values on the left.

10. Read the specific gravity value at the line where light and dark meet.

11. Record the value on the laboratory report form.

12. Sanitize and disinfect the refractometer and the dropper. Put them away when they are dry.

13. Clean and disinfect the work area.

14. Remove the gloves and wash your hands.

15. Record the value in the patient's chart.

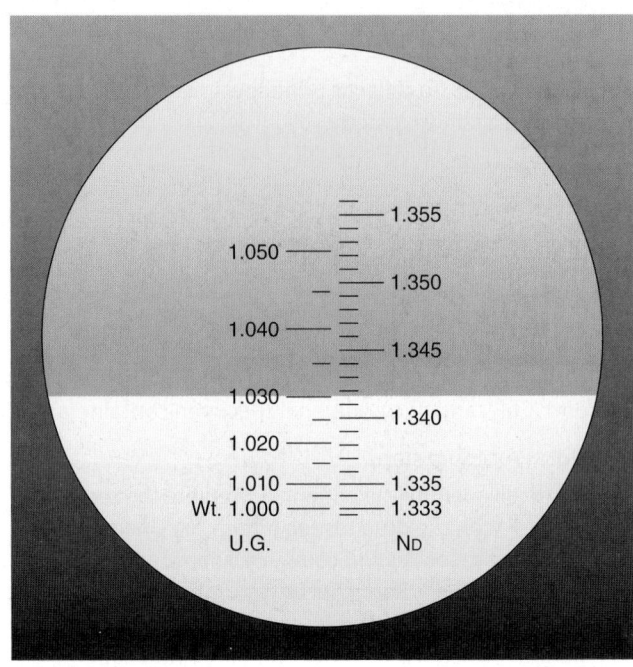

FIGURE Procedure 47-4 Step 9 A refractometer uses light refraction to measure specific gravity.

PROCEDURE 47-5 Performing a Reagent Strip Test

Procedure Goal: To perform chemical testing on urine specimens to screen for the presence of various elements, including leukocytes, nitrite, urobilinogen, protein, pH, blood, specific gravity, ketones, bilirubin, and glucose.

OSHA Guidelines:

Materials: Urine specimen, laboratory report form, reagent strips, paper towel, and a timer.

Method: Procedure steps.

1. Wash your hands and don personal protective equipment.

2. Check the specimen for proper labeling and examine it to make sure there is no visible contamination. Perform the test as soon as possible after collection. Refrigerate the specimen if testing will take place more than 1 hour later. Bring the refrigerated specimen back to room temperature prior to testing.

3. Check the expiration date on the reagent strip container and check the strip for damaged or discolored pads.
   RATIONALE: To ensure the reagent strip is still valid.

4. Swirl the specimen.
   RATIONALE: To mix the specimen thoroughly.

5. Remove a small amount (aliquot) of the urine with a pipette and place it into a secondary container.

RATIONALE: In the event that a urine culture is needed, the entire sample is not contaminated by chemicals on the reagent pads. These chemicals could interfere with a urine culture test.

Dip a urine strip into the aliquoted specimen, making sure each pad is completely covered. Briefly tap the strip sideways on a paper towel. *Do not blot* the test pads.
RATIONALE: Excess urine could migrate to the other pads and alter the test results.

6. Read each test pad against the chart on the bottle at the designated time.
   Note: It is important to read each pad at the appropriate time. Most reagent strip results are invalid after 2 minutes.

FIGURE Procedure 47-5 Step 6 Read the reagent strip by the time indicated in the manufacturer's instructions.

RATIONALE: Test pads read at inappropriate times will yield inaccurate results.

7. Record the values on the laboratory report form.
8. Discard the used disposable supplies.
9. Clean and disinfect the work area.
10. Remove your gloves and wash your hands.
11. Record the result in the patient's chart.

PROCEDURE 47-6 Pregnancy Testing Using the EIA Method

Procedure Goal: To perform the enzyme immunoassay in order to detect HCG in the urine (or serum) and to interpret results as positive or negative.

OSHA Guidelines:

Materials: Gloves, urine specimen, timing device, surface disinfectant, pregnancy control solutions, and pregnancy test kits.

Method: Procedure steps.

1. Wash your hands and don exam gloves.
2. Gather the necessary supplies and equipment.
3. If materials have been refrigerated, allow all materials to reach room temperature prior to conducting the testing.
4. Label the test chamber with the patient's name or identification number; label one test chamber for a negative and positive control.
5. Apply the urine (or serum) to the test chamber per the manufacturer's instructions.
   RATIONALE: Different tests may have slightly different instructions.
6. At the appropriate time, read and interpret the results.
   RATIONALE: Most tests are invalid after 10 minutes.

FIGURE Procedure 47-6 Step 6 A positive pregnancy test (top) and a negative control (bottom).

7. Document the patient's results in the chart; document the quality control results in the appropriate log book.
8. Dispose of used reagents in a biohazard container.
9. Clean the work area with a disinfectant solution.
10. Remove your gloves and wash your hands.

PROCEDURE 47-7 Processing a Urine Specimen for Microscopic Examination of Sediment

Procedure Goal: To prepare a slide for microscopic examination of urine sediment.

OSHA Guidelines:

Materials: Fresh urine specimen, two glass or plastic test tubes, water, centrifuge, tapered pipette, glass slide with coverslip, microscope with light source, and laboratory report form.

Method: Procedure steps.

1. Wash your hands and don exam gloves.
2. Check the specimen for proper labeling and examine it to make sure there is no visible contamination and that no more than 1 hour has passed since collection (or since the specimen has been removed from the refrigerator and brought back to room temperature).

3. Swirl the urine specimen.
   RATIONALE: To mix the specimen thoroughly.

4. Pour approximately 10 mL of urine into one test tube and 10 mL of plain water into the balance tube.

FIGURE Procedure 47-7 Step 4   Fill one test tube with approximately 10 mL of urine and the other with 10 mL of water.

5. Balance the centrifuge by placing the test tubes on either side.
   RATIONALE: An unbalanced tube could "walk" or wobble off the table.

FIGURE Procedure 47-7 Step 5   The centrifuge must be balanced by placing one test tube on each side.

6. Make sure the lid is secure and set the centrifuge timer for 5 to 10 minutes.
   RATIONALE: Spinning the urine will force the solids (cells, casts, and crystals) to the bottom of the tube.

FIGURE Procedure 47-7 Step 6   Set the centrifuge timer for 5 to 10 minutes.

7. Set the speed as prescribed by your office's protocol (usually 1500 to 2000 revolutions per minute) and start the centrifuge.

8. After the centrifuge stops, lift out the tube containing the urine and carefully pour most of the liquid portion—called the **supernatant**—down the sink drain.

FIGURE Procedure 47-7 Step 8   Make sure you do not lose any sediment when you pour off the urine.

9. A few drops of urine should remain in the bottom of the test tube with any sediment. Mix the urine and sediment together by gently tapping the bottom of the tube on the palm of your hand.
   RATIONALE: To resuspend the solid material.

10. Use the tapered pipette to obtain a drop or two of urine sediment. Place the drops in the center of a clean glass slide.

11. Place the coverslip over the specimen, allow it to settle, and place it on the stage of the microscope.

12. Correctly focus the microscope as directed in the *Microbiology and Disease* chapter.

    Note: Most medical assistants are trained to perform this procedure only up to this point. After this, the physician usually examines the specimen. You may, however, be asked to clean the items after the examination is completed. The remaining steps are provided for your information.

13. Use a dim light and view the slide under the low-power objective. Observe the slide for casts (found mainly around the coverslip's edges) and count the casts viewed.

14. Switch to the high-power objective. Identify the casts. Identify any epithelial cells, mucus, protozoa, yeasts, and crystals. Adjust the slide position so you can view and count the cells, protozoa, yeasts, and crystals from at least 10 different fields. Turn off the light after the examination is completed.

15. Record the observations on the laboratory report form.

16. Properly dispose of used disposable materials.

17. Sanitize and disinfect nondisposable items; put them away when they are dry.

18. Clean and disinfect the work area.

19. Remove the gloves and wash your hands.

20. Record the observations in the patient's chart.

PROCEDURE 47-8 Fecal Occult Blood Testing Using the Guaiac Testing Method

Procedure Goal: To test for the presence of blood in a fecal sample.

OSHA Guidelines:

Materials: Fecal occult blood testing cards or slides, fecal collection spoon or other device, written patient instructions, and testing reagents.

Method: Procedure steps.

1. Confirm the patient's identity and ensure all forms are completed correctly.

2. Label the occult blood testing card or slide with the patient's name and date of birth. Give the patient the test card or slide and collecting spoon or applicator.

3. Give the patient pretest and collection instructions, including

   a. Do not collect sample if you are menstruating or if visible blood is seen in the feces or toilet.

   b. For three days prior to collecting the sample, avoid red meats (beef, veal, and lamb), horseradish, vitamin C supplements, certain fruits and vegetables such as cabbage, cucumbers, broccoli, carrots, beets, radishes, mushrooms, and citrus fruits, aspirin or other nonsteroidal anti-inflammatory drugs, and other medications including corticosteroids. (Consult the specific test instructions for dietary and medication restrictions as these may vary from test to test.)

   RATIONALE: Some foods and medications may cause a false-positive or a false-negative test result.

   c. Collect the samples (depending on the specific test) on two or three different days.

   d. Collect the specimen before it comes into contact with the toilet water. (The patient may use a clean container or a specimen collection hat.)

   RATIONALE: Chemicals in the toilet could interfere with the test.

   e. Place a small amount of fecal material on each slide or test card window with the applicator. The sample should be thinly smeared in the sample area.

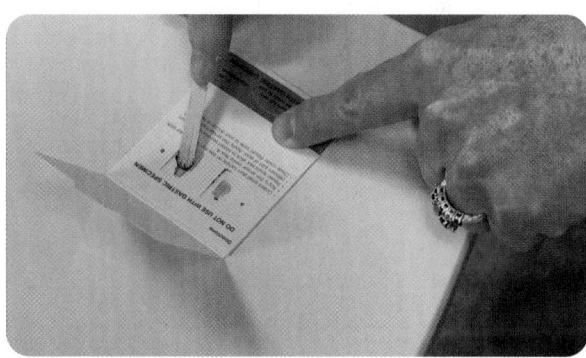

FIGURE Procedure 47-8 Step 3e   The patient should apply a thin smear of fecal material on each window of the test card.

   f. Close the card window or place the slide in the provided container and write the collection date on the card or slide.

   g. Return the card or slide to the office.

Processing the Test

4. Wash your hands and don gloves.

5. Open the back of the card. Add the recommended amount of developing reagent directly over the smeared area

on the back side of the paper and over the positive and negative controls, if present, on the card.
RATIONALE: To ensure that the test is working correctly.

6. Read the test results at the appropriate time according to the manufacturer's instructions (usually within 60 seconds). There will be a blue color on the guaiac paper if blood is present.

7. Dispose of the testing card according to OSHA regulations.

8. Remove your gloves and wash your hands.

9. Document the results in the patient's chart.

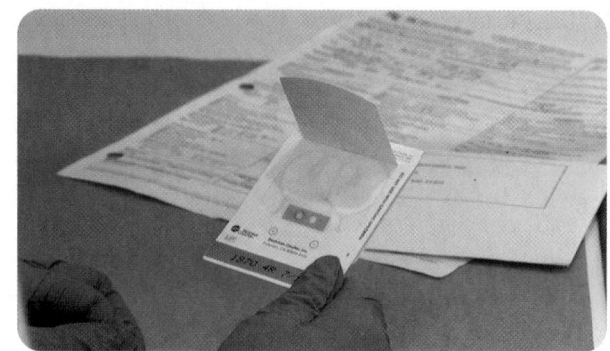

FIGURE Procedure 47-8 Step 6 Read the card by the time indicated in the manufacturer's instructions.

SUMMARY OF LEARNING OUTCOMES

LEARNING OUTCOMES	KEY POINTS
47.1 Discuss the role of the medical assistant in collecting, processing, and testing urine and stool samples.	Your role as a medical assistant includes collecting, processing, and testing urine samples and processing and testing stool samples. You also will be responsible for teaching patients proper collection methods for urine and stool samples.
47.2 Carry out procedures for following guidelines when collecting urine specimens.	The general guidelines for collecting a urine specimen include following the procedure specified for the urine test that will be performed; using the type of specimen container indicated by the laboratory; properly labeling the specimen container; explaining the procedure to the patient when assisting in the collection process; washing your hands before and after the procedure and wearing gloves during the procedure; and complete all necessary paperwork.
47.3 Describe the process of urinalysis and its purpose.	Urinalysis is the evaluation of urine by various types of testing methods to obtain information about body health and disease.
47.4 Carry out the proper procedure for collecting and processing a stool sample for fecal occult blood testing.	The general guidelines for collecting a stool specimen include instructing the patient about the need to follow all collection procedures including when to collect, how to collect, and how to return the specimen to the office; following the testing procedure for fecal occult blood testing, using Standard Precautions when performing the test; and documenting the test and results in the patient's chart.

CASE STUDY CRITICAL THINKING

Recall Ken Washington from the beginning of the chapter. Now that you have completed the chapter, answer the following questions regarding his case.

1. What instructions will you give Ken in collecting the urine sample for reagent testing?

2. What tests are included in a reagent test?

3. Describe the instructions you will need to give Ken regarding his 24-hour urine collection.

1. (LO 47.2) Which of the following catheters is used after plastic repair of the ureter?
   a. Indwelling
   b. Urinary
   c. Drainage
   d. Splinting
   e. Permanent

2. (LO 47.3) The average adult urinary output is
   a. 650 mL
   b. 1000 mL
   c. 1250 mL
   d. 1500 mL
   e. 2000 mL

3. (LO 47.3) A urine sample that is turbid is said to be
   a. Cloudy
   b. Clear
   c. Odorous
   d. Dark
   e. Dilute

4. (LO 47.3) What is the specific gravity of distilled water?
   a. 0.00
   b. 1.000
   c. 1.001
   d. 1.010
   e. 1.100

5. (LO 47.3) Which of the following is (are) normally found in a urine sample?
   a. Cholesterol
   b. Tyrosine
   c. Ketone bodies
   d. Amorphous phosphates
   e. Glucose

6. (LO 47.4) A test for the presence of hidden blood in a stool sample is which of the following?
   a. SGOT
   b. FOBT
   c. Bilirubin
   d. EIA
   e. Urobilinogen

7. (LO 47.3) Calcium carbonate, calcium oxalate, and triple phosphate are types of which kind of structure sometimes present in urine?
   a. Casts
   b. Blood cell components
   c. Bence Jones proteins
   d. Vitamins
   e. Crystals

8. (LO 47.3) Which of the following is a chemical component of urine?
   a. Color
   b. Volume
   c. Blood
   d. Specific gravity
   e. Clarity

9. (LO 47.2) The most common type of urine sample is
   a. First morning
   b. 24-hour
   c. Timed
   d. Random
   e. Midstream

10. (LO 47.3) The term meaning insufficient production of urine is
    a. Anuria
    b. Oliguria
    c. Polyuria
    d. Proteinuria
    e. Hematuria

Go to CONNECT to see activities about *Ordering a Test, Recording Test Results,* and *Processing Test Results.*

CASE STUDY

PATIENT INFORMATION		
Patient Name	**Gender**	**DOB**
Sylvia Gonzales	Female	9/1/19XX
Attending	**MRN**	**Allergies**
Alexis N. Whalen, MD	341-73-792	PCN

Sylvia Gonzales, a 51-year-old female, is at the office for a 3-month return check for her newly diagnosed Type II diabetes. She states that she has taken the medication she received for her "sugar" and she knows the doctor wants to a do a special "sugar test" this time. Her medication list includes Januvia 100 mg daily. The physician has ordered a fasting blood sugar (FBS) and a hemoglobin A1C blood test. You will need to perform both of these waived tests in your office lab. You will be drawing the blood by dermal puncture.

Keep Sylvia in mind as you study this chapter. There will be questions at the end of the chapter based on the case study. The information in the chapter will help you answer these questions.

LEARNING OUTCOMES

After completing Chapter 48, you will be able to:

48.1 Discuss the role of the medical assistant when collecting, processing, and testing blood samples.

48.2 Carry out the procedure for collecting a blood specimen.

48.3 Summarize ways to respond to patients' needs when collecting blood.

48.4 Carry out the procedure for performing blood tests.

KEY TERMS

anticoagulants
automatic puncturing devices
buffy coat
butterfly system
capillary puncture
complete blood (cell) count
EDTA (Ethylenediamine-tetraacetic acid)
erythrocyte sedimentation rate (ESR)

formed elements
hematoma
hemolysis
lancet
micropipette
morphology
packed red blood cells
phlebotomy
serum separators
tourniquet
venipuncture
whole blood

I. P (2)   Perform Venipuncture

I. P (3)   Perform capillary puncture

I. P (12) Perform CLIA waived hematology testing

I. P (13) Perform CLIA waived chemistry testing

I. P (15) Perform CLIA waived immunology testing

I. P (16) Screen test results

II. P (2) Maintain laboratory test results using flow sheets

III. P (3) Select appropriate barrier/personal protective equipment (PPE) for potentially infectious situations

III. A (1) Display sensitivity to patient rights and feelings in collecting specimens

III. A (3) Show awareness of patients' concerns regarding their perceptions related to the procedure being performed

3. **Medical Terminology**

   Graduates:

   d. Recognize and identify acceptable medical abbreviations

9. **Medical Office Clinical Procedures**

   Graduates:

   f. Screen and follow up patient test results

   i. Use standard precautions

   q. Instruct patients with special needs

10. **Medical Laboratory Procedures**

    Graduates:

    a. Practice quality control

    b. Perform selected CLIA-waived tests that assist with diagnosis and treatment

       (2) Hematology testing

       (3) Chemistry testing

       (4) Immunology testing

    c. Dispose of biohazardous materials

    d. Collect, label, and process specimens

       (1) Perform venipuncture

       (2) Perform capillary puncture

▶ Introduction

In many healthcare settings, the medical assistant is responsible for collecting blood specimens from patients and sometimes performing waived testing. In this chapter, you will be introduced to venipuncture and capillary collection procedures and you will learn the appropriate supplies and equipment needed to perform these procedures. You also will learn techniques for dealing with different types of patients and how to obtain blood samples efficiently and effectively. Additionally, you will receive instruction on the performance and screening of common blood tests.

▶ The Role of the Medical Assistant   LO 48.1

The examination of blood can provide extensive information about a patient's condition. You may be asked to collect and process blood specimens for examination in your work as a medical assistant. A basic understanding of the anatomy and physiology of the circulatory system will help you properly perform these tasks. You also will need a working knowledge of the functions of blood and the kinds of cells that make up blood tissue. (See *The Cardiovascular System* and *The Blood* chapters for more information.)

You will use several techniques to obtain blood specimens. **Phlebotomy** is the insertion of a needle or cannula (small tube) into a vein for the purpose of withdrawing blood. Phlebotomists receive special training in phlebotomy; drawing blood is the main task in their work. Smaller blood samples may be obtained by using a small, disposable instrument to pierce surface capillaries. You must be able to perform such procedures accurately so the sample is appropriate for the ordered tests. You also must be skilled in putting the patient at ease during this procedure. Your reassuring manner, ability to handle technical problems, and careful preparation for answering many kinds of questions will be important to your success in this area.

In addition to your many duties as a medical assistant, you must understand how to process blood specimens and conduct various blood tests, particularly if you work in a laboratory. You also must be able to complete the necessary paperwork to ensure that test results are handled efficiently and accurately. All these skills are essential, regardless of whether you collect blood specimens in a physician's office laboratory (POL), hospital, or laboratory drawing station.

www.mhhe.com/BoothMA8

Ordering Laboratory Tests

▶ Collecting Blood Specimens   LO 48.2

Following the steps in the standard process for drawing blood specimens will enable you to perform the procedure smoothly, accurately, and safely while ensuring properly completed documentation.

Reading and Interpreting the Test Order

The first steps in preparing to draw blood for testing are to review the written testing request and to assemble the equipment and supplies. The patient should arrive with a laboratory request form if you are working in a physician's office laboratory or a laboratory drawing station.

Reviewing the Test Order It is essential to first review the patient's blood-collection order to determine what tests will be run. Many tests require expedited or special handling to ensure accurate results.

Your office will have specific collection procedures for each type of test. If you have any questions about these procedures, ask your supervisor. If you will be sending the blood specimen to a reference laboratory for testing, make sure you know its requirements. The cost of reprocessing a test far surpasses the extra time needed to be sure of the process requirements.

When reviewing the test order, you will need to know the meaning of certain abbreviations. Many abbreviations used in laboratory work and their meanings are presented in Table 48-1. If you are ever in doubt or if the resources in your office or laboratory do not provide the answers you need, ask the doctor or your supervisor.

Assembling the Equipment and Supplies Specific blood-drawing equipment and collection devices vary with the type of test. Make sure you have the appropriate

TABLE 48-1	Abbreviations Routinely Used in Blood Tests			
Ab	Antibody		COHb	Carboxyhemoglobin
ABO	Classification system for four blood groups		CPK	Creatine phosphokinase
AcAc	Acetoacetate		CRCL	Creatinine clearance
ACE	Angiotensin-converting enzyme		Cre	Creatinine
ACT	Activated coagulation time		DHEA-SO4	Dehydroepiandrosterone sulfate
ACTH	Adrenocorticotropic hormone		Dif	Differential (blood cell count)
ADH	Antidiuretic hormone		EBNA-IgG	Epstein-Barr virus nuclear antigen
AFB	Acid-fast bacillus		EBV	Epstein-Barr virus
AFP	Alpha-fetoprotein		EDTA	Ethylenediaminetetraacetic acid
Ag	Antigen		ELP	Electrophoresis, protein
AG	Anion gap		Eos	Eosinophil
A/G R	Albumin-globulin ratio		Eq	Equivalent
ALB	Albumin		ESR	Erythrocyte sedimentation rate
ALP; alk phos	Alkaline phosphatase		ETOH	Alcohol
ALT	Alanine aminotransferase		FBS	Fasting blood sugar
ANA	Antinuclear antibody		Free T_4	Free thyroxine
APAP	Acetaminophen		FSH	Follicle-stimulating hormone (follitropin)
APTT	Activated partial thromboplastin time		FTI	Free thyroxine index
ASA	Acetylsalicylic acid (aspirin)		GFR	Glomerular filtration rate
AST	Aspartate aminotransferase		GH	Growth hormone
AT-III	Antithrombin III		GHRH	Growth hormone-releasing hormone
B	Blood (whole blood)		GnRH	Gonadotropin-releasing hormone
Baso	Basophil		GTT	Glucose tolerance test
BCA; BRCA	Breast cancer antigen		HA	Hemagglutination
BJP	Bence Jones protein		HAI	Hemagglutination inhibition test
BT	Bleeding time		HAV	Hepatitis A virus
BUN	Blood urea nitrogen		Hb; Hgb	Hemoglobin
Ca; Ca^{++}	Calcium		HbCO	Carboxyhemoglobin
CA	Cancer antigen		HBV	Hepatitis B virus
CBC	Complete blood (cell) count		HCG; hCG	Human chorionic gonadotropin
CEA	Carcinoembryonic antigen		Hct	Hematocrit
CHS	Cholinesterase test		HCV	Hepatitis C virus
CMV	Cytomegalovirus		HDL	High-density lipoprotein
CO	Carbon monoxide		HDV	Hepatitis delta virus
CO_2	Carbon dioxide		HGH; hGH	Human growth hormone

TABLE 48-1 *(concluded)*

HIV	Human immunodeficiency virus	PMN	Polymorphonuclear (leukocyte; neutrophil)
HLA	Human leukocyte antigen	PRL	Prolactin
HPV	Human papilloma virus	PSA	Prostate-specific antigen
HSV	Herpes simplex virus	PT	Prothrombin time
HTLV	Human T-cell lymphotrophic virus	PTH	Parathyroid hormone
Ig	Immunoglobulin	PTT	Partial thromboplastin time
IgE	Immunoglobulin E	PZP	Pregnancy zone protein
INH	Inhibitor	RAIU	Thyroid uptake of radioactive iodine
IV	Intravenous	RBC	Red blood cell; red blood (cell) count
L	Liver	RBP	Retinol-binding protein
LD; LDH	Lactate dehydrogenase	RDW	Red cell distribution of width
LDL	Low-density lipoprotein	Retic	Reticulocyte
LH	Luteinizing hormone	RF	Rheumatoid factor; relative fluorescence unit
LMWH	Low-molecular-weight heparin	Rh	Rhesus factor
Lytes	Electrolytes	RIA	Radioimmunoassay
MCH	Mean corpuscular hemoglobin	rT_3 or $REVT_3$	Reverse triiodothyronine
MCHC	Mean corpuscular hemoglobin concentration	S	Serum
MCV	Mean corpuscular volume	Segs	Segmented polymorphonuclear leukocyte
MHb	Methemoglobin	SPE	Serum protein electrophoresis
MONO	Monocyte	T_3	Triiodothyronine
MPV	Mean platelet volume	T_4	Thyroxine
msAFP	Maternal serum alpha-fetoprotein	TBG	Thyroxine-binding globulin
NE	Norepinephrine	TBV	Total blood volume
OGTT	Oral glucose tolerance test	TG	Triglyceride
P	Plasma	TRH	Thyrotropin-releasing hormone
PBG	Porphobilinogen	TSH	Thyroid-stimulating hormone
PCT	Prothrombin consumption time	VDRL	Venereal Disease Research Laboratory (test for syphilis)
PCV	Packed cell volume (hematocrit)	VLDL	Very low-density lipoprotein
Pi	Inorganic phosphate	WB	Western blot
PKU	Phenylketonuria	WBC	White blood cell; white blood (cell) count
PLT	Platelet		

Source: http://labtestsonline.org/.

equipment to collect all necessary samples if more than one test are ordered. All specimen-collection tubes, slides, and other containers should be labeled immediately after collection with the patient's name, the date and time of collection, the initials of the person collecting the specimen, and other information as required by the test procedure or your office. Some offices use an identification code for each patient.

Alcohol and cotton balls or alcohol wipes, sterile gauze, and adhesive bandages are standard supplies for procedures during which blood is drawn from a vein or capillaries. Alcohol causes inaccurate results for certain tests, however, so for these tests, povidone-iodine or benzalkonium chloride is used. You will need a **tourniquet** (a flat, broad length of vinyl or rubber or a piece of fabric with a Velcro closure) for **venipuncture**, the puncture of a vein—performed with a needle for the purpose of drawing blood.

Preparing Patients

After you review the test order and assemble the necessary equipment and supplies, take a moment to relax, gather your thoughts, and consider your purpose. This may strike you as odd advice, but your calm and positive demeanor helps establish the best possible relationship with a patient who may be uneasy about having blood drawn. The moment you use to relax and focus may save you time and save patients unnecessary discomfort by contributing to a quick, efficient procedure.

Greeting and Identifying Patients Greet patients pleasantly, introduce yourself, and explain that you will be drawing some blood. It is essential to identify patients correctly before you begin the procedure. Ask patients to state their full name and be sure you hear both the first and last names correctly.

Verify that the name the patient gives is the name on the order. (In some facilities, the phlebotomist may ask for a date of birth, patient ID, or chart number to further identify the patient.)

Confirming Pretest Preparation The presence and level of certain substances in blood are affected by food and fluid intake or by other daily life activities. Some tests, like the glucose tolerance test, require the patient to follow certain pretest restrictions to minimize the influence of the restricted food on the blood, or to stress the body to see how it responds, as indicated by the blood.

The glucose tolerance test measures a patient's ability to metabolize carbohydrates and is used to detect hypoglycemia and diabetes mellitus. Instruct the patient to eat a high-carbohydrate diet for 3 days before the test and to fast for 8 to 12 hours before the appointment. After initial blood and urine samples are taken, the patient ingests a measured dose of glucose solution. Blood and urine samples are then taken at prescribed intervals as ordered by the physician. The glucose levels in the samples are often graphed for the physician's review.

Before you draw blood for any test, determine whether the patient has complied with pretest instructions. If the patient has not complied, explain that the test cannot be performed. Make a note on the order and report the information to the physician or your supervisor.

Explaining the Procedure and Safety Precautions Explain to the patient the procedure you will use to obtain the blood specimen for testing. Be clear and brief when you describe what you will do; too much detail leaves some patients queasy. You must follow Standard Precautions during all phlebotomy procedures, as described in the Caution: Handle with Care section. These precautions may be second nature to you, but they may raise concerns in the patient. Explain the need for each of the preventive measures in language the patient can understand. Assure the patient that these measures protect against exposure to infection.

Establishing a Chain of Custody You will need to follow specific guidelines to establish a chain of custody for blood samples drawn for drug and alcohol analysis. Because donating a specimen for drug and alcohol testing is potentially self-incriminating, the patient must sign a consent form for the testing. The *Processing and Testing Urine and Stool Specimens* chapter explains general chain of custody procedures.

Handling an Exposure Incident When you adhere to Standard Precautions, the risk of exposure to bloodborne pathogens is very small. Accidents can occur, however. If you suffer a needlestick or other injury that results in exposure to blood or blood products from another person, you

CAUTION: HANDLE WITH CARE
Phlebotomy and Personal Protective Equipment

The Centers for Disease Control and Prevention (CDC) has classified all phlebotomy procedures as a risk for exposure to contaminated blood or blood products. You must use appropriate personal protective equipment (PPE) during all phlebotomy procedures. Remember, it is up to you to protect yourself and the patient.

Gloves
Gloves—which protect against spills and splashing of contaminated blood—are the first line of defense during a phlebotomy procedure. Wash your hands and don clean exam gloves that fit snugly before you work with each patient. Remove the gloves, dispose of them in a biohazardous waste container, and wash your hands after working with each patient.

Garments
Garments like laboratory coats and aprons can protect your clothing from spills and splashes and provide a measure of protection from contaminated materials. Some garments are designed to resist penetration by blood or blood products. You may find it necessary to wear such garments when drawing blood or performing blood tests.

Masks and Protective Eyewear
Mucous membranes are especially vulnerable to invasion by infectious agents. Use masks and protective eyewear to help safeguard mucous membranes in your mouth, nose, and eyes from infection.

Masks help protect your mouth and nose from splashes or sprays of blood or blood products. You cannot predict when exposure to blood may occur. Accidental puncture of an artery during a phlebotomy procedure could result in a spray of blood, or blood may spray or splash accidentally during testing protocols. Most medical assistants do not routinely wear masks for phlebotomy procedures once they have achieved proficiency in performing them.

Goggles can protect your eyes from splashing and spraying during blood drawing or testing. Healthcare workers in dental offices often wear goggles because patient treatments can easily expose workers to contaminated blood or bloody saliva.

Clear plastic face shields combine the protection of masks and goggles and are often used during major surgical procedures. You may use a face shield if you do extensive testing on blood specimens, but face shields are not usually worn when drawing blood.

PPE works two ways: it protects you from a patient's contaminated blood and it also protects the patient from infectious agents you may be carrying. By using PPE correctly, you will make your workplace a safer place for you and the patients.

must report the incident to the appropriate staff members immediately. Wash the injured area carefully and apply a sterile bandage. Record the time and date of the incident, the names of the people involved, and the nature of the exposure. Depending on the situation, you may receive medications. You and the other person involved will be asked to undergo blood testing and be involved in follow-up studies. The Occupational Safety and Health Administration (OSHA) requires every employer to have an established procedure for handling exposure incidents. (See the *Basic Safety and Infection Control* chapter for more information.)

Drawing Blood

Some states permit medical assistants to obtain blood samples. Your office will clarify which phlebotomy-related duties, if any, you may perform. If your duties include collecting blood samples, you will obtain them through either venipuncture or capillary puncture. You must understand when these techniques are used and know how to perform them. Procedure 48-1, at the end of this chapter, details quality control procedures for collecting blood specimens.

Go to CONNECT to see a video about *Quality Control Procedures for Blood Specimen Collection.*

Venipuncture Venipuncture requires puncturing a vein with a needle and collecting blood into either a tube or a syringe. The most common sites for venipuncture are the median cubital and cephalic veins of the forearm, although other sites may be used if the primary site is unacceptable. Figure 48-1 shows the veins in the antecubital fossa (the small depression inside the bend of the elbow) and the forearm that are used for venipuncture.

Various instruments are used to perform venipuncture. Practice using the devices so your technique is smooth, steady, and competent.

Evacuation Systems Evacuation systems—the most common is the VACUTAINER system (manufactured by Becton Dickinson VACUTAINER Systems, Franklin Lakes, New Jersey)—use a special double-pointed needle, a plastic needle holder/adapter, and collection tubes (Figure 48-2). The collection tubes are sealed to create a slight vacuum. You insert the covered inner point of the needle into one end of the holder/adapter and the first collection tube into the other end. Procedure 48-2, at the end of this chapter, explains how to use an evacuation system to draw a blood sample.

An evacuation system has several advantages over other methods of blood collection. It is easy to collect several samples from one venipuncture site using the interchangeable vacuum collection tubes, which are calibrated by evacuation to collect the exact amount of blood required. Some collection tubes are prepared with additives needed to correctly process the blood sample for testing, such as anticoagulants. Finally, because there is no need to transfer blood from a collection syringe to a sample tube, the potential for exposure to contaminated blood is reduced.

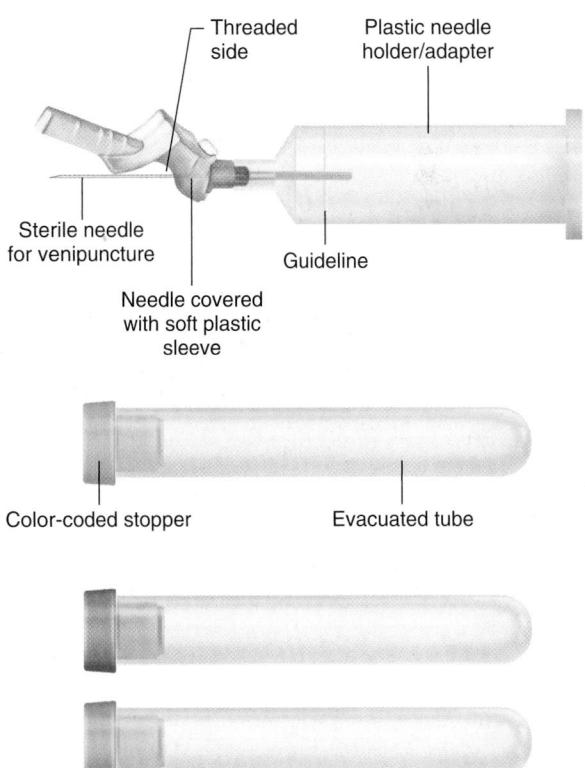

FIGURE 48-2 The VACUTAINER system uses interchangeable collection tubes that allow you to draw several blood specimens from the same venipuncture site.

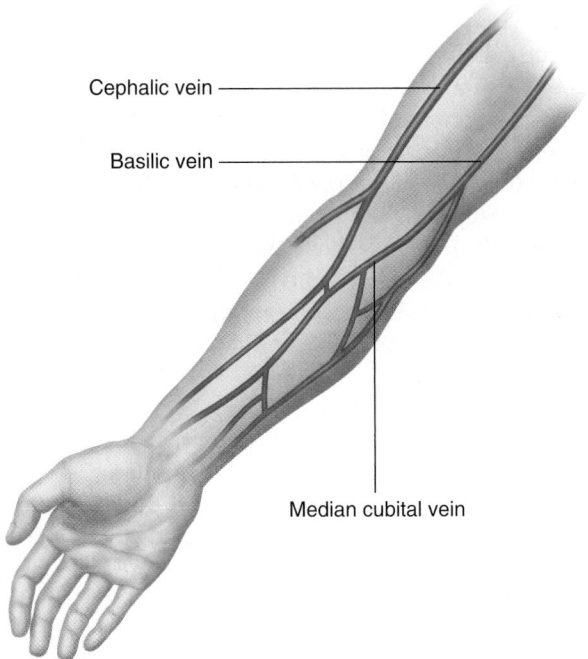

FIGURE 48-1 Veins commonly used for venipuncture include the cephalic vein, the basilic vein, and the median cubital vein.

Needle and Syringe Systems An evacuation system is not the best choice for drawing blood in every case. For example, if the patient has small or fragile veins, the vacuum created when the collection tube is pressed over the needle point can cause the veins to collapse. You may collect blood using a sterile needle and syringe assembly when an evacuation system is not suitable, such as when the patient is difficult to stick. You can use a smaller needle—no smaller than 23-gauge to avoid hemolyzing the blood—and control the vacuum in the syringe by pulling the plunger back slowly. Other aspects of the procedure are essentially the same, except that the blood sample is collected in the syringe and must immediately be transferred to a collection tube.

Butterfly Systems You also may use a **butterfly system**, or winged infusion set, when you work with patients who have small or fragile veins. Flexible wings attached to the needle simplify needle insertion. A length of flexible tubing (either 5 or 12 inches, approximately) connects the needle to the collection device. The inserted needle remains completely undisturbed while the collection device is manipulated. Because it is motionless, the needle causes less trauma to the vein and surrounding tissue than other venipuncture systems. A butterfly system also generally uses a smaller needle (23-gauge) than other venipuncture techniques and can be used with an evacuated collection tube or a syringe (Figure 48-3).

Butterfly

Tubing

Adapter

Holder

Evacuated tube

FIGURE 48-3 Once inserted, the needle of a butterfly system remains undisturbed during specimen collection.

FIGURE 48-4 Special color-coded stoppers on collection tubes indicate which additives are present and, therefore, which types of laboratory tests may be performed on each blood specimen.

Collection Tubes No matter which method is used to collect blood, the samples must immediately be mixed with the appropriate additives in the correct collection tubes before they are transported to the laboratory for testing. The tube stoppers are different colors, each color identifying the type of additives (if any) they contain (Figure 48-4). These additives must be compatible with the laboratory process the sample will undergo. Each laboratory may choose which tubes to use for a particular test.

Additives include anticoagulants, like **EDTA (Ethylenediaminetetraacetic acid)** and other materials that help preserve or process a sample for particular types of testing. When you collect a blood sample, double-check that you are using the appropriate collection tubes for the tests ordered. You also must fill the tubes in a specific order to preserve the blood sample's integrity by preventing carryover of tube additives from one tube to the next. Each laboratory requires a specific order of draw for collection tubes. The National Committee for Clinical Laboratory Standards also publishes its recommended order of draw. Table 48-2 identifies collection tube stopper colors, additives present in the tubes, and types of tests, in a typical order of draw. Additional information regarding drawing blood for cultures is found in the Points on Practice: Collecting a Blood Culture Specimen box.

Engineered Safety Devices In response to the Needlestick Safety and Prevention Act, a number of engineered safety devices have been developed to reduce the possibility of needlestick injuries (Figure 48-5). According to the National Institute for Occupational Safety and Health (NIOSH), desired characteristics of engineered safety devices include:

- The performance of the device is reliable.
- The device is easy to use, safe, and effective.
- The device should be needleless when possible.

Stopper Color		Additive	Test Types
Yellow	○	Sodium polyanetholsulfonate	Blood cultures
Light blue	○	Sodium citrate	Coagulation studies
Red	●	Clot activator Silicone coated	Blood chemistries, HIV/AIDS antibody, viral studies, and serologic tests
Gold or red/gray	○ ●	Clot activator Silicone serum separator	Tests requiring blood serum, routine blood donor screening, and infectious disease testing
Green	●	Heparin	Electrolyte studies and arterial blood gases
Lavender	○	Ethylenediaminetetraacetic acid (EDTA) (anticoagulant)	Hematology studies
Gray	●	Potassium oxalate or sodium fluoride (anticoagulant)	Blood glucose

TABLE 48-2   Blood Collection Tubes

Note: Tubes are listed in the order they should be collected (order of draw).

POINTS ON PRACTICE
Collecting a Blood Culture Specimen

Blood culture specimens are collected to test for the presence of bacteria in the blood. When collecting blood for a culture it is important that no skin organisms contaminate the specimen. Skin organisms like staphylococci and streptococci can cause a false positive blood culture test result. For this reason, proper aseptic technique is essential. Pay special attention to keeping the collection bottle, syringe, and needle sterile and properly cleansing the skin. If you are drawing additional specimens for other tests, always draw the blood culture first. This eliminates the possibility of contaminating the culture with additives from other tubes. When collecting a blood culture specimen you should follow these steps:

1. Select the appropriate site for venipuncture.
2. Cleanse the skin with isopropyl alcohol.
3. Cleanse the skin again with an iodine or chlorhexidine solution applied in an outward circular pattern (cleansing from inside to outside).
4. Allow the iodine solution to air dry.
5. Remove the plastic top from the collection bottle and wipe with a sterile alcohol pad.
6. Allow the alcohol to air dry.
7. Draw the blood from the selected site.
8. Properly label the specimens.

Separate blood specimens are put into two collection bottles, one for aerobic and one for anaerobic culture. You may be asked to draw a second set of specimens from another vein. Use the same technique for each specimen and make sure they are properly identified.

FIGURE 48-5   Various venipuncture and capillary puncture safety devices.

- The device should either not have to be activated by the user or may be activated using only one hand.
- Once the safety feature is activated, it cannot be deactivated.

In certain circumstances, some of these characteristics are not feasible. Drawing blood from an artery or a vein is not possible without the use of a needle. Several types of safety devices for collecting blood specimens have been developed. These include:

- Retracting needles.
- Hinged or sliding shields that cover phlebotomy and winged-steel (butterfly) needles.

- Self-blunting phlebotomy and winged-steel needles.
- Retractable lancets.

Studies show that these devices, when used properly, have reduced needlestick injuries. NIOSH reports a 76% reduction of injuries with self-blunting needles, a 66% reduction with hinged needle shields, and a 23% reduction with sliding shields. Refer to the *Basic Safety and Infection Control* chapter for more information on engineered safety devices.

Capillary Puncture **Capillary puncture** requires a superficial puncture of the skin with a sharp point. Compared with venipuncture, capillary puncture releases a smaller amount of blood. The blood may be collected in small, calibrated glass tubes; collected on glass microscope slides; or applied directly to reagent strips (or dipsticks), which are specially treated paper or plastic strips used in specific diagnostic tests. Blood also may be collected on special cards or paper and sent to an outside laboratory for special screening tests such as PKU. For more information about PKU testing see the Points on Practice: Testing for Phenylketonuria box.

Capillary puncture in adults and children is usually performed on the great (middle) finger or the ring finger. (Use the patient's nondominant hand for this procedure if possible.) The puncture should be made slightly off center on the pad of the fingertip, as the pad's center is usually more sensitive. Capillary puncture in infants is usually performed on one of the outer edges of the underside of the heel (Figure 48-6). An alternate site for both children and adults is the lower part of the earlobe, unless the patient's ear is pierced.

Lancets Lancets are used in the capillary puncture technique. This technique is employed when the amount of blood required for a specific procedure is not very large or when technical difficulties prevent use of the venipuncture technique. A **lancet** is a small, disposable instrument with a sharp point used to puncture the skin and make a shallow

POINTS ON PRACTICE
Testing for Phenylketonuria (PKU)

Phenylketonuria (PKU) is a rare metabolic disorder. It is caused by a mutation in a gene that is responsible for creating an enzyme that breaks down phenylalanine, an amino acid found in protein-rich foods. If this amino acid is not broken down, it accumulates in the body and causes brain damage. Screening newborns for PKU is required in all states.

The screening test is a qualitative test for the presence of phenylalanine and related substances and is usually done 24–48 hours after birth. The newborn must ingest proteins prior to the test to ensure accuracy. Though this test is usually done in the hospital prior to discharge, there may be occasions when it is done in the physician's office.

To perform the test you will perform a capillary puncture on the infant's heel. Collect drops of the infant's blood, usually three or four, on a special card or paper. Make sure the information on the card is complete, including:

- Mother's name and address.
- Ordering physician's name and contact information.
- Baby's name, date of birth and weight.
- Gestational age.
- Date and time of the collection.

incision (between 2.0 and 3.0 mm deep for an adult and no deeper than 2.4 mm for an infant). The blood welling up from the incision is then collected.

Automatic Puncturing Devices **Automatic puncturing devices** are loaded with a lancet. Because the depth to which they puncture the skin is mechanically controlled, they are more accurate and comfortable than the traditional

(a)

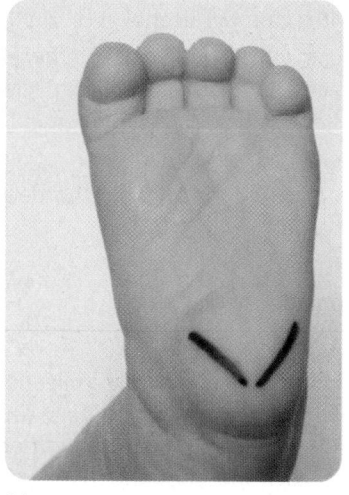

(b)

FIGURE 48-6 Capillary puncture sites for (a) an adult and (b) an infant.

lancet method. These spring-loaded devices have disposable platforms that rest on the finger. Different platforms are used, depending on the desired depth of the puncture. Both the lancet and the platform should be discarded after use. Pen-like devices also can hold a lancet inside. This device is held against the skin and activated by pushing a button. The advantages of these devices are that they are easy to use, the puncture depth can be easily adjusted, and there is an automatic ejection button for lancet disposal. Some companies also manufacture completely disposable devices, which come individually wrapped and are used only once.

Micropipettes A pipette is a calibrated glass tube for measuring fluids. A **micropipette** is a small pipette that holds a small, precise volume of fluid. You will use micropipettes to collect capillary blood for some tests. Capillary tubes, with a single calibration mark, are also used to collect capillary blood for certain tests. Procedure 48-3, at the end of this chapter, explains how to perform a capillary puncture and collect a sample of capillary blood.

MICROTAINER Tubes MICROTAINER tubes (manufactured by Becton Dickinson VACUTAINER Systems) are small plastic tubes with a wide-mouthed collector, similar to a funnel, that allows blood to flow quickly and freely into the tube. Like collection tubes in an evacuation system, MICROTAINER tubes have different colored tops indicating the additives, if any, they contain.

Reagent Products Several common tests do not require processing of fluid blood samples. For these tests, you may apply droplets of freshly collected blood to chemically treated paper or plastic reagent strips (dipsticks) or add freshly collected blood droplets to small containers holding chemicals that react in the presence of specific substances or microorganisms. Some of the blood tests performed in this way detect blood glucose levels, sickle cell anemia, infectious mononucleosis, and rheumatoid arthritis.

Smear Slides You may need to apply a drop of freshly collected blood to a prepared microscope slide for some tests. More commonly, a smear slide is prepared in the laboratory from a blood sample containing an anticoagulant, for examination under a microscope.

▶ Responding to Patient Needs LO 48.3

Many patients are anxious when they have a blood test, and some patients have special needs or present special problems that make drawing blood challenging. Anxiety about blood tests may stem from a variety of concerns. Special needs may be related to a patient's age group or a medical condition. Some problems involve difficulty obtaining a blood sample or the patient's physiological or emotional response to a procedure. Being aware of possible sources of patient anxiety and understanding a wide range of special concerns can help you respond to patient needs with sensitivity and competence.

Patient Fears and Concerns

Some patients express their fears or concerns directly. Other patients ask questions that highlight their fears. Providing more information or a complete understanding is reassuring to many patients. For others, the information serves only to confuse, overwhelm, or create more fear. You must decide how much information to give each patient and be prepared to answer questions.

Patients sometimes ask questions that are not appropriate for you to answer. A patient may ask you about his prognosis, medical condition, blood type, or other medical information. It is not appropriate for you to discuss these topics with the patient. Encourage the patient to discuss these issues with the physician. Some commonly expressed fears and concerns to which you should respond, however, are covered in the following paragraphs.

Pain The question medical assistants performing phlebotomy probably hear most often is, "Will this hurt"? Never lie to a patient who asks this question. Inform the patient that he will feel a stick just as the lancet or point of the needle is inserted but that this pain goes away almost immediately. Tell a patient who seems particularly nervous to take a deep breath and let it out slowly. Also suggest the patient focus on something else in the room or close his eyes and relax during the procedure.

A patient may express concern and report a previous unpleasant experience with blood testing. Listen to the patient's concerns. Describe what you will do to reduce discomfort and what the patient can do to be more at ease. Let the patient know you will help him sit comfortably or lie down while the blood sample is being obtained. Tell the patient to let you know if he begins to feel light-headed. You might also ask the patient whether one arm is better to use than the other. Many patients have had blood drawn before and can tell you which sites were successful. Consulting the patient helps the patient feel more in control and provides you with important information.

Bruises or Scars Some patients may express fear of getting a bruise or scar from a blood test. Explain that some bruising is possible but that it will fade within a few days. Most bruising is caused by a hematoma, which occurs when blood leaks out of the vein and collects under the skin. Hematomas can be prevented by releasing the tourniquet before withdrawing the needle and applying proper pressure over the puncture site after the needle has been withdrawn. Bruising is common with fair-skinned patients. Scars, on the other hand, are unlikely.

Serious Diagnosis Patient fears are not always rational. One fear patients express is that the more tubes of blood you require, the more serious their condition must be. Patients also may fear that a blood test is being done to help the doctor diagnose an extremely serious disease.

You can help relieve a patient's fears by explaining that a blood test is one of the best ways to obtain an overall picture of health (emphasize health, not disease). Note that blood tests show what is normal about the blood as well as any abnormalities. You might also explain that several samples are being taken because the blood used in blood tests is processed in different ways; the blood collected for one test cannot be used in another.

Blood testing also may be done to determine how well and at what levels medications are acting in the blood. Explain that the doctor may want to see how much medication is in the blood to better manage the prescribed dosage. When a patient needs repeated tests for drug levels, explain that the tests show how the body is using the medication.

Contracting a Disease from the Procedure Probably the greatest fear of patients undergoing blood tests is contracting HIV/AIDS or hepatitis B virus (HBV). Although many people are now well informed about how HIV/AIDS and other serious diseases are contracted, it is understandable for a patient to worry about bloodborne pathogens. Do not dismiss the patient's concerns and do not downplay the importance of following Standard Precautions.

Explain the precautions you will take to prevent the spread of infection. Allow the patient to see you wash your hands and put on new gloves before you begin to take the blood sample. Stress that the needle is sterile. Explain that you have not touched the needle and that it will be discarded when you finish. Let the patient see you put the needle in the sharps container.

Use this opportunity to educate the patient about the transmission of HIV/AIDS. Emphasize that HIV/AIDS, and other infections transmitted by blood, can be transmitted only when there is direct contact with contaminated blood or other body fluids. Explain that your gloves protect both you and the patient by providing a barrier to infection transmission from one person to another. Explain that your other protective equipment, such as goggles or a mask, also helps prevent the spread of infection.

Special Considerations

As you collect blood specimens, you will encounter a variety of patients, some of whom have special needs. You will find yourself in many different situations, some of them problematic. Some special needs and problematic situations are fairly common, and you must be prepared to deal with them.

Patients at Risk for Uncontrolled Bleeding Patients who have hemophilia or are taking blood-thinning medications are at risk for uncontrolled bleeding at the collection site. (Hemophilia is a disorder in which the blood does not coagulate at a wound or puncture site.) Be especially careful and alert as you follow the standard procedures for collecting a blood specimen. In addition, hold several gauze squares over the puncture site for at least 5 minutes to make sure bleeding has stopped completely. If uncontrolled bleeding does occur, call the physician immediately.

Difficult Patients You may encounter a particular challenge in working with a patient either because of technical problems or because of personality issues. Being prepared for these situations is the best method for coping with them.

The Difficult Venipuncture There will be times when you simply cannot get a good blood sample. If your first attempt at drawing blood fails, try again at another site. Give the patient (and yourself) a short break and make an attempt on the other arm, for instance. Sometimes the veins in one arm

FIGURE 48-7 Venipuncture chairs are designed to make blood drawing easier and to prevent patients from falling if they should faint.

are easier to work with than the veins in the other arm. If you cannot get a good sample on the second try, stop. Ask for assistance from your supervisor or the doctor.

Fainting Patients It is impossible to predict which patients will have a reaction to a blood-drawing procedure. Generally, however, an ill patient is more likely to experience a reaction than a well patient. The best way to deal with this potential problem is to position every patient so that, if fainting does occur, no injury will result. Have patients sit in a special venipuncture chair (Figure 48-7), designed to help prevent patients from sliding to the floor in the event of fainting. If your office is not equipped with a venipuncture chair, have patients lie down on an examining table. A patient who has a history of fainting or feels ill should lie down with feet elevated or knees drawn up while you complete the procedure. Sometimes just talking with the patient, asking him or her simple questions, will help keep the patient from fainting.

If a patient does faint and the needle is still in the vein, release the tourniquet and withdraw the needle quickly and steadily. Apply pressure to the site. Most people revive promptly and no other action is required. Do not leave the patient alone. Notify the doctor the patient fainted and ask the doctor whether you should continue with the procedure.

If there is a more severe reaction, notify the appropriate staff member and remain with the patient. If the patient is in a chair and begins to slide out, raise the safety arm and gently lower the patient to the floor. Protect the patient's head at all times and make sure the patient is breathing. The doctor should examine the patient before the patient is moved. Follow the doctor's instructions.

When the patient begins to recover, assist the patient into a sitting position and then to a chair or couch. The patient should rest until feeling strong enough to walk—usually about 15 minutes. When the patient feels steady, take the patient to another area of the office, such as the patient reception area. At this point, another staff member usually becomes responsible for the patient's care and determines when it is safe for the patient

CAUTION: HANDLE WITH CARE

Venipuncture Complications

Venipuncture is, in general, a safe procedure. Most of the complications you encounter are mild and more of a nuisance than anything. Venipuncture can have some serious complications, but they are rare. You must be aware of possible complications and ways to avoid them, and you should understand how to deal with them if they occur. Some of the more serious complications you may encounter are:

- **Hematoma.** A collection of blood will sometimes form under the skin. This is especially a problem in patients who have bleeding disorders, are elderly, or are taking anticoagulants. To avoid hematomas, hold the needle as still as possible while filling and changing the tubes. You may need to use a butterfly collection device. Hold pressure on the venipuncture site as soon as you remove the needle. Have the patient elevate her arm but not bend the elbow. If a hematoma does form, apply extra gauze to the puncture site and wrap with stretch bandage. Watch the patient and alert the doctor if necessary.

- *Latex allergy.* Some patients may have an allergy to latex. Make sure you ask the patient if he has any allergies before you begin the procedure. If the patient has a latex allergy, make sure you use nonlatex gloves, tourniquet, and bandages. If the patient has an unexpected allergic reaction to latex, alert the physician and follow her instructions.

- *Nerve injury.* It is essential that you know the anatomy of the antecubital fossa so you can accurately locate the proper veins for venipuncture. Inserting a needle into a nerve can cause nerve damage. Permanent sensory and/or motor damage to the arm and hand can occur if the venipuncture is done incorrectly. If you suspect you have stuck the patient's nerve, withdraw the needle immediately and alert the physician.

- *Infections.* Though quite rare, infections after venipuncture do occur and can be very serious. Use only approved single-use venipuncture equipment. Cleanse the venipuncture site well before the procedure. An infection at the venipuncture site may not be evident for several days after the procedure. If the patient calls complaining of redness, heat, or drainage at the site, have her return to the office to see the physician. A more serious blood infection (sepsis) may first seem like the patient has the flu, as fever and chills are the first symptoms. A patient with a blood infection can go into shock if left untreated. If you suspect the patient has a blood infection, have her see the physician immediately.

---

to leave. Additional information about venipuncture complications is found in the Caution: Handle with Care section.

Angry or Violent Patients Some patients are extremely resistant to having blood drawn. Although their objections may seem illogical, remember, people often do not think as clearly in moments of high emotion as they normally do.

Encourage a patient who is mildly upset and wants to argue about the need for the blood test to let you take the sample and then discuss the situation with the doctor. If you convince the patient to submit to the test, complete the procedure quickly and accurately. Avoid arguing with the patient.

Do not force the issue with a patient who becomes violent or refuses outright to submit to the procedure. A patient does have the right to refuse testing or treatment. Under no circumstances should you attempt to physically force a patient to give a blood sample. Never endanger yourself, other patients, or your colleagues by refusing to back down from an angry or violent patient. Report the problem to the appropriate staff, make a note on the order, and follow other established procedures.

▶ Performing Common Blood Tests LO 48.4

Many blood tests are routinely ordered as part of a complete general exam to determine a patient's overall health. The results of individual tests can provide information that aids in the diagnosis of specific conditions, diseases, and disorders, as noted in Table 48-3.

The number of blood tests routinely performed in POLs has declined since the implementation of Clinical Laboratory Improvement Amendments of 1988 (CLIA '88) regulations. Many POLs now perform only waived tests. Each POL is different, however, and regulations do change. Check with your employer about what tests your office performs regularly. You should be familiar with a wide range of tests and the steps involved with each even if you do not anticipate performing them.

Given that some testing can occur in the POL, you may encounter several chemical substances while performing your responsibilities in the laboratory. Chemicals you might encounter in laboratory work include the following:

- **Anticoagulants**, which cause the blood to remain in a liquid, uncoagulated state.

- **Serum separators**, which form a gel-like barrier between serum and the clot in a coagulated blood sample.

- Stains, which color particular cells, making microscopic studies easier to complete.

Anticoagulants or serum separators are always present in blood-collection tubes and do not need to be added to the sample.

You must be absolutely clear about which chemicals are used for which tests and the precise amounts involved. It is also important to understand the purpose of blood tests so you can educate patients. You must, in addition, know the range of normal test values so you can be aware of potential problems and note them for the doctor's attention. Table 48-4 shows the normal ranges for a variety of blood tests.

TABLE 48-3   Common Blood Tests and the Conditions They Help Identify

Substance Identified or Quantified	Stopper Color and Additive	Part of Blood Tested	Indication, Disease, or Disorder
Alanine aminotransferase (ALT)	Clot activator / Silicone serum separator	Serum	Liver disorders
Alpha-fetoprotein (AFP)	Clot activator / Silicone serum separator	Fetal serum	Fetal liver and gastrointestinal tract status, and hepatitis
Amylase	Clot activator / Silicone serum separator	Serum	Drug toxicity and parotid or pancreas disorders
Angiotensin-converting enzyme (ACE)	Clot activator / Silicone serum separator	Serum	Lung cancer, sarcoidosis, and acute or chronic bronchitis
Antidiuretic hormone (ADH)	EDTA	Plasma	Syndrome of inappropriate ADH, Guillain-Barré syndrome, and brain tumor
Aspartate aminotransferase (AST)	Clot activator / Silicone serum separator	Serum	Liver disease (including viral hepatitis), infectious mononucleosis, and damaged heart or skeletal muscle
Bilirubin	Clot activator / Silicone serum separator	Serum	Liver disease, fructose intolerance, and hypothyroidism
Blood urea nitrogen (BUN)	Clot activator / Silicone serum separator	Serum	Kidney disorders
Calcium, total (fasting)	Clot activator / Silicone serum separator	Serum	Hyperparathyroidism and malignant disease with bone involvement
Cancer antigens (numbers 125, 15-3, 549, 72-4), tumor-associated glycoprotein (TAG)	Clot activator / Silicone serum separator	Serum	Specific cancers identified, depending on antigen tested
Carbon dioxide, total	Clot activator / Silicone serum separator	Venous serum	Acidosis or alkalosis (acid-base balance)

TABLE 48-3 *(concluded)*

Substance Identified or Quantified	Stopper Color and Additive	Part of Blood Tested	Indication, Disease, or Disorder
Cholesterol, total	Clot activator	Serum	Hyperlipoproteinemia, coronary artery disease, and atherosclerosis
	Silicone serum separator		
Creatine kinase (CK)	EDTA	Serum	Muscular dystrophies, Reye's syndrome, heart disease, shock, and some neoplasms
Erythrocyte count (RBC)	EDTA	Whole blood	Anemia
Erythrocyte sedimentation rate (ESR)	EDTA	Whole blood	Inflammation, infectious diseases, malignant neoplasms, and sickle cell anemia
Glucose (fasting)	Potassium oxalate or sodium fluoride	Whole blood	Pancreatic function and ability of intravenous insulin to offset diet in diabetes mellitus
Glucose (fasting—tolerance test)	Potassium oxalate or sodium fluoride	Serum	Diabetes mellitus and hypoglycemia
Lactate dehydrogenase (LD)	Clot activator	Serum	Anemia, viral hepatitis, shock, hypoxia, and hyperthermia
	Silicone serum separator		
Leukocyte count (WBC)	EDTA	Whole blood	Leukemia, infection, and leukocytosis
Phenylalanine	Heparin or newborn screening card	Plasma	Hyperphenylalaninemia, obesity, and phenylketonuria
Potassium (K+) and sodium (Na+)	Clot activator	Serum	Fluid-electrolyte balance
	Silicone serum separator		
Prostate specific antigen (PSA)	Clot activator	Serum	Prostate cancer and BPH
	Silicone serum separator		
Sickle cells	EDTA	Whole blood	Sickle cell anemia
Thyroid-stimulating hormone (TSH), triiodothyronine (T_3), thyroxine (T_4)	Clot activator	Serum	Thyroid function
	Silicone serum separator		
Uric acid	Clot activator	Serum	Gout and leukemia
	Silicone serum separator		

Note: Various laboratories may have different testing protocols and require other tube tops than those represented in this table. Consult your laboratory procedures manual for additional information regarding required collection tubes.

TABLE 48-4 Normal Ranges for Blood Tests

Blood Test	Stopper Color and Additive*	Blood Component Tested	Normal Range**
Blood Counts			
Red blood cells (erythrocytes)		EDTA	
Men		Whole blood	$4.7–6.1 \times 10^6$ cells/mcL
Women		Whole blood	$4.2–5.4 \times 10^6$ cells/mcL
White blood cells (leukocytes)		EDTA Whole blood	$4.5–11.0 \times 10^3$ cells/mcL
Platelets		Whole blood	$150–400 \times 10^3$ cells/mcL
Differential			
Neutrophils		Whole blood	40%–60%
Eosinophils		Whole blood	1%–4%
Basophils		Whole blood	0.5%–1%
Lymphocytes		Whole blood	20%–40%
Monocytes		Whole blood	2%–8%
Hematocrit (Hct)		EDTA Whole blood	
Men			40.7%–50.3%
Women			36.1%–44.3%
Hemoglobin (Hb, Hgb)		EDTA Whole blood	
Men			13.8–17.2 g/dL
Women			12.1–15.1 g/dL
Erythrocyte Sedimentation Rate (ESR)			
Wintrobe		EDTA Whole blood	
Men			0–5 mm/hour
Women			0–15 mm/hour
Westergren		Whole blood	
Men			0–15 mm/hour
Women			0–20 mm/hour
Coagulation Tests			
Prothrombin time (PT)		Sodium citrate	Plasma	11–15 seconds
Bleeding time		Sodium citrate	Whole blood	2–7 minutes
Electrolytes			
Bicarbonate (HCO_3^-)		Clot activator	Arterial plasma	21–28 mEq/L
			Venous plasma	27–29 mEq/L
Calcium (Ca^{++})			Serum	8.6–10.0 mEq/L
Chloride (Cl^-)			Serum, plasma	98–108 mEq/L
Potassium (K^+)		Silicone serum separator	Serum	3.5–5.1 mEq/L
Sodium (Na^+)			Serum	136–145 mEq/L
Chemical and Serologic Tests			
Alanine aminotransferase (ALT)		Clot activator	Serum	
Men		Silicone serum separator		10–40 U/L
Women				7–35 U/L
Alpha-fetoprotein (AFP)		Clot activator	Serum	
Fetal, first trimester		Silicone serum separator		20–400 mg/dL
Adult				<15 ng/mL

TABLE 48-4 (continued)

Blood Test	Stopper Color and Additive*		Blood Component Tested	Normal Range**
Aspartate aminotransferase (AST, formerly SGOT)		Clot activator	Serum	
Men				11–26 U/L
Women		Silicone serum separator		10–20 U/L
Bilirubin, total direct		Clot activator	Serum	0.3–1.2 mg/dL
		Silicone serum separator		
Blood urea nitrogen (BUN)		Clot activator	Serum, plasma	6–20 mg/dL
		Silicone serum separator		
Carcinoembryonic antigen (CEA)		Clot activator	Serum	<5.0 ng/mL
		Silicone serum separator		
Cholesterol, total		Clot activator	Serum, plasma	
Men				158–277 mg/dL
Women				162–285 mg/dL
High-density lipoproteins (HDLs)			Serum, plasma	
Men				28–63 mg/dL
Women				37–92 mg/dL
Low-density lipoproteins (LDLs)			Serum, plasma	
Men		Silicone serum separator		89–197 mg/dL
Women				88–201 mg/dL
Creatine kinase (CK)		EDTA	Serum, plasma	
Men				38–174 U/L
Women				26–140 U/L
Creatinine		Clot activator	Serum, plasma	
Men				0.9–1.3 mg/dL
Women		Silicone serum separator		0.6–1.2 mg/dL
Cytomegalovirus (CMV)		Clot activator	Serum	None
		Silicone serum separator		
Epstein-Barr virus (EBV)		Clot activator	Whole blood	None
		Silicone serum separator		
Fibrinogen		Sodium citrate	Plasma	200–400 mg/dL
Glucose (fasting blood sugar, FBS)		Potassium oxalate or sodium fluoride	Serum	74–120 mg/dL

(continued)

TABLE 48-4 *(concluded)*

Blood Test	Stopper Color and Additive*	Blood Component Tested	Normal Range**
Group A beta-hemolytic streptococci	Clot activator	Serum	None
	Silicone serum separator		
Human immunodeficiency virus (HIV) antibodies	Clot activator	Serum, plasma	None
	Silicone serum separator		
Insulin	Clot activator	Serum	<17 micro U/mL
	Silicone serum separator		
Iron, total	Clot activator	Serum	
Men			65–175 micrograms/dL
Women	Silicone serum separator		50–170 micrograms/dL
Lactate dehydrogenase (LD)	Clot activator	Serum, plasma	140–280 U/L
	Silicone serum separator		
pH	Clot activator	Arterial blood	7.35–7.45
		Venous blood	7.32–7.43
	Silicone serum separator		
Proteins	Clot activator	Serum	
Total			6.2–8.0 g/dL
Albumin	Silicone serum separator		3.4–4.8 g/dL
Uric acid	Clot activator	Serum	
Men Women			4.4–7.6 mg/dL 2.3–6.6 mg/dL
	Silicone serum separator		

*Various laboratories may have different testing protocols and require other tube tops than those represented in this table. Consult your laboratory procedures manual for additional information regarding required collection tubes.

**Reference Ranges for Normal Values may be slightly different in different labs. Consult the reference ranges provided by your individual lab for each test.

Hematologic Tests

Hematologic tests—including blood cell counts, morphologic studies, coagulation tests, and the nonautomated erythrocyte sedimentation rate test—are commonly performed in routine blood testing. These tests can be performed on venous or capillary whole blood samples.

Blood Counts **Whole blood** contains **formed elements** (RBCs, WBCs, and platelets) and a fluid portion (plasma). The total number of blood cells and the percentage of the whole sample each type represents can tell the physician a great deal about a patient's condition. A physician can order an individual test or a **complete blood (cell) count** (CBC), which includes the following tests:

- Red blood (cell) count—the total number of RBCs in a sample.
- White blood (cell) count—the total number of WBCs in a sample.
- Differential WBC count—the percentage of each type of WBC (basophils, eosinophils, neutrophils, lymphocytes, and monocytes) in the first 100 leukocytes of a sample.
- Platelet count (automated)—the number of platelets in a sample, or a platelet estimate, which indicates whether the amount of platelets is adequate.
- Hematocrit determination—identifies how much of a sample's volume (expressed as a percentage) is made up of RBCs after the sample has spun in a centrifuge.

- Hemoglobin determination—measures the amount of hemoglobin by weight per volume in the sample.

Most POLs use automated equipment for performing blood counts, but you need to understand how to perform blood counts manually. Check your state regulations and office policy to find out if you are allowed to perform differential blood counts. Knowing how to perform blood counts manually provides a backup for the automated instrumentation and puts you in a better position to recognize unusual findings among automated results. All manual counts are estimates. The types of blood cell counts differ in sample preparation and in the equipment and methods used.

Differential Cell Counts You will prepare a blood smear slide and stain the smear for a differential cell count. Procedure 48-4, at the end of this chapter, details preparation of a blood smear slide. When you carry out this process correctly, there will be a region of the slide where blood cells are dense but lie in a single plane (not stacked or bunched together). This is the region where the cells are counted.

A polychromatic (multicolored) stain like Wright's stain simplifies a differential cell count. The blue and red-orange dyes (methylene blue and eosin, respectively) stain cell structures in ways that identify each of the five WBC types. The staining characteristics of each WBC type are listed below:

- Neutrophils—dark purple nucleus and pale pink cytoplasm containing fine pink or lavender granules.
- Basophils—purple nucleus and light purple cytoplasm containing large, blue-black granules.
- Eosinophils—purple nucleus and bright orange granules in pink cytoplasm.
- Lymphocytes—large, dark purple nucleus surrounded by a small amount of blue cytoplasm.
- Monocytes—the largest WBC, has gray-blue cytoplasm.

There are several types of blood staining kits. Follow the manufacturer's instructions when performing this procedure.

Figure 48-8 shows the zigzag pattern for counting leukocytes visible in the field when using the microscope's oil-immersion objective. A total of 100 leukocytes are counted and recorded on a differential counter. Each cell type is expressed as a percentage of the 100 leukocytes counted. The platelet count is averaged in 10 to 15 fields.

Go to CONNECT to see a video about *Preparing a Blood Smear Slide.*

Hematocrit You measure a patient's hematocrit percentage by collecting a small sample of the patient's blood in a microhematocrit tube, sealing the tube, and spinning it in a centrifuge. This process is described in Procedure 48-5, at the end of this chapter. During this process, heavier RBCs move to one end of the tube and lighter plasma moves to the other end. Between the RBCs, or **packed red blood cells**, and the plasma is the buffy coat (Figure 48-9). The **buffy coat** contains the WBCs and platelets.

Feather edge | Counting area | Thick end | Frosted end

John Smith 11/25/XX

FIGURE 48-8 Follow this pattern when counting leukocytes visible in the field under the oil-immersion objective of the microscope.

Microhematocrit tube

Plasma

Buffy coat

Packed red blood cells

Sealing clay

FIGURE 48-9 Blood in a centrifuged microhematocrit tube separates into packed red blood cells, the buffy coat, and plasma.

Always run two samples of the patient's blood specimen. After removing each sample from the centrifuge, compare the column of packed RBCs with a standard hematocrit gauge. Read on the gauge the percentage of total blood volume represented by the RBCs. Average the readings of the two patient samples. (The samples should be within 2% of each other. If they are not, repeat the test.)

Go to CONNECT to see a video about *Measuring Hematocrit Percentage after Centrifuge.*

Automated Hematocrit Readers You also may use a hand-held device to obtain hematocrit readings. Devices like the UltraCrit® are CLIA-waived testing devices for rapid and accurate measurement of hematocrit. The test may be completed on venous or capillary blood and results are obtained in less than one minute. These devices are often used by blood banks to rapidly screen donors for eligibility to donate.

Hemoglobin Hemoglobin resides within the RBCs. You will determine the concentration of hemoglobin in the blood by lysing (rupturing) the RBCs (**hemolysis**) and evaluating the color of the sample. This procedure may be done with a hemoglobinometer—a handheld device that makes color evaluation less subjective (open for interpretation) than older methods of visually matching with color samples. Older testing methods had to be read by the human eye, leaving test interpretation up to the individual eye. Any change in color perception by the person reading the test could affect the test result reading. Blood specimens mixed with a reagent, such as Drabkin's reagent, undergo a color reaction that can be quantified by reading color intensity in a photoelectric colorimeter (an instrument that uses light to read color).

Several automated hemoglobin analyzers are now included on the CLIA '88 waived list. These analyzers measure the amount of hemoglobin in a whole blood sample using a photometer (an instrument used to measure absorbed light). The blood sample can be obtained from either a finger stick or venous blood. Examples of automated hemoglobin analyzers are HemoCue HB 301 Analyzer® (HemoCue AB) and the HemoPoint H2 Hemoglobin Measurement System® (Stanbio Laboratory). Follow the manufacturer's instructions when performing these tests.

Morphologic Studies **Morphology** is the study of the shape or form of objects, which is often performed just after the differential count and platelet estimate on the same blood smear slide. A morphologic study of a blood sample can provide important information about a patient's condition. It examines a blood smear sample and records the appearance and shape of cells for abnormal size, shape, or content and abnormal cell organization. Morphologic studies require special training and are not routinely done by medical assistants.

Coagulation Tests A physician may order coagulation tests to identify potential bleeding problems before surgical procedures or to monitor therapeutic drug levels when a patient is receiving medications like heparin or warfarin (Coumadin). Coagulation studies include the prothrombin time (PT) and partial thromboplastin time (PTT) tests. These tests are usually performed using automated devices like the Coaguchek XS System® (Roche Diagnostics) or the Alere IN-Ratio System® (Alere). These systems monitor the changing pattern of light transmission through the sample as coagulation occurs and calculate the INR (International Normalized Ratio). The INR—used to evaluate patients who are taking blood thinners like warfarin—measures the amount of time it takes for the test sample to clot and compares it to a reference average. The World Health Organization (WHO) developed the INR method so samples from different labs can be compared. Medical assistants sometimes perform these studies.

Erythrocyte Sedimentation Rate The nonautomated **erythrocyte sedimentation rate (ESR)** test measures the rate at which RBCs, the heaviest blood component, settle to the bottom of a blood sample. It is used as a diagnostic tool for inflammatory disease, cancer, and thyroid disease. To run this test, you will transfer freshly collected, anticoagulated blood to a calibrated tube and place the tube in a sedimentation rack (Figure 48-10). You examine the tube an hour later to determine how far the RBCs have fallen. Test results are recorded as millimeters per hour (mm/hr). Several standard testing systems are used, including the Westergren and Wintrobe systems. You must adhere closely to each manufacturer's instructions when using these systems. When performing an ESR, follow these general guidelines to ensure its validity:

- Use only a fresh sample of blood.
- Draw the blood into a tube with anticoagulant additives.
- Temperature, either too hot or too cold, will affect the test. Maintain laboratory temperatures near 70°F.
- Precisely position the sample tubes vertically in the rack. They must not be leaning.
- Avoid vibrating or bumping the rack during the test.
- Avoid introducing bubbles into the sample when transferring blood into the tube.
- Carefully watch the time and read the results at exactly one hour.

FIGURE 48-10 The sedimentation rack holds blood specimens steady and level for the ESR test.

Chemical Tests

Blood chemistry analysis examines several dozen chemicals found in human blood. Tables 48-3 and 48-4 include many of these chemical tests. Highly detailed studies are rarely performed in the POL because they require expensive, sophisticated equipment and techniques. Complex testing is also subject to strict CLIA '88 regulations that increase the administrative work and the need for more highly trained personnel. So, these types of tests are commonly performed at an independent test laboratory. Automated equipment for analyzing blood chemistry, however, is becoming more available, less expensive, and simpler to operate than it was in the past. New waived tests for an increasing array of chemicals in the blood are developed each year, making it more likely that you may use automated equipment to perform some blood chemistry tests. Keeping abreast of new developments will help prepare you for possible changes in your laboratory duties.

Blood Glucose Monitoring Some blood chemistry tests routinely conducted in the POL include blood glucose monitoring, which is often performed by a medical assistant or by a patient. Glucose monitoring systems require sterile lancets to perform a capillary puncture. You will collect the blood on reagent strips that change color in accordance with glucose levels present in the blood. The level is determined either by comparing the color on the strip with color standards provided with the reagent strips or by feeding the strip into a handheld reading device. You will teach patients to perform this kind of test at home. Be sure to stress the importance of following the manufacturer's guidelines for correct operation. Procedure 48-6, at the end of this chapter, outlines the general steps for measuring blood glucose using a handheld glucometer.

You also will teach patients and their families how to manage diabetes. This will include performing the blood glucose test, managing diet and exercise, self-monitoring for complications associated with diabetes, and providing additional resources for further education. See the Educating the Patient feature.

Go to CONNECT to see a video about *Measuring Blood Glucose Using a Handheld Glucometer.*

Hemoglobin A1c Another test used to monitor the health of diabetic patients is the hemoglobin A1c test, which measures the amount of glycosylated hemoglobin (hemoglobin with glycosal groups attached) in the blood. When blood glucose levels are elevated, the glucose molecules bind with hemoglobin to form hemoglobin A1c (HgBA1c). Once HgBA1c is formed, it remains for the RBC's life (90 to 120 days), making it a useful tool for monitoring the overall stability of the patient's blood glucose.

It is important for a patient to maintain a normal blood glucose level. Large fluctuations in blood sugar are problematic in patients with diabetes and can cause complications such as eye disease, stroke, renal failure, and cardiovascular disease. The HgBA1c test gives the physician a good overall picture of

the patient's compliance to and the effectiveness of diabetes treatment.

Several options for performing this test include:

- Sending it to an outside reference laboratory. Results are available in 1 to 7 days.
- Performing it in the office laboratory if the necessary equipment is available. Results are usually available in less than 10 minutes.
- Taking the test at home. Several home tests are available, allowing the patient to monitor his own HgBA1c levels and therefore, the efficiency of his diabetes treatment.

Testing of HgBA1c should always be done in conjunction with routine blood glucose monitoring. Daily monitoring of blood glucose helps the patient with insulin therapy and diet maintenance. HgBA1c monitoring is important in assessing the patient's overall glucose levels. The advantages of this testing include:

- No pretesting preparation. The test may be done without regard to meals.
- Better overall assessment of long-term blood glucose control. Blood glucose testing gives information about glucose levels at one point in time. HgBA1c gives information over a period of 2 to 3 months.

Patients should have their HgBA1c levels checked two to four times per year. The target range for HgBA1c levels is less than 7%. Patients whose HgBA1c levels exceed 8% are at a greater risk for diabetes-associated complications.

Cholesterol Tests Blood cholesterol tests are performed on a routine basis in the POL. Several automated devices can be used for metabolic chemistry testing both in the POL and at home. These analyzers test a variety of blood chemicals, including glucose, total cholesterol, HDL cholesterol, and triglycerides. The sample required is minimal and can be obtained with a capillary puncture.

FDA-approved waived tests include:

- Polymer Technology Systems CardioChek Analyzer® (Polymer Technology Systems, Inc.)
- SpotChem HDL, Total Cholesterol, and Triglyceride® (Arkray, Inc.)
- Piccolo Lipid Panel Plus Reagent Disc® (Abaxis, Inc.)

Serologic Tests

Serologic tests detect the presence of specific substances in a blood sample. The terms *serologic test* and *immunoassay* refer to the introduction of an antigen or antibody into the specimen and the detection of a specific reaction to the antigen or antibody. Serologic testing methods can be used to detect disease antibodies, drugs, hormones, and vitamins in the blood and to determine blood types. They also are used to test urine and other body fluids.

Immunoassays Although medical assistants usually do not perform immunoassays, you should be familiar with

Managing Diabetes

Diabetes affects an estimated 6 percent of the population, with more than 1 million newly diagnosed cases each year. In order to reduce the complications associated with diabetes, patients need to maintain stable blood sugar. Proper patient education and medical care will help patients achieve this goal. As a medical assistant, you can assist patients and their families by providing them with information about diabetes that includes:

1. The risks and consequences associated with uncontrolled blood sugar. Patients whose blood sugar is unstable are at greater risk of developing the following conditions:
   - Loss of vision
   - Kidney failure
   - Heart disease
   - Nerve damage
   - Stroke

2. The patient's type of diabetes. Patients need to know the type of diabetes they have so they can understand the type of treatment prescribed. The types of diabetes are:
   - Type 1 diabetes—An autoimmune disorder characterized by the body's inability to make enough insulin. Insulin is required for glucose utilization. Patients with Type I diabetes will need to take insulin daily.
   - Type 2 diabetes—The most common type of diabetes. Insulin is still being produced at normal levels but can no longer be utilized by the body's cells. This causes a buildup of unused glucose in the blood. This type of diabetes is often controlled with careful diet management and increased exercise. A number of oral medications also can be used.
   - Gestational diabetes—Develops only during pregnancy. This type of diabetes is generally managed through proper diet and exercise. Careful monitoring is important to reduce the risk of fetal complications. Women who have had gestational diabetes have an increased risk of developing Type 2 diabetes.

3. Maintaining proper diet and exercise, including:
   - Making proper food choices.
   - Keeping a food diary.
   - Reading food labels.
   - Choosing proper food exchanges.
   - Creating and implementing a routine exercise program.

4. Routine self-monitoring of blood sugar and hemoglobin A1c levels. Information should include:
   - The types of blood glucose monitors available. Figure 48-11 illustrates one type—a glucometer.
   - Instructions on obtaining monitoring supplies.
   - The number of times and the specific intervals at which blood sugar should be checked, based on individual needs and the physician's recommendations.

FIGURE 48-11 A handheld glucometer is an important tool in helping patients manage diabetes.

   - Instructions on performing blood glucose testing.
   - Guidelines on how to maintain a chart of blood glucose levels, including the time of day, associated meals and activities, and actual blood sugar values.
   - Hemoglobin A1c monitoring. The patient should understand what hemoglobin A1c is and why it is important to monitor these values.
   - Normal (target) values for blood glucose and hemoglobin A1c:
     - Blood glucose levels should remain between 70 and 130 mg/dL before meals and less than 180 mg/dL for 1 to 2 hours after meals. Target ranges may be different for each patient. Consult with the physician about individual blood glucose levels.
     - Hemoglobin A1c is a test that shows the average amount of glucose in the blood over a three-month period. Ideally, this value should be less than 7%.

5. Symptoms of uncontrolled blood sugar. Patients need to be aware of the symptoms of both high and low blood sugar—both require immediate attention. Patients should test their blood sugar if any of the following occur:
   - Nausea, vomiting, or abdominal pain.
   - Feeling tired all the time.
   - Excessive thirst or dry mouth.
   - Flushed skin.
   - Confusion or difficulty thinking.

6. Self-screening for diabetes complications. Patients should be aware of the complications associated with diabetes and how to recognize them, and should be instructed to do the following:
   - Perform a daily foot inspection for sores.
   - Recognize changes in vision.

- Recognize the symptoms of kidney failure, which include nausea, vomiting, yellow skin, and swelling of the hands and feet.
- Recognize early signs of nerve damage, which include numbness and tingling of the arms, hands, feet, or legs; dizziness; double vision; and drooping of the eyelid or lip.

7. **Additional sources of information.** Encourage patients to continue their education about diabetes. Providing patients with additional information encourages them to take an active role in controlling their diabetes. Additional information sources include:

- American Association of Diabetes Educators 1-800-338-DMED
- American Diabetes Association 1-800-DIABETES
- American Dietetic Association 1-800-366-1665
- Centers for Disease Control and Prevention Diabetes Public Health Resource, 1-800-CDC-INFO (232-4636)
- Juvenile Diabetes Research Foundation International 1-800-223-1138
- National Institute of Diabetes and Digestive and Kidney Diseases: National Diabetes Information Clearinghouse, 1-800-860-8747

several immunoassay methods that have common applications. These methods include:

- Western blot, in which antigens are blotted onto special filter paper for examination. Western blot tests are generally used to confirm HIV infection diagnosis.
- Radioimmunoassay (RIA), in which radioisotopes are used to "tag" antibodies. RIA tests are extremely sensitive and are generally performed in a reference laboratory.
- Enzyme-linked immunosorbent assay (ELISA), in which enzyme-labeled antigens and substances that can absorb antigens generate reactions to specific antibodies. These reactions are identified through visual or photoelectric color detection. HIV infection is diagnosed using an ELISA test.
- Immunofluorescent antibody (IFA) test, in which dye, visible when the sample is examined under a fluorescent microscope, colors specific antibodies.

Rapid Screening Tests Several serologic tests have been developed for quick processing. Some, like early pregnancy tests performed on urine, are available for home use. There

are also rapid screening tests for detecting antibodies to certain infections, including

- Infectious mononucleosis
  - LifeSign Status Mono (Princeton Boimeditech Corp.)
  - BioStar Acceava Mono II (Acon Laboratories, Inc.)
- HIV
  - Clearview HIV—Stat-Pak (Chembio Diagnostic Systems, Inc.)
  - Uni-gold Recombigen HIV Test (Trinity Biotech plc)
- *Helicobacter pylori*
  - Rapid Response *H. pylori* Rapid Test Device (Acon Laboratories, Inc.)
  - Beckman Coulter ICON HP Test (Princeton Biomed-tech Corp.)

When you use tests of these types or explain their use to a patient, keep in mind that the manufacturer's guidelines must be carefully followed to ensure accurate results. Procedure 48-7, at the end of this chapter, outlines the steps for performing a rapid mononucleosis test.

PROCEDURE 48-1 Quality Control Procedures for Blood Specimen Collection

Procedure Goal: To follow proper quality control procedures when taking a blood specimen.

OSHA Guidelines:

Materials: Necessary sterile equipment, specimen-collection container, paperwork related to the type of blood test the specimen is being drawn for, requisition form, marker, and proper packing materials for transport.

Method: Procedure steps.

1. Review the request form for the test ordered, verify the procedure, prepare the necessary equipment and paperwork, and prepare the work area.
2. Identify the patient and explain the procedure. Confirm the patient's identification. Ask the patient to spell her name. Make sure the patient understands the procedure to be performed, even if she has had it done before.

3. Confirm the patient has followed any pretest preparation requirements such as fasting, taking any necessary medication, or stopping a medication. For example, if a fasting specimen is being taken, the patient should not have eaten anything after midnight of the day before. Some doctors' offices will let the patient drink water or black coffee, however. It often depends on the type of specimen being taken.

   RATIONALE: The test may be invalid if the patient did not follow the pretest instruction.

4. Collect the specimen properly. Collect it at the right time intervals if that applies. Use sterile equipment and proper technique.

5. Use the correct specimen-collection containers and the right preservatives, if required. For example, blood collected into a test tube with additives should be mixed immediately.

   RATIONALE: To prevent clotting.

6. Immediately label the specimens. The label should include the patient's name, the date and time of collection, the test's name, and the name of the person collecting the specimen. Do not label the containers before collecting the specimen.

   RATIONALE: To keep from wasting tubes if there is a problem drawing the blood.

7. Follow correct procedures for disposing of hazardous specimen waste and decontaminating the work area. Used needles, for instance, should immediately be placed in a biohazard sharps container.

8. Thank the patient. Keep the patient in the office if any follow-up observation is necessary.

9. If the specimen is to be transported to an outside laboratory, prepare it for transport in the proper container for that type of specimen, according to OSHA regulations. Place the container in a clear plastic bag with a zip closure and dual pockets with the international biohazard label imprinted in red or orange. The requisition form should be placed in the bag's outside pocket. This ensures protection from contamination if the specimen leaks. Have a courier pick up the specimen and place it in an appropriate carrier (like an insulated cooler) with the biohazard label. Place specimens to be sent by mail in appropriate plastic containers, and then place the containers inside a heavy duty plastic container with a screw-down, nonleaking lid. Then place this container in either a heavy-duty cardboard box or a nylon bag. The words *Human Specimen* or *Body Fluids* should be imprinted on the box or bag. Seal with a strong tape strip.

   RATIONALE: To protect the courier or anyone who handles the package from exposure to bloodborne pathogens.

PROCEDURE 48-2 Performing Venipuncture Using an Evacuation System

Procedure Goal: To collect a venous blood sample using an evacuation system.

OSHA Guidelines:

Materials: VACUTAINER components (safety needle, needle holder/adapter, collection tubes), antiseptic and cotton balls or antiseptic wipes, tourniquet, sterile gauze squares, and sterile adhesive bandages.

Method: Procedure steps.

1. Review the laboratory request form and make sure you have the necessary supplies.

2. Greet the patient, confirm the patient's identity, and introduce yourself.

3. Explain the purpose of the procedure and confirm that the patient has followed the pretest instructions.

   RATIONALE: To ensure the test will be valid.

4. Make sure the patient is sitting in a venipuncture chair or is lying down.

5. Wash your hands. Don exam gloves.

6. Prepare the safety needle holder/adapter assembly by inserting the threaded side of the needle into the adapter and twisting the adapter in a clockwise direction. Push the first collection tube into the other end of the needle holder/adapter until the outer edge of the collection tube stopper meets the guideline.

   RATIONALE: So the tube is stabilized but not completely punctured.

7. Ask the patient whether one arm is better than the other for the venipuncture. The chosen arm should be positioned slightly downward.

FIGURE Procedure 48-2 Step 7   The patient's arm should be positioned slightly downward for a venipuncture.

8. Apply the tourniquet to the patient's upper arm midway between the elbow and the shoulder. Wrap the tourniquet around the patient's arm and cross the ends. Holding one end of the tourniquet against the patient's arm, stretch the other end to apply pressure against the patient's skin. Pull a loop of the stretched end under the end held tightly against the patient's skin, as shown in the figure below. The tourniquet should be tight enough to cause the veins to stand out but should not stop the flow of blood. You should still be able to feel the patient's radial pulse.
RATIONALE: To make the veins in the forearm stand out more prominently.

FIGURE Procedure 48-2 Step 8   Applying a tourniquet makes it easier to find a patient's vein when you are drawing blood.

9. Palpate the proposed site and use your index finger to locate the vein, as shown in the figure. The vein will feel like a small tube with some elasticity. If you feel a pulsing beat, you have located an artery. Do not draw blood from an artery. If you cannot locate the vein within 1 minute, release the tourniquet and allow blood to flow freely for 1 to 2 minutes. Then reapply the tourniquet and try again to locate the vein.

FIGURE Procedure 48-2 Step 9   Use your index finger to locate the vein.

10. After locating the vein, clean the area with an antiseptic wipe. Use a circular motion to clean the area, starting at the center and working outward. Allow the site to air-dry.
RATIONALE: The alcohol could interfere with some of the tests.

11. Remove the plastic cap from the outer point of the needle cover and ask the patient to tighten the fist. Hold the patient's skin taut below the insertion site.
RATIONALE: To anchor the vein so it does not roll.

12. With a steady and quick motion, insert the needle—held at a 15-degree angle, bevel side up, and aligned parallel to the vein—into the vein. You will feel a slight resistance as the needle tip penetrates the vein wall. Penetrate to a depth of ¼ to ½ inch. Grasp the holder/adapter between your index and great (middle) fingers. Using your thumb, seat the collection tube firmly into place over the needle point, puncturing the rubber stopper. Blood will begin to flow into the collection tube.

FIGURE Procedure 48-2 Step 12   When performing venipuncture, hold the needle at a 15-degree angle.

13. Fill each tube until the blood stops running to ensure the correct proportion of blood to additives. Switch tubes as needed by pulling one tube out of the adapter and inserting the next in a smooth and steady motion. (The soft plastic cover on the inner point of the needle retracts as each tube is inserted and recovers the needle point as each tube is removed.)

14. Once blood is flowing steadily, ask the patient to release the fist and untie the tourniquet by pulling the end of the tucked-in loop. The tourniquet should, in general, be left on no longer than 1 minute.
    RATIONALE: Longer periods may cause hemoconcentration, an increase in the blood-cell-to-plasma ratio, and invalidate test results.
    You must remove the tourniquet before you withdraw the needle from the vein.
    RATIONALE: Removing the tourniquet releases pressure on the vein.

15. As you withdraw the needle in a smooth and steady motion, place a sterile gauze square over the insertion site. Immediately activate the safety device on the needle if it is not self-activating. Properly dispose of the needle immediately. Instruct the patient to hold the gauze pad in place with slight pressure. The patient should keep the arm straight and slightly elevated for several minutes.
    RATIONALE: To reduce the possibility of a hematoma.

16. If the collection tubes contain additives, you will need to invert them slowly several times.

FIGURE Procedure 48-2 Step 15   Place a sterile gauze square over the insertion site as you withdraw the needle.

RATIONALE: To mix the chemical agent and the blood sample.

17. Label specimens and complete the paperwork.

18. Check the patient's condition and the puncture site for bleeding. Replace the sterile gauze square with a sterile adhesive bandage.

19. Properly dispose of used supplies and disposable instruments and disinfect the work area.

20. Remove the gloves and wash your hands.

21. Instruct the patient about care of the puncture site.

22. Document the procedure in the patient's chart.

PROCEDURE 48-3 Performing Capillary Puncture

Procedure Goal: To collect a capillary blood sample using the finger puncture method.

OSHA Guidelines:

Materials: Capillary puncture device (safety lancet or automatic puncture device like an Autolet or Glucolet), antiseptic and cotton balls or antiseptic wipes, sterile gauze squares, sterile adhesive bandages, reagent strips, micropipettes, and smear slides.

Method: Procedure steps.

1. Review the laboratory request form and make sure you have the necessary supplies.

2. Greet the patient, confirm the patient's identity, and introduce yourself.

3. Explain the purpose of the procedure and confirm that the patient has followed the pretest instructions, if indicated.
   RATIONALE: The test may be invalid if the patient did not follow the pretest instructions.

4. Make sure the patient is sitting in the venipuncture chair or is lying down.

5. Wash your hands. Don exam gloves.

6. Examine the patient's hands to determine which finger to use for the procedure. Avoid fingers that are swollen, bruised, scarred, or calloused. Generally, the ring and great (middle) fingers are the best choices. If you notice the patient's hands are cold, you may want to warm them between your own, have the patient put them in a warm basin of water or under warm running water, or wrap them in a warm cloth.
   RATIONALE: Warming the patient's hands improves circulation.

7. Prepare the patient's finger with a gentle "massaging" or rubbing motion toward the fingertip. Keep the patient's

hand below heart level so that gravity helps the blood flow.

8. Clean the area with a cotton ball moistened with antiseptic or an antiseptic wipe. Allow the site to air-dry.
   RATIONALE: The alcohol may interfere with some tests.

9. Hold the patient's finger between your thumb and forefinger. Hold the safety lancet or automatic puncture device at a right angle to the patient's fingerprint, as shown in the figure below. Puncture the skin on the pad of the fingertip with a quick, sharp motion. The depth to which you puncture the skin is generally determined by the length of the lancet point. Most automatic puncturing devices are designed to penetrate to the correct depth.

FIGURE Procedure 48-3 Step 9 Hold the lancet or automatic puncture device at a right angle to the patient's fingerprint.

10. Allow a drop of blood to form at the end of the patient's finger. If the blood droplet is slow in forming, apply steady pressure. Avoid milking the patient's finger.
    RATIONALE: It dilutes the blood sample with tissue fluid and causes hemolysis.

FIGURE Procedure 48-3 Step 10 Apply steady pressure to the patient's finger, but do not milk it.

11. Wipe away the first droplet of blood. (This droplet is usually contaminated with tissue fluids released when the skin is punctured.) Then fill the collection devices, as described.

    Micropipettes: Hold the tip of the tube just to the edge of the blood droplet. The tube will fill through capillary action. If you are preparing microhematocrit tubes, you need to seal one end of each tube with clay sealant. (See Procedure 48-5 for this process.)

FIGURE Procedure 48-3 Step 11 Touch the tube to the drop of blood to fill it.

    Reagent strips: With some reagent strips (dipsticks), you must touch the strip to the blood drop but not smear it; with other strips, you must smear it. Follow the manufacturer's guidelines.

    Smear slides: Gently touch the blood droplet to the smear slide and process the slide as described in Procedure 48-4.

12. After you have collected the required samples, dispose of the lancet immediately. Then wipe the patient's finger with a sterile gauze square. Instruct the patient to apply pressure to stop the bleeding.

FIGURE Procedure 48-3 Step 12 Use a sterile gauze square to wipe remaining blood from the patient's finger.

13. Label specimens and complete the paperwork. Some tests, such as glucose monitoring, must be completed immediately.

14. Check the puncture site for bleeding. If necessary, replace the sterile gauze square with a sterile adhesive bandage.

15. Properly dispose of used supplies and disposable instruments and disinfect the work area.

16. Remove the gloves and wash your hands.

17. Instruct the patient about care of the puncture site.

18. Document the procedure in the patient's chart. (If the test has been completed, include the results.)

PROCEDURE 48-4   Preparing a Blood Smear Slide

Procedure Goal: To prepare a blood specimen to be used in a morphologic or other study.

OSHA Guidelines:

Materials: Blood specimen (from either a capillary puncture or a specimen tube containing anticoagulated blood), capillary tubes, sterile gauze squares, slide with frosted end, and wooden applicator sticks.

Method: Procedure steps.

1. Wash your hands and don exam gloves.

2. If using blood from a capillary puncture, follow the steps in Procedure 48-3 to express a drop of blood from the patient's finger. If using a venous sample, check the specimen for proper labeling, carefully uncap the specimen tube, and use wooden applicator sticks to remove any coagulated blood from the inside rim of the tube. You may use a special safety transfer device if available.
   RATIONALE: Uncapping the specimen tube puts you at risk of exposure to bloodborne pathogens. The blood can spray or splatter or the tube could break. The safety device decreases the likelihood of exposure.

3. Touch the tip of the capillary tube to the blood specimen either from the patient's finger or the specimen tube. The tube will take up the correct amount through capillary action.

4. Pull the capillary tube away from the sample, holding it carefully to prevent spillage. Wipe the outside of the capillary tube with a sterile gauze square.
   RATIONALE: To remove excess blood.

5. With the slide on the work surface, hold the capillary tube in one hand and the frosted end of the slide against the work surface with the other.

6. Apply a drop of blood to the slide, about ¾ inch from the frosted end, as shown in the figure below. Place the capillary tube in the sharps container.

FIGURE Procedure 48-4 Step 6   Apply a drop of blood to the slide about ¾ inch from the frosted end.

7. Pick up the spreader slide with your dominant hand. Hold the slide at approximately a 30- to 35-degree angle. Place the edge of the spreader slide on the smear slide close to the unfrosted end. Pull the spreader slide toward the frosted end until the spreader slide touches the blood drop. Capillary action will spread the droplet along the edge of the spreader slide.
   RATIONALE: So the sample can be thinly spread on the slide.

FIGURE Procedure 48-4 Step 7   Hold the spreader slide at a 30-degree to 35-degree angle. Pull the spreader slide toward the frosted end until it touches the drop of blood.

8. As soon as the drop spreads out to cover most of the spreader slide edge, push the spreader slide back toward the unfrosted end of the smear slide, pulling the sample across the slide behind it, as shown in in the figure below. Maintain the 30- to 35-degree angle.

FIGURE Procedure 48-4 Step 8   When the drop covers most of the spreader slide edge, push the spreader slide back toward the unfrosted end of the smear slide.

9. Continue pushing the spreader until you come off the end, still maintaining the angle, as shown in the figure. The resulting smear should be approximately 1½ inches long, preferably with a margin of empty slide on all

sides. The smear should be thicker on the frosted end of the slide.

FIGURE Procedure 48-4 Step 9   Push the spreader slide off the end of the smear slide, maintaining a 30-degree to 35-degree angle. The smear should be thicker on the frosted end of the slide.

10. Properly label the slide, allow it to dry, and follow the manufacturer's directions for staining it for the required tests.
11. Properly dispose of used supplies and disinfect the work area.
12. Remove the gloves and wash your hands.

PROCEDURE 48-5   Measuring Hematocrit Percentage after Centrifuge

Procedure Goal: To identify the percentage of a blood specimen represented by RBCs after the sample has been spun in a centrifuge.

OSHA Guidelines:

Materials: Blood specimen (from either a capillary puncture or a specimen tube containing anticoagulated blood), micro-hematocrit tube, sealant tray containing sealing clay, centrifuge, hematocrit gauge, wooden applicator sticks, and gauze squares.

Method: Procedure steps.

1. Wash your hands and don exam gloves.
2. If using blood from a capillary puncture, follow the steps in Procedure 48-3 to express a drop of blood from the patient's finger. If using a venous blood sample, check

the specimen for proper labeling, carefully uncap the specimen tube, and use wooden applicator sticks to remove any coagulated blood from the inside rim of the tube. Alternately, use a special safety transfer device if available.
   RATIONALE: The safety device decreases the likelihood of exposure to bloodborne pathogens.
3. Touch the tip of one of the microhematocrit tubes to the blood sample, as shown in the figure below. The tube will take up the correct amount through capillary action.

FIGURE Procedure 48-5 Step 3   Touch the tip of one of the microhematocrit tubes to the blood specimen.

4. Pull the microhematocrit tube away from the sample, holding it carefully to prevent spillage. Wipe the outside of the microhematocrit tube with a gauze square.

   RATIONALE: To remove excess blood so it is not splashed or splattered on the inside of the centrifuge.

5. Hold the microhematocrit tube in one hand and press the other end of the tube gently into the clay in the sealant tray. You may need to place a gloved finger over the other end of the tube to prevent leakage. The clay plug must completely seal the end of the tube.

   RATIONALE: The tube must be sealed to prevent the sample from being forced out of the tube during the spinning process.

FIGURE Procedure 48-5 Step 5   Press the end of the tube into the clay in the sealant tray.

6. Repeat the process to fill another microhematocrit tube. Tubes must be processed in pairs.

   RATIONALE: To maintain a balance in the centrifuge.

7. Place the tubes in the centrifuge, with the sealed ends pointing outward. If you are processing more than one sample, record the position identification number in the patient's chart to track the sample.

FIGURE Procedure 48-5 Step 7   Be sure to place the tubes in the centrifuge so the sealed ends are pointing outward or downward.

8. Seal the centrifuge chamber.

9. Run the centrifuge for the required time, usually between 3 and 5 minutes. Allow the centrifuge to come to a complete stop before unsealing it.

10. Determine the hematocrit percentage by comparing the column of packed RBCs in the microhematocrit tubes with the hematocrit gauge, as shown in the figure below. Position each tube so the boundary between sealing clay and RBCs is at zero on the gauge. Some centrifuges are equipped with gauges, but others require separate handheld gauges.

(a)

(b)

FIGURE Procedure 48-5 Step 10   Read the column of packed red blood cells using the microhematocrit gauge (a) or reader (b) to determine the hematocrit percentage.

11. Record the percentage value on the gauge that corresponds to the top of the column of RBCs for each tube. Compare the two results. They should not vary by more than 2%. If you record a greater variance, at least one of the tubes was filled incorrectly and you must repeat the test.

12. Calculate the average result by adding the two tube figures and dividing that number by 2.

13. Properly dispose of used supplies and clean and disinfect the equipment and the area.

14. Remove the gloves and wash your hands.

15. Record the test result in the patient's chart. Be sure to identify abnormal results.

PROCEDURE 48-6 Measuring Blood Glucose Using a Handheld Glucometer

Procedure Goal: To measure the amount of glucose present in a blood sample.

OSHA Guidelines:

Materials: Safety engineered capillary puncture device (automatic puncture device or other safety lancet), antiseptic and cotton balls or antiseptic wipes, sterile gauze squares, sterile adhesive bandages, handheld glucometer, and reagent strips appropriate for the device.

Method: Procedure steps.

1. Wash your hands and don exam gloves.
2. Review the manufacturer's instructions for the specific device used.
3. Check the expiration date on the reagent strips.
   RATIONALE: To make sure they are not outdated.
4. Code the meter to the reagent strips if required.
   RATIONALE: Some machines will need to be coded to account for small differences in the strips that occur during the manufacturing process.
5. Turn the device on according to the manufacturer's instructions.
6. Perform the required quality control procedures.
   RATIONALE: To ensure the machine is working as expected.
7. Insert the strip into the meter following the manufacturer's instructions.
8. Perform a capillary puncture following the steps outlined in Procedure 48-3.
9. Touch the drop of blood to the reagent strip, allowing it to be taken up by the strip.
10. Read the digital result after the required amount of time.
11. Discard the reagent strip and used supplies according to OSHA standards.
12. Record the time of the test and the result on the laboratory slip.
13. Disinfect the equipment and area.
14. Remove the gloves and wash your hands.
15. Document the test results in the patient's chart. Record the quality control tests in the laboratory control log.

PROCEDURE 48-7 Performing a Rapid Infectious Mononucleosis Test

Procedure Goal: To determine the presence of antibodies associated with infectious mononucleosis using whole blood, serum, or plasma.

OSHA Guidelines:

Materials: Infectious mononucleosis test kit, patient blood sample, and a watch or timer.

Method: Procedure steps.

1. Review the laboratory request form and gather the necessary supplies.
2. Greet the patient, confirm the patient's identity, and introduce yourself.
3. Explain the procedure.
4. Wash your hands and don required PPE.
5. Obtain a sample of the patient's blood using appropriate venipuncture technique.
6. Process the blood sample to obtain whole blood, plasma, or serum as required by the testing procedure.
7. Open the test kit and check the expiration date.
8. Run the recommended controls according to the manufacturer's instructions.
   RATIONALE: To ensure the test is working correctly.
9. Place the required amount of blood, serum, or plasma onto the testing device, following the manufacturer's instructions.
10. Add testing reagent or reagents to the testing device, according to the manufacturer's instructions.
11. Wait the required amount of time. Do not go over the recommended time.
    RATIONALE: Reading the test too early can result in a false negative and reading the test too long after the recommended time could result in a false positive.

12. Read the results and record them in the patient's chart.
13. Discard the testing supplies according to OSHA regulations.
14. Disinfect the work area.
15. Remove your PPE and wash your hands.
16. Document the results in the patient's chart.

SUMMARY OF LEARNING OUTCOMES

LEARNING OUTCOMES	KEY POINTS
48.1 **Discuss the role of the medical assistant when collecting, processing, and testing blood samples.**	As a medical assistant, you will collect and process blood specimens for examination, make sure the test results are handled efficiently and accurately, and complete the necessary paperwork before and after each test.
48.2 **Carry out the procedure for collecting a blood specimen.**	Blood is collected by one of two means: venipuncture and capillary puncture. Venipuncture is the process of obtaining a blood sample from a vein. Capillary puncture is the process of obtaining blood from a superficial skin puncture. When collecting blood specimens, it is essential that you confirm the patient's identity before the sample is collected, cleanse the skin prior to collection, follow standard precautions, collect the sample needed in the appropriate tube or container, and ensure the patient's safety at all times.
48.3 **Summarize ways to respond to patients' needs when collecting blood.**	Patients are often concerned about pain, bruising, and scarring when having blood drawn. They are sometimes afraid they may have a serious disease, especially if large amounts of blood are drawn. Good communication by the medical assistant is the key to easing these fears. There are always patients who will have special needs, including children, the elderly, patients who have bleeding disorders, and difficult patients. Each patient will present a special set of challenges and should be treated with the utmost care and concern.
48.4 **Carry out the procedure for performing blood tests.**	Hematologic, chemical, and serologic tests require special care when performing them. The medical assistant should review the manufacturer's instructions carefully for important information about correctly performing each test.

CASE STUDY CRITICAL THINKING

Recall Sylvia Gonzales from the beginning of the chapter. Now that you have completed the chapter, answer the following questions regarding her case.

1. Compare a fasting blood sugar test to a hemoglobin A1c test.

2. What steps will you take to perform a dermal puncture?

3. If Sylvia tells you that she ate breakfast before coming in for the test, what should you do?

1. (LO 48.2) The small depression inside the bend of the elbow is the
   a. Cephalic space
   b. Median cubital depression
   c. Basillic area
   d. Axillary depression
   e. Antecubital fossa

2. (LO 48.4) The rupturing of erythrocytes is known as
   a. Hemolysis
   b. Hemoglobin
   c. Hematopoiesis
   d. Hemorrhage
   e. Erythrocytosis

3. (LO 48.2) A lavender-topped venipuncture collection tube contains which of the following?
   a. Sodium citrate
   b. Heparin
   c. EDTA
   d. SST
   e. Potassium oxalate

4. (LO 48.4) What is contained within the buffy coat?
   a. Plasma
   b. White blood cells
   c. Red blood cells
   d. Fibrinogen
   e. Serum

5. (LO 48.4) Which of the following tests gives the physician an overall picture of a patient's compliance with diabetes diet and treatment?
   a. Blood glucose
   b. Hemoglobin A1c
   c. Cholesterol
   d. CBC
   e. Fasting blood sugar

6. (LO 48.2) A flat, broad length of vinyl or rubber used to apply pressure to the forearm so the underlying veins stick out is a
   a. Drain
   b. Velcro closure
   c. Butterfly
   d. Tubing
   e. Tourniquet

7. (LO 48.2) The abbreviation for the classification of blood groups is
   a. AcAc
   b. ACE
   c. AST
   d. ABO
   e. AFB

8. (LO 48.4) Which of the following keeps blood from clotting?
   a. Serum separator
   b. Anticoagulant
   c. Antibody
   d. Silicone
   e. Clot activator

9. (LO 48.4) Which of the following tests is most likely used to test for inflammation, infectious diseases, and malignant neoplasms?
   a. Erythrocyte sedimentation rate
   b. RBC count
   c. AST
   d. Amylase
   e. FBS

10. (LO 48.2) Which of the following represents the correct "order of draw" from first venipuncture collection tube to last?
    a. Gold, light blue, green, lavender, yellow
    b. Light blue, green, gold, yellow, lavender
    c. Yellow, light blue, gold, green, lavender
    d. Green, yellow, lavender, gold, light blue
    e. Yellow, lavender, gold, light blue, green

Go to CONNECT to see activities about *Sending a Patient's Test Report* and *Creating a Patient Order Form*.

Access the OLC to practice ordering several laboratory tests in a live EHR program. Refer to the EHR Appendix IV at the end of the book for more information and directions.

49 Electrocardiography and Pulmonary Function Testing

LEARNING OUTCOMES

After completing Chapter 49, you will be able to:

49.1 Discuss the medical assistant's role in electrocardiography and pulmonary function testing.

49.2 Explain the basic principles of electrocardiography and how it relates to the conduction system of the heart.

49.3 Identify the components of an electrocardiograph and what each does.

49.4 Carry out the steps necessary to obtain an ECG.

49.5 Summarize exercise electrocardiography and echocardiography.

49.6 Explain the procedure of Holter monitoring.

49.7 Carry out the various types of pulmonary function tests.

49.8 Describe the procedure for performing pulse oximetry testing.

KEY TERMS

calibration syringe	Holter monitor
cardiac cycle	hypoxemia
deflection	lead
depolarization	polarity
echocardiography	pulmonary function test
electrocardiogram (ECG)	repolarization
electrocardiograph	sleep apnea
electrocardiography	spirometer
electrode	spirometry
forced vital capacity (FVC)	stylus

I. C (9)   Describe implications for treatment related to pathology

I. P (4)   Perform pulmonary function testing

I. P (5)   Perform electrocardiography

III. A (3) Show awareness of patients' concerns regarding their perceptions related to the procedure being performed

IV. P (6) Prepare a patient for procedures and/or treatments

2. **Anatomy and Physiology**
   Graduates:
   c. Assist the physician with the regimen of diagnostic and treatment modalities as they relate to each body system

8. **Medical Office Business Procedures Management**
   Graduates:
   y. Perform routine maintenance of administrative and clinical equipment
   ll. Apply electronic technology

9. **Medical Office Clinical Procedures**
   Graduates:
   b. Apply principles of aseptic techniques and infection control
   f. Screen and follow up patient test results
   k. Prepare and maintain examination and treatment area
   o. Perform
      (1) Electrocardiograms
      (2) Respiratory testing

▶ Introduction

It is not uncommon for patients to have cardiovascular or respiratory problems when they consult physicians. As a medical assistant, you may be responsible for performing screening and/or diagnostic testing in the physician's office. To correctly perform cardiac and respiratory testing, you need to review the anatomy and physiology of the heart and the respiratory system. (Refer to *The Cardiovascular System* and *The Respiratory System* chapters.) This chapter introduces you to the electrocardiograph instrument and how to administer an electrocardiogram. You also will learn how to apply electrocardiograph electrodes and wires, operate the instrument, and troubleshoot problems that can occur while recording the heart's electrical activity. Because many physicians perform more complex cardiac diagnostic testing, you also will learn about Holter monitors and stress testing. Pulmonary function testing is a procedure performed in physicians' offices, and this chapter introduces you to the basics of performing respiratory procedures like spirometry, peak flow, and pulse oximetry.

▶ The Medical Assistant's Role in Electrocardiography and Pulmonary Function Testing   LO 49.1

Electrocardiography and pulmonary function testing are two procedures you may be required to perform in a medical office. **Electrocardiography** is the process by which a graphic pattern is created from the electrical impulses generated within the heart

as it pumps. It is often performed to evaluate symptoms of heart disease, to detect abnormal heart rhythms, to evaluate a patient's progress after a myocardial infarction (MI), or to check the effectiveness or side effects of certain medications. Electrocardiography is sometimes performed as part of a general examination.

Pulmonary function tests (PFTs) measure and evaluate a patient's lung capacity and volume. Such tests are commonly performed when a person suffers from shortness of breath, but they also may be performed as part of a general examination. Pulmonary function tests can help detect and diagnose pulmonary problems. They also are used to monitor certain respiratory disorders and to evaluate the effectiveness of treatment.

▶ Basic Principles of Electrocardiography   LO 49.2

Weak or strong, fast or slow, each heartbeat produces an electrical current that can be measured with an electrocardiograph. Measuring and recording each heartbeat gives the doctor a "picture" of how the heart's electrical system is working. Understanding the basics of the conduction system and how it appears on the ECG tracing is essential when performing electrocardiography.

Conduction and Electrocardiography

Electrocardiography records the transmission, magnitude, and duration of the heart's various electrical impulses. Before you can understand how electrocardiography works, you must understand **polarity**, the condition of having two separate poles, one of which is positive and the other negative. Similar to a bar magnet with

TABLE 49-1	Parts of the Conduction System
Part	**Function**
Sinoatrial (SA) node (pacemaker)	Initiates heartbeat at a rate of 60 to 100 beats per minute with an electrical impulse that causes depolarization.
Atrioventricular (AV) node	Delays the electrical impulse to allow for the atria to complete their contraction and ventricles to fill before the next contraction.
Bundle of His (AV bundle)	Conducts electrical impulses from the atria to the ventricles.
Bundle branches	Conduct impulses down both sides of the interventricular septum.
Purkinje fibers (network)	Distribute the electrical impulses through the right and left ventricles.

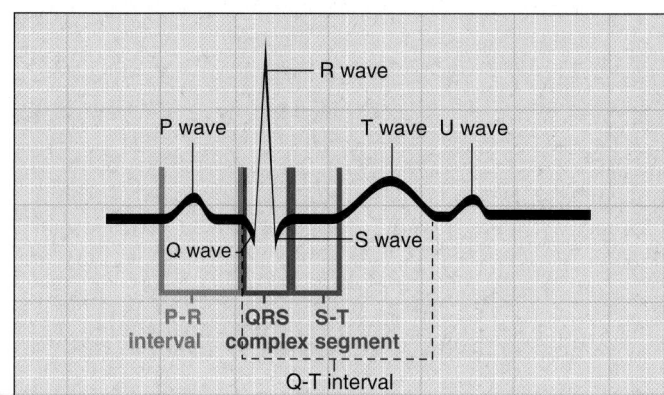

FIGURE 49-1 This ECG tracing shows the pattern of one cardiac cycle in a normal heart. These specific electrical impulses (top) represent the cycle of cardiac contraction and relaxation. The waves and lines (bottom) represent specific parts of the pattern.

one end north and one south, a resting cardiac cell is polarized; that is, it has a negative charge inside and a positive charge outside. When the cardiac cell loses its polarity (a natural occurrence), depolarization occurs. **Depolarization** is the electrical impulse that initiates a chain reaction resulting in contraction. This wave of depolarization flows from the SA node to the ventricles and can be detected by **electrodes**, or electrical impulse sensors, placed on specific areas on the surface of the body. During electrocardiography, electrodes detect and record the heart's electrical activity, including disturbances or disruptions in its rhythm.

Depolarization is always followed by a period of electrical recovery called **repolarization**, when polarity is restored. Following repolarization, the heart returns to a resting, polarized state. The electrical cycle is then repeated, leading to another **cardiac cycle**—sequence of contraction and relaxation. See Table 49-1, Parts of the Conduction System.

The Basic Pattern of the Electrocardiogram

The waves of electrical impulses responsible for the cardiac cycle produce a series of waves and lines on an **electrocardiogram** (abbreviated **ECG** or EKG), which is the tracing made by an **electrocardiograph**, an instrument that measures and displays these impulses (Figure 49-1). These peaks and valleys, called waves or **deflections**, are labeled with the letters P, Q, R, S, T, and U. Each letter represents a specific part of the pattern, as explained in Table 49-2. The recognition of abnormalities in the

TABLE 49-2	Parts of the ECG	
Name	**Appearance**	**Represents**
P wave	Small upward curve	Sinoatrial node impulse, wave of depolarization through atria, and resultant contraction.
QRS complex	Includes Q, R, and S waves	Contraction (following depolarization) of ventricles; QRS complex is larger than P wave because ventricles are larger than atria.
Q wave	Downward deflection	Impulse traveling down septum toward Purkinje fibers.
R wave	Large upward spike	Impulse going through left ventricle.
S wave	Downward deflection	Impulse going through both ventricles.
T wave	Upward curve	Recovery (repolarization of ventricles); repolarization of atria is not obvious because it occurs while ventricles are contracting and producing QRS complex.
U wave	Small upward curve sometimes found after T wave.	May be seen in normal individuals, in patients who experience slow recovery of Purkinje fibers, or in patients who have low potassium levels or other metabolic disturbances.
P-R interval	Includes P wave and straight line connecting it to the QRS complex.	Time it takes for electrical impulse to travel from SA node to AV node.
Q-T interval	Includes QRS complex, S-T segment, and T wave.	Time is takes for ventricles to contract and recover, or repolarize.
S-T segment	Connects end of QRS complex with beginning of T wave.	Time between contraction of ventricles and recovery.

size of the waves or the various time intervals can aid in the diagnosis of certain types of heart problems.

▶ The Electrocardiograph

Each type of electrocardiograph works in the same way. The electrical impulses produced by the heart can be detected through the skin; these impulses are measured, amplified, and recorded on the ECG. Detection begins with electrodes that conduct and transmit the electrical impulses to the electrocardiograph through insulated wires. An amplifier increases the signal, making the heartbeat visible.

The **stylus**, a penlike instrument, records this movement on the ECG paper. The impulses received through various combinations of electrodes constitute different **leads**, or views of the electrical activity of the heart, that are recorded on the ECG.

Types of Electrocardiographs

Several different types of electrocardiographs are in use today. Two types are shown in Figure 49-2. The standard machine is a 12-lead electrocardiograph, which records the electrical activity

FIGURE 49-2 Single-channel (top) and multichannel (bottom) electrocardiographs are used to obtain an ECG.

of the heart simultaneously from 12 different views. A single-channel electrocardiograph records the electrical activity of one lead and, consequently, one view of the heart's electrical activity at a time. The record is printed on a long, thin strip of ECG paper. The most common single-channel units allow you to attach all electrodes at the same time and obtain a manual or automatic printout of individual leads—sometimes referred to as a *rhythm strip*. The multichannel units record more than one lead at a time. These machines use wider paper and more than one stylus to record the leads. Some models of multichannel ECGs provide a diagnosis or an interpretation of the electrocardiogram. The interpretive option can be turned on or off. Even though the interpretive electrocardiograph can provide a diagnosis, the physician will review the tracing and confirm the diagnosis before treatment is ordered. Larger medical facilities may use an electronic health records (EHR) software program so electrocardiograms can be inserted into the patient medical record and transmitted to specialists to interpret. Electrocardiograms can be transmitted by fax or telephone, depending on the software and model of the electrocardiograph.

Electrodes and Electrolyte Products

Electrodes are attached to the patient's skin during electrocardiography. Disposable electrodes (Figure 49-3) are the most widely used.

Because the skin does not conduct electricity well, an electrolyte (a substance that enhances transmission of electric current) is needed with each electrode. Disposable electrodes come with an electrolyte preparation in place.

When performing routine electrocardiography, you place electrodes on 10 areas of the body: one each on the right arm (RA), left arm (LA), right leg (RL), and left leg (LL) and six on specific locations on the chest wall. The right leg is designated as the ground. These 10 electrodes are used to evaluate 12 different pathways of the heart's electrical activity (leads). This is why it is called a 12-lead ECG. Evaluating different leads—the

FIGURE 49-3 Disposable electrodes are available in several varieties.

electrical activity measured through various combinations of electrodes—enables the physician to pinpoint the origin of certain problems like arrhythmias and heart block.

Leads

Each lead provides an image of the heart's electrical activity from a different angle. Together, the images give the doctor a full picture of electrical activity moving up and down, left and right, and forward and backward through the heart. Monitoring the electrodes on the arms and legs in two different ways produces six leads that record electrical impulses that move up and down and left and right. The electrodes placed on the chest provide six more leads, showing electrical activity moving forward and backward (from the front of the body toward the back and vice versa). Each lead is given a specific designation and code. The 12 leads are usually marked automatically on the ECG.

Limb Leads Of the six leads that directly monitor electrodes on the arms and legs, three are standard and three are augmented. Each of the standard leads monitors two limb electrodes, recording electrical activity between them. These leads are also called *bipolar leads* because they monitor two electrodes. The augmented leads monitor one limb electrode and a point midway between two other limb electrodes, recording electrical activity between the monitored electrode and the midway point. Because they directly monitor only one electrode, augmented leads are also called *unipolar leads*. The electrical activity recorded by these leads is very slight, requiring the machine to augment (amplify) the tracings to produce readable waves and lines on the ECG paper. The standard limb leads appear on the ECG as I, II, and III and the augmented limb leads appear as aVF (augmented voltage-foot), aVR (augmented voltage-right), and aVL (augmented voltage-left).

Precordial Leads The six precordial, or chest, leads are unipolar leads. The electrodes are placed across the chest in a precise specific pattern (Figure 49-4). Each precordial lead monitors one electrode and a point within the heart. The precordial leads are each designated by a letter and a number: V_1 through V_6. The designations for the 12 leads of a routine ECG are shown in Table 49-3. The table also indicates which electrodes and points are monitored by each lead.

ECG Paper

ECG paper is provided in a long, continuous roll or pad. If the paper is designed for use with a single-channel electrocardiograph, it is just wide enough for a single trace. Other ECG papers can accommodate several traces at once; these papers are used with multichannel electrocardiography. ECG paper consists of two layers and is both heat- and pressure-sensitive. The heated stylus on the electrocardiograph serves as a "pen" that records the ECG pattern on the paper. Handle the paper carefully to reduce the likelihood of making errant marks that might affect the tracing.

V_1 Fourth intercostal space (between the ribs), to the right of the sternum (breastbone)
V_2 Fourth intercostal space, to the left of the sternum
V_4 Fifth intercostal space, on the left midclavicular line
V_3 Fifth intercostal space, midway between V_2 and V_4
V_6 Fifth intercostal space, on the left midaxillary line
V_5 Fifth intercostal space, midway between V_4 and V_6

FIGURE 49-4 Six precordial electrodes are arranged in specific positions on the chest. Notice that electrode V_4 must be positioned before V_3 and V_6 before V_5.

ECG paper (Figure 49-5) is marked with light and dark lines or with dots and lines—a standardized pattern that permits uniform interpretation by any physician. Each small square, or square area delineated by dots, measures 1 mm by 1 mm. Each large square measures 5 mm by 5 mm.

The vertical, or short, axis of the paper records the voltage, or strength of the impulse; the horizontal axis measures time. Normally, the paper moves through the machine at a speed

TABLE 49-3	ECG Lead Designations
Lead	**Electrodes and Points Monitored**
Standard limb	
I	RA and LA
II	RA and LL
III	LA and LL
Augmented limb	
aVR	RA and (LA and LL)
aVL	LA and (RA and LL)
aVF	LL and (RA and LA)
Precordial	
V_1	V_1 and (LA − RA − LL)*
V_2	V_2 and (LA − RA − LL)*
V_3	V_3 and (LA − RA − LL)*
V_4	V_4 and (LA − RA − LL)*
V_5	V_5 and (LA − RA − LL)*
V_6	V_6 and (LA − RA − LL)*

*The point within the heart is identified by averaging the readings from the electrodes.

FIGURE 49-5 The pattern and spacing of lines or lines and dots on ECG paper are standardized and represent specific units of voltage and time.

of 25 mm per second. This means the distance across 1 small square represents 0.04 second. The distance across 1 large square represents 0.2 second. The distance across 5 large squares represents 1.0 second. In 1 minute (60 seconds), the paper advances 300 large squares, or 1500 mm (150 cm).

Each electrocardiograph is standardized before use so that one small square represents 0.1 millivolt (mV). One large square represents 0.5 mV\, and two large squares represent 1.0 mV.

Electrocardiograph Controls

The location of certain knobs and buttons on an electrocardiograph may vary from model to model. However, certain features are common to most machines, including the standardization control, speed selector, sensitivity control, lead selector, centering control, stylus temperature control, marker control, and on/off switch.

On/Off Switch The on/off switch turns the machine on and off. Most machines have an indicator light that signals when the power is on.

Standardization Control Before you obtain an ECG, you must correctly standardize the machine. The standardization control uses a 1-mV impulse to produce a standardization mark on the ECG paper. When you press the standardization control, the stylus should move up ten small squares, or 10 mm (1 cm) and remain there for 0.08 second (two small

squares, or 2 mm). If it does not, the instrument must be adjusted before you use it. Most newer machines standardize automatically; check the manufacturer's instructions to ensure standardization.

Speed Selector The paper is normally set to run at 25 mm per second for adults. When you run an ECG on infants and children or on adults with a rapid heartbeat, the deflections may appear too close together. In these cases, you may need to adjust the speed to 50 mm per second to separate the peaks and create a tracing that is easier to read. If you must set the speed at 50 mm per second, note it on the strip. Otherwise, a speed of 25 mm per second is assumed. In any case, do not change the speed selection unless the doctor directs you to do so.

Sensitivity Control The sensitivity control—normally set on 1—adjusts the height of the standardization mark and the tracing. When an ECG tracing's height is too high to fit completely on the paper, however, adjust this control to ½ to reduce the size of both the standardization mark and the tracing by one half. For tracings that have very low peaks, set this control on 2 to double the standardization mark and the height of the tracing. Note this change on the ECG. Digital machines standarize the wave output height (gain) automatically and a standardization mark may be seen on the tracing.

Lead Selector Most electrocardiographs have a setting that enables a standard 12-lead tracing to run automatically. All machines have a lead selector that allows you to run each lead individually, in case you need to repeat a strip containing artifacts (erroneous marks or defects).

Centering Control The centering control allows you to adjust the position of the stylus, which must be centered on the paper. Centering the stylus simplifies the process of measuring wave heights for the person who interprets the ECG.

Line Control Another control allows you to adjust the temperature of the stylus. A higher temperature results in a heavier line, whereas a lower temperature results in a lighter, thinner line. The line should be clear without being so dark that it bleeds or smears on the ECG paper. Newer ECG machines do not have a temperature control but may have an adjustment to change the line. Check the manufacturer's directions.

▶ Performing an ECG
LO 49.4

You must obtain a good-quality tracing when performing electrocardiography. To do so, you must be able to recognize an artifact or a generally defective ECG tracing when you see one. Proper technique is also essential to help you obtain the best-quality tracing. The following sections guide you through the process. The steps in obtaining a standard 12-lead ECG using a single-channel electrocardiograph are listed in Procedure 49-1, at the end of this chapter.

Preparing the Room and Equipment

Be sure the room and equipment are properly set up before you begin to administer an electrocardiogram. The accuracy of an ECG can sometimes be affected by electric currents emitted from nearby machines. Although some electrocardiographs have filters to minimize outside electrical interference, it is always a good idea to perform electrocardiography in a room where all other electrical equipment—air conditioners, refrigerators, fans, and laboratory and diagnostic equipment—is turned off.

The room should be in a quiet, private location, protected from interruptions. Because the patient must partially disrobe, adjust the room temperature to a comfortable level.

The examining table should be sturdy and comfortable. Make sure the table paper is fresh and the table is disinfected after each patient's use.

Before using the electrocardiograph, check the date of its last inspection. Each machine should be periodically inspected and certified safe to use for a specific period of time. Using a machine only within this time period helps ensure both your and the patient's safety. Be sure to turn the machine on ahead of time to allow the stylus to warm up. It is good practice to check the ECG paper and ECG electrodes prior to preparing the patient, restocking these supplies if necessary, as this will save time for you and the physician.

Preparing the Patient

Introduce yourself to the patient, explain the procedure, and answer any questions the patient has. Follow the steps described in Procedure 49-1, at the end of this chapter, as you prepare the patient for electrocardiography. Keep in mind, some patients are apprehensive about undergoing electrocardiography. Anxiety often stems from the fear of receiving an electric shock from the machine. See the Caution: Handle with Care section for ways to allay a patient's anxiety about having an ECG.

CAUTION: HANDLE WITH CARE

Allaying Patient Anxiety About Having Electrocardiography

The most common reason for a patient's anxiety is not knowing what to expect from electrocardiography. The patient may be fearful of being hooked up to an electrical device and worried about receiving an electric shock.

Calmly and simply explain the procedure in detail, both before you begin and while you prepare the patient for the test. Assure her it is a safe procedure that will last about 10 to 15 minutes. Explain that the machine measures the heart's electrical activity and that no outside electricity will pass through the body. It is also helpful to explain why the doctor has ordered the procedure, without giving any diagnosis or prognosis.

Above all, talk to and listen to the patient. Encourage her to express her concerns and ask questions. Respond to the patient's concerns and questions calmly, fully, and respectfully.

Ensuring Patient Comfort

Ensuring that the patient is comfortable will help her feel more at ease. It also will result in less body movement and a more accurate ECG.

Each patient is an individual. You will need to find out from the patient what is and is not comfortable for her. First, make sure the room temperature is right for the patient. If she says the room feels too cool, provide an extra blanket to prevent chills, as this can make a patient shiver and increase her anxiety. Shivering can cause muscle tremor artifacts. Next, ensure the patient is comfortable on the examining table. Placing a small pillow under the head can help, but make sure it does not touch the shoulders or raise them off the table. For most patients, placing a pillow under the knees helps relax the abdomen and lower extremities and prevents lower back pain. Try this arrangement and let the patient decide if this feels comfortable. If the patient has trouble breathing, shift her into a Fowler's or semi-Fowler's position. Ask the patient which position is more comfortable and use the position she chooses. If the patient chooses a position other than supine, be sure to note the position in her chart.

Applying the Electrodes and the Connecting Wires

You must prepare the patient's skin before applying the electrodes. Proper contact between an electrode and the skin allows for proper conduction of the impulses. Follow the steps described in Procedure 49-1, at the end of this chapter, as you prepare the patient's skin. Depending on your office policy, you may be required to trim chest or leg hair if it is dense to ensure proper contact.

Electrodes Disposable electrodes—which come with the electrolyte product already applied—are the most commonly used type of electrode. Simply remove the adhesive backing and press the electrode firmly into place on the skin. Because the electrolyte gel is prepackaged and measured, artifacts occurring from the placement of unequal amounts of electrolyte are minimized.

Positioning the Electrodes You must position electrodes at 10 locations on the body (Figure 49-6). If the electrocardiograph has only five electrodes, you will need to move the fifth electrode to six different positions on the patient's chest to obtain the necessary tracings.

Limb Electrodes Limb electrodes are most commonly placed on the inside of the fleshy part of the calf muscle and on the outside of the upper arm. Sometimes they are placed on the thigh, abdomen, and above the wrist. Follow office policy on limb placement, but remember, a consistent technique will ensure that all ECGs will be standardized, even with different equipment models. It is generally better to place arm electrodes on the upper arm because this reduces the amount of artifact caused by arm movement. Attach the electrodes to a smooth and fleshy part of each limb to ensure optimal conduction of impulses. Limb electrodes must always be placed at the same level on both arms and on both legs. If a patient has had a leg amputated, both leg electrodes should be placed on the thighs or abdomen, parallel to each other. If the patient has had an arm amputated, place both electrodes at shoulder level. Note the alternate electrode placement in the patient's chart and the ECG tracing, because differences in placement can cause changes in the ECG tracing.

Precordial Electrodes Unlike the limb electrodes, the precordial electrodes must be placed at precise, specific locations on the chest to obtain accurate readings. These locations specify intercostal spaces—the spaces between the ribs—which are numbered from top to bottom. Refer to Figure 49-4 for the exact description of each location.

Determine the position for the first precordial electrode (V_1) by counting to the fourth intercostal space to the right of the sternum (breastbone). The V_1 electrode should be placed over this space, directly adjacent to the sternum. After you have this electrode in place, use it as a guide to position the other electrodes.

Place the V_2 electrode in the fourth intercostal space to the left of the sternum in the same manner. Note that the V_1 and V_2 positions may not line up exactly; one may be higher than the other. Perfect symmetry is rare in the human body.

Next, place the V_4 electrode in the fifth intercostal space, where it intersects an imaginary line drawn straight down from the middle of the clavicle (midclavicular line). When the V_4 electrode is in place, place the V_3 electrode midway between V_2 and V_4 in the fifth intercostal space.

Place the V_6 electrode in the fifth intercostal space directly below the middle of the armpit (midaxillary line). Place the last electrode (V_5) in the fifth intercostal space midway between V_4 and V_6.

Attaching the Wires After placing the electrodes, attach the wires that connect the electrodes to the electrocardiograph. Numbers and letters on the wires correspond to numbers and letters for the electrodes. For example, RA stands for right arm, LL stands for left leg, and so on. The precordial electrode wires are labeled V_1 through V_6. Connect the limb wires first, then the precordial wires, in the sequence already described. Some wires are also color-coded.

RA (right arm)

LA (left arm)

Electrocardiograph

RL (right leg)

LL (left leg)

FIGURE 49-6 There are 10 electrode positions for electrocardiography.

Depending on the type of electrodes you use, connect the wires to the electrodes by snapping, clipping, or screwing the wire tips tightly in place. Wires should follow the patient's body contours and lie flat against the body. Drape the wires over the patient to avoid putting tension on the electrodes, which could cause interference. You also may bundle the wires together to form a single cable.

Operating the Electrocardiograph

Before running the ECG, remind the patient to remain as still as possible and not to talk. Be sure the patient is comfortable. A comfortable patient is less likely to move around and cause artifacts on the ECG tracing.

Standardizing the Electrocardiograph Follow the steps described in Procedure 49-1, at the end of this chapter, if you need to standardize the electrocardiograph. Some machines have automatic standardization. The stylus should move upward above the baseline 10 mm (two large squares) when you press the standardization button. If it does not, you must see to it that the instrument is adjusted before continuing.

Running the ECG You can now run the ECG. On most machines, turning the lead selector to the automatic mode produces a standard 12-lead strip. Because each lead provides a specific view of the heart's electrical activity, each of the 12 leads has a characteristic tracing (Figure 49-7).

Manual ECGs If your office has a machine without an automatic setting, you must manually run the ECG for each of the 12 leads. You also may be required to repeat certain leads manually if artifacts are detected. Most ECG machines can run single-channel or multichannel ECGs.

To run a manual ECG, standardize the machine as already outlined. Then turn the lead selector to standby mode. Some older machines may require you to stop the paper before selecting the first lead (I) using the lead selector. Push the marking button on the machine to indicate the lead if the machine does not do this automatically. Allow the strip to run for four to five cardiac cycles, taking about 3 to 5 seconds. Turn the machine back to the standby mode; stop the paper if necessary; and repeat the procedure for leads II and III, the augmented leads, and the precordial leads. Remember, standardize the machine for consistency before running each lead.

Many physicians request another strip on lead II to assess for rhythm. Some physicians choose a different lead for the rhythm strip. Run the rhythm strip on the requested lead to produce a strip at least 2 feet long so rhythmic abnormalities can be easily recognized.

Multiple-Channel Electrocardiographs Some electrocardiographs have multiple channels that can record three, four, or six leads simultaneously (Figure 49-8). Electrode placement is the same as for single-channel electrocardiographs.

Checking the ECG Tracing After running the 12 leads and before disconnecting the patient from the machine, check all tracings to make sure they are clear and free of artifacts. If any of the leads do not appear on a tracing, it may

FIGURE 49-7 The tracing from each lead will differ. The long tracing of a single lead along the bottom is the rhythm strip.

Source: Courtesy of Cardiac Science Corporation, Milton, Wisconsin.

FIGURE 49-8 Some electrocardiographs allow you to run six leads at the same time.

Source: Courtesy of Cardiac Science Corporation, Milton, Wisconsin.

mean a wire has come loose. In this case, reconnect the wire and repeat the tracing. Repeat any unclear tracings.

Also, check that all tracings are contained within the paper's boundaries and that no waves peak above its edges. If this happens, recenter the stylus if it is positioned too high, or set the sensitivity selector to ½ before repeating the tracing. In the reverse situation—where very low peaks appear—set the sensitivity selector to 2 to increase the height of the peaks.

If the peaks in a tracing are too close together, increase the paper speed to 50 mm per second. Increasing the speed separates the peaks and makes the tracing easier to read.

Make a note on the ECG tracing whenever it is necessary to adjust sensitivity or speed settings. This information is vital to the interpretation of the test.

Troubleshooting: Artifacts and Other Problems

To ensure high-quality tracings, it is essential to recognize artifacts and identify sources of interference. You also must know how to correct them.

Artifacts Improper technique, poor conduction, outside interference, or improper handling of a tracing can cause artifacts. If artifacts are present on an ECG tracing, the doctor may not be able to make an accurate diagnosis of the patient's condition.

There are several types of artifacts. Among the common ones you may see are a wandering baseline or a flat line. Recognizing the presence of an artifact in the baseline during setup allows you to correct the problem before the tracing is

recorded. You also may see marks that are not characteristic of a tracing; large, erratic spikes; or uniform, small spikes. Table 49-4 outlines these artifacts and summarizes possible causes and solutions.

Wandering Baseline A wandering baseline, shown in Figure 49-9, is identified by a shift in the baseline from the center position for that lead. Causes include somatic interference and a variety of mechanical problems. Mechanical problems may be an inadequately warmed stylus, improper application of electrodes (too loose or incorrectly placed), tension on electrodes caused by a dangling wire, inadequate electrolyte, inadequate skin preparation, or the presence of creams or lotions on the skin.

Having the patient lie still can reduce somatic interference. Proper skin preparation and electrode placement are also essential. When the electrocardiography appointment is made, instruct the patient to use no creams or lotions, deodorant, perfume, or powder. Be sure to include specific instructions in patient education materials and ask the patient whether any of these substances were used before the procedure. If so, clean each area of electrode placement thoroughly with alcohol to avoid conduction disturbances.

Flat Line A flat line on one of the lead's tracings (Figure 49-10) is typically caused by a loose or disconnected wire. If flat lines occur on more than one lead, two of the wires may have been switched. If flat lines occur on all leads, the patient cable may be loose or disconnected, or there may be a break (short)

TABLE 49-4   Correcting ECG Artifacts

Problem	Possible Causes	Solutions
Wandering baseline	Inadequately warmed stylus	Allow electrocardiograph to warm up.
	Poor skin preparation	Repeat skin preparation and lead placement.
	Loose electrode	Reapply electrode.
	Improper electrode placement	Reapply electrode.
	Dirty or corroded electrode	Clean and reapply electrode/replace electrode.
	Somatic interference	Help patient relax and be comfortable.
	Pickup of breathing movement	Reposition electrode.
	Tension on electrode	Drape wires over patient.
Flat line	Detached/loose wire or cable	Reattach wires or cable.
	Wrong selector switch setting	Check/change selector switch setting.
	Crossed wires	Check/switch wires.
	Short circuit in wires	Check/replace broken equipment.
	Cardiac arrest	Check pulse/respiration; begin CPR.
Marks not part of tracing	Careless handling	Handle carefully.
	Use of paper clips	Use a rubber band.
	Wet hands	Ensure that hands are dry.
	Improper mounting	Mount properly.
Uniform, small spikes	AC interference	Turn off/unplug other electrical equipment; remove patient's watch.
	Improper electrode placement	Reapply electrode.
	Inadequate grounding	Check grounding.
	Dirty electrode	Clean and reapply electrode.
Large, erratic spikes	Somatic interference	Help patient relax and be comfortable.
	Loose/dry electrode	Reapply electrode.
	Electrode placed over bone	Reposition electrode.

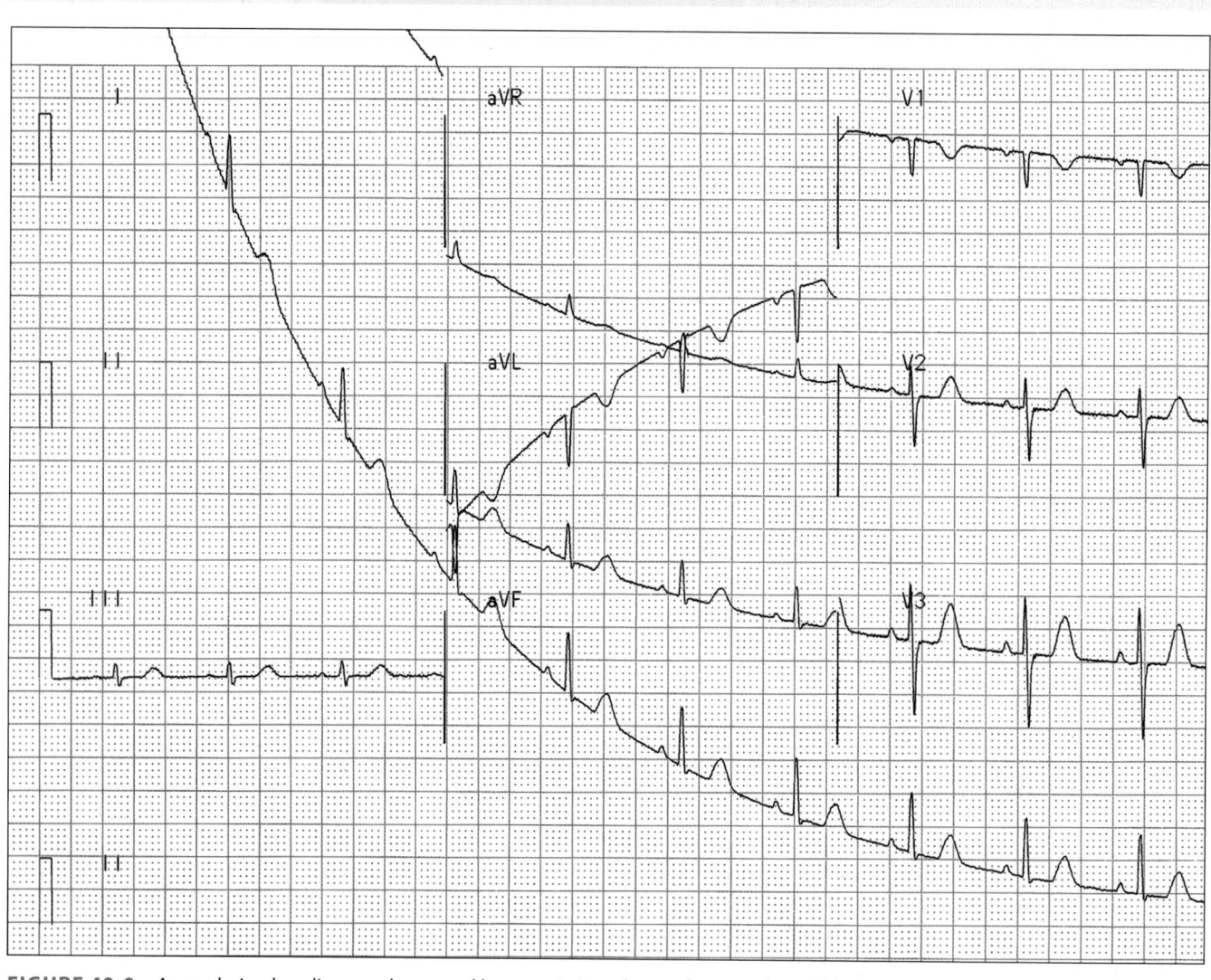

FIGURE 49-9   A wandering baseline may be caused by somatic interference or a mechanical problem.

Source: Courtesy of Cardiac Science Corporation, Milton, Wisconsin.

FIGURE 49-10   A flat line on one of the leads is caused by a loose or disconnected wire.

Source: Courtesy of Cardiac Science Corporation, Milton, Wisconsin. (ECG tracing represents earlier model from Burdick, Inc.)

somewhere in the unit. On the other hand, a flat line on all leads can indicate cardiac arrest. In this case, always assess the patient's pulse and respiration first.

Extraneous Marks   Because ECG graph paper is heat- and pressure-sensitive, it can easily be damaged. Careless handling, like using paper clips to hold the tracing together or handling the tracing with wet hands, can cause extraneous marks on the paper.

Causes of Artifacts   You can use the line of the tracing to identify the cause of artifacts. Then you can take steps to eliminate the particular type of interference involved.

Alternating Current (AC) Interference   AC interference occurs when the electrocardiograph picks up a small amount of electric current given off by another piece of electrical equipment. The tracing's line will be jagged, consisting of a series of uniform, small spikes (Figure 49-11). Many newer

FIGURE 49-11   This type of artifact is caused by AC interference.

Source: Courtesy of Cardiac Science Corporation, Milton, Wisconsin.

electrocardiographs have filters to reduce or eliminate most of this interference, and it often can be eliminated by turning off or unplugging other appliances in the room. Keeping the examining table away from the wall also can help, as wiring in the wall can contribute to AC interference. If the wires are crossed and the lead wires are not following the patient's body contour, this can cause AC interference. Make sure the ECG cable is not underneath the examination table. If these remedies do not work, check to see whether the electrodes are dirty or attached improperly or whether the machine is incorrectly grounded.

Somatic Interference Muscle movement—tensing of voluntary muscles, shifting of body position, tremors, or even talking (which requires muscular contractions that generate electrical impulses)—causes somatic interference. A sensitive electrocardiograph detects these impulses, resulting in erratic stylus movement during the tracing, leading to large, erratic spikes and a shifting baseline (Figure 49-12).

Eliminate this type of interference by reminding the patient to remain still and to refrain from talking. To reduce the chance of the patient shivering, shifting, and moving, be sure the room temperature is comfortable for the patient.

Placing the limb electrodes closer to the body's trunk—on the upper arms, close to the shoulder, and on the upper thighs—can reduce interference. Reducing patient anxiety by explaining the procedure also can help reduce somatic interference.

Certain nervous system disorders, like Parkinson's disease, cause patients to experience involuntary movements that can cause interference. So, although placing the limb electrodes closer to the body's trunk is often helpful, it may be necessary to interrupt the tracing until the tremors subside.

Identifying the Source of Interference The source of interference on an ECG often can be identified by checking the tracings obtained on leads I, II, and III. If there is a problem with a particular limb electrode, the interference will be prominent in two leads. For prominent interference in the following pairs of leads, check the limb electrode indicated:

- Leads I and II, right arm electrode.
- Leads I and III, left arm electrode.
- Leads II and III, left leg electrode.

If the cause of the artifact or the source of interference cannot be determined, stop the machine and notify your supervisor or the physician. Do not disconnect the patient from the electrocardiograph.

Completing the Procedure

When you are sure the quality of all ECG tracings is acceptable, disconnect the patient from the machine. First, remove the tracing from the machine and label it with the patient's name, the date, and your initials. If using a single-channel ECG, loosely roll long tapes from single-channel machines with the printed side facing in and secure them with a rubber band. Remember, do not use paper clips; they can cause extraneous marks.

Next, disconnect the wires from the electrodes and remove the electrodes from the patient. Wipe excess electrolyte from the patient's skin with a moist towel. Assist the patient to a sitting position, allowing a moment's rest before assisting the patient from

FIGURE 49-12 The somatic interference in this ECG was caused by patient tremors.

Source: Courtesy of Cardiac Science Corporation, Milton, Wisconsin.

the table. Help the patient dress if necessary, or allow the patient privacy to dress. Remove disposable paper covers from the table and pillows, clean surfaces according to OSHA guidelines, and discard all disposable materials in a biohazardous waste container.

Mounting the Tracing Several types of ECG mounts or holders are available for single-channel ECG tracings, including slotted folders and folders with self-adhesive surfaces. These mounts form a permanent record of the ECG and allow the doctor to read tracings from all 12 leads at once. Mounts are not typically necessary for multiple-channel ECG tracings because these are compact records of several leads.

Interpreting the ECG Although you are not responsible for interpreting an ECG as a medical assistant, knowing something about how ECGs are interpreted may allow you to recognize an urgent problem. Some of the features assessed by an ECG include heart rhythm, heart rate, the length and position of intervals and segments, and wave changes. A series of ECGs are often taken before a physician makes a diagnosis. The tracings are compared for changes in a patient's condition, progress, or response to a specific medication.

Heart Rhythm The ECG is the best way to assess heart rhythm—the regularity of the heartbeat. A normal heart rhythm is indicated on the ECG by regularly spaced complexes. In a regularly spaced complex, the distance between one P wave and the next P wave—or one R wave and the next R wave—is consistent. The physician assesses the patient's rhythm by viewing the rhythm strip you obtain from lead II.

Heart Rate The heart rate can easily be determined by counting the number of QRS complexes in a 6-second strip of the tracing (30 large squares at 25 mm per second) and multiplying by 10. Heart rate irregularities may result from conduction abnormalities or reactions to certain drugs.

Intervals and Segments Variations in the length and position of the intervals and segments can indicate many heart conditions, including conduction disturbances and myocardial infarction. For example, following a myocardial infarction, the ST segment will be elevated in the tracing for a period of time. Thus, the ECG can be used to determine not only the occurrence of a myocardial infarction but also the approximate time it occurred. Electrolyte disturbances in the blood and drug reactions also can affect intervals and segments.

Wave Changes The direction of certain waves may vary, depending on which lead is being viewed. Normally, each wave should have a similar appearance in each of the leads. Changes in the height, width, or direction of a wave may indicate a problem. During the early stages of a myocardial infarction, for example, the T wave forms a large peak. Not long afterward, the T wave inverts and appears below the baseline.

Cardiac Arrhythmias Irregularities in heart rhythm are called *arrhythmias*. Although some arrhythmias do not cause problems, many of them can be dangerous, so it is important to detect these irregularities with an ECG.

Ventricular Fibrillation (V-Fib) Ventricular fibrillation, commonly referred to as *v-fib*, is a life-threatening heart condition in which the ventricles of the heart appear to "quiver" and there is no cardiac output. The patient will quickly lose consciousness, and cardioversion (defibrillation) must be used to stop the arrhythmia. Ventricular fibrillation is seen in patients experiencing a myocardial infarction. The tracing is often described as a "saw tooth" image (Figure 49-13).

Premature Ventricular Contractions (PVCs) Premature ventricular contractions (PVCs) are premature heartbeats that originate from the heart's ventricles. A PVC is identified as a beat that occurs early in the cycle, followed by a pause before the next cycle (Figure 49-14). PVCs are premature because they occur before the regular heartbeat. These heartbeats are the result of an irritability of the heart muscle in the ventricles and can be caused by myocardial infarctions, electrolyte imbalances, lack of oxygen, or certain medications. A PVC appears on the ECG as having no P wave, a wide QRS complex, and T waves that deflect in the opposite direction from the R wave.

Atrial Fibrillation Atrial arrhythmias occur because of electrical disturbances in the atria and/or the AV node, which leads to fast heartbeats (tachycardia). Atrial fibrillation is a common atrial arrhythmia that causes speedy, multiple electrical signals that fire rapidly from different areas in the atria rather than from the SA node. Causes of atrial fibrillation include myocardial infarction; hypertension; heart failure; mitral valve diseases, such as MVP; overactive thyroid;

FIGURE 49-13 Ventricular fibrillation resembles and is sometimes referred to as a "saw tooth" pattern.

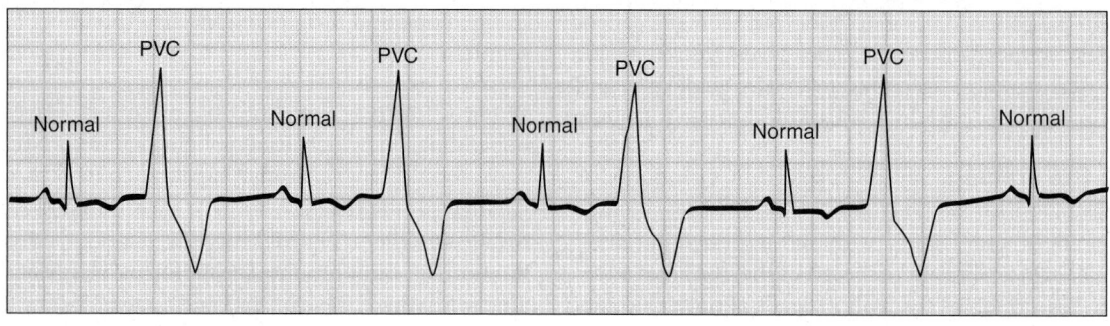

FIGURE 49-14 This rhythm strip compares a normal deflection to a premature ventricular contraction (PVC).

FIGURE 49-15 Atrial fibrillation.

pulmonary embolisms (blood clots); excessive alcohol consumption; emphysema; and pericarditis. Atrial fibrillation is seen on the ECG as small, irregular, uncoordinated complexes that are difficult to interpret because the P waves cannot be identified (Figure 49-15).

Go to CONNECT to see a video about *Obtaining an ECG.*

▶ Exercise Electrocardiography (Stress Testing) and Echocardiography LO 49.5

The resting ECG does not always provide a doctor with enough information to diagnose a problem. There are several additional tests a doctor can use for diagnosing heart diseases and disorders. Exercise electrocardiography, more commonly known as a *stress test*, assesses the heart's conduction system during exercise, when the demand for oxygen increases. This test measures a patient's response to a constant or increasing workload. **Echocardiography** uses ultrasound to view the heart in motion. This can be done at rest or after strenuous activity like riding a bike or walking on a treadmill.

Exercise Electrocardiography

A stress test may be performed on a patient who has had surgery or a myocardial infarction to determine how the heart is functioning. It is sometimes used to screen a patient for heart disease and to determine a patient's ability to undertake an exercise program.

During the procedure, the patient is required to walk on a treadmill, pedal a stationary bicycle, or walk on a stair-stepping ergonometer while ECG readings are taken (Figure 49-16). An

FIGURE 49-16 During a stress test, the patient exercises on special equipment to see how well the heart handles increased physical demands.

ergonometer measures work performed. You are responsible for preparing the patient for electrocardiography and monitoring blood pressure throughout the procedure. The test continues until the patient reaches a target heart rate, experiences chest

Ensuring Patient Safety during Stress Testing

Some risk is involved in exercise electrocardiography because patients who most commonly undergo the test may either already have cardiac problems or be suspected of having them. The risk of having a myocardial infarction during a stress test, however, is less than 1 in 500, and the risk of death is less than 1 in 10,000. Still, some patients may be apprehensive about the procedure because of the risks.

You can help educate and prepare patients for stress tests and assist them during the procedure. One way to help is to ask patients to wear comfortable shoes and clothes. In addition, there are several ways to help these patients be less fearful of the procedure while helping to ensure their safety.

A patient who has recently suffered a myocardial infarction may be particularly afraid to undergo stress testing. However, this test may be the only way the physician can accurately determine the functional ability of the patient's heart and assess his physical limitations. This information is vital to preventing future myocardial infarctions.

When you inform the patient of what symptoms he may expect during the test—including fatigue, slight breathlessness,

an increased heart rate, and increased perspiration—the patient will be better able to cope with the test. Make it clear that an advance warning of adjustments in the procedure, such as an increased workload, will be given.

Assure the patient that there are few risks associated with the test and that the test may be stopped if he experiences chest pain or extreme fatigue. Patients will relax and follow instructions better when they know the procedure can be controlled. Also, tell the patient that both you and the physician will be monitoring his vital signs during and after the procedure and that all safety precautions will be taken. Explain the presence of the safety equipment—for example, the crash cart with medication, equipment, and supplies.

During the test, remember to talk to and listen to the patient. Even symptoms not related to cardiac symptoms should be reported, and the patient should be encouraged to report any symptoms. Observe the patient for signs of distress and inform the physician immediately if such symptoms appear.

---

pain or fatigue, or develops complications, such as tachycardia or dysrhythmia.

A patient who undergoes stress testing is often suspected of having a heart problem or is recovering from a myocardial infarction or surgery. Consequently, there may be a risk of cardiac distress, myocardial infarction, or cardiac arrest during testing. Because of the risks, the patient must sign an informed consent form before the procedure and a physician must monitor the patient throughout the test. Emergency medication and equipment, like a defibrillator, must always be present in the room. Because of the potential risk, patients may be apprehensive about the test. As a medical assistant, you can be instrumental in helping them feel comfortable about undergoing the procedure and in making the procedure as safe as possible for them. See the Caution: Handle with Care section for ways to help a patient safely undergo stress testing.

Echocardiography

The ability to view the moving heart is essential to understanding how the structures within the heart are functioning. An echocardiogram produces a video image of the working heart valves and chambers and how well blood moves through these structures. There are several types of echocardiograms:

- Transthoracic—the ultrasound transducer is moved around on the chest and or abdomen to produce heart images.
- Transesophageal—the transducer is passed into the esophagus, where it produces clearer images of the heart because it is closer to the heart and the sound waves do not have to penetrate the ribs.
- Doppler—uses a special type of ultrasound to look at blood flow through the heart. The direction and speed of blood

flow through the heart are assessed with this type of test, giving the physician information about coronary artery blockage and heart valve damage.

- Stress echo—echocardiography is done before and after exercise or injection of a drug that makes the heart work faster and harder. This is usually done in conjunction with an electrocardiogram to assess how well the heart responds to increased demand.

Pretest Preparation There is usually no special pretest preparation for transthoracic and doppler echocardiography. The patient should not eat a heavy meal prior to a stress echo. Since patients having transesophageal echocardiography receive a sedative and the transducer is passed into the esophagus, they should not eat for at least 6 hours prior to the test. Make sure you carefully explain all pretest instructions verbally and in writing and give the patient an opportunity to ask any questions. Reassure the patient of the limited risk during the procedure. Finally, have the patient sign a consent form prior to having the echocardiogram.

▶ Ambulatory Electrocardiography (Holter Monitoring) LO 49.6

Patients who experience intermittent chest pain or discomfort may have a normal resting ECG and a normal stress test. When this is the case, the electrical activity of the patient's heart can be monitored over a 24-hour period of normal activity to help diagnose the problem. A special monitor, the Holter monitor, is used for this purpose.

FIGURE 49-17 The Holter monitor is used to determine electrical activity of a patient's heart over a 24-hour period. This Burdick Vision Holter is one type of monitor.

Source: Reprinted with permission of Cardiac Science Corporation.

Function of the Holter Monitor

The **Holter monitor** is an electrocardiography device that includes a small cassette or microchip recorder worn around a patient's waist or on a shoulder strap to record the heart's electrical activity. The monitor is connected to electrodes on the patient's chest (Figure 49-17). During the testing period, the patient is asked to perform usual daily activities and to keep a written log of activities undertaken and of stress or symptoms experienced. To aid in the diagnosis, some monitors allow patients to press an event button to mark the area on the recording whenever symptoms appear.

The patient returns to the office at the end of the 24-hour test period to have the monitor and electrodes removed. The recording is analyzed by a computer in the office or at a reference laboratory and a printout of the results is prepared. When the tracing has been evaluated, the doctor can correlate cardiac irregularities, like arrhythmias or ST segment changes, with the activities and symptoms listed in the patient's diary.

In addition to its role as a diagnostic tool, Holter monitoring can be used to evaluate the status of a patient who is recovering from a myocardial infarction. It can indicate progress or the need to change therapy or modify the rehabilitation plan.

Patient Education

It is absolutely essential that the patient continue normal activities during Holter monitoring. Give the patient the following additional instructions:

- Record all activities, emotional upsets, physical symptoms, and medications taken.
- Wear loose-fitting clothing that opens in the front while wearing the monitor.
- Avoid going near magnets, metal detectors, and high-voltage areas and avoid using electric blankets during the monitoring period. These devices and areas can interfere with the recording.

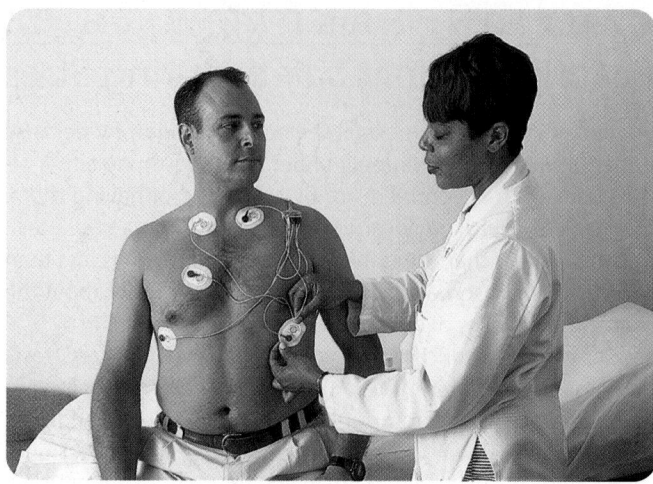

FIGURE 49-18 Taping the wires to the patient's chest reduces the chance that tension on a wire or electrode will produce artifacts on the ECG.

- Avoid getting the monitor wet. Do not take a bath or shower. A sponge bath is permissible.
- Show the patient how to check the monitor to make sure it is working properly. This step is particularly important if any of the electrodes seem loose. Instruct the patient to inform the office if there are any problems.

Connecting the Patient

Holter monitors have either three or five electrodes, depending on the unit. As with a resting ECG, correct placement of the electrodes is necessary for accurate readings. Before connecting the patient to the Holter monitor, make sure he has signed an informed consent form and explain that you need to attach electrodes to the patient's skin.

Because the electrodes must stay in place for 24 hours, you may need to shave the areas where the electrodes are attached to permit optimum adherence. The wires may be connected to the electrodes before they are attached to minimize patient discomfort.

After the electrodes and wires are attached and the monitor is in place, tape the wires to the patient's chest to eliminate tension on the wires or electrodes (Figure 49-18). Be sure the unit has a fresh battery, that a cassette tape or other data storage device has been inserted if necessary, and that the unit is turned on. The steps in performing Holter monitoring are outlined in Procedure 49-2, at the end of this chapter. Go to CONNECT to see a video about *Holter Monitoring.*

▶ Pulmonary Function Testing   LO 49.7

Pulmonary function tests (PFT) help the doctor evaluate ventilatory function of the lungs and chest wall. They evaluate lung volume and capacity and are commonly used to evaluate shortness of breath and to help detect and classify pulmonary disorders. They also may be performed as part of a general examination. PFTs are used to monitor conditions such as asthma, certain allergies, cystic fibrosis, and chronic obstructive pulmonary disease (COPD), a chronic lung disorder. The tests are also used to evaluate the effectiveness of particular treatments on a patient's lung function.

Spirometry

Spirometry is a test used to measure breathing capacity. An instrument called a **spirometer** measures the air taken in by and expelled from the lungs. Several different measurements related to lung volume and capacity can be made with a spirometer. Some of these measurements are made directly by the spirometer; others are calculated. For more information about lung volumes and capacities see the *Respiratory System* chapter.

Forced Vital Capacity

Many measurements can be obtained during one particular maneuver—obtaining the **forced vital capacity (FVC)**, the greatest volume of air that can be expelled when a person performs rapid, forced expiration. To obtain the FVC, ask the patient to take as deep a breath as possible and to exhale into the spirometer as quickly and completely as possible. You can determine the lung's ability to function by taking into account the volume of air expelled and the time it takes to perform this maneuver.

Types of Spirometers

Many models of computerized spirometers are used in physicians' offices. Each consists of a mouthpiece or a mouthpiece and a tube to carry air to the machine, a mechanism to measure the volume or flow of air, and a means of calculating and printing the results.

Computerized spirometers measure air volume and airflow, perform various calculations, and print a graphic representation of the information. Figure 49-19 shows a computerized spirometer.

Performing Spirometry

The technique for performing pulmonary function testing is similar for all types of spirometers. Successful spirometry

FIGURE 49-19 This computerized spirometer measures air volume and airflow.

depends on proper patient preparation and consistent technique in performing the procedure and analyzing the results. The steps involved in measuring forced vital capacity using a spirometer are described in detail here and outlined in Procedure 49-3, at the end of this chapter.

Patient Preparation When patients are scheduled for pulmonary function tests, inform them that the following conditions and activities may affect the test's accuracy:

- Viral infection or acute illness within the previous 2 to 3 weeks.
- Serious medical condition, like a recent myocardial infarction.
- Recent use of a prescribed medication if the test order calls for spirometry before and after prescribed medication.
- Use of a sedative or opioid substance before the test.
- Smoking or eating a heavy meal within 1 hour of taking the test.

Review the conditions and activities with patients again on the day of the test to ensure that none apply. If there are no contraindications, weigh and measure patients. Use simple terms to explain the procedure and its purpose. Have them loosen tight clothing so they will be comfortable and their breathing will not be restricted in any way. The procedure is performed with patients sitting down. Make sure their legs are not crossed and that both feet are flat on the floor.

Explain that they need to wear a nose clip or hold the nose tightly closed to be sure they will inhale and exhale through the mouth. The mouthpiece of the unit may be a disposable cardboard tube or a reusable rubber one that can be disinfected after use. If disposable mouthpieces are used, instruct patients to avoid biting down on them, as that will obstruct airflow. Be sure patients form a tight seal around the mouthpiece with their lips. Dentures normally help maintain a tight seal; however, they should be removed if they hinder the process.

Proper Positioning Instruct patients to keep their chin and neck in the correct position during the procedure. The chin should be slightly elevated and the neck slightly extended. Bending the chin to the chest tends to restrict airflow and should be avoided (Figure 49-20). Some bending at the waist is acceptable.

Explaining and Demonstrating the Procedure Tell patients to take the deepest breath possible, insert the mouthpiece into the mouth, form a tight seal, and then blow into the mouthpiece as hard and as fast as possible to completely exhale. Tell them to exhale as long as they can to force air from the lungs. Remind them that the initial force of their exhalation must be strong to get a valid reading. Demonstrate the procedure to show how to do the test correctly.

Performing the Maneuver You can improve patients' performance during the maneuver by actively and forcefully coaching them. Urge patients to blow hard and to continue blowing. After a maneuver, give them feedback on their

(a)

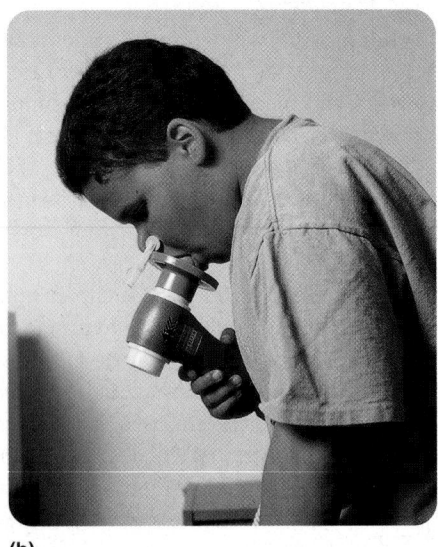

(b)

FIGURE 49-20 During a pulmonary function test, the patient must maintain the proper position. (a) The chin should be slightly elevated and the neck slightly extended. (b) The chin should not approach the chest.

FIGURE 49-21 These spirometry tracings show air volume per second before and after use of a medication.

performance and indicate corrective actions they can take to improve the next maneuver.

Some spirometers indicate whether a particular maneuver was of adequate force and duration to be measured. However, adequate force does not indicate the maneuver was acceptable. An acceptable maneuver must have the following five features:

1. No coughing, particularly during the first second.
2. A quick and forceful start.
3. An adequate length of time (a minimum of 6 seconds).
4. A consistent and fast flow with no variability.
5. Consistency with other maneuvers.

Spirometry tracings plot volume and time. You will need to obtain three acceptable maneuvers, which may require more than three attempts. Observe the patient for signs of breathing

difficulty, dizziness, light-headedness, or changes in pulse and blood pressure. If necessary, allow the patient to rest briefly before continuing. Notify the physician immediately if symptoms are severe.

Determining the Effectiveness of Medication
Spirometry is often used to determine the effectiveness of certain medications a patient is taking. You will perform two sets of maneuvers if this determination is required. Instruct the patient to refrain from taking the prescribed medication on the day of the test. Before performing the test, confirm that the patient has followed this instruction. Conduct the first set of maneuvers, ensuring that they are acceptable. After obtaining the results, instruct the patient to take the prescribed medication. Allow the medication to take effect, and then perform a second set of maneuvers. Comparing the two sets of readings shows whether the medication has effectively improved the patient's lung function. Some computerized spirometers can graph both sets of readings together to simplify the comparison (Figure 49-21).

Special Considerations On occasion, you may have to deal with an uncooperative patient, one who cannot understand or follow directions, or one who cannot perform the procedure. In these situations, patience and skill are essential for obtaining an acceptable spirometry tracing.

The doctor may be able to convince an uncooperative patient to perform the maneuver. You can help by taking a no-nonsense

FIGURE 49-22 A calibration syringe delivers a fixed volume of air.

approach, perhaps stating that the doctor needs these test results to help the patient. Patients who cannot understand or follow directions—the very young, the very old, those who have limited proficiency in English, or those with a hearing impairment—may need extra attention and patience to obtain acceptable results. Explain the procedure in simple terms and repeat instructions as necessary. If, after eight attempts, the patient is unable to perform the procedure, stop and report the situation to the doctor.

The Importance of Calibration Spirometers should be calibrated each day they are used to ensure accurate readings. You may be responsible for this procedure, which requires the use of a standardized measuring instrument called a **calibration syringe** (Figure 49-22). When the plunger is pulled back, this syringe contains a fixed volume of air. Connect the syringe to the patient tubing (this tubing runs from the mouthpiece to the machine) and depress the plunger to inject the entire volume of air. The spirometer reading should be within 3% of the stated volume. Keep a calibration logbook for each spirometer.

While calibrating the spirometer, you can detect leaks by checking the volume/time graph. The volume should remain at a steady reading; if it declines with time, a leak exists in the system.

Infection Control After a patient completes the pulmonary function test, you must clean the spirometer and other pulmonary function devices thoroughly to prevent transmission of microorganisms. If disposable mouthpieces, nose clips, and patient tubing are used, discard them in a biohazardous waste container. If reusable mouthpieces, nose clips, and tubing are used, clean and disinfect them between patients. Most important, wash your hands thoroughly before and after performing a pulmonary function test.

Go to CONNECT to see a video about *Measuring Forced Vital Capacity Using Spirometry.*

Peak Expiratory Flow Rate (PEFR)

A peak expiratory flow rate (PEFR) is a measurement taken to determine the amount of air that can be quickly forced from the

FIGURE 49-23 Peak expiratory flow meter markings will determine the patient's treatment based on accurate readings.

lungs. A peak flow meter—a small handheld device that can be used in the medical office or the patient's home (Figure 49-23)—is often used to obtain a PEFR. Patients who suffer from asthma are commonly asked to monitor their asthma by using a peak flow meter and recording their results. During an asthma flare-up, the large airways of the lungs begin to narrow, which slows the speed of air leaving the lungs. A peak flow meter, when used properly, can reveal narrowing of the airways in advance of an asthma attack. Peak flow meters can help determine:

- When to seek emergency medical care.
- The effectiveness of an asthma management treatment plan.
- When to stop or add medication as directed by a physician.
- Asthma triggers, like stress or exercise.

Procedure 49-4, at the end of this chapter, explains the procedure for obtaining a peak expiratory rate using a peak flow meter.

Peak Flow Zones After obtaining a peak expiratory flow rate, the type of patient care given will be determined based on the individual's results. The physician will instruct the patient about the peak flow zones and how to respond to each zone. Peak flow zones are different for each patient and will be determined by the physician. The three peak flow zones are green, yellow, and red.

Green Zone The green zone indicates good control of asthma, with peak flow rates of 80% to 100% of the highest peak flow rate. Measurements in this zone indicate that air moves well through the large airways and the patient's usual activities can be continued.

Yellow Zone Peak flow rates in the yellow zone range from 50% to 80% of the highest peak flow rate. Measurements in this zone indicate that the large airways are beginning to narrow and medication is needed. Patient symptoms include tiredness and tightening of the chest.

Red Zone Peak flow rates in the red zone are less than 50% of the highest or best personal reading recorded. Narrowing of the largest airways has occurred and is considered a medical emergency. Medical treatment should be sought immediately. Patients are usually directed to take a bronchodilator or other medication that will open the airway and call their physician. Symptoms include wheezing, shortness of breath, and trouble walking and talking.

Go to CONNECT to see a video about *Obtaining a Peak Expiratory Flow Rate.*

▶ Pulse Oximetry

LO 49.8

Pulse oximetry is a noninvasive test that measures the saturation of oxygen in a patient's arterial blood. A sensor is placed on a patient's finger, earlobe, toe, or bridge of the nose (Figure 49-24). A red infrared light is shone through one side of the appendage to the other. The amount of light absorbed by the hemoglobin is detected by the pulse oximeter. Any reading less than 95% indicates **hypoxemia** (low blood oxygen). Pulse oximetry is performed on patients with pulmonary or cardiac

FIGURE 49-24 A pulse oximeter is a portable, handheld device used by many medical facilities.

conditions and during post-operative patient observation. It is also used to help diagnose **sleep apnea,** a condition characterized by pauses in breathing during sleep. The pauses are often long enough to cause a drop in blood oxygen levels. Some medications after surgery can slow breathing rates and it is important that their blood oxygen levels be carefully monitored. Procedure 49-5, at the end of this chapter, explains the process of obtaining a pulse oximetry reading.

Go to CONNECT to see a video about *Obtaining a Pulse Oximetry Reading.*

PROCEDURE 49-1 Obtaining an ECG

Procedure Goal: To obtain a graphic representation of the electrical activity of a patient's heart.

OSHA Guidelines:

Materials: Electrocardiograph, ECG paper, electrodes, electrolyte preparation, wires, patient gown, drape, blanket, pillows, gauze pads, alcohol, moist towel, and scissors for trimming hair (if needed).

Method: Procedure steps.

1. Turn on the electrocardiograph and, if necessary, allow the stylus to heat up.
2. Identify the patient, introduce yourself, and explain the procedure.
3. Wash your hands.
4. Ask the patient to disrobe from the waist up and remove jewelry, socks or stockings, bra, and shoes. If the electrodes will be placed on the patient's legs, have the patient roll up his or her pant legs. Sometimes the electrodes are placed on the sides of the lower abdomen—check the manufacturer's instructions.

Provide a gown if the patient is female and instruct her to wear the gown with the opening in front.
   RATIONALE: Making sure the patient knows exactly what clothing to remove and the correct way to put on the gown will make the process more efficient.

5. Assist the patient onto the table and into a supine position. Cover the patient with a drape (and a blanket if the room is cool). If the patient experiences difficulty breathing or cannot tolerate lying flat, use a Fowler's or semi-Fowler's position, adjusting with pillows under the head and knees for comfort if needed.

6. Tell the patient to rest quietly and breathe normally. Explain the importance of lying still to prevent false readings.

7. Wash the patient's skin, using gauze pads moistened with alcohol. If needed, rub it vigorously with dry gauze pads to promote better contact of the electrodes.
   RATIONALE: If a patient has applied lotion in the areas where electrodes are placed, it may cause conduction problems.

8. If the patient's leg or chest hair is dense, use a small pair of scissors to closely trim the hair where you will attach the electrode. (Shaving is not recommended because of the risk of bleeding and infection.)

9. Apply electrodes to fleshy portions of the limbs, making sure the electrodes on one arm and leg are placed similarly to those on the other arm and leg. Attach electrodes to

areas that are not bony or muscular. The arm lead tabs on the electrode point downward and the electrode tabs for the leg leads point upward. Peel off the backings of the disposable electrodes and press them into place.

RATIONALE: Using the correct tab position will reduce tension on the limb wires. Artifacts can occur when electrodes are placed on bones and muscles.

FIGURE Procedure 49-1 Step 9   Place electrodes at the specified locations on the chest, arms, and legs.

10. Apply the precordial electrodes at specified locations on the chest. Precordial electrode tabs point downward.
11. Attach wires and cables, making sure all wire tips follow the patient's body contours.
12. Check all electrodes and wires for proper placement and connection; drape wires over the patient to avoid creating tension on the electrodes that could result in artifacts.

FIGURE Procedure 49-1 Step 12   Attach wires and cables, draping wires over the patient to avoid tension that can result in artifacts.

13. Enter the patient data into the electrocardiograph. Press the on, run, or record button. Standardize the machine, if necessary, by following these steps:
    a. Set the paper speed to 25 mm per second or as instructed.
    b. Set the sensitivity setting to 1 or as instructed.
    c. Turn the lead selector to standardization mode.
    d. Adjust the stylus so the baseline is centered.
    e. Press the standardization button. The stylus should move upward above the baseline 10 mm (two large squares).
14. Run the ECG.
    a. If the machine has an automatic feature, set the lead selector to automatic.
    b. For manual tracings, turn the lead selector to standby mode. Select the first lead (I) and record the tracing. Switch the machine to standby and then repeat the procedure for all 12 leads.
15. Check tracings for artifacts.
16. Correct problems and repeat any tracings that are not clear.
17. Disconnect the patient from the machine.
18. Remove the tracing from the machine and label it with the patient's name, the date, and your initials.
19. Disconnect the wires from the electrodes and remove the electrodes from the patient.
20. Clean the patient's skin with a moist towel.
21. Assist the patient into a sitting position.
22. Allow a moment for rest and then assist the patient from the table.
    RATIONALE: Some patients may experience postural hypotension after lying and may feel dizzy.
23. Assist the patient in dressing if necessary, or allow the patient privacy to dress.
24. Wash your hands.
25. Record the procedure in the patient's chart.
26. Properly dispose of used materials and disposable electrodes.
27. Clean and disinfect the equipment and the room according to OSHA guidelines.

PROCEDURE 49-2   Holter Monitoring

Procedure Goal: To monitor the electrical activity of a patient's heart over a 24-hour period to detect cardiac abnormalities that may go undetected during routine electrocardiography or stress testing.

OSHA Guidelines:

Materials: Holter monitor, battery, cassette tape if applicable, patient diary or log, alcohol, gauze pads, disposable shaving supplies, disposable electrodes, hypoallergenic tape, drape, and electrocardiograph.

Method: Procedure steps.

1. Identify the patient, introduce yourself, and explain the procedure.
2. Ask the patient to remove clothing from the waist up; provide a drape if necessary.

3. Wash your hands and assemble the equipment.

4. Assist the patient into a comfortable position (sitting or supine).

5. If the patient's body hair is particularly dense, don examination gloves and trim the areas where the electrodes will be attached.
   RATIONALE: Trimming the area will ensure the electrodes will stay secure during the 24-hour period.

6. Clean the electrode sites with alcohol and gauze.

7. Rub each electrode site vigorously with a dry gauze square.
   RATIONALE: To help electrodes adhere to the skin.

8. Attach wires to the electrodes and peel off the paper backing on the electrodes. Apply as indicated in the figure below, pressing firmly to ensure that each electrode is securely attached and is making good contact with the skin.
   RATIONALE: Good skin contact is essential to obtain an accurate reading.

FIGURE Procedure 49-2 Step 8   Correctly connecting the patient to the Holter monitor is essential.

9. Attach the patient cable.

10. Insert a fresh battery, and position the unit.

FIGURE Procedure 49-2 Step 10   Make sure the monitor has a fresh battery and cassette tape if one is used.

11. Tape wires, cable, and electrodes as necessary to avoid tension on the wires as the patient moves.

12. Insert the cassette tape, if necessary, and turn on the unit.

13. If the unit uses a cassette tape, confirm that the tape is actually running. Indicate the start time in the patient's chart.
    RATIONALE: If the cassette tape is not running, results will not be recorded and the test will have to be repeated.

FIGURE Procedure 49-2 Step 13   Observe the cassette to make sure the tape is moving through the recording unit. Check digital recorders to make sure they are working.

14. Instruct the patient on proper use of the monitor and how to enter information in the diary. Caution the patient not to alter any diary entries; it is crucial to know what the patient is doing at all times.

15. Schedule the patient's return visit for the same time on the following day.

16. On the following day, remove the electrodes, discard them, and clean the electrode sites.

17. Wash your hands.

18. Remove the cassette tape and obtain a printout of the tracing OR transfer the data from the monitor to patient's electronic chart according to office procedure and the manufacturer's directions. Document all parts of the procedure.

> Holter monitoring placed at 0900. Patient instructed how to maintain diary during monitoring period and to return to clinic on 10/28/14. Patient stated she understood and had no questions. _____
> _____ *K. Booth RMA (AMT)*

PROCEDURE 49-3 Measuring Forced Vital Capacity Using Spirometry

Procedure Goal: To determine a patient's forced vital capacity using a volume-displacing spirometer.

OSHA Guidelines:

Materials: Adult scale with height bar, spirometer, patient tubing (tubing that runs from the mouthpiece to the machine), mouthpiece, nose clip, and disinfectant.

Method: Procedure steps.

1. Prepare the equipment. Ensure that the paper supply in the machine is adequate.
2. Calibrate the machine as necessary.
3. Identify the patient and introduce yourself.
4. Check the patient's chart to see whether there are special instructions to follow.
5. Ask whether the patient has followed instructions.
6. Wash your hands and don examination gloves.
7. Measure and record the patient's height and weight.
8. Explain the proper positioning.
9. Explain the procedure.
10. Demonstrate the procedure.
    RATIONALE: Explanations and demonstrations are effective patient teaching methods.
11. Turn on the spirometer and enter applicable patient data and the number of tests to be performed.
12. Ensure the patient has loosened any tight clothing, is comfortable, and is in the proper position. Apply the nose clip.

FIGURE Procedure 49-3 Step 12   The nose clip is applied over the fleshy part of the nose.

13. Have the patient perform the first maneuver, coaching when necessary.

FIGURE Procedure 49-3 Step 13   You may need to coach the patient while performing the maneuver.

14. Determine whether the maneuver is acceptable.
15. Offer feedback to the patient and recommendations for improvement if necessary.
16. Have the patient perform additional maneuvers until three acceptable maneuvers are obtained.
17. Record the procedure in the patient's chart and place the chart and the test results on the physician's desk for interpretation.
18. Ask the patient to remain until the physician reviews the results.
    RATIONALE: The physician may want to speak with the patient regarding results or may want to order additional testing.
19. Properly dispose of used materials and disposable instruments.
20. Sanitize and disinfect patient tubing, reusable mouthpiece, and nose clip.
21. Clean and disinfect the equipment and room according to OSHA guidelines.

PROCEDURE 49-4 Obtaining a Peak Expiratory Flow Rate

Procedure Goal: To determine a patient's peak expiratory flow rate.

OSHA Guidelines:

Materials: Peak flow meter and a disposable mouthpiece.

Method: Procedure steps.

1. Assemble all necessary equipment and supplies for the test.
2. Wash your hands and identify the patient.
3. Explain and demonstrate the procedure to the patient.
   RATIONALE: Patient education and understanding are crucial for getting accurate test results.
4. Position the patient in a sitting or standing position with good posture. Make sure any chewing gum or food is removed from the patient's mouth.
5. Set the indicator to zero.
   RATIONALE: Helps to ensure accurate results.
6. Ensure the disposable mouthpiece is securely placed onto the peak flow meter.

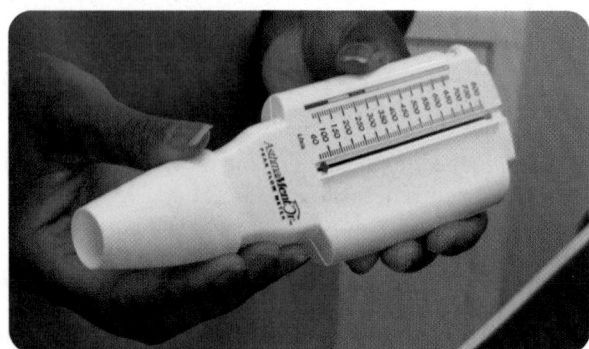

FIGURE Procedure 49-4 Step 6   A disposable mouthpiece is securely fastened to the peak flow meter.

7. Hold the peak flow meter with the gauge uppermost and ensure your fingers are away from the gauge.
8. Instruct the patient to take as deep a breath as possible.

9. Instruct the patient to place the mouthpiece into his mouth and close his lips tightly around the mouthpiece, sealing his lips around it.

FIGURE Procedure 49-4 Step 9   Have the patient close his lips tightly around the mouthpiece so no air escapes.

10. Instruct the patient to blow out as fast and as hard as possible.
    RATIONALE: A fast blast is better than a slow blow.
11. Observe the reading where the arrowhead is on the indicator.
12. Reset the indicator to zero and repeat the procedure two times, for a total of three readings. You will know the technique is correct if the reading results are close. If coughing occurs during the procedures, repeat the step.
13. Document the readings into the patient's chart. The highest reading will be the peak flow rate.
    RATIONALE: The highest reading represents the personal best reading for the patient, and future measurements are based upon this result. Do not average the results.
14. Dispose of the mouthpiece in a biohazardous waste container.
15. Disinfect or dispose of the peak flow meter per office policy.
16. Wash your hands.

PROCEDURE 49-5   Obtaining a Pulse Oximetry Reading

Procedure Goal: To obtain a pulse oximetry reading.

OSHA Guidelines:

Materials: Pulse oximeter.

Method: Procedure steps.

1. Assemble all the necessary equipment and supplies.
2. Wash your hands and correctly identify the patient.
3. Select the appropriate site to apply the sensor to by assessing capillary refill in the patient's toe or finger.
   RATIONALE: If the patient has poor circulation in his fingers or toes, use the bridge of his nose or an earlobe.
4. Prepare the selected site, removing nail polish or earrings if necessary. Wipe the selected site with alcohol and allow it to air dry.

RATIONALE: Nail polish can alter the test results.

5. Attach the sensor to the site (if a finger is used, placed in the clip).
6. Instruct the patient to breathe normally.
7. Attach the sensor cable to the oximeter. Turn on the oximeter and listen to the tone.
8. Set the alarm limits for high and low oxygen saturations and high and low pulse rates, as directed by the physician's order, and turn on the oximeter.
9. Read the saturation level and document it in the patient's chart. Report to the physician readings that are less than 95%. Manually check the patient's pulse and compare it to the pulse oximeter. Document all the readings and the application site in the patient's medical chart.
10. Wash your hands.
11. Rotate the patient's finger sites every four hours if using a pulse oximeter long-term.

LEARNING OUTCOMES	KEY POINTS
49.1 Discuss the medical assistant's role in electrocardiography and pulmonary function testing.	As a medical assistant, you will be responsible for preparing the patient for ECG and pulmonary function tests, maintaining the equipment used for these tests, and performing them.
49.2 Explain the basic principles of electrocardiography and how it relates to the conduction system of the heart.	The heart's conduction system is responsible for the electrical pathway that occurs during a heartbeat. The pathway begins with the SA node, travels through the AV node—bundle of HIS—right and left bundle branches, and ends with the Purkinje fibers. This electrical energy pathway is measured with an electocardiograph and a tracing of the impulses is produced. The electrical impulses are represented in wave forms or deflections. Each deflection is labeled by letters PQRSTU and represents a part of the pattern.
49.3 Identify the components of an electrocardiograph and what each does.	The electrocardiograph consists of the following components: electrodes, which detect and conduct electrical impulses to the electrocardiograph; amplifier, which increases the signal, making the heartbeat visible; stylus, which records the movement on the ECG paper; leads, combinations of electrodes each providing different views of the electrical activity of the heart; and ECG paper, special heat-sensitive paper used for recording the ECG tracing.
49.4 Carry out the steps necessary to obtain an ECG.	The steps in obtaining an accurate ECG include preparing the room and equipment, identifying the patient, properly placing the limb and chest electrodes, attaching the lead wires, entering the patient data into the ECG machine, running the tracing, checking the tracing for artifacts, disconnecting the patient from the lead wires and removing the electrodes, and assisting the patient as required.
49.5 Summarize exercise electrocardiography and echocardiography.	Exercise electrocardiography is referred to as *stress testing*. This measures the efficiency of the heart during constant or increasing workload. Echocardiography uses ultrasound to create a picture of the moving heart. This can be done while the patient is resting or after exercise.
49.6 Explain the procedure of Holter monitoring.	A Holter monitor is used to measure the heart's activity over a 24-hour period. This is used when the patient has intermittent chest pain or discomfort and a normal ECG and stress test.
49.7 Carry out the various types of pulmonary function tests.	Forced vital capacity is the measurement of the greatest volume of air expelled when a patient performs a rapid, forced expiration. The lung's ability to function is measured by the volume of air expelled and the time taken to perform the maneuver. Accurate spirometry testing includes proper patient positioning, coaching the patient during the procedure, obtaining three acceptable maneuvers, and recording the results in the patient's chart. A peak expiratory flow rate is obtained by having the patient sit or stand using good posture, take in as deep a breath as possible, and blow out through the peak flow meter as fast and as hard as possible three times. The highest reading of the three is the peak flow rate and should be recorded in the patient's chart.
49.8 Describe the procedure for performing pulse oximetry testing.	Pulse oximetry testing is performed by applying the pulse oximeter to the patient's finger or toe, attaching the sensor cable to the oximeter, turning the oximeter on, setting the alarm limits for high and low oxygen saturations, and reading the patient's oxygen saturation levels. The oxygen saturation levels should be recorded in the patient's chart.

Recall John Miller from the beginning of the chapter. Now that you have completed the chapter, answer the following questions regarding his case.

1. Explain to John the difference between an ECG and an echocardiogram.

2. John expresses concern about having a heart attack during the procedure. How can you alleviate his fear?

3. You must perform an ECG on this patient. Describe the steps in the procedure.

1. (LO 49.2) Which of the following initiates the heartbeat?
   a. AV node
   b. SA node
   c. Bundle of His
   d. Purkinje fibers
   e. Bundle branch

2. (LO 49.4) The ECG tracing is showing somatic interference. What can be done?
   a. Turn off or unplug appliances in the room
   b. Remove oil from the patient's skin
   c. Connect a loose wire
   d. Remind the patient to remain still
   e. Reschedule the test

3. (LO 49.8) What does a pulse oximeter measure?
   a. Oxygen saturation of the blood
   b. Oxygen saturation of the skin
   c. Electrical activity of the heart
   d. Forced vital capacity
   e. Lung capacity

4. (LO 49.7) When obtaining a peak flow rate, you should _____ the _____ reading(s).
   a. Average, two
   b. Average, three
   c. Add, two
   d. Document, three
   e. Document, two

5. (LO 49.4) Which of the following irregularities on an ECG would be considered the most severe?
   a. PVC
   b. V-fib
   c. A-fib
   d. AC interference
   e. Tachycardia

6. (LO 49.3) The precordial ECG leads are also called
   a. AVR leads
   b. Ground leads
   c. Chest leads
   d. Augmented leads
   e. Limb leads

7. (LO 49.4) When standardizing the ECG machine, the stylus should move
   a. 1 small block above the baseline
   b. Below the baseline
   c. 1 large block below the baseline
   d. Only slightly
   e. 2 large blocks above the baseline

8. (LO 49.4) Turning off unnecessary electrical equipment in the room when performing an ECG is helpful in reducing which type of artifact?
   a. Extraneous marks
   b. Flat line
   c. Somatic interference
   d. AC artifact
   e. Wandering baseline

9. (LO 49.8) Low blood oxygen is known as
   a. Hypoxemia
   b. Sleep apnea
   c. Hyperpnea
   d. Oximetry
   e. COPD

10. (LO 49.7) The greatest volume of air that can be expelled when a person performs rapid, forced expiration is
   a. Peak expiratory flow
   b. Total lung capacity
   c. Maximum voluntary ventilation
   d. Forced vital capacity
   e. Tidal volume

Diagnostic Imaging

CASE STUDY

PATIENT INFORMATION	Patient Name	Gender	DOB
	Raja Lautu	F	2/23/19XX
	Attending	**MRN**	**Allergies**
	Elizabeth H. Williams, MD	224-86-564	Benzalkonium chloride

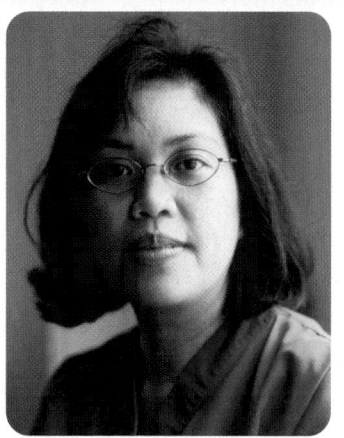

Raja Lautu, a 42-year-old woman, has arrived at the office for her annual gynecological physical. After her physical exam, she is scheduled for her annual digital mammogram. The digital mammogram results reveal a small, abnormal density close to the chest wall on the right breast. Stereotactic fine-needle breast biopsy reveals a grade II infiltrating ductal carcinoma (IDC). Dr. Williams refers Ms. Lautu to a radiation oncologist for treatment. She will most likely be treated with brachytherapy.

Keep Raja in mind as you study this chapter. There will be questions at the end of the chapter based on the case study. The information in the chapter will help you answer these questions.

LEARNING OUTCOMES

After completing Chapter 50, you will be able to:

50.1 Explain what X-rays are and how they are used for diagnostic and therapeutic purposes.

50.2 Compare invasive and noninvasive diagnostic procedures.

50.3 Carry out the medical assistant's role in X-ray and diagnostic radiology testing.

50.4 Discuss common diagnostic imaging procedures.

50.5 Describe different types of radiation therapy and how they are used.

50.6 Explain the risks and safety precautions associated with radiology work.

50.7 Relate the advances in medical imaging to EHR.

KEY TERMS

arthrography
barium enema
barium swallow
brachytherapy
cholangiography
contrast medium
diagnostic radiology
intravenous pyelography (IVP)
invasive
KUB radiography

mammography
MUGA scan (nuclear ventriculography)
myelography
noninvasive
nuclear medicine
PET
radiation therapy
retrograde pyelography
SPECT
teletherapy

I. C (9) Describe implications for treatment related to pathology

III. A (2) Explain the rationale for performance of a procedure to the patient

III. A (3) Show awareness of patients' concerns regarding their perceptions related to the procedure being performed

2. **Anatomy and Physiology**
   Graduates:
   c. Assist the physician with the regimen of diagnostic and treatment modalities as they relate to each body system

8. **Medical Office Business Procedures Management**
   Graduates:
   y. Perform routine maintenance of administrative and clinical equipment
   ll. Apply electronic technology

9. **Medical Office Clinical Procedures**
   Graduates:
   b. Apply principles of aseptic techniques and infection control
   f. Screen and follow up patient test results

▶ Introduction

Diagnostic radiology has evolved immensely since the discovery of the simple X-ray beam, which has become a valuable screening and clinical diagnosis tool for physicians. In this chapter, you will learn the basics of noninvasive and invasive radiology along with your role as a medical assistant in this testing. Safety issues for the administration of radiologic testing are discussed, as are the proper handling and storage of the actual films. In addition, you will learn about preparing and instructing patients for the more common radiology procedures.

▶ Brief History of the X-Ray   LO 50.1

In 1895, Wilhelm Konrad Roentgen (1845–1923) discovered the X-ray, or roentgen ray, a type of electromagnetic wave. It has a high energy level, traveling at the speed of light (186,000 miles per second), and an extremely short wavelength (one-billionth of an inch) that can penetrate solid objects. X-rays react with photographic film to produce a permanent record (X-ray, or radiograph). The X-ray image is lightest where the film is struck by the most X-ray energy. Differences in tissue densities produce the X-ray image, with the least dense being lightest and the most dense being darkest on the film.

Today, X-rays and radioactive substances have both diagnostic —like a wrist X-ray to diagnose a fracture—and therapeutic— like radiation treatment for cancerous tumors—uses. Radiologic technologists are trained medical personnel, certified to perform certain radiologic procedures upon completion of a 2- to 4-year radiology curriculum. Some radiologic technologists receive further training in radiology subspecialties, like ultrasound, mammography, magnetic resonance imaging, and nuclear medicine. Radiographers, sonographers, radiation therapists, and nuclear medicine technologists are all radiologic technologists. Invasive radiologic procedures or procedures requiring a high degree of expertise are nearly always performed by a radiologist—a physician who specializes in radiology. A radiologist is also the physician who interprets the films for other physicians. Other specialists who perform radiologic procedures, either alone or with a radiologist's assistance, include cardiologists, orthopedists, obstetricians, and oncologists.

▶ Diagnostic Radiology   LO 50.2

Diagnostic radiology is the use of X-ray technology for diagnostic purposes. Radiologic tests sometimes use contrast media as well as special techniques or instruments for viewing internal body structures and functions. A **contrast medium** is a substance that makes internal organs denser and blocks the passage of X-rays to the photographic film. Introducing contrast media into certain structures or areas of the body can provide a clearer image of organs and tissues and an indication of how well they are functioning. Contrast media include gases (air, oxygen, or carbon dioxide); heavy metal salts (barium sulfate or bismuth carbonate); paramagnetic compounds (substances that are attracted to a magnetic field), which are used for MRI contrast (gadolinium); and iodine compounds. They can be administered orally, parenterally (for example, intravenously), or by routes that introduce them into an organ or body cavity (for example, by insertion). Types of diagnostic imaging include X-rays, computed tomography (CT), nuclear medicine, magnetic resonance imaging (MRI), and ultrasound.

Invasive Procedures

Diagnostic tests can be invasive or noninvasive. An **invasive** procedure, such as angiography, requires a radiologist to insert a catheter, wire, or other testing device into a patient's blood vessel or organ through the skin or a body orifice. All invasive tests require surgical aseptic technique. Some procedures, including angiography, are performed in a hospital or same-day surgical

FIGURE 50-1 A standard X-ray is one of the most frequently performed radiologic tests.

facility. The patient may need general anesthesia for some procedures. The anesthetist must closely monitor the patient, who is under anesthesia during and after the test, for life-threatening complications like anaphylaxis.

Noninvasive Procedures

Noninvasive procedures, such as standard X-rays or ultrasonography, use other technologies to view internal structures. They do not require inserting devices, breaking the skin, or the degree of monitoring needed with invasive procedures.

The most familiar equipment used for diagnostic imaging is the conventional X-ray machine, as shown in Figure 50-1. This machine consists of a table, an X-ray tube, a control panel, and a high-voltage generator. The image produced by a conventional X-ray may be developed on standard X-ray film or captured digitally on special equipment. Digital radiography is discussed later in the chapter. Other equipment used for diagnostic radiology includes instruments specifically designed for the test. Examples are a mammography unit, a scanner for CT, and a transducer for ultrasound.

▶ The Medical Assistant's Role in Diagnostic Radiology

LO 50.3

As a medical assistant, you may work with diagnostic radiology in a radiology facility or in a medical office. Your duties in a radiology facility will include assisting a radiologic technologist or a radiologist in performing diagnostic radiologic procedures. Depending on the scope of practice in your state, you may be allowed to learn how to operate certain X-ray equipment. Even if you are not allowed to assist with an X-ray procedure or to operate X-ray equipment, you will probably provide preprocedure and postprocedure patient care. Your duties in an orthopedic office may include assisting a radiologic technologist in performing X-ray procedures. In an obstetric practice, you might assist a physician in performing an ultrasound examination of a pregnant woman. Even if you work in a medical office that does not perform radiologic testing, you must still provide a certain amount of preprocedure care and education. In order to properly explain a test to a patient and to assist a radiologic technologist or radiologist in performing a test, you must have a basic understanding of X-ray technology. You also may need inservice training to ensure accuracy and patient safety for some procedures. See the Educating the Patient feature on Providing Patient Instruction for Radiologic Procedures.

Preprocedure Care

Preprocedure care varies somewhat, depending on the test. In general, however, you may do the following:

- Schedule the patient's appointment, if necessary. Inform the patient of the location, date, and time of the procedure.
- Provide preparation instructions. Advise the patient about diet restrictions or requirements (like fasting or drinking liquids) as well as medication requirements (like taking a laxative). Always check with the radiology facility for specific requirements and be sure the patient receives this information.
- Explain the procedure to the patient briefly and clearly. Use proper terminology and nontechnical language. Reinforce the doctor's reason for requesting the procedure and provide any available written information about the test. Inform the patient about the length of the examination, possible side effects or safety precautions and warnings, and injections or uncomfortable steps. Check for clarity and understanding by using the mirroring communication technique when communicating with the patient. You must ensure that the patient understands the preprocedure directions.
- Ask pertinent questions. Obtain a medication history from the patient, because current medications could interfere with some procedures. If the patient is a woman of childbearing age, ask whether she is pregnant or if there is any chance she could be pregnant. Report the answers to the physician in a medical office or to the radiologic technologist in a radiology facility.

Care during and after the Procedure

If you work in a radiology facility, your responsibilities include preparing and guiding the patient through the procedure. You also may assist the radiologic technologist or the radiologist in performing the procedure by placing, removing, and developing film in the X-ray machine. Procedure 50-1, at the end of this chapter, describes the general process of assisting with a radiologic procedure.

FIGURE 50-2 These are X-ray pathways and resulting projections for the most common types of X-rays.

You may care for a patient and assist the radiologic technologist or radiologist during a wide variety of X-ray and other diagnostic imaging tests. While requirements of different procedures vary, you will probably be asked to perform many of the duties described in Procedure 50-1. Although you are unlikely to position the patient, you should know that the position relative to the X-ray source determines the path of the X-rays and the resulting images. Figure 50-2 illustrates common X-ray pathways and the images produced.

Verifying Insurance for Radiologic Procedures

Managed care health insurance plans are the most common type of insurance you will encounter in the office. Patients with

HMOs are often required to use the services of certain radiology facilities. Because managed care plans often have facilities with which they are contracted, be sure the patient is sent to a radiology facility that is contracted with his or her health insurance. If needed, verify and complete the necessary referrals for all radiology testing. Make insurance verification a regular step in preprocedure care.

Storing and Filing X-Rays

Many X-rays are now stored digitally, but there may be some instances where an actual X-ray film is produced. In this case, you may be responsible for storing X-ray films if you work in a radiology facility. Follow these guidelines for proper X-ray storage:

- Keep fresh film on hand at all times.
- Maintain new and exposed films in as good a condition as possible by keeping them at a temperature between 50°F and 70°F (between 10°C and 20°C) and a relative humidity between 30% and 50%. Radiology facilities usually have one or more special rooms for films.
- Prevent pressure marks and keep expiration dates visible by storing packages on end; do not stack them on top of each other.
- Use a first-in, first-out method for using film (that is, use the oldest film first).
- Open film packages or boxes only in the darkroom.
- Do not store film near acid or ammonia vapors.

You also will be responsible for providing accurate record-keeping of X-rays. See Procedure 50-2, at the end of this chapter, for guidelines on documentation and filing techniques.

Remember, actual X-ray films are the property of the radiology facility or the doctor's office where they are taken. Although the films may be sent (or taken by the patient) to a hospital or another doctor for consultation, they should be returned to the original facility (for example, the radiologist's office). In some facilities, the images are stored on a computer and the patient receives an electronic copy to take to another doctor or medical facility. The information, however, is the patient's property, so the patient need not return reports.

▶ Common Diagnostic Radiologic Tests

LO 50.4

A variety of radiologic imaging tests are available. Table 50-1 identifies some of the most frequently ordered tests and the disorders they are used to diagnose.

Contrast Media in Diagnostic Tests

Various procedures involve the use of contrast media to see body structures and observe their function. These procedures include angiography, arthrography, barium enema, barium swallow, cholangiography, cholecystography, cystography, fluoroscopy, intravenous pyelography, magnetic resonance imaging (sometimes), myelography, nuclear medicine studies, and retrograde pyelography.

As mentioned, contrast media can be administered by mouth, by needle or catheter into a blood vessel, or by a route that introduces the medium into an organ or body cavity (for example, into the colon). A contrast medium can cause adverse effects in some patients. Common adverse effects with oral agents include mild and transient abdominal cramping, constipation, nausea, vomiting, diarrhea, skin rashes, itching, heartburn, dizziness, and headache. Intravenous agents cause some of the same adverse effects as well as localized injection-site reactions and more serious reactions like anaphylaxis. Because many contrast media contain iodine, a common allergen, patients should be questioned about known allergies to iodine or shellfish, which contain iodine, before procedures involving the use of contrast media. All patients should be observed during such procedures for signs of allergic reaction.

Fluoroscopy

X-rays can cause certain chemicals to fluoresce, or emit visible light. When X-rays penetrate a body structure and are directed onto a fluorescent screen, they produce an image the radiologist can view either directly or through special glasses. Usually, a radiologist, rather than a radiology technician or medical assistant, performs fluoroscopic procedures.

Many diagnostic procedures involve fluoroscopy, which allows viewing of internal organ movement or the movement of a contrast medium, like barium sulfate, while the contrast medium travels through the alimentary canal. Fluoroscopy also guides the radiologist in locating a precise internal area that needs to be recorded on film or digitally.

Fluoroscopic images are sometimes photographed for further study. Photofluorography is a series of these photographs that records the body's internal movements over time. Cinefluorography is a motion picture of the internal movements of the body.

Hysterosalpingography

Hysterosalpingography, also called uterosalpingography, is a radiologic examination of a women's uterus and fallopian tubes using fluoroscopy. This procedure is used to examine women who have difficulty becoming pregnant. It is sometimes ordered when the woman has a history of miscarriages that result from congenital abnormalities of the uterus or as part of a fertility exam. It is also used to determine the presence and severity of tumor masses or adhesions, uterine fibroids, and fallopian tube adhesions or obstructions. A hysterosalpingogram (Figure 50-3) assists the radiologist in evaluating the shape and structure of

TABLE 50-1   Common Radiologic Tests and Disorders Diagnosed

Test	Disorders Diagnosed/Treated
Angiography	
Cardiovascular	Status of blood flow, collateral circulation, malformed vessels, aneurysms, narrowing or blockages of vessels, and presence of hemorrhage
Cerebral	Aneurysm, hemorrhage, evidence of cerebrovascular accident, and arteriosclerosis
Gastrointestinal (GI)	Upper gastrointestinal bleeding
Pulmonary	Pulmonary emboli (especially when lung scan is inconclusive) and evaluation of pulmonary circulation in some heart conditions before surgery
Renal	Abnormalities of blood vessels in urinary system
Arthrography	Joint conditions
Barium enema (lower GI series)	Obstructions, ulcers, polyps, diverticulosis, tumor, and motility problems of colon or rectum
Barium swallow (upper GI series)	Obstructions, ulcers, polyps, diverticulosis, tumor, and motility problems of esophagus, stomach, duodenum, and small intestine
Cholangiography, cholecystography	Gallstones, gallbladder, or common bile duct stones or obstructions; ability of gallbladder to concentrate and store dye
Computed tomography (CT)	Aortic and heart aneurysms, disorders of liver and biliary systems, renal and pulmonary tumors, brain abnormalities (tumors, blood clots, evidence of cerebrovascular accident, outlines of brain ventricles), GI tract lesions, GI disorders (acute pseudocyst of pancreas, abdominal abscesses, biliary obstruction), breast diseases and disorders, and spinal disorders; and to guide biopsy procedures
Fluoroscopy	Structure, process, and function of organs in motion to detect abnormalities
Intravenous pyelography (IVP) (excretory urography)	Urinary system abnormalities, including renal pelvis, ureters, and bladder (for example, kidney stones); abnormal size, shape, or structure of kidneys, ureters, or bladder; space-occupying lesions; pyelonephrosis; hydronephrosis; and trauma to the urinary system
KUB (kidneys, ureters, bladder) radiography	Size, shape, and position of urinary organs; urinary system diseases or disorders; and kidney stones
Magnetic resonance imaging (MRI)	Cancerous tissue, atherosclerotic tissue, blood clots, tumors, and deformities, particularly of the heart valves, brain, spine, and joints
Mammography	Breast tumors and lesions
Myelography	Irregularities or compression of spinal cord
Nuclear medicine (radionuclide imaging)	Abnormal function (defects), lesions, or disorders of bone, brain, lungs, kidneys, liver, pancreas, thyroid, and spleen
Radiation therapy	Treatment of cancer
Retrograde pyelogram	Obstruction of ureters, bladder, or urethra (including tumors, stones, strictures, or blood clots); and perinephritic abscess
Ultrasound	Abnormalities of gallbladder, liver, spleen, heart, kidneys, gonads, blood vessels, and lymph system; and fetal conditions (including number of fetuses; age and sex of fetus; fetal development, position, and deformities)

the uterus, the openness (patency) of the fallopian tubes, and any scarring within the fallopian tubes and peritoneal cavity. Hysterosalpingography is usually performed on an outpatient basis.

Angiography

Angiography requires a physician (usually a radiologist) to insert a catheter into the patient's vein (venography) or artery (arteriography). The test—used to evaluate the heart vessels (coronary angiography), the brain (cerebral angiography), and the femoral, brachial, or carotid artery—may be performed jointly by a radiologist and a vascular surgeon or other specialist. The physician first guides the catheter tip to the vessel being examined, then injects a contrast medium through the catheter and takes a series of X-rays to assess the vessel's blood flow and condition (Figure 50-4).

Because this procedure requires insertion of a catheter into a blood vessel and the use of local anesthesia, the patient is admitted to a hospital or same-day surgical facility. The physician who performs the examination provides the patient with

FIGURE 50-3   A hystersalpingogram of the uterus and fallopian tubes.

instructions immediately before the procedure. You will, however, schedule the procedure, and you can encourage the patient

FIGURE 50-4 Carotid angiogram: an intra-arterial catheter is inserted and a contrast medium is injected to create an image of the arteries.

to ask questions. Radiology facilities usually have information sheets for each procedure. If the patient has questions you cannot answer or if you have any doubt about preprocedure instructions, check with your supervisor.

Arthrography

Arthrography is performed by a radiologist, who uses a contrast medium and fluoroscopy to help diagnose abnormalities or injuries in the cartilage, tendons, or ligaments of the joints—usually the knee or shoulder. Although MRI is used more often to evaluate soft-tissue injuries in joints, arthrography can provide an image while the patient moves the joint. When preparing patients for arthrography or assisting with the procedure, follow these guidelines:

- Describe the procedure to patients and inform them the examination will take about 1 hour. Ask patients about possible allergies to contrast media, iodine, or shellfish. If they have any of these allergies, inform the radiologist immediately.
- Explain to patients that no special preprocedure preparations are necessary.
- Tell patients the doctor will first inject a local anesthetic to numb the area being examined. Then the doctor will inject the contrast medium (dye, air, or both) into the joint

and will use a fluoroscope to evaluate the joint's function. Inform patients who are having a knee examined that the doctor may ask them to walk a few steps to spread the contrast medium.

- After the test is completed, advise patients that for 1 or 2 days they may experience some pain or swelling, particularly if the joint is exercised. Tell them to rest and avoid putting strain on the joint.

Barium Enema (Lower GI Series)

A **barium enema** is performed by a radiologist, who instills barium sulfate through the anus into the rectum and then into the colon, to help diagnose and evaluate obstructions, ulcers, polyps, diverticulosis, tumors, or motility problems of the colon or rectum. This procedure is called a *lower GI (gastrointestinal) series*—a series of X-rays of the colon and rectum. The two types of barium enema techniques are single-contrast, in which only barium is instilled into the colon, and double-contrast, in which air is forced into the colon to distend or inflate the tissue. The air may be added while the barium is present, after it has been expelled, or both. The double-contrast technique makes structures more visible by fluoroscopy and allows identification of small lesions. The digestive tract must be totally empty, requiring the patient to thoroughly cleanse the tract with a series of preparatory steps and to have nothing by mouth for 8 hours before the test, except for one cup of clear liquid on the morning of the test. In most facilities, a radiologic technologist assists with a barium enema, but you may assist the patient before and after the procedure. If you do assist with a barium enema, you will have various responsibilities before, during, and after the procedure.

Before the Procedure Schedule the patient's appointment in the morning so he can sleep through most of the period during which his digestive tract must be empty and thus avoid experiencing hunger unnecessarily. Include the following items when you instruct a patient about the preparation for a barium enema:

- Describe the procedure and tell the patient the examination will take 1 to 2 hours.
- Ask about possible allergies to contrast media, iodine, or shellfish and report such allergies to the radiologist.
- Explain the importance of following the preparation instructions so the colon and rectum are free of residual material. Residual material in the colon or rectum could cause blockages or shadows, resulting in an inaccurate test.
- Preprocedure preparation on the day before the examination includes following a clear liquid diet beginning in the morning (coffee, tea, carbonated beverages, clear gelatin, strained fruit juice, bouillon, or clear broths; milk is not permitted) and taking prescribed amounts of electrolyte solution or other laxative preparations and fluids on a specified schedule).
- Tell the patient he may have one cup of coffee, tea, or water on the morning of the examination.

During the Procedure Follow these steps when assisting during a barium enema:

1. Have the patient undress and put on a gown.

2. Tell the patient to expect some discomfort during the examination, as well as frequent side-to-side turning.

3. Have the patient lie on his side. The radiologist inserts the enema tip, designed to help the patient hold the liquid, into the rectum and instills the barium sulfate into the colon. If the patient experiences cramping or the urge to defecate during instillation of the barium, instruct him to relax the abdominal muscles by breathing slowly and deeply through the mouth.

4. Instruct the patient to remain still and hold his breath when X-rays are taken. Using a fluoroscope, the doctor observes the barium as it flows through the lower bowel and periodically takes X-rays while the patient is placed in various positions. You may be asked to assist with placing the patient in these positions.

5. If a double-contrast study is being performed, tell the patient that air will be introduced into the colon to expand the colon tissue. Explain that the combination of air and barium provides a clearer view of structures than only one contrast medium would provide and allows possible identification of small lesions if they are present.

6. When the doctor has completed the barium portion of the examination, including X-rays with both barium and air, tell the patient to use the toilet and expel as much barium as possible. Explain that if enough barium is expelled, the doctor may take a final X-ray of the empty colon.

7. Have the patient wait to dress until the doctor tells you that no additional X-rays are needed.

After the Procedure After the radiologist has completed the barium enema, instruct the patient in postprocedure care. Tell the patient the following:

- He may now have a regular meal.
- The residual barium may make his stools appear whitish or lighter than usual, but this is normal.
- The barium may cause constipation, so he should drink extra water to help relieve constipation and to eliminate the remaining barium sulfate. The physician may order a laxative to be taken if constipation is not relieved within 1 or 2 days.

Barium Swallow (Upper GI Series)

A **barium swallow** involves oral administration of a barium sulfate drink to help diagnose and evaluate obstructions, ulcers, polyps, diverticulosis, tumors, or motility problems of the esophagus, stomach, duodenum, and small intestine. This test is called an *upper GI series*. In preparation for this test, the patient can have nothing by mouth for at least 8 hours before the test. You will have various responsibilities before, during, and after the procedure.

Before the Procedure Schedule the patient's appointment in the morning so she can sleep through most of the period during which her digestive tract is empty and thus avoid experiencing hunger unnecessarily. When instructing a patient about the preparation for an upper GI series, include the following items:

- Describe the procedure and tell the patient the examination will take about 1 hour. If X-rays of the small bowel are needed, the test may take several hours.
- Ask about possible allergies to contrast media, iodine, or shellfish and report such allergies to the radiologist.
- Explain the importance of following the preparation instructions so the stomach is empty. Preprocedure requirements include having nothing by mouth (food or liquids) after midnight the night before and no breakfast the morning of the examination. If the patient's small bowel is to be evaluated, also tell her to take the prescribed laxative preparation between 2:00 and 4:00 p.m. the day before the examination.
- Instruct the patient not to swallow water when brushing her teeth or rinsing her mouth and, if applicable, to stop smoking because nicotine stimulates gastric secretions and can affect the test results.

During the Procedure When assisting during an upper GI series, take the following steps:

1. Have the patient undress and put on a gown.

2. Explain that she will be drinking a barium sulfate drink that tastes chalky and resembles a milk shake.

3. Have the patient stand and drink part of the barium.

4. The radiologist will use a fluoroscope to observe the flow of the barium and to assess the functioning of the esophagus, stomach, duodenum, and small intestine as the barium passes through the structures. (The doctor will then direct the patient to drink additional barium and continue to observe the function of the various structures.)

5. Place the patient on the X-ray table and move her into different positions (if medical assistants are permitted to do so in your state), as instructed by the doctor, to allow X-rays to be taken of the upper digestive tract. Instruct the patient to remain still and hold her breath when X-rays are taken.

After the Procedure After the physician completes the upper GI series, instruct the patient in postprocedure care. Give the patient the following information:

- She may now have a regular meal.
- Her stools may appear whitish or lighter than usual as the barium is eliminated, but this is normal.
- Sometimes, another examination may be required after 24 hours to determine whether the barium has moved into the large intestine. If this test is indicated, tell the patient to follow a clear liquid diet (coffee, tea, carbonated beverages, clear gelatin, strained fruit juices, bouillon, or clear broths; milk is not permitted) and to return in 24 hours.

Cholecystography and Cholangiography

Two similar tests performed by a radiologist are cholecystography and cholangiography. Both tests involve use of a contrast medium to view parts of the gallbladder.

Cholecystography A radiologist uses cholecystography to detect gallstones and other gallbladder abnormalities, usually when ultrasound does not provide enough information for a diagnosis. The doctor X-rays the patient's gallbladder after the patient has ingested an oral contrast medium. You will be responsible for preparing the patient for the procedure and assisting during the procedure.

Before the Procedure Schedule the patient's appointment in the morning so he can sleep through most of the period during which his digestive tract is empty and thus avoid experiencing hunger unnecessarily. When instructing a patient about preparing for a cholecystography, follow these guidelines:

- Describe the procedure and explain that the examination will take about 1 to 2 hours.
- Ask the patient about possible allergies to contrast media, iodine, or shellfish and report them to the radiologist.
- Explain the diet restrictions necessary to prepare for the test. Tell the patient to have a fat-free dinner (dry toast, tea, fruit, gelatin dessert) the evening before the examination. He should not smoke or have any food or liquids after midnight and should have no breakfast the morning of the examination.
- Instruct the patient to take the oral contrast medium (usually in tablet form) beginning about 2 hours after dinner or as prescribed by the doctor. The tablets should be taken one at a time, normally 5 minutes apart (time may vary depending on the contrast agent), with a small amount of water, until six tablets have been taken. Explain that the contrast agent may cause nausea or diarrhea but that nothing should be taken for these conditions. In the case of severe nausea, the doctor may prescribe an antiemetic; diarrhea is an expected result of the contrast medium used for this test.
- Some doctors also order a laxative for the patient to take the day before the examination.

During and after the Procedure When assisting during a cholecystography, take the following steps:

1. Have the patient undress and put on a gown.
2. Have the patient lie on the X-ray table in the supine position (face up).
3. Explain that the radiologist will take X-rays of the gallbladder, which will be filled with the contrast medium the patient took the night before. Then the radiologist will use a fluoroscope to study the gallbladder's function. A functioning gallbladder absorbs the contrast agent properly.
4. Next, give the patient a specially prepared fatty meal, which should stimulate the gallbladder to empty bile into the duodenum. After about 1 hour, the doctor takes more X-rays to study the gallbladder's function. A functioning gallbladder empties the contrast medium properly. A non-functioning gallbladder may indicate, for example, the presence of gallstones or obstruction of the bile ducts.
5. After the examination, advise the patient to return to a normal diet and to drink plenty of fluids to replace those lost through diarrhea.

Cholangiography Cholangiography, similar to cholecystography, is performed by a radiologist to evaluate the function of the bile ducts. It involves injection of the contrast medium directly into the common bile duct (during gallbladder surgery) or through a T tube (after gallbladder surgery or during radiologic testing). X-rays are taken immediately after injection. Use the guidelines for cholecystography. Instruct the patient as follows:

- Describe the procedure to the patient and tell him the examination will take about 2 to 3 hours. Ask the patient about possible allergies to contrast media, iodine, or shellfish and report them to the radiologist.
- Explain the preparation instructions. Tell the patient to eat a light evening meal the night before the examination, to take a laxative (as prescribed by the doctor), and to have no food or liquids after midnight. He also should have no solid food the morning of the examination.

Conventional Tomography and Computed Tomography

Conventional tomography produces tomograms, and computed tomography produces CT scans. These two techniques are frequently confused. Computers are involved in producing both kinds of images, but the computers are different and have different functions.

Conventional tomography uses a computerized X-ray camera that moves back and forth in an arc over the patient to produce a series of views of a body part. The computer sets the angle and layer for each arc, and the camera produces one view per arc.

In CT scans produced by computed tomography, the X-ray camera rotates completely around the patient and the computer compiles one cross-sectional view from each rotation of the camera. The patient is lying on a special table that gradually moves through the doughnut-shaped machine containing the rotating camera.

The preparation is essentially the same for the two procedures. Reassure the patient that he will not be inserted into an enclosed space, as is the case in magnetic resonance imaging. The patient will be able to see around the room during the test.

Tomograms and CT scans are used to diagnose abnormalities in almost all body structures, including the head, kidneys, heart, chest, liver, biliary tract, pancreas, GI tract, spine, pelvis, bones, and breast. When preparing the patient for a tomogram or a CT scan, use the following guidelines:

- Ask the patient about possible allergies to contrast media, iodine, or shellfish and report them to the radiologist.

- Tell the patient he will be placed on a table that moves through the scanner for CT scans or on an X-ray table for tomograms.
- Inform the patient that the procedure will last about 45 to 90 minutes and that he must lie still while the scans are taken. The patient may breathe normally while the CT scans are taken but must hold his breath for each of the tomograms.
- If a contrast medium will be used, advise the patient that it will be injected into a vein in the arm or on the back of the hand (except with a CT scan of the spine) to enhance detail of the structure being evaluated.
- If the patient is having a CT scan of the head or chest, instruct him not to eat anything for 4 hours or drink any liquids for 2 hours before the examination. Explain that he may experience mild nausea after injection of the contrast medium if the stomach is too full.
- If the patient is having tomograms or a CT scan of the abdomen or pelvis, tell him to obtain a preparation kit from the office or hospital the day before the examination. This kit includes a special drink the patient must take the night before the examination that helps outline the intestines. Inform the patient that the drink should not produce a laxative effect or any discomfort.
- Tell the patient to remove metallic objects that could interfere with the path of the X-rays. Also, ask if the patient has skin staples or metallic prostheses that could interfere.
- Inform the patient that a written report of the results should be available within 24 hours of the test and that a report will be sent to his primary care physician (or the referring physician).

Heart X-Ray

An X-ray of the heart, using a contrast medium, may be necessary to show the heart's configuration and to reveal cardiac enlargement and aortic dilation. Angiography of the heart is called angiocardiography, in which a contrast medium is injected into a major blood vessel. X-rays are taken while the medium flows through the heart, lungs, and major vessels. Coronary arteriography uses a dye inserted through a catheter that has been passed through an artery to the heart. Both procedures require hospital admission, usually in a day surgery or ambulatory surgery unit.

Intravenous Pyelography

Also known as *excretory urography*, **intravenous pyelography (IVP)** is performed by a radiologist who injects a contrast medium into a vein. The doctor then takes a series of X-rays as the contrast medium travels through the kidneys, ureters, and bladder. IVP is used to evaluate urinary system abnormalities or trauma to the urinary system. In most facilities, a radiologic technologist assists with IVP, but you may assist the patient before the procedure. If you assist with IVP, you will have several responsibilities both before and during the procedure.

Before the Procedure Schedule the patient's appointment in the morning so she can sleep through most of the period during which her digestive tract is empty and thus avoid experiencing hunger unnecessarily. When instructing a patient about the preparation for an IVP, include the following information:

- Describe the procedure and tell the patient the examination will take about 1½ hours.
- Ask the patient about possible allergies to contrast media, iodine, or shellfish and report such allergies to the radiologist.
- Explain the importance of adhering to the preparation instructions, so the bowel is free of any material that could obstruct the view of the urinary organs.
- Tell the patient to follow a liquid diet (coffee, tea, carbonated beverages, clear gelatin, strained fruit juice, bouillon, or clear broths, but no milk) the day before the examination. The patient may be given a laxative preparation to take the night before the examination.
- No food or liquids are allowed after midnight and no breakfast the morning of the examination. Some physicians also order an enema to be taken about 2 hours before the examination.

During and after the Procedure When assisting during an IVP, you will generally proceed in this manner:

1. Have the patient undress and put on a gown.
2. Explain that a contrast medium will be injected into her vein (usually in the arm). Instruct her to inform the physician if she notices shortness of breath or itching after injection of the dye because this can indicate an allergic reaction.
3. Have the patient lie on the X-ray table and move her into different positions, as instructed by the physician, to allow X-rays to be taken of the urinary tract as the contrast medium is excreted. Instruct the patient to remain still and hold her breath when X-rays are taken.
4. Note that some physicians place a compression device on the abdomen, which helps hold the contrast medium in the kidneys and ureters by exerting moderate pressure.
5. After the physician takes the series of X-rays to evaluate urinary system function, ask the patient to urinate and explain that a final X-ray will be taken.
6. Inform the patient that she may resume a normal diet after the test and that the contrast medium will be eliminated in the urine.

Retrograde Pyelography

Retrograde pyelography is similar to the IVP, except that the doctor injects the contrast medium through a urethral catheter. This procedure, which evaluates function of the ureters, bladder, and urethra, is often used for patients with poor kidney function. Follow the same preparation and assistance instructions as for the IVP.

Kidneys, Ureters, and Bladder (KUB) Radiography

Also called a *flat plate of the abdomen*, **KUB radiography** is an X-ray of the abdomen used to assess the size, shape, and position of the urinary organs; to evaluate urinary system diseases or disorders; and to determine the presence of kidney stones. It also can be helpful in determining the position of an intrauterine device (IUD) or in locating foreign bodies in the digestive tract. No patient preparation is required. A radiologic technologist takes a KUB X-ray; thus, you follow the guidelines you would use for a patient having any type of standard, noninvasive X-ray.

Magnetic Resonance Imaging (MRI)

Nonionizing radiation (radio frequency signals) and a strong magnetic field are combined in magnetic resonance imaging to allow the physician to examine internal structures and soft tissues of any body area. The combination of nonionizing radiation and magnetic field, which allows the MRI scanner to produce images based primarily on the water content of tissues, appears to have no harmful effects on the patient. The test may be performed with or without contrast. You will be responsible for preparing the patient for an MRI and assisting with the procedure.

High-speed MRI scanners scan four times faster than other MRIs, which makes the procedure more tolerable for the patient and produces clear, high-resolution images that help physicians improve diagnoses for conditions like common knee and shoulder conditions and abdominal and brain disorders.

Before the Procedure When instructing a patient about preparing for an MRI, include the following steps:

- If a contrast medium is going to be used, ask the patient and inform the radiologist about possible allergies to contrast media, iodine, or shellfish.

- Screen the patient to determine whether any internal metallic materials are present. (This is especially important because a strong magnetic field is involved in creating the image.) Ask about a pacemaker, brain or aneurysm clips, brain or heart surgery, shunts and heart valves, other surgeries, and shrapnel or metal fragments (particularly in an eye).

- Ask the patient whether he is or has been a metalworker. If so, he may carry metal slivers, chips, or filings under his nails or skin.

- Instruct women not to wear eye makeup the day of the examination, as it often contains metallic ingredients.

- Describe the procedure to the patient and explain that the examination will take between 45 minutes and 2 hours.

- Inform the patient that he may wear street clothing during the test, but to avoid wearing clothing with metallic thread, metal stays or grippers, or thick elastic. Tell the patient he will probably be asked to undress, however, and put on a gown.

- Tell the patient he does not need to fast before the examination or follow any preprocedure diet, unless he is having an MRI of the pelvis. In that case, instruct him to have no solid food for 6 hours and no liquids for 4 hours before the examination. Inform the patient that he may take prescription medications.

- Explain that he will not be required to drink an oral contrast preparation but should avoid caffeine for 4 hours before the examination. Tell the patient he will probably have no side effects from the examination but that some nausea may occur as a result of the contrast medium.

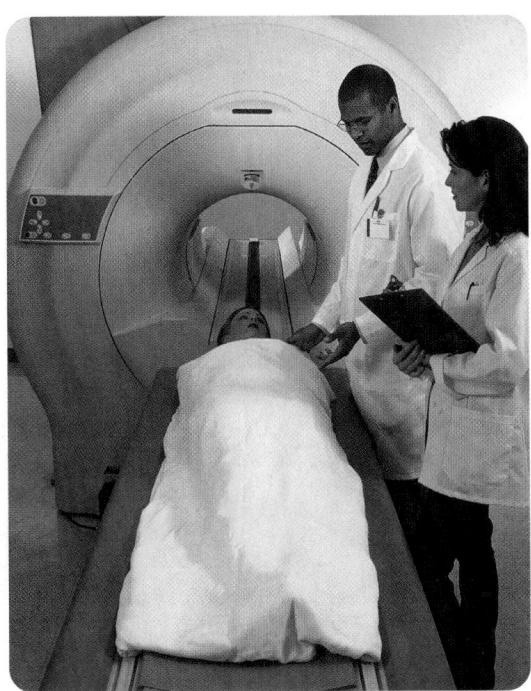

FIGURE 50-5 A patient who is claustrophobic or unable to lie still may require sedation during an MRI.

During and after the Procedure When assisting during an MRI, you will need to follow these specific steps:

1. Have the patient lie on the padded table.

2. Explain that the table will be placed inside a long, narrow tube about 22 inches in diameter and that he will hear a loud knocking noise as the machine scans. Offer the patient hearing protection devices (ear plugs or headphones) during the test. Warn the patient to remain still to avoid blurring the image and the consequent need for a retake. Note that physicians may order sedation for patients who are claustrophobic or cannot lie still for a long period (Figure 50-5).

3. Advise the patient that although the technician will not be in the scanning room during the examination, she will maintain contact with a camera and a microphone. The patient may speak to the technician at any time in case of a problem, but he is encouraged to be still for each series.

4. Inform the patient that his primary care physician or referring doctor should have a preliminary report of test results within about 24 hours.

Mammography

Mammography, the X-ray exam of the internal breast tissues, helps in diagnosing breast abnormalities (Figure 50-6). A specially trained radiologic technologist takes mammograms.

You will have several responsibilities during both setup and patient care before and after mammography. However, a medical assistant does not assist during mammography in most states. Instead, you will prepare the patient for the procedure and ease her fears. The Educating the Patient section provides information on this topic.

FIGURE 50-6 Mammograms can reveal the presence of tumors that are not detected by other means. The mammogram on the right indicates normal breast tissue, whereas the one on the left suggests a malignancy.

Mammotest Biopsy Procedure

When a mammogram reveals an abnormality in the breast tissue, it is often treated in one of two ways—either the abnormality is followed for a period of time to see if there are any significant changes, or a surgical excision biopsy is performed. Because so many abnormalities revealed by mammography are benign and present no health risk, physicians now perform *stereotactic breast biopsies*, which are less painful and less invasive than conventional excisional biopsies. The procedure is performed by a physician and a radiologic technologist and is similar to mammography except that the patient is usually lying face down or sitting rather than standing. The breast is compressed with a compression paddle to confirm that the area of the breast with the lesion is correctly centered in the paddle window. A computer is used to help determine the exact positioning of the biopsy needle and the physician takes a small sample of tissue to be examined by a pathologist for the presence of malignant cells. The attending physician later contacts the patient with the test results.

Myelography

Although MRI is used more often to evaluate the spinal cord and spinal nerves, **myelography** is a kind of fluoroscopy of the

---

EDUCATING THE PATIENT

Preprocedure Care for Mammography

A patient who is scheduled for mammography must know the guidelines to follow before the exam. You can help educate the patient by instructing her in the following preprocedure care:

- The mammography should be scheduled for the first week after the patient's menstrual cycle. This timing helps minimize discomfort from compression of the breasts and ensures that the breasts are in their most normal state.

- No special preprocedure diet or medication requirements are necessary, but the patient should consider avoiding caffeine for 7 to 10 days before the exam (in some patients, caffeine may cause swelling and soreness that would heighten discomfort during the procedure). Have the patient decrease caffeine intake gradually, however, to avoid getting headaches.

- The patient should shower or bathe as close as possible to the time of the mammography and wear loose, easy-to-remove clothing. A blouse and pants or skirt work best to allow undressing only to the waist.

- The patient should not use deodorants, powders, or perfumes on the breasts or underarm areas before the examination because these products could produce a false result on the X-ray.

- Inform the patient that the radiologist will want films from a prior mammogram if the mammogram was obtained from a different facility. Some radiologists may not read the films for an impression if a comparison study is not possible.

In addition to providing these instructions, you may need to reassure a patient who is fearful about mammography. Explain that although mammography is uncomfortable, it is usually not painful. Describing how the procedure is performed may alleviate the patient's fears. Provide the patient with the following information:

- The procedure may take up to 20 minutes. The patient removes everything above her waist (including jewelry) and wears a gown with the opening in the front. Most current mammogram procedures do not require lead shielding during the procedure.

- The patient will be positioned in front of the machine. The technician will compress the left breast between the machine plates and take two X-rays—one horizontal view and one vertical view—of the left breast.

- The technician will then position and compress the right breast between the machine plates. Two X-rays will be taken of the right breast.

- If needed, a mild pain reliever may be used to alleviate discomfort or aching after the procedure.

spinal cord used when MRI is not practical—if a patient has a pacemaker or other medical device that prevents the patient from undergoing MRI. The physician performs a lumbar puncture, removes some cerebrospinal fluid (CSF), and instills a contrast medium to evaluate spinal abnormalities, like compression of the spinal cord. Sometimes the physician performs pneumoencephalography, which involves instilling air after removal of the CSF to allow viewing of the cerebral cavities.

The physician who performs myelography or pneumoencephalography must be skilled in performing lumbar puncture—most likely a radiologist, neurologist, neuro-surgeon, or anesthetist. A radiologic technologist is typically the only other person present for the test. Although myelography is not used as frequently as it was before the invention of CT and MRI, it is still performed when these newer techniques do not provide enough information about the spinal canal. Myelography may be reserved for cases in which the clinical findings are unusual or the scanning results uncertain.

Nuclear Medicine

Also known as *radionuclide imaging*, **nuclear medicine** involves use of radionuclides, or radioisotopes (radioactive elements or their compounds). The radionuclides are administered orally, intravenously, or through routes that introduce them into organs or body cavities. The purpose is to evaluate the bone, brain, lungs, kidneys, liver, pancreas, thyroid, or spleen. Sometimes, the entire body is scanned for "hot spots," or places where the radioisotope is concentrated.

For common nuclear medicine scans, the technician uses a scanner called a *gamma camera*. This scanner detects radiation from the radioisotope and converts it into an image (called a *scintiscan* or *scintigram*) to be photographed or displayed on a screen (see Figure 50-7). Some images are produced immediately, whereas others may take up to several days. Radionuclide imaging exposes patients to lower doses of radiation than some radiologic techniques because the amount of ionizing radiation in the isotope is less than that emitted from X-ray cameras. Other nuclear medicine procedures include single photon emission computed tomography (SPECT), positron emission tomography (PET), and MUGA (multiple gated acquisition) scan.

- **SPECT** is often used to locate and determine the extent of brain damage from a stroke. The gamma camera detects signals induced by gamma radiation and a computer converts these signals into either two- or three-dimensional images that are displayed on a screen.

- **PET** entails injecting isotopes combined with other substances involved in metabolic activity, like glucose. These special isotopes emit positrons, which a computer processes and displays on a screen. PET is especially useful for diagnosing brain-related conditions like epilepsy, mental illnesses, and Parkinson's disease.

- **Nuclear ventriculography—MUGA scan**—evaluates the condition of the heart's myocardium. It can be done while the patient is at rest or in stress (exercise) and involves the injection of radioisotopes that concentrate in the myocardium.

FIGURE 50-7   This bone scan shows the uptake of the radioactive contrast medium.

The gamma camera allows the physician to measure ventricular contractions to evaluate the patient's heart wall.

When preparing a patient for a nuclear medicine procedure, describe the procedure and explain how long it will take. Also, explain any preparation requirements and other special instructions and tell the patient she will need to wait the required length of time for the uptake of the radioisotope. Length of examination and requirements for common scans are as follows:

- A bone scan lasts about 1 hour; it is done 2 to 3 hours after a 15-minute injection; the patient drinks 1 quart of liquid between the injection and the scan; a normal diet is permitted.

- A liver/spleen or lung scan lasts approximately 1 hour; there are no diet restrictions.

- A kidney scan lasts about 2 hours; there are no diet restrictions.

- A thyroid uptake and scan test usually requires 2 days; the patient takes a capsule of contrast medium in the morning and has the scan on the first day; the patient returns 24 hours later for the second scan; there are no diet restrictions, except the patient must have no fish because of its natural iodine content.

Ultrasound

Ultrasound directs high-frequency sound waves through the skin over the area of the body being examined and produces an image based on the echoes. A radiologist or an ultrasound

FIGURE 50-8 Ultrasound is commonly used to evaluate the health of a developing fetus.

sonographer coats the body area with a special gel and passes a transducer (instrument similar to a microphone) over the area. As the transducer passes back and forth, it picks up echoes from the sound waves, which a computer converts into an image—sometimes called a sonogram—on a screen. Ultrasound is used to detect abnormalities in the gallbladder, liver, spleen, heart, and kidneys. It is also safe to use in obstetrics to evaluate the developing fetus or to detect multiple fetuses because it does not expose the patient (or the fetus) to radiation (Figure 50-8). In this case, the obstetrician may perform the test in the office.

One form of ultrasound—Doppler echocardiography—involves sound waves that echo against the flow of blood through vessels. Doppler echocardiography is usually performed by a cardiologist to determine whether blood flow is laminar (normal) or turbulent (disturbed).

Echocardiography, a type of ultrasound test, is used to study the structure and function of the heart. The test is usually performed while the patient is resting and again after exercising on a treadmill or bicycle. Images of the heart before and after exercise help the physician diagnose abnormalities of the structure and function of the heart and heart valves.

When preparing the patient for an ultrasound or assisting with the examination, follow these guidelines:

- Describe the procedure to the patient and inform her that the examination will take about 1½ to 2 hours, depending on the type of ultrasound. For example, a cardiac ultrasound takes about 1½ hours; pelvic, 1 to 2 hours; and abdominal, ½ to 1 hour.

- Explain the preparation requirements, which vary according to the type of ultrasound. Tell a patient who is having a gallbladder or liver ultrasound not to eat for several hours before the test. Tell a pregnant patient to drink the prescribed amount of water 1 hour before the examination and not to void. Advise a patient having a pelvic ultrasound to take the prescribed laxative (if indicated), drink three to four glasses of water within 1 hour, and not to void within 1 hour of the

test. If the patient is having an abdominal ultrasound, instruct her to take a laxative the night before the examination and not to have any food or fluids for 8 hours before the test.

- Advise the patient to wear loose, easy-to-remove clothing.

▶ Common Therapeutic Uses of Radiation

LO 50.5

Used therapeutically, radiology is called **radiation therapy,** which is used to treat cancer by preventing cellular reproduction. The two types of radiation therapy are teletherapy and brachytherapy. **Teletherapy,** also called external beam radiotherapy, is the most common form of radiation therapy and is done on an outpatient basis. It allows deep penetration of tissues and is used primarily for deep tumors. The patient experiences minimal side effects, which may include a "sunburn" effect at the treatment site, mild swelling and tenderness, and sometimes mild fatigue. Generally, the superficial tissues are not permanently damaged.

Stereotactic radiosurgery is a type of teletherapy that uses CT or MRI scanning in conjunction with radiation to treat brain tumors, acoustic neromas, and arteriovenous malformations—defects in connections between arteries and veins—deep in the brain. In some cases, liver, prostate, and lung tumors are also treated with stereotactic radiosurgery. This method allows for very precise delivery of radiation to areas of the brain or other organs that are normally inaccessible with traditional surgical techniques, helping spare precious healthy tissue while still treating the tumor.

For a patient having stereotactic radiosurgery for brain tumors, first a neurosurgeon temporarily fastens a stereotactic frame to the patient's head using local anesthesia. The frame helps guide the physician to precisely locate the treatment. A CT or MRI scan is then performed to locate the tumor or malformation. Once the frame is in place and the imaging scan is complete, a radiation oncologist and a neurosurgeon use a special computer program to plan the patient's treatment. The patient undergoes treatment based on this plan, has the stereotactic frame removed, and, in most cases, can go home the same day.

Localized cancers are treated with **brachytherapy.** In this technique, the radiologist places temporary radioactive implants close to or directly into cancerous tissue. This technique limits radiation exposure to healthy tissue, targeting only the area where the tumor is located. During brachytherapy, both the staff and patient are subject to radiation exposure, so radiation safety precautions must be closely followed. When preparing the patient for radiation therapy, follow these guidelines:

- Describe the procedure and explain how long it will take, as determined by the radiologist and oncologist according to the patient's diagnosis and condition.

- Encourage patients to tell the physician about all medications, vitamins, or supplements they are taking.

- Inform the patient that the radiologist or oncologist will explain the treatment's possible side effects. Common side effects include nausea, vomiting, hair loss, ulceration of mucous membranes, weakness, and malaise. Other possible effects include localized burns on tissue and damage to organs in the treatment path. Encourage the patient to discuss with the doctor (or the oncology nurse specialist) measures to relieve or minimize stress and discomfort.

- Advise the patient to immediately report any other symptoms to the doctor.
- Encourage the patient to get plenty of rest, eat a balanced diet, and drink plenty of fluids.

▶ Radiation Safety and Dose   LO 50.6

For many years after the X-ray's discovery, the seriousness of radiation hazards was not addressed. In the 1920s, the government of Great Britain took the first steps to limit X-ray exposure. Since World War II, studies have been performed, mostly on the effects of high-dose radiation.

Other studies on the effects of background radiation and nonradiologic versus radiologic (X-ray-related) risks have enabled scientists to assess diagnostic X-ray risks. Results from these studies show the risk of excess radiation from routine X-rays to be minimal.

Reducing Patient Exposure

Advances in diagnostic imaging technology, and limits to radiation exposure, have helped reduce the dose of radiation to which a patient is exposed during a diagnostic procedure. Another way to reduce excessive radiation exposure risk lies with the physician, who must assess the benefit-to-risk ratio when recommending a diagnostic radiology procedure. Because radiation has a cumulative effect, the physician must have valid medical reasons for ordering the test, particularly if the patient has recently had other X-rays. Some types of X-rays, like mammograms, should be repeated regularly, however, because of their potential to prevent or promote treatment of life-threatening disorders.

According to a 1993 report by the National Council on Radiation Protection and Measurements (NCRP), titled *Limitation of Exposure to Ionizing Radiation*, one of the earliest pieces of legislation in the United States to limit occupational radiation exposure was enacted in the 1930s. The first legislation to limit public exposure, however, was not enacted until the 1950s. The 1993 NCRP report set guidelines for protection from radiation in and out of the workplace. The two primary objectives outlined in the report are to prevent serious general tissue damage from radiation by limiting radiation dose to levels below known thresholds for such damage and to reduce the risk of cancer and genetic effects to a level balanced by potential benefits to the individual and society.

Because radiation exposure always poses some degree of risk, the NCRP recommends that any activity involving radiation exposure be justified, or balanced against the expected benefits to society. Furthermore, the NCRP recommends the cost, or detriment, to society from such activities be kept *as low as reasonably achievable* (ALARA) and that individual dose limits be applied to ensure that justification and ALARA principles do not result in unacceptable risk levels for individuals or groups.

The NCRP has developed detailed lists on radiation doses to achieve the primary objectives stated in the report. Separate specific limits exist for occupational and public exposure.

Safety Precautions

Understanding and following standard safety precautions are crucial for protection from radiation exposure and are essential to the health and safety of both medical personnel and patients.

Personnel Safety If you work in a medical facility that performs radiologic tests, you are at risk for excessive radiation exposure. To protect yourself from exposure, you must adhere to the following specific guidelines:

- You (and other members of the medical staff) must always wear a radiation exposure badge, or dosimeter, which is a sensitized piece of film in a holder (Figure 50-9). You must have the badge checked regularly by specially qualified personnel, who measure the degree of radiation uptake on the film to determine the amount of radiation to which you have been exposed.
- Make sure all equipment is in good working order and is checked routinely for radiation leakage and any other problems.
- Be aware that the technician and any other staff members present when equipment is operating should always wear a garment that contains a lead shield.

Patient Safety You must follow all rules governing patient safety from radiation exposure. The Educating the Patient section explains safety measures and information that help protect a patient from exposure to unnecessary radiation.

FIGURE 50-9 A radiation exposure badge contains a film that registers the levels of radiation to which a medical staff member is exposed at work.

Safety with X-Rays

You are responsible for teaching the patient about X-ray safety. In this role, you will need to obtain pertinent patient history data, answer questions, and provide basic information on X-rays, possible side effects, and other important guidelines. Consider the following points when teaching the patient about X-ray safety.

Patient History

- Ask the patient about X-rays received in the past, including how many and what type, and about the possibility of exposure to radiation in the home, school, or workplace. Explain that the effects of radiation exposure are cumulative; that is, the effects are related to total exposure over the lifetime as well as to exposure from each procedure.

- Ask a female patient about the possibility of pregnancy. Use the 10-day rule—take an X-ray only within 10 days of the last menstrual period to avoid taking an X-ray of a patient who is unknowingly pregnant. If the patient knows she is pregnant, do not schedule an X-ray unless approved by the radiologist.

- Inform the patient about possible radiation exposure side effects, which include fetal abnormality or genetic mutation in a fetus (when a patient is pregnant) and the depression of bone marrow activity, which decreases the production of red blood cells and white blood cells.

Patient Questions

- Always answer questions in simple, easy-to-understand language; make explanations brief and clear. Do not use complex medical terms; however, do include proper terminology. Offer written information about the test, if available.

- Answer fully any questions about examinations, including descriptions of procedures; the doctor's reason for ordering them; their length, side effects, injections, or other uncomfortable aspects; preprocedure requirements; cost and insurance issues; and availability of test results.

- Help reduce the patient's fear or anxiety surrounding the scheduled test and help her feel comfortable and informed about the procedure.

General X-Ray Information

- Be aware of the most current guidelines established by the American College of Radiology. Always keep up with new studies on radiation exposure risks.

- Encourage the patient to ask questions about the need for X-rays ordered by the doctor and risks associated with those X-rays.

- If the patient's employer requires annual X-rays or a potential employer asks for preemployment X-rays, advise the patient to question the necessity of these tests. Suggest that the patient find out whether the doctor has submittable X-rays on file.

- Advise the patient to discuss testing options with the doctor. For instance, if the doctor orders fluoroscopy, the patient might ask whether standard X-rays can be taken instead, as fluoroscopy, and often mobile X-ray exams, usually carry a higher radiation exposure risk than standard X-rays. Advise the patient to ask questions about X-ray safety standards in the office or hospital in which the tests are to take place.

- Tell the patient to avoid dental X-rays performed with wide-beamed plastic cones; narrow-beamed cones are more exact and less dangerous. In addition, educate the patient about the opinions of the American Dental Association and the National Conference of Dental Radiology, both of which believe X-rays should not be performed solely for insurance claim purposes. Advise the patient to always ask for a lead apron over organs not being studied. Tell the patient to avoid retakes of X-rays because of blurriness or shadows (which are caused by movements or breathing) by remaining still when instructed to do so during X-ray exams.

- Explain the importance of X-rays in proper diagnosis of disorders. Inform the patient about the constant improvements in equipment and X-ray procedures and the much lower doses of radiation now used in these procedures.

- Advise the patient to keep a family record of X-ray exams.

- Educate a female patient without breast disease on the correct schedule for mammography exams. The patient should have a baseline mammogram between ages 35 and 40; a mammogram every 1 to 2 years between ages 40 and 49; and an annual mammogram after age 50.

- Also, tell the patient to see a doctor immediately if she notices a breast mass, lump, or nipple discharge.

▶ Electronic Medicine   LO 50.7

Recent major advances in telemedicine technology, including rapid video and computer-based communications of medical information, enable physicians to "examine" a patient in another city or country, view highly detailed medical images, consult with specialists in other cities, and supervise complex medical procedures. In addition, healthcare personnel, including medical assistants, can participate in interactive teaching conferences by means of closed-circuit television.

In some cities, emergency medical technicians (EMTs) can transmit an electrocardiogram (ECG) electronically to

FIGURE 50-10   A digital lateral MRI image of the brain.

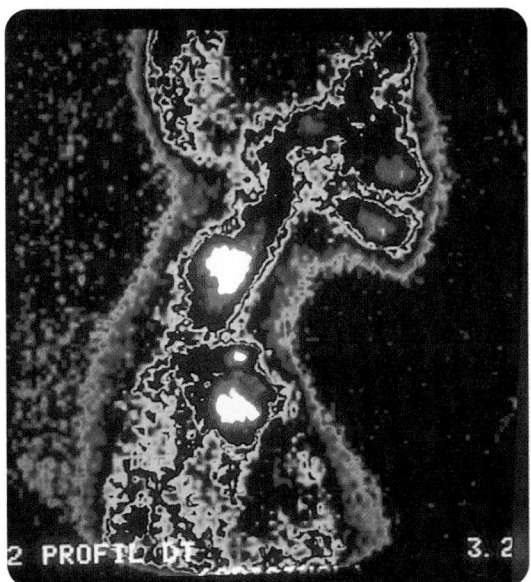

FIGURE 50-11   A digital bone scan of the neck and skull showing malignant tumors.

an emergency room physician to obtain life-saving directives from the physician. These directives may involve administration of drugs or other measures the EMTs would not be permitted to perform without a physician's order. Similarly, cardiologists monitor some patients by the transmission of daily ECGs through telephone lines to the cardiologist's office.

Digital Imaging and the EHR

With the emergence of electronic health records (EHR), technology in healthcare is expanding rapidly. However, no department is affected more than radiology because it is the only completely technology-driven specialty. Digital radiology (DR) devices are integrated with the EHR system to provide quality images and rapid access and to eliminate the time and equipment associated with film processing and development (Figure 50-10).

Digital Radiography

Conventional, film-based radiography is quickly being replaced by digital imaging techniques. Digital radiography uses a digital reader to "capture" or digitize the X-ray image instead of exposing traditional film. Using digital radiography has several advantages, including:

- Better image consistency and quality.
- Faster results.
- Decreased radiation to patient.
- Easier X-ray file sharing.
- Simpler storage.
- Environmentally safer (producing the image requires no chemicals).

Digital Imaging and Communications in Medicine (DICOM)   Digital Imaging and Communications is a communications protocol or standard for handling, storing, printing, and transmitting information in medical imaging.

DICOM was designed as part of the Integrating the Healthcare Enterprise (IHE) initiative that makes it easier for medical systems to share information. A Picture Archive and Communication System (PAC) is the digital storage area where digital images are sent and stored for diagnostic viewing and electronic image storage and distribution (Figure 50-11).

Advances in Radiology

As radiology continues to experience technological changes, more advances are occurring to enhance digital imaging quality. Some major advances include 3D/4D ultrasound, which provides "live-action" images that allow physicians to observe fetal movement, study body organs, and guide needle biopsies (Figure 50-12).

FIGURE 50-12   A 3D ultrasound shows the fetus in great detail.

PROCEDURE 50-1 Assisting with an X-Ray Examination

Procedure Goal: To assist with a radiologic procedure under the supervision of a radiologic technologist.

OSHA Guidelines: This procedure does not involve exposure to blood, body fluids, or tissue. You must wear a radiation exposure badge (dosimeter), however, and will be required to wear a garment containing a lead or approved nonlead shield if you remain in the room during the operation of X-ray equipment.

Materials: X-ray examination order, X-ray machine, X-ray film and holder, X-ray film developer, drape, and patient shield.

Method: Procedure steps.

1. Check the X-ray examination order and equipment needed.
2. Identify the patient and introduce yourself.
3. Determine whether the patient has complied with the preprocedure instructions. Do not depend on the patient to inform you, but ask the patient if and how he prepped for the procedure.
   RATIONALE: If a patient has not been compliant with preprocedural directions, then the test ordered may not be as effective as it should and will need to be rescheduled.
4. Explain the procedure and the purpose of the examination to the patient.
5. Instruct the patient to remove clothing and all metals (including jewelry) as needed, according to the body area to be examined, and to put on a gown. Explain that metals may interfere with the image. Ask whether the patient has any surgical metal or a pacemaker and

report this information to the radiologic technologist. Leave the room to ensure patient privacy.

Note: Steps 6 through 11 are nearly always performed by a radiologic technologist.

6. Position the patient according to the X-ray view ordered.
7. Drape the patient and place the patient shield appropriately.
8. Instruct the patient about the need to remain still and to hold the breath when requested.
9. Leave the room or stand behind a lead shield during the exposure.
10. Ask the patient to assume a comfortable position while the films are developed. Explain that X-rays sometimes must be repeated.
11. Develop the films.
12. Determine if the X-ray films are satisfactory by allowing the radiologist to review the films.
    RATIONALE: The radiologist may want another film or view.
13. Instruct the patient to dress and tell the patient when to contact the physician's office for the results.
14. Label the dry, finished X-ray films; place them in a properly labeled envelope; and file them according to your office's policies.
15. Record the X-ray examination, along with the final written findings, in the patient's chart.

> AP and lateral chest X-rays completed. Results placed in chart. _____
> _____ _K. Booth RMA (AMT)_

PROCEDURE 50-2 Documentation and Filing Techniques for X-Rays

Procedure Goal: To document X-ray information and file X-ray films properly.

OSHA Guidelines: This procedure does not involve exposure to blood, body fluids, or tissues.

Materials: X-ray film(s), patient X-ray record card or book, label, film-filing envelopes, film-filing cabinet, inserts, and a marking pen.

Method: Procedure steps.

1. Document the patient's X-ray information on the patient record card or in the record book. Include the patient's

name, the date, the type of X-ray, and the number of X-rays taken.

2. Verify that the film is properly labeled with the referring doctor's name, the date, and the patient's name. To note corrections or unusual positions or to identify a film that does not include labeling, attach the appropriate label and complete the necessary information. Some facilities also record the name of the radiologist who interpreted the X-ray.
   RATIONALE: To reduce the likelihood of misidentifying a patient's X-ray.

3. Place the processed film in a film-filing envelope. File the envelope alphabetically or chronologically (or according to your office's protocol) in the filing cabinet.

4. If you remove an envelope for any reason, put an insert or an "out card" in its place until it is returned to the cabinet.
   RATIONALE: Proper filing techniques save time and prevent litigation.

X-RAY EXAMINATIONS RECORD

Patient	Date	Type X-Ray	No. Taken	Referring Doctor	Comments
Jill Cabot	2/16	Chest	4	Wapnir	
M. C. Gaines	2/16	Right knee	8	Wright	
J. Hale	2/19	Right wrist	6	McCarthy	
L. Becker	2/23	Left hip	4	Wright	
R. Bell	2/24	Chest	4	Wapnir	
Donna Lin	2/24	Sinuses	6	Harris	
Jon Carey	2/26	Right hand	2	Cohen	

FIGURE Procedure 50-2 Step 1 Keeping accurate records of patient X-ray information is an important duty of the medical assistant.

LEARNING OUTCOMES	KEY POINTS
50.1 **Explain what X-rays are and how they are used for diagnostic and therapeutic purposes.**	An X-ray is a high-energy electromagnetic wave that travels at the speed of light and can penetrate solid objects. X-rays can be used for diagnosis by producing images of internal body structures. Therapeutically, X-rays are used to treat cancer by preventing cellular reproduction.
50.2 **Compare invasive and noninvasive diagnostic procedures.**	Invasive procedures require a radiologist to insert a catheter, wire, or other testing device into a patient's blood vessel or organ through the skin or a body orifice. Noninvasive diagnostic procedures do not require inserting devices, breaking the skin, or the degree of monitoring needed with invasive procedures.
50.3 **Carry out the medical assistant's role in X-ray and diagnostic radiology testing.**	A medical assistant can work directly with a radiology facility to assist the radiologist or technicians in performing diagnostic procedures. Providing preprocedure and postprocedure care are duties a medical assistant can perform in a medical or radiology facility.
50.4 **Discuss common diagnostic imaging procedures.**	Numerous diagnostic imaging procedures are used in medicine today including angiography, fluoroscopy, MRI, CT, arthrography, IVP, KUB, mammography, upper and lower GI series, ultrasound, and cholangiography.
50.5 **Describe different types of radiation therapy and how they are used.**	The two basic types of radiation therapy are teletherapy and brachytherapy. Teletherapy is also called external beam radiotherapy because an external beam of radiation is used to penetrate deep tumors. Brachytherapy uses temporary radioactive implants positioned close to or directly into cancerous tissue to treat the tumor and spare healthy tissue.
50.6 **Explain the risks and safety precautions associated with radiology work.**	The greatest risk associated with a radiology facility is the potential for radiation exposure to patients and healthcare workers. To eliminate this risk, certain safety precautions should be followed. These include careful evaluation by the physician to determine the medical necessity of radiology testing, avoidance of X-rays altogether if a patient is pregnant, and the requirement that all personnel who work in a radiology facility wear a dosimeter.
50.7 **Relate the advances in medical imaging to EHR.**	Major advances in telemedicine technology, including rapid video and computer-based communications of medical information, enable physicians to "examine" a patient in another city or country, view highly detailed medical images, consult with specialists in other cities, and supervise complex medical procedures. Sharing records including actual radiographic images between facilities is easier with the advent of digital radiographic procedures and the electronic health record.

Recall Raja Lautu from the beginning of the chapter. Now that you have read the chapter, answer the following questions regarding her case.

1. What is the difference between brachytherapy and teletherapy?
2. What should you tell Raja to help prepare her for her radiation treatment?

E X A M   P R E P A R A T I O N   Q U E S T I O N S

1. (LO 50.3) Which of the following would the medical assistant least likely perform?
   a. Using a mammotest
   b. Filing X-rays
   c. Providing preprocedure instruction for a mammogram
   d. Advising the patient to report symptoms after radiation treatment
   e. Assisting with an ultrasound

2. (LO 50.6) A dosimeter is used to:
   a. Prevent radiation exposure
   b. Measure radiation exposure
   c. Measure the dose of medicine given during radiation treatments
   d. Monitor fluctuations in radiation exposure
   e. Determine how much radiation is needed to obtain an image

3. (LO 50.2) Which of the following is considered invasive?
   a. Chest X-ray
   b. Mammogram
   c. MRI
   d. Fluoroscopy
   e. Angiogram

4. (LO 50.4) What organs are evaluated with a KUB?
   a. Kidneys, ureters, bladder
   b. Kidneys, urethra, bladder
   c. Kidneys, ureters, bowels
   d. Kidneys, urethra, bowels
   e. Kidneys and urethra for blood

5. (LO 50.3) Which step in the X-ray procedure would most likely be performed by a medical assistant?
   a. Develop the films
   b. Evaluate the films
   c. Label the films
   d. Position the patient
   e. Set up the X-ray machine

6. (LO 50.2) A substance that makes internal organs denser and blocks the passage of X-rays to the photographic film is a
   a. Shielding material
   b. Dosimeter
   c. Radiolucent medication
   d. Digital reader
   e. Contrast medium

7. (LO 50.4) Which of the following is used to detect gallstones?
   a. Angiography
   b. Cholecystography
   c. MUGA scan
   d. Lower GI series
   e. IVP

8. (LO 50.4) Hysterosalpingography is used to determine which of the following?
   a. Position of the kidneys
   b. Presence of gallstones
   c. Liver abscess
   d. Patency of the fallopian tubes
   e. Development of the fetus

9. (LO 50.5) Which of the following is used to treat tumors deep in the brain while sparing healthy tissue?
   a. Stereotactic radiosurgery
   b. Chemotherapy
   c. MRI
   d. Cerebral angiography
   e. Paramagnetic contrast

10. (LO 50.1) Wilhelm Konrad Roentgen is credited with discovering
    a. X-rays
    b. Photographic film
    c. Radiation therapy
    d. Magnetic resonance imaging
    e. SPECT scanning

Principles of Pharmacology

Malik Katahri, CMM, the office manager, has been happy with the performance of Kaylyn Haddix, RMA (AMT), and gives her the responsibility of maintaining the sample drug inventory and office medications. The office has a space dedicated to the samples and office medications, but the area is very disorganized. The first task is to organize and implement an inventory system for the drugs. Kaylyn is concerned about her abilities since she has only been working for BWW Associates for a couple of months.

Keep Kaylyn Haddix, RMA (AMT), in mind as you study the chapter. There will be questions at the end of the chapter based on the case study. The information in the chapter will help you answer these questions.

LEARNING OUTCOMES

After completing Chapter 51, you will be able to:

51.1 Identify the medical assistant's role in pharmacology.

51.2 Recognize the five categories of pharmacology and their importance to medication administration.

51.3 Differentiate the major drug categories, drug names, and their actions.

51.4 Classify over-the-counter (OTC), prescription, and herbal drugs.

51.5 Use credible sources to obtain drug information.

51.6 Carry out the procedure for registering or renewing a physician with the Drug Enforcement Administration (DEA) for permission to administer, dispense, and prescribe controlled drugs.

51.7 Identify the parts of a prescription, including commonly used abbreviations and symbols.

51.8 Discuss nonpharmacological treatments for pain.

51.9 Describe how vaccines work in the immune system.

KEY TERMS

administer	opioid
controlled substance	package insert
dispense	pharmacodynamics
efficacy	pharmacognosy
e-prescribing	pharmacokinetics
generic name	pharmacology
indication	pharmacotherapeutics
labeling	prescribe
magnetic therapy	toxicology
narcotic	trade name

I. C (11) Identify the classifications of medications, including desired effects, side effects and adverse reactions

I. C (12) Describe the relationship between anatomy and physiology of all body systems and medications used for treatment in each

II. C (6) Identify both abbreviations and symbols used in calculating medication dosages

IV. P (3) Use medical terminology, pronouncing medical terms correctly, to communicate information, patient history, data and observations

V. P (7) Use internet to access information related to the medical office

IX. C (13) Discuss all levels of governmental legislation and regulation as they apply to medical assisting practice, including FDA and DEA regulations

3. **Medical Terminology**

   Graduates:

   d. Recognize and identify acceptable medical abbreviations

4. **Medical Law and Ethics**

   Graduates:

   f. Comply with federal, state, and local health laws and regulations

6. **Pharmacology**

   Graduates:

   b. Properly utilize *PDR*, drug handbook, and other drug references to identify a drug's classification, usual dosage, usual side effects, and contraindications

   c. Identify and define common abbreviations that are *accepted* in prescription writing

   d. Understand legal aspects of writing prescriptions, including federal and state laws

   e. Comply with federal, state, and local health laws and regulations

8. **Medical Office Business Procedures Management**

   Graduates:

   jj. Perform fundamental writing skills including correct grammar, spelling, and formatting techniques when writing prescriptions, documenting medical records, etc.

   ll. Apply electronic technology

9. **Medical Office Clinical Procedures**

   Graduates:

   g. Maintain medication and immunization records

▶ Introduction

Pharmacology—the science of drugs—is a great responsibility of allied health professionals. Medication mistakes can injure or even cause the death of a patient. Before you administer drugs, it is important to begin with a good working knowledge of the foundations of pharmacology including how medications work, how they should be taken, and what problems can occur when medication is taken. This chapter provides an overview of the role of drugs in ambulatory healthcare facilities.

▶ The Medical Assistant's Role in Pharmacology   LO 51.1

As a medical assistant, you will be expected to have a basic knowledge of medications. This includes knowledge of prescription drugs and over-the-counter (OTC) drugs. Prescription drugs require a physician's written order to authorize the dispensing (and, sometimes, administering) of drugs to a patient. OTC drugs—available in pharmacies and supermarkets—are

purchased by people to treat themselves for ailments ranging from arthritis to colds to stomach ulcers. As a medical assistant you will need to

- Be attentive to ensure the physician is aware of all medications a patient is taking, both prescription and OTC.

- Ask each patient about alcohol and recreational drug use (both past and present) as well as herbal remedies.

- Assist in managing and renewing medication prescriptions.

- Educate the patient, using guidelines provided by the licensed practitioner, about the purpose of a drug and how to take the drug for maximum effectiveness and minimum adverse effects.

As your state and scope of practice permit, you also may be asked to enter medication orders and give drugs to a patient. Safe and effective drug therapy requires additional knowledge and special skills. To handle these important functions, you must understand pharmacologic principles and sources of drug information, be able to translate prescriptions, and be prepared to answer basic patient questions (Figure 51-1). You also must

FIGURE 51-1 A medical assistant may need to be prepared to answer the patient's questions about a drug the doctor is prescribing.

FIGURE 51-2 The foxglove plant, shown here, is the natural source for the medication digitoxin.

adhere to legal requirements and keep accurate records. Additionally, the Centers for Medicare and Medicaid Services (CMS) ruled in September of 2012 that credentialed medical assistants may enter medication orders into a computerized order entry system. Another excellent reason to become a credentialed medical assistant once you complete your program.

▶ Pharmacology

LO 51.2

A drug is a chemical compound used to prevent, diagnose, or treat a disease or other abnormal condition. The study of drugs is called **pharmacology.** A specialist in pharmacology is called a *pharmacologist.* Included in pharmacology are

- **pharmacognosy** (the study of characteristics of natural drugs and their sources).
- **pharmacodynamics** (the study of what drugs do to the body).
- **pharmacokinetics** (the study of what the body does to drugs).
- **pharmacotherapeutics** (the study of how drugs are used to treat disease).
- **toxicology** (the study of poisons or poisonous effects of drugs).

According to the Department of Justice's Drug Enforcement Administration (DEA) guidelines, a doctor **prescribes** a drug when he gives a patient a prescription to be filled by a pharmacy. To **administer** a drug is to give it directly by injection, by mouth, or by any other route that introduces the drug into a patient's body. A healthcare professional **dispenses** a drug by distributing it, in a properly labeled container, to a patient who is directed to use it.

Sources of Drugs (Pharmacognosy)

Many drugs originate as natural products. Other drugs originate in the chemical laboratory, as chemists seek to improve existing drugs.

Natural Products Most often, drugs originate as substances from natural products, such as plants, animals, minerals, bacteria, or fungi. For hundreds of years, drugs have been made from seeds, bulbs, roots, stems, buds, leaves, or other parts of plants. Two examples of plant-derived drugs are digitoxin, which comes from the foxglove plant (see Figure 51-2), and quinine, which comes from cinchona tree bark. Digitoxin is used to treat heart failure and abnormal heart beats. Quinine is used to treat malaria.

Animals also are used as a source of drugs. Certain animal substances have been shown to be compatible with human physiology. Some examples of animal substances used as drugs include glandular substances, such as insulin and thyroid hormones; fats and oils, such as cod-liver oil; enzymes, such as pancreatin and pepsin; and antiserums and antitoxins for vaccines.

Mineral sources yield various substances that can be used as they occur naturally or mixed with other substances. Two drugs derived from mineral sources are potassium chloride and mineral oil. Simple organisms, like bacteria and fungi, produce substances that are used to make certain antibiotics, such as cephalosporins and penicillins (see Figure 51-3).

Chemical Development A chemist conducts investigations that lead to the synthesis (chemical duplication) of one or more drugs, based on a natural substance's chemical properties. Some drugs are synthesized by strictly chemical methods. Others are duplicated by manipulating genetic information in a host organism. For example, human insulin is produced by these means, also known as *recombinant deoxyribonucleic acid (DNA)* techniques.

FIGURE 51-3 Bacteria, fungi, and yeasts are natural sources for antibiotics.

Pharmacodynamics

Pharmacodynamics is the study of the mechanism of action, or how the drug works to produce a therapeutic effect. Drugs are placed in categories based on their mechanism of action. Pharmacodynamics includes the interaction between the drug and target cells or tissues and the body's response to that interaction. For example, when a patient with diabetes takes insulin, the drug acts by allowing the movement of glucose across cell membranes. This movement makes the glucose available to cells to use as an energy source. The end result is a decrease in the blood glucose level.

Go to CONNECT to see an animation about *Pharmacokinetics vs. Pharmacodynamics.*

Pharmacokinetics

Pharmacokinetics is what the body does to a drug—that is, how the body absorbs, distributes, metabolizes, and excretes the drug. It is important to understand these processes so you will be able to explain to patients the reasons for taking a particular drug with food or for drinking plenty of water while taking a drug. These four processes can be remembered by using the acronym ADME: **A**bsorption–**D**istribution–**M**etabolism–**E**limination.

Absorption Absorption is the process of converting a drug from its dose form, like a tablet or capsule, into a form the body can use. For example, tablets or capsules are absorbed

through the stomach or intestines into the bloodstream. Water, food, or a particular food may either hinder or assist the absorption of a specific drug through the stomach or intestines. Some drugs may irritate the digestive organs if they are taken without food or water. Because of such possible reactions, patients must precisely follow instructions for taking a drug with plenty of water, with food, or without food.

Injected drugs are absorbed through the skin (intradermally), through the tissue just beneath the skin (subcutaneously), or through muscle (intramuscularly), depending on the method of injection. Absorption allows the drug to enter the bloodstream and pass into tissues. The extent and rate of drug absorption depend on several factors, including the route of administration. When the drug is administered by mouth, for example, coatings on tablets or capsules and the amount and type of food consumed with the drug may affect absorption. Drugs administered intravenously do not require absorption; they are directly available to target cells from the bloodstream.

Distribution Distribution is the process of transporting a drug from its administration site, such as the muscle of an injection site, to its site of action. Distribution also pertains to the length of time a drug takes to achieve maximum or peak plasma levels; that is, the length of time between dosing and availability in the bloodstream.

Metabolism Drug metabolism is the process by which drug molecules are transformed into simpler products called *metabolites.* This transformation usually occurs in the liver, where enzymes break down the drug. Some drugs, however, are metabolized in the kidneys. Metabolism can be affected by disease, a patient's age or genetic makeup, a drug's characteristics, or other factors. When drugs metabolized in the liver are prescribed for either children or the elderly, the dose is likely to be lower than that prescribed for young adults. Metabolism in children and the elderly is different from metabolism in other patients; the drugs may remain in the body longer and possibly reach harmful levels. The same concern holds true for any patient with impaired liver or kidney function if prescribed drugs are metabolized in the affected organ.

Excretion Excretion describes the manner in which a drug is eliminated from the body. Most drugs are eliminated in urine. Drugs also may be excreted in feces, perspiration, saliva, bile, exhaled air, and breast milk.

Go to CONNECT to see animations about *Medication Absorption, Medication Distribution, Medication Metabolism,* and *Medication Excretion.*

Pharmacotherapeutics

Pharmacotherapeutics is the study of how drugs are used to treat disease. This area of pharmacology is sometimes called *clinical pharmacology.* Pharmacotherapeutics includes topics such as drug categories (discussed in the next section), drug indications and labeling, safety, **efficacy** (therapeutic value), and kinds of therapy.

Indications and Labeling An **indication** is the purpose or reason for using a drug. The Food and Drug Administration (FDA) must approve indications before they can become part of a drug's labeling. The FDA is an agency of the Department of Health and Human Services. It regulates the manufacture and distribution of every drug used in the United States. **Labeling** also includes the form of the drug, such as tablet or liquid. Regardless of category, some drugs may be used to treat several different conditions. Multiple uses are possible if the drug affects several body systems at once or if the drug's primary effect produces significant secondary effects in other body systems.

When a drug is used for multiple indications, one or more indications may not be in its labeling. Off-label prescribing is legal. For example, Benadryl (diphenhydramine) is an antihistamine used to treat allergic symptoms in both children and adults. Because it tends to make a patient sleepy but is safe for children, a pediatrician may use a low dose of Benadryl as a temporary sedative for a young child. Its use as a sedative, however, is not part of the labeling for Benadryl. Another example of a drug with multiple uses is minoxidil. As a trade-name tablet, it is known as the antihypertensive Loniten®; as a trade-name topical solution, it is known as the hair-growth stimulant Rogaine®. In the case of minoxidil, both indications are approved, but the tablet labeling is for hypertension and the topical solution labeling is for hair growth. It is important to be aware of these labeling considerations when dealing with questions from patients. Never assume a drug is appropriate for only one use or administered in only one form. Always consult the physician or other approved source of drug information before answering a patient's question.

Safety The safety of a drug is determined by how many and what kinds of adverse effects are associated with it. Some adverse effects are common, whereas others are rare. An adverse effect may require immediate attention. It is not uncommon for a patient to call the physician's office with complaints of new symptoms soon after beginning therapy with a drug. Be alert for such complaints because they could be signs of an adverse reaction to the drug or an interaction with another medication. These calls should be brought to the physician's attention.

Efficacy A patient may complain that a newly prescribed drug is not doing what the doctor said it would. There are a variety of possible explanations for such a complaint, including

- The drug is working adequately, but the patient does not understand how it works.
- The dosage (size, frequency, and number of doses) needs to be adjusted.
- The patient is not taking the medication according to the directions.
- The drug has not yet reached a therapeutic level in the bloodstream.

- The wrong drug was prescribed, or the wrong drug was dispensed by the pharmacy (this is rare, but possible).
- Some drugs work better in some patients than in others; not every drug is for everyone (this is particularly true of antihistamines).
- Some forms of a drug work better than others, such as tablets versus injection.
- The generic drug does not work, but the trade name drug does.

Kinds of Therapy There are several descriptive terms for drug therapy. Depending on a patient's condition, the physician may use drugs for any of the following kinds of therapy:

- Acute: Drug is prescribed to improve a life-threatening or serious condition, such as epinephrine for severe allergic reaction.
- Empiric: Drug is prescribed according to experience or observation until blood or other tests prove another therapy to be appropriate, such as penicillin for suspected strep throat.
- Maintenance: Drug is prescribed to maintain a condition of health, especially in chronic disease, such as an anti-inflammatory medication for inflammatory bowel disease.
- Palliative: Drug is prescribed to reduce the severity of a condition or its accompanying pain, such as morphine for cancer.
- Prophylactic: Drug is prescribed to prevent a disease or condition, such as immunizations or birth control drugs.
- Replacement: Drug is prescribed to provide chemicals otherwise missing in a patient, such as hormone replacement therapy for a woman in menopause.
- Supportive: Drug is prescribed for a condition other than the primary disease until that disease resolves, such as a corticosteroid for severe allergic reactions.
- Supplemental: Drug or nutrients are prescribed to avoid deficiency, such as iron for a woman who is pregnant.

Toxicology

Toxicology is the study of the poisonous effects, or toxicity, of drugs, including adverse effects and drug interactions. In addition to immediate toxic effects that can occur when drugs are administered, you must be aware of some possible toxic effects that may not be apparent right away:

- An adverse effect on a fetus when the drug crosses the placenta.
- An adverse effect on infants when the drug passes easily into breast milk.
- Adverse reactions reported in clinical trials, such as headache, drowsiness, gastric upset, or other effects.
- An adverse effect in immunocompromised patients who are unable to metabolize a drug normally.
- An adverse effect in pediatric or elderly patients or in patients with hypertension, diabetes mellitus, or other serious chronic conditions.

- An adverse drug interaction when the drug is taken with another drug or food that is incompatible.
- A carcinogenic (cancer-causing) effect in some patients.

Nearly always, an adverse effect is encountered during the clinical trials of a drug, and there will be mention of the adverse effect under that heading in the package insert or in accepted drug reference works. In the reports of clinical trials, the drug company must report all adverse effects noted during testing. As a result, effects that, at least theoretically, could be caused by the drug are included. In dealing with patients who are about to begin drug therapy, use discretion when mentioning specific adverse effects associated with drugs. The patient must be informed; however, you do not want to cause undue alarm or discourage patients from taking the needed medication. Always ask patients if they have any questions and have the doctor answer patients' drug-related questions. Because patients will receive lists of adverse effects from the pharmacist, encourage them to discuss concerns with the pharmacist or to call the doctor's office. Also encourage patients to inform the doctor of adverse effects they experience after beginning drug therapy.

Drug Names and Categories · LO 51.3

One drug may have several different names, including the drug's official name (also known as the **generic name**), international nonproprietary name, chemical name, and **trade name** (brand or proprietary name). To demonstrate, the trade name antibacterial drug prescribed by physicians as Keflex® or Biocef is also identified by the following names:

- Cephalexin (generic name)
- Cefalexin (international nonproprietary name)
- 7-(D-α-amino-α-phenylacetamido)-3-methyl-3-cephem-4-carboxylic acid monohydrate (chemical name)

As a medical assistant, you will probably need to use only generic and trade names. In general, think of the generic name of a drug as a simple form of its chemical name. For each new drug marketed by a drug manufacturer, the United States Adopted Names (USAN) Council selects a generic name. This name is nonproprietary, meaning it does not belong to any one manufacturer. A generic name is also considered a drug's official name, which is listed in the United States Pharmacopeia/ National Formulary.

A drug's manufacturer selects the drug's trade name, which is protected by copyright and is the property of the manufacturer. When a new drug enters the market, its manufacturer has a patent on that drug, which means that no other manufacturer can make or sell the drug for 17 years. When the patent runs out, any manufacturer can sell the drug under the generic name or a different trade name. The original manufacturer, however, is the only one allowed to use the drug's original trade name. For example, the antibiotic cephalexin has two trade names, Keflex® and Biocef. Different manufacturers own these names.

A physician may prescribe a drug by its generic or trade name. Because generic drugs are usually less expensive, most physicians try to prescribe them if possible. Many states allow pharmacists to substitute a generic drug for a trade name drug unless the physician specifies otherwise. In fact, most health insurance prescription plans now require the substitution of generic drugs for trade name drugs (unless otherwise specified by a physician). Frequently, they also require the pharmacy to charge a higher copay amount for trade name drugs than for generic drugs. Some prescription plans now offer a mail-in pharmacy through which a patient can obtain generic drugs with a reduced copayment or without any copayment.

Drugs are categorized by their action on the body, general therapeutic effect, or the body system affected. Table 51-1 lists a variety of drug categories, their actions, and common drugs, including drugs from the top 200 drugs most commonly prescribed in the year 2010.

FDA Regulation and Drugs · LO 51.4

The Food and Drug Administration (FDA) requires that drug manufacturers perform clinical tests on new drugs before humans use the drugs. These tests include toxicity tests in laboratory animals, followed by clinical studies (clinical trials) in controlled groups of volunteers. Some volunteers are patients; others are healthy subjects. Clinical tests are designed to consider the ratio of benefits to the risk of adverse side effects. If the clinical tests prove the drug is safe and effective, the FDA approves it for marketing. The manufacturer must continue to demonstrate the drug's safety and efficacy and must submit reports whenever it discovers unexpected adverse reactions. The FDA can withdraw a drug from the market at any time if evidence suggests it is no longer safe or effective. This is known as a *recall*.

The FDA also regulates drug manufacturing. It ensures that drugs shipped between states have the proper identity, strength, purity, and quality. Each manufacturer must consistently identify each drug by a particular color, form, shape, size, and label. It must produce every dose at the same tested strength, using the exact formula approved by the FDA. The manufacturer also must use high-quality, contaminant-free ingredients. The FDA regulates all drugs in one way or another, including over-the-counter, prescription, and even complementary and alternative therapies (CAM). See Points on Practice: The FDA and CAM Therapies.

Over-the-Counter Drugs

A nonprescription, or over-the-counter (OTC), drug is one the FDA has approved for use without a licensed healthcare practitioner's supervision. The consumer must follow the manufacturer's directions to use the drug safely. Some drugs, like aspirin and vitamin supplements, have been OTC drugs for many years. The number of prescription drugs granted OTC status is increasing. Although OTC drugs are safe when used as directed on the package, patient education contributes significantly to their safe use.

TABLE 51-1   Drug Categories and Actions for Commonly Prescribed Drugs

Drug Category	Action of Drug	Examples* Generic Name (Trade Name)
Analgesic	Relieves mild to severe pain	Acetaminophen (Tylenol®)*; Acetylsalicylic acid, or aspirin; morphine sulfate (MS Contin®)*; oxycodone HCl (Percocet®)*
Anesthetic	Prevents sensation of pain (generally, locally, or topically)	Lidocaine HCl (Xylocaine®, Lidoderm®)*; tetracaine HCl (Pontocaine®)
Antacid/Antiulcer	Neutralizes stomach acid	Calcium carbonate (Tums®); esomeprazole (Nexium®); lansoprazole (Prevacid®); pantoprazole sodium (Protonix®)*
Anthelmintic	Kills, paralyzes, or inhibits the growth of parasitic worms	Mebendazole (Vermox®); pyrantel pamoate (Combantrin®, Antiminth®)
Antiarrhythmic	Normalizes heartbeat in cases of certain cardiac arrhythmias	Disopyramide phosphate (Norpace®); propafenone HCl (Rythmol®); propranolol HCl (Inderal®)*
Antiasthmatic	Treats or prevents asthma attacks	Montelukast (Singulair®)*; fluticasone propionate/salmeterol (Advair Diskus®)*; albuterol (ProAir HFA®)*
Antibiotics (antibacterial)	Kills bacterial microorganisms or inhibits their growth	Amoxicillin (Amoxil®)*; azithromycin (Zithromax®)*; cefprozil (Cefzil®)*; ciprofloxacin (Cipro®)*; clarithromycin (Biaxin® XL)*; levofloxacin (Levaquin®)*
Anticholinergic	Blocks parasympathetic nerve impulses	Atropine sulfate (Isopto® Atropine); dicyclomine HCl (Bentyl®); ipratropium (Atrovent®)
Anticoagulant	Prevents blood from clotting	Enoxaparin sodium (Lovenox®); heparin sodium (Hep-Lock®); warfarin sodium (Coumadin®)*
Anticonvulsant	Relieves or controls seizures (convulsions)	Clonazepam (Klonopin®)*; divalproex (Depakote®)*; phenobarbital sodium (Luminol® Sodium)*; phenytoin (Dilantin®)*
Antidepressant (four types) Tricyclic Monoamine oxidase inhibitor (MAOI) Selective serotonin reuptake inhibitor (SSRI) Serotonin-norepinephrine reuptake inhibitor (SNRI)	Relieves depression	Amitriptyline HCl (Elavil®)*; doxepin HCl (Sinequan®)* Phenelzine sulfate (Nardil®); tranylcypromine sulfate (Parnate®) Escitalopram (Lexapro®)*; fluoxetine HCl (Prozac®)*; paroxetine (Paxil®)*; sertraline HCl (Zoloft®)* Venlafaxine HCl (Effexor XR®)*; duloxetine HCl (Cymbalta®)*
Antidiabetic	Treats diabetes by reducing glucose	Metformin (Glucophage®)*; glipizide (Glucotrol®)*; glyburide (Micronase®)*; pioglitazone HCl (Actos®)
Antidiarrheal	Relieves diarrhea	Bismuth subsalicylate (Pepto-Bismol®); kaolin and pectin mixtures (Kaopectate®); loperamide HCl (Imodium®)
Antiemetic	Prevents or relieves nausea and vomiting	Prochlorperazine (Compazine®); promethazine (Phenergan®)*; trimethobenzamide HCl (Tigan®)
Antifungal	Kills or inhibits growth of fungi	Amphotericin B (Fungizone®); fluconazole (Diflucan®)*; nystatin (Mycostatin®)*; terbinafine (Lamisil®)*
Antihistamine	Counteracts effects of histamine and relieves allergic symptoms	Cetirizine HCl (Zyrtec®)*; diphenhydramine HCl (Benadryl®); fexofenadine (Allegra®)*; desloratadine (Clarinex®)*
Antihypertensive	Reduces blood pressure	Amlodipine (Norvasc®)*; diltiazem HCl (Cartia XL®); quinapril (Prinivil®)*; metoprolol succinate (Toprol XL®)*; valsartan (Diovan®)*
Anti-inflammatory (two types) Nonsteroidal (NSAIDs) Steroids	Reduces inflammation	Naproxen (Aleve); colchicine* (Colcrys®); ibuprofen (Motrin®, Advil®); celecoxib (Celebrex®)* Dexamethasone (Decadron®); methylprednisolone (Medrol®)*; prednisone (Deltasone™)*; triamcinolone (Kenalog®)
Antilipemic (antilipidemic)	Lowers blood lipids such as triglycerides	Gemfibrozil (Lopid®); atorvastatin (Lipitor®)*; fenofibrate (TriCor®)*; ezetimibe/simvastatin (Vytorin®)*; ezetimibe (Zetia®)*; rosuvastatin (Crestor®)*
Antineoplastic	Poisons cancerous cells	Bleomycin sulfate (Blenoxane®); dactinomycin (Cosmegen®); paclitaxel (Taxol®); tamoxifen citrate (Nolvadex®)*
Antipsychotic	Controls psychotic symptoms	Chlorpromazine HCl (Thorazine®); clozapine (Clozaril®); haloperidol (Haldol®); risperidone (Risperdal®); thioridazine HCl (Mellaril®)

TABLE 51-1 *(concluded)*

Drug Category	Action of Drug	Examples* Generic Name (Trade Name)
Antipyretic	Reduces fever	Acetaminophen (Tylenol®); acetylsalicyclic acid, or aspirin
Antiseptic	Inhibits growth of microorganisms	Isopropyl alcohol; 70% povidone-iodine (Betadine®); chlorhexidine gluconate (PerioChip)
Antitussive	Inhibits cough reflex	Codeine; dextromethorphan hydrobromide (component of Robitussin® DM)
Bronchodilator	Dilates bronchi (airways in the lungs)	Albuterol (Proventil®)*; epinephrine (Epinephrine Mist); salmeterol (Serevent®)
Cathartic (laxative)	Induces defecation, alleviates constipation	Bisacodyl (Dulcolax®); casanthranol (Peri-Colace®); magnesium hydroxide (Milk of Magnesia®)
Contraceptive	Reduces risk of pregnancy	Ethinyl estradiol and norgestimate (Ortho Tri-Cyclen®)*; norethindrone and ethinyl estradiol (Ortho-Evra®)*; norgestrel (Ovrette®)
Decongestant	Relieves nasal swelling and congestion	Oxymetazoline HCl (Afrin®); phenylephrine HCl (Neo-Synephrine®); pseudoephedrine HCl (Sudafed®)
Diuretic	Increases urine output, reduces blood pressure and cardiac output	Bumetanide (Bumex®); furosemide (Lasix®)*; hydrochlorothiazide (HydroDIURIL®)*; mannitol (Osmitrol®)
Expectorant	Liquefies mucus in bronchi; allows expectoration of sputum, mucus, and phlegm	Guaifenesin (Mucinex®)
Hemostatic	Controls or stops bleeding by promoting coagulation	Aminocaproic acid (Amicar®); phytonadione or vitamin K$_1$ (Mephyton®); thrombin (Thrombogen)
Hormone replacement	Replaces or resolves hormone deficiency	Insulin (Humulin®)* for pancreatic deficiency; levothyroxine sodium (Synthroid®)* for thyroid deficiency; conjugated estrogens (Premarin Tabs®)*
Hypnotic (sleep-inducing) or sedative	Induces sleep or relaxation (depending on drug potency and dosage)	Chloral hydrate (Noctec®); secobarbital sodium (Seconal® Sodium); zolpidem (Ambien®)*
Muscle relaxant	Relaxes skeletal muscles	Carisoprodol (Rela or Soma®); cyclobenzaprine HCl (Flexeril®)*
Mydriatic	Constricts vessels of eye or nasal passage, raises blood pressure, dilates pupil of eye in ophthalmic preparations	Atropine sulfate (Atropisol) for ophthalmic use; phenylephrine HCl (Alcon Efrin) for ophthalmic use or (Neo-Synephrine®) for nasal use
Stimulant (central nervous system)	Increases activity of brain and other organs, decreases appetite	Amphetamine sulfate (Benzedrine); caffeine (No-Doz®); also a component of many analgesic formulations and coffee
Vasoconstrictor	Constricts blood vessels, increases blood pressure	Dopamine HCl (Intropin); norepinephrine bitartrate (Levophed®)
Vasodilator	Dilates blood vessels, decreases blood pressure	Enalapril (Vasotec®); lisinopril (Prinivil®)*; nitroglycerin (Nitrostat®*, NitroQuick®)

*Indicates top 200 commonly prescribed drug in the year 2011.

Sources: *Physicians' Desk Reference (PDR) 2012*, www.pdr.net, and RXList, www.rxlist.com.

Prescription Drugs

A prescription drug is one that can be used only by order of a physician and must be dispensed by a licensed healthcare professional, such as a pharmacist, physician, podiatrist, or licensed midwife. Some prescription drugs are dispensed as OTC medications at much lower strengths.

Pregnancy Categories

Because clinical trials are not typically done on pregnant women, most of the data about the effect of medications on pregnant women is obtained after FDA approval. Some drugs can cause physical defects to the fetus if the mother takes them during pregnancy, especially during the first trimester. To assist physicians who are prescribing medications for pregnant women, the FDA has created the categories A, B, C, D, and X based upon the degree to which available information has ruled out risk to the fetus. See Table 51-2. Most medications are typically Category C, although a medication can change categories after approval based upon adverse reactions. Also, some medications are placed into different categories based upon the trimester of the pregnancy.

POINTS ON PRACTICE
The FDA and CAM Therapies

Complementary and alternative therapies such as dietary supplements, herbal products, and the use of other natural but as yet scientifically unproven therapies are increasing in use. Many physicians prescribe these therapies and even more patients take them on their own with success. There is one important difference between dietary supplements and medications. Medications must meet approval of the FDA prior to being marketed and sold. Drug manufacturers must provide scientific documentation of the effectiveness of a drug before it can be marketed. On the other hand, manufacturers of dietary supplements do not have to provide evidence of effectiveness or safety. Of course, they are not permitted to market or sell a product that is proven unsafe. However, once a supplement is marketed, the FDA must prove that the product is not safe to have it taken from the market. Additionally, dietary supplements are not standardized between batches or among manufacturers. Standardization is a process that ensures the consistency and quality of each batch of supplement produced. Thus, the amount and quality of a dietary supplement may differ between batches by one manufacturer or between the same supplement made by two different manufacturers. FDA-approved medications must be standardized and will always be consistent between batches and manufacturers.

The FDA does require that certain information appear on dietary supplement labels. Dietary supplements may include claims on their labels that describe the effect of a substance in maintaining the body's normal structure or function. For example, a label might state, "Promotes healthy joints and bones." The FDA does not review or authorize this claim, so the manufacturer is required to also place a disclaimer on the product. This disclaimer is a statement indicating that the claims have not been evaluated by the FDA. For example, the disclaimer for the claim above would be: "This statement has not been evaluated by the Food and Drug Administration. This product is not intended to diagnose, treat, cure, or prevent disease." Figure 51-4 shows an example of a label that meets the FDA's labeling requirements.

Anatomy of the Requirements for Dietary Supplement Labels (Effective March 1999)

Statement of identity

Net quantity of contents

Structure-function claim

Directions

Supplement Facts panel

Other ingredients in descending order of predominance and by common name or proprietary blend

Name and place of business of manufacturer, packer, or distributor; this is the address to write for more product information

FIGURE 51-4 The Food and Drug Administration provides specific guidelines for the information found on a dietary supplement label.

TABLE 51-2	Categories for Drug Use in Pregnancy
Category	**Description**
A	*Controlled studies show no risk.* Adequate, well-controlled studies in pregnant women have not shown an increased risk of fetal abnormalities.
B	*No evidence of risk in humans.* Either animal findings show risk while human findings do not, or, if no adequate human studies have been done, animal findings are negative.
C	*Risk cannot be ruled out.* Human studies are lacking, and animal findings are either positive for fetal risk or lacking as well. Potential benefits may outweigh the risks.
D	*Positive evidence of risk.* Studies in pregnant women, either adequate and well-controlled or observational, have demonstrated a risk to the fetus. Potential benefits may outweigh the risks.
X	*Contraindicated in pregnancy.* Studies in animals or pregnant women, either adequate and well-controlled or observational, have demonstrated positive evidence of fetal abnormalities.
NR	*No rating is available.*

▶ Sources of Drug Information   LO 51.5

Having access to up-to-date and credible sources of drug information in the office for when you or the physician need detailed information about a specific drug is essential. The most up-to-date resources are found online or through smartphone or other electronic applications. Books are available, but resource books are also available online. The *Physicians' Desk Reference* (Figure 51-5), *United States Pharmacopeia/National Formulary*, American Hospital Formulary Service (AHFS®), and Epocrates® are credible sources of drug information. Package inserts and drug labels are also valuable drug information sources.

Physicians' Desk Reference (PDR)

The *Physicians' Desk Reference®*, or *PDR*, is published annually, along with supplements twice a year. It is sent free to doctors' offices and sold through bookstores. PDR Network, the company that publishes the *PDR*, also publishes separate editions for generic, nonprescription, and ophthalmologic drugs, as well as a guide to drug interactions, adverse effects, and indications. It is also available online. The *PDR* presents information provided by pharmaceutical companies about more than 2500 prescription drugs. It has the following sections:

- Section 1—Manufacturer's index (color-coded white), which includes the pharmaceutical company's name, address, emergency telephone number, and available products.
- Section 2—Brand- and generic-name index (color-coded pink).
- Section 3—Product category index (color-coded blue).
- Section 4—Product identification guide with full-color photos of more than 2400 actual medications.

- Section 5—Product information.
- Section 6—Diagnostic product information.

The product information section is divided according to manufacturer, and the drugs are then grouped alphabetically within each manufacturer's subsection. The information is provided for the *PDR* by the manufacturer and is either the drug package insert or a similar document.

After the large product information section, various smaller other sections are provided, which include diagnostic product information, state drug information centers, ratings for drug use in pregnancy, a state DEA directory, state-aided drug-assistance programs, patient assistance programs, drugs that should not be crushed, dosing instructions in Spanish, and the system for reporting adverse reactions to medications. All of these plus the *PDR* Internet site and *PDR* electronic library that come with the *PDR* are important resources for drug information.

United States Pharmacopeia/National Formulary

The United States Pharmacopeia/National Formulary, or USP-NF, is the official source of drug standards in the United States, published about every 5 years. As the official public standards-setting authority for all prescription medications, OTC drugs, dietary supplements, and other healthcare products, by law, every product sold under a name listed in the USP-NF must meet the USP's strict standards.

The USP-NF describes each product approved by the federal government and lists its standards for purity, composition, and strength as well as its uses, dosages, and storage. The NF portion of the book provides the chemical formulas of the drugs. The USP-NF is available online.

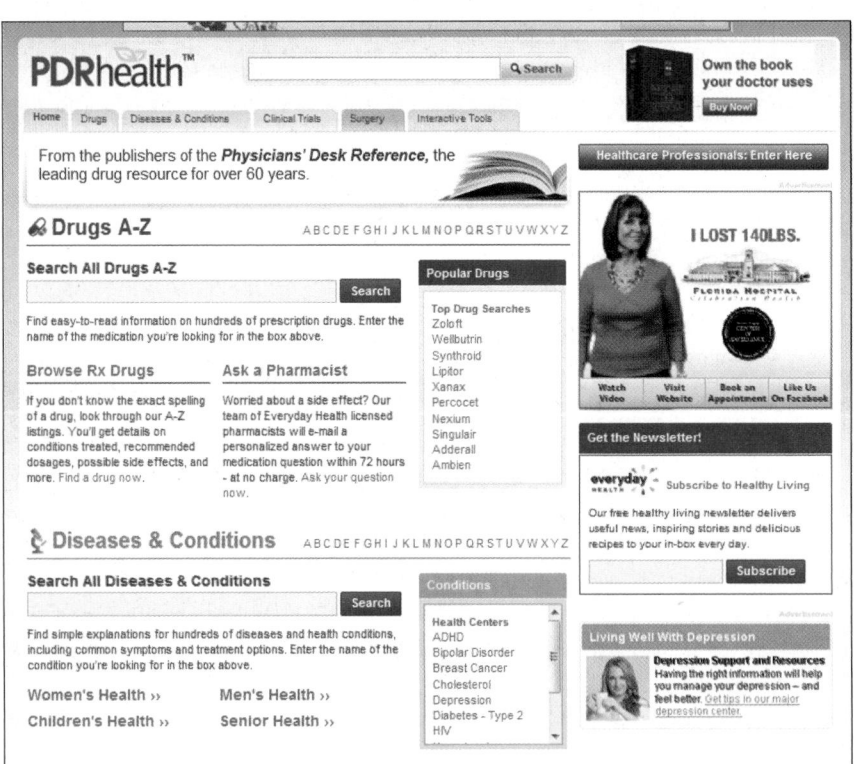

FIGURE 51-5   PDRhealth, found at www.PDRhealth.com, is a consumer and patient website with up-to-date drug and patient information.

American Hospital Formulary Service (AHFS®)

The American Society of Hospital Pharmacists in Bethesda, Maryland, publishes the American Hospital Formulary Service, or AHFS®. It sells the two-volume set by subscription and provides four to six supplements each year. The AHFS lists generic names and is divided into sections based on drug actions. The AHFS® is also available online.

Epocrates®

Epocrates® is a software program that can be loaded on to a smartphone or other personal digital assistant. Epocrates® includes more than 3,300 brand and generic drugs, alternative medicines, a drug-drug interaction checker, an IV compatibility checker, health insurance Medicare Part D formularies, and an infectious disease treatment guide.

Package Insert

The **package insert** for each drug describes the drug, its purpose and effects (clinical pharmacology), indications, contraindications (conditions under which the drug should not be administered), warnings, precautions, adverse reactions, drug abuse and dependence, overdosage, dosage and administration, and how the drug is supplied (for example, tablets in different doses, or liquid). The package insert, whether it is part of the *PDR* or found in the medication package, is a valuable resource for drug information. See Figure 51-6.

FIGURE 51-6 Use the package insert to become familiar with a drug's indications, contraindications, dosage, and adverse effects. Here is the format for a package insert for an injectable drug.

Drug Labels

To prepare and administer drugs, you must understand information that appears on drug labels, including the drug name, form, dosage strength, total amount in the container, route of administration, warnings, storage requirements, and manufacturing information. See Figure 51-7. By law, the generic name, as determined by the USP-NF, must appear on the drug's label. The drug label also may include the trade (brand) name used to market the drug. The trade name is typically indicated by a registered trademark symbol ®. The form of the drug is included, such as a tablet, capsule, liquid for oral administration or an injection. Drug labels include information about the amount of the drug present. This amount, combined with information about the form of the drug, identifies the drug's dosage strength.

On the label, the dosage strength is stated as the amount of drug per dosage unit. In most cases, the amount of the drug is listed in grams (g), milligrams (mg), or micrograms (mcg). In some cases, a drug may be a combination drug, meaning more than one drug is included. If a container holds more than one dose of medication, then the total number or volume of medication is listed on the label. The label also should include the route of administration, especially if it is a liquid. Warnings, such as "May be habit forming," are included, as well as storage information. Storage information indicates the specific conditions under which a medication must be stored. Manufacturer's information is always included. Information about how to mix or reconstitute a medication also may be found on the medication label.

FIGURE 51-7 (a) Check the medication label carefully. (b) Always read label warnings and storage information. (c) Amoxicillin and clavulanate potassium is a combination medication.

Controlled Substances

LO 51.6

A **controlled substance** is a drug or drug product categorized as potentially dangerous and addictive. The greater the potential for abuse, the more severe the limitations on prescribing it. Federal laws strictly regulate use of these controlled drugs. States, municipalities, and institutions must adhere to these laws but may also impose their own regulations.

Comprehensive Drug Abuse Prevention and Control Act

The Comprehensive Drug Abuse Prevention and Control Act, also known as the Controlled Substances Act (CSA) of 1970, is the federal law that created the DEA and strengthened drug enforcement authority. The CSA designates five schedules, according to degree of potential for a substance to be abused or used for a nontherapeutic effect. Schedule I drugs do not have a medical use. Schedule II drugs include **opioids**, which are natural or synthetic drugs that produce opium-like effects. Examples of Schedule II drugs include codeine, morphine, and meperidine (Demerol®). Government agencies use the popular term **narcotics** for opioids.

Sometimes the DEA reclassifies drugs. For example, a Schedule III drug may eventually be found to be less addictive than originally determined and therefore reclassified as a Schedule IV drug. The five schedules and examples of substances in each are outlined in Table 51-3.

Controlled Substance Labeling

The CSA also set up a labeling system to identify controlled substances. An example of this label is shown in Figure 51-8. The large C means the drug is a controlled substance and the Roman numeral inside the C corresponds to the drug's DEA schedule.

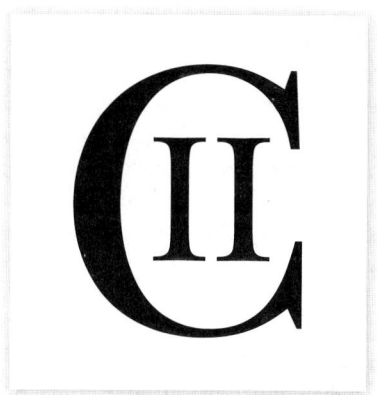

FIGURE 51-8 This symbol indicates that the drug is a Schedule II controlled substance.

TABLE 51-3   Schedule of Controlled Substances

Schedule	Description	Prescription and Legal Considerations	Examples
I	High abuse potential (no accepted medical use)	No prescriptions written.	GHB, heroin, LSD, mescaline
II	High abuse potential (accepted medical use; abuse may lead to dependence)	• Must be written by DEA-licensed physician and include DEA number.	Opioids: morphine (MS-Contin®), meperidine (Demerol®), fentanyl (Duragesic®)
		• Multiple and/or special forms may be required.	Barbiturates: secobarbital
		• Must be filled in 7 days and cannot be refilled.	Amphetamines: Methylphenidate (Ritalin®)
		• Must be stored under lock and key.	
		• Dispensing records are kept for two years.	
III	Lower abuse potential than Schedule I and II drugs (accepted medical use; abuse may lead to moderate dependence)	• Five refills are allowed in 6 months.	Anabolic steroids
		• Handwritten by physician.	Analgesic: hydrocodone/codeine (Vicodin®, Tylenol 3®)
		• Can only be telephoned by physician.	Barbiturate: talbutal
			Antidiarrheal: Paregoric
IV	Lower abuse potential than Schedule III drugs (accepted medical use; abuse may lead to limited dependence)	• Five refills are allowed in 6 months.	Benzodiazepines: alprazolam (Xanax®), chloridiazepoxide (Librium®), diazepam (Valium®), zolpidem (Ambien®), pentazocine (Talwin®)
		• Must be signed by physician.	
		• Refills may be authorized over the phone.	
		• Inventory records must be kept on these drugs.	
V	Lower abuse potential than Schedule IV drugs (accepted medical use; very limited physical dependence)	• Inventory records must be kept on these drugs.	Antitussive and antidiarrheals that combine small amounts of opioids, including Lomotil®, Kaolin, and Robitussin AC®
		• Five refills are allowed in 6 months.	
		• Must be signed by physician.	
		• Refills may be authorized over the phone.	

Source: U.S. Department of Justice, Drug Enforcement Administration, Office of Diversion Control, www.deadiversion.usdoj.gov.

Doctor Registration and Drug Ordering

Doctors who administer, dispense, or prescribe any controlled substance must register with the DEA and have a current state license to practice medicine and, if required, a state controlled substance license. They also must comply with all aspects of the CSA. This includes registration, renewal, and ordering of controlled substances, as outlined in Procedure 51-1, at the end of this chapter.

Drug Security

Drugs that are controlled substances must be kept in a locked cabinet or safe. If required by state law, use double locks for opioids. The physician or other licensed practitioner should keep the key(s) at all times, except when asking you to add to or take from the stock (if this is a task medical assistants are permitted to perform in your state). If controlled drugs are stolen from the physician's office, call the regional DEA office at once. Also, notify the state bureau of narcotic enforcement and the local police. File all reports required by the DEA and other agencies as a follow-up.

Recordkeeping

A physician who administers or dispenses (as opposed to prescribing) controlled drugs to patients must maintain two types of records: dispensing records and inventory records. Note that these requirements do not apply to physicians who prescribe drugs but who do not administer or dispense controlled drugs.

Dispensing Records The dispensing record for Schedule II drugs must be kept separate from the patient's regular medical record. Each time a drug is administered or dispensed, the doctor must note the date, the patient's name and address, the drug, and the quantity dispensed. The dispensing record for drugs on Schedules III through V must include the same information. The record for these drugs may be kept in the patient's medical record unless the physician charges for the drugs dispensed. All dispensing records must be kept for 2 years and are subject to inspection by the DEA.

Inventory Records A physician who regularly dispenses controlled drugs also must keep inventory records of all stock on hand. This regulation applies to all scheduled drugs. To take an inventory, count the amount of each drug on hand. Compare this amount with the amount of the drug ordered and the amount dispensed to patients. The controlled drug inventory must be repeated every 2 years. You must include copies of invoices from drug suppliers in the inventory record. All Schedule II drug inventories and records must be kept separate from other records.

Inventories and records of other controlled drugs must be separate or easily retrievable from ordinary business and professional records. All records on controlled drugs must be retained for 2 years and made available for inspection and copying by DEA officials if requested.

Disposing of Drugs If the doctor asks you to dispose of any outdated, noncontrolled drugs, you will most likely use the disposal company that takes your biohazardous waste. The DEA does not allow businesses to flush any medications and medications should not be placed in the trash. In some cases, you may work with a larger healthcare facility or pharmacy to ensure proper disposal so medications do not pollute the environment or end up in the trash where someone may take them. If the physician needs to dispose of controlled drugs, like expired samples, obtain DEA Form 41, called Registrants Inventory of Drugs Surrendered, which is available from the nearest DEA office or on the Internet. Complete the form in quadruplicate, have the doctor sign it, and call the DEA to obtain instructions for disposal of the drugs. If you must ship them, use registered mail. After the drugs have been destroyed, the DEA will issue the physician a receipt, which you should keep in a safe place. If physicians terminate their medical practice, they must return their DEA registration certificate and any unused copies of DEA Form 222 to the nearest DEA office. To prevent unauthorized use, write the word VOID across the front of these forms. Regional DEA offices will tell the physicians how to dispose of any remaining controlled drugs.

▶ Prescriptions
LO 51.7

Any drug not available over the counter requires a prescription. As a medical assistant, you should be able to interpret a prescription in order to discuss it with the patient, authorized prescriber, or pharmacist. You must become familiar with the doctor's style of writing or the electronic prescription process at your facility.

Interpreting a Prescription

Prescriptions for new or renewed medications are completed or approved by the physician. A prescription has specific parts that must be present before it can be filled or renewed (Figure 51-9).

The basic components of a prescription are

- *Prescriber information:* Name, address, telephone number, and other information identifying the prescriber.
- *Patient information:* Date, patient's full name, date of birth, address, and other information to identify the patient.
- *Medication prescribed:* Includes generic or brand name, strength, and quantity. This is sometimes called the inscription and is found after the Rx.
- *Subscription:* Instructions to the pharmacist dispensing the medication. This may include generic substitution and refill authorization.
- *Signa:* Also known as the transcription; refers to patient instructions. These instructions generally follow the abbreviation Sig, which means *mark*.
- *Signature:* Prescriber's signature for handwritten prescriptions. The prescriber's signature must be in ink, but it cannot be a stamped signature. A digital signature is used if it is secure; otherwise, the prescription must be printed and then signed or otherwise authorized.
- *DEA number:* This is required for prescriptions of Schedules II, III, IV, and V medications only.

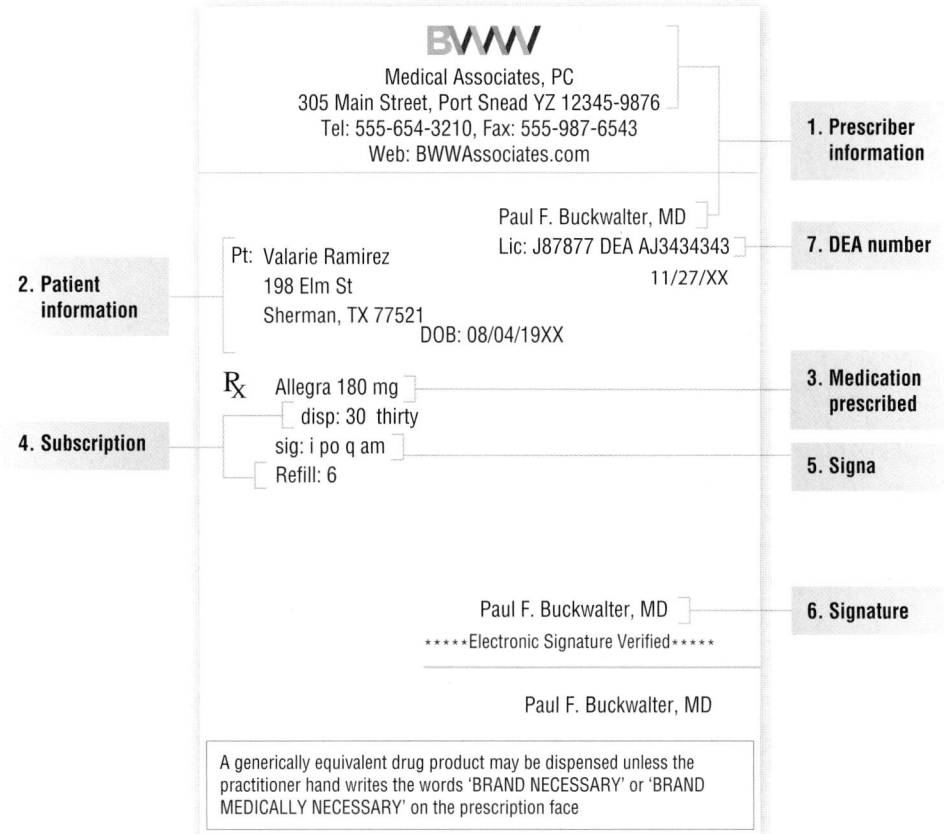

FIGURE 51-9 Parts of a prescription.

Many terms and abbreviations are used in prescriptions. See Table 51-4 for examples. Abbreviations for drug names should not be used because there are similar abbreviations for multiple drugs. Certain other abbreviations are not to be used, as discussed in the *Patient Interview and History* chapter, because they tend to cause errors.

A medical assistant must be able to interpret a prescription with accuracy. Refer to Procedure 51-2, Interpreting a Prescription, at the end of this chapter.

Managing Prescriptions Prescriptions may be printed or handwritten on a prescription blank. They also may be entered electronically and printed, or entered electronically and transmitted directly to a pharmacy. When the information is entered electronically and transmitted directly, this is known as **e-prescribing**. With e-prescribing, the medication information is received at the pharmacy and the actual prescription is never in the patient's hands. This is the most secure and efficient way for prescriptions to be completed. See Points on Practice: E-Prescribing.

POINTS ON PRACTICE
E-Prescribing

On July 15, 2008, Congress enacted the Medicare Improvements for Patients and Providers Act of 2008 (MIPPA) and it became law. MIPPA provides positive incentives for practitioners who use electronic prescribing in 2009 through 2013. E-prescribing is intended to bring greater safety to patients by providing for automatic drug and allergy interaction checking and the elimination of medication errors due to poor handwriting. E-prescribing also is designed to bring a greater efficiency to the prescribing process for providers, as it dramatically decreases communication from pharmacies requesting prescription clarifications.

Surescripts is the national clearinghouse for e-prescribing. The company electronically connects physicians, pharmacists, and payers nationwide, enabling them to exchange health information and prescribe without paper. Surescripts collaborates with national EHR vendors, pharmacies, and health plans to support physicians using EHR software. With this network in place, healthcare providers can electronically access prescription information from pharmacies, health plans, and other providers to see the patient's total prescription history from all sources. Through e-prescribing, EHRs are providing meaningful improvements in cost, quality, and patient safety. For example, when a medication is taken off the market, a record of all patients who have been prescribed this medication can be queried electronically and the physicians and patients notified of the change.

TABLE 51-4 Abbreviations Used in Prescriptions

Abbreviation	Meaning	Abbreviation	Meaning
a	Before	min	Minute, minimum
aa	Of each	mL	Milliliters
ac	Before meals	mm	Millimeters
AM	Morning	neb	Nebulizer
amp	Ampule	noct	Night
apl	Applicatorful	NPO	Nothing by mouth
aq	Water	nr	No refills
bid	Twice daily	oz	Ounce
c̄	With	pc	After meals
cap	Capsule	per	By means of; through
cd	Cycle day (menstrual cycle)	PM	Evening or nighttime
cmpd	Compound	po, PO	By mouth
cr	Cream	PR, pr	Rectally
d	Daily or day	q	Every
DAW	Dispense as written (no generic)	qam	Every morning
disp	Dispense	q4h	Every 4 hours
ds	Double strength	qid	Four times daily
dx	Diagnosis	qs	Sufficient amount
elix	Elixir	r, rec	Rectally
eq	Equivalent	rept	Repeat
g, gm	Gram	rf	Refill(s)
gen	Generic	s̄	Without
gr	Grain (60 to 65 mg)	stat	Immediately
gtt	Drop(s)	subcut	Subcutaneously
h, hr	Hour	sup	Suppository
H_2O	Water	susp	Suspension
IM	Intramuscularly	sx	Symptoms
inj	Inject, injection	syr	Syrup
IV	Intravenously	tab	Tablet(s)
kg	Kilogram	tbsp	Tablespoon
L	Liter	tsp	Teaspoon
liq	Liquid	tx	Treatment
lot	Lotion	ud, utd	As directed
MDI	Metered dose inhaler	ung	Ointment
mEq	Milliequivalent	vag	Vaginally, into vagina
mg	Milligram(s)	YO	Years old

In rare cases, preprinted prescription blanks are used that include the physician's name, address, telephone number, state license number, and DEA registration number plus blank space for writing the patient's name and address, the date, and other information. To prevent unauthorized use of prescription blanks, never leave them unattended. Most frequently, prescriptions are entered into an EHR, then printed and signed for patients to take with them to the pharmacy. If something about a prescription arouses suspicion, the pharmacist who receives a prescription may call the physician's office to verify it. You should be able to check the patient's records and tell the pharmacist whether the doctor wrote a prescription for that patient. If the prescription is a forgery, notify the physician and, if she gives you authorization, notify the DEA.

Telephone Prescriptions If requested by the physician, you may telephone a new or renewal prescription to the patient's pharmacy. You may not, however, telephone a prescription for a Schedule II drug. In an emergency situation, when a patient needs a drug immediately and no alternative is available, the doctor may telephone a prescription for a Schedule II drug. The amount must be limited to the period of emergency and a written prescription must be sent to the pharmacist within 72 hours. The pharmacist must notify the DEA if a written prescription does not arrive within the specified time.

Patient requests for prescription renewals occur daily. The renewal requests may be called in to the receptionist or left on a designated phone or mail system. It is the medical assistant's responsibility, if asked, to handle the prescription renewals/refills in an appropriate manner.

Go to CONNECT to see a video about *Interpret a Prescription.*

▶ Nonpharmacologic Pain Management

LO 51.8

Because of drug interactions, adverse effects, or the risk of dependence, many patients may either prefer not to or should not take drugs to relieve chronic pain. The overuse and abuse of pain medications can be a problem for patients. Pain frequently motivates these patients to use complementary and alternative medicine (CAM). Some examples include

- Chiropractors use spinal adjustments to treat chronic back or neck pain.
- Massage is used to treat headache or arthritis and to promote healing through relaxation.
- An acupuncture procedure in which very small amounts of electrical current are applied through needles has been used successfully to block the pain of surgery without anesthesia.
- Yoga uses postures to exercise the spine and stimulate the lymphatic system, helping to remove from the body toxins that may cause pain and stiffness in muscles and joints.
- Meditation is said to balance a person's physical, emotional, and mental states and is used as an aid in treating stress, anxiety, and pain.
- Hypnotism may be used to help patients overcome pain caused by stress-induced migraine headaches.
- Glucosamine chondroitin, a dietary supplement, is taken to treat osteoarthritis by reducing pain and slowing down joint cartilage damage.
- **Magnetic therapy** involves the use of magnets of varying sizes and strengths placed on the body to relieve pain or treat disease.

- Biofeedback can help a patient learn to evoke relaxation, which helps block pain perception.

CAM approaches and therapies have become more common in recent years. Some physicians and patients are seeking agents and treatments to manage health problems, like chronic pain, that are less expensive, have fewer side effects, and are more accessible than traditional medical interventions. Pain clinics that use multiple pain management techniques are common.

▶ Vaccines

LO 51.9

A vaccine is a special preparation made from microorganisms and administered to a person to produce reduced sensitivity to, or increased immunity to, an infectious disease. Vaccines are stored with the office supply of drugs and require similar handling. If you work in a pediatrician's office, you will handle the vaccines for childhood diseases. In an adult practice, you can expect to see influenza and pneumonia vaccines and vaccines for diseases to which patients might be exposed in foreign travel. It is important to know how vaccines work in the immune system. Through the immune system's action, a patient can be protected from—or made not susceptible to—a disease. This immunity results from the formation of antibodies that destroy or alter disease-causing agents. You should review information about immunity discussed in *The Lymphatic and Immune Systems* chapter.

Antibody Formation

The human body creates antibodies in response to an invasion by an antigen (foreign substance). When an antigen enters the body, specialized white blood cells (lymphocytes) produce antibodies, which in turn combine with the antigens to neutralize them. This action arrests or prevents the reaction or disease the antigen otherwise would cause. Specific antibodies always fight specific antigens. Antigens can be bacteria, viruses, or other organisms that enter the body in spite of its natural defenses. Toxins, pollens, and drugs also can be antigens if the body reacts to them by forming antibodies. (Allergens are antigens that induce an allergic reaction.)

Vaccines contain organisms that have been killed or attenuated (weakened) in a laboratory. Because the organisms have been weakened, they stimulate antibody formation but do not overpower the body and cause disease. They may, however, still be strong enough to cause a fever and slight inflammation at the injection site. Some vaccines, like those for influenza, may even produce some of the lesser effects of the disease against which they provide protection.

Immunizations made from organisms are called *vaccines.* Those made from the toxins of organisms are called *toxoids.* Some immunizations, such as the polio vaccine, last a lifetime. Others, like tetanus toxoid, do not. In the latter case, booster immunizations must be used to stimulate the lymphocytes to produce antibodies again.

Immunizations

The Advisory Committee on Immunization Practices, the American Academy of Pediatrics, and the American Academy of Family Physicians jointly publish immunization schedules, which are found in the *Assisting in Pediatrics* chapter. These schedules cover children from infancy through 18 years of age. Just as children receive immunizations before exposure to disease, adults may receive immunizations for influenza, pneumonia, or other diseases, including those to which an adult could be exposed during travel. Figure 51-10 displays the adult immunization schedule.

Patients are sometimes immunized after exposure. For example, if patients have been exposed to a serious disease and there is too little time for them to produce antibodies, they may receive an antiserum containing antibodies to the disease-carrying organism. These immunizations are made from human or animal serum. If bacterial toxins (rather than bacteria) cause the disease, the patient may receive an antitoxin.

Antiserums and antitoxins must be used cautiously and are usually reserved for life-threatening infectious diseases. Because patients can be allergic to substances in animal antiserums and antitoxins, human serums are usually preferred. An example of a post-exposure immunization is one given to a patient who has been exposed to hepatitis B virus (HBV). This patient should be given the antiserum hepatitis B immune globulin (HBV-Ig) within 7 days after exposure and again 28 to 30 days later. Because HBV-Ig is made from human serum, it causes relatively few adverse reactions. Another example involves a patient who may have been exposed to tetanus (lockjaw) organisms as the result of an injury like a puncture wound. This patient may receive tetanus immune globulin (T-Ig, a human product) or tetanus antitoxin. Because tetanus antitoxin is made from horse serum, it may cause serious reactions in patients who are allergic to horses or horsehair.

For every vaccine in your medical office, you must be familiar with the indications, contraindications, dosages, administration routes, potential adverse effects, and methods of storage and handling. You must carefully read the package insert provided with each vaccine and, when necessary, consult drug reference books for further information. Knowledge of correct administration techniques is required and will be discussed in the *Medication Administration* chapter.

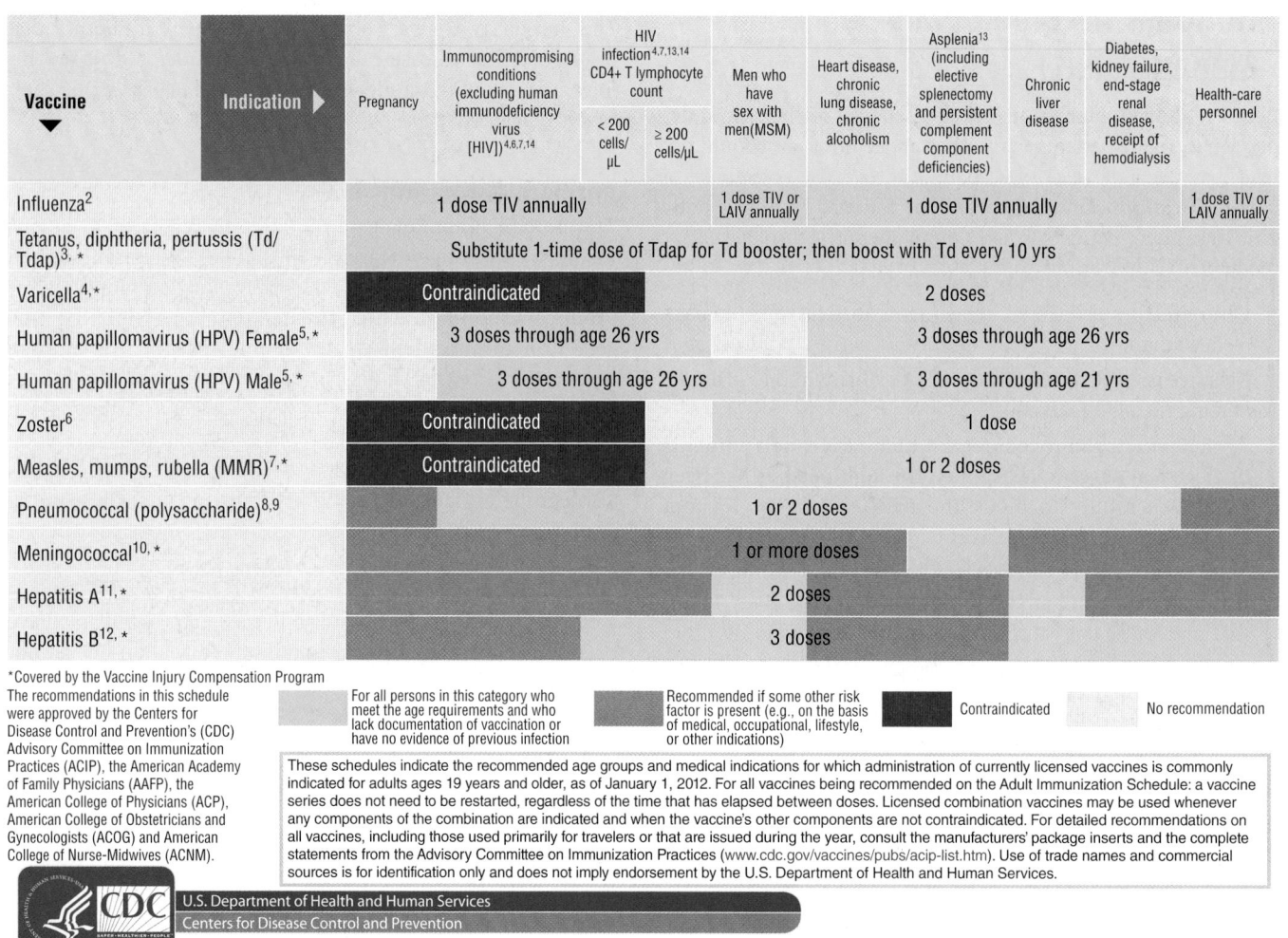

FIGURE 51-10 Adult immunization schedule.

PROCEDURE 51-1 Helping the Physician Comply with the Controlled Substances Act of 1970

Procedure Goal: To comply with the Controlled Substances Act of 1970.

OSHA Guidelines: This procedure does not involve exposure to blood, body fluids, or tissues.

Materials: DEA Form 224, DEA Form 222, DEA Form 41, computer or a pen (available in the workbook that accompanies this textbook or online at the U.S. Department of Justice's website).

Method: Procedure steps.

1. Use DEA Form 224 to register the physician with the Drug Enforcement Administration. Be sure to register each office location at which the physician administers or dispenses drugs covered under Schedules II through V. Renew all registrations every 3 years using DEA Form 224a. Form 224 can be printed from the U.S. Department of Justice website. The renewal application (Form 224a) can be completed through registration at this site.

2. Order Schedule II drugs using DEA Form 222, as instructed by the physician. (Stocks of these drugs should be kept to a minimum.)

RATIONALE: Accurate instruction from the physician is necessary to ensure safety.

3. Include the physician's DEA registration number on every prescription for a drug in Schedules II through V.
   RATIONALE: The DEA number is required or prescriptions will not be accepted.

4. Complete an inventory of all drugs in Schedules II through V every 2 years (as permitted in your state; this task may be reserved for other healthcare professionals).

5. Store all drugs in Schedules II through V in a secure, locked safe or cabinet (as permitted in your state).
   RATIONALE: To prevent theft.

6. Keep accurate dispensing and inventory records for at least 2 years.

7. Dispose of expired or unused drugs according to the DEA regulations. Always complete DEA Form 41 when disposing of controlled drugs.

PROCEDURE 51-2 Interpreting a Prescription

Procedure Goal: To read and accurately interpret a prescription.

OSHA Guidelines: This procedure does not involve exposure to blood, body fluids, or tissues.

Materials: Prescription (use Figure 51-9), Table 51-4 Abbreviations Used in Prescriptions, and a method of recording (pen or electronic).

Method: Procedure steps.

1. Verify the prescriber information. This is especially important in a multiphysician practice or electronic health record.

2. Ensure that patient information is accurate, including correct spelling of name, date of birth, and address. For written prescriptions, check legibility.

3. Confirm the date of the prescription.

4. Check the medication name and double-check spelling.

5. Verify that instructions to the pharmacist are complete and include refill authorization and generic substitution.

6. Translate the instructions to the patient using Table 51-4.

7. Make sure that the prescription is signed in ink for handwritten prescriptions and digitally for electronic prescriptions.

SUMMARY OF LEARNING OUTCOMES

LEARNING OUTCOMES	KEY POINTS
51.1 **Identify the medical assistant's role in pharmacology.**	The role of the medical assistant in pharmacology includes being attentive to ensure the physician is aware of all medications, both prescription and OTC, that a patient is taking; asking each patient about alcohol and recreational drug use (both past and present), as well as herbal remedies; assisting in managing and renewing medication prescriptions; and educating the patient, using guidelines provided by the licensed practitioner, about the purpose of a drug and how to take the drug for maximum effectiveness and minimum adverse effects.

LEARNING OUTCOMES	KEY POINTS
51.2 Recognize the five categories of pharmacology and their importance to medication administration.	The five categories of pharmacology include pharmacognosy, pharmacokinetics, pharmacodynamics, pharmacotherapeutics, and toxicology. It is important to understand each of these in order to carry out the medical assistant's role in pharmacology.
51.3 Differentiate the major drug categories, drug names, and their actions.	Drug categories are sometimes named based on their action; for example, anticonvulsants are used to treat convulsions (seizures). The major drug categories and their actions are outlined in Table 51-1.
51.4 Classify over-the-counter (OTC), prescription, and herbal drugs.	Nonprescription drugs, including herbal and OTC drugs, can be obtained without a physician's order. For prescription drugs, patients must have a physician's written (or oral) order.
51.5 Use credible sources to obtain drug information.	Credible sources for drug information are the *Physicians' Desk Reference® (PDR)*, United States Pharmacopeia/National Formulary, and the American Hospital Formulary Service (AHFS®). You also may access medication information from package inserts, drug labels, and other reliable Internet sites.
51.6 Carry out the procedure for registering or renewing a physician with the Drug Enforcement Administration (DEA) for permission to administer, dispense, and prescribe controlled drugs.	The medical assistant should assist the physician with registration, renewal, and ordering of controlled substances, as outlined in the Controlled Substances Act of 1970 and Procedure 51-1.
51.7 Identify the parts of a prescription, including commonly used abbreviations and symbols.	A prescription must be complete to be filled. The medical assistant must be able to interpret a prescription in order to manage new and refilled medications. Procedure 51-2 and Table 51-4 will assist the medical assistant in performing these tasks.
51.8 Discuss nonpharmacological treatments for pain.	Multiple nonpharmacologic methods are used to treat pain, including CAM therapies such as massage, yoga, biofeedback, chiropractic, acupuncture, magnetic therapy, hypnotism, and glucosamine chondroitin.
51.9 Describe how vaccines work in the immune system.	Immunizations usually contain killed or weakened organisms. When given, they stimulate the body to build up a resistance to the organism. They are used to provide immunity against specific diseases.

CASE STUDY CRITICAL THINKING

Recall Kaylyn Haddix, RMA (AMT), from the beginning of the chapter. Now that you have completed the chapter, answer the following questions regarding her case.

1. Detail the steps Kaylyn should take to design and implement an inventory system.
2. What are some credible sources of drug information Kaylyn can use to complete her task?

1. (LO 51.3) Which drug may prevent an asthma attack?
   a. ProAir HFA®
   b. Elavil®
   c. Lovenox®
   d. Levaquin®
   e. Lipitor®

2. (LO 51.5) Which source of medication information is divided into six sections?
   a. American Hospital Formulary Service (AHFS®)
   b. United States Pharmacopeia/National Formulary
   c. *Physicians' Desk Reference® (PDR)*
   d. Epocrates®
   e. RXList.com

3. (LO 51.6) Which of the following medications has the highest potential for addiction?
   a. Lomotil®
   b. Vicodin®
   c. Valium®
   d. Demerol®
   e. Ambien®

4. (LO 51.6) What method is used for disposing of controlled drugs?
   a. Discard drugs, then complete DEA Form 41
   b. Use the disposal company that takes your biohazardous waste
   c. Turn drugs over to a larger healthcare facility
   d. Complete DEA Form 41 and call the DEA for disposal instructions
   e. Complete DEA Form 222, then dispose of drugs with biohazardous waste

5. (LO 51.4) An example of an OTC medication is
   a. Glucophage®
   b. Lasix®
   c. Coumadin®
   d. Darvocet®
   e. Prevacid®

6. (LO 51.7) The Sig line of a prescription reads: " i tab po qd." What does it mean?
   a. Take one tablet by mouth twice a day
   b. The order is not accurate and cannot be used
   c. Take 1 tablet by mouth daily
   d. Take ½ tablet daily
   e. Take daily one tablet

7. (LO 51.8) A patient would like to know more about non-pharmacologic treatments for pain. Which of the following would you *least* likely discuss with this patient?
   a. Massage therapy
   b. Biofeedback therapy
   c. Acupuncture
   d. Glucosamine chondroitin
   e. Opioids

8. (LO 51.1) Which of the following would *least* likely be the medical assistant's role?
   a. Make sure the physician is aware of all medications a patient is taking
   b. Ask each patient about alcohol and recreational drug use
   c. Prescribe and dispense certain medications
   d. Manage and renew medication prescriptions
   e. Educate the patient according to physician guidelines

9. (LO 51.9) Which of the following is made from microorganisms and administered to a person to produce reduced sensitivity to an infectious disease?
   a. Controlled substance
   b. Immunity
   c. Vaccine
   d. Antibiotic
   e. Pharmaceutical

10. (LO 51.2) Which of the following is the category of pharmacology that is also called *clinical pharmacology*?
    a. Pharmacodynamics
    b. Pharmacognosy
    c. Pharmacokinetics
    d. Pharmacotherapeutics
    e. Toxicology

52

Dosage Calculations

L E A R N I N G   O U T C O M E S

After completing Chapter 52, you will be able to:

52.1 Explain the role of the medical assistant to ensure safe dosage calculations.

52.2 Identify systems of measurements and their common uses.

52.3 Convert among systems of measurements.

52.4 Execute dosage calculations accurately.

52.5 Calculate dosages based upon body weight and body surface area.

K E Y   T E R M S

body surface area (BSA)

formula method

nomogram

proportion method

volume

weight

II. C (1)   Demonstrate knowledge of basic math computations

II. C (2)   Apply mathematical computations to solve equations

II. C (3)   Identify measurement systems

II. C (4)   Define basic units of measurement in metric, apothecary and household systems

II. C (5)   Convert among measurement systems

II. P (1)   Prepare proper dosages of medication for administration

II. A (1)   Verify ordered doses/dosages prior to administration

6. Pharmacology

Graduates:

a. Demonstrate accurate occupational math and metric conversions for proper medication administration

Introduction

Depending upon the facility and state where you work as a medical assistant, you may be called upon to administer medications. All aspects of this skill require close attention to detail for the safety of the patient. Before you administer a drug you may need to calculate the dose prescribed by the physician. You should also be familiar with the equipment you will be using. You must execute all dosage calculations carefully and accurately in order to prevent medication errors. To do so, you must perform basic math, understand various systems of measurement, and be able to convert from one measurement system to another or within a system. You also may need to know calculations for special patient populations. This chapter will provide the basics of safe dosage calculations. Remember to check the scope of practice in your state and at your place of employment before working with dosages.

Ensuring Safe Dosage Calculations   LO 52.1

In order to be able to calculate dosages, you must understand and be able to perform basic math accurately. Whether you are using a calculator or doing it by hand, accuracy is key. Remember that a minor mistake in basic math can mean major errors in the patient's medication. When you perform any calculation, think about the answer you obtain and determine if it is reasonable.

Consider this example: While performing a calculation, a medical assistant adds the following numbers: 21¾, 12½, and 1½. He calculates an answer of 49¼. Before he accepts this answer as correct, however, he asks himself, "Is this reasonable?" In order to answer this question, he does a quick estimation. First, he adds the whole numbers from each of the mixed numbers in the problem: 21 + 12 + 1 = 34. Then he rounds each mixed number up to a whole number and adds them: 22 + 13 + 2 = 37. He recognizes that the correct answer to the problem must be between 34 and 37, so his original answer is incorrect. He probably entered one of the numbers

into his calculator incorrectly. When he repeats the original calculation, he now comes up with an answer of 35¾. This is between the values that he expected based on his estimate, so it is a reasonable answer to the problem.

Think about the example. When performing calculations, there are many steps in which an error might be made. In this case, a number had been entered incorrectly into a calculator. While errors like this can happen to anyone, they can usually be detected by performing a quick check to see if the answer is reasonable. You should develop the habit of asking yourself the same question *every time you perform a calculation*. When performing a calculation, analyze the problem and try to estimate a reasonable range for the answer. This critical thinking skill can help you to detect errors and should become a part of every calculation you perform.

Measurement Systems   LO 52.2

Three systems of measurement are used in the United States for pharmacology and drug administration. These include metric, apothecary, and household systems. Metric is the most commonly used system. Although apothecary and household systems are rarely used, basic knowledge of these systems may be needed.

To understand drug measurement, focus primarily on remembering the basic unit of volume and weight. **Volume** refers to the amount of space a drug occupies. **Weight** refers to its heaviness. Length, which is also a basic unit, is discussed in the *Vital Signs and Measurements* chapter.

Metric System

Like the decimal system, the metric system is based on multiples of 10. The greater confidence you have working with decimals, the more comfortable you will be working with metric units. See the Caution: Handle with Care feature Working with Decimals. The basic units of volume and weight in the decimal-based metric system are liters (L) to measure volume and grams (g) to measure weight. Prefixes are added to these basic units of

CAUTION: HANDLE WITH CARE
Working with Decimals

Consider the following when working with decimals to prevent errors in dosage calculations.

1. Writing decimals:
   - Write the whole-number part of the decimal to the left of the decimal point.
   - Write the decimal fraction part to the right of the decimal point. Decimal fractions are equivalent to fractions that have denominators of 10, 100, 1000, and so forth.
   - Use zero as a placeholder to the right of the decimal point just as you use zero for whole numbers. The decimal number 1.203 represents 1 ones, 2 tenths, 0 hundredths, and 3 thousandths.

2. Using zeros:
   - Always write a zero to the left of the decimal point when the decimal number has no whole-number part. Using the zero makes the decimal point more noticeable.
   - Never place a trailing zero after the decimal point when working with medication dosages.

3. Rounding decimals:
   - Underline the place value to which you want to round.
   - Look at the digit to the right of this target place value. If this digit is 4 or less, do not change the digit in the target place value. If this digit is 5 or more, round the digit in the target place value up one unit.
   - Drop all digits to the right of the target place value.

TABLE 52-1	Common Metric Units				
Prefix	**Kilo-**	**Base Unit**	**Centi-**	**Milli-**	**Micro-**
Value	× 1000	—	÷ 100	÷ 1000	÷ 1,000,000
Weight	kilogram (kg) 1000 g	gram (g) 1 g	centigram (cg) 0.01 g	milligram (mg) 0.001 g	microgram (mcg) 0.000001 g
Volume	kiloliter (kL) 1000 L	liter (L) 1 L	centiliter (cL) 0.01 L	milliliter (mL) 0.001 L	microliter (mcL) 0.000001 L

measurement to indicate multiples, such as kilogram (kg), or fractions, such as milliliter (mL) or microgram (mcg). Common metric units and equivalents are presented in Table 52-1. Note that a cubic centimeter (cc) is the amount of space occupied by 1 mL. Although these two measurements are equal, the accepted medical abbreviation is mL. Do not use the abbreviation "cc," even though you may sometimes see it in practice. Additionally, note that the abbreviation for liters is a capital L instead of a small l. The small l can be confused with the numeral 1.

Apothecary and Household Systems

Although the metric system is preferred for dosage calculations, as a medical assistant you should have basic knowledge of the much older apothecary system, as well as the commonly known household system. The apothecary system uses units such as fluid ounces, fluid drams, pints, and quarts for volume, and drams, ounces, and pounds for weight. The only household units used for measurement are units of volume. They include drops, teaspoons, tablespoons, ounces, cups, pints, quarts, and gallons. Keep in mind that units of measurement found in both the apothecary and the household systems are equal: an apothecary ounce equals a household ounce. Apothecary and household units and equivalents you may come across in practice are outlined in Table 52-2 and Table 52-3.

TABLE 52-2	Apothecary Units and Equivalents
Apothecary Units	**Equivalent**
Measures of Volume	
8 fluid drams (fl dr) =	1 fluid ounce (fl oz)
16 fl oz =	1 pint (pt)
2 pt =	1 quart (qt)
4 qt =	1 gallon (gal)
Measures of Weight	
60 gr =	1 dram (dr)
8 dr =	1 ounce (oz)
16 oz =	1 pound (lb)

TABLE 52-3	Household Units and Equivalents
Household Units	**Equivalent**
Measures of Volume	
60 drops* (gtt) =	1 teaspoon (tsp)
3 tsp =	1 tablespoon (tbsp)
6 tsp =	1 ounce (oz) or 2 tbsp
8 oz =	1 cup (c)
2 c =	1 pint (pt)
4 c =	1 quart (qt) or 2 pt

*Droppers may vary.

Conversions within and between Measurement Systems

LO 52.3

Frequently you will need to convert units of measure within a system of measure or between systems of measure. Most commonly you will convert within the metric system. For example, you may need to determine how many milligrams of medication to give a patient when the medication only comes in grams. Sometimes you may need to convert from one measurement system to another. For example, a patient may need to take five milliliters of medication and the only device she has is a teaspoon.

Converting within the Metric System

Converting one metric unit of measurement to another is similar to multiplying and dividing decimal numbers. When you convert a quantity from one unit of metric measurement to another, you should follow these rules:

1. Move the decimal point to the right when you convert from a larger to a smaller unit. This is dividing.
2. Move the decimal point to the left when you convert from a smaller to a larger unit. This is multiplying.

Use Table 52-1 and Figure 52-1 to help determine both the direction and the number of places to move the decimal point when you convert between units of metric measurement. For example, milliliter is three decimal places to the right of liter, the basic unit. To convert a quantity from liters (larger) to milliliters (smaller), move the decimal point three places to the right, or three steps down the stairs shown in Figure 52-1.

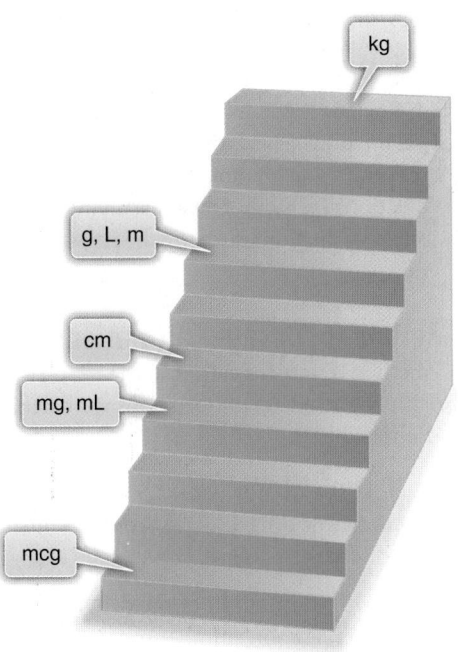

FIGURE 52-1 Use the metric steps to convert between units in the metric system.

Similarly, to convert a quantity from grams (smaller) to kilograms (larger), move the decimal point three places to the left, or three steps up the stairs.

Let's try these examples.

Example A You need to change the patient's weight from grams to kilograms to determine how much medication should be given based upon the patient's weight. An infant weighs 9600 grams (g). How many kilograms (kg) does she weigh? A gram is smaller than a kilogram, so you need to move the decimal point to the left three steps, or divide by 1000.

$$9600 \text{ g} \div 1000 = 9.6 \text{ kg}$$

Example B The physician orders a patient to have a one-gram dose of amoxicillin. The medication is supplied in 1000 mg tablets. You will need to determine how many milligrams are in a gram. A gram is larger than a milligram, so you need to move the decimal point to the right three steps, or multiply by 1000.

$$1.000. \text{ gram} \times 1000 = 1000 \text{ mg}$$

Your Turn A patient takes a daily dose of Synthroid 100 mcg (micrograms). How many mg (milligrams) does he take?

First determine how many mg are in a mcg. A microgram is smaller than a milligram, so you need to move the decimal point to the left three steps, or divide by 1000. The answer is 0.1 mg.

Converting between Systems of Measurement

When performing dosage calculations, sometimes it will be necessary to convert units from one system to another. In order to do this, you must become familiar with their equivalent measures. Because of the difference in basic units of measure, you must remember that conversions between systems are only approximate equivalents. If you use a conversion chart, read it carefully before administering a drug. Check it several times and place a ruler under the line you are reading to be absolutely sure you are reading the chart properly. Table 52-4 provides equivalent measures for the metric, apothecary, and household systems.

In some cases, you may need to convert between systems of measurement by doing a calculation. You can use the **proportion method** to calculate these conversions. Let's try these examples.

TABLE 52-4	Common Equivalent Measures for the Metric, Apothecary, and Household Systems*	
1 teaspoon = 5 mL	1 tablespoon = 15 mL	1 fl oz = 30 mL
1 pint = 480 mL	1 kg = 2.2 lbs	1 fl oz = 2 tbsp

*Equivalent measures are approximates.

Example A Suppose the physician orders 5 milliliters (mL) of Benadryl elixir. However, there is only a teaspoon (tsp) available to measure the dose. To make this conversion, follow these steps.

1. Set up a fraction with the ordered dose on the top and the unknown amount on the bottom:

$$\frac{5 \text{ mL}}{x}$$

2. Next set up a fraction with the standard equivalent. See Table 52-4. Make sure that for this fraction you use units of measure on the top and the bottom that match the units of measure on the top and the bottom of the first fraction:

$$\frac{5 \text{ mL}}{1 \text{ tsp}}$$

3. Then set up a proportion with both fractions:

$$\frac{5 \text{ mL}}{x} = \frac{5 \text{ mL}}{1 \text{ tsp}}$$

4. Now cross multiply. Multiply the bottom left number by the top right number, and multiply the top left number by the bottom right number:

$$x \times 5 \text{ mL} = 5 \text{ mL} \times 1 \text{ tsp}$$

5. To solve for *x,* divide both sides of the equation by 5 mL, then do the arithmetic, canceling out like terms in the top and bottom of each fraction:

$$\frac{x \times \cancel{5 \text{ mL}}}{\cancel{5 \text{ mL}}} = \frac{\cancel{5 \text{ mL}} \times 1 \text{ tsp}}{\cancel{5 \text{ mL}}}$$

$$x = 1 \text{ tsp}$$

Example B Suppose the medication is ordered based upon the patient's weight in kilograms. You know the patient's weight is 168 lbs. To make this conversion, follow these steps:

1. Set up a fraction with the weight in pounds on top and the unknown weight in kilograms on the bottom:

$$\frac{168 \text{ lbs}}{x \text{ kg}}$$

2. Next set up a fraction with the standard equivalent. See Table 52-4. Make sure that for this fraction you use units of measure on the top and the bottom that match the units of measure on the top and the bottom of the first fraction:

$$\frac{2.2 \text{ lbs}}{1 \text{ kg}}$$

3. Then set up a proportion with both fractions:

$$\frac{168 \text{ lbs}}{x \text{ kg}} = \frac{2.2 \text{ lbs}}{1 \text{ kg}}$$

4. Now cross multiply. Multiply the bottom left number by the top right number, and multiply the top left number by the bottom right number:

$$x \times 2.2 \text{ lbs} = 168 \text{ lbs} \times 1 \text{ kg}$$

5. To solve for *x,* divide both sides of the equation by 2.2 lbs, then do the arithmetic, canceling out like terms in the

top and bottom of each fraction and then dividing 168 by 2.2:

$$\frac{x \times \cancel{2.2 \text{ lbs}}}{\cancel{2.2 \text{ lbs}}} = \frac{168 \cancel{\text{ lbs}} \times 1 \text{ kg}}{2.2 \cancel{\text{ lbs}}}$$

$$x = 76.36 \text{ kg}$$

Your Turn You need to prepare a solution for the physician to clean a wound. He asks for 3½ ounces (oz) of saline to be placed in sterile bowl. Your container of saline is marked in milliliters (mL). Use these steps to make the conversion.

1. Set up a fraction with the ordered dose on the top and the unknown amount on the bottom.

2. Next, set up a fraction with the standard equivalent. See Table 52-4. Make sure that for this fraction you use units of measure on the top and the bottom that match the units of measure on the top and the bottom of the first fraction.

3. Then set up a proportion with both fractions.

4. Now cross multiply. Multiply the bottom left number by the top right number, and multiply the top left number by the bottom right number.

5. To solve for *x,* divide both sides of the equation by 1, then do the arithmetic, canceling out like terms in the top and bottom of each fraction.

If you followed each step correctly, you will find that you need 105 mL of saline.

▶ Dosage Calculations
LO 52.4

As a medical assistant you may be called upon to calculate medication doses. Remember to follow your scope of practice. You may be able to calculate these using either the proportion method or a **formula method**. No matter what method you use, you must be aware that the patient's health or life can depend on your calculations. Always take the time to check and recheck your arithmetic. For a quick review of basic math, see Points on Practice: Math Review. If you have a question or you are not sure about your calculations, check the problem again and then have a coworker check. If you are not 100% sure you know how to do dosage calculations correctly, consider buying and using a dosage calculation workbook or searching the Internet for extra practice.

Proportion Method for Dosage Calculations

The proportion method described earlier in the chapter for unit conversion also can be used to perform dosage calculations. Let's try some examples.

Example A Suppose the doctor orders 500 mg of ampicillin, but each tablet contains only 250 mg. To calculate how to provide this dose, follow these steps:

1. Set up a fraction with the amount of the drug ordered over the unknown (in this case, the number of tablets).

$$\frac{500 \text{ mg}}{x \text{ tab}}$$

POINTS ON PRACTICE

Math Review

Recall the following math rules while performing dosage calculations.

1. Order of operations: When solving a math problem, first divide or multiply from left to right, then add or subtract from left to right. For example: For the equation $\frac{650}{325} \times 3 = x$, you would need to divide 650 by 325 first. This equals 2.

$$2 \times 3 = x$$

Now multiply second: $6 = x$.

2. Proportions: Proportions are two fractions that are equal to each other. When 3 of the 4 values in a proportion are known, the unknown value can be calculated. Proportions using fractions are solved by cross multiplying. For example: To solve for the unknown in $2/3 = x/12$, cross multiply ($3 \times x = 2 \times 12$) and then solve for the unknown ($x = 8$).

3. Rounding: When rounding, you must look at the first digit to the right of the place value that you are rounding to. If this digit is 5 or more, round up. If it is less than 5, round down. For example, to round 2.7384 to the hundredths place, you look at the digit to the right of the 3. This digit, 8, is greater than 5, so you round the number up to 2.74.

2. Next, set up a fraction with the amount of drug in a single tablet (dose on hand) over one tablet (dosage unit).

$$\frac{250 \text{ mg}}{1 \text{ tab}}$$

3. Now set up the proportion with both fractions, making sure the same units of measure are on the top and bottom of each side of the proportion.

$$\frac{500 \text{ mg}}{x \text{ tab}} = \frac{250 \text{ mg}}{1 \text{ tab}}$$

4. Cross multiply. Multiply the bottom left number by the top right number, and multiply the top left number by the bottom right number:

$$x \text{ tab} \times 250 \text{ mg} = 500 \text{ mg} \times 1 \text{ tab}$$

5. To solve for x, divide both sides of the equation by 250 mg, then do the arithmetic, canceling out like terms in the top and bottom of each fraction:

$$\frac{x \times 250 \text{ mg}}{250 \text{ mg}} = \frac{500 \text{ mg} \times 1 \text{ tab}}{250 \text{ mg}}$$
$$x = \frac{500 \text{ tabs}}{250}$$
$$x = 2 \text{ tabs}$$

The patient will receive 2 tablets.

Example B The doctor orders 30 mg of Adalat, but each capsule (cap) contains only 10 mg. To calculate the prescribed drug dose using the proportion method, you would follow these steps.

1. Set up a fraction with the amount of the drug ordered over the unknown amount (in this case, the number of capsules).

$$\frac{30 \text{ mg}}{x \text{ cap}}$$

2. Next set up a fraction with the amount of drug in a single tablet (dose on hand) over one capsule (dosage unit).

$$\frac{10 \text{ mg}}{1 \text{ cap}}$$

3. Now set up the proportion using both fractions, making sure the same units of measure are on the top and bottom of each side of the proportion.

$$\frac{30 \text{ mg}}{x \text{ cap}} = \frac{10 \text{ mg}}{1 \text{ cap}}$$

4. Cross multiply. Multiply the bottom left number by the top right number, and multiply the top left number by the bottom right number:

$$x \text{ cap} \times 10 \text{ mg} = 30 \text{ mg} \times 1 \text{ cap}$$

5. To solve for x, divide both sides of the equation by 10 mg, then do the arithmetic, canceling out like terms in the top and bottom of each fraction:

$$\frac{x \times 10 \text{ mg}}{10 \text{ mg}} = \frac{30 \text{ mg} \times 1 \text{ cap}}{10 \text{ mg}}$$
$$x = \frac{30 \text{ caps}}{10}$$
$$x = 3 \text{ caps}$$

The patient will receive 3 capsules.

Example C Now let's try a liquid medication. The physician wants a patient to have 250 mg of Zithromax®. You have on hand a bottle of Zithromax® oral suspension. See the label in Figure 52-2. Follow these steps:

FIGURE 52-2 Zithromax® oral suspension.

1. Set up a fraction with the amount of the drug ordered over the unknown amount (in this case, the amount of liquid in mL).

$$\frac{250 \text{ mg}}{x \text{ mL}}$$

2. Next set up a fraction with the amount of drug in a single dose (dose on hand) over the number of mL in a single dose (dosage unit).

$$\frac{100 \text{ mg}}{5 \text{ mL}}$$

3. Now set up the proportion using both fractions, making sure the same units of measure are on the top and bottom of each side of the proportion.

$$\frac{250 \text{ mg}}{x \text{ mL}} = \frac{100 \text{ mg}}{5 \text{ mL}}$$

4. Cross multiply. Multiply the bottom left number by the top right number, and multiply the top left number by the bottom right number:

$$x \times 100 \text{ mg} = 250 \text{ mg} \times 5 \text{ mL}$$

5. To solve for x, divide both sides of the equation by 100 mg, then do the arithmetic, canceling out like terms in the top and bottom of each fraction and then multiplying 250×5 and dividing by 100:

$$\frac{x \times \cancel{100 \text{ mg}}}{\cancel{100 \text{ mg}}} = \frac{250 \cancel{\text{ mg}} \times 5 \text{ mL}}{100 \cancel{\text{ mg}}}$$

$$x = \frac{250 \times 5 \text{ mL}}{100}$$

$$x = 12.5 \text{ mL}$$

The patient will receive 12.5 mL of medication.

Your Turn The physician wants a patient with chest pain to have 0.8 mg of Nitrostat® sublingually (under his tongue). You have on hand the bottle of Nitrostat® shown in Figure 52-3. Follow the steps below to determine how much medicine the patient should receive.

1. Set up a fraction with the amount of the drug ordered over the unknown (in this case, the number of tablets).

2. Next, set up a fraction with the amount of drug in a single tablet (dose on hand) over one tablet (dosage unit).

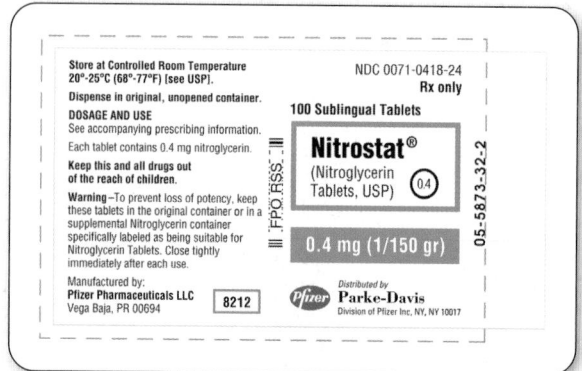

FIGURE 52-3 Nitrostat® sublingual tablets.

3. Now set up the proportion with both fractions making sure the same units of measure are on the top and bottom of each side of the proportion.

4. Cross multiply. Multiply the bottom left number by the top right number, and multiply the top left number by the bottom right number.

5. To solve for x, divide both sides of the equation by 0.4 mg, then do the arithmetic, canceling out like terms in the top and bottom of each fraction.

If you did the problem correctly, you will discover that the patient needs two tablets.

Formula Method for Dosage Calculations

In some instances, you can use a basic formula to calculate drugs that have the same label as the dose ordered—such as milligrams and milligrams—and therefore do not require a conversion. When you use the formula method, you substitute the correct numbers for what each of the letters represents. The basic formula that you would use looks like this:

$$D/H \times Q$$

Using this formula, you will need to know the following:

D = Desired dose or the amount of medication the physician has ordered the patient to take.

H = Dose on hand or the amount of medication in each unit of the drug; for example, the number of mcg, mg, or g in each unit dose.

Q = Quantity of the dose on hand or dosage unit; for example, a pill or an amount of liquid.

Let's try some examples.

Example A Suppose that the physician orders acetaminophen, 650 milligrams (mg). This is the desired dose (D). However, all that the office has on hand are 325 mg Tylenol tablets (tabs). The dose on hand (H) is 325 mg, and the quantity (Q) or dosage unit is 1 tablet. Follow these steps to perform the calculation:

1. Use the formula, inserting each number, and label all the parts:

$$D/H \times Q$$

$$\frac{650 \text{ mg}}{325 \text{ mg}} \times 1 \text{ tablet (tab)}$$

2. Cancel and solve:

$$\frac{650 \cancel{\text{ mg}}}{325 \cancel{\text{ mg}}} \times 1 \text{ tablet (tab)}$$

$$\frac{650}{325} \times 1 \text{ tab} = 2 \text{ tablets}$$

Two tablets need to be given to the patient. See the *Medication Administration* chapter for the correct procedure for administering a medication.

CAUTION: HANDLE WITH CARE
Preventing Errors during Dosage Calculations

Medication errors are a serious problem in healthcare. The possibility of error occurs several times during medication administration. Error can occur when performing calculations, when selecting the medication to administer, and when reading the label to perform the calculation. Always pay close attention to the dose and the route of administration (how the medication is given). You must check and recheck the ordered form of the drug as well as the amount of drug per dose of the drug. In the following example, this crucial relationship is illustrated.

Prochlorperazine (Compazine) is an antiemetic drug for acute nausea and vomiting. It is given to both children and adults. When the vomiting is so severe that a tablet or capsule cannot be swallowed, the drug is administered in injectable or suppository form. This drug is available in multiple forms:

- 10 mL multidose vials with 5 mg of drug per mL, written as 5 mg/mL
- 2 mL single-dose vials with 5 mg/mL
- 4 fl oz bottles of syrup with 5 mg/5 mL (5 mg/1 tsp)
- 5 mg tablets
- 10 mg tablets
- 2 mL prefilled disposable syringes with 5 mg/mL
- 2½ mg suppositories
- 5 mg suppositories
- 25 mg suppositories
- 10 mg extended release capsules
- 15 mg extended release capsules

Because so many forms of this drug are available, there is a high risk of error in choosing the correct form. In addition, the route of administration can determine how much drug is delivered in one dose. For example, note that suppositories are available in 2½ mg, 5 mg, and 25 mg forms. If the 2½ mg dose were written as 2.5 mg, there might be confusion with the 25 mg dose suppository. Thus, the 2½ mg suppository is always written this way, even in the *PDR*. This clarification helps prevent a child from receiving the adult dose of 25 mg, which could result in serious complications to the central nervous system. This possible confusion is one example of how much difference a decimal point can make.

Note also that in the syrup there is a 5 mg dose of drug per 5 mL (1 tsp), whereas in the other liquid forms (vials and prefilled syringes), there is a 5 mg dose of drug per 1 mL. The injectable form is five times more concentrated than the syrup. Therefore, if you were to administer the same amount of injectable liquid as syrup to a patient, you would give the patient five times more drug than in the syrup. Just as a child could be endangered with the 25 mg suppository, an adult could be endangered with the wrong form of liquid. Because elderly patients often receive syrup forms of medication, this instruction could be particularly confusing.

Example B Now let's say the physician asks you to administer and inject 10 mg of Compazine. Ten (10) mg is the desired dose (D). According to the Compazine label, the liquid contains 5 mg/mL, which means there are 5 milligrams (mg) of Compazine in every 1 milliliter (mL) of liquid, so 5 mg is the dose on hand (H) and 1 mL is the quantity (Q) or dosage unit. Always read the labels carefully to determine the dose on hand and the quantity or dosage unit. See the Caution: Handle with Care feature Preventing Errors during Dosage Calculations. Follow the same steps to perform the calculation:

1. Use the formula, inserting each number in the correct place, and label all the parts:

$$\text{D/H} \times \text{Q}$$

$$\frac{10 \text{ mg}}{5 \text{ mg}} \times 1 \text{ mL}$$

2. Cancel and solve:

$$\frac{10 \text{ mg}}{5 \text{ mg}} \times 1 \text{ mL}$$

$$\frac{10}{5} \times 1 \text{ mL} = 2 \text{ mL}$$

Two (2) mL needs to be injected into the patient. See the *Medication Administration* chapter for the correct procedure for administering a medication.

Example C The physician wants a pediatric patient to have 200 mg of Biaxin® liquid. The label of the only bottle you have on hand is pictured in Figure 52-4.

FIGURE 52-4 Biaxin oral suspension.

1. Use the formula, inserting each number, and label all the parts:

$$D/H \times Q$$

$$\frac{200 \text{ mg}}{250 \text{ mg}} \times 5 \text{ mL}$$

2. Cancel and solve:

$$\frac{200 \text{ mg}}{250 \text{ mg}} \times 5 \text{ mL}$$

$$\frac{200}{250} \times 5 \text{ mL} = 4 \text{ mL}$$

The patient should receive 4 mL of oral suspension. See the *Medication Administration* chapter for the correct procedure for administering an oral medication.

Your Turn The physician orders 500 mg of Amoxicillin Suspension. You have on hand the medication shown in Figure 52-5. How much medication should the patient receive?

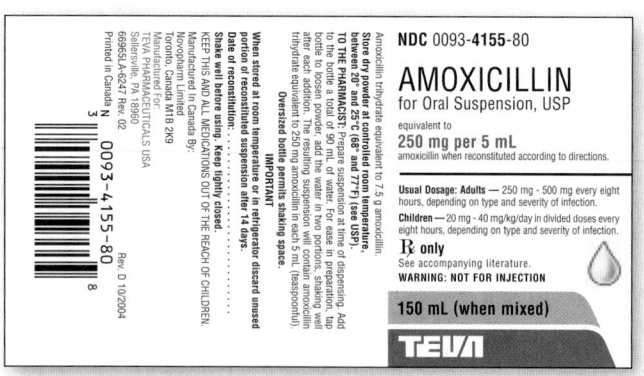

FIGURE 52-5 Amoxicillin Oral Suspension.

1. Use the formula, inserting each number, and label all the parts.
2. Cancel and solve.

The patient should receive 10 mL of medication. If you only have a teaspoon available, you would administer 2 teaspoons. See the *Medication Administration* chapter for the correct procedure for administering an oral medication.

▶ Body Weight and Body Surface Area Calculations

LO 52.5

In certain cases, a drug dose is determined based on the **body surface area (BSA)** or the weight of the patient. This is more common with pediatric and geriatric patients. These patients are at greater risk of harm from medication because of the way they break down and absorb medications. Calculations for these individuals must be precise. Although BSA and weight dosage calculations are usually done by the physician or other licensed healthcare personnel, you may be asked to perform calculations, depending on your area of practice.

Dosages Based upon Weight

An order based on weight often states the amount of medication per weight of the patient per unit of time. For example, an order for a 34 lb child may read "Erythromycin 40 mg/kg/day po q4h." This means that over the course of a day, the patient should receive 40 mg of medication for every kilogram (kg) he or she weighs. It is to be given every four (4) hours or six (6) times during a 24-hour period. You will need to calculate the patient's weight in kilograms, the total medication to administer in 24 hours, and the amount of medication to administer in each dose. Use these steps.

1. Calculate the weight in kilograms using the proportion method. For accuracy, round the results to the nearest hundredth (two places after the decimal point).

   a. Set up the proportion. Recall from Table 52-4 that 2.2 lb = 1 kg.

   $$\frac{34 \text{ lb}}{x \text{ kg}} = \frac{2.2 \text{ lb}}{1 \text{ kg}}$$

   b. Cross multiply. Remember to multiply the bottom left number by the top right number, and multiply the top left number by the bottom right number.

   $$x \text{ kg} \times 2.2 \text{ lbs} = 34 \text{ lb} \times 1 \text{ kg}$$

   c. Solve for x (the unknown).

   $$x = \frac{34}{2.2} \text{ kg} = 15.45 \text{ kg}$$

2. Calculate the desired dose (D) for 24 hours by multiplying the dose ordered by the weight in kilograms.

   $$40 \text{ mg} \times 15.45 \text{ kg} = \text{desired dose (D) for 24 hours}$$

   618 mg = D (the amount of medication to be given in 24 hours)

3. Calculate the desired dose (D) for the one dose you have been asked to administer. This is done by dividing the amount to be received in 24 hours by the number of times the medication will be received in 24 hours. In this case, the medication is to be given six times in 24 hours.

   $$618 \text{ mg} \div 6 = 103 \text{ mg} \text{ (the desired dose for one dose)}$$

4. Calculate the amount to administer. On hand you have the medication shown in Figure 52-6.

   a. Set up the equation. You want to give 103 mg of medication, and the label shows there are 200 mg in 5 mL of medication.

   $$\frac{103 \text{ mg}}{x \text{ mL}} = \frac{200 \text{ mg}}{5 \text{ mL}}$$

   b. Cross multiply. Remember to multiply the bottom left number by the top right number, and multiply the top left number by the bottom right number.

   $$x \text{ mL} \times 200 \text{ mg} = 103 \text{ mg} \times 5 \text{ mL}$$

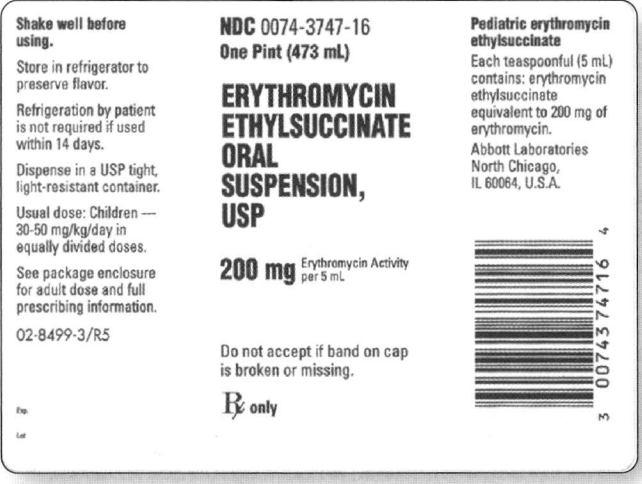

FIGURE 52-6 Erythromycin ethylsuccinate oral suspension.

c. Solve for *x* to determine the amount of liquid medication to administer to this patient.

$$x \text{ mL} = 103 \times \frac{5}{200}$$

$$\text{mL} = 2.575$$

$$\text{mL} = 2.6 \text{ (rounded to the nearest tenth)}$$

Now that you have determined the amount, refer to the *Medication Administration* chapter before you give the medication to the patient.

Dosages Based upon Body Surface Area

The total surface area of the body, or body surface area (BSA), is used to calculate very precise medication dosages. Pediatric patients, as well as burn victims or patients undergoing chemotherapy or radiation therapy, may need BSA dosage calculations. A complex formula or a nomogram, shown in Figure 52-7, may be used to determine the BSA. A **nomogram** is a set of scales arranged so that a ruler aligned with two of the values shows the corresponding value on the third scale. In Figure 52-7, aligning the ruler with a person's height and weight shows the body surface area.

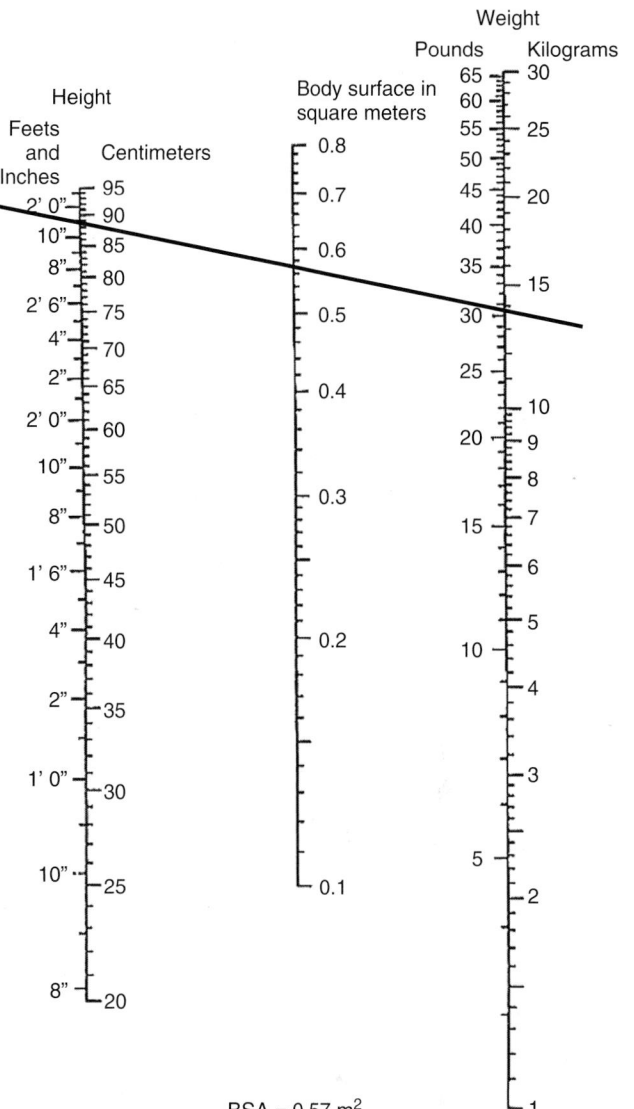

BSA = 0.57 m²

FIGURE 52-7 A nomogram is used to determine the BSA in order to calculate a medication dose. In this metric nomogram, the child weighs 13.9 kg and is 89 cm tall.

SUMMARY OF LEARNING OUTCOMES	
LEARNING OUTCOMES	**KEY POINTS**
52.1 **Explain the role of the medical assistant to ensure safe dosage calculations.**	A medical assistant must be proficient in math and determine if the answer to every calculation he performs is reasonable.
52.2 **Identify systems of measurements and their common uses.**	The metric system is based on 10 and is the most common system of measurement for dosage calculations. Metric units commonly used for dosage calculations include g, mg, mcg, and mL. The apothecary and household systems have some equal measures, but they are used rarely.
52.3 **Convert among systems of measurements.**	To convert among systems of measurements, you can refer to a conversion chart or perform a proportion method calculation. Keep in mind that measurements between the metric and the apothecary and household systems are only approximations.

LEARNING OUTCOMES	KEY POINTS
52.4 **Execute dosage calculations accurately.**	Use the formula method or proportion method to perform dosage calculations. *Formula Method* $D/H \times Q$ D = Desired dose or the amount of medication the physician has ordered the patient to take. H = Dose on hand or the amount of medication in each unit of the drug. Q = Quantity of the dose on hand or dosage unit. *Proportion Method* 1. Set up a fraction with the amount of the drug ordered over the unknown amount. 2. Set up a fraction with the amount of drug in a single dose (dose on hand) over the dosage unit. 3. Set up the proportion using both fractions, making sure the same units of measure are on the top and bottom of each side of the proportion. 4. Cross multiply. 5. To solve for *x*, do the arithmetic, then cancel out like terms in the top and bottom of each fraction.
52.5 **Calculate dosages based upon body weight and body surface area.**	Dosages based on body weight and BSA are used when precise amounts of medication must be administered. Body weight calculations are usually ordered in mg/kg/day. BSA calculations use special formulas or a nomogram.

CASE STUDY / CRITICAL THINKING

Recall Valarie Ramirez from the beginning of the chapter. Now that you have completed the chapter, answer the following questions.

1. The medication must be administered based upon Valarie's weight. What is her weight in kilograms?

2. You perform the calculation for Valarie's medication and determine she needs 2.95 mL of medication, but the syringe in marked in tenths. How much medication should you give?

3. Name at least three things you can do to ensure that Valarie receives a safe and accurate dose of medication.

EXAM PREPARATION QUESTIONS

There may be more than one correct answer. Circle the *best* answer.

1. (LO 52.1) As a medical assistant, how can you *best* ensure safe dosage calculations?
   a. Use a calculator for every calculation
   b. Check with a co-worker for every calculation you perform
   c. Do not use the unit of measurement when performing calculations
   d. Use a trailing zero after the decimal point for whole numbers
   e. Check your calculation by determining if the results are reasonable

2. (LO 52.2) What do the following metric prefixes represent in comparison to the base unit kilo, milli, micro?
   a. × 1000, ÷ 100, ÷ 1,000,000
   b. × 100, ÷ 1000, ÷ 1,000,000
   c. ÷ 1,000,000, × 1000, ÷ 1000
   d. × 1000, ÷ 1000, ÷ 1,000,000
   e. ÷ 1000, × 1000, ÷ 1,000,000

3. (LO 52.4) How much medication should be given if the physician ordered Keflex 500 mg and you have on hand Keflex 250 mg per 5 mL?
   a. 5 mL
   b. 250 mg
   c. 500 mg
   d. 10 mL
   e. 125 mL

4. (LO 52.4) How much medication would be in the syringe if the physician ordered Decadron 6 mg IM now and you have on hand Decadron 4 mg per mL?
   a. 1.5 mg
   b. 1.5 mL
   c. 4 mL
   d. 1 mL
   e. 3 mL

5. (LO 52.4) The doctor orders 5 mg of glyburide, but each tablet contains only 1.25 mg. How many tablets should the patient take?
   a. 3
   b. 1.25
   c. 5
   d. 1
   e. 4

6. (LO 52.4) You need to give Engerix-B® 10 mcg IM now. You have on hand the medication pictured below. How much medication would you administer?

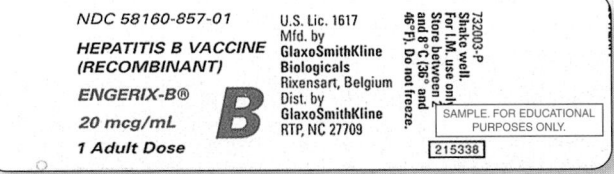

   a. 0.5 mcg
   b. 1 mL
   c. 0.5 mL
   d. 2 mL
   e. 1 mcg

7. (LO 52.3) The physician orders Ceclor 0.375 g PO bid. You have on hand Ceclor oral suspension 187 mg per 5 mL. How many mg of Ceclor are ordered?
   a. 187
   b. 5
   c. 0.375
   d. 375
   e. 0.187

8. (LO 52.4) The physician orders Ceclor 0.375 g PO bid. You have on hand Ceclor oral suspension 187 mg per 5 mL. How many mL of Ceclor do you need to give?
   a. 10
   b. 5
   c. 187
   d. 2.5
   e. 0.375

9. (LO 52.4) The physician wants you to give the patient an IM injection of 500 mcg of Cyanocobalamin. You have on hand the medication pictured below. How many mL of medication would you inject?

   a. 2 mL
   b. 500 mcg
   c. 0.5 mL
   d. 1000 mcg
   e. 0.5 mcg

10. (LO 52.5) A 5-year-old child weighs 44 lbs. The physician orders him to receive Zinacef 50 mg/kg/day IM q6h. How many milligrams of medication should the child receive in one dose?
    a. 1000 mg
    b. 167 mg
    c. 20 kg
    d. 250 mg
    e. 50 mg

Medication Administration

LEARNING OUTCOMES

After completing Chapter 53, you will be able to:

53.1 Describe rules and responsibilities regarding drug administration and the initial preparation for the drug administration.

53.2 List the rights of drug administration.

53.3 Recognize the correct equipment to use for administering medications.

53.4 Carry out the procedures for administering oral medications.

53.5 Carry out procedures for administering parenteral medications by injection.

53.6 Carry out procedures for administering parenteral medications by other routes.

53.7 Relate special considerations required for medication administration to pediatric, pregnant, breast-feeding, and geriatric patients.

53.8 Outline patient education information related to medications.

53.9 Implement accurate and complete documentation of medications.

KEY TERMS

buccal
diluent
douche
infusion
intradermal (ID)
intramuscular (IM)
intravenous (IV)

ointment
scored
solution
subcutaneous (subcut)
sublingual
transdermal
Z-track method

CAAHEP

I. P (7) Select proper sites for administering parenteral medication

I. P (8) Administer oral medications

I. P (9) Administer parenteral (excluding IV) medications

II. C (6) Identify both abbreviations and symbols used in calculating medication dosages

II. P (1) Prepare proper dosages of medication for administration

II. A (1) Verify ordered doses/dosages prior to administration

IV. P (5) Instruct patients according to their needs to promote health maintenance and disease prevention

IX. P (7) Document accurately in the patient record

ABHES

2. Anatomy and Physiology
   Graduates:
   c. Assist the physician with the regimen of diagnostic and treatment modalities as they relate to each body system

6. Pharmacology
   Graduates:
   b. Properly utilize PDR, drug handbook and other drug references to identify a drug's classification, usual dosage, usual side effects, and contradictions

9. Medical Office Clinical Procedures
   Graduates:
   g. Maintain medication and immunization records
   j. Prepare and administer oral and parenteral medications as directed by physicians

11. Career Development
    b. Demonstrate professionalism by:
       9 Conducting work within scope of education, training, and ability

Introduction

Drug administration is one of the most important and most dangerous duties for a medical assistant. By following the procedures for proper drug administration, you can help restore patients to health. If you calculate dosages inaccurately, measure drugs incorrectly, or administer drugs improperly, patients' medications may have no therapeutic effect, may worsen their disease or abnormal condition, or may even cause them to die.

To administer drugs safely and effectively to all patient groups, including pediatric, pregnant, and elderly patients, you must know and understand the principles of pharmacology (see the *Principles of Pharmacology* chapter) and how to perform dosage calculations (see the *Dosage Calculation* chapter). This chapter prepares you to understand the fundamentals of drug administration, including the following:

* Rules and responsibilities of drug administration.
* Rights of drug administration.
* Routes of medication administration.
* Techniques needed to administer drugs.
* Special patient considerations.
* Patient education.

Your role may vary depending upon the state and practice where you are employed. Many states have medical practice acts that define the exact duties of medical assistants in drug administration. For example, an act may specify which drugs you are allowed to administer and by which routes. Because state laws vary, you need to research the scope of practice for medical assistants in the state where you will work.

Preparing to Administer a Drug   LO 53.1

To administer drugs, you should know the uses, contraindications, interactions, and adverse effects of common drugs. You should be familiar with the medications frequently prescribed in your practice. Furthermore, to be able to assume a role in patient education, you must be comfortable with all aspects of drug administration so that you can instruct patients about the drugs prescribed to them.

Although the physician gives the order to administer a drug, the medical assistant has a lot of responsibility before a medication can be administered. As a medical assistant, you will often interview the patient. You must be alert to—and inform the doctor of—any change in the patient's condition that could affect drug therapy. Some preparation tasks are related to the drugs and drug allergies, administration site, patient condition, and patient consent.

Drugs and Drug Allergies

Before any medication is given, the physician should be aware of the current medications the patient is taking. As you learned in the *Principles of Pharmacology* chapter, some medications, including herbal medications, can interact in a negative way, so the physician needs to know everything the patient is taking before he orders a medication. The medical assistant is responsible for ensuring that a complete and accurate medication list is maintained on the patient's chart. This medication list must be updated every time the patient comes for an appointment. While asking about medications, you also must ask the patient about any drug allergies. Even though you may see a patient on a regular basis, be in the habit of asking about drugs and drug allergies at every patient visit. Patients often see other physicians or specialists, who may have prescribed different medications. A patient could have had a drug reaction to a medication that has been prescribed by another physician. If applicable, document in the patient chart "NKDA" or "no known drug allergies." See Figure 53-1.

Administration Site

Drugs may be administered for either local or systemic effects. Generally, drugs that have local effects are applied directly to the skin, tissues, or mucous membranes. Drugs that produce systemic effects are administered by routes that allow the drug to be absorbed and distributed in the bloodstream throughout the body. These various routes are discussed in the Drug Routes and Equipment section of this chapter. Before you administer a drug, you must check the site of administration. For example, if you are asked to give an oral medication, you would make sure the patient can take the medication. You may ask if the patient is nauseated, can swallow a pill, or has had anything to eat or drink, depending upon the medication.

For an injection, you must locate and inspect the injection site. Find the appropriate injection site by using anatomical landmarks. Inspect the skin by checking for the following conditions, which may eliminate the site:

- Moles
- Scars
- Birthmarks
- Traumatic injury
- Redness
- Rash
- Edema
- Cyanosis
- Burns
- Tattoos
- Side of a mastectomy
- Paralyzed areas
- Warts

If you are unsure about any of these conditions, inform the physician.

Patient Condition

Before administering a drug, assess the patient's overall condition. For example, does the patient have a viral infection? Vaccines are not recommended if the patient has a viral infection such as a common cold. In addition, review the patient's drug list to ensure that any medications already being taken will not interfere with the ordered drug or route of administration. Also,

verify again that the ordered dose is appropriate for the patient's age and weight.

Patient Consent Form

Many physicians require that a patient sign a consent form before receiving an injection. A consent is necessary for vaccines, for example. This form provides general information regarding the medication or vaccine and lists the possible side effects or adverse reactions. If a consent form is needed, make sure that the patient signs the form and that you have answered any questions prior to giving the injection.

General Rules for Drug Administration

No matter what drug or administration route is ordered, follow these general rules when administering drugs.

- Give only the drugs the physician has ordered. Written orders are preferable, but oral orders are appropriate for emergencies. If you are unfamiliar with any aspect of a drug the physician orders, consult a credible drug reference.
- Wash your hands before handling the drug. Prepare the drug in a well-lit area, away from distractions. Focus only on the task at hand.
- Perform a *"Triple Check"* by checking the medication three times. Check the medication three times even if the dose is prepackaged, labeled, and ready to be administered.
  - *1st check*—when you take it from the storage container and match it to the medication administration record (MAR).
  - *2nd check*—when you prepare it.
  - *3rd check*—before you close the storage container or just before you administer the medication to the patient.
- Calculate the dose if necessary. See the *Dosage Calculation* chapter. Remember, if you are unsure of your computation, ask another medical assistant or a licensed practitioner to check it.
- Avoid leaving a prepared drug unattended and never administer a drug that someone else has prepared.
- Ask the patient to state his name and date of birth to ensure correct identification. Double-check with the patient about possible drug allergies. Do not rely on documentation in his chart; he may have developed a new allergy that has not yet been added to the record.
- Be sure the physician is in the office when you administer a drug or vaccine. If the patient develops an anaphylactic reaction (sudden, severe allergic reaction) to the drug or vaccine, the physician must administer epinephrine.
- After administering the drug, ask the patient to remain in the facility for 10 to 20 minutes so that you can observe the patient for any unexpected effects.
- Give the patient specific instructions about the effects of the drug as well as general information about drug use.
- If the patient refuses to take the drug, discard it according to your facility policy. Do not flush it down the toilet or return it to the original container. Be sure to document the refusal in the patient's record and tell the physician.

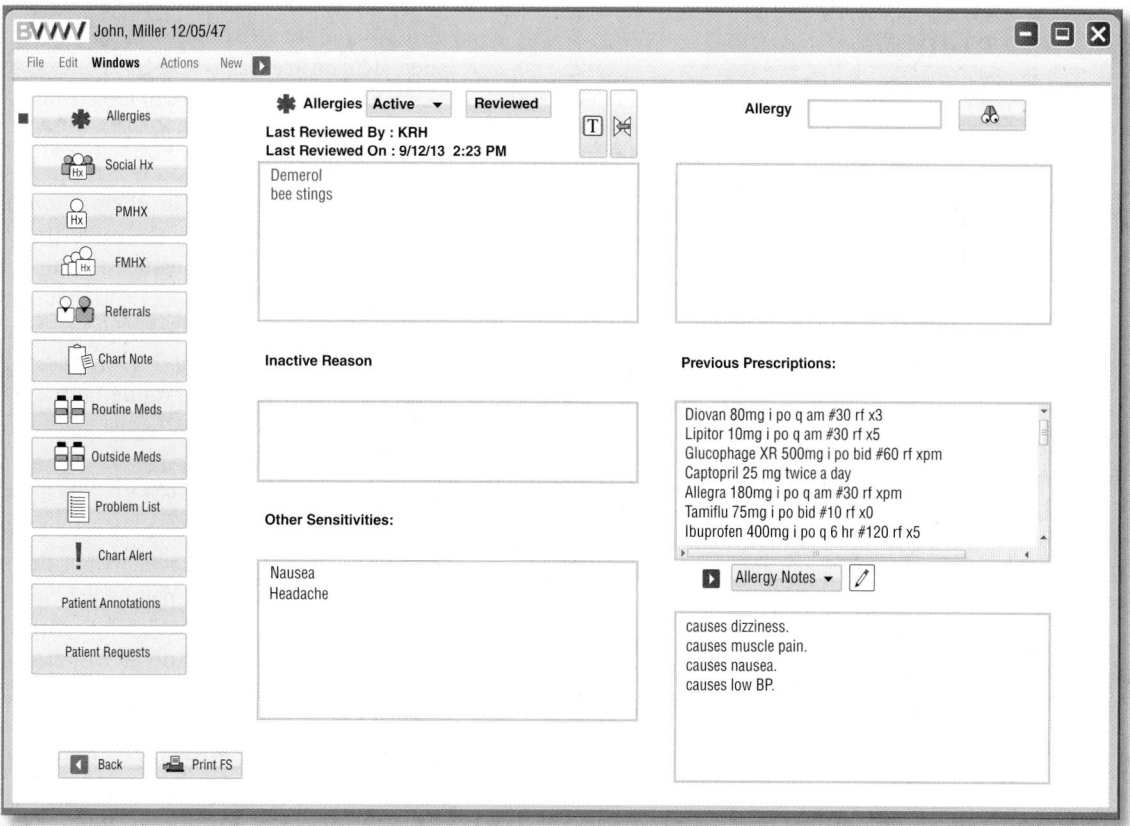

(a)

(b)

FIGURE 53-1 (a) Each time a patient visits the clinic, update the medication list as needed. (b) Be certain to ask about allergies and record these in the allergy window in the electronic health record.

Source: Screen captures of SpringCharts™ Electronic Health Records software are reprinted with permission from Spring Medical Systems, Inc. All rights reserved.

Handling Medication Errors

Medication errors are a serious, yet inevitable, problem. Great care should always be taken to prevent them. However, if an error does occur, no matter the cause, it must be reported. Immediately tell the licensed practitioner. Not reporting an error is unethical and in some cases illegal, especially if a serious consequence occurs. Most facilities require that an incident report be completed. This form documents the error. It is completed and then signed by everyone involved, as well as your supervisor. Errors also are reported online through an online program developed by the U.S. Pharmacopeia and the Institute for Safe Medical Practices. Reporting errors at these sites provides information to assist in the prevention of errors.

- If you make an error in drug administration, tell the physician immediately. See the Caution: Handle with Care feature Handling Medication Errors.
- Document immediately the drug and dose administered; never document administration before giving medicine.

▶ Rights of Medication Administration

LO 53.2

The rights of medication administration are a set of safety checks the medical assistant should follow to prevent a medication administration error. When administering medications, the medical assistant must observe the rights of medication administration (see Table 53-1) to avoid errors and ensure patient safety. The six basic rights of medication administration include right patient, right drug, right dose, right route, right time, and right documentation. A violation of any of the six basic rights constitutes a medication error. Additional rights include right reason, right to know, right to refuse, and right technique.

Right Patient

Always check the name and date of birth on the order for a drug or vaccine in the patient's chart, then compare to the name and date of birth that the patient tells you. Do not call the patient by name because a forgetful or confused patient might answer to

TABLE 53-1	The Rights of Medication Administration
Basic Rights	**Additional Rights**
1. Right patient	7. Right reason
2. Right drug	8. Right to know
3. Right dose	9. Right to refuse
4. Right route	10. Right technique
5. Right time	
6. Right documentation	

FIGURE 53-2 Check the label for the expiration date before administering a drug.

any name. Have an attending caregiver or family member state the name and date of birth if the patient is unable.

Right Drug

Carefully compare the name of the prescribed drug or vaccine in the patient's chart with the label on the drug container. As you check the drug name on the label, look at the expiration date. Never use a drug that has passed this date (Figure 53-2). If you are unfamiliar with the drug, look it up in a credible drug reference. Also, never prepare a drug from a container with a damaged or handwritten label. Always perform the "triple check" every time you prepare a medication.

Right Dose

Compare the dose on the order in the patient's chart with the dose you prepare. To obtain the right dose, read the label closely and calculate accurately. Do not confuse the dose contained in one tablet with the number of tablets in the container.

Right Route

Double-check to make sure the administration route you are preparing to use matches the route the doctor ordered. Also check that the medication you are using can be administered by the route ordered. For example, do not confuse ear (otic) drops with eye (optic) drops. Check that the patient can receive the drug by this route and that the route seems appropriate. For example, if the patient has an injury at the specified injection site, consult the doctor for a possible alternative site or a different route.

Right Time

Be sure to give the drug at the right time. If it must be given after meals, make sure the patient has eaten recently. For certain drugs, you must ensure that it is the correct time of day and the correct time in a series of doses. For example, timing is crucial with allergy shots because of possible reactions.

Right Documentation

Document the procedure immediately after administering the drug or vaccine to the patient. Do not wait until later and do not document before administration. Be sure to include the date, time, drug or vaccine name, lot number, dose, administration route, patient reaction, patient education about the drug, and your first initial and last name. If the drug is a controlled substance, also document it on the controlled substance inventory record. Always double-check your entry for computer documentation before submitting. Use neat handwriting for written documentation.

Go to CONNECT to see a video about *Record a Medication in a Patient's Chart.*

Right Reason

The person who administers the medication should know the reason the medication is being given.

Right to Know

All patients have the right to be educated about the medications they are receiving. This should include the reason, the effect, and the side effects of medications.

Right to Refuse

Every patient has the right to refuse a medication. If a patient does refuse a medication or vaccine, you should report this to the physician who ordered the medication. A refusal of medication by a patient should be documented in the patient's medical record.

Right Technique

Always use the proper administration technique. If you have not given a drug or vaccine by the ordered route recently, review the technique before administering the drug.

▶ Drug Routes and Equipment   LO 53.3

The physician may ask you to administer drugs by one of the routes outlined in Table 53-2. Most patients take a prescription to a pharmacy to be filled and then take oral drugs at home, so you may not need to administer these drugs in the office very often. However, you are likely to be asked to do the following:

- Place drugs in the patient's mouth between the cheek and gum or under the tongue.
- Administer a drug by any means other than by mouth (if permitted by your scope of practice and state laws).
- Demonstrate how to use an inhaler.
- Apply topical drugs (those applied to the skin).
- Administer or assist in administering drugs into the urethra, vagina, or rectum.
- Administer medications to the eye or ear, as discussed in the *Assisting with Eye and Ear Care* chapter.

These duties require you to master a variety of techniques to give drugs safely by any route.

▶ Medications by Mouth   LO 53.4

Medications that are put in the mouth are usually swallowed. This is called *oral administration.* Medications that are not meant to be swallowed also may be placed in the mouth. These methods include buccal and sublingual administration.

Oral Administration

Drugs that are swallowed are absorbed relatively slowly as they travel along the gastrointestinal (GI) tract. Drugs for oral administration include tablets, capsules, lozenges, and liquids. One special type of tablet you should be aware of is a **scored** tablet. See Figure 53-3. This means that the medication can be broken into pieces along a scored (indented) line on the tablet.

Oral administration is contraindicated in patients who have severe nausea, are comatose, or cannot swallow. Certain drugs are ineffective when administered orally because the digestive process changes them chemically to an ineffective form or does not deliver them to the bloodstream quickly enough.

Many drugs, however, are most effective when given orally. These include antibiotics, vitamins, throat lozenges, and cough syrups. Although these drugs are familiar to most people, as a medical assistant, you must follow certain steps to ensure that the patient understands the drug and that the drug is administered safely and effectively. The steps for oral administration are outlined in Procedure 53-1, at the end of this chapter.

Buccal and Sublingual Administration

Although **buccal** and **sublingual** drugs are placed in the mouth, they do not continue along the GI tract. Instead, they dissolve and are absorbed in the buccal area (between the cheek and gum) or the sublingual area (under the tongue), where they are placed. The medication is absorbed through tissue that is rich in capillaries and the drug enters the bloodstream directly. Because the drug does not pass into the stomach or intestines before absorption, it produces a therapeutic effect more quickly than do oral drugs.

Specially formulated tablets may be given by the buccal or sublingual routes. When you administer buccal or sublingual medications, your role usually includes teaching the patient

FIGURE 53-3 Scored tablets can be broken along the scored line.

TABLE 53-2 Routes and Methods of Drug Administration

Route and Drug Forms	Method
Buccal route Tablets	Place drug between the patient's gum and cheek. To ensure absorption, tell the patient to leave the tablet there until it dissolves and not to chew or swallow it. Tell the patient not to eat, drink, or smoke until the tablet is completely dissolved.

Inhalation therapy (nasal or oral)
  Aerosols
  Sprays
  Mists or steam
	Administer the drug by inhalation to reach the respiratory tract. The drug will be absorbed in 7 to 20 seconds.

Intradermal route
  Solutions
  Powders for reconstitution
	Administer the drug by injection between the upper layers of the patient's skin.

Intramuscular route
  Solutions
  Powders for reconstitution
	Administer the drug by injection into the muscle. The drug will be absorbed in 3 to 5 minutes.

Intravenous route
  Solutions (often in bags of 250, 500, or 1000 mL)
  Powders for reconstitution
  Blood and blood products
	Administer the drug by injection or infusion into a vein. The drug will be absorbed in 15 to 30 seconds.

Ophthalmic (eye) or otic (ear) route
  Solutions
  Ointments
	Apply the drug, usually as drops, in the patient's eye or ear.

Oral route
  Tablets
  Capsules
  Liquids
  Lozenges
	Give the drug to the patient to swallow. The drug will be absorbed in 20 minutes to 3 hours, depending on food and drug ingestion.

Rectal route
  Suppositories
  Solutions
	Insert a suppository into the patient's rectum. Administer a solution as an enema, using a tube and nozzle.

Subcutaneous route
  Solutions
  Powders for reconstitution
	Administer the drug by injection into the subcutaneous layer of skin. The drug will be absorbed in 3 to 5 minutes.

Sublingual route
  Tablets
  Sprays
	Place the drug under the patient's tongue. To ensure absorption, tell the patient to leave the tablet there until it dissolves and not to chew or swallow it. Tell the patient not to eat, drink, or smoke until the tablet is completely dissolved.

Topical route
  Ointments
  Lotions
  Creams
  Tinctures
  Powders
  Sprays
  Solutions
	Apply the drug to the patient's skin or rub it into the skin.

Transdermal route Patches	Apply the drug to a clean, dry, nonhairy area of the patient's skin.
Urethral route Solutions	Administer the drug by instilling it in the patient's bladder, using a catheter.

Vaginal route
  Solutions
  Suppositories
  Ointments
  Foams
  Creams
	Administer a solution as a douche, using a tube and nozzle.
	Administer other forms by inserting them into the vagina with an applicator.

how to administer these medications at home. See Procedure 53-2, Administering Buccal or Sublingual Drugs, at the end of this chapter.

Go to CONNECT to see a video about *Administering Drugs by Mouth.*

▶ Medications by Injection
LO 53.5

Medications given by injection are called *parenteral medications*. Parenteral administration is the administration of a substance such as a drug by muscle, vein, or any means other than through the GI tract. Although the parenteral route offers the advantage of rapid drug action, it has several potential drawbacks. Parenteral administration poses more safety risks for the patient because after the drug has been injected, it cannot be retrieved.

Parenteral administration also increases your risk of potential exposure to bloodborne pathogens when you perform injections and dispose of used needles. To minimize risks, follow Standard Precautions during injections. Also adhere to Occupational Safety and Health Administration (OSHA) and Environmental Protection Agency (EPA) regulations for disposing of contaminated needles and other sharp items. Offices must provide a rigid, puncture-proof container for collecting disposable sharp instruments. This container must be self-sealing and must have a lock-tight cap and a safety neck.

After using a needle, lancet, or syringe, engage the safety mechanism, then immediately place it in the sharps container. See Figure 53-4. To avoid puncturing yourself, always ensure the safety mechanism is engaged and do not force the needle, lancet, or syringe into the container. If you do accidentally stick yourself, notify the physician at once so you can be treated.

FIGURE 53-4 To prevent needlestick injuries, engage the safety mechanism and place all needles in a sharps container like this one immediately.

OSHA requires medical follow-up for all workers who have been accidentally punctured.

Never let a sharps container become full. When the container is two-thirds full, seal it and follow your office procedure for container disposal.

Needles

When you administer a parenteral drug, you must select the appropriate needle, syringe, and drug form to use on the basis of the type of injection. The following are methods of injection:

- Intradermal (ID), or within the upper layers of the skin.
- Subcutaneous (subcut), or beneath the skin.
- Intramuscular (IM), or within a muscle.
- Intravenous (IV), or directly into a vein.

See Figure 53-5.

FIGURE 53-5 Injection needles are placed into separate areas under the skin: (a) intradermal (ID), (b) intramuscular (IM), (c) subcutaneous (subcut), and (d) intravenous (IV).

(a)

FIGURE 53-6 Understanding the parts of a needle will help you use it correctly.

Needles consist of a hub, hilt, shaft, lumen, point, and bevel (Figure 53-6). The hub of the needle fits onto the syringe. The needle tip is beveled (sloped at the opening). The bevel helps the needle cut through the skin with minimum trauma.

Needles are available in various gauges (inside diameters) and lengths (Figure 53-7). A needle's gauge is expressed with numbers. The smaller the number, the larger the gauge. For example, a 25-gauge needle is smaller than an 18-gauge needle. Use the right gauge for the type of injection and the viscosity (thickness) of the drug to be administered. For example, use a large-gauge needle for a highly viscous drug.

When selecting a needle, also consider its length. It must be long enough to penetrate the appropriate layers of tissue, but not so long as to go too deep. Choose the correct needle length on the basis of the type of injection as well as the patient's size, amount of fatty tissue, and injection site. Table 53-3 lists the approximate ranges of needle gauge and length that are typically used for intradermal, subcutaneous, and intramuscular injections.

Syringes

Syringes have two basic parts: a barrel and a plunger. The barrel is the calibrated cylinder that holds the drug. The plunger forces

(b)

FIGURE 53-7 (a) The gauge of the needle relates to the diameter. Notice the larger the number, the smaller the needle diameter. (b) Always choose a needle with a length and gauge appropriate to the type of injection, the drug being injected and the patient receiving the injection.

				Maximum	
Type	**Age**	**Needle Size**	**Needle Length**	**Injection Amount**	**Location**
Intradermal (ID)					
ID	All ages	25 to 26 gauge	⅜ to ½ inch	0.1 mL	Interior aspect of forearm (most common)
Subcutaneous (Subcut)					
Subcut	1 to 12 months	23 to 27 gauge	⅝ inch	1 mL	Fatty tissue over anterior lateral thigh muscle
Subcut	> 12 months to adult	23 to 27 gauge	½ to ¾ inch; ⅝ is most common	1 mL	Fatty tissue over anterior lateral thigh muscle or over triceps
Intramuscular (IM)					
IM	1 to 28 days	18 to 23 gauge	⅝ inch	1 mL	Anterolateral thigh muscle
IM	1 to 12 months	18 to 23 gauge	1 inch	1 mL	Anterolateral thigh muscle
IM	1 to 2 years	18 to 23 gauge	1 to 1¼ inch ⅝ to 1 inch	1 mL	Anterolateral thigh muscle Deltoid muscle of arm
IM	3 to 18 years	18 to 23 gauge	⅝ to 1 inch 1 to 1¼ inch	2 mL	Deltoid muscle of arm Anterolateral thigh muscle
IM	All adults ≥ 19 years < 130 lb	18 to 23 gauge	⅝ to 1 inch	3 mL	Deltoid muscle of arm
IM	All adults ≥ 19 years Female 130 to 200 lb Male 130 to 260 lb	18 to 23 gauge	1 to 1½ inch	3 mL	Deltoid muscle of arm
IM	Male Adults ≥ 19 years Female 200 + lb Male 260 + lb	18 to 23 gauge	1½ inch	3 mL	Deltoid muscle of arm

TABLE 53-3 Suggested Needle Gauge, Length, Injection Amount, and Location

(d) Plunger
(c) Barrel
(b) Syringe hub
(a) Needle
(e) Trailing ring
(f) Leading ring
(g) Needlestick prevention safety device

FIGURE 53-8 The parts of a standard syringe include (a) the needle; (b) the syringe hub; (c) the barrel that contains the liquid; (d) the plunger; (e) the trailing ring; (f) the plunger tip, also called the leading ring; and (g) the needlestick prevention safety device.

the drug through the barrel and out the needle. The syringe may be packaged with the needle attached and a guardcap over the needle, or the syringe and needle may be packaged separately. All syringes must include a needlestick prevention safety device. See Figure 53-8.

Syringes come in many sizes and are calibrated according to how the syringe will be used. For example, the common 3-mL syringe is divided into tenths of a milliliter. It is used to measure most drugs. A tuberculin (TB) syringe holds 1 mL and is calibrated in hundredths of a milliliter. Insulin syringes are calibrated in units (U), commonly either 50 U or 100 U (Figure 53-9). Unlike other syringes, insulin syringes have permanently attached needles and no dead space (fluid remaining in the needle or syringe after the plunger is depressed fully). These differences help the patient self-administer the correct amount of insulin.

Forms of Packaging for Parenteral Drugs

Parenteral drugs are supplied in the forms shown in Figure 53-10. They include cartridges, ampules, and vials.

- A cartridge is a small barrel prefilled with a sterile drug. It slips into a special, reusable syringe assembly.

- An ampule is a small glass or plastic container that is sealed to keep its contents sterile. It must be opened and used with care, as described in Procedure 53-3, at the end of this chapter.

- A vial is a small bottle with a rubber diaphragm that can be punctured by needle. A vial contains a liquid or powder, which must first be reconstituted with a **diluent** (liquid used to dissolve and dilute a drug), as described in Procedure 53-4, at the end of this chapter. It may contain a single or multiple doses. This procedure requires two needles and syringe sets—one for inserting the diluent into the vial and another to draw and administer the reconstituted drug—to avoid using a contaminated needle. The first needle is considered contaminated when you set it down to mix the diluent and the drug.

Go to CONNECT to see videos about *Drawing a Drug from an Ampule* and *Reconstituting and Drawing a Drug for Injection.*

50 unit Lo-Dose syringe
Standard 100 unit syringe

Each large mark indicates 5 units
Each small mark indicates 1 unit

Each large mark indicates 10 units
Each small mark indicates 2 units

FIGURE 53-9 Insulin syringes: Always check the calibrations carefully because the marks on syringes of different sizes use different scales.

FIGURE 53-10 Injectable drugs may come in a cartridge (left), an ampule (center), or a vial (right).

Methods of Injection

Injections are the most common method of drug administration in a medical office. You need to be knowledgeable about all injection methods: intradermal, subcutaneous, intramuscular, and intravenous.

Intradermal An **intradermal (ID)** injection is administered into the upper layer of skin at an angle almost parallel to the skin, as described in Procedure 53-5, at the end of this chapter. Common sites for intradermal injections are the forearm and back. Intradermal injections are usually used to administer a skin test, such as an allergy test or a TB test. When choosing an injection site on patients, avoid scarred, blemished, or hairy areas because those features interfere with your ability to interpret test results on the skin.

The drug is injected under the top skin layer and a little bubble or wheal is raised. If the body reacts to the drug, erythema (redness) and induration (hardening) occur. This reaction generally takes place 15 to 20 minutes after an allergy test and from 48 to 72 hours after a TB test.

Go to CONNECT to see a video about *Giving an Intradermal Injection.*

Subcutaneous A **subcutaneous (subcut)** injection provides a slow, sustained release of a drug and a relatively long duration of action. Generally, 1 mL or less of a drug can be delivered by a subcut injection (Procedure 53-6, at the end of this chapter). Various drugs, such as insulin and heparin, are commonly administered by a subcut injection. Common subcutaneous injection sites include an area on the back between the shoulder blades, the outer sides of the upper arms and thighs, and the abdomen (except for a 2-inch area around the umbilicus).

To prepare for a subcut injection, select a site away from bones and blood vessels. Do not use an area that is edematous (swollen), scarred, or hardened or one that has a large amount of fat because these areas may not have the capillary network needed for absorption. When patients need regular subcut injections, remember to rotate injection sites systematically. Begin the rotation pattern by giving injections in rows in the same area of the body (such as the abdomen). After all those sites have been used once, proceed to the next area on the body (such as the right leg) and follow a similar pattern there. Rotating sites promotes drug absorption and prevents hard subcutaneous lumps from forming. At the injection site, ensure that you can pinch at least a 1-inch skin fold for the injection. If a patient is frail, dehydrated, or thin, you may need to use a site other than the back or abdomen to provide the necessary fold of skin.

Go to CONNECT to see a video about *Giving a Subcutaneous Injection.*

Intramuscular When a patient requires rapid drug absorption, you may be asked to administer an **intramuscular (IM)** injection, as described in Procedure 53-7, at the end of this chapter. An IM injection usually irritates a patient's tissues less than a subcut injection and allows administration of a larger amount of drug.

Common IM injection sites include the ventrogluteal, vastus lateralis, and deltoid muscles, illustrated in Figure 53-11. The dorsogluteal is rarely used because of the chance of hitting the sciatic nerve. Before giving an IM injection, identify the site carefully to prevent injury to blood vessels and nerves in the area. As with subcut injections, rotate sites if the patient must receive regular or multiple IM injections.

FIGURE 53-11 For intramuscular injection in an adult, use (a) the ventrogluteal site, (b) the deltoid site, or (c) the vastus lateralis site.

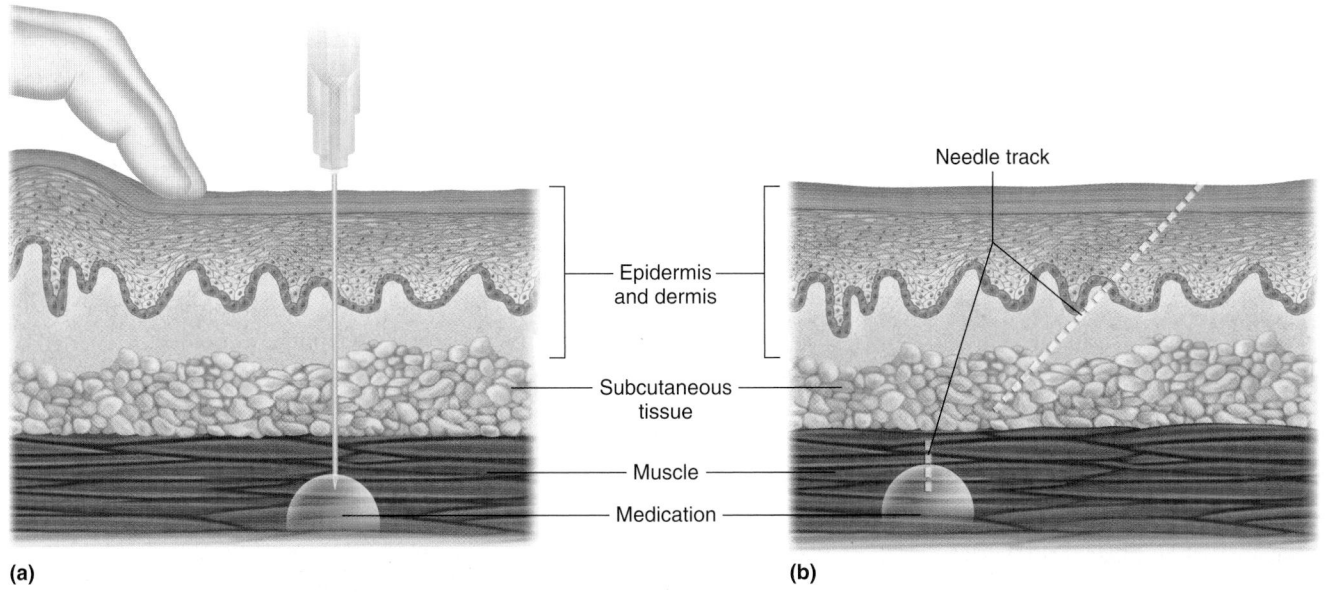

FIGURE 53-12 Use the Z-track method for IM injection of irritating solutions. (a) Pull the skin to one side before inserting the needle. (b) After injecting the drug, release the skin to seal off the needle track.

Take into consideration the patient's layer of fat when choosing an IM injection site. You want the injection to penetrate beyond the fat layer to muscle. If, for example, a patient is heavy in the buttocks and thighs, the deltoid may be the best site for administering an IM injection.

When injecting an IM drug that can irritate subcutaneous tissues, such as iron dextran (Imferon), use the **Z-track method**, illustrated in Figure 53-12. To do this, pull the skin and subcutaneous tissue to the side before inserting the needle at the site. After the drug is injected, release the tissue. This technique creates a zigzag path in the tissue layers, which prevents the drug from leaking into the subcutaneous tissue and causing irritation.

Go to CONNECT to see a video about *Giving an Intramuscular Injection.*

Intravenous Although **intravenous (IV)** injections are not commonly performed in a medical office or by medical assistants, certain drugs may be administered this way. Drugs also may be mixed and dissolved into a **solution** (a homogeneous mixture of a solid, liquid, or gaseous substance in a liquid) and given by IV **infusion** (slow drip) into a vein. Examples of IV drugs include powerful antibiotics, chemotherapeutic drugs, emergency drugs, and electrolytes. Because these drugs are introduced directly into the bloodstream, they produce an almost immediate effect. They also can cause sudden adverse reactions.

Although in most cases a licensed practitioner must administer an IV drug, you may assist by laying out supplies and equipment. When assisting with any intravenous medications, gather the ordered drug and a tourniquet, bedsaver pad, gloves, iodine and alcohol swabs, venipuncture device, tape, and gauze pad, as ordered. Obtain other supplies and equipment depending on the specific type of infusion or injection being administered.

Other Medication Routes LO 53.6

Additional parenteral routes of administration include inhalation therapy (sometimes called respiratory therapy); topical application; and urethral, vaginal, and rectal administration.

Inhalation Therapies

Inhalation therapy is medication that is delivered into the respiratory system during inhalation. This medication can be administered through the mouth or nose. There are a number of disorders for which the physician may order an inhaler or aerosol form of medication. For example, an oral inhaler is frequently used by patients with asthma, whereas a nasal inhaler is frequently used for local treatment of nasal congestion. Nasal inhalers also are used to administer medicines for systemic effect, such as a vasopressin derivative for nocturnal bedwetting. Some types of influenza vaccines are now delivered by nasal inhalation. Always read the inserts for inhaled drugs for a detailed description of the exact procedure for the type of inhalation you will be administering. Procedure 53-8, at the end of this chapter, provides the basic steps of the procedure, as well as needed patient education.

Topical Application

Topical application is the direct application of a drug on the skin. Topical drugs can take the form of creams, lotions, **ointments** (salves), tinctures, powders, sprays, and solutions, which are used for their local effects. They include antibacterial and antifungal drugs, as well as corticosteroids.

To apply a cream, lotion, or ointment, use long, even strokes with a cotton-tipped applicator and/or a gloved finger when rubbing it into the skin. Follow the direction of the hair growth to avoid irritating the hair follicles and skin. To apply a powder, shake it on but do not rub it in.

A specialized type of topical administration that produces a systemic effect is the **transdermal** system (or patch).

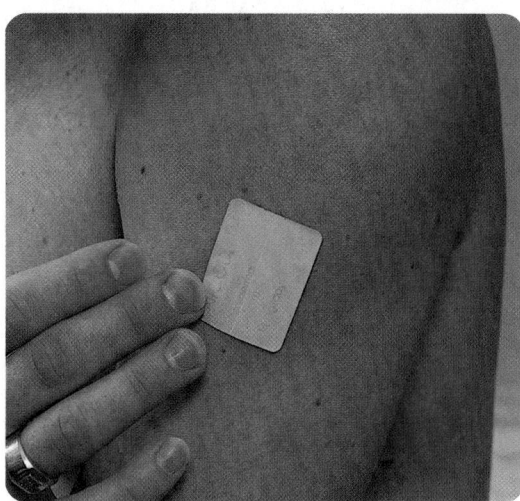

FIGURE 53-13 Application of a transdermal patch; date, time, and signature will be added to the patch.

See Figure 53-13. A drug administered through the transdermal patch is absorbed through the skin directly into the bloodstream. The patch slowly and evenly releases a systemic drug, such as scopolamine, nitroglycerin, estrogen, or fentanyl, through the skin. The patient receives a timed-release dose, usually over a day or several days. See Procedure 53-9, at the end of this chapter.

Urethral Administration

The urethral route is used when antibiotic and antifungal drugs are needed locally—that is, at the site of infection—for some urinary tract infections. Depending on the nature of the infection and the duration of drug action, the physician or a nurse may instill liquid drugs only one time or several times a day for a week. Urethral administration is used in both men and women.

Urethral drug administration requires passing a small-diameter urinary catheter into the bladder, instilling a drug through it, and clamping the catheter to let the drug bathe the urinary bladder walls. See Procedure 53-10, at the end of this chapter.

Vaginal Administration

Physicians usually prescribe vaginal drugs to treat local fungal infections. The drugs also may be used for local bacterial infections. They are usually packaged as suppositories (the most common form), solutions, creams, ointments, and foams. The liquid form of vaginal medication is administered by performing a **douche** (vaginal irrigation). This process is similar to giving a urethral drug, but it requires a special irrigating nozzle. Patients frequently ask about administering vaginal medications, and they usually administer such medications at home. Therefore, you must be prepared to provide detailed patient education for this route of administration. The physician may ask you to administer the first dose as a means of teaching a patient the method to use at home, or you may be asked to administer a one-time-only dose. See Procedure 53-11, at the end of this chapter.

Rectal Administration

Certain medications, such as drugs used to treat constipation, nausea, and vomiting, may be administered by the rectal route.

These medications may be given in the form of suppositories or enemas and may produce local or systemic effects. See Procedure 53-12, at the end of this chapter.

▶ Special Considerations

LO 53.7

Pediatric, pregnant, breast-feeding, and geriatric patients require special considerations when administering medications. Note: Geriatric considerations are discussed in the *Assisting in Geriatrics* chapter. When giving a drug to these patients, you must adjust patient care and technique as needed.

Pediatric Patients

Children pose special challenges in drug administration and use. Their physiology and immature body systems may make drug effects less predictable because drugs are absorbed, distributed, metabolized, and excreted differently in children than in adults. Therefore, plan to observe a pediatric patient closely for adverse effects and interactions.

A child's small size increases the risk of overdose and toxicity. These factors require dosage adjustments and careful measurement of small doses. To help administer drugs safely to pediatric patients, always check your calculations for providing a prescribed dose, and then ask a licensed practitioner to double-check them.

Administration sites and techniques for a child may differ from those for an adult. For example, fewer IM injection sites can be used for a young child. Also, the technique for eardrop administration varies slightly (see the *Assisting with Eye and Ear Care* chapter).

When dealing with an infant or young child, teach the parents—not the patient—about the drug. With an older child, include parents and patient in the teaching session. Be sure to use age-appropriate language when speaking to children.

Patience and sensitivity are important when working with pediatric patients. The first memorable exposure to an office visit may often determine how the child will react to physician visits for years to come. Infants and children can sense when you are irritated or annoyed. Pay close attention to your nonverbal communication as well as your verbal communication. New mothers are often apprehensive about invasive procedures when it concerns their children and this apprehension is often reflected in the child. Empathy and compassion are needed to ensure that the office visit is a pleasant one.

Administering medications to a pediatric patient may become a challenge if the child is not cooperative. It is important to ensure that the child receives the full dose as ordered.

Oral Medications When administering oral medications to children, follow these guidelines:

- Use a calibrated dropper or spoon device to measure the ordered dose. See Figure 53-14.
- Administer the medication to the side of the tongue; this method prevents the child from spitting out the medication.
- Hold the child until you are sure the medication is swallowed. In some cases you may gently hold the child's mouth closed to ensure that the medication is swallowed.

(a)

(b)

FIGURE 53-14 (a) Droppers come in various sizes with different calibrations. (b) Calibrated spoons.

- If a small amount dribbles from the mouth, do not attempt to give more medication to the child.
- If the child vomits within 5 minutes and you can see the medication in the vomit, you should readminister the medication after the child is calm. If you are unsure of readministering medication, consult with the physician.
- If the medication comes only in tablet form and the child is unable to swallow a tablet or capsule, check a creditable drug reference to see if the medication can be crushed and given with food, such as applesauce.

Injections Stress and anxiety will differ from child to child. When giving injections to pediatric patients, the following steps will help ensure a smooth procedure:

- Distract the patient. Talk to the child while giving the injection. Don't ask permission. Often the injection is performed and over before the child realizes it.
- Use an anesthetic topical agent prior to the injection. This can be applied in the office or at home before the patient arrives in the office.
- Try not to allow the child to see the syringe before giving the injection.

- Be swift. Do not allow a lot of time to pass before giving the injection. The faster the better.
- Praise the child. Say things that promote maturity and self-esteem.

Pediatric Injection Sites Pediatric patients have less muscle development than adults do, which limits the sites for intramuscular injections. The deltoid muscle is not developed enough for an injection and can be painful for the child. The sciatic nerve is larger in children; dorsogluteal injections are therefore not recommended because of the danger of hitting the sciatic nerve.

The vastus lateralis and ventrogluteal sites are recommended for infants and children. The vastus lateralis site is good because it is a large and thick muscle that is developed before the child begins to walk. It is also the most desirable site for infants and children because it is not near major nerves and blood vessels. For a child who has been walking for about a year, you can use the ventrogluteal or dorsogluteal site. For an older, well-developed child, use any adult site. The vastus lateralis site is an easier site if you need to incorporate restraining methods.

The most common injections given to pediatric patients are vaccines. Most vaccines are given intramuscularly with a 25-gauge, ⅝-inch needle. The gauge and length vary based on the size of the patient. Use the shortest length needle that will allow you to reach muscle, usually ⅝ to 1 inch.

In many cases, pediatric patients require more than one vaccine injection in a single limb (vastus lateralis). When this is the case, the injections should be at least one inch apart on the site and the specific location of each vaccine should be documented.

Restraining Methods Sometimes a pediatric patient will need to be restrained in order for you to administer an injection. Two medical assistants may be needed to safely restrain a child while giving an injection. Common restraining methods include the following:

- Have the child "hug the mother." The mother holds the child in front of her, with the child's thighs extended on either side of her torso. As the mother is talking to her child, make the injection in the vastus lateralis.
- Weight-bearing restraining is better than muscular control. Have the child sit on the edge of the examining table and use your weight to immobilize the child's legs against the table.

Pregnant Patients

When dealing with pregnant patients, remember that you are caring for two patients at once: the mother and her fetus. When you give the mother a drug, you also may be giving it to the fetus. Some drugs can cause physical defects in the fetus if the mother takes them during pregnancy (especially in the first trimester). It is extremely important to double-check the drug in a credible drug reference for toxicology or pregnancy warnings. After administering the drug, assess the patient carefully for therapeutic and adverse effects of the drug. If the physician orders a drug for a pregnant patient, double-check the order against the pregnancy drug risk categories discussed in the *Principles of Pharmacology* chapter. If it is a high-risk drug, check with the physician before administering the drug.

Patients Who Are Breast-Feeding

Some drugs are excreted in breast milk and can thus be ingested by a breast-feeding infant. This ingestion can be dangerous because infants have immature body systems and cannot metabolize and excrete drugs that are safe for the mother. Some drugs, such as sedatives, diuretics, and hormones, can reduce the mother's flow of breast milk.

Whenever a drug is ordered for a patient who is breast-feeding, check a drug reference to see whether the drug is contraindicated during lactation. If so, consult the doctor. If not, teach the mother to recognize signs of adverse drug effects in her infant. If a mother must take a drug that affects lactation, advise her to supplement breast-feedings with infant formula.

▶ Patient Education about Medications

LO 53.8

As a medical assistant, you have an important role in patient instruction about medications. This role may vary depending upon your state, training, or place of employment, but the importance of drug education should not be underestimated. Specific instructions should be given about all the drugs a patient is taking, whether prescription or over-the-counter (OTC). Patients also should know how to take and record their medications safely and correctly.

Over-the-Counter Drugs

Even though patients can obtain OTC drugs without a prescription, they need to know several important facts to use them safely. Patients should not treat themselves with OTC drugs as a way to avoid medical care. For example, OTC drugs are available to treat recurrent yeast infections. Nonetheless, a patient should consult a doctor the first time she develops an infection.

Patients also should know that OTC drugs may not produce enough therapeutic benefit in some cases or be dangerous when used in combination with other substances. For example, a combination of the OTC medication acetaminophen (Tylenol®) and alcohol can cause liver damage. In addition, some OTC drugs may even mask symptoms or aggravate a problem.

Many OTC drugs contain more than one active ingredient. These extra ingredients, such as aspirin, acetaminophen, or caffeine, can cause allergic reactions or other undesirable effects. Excess caffeine can cause elevated heart rates. Too much acetaminophen (Tylenol®)—over 4 grams in 24 hours—can inadvertently be taken, causing severe liver damage.

Prescription Drugs

Before patients begin drug therapy, they should be informed of certain considerations (such as when and how to take the drug)

BWW Medical Associates, PC
305 Main Street
Port Snead, YZ 12345-9876

Patient Name: Mohammad Nassar

RX#: 711428172

Drug: Albuterol Inhalation Aerosol

COMMON USES:

To treat asthma, bronchitis, and other lung diseases.

HOW SHOULD I USE IT?

Follow your doctor's and/or the package instructions. Shake well before each use. Rinse mouth after each inhalation to avoid dryness. If breathing has not improved in 20 minutes, call doctor.

ARE THERE ANY SIDE EFFECTS?

Very unlikely, but report: Flushing, trembling, headache, nausea, vomiting, rapid heartbeat, chest pain, weakness, dizziness.

HOW DO I STORE THIS?

Store at room temperature away from moisture and sunlight. Do not puncture. Do not store in the bathroom. Rinse and clean inhaler regularly as described in package instructions.

FIGURE 53-15 Drug information sheets, like this one, are important for consumers to understand the medications they are taking.

and drug safety precautions. First you must check a credible drug information resource about any drug with which you are not familiar.

As part of your patient education, provide instructions orally and, if possible, in writing. For commonly prescribed medications, you can obtain preprinted information sheets or create one using an electronic health record (EHR) program. Most pharmacies now routinely provide these with each dispensed drug. See Figure 53-15.

An important aspect of this kind of information is teaching the patient how to read a prescription drug label. Instruct the patient to be particularly alert for special instructions and warning labels, such as those shown in Figure 53-16.

Interactions

Interactions may occur between two prescription or nonprescription drugs or between a drug and food and may cause serious effects. The greater the number of drugs the patient takes, including over-the-counter medications or supplements, the greater the chance of a drug interaction.

FIGURE 53-16 Teach the patient to heed warning labels and instructions on drug bottles.

Drug-Drug Interactions When two drugs are taken at the same time, there are several possible interactions. In some cases, the effects of both drugs are increased, causing either a toxic or beneficial effect. For example, when alcohol is combined with diazepam (Valium), there is the potential toxic effect of severe central nervous system depression because one drug intensifies the effect of the other. An example of a beneficial effect is the combination of acetaminophen and codeine, which increases the activity of both drugs, allowing the physician to prescribe a lower dose of each. In fact, this combination of drugs is available in one tablet (Tylenol® with codeine).

In other cases, the effects of both drugs are decreased, or one drug cancels out the effect of the other. For example, combining propranolol (Inderal®) with albuterol (Proventil®) causes each drug to lose its effectiveness.

In still other cases, the effect of one of the drugs is increased by the other. For example, the effect of digoxin (Lanoxin®) is increased by the presence of furosemide (Lasix®), but the furosemide still works at the same degree of effectiveness as when administered alone.

Drug interactions can lead to adverse reactions. For example, a patient who takes the prescription blood modifier (anticoagulant) warfarin (Coumadin®) to prevent blood clots must avoid taking aspirin for pain relief. Taking these drugs together increases the risk of uncontrolled bleeding.

To help prevent unintentional drug interactions, thoroughly check the patient's medication use. Be sure to ask about medications prescribed by specialists as well as OTC drugs and supplements. Question the patient about past and present use of alcohol and recreational drugs as well as herbal remedies. Update the chart as needed. If you detect a potential for drug interactions, notify the physician. Drug interaction checkers are available online.

Also teach patients about possible drug interactions and how to avoid or minimize them. For example, patients may need to take certain drugs at least 4 hours apart. As an example, the hormone replacement drug Synthroid® and calcium should not be taken together. Instruct patients to call the office if they think their drugs are interacting adversely.

Drug-Food Interactions Interactions between a drug and food can alter a drug's therapeutic effect. For example, taking tetracycline with milk can reduce the drug's effectiveness because of decreased absorption from the GI tract. The drug-food interaction between a monoamine oxidase (MAO) inhibitor (such as Parnate®, an antidepressant drug) and aged cheese or meat or other foods containing high levels of tyramine can produce a toxic effect. This interaction can cause a dangerous hypertensive crisis in which the patient's blood pressure rises quickly to dangerous levels, possibly leading to stroke and death.

A food that may interact with drugs is grapefruit and grapefruit juice. Interactions with some heart or blood pressure medications, such as Nifedipine, might cause irregularities in heartbeat, called arrhythmia.

Some drug-food interactions can affect the body's use of nutrients. For example, the cholesterol-lowering drugs cholestyramine resin (Locholest®) and colestipol HCl (Colestid®) may reduce the body's absorption of fat-soluble vitamins (A, D, E, and K) from food.

When teaching a patient about drug-food interactions, specify exactly which foods to avoid and when. For example, a patient may drink milk or eat food several hours before or after taking tetracycline, whereas a patient taking an MAO inhibitor must avoid foods that contain high levels of tyramine at all times. Explain what to expect if an interaction occurs and describe how to deal with it.

Adverse Effects

Adverse effects or reactions associated with a drug and reported are somewhat predictable and range from mild adverse reactions, such as stomach upset, to severe or life-threatening allergic responses. For example, certain cholesterol-lowering medications, called statins (e.g., Lipitor®), can increase the likelihood of painful muscle disorders. Unpredictable adverse effects also can occur; they are unique to each patient.

Elderly patients and patients with liver or kidney disease are more susceptible than others to adverse effects because these conditions affect drug metabolism and excretion. When drugs are not metabolized properly or excreted from the body quickly enough, drugs can reach toxic levels, even with normal doses.

To help prevent adverse effects, teach the patient to take the drug at the right time, in the right amount, and under the right circumstances. For example, the patient may need to take a cephalosporin with food to avoid nausea and diarrhea. Also teach the patient to recognize significant adverse effects and to call the office if any of them occur. The patient also should report any change in overall health because that change could be drug-related.

Tell patients to inform each of their doctors of any adverse reactions (including allergic reactions) they have had to drugs. Previous adverse reactions may prompt a doctor to adjust a dosage or select a different drug. A history of drug allergies may contraindicate the use of a particular drug.

Complete Medication List

Patients must inform the doctor of all substances they use regularly or periodically. This includes prescription and OTC drugs, plus herbals and supplements. It also includes past and present use of alcohol and recreational drugs. When patients have more than one doctor, tell them to inform each doctor about all medications they are taking. Encourage them to keep up-to-date medication lists with dosages (some patients keep this information on their home computers). This information can help patients and healthcare professionals prevent and monitor for drug interactions. The list should be kept on the patient chart and updated with every visit to the physician's office.

Patient Compliance

To help ensure that patients comply with instructions, confirm that they completely understand the name, dosage, and purpose of each drug prescribed for them. If patients must take more than one drug at a time, be sure they know the correct and relevant information for each one. In addition, cover each of the following points when educating patients about drugs:

- Explain how and when to take each drug to ensure its safety and effectiveness. Some drugs should be taken with food to minimize gastrointestinal irritation. Others should be taken on an empty stomach for proper absorption and metabolism. Some drugs must be taken once a day in the morning; others should be taken three or four times a day. If patients' medication schedules are complex, suggest that they create an alarm, chart, calendar, or diary to remind them of what drug to take and when, or create a schedule for them.

- Tell patients how long to take each drug. In the case of antibiotics, advise them to take the entire course of the drug as scheduled, even if they feel better before finishing it. In the case of medicines prescribed for chronic disease, advise patients that they will need to continue taking the medication unless the doctor tells them to stop. Be aware that some drugs, such as prednisone, must be tapered off slowly to prevent adverse reactions.

- Explain how to identify possible adverse effects of each drug and safety measures related to adverse effects. For example, instruct patients to avoid certain activities, such as driving or operating machinery, while taking a drug that causes drowsiness. If appropriate, inform patients that misuse of the drug may lead to dependence, and mention the dangers of drug dependence.

- Tell patients not to save medications that are over one year old or share them with anyone else. Old medications and those taken by people other than the patient for whom they were prescribed can cause severe, unexpected adverse effects. Advise patients to check the expiration date on all drugs and to discard them by wrapping in a tightly sealed container and placing in the trash. Flushing is not recommended due to possible water contamination. Some pharmacies will also dispose of medications for patients.

- Suggest that patients avoid alcohol when taking certain drugs. Alcohol interacts with some drugs, causing adverse effects such as lethargy, confusion, or coma.

- Tell patients to ask their pharmacists where to store each medication. Some drugs must be refrigerated. Others should be kept in a dry, cool area. Drugs should not usually be kept in a hot, damp place, such as a bathroom. They must always be kept out of the reach of children.

- Tell patients to take their drugs in a well-lit area so they can read each drug label carefully before taking each dose. They should never assume that they are taking the right medication without reading the label on the container. If patients have poor vision, print the name of the drug and the dosage schedule clearly on a separate piece of paper or card to attach to the medication container.

- Instruct patients to call the doctor if they have any questions about their drug therapy.

▶ Charting Medications
LO 53.9

Whenever a patient receives some form of treatment, such as medication, a record is kept of that treatment. Special problems or circumstances are also recorded, such as new symptoms, the patient's own statements, and how the patient tolerated the medications or treatment. Most charting in the physician's office is documented on a progress note or a medication administration record (MAR). These documents are essential to serve as communication tools for all healthcare members who are connected to that patient. The medical record is considered a legal document and is taken as proof that medication or treatment was administered to the patient.

All chart entries must be factual, accurate, complete, current, organized, and confidential. Avoid using words or statements that can be interpreted as your opinion. For example, if a patient gags and spits up cough syrup that you just administered, you would not write that the patient did not like the taste of the medication; you would simply state, "patient experienced difficulty in swallowing medication and expelled medication." Avoid terms like "appear" or "seems," which can lead you to draw assumptions without objective data to support them. Be specific. Chart what the patient said or did, not what you think. Use abbreviations when appropriate because they allow you to say a great deal in a small space.

Review your office's medical records to keep consistent with the charting methods used in them. Follow these few simple rules:

- Before you begin, make sure you have the right chart and the right location in the chart.
- Chart medications directly from the physician order.
- Be specific. Do not write, "Gave Demerol for pain in the evening." Instead, write, "(Date), Demerol 100 mg given IM in right upper outer quadrant of gluteus maximus for c/o sharp pain, rated 7 on a scale of 10, in left arm, lot number, expiration date, initials."
- If using paper charts, do not leave gaps or skip lines. If an entry does not fill a complete line, draw a straight line to fill the gap. Put your signature or first initial and last name and title at the right side directly after the note.

- If you make an error, do not erase it. Draw a line through the mistake. The mistake should still be visible, so do not black it out. Initial it and then rechart the information correctly. Follow the specific procedure for making corrections in an electronic health record.
- Never use ditto marks.
- Write neatly in longhand or carefully enter into the electronic chart and check your note before submitting it. Ensure that your spelling is accurate.
- Use abbreviations and correct symbols. Most facilities have an approved abbreviation list to use as a reference.
- If you are unsure about charting, check with your supervising licensed practitioner. See Figure 53-17 for an example of complete and accurate charting.

Date	Patient Name: Valarie Ramirez	DOB 12/12/XX	Progress Note
11/29/XX	PPD, 0.1cc given ID, Rt. Forearm, Lot # 222-01, Exp. Date 12/11, ABC Pharmaceutical Co. Pt to return to office in 48–72 hours for screening results Patient tolerated well _____ Kaylyn Haddix RMA (AMT)		

FIGURE 53-17 Charting medication administration.

PROCEDURE 53-1 Administering Oral Drugs

Procedure Goal: To safely administer an oral drug to a patient.

OSHA Guidelines: This procedure does not involve exposure to blood, body fluids, or tissues.

Materials: Drug order (in patient chart), container of oral drug, small paper cup (for tablets, capsules, or caplets) or plastic calibrated medicine cup (for liquids), glass of water or juice, straw (optional), package insert or drug information sheet.

Method: Procedure steps.

1. Identify the patient and wash your hands.
2. Select the ordered drug (tablet, capsule, or liquid).
3. Check the rights, comparing information against the drug order.
   RATIONALE: To ensure necessary accuracy.
4. If you are unfamiliar with the drug, check a drug reference, read the package insert, or speak with the physician. Determine whether the drug may be taken with or followed by water or juice.
5. Ask the patient about any drug or food allergies. If the patient is not allergic to the ordered drug or other ingredients used to prepare it, proceed.
   RATIONALE: To prevent a reaction to the medication.
6. Perform any calculations needed to provide the prescribed dose. If you are unsure of your calculations, check them with a coworker or the physician.

If You Are Giving Tablets or Capsules

7. Open the container and tap the correct number into the cap. Do not touch the inside of the cap because it is sterile. If

you pour out too many tablets or capsules and you have not touched them, tap the excess back into the container.

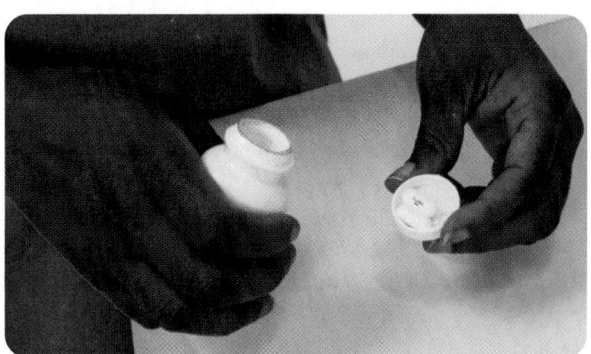

FIGURE Procedure 53-1 Step 7 Tap tablets gently into the cap.

8. Tap the tablets or capsules from the cap into the paper cup.

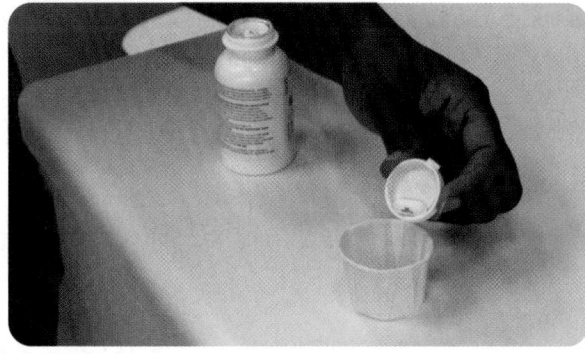

FIGURE Procedure 53-1 Step 8 Tap tablets from the cap into the paper cup.

9. Recap the container immediately.
   RATIONALE: Recapping immediately protects the medication from exposure to air, which can break down the medication.

10. Give the patient the cup along with a glass of water or juice. If the patient finds it easier to drink with a straw, unwrap the straw and place it in the fluid. If patients have difficulty swallowing pills, have them drink some water or juice before putting the pills in the mouth.
    RATIONALE: Additional fluid makes the pills float in the mouth and allows patients to swallow easier.

If You Are Giving a Liquid Drug

11. If the liquid is a suspension, shake it well.

12. Locate the mark on the medicine cup for the prescribed dose. Keeping your thumbnail on the mark, hold the cup at eye level and pour the correct amount of the drug. Keep the label side of the bottle on top as you pour or put your palm over it.
    RATIONALE: To prevent liquid drips from obscuring the label.

13. After pouring the drug, place the cup on a flat surface and check the drug level again. At eye level the base of the meniscus (the crescent-shaped form at the top of the liquid) should align with the mark that indicates the prescribed dose. If you poured out too much, discard it.
    RATIONALE: Do not return it to the container because medicine cups are not sterile.

Meniscus

FIGURE Procedure 53-1 Step 13   Looking at eye level, find the base of the meniscus, or the crescent-shaped form at the top of the liquid, for the correct measure.

14. Give the medicine cup to the patient with instructions to drink the liquid. If indicated, offer a glass of water or juice to wash down the drug.

After You Have Given an Oral Drug

15. Wash your hands.

16. Give the patient an information sheet about the drug. Discuss the information with the patient and answer any questions she may have. If the patient has questions you cannot answer, refer her to the physician.

17. Document the drug administration in the patient's chart with the date, time, drug name, dosage, expiration date, lot number, manufacturer, route, site, significant patient reactions, and any patient education.

PROCEDURE 53-2 Administering Buccal or Sublingual Drugs

Procedure Goal: To safely administer a buccal or sublingual drug to a patient.

OSHA Guidelines: This procedure does not involve exposure to blood, body fluids, or tissues.

Materials: Drug order (in patient chart), container of buccal or sublingual drug, small paper cup, package insert or drug information sheet.

Method: Procedure steps.

1. Identify the patient and wash your hands.

2. Select the ordered drug.

3. Check the rights, comparing information against the drug order.
   RATIONALE: To ensure necessary accuracy.

4. If you are unfamiliar with the drug, check the *PDR* or other creditable drug reference, read the package insert, or speak with the physician.

5. Ask the patient about any drug or food allergies. If the patient is not allergic to the ordered drug or other ingredients used to prepare it, proceed.
   RATIONALE: To prevent a reaction to the medication.

6. Perform any calculations needed to provide the prescribed dose. If you are unsure of your calculations, check them with a coworker or the physician.

7. Open the container and tap the correct number into the cap. Do not touch the inside of the cap because it is sterile. If you pour out too many tablets or capsules and you have not touched them, tap the excess back into the container.

8. Tap the tablets or capsules from the cap into the paper cup.

9. Recap the container immediately.
   RATIONALE: Recapping immediately protects the medication from exposure to air, which can break down the medication.

If You Are Giving Buccal Medication

10. For a *buccal* drug, provide patient instruction, including
    - Tell the patient not to chew or swallow the tablet.
    - Place the medication between the cheek and gum until it dissolves.

    RATIONALE: This area is rich in blood supply to promote rapid absorption of the drug.

    - Instruct the patient not to eat, drink, or smoke until the tablet is completely dissolved.

    RATIONALE: Food and fluids wash the drug into the gastrointestinal (GI) tract, slowing absorption or allowing gastric juices to destroy it. Smoking increases salivation, causing impaired absorption of the drug.

FIGURE Procedure 53-2 Step 10 Place a buccal drug between the cheek and gum.

If You Are Giving a Sublingual Drug

11. For a *sublingual* drug, provide patient instruction, including
    - Tell the patient not to chew or swallow the tablet.
    - Place the medication under the tongue until it dissolves.

    RATIONALE: The capillaries in this area promote rapid absorption of the drug.

- Instruct the patient not to eat, drink, or smoke until the tablet is completely dissolved.

  RATIONALE: Food and fluids wash the drug into the GI tract, slowing absorption or allowing gastric juices to destroy it. Smoking increases salivation, causing impaired absorption of the drug.

FIGURE Procedure 53-2 Step 11 Place a sublingual drug under the tongue.

After You Have Given a Buccal or Sublingual Medication

12. Remain with the patient until the tablet dissolves to monitor for possible adverse reaction and to ensure that the patient has allowed the tablet to dissolve in the mouth instead of chewing or swallowing it.
13. Wash your hands.
14. Give the patient an information sheet about the drug. Discuss the information with the patient and answer any questions she may have. If the patient has questions you cannot answer, refer her to the physician.
15. Document the drug administration in the patient's chart with the date, time, drug name, dosage, expiration date, lot number, manufacturer, route, site, significant patient reactions, and any patient education.

PROCEDURE 53-3 Drawing a Drug from an Ampule

Procedure Goal: To safely open an ampule and draw a drug, using sterile technique.

OSHA Guidelines:

Materials: Ampule of drug, alcohol swab, 2 × 2 gauze square, small file (provided by the drug manufacturer), sterile filtered needle, sterile needle, and a syringe of the appropriate size.

Method: Procedure steps.

1. Wash your hands and put on exam gloves.
2. Gently tap the top of the ampule with your forefinger to settle the liquid to the bottom of the ampule.
3. Wipe the ampule's neck with an alcohol swab.

4. Wrap the 2 × 2 gauze square around the ampule's neck, then snap the neck away from you. If it does not snap easily, score the neck with the small file and snap it again.

FIGURE Procedure 53-3 Step 4   To prevent possible injury, wrap the neck of the ampule with gauze before snapping.

5. Insert the filtered needle into the ampule without touching the side of the ampule.
   RATIONALE: A filtered needle will prevent contamination of the medication.
6. Pull back on the plunger to aspirate (remove by vacuum or suction) the liquid completely into the syringe.
7. Replace with the regular needle and push the plunger on the syringe until the medication just reaches the tip of the needle. The drug is now ready for injection.

PROCEDURE 53-4 Reconstituting and Drawing a Drug for Injection

Procedure Goal: To reconstitute and draw a drug for injection, using sterile technique.

OSHA Guidelines:

Materials: Vial of drug, vial of diluent, alcohol swabs, two disposable sterile needle and syringe sets of appropriate size, sharps container.

Method: Procedure steps.
1. Wash your hands and put on exam gloves.
2. Place the drug vial and diluent vial on the countertop. Wipe each rubber diaphragm with a fresh alcohol swab.
3. Remove the cap from the needle and the guard from the syringe. Pull the plunger back to the mark that equals the amount of diluent needed to reconstitute the drug ordered.
   RATIONALE: This action aspirates air into the syringe.
4. Puncture the diaphragm of the vial of diluent with the needle and inject the air into the diluent.

FIGURE Procedure 53-4 Step 4   Injecting air into the diluent.

RATIONALE: This action creates positive pressure that lets you draw the diluent easily. If you do not add air, a vacuum forms, making it difficult to draw the diluent.

5. Invert the vial and aspirate the diluent.
6. Remove the needle from the diluent vial, inject the diluent into the drug vial, and withdraw the needle. Properly dispose of this needle and syringe.
7. Roll the vial between your hands to mix the drug and diluent thoroughly. Do not shake the vial unless so directed on the drug label. When completely mixed, the solution in the vial should have no flakes. The solution may be clear or cloudy when completely mixed (depending on the drug).
8. Remove the cap and guard from the second needle and syringe.
9. Pull back the plunger to the mark that reflects the amount of drug ordered. Inject the air into the drug vial.
10. Invert the vial and aspirate the proper amount of the drug into the syringe. The drug is now ready for injection.

FIGURE Procedure 53-4 Step 10   Aspirating the drug into the syringe.

PROCEDURE 53-5 Giving an Intradermal Injection

Procedure Goal: To administer an intradermal injection safely and effectively, using sterile technique.

OSHA Guidelines:

Materials: Drug order (in patient chart), alcohol swab, disposable needle and syringe of the appropriate size filled with the ordered dose of drug, sharps container.

Method: Procedure steps.

1. Identify the patient. Wash your hands and put on exam gloves.
2. Check the rights, comparing information against the drug order.
   RATIONALE: To ensure necessary accuracy.
3. Identify the injection site on the patient's forearm. To do so, rest the patient's arm on a table with the palm up. Measure 2 to 3 finger-widths below the antecubital space and a hand-width above the wrist. The space between is available for the injection.

FIGURE Procedure 53-5 Step 3   This space is available for intradermal injection sites.

4. Prepare the skin with the alcohol swab, moving in a circle from the center out.
5. Let the skin dry before giving the injection.
   RATIONALE: To prevent you from introducing antiseptic under the skin, which could cause irritation and falsify intradermal test results.
6. Hold the patient's forearm and stretch the skin taut with one hand.
7. With the other hand, place the needle—bevel up— almost flat against the patient's skin. Press the needle against the skin and insert it.

FIGURE Procedure 53-5 Step 7   Inserting the needle for an intradermal injection.

8. Inject the drug slowly and gently. You should see the needle through the skin and feel resistance. As the drug enters the upper layer of skin, a wheal (raised area of the skin) will form.

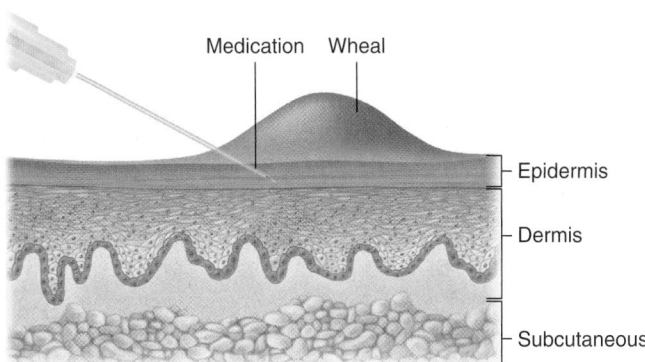

FIGURE Procedure 53-5 Step 8   Medication collects under the skin, forming a wheal, during an intradermal injection.

9. After the full dose of the drug has been injected, withdraw the needle. Properly dispose of used materials and the needle and syringe immediately.
10. Remove the gloves and wash your hands.
11. Stay with the patient to monitor for unexpected reactions.
12. Document the injection in the patient's chart with the date, time, drug name, dosage, expiration date, lot number, manufacturer, route, site, significant patient reactions, and any patient education.

PROCEDURE 53-6 Giving a Subcutaneous (Subcut) Injection

Procedure Goal: To administer a subcutaneous injection safely and effectively, using sterile technique.

OSHA Guidelines:

Materials: Drug order (in patient's chart), alcohol swabs, sterile 2 × 2 gauze or cotton ball, container of the ordered drug, disposable needle and syringe of the appropriate size, sharps container.

Method: Procedure steps.

1. Identify the patient. Wash your hands and put on exam gloves.
2. Check the rights, comparing information against the drug order.
   RATIONALE: To ensure necessary accuracy.
3. Prepare the drug and draw it up to the mark on the syringe that matches the ordered dose.
4. Choose a site and clean it with an alcohol swab, moving in a circle from the center out. Let the area dry.

FIGURE Procedure 53-6 Step 4   Many sites are available for subcutaneous injection.

5. Pinch the skin firmly to lift the subcutaneous tissue.
6. Position the needle—bevel up—at a 45- to 90-degree angle to the skin.
   RATIONALE: The angle of the needle helps ensure that the medication is administered into the correct location. A 90-degree angle is used when you can pinch at least two inches. A 45-degree angle is used when you can only pinch one inch of skin.

(a)

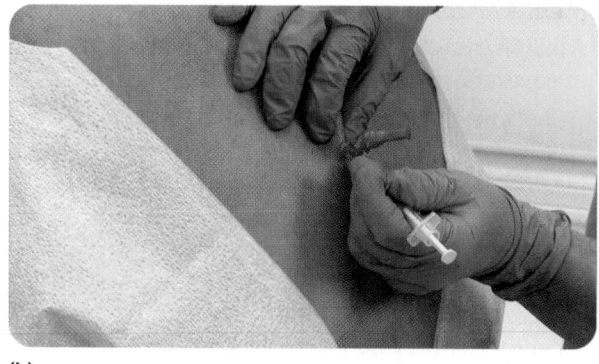

(b)

FIGURE Procedure 53-6 Step 6   Positioning the needle for subcutaneous injection: (a) 90-degree angle; (b) 45-degree angle.

7. Insert the needle in one quick motion, then release the skin and inject the drug slowly. With some medications, you will check the placement of the needle by pulling back on the plunger before injecting. If blood is seen in the hub, you should withdraw the needle and start with a fresh needle and syringe. If no blood is seen, inject the medication slowly.
8. After the full dose of the drug has been injected, place a 2 × 2 gauze over the site and withdraw the needle at the same angle you inserted it.
9. Apply pressure at the puncture site with the gauze or cotton ball.
10. Massage the site gently to help distribute the drug, if indicated. Do not massage insulin, heparin, or other anticoagulant medications.
    RATIONALE: Massaging a site for heparin can cause bruising.
11. Properly dispose of the used materials and the needle and syringe.
12. Remove the gloves and wash your hands.
13. Stay with the patient to monitor for unexpected reactions.
14. Document the injection in the patient's chart with the date, time, drug name, dosage, expiration date, lot number, manufacturer, route, site, significant patient reactions, and any patient education.

PROCEDURE 53-7 Giving an Intramuscular Injection

Procedure Goal: To administer an intramuscular injection safely and effectively, using sterile technique.

OSHA Guidelines:

Materials: Drug order (in patient's chart), alcohol swabs, sterile 2 × 2 gauze or cotton ball, container of the ordered drug, disposable needle and syringe of the appropriate size, sharps container.

Method: Procedure steps.

1. Identify the patient. Wash your hands and put on exam gloves.
2. Check the rights, comparing information against the drug order.
   RATIONALE: To ensure necessary accuracy.
3. Prepare the drug and draw it up to the mark on the syringe that matches the ordered dose.
4. Choose a site and gently tap it. Tapping stimulates the nerve endings and reduces pain caused by the needle insertion.

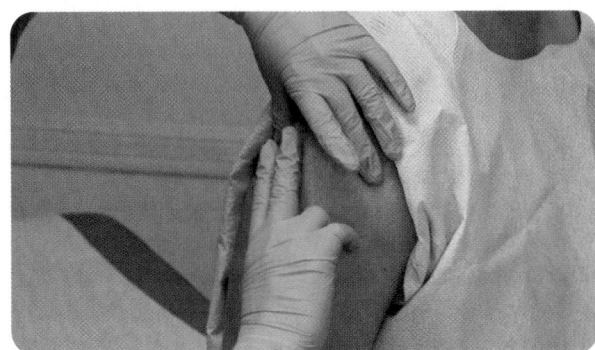

FIGURE Procedure 53-7 Step 4   Gently tap the site to stimulate the nerve endings.

5. Clean the site with an alcohol swab, moving in a circle from the center out. Let the site dry.
6. Stretch the skin taut over the injection site between the thumb and forefinger. For the pediatric and geriatric patients you may grasp the tissue and "bunch up" the muscle. For a Z-track stretch and hold the skin and fat laterally.
7. Hold the needle and syringe at a 90-degree angle to the skin, then insert the needle with a quick, dart-like thrust.
   RATIONALE: The angle of the needle helps ensure that the medication is administered into the correct location.
8. Release the skin and aspirate by pulling back slightly on the plunger to check the needle placement. If pulling back on the plunger produces blood, placement is incorrect and you must begin again with a fresh needle and syringe. If pulling back on the plunger produces no blood, placement is correct. Inject the drug slowly.
   RATIONALE: Injecting an intramuscular drug into the bloodstream can cause severe side effects for the patient.
9. After the full dose of the drug has been injected, place a 2 × 2 gauze over the site, then quickly remove the needle at a 90-degree angle.
10. Use the 2 × 2 gauze to apply pressure to the site and massage it, if indicated.
11. Properly dispose of used materials and the needle and syringe.
12. Remove the gloves and wash your hands.
13. Stay with the patient to monitor for unexpected reactions.
14. Document the injection in the patient's chart with the date, time, drug name, dosage, expiration date, lot number, manufacturer, route, site, significant patient reactions, and any patient education.

PROCEDURE 53-8 Administering Inhalation Therapy

Procedure Goal: To administer inhalation therapy safely and effectively.

OSHA Guidelines: This procedure does not involve exposure to blood, body fluids, or tissues.

Materials: Drug order (in patient's chart), container of the ordered drug, tissues, package insert or patient education sheet about medication.

Method: Procedure steps.

1. Identify the patient. Wash your hands.
2. Check the rights, comparing information against the drug order. Make sure you have the correct type of inhaler based upon the order (oral or nasal).
   RATIONALE: To ensure necessary accuracy.
3. Prepare the container of medication as directed. Use the package insert and show the directions to the patient.
4. Shake the container as directed and stress this step to the patient.
   RATIONALE: The drug must be evenly distributed in the inhaler to ensure its effectiveness.

For a Nasal Inhaler

5. Instruct the patient to complete the following steps:
   - Have the patient blow the nose to clear the nostrils.
   - Tilt the head back and, with one hand, place the inhaler tip about ½ inch into the nostril.
   - Point the tip straight up toward the inner corner of the eye.

RATIONALE: Angling the inhaler downward makes the drug run down the back of the throat, causing a burning sensation.

- Use the opposite hand to block the other nostril.
- Inhale gently while quickly and firmly squeezing the inhaler.
- Remove the inhaler tip and exhale through the mouth.
- Shake the inhaler and repeat the process in the other nostril.
- If indicated in the package insert, instruct patients to keep the head tilted back and not to blow their nose for several minutes.

For an Oral Inhaler

6. Instruct the patient to complete the following steps:
   - Warm the canister by rolling it between the palms of your hands.
   - Uncap the mouthpiece and assemble the inhaler as directed on the package insert.
   - Hold the mouth open and place the canister in the mouth or about 1 inch from the mouth. Check the package insert for the proper placement.
   - Exhale normally and inhale through the canister as he or she depresses it. The medication must be inhaled.
   - Breathe in until the lungs are full and hold the breath for 10 seconds.
   - Breathe out normally.

After You Have Given an Inhalation Medication

7. Remain with the patient to monitor for changes and possible adverse reaction.
8. Recap and secure the medication container. Instruct the patient in this procedure.
9. Wash your hands.
10. Give the patient an information sheet about the drug. Discuss the information with the patient and answer any questions she may have. If the patient has questions you cannot answer, refer her to the physician.
11. Document the drug administration in the patient's chart with the date, time, drug name, dosage, expiration date, lot number, manufacturer, route, site, significant patient reactions, and any patient education.

PROCEDURE 53-9 Administering and Removing a Transdermal Patch and Providing Patient Instruction

Procedure Goal: To safely administer a transdermal patch drug to and remove it from a patient.

OSHA Guidelines: This procedure does not involve exposure to blood, body fluids, or tissues.

Materials: Drug order (in patient chart), transdermal patch medication, gloves, package insert or drug information sheet, patient chart.

Method: Procedure steps.

1. Identify the patient, wash your hands, and put on gloves.
   RATIONALE: Gloves prevent the medication from being absorbed through your skin.
2. Select the ordered transdermal patch and check the rights, comparing information against the drug order.
   RATIONALE: To ensure necessary accuracy.
3. Ask the patient about any drug or food allergies. If the patient is not allergic to the ordered drug or other ingredients used to prepare it, proceed.
   RATIONALE: To prevent a reaction to the medication.
4. If you are unfamiliar with the drug, check the *PDR* or other credible drug reference, read the package insert, or speak with the physician. The package insert is extremely detailed for transdermal medications and should be used when applying the medication and/or doing patient teaching.
5. Perform any calculations needed to provide the prescribed dose. If you are unsure of your calculations, check them with a coworker or the physician.

Applying the Transdermal Medication

6. Remove the patch from its pouch. The plastic backing is easily peeled off once the patch is removed from the pouch. For patches without a protective pouch, bend the sides of the transdermal unit back and forth until the clear plastic backing snaps down the middle.
7. For either type of patch, demonstrate how to peel off the clear plastic backing to expose the sticky side of the patch.
8. Apply the patch to a reasonably hair-free site, such as the abdomen. Note that estrogen patches are usually placed on the hip.
9. Instruct the patient on how to apply the patch. Advise the patient to avoid using the extremities below the knee or elbow, skin folds, scar tissue, or burned or irritated areas.
   RATIONALE: These areas do not absorb the medication as well because of the reduced blood supply.

Step 1

Step 2

Step 3

FIGURE Procedure 53-9 Step 8 To apply a transdermal patch, first (1) either remove it from the pouch or bend the sides back and forth until the backing snaps; then (2) peel the backing off the patch and (3) apply the patch, sticky side down, to a clean, relatively hairless site.

Removing the Transdermal Patch

10. Gently lift and slowly peel the patch back from the skin. Wash the area with soap and dry it with a towel. Instruct the patient on this technique.

11. Explain to the patient that the skin may appear red and warm, which is normal. Reassure the patient that the redness will disappear. In some cases, lotion may be applied to the skin if it feels dry.

12. Instruct the patient to notify the doctor if the redness does not disappear in several days or if a rash develops.

13. *Never* apply a new patch to the site just used. It is best to allow each site to rest between applications. Some transdermal systems call for waiting 7 days before using a site again. Be sure to check the package directions regarding site rotation.

After You Have Applied and/or Removed the Transdermal Patch

14. Wash your hands and instruct the patient to do the same after applying or removing a transdermal system at home.

15. Give the patient an information sheet about the drug. Discuss the information with the patient and answer any questions she may have. If the patient has questions you cannot answer, refer her to the physician.

16. Document the drug administration in the patient's chart with the date, time, drug name, dosage, expiration date, lot number, manufacturer, route, site, significant patient reactions, and any patient education.

PROCEDURE 53-10 Assisting with Administration of a Urethral Drug

Procedure Goal: To assist with a urethral administration.

OSHA Guidelines:

Materials: Urinary catheter kit, either a syringe without a needle or tubing and a bag (depending on the amount of drug to be administered), sterile gloves, the prescribed drug, a drape, and a bedsaver pad.

Method: Procedure steps.

1. Wash your hands and use sterile technique to assemble the equipment.

2. Check the rights, comparing information against the drug order, and explain the procedure and the drug order to the patient.
   RATIONALE: To ensure necessary accuracy.

3. Assist the patient into the lithotomy position and drape her to preserve her modesty while exposing the vulva.

FIGURE Procedure 53-10 Step 3 Use the stirrups to place the patient in the lithotomy position. Clothing should be removed and a drape applied.

4. Place a bedsaver pad under the buttocks.
5. Open the catheter kit.
6. Put on sterile gloves.
7. Cleanse the vulva as you would to perform catheterization, using the materials in the kit. As you sweep down with the antiseptic swab, watch for the urethral opening to "wink."

RATIONALE: The wink helps you accurately locate the urethral opening.

8. The physician or nurse will insert the lubricated catheter. Tell the patient that she should feel pressure, not pain, and that the physician or nurse is going to attach the syringe to the catheter and insert the drug (or attach the tubing and bag to the catheter and let the drug run in by gravity).

9. After instilling the drug, the physician or nurse will clamp the catheter and leave the drug in place for the ordered amount of time.

10. Stay with the patient not only to ensure that she remains still but also to reassure her that the full feeling in the bladder is normal. She also may say she feels the need to urinate. Advise her that this feeling, too, is normal and is caused by the catheter.

11. When the time is up, unclamp the catheter, gently remove it, and allow the patient to urinate. Assist the patient as needed.

12. While the patient is dressing, immediately document the drug instillation with date, time, drug, dose, route, and any significant patient reactions.

PROCEDURE 53-11 Administering a Vaginal Medication

Procedure Goal: To safely administer a vaginal medication with patient instruction.

OSHA Guidelines:

Materials: Prescription or drug order in the patient's chart, a cloth or paper drape, a bedsaver pad, gloves, cotton balls, water-soluble lubricant, and the prescribed drug.

Method: Procedure steps.

1. Wash your hands.
2. Check the rights, comparing information against the drug order, and explain the procedure and the drug order to the patient.
   RATIONALE: To ensure necessary accuracy.
3. Give the patient the opportunity to empty her bladder before beginning.
4. Assist the patient into the lithotomy position and drape her.
   RATIONALE: To preserve her modesty while exposing the vulva.

5. Place a bedsaver pad under the buttocks.
6. Put on gloves.
7. Cleanse the perineum with soap and water, using one cotton ball per stroke, and cleanse the center last, while spreading the labia.
   RATIONALE: This technique prevents contamination of areas already cleaned.
8. Lubricate the vaginal suppository applicator in lubricant spread on a paper towel. For vaginal drugs in the form of creams, ointments, gels, and tablets, use the appropriate applicator, preparing it according to the package insert.
9. While spreading the labia with one hand, insert the applicator with the other (the applicator should be about 2 inches into the vagina and angled toward the sacrum).
10. Release the labia and push the applicator's plunger to release the suppository into the vagina.
11. Remove the applicator and wipe any excess lubricant off the patient.
12. Help her to a sitting position and assist with dressing if needed.
13. Document the administration with date, time, drug, dose, route, and any significant patient reactions.

PROCEDURE 53-12 Administering a Rectal Medication

Procedure Goal: To safely administer a rectal medication.

OSHA Guidelines:

Materials: Prescription or drug order in the patient's chart, a cloth or paper drape, a bedsaver pad, gloves, water-soluble lubricant, and the prescribed drug.

Method: Procedure steps.

1. Check the rights, comparing information against the drug order.
   RATIONALE: To ensure necessary accuracy.
2. Explain the procedure and the drug order to the patient.
3. Give the patient the opportunity to empty the bladder before beginning.
4. With the patient in a gown, help the patient into Sims' position and use a drape to prevent exposing the patient. Place a bedsaver pad under the patient.

FIGURE Procedure 53-12 Step 4   Place the patient into Sims' position. The patient should be in a gown with a drape in place.

5. Lift the patient's gown to expose the anus.
6. Wash your hands, put on gloves, and prepare the medication.

When Administering a Suppository

7. Lubricate the tapered end of the suppository with about 1 tsp of lubricant.
8. While spreading the patient's buttocks with one hand, insert the suppository—tapered end first—into the anus with the other hand.
9. Gently advance the suppository past the sphincter with your index finger. Before it passes the sphincter, the suppository may feel as if it is being pushed back out the anus. When it passes the sphincter, it seems to disappear.
10. Use tissues to remove excess lubricant from the area.

11. Remove your gloves and ask the patient to lie quietly and retain the suppository for at least 20 minutes. When the treatment is completed, help the patient to a sitting, then standing, position.
    RATIONALE: To ensure the maximum effectiveness of the medication.

When Administering a Retention Enema

7. Place the tip of a syringe into a rectal tube. Let a little rectal solution flow through the syringe and tube. While holding the tip up, clamp the tubing.
8. Lubricate the end of the tube, spread the patient's buttocks, and slide the tube into the rectum about 4 inches.
9. Slowly pour the rectal solution into the syringe, release the clamp, and let gravity move the solution into the patient. When you have administered the ordered amount of solution, clamp the tube and then remove it.
10. Using tissues, apply pressure over the anus for 20 seconds to stifle the patient's urge to defecate, and then wipe any excess lubricant or solution from the area. Encourage the patient to retain the enema for the time ordered.
    RATIONALE: To ensure the maximum effectiveness of the medication.
11. When the time has passed, help the patient use a bedpan or direct the patient to a toilet to expel the solution.

After the Administration Is Complete

12. Remove your gloves and wash your hands.
13. Immediately document the drug administration with date, time, drug, dose, route, and any significant patient reactions.

SUMMARY OF LEARNING OUTCOMES

LEARNING OUTCOMES	KEY POINTS
53.1 **Describe the rules and responsibilities regarding drug administration and the initial preparation for the drug administration.**	Before administering a medication, you should check the patient for allergies and also evaluate any drug-drug interactions. You should check all injection sites for abnormalities such as scars, bruises, burns, rash, edema, moles, birthmarks, traumatic injuries, redness, cyanosis, tattoos, warts, side of a mastectomy, and paralyzed areas. Additionally, you should be aware of the patient's condition and have the patient sign a consent form if necessary.
53.2 **List the rights of drug administration.**	The rights of drug administration include the right patient, right drug, right dose, right route, right time, right documentation, right reason, right to know, right to refuse, and right technique.
53.3 **Recognize the correct equipment to use for administering medications.**	Drugs may be administered for either local or systemic effects. Generally, drugs that have local effects are applied directly to the skin, tissues, or mucous membranes. Drugs that produce systemic effects are administered by routes that allow the drug to be absorbed and distributed in the bloodstream throughout the body. Table 53-2 outlines the many drug administration routes.

LEARNING OUTCOMES	KEY POINTS
53.4 **Carry out the procedures for administering oral medications.**	Oral medications typically are swallowed and absorbed through the digestive tract. Sublingual medications go under the tongue and buccal medications go between the cheek and gum.
53.5 **Carry out procedures for administering parenteral medications by injection.**	The three most common injection routes are ID, subcut, and IM. IV is less frequently used in a medical office. All injections are given using aseptic technique. Intradermal (ID) injections are administered between the upper layers of skin and create a wheal. Subcutaneous (SQ/SC/SubQ) injections are administered just under the skin, and intramuscular (IM) injections are administered into a muscle.
53.6 **Carry out procedures for administering parenteral medications by other routes.**	Other medication routes include inhalants (respiratory), topical (including transdermal), urethral, vaginal, and rectal.
53.7 **Relate special considerations required for medication administration to pediatric, pregnant, breast-feeding, and geriatric patients.**	Certain special considerations must be made when caring for pediatric, pregnant, and breastfeeding patients. Pediatric patients require extreme care when calculating doses due to the differences in how their bodies absorb, metabolize, eliminate, and distribute the medications. Treat pediatric patients with special care and communication to make the experience as positive as possible. Restraining may be necessary. Checking medications given to pregnant and breast-feeding patients for possible adverse effects is essential. Geriatric considerations are discussed in the *Assisting in Geriatrics* chapter.
53.8 **Outline patient education information related to medications.**	Patients should be educated about why, when, and how they should take medications. This includes instruction to ensure patient compliance regarding nonprescription and prescription drugs as well as herbal remedies and supplements. Patients also should be instructed about the dangers of medication combinations, the importance of reporting an adverse effect, and maintaining a complete medication list.
53.9 **Implement accurate and complete documentation of medications.**	Documentation of medication administered should occur immediately after the medication is given and should include the name, date, time, medication administered, dose, route, location, lot #, and how the patient tolerated it.

CASE STUDY CRITICAL THINKING

Recall John Miller from the beginning of the chapter. Now that you have completed this chapter, answer the following questions regarding his case.

1. What questions do you need to ask Mr. Miller during his initial interview regarding his medications?

2. When you get ready to administer the pneumococcal immunization, Mr. Miller states that he had a bad reaction the last time he received a shot. What should you do?

3. If the site of the injection from his last visit was just irritated due to the medication, what could be done to reduce the irritation for his next IM injection?

1. (LO 53.3) Which of the following would you expect to be absorbed in the least amount of time?
   a. 200 mL of D5W IV
   b. 5 mL of Compazine IM
   c. 325 mg of ASA orally
   d. ii puffs of albuterol by oral inhalation
   e. PPD subcut injection

2. (LO 53.2) Which of the following is *not* a basic right of medication administration?
   a. Right dose
   b. Right drug
   c. Right to refuse
   d. Right patient
   e. Right time

3. (LO 53.8) Which of the following patients has the greatest risk of overdose and toxicity from a medication?
   a. A 35-year-old woman
   b. A 6-year-child with the flu
   c. A 50-year-old male with hypertension
   d. A 16-year-old Hispanic girl with mononucleosis
   e. A 25-year-old man with diabetes

4. (LO 53.1) When performing a triple check, which of the following would you *least* likely do?
   a. *1st check*—when you take it from the storage container and match it to the MAR
   b. *2nd check*—when you prepare it
   c. *3rd check*—before you close the storage container
   d. *3rd check*—just after you administer the drug
   e. *3rd check*—just before you administer the drug

5. (LO 53.4) A patient is taking a nitroglycerin tablet under his tongue. What route of administration is this?
   a. Urethral
   b. Topical
   c. Inhalant
   d. Sublingual
   e. Buccal

6. (LO 53.5) You are injecting a medication ID; what would best let you know that you have done it correctly?
   a. The patient does not have pain
   b. There is a wheal on the skin at the site
   c. The angle of the needle is at 90 degrees
   d. The medication went into a muscle
   e. The medication went under the skin

7. (LO 53.6) You are administering a suppository. What route of administration are you most likely performing?
   a. Oral
   b. Vaginal
   c. Respiratory
   d. IV
   e. Topical

8. (LO 53.7) An infant needs an immunization subcut. What site and what needle would be your best choice?
   a. Vastus lateralis, 20 gauge, ⅝ inch
   b. Vastus lateralis, 25 gauge, 1½ inch
   c. Ventrogluteal, 25 gauge, ⅝ inch
   d. Dorsogluteal, 23 gauge, 1 inch
   e. Vastus lateralis, 25 gauge, ⅝ inch

9. (LO 53.8) Which of the following would be done to improve patient compliance?
   a. Have patients with multiple meds create an alarm, calendar, or chart
   b. Remind patients taking antibiotics to stop once they are feeling better
   c. To avoid waste, encourage patients to share medication if they have too much
   d. Dispose of expired drugs one year after the expiration date on the medication
   e. Encourage anxious patients to have at least three servings of alcohol each day

10. (LO 53.9) Which of the following is the most complete medication documentation?
    a. Gave Demerol for pain at 2 pm
    b. Demerol 100 mg IM in deltoid
    c. 4/12/XX Demerol IM in left deltoid
    d. 4/12/XX Phenergan 200 mg PO for nausea
    e. Phenergan PO for nausea—Kaylyn R. Haddix RMA(AMT)

54 Physical Therapy and Rehabilitation

CASE STUDY

PATIENT INFORMATION

Patient Name	Gender	DOB
Shenya Jones	Female	11/3/19XX

Attending	MRN	Allergies
Elizabeth H. Williams, MD	124-86-564	cinnamon, peanuts

Shenya Jones, a 34-year-old female, arrives at the office with swelling and a red pustule on her face. She states that the problem started two days ago as a small pimple near her nose. It became irritated then extremely swollen and painful overnight. Now this AM, there was yellow drainage noted at the lesion site and the swelling has increased. The area of drainage is approximately 1 cm in diameter. The upper lip, side of the face, and nose are all swollen. You have taken her vital signs but must ask her about her level of pain and measure the area of drainage. She rates the pain in her face as a 7 out of 10. The physician thinks the condition may be impetigo or MRSA. A wound culture is obtained and the patient is prescribed Augmentin XR 100 mg 1 BID X 14 days and Bactrim DS 800 mg 1 BID X 14 days. In addition, the physician instructs Shenya to take OTC pain relievers and apply moist heat to the area twice a day.

Keep Shenya in mind as you study this chapter. There will be questions at the end of the chapter based on the case study. The information in the chapter will help you answer these questions.

LEARNING OUTCOMES

After completing Chapter 54, you will be able to:

54.1 Discuss the general principles of physical therapy.

54.2 Relate various cold and heat therapies to their benefits and contraindications.

54.3 Recall hydrotherapy methods.

54.4 Name several methods of exercise therapy.

54.5 Describe the types of massage used in rehabilitation therapy.

54.6 Compare different methods of traction.

54.7 Carry out the procedure for teaching a patient to use a cane, a walker, crutches, and a wheelchair.

54.8 Model the steps you should take when referring a patient to a physical therapist.

KEY TERMS

cryotherapy
diathermy
erythema
fluidotherapy
gait
goniometer
hydrotherapy

mobility aid
physical therapy
posture
range of motion (ROM)
therapeutic team
thermotherapy
traction

I. P (10) Assist physician with patient care

I. A (1) Apply critical thinking skills in performing patient assessment and care

IV. P (6) Prepare a patient for procedures and/or treatments

XI. C (10) Identify principles of body mechanics and ergonomics

2. **Anatomy and Physiology**

Graduates:

c. Assist the physician with the regimen of diagnostic and treatment modalities as they relate to each body system

5. **Psychology of Human Relations**

Graduates:

b. Identify and respond appropriately when working/caring for patients with special needs

9. **Medical Office Clinical Procedures**

Graduates:

l. Prepare patient for examinations and treatments

m. Assist physician with routine and specialty examinations and treatments

q. Instruct patients with special needs

▶ Introduction

Applying cold and heat therapy and assisting patients with ambulation (walking around) are common responsibilities of a medical assistant. These activities are part of the physical therapy field. For a full program of physical therapy, a physician generally refers a patient to a licensed physical therapist. However, a physician may request that you assist with some forms of physical therapy, including:

- Applying cold and heat.
- Teaching basic exercises.
- Demonstrating how to use a cane, walker, and crutches.
- Demonstrating how to use a wheelchair.
- Discussing with the patient specific therapies for use at home.

▶ General Principles of Physical Therapy
LO 54.1

Physical therapy is a medical specialty for the treatment of musculoskeletal, nervous, and cardiopulmonary disorders. A physical therapist uses a variety of treatments, including cold, heat, water, exercise, massage, and traction. Some physical therapy regimens combine two or more treatments. Exercising in a pool, for example, combines the use of water and exercise. In addition, the physical therapist actively promotes patient education and rehabilitation programs.

Physical therapy benefits patients in several ways. It restores and improves muscle function, builds strength, increases joint mobility, relieves pain, and increases circulation. Physical therapy is used to treat various disorders, including arthritis, stroke, lower back pain, muscle spasms, muscle injuries or diseases, pressure sores, skin disorders, and burns.

Assisting within a Therapeutic Team

Many people who require physical therapy are recovering from traumatic injuries or dealing with chronic illnesses, so they may be receiving therapeutic attention from several different specialists. Physicians, nurses, medical assistants, and other specialists who work with patients dealing with chronic illness or recovery from major injuries make up a **therapeutic team**. When you work with such patients, your responsibilities may include:

- Coordinating the patient's schedule of sessions with different specialists.
- Making referrals, as directed by the physician.
- Explaining a specialist's treatment approach to the patient.
- Communicating the physician's findings to the specialist.
- Documenting the specialist's treatments and findings for the physician.
- Reinforcing the specialist's instructions for the patient.
- Answering the patient's questions.

To fulfill these responsibilities, you must have a working knowledge of therapy techniques. If, for example, the physician refers a patient to an art therapist, you would set up an art therapy appointment and explain in general terms what the patient can expect. The Educating the Patient section offers basic information about various specialized therapies.

Besides learning the basic information you need to know about physical therapy, you will want to keep up-to-date on emerging techniques. You may want to become proficient in some of these new techniques. By expanding your knowledge and skills, you increase your value as a member of the therapeutic team.

Specialized Therapies and Their Benefits

Healthcare professionals recognize the contribution of specialized therapies to a patient's recovery. Because many people do not know about these specialized therapies, you may be called on to explain them to patients. You can educate patients about potential benefits of art therapy or other specialized therapies. When specialized therapies are ordered, patients will be more at ease if they know what to expect. You can help when necessary by explaining the following types of therapies and their advantages.

- In art therapy, patients learn to express themselves visually through drawing, painting, and sculpture. Art therapy aids both physical and mental healing, provides a recreational outlet, improves mobility and fine motor coordination, provides an outlet for expressing fears or other emotions patients may be unaware of or unable or unwilling to express verbally, helps relieve anxiety, allows patients to focus on something other than their physical condition, and encourages patients to take better care of themselves. To aid in the art therapy process, encourage patients to relax and give this approach time to work. Although the benefits of art therapy may be evident immediately, they are just as likely to be perceived only after the course of therapy is well under way.

- In music therapy, patients listen to and create music to help them relax and alleviate anxiety. This therapy is often used with surgical patients and patients with chronic pain.
- In dance therapy, patients participate in dance to improve balance, flexibility, strength, and quality of life.
- In writing therapy, patients express themselves through a chosen form of writing, like composing poetry or keeping a journal.
- In crafts therapy, patients express themselves by using a variety of media to create handiworks.
- In pet therapy, patients play with, groom, or walk a pet. Pets provide companionship and the opportunity to nurture.
- In aquatic therapy, patients swim in a therapeutic pool equipped with a ramp and a lift so that it is accessible to all. Many patients who cannot walk on land can move their legs remarkably well in water.
- In horticultural therapy, patients work with plants and flowers to bring beauty into their daily lives and to help improve their balance, strength, memory, and socialization skills.
- In equestrian therapy, patients ride horses to help develop strength, coordination, and muscle tone, and to improve balance.

Assisting with Patient Assessment

Before the doctor prescribes physical therapy, she assesses the patient's physical abilities and condition. She inspects and palpates the patient's joints and muscles and tests the patient's joint mobility, muscle strength, gait, and posture. You will typically assist with these tests. In some cases, the doctor may direct you to perform them.

Joint Mobility Testing People usually assume their joints are mobile until stiffness or injury limits them. When a patient complains of these difficulties, the doctor may ask you to assist in testing range of motion. **Range of motion (ROM)** is the degree to which a joint is able to move, measured in degrees with a protractor device called a universal **goniometer** (Figure 54-1). The measurement of joint mobility, known as *goniometry*, is a noninvasive test frequently performed in doctors' offices, requiring the patient to move each major joint in various ways. The specific movements evaluated are described in Figure 54-2. Review the chapter *The Muscular System* for more information about body movement. The doctor may ask you to assist with goniometry and, after special training, you may be asked to perform it. When performing goniometry, you measure the joints from the head to the feet, comparing each joint measurement with a standard measurement (in degrees of movement) for that joint.

Muscle Strength Testing The physician tests muscle strength to determine the amount of force the patient is able

to exert with a muscle or group of muscles. This test—usually done at the same time as ROM testing—may be performed by the physician with your assistance or, once you have had special training, the physician may ask you to perform it yourself.

Like the ROM test, the muscle strength test is usually done from head to foot. The patient is asked to resist the pressure that

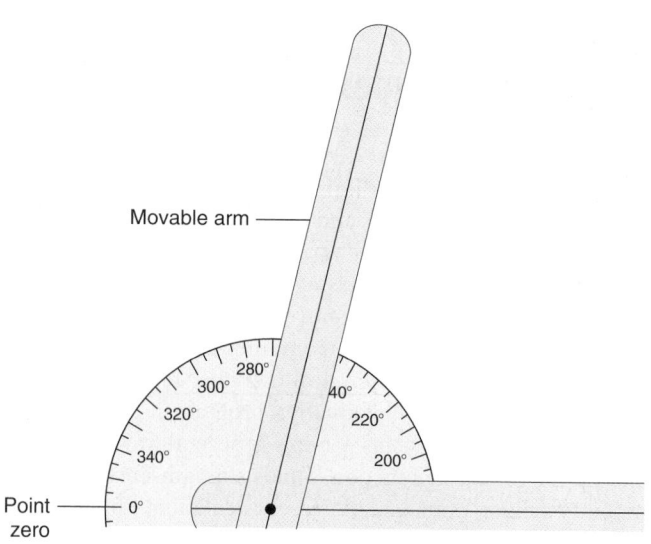

FIGURE 54-1 A universal goniometer is a protractor with a movable pointer that measures degrees of joint movement.

you or the physician applies to each muscle or group of muscles (usually near a joint). Strength is rated on a five-point scale.

Typically, a patient can move a joint a certain distance and can easily resist the pressure you apply. The patient usually has equal strength on both sides of the body. If there is weakness, however, a medical problem may be indicated. The physician must be made aware of weaknesses so he can use this information to develop a treatment plan.

Gait Testing Gait is the way a person walks. Generally, a physician or physical therapist assesses a patient's gait. To do so, the physician asks the patient to walk away, turn around, and

walk back. Assessment of gait includes an appraisal of the patient's length of stride, balance, coordination, direction of knees (inward or outward), and direction of feet (inward or outward).

Posture Testing Posture is body position and alignment. The doctor assesses posture by looking at the patient's spinal curve from the sides, back, and front. Normally, the thoracic spine has a convex (outward) curve and the lumbar spine has a concave (inward) curve. The doctor also notes the symmetry of alignment of the shoulders, knees, and hips.

To assess alignment and degree of straightness of the spine, the doctor asks the patient to bend at the waist and let the arms

FIGURE 54-2 When you measure joint ROM, begin at the head and work down to the feet. *(continued)*

FIGURE 54-2 *(concluded)*

dangle freely. To assess knee position, the doctor asks the patient to stand with both feet together to determine whether the knees are at the same height, facing forward, and symmetrical.

▶ Cryotherapy and Thermotherapy LO 54.2

Applying cold to a patient's body for therapeutic reasons is called **cryotherapy**. This type of therapy can be administered in a number of ways. Treatments may be dry or wet, and they may be chemical or natural. Examples of dry cold applications are ice bags and ice packs. Wet cold applications include cold compresses and ice massage.

Applying heat to a patient's body for therapeutic reasons is called **thermotherapy**. As with cryotherapy, thermotherapy can be administered in a variety of ways. Examples of devices used in dry heat treatments are electric heating pads, hot-water bottles, and heat lamps. Moist heat treatments include hot soaks and the use of hot compresses and hot packs.

Factors Affecting the Use of Cryotherapy and Thermotherapy

To choose a cold or heat therapy for a patient, the physician considers the therapy's purpose, the location and condition of

TABLE 54-1 Contraindications, Precautions, and Side Effects Related to Cold and Heat

Therapy	Precautions	Contraindications	Side Effects
Dry and moist cold applications	Poor circulation, extreme age or youth, arthritis, and impaired sensation (insensitivity to cold)	Severe circulatory problems, inability to tolerate weight of device, and pain caused by application (more common with moist cold)	Numbness, pain, very pale or bluish skin, and blood clots (rare)
Dry and moist hot applications	Impaired kidney, heart, or lung functions; atherosclerosis; impaired sensation (insensitivity to heat); extreme age or youth; and pregnancy	Possibility of hemorrhage, malignancy; acute inflammation, like appendicitis; severe circulation problems; and pain caused by the weight of the device	Burns (especially with heat lamps), increased respiratory rate, and lowered blood pressure

the affected area, and the patient's age and general health. After choosing a therapy, the physician may direct you to apply the cold or heat treatment and to teach the patient and family how to continue the therapy at home.

Performed correctly, cold and heat therapies generally promote healing. These therapies can, however, cause side effects in some patients, so you need to exercise caution when applying the therapies. Cold therapy can cause damage to underlying nerves and tissues if applied incorrectly or for too long. Heat therapy can cause burns to the skin and underlying tissues if incorrectly applied. Monitor the patient carefully for signs of tissue damage, which include extreme blanching, redness, or blistering of the skin. You also need to be aware of conditions that contraindicate (make inadvisable) cold or heat therapies. Table 54-1 summarizes circumstances that warrant precautions or contraindications for the therapies and possible side effects. When performing any cold or heat therapy, you should consider the patient's age, treatment location, any patient problems with circulation or sensation, and individual temperature tolerance.

Treatment Location Thin-skinned areas often covered with clothing (like the back, chest, and abdomen) are more sensitive to cold and heat therapies than other areas, like the face and hands. Use caution around any broken skin (as with a wound) because it is susceptible to further tissue damage from cryotherapy or thermotherapy.

Circulation or Sensation Impairment Patients with diabetes or cardiovascular disease may have impaired circulation or sensory perception. These impairments may prevent such patients from sensing that a treatment is too cold or too hot. These patients require close monitoring during cryotherapy or thermotherapy. Carefully observe their skin to determine the treatment's therapeutic effect.

Temperature Tolerance Tolerance of temperature extremes varies greatly from person to person. Some people are unusually sensitive to cold or to heat. Listen carefully to patients for any indication of temperature intolerance during treatment. Cases of intolerance should be reported to the physician, who may decide to change the treatment.

Elderly Patients' Sensitivity to Cold and Heat

Age is an important consideration when using cryotherapy and thermotherapy. Elderly patients are usually more sensitive than others to cold and heat. They may have poor circulation; arthritis; impaired sensation; kidney, heart, or lung disease; or atherosclerosis. They also may have impaired skin integrity—thinning of the skin resulting in increased risk of skin tear, bruising, and burning. When administering cryotherapy or thermotherapy, stay with an elderly patient during its application to check the patient's skin frequently for excessive paleness or redness.

Principles of Cryotherapy

The application of cryotherapy causes blood vessels to constrict and involuntary muscles of the skin to contract. These physiologic responses can have the following results:

- Prevention of swelling by limiting edema, or fluid accumulation in body tissue.
- Control of bleeding by constricting blood vessels.
- Reduction of inflammation by slowing blood and fluid movement in the affected area.
- Provision of an anesthetic effect for pain by reducing inflammation.
- Reduction of pus formation by inhibiting microorganism activity.
- Lowering of body temperature.

Administering Cryotherapy

Cryotherapy is highly effective in alleviating swelling, pain, inflammation, and bleeding caused by various types of injuries. For best results, cryotherapy should be used frequently (about 20 minutes every hour) for the first 48 hours after an injury. As cold is applied, the skin becomes cool and pale because blood vessels constrict, decreasing the blood supply to the area. The decreased blood supply also reduces tissue metabolism, oxygen use, and waste accumulation.

Dry Cold Applications Dry cold applications include ice bags, ice collars, and chemical ice packs. An ice bag is a rubber or plastic bag with a locking lid. An ice collar is a rubber or plastic kidney-shaped bag, specially curved to fit around the back of the neck. A chemical ice pack is usually a flat plastic bag containing a semifluid chemical (Figure 54-3). Ice packs come in various sizes and types; some are disposable and others can be stored in a freezer and reused. The chemical prevents them from freezing solid, allowing them to be molded to the area to be treated. Chemical ice packs may

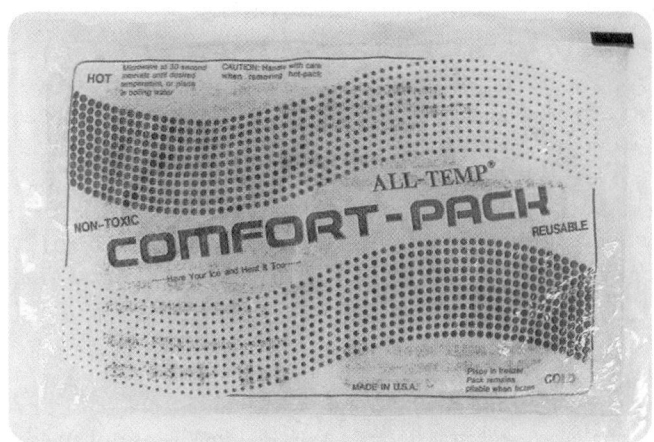

FIGURE 54-3 This chemical pack can be frozen, boiled, or microwaved for cold and heat therapy.

require squeezing or shaking to activate the cooling action. Most packs remain cold for 30 to 60 minutes. Some ice packs come with a soft covering; others must be wrapped in a cloth before they are applied to the skin.

Wet Cold Applications Wet cold applications include cold compresses and ice massage. A cold compress is a cloth or gauze pad moistened with ice water. It may be used to treat the pain associated with a toothache, tooth extraction, eye injury, or headache. The ice used in ice massage may be a cube wrapped in a plastic bag or water frozen in a paper cup. The combination of the cold temperature and the motion of the massage can provide therapeutic relief for the localized pain resulting from a sprain or strain. Although cold causes muscles to contract, the pain-relieving effect can help a patient relax. The procedure for administering cryotherapy is outlined in Procedure 54-1, at the end of this chapter.

Principles of Thermotherapy

The application of thermotherapy causes blood vessels to dilate (expand), which increases the blood supply to the area. Increased blood supply brings about an increased tissue metabolism that carries oxygen and nutrients to the cells of the area being treated. Increased metabolism carries toxins and wastes away from the cells. During thermotherapy, the treated skin becomes warm and develops **erythema** (redness) as the capillaries in the skin's deep layers fill with blood. These physiologic responses can have the following results:

- Relief of pain and congestion.
- Reduction of muscle spasms.
- Muscle relaxation.
- Reduction of inflammation.
- Reduction of swelling by increasing the fluid absorption from the tissues.

Administering Thermotherapy

Thermotherapy is highly effective in relieving pain, congestion, muscle spasms, and inflammation and promoting muscle relaxation. However, if heat is applied for too long, it may increase skin secretions that soften the skin and lower resistance. Heat that is too extreme can burn the skin or increase edema. Always monitor patients receiving thermotherapy, particularly children and elderly patients. The three basic types of thermotherapy are dry heat, moist heat, and diathermy. The general principles for administering the following types of thermotherapy are outlined in Procedure 54-2, at the end of this chapter.

Dry Heat Therapies Several types of dry heat therapy are available. They include the use of chemical hot packs, heating pads, hot-water bottles, heat lamps with infrared or ultraviolet bulbs, and fluidotherapy.

Chemical Hot Pack A chemical hot pack is a disposable, flexible pack of chemicals that becomes hot when you activate it by kneading or slapping it. After activating the pack, cover it with a cloth and place it on the patient's skin in the area being treated. Chemical hot packs are pliable and conform to body contours. For best results, follow the manufacturer's directions.

Heating Pad A heating pad is a flat pad with electrical coils between layers of soft fabric. When turned on, the coils provide localized heat. The physician should specify the heating pad temperature (low, medium, or high) and the length of time the pad should be applied.

Before applying a heating pad, cover it with a pillowcase or towel, check to be sure the cord is not frayed, and plug it into an electrical outlet. Make sure the patient's skin is dry. Then turn on the pad and set the temperature selector switch to the specified temperature. The patient should never lie on top of a heating pad, as burns could result.

Hot-Water Bottle A hot-water bottle is a flat, flexible, plastic or rubber bottle with a stopper. Fill the bottle with hot water, using a thermometer to make sure the water temperature does not exceed 125°F. For children under the age of 2 years and for elderly patients, the temperature should range from 105° to 115°F. For older children, a safe temperature is 115° to 125°F. Fill the bottle halfway; then compress it to expel air. The half-filled bottle can conform to the area to be treated. A half-filled bottle is also lighter than a full one so it is more comfortable for the patient. Cover the bottle with a cloth or pillowcase before you apply it.

After you apply the hot-water bottle, check with the patient to make sure the temperature is not too hot. Check the temperature frequently and replace the hot water as needed. Each time you remove the bottle, check the patient's skin to make sure it is merely warm to the touch.

Heat Lamp A heat lamp uses an infrared or ultraviolet bulb to provide heat. When the lamp is turned on, infrared rays heat and penetrate the skin's surface to a depth of 3 to 5 millimeters. To avoid burning the skin, place an infrared heat lamp 2 to 4 feet from the area being treated. Treatment usually lasts for 20 to 30 minutes or as directed by the physician.

Although ultraviolet rays produce little heat, they can burn the skin and damage the eyes. Ultraviolet rays are used to kill bacteria and promote vitamin D formation. They stimulate epithelial cells and cause blood vessels to overfill, increasing the skin's defenses against bacterial infections. Ultraviolet lamps are used to treat psoriasis, pressure sores, and wound infections.

Before recommending the use of an ultraviolet lamp, the physician assesses the patient's sensitivity and determines the treatment duration, which usually ranges from 30 seconds to a few minutes. The duration is usually increased in 10-second intervals. Because ultraviolet rays can burn the skin, monitor the patient closely. Do not leave the room during treatment. Both you and the patient must wear goggles to protect the eyes.

Fluidotherapy **Fluidotherapy** is a technique for stimulating healing, particularly in the hands and feet. The patient places the affected body part in a container of glass beads that are heated and agitated with hot air. Although the therapy is dry, its effect is similar to that of a therapy using water.

Moist Heat Applications Moist heat is often used to increase circulation and decrease pain to specific body areas, especially muscles and tendons. Moist heat applications include hot soak, hot compress, hot pack, and paraffin bath.

Hot Soak With hot-soak therapy, the patient places the affected body part—usually an arm or leg—in a container of plain or medicated water that has been heated to no more than 110°F. A hot soak should last about 15 minutes.

Hot Compress A compress is a piece of gauze or cloth suitable for covering a small area. After soaking the compress in hot water, wring it out and apply it to the area to be treated. Keep the compress warm either by placing a hot-water bottle on top of it or by frequently rewarming the compress in hot water.

Hot Pack A hot pack is a large canvas bag filled with a heat-retaining gel that is used on a large body area. Like a hot compress, a hot pack retains heat after being placed in hot water.

Paraffin Bath A paraffin bath is a receptacle of heated wax and mineral oil. It is used to reduce pain, muscle spasms, and stiffness in patients with arthritis and similar disorders. The patient's affected area should first be washed. Then it is dipped repeatedly into the mixture until the area is covered with a thick coat of wax. The wax remains on the area for about 30 minutes and then is peeled off. Particularly useful for joints, especially the hands and feet, the paraffin bath has the added benefit of leaving the skin warm, flexible, and soft. Some erythema may result.

Alternating Hot and Cold Packs A physician may order application of a hot pack followed by a cold pack. This increases circulation to the area by dilating and constricting the blood vessels. Be sure to apply the hot pack first. Applying the cold pack first can numb the skin and keep the patient from recognizing a hot pack is too hot. This can result in serious skin burns.

Diathermy **Diathermy** is a type of heat therapy in which a machine produces high-frequency waves that achieve deep heat penetration in muscle tissue. The heat helps decrease joint stiffness, dilate blood vessels, relieve muscle spasms, and reduce discomfort from sprains and strains. Three types of diathermy are ultrasound, shortwave, and microwave. Equipment for these therapies is continually being improved. Be sure to familiarize yourself with the manufacturer's instructions regarding the specific equipment in your office.

Ultrasound Ultrasound is the most common type of diathermy, used to treat sprains, strains, and other acute ailments. It projects high-frequency sound waves that are converted to heat in muscle tissue.

Ultrasound diathermy may be administered by rubbing a gel-covered transducer over the skin in circular patterns. It also may be administered to a body part under water. Do not use ultrasound in areas where bones are near the skin's surface as this could cause bone damage.

Shortwave Shortwave diathermy uses radio waves that travel through the body between two condenser plates and are converted to heat in the tissues. This type of diathermy is used to treat acute, subacute, and chronic inflammation. Treatment typically ranges from 20 to 30 minutes. Do not use shortwave diathermy on a patient who has a pacemaker.

Microwave Microwave diathermy uses microwaves to provide heat deep in body tissues. Contraindications include use on patients with pacemakers, use in combination with wet dressings, or use in high dosages on patients with swollen tissue. Also, never use microwave diathermy near metal implants because the reaction between metal and microwaves could cause burns.

▶ Hydrotherapy   LO 54.3

Hydrotherapy is the use of water to treat physical problems. It is typically performed in the physical therapy department of a hospital, in an outpatient clinic, or at home. Common forms of hydrotherapy include the use of whirlpools and contrast baths and underwater exercises.

Whirlpools

Whirlpools are tanks in which water is agitated by jets of air under pressure. Whirlpools vary in size from small (capable of accommodating only one body part) to very large (capable of accommodating a wheelchair or full-body submersion). The agitated water's action in a whirlpool generates a hydromassage, which relaxes muscles and increases circulation. Whirlpools also are used to cleanse and debride (remove foreign matter and dead tissue from) the skin of patients with wounds, ulcers, or burns.

Contrast Baths

Contrast baths are separate baths, one filled with hot water and the other with cold water. The patient alternately moves the treated body part quickly from one bath to the other. This treatment induces relaxation, stimulates improved circulation (which speeds up healing), and results in greater mobility.

Underwater Exercises

Underwater exercises—prescribed for patients with joint injuries, burns, and arthritis—are usually performed in a warm swimming pool. Because the water's buoyancy takes pressure off the joints, these exercises are particularly useful for patients with painful or limited movement. Combined with the movement of the water around the body, the exercises promote relaxation and increased circulation.

▶ Exercise Therapy   LO 54.4

For many patients, exercise is as important as medications or other treatments and offers both preventive and therapeutic benefits. As a patient ages, exercise helps promote flexibility, mobility, muscle tone, and strength. Exercise is a primary treatment for fractures, arthritis, and some respiratory disorders; it can minimize symptoms or help slow disease progression. For patients who have had surgery, stroke, burns, or amputation, regular exercise therapy can help prevent problems caused by inactivity.

A doctor orders exercise therapy for many reasons. Exercise improves or restores general health and is especially therapeutic when a patient is weak from illness. Explain to patients that exercise will help them to

- Improve muscle tone and strength.
- Regain ROM after an injury.
- Prevent ROM from diminishing in chronic conditions.
- Prevent or correct physical deformities.
- Promote neuromuscular coordination.
- Improve circulation.
- Relieve stress.
- Lower cholesterol levels.
- Aid in the resumption of normal daily activities.

Commonly used for treating sports injuries, exercise therapy for injured athletes is described in the Educating the Patient section. This type of therapy focuses primarily on regaining muscle strength and flexibility in the injured area.

Role of the Medical Assistant

As a medical assistant, you may have several roles in exercise therapy. As an information resource for the patient and family, you must understand various types of exercise programs and the patient's specific treatment plan. You also may serve as a source of support and encouragement when exercise programs are long and difficult. You may, for example, assist with ROM exercises and teach the patient and family how to perform them at home.

When teaching patients about exercises, give them illustrations of the exercises. Include with each illustration written instructions on the number of times to perform the exercise, as prescribed by the doctor.

After demonstrating each exercise, have patients perform it while you watch and give direction. Patients are more likely to perform exercises properly at home if they can perform them correctly in your presence. It is also helpful for patients' caregivers or family members to watch and perform the exercises to become familiar with them.

Types of Exercise

Before a patient begins an exercise program, the doctor evaluates the patient's heart and lung function and overall physical condition. The doctor adjusts the level of exercise accordingly and may prescribe other forms of physical therapy, like cryotherapy, thermotherapy, or hydrotherapy. Careful preparation by the doctor and patient before beginning an exercise therapy program helps prevent injuries. Some measures to prevent and treat common exercise therapy problems are outlined in Table 54-2. A doctor may also refer a patient to a physical therapist, who will develop an exercise program specifically for that patient. Types of exercises in therapeutic programs include active mobility, passive mobility, aided mobility, active resistance, isometric, and ROM.

Active Mobility Exercises Active mobility exercises are self-directed exercises the patient performs without assistance to increase muscle strength and function. They often require equipment like a stationary bicycle or a treadmill.

Passive Mobility Exercises In passive mobility exercises, the physical therapist or a machine moves a patient's body part. The patient does not actively assist in these exercises. Patients who require passive mobility exercises may have neuromuscular disability or weakness. These exercises can help retain patients' ROM and improve their circulation.

Aided Mobility Exercises Aided mobility exercises are self-directed exercises. The patient performs them with the aid of a device like an exercise machine or a therapy pool. Aided mobility exercises help retain or increase patients' ROM.

TABLE 54-2	Preventing and Treating Common Problems of Exercise Therapy	
Problem	**Prevention Methods**	**Treatment**
Muscle strain	Beginning with gentle warm-up exercises	Rest and application of heat followed by ice
Muscle aches	Keeping track of the number of repetitions and amount of weight (resistance), if used; increasing the number of repetitions or amount of weight slowly	Rest and soaking in hot bath to relieve aches
Impatience with slowness of progress	Discussing expectations with patient; setting realistic goals with patient; stressing necessity of avoiding recurrent injury, which would prolong recovery	Creation of goal sheet, noting small successes as therapy progresses

The Injured Athlete

The risk of injury is associated with most sports, but some sports carry a greater risk of serious injury than others. Many sports-related injuries affect joints in the neck, shoulders, elbows, wrists, hands, knees, ankles, or feet.

You may be called on to educate injured athletes and to start them on the road to recovery. To do so, you need to understand the mind of the athlete. Why do many athletes get injured in the first place? Here are some reasons:

- The sport they participate in has a high injury rate.
- They return to a sport before their injuries are completely healed.
- They become impatient with a physical therapy regimen.
- They do not work at gradual muscle strengthening.

When does your job begin? After diagnosing the injury, the physician will probably refer the athlete to a sports medicine center or other physical therapy setting, where an individualized program will be set up. As a medical assistant, you will often be responsible for counseling an athlete about the physical therapy program she will be entering. Here are some basic rules you can communicate:

- Follow the physical therapy regimen set up by the physician or physical therapist—even if it is tedious or time-consuming.
- Use only the equipment specified by the therapist: free weights, weight-training equipment, stationary bike, other aerobic equipment, or swimming pool. The physical therapist recommends the designated equipment based on the type of injury. Using other equipment could cause further injury or interfere with healing.

- Do not rush the therapy in an attempt to recover more quickly.
- Work slowly to strengthen muscles and improve flexibility.
- Continue exercises at home as instructed.
- Be patient.

Explain to the athlete how the physical therapy program will be presented. Knowing what to expect from the physical therapist can improve the athlete's compliance. Here are some explanations you might offer:

- The therapist will demonstrate exercises and then watch you perform them.
- The therapist may increase the number of repetitions or the amount of resistance (weight) but probably not both at the same time.
- The therapist will provide handouts illustrating the exercises, along with instructions on how to perform them.
- The therapist may provide an activity log to help you chart your progress.

An athlete who is impatient with a physical therapy regimen and returns to a sport before an injury has completely healed has an increased risk of repeated injury. Impress on the athlete the importance of the physical therapy process. Emphasize the need for gradual strengthening and healing over a period of time. To help the athlete in the long run, focus on recovery from injury and on the need to prevent recurrent injury.

Active Resistance Exercises In active resistance exercises, the patient works against resistance (counter-pressure) to increase muscle strength. Resistance is provided manually by the therapist or mechanically by an exercise machine.

Isometric Exercises During isometric exercises, the patient relaxes and then contracts the muscles of a body part while in a fixed position. Isometric exercises can maintain the patient's muscle strength when a joint is temporarily or permanently immobilized.

ROM Exercises ROM exercises move each joint through its full range of motion. These exercises should be done slowly and gently. Doing them too quickly or too soon after an injury can cause pain, fracture, or bleeding into the joint. For this reason, a physical therapist assesses the patient and determines a recommended regimen of ROM exercises. You may be asked to educate the patient and caregiver or family about the regimen.

ROM exercises are typically prescribed after a joint injury. The physical therapist may recommend that the joint be moved

in its full range of motion three times, twice a day. ROM exercises are also recommended for elderly people, to improve circulation and muscle function. The therapist will prescribe one of three types of ROM exercises for patients:

1. Active range of motion exercises: performed by the patient without assistance.
2. Assisted range of motion exercises: performed by the patient with the help of another person or a machine.
3. Passive range of motion exercises: performed by another person or a machine

ROM exercises do not build muscle strength but do improve flexibility and mobility. Typical ROM exercises are illustrated in Figure 54-4.

Electrical Stimulation

Electrical stimulation helps prevent atrophy in muscles that cannot move voluntarily by causing the muscles to contract involuntarily (on impulse) and relax. Electrical stimulators deliver controlled amounts of low-voltage electric current to motor and sensory nerves to stimulate muscles. Frequent and regular

FIGURE 54-4 A medical assistant helps a patient perform typical ROM exercises: (a) shoulder abduction, (b) back rotation, (c) hip flexion, and (d) toe abduction.

electrical stimulation also aids in healing injured joints and in revitalizing muscles.

Electrical stimulation can help retrain a patient to use injured muscles by creating a perceivable connection between the stimulus (muscle movement) and the area of the brain that controls those muscles. If a limb does not function because of injury or disease, this therapy can give the patient hope that injured muscles are not dead. Hope often encourages a patient to work harder and to cooperate in the physical therapy regimen, which can be long and arduous. Wearable electrical stimulation units are being developed for people with spinal cord injuries to help them retrain affected muscles.

▶ Massage   LO 54.5

The practice of massage uses pressure, kneading, stroking, vibration, and tapping to positively affect patients' health and well-being. Massage helps the patient relax and counteracts the effects of stress. During massage, the heart rate and blood pressure are lowered and blood circulation and lymph flow are increased. Massage helps reduce pain caused by tight muscles and helps relax muscle spasms.

Massage benefits the mind as well as the body: It helps improve concentration, promotes restful sleep, and helps the mind relax. Many patients find they handle daily stresses better when

FIGURE 54-5 An example of Swedish massage. Massage uses kneading, pressure, stroking, and human touch to alleviate pain and promote healing through relaxation.

they have regular massage. People who get massages on a regular basis find they become ill less often and less severely and they feel less stressed and tense. Some patients notice their muscles beginning to tighten and are aware that if they get a massage, it will decrease muscle tension before it becomes severe.

Swedish Massage

Swedish massage is one of the best-known and most frequently taught massage techniques. It stimulates circulation and lymph flow with five basic strokes that manipulate the body's soft tissues. The strokes include pétrissage (kneading), effleurage (stroking), tapotement (percussion), vibration, and friction. Oils and/or lotions are used to reduce friction on the patient's skin. One type of Swedish massage is done on warm muscles immediately after exercise. Another type is a stress-reduction massage that is done with the same basic strokes on patients who have not been exercising (Figure 54-5).

Neuromuscular Massage

Neuromuscular massage is applied to specific muscles and helps release tension and knots, relieve pain and release pressure on nerves, and increase blood flow. Trigger point therapy is one type of neuromuscular massage in which strong finger pressure is applied to trigger points in the muscles.

▶ Traction   LO 54.6

Traction is the pulling or stretching of the musculoskeletal system to treat fractured bones and dislocated, arthritic, or other diseased joints. It is traditionally performed by a therapist in a specially equipped setting. A physical therapist may set up traction in the patient's home and visit regularly to ensure that the equipment is used and maintained properly. Traction may be used to

- Create and maintain proper bone alignment.
- Reduce or prevent joint stiffening and abnormal muscle shortening.

- Correct deformities.
- Relieve compression of vertebral joints.
- Reduce or relieve muscle spasms.

Although you will not be setting up or performing traction, you should know about its types and uses. This information will prepare you to answer basic questions from patients and family members.

Manual Traction

The physical therapist performs manual traction by using his hands to pull a patient's limb or head gently. Pulling stretches the muscles and separates the joints, allowing for greater motion and less stiffening. Manual traction is used with patients who have muscle spasms, stiffness, and arthritis.

Static Traction

To perform static traction, or weight traction, the therapist places a patient's limb, pelvis, or chin in a harness. The harness is then attached to weights through a pulley system. This type of traction is commonly used to relieve muscle spasms.

Skeletal Traction

Skeletal traction is performed in inpatient facilities on patients whose injuries require long traction time and heavy weights. During surgery, a surgeon inserts pins, wires, or tongs into bones. After surgery, the pins, wires, or tongs are attached to pulleys and weights to provide continuous traction.

Mechanical Traction

Mechanical traction uses a special device that intermittently pulls and relaxes a prescribed body part, such as the neck. The therapist sets the time intervals between contractions and relaxations. Mechanical traction is used to promote relaxation.

▶ Mobility Aids   LO 54.7

Mobility aids (also called *mobility assistive devices*) are designed to improve patients' ability to ambulate, or move from one place to another. These include canes, walkers, crutches, and wheelchairs.

The appropriate aid depends on the patient's disability, muscle coordination, strength, and age. The patient may need a device temporarily—perhaps crutches after a sprain—or permanently—like a wheelchair in the case of permanent paralysis.

Canes

Canes provide support and help patients maintain balance. They come in several styles, including standard, tripod, and quad-base (Figure 54-6), which are all lightweight, are made of wood or aluminum, and have a rubber tip or tips at the bottom. Canes are especially useful for patients with weaknesses on one side of the body (possibly due to a stroke), joint disability, or neuromuscular defects.

A standard cane is best for a patient who needs only a small amount of support. Its curved handle is convenient, allowing the patient to hang it from a pocket or a doorknob. When the

FIGURE 54-6 Shown here are three styles of canes: (a) standard, (b) tripod, and (c) quad-base.

Source: Borrowed from *McGraw-Hill Health Care Science Technology* by Booth, 2004.

FIGURE 54-7 A standard walker.

patient uses a standard cane, however, the curved handle concentrates most of the patient's weight in one small area of the hand. To avoid stressing the hand in this way, some standard canes have a T-shaped handle, which distributes pressure on the hand more evenly. Tripod canes have three legs, and quad-base canes have four. The multiple legs create a wide base of support, making them more stable than a standard cane. Tripod and quad-base canes can stand alone, freeing up the patient's hands when she sits down. These canes are bulkier and more difficult to pick up and put down than a standard cane, however. Both styles have T-shaped handles.

After determining the most suitable cane for the patient, the physical therapist adjusts the cane's height. When the cane is the correct height, the patient's elbow is flexed at 20 to 25 degrees and the patient stands tall while using the cane (instead of leaning on it for support). The therapist makes sure the handle is the right size for the patient's hand and instructs the patient on how to use the cane. If directed, you may do the teaching or reinforce it, as discussed in Procedure 54-3, at the end of this chapter.

Walkers

A walker is a lightweight, easy-to-use aluminum frame that is open on one side and has four widely placed, adjustable, rubber-tipped legs that can be adjusted to various heights (Figure 54-7). Some models are designed to fold up for storage. To use a walker, the patient stands within the frame and leans on the upper bar, which has a handgrip on each side.

Typically, older patients who are too weak to walk unassisted or who have balance problems use a walker. The walker is designed to give these patients a sense of stability as they ambulate. In tight spaces or in areas with throw rugs, however, a walker may be difficult to manage. A patient who is too weak to pick up the walker may use a walker on wheels. Wheeled walkers have brakes for safety. Patients should never slide a walker that does not have wheels because the movement could easily result in a fall.

A physical therapist selects a walker that suits the patient's abilities and height. A walker should reach the patient's hipbone. See Table 54-3 for more information about different types of walkers. Although the physical therapist usually trains the

TABLE 54-3	**Types of Walkers**		
Walker	**Features**	**Advantages**	**Disadvantages**
Standard	No wheels, adjustable legs	Very stable on flat surfaces; easier to use than crutches	Requires upper-body strength to use
Standard folding	No wheels, sides fold in	Easy to transport and store	Requires upper-body strength to use, requires pressing a tab to release and fold
Rolling	Front wheels	Requires less upper-body strength to use	Not as stable as a standard walker
Rolling with brakes	Front wheels and brakes	Disengages wheels when weight from upper body is applied	Not as stable as a standard walker
Three-wheel rolling with brakes	Bicycle-style hand brakes	Better maneurverability; folds for transport and storage	Requires better balance than other walkers
Reciprocal	Each side of walker moves alternately	Allows for more natural gait	Requires better balance and coordination than other walkers; catches on some floor surfaces

patient in the use of a walker, you may be asked to do this, or you may need to reinforce the information presented in Procedure 54-4, at the end of this chapter.

Crutches

Crutches allow a patient to walk without putting weight on the feet or legs by transferring that weight to the arms. Crutches are made of aluminum or wood. Aluminum crutches are lighter and usually more expensive than those made of wood. Pediatric crutches are available for children. The two basic types of crutches are axillary and Lofstrand. Procedure 54-5, at the end of this chapter, provides the steps for teaching patients how to use crutches.

Axillary crutches reach from the ground to the armpit. Each crutch has a rubber tip on the bottom to prevent slipping. This type of crutch is designed for short-term use by patients with injuries such as a sprained ankle.

Lofstrand, or Canadian, crutches reach from the ground to the forearm, and each one has a rubber tip on the bottom to prevent slipping. For additional support, this type has a handgrip extension attached at a 90-degree angle and a metal cuff that fits securely around the patient's forearm. Lofstrand crutches are geared for long-term use by patients with disorders such as paraplegia (Figure 54-8).

Measuring the Patient for Crutches To prevent back pain and nerve injury to the armpits and palms, crutches must be measured to fit each patient. Axillary crutches that are too long can put pressure on nerves in the armpit, causing a condition called crutch palsy (muscle weakness in the forearm, wrist, and hand). They also can force the patient's shoulders forward, causing strain on the back and making ambulation difficult. Crutches that are too short force the patient to bend forward during ambulation, causing back pain or imbalance, which can lead to falls.

Before a patient who uses crutches leaves the office, make sure the crutches fit properly and that the patient is comfortable walking with them. To confirm a correct fit, check for the following conditions (see Figure 54-9):

- The patient is wearing the type of shoes he will wear when walking.
- The patient is standing erect with feet slightly apart.
- The crutch tips are positioned 2 to 6 inches in front of the patient's feet and 4 to 6 inches to the side of each foot.
- The axillary supports allow 2 to 3 finger-widths between supports and armpits. (Use wing nuts and bolts to adjust crutches.)
- The handgrips are positioned to create 30-degree flexion at the elbows. (Use wing nuts and bolts to adjust; use a goniometer to check flexion.)

Crutch Gaits To teach a patient how to stand and walk with crutches, you must learn the crutch gaits, or walks. First, show the patient the standing, or tripod, position. To do this, have the patient stand erect and look straight ahead. The patient should place the crutch tips 4 to 6 inches in front of her feet and 4 to 6 inches away from the side of each foot. See Figure 54-10.

Go to CONNECT to see a video about *Teaching a Patient How to Use Crutches.*

FIGURE 54-8 A child using Lofstrand crutches.

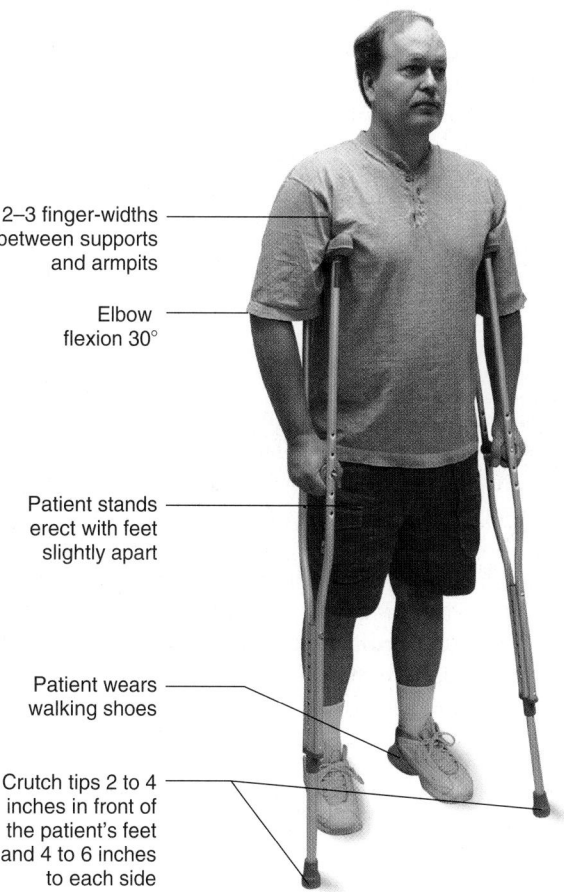

2–3 finger-widths between supports and armpits

Elbow flexion 30°

Patient stands erect with feet slightly apart

Patient wears walking shoes

Crutch tips 2 to 4 inches in front of the patient's feet and 4 to 6 inches to each side

FIGURE 54-9 Use these guidelines when measuring a patient for crutches.

FIGURE 54-10 This is the correct beginning position for the patient's feet and crutches when you are teaching a patient to walk with crutches.

Source: Borrowed from *McGraw-Hill Health Care Science Technology* by Booth, 2004.

To determine the proper gait for a patient, you will make a preteaching assessment of the patient's muscle coordination and physical condition. In general, instruct a patient to use a slow gait in crowded areas or when feeling tired. The patient can use a faster gait in open places or when feeling more energetic. Using various gaits and speeds enables the patient to exercise different muscle groups and improve overall conditioning.

Four-Point Gait The four-point gait is a slow gait used only when a patient can bear weight on both legs. Because this gait has three points of contact with the ground at all times, it is stable and safe. It is especially useful for patients with leg muscle weakness, spasticity, or poor balance or coordination. To teach this gait, have the patient start in the tripod position. Then outline the following steps, as illustrated in Figure 54-11a:

1. Move the right crutch forward.
2. Move the left foot forward to the level of the left crutch.
3. Move the left crutch forward.
4. Move the right foot forward to level of the right crutch.

Three-Point Gait The three-point gait is used when a patient cannot bear weight on one leg but can bear full weight on the unaffected leg. This gait allows the patient's weight to be carried alternately by the crutches and by the unaffected leg. It is appropriate for amputees, patients with tissue or musculoskeletal trauma (like a fractured or sprained leg), and those recovering from leg surgery. The patient must have good muscle coordination and arm strength, however. To teach this gait, have the patient start in the tripod position. Then give the patient the following instructions, as illustrated in Figure 54-11b:

1. Move both crutches and the affected leg forward.
2. Move the unaffected leg forward while weight is balanced on both crutches.

Two-Point Gait The two-point gait is faster than the four-point gait and is used by patients who can bear some weight on both feet and have good muscle coordination and balance. To

(a)

(b)

(c)

FIGURE 54-11 Crutch gaits include (a) a four-point gait, (b) a three-point gait, and (c) a two-point gait.

(a)　　　　**(b)**

FIGURE 54-12 Patients with severe disabilities may walk with crutches using (a) the swing-to gait or (b) the swing-through gait.

teach this gait, have the patient start in the tripod position. Then outline the following steps, as illustrated in Figure 54-11c:

1. Move the left crutch and the right foot forward at the same time.
2. Move the right crutch and the left foot forward at the same time.

Swing Gaits Patients with severe disabilities, like leg paralysis or deformity, may use one of two swing gaits: the swing-to gait or the swing-through gait (Figure 54-12a and b). To teach the swing-to gait, have the patient start in the tripod position. Then outline the following steps:

1. Move both crutches forward at the same time.
2. Lift the body and swing to the crutches.
3. End with the tripod position again.

To teach the swing-through gait, have the patient start in the tripod position. Then review the following steps:

1. Move both crutches forward.
2. Move the body and swing past the crutches.

Wheelchairs

Wheelchairs range from small, folding models to large, motorized ones. The physical therapist will select an appropriate wheelchair depending on the patient's disability and the length of time the wheelchair will be needed.

When patients come to the medical office in a wheelchair, the doctor may not be able to examine them adequately if they remain in the wheelchair. If this is the case, you will be responsible for transferring the patients from the wheelchair to the examining table and back to the wheelchair after the exam. To ensure their safety and yours, see the *Assisting with a General Physical Examination* chapter for more information about transferring patients from a wheelchair. Here are some reminders on preventing injury:

- Ask for help if the patient is weak, heavy, or unstable.
- Explain to the patient the steps of transfer you will use.
- Before starting the transfer, make sure the wheelchair is in the locked position and the patient is sitting at the front of the wheelchair seat.
- When you lift, use the large muscles in your thighs, which are stronger than your back muscles.
- When lifting, bend from the knees and keep your back straight.
- Count to 3 and enlist the patient's help on the count of 3.

▶ Referral to a Physical Therapist　　LO 54.8

If the doctor refers the patient to a physical therapist or other specialist, you may be asked to contact the specialist directly or to give the patient a written order and information about contacting the specialist. Keep a file with information about the therapists your office uses. In the file, note the forms and information each therapist requires. If you speak to the therapist, be sure to inform the doctor and to document the referral in the patient's chart. The therapist may be an independent practitioner or may be employed by a hospital, clinic, or home healthcare agency.

In addition to physical therapy, some patients may decide to try alternative therapies, like acupuncture, chiropractic, or biofeedback training. These therapies are acknowledged by many healthcare professionals and often provide relief for people with chronic pain or other debilitating conditions.

PROCEDURE 54-1　Administering Cryotherapy

Procedure Goal: To reduce pain and swelling by safely and effectively administering cryotherapy.

OSHA Guidelines:

Materials: Gloves, cold application materials required as ordered: ice bag, ice collar, chemical cold pack, washcloth or gauze squares, or ice.

Method: Procedure steps.

　　1. Double-check the physician's order. Be sure you know where to apply therapy and how long it should remain in place.

2. Identify the patient and explain the procedure and its purpose. Ask if the patient has any questions.

3. Have the patient undress and put on a gown, if required; provide privacy or assistance as needed.

4. Wash your hands and don gloves.

5. Position the patient comfortably and drape appropriately.
RATIONALE: The patient should be able to relax during the therapy.

6. Prepare the therapy as ordered.
- Ice bag or collar
  a. Prior to use, check the ice bag or collar for leaks.
  b. Fill the ice bag or collar two-thirds full with ice chips or small ice cubes. Compress the container to expel any air and then close it.
RATIONALE: Ice will not conform to the patient if there is air in the bag.
  c. Dry the bag or collar completely and cover it with a towel. This will absorb moisture and provide comfort.
- Chemical ice pack
  a. Check the pack for leaks.
RATIONALE: To avoid the chemicals coming in contact with the patient.
  b. Shake or squeeze the pack to activate the chemicals, or use a cold chemical pack taken from a refrigerator or freezer.
RATIONALE: Pack will not be cold if it is not activated.
  c. Cover the pack with a towel.
RATIONALE: To keep the patient comfortable and avoid cold burn.

- Cold compress
  a. Place the washcloth or gauze squares under a stream of running water.
  b. Wring them out.
  c. Rewet at frequent intervals.

7. Place the device on the patient's affected body part. If you are using a compress, place an ice bag on it, if desired, to keep it colder longer.

8. Ask the patient how the device feels.
RATIONALE: To prevent cold burn of the skin.

9. Explain the cold is of great benefit, although it may be somewhat uncomfortable.

10. Leave the device in place for the length of time ordered by the physician. Periodically check the skin for color, feeling, and pain. If the area becomes excessively pale or blue, numb, or painful, remove the device and have the physician examine the area. For cold application using ice, limit application time to 20 minutes.
RATIONALE: To reduce the possibility of cold burn.

11. Remove the application and observe the area for reduced swelling, redness, and pain. If the patient has a dressing, replace it at this time.

12. Help the patient dress, if needed.

13. Remove equipment and supplies, properly discarding used disposable materials; sanitize, disinfect, and/or sterilize reusable equipment and materials as needed.

14. Remove the gloves and wash your hands.

15. Document the treatment and your observation in the patient's chart. If you teach the patient or the patient's family how to use the device, document your instructions.

PROCEDURE 54-2 Administering Thermotherapy

Procedure Goal: To administer thermotherapy safely and effectively.

OSHA Guidelines:

Materials: Gloves, towels, blanket, heat application materials required for order: chemical hot pack, heating pad, hot-water bottle, heat lamp, container and medication for hot soak, and container and gauze for hot compress.

Method: Procedure steps.

1. Double-check the physician's order. Be sure you know where to apply therapy, the proper temperature for the application, and how long it should remain in place.

2. Identify the patient and explain the procedure and its purpose. Ask if the patient has any questions.

3. Have the patient undress and put on a gown, if required; provide privacy or assistance as needed.

4. Wash your hands and don gloves.

5. Position the patient comfortably and drape appropriately.
RATIONALE: The patient should be able to relax during the therapy.

6. If the patient has a dressing, check the dressing for blood and change as necessary. Alert the physician and ask if treatment should continue.
RATIONALE: If the wound is actively bleeding, heat application could cause increased bleeding.

7. Check the temperature by touch and look for the presence of adverse skin conditions (excessive redness, blistering, or irritation) on all applications before and during the treatment.
RATIONALE: To avoid patient burn injuries.

8. As necessary, reheat devices or solutions to provide therapeutic temperatures and then reapply them.

9. Prepare the therapy as ordered.
- Chemical hot pack
  a. Check the pack for leaks.
RATIONALE: To avoid the chemicals coming in contact with the patient.

b. Activate the pack. (Check manufacturer's directions.)

RATIONALE: The pack will not get hot if it is not activated.

c. Cover the pack with a towel.

- Heating pad
  a. Turn the heating pad on, selecting the appropriate temperature setting.
  b. Cover the pad with a towel or pillowcase.
  c. Make sure the patient's skin is dry and do not allow the patient to lie on top of the heating pad.

RATIONALE: To avoid burns.

- Hot-water bottle
  a. Fill the bottle one-half full with hot water of the correct temperature—usually 110°F to 115°F. Use a thermometer. The physician can provide information on the ideal temperature water that should be used, which will depend on the area being treated.
  b. Expel the air and close the bottle.

RATIONALE: The bottle should conform to the body part.

  c. Cover the bottle with a towel or pillowcase.

RATIONALE: To avoid burns.

- Heat lamp
  a. Place the lamp 2 to 4 feet away from the treatment area. (Check manufacturer's directions.)
  b. Follow the treatment time as ordered.

- Hot soak
  a. Select a container of the appropriate size for the area to be treated.
  b. Fill the container with hot water that is no more than 110°F. Use a thermometer. Add medication to the container if ordered.

- Hot compress
  a. Soak a washcloth or gauze in hot water. Wring it out.
  b. Frequently rewarm the compress to maintain the temperature.

10. Place the device on the patient's affected body part, or place the affected body part in the container. If you are using a compress, place a hot-water bottle on top, if desired, to keep it warm longer.

11. Ask the patient how the device feels. During any heat therapy, remember, dilated blood vessels cause heat loss from the skin and this heat loss may make the patient feel chilled. Be prepared to cover the patient with sheets or blankets.

12. Leave the device in place for the length of time ordered by the physician. Periodically check the skin for redness, blistering, or irritation. If the area becomes excessively red or develops blisters, remove the patient from the heat source and have the physician examine the area.

13. Remove the application and observe the area for inflammation and swelling. Replace the patient's dressing if necessary.

14. Help the patient dress, if needed.

15. Remove equipment and supplies, properly discarding used disposable materials, and sanitize, disinfect, and/or sterilize reusable equipment and materials as needed.

16. Remove the gloves and wash your hands.

17. Document the treatment and your observation in the patient's chart. If you teach the patient or the patient's family how to use the device, document your instructions.

PROCEDURE 54-3 Teaching a Patient How to Use a Cane

Procedure Goal: To teach a patient how to use a cane safely.

OSHA Guidelines: This procedure does not involve exposure to blood, body fluids, or tissues.

Materials: A cane suited to the patient's needs.

Method: Procedure steps.

Standing from a Sitting Position

1. Instruct the patient to slide his buttocks to the edge of the chair.

2. Tell the patient to place his right foot slightly behind and inside the right front leg of the chair and his left foot slightly behind and inside the left front leg of the chair. (This provides him with a wide, stable stance.)

3. Instruct the patient to lean forward and use the armrests or seat of the chair to push upward. Caution the patient not to lean on the cane.

4. Have the patient position the cane for support on the uninjured or strong side of his body, as indicated.

Walking

1. Teach the patient to hold the cane on the uninjured or strong side of her body with the tip(s) of the cane 4 to 6 inches from the side and in front of her strong foot. Remind the patient to make sure the tip is flat on the ground.

RATIONALE: To reduce the risk of the patient falling.

2. Have the patient move the cane forward approximately 8 inches and then move her affected foot forward, parallel to the cane.

3. Next, have the patient move her strong leg forward past the cane and her weak leg.

4. Observe as the patient repeats this process.

Ascending Stairs

1. Instruct the patient to always start with his uninjured or strong leg when going up stairs.

2. Advise the patient to keep the cane on the uninjured or strong side of his body and to use the wall or rail, if available, for support on the weak side. If a rail is not available, the patient may need assistance for safety.

3. After the patient steps on the strong leg, instruct him to bring up his weak leg and then the cane.

4. Remind the patient not to rush.

Descending Stairs

1. Instruct the patient to always start with her weak leg when going down stairs.

2. Advise the patient to keep the cane on the uninjured or strong side of her body and to use the wall or rail, if available, for support on the weak side. If a rail is

not available, the patient may need assistance for safety.

3. Have the patient use the uninjured or strong leg and wall or rail to support her body, put the cane on the next step, and bend the strong leg as she lowers the weak leg to the next step.

4. Instruct the patient to step down with the strong leg.

Walking on Snow or Ice

Suggest the patient try a metal ice-gripping cane or a ski pole. These can be dug into the snow or ice to prevent slipping. Instruct the patient to avoid walking on ice unless absolutely necessary.

PROCEDURE 54-4 Teaching a Patient How to Use a Walker

Procedure Goal: To teach a patient how to use a walker safely.

OSHA Guidelines: This procedure does not involve exposure to blood, body fluids, or tissues.

Materials: A walker suited to the patient's needs.

Method: Procedure steps.

Walking

1. Instruct the patient to step into the walker.

2. Tell the patient to place her hands on the handgrips on the sides of the walker.

3. Make sure the patient's feet are far enough apart so she feels balanced.
   RATIONALE: A wider base provides for better balance.

4. Instruct the patient to pick up the walker and move it forward about 6 inches.

5. Have the patient move one foot forward and then the other foot.

6. Instruct the patient to pick up the walker again and move it forward. If the patient is strong enough, explain that

she may advance the walker after moving each leg rather than waiting until she has moved both legs.

Sitting

1. Teach the patient to turn his back to the chair or bed.

2. Instruct the patient to take small, careful steps and to back up until he feels the chair or bed at the back of his legs.

3. Instruct the patient to keep the walker in front of himself, let go of the walker, and place both his hands on the arms or seat of the chair or on the bed.

4. Teach the patient to balance himself on his arms while lowering himself slowly to the chair or bed.

5. If the patient has an injured or affected leg, he should keep it forward while bending his unaffected leg and lowering his body to the chair or bed.

Ascending and Descending Stairs

If a patient needs to use a walker on stairs, refer him to a physical therapist for additional training.

PROCEDURE 54-5 Teaching a Patient How to Use Crutches

Procedure Goal: To teach a patient how to use crutches safely.

OSHA Guidelines: This procedure does not involve exposure to blood, body fluids, or tissues.

Materials: A pair of crutches suited to the patient's needs.

Method: Procedure steps.

1. Verify the physician's order for the type of crutches and gait to be used.

2. Wash your hands, identify the patient, and explain the procedure.

3. Elderly patients or patients with muscle weakness should be taught muscle strength exercises for their arms.

4. Have the patient stand erect and look straight ahead.

5. Tell the patient to place the crutch tips 2 to 6 inches in front of and 4 to 6 inches to the side of each foot.

6. When instructing a patient to use an axillary crutch, make sure the patient has a 2-inch gap between the axilla and the axillary bar and that each elbow is flexed 25 to 30 degrees.
   RATIONALE: To reduce the incidence of nerve injury to the axilla.

FIGURE Procedure 54-5 Step 6   The patient's elbow should be flexed 25 to 30 degrees.

7. Teach the patient how to get up from a chair:
   a. Instruct the patient to hold both crutches on his affected or weaker side.
   b. Have the patient slide to the edge of the chair.
   c. Tell the patient to push down on the arm or seat of the chair on his stronger side and use his strong leg to push up. If indicated, keep the affected leg forward.

FIGURE Procedure 54-5 Step 7c   The patient should push up from his stronger side.

   d. Advise the patient to put the crutches under his arms and press down on the hand grips with his hands.
8. Teach the patient the required gait. Which gait the patient will use depends on the patient's muscle strength and coordination. It also depends on the type of crutches, the injury, and the patient's condition. Check the physician's orders, and see Figures 54-11 and 54-12 for examples.
9. Teach the patient how to ascend stairs:
   a. Start the patient close to the bottom step and tell him to push down with his hands.
   b. Instruct the patient to step up on the first step with his good foot.

FIGURE Procedure 54-5 Step 9b   The patient should lead with his unaffected leg when ascending stairs.

   c. Tell the patient to lift the crutches to the same step and then lift his other foot. Advise the patient to keep his crutches with his affected limb.
   d. Remind the patient to check his balance before he proceeds to the next step.
10. Teach the patient how to descend stairs:
   a. Have the patient start at the edge of the steps.
   b. Instruct the patient to bring his crutches and then the affected foot down first. Advise the patient to bend at the hips and knees to prevent leaning forward, which could cause him to fall.

FIGURE Procedure 54-5 Step 10b   The patient should lead with the affected foot when descending stairs.

   c. Tell the patient to bring his unaffected foot to the same step.
   d. Remind the patient to check his balance before he proceeds. In some cases, a handrail may be easier and can be used with both crutches in one hand.
11. Give the patient the following general information related to the use of crutches:
   a. Do not lean on crutches.
   b. Report to the physician any tingling or numbness in the arms, hands, or shoulders.

c. Support body weight with the hands.

d. Always stand erect to prevent muscle strain.

e. Look straight ahead when walking.

f. Generally, move the crutches not more than 6 inches at a time to maintain good balance.

g. Check the crutch tips regularly for wear; replace the tips as needed.

h. Check the crutch tips for wetness; dry the tips if they are wet.

i. Check all wing nuts and bolts for tightness.

j. Wear flat, well-fitting, nonskid shoes.

k. Remove throw rugs and other unsecured articles from traffic areas.

l. Report any unusual pain in the affected leg.

SUMMARY OF LEARNING OUTCOMES

LEARNING OUTCOMES	KEY POINTS
54.1 **Discuss the general principles of physical therapy.**	Physical therapy is a medical specialty for the treatment of musculoskeletal, nervous, and cardiopulmonary disorders using a variety of treatments, including cold, heat, water, exercise, massage, and traction.
54.2 **Relate various cold and heat therapies to their benefits and contraindications.**	There are various types of cold and heat therapies, including dry and wet cold and heat applications. Cold and heat therapy promote healing and increase patient comfort. Contraindications to cold and heat therapies include circulation problems, pain, and hemorrhage.
54.3 **Recall hydrotherapy methods.**	Various types of hydrotherapy used to treat physical problems include whirlpools, contrast baths, and underwater exercises.
54.4 **Name several methods of exercise therapy.**	There are several methods of exercise therapy, including active mobility, passive mobility, aided mobility, and active resistance.
54.5 **Describe the types of massage used in rehabilitation therapy.**	The two major types of massage used in rehabilitation therapy are Swedish and neuromuscular. Swedish massage uses 5 basic strokes to manipulate soft tissues. Neuromuscular massage is applied to specific muscles and helps release tension and knots, relieve pain and release pressure on nerves, and increase blood flow. Trigger point therapy is commonly used during neuromuscular massage.
54.6 **Compare different methods of traction.**	The different methods of traction used to treat physical problems include manual, static, skeletal, and mechanical.
54.7 **Carry out the procedure for teaching a patient to use a cane, a walker, crutches, and a wheelchair.**	The various mobility aids include canes, walkers, crutches, and wheelchairs. Specific instructions for each of these aids must be followed to reduce the possibility of patient injury during their use.
54.8 **Model the steps you should take when referring a patient to a physical therapist.**	You may be asked to contact the specialist directly or to give the patient a written order and information about contacting the specialist. Keep a file with information about the therapists your office uses, noting the forms and information each therapist requires.

Recall Shenya Jones from the beginning of the chapter. Now that you have completed the chapter, answer the following questions regarding her case.

1. Why is thermotherapy used?

2. What is the best way for Shenya to keep the compress warm while applying it?

3. What should you tell Shenya to watch for while administering hot compresses to her face?

1. (LO 54.1) Which of the following is an example of inversion?
a. Flexing the foot
b. Pointing the foot upward
c. Turning the sole of the foot inward
d. Rotating the foot back and forth
e. Turning the sole of the foot downward

2. (LO 54.1) Body position and alignment are known as
a. Posture
b. Gait
c. Range of motion
d. Flexion
e. Extension

3. (LO 54.4) Which of the following is a type of exercise whereby the patient relaxes and contracts the muscles of a specific body part without moving the body part?
a. ROM
b. Passive mobility
c. Active resistance
d. Isometric
e. Aided mobility

4. (LO 54.6) Another name for weight traction is
a. Static
b. Skeletal
c. Mechanical
d. Manual
e. Harness

5. (LO 54.7) Which of the following crutch gaits is the best for someone with leg paralysis?
a. Two-point
b. Three-point
c. Swing-to
d. Four-point
e. Crutches are never used by people with leg paralysis

6. (LO 54.2) Which of the following therapies causes blood vessels to constrict?
a. Neuromuscular massage
b. Thermotherapy
c. ROM
d. Active resistance exercise
e. Cryotherapy

7. (LO 54.5) In Swedish massage, which of the following strokes is a percussive stroke?
a. Pétrissage
b. Effleurage
c. Vibration
d. Tapotement
e. Friction

8. (LO 54.4) Riding a stationary bicycle is an example of a(n)
a. Active mobility exercise
b. Isometric exercise
c. Passive mobility exercise
d. Active range of motion exercise
e. Aided mobility exercise

9. (LO 54.7) Which of the following crutch gaits is considered the slowest?
a. Two-point
b. Swing-through
c. Three-point
d. Swing-to
e. Four-point

10. (LO 54.1) A goniometer is used to measure
a. Pain
b. The effectiveness of cold therapy
c. Range of motion
d. Muscle contraction
e. The type of traction needed.

Nutrition and Health

PATIENT INFORMATION

Patient Name	Gender	DOB
Mohammad Nassar	Male	5/17/XX

Attending	MRN	Allergies
Elizabeth H. Williams, MD	423-90-687	NKA

A 16-year-old male patient is brought to BWW Associates by his parents. As the medical assistant, you take his history and physical, noting that he has a past history of mild asthma. The patient mentions that he is avoiding food because he is being "careful not to eat too many calories" so he can keep his weight down and have a chance to fight in the lightest weight class. He tells you he hopes to get a scholarship for wrestling so he can attend college next fall. You note that his vital signs are blood pressure: 100/60 Height: 5' 10" Weight: 131 lbs. Pulse rate: 50. He appears dehydrated and exhibits signs of muscle weakness.

Keep Mohammad Nassar in mind as you study the chapter. There will be questions at the end of the chapter based on the case study. The information in the chapter will help you answer these questions.

L E A R N I N G   O U T C O M E S

After completing Chapter 55, you will be able to:

55.1 Relate daily energy requirements to the role of calories.

55.2 Identify nutrients and their role in health.

55.3 Implement a plan for a nutritious, well-balanced diet and healthy lifestyle using the USDA's guidelines.

55.4 Describe methods used to assess a patient's nutritional status.

55.5 Explain reasons why a diet may be modified.

55.6 Identify types of patients who require special diets and the modifications required for each.

55.7 Describe the warning signs, symptoms, and treatment for eating disorders.

55.8 Educate patients about nutritional requirements.

K E Y   T E R M S

amino acid	dehydration
anabolism	fiber
anorexia nervosa	food exchange
antioxidant	gluten
behavior modification	protein
bulimia	mineral
calorie	parenteral nutrition
catabolism	saturated fat
cholesterol	unsaturated fat
complex carbohydrate	vitamin

I. C (8) Discuss implications for disease and disability when homeostasis is not maintained

IV. P (5) Instruct patients according to their needs to promote health maintenance and disease prevention

IV. P (9) Document patient education

IX. P (7) Document accurately in the patient record

2. Anatomy and Physiology

Graduates:

a. Comprehend and explain to the patient the importance of diet and nutrition. Effectively convey and educate patients regarding the proper diet and nutrition guidelines. Identify categories of patients that require special diets or diet modifications.

9. Medical Office Clinical Procedures

Graduates:

r. Teach patients methods of health promotion and disease prevention

▶ Introduction

Nutrition is the process of how the body takes in and utilizes food and other sources of nutrients. It is a five-part process that includes intake, digestion, absorption, metabolism, and elimination.

You need to know what effect nutrition has on health so that you can help patients meet their dietary requirements. Food is the body's source of nutrients, or substances the body needs to function properly. As you study this chapter, you will learn how the body uses nutrients and the importance of a well-planned diet to health. People need specific types of foods to stay healthy or to regain their health after illness or surgery. People with specific conditions also may need to follow special diets. As a medical assistant, you will work closely with the rest of the healthcare team to ensure that patients understand the role of diet in health and that they adhere to any diet prescribed by their physician or dietitian.

▶ Daily Energy Requirements　LO 55.1

The human body requires the nutrients in food for three major purposes:

- To provide energy
- To build, repair, and maintain body tissues
- To regulate body processes

A person's daily energy requirements depend on many factors. To understand the relationship of food to good health, you need to understand how the body uses food.

Metabolism

Food must be broken down before the body can use it. This process is an integral part of metabolism. Metabolism is the sum of all the cellular processes that build, maintain, and supply energy to living tissue. During metabolism, body tissue is built up and broken down, and heat and energy are produced.

Metabolism takes place in two phases. In **anabolism**, substances such as nutrients are changed into more complex substances and used to build body tissues. In **catabolism**, complex substances, including nutrients and body tissues, are broken down into simpler substances and converted into energy. The body uses this energy to maintain and repair itself. Of the energy people get from the food they eat, about 25% is directly used for bodily functions, and the rest becomes heat.

Each person's body requires a minimal amount of nutrients to carry on a basic level of metabolism to live. Each person's daily nutritional requirements vary with age, weight, percentage of body fat, activity level, state of health, and other variables. The body's metabolic rate, or speed of metabolism, also can be affected by many factors, such as pregnancy, malnutrition, and disease.

Calories

The amount of energy a food produces in the body is measured in kilocalories. A kilocalorie, commonly called a **calorie**, is the amount of energy needed to raise the temperature of 1 kilogram of water by 1°C. Foods differ in the number of calories they contain. The more calories in a food, the more available energy it has. Calories also are used to measure the energy the body uses during all activities and metabolic processes.

As mentioned, people's daily nutritional needs differ, depending on variables of age, weight, percentage of body fat, activity level, and state of health. If people eat an excess of calories—more than the body can use—the excess is stored as fat in the body. Conversely, lowering caloric intake causes the body to burn off stored fat for energy.

Depending on the food's weight (in grams) or volume, each food has a value in calories. Therefore, you can count the number of calories a person consumes by monitoring food intake and adding up the calories in each food serving. You can use a food calorie counter, such as those often found in books or software applications, to look up caloric values. A calorie counter tells you, for instance, that 1 cup of cooked carrots contains 50 calories or that 1 cup of cooked corn kernels contains 130 calories. Calories also are listed on the labels of food packages. You can estimate the number of calories a person burns during certain activities by consulting a chart similar to Table 55-1.

TABLE 55-1 Calories Burned per Hour in Selected Activities

Moderate Physical Activity	Approximate Calories/Hr for a 154-lb Person*
Hiking	370
Light gardening/yard work	330
Dancing	330
Golf (walking and carrying clubs)	330
Bicycling (<10 mph)	290
Walking (3.5 mph)	280
Weight lifting (general light workout)	180

Vigorous Physical Activity	Approximate Calories/Hr for a 154-lb Person*
Running/jogging (5 mph)	590
Bicycling (> 10 mph)	590
Swimming (slow freestyle laps)	510
Aerobics	480
Walking (4.5 mph)	460
Heavy yard work (chopping wood)	440
Weight lifting (vigorous effort)	440
Basketball (vigorous)	440

*Calories burned per hour will be higher for people who weigh more than 154 lb (70 kg) and lower for people who weigh less.

Source: U.S. Department of Health and Human Services, U.S. Department of Agriculture, Dietary Guidelines for Americans 2010, www.healthierus.gov/dietaryguidelines.

▶ Nutrients
LO 55.2

The body needs a variety of nutrients for energy, growth, repair, and basic processes. Seven basic food components provide these nutrients and work together to help keep the body healthy:

1. Proteins
2. Carbohydrates
3. Fiber
4. Lipids
5. Vitamins
6. Minerals
7. Water

As the body digests foods that contain these components, it breaks them down so that it can use them. Of the seven components, only proteins, carbohydrates, and fats contain calories and provide the body with energy. The rest perform a variety of other essential functions.

Proteins

Protein is the most essential nutrient for building and repairing cells and tissue. Therefore, it is especially important for people to get enough protein during illness and healing. Other major functions of protein are to

- Help maintain the body's water balance.
- Assist with antibody production and disease resistance.
- Help maintain body heat.

The optimal level of protein in a healthy person's diet is 10% to 35% of total caloric intake. A variety of lean proteins are best. More protein may be required during illnesses and recovery from injury. A deficiency in protein leads to weight loss and fatigue, malnutrition, extremely dry skin, lowered resistance to infection, and interference with normal growth processes.

The body makes protein out of **amino acids,** which are natural organic compounds found in plant and animal foods. Besides being used to build and maintain tissue, protein can be broken down to produce energy, especially if other energy sources are low. Each gram of protein contains 4 calories. Excess protein is broken down by the body and contributes to fat stores.

Amino acids are found in animal sources such as meats, milk, fish, and eggs, as well as in plant sources such as soy, beans, legumes, nut butters, and some grains (such as wheat germ). Individuals do not need to eat animal products to get all the protein they need in their diet. See Figure 55-1.

(a)

(b)

FIGURE 55-1 Protein foods supply essential, nonessential, and conditional amino acids. (a) Individuals who eat animal products should select lean proteins and have seafood at least once a week. (b) Individuals who do not eat animal products can get protein from these foods.

Amino acids are classified into three groups:

- *Essential amino acids* cannot be made by the body and must be supplied by food. They do not need to be eaten at one meal. The balance over the whole day is more important. There are nine essential amino acids.
- *Nonessential amino acids* are made by the body from essential amino acids or in the normal breakdown of proteins. There are four nonessential amino acids.
- *Conditional amino acids* are usually not essential, except in times of illness and stress. There are at least eight conditional amino acids.

Go to CONNECT to see an animation about *Protein Synthesis*.

Carbohydrates

Carbohydrates in food provide about two-thirds of a person's daily energy needs. Carbohydrates also provide heat, help metabolize fat, and help reserve protein for uses other than supplying energy. Each gram of carbohydrate contains 4 calories. The daily requirement for carbohydrates is 45% to 65% of total caloric intake. Carbohydrate deficiency leads to weight loss, protein loss, and fatigue.

There are two basic types of carbohydrates:

- *Simple carbohydrates* (sugars), found in fruits, some vegetables, milk, and table sugar.
- *Complex carbohydrates*, found in grain foods, such as breads, pastas, cereals, and rice; in some fruits and vegetables, such as potatoes, corn, broccoli, apples, and pears; and in legumes, such as peas, peanuts, and beans.

Simple sugars are small molecules that consist of 1 or 2 sugar (saccharide) units. **Complex carbohydrates,** or polysaccharides, are long chains of sugar units. Starch is a type of complex carbohydrate that is a major source of energy from foods of plant origin. Fiber, another type of complex carbohydrate, is discussed in the next section.

Carbohydrates used for immediate fuel are converted to glucose, a simple sugar that cells use for energy. An excess of carbohydrates is either stored in the liver and muscle cells as glycogen (long chains of glucose units—the animal equivalent of starch) or converted into and stored as fat. After the body's carbohydrate reserves are depleted, it starts burning fat. Healthful, nutritive sources of carbohydrates include fruits and vegetables, whole-grain pasta and cereal, and potatoes (Figure 55-2). The American Dietetic Association suggests these sources of carbohydrates with an emphasis on complex carbohydrates such as vegetables, legumes, and whole-grain breads and cereals. Sugary foods, such as sweet desserts, candy, and soft drinks, also contain carbohydrates, but they are high in calories and low in nutritional value.

Fiber

Fiber is in a separate category, although it is a type of complex carbohydrate. Fiber does not supply energy or heat to the body.

FIGURE 55-2   Healthful sources of carbohydrates are plentiful.

It is the tough, stringy part of vegetables and grains. Fiber is not absorbed by the body, but it serves these important digestive functions:

- Increasing and softening the bulk of the stool, thus promoting normal defecation.
- Absorbing organic wastes and toxins in the body so that they can be expelled.
- Decreasing the rate of carbohydrate breakdown and absorption.

Therapeutically, fiber can help treat and prevent constipation, hemorrhoids, diverticular disease, and irritable bowel syndrome. It is linked to reduced blood cholesterol levels, reduction of gallstone formation, control of diabetes, and reduction in the risk of certain types of cancer and other diseases. Too little fiber can result in an increased risk of colon cancer, hypercholesterolemia (high blood cholesterol), and increased blood glucose levels after eating. Too much fiber can cause constipation, diarrhea, and other gastrointestinal disorders and can impair mineral absorption.

The recommended amount of fiber for adults is 14 grams for every 1000 calories you eat per day. So if you eat 2000 calories each day, you should have 28 grams of fiber. Because fiber works in conjunction with other substances and nutrients, it is advisable to get dietary fiber from a variety of food sources (Figure 55-3). Adequate water intake is especially important for fiber to work properly.

Fiber can be classified as soluble or insoluble. Soluble fiber, found in foods such as oats, dry beans, barley, and some fruits and vegetables, is the type that tends to absorb fluid and swell when eaten. It slows the absorption of food from the digestive tract, helps control the blood sugar level of diabetics, lowers blood cholesterol levels, and softens and increases the bulk of stools. Insoluble fiber, found in the bran in whole wheat bread and brown rice, for example, promotes regular bowel movements by contributing to stool bulk.

FIGURE 55-3 Dietary fiber serves many functions in the human body and is considered a basic food component.

FIGURE 55-4 Foods that contain saturated fats include meat and butter. Most vegetable oils contain unsaturated fats.

Lipids

Lipids in the diet include dietary fats and fat-related substances. Fats are a concentrated source of energy that the body can store in large amounts. Each gram of fat contains 9 calories (more than twice the calorie content of proteins and carbohydrates). About 95% of the lipids from plant and animal sources of food are fats. These simple lipids, or triglycerides, consist of glycerol (an alcohol) and three fatty acids. Chemical qualities of the fatty acids in a triglyceride determine the fat's characteristic flavor and texture. About 5% of dietary lipids are compound lipids such as cholesterol. Compound lipids are fat-related substances that are important components of cell membranes, nervous tissue, and some hormones. Compound lipids are vital to the transport of all fatlike substances within the body. Lipids assist with important body functions and are essential to growth and metabolism. Among this nutrient's jobs are the following:

 Providing a concentrated source of heat and energy.
 Transporting fat-soluble vitamins.
 Storing energy in the form of body fat, which insulates and protects the organs.
 Providing a feeling of satiety, or fullness, because it is digested more slowly than other nutrients.

A lipid deficiency can interfere with the body's absorption and utilization of vitamins and can cause fatigue and dry skin. However, an excess of lipids, particularly some dietary fats, can lead to increased levels of triglycerides and cholesterol in the blood and an increased risk of heart and artery disease and other diseases. It is recommended that adults obtain no more than 20 to 30% of their daily calories from fat sources. Cholesterol intake should be limited to 300 milligrams per day. People with heart disease and certain other diseases or risks may benefit from even lower levels of lipid intake.

Saturated and Unsaturated Fats The fats in food can be classified as either saturated fats or unsaturated fats

(Figure 55-4). **Saturated fats** are derived primarily from animal sources and are usually solid at room temperature. They are found in meats and animal products such as butter, egg yolks, and whole milk. Coconut oil and palm oil are also saturated fats. Consumption of saturated fats should be restricted because these fats tend to raise blood cholesterol levels.

Unsaturated fats are usually liquid at room temperature. They include most vegetable oils. Unsaturated fats can be divided into two classes:

 Polyunsaturated fats, such as corn, soya, safflower, and sunflower oils.
 Monounsaturated fats, such as peanut, canola, and olive oils.

The body needs essential fatty acids (primarily linoleic acid) for building and maintaining tissues. Because the body cannot produce these fatty acids, they must be supplied by food. Saturated fats in butter, egg yolks, and milk and unsaturated fats in corn, canola, sunflower, and safflower oils are good sources of essential fatty acids.

Trans Fats Also known as trans fatty acids, trans fats are a specific type of fat that is formed when hydrogen is added to vegetable oil through a process called *hydrogenation*. Hydrogenation is a process that turns liquid oils into solid fats. Trans fats can be found in vegetable shortenings, some margarines, crackers, candy, cookies, snack foods, fried foods, baked goods, and other processed foods. The U.S. Food and Drug Administration (FDA) recommends that individuals consume as close to zero grams as possible on a daily basis. The FDA currently requires that the amount of trans fat be displayed on all food labels.

Cholesterol **Cholesterol** is a fat-related substance produced by the liver that also can be obtained through dietary sources. Only animal-based foods contain cholesterol. It is essential to health because it

- Serves as an integral part of cell membranes.
- Provides the structural basis for all steroid hormones and vitamin D.
- Serves as a constituent of bile, which aids in digestion.

Lipid Levels in the Blood Lipids, like other nutrients, are carried throughout the body in the bloodstream. When blood lipid levels become excessive, however, they pose certain risks. Doctors often order blood tests to determine the level of triglycerides and cholesterol in their patients' blood as a measure of overall health. High levels of cholesterol, especially if accompanied by high levels of triglycerides, may indicate an increased risk of heart disease, stroke, and peripheral vascular disease.

Lipids are not soluble in water; fats (or oil) and water do not mix. Because the fluid portion of blood is 90% water, lipids are encased in large molecules that are fat-soluble on the inside and water-soluble on the outside. These large molecules, called lipoproteins, carry lipids such as cholesterol and triglycerides through the bloodstream.

Low-density lipoproteins (LDLs) and high-density lipoproteins (HDLs) are the two main types of lipoproteins. Cholesterol in blood is identified as HDL or LDL, depending on which type of lipoprotein carries it. High levels of LDL cholesterol in blood are a primary risk factor for heart attacks. High levels of LDL cholesterol occur in people whose diets are high in saturated fats. HDL cholesterol, commonly referred to as good cholesterol, carries excess cholesterol away from arteries and back to the liver for breakdown and elimination. Patients often can reduce elevated cholesterol levels by increasing exercise and intake of soluble fiber and decreasing the dietary intake of saturated fats. These measures tend to elevate the level of HDL cholesterol in the bloodstream and reduce the level of LDL cholesterol. Table 55-2 lists the saturated fat and cholesterol contents of various foods.

Vitamins

Vitamins are organic substances that are essential for normal body growth and maintenance and resistance to infection. Vitamins also help the body use other nutrients and assist in various body processes.

Most vitamins are absorbed directly through the digestive tract. Some vitamins are water-soluble and others are fat-soluble. Water-soluble vitamins, such as vitamin C and the B vitamins, are not stored by the body and therefore must be replaced every day. Fat-soluble vitamins, such as vitamins A, D, E, and K, are stored for longer periods.

The amounts of vitamins the body needs are relatively small; however, a vitamin deficiency through lack of ingestion or absorption can lead to disease. Some vitamins also can cause health problems if taken in excess. Toxic levels of vitamin A, for example, can produce effects ranging from headache to liver damage. Because the level of vitamin intake is so essential to

TABLE 55-2	Saturated Fat and Cholesterol Contents of Various Foods	
Food	Saturated Fat (g)	Cholesterol (mg)
Cheddar cheese (1 oz)	6.0	30
Mozzarella, part skim (1 oz)	3.1	15
Whole milk (1 c)	5.1	33
Skim milk (1 c)	0.3	4
Butter (1 tbsp)	7.1	31
Mayonnaise (1 tbsp)	1.7	8
Tuna in oil (3 oz)	1.4	55
Tuna in water (3 oz)	0.3	48
Lean ground beef, broiled (3 oz)	6.2	74
Leg of lamb, roasted (3 oz)	5.6	78
Bacon (3 slices)	3.3	16
Chicken breast, roasted (3 oz)	0.9	73

Source: U.S. Department of Agriculture.

health, the Food and Nutrition Board of the National Research Council has established recommended dietary allowances (RDAs) for vitamins. For detailed information on specific vitamins, see Table 55-3.

Eating a well-balanced, nutritious diet minimizes the likelihood of vitamin deficiency. Many manufactured foods are also vitamin-fortified. Even so, some people choose to augment their diets with vitamin supplements (Figure 55-5). A physician or other member of the medical team may, in some instances, prescribe vitamin supplements for patients.

Minerals

Minerals are natural, inorganic substances the body needs to help build and maintain body tissues and carry on life functions. Minerals are classified according to the relative amounts the body requires:

- Major minerals are those that the body needs in fairly large quantities, including calcium, magnesium, and phosphorus.
- Trace minerals are those that the body needs in tiny amounts, including iron, iodine, zinc, selenium, copper, fluoride, chromium, manganese, and molybdenum.

Most minerals are absorbed in the intestines and any excess is eliminated. Calcium, iron, and iodine are the minerals in which people are most often deficient.

Minerals with Recommended Dietary Allowances

There are several minerals for which RDAs have been established. These minerals are calcium, iron, iodine, zinc, magnesium, phosphorus, and selenium.

Calcium Calcium builds healthy bones and teeth, aids in blood clotting, and helps nerves and muscles function properly. It is found in dairy products, green leafy vegetables,

TABLE 55-3   Vitamins

Vitamin	Functions	Adult RDA*	Food Sources	Deficiencies and/or Toxicities
Vitamin A (retinol, provitamin, carotene)	Aids in night vision; cell growth and maintenance; normal reproductive function; health of skin, mucous membranes, and internal tracts	Males: 900 mcg retinol equivalents Females: 700 mcg retinol equivalents	Milk fat; butter; egg yolks; meat; fish liver oil; liver; green, yellow, and orange leafy vegetables; yellow and orange fruits	Deficiency: night blindness; dry, rough skin; risk of internal infection Toxicity: headache, vomiting, joint pain, hair loss, jaundice, liver damage
Vitamin B₁ (thiamine)	Aids enzymes in breaking down and using carbohydrates; helps the nerves, muscles, and heart function efficiently	Males: 1.2 mg Females: 1.1 mg	Whole grains, brewer's yeast, organ meats, lean pork, beef, liver, legumes, seeds, nuts	Deficiency: beriberi with appetite loss, digestive problems, muscle weakness and deterioration, nervous disorders, heart failure
Vitamin B₂ (riboflavin)	Aids enzymes in metabolism of fats and proteins	Males: 1.3 mg Females: 1.1 mg	Dairy products, organ meats, green leafy vegetables, enriched and fortified grain products	Deficiency: cracks at lip corners, irritations at nasal angles, inflammation of the tongue, seborrheic dermatitis, anemia
Vitamin B₃ (niacin)	Aids enzymes in metabolism of carbohydrates and fats	Males: 16 mg Females: 14 mg	Meat, fish, poultry, enriched and fortified grain products	Deficiency: pellagra with dermatitis, diarrhea, inflammation of mucous membranes, dementia Toxicity: dilation of blood vessels; if sustained, abnormal liver function
Vitamin B₆ (pyridoxine)	Aids enzymes in synthesis of amino acids	Males: 1.7 mg Females: 1.3–1.5 mg	Chicken, fish, pork, liver, kidney, some vegetables, grains, nuts, legumes	Deficiency: convulsions, dermatitis, anemia Toxicity: loss of muscle coordination, severe sensory neuropathy
Folate (compounds)	Works with cobalamins in nucleic acid synthesis and metabolism of amino acids; maintains red blood cells	Males: 400 µg Females: 400 µg	Liver, yeast, legumes, green leafy vegetables, some fruits	Deficiency: glossitis, diarrhea, anemia, lethargy
Vitamin B₁₂ (cobalamins)	Works with folate in nucleic acid synthesis and metabolism of amino acids; coenzyme in metabolism of fatty acids	2.4 µg	Seafood, meat, milk, eggs, cheese, brewer's yeast, blackstrap molasses	Deficiency: pernicious anemia, irreversible liver damage
Vitamin C (ascorbic acid)	Coenzyme involved in collagen production, capillary integrity, use of iron in hemoglobin, and synthesis of many hormones; improves absorption of iron; is an antioxidant	Males: 90 mg Females: 75 mg	Citrus fruits, mangoes, strawberries, green peppers, broccoli, potatoes, green leafy vegetables	Deficiency: scurvy with hemorrhages, loose teeth, poor wound healing Toxicity: stomachache, diarrhea
Vitamin D (calciferol)	Builds bones and teeth; helps maintain calcium-phosphorus balance in blood	5–15 µg	Egg yolks, butter, liver, fortified milk, margarine, and prepared cereals	Deficiency: rickets in children, osteomalacia in adults Toxicity: excess blood calcium and phosphorus, calcium deposits in soft tissue, bone pain, irreversible kidney and cardiovascular damage
Vitamin E (group)	Is an intracellular antioxidant; maintains cell structure; aids in formation of red blood cells	15 mg	Vegetable oils, margarine, shortening, wheat germ, nuts, green leafy vegetables	Deficiency: damage to cells, hemolytic anemia
Vitamin K (compounds)	Aids in blood clotting and bone growth	Males: 120 µg Females: 90 µg	Green leafy vegetables, milk, dairy products, meat, eggs, cereals, fruits, vegetables	Deficiency: slow blood clotting; hemorrhagic disease in newborns

*RDAs may vary for different age groups.

Source: Adapted from the Institute of Medicine of the National Academies, http://www.iom.edu (accessed April 2012), and Office of Dietary Supplements, National Institutes of Health, http://ods.od.nih.gov (accessed April 2012).

FIGURE 55-5 Some people use supplements to augment their dietary intake of vitamins and minerals.

broccoli, legumes, and the soft bones of sardines and salmon (Figure 55-6).

Calcium deficiency can cause poor bone growth and tooth development in children, osteoporosis in adults, and poor blood clotting. The normal requirement is 800 to 1200 milligrams per day.

FIGURE 55-6 These foods are excellent sources of calcium, a mineral that is necessary for strong bones and teeth.

FIGURE 55-7 Iron, a mineral that is needed in small amounts, is found in a wide variety of foods.

Iron Iron, one of the most important nutrients, is essential for the production of red blood cells, which transport oxygen throughout the body. It is also a component of enzymes needed for energy production. Although iron is found in a wide variety of foods, it is the most frequently deficient nutrient in people's diets. Liver, meat, poultry, fish, egg yolks, fortified breads and cereals, dark green vegetables, and dried fruits are good dietary sources of iron (Figure 55-7), although less than 20% of it is usually absorbed.

Iron deficiency can cause anemia, a blood disorder that results in fatigue, weakness, and impaired mental abilities. At toxic levels, iron may increase the risk of coronary heart disease (CHD). The daily requirement is 10 to 15 milligrams.

Iodine Iodine plays a vital role in the activities of the thyroid hormones, which are involved in reproduction, growth, nerve and muscle function, and the production of new blood cells. Deficiency can cause an enlarged thyroid gland, known as *goiter*. Iodine can be obtained in seafood, iodized salt, and seaweed products. The daily requirement is 150 micrograms.

Zinc Zinc promotes normal growth and wound healing and participates in many cell activities that involve proteins, enzymes, and hormones. It is found in liver, lamb, beef, eggs, oysters, and whole grain breads and cereals, although it is not always easily absorbed. Deficiency can result in growth retardation, impaired taste and smell, and reduced immune function. The daily requirement is 12 to 15 milligrams.

Magnesium Magnesium activates cell enzymes, helps metabolize proteins and carbohydrates, maintains the structural integrity of the heart and other muscles, and aids in muscle contraction. Good sources include green leafy vegetables, nuts, legumes, bananas, and whole grain products.

A deficiency may result from persistent vomiting or diarrhea, kidney disease, general malnutrition, alcoholism, and the use of certain medications. The daily requirement is 280 milligrams for women and 350 milligrams for men.

Phosphorus Phosphorus is involved in bone and tooth formation, chemical reactions in the body, and energy production. It is found in dairy foods, animal foods, fish, cereals, nuts, and legumes. A deficiency of phosphorus can cause gastrointestinal, blood cell, and other disorders. Toxicity is harmful as well. The daily requirement is 800 milligrams for adults 25 and over.

Selenium Selenium works with vitamin E to aid metabolism, growth, and fertility. It is found in seafood, kidney, liver, meats, grain products, and seeds. A daily dietary intake of 55 micrograms for women and 70 micrograms for men is recommended.

Minerals with Estimated Safe and Adequate Dietary Intakes When data were sufficient to estimate a range of requirements—but insufficient for developing an RDA—the Food and Nutrition Board established a category of safe and adequate intakes for essential nutrients. The minerals in this category are copper, fluoride, chromium, manganese, and molybdenum.

Copper Copper interacts with iron to form hemoglobin and red blood cells. It can be obtained through a wide variety of foods, such as liver, seafood, nuts and seeds, and whole grain products. Copper deficiency can cause anemia and central nervous system problems. The safe and adequate range of dietary copper for adults is 1.5 to 3.0 milligrams per day.

Fluoride Fluoride is another contributor to bone and tooth formation, and it protects against tooth decay. Many municipal water supplies are fluoridated, and the mineral is also contained in saltwater fish, tea, and fluoridated toothpaste. Fluoride deficiency may predispose people to cavities and osteoporosis. Excess fluoride can cause discoloration and pitting of the teeth as well as other conditions. The range of safe and adequate intake for adults is 1.5 to 4.0 milligrams per day.

Chromium Chromium is essential for the body to use glucose, the primary food of cells. Foods containing chromium include calf's liver, American cheese, and wheat germ. A range of intakes between 50 and 200 micrograms per day is considered safe and adequate for adults.

Manganese Manganese is part of several cell enzymes. It is also essential for bone formation and maintenance, insulin production, and nutrient metabolism. It is found in whole grain products, fruits, vegetables, and tea. A daily dietary intake of 2 to 5 milligrams for adults is recommended.

Molybdenum Molybdenum helps in the metabolism of the mineral sulfur and the production of uric acid. The best sources are legumes, whole grains, milk, and organ meats such as liver and kidneys. The recommended range for dietary intake is 75 to 250 micrograms per day for adults.

Water

Water has no caloric value, but it contributes about 65% of body weight and is essential to the body's normal functioning. In general, water helps provide the body with other nutrients it needs and helps rid the body of what it does not need. Water has many functions, including these:

- Helping to maintain the balance of all the fluids in the body.
- Lubricating the body's moving parts.
- Dissolving chemicals and nutrients.
- Aiding in digestion.
- Helping to transport nutrients and secretions throughout the body.
- Flushing out wastes.
- Regulating body temperature through perspiration.

The amount of water in the body directly affects the concentration and distribution of body fluids and all the functions related to them. The body maintains a careful balance between water consumed (in foods and beverages) and water lost (through urination, perspiration, and respiration). In a healthy fluid balance, water input equals water output. Measuring an ill person's level of water intake and output can help determine the best fluid replacement regimen to use.

People obtain most of their water from beverages such as tap water, milk, and fruit juices as well as coffee, tea, and soft drinks. On average, a person needs to drink six to eight glasses of water a day to maintain a healthy water balance. The daily need for water varies with size and age, the temperatures to which someone is exposed, the degree of physical exertion, and the water content of the foods one eats. Someone who is eating mostly foods with a high water content, such as fruits and vegetables, can drink a little less water than someone who is eating mostly foods with a low water content.

If people get too little water or lose too much water through vomiting, diarrhea, burns, or perspiration, they become dehydrated. Signs and symptoms of **dehydration** include dry lips and mucous membranes, weakness, lethargy, decreased urine output, and increased thirst. Severe dehydration can lead to hypovolemia, a reduction in the volume of blood in the body. Severe hypovolemia can result in inadequate blood pressure that affects the functioning of the heart, central nervous system, and various organs—a condition known as hypovolemic shock. If dehydration progresses so that water is lost from body cells, death usually occurs within a few days. Patients should know whether they are to drink extra fluids to replace fluids lost in an illness or to help rid the body of waste.

Principal Electrolytes and Other Nutrients of Special Interest

The principal electrolytes are essential to normal body functioning. Other nutrients, such as antioxidants, also merit special mention.

Principal Electrolytes Although the principal electrolytes in the body—sodium, potassium, and chloride—are often excluded from lists of nutrients, they are essential dietary components. Electrolytes play an important role in maintaining body functions, such as normal heart rhythm.

Sodium Sodium (Na) maintains fluid and acid-base balances, assists in the transport of glucose, and maintains normal conditions inside and outside cells. Salt is the main dietary source of sodium, and high salt intakes are normally associated with a diet high in processed foods. Too much sodium can be associated with high blood pressure in salt-sensitive individuals. Although many Americans consume far more, it is recommended that daily sodium intake be limited to 2.4 grams or less.

Potassium Potassium (K) is a crucial element in the maintenance of muscle contraction and fluid and electrolyte balance. It contributes to acid-base balance and the transmission of nerve impulses. Its role in fluid balance helps regulate blood pressure. Potassium occurs in unprocessed foods, particularly in fruits such as bananas, raisins, and oranges; many vegetables; and fresh meats (Figure 55-8). The minimum requirement is 1600 to 2000 milligrams per day.

Chloride Chloride (Cl) is essential in maintaining fluid and electrolyte balance, and it is a necessary component of hydrochloric acid, secreted into the stomach during digestion of food. Because dietary chloride comes almost entirely from sodium chloride, sources are essentially the same as those of sodium.

Antioxidants Antioxidants are chemical agents that fight certain cell-destroying chemical substances called

FIGURE 55-8 These foods are a good source of potassium.

FIGURE 55-9 Antioxidants are substances in food that may offer protection against certain chronic diseases. Foods rich in beta-carotene, vitamin C, vitamin E, and selenium contain antioxidants.

free radicals. In fact, antioxidants may help ward off cancer and heart disease by neutralizing free radicals, which are byproducts of normal metabolism that also may form as a result of exposure to various damaging factors such as cigarette smoke, alcohol, or x-rays. Antioxidants may be added to foods and cosmetics as preservatives. The nutrients beta-carotene, vitamin C, vitamin E, and selenium are natural antioxidants (Figure 55-9).

▶ Dietary Guidelines LO 55.3

Dietary guidelines exist to help people get proper nutrition, reduce the occurrence of disease, and control their weight. These recommendations are designed to encourage healthy eating habits.

Dietary guidelines suggest the types and quantities of food that people should eat each day. They also may contain recommendations about which types of foods to limit and which types of foods to increase.

USDA Dietary Guidelines for Americans

The U.S. Department of Agriculture and the U.S. Department of Health and Human Services updated their Dietary Guidelines for Americans in 2010. These guidelines encourage people to eat a balanced diet, limit consumption of less nutritious foods, increase physical activity, and make good nutritional decisions consistently.

Key Recommendations The 2010 USDA Dietary Guidelines recommend that you balance the food you eat with physical activity. They also recommend that you maintain or improve your weight to help reduce your chances of high blood pressure, heart disease, stroke, some types of cancer, and diabetes. Specific recommendations are included in Table 55-4.

TABLE 55-4	USDA 2010 Dietary Guidelines Key Recommendations
Balancing calories to manage weight	• Promote healthy weight through improved eating and physical activity behaviors.
	• Control total calorie intake to manage body weight. For people who are overweight or obese, this will mean consuming fewer calories from foods and beverages.
	• Maintain appropriate calorie balance during each stage of life: childhood, adolescence, adulthood, pregnancy and breastfeeding, and older age.
Foods and food components to reduce	• Reduce daily sodium intake to less than 2,300 milligrams (mg). Further reduce intake to 1,500 mg among people who are 51 and older and those of any age who are African American or have hypertension, diabetes, or chronic kidney disease.
	• Consume less than 10 percent of calories from saturated fatty acids by replacing them with monounsaturated and polyunsaturated fatty acids.
	• Consume less than 300 mg per day of dietary cholesterol.
	• Keep trans fatty acid consumption as low as possible by limiting foods that contain synthetic sources of trans fats and by limiting other solid fats.
	• Reduce the intake of calories from solid fats and added sugars.
	• Limit the consumption of foods that contain refined grains, especially refined grain foods that contain solid fats, added sugars, and sodium.
	• If alcohol is consumed, it should be consumed in moderation (up to one drink per day for women and two drinks per day for men) and only by adults of legal drinking age.
Food and nutrients to increase (within calorie needs)	• Increase vegetable and fruit intake.
	• Eat a variety of vegetables, especially dark green, red and orange, beans, and peas.
	• Consume at least half of all grains as whole grains.
	• Increase intake of fat-free or low-fat milk and milk products.
	• Choose a variety of protein foods, which include seafood, lean meat and poultry, eggs, beans and peas, soy products, and unsalted nuts and seeds.
	• Increase the amount and variety of seafood consumed by choosing seafood in place of some meat and poultry.
	• Replace protein foods that are higher in solid fats with choices that are lower in solid fats and calories and/or are sources of oils.
	• Use oils to replace solid fats where possible.
	• Choose foods that provide more potassium, dietary fiber, calcium, and vitamin D, which are nutrients of concern in American diets.
Building healthy eating patterns	• Select an eating pattern that meets nutrient needs at an appropriate calorie level.
	• Monitor foods and beverages consumed, and their fit within a healthy eating pattern.
	• Follow food safety recommendations when preparing and eating foods.

USDA Choose MyPlate Guidelines

MyPlate is an initiative based on the 2010 Dietary Guidelines for Americans discussed above. MyPlate is designed to remind Americans to eat healthfully and includes the following selected messages. See Figure 55-10.

Balancing Calories
- Enjoy your food, but eat less.
- Avoid oversized portions.

Foods to Increase
- Make half your plate fruits and vegetables.
- Make at least half your grains whole grains.
- Switch to fat-free or low-fat (1%) milk.

Foods to Reduce
- Compare sodium in foods such as soup, bread, and frozen meals—and choose foods with lower numbers.
- Drink water instead of sugary drinks.

You can assist patients through education in making better food choices by following the latest guidelines and using the SuperTracker and other tools found at www.choosemyplate.gov.

FIGURE 55-10 MyPlate is designed to remind Americans to make healthful food choices.
Source: www.choosemyplate.gov.

ACS Recommendations for Individual Choices	
Achieve and maintain a healthy weight throughout life	• Be as lean as possible throughout life without being underweight. • Avoid excess weight gain at all ages. For those who are overweight or obese, losing even a small amount of weight has health benefits and is a good place to start. • Get regular physical activity and limit intake of high-calorie foods and drinks as keys to help maintain a healthy weight.
Be a physically active	• Adults: Get at least 150 minutes of moderate intensity or 75 minutes of vigorous intensity activity each week (or a combination of these), preferably spread throughout the week. • Children and teens: Get at least 1 hour of moderate or vigorous intensity activity each day, with vigorous activity on at least 3 days each week. • Limit sedentary behavior such as sitting, lying down, watching TV, and other forms of screen-based entertainment. • Doing some physical activity above usual activities, no matter what one's level of activity, can have many health benefits.
Eat a healthy diet, with an emphasis on plant foods	• Choose foods and drinks in amounts that help you get to and maintain a healthy weight. • Limit how much processed meat and red meat you eat. • Eat at least 2½ cups of vegetables and fruits each day. • Choose whole grains instead of refined grain products.
If you drink alcohol, limit your intake	• Drink no more than 1 drink per day for women or 2 per day for men.

American Cancer Society Nutritional and Physical Activity Guidelines

The American Cancer Society updated their nutritional and physical activity guidelines in 2011 to aid in the prevention of cancer. A summary of their guidelines are found in Table 55-5. For more information visit their website at www.cancer.org.

Assessing Nutritional Levels   LO 55.4

Doctors assess a patient's nutritional status by analyzing age, health status, height, weight, type of body frame, body circumference, percentage of body fat, body mass index, nutritional and exercise patterns, and energy needs. They accomplish this assessment through direct measurement as well as through questionnaires and interviews. During the analysis, doctors take into account individual factors such as culture, beliefs, lifestyle, and education.

Body mass index (BMI) is a measure of body fat based on height and weight that applies to adult men and women. Body mass index calculators are available online. One example is at the National Heart, Lung, and Blood Institutes website. BMI is discussed in the *Vital Signs and Measurements* chapter.

To measure fat as a percentage of body weight, doctors may perform a *skinfold test*, measuring the thickness of a fold of skin with a caliper (Figure 55-11). This measurement is often made on the triceps, midway between the shoulder and elbow. The test indicates the total percentage of fat because about 50% of body fat is just below the skin and the volume of fat below the skin is related to the volume of inner fat. A trained individual must perform this test, which must be precise to be reliable.

The optimal percentage of body fat differs between men and women. For males younger than age 50, it is 10% to 14%; age 50 and older, 12% to 19%. In females younger than age 50, it is 14% to 23%; age 50 and older, 16% to 25%. Aging usually changes the ratio a bit because some muscle tissue is replaced by fat, even if weight remains constant.

Modified Diets   LO 55.5

A person's diet has a significant effect on health, appearance, and recovery from disease. After a physician or dietitian has established a patient's nutritional status, any necessary or beneficial dietary adjustments can be instituted. Dietary modification may be used alone or in combination with other therapies to prevent or treat illness.

Physicians work with dietitians to determine the best diet therapy to initiate for individual patients. Diet therapy is based on many factors, including particular foods and nutrients associated with different diseases or body states. Specific types of diet modifications include changes in texture, nutrient level, frequency and timing of meals, and exclusions.

Texture

A patient may need changes in food consistency as a result of swallowing, chewing, or other gastrointestinal problems or to fulfill short-term needs that result from events such as laboratory tests or surgical procedures. The following special diets are based on texture:

• A *clear-liquid diet* consists solely of foods that you can see through, such as tea, broth, noncitrus juices, clear carbonated

Triceps (back of arm)

Subscapular (below shoulder blade)

Suprailiac (above hipbone)

Thigh (front)

FIGURE 55-11 To estimate an individual's body fat percentage, a professional uses a tool called a caliper to measure the thickness of a fold of skin at one or more points on the body.

beverages, popsicles, and gelatin. A full-liquid diet is less restrictive and includes strained cooked cereals, plain ice cream, sherbet, pudding, and strained soups.

- A *soft diet* includes foods that are easy to chew, swallow, and digest. Foods that patients cannot tolerate and those high in fiber are eliminated from this diet.

- All foods in a *pureed diet* are put through a strainer so that they are in the form of a semisolid. Pureed foods are easy to chew and swallow.

- A *high-fiber diet* contains large amounts of fiber (more than 40 grams) from sources such as fresh fruits, vegetables, and bran cereal. Physicians may prescribe this diet for patients with conditions such as diverticulosis and constipation. The diet increases the bulk of fecal matter

and stimulates peristalsis (waves of alternating contraction and relaxation of the intestine that move contents through the intestine).

Nutrient Level

Doctors may make nutrient-level modifications in patients' diets before or after surgical or medical procedures or for patients who have specific conditions. Some of these types of diets are discussed in more detail in the next section. The following special diets are based on nutrient levels:

- Doctors may prescribe *low-sodium diets* for patients who suffer from many disease conditions such as those affecting the cardiovascular or urinary system, liver, pancreas, and gallbladder, including edema and hypertension. Dietary Approaches to Stop Hypertension (DASH) is one eating plan that includes lowering sodium. The typical American diet contains 2 to 5 grams of sodium daily. Following are sodium-restricted diet levels:

  - Mild restriction, 2 to 3 grams: reduce salt in cooking, add no salt at the table, and avoid processed foods.

  - Moderate restriction, 1 gram per day: add no salt in cooking or at the table and limit high-sodium vegetables, meat, and milk.

  - Severe restriction, 500 milligrams per day: greatly limit high-sodium vegetables, meat, milk, and eggs.

- Doctors recommend *low-cholesterol diets* for patients with high blood cholesterol levels. Such diets involve replacing saturated fats with unsaturated fats, using low-fat or nonfat cooking methods, and restricting fatty foods.

- Doctors may prescribe *reduced-calorie diets* to promote weight loss in patients who are overweight.

- Doctors may recommend *low-tyramine diets* for patients who have migraine headaches and patients who are taking certain antidepressant drugs. The compound tyramine is found in aged cheeses, red wine, beer, cream, chocolate, and yeast.

- Doctors may order *high-calorie, high-protein diets* for patients who have infections, are recovering from burns or surgery, or have had weight loss caused by a severe illness. Food intake is increased to provide 3000 to 5000 calories per day. Protein usually accounts for the greatest caloric increase in these diets.

- Doctors may prescribe *high-carbohydrate diets* for patients with kidney diseases and some cardiac conditions.

You can help patients who need to make nutrient-level modifications by teaching them how to read food labels. All packaged foods carry a Nutrition Facts label that contains information on the ingredients, major nutrients, and recommended amounts of key nutrients in daily diets. Procedure 55-1, at the end of this chapter, explains how to educate patients about reading food labels. You also can teach patients how to interpret the terms on food labels (Table 55-6). Understanding marketing terms simplifies the process of buying the right foods to meet special dietary needs.

TABLE 55-6 Food Label Terms and Definitions

Term	Definition
Low calorie	Less than or equal to 40 calories per serving
Reduced calorie	At least 25% fewer calories per serving than the food it replaces
Cholesterol free	Less than or equal to 2 mg cholesterol per serving
Low cholesterol	Less than or equal to 20 mg cholesterol per serving
Reduced cholesterol	At least 25% less cholesterol per serving than the food it replaces
Low fat	Less than or equal to 3 g fat per serving
Reduced fat	At least 25% less fat per serving than the food it replaces
Sodium free	Less than or equal to 5 mg sodium per serving
Very low sodium	Less than or equal to 35 mg sodium per serving
Low sodium	Less than or equal to 140 mg sodium per serving
Reduced sodium	At least 25% less sodium per serving than the food it replaces

Source: U.S. Department of Health and Human Services, Food and Drug Administration.

Frequency and Timing of Meals

A patient's diet also may be modified by adjusting the standard three-meal pattern. The goal may be to eat six small meals rather than three large meals to minimize stress on organs affected by disease conditions—as in patients with an ulcer or hiatal hernia. Six small meals also may be recommended to help regulate the blood sugar for patients with hypoglycemia, or low blood glucose. In other cases, meals may simply be timed to follow tests or therapeutic procedures.

Exclusion of Certain Foods

Physicians may order that specific foods be omitted from patients' diets for health reasons.

- In a *bland diet,* specific foods that cause irritation are eliminated, along with caffeine, alcohol, nicotine, aspirin, and some spices. A typical bland diet includes easily digested foods such as mashed potatoes and gelatins. Raw fruits and vegetables, whole grain foods, and very hot or cold items are among foods to avoid. A physician may prescribe this type of diet for a patient with a peptic ulcer, for example. A patient with diverticulosis may be on a bland diet and be restricted from eating nuts and seeds. In *diverticulosis* there are small pockets in the intestine that can get blocked with food, causing pain and inflammation in the abdomen.

- *Exclusion diets* are prescribed for patients who have food intolerances. These diets must eliminate foods that contain the offending substances but still provide the nutrients needed for good health. Intolerance to lactose, the sugar in milk, is fairly common. Intolerance to the amino acid phenylalanine—a condition present at birth—is fairly rare but very serious. Infants born in hospitals in the United States are tested for this intolerance because if these infants were to receive a standard diet, they would develop severe mental

retardation. People with this condition, known as phenylketonuria (PKU), must be vigilant about checking labels on prepared foods as well as knowledgeable about the phenylalanine content of fresh foods. Intolerance to gluten can range from mild to severe. **Gluten** is a protein substance found in wheat, rye, and barley. Mild intolerance can cause intestinal symptoms such as bloating and nausea. Severe intolerance is known as *celiac disease*. After eating gluten, the patient with celiac disease experiences damage to his small intestine that causes reduction in the absorption of nutrients from foods. Only gluten-free foods should be eaten.

▶ Patients with Specific Nutritional Needs LO 55.6

Patients may have a variety of conditions that require special diets or nutrients. In situations such as those that follow, you may need to educate patients about their diets and answer their questions. You may need to provide encouragement and emotional support and teach patients' caregivers how to perform physical tasks, such as holding utensils for patients during meals.

Patients with Allergies

Some patients have food allergies. Usually specific foods must be eliminated from or restricted in an allergic patient's diet. Procedure 55-2, at the end of this chapter, provides information on discussing with the patient potential dangers of common foods and reactions to those foods.

Some of the most common food allergens are wheat, milk, eggs, shellfish, peanuts, and chocolate. The doctor may confirm an allergy by eliminating and then reintroducing the patient's suspect foods one by one. The patient's allergy may decrease over time through systematic desensitization by means of allergy shots and other regimens.

If a food that is being eliminated or restricted was a primary source of nutrients for the patient, then the doctor must adjust the diet to include another source of those nutrients. For example, for a baby who is allergic to milk, the doctor may recommend a milk-substitute formula.

Patients with Anemia

Iron deficiency anemia, the most common type of anemia, is usually caused by chronic blood loss, a lack of iron in the diet, impaired intestinal absorption of iron, or an increased need for iron, as in pregnancy. A patient may need to take iron supplements and ingest more dietary iron as part of the treatment for this disorder. Foods high in iron include liver, egg yolks, dark green vegetables, beans, some dried fruits, and fortified breads and cereals.

Patients with Cancer

Many patients being treated for cancer undergo weight loss resulting both from the cancer and from treatments involving radiation or chemotherapy. To help their bodies fight off the cancer, it is especially important that they get enough protein because protein is needed to regenerate cells to replace the cells destroyed by the cancer and cancer treatments. These patients also may need to increase their intake of B vitamins and vitamins A, C, D, and E to support tissue growth and repair and promote efficient metabolism and use of all nutrients in the diet.

Encourage patients with cancer to follow the diet the physician sets for them. Patients may find this difficult because cancer often produces loss of appetite. They also may experience nausea and vomiting. Educate patients about ways to make food more appealing and easier to digest. Consuming small meals at frequent intervals may help. Patients also may follow a liquid diet. Bringing food to room temperature or chilling it slightly may reduce food odors that can trigger nausea. In some cases, especially during cancer treatment, the physician will prescribe medications to reduce the nausea and thus increase the patient's appetite.

Patients with Diabetes

A special diet is one of the foundations of treatment for diabetes. Dietary guidelines for patients with diabetes must not only provide them with adequate nutrition, but also keep their blood sugar level under control and interact appropriately with medication.

The diet a physician or dietitian prescribes for someone with diabetes includes a specific number of calories, meals per day, amount of carbohydrates, and amounts of other nutrients. As a way to simplify the diet, a system of **food exchanges** is used. All food exchanges in a particular food category provide the same amounts of protein, fat, and carbohydrates.

The list of exchanges is divided into seven categories—nonstarchy vegetables, fruits, starches, meats/meat alternatives, fats, milk, and sweets—and indicates how large a portion of each food in a category is equal to one "exchange" of food in that category. This information tells patients what portions of specific foods are interchangeable and whether they are eating the correct amounts of those foods. The list includes a variety of foods from which patients make their selections. It is important that patients with diabetes not skip a meal because skipping meals disturbs the balance of blood sugar and metabolism. Table 55-7 provides example food exchanges recommended for diabetics. These lists also can be obtained to provide for patients from a registered dietitian or the American Diabetes Association.

Patients with diabetes who are dependent on insulin should eat regular meals at consistent times. Skipping or delaying meals can result in hypoglycemia or an insulin reaction. The healthcare team specifies the proportion of carbohydrates and calories in meals, depending on the type of insulin each patient uses and the timing of injections.

Fiber is also important for patients who have diabetes. Fiber can sometimes prevent a sharp rise in blood glucose after a meal and may reduce the amount of insulin needed. It is therefore recommended that people with diabetes gradually increase their fiber intake until it is at about 45 grams per day.

Patients with Heart Disease

Coronary heart disease that is caused by atherosclerosis usually results from hyperlipidemia, or an excess of lipids in the bloodstream. Left untreated, this condition can lead to angina, heart attack, or stroke.

Patients can significantly lower their risk by reducing their blood cholesterol levels and losing weight if they are overweight. Patients who have coronary heart disease usually must reduce their consumption of fats to a level that provides less than 30% of their total caloric intake. Saturated fats should provide less than 10% of their caloric intake. Patients who have had a heart attack or are at increased risk for a heart attack are also encouraged to increase their consumption of soluble fiber.

As a medical assistant, your role with these patients is to encourage them to follow the nutritional regimen prescribed by the doctor.

Patients with Hypertension

Hypertension (high blood pressure) is a condition that affects more than 20% of American adults. Nutritional therapy for patients with hypertension involves the following:

- Restricting sodium intake to 2 to 3 grams per day, especially in salt-sensitive individuals.
- Increasing potassium intake through consumption of fresh fruits and vegetables, especially when taking certain medications.
- Ensuring adequate calcium intake to meet an RDA of 800 milligrams.
- Eliminating or reducing alcohol use.
- Decreasing total fat intake and obtaining no more than 10% of calories from saturated fats.

Patients with Lactose Sensitivity

Lactose is the sugar contained in human and animal milk. It must be broken down in the body by the enzyme lactase to enable the body to digest dairy products. In people from some parts of the world, lactase is present in the body until age 3 or 4, after which it all but disappears. As a result, after early childhood many people have trouble digesting foods that contain lactose and eliminate these foods from their diets. People who are especially sensitive to dietary lactose are often referred to as *lactose intolerant.*

Chemical preparations can help a person digest lactose. Those preparations may be added to certain foods, such as ice cream, for lactose-sensitive people. If people with a lactose sensitivity choose to avoid dairy products, they need to be sure to obtain protein and calcium from other sources.

Go to CONNECT to see an animation about *Digestion: Lactose Intolerance.*

Patients Who Are Overweight

More than one-third of American adults are obese. Seventeen percent of children age 2 to 19 are obese. Overweight patients weigh 10% to 20% more than is recommended for their height and gender. Patients who are more than 20% overweight are

TABLE 55-7 Diabetic Food Exchange Table

Food Exchange	U.S. Unit	Comments
Starches		
15g Carb, 3g Protein, 1g Fat		
• English muffin	½	• Most starches are a good source of B vitamins
• Graham crackers (2 ½-inch squares)	3	• Choose whole grain foods such as 100% whole wheat bread and flour, brown rice, tortillas, etc., for nutrients and fiber
• Bagel, large (4 ounces)	¼ (1 oz)	
• Bread, pumpernickel, rye, white, whole-grain	1 slice (1 oz)	• Combine beans (starch and meat) with grains (starch) for their complementary proteins and fiber
• Bread, reduced calorie	2 slices (1½ oz)	
• Cereal: bran, oats, spoon-size shredded wheat, frosted cereals	½ cup	• Combine grains (starch) with milk (milk) or cheese (meat) to complement proteins
• Cereal: unsweetened	¾ cup	• Add 1 fat exchange for starchy foods prepared with fat
• Grits, cooked	½ cup	
• Tabbouleh, prepared	½ cup	
• Pasta, cooked	⅓ cup	
• Wild rice, cooked	½ cup	
• Corn	½ cup	
• Popcorn, popped	3 cups	
• Potato (large, baked with skin)	¼ (3 oz)	
• Potato, mashed	½ cup	
• Sweet potato	½ cup (4 oz)	
• Squash, acorn, butternut	1 cup	
Add 1 meat exchange for the following starches:		
• Baked beans	⅓ cup	
• Beans, cooked: black, garbanzo, kidney, lima, pinto, navy, white	½ cup	
• Peas, cooked: black-eyed, green	½ cup	
• Refried beans, canned	½ cup	
Vegetables (3–5 exchanges)		
5g Carb, 2g Protein		
• Raw vegetables	1 cup	• Choose more dark green leafy and deep yellow vegetables such as spinach, broccoli, carrots, and peppers
• Cooked vegetables	½ cup	
Fruit (2–4 exchanges)		
15g Carb		
Fresh fruit:		• Choose whole fruits for fiber
• Apple, small (2 inches across)	1 (4 oz)	• Choose citrus fruits such as oranges, grapefruits, or tangerines
• Berries: blackberries, blueberries	¾ cup	
• Grapefruit, large	½	
• Mango, cubed	½ cup	
• Orange, small	1 (6 oz)	
• Strawberries	1¼ cup (13½ oz)	
Dried fruit:		
• Apple	4 rings	
• Prunes	3	
• Raisins	2 tbsp	
Canned fruit, unsweetened:		
• Applesauce, apricots, cherries, peaches, pears, pineapple, plums	½ cup	
• Grapefruit	¾ cup	
• Mandarin oranges	¾ cup	
Fruit juice, unsweetened: Apple, grapefruit, orange, pineapple	½ cup (4 fl oz)	

(continued)

TABLE 55-7 (concluded)

Food Exchange	U.S. Unit	Comments
Meat & Substitutes (5–7 exchanges)		
7g Protein, 0–13g Fat		
• Beef	1 oz	• Choose leaner meats such as chicken, fish, and lean cuts of meat; add fat exchange for higher-fat meats and substitutes
• Cheese	1 oz	• Remove skin from poultry
• Cottage cheese	¼ cup	• Limit frying or adding fat
• Egg whites	2	• Have 2 servings of fish per week for Omega 3 fatty acid
• Egg substitutes	¼ cup	
• Fish, fresh or frozen	1 oz	
• Pork	1 oz	
• Bacon	2 slices	
• Poultry	1 oz	
• Peanut butter	1 tbsp	
• Tofu	½ cup	
Milk (2–3 exchanges)		
12g Carb, 8g Protein, 0–8g Fat		
• Milk	1 cup	• Choose lower-fat milks; add fat exchange for higher-fat milk
• Soy milk	1 cup	
• Rice drink, low-fat, flavored	1 cup (8 fl oz)	
• Yogurt, low-fat with fruit	⅔ cup (6 oz)	
Fat (use sparingly)		
5g Fat		
• Almonds	6	• Eat less fat
• Coconut, shredded	2 tbsp	• Eat less saturated fat, such as animal fat found in fattier meat, cheese, and butter; also eat less hydrogenated fat
• Oil: canola, olive, peanut, corn, safflower, soybean, sunflower	1 tsp	• Check Nutrition Facts on food labels; 5g Fat = 1 Fat exchange
• Mayonnaise	1 tsp (1 tbsp if reduced-fat)	
• Cream cheese	1 tbsp (1½ if reduced-fat)	
• Salad dressing	1 tbsp (2 tbsp if reduced-fat)	
• Peanuts	10	
• Avocado	2 tbsp (1 oz)	
• Butter or margarine	1 tsp	

Sources: Mayo Clinic, www.mayoclinic.com/health/diabetes-diet/DA00077, and American Diabetes Association, www.americandiabetes.com/living-diabetes/diabetes-nutrition-articles/using-exchange-lists-diabetes-meal-planning (accessed May 21, 2012).

considered obese. Morbid obesity is when someone is more than 100 pounds overweight. Obesity can lead to medical complications such as elevated blood cholesterol levels, hypertension, diabetes, joint problems, respiratory problems, and heart disease.

Approaches to Weight Loss Weight reduction may be approached with dietary modification alone, but an exercise program is usually included. Behavior modification is also a common element of weight-loss programs. In a weight-loss program, foods should be proportioned in accordance with dietary guidelines and the diet should be appealing and enjoyable. The goal is to have the patient decrease daily caloric intake and increase physical activity at an appropriate rate while remaining comfortable and healthy.

Weight loss will not occur unless patients expend more energy than they consume. Calculators are available online and for smartphone devices that help individuals determine how much they can eat and how much exercise will result in weight loss. Foods that are high in nutrients but low in calories are desirable.

The **behavior modification** facet of weight loss includes such methods as keeping a food diary to pinpoint overeating patterns, controlling the stimuli associated with overeating, and providing rewards for successful behavior. Weight loss behaviors are important to maintain for a lifetime.

You can help overweight patients in their weight-loss efforts by teaching them to

- Eat slowly because the message that the stomach is full takes 20 minutes to register with the brain.
- Eat five or six small meals daily.
- Be patient—reliable weight loss occurs over time, not immediately.

Motivation and Education Patients who are trying to lose weight may have trouble with motivation. You may be able to introduce the patient to low-calorie or low-fat recipes, for instance, and positively reinforce the patient's efforts by complimenting small, gradual successes.

Tell patients that fad weight-loss methods can lead to vitamin, mineral, and protein deficiency; serious medical disorders; and even death. Use the following criteria to identify fad diets:

- They promise ease and comfort in weight loss.
- They include only a few foods, such as grapefruit or low-protein foods.
- They require the purchase of some secret ingredient or pill.
- They are often published in a book or magazine.

Truly effective weight-loss regimens usually possess the following qualities:

- They include a variety of foods that contain adequate nutrients.
- They include an activity component.
- They may be safely followed over a long period of time.

An effective program is one in which the patient is able to lose weight (including fat) gradually and constantly, with some plateaus, and then maintain the loss indefinitely afterward. You can help patients with the challenge of maintaining their weight loss by recommending a reputable weight-loss group or support group that will help them make the necessary lifestyle changes and remain motivated.

Go to CONNECT to see an animation about *Obesity*.

Pediatric Patients

During the first year of life, an infant experiences the most rapid period of growth and development that occurs during the life span. Breast milk is the best food for an infant up to six months of age. It contains the right amount of fat, sugar, water, and protein for an infant's growth and development. Breast-feeding saves time and money and helps the mother recover as well as reduces the risk of breast and ovarian cancers. If breast-feeding is not an option, infant formula is recommended by the physician. Regular, full-fat cow's milk should not be given to a child until after his or her first birthday.

Solid foods are introduced gradually starting at age four to six months. Infants should be able to hold their head up while sitting, open their mouth, swallow, and have an interest in food. The following are some basic guidelines for introducing foods to infants and toddlers:

- About 4 to 6 months: Iron-fortified, single-grain baby cereal; strained/pureed vegetables and fruit.
- 6 to 9 months: Strained meats/poultry; mixtures of strained vegetables and fruits; chunky, soft prepared baby foods; egg yolk; yogurt; and cottage cheese.
- 9 to 12 months: Soft, finely chopped foods; soft combination foods such as casseroles; macaroni and cheese; spaghetti; cheese; beans.
- Over 12 months: Toddler foods; family foods; fiber foods; whole cow's milk.

Additional detailed information is available about the nutritional requirements for infants and children at the U.S. Department of Agriculture website, http://www.usda.gov. Parents should be educated about these guidelines during their visits to the pediatrician's office.

The pace of growth is steadier and slower during childhood, with growth spurts throughout. Nutritional needs change to reflect growth, maturation, and increasing activity levels. Vitamin D and calcium are critical to tooth and bone formation, and fluoride strengthens teeth. Hunger regulates food intake in young children, but forcing children to eat can promote eating habits that lead to obesity.

Patients Who Are Pregnant or Lactating

Nutrition is especially important during pregnancy, when it provides for normal growth and health of the baby as well as the health of the pregnant woman. Doctors recommend that pregnant women gain a certain amount of weight during each trimester of pregnancy, with a total weight gain of about 25 to 35 pounds. The rate of weight gain should be 2 to 5 pounds in the first trimester and about 1 pound per week after that. Gaining too little or too much weight during pregnancy can result in serious complications. See Figure 55-12.

Here are some nutritional suggestions for pregnant women:

- An additional 10 to 15 grams of protein a day in the form of meat, poultry, fish, eggs, and dairy products.
- 1200 milligrams of calcium a day, preferably in the form of low-fat dairy products such as skim milk.
- 30 milligrams of iron a day through meat, liver, egg yolks, grains, leafy vegetables, nuts, dried fruits, legumes, and supplements (it is difficult to meet the daily need with food alone).
- Folic acid intake of 400 micrograms a day through leafy vegetables, yeast, and liver as well as supplements.
- Adequate fiber intake to prevent the constipation that often accompanies pregnancy.

Breast-feeding has specific nutritional and dietary requirements as well because breast milk is nutrient-rich and the body requires considerable energy and nutrients to produce it. The infant depends on this milk for the extensive

FIGURE 55-12 Pregnant patients should follow special nutritional guidelines to help ensure a healthy baby and mother.

growth that takes place during the first months of life. Lactating women need to consume an additional 500 calories and an additional 12 to 19 grams of protein per day as well as 260 to 280 micrograms of folic acid and 1200 milligrams of calcium.

Patients Requiring Supplements and/or Parenteral Nutrition

When a patient has a loss or lack of appetite or cannot tolerate a normal meal, the doctor may prescribe a specially formulated food supplement that provides protein, carbohydrates, fat, vitamins, and minerals. A patient who is chronically ill, underweight, or anemic or who has just undergone surgery may take supplements orally or through a tube to the stomach or small intestine. If the supplement is being taken orally, encourage the patient to follow the prescribed directions.

When patients cannot tolerate receiving supplements enterally (by way of the digestive tract), they may be fed parenterally. **Parenteral nutrition** is provided to patients as specially prepared nutrients injected directly into their veins rather than given by mouth. Because a parenteral feeding bypasses the digestive system, the nutrients it contains must already be in a form the body can use as they enter the blood.

Patients Undergoing Drug Therapy

Drugs may change a patient's nutritional status and needs. Long-term drug therapy and multiple prescriptions make close nutritional monitoring a high priority.

Drug therapy can cause a change in food intake, a change in the body's absorption of a nutrient, or both. Likewise, foods can interfere with the metabolism and action of a drug. For example, laxatives and certain other types of drugs may suppress the appetite. Antihistamines, alcohol, insulin, thyroid hormones, and some other drugs can stimulate appetite. Anesthetics can interfere with taste. Calcium in milk can diminish the absorption of some antibiotics. Be sure to discuss any possible interactions with the physician or dietitian before discussing diet and drug regimens with a patient.

▶ Eating Disorders   LO 55.7

Eating disorders, characterized by extremely harmful eating behavior, can lead to health problems. These disorders can damage the body and even cause death. They are most common in adolescent girls and young women, although 10% to 15% of patients with eating disorders are male. Refer to the Points on Practice feature to identify the signs and symptoms of common eating disorders.

Anorexia Nervosa

Anorexia nervosa is an eating disorder in which people starve themselves. They fear that if they lose control of eating, they will become grossly overweight. They lose an excessive amount of weight and become malnourished, and women often stop menstruating. The typical patient with anorexia nervosa is a high-achieving, white female in her teens or early 20s. The numbers of children and middle-aged women who suffer from the disorder, however, have been increasing. The cause of anorexia remains unknown, but risk factors include the following:

- Coming from a family that has problems with alcoholism.
- Suffering a childhood trauma, such as sexual abuse (20% to 50% of patients were sexually abused).
- Having a high stress level.
- Suffering from depression.
- Suffering from shame and low self-esteem.
- Having an extreme need to be in control.

It also has been noted that anorexia tends to run in families. The victim of anorexia often uses food as a way to deal with the psychological effects of trauma by numbing the emotions or as a means of getting some measure of control in life. Anorexia can be precipitated by any major life change.

This disorder can be fatal. The first stage of treatment is to restore normal nutrition. Patients may need to be hospitalized and fed intravenously or by nasogastric tube, which enters through the nose and delivers food into the stomach. Hospitalization may be necessary because patients with excessive weight loss may develop cardiac and other medical disorders. These patients also may be at risk for suicide. The hospital stay may eventually provide patients with the structure and support they need to establish healthy eating patterns.

Psychotherapy is essential and involves a combination of one-on-one and group therapy. Therapy groups that are single-sex rather than coed are preferable because of the different gender and peer group issues men and women face. Doctors may prescribe medication for depression and anxiety. The later

Recognizing the Signs and Symptoms of Common Eating Disorders

As a medical assistant, one of your primary responsibilities is to interview patients about their medical histories. It is important to know signs and symptoms of eating disorders in order to accurately form questions to gain complete medical information for the physician.

Anorexia Nervosa

- Unexplained weight loss of at least 15%.
- Self-starvation.
- Excessive fear of gaining weight.
- Malnourishment.
- Cessation of menstruation in women.
- Drastic reduction in food consumption.
- Denial of feeling hungry.
- Ritualistic eating habits.
- Overexercising.
- Unrealistic self-image as being obese.
- Extremely controlled behavior.

Bulimia

- Eating large quantities of food in a short period, followed by purging.
- Pretexts for going to the bathroom after meals.
- Using laxatives or diuretics to control weight.
- Buying and consuming large quantities of food.
- Feeling out of control while eating.
- Maintaining a constant weight while eating a large amount of fattening foods.
- Mood swings.
- Awareness of having a disorder, but fear of not being able to stop.
- Depression, self-deprecation, and guilt following the episodes.

Binge Eating

- Bingeing on food, not followed by purging.
- Weight gain.

stages of treatment include teaching patients and their families about nutrition concepts.

Bulimia

Bulimia is an eating disorder in which people eat a large quantity of food in a short time (bingeing) and then attempt to counter the effects of bingeing by self-induced vomiting, use of laxatives or diuretics, and/or excessive exercise. People with bulimia may use such behavior to try to gain control of their lives and weight.

Bulimia can be triggered when a slightly overweight person diets but fails to achieve the goal. Episodes are usually frequent, rapid, and uncontrollable. The behavior may occur only during periods of stress.

People with bulimia often diet when not bingeing. Psychologically, they believe their worth depends on being thin. Behind their cheerful exterior, they usually feel depressed, lonely, ashamed, and empty.

Most bulimics who seek help are in their early 20s and report that they have been bulimic for 4 to 6 years. Because they are more likely to want and seek help, they are slightly easier to treat than anorexics are.

Bulimia is usually not life-threatening, but it can cause the following serious health problems:

- Erosion of tooth enamel
- Enlarged salivary glands
- Lesions in the esophagus
- Stomach spasms
- Chemical and hormonal imbalances

As with anorexia, treatment for bulimia involves a combination of psychotherapy and medication. Dental work, medication for depression and anxiety, nutritional counseling, and support groups may be used. The goal is to establish a healthy weight and good eating patterns as well as to resolve the psychosocial triggers.

Getting Help

Studies show an unsatisfactory rate of recovery from eating disorders; only about half of anorexic patients fully recover. The disorders can become chronic, with periods of remission and relapse. Chronic anorexia can be fatal, and many people who do recover from eating disorders remain preoccupied with food.

If you suspect that a patient has an eating disorder, be alert for the following eating or activity patterns that the patient might mention in conversation:

- Skipping two or more meals a day or limiting caloric intake to 500 or fewer calories a day.
- Eating a very large amount of food in an uncontrollable manner over the course of 2 hours.
- Eating large quantities of food without being hungry.
- Using laxatives, excessive exercise, vomiting, diuretics, or other purges for weight control.
- Avoiding social situations because they may interfere with a diet or exercise.
- Feeling disgust, depression, and guilt after a binge.
- Feeling that food controls life.

▶ Patient Education

LO 55.8

Whenever you teach patients about nutrition and diet, you help them take steps to improve their health. In most instances, a physician or dietitian gives the patient instructions, which you then reinforce. Patients may feel more comfortable asking you questions about their diet than asking other members of the healthcare team. They may think their concerns are too trivial or simple for the physician or dietitian.

Because of your frequent contact with patients, you can play a major role in education. You can teach patients about the role of nutrition in helping to prevent specific medical conditions. You also can teach patients how to be wise consumers when they shop by reading food package labels. You will be better equipped to educate patients and answer their questions if you have a solid knowledge of diet and nutrition and if you stay current with recent research findings. See the Educating the Patient section for information on the relevance of such research. Before discussing a diet with any patient, be sure you understand the regimen the physician or dietitian is recommending as well as how to implement it.

If you are unsure of answers to any patient's questions, always ask the physician. Refer patients who have questions about meal patterns and food selections to the registered dietitian, if one is available.

Your Role in Patient Education

When discussing dietary requirements with a patient, keep in mind that the patient is always the focus of nutritional care. Specific factors to take into account include the following:

- Any psychological or lifestyle factors that affect food choices and behaviors. Learn about the patient's dietary likes and dislikes, as well as religious or cultural restrictions, before you suggest the use of specific foods in meeting dietary requirements.
- The patient's age and family circumstances. For example, parents need to know the specifics about an infant's or a child's diet. An elderly person's diet needs to be physically and economically manageable as well as nutritious.
- Diseases and disorders. For example, if the patient has chewing or breathing problems or is nauseous, the doctor will have to prescribe treatments or medications to address those problems.
- The patient's psychological condition. You can learn a great deal about psychological status through discussion and nonverbal cues. For instance, you might look for signs that the patient is frustrated with the dietary changes or is in denial about a problem. The greater the rapport you develop with a patient, the more you will be able to help.

Remind patients that eating healthfully will help them feel and look better and help their bodies work better. When the doctor prescribes therapeutic diets, be sure patients are fully aware of the reasons they must follow the diets. Help patients set realistic goals and praise them for even the smallest accomplishments. Offer positive reinforcement for current and new good food habits.

As with all patient education, teaching methods such as role playing, repetition of concepts, and the use of literature and other media reinforce your discussion. Use printed and audiovisual materials. Patient education sessions can be formal or informal and can take place at any appropriate time and place, such as in the office, over the telephone, or during a treatment or procedure. If possible, let patients decide which arrangements they prefer, or let them know the schedule in advance.

Patients need your support and empathy in working toward diet and nutrition goals, whether preventive or therapeutic. Follow these guidelines for best results when discussing diets with patients:

- Treat each patient as an individual with unique eating habits, knowledge of nutrition, and ability to learn.
- Teach a small amount of material at a time; 15- to 30-minute sessions are better than hour-long ones.
- Keep explanations at the level of the patient's understanding and vocabulary.
- Emphasize the patient's good eating behavior to reinforce it.
- Let the patient play an active role in the learning process—for example, by helping to plan the diet.
- Give the patient a written diet plan to take home as well as any other helpful materials you have to offer.
- Suggest that the patient contact local support groups for people who are trying to maintain the same kind of diet.

Nutritional education is part of preventative health care. Documentation is necessary to ensure payment by managed care and other health insurance providers. Failure to document can jeopardize a patient's insurance coverage. Document all patient education including the specific topic, the amount of involvement by the patient, what type of materials were used, and if follow-up is planned. See below for an example of nutritional documentation.

4/30/20XX Discussed low-calorie diet, exercise, and weight loss with patient. Patient encouraged to ask questions. 1800-calorie diet menu provided. Contact information provided for Weight Watchers. Patient scheduled for follow-up appointment in 6 weeks. ⸻

⸻ *Kaylyn R. Haddix RMA (AMT)*

Cultural Considerations

Eating is a personal and social activity, and cultural issues play an especially important part in diet and nutrition. A person's cultural heritage, religious background, family traditions, socioeconomic status, and personal beliefs help determine eating habits and preferences. Culture and lifestyle also help shape food purchasing and serving habits, likes and dislikes, meal timing and frequency, attitude toward food supplements, and tendency to snack.

Dietitians and nutritionists who design diets and recipes for patients know that to design successful diets, they must take into account cultural and lifestyle factors. You can increase the effectiveness of your patient education if you become familiar with the food habits and beliefs common to your patients' cultural backgrounds. Learn to recognize the eating patterns belonging to different cultures and make a special effort to familiarize yourself with the food preferences of the ethnic groups most commonly represented among the patients in the practice where you work.

Changes in Nutritional Recommendations

In the field of nutrition—as in other scientific fields—research continues to provide people with additional information. You can help answer patients' questions about the potential usefulness of new information by understanding the difference between initial research findings and those evaluated and endorsed by the government. In many cases, information is not officially released or endorsed until the government has studied the facts and determined that they are accurate and concrete enough for public consideration. For example, initial findings have suggested the following information:

- Beta-carotene supplements may provide no benefit and may even be harmful.
- Certain fruit-derived flavonoids—pigmented antioxidants—may help halt the growth of cancer cells.
- Vitamin D may reduce the risk of certain cancers.

Patients may read about research studies and ask whether they should make whatever dietary changes the findings suggest. You need to explain that such findings are preliminary and not formally approved by a government agency. Although the approval process is lengthy—requiring a significant amount of data and test results—it provides a system for protecting consumers from false nutritional claims.

Tell patients that once the government determines that a nutritional recommendation is warranted, it often acts on it. One example is the case of folate. Since the 1960s a number of studies have been conducted on the importance of folate in the diet. Over the years, those studies have yielded the following results:

- Folate offers protection from neural tube defects in unborn babies.
- Folate can reverse certain anemias.
- Folate may reduce the risk of cervical dysplasia.
- Folate appears to lower the likelihood of heart attacks.

As a result of these studies, the Department of Health and Human Services' Food and Drug Administration considered folate to be so important to all people that it approved the addition of folate to flour. Several nutrients have long been added to certain products to improve the products' nutritional value and to increase people's intake of important nutrients lacking in the general diet:

- Vitamin A and vitamin D, added to dairy products.
- Iodine, added to salt.
- Niacin, added to milled grain products.
- Various vitamins and minerals, added to processed cereals.

Explain to patients that nutritional recommendations change as scientists learn more about the ways various foods affect the human body and the exact amount of nutrients the body requires. Keep up-to-date on nutrition research so you can provide patients with the latest information and help them steer clear of unsubstantiated claims.

Organizations such as the American Dietetic Association, American Heart Association, and many others have excellent Internet sites. Websites such as www.health.gov are available to you and your patients.

PROCEDURE 55-1 Teaching Patients How to Read Food Labels

Procedure Goal: To explain how patients can use food labels to plan or follow a diet.

OSHA Guidelines: This procedure does not involve exposure to blood, body fluids, or tissues.

Materials: Food labels from products.

Method: Procedure steps.

1. Identify the patient and introduce yourself.
2. Explain that food labels can be used as a valuable source of information when planning or implementing a prescribed diet.
3. Using a label from a food package, such as the ice-cream label on the next page, point out the Nutrition Facts section.
4. Describe the various elements on the label—in this case, the ice cream label.
   - Serving size is the basis for the nutrition information provided. One serving of the ice cream is ½ cup. There are 14 servings in the package of ice cream.

RATIONALE: Paying close attention to the serving size and how many servings are in a container helps determine how many servings are being consumed.

- Calories and calories from fat show the proportion of fat calories in the product. One serving of the ice cream contains 180 calories; more than 41% of the calories come from fat.
- The % Daily Value section shows how many grams (g) or milligrams (mg) of a variety of nutrients are contained in one serving. Then the label shows the percentage (%) of the recommended daily intake of each given nutrient (assuming a diet of 2000 calories a day). The ice cream contains 28% of a person's recommended daily saturated fat intake and no dietary fiber.
- Recommendations for total amounts of various nutrients for both a 2000-calorie and a 2500-calorie diet are shown in chart form near the bottom of the label. These numbers provide the basis for the daily value percentages.

Cookie Dough

Nutrition Facts

Serving Size: 1/2 Cup (65g)
Servings Per Container: 14

Amount Per Serving

Calories 180   Calories from Fat 80

% Daily Value*

Total Fat 9g	13%
Saturated Fat 6g	28%
Trans Fat 0g	
Cholesterol 25mg	9%
Sodium 55mg	2%
Total Carbohydrate 21g	7%
Dietary Fiber 0g	0%
Sugars 15g	
Protein 3g	

Vitamin A   8%   •   Vitamin C 0%

Calcium   6%   •   Iron   2%

*Percent Daily Values are based on a 2,000 calorie diet. Your daily values may be higher or lower depending on your calorie needs.

	Calorie	2,000	2,500
Total Fat	Less than	65g	80g
Sat Fat	Less than	20g	25g
Cholesterol	Less than	300mg	300mg
Sodium	Less than	2400mg	2400mg
Total Carbohydrate		300g	375g
Dietary Fiber		25g	30g

MANUFACTURED BY
EDY'S GRAND ICE CREAM
HOME OFFICE: 5929 COLLEGE AVE.
OAKLAND, CA 94618

KEEP FROZEN UNTIL SERVED
S950603

FIGURE Procedure 55-1 STEP 3   Food labels are a source of nutrition information. This label provides facts on the nutrients and ingredients contained in this regular ice cream.

Nutrition Facts

Serving Size: 1/2 Cup (62g)
Servings Per Container: 14

Amount Per Serving

Calories 120   Calories from Fat 45

% Daily Value*

Total Fat 5g	8%
Saturated Fat 2g	10%
Trans Fat 0g	
Cholesterol 10mg	3%
Sodium 80mg	3%
Total Carbohydrate 15g	5%
Dietary Fiber 2g	8%
Sugars 3g	
Sugar Alcohol 4g	
Protein 3g	

Vitamin A   6%   •   Vitamin C 0%

Calcium   10%   •   Iron   0%

* Percent Daily Values are based on a 2,000 calorie diet. Your daily values may be higher or lower depending on your calorie needs.

	Calories:	2,000	2,500
Total Fat	Less than	65g	80g
Sat Fat	Less than	20g	25g
Cholesterol	Less than	300mg	300mg
Sodium	Less than	2400mg	2400mg
Total Carbohydrate		300g	375g
Dietary Fiber		25g	30g

FIGURE Procedure 55-1 STEP 5   By reading this label, a patient would learn that this light, no-sugar-added ice cream contains less sugar and fewer calories than regular ice cream.

- Ingredients are listed in order from largest quantity to smallest quantity. In this half-gallon of ice cream, skim milk, cream, and cookie dough are the most abundant ingredients.

5. Inform the patient that a variety of similar products with significantly different nutritional values are often available. Explain that patients can use nutrition labels to evaluate and compare such similar products. Patients must consider what a product contributes to their diets, not simply what it lacks. To do this, patients must read the entire label. Compared with the regular ice cream, the "light, no sugar added" ice cream (see label) contains less fat, fewer carbohydrates, and two grams of dietary fiber, but it contributes an additional 25 milligrams of sodium and contains sugar alcohol, which is an artificial sweetener.

6. Ask the patient to compare two other similar products and determine which would fit in better as part of a healthful, nutritious diet that meets that patient's individual needs.

7. Document the patient education session in the patient's chart, indicate the patient's understanding, and initial the entry.

Example documentation:

> 5/23/20XX Patient education session for low-fat diet. Patient given a written pamphlet. Patient stated knows the reason for a low-fat diet but may have trouble staying on the diet because she likes to eat ice cream. Shown ice cream food labels and practiced identifying type of ice cream with least amount of fat. Patient had no questions. _____
> _____ _K. Booth RMA (AMT)_

RATIONALE: Many insurance companies require evidence of preventative health counseling, and documentation is an important aspect of patient insurance coverage.

PROCEDURE 55-2 Alerting Patients with Food Allergies to the Dangers of Common Foods

Procedure Goal: To explain how patients can eliminate allergy-causing foods from their diets.

OSHA Guidelines: This procedure does not involve exposure to blood, body fluids, or tissues.

Materials: Results of the patient's allergy tests, patient's chart, pen, patient education materials.

Method: Procedure steps.

1. Identify the patient and introduce yourself.
2. Discuss the results of the patient's allergy tests (if available), reinforcing the physician's instructions. Provide the patient with a checklist of the foods that the patient has been found to be allergic to and review this list with the patient.
3. Discuss with the patient the possible allergic reactions those foods can cause.
   RATIONALE: The patient should know what signs to look for in the event an allergic reaction to food occurs so that he or she can react quickly and appropriately.
4. Discuss with the patient the need to avoid or eliminate those foods from the diet. Point out that the patient needs to be alert to avoid the allergy-causing foods not only in their basic forms but also as ingredients in prepared dishes and packaged foods. (Patients allergic to peanuts, for example, should avoid products containing peanut oil as well as peanuts.)
5. Tell the patient to read labels carefully and to inquire at restaurants about the use of those ingredients in dishes listed on the menu.
6. With the physician's or dietitian's consent, talk with the patient about the possibility of finding adequate substitutes for the foods if they are among the patient's favorites. Also discuss, if necessary, how the patient can obtain the nutrients in those foods from other sources (for example, the need for extra calcium sources if the patient is allergic to dairy products). Provide these explanations to the patient in writing, if appropriate, along with supplementary materials such as recipe pamphlets, a list of resources for obtaining food substitutes, and so on.
7. Discuss with the patient the procedures to follow if the allergy-causing foods are accidentally ingested.
   RATIONALE: Do not assume a patient will know what to do in the event of an allergic reaction.
8. Answer the patient's questions and remind the patient that you and the rest of the medical team are available if any questions or problems arise later on.
9. Document the patient education session or interchange in the patient's chart, indicate the patient's understanding, and initial the entry.
   RATIONALE: Many insurance companies require evidence of preventative health counseling, and documentation is an important aspect of patient insurance coverage.

Example documentation:

> 8/30/20XX Patient tested positive for peanut allergy. Explained the dangers of exposure to peanuts as well products cooked in peanut oils. Instructed to read package and inquire at restaurants before eating foods. Patient restated how to use EpiPen and other emergency actions in case an exposure to peanuts occurs. Education brochure provided to patient. _____
> _____ _K. Booth RMA (AMT)_

LEARNING OUTCOMES	KEY POINTS
55.1 Relate daily energy requirements to the role of calories.	The body uses food for three major purposes: to provide energy; to build, repair, and maintain body tissues; and to regulate body processes. Calories provide energy for the body. Calories are measured in the foods we eat. We also can estimate the amount of calories used by the body during activity.
55.2 Identify nutrients and their role in health.	The body needs a variety of nutrients for energy, growth, repair, and basic processes. Several food components provide nutrients. These are proteins, carbohydrates, fiber, lipids, vitamins, minerals, and water.
55.3 Implement a plan for a nutritious, well-balanced diet and healthy lifestyle using the USDA's guidelines.	Dietary guidelines suggest the types and quantities of food that people should eat each day. They also may contain the recommendations about which types of foods to limit and which types of foods to increase. MyPlate provides recommendations for eating a variety of nutrients and maintaining physical activity. Using MyPlate recommendations promotes a well-balanced diet and healthy lifestyle.
55.4 Describe methods used to assess a patient's nutritional status.	Calipers are used to perform a skinfold test that determines the percentage of body fat. BMI is the body mass index. Both measurements, along with other factors, may be used to assess a patient's nutritional status.
55.5 Explain reasons why a diet may be modified.	Dietary modifications may be used alone or in combination with other therapies to prevent or treat illness.
55.6 Identify types of patients who require special diets and the modifications required for each.	Patients with allergies, anemia, cancer, diabetes, heart disease, hypertension, lactose sensitivity, and obesity need special diets. In addition pediatric, pregnant, lactating, and debilitated patients as well as those undergoing drug therapy need modifications to their diet.
55.7 Describe the warning signs, symptoms, and treatment for eating disorders.	You should know the signs and symptoms of eating disorders in order to evaluate for these disorders during the patient interview. Some of the more common signs and symptoms for each include • Anorexia nervosa—unexplained weight loss, self-starvation, and fear of weight gain. • Bulimia—eating large quantities of food in a short period of time, going to the bathroom immediately after eating, and using laxatives to excess. • Binge eating—eating large quantities of food, not followed by purging, and weight gain.
55.8 Educate patients about nutritional requirements.	Patients need to be educated about special diets and how to implement dietary changes as instructed by physicians and dietitians. Knowledge of basic nutritional principles and current nutritional findings is necessary. Documentation is required to help ensure payment by managed care and other health insurance companies.

Recall Mohammad Nassar from the beginning of this chapter. Now that you have completed this chapter, answer the following questions:

1. What is the patient's probable diagnosis?
2. Do you think that the patient's attention to calorie intake is simply, as he says, preparation for wrestling competition?
3. Why is this patient experiencing muscle weakness?

E X A M   P R E P A R A T I O N   Q U E S T I O N S

1. (LO 55.6) What is the most highly recommended food for a patient less than 6 months old?
   a. Single-grain baby cereal
   b. Iron-fortified infant formula
   c. Breast milk
   d. Whole milk
   e. Two percent milk

2. (LO 55.5) Which of the following foods should not be given to a patient with lactose sensitivity?
   a. Cheese
   b. Broccoli
   c. Chicken
   d. Eggs
   e. Bananas

3. (LO 55.3) Which of the following is a key recommendation of the USDA Dietary Guidelines?
   a. Reduce physical activity to less than 2 days per week
   b. Reduce sodium intake to less than 2300 mg a day
   c. Consume no more than three alcoholic beverages a day
   d. Consume at least 500 mg of cholesterol a day
   e. Avoid oils and use solid fats for cooking

4. (LO 55.2) On average, an adult should drink _____ glasses of water a day.
   a. 2 to 8
   b. 6 to 8
   c. 4 to 10
   d. 4 to 6
   e. 2 to 6

5. (LO 55.2) Which of the following statements about protein is correct?
   a. Protein decreases the rate of carbohydrate breakdown and absorption
   b. Protein serves as a constituent of bile, which aids in digestion

   c. Protein assists with antibody production and disease resistance
   d. Protein provides a concentrated source of heat and energy
   e. Protein flushes out wastes

6. (LO 55.4) Which of the following best describes the skin-fold test?
   a. Measure of body fat based on height and weight that applies to adult men and women
   b. Provides the same amounts of protein, fat, and carbohydrates
   c. Pinching of the skin with a caliper to determine the weight of a patient
   d. Measure of fat as percentage of body weight
   e. Requires a formula to be determined

7. (LO 55.1) Which of the following is *not* a part of the process of nutrition?
   a. Absorption
   b. Elimination
   c. Intake
   d. Metabolism
   e. Indigestion

8. (LO 55.8) Which of the following guidelines would you *least* likely use when educating a patient about nutrition?
   a. Treat each patient as an individual with unique eating habits, knowledge of nutrition, and ability to learn
   b. Teach an eating plan that you have developed using specific dietary guidelines
   c. Teach a small amount of material at a time; 15- to 30-minute sessions are better than hour-long ones
   d. Keep explanations at the level of the patient's understanding and vocabulary
   e. Emphasize the patient's good eating behavior to reinforce it

9. (LO 55.7) The patient is 5′6″ and weighs 145 lbs, which is the same as her last visit 6 months ago. She says she can easily eat at least one dozen donuts for breakfast and her mother is always telling her she is moody. You know you need to report this information to the physician because it is possible the patient has
   a. Anorexia
   b. Lactose intolerance
   c. Bulimia
   d. Binge eating
   e. Hypertension

10. (LO 55.5) The DASH eating plan would be used by someone who has
   a. Diabetes
   b. Obesity
   c. Hypothyroidism
   d. Hypertension
   e. Lactose intolerance

Practice Management

PATIENT INFORMATION

Patient Name	Gender	DOB
Cindy Chen	F	07/15/19XX
Attending	**MRN**	**Allergies**
Alexis N. Whalen, MD	324-86-542	NKA

Cindy Chen is a 28-year-old HIV positive female who is a patient of Dr. Whalen. Cindy has recently completed a phlebotomy course at the local community college—in fact, she did her externship at BWW Medical Associates and did very well. There is an opening at BWW for a phlebotomist and Cindy has applied for the position. The staff all like Cindy and would like to be part of her "new lease on life."

Keep Cindy in mind as you study the chapter. There will be questions at the end of the chapter based on the case study. The information in the chapter will help you answer these questions.

LEARNING OUTCOMES

After completing Chapter 56, you will be able to:

56.1 Explain the basic organizational designs of the medical office and the relationship of the physician and the medical assistant with the practice manager and direct supervisors.

56.2 Describe the responsibilities of the practice manager.

56.3 Summarize the basic human relations functions in practice management.

56.4 Distinguish the four traits of someone with leadership skills and the importance of these skills to the healthcare team.

56.5 Compare risk management and quality assurance in a medical facility.

56.6 Calculate an employee's gross earnings, deductions, and net earnings for a pay period.

56.7 Describe the tax forms commonly used in the medical office and the purpose of the office tax liability account.

KEY TERMS

agenda
budget
chain of command
employee handbook
Federal Unemployment Tax Act (FUTA)
Form I-9
Form W-2
Form W-4
grievance process
incident report

labor relations
mediation
midlevel provider
net earnings
organizational chart
policies and procedures (P&P)
probationary period
sexual harassment
tax liability account

IV. P (4) Explain general office policies

IV. A (1) Demonstrate empathy in communicating with patients, family and staff

IV. A (2) Apply active listening skills

V. P (6) Use office hardware and software to maintain office systems

V. A (2) Implement time management principles to maintain effective office function

IX. C (2) Explore issue of confidentiality as it applies to the medical assistant

IX. C (3) Describe the implications of HIPAA for the medical assistant in various medical settings

IX. C (12) List and discuss legal and illegal interview questions

IX. P (1) Respond to issues of confidentiality

IX. P (6) Complete an incident report

IX. A (3) Recognize the importance of local, state and federal legislation and regulations in the practice setting

X. C (5) Identify the effect personal ethics may have on professional performance.

4. **Medical Law and Ethics**
   Graduates:
   f. Comply with federal, state and local health laws and regulations

8. **Medical Office Business Procedures/Management**
   Graduates:
   l. Establish and maintain a petty cash fund
   x. Maintain medical facility
   dd. Serve as liaison between physician and others
   ff. Interview effectively

11. **Career Development**
    Graduates:
    b. Demonstrate professionalism by:
        (1) Exhibiting dependability, punctuality, and a positive work ethic
        (3) Maintaining confidentiality at all times

▶ Introduction

In previous chapters, you have explored many of the complex systems, procedures, requirements, and roles required in the modern medical office. Today, it is much more difficult for the physician to care for patients and manage the office as he or she may have done in the past. While the healthcare facility's management differs by ownership, size, and other variables (addressed in the *Legal and Ethical Issues* chapter), one person is generally in charge of overseeing the day-to-day operations, working closely with the practice physicians to keep the practice running smoothly and its staff working at its professional peak (Figure 56-1). The title of this person has varying names like *practice* or *office manager*, *executive*, or *director*; or *healthcare administrator*. This chapter discusses this person's position, responsibilities, and relationship with the physician and medical assistant. The terms "medical practice manager" and "office manager" represent the role. Employee management functions, including human resources and facility management, also are discussed in this chapter.

▶ Organizational Design   LO 56.1

Every medical office has an organizational design that may or may not be represented by a formal **organizational chart**. The design and chart show the supervisory structure and reporting relationships between different functions and positions—in other words, who is responsible for whom and for what. In most

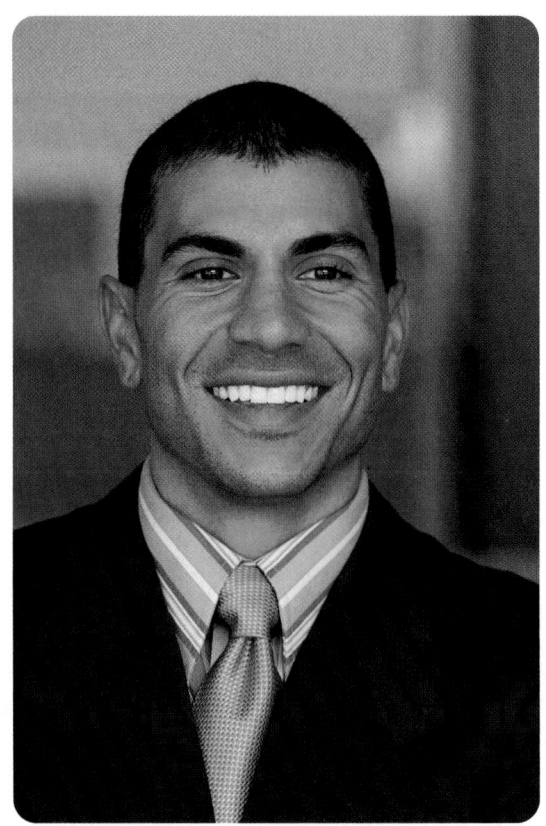

FIGURE 56-1 As the practice manager, Malik Katahri keeps the practice running smoothly.

states, the medical assistant is required to be under the direct supervision of the physician, physician assistant, or nurse practitioner for direct patient care activities. However, the practice manager or that person's designee is usually responsible for interviewing, hiring, firing, evaluating, and ensuring training and credentialing, which are all considered administrative and not direct patient care functions. Both physician-owned and company-owned medical practices rely on some form of organizational design in order to function effectively.

Physician-Owned Medical Practice

Figure 56-2 represents a physician-owned practice's simplified organizational chart. As you learned in the *Legal and Ethical Issues* chapter, a physician-owned medical practice sometimes obtains the legal designation of a professional corporation (PC). The owner is usually an individual doctor or group of physicians. The placement of the boxes and lines shows that the physician carries the ultimate responsibility but designates it to the person below him—the practice manager. The practice manager reports to the physician who also pays his or her salary. The manager is the physician's employee who oversees the daily operations and the administrative functions of the entire office and staff, including the medical assistants. The solid line from the physician to the medical assistant demonstrates that the physician also has direct responsibility for the medical assistants. As mentioned previously, this responsibility involves direct patient

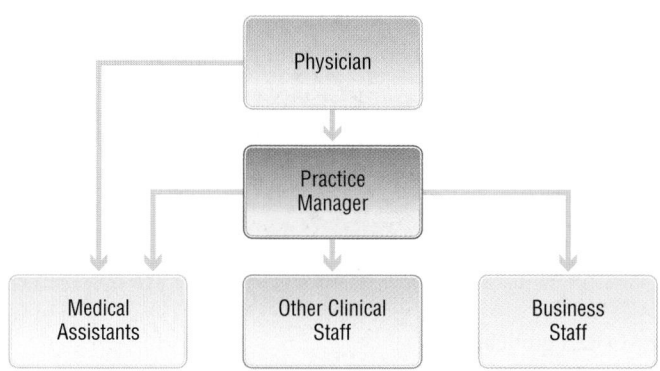

FIGURE 56-2 Practice organizational chart for a physician-owned practice.

care. Depending on the size of the practice, other supervisory personnel might report to the practice manager. Each supervisor would then have staff reporting directly to him or her. In multispecialty organizations, supervisors may be designated by specialty such as pediatrics, internal medicine, and cardiology.

Company-Owned Medical Practice

Figure 56-3 represents a simplified organizational chart of a company-owned medical facility. The company may be non-profit, like a community health center, or for-profit, like Cigna HealthCare. The president or chief executive officer (CEO) has the ultimate responsibility. However, again, the practice manager is in charge of the day-to-day operations with the exception of the direct patient care functions. The medical director is in charge of the patient care end of the practice, overseeing the physicians, nurses, **midlevel providers** (physician assistants and nurse practitioners), and medical assistants. The dotted lines between the practice manager and the medical director indicate they are equal in rank and collaborate with each other. The dotted line from the practice manager to the other physicians indicates collaboration. For example, the practice manager may ensure that the physicians are properly credentialed, but the medical director has the majority of the responsibility for the providers, including their schedules and periodic evaluations. The president, practice manager, medical director, and other physicians and staff are paid employees of the company. A board of directors is ultimately responsible for the practice, through the CEO, but this board is not involved in the company's daily operations.

The Chain of Command

The phrase **chain of command** began in the military to demonstrate how each rank is accountable to those directly superior and how the authority passes from one link in the chain to the next from bottom to top or top to bottom. For example, in the military, a private is accountable to the sergeant, who is accountable to the lieutenant, and so on. The lieutenant would give an order to the sergeant, who gives it to the private. Each level of the chain has many steps, including the determination of the equipment, training, and strategies needed to carry out the order or mission. The majority of today's businesses, including medical practices, operate using this approach.

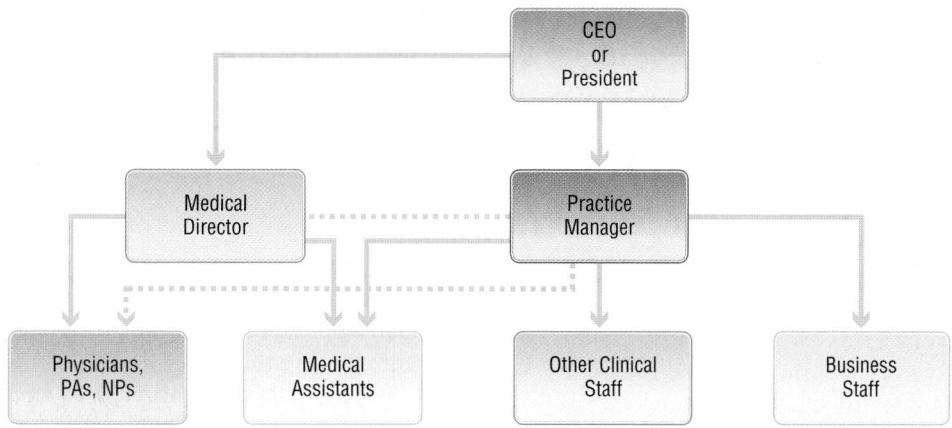

FIGURE 56-3 Practice organizational chart for a company-owned medical practice.

It is important to understand the chain of command in your facility and to understand who your supervisor is. Since medical assistants work closely with physicians, the tendency may be to go to the physician with requests such as asking for time off. If the physician is not your supervisor, it is inappropriate to "go over your supervisor's head" and make the request of the physician as he may not have the authority to grant your request. It is also inappropriate to go outside the chain of command with a complaint, even if the complaint is about your supervisor. First, address the issue with your supervisor. If this issue is not resolved, then go to the next person in the chain of command, such as the practice manager. Most offices have policies and procedures for handling complaints. Should you seek other employment, that organization will contact your previous supervisor for references. No matter how friendly or informal the medical practice is, stay within the chain of command.

▶ Managing the Medical Practice LO 56.2

The practice manager's role includes providing communication avenues for all medical team members as well as communicating with members of the community outside the medical practice. The practice manager is also responsible for ensuring that legal, business, health, and safety requirements are in compliance; guaranteeing the adequacy of the technology and physical plant; providing for the practice's financial viability; and monitoring risk management and customer care and satisfaction. Sometimes, the manager also may be in charge of multiple satellite offices.

Communication Skills of the Practice Manager

The *Interpersonal Communication* chapter described general communication techniques used in communication with patients, persons with special needs, and coworkers. The *Written and Electronic Documents* chapter outlined the general practices for producing effective and professional written communication. The practice management position requires exceptional verbal and written communication skills and excellent interpersonal skills. Listed are some of the routine individuals and groups with whom the practice manager communicates on a regular basis:

- Staff
- Patients
- Physicians (within practice and in other practices)
- Hospitals
- Insurers
- Vendors
- Employers
- Contractors
- Governmental agencies
- Other regulatory and professional agencies
- Educational facilities
- Bankers
- Attorneys
- Community organizations

Communicating with each individual and group requires knowledge of the business or situation and, often, excellent problem-solving techniques. The manager's role is also to ensure that all communication is appropriate, respectful, timely, and HIPAA compliant. Many offices have policies and procedures related to communication, especially electronic communication.

The Policies and Procedures Manual

The **policies and procedures (P&P)** manual is a key written communication tool in the medical office. No discussion of communication in the medical office would be complete without a description of this important document. Both permanent and temporary employees use this manual, which covers all office policies for administrative and clinical procedures. The physician (or physicians), practice manager, and staff (often including the medical assistant) usually develop this manual as a joint effort. See Figure 56-4.

Policies are rules or guidelines that dictate an office's day-to-day workings. Although individual policies vary from office to office, most medical office manuals describe the following policy areas:

- Office purposes, objectives, and goals as set by the physician(s).
- Rules and regulations.
- Job descriptions and duties of staff personnel.
- Office hours.
- Dress code.
- Insurance and other benefits.
- Vacation, sick leave, FMLA, and other time away from the office.
- Salary and performance evaluations.
- Maintenance of equipment and supplies.
- Mailings.
- Bookkeeping.
- Scheduling of appointments and maintenance of patient records.
- OSHA guidelines.

Policies This section of the manual typically includes the previously described chain of command for the office and/or the person to whom each employee reports. The policy section often also includes the statement of intent or goal intended, resulting in the procedures that follow.

Procedures The procedure—the map for reaching the goal—incorporates the correct manner for carrying out each individual policy. For example, the policy might state that OSHA guidelines for bloodborne pathogens will be maintained by all staff at all times. The accompanying procedure would describe the steps expected to maintain bloodborne pathogen guidelines. Facilities may have more than one P&P manual, such as one for human resources, one for safety, one for clinical procedures, and one for administrative procedures. The practice manager must stay current with new practices and standards of the community and all applicable professional organizations, updating the office manual as

BWW Medical Associates, PC
305 Main Street, Port Snead YZ 12345-9876
Tel: 555-654-3210, Fax: 555-987-6543
Web: BWWAssociates.com

Paul F. Buckwalter, MD
Alexis N. Whalen, MD
Elizabeth H. Williams, MD

POLICY AND PROCEDURE

Subject: Competency of Staff

Date of Issue: Sept. 25, 20XX

Policy # 1001

Effective Date: Oct. 1, 20XX

I. POLICY

It is the policy of BWW Medical Associates, PC that all employees meet the standards of competency as defined by its various policies and the requirements of TJC and other regulatory and credentialing agencies.

II. PURPOSE

The competence of staff members is (a) defined by job descriptions designed by the director; (b) assessed initially during the orientation process; (c) maintained through educational updates; and (d) evaluated periodically in conjunction with the performance appraisal process.

III. IMPLEMENTATION

a. Job Descriptions
i. The office manager will write and/or review each job description annually. Each job description will reflect the educational experience and training needed for the position and include competency-based performance standards.

FIGURE 56-4 Sample from BWW Medical Associates' policies and procedures manual.

required. In addition, new laws and requirements of governmental agencies like OSHA and CMS must be monitored and incorporated. Reading the policies and procedure manual(s) is typically part of new employee orientation. Each employee should know the location of the policies and procedures manual; an employee should look here if he or she is unsure about a specific duty or task.

The clinical procedures manual should include instructions regarding the following for each test performed:

- Purpose of the test, clinical application, and usefulness.
- Specimen required and collection method; special patient preparation or restrictions.
- Reagents, standards, controls, and media used; special supplies.
- Instrumentation, including calibration and schedules.
- Step-by-step directions.

The administrative procedure manual may include instructions regarding the following procedures:

- Appropriate telephone procedures for emergency and non-emergency calls.
- Releasing of patient PHI.

- Guidelines for submission of "clean" claims for each provider.
- Templates for frequently created communications like normal lab and X-ray results.

Licenses, Certifications, and Contracts

The medical practice includes many positions and facets that require federal, state, or local approval. Approvals may be in the form of a license, certification, or other credential or contract. Some are simple procedures; others are more expensive and complicated. Common responsibilities include ensuring that

- Physicians and midlevel providers are properly licensed and credentialed with CMS and other payers as required and that the credentialing is up-to-date.
- Physician and midlevel provider DEA forms are up-to-date.
- Medical assistants, phlebotomists, coders, and other personnel are properly trained and certified or credentialed according to federal, state, and professional standards.
- Required licenses to operate the facility, like local business licenses, are up-to-date.
- Insurance requirements like malpractice and liability contracts are up-to-date and reflect current values.

- Health insurance companies, laboratories, attorneys, and service contracts necessary to conduct business are current.
- The practice is compliant with required reporting to authorities such as that for reporting communicable diseases.

Depending on the healthcare organization's size, the manager may have other employees involved in carrying out these duties. However, the manager has the ultimate responsibility to guarantee that these tasks are completed in a proper and timely fashion.

Budget and Overall Finances

With the exception of large organizations that have a chief financial officer (CFO), the responsibility for the practice finances is part of the manager's extensive role. A **budget** is created annually and reviewed at least monthly. The budget predicts the expenses and revenues related to operations over a given period of time. First, the manager must know the total expenses. Salaries are usually the biggest budget expense. The manager reviews the healthcare insurance and governmental agencies' patient care contracts and other sources of income. Sometimes the manager must renegotiate the contract if costs have risen. If revenues are lower than expected and costs are higher, the manager must make unpopular budget cuts so the practice remains profitable and able to continue to provide care for the community it serves.

As the office medical assistant, be mindful that financial responsibility is the role of every employee. In a very real sense, even something as seemingly inconsequential as taking pens home from the office can have an impact on the practice. The immediate thought may be, "it's just a pen," but the reality is, you did not purchase the pen—the practice did—and if every member of the staff took "only a pen or two," soon there would not be enough pens in the practice. Part of the ethics and integrity of being in the medical profession is your professional behavior—particularly "when no one is looking."

Managing Petty Cash Another budget function, often managed by the medical assistant with oversight by the practice manager, is the petty cash fund. This fund is used to make small (petty) cash disbursements for minor expenses like postage-due fees or holiday decorations (Figure 56-5).

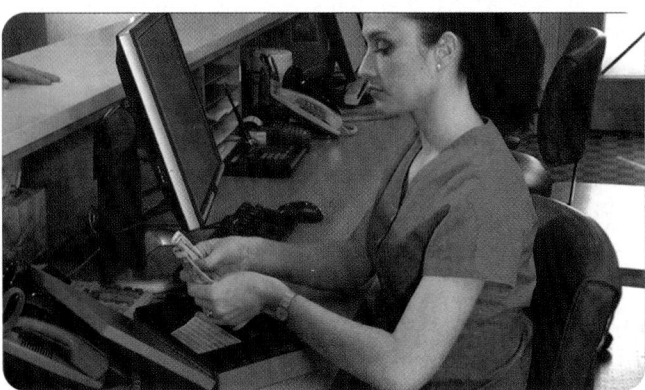

FIGURE 56-5 Managing petty cash is often the task of the medical assistant.

To avoid writing checks for such small amounts, you may pay for them from the petty cash fund (also known as the revolving fund)—cash kept on hand in the office for small purchases. The practice manager often determines the amount of the petty cash account (usually $50) and the minimum amount of cash to be kept on hand (such as $15).

Starting and Maintaining a Petty Cash Fund To start the fund with $50, write a check to "Petty Cash" or "Cash" for that amount. Enter the check in the miscellaneous column of the monthly disbursements journal (refer to the *Financial Management* chapter). Then, cash the check. Because this money will be used for small disbursements, be sure to get some of it in pennies, nickels, dimes, quarters, and dollar bills. Put this money in a special petty cash box, along with a stack of petty cash vouchers.

For each payment from the petty cash fund, obtain a receipt or create a petty cash voucher. The voucher should record the transaction number, date, amount paid, purpose of the expense, your signature (as the person issuing the money), and the signature of the person receiving it. Keep the receipt for any item purchased, along with the completed voucher, in the petty cash box to verify expenses later.

Also, document each petty cash withdrawal on a petty cash record form. Include the transaction number, date, payee, a brief description, amount, and type of expense (such as office expense, auto expense, or miscellaneous expense). If a space is provided, calculate and record the new balance in the petty cash fund.

Replenishing the Petty Cash Fund At the end of the month (or whenever the fund is low), compare the latest petty cash balance to the money in the petty cash box. If you have not kept a running balance, total the receipts and vouchers, then count the cash on hand. Subtract the total amount on the receipts and vouchers (for example, $35) from the original balance (for example, $50). The difference ($15) should equal the cash on hand in the petty cash box ($15).

To replenish the account, write a check to "Cash" or "Petty Cash" for the amount spent ($35). Cash the check and add the money to the box, bringing the total back up to the original amount of $50. Record the check for $35 in the disbursements journal. Also, total the receipts and vouchers by expense category. Record those totals in the appropriate columns on the disbursement record.

Go to CONNECT to see a video about *Petty Cash.*

Scheduling and Travel

Ensuring that adequate staff members are on duty at all times for the business to function properly is an additional aspect of the practice manager's role. Scheduling is a job that may be delegated to a supervisor or other person, depending on the practice's size, but the practice manager monitors it. When office staff members are absent due to vacation, extended illness, or educational purposes, rearranging remaining staff member schedules to provide coverage may be necessary. If physicians are not available to see patients, the office may be closed during their absence.

Sometimes, physicians and other staff, like medical assistants, travel for educational purposes with expenses covered by the practice, in which case work-related expenses may be reimbursed if the appropriate receipts are kept and an expense report is completed (Figure 56-6). Procedure 56-1, at the end of this chapter, provides you with practice in completing a travel expense report.

Other Business Functions

The contemporary medical office relies on technology for communication, appointment scheduling, coding, billing, diagnostic test ordering and reporting, prescription refills, and the electronic health record. The office manager evaluates and purchases the systems that fit the practice's needs and budget, facilitates the installation and staff training, then oversees the ongoing operations through an in-house technical support person or through a service contract. Other managerial functions include ensuring availability of mailing and shipping services,

BWW

BWW Medical Associates, PC
305 Main Street, Port Snead YZ 12345-9876
Tel: 555-654-3210, Fax: 555-987-6543
Web: BWWAssociates.com

Paul F. Buckwalter, MD
Alexis N. Whalen, MD
Elizabeth H. Williams, MD

TRAVEL EXPENSE REPORT
(Travel with estimated expenses must be approved prior to the event)

Applicant's name: _____ Date: _____

Applicant's address: _____

Applicant's cell phone and home phone: _____

Name of activity and type (example: professional meeting, conference; attach Web or brochure

information): _____

Purpose of travel: _____

Location of activity: _____

Registration fee	$
Transportation: *indicate major mode of travel	$
Airport shuttle or parking	$
Taxi	$
Lodging (daily rate _____ × _____ number of days)	$
Meals ($30 per day × _____ number of days)	$
Other (explain)	$
Total	$

Did you miss work days: [ ] NO [ ] YES (If "YES" include dates and number of days)

Dates: _____ Number of days: _____

Signature: _____

*If using your own vehicle, mileage is reimbursed at the current rate. Check with your supervisor prior to travel.

This form must be submitted with receipts in 10 working days upon return. Noncompliance may result in denial of reimbursement or if funds were previously awarded, payroll deduction may occur to recover the amount.

For Management Use Only

[ ] Not approved [ ] Approved Amount: _____

Name (print): _____ Date: _____

Signature: _____

FIGURE 56-6 Typical travel expense report to be submitted with appropriate receipts to allow for reimbursement of business-related travel expenses.

inventory and supply purchases, and appropriate marketing and public relation strategies, which may include websites, brochures, and community event sponsorship.

▸ Human Relations and Practice Management

LO 56.3

The practice manager's role includes the human resources (HR) component of the medical office. This area of the organization is probably the only one that does not involve the patient. If the practice or facility is large, it may have its own human relations coordinator or supervisor who reports to the practice manager. If the practice is smaller, the practice manager often functions as the human resources "department." In the business world, human resources directly concerns employee-related issues like hiring (and terminating), training, benefits, and labor relations. Other names for HR include personnel services, personnel department, or people services. Within this section of the chapter, we will follow Miguel A. Perez's experience with the hiring process at BWW Medical Associates.

The Hiring Process

As discussed in the *Legal and Ethical Issues* chapter, federal, state, and local governments regulate many hiring practices, including the Equal Employment Opportunity Commission (EEOC—Figure 56-7), Fair Labor Standards Act, Equal Pay Act, Age Discrimination in Employment Act, and Americans with Disabilities Act (ADA), as well as the Family Medical Leave Act (FMLA), which allows employees up to 12 job-protected weeks of unpaid leave for approved medical needs for the employee and certain family members. Violations can result in monetary and other penalties. Understanding and staying current with these often complex laws is a major HR role. Table 56-1 outlines some legal versus illegal questions that may be asked during the interview process. Keep in mind, one of the best techniques may be to ask a legal question and then remain quiet. Most people

FIGURE 56-7 The EEOC prevents discrimination based on race, color, religion, sex, or national origin.

get nervous during silent moments and often end up giving you more information than you asked for.

In addition to understanding the laws surrounding the hiring process, it is always best to stress competencies like teamwork, policies and procedures, and cross-training during the interview process and during orientation. Potential employees should understand the qualities that are important to the practice at which they are seeking employment—they need to know if they will be a good fit in the practice and if the practice will be a good fit for them. Employee orientation is essential in the personnel management phase. During this process, the new hire gets to see and meet important people within the organization. He or she also gets to know what is expected of the position, as well as gain information about company benefits.

The basics of hiring a successful employee are

- Always try to find the most qualified person for the job.
- Scrutinize and check references carefully.
- Have a salary range so you can negotiate successfully and pay for the "most qualified" person.
- Discuss policies and procedures (and expectations) early.
- Train properly and retrain when new technology arrives.

When BWW Medical Associates decided to hire an administrative medical assistant, a job description was written that consisted of the following:

- Name of organization
- Name of the position
- Employment grade
- Summary of the position
- Job responsibilities
- Requirements and qualifications
- Title of the supervisor

One of the job description requirements was that the applicant have a current CMA (AAMA) or a RMA (AMT) certification. The next step was to recruit qualified candidates. Miguel A. Perez was a CMA (AAMA) who applied for the position and his application was one of those selected. He interviewed very well and after his references were checked, Miguel was offered the position with an appropriate salary. HR maintains a personnel file for every employee. Malik Katahri, the office manager at BWW, initiated an HR file for Miguel.

Orientation and Staff Development

The human resource department provides orientation for new employees and facilitates training and staff development for established employees. Orientation has three overarching sections: the organization; health and safety; and the employee's job. The US Department of Labor (DOL) publishes and provides online copies of the Employment Law Guide that addresses many aspects of each of these sections. An **employee handbook** provides a synopsis of the HR policies and procedures. Employee handbooks and HR policies should address **sexual harassment**, which is a violation of federal and some

TABLE 56-1	Legal versus Illegal Interview Questions	
Topic	**Illegal Questions**	**Legal Questions**
Reliability/attendance	Number of children?	What hours and days can you work?
	Who is going to baby-sit?	Are there specific times that you cannot work?
	What religion are you?	Do you have responsibilities other than work that will interfere with specific
	Do you have preschool-age children at home?	job requirements such as traveling?
	What is your marital status?	
	Do you have a car?	
Citizenship/national origin	What is your national origin?	Are you legally eligible for employment in the United States?
	Where are your parents from?	
References	What is your maiden name?	Have you ever worked under a different name?
	What is your father's surname?	
	What are the names of your relatives?	
Arrests/convictions	Have you ever been arrested?	Have you ever been convicted of a crime? If so, when, where, and what was the disposition of the case?
Disability	Do you have any disabilities?	Can you perform the duties of the job you are applying for?
Birth date	What is your date of birth?	If hired, can you furnish proof that you are over age 18?
Emergency contact	What is the name and address of the relative to be notified in case of an emergency?	What is the name and address of the person to be notified in case of an emergency? (Request only after the individual has been employed.)
Credit history	Do you own your own home?	Credit references may be used if in compliance with the Fair Credit Reporting
	Have your wages ever been garnished?	Act of 1970 and the Consumer Credit Reporting Reform Act of 1996.
	Have you ever declared bankruptcy?	
Military service	What type of discharge did you receive?	What type of education, training, or work experience did you receive while in the military?
Languages	What is your native language?	Inquiry into languages applicant speaks and writes fluently (if the job requires
	Inquiry into how applicant acquired the ability to read, write, or speak a foreign language.	additional languages).
Organizations	List all clubs, societies, and lodges to which you belong.	Inquiry into applicant's membership in organizations that the applicant
	Are you a union member?	considers relevant to his or her ability to perform the job.
Race/color	Complexion or color of skin.	None
	Coloring.	
W/C	Have you ever filed for workers' compensation?	None
	Have you had any prior work injuries?	
Religion/creed	Inquiry into applicant's religious denomination, religious affiliations, church, parish, pastor, or religious holidays observed.	None
Gender	Do you wish to be addressed as Mr., Mrs., Miss, or Ms.?	None
Address	What was your previous address?	None
	How long did you reside there?	
	How long have you lived at your current address?	
	Do you own your own home?	
Education	When did you graduate from high school or college?	Do you have a high school diploma or equivalent?
		Do you have a university or college degree?
Personal	What color are your eyes, hair?	Only permissible if there is a bona fide occupational qualification.
	What is your weight?	

TABLE 56-2 Typical Topics Found in an Employee Handbook

Welcome message	EEOC statement	Personal communications
Organization mission statement	Employment application	Personnel records
Orientation	Equipment and facility use	Probationary periods
Attendance policies	Electronic communication and device use	Performance reviews and improvement plans
Benefits	Job descriptions	Safety and security
Disability benefits	Grievance process	Risk management and incident reports
Leaves of absence	On-the-job injuries	Sexual harassment guidelines
Bereavement policies	OSHA	(Non) Smoking policy
Holidays	Overtime policies	Substance abuse
Jury duty	Payroll periods	Subpoenas
Confidentiality and HIPAA	ADA statements	Wage increases and adjustments
Continuing education and tuition reimbursement	Disaster preparedness and emergency response	Schedules, accountability, and time-off requests
Dress code	Drug testing	

state laws. The legal definition is *unwelcome verbal, visual, or physical conduct of a sexual nature that is severe or pervasive and affects working conditions or creates a hostile work environment.* Other topics in a typical employee handbook are found in Table 56-2.

When Miguel began his employment, he, like all new employees, was on a 90-day **probationary period** or *trial period.* During this time frame, the HR department begins to facilitate staff development and training. Miguel, along with other staff members, attended training for the new electronic health record system the practice is implementing. Other training may include new policies and procedures, cultural diversity and sensitivity, CPR certification, new equipment, and wellness topics like stress management.

The trial period allows both the new employee and the organization an opportunity to decide if they are a "good fit." During the probationary period, the employer may terminate the new employee without cause. Likewise, the employee can also decide to leave the new position with little or no notice.

BWW Medical Associates conducts employee performance reviews at the end of the probationary period and then annually. The performance review typically includes the responsibilities in the job description and a form that includes the professional behaviors discussed throughout this textbook. Salary increases are usually based on the review rating.

Many medical practices also provide tuition reimbursement and reimburse expenses for employees who attend conferences that provide continuing education units so the employee may maintain the appropriate credentials for his or her position. Copies of all training and staff development activities and certificates are maintained in the employee's personnel file.

Staff Communication

The effective manager ensures convenient two-way, open, and consistent avenues of communication with the staff. The following modalities are often used:

- Staff meetings. Staff meetings should be at a consistent time each month when patients are not seen. The time is blocked off in the appointment matrix. The location should allow privacy. An **agenda,** which is the list of meeting topics and the order they will be addressed, should be used (Figure 56-8). See Procedure 56-2, Preparing an Agenda, located at the end of this chapter. Formal minutes (the meeting record) may or may not be kept, but at least meeting notes should be maintained by the practice manager that contain the date and time, who was present and absent, what was discussed, and who was

BWW Medical Associates, PC: Staff Lounge
Staff Meeting Agenda
October 1, 20XX, 12:00 to 1:30 p.m.

Lunch provided

Introductions	Malik Katahri
Staff News	All
Quality Assurance Report	Kalyn Haddix
Policies and Procedures Update	Malik Katahri
EHR Committee Report	Miguel Perez
Report from AAMA Conference	Miguel Perez

Old Business:
- Extending office hours — Paul Buckwalter, MD
- Upcoming flu shot clinic — Kalyn Haddix

New Business:
- Holiday Party — Malik Katahri
- Volunteers for Flu Preparedness Committee — Alexis Whalen, MD

Other

Adjournment

Next meeting November 3, 20XX, 12:00 to 1:30 p.m.

FIGURE 56-8 Sample of a staff meeting agenda.

responsible for any follow-up actions. These minutes may be needed for credentialing and licensing agencies or as proof of educational and informational topics addressed and as a tool for staff evaluations.

- E-mail. A large number of offices have e-mail for each employee or group of employees. Electronic communication is rapid and convenient but should be read and edited carefully. Staff and management messages should maintain a professional tone and responses provided in a reasonable time.

- Newsletters. Larger practices may have a monthly or quarterly electronic or hard-copy newsletter that may be the responsibility of the practice manager. The content usually provides information on what is going on in the practice, new policies and procedures or requirements, accomplishments and awards, and internal and community events, and often highlights staff members or departments.

- Bulletin boards. Usually located in the staff lounge, these boards should not contain any confidential or sensitive information since janitorial staff and others outside of the practice may have access.

- Open-door policy. This policy, maintained by many practice managers, gives staff the freedom to come talk any time the manager's office door is open. Staff should be respectful of the manager's time and, if the topic is involved and lengthy, schedule an appointment.

- Suggestion boxes. In some facilities, staff and sometimes patients are encouraged to place ideas in a suggestion box; they can submit the suggestion with a name or anonymously. If the suggestion is implemented, some organizations provide a monetary or other award.

Labor Relations

Labor relations is an HR role and refers to issues that arise between employees and management. When most people hear the term "labor relations," they tend to think of the process of hiring and terminating employees, but other functions relate to labor relations. For instance, overseeing the **grievance process** if the employee feels he or she was unjustly treated would come under the heading of labor relations. HR also may mediate or arrange **mediation** for differences between employees, groups of employees, or employees and management. The mediator's role is to facilitate communication between the parties, assist them in focusing on the real issues of the disagreement in a nonadversarial manner, and attempt to reach conflict resolution.

The practice manager's role is not easy but carries the opportunity for many personal and professional rewards. Seeing the healthcare organization provide excellent patient care in a safe, financially sound environment where staff members are happy to come to work is an accomplishment of much pride and satisfaction. To create or sustain this environment, the manager, as all positions in healthcare, must stay current in the field by reading appropriate journals and books; attending seminars and courses; maintaining membership in his or her professional organizations; and networking with local, state, and national managers. When you experience your applied training, sometimes called an externship or practicum, think about the practice manager's many jobs.

▶ Being a Leader — LO 56.4

Think about someone you admire and the reasons you admire that person. Now think of three words that describe that person. It will not be surprising if words like confident, integrity, responsible, and organized come to mind. These are terms, along with others, that describe leaders. Leaders are people who can influence other people to work toward a common goal . . . to build a team to accomplish those goals. Do not confuse leadership with supervising. There are many excellent leaders who are not supervisors and probably just as many supervisors who are not effective leaders. Let's look at why leadership, particularly in the healthcare field, is important and how you can become a leader as a medical assistant.

Becoming a Leader

It may sound strange, but to be a good leader, you must first be a good follower; to learn to lead, you must first understand how to be supervised and have a willingness to follow directions. How would you be able to ask someone to follow your directions if you consistently show an unwillingness to follow your own superior's direction? Other traits of effective leaders include

- A desire to achieve both personal and organizational goals.
- Confidence that is based on a good understanding of the situation at hand.
- An ability to be a team member and influence other members of the team to accomplish stated goals.
- Excellent communication skills (oral and written).
- An ability and willingness to accommodate change.
- Integrity.
- Willingness, even eagerness, to accept responsibility.
- Realization that goals are best achieved through the efforts of many.
- Giving genuine recognition to others that assist in achieving goals.

Building Your Team Good leaders know that effective teams accomplish goals by capitalizing on each member's strengths. But how do you go about building a team when often, in the office setting, healthcare workers often have jobs that mean each member has to pretty much focus on his or her area of expertise so that the office runs smoothly? The key is participation. It is up to the leader to create an atmosphere that values and *encourages* teamwork. To do this, an effective leader

- Ensures that each team member really knows his or her job and performs those tasks to the best of the individual's ability.
- Values each team member and encourages each member's contributions.
- Uses excellent communication skills to build trust between the team members.
- Assists each member of the team to set worthwhile and attainable goals.

Setting Goals Most people will say they achieve more when they know what is expected of them. Setting goals allows team members to know and understand those expectations and also provides a method to measure progress and identify areas that require attention. When setting goals, it is important to remember some key points:

- Make goals challenging, but not so much so that the goal is impossible to attain.

- Allow team members to contribute their ideas regarding personal and team goals.

- Make sure that the goal is measurable in some way so that success can be *seen*.

- When the goal has been set, make sure to have an action plan to reach the goal. The plan itself should outline what is to be done, the responsible person, and a time frame for completion of the task.

- The team leader should meet with individuals and teams to evaluate progress. If the goal was met, did it meet expectations? What is working and what needs improving? These evaluations provide the basis for the next goal-setting session.

Diversity and Leadership

We have all heard the sayings "Opposites attract" and "It takes all kinds." Both are true, and truly understanding that and respecting differences will make you a better leader. Keep in mind that if you feel that someone is "different," it is very likely that person is thinking the same thing about you! Diversity can include differences in all manner of identities, age, sex, race, physical abilities, ethnicity, religious beliefs, values and mores, sexual orientation, and personalities. Open communication among people who are different from each other leads to understanding and respect for those differences. It does not mean you must agree with all the differences or beliefs, but you will develop a respect and acceptance of the right of people to be "different." Listed below are some suggestions to help you increase your understanding and respect for diversity:

- Communicate openly to increase your awareness of diversity. This will increase your knowledge of similarities and differences among individuals.

- Examine your own feelings. No one is immune to biases and people tend to stereotype others, which leads to discrimination—the exact opposite of accepting diversity. What are your biases? Are they realistic or are they hurting your ability to effectively communicate with others? Be honest with yourself.

- Look at each person as an individual and not as part of a "group." By learning and communicating with individuals, biases and "walls" begin to come down.

- Learn to value each person's uniqueness. Every person on the team is valuable and has a contribution to make. Be open to each person's insight and contribution.

- Keep in mind that in healthcare you must be open and respectful of diversity in order to provide quality care to each patient. This respect must carry over to all members of the healthcare team as well.

Think back to the beginning of this section and the person that you admire. Does he or she possess traits you would like to emulate? Many effective leaders learn from their mentors. They also learn not only from their successes, but also from their failures. Anyone can make a mistake . . . the trick is to not make the same mistake repeatedly. "You get what you get, when you do what you do." If you do not like the result of something, change how or what you are doing and the result also will change. There is almost always more than one way to accomplish a task; be open to listening to everyone in the office and trying new ideas. When you do, you are on your way to not only being a team member, but also a team leader.

▶ Risk Management and Quality Assurance   LO 56.5

The term *risk management* (RM) is defined as plans and processes that continually identify, assess, correct, and monitor functions of the medical office to prevent negative outcomes and minimize exposure to risk and consequent liability. Immediately recognizing and addressing potential problems is everyone's focus. Risk management also identifies opportunities for improvement. A simple example of risk management is the procedure you learned for opening and closing the office, discussed in the *Patient Reception* chapter. On the other hand, quality assurance (QA) procedures ensure that the services provided in the medical practice meet or exceed the requirements and standards. Quality assurance also encompasses *utilization review* (UR), which is ensuring that the treatment plan and services are appropriate and cost-effective. Determining medical necessity is usually required. These areas include almost every aspect of the practice manager's role and are a huge responsibility. The Joint Commission (TJC) and the National Committee on Quality Assurance (NCQA) review the office's RM and QA plans and outcomes during accreditation visits. They look for a problem-solving model that follows the issue to resolution. This is referred to as *closing the loop*. The following is an example of a typical five-step problem-solving model (Figure 56-9):

1. Identification
2. Assessment

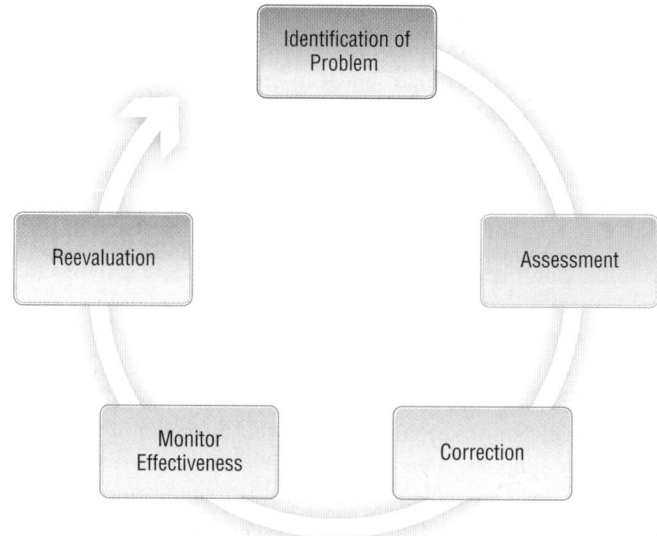

FIGURE 56-9   The problem-solving process.

3. Correction (design and implementation of an improvement plan)
4. Monitoring to ensure effectiveness of the plan
5. Reevaluation

A simple example would be that Malik, the practice manager at BWW Medical Associates, PC, notices the carpet in the reception area is torn. Patients and staff are placed at risk of falling (identification). He examines the tear and the entire carpet (assessment). Malik places tape over the tear and orders replacement carpeting (correction). The staff members are made aware and asked to be observant for other tears and similar problems (monitoring of effectiveness). Malik will reevaluate the condition of the carpet at intervals to ensure it is not a risk for tripping and falling, until the new carpeting is installed.

Incident Reports

An **incident report** (Figure 56-10), or occurrence report, is a special form required by a facility when an adverse outcome or event with risk of liability occurs. Refer to Procedure 56-3, Completing an Incident Report, at the end of this chapter. A fall caused by the torn carpeting would have required an incident report.

The report contains only factual information. Opinions and assumptions are omitted. Incident reports are not placed in a

BWW

BWW Medical Associates, PC
305 Main Street, Port Snead YZ 12345-9876
Tel: 555-654-3210, Fax: 555-987-6543
Web: BWWAssociates.com

Paul F. Buckwalter, MD
Alexis N. Whalen, MD
Elizabeth H. Williams, MD

Incident Report
(Only for Internal Use)

Date/time of incident: _____ Location: _____

Name of injured or at-risk party: _____

Circle one: Patient   Staff Member   Other (complete blank) _____

Address of above party: _____

Phone numbers of above party: home _____ cell _____

Describe the incident (use back of sheet if additional space needed): _____

_____

_____

Describe action(s) taken and by whom: _____

_____

_____

Name(s)/contact information of witnesses: _____

_____

_____

Name(s)/time of all parties notified: _____

_____

Name of person completing report: _____ Date/time: _____

Report submitted to: _____ Date/time: _____

(Submit form to immediate supervisor of area where the incident occurred)

FIGURE 56-10 Typical incident report form.

patient's medical record and some institutions prefer that the actual incident report not be completed in the presence of the injured party. The standard practice is that no copies of an incident report are made and only the original is maintained in a dedicated risk management file. As part of risk management, the practice manager routinely monitors and identifies any trends in incident reports to work on reducing risk. While risk management includes anyone who enters the medical office, quality assurance generally involves the patient and his or her care.

Go to CONNECT to see a video about *Completing an Incident Report.*

▶ Handling Payroll
LO 56.6

As a medical assistant, you may be responsible for handling the office payroll (Table 56-3). If so, your duties may include

- Obtaining tax identification numbers.
- Creating employee payroll information sheets.
- Calculating employees' earnings.
- Subtracting taxes and other deductions.
- Writing paychecks.
- Creating employee earnings records.
- Preparing a payroll register.
- Submitting payroll taxes.

Applying for Tax Identification Numbers

Every employer—whether a single physician or a corporate practice—must have an employer identification number (EIN). An EIN is required by law for federal tax accounting purposes. To obtain an EIN, complete Form SS-4 (Application for Employer Identification Number) from www.federaltaxid.us and submit it to the Internal Revenue Service (IRS) at www.irs.gov. Some states also require employer tax reports, for which the practice must have a state identification number, obtained from the proper state agency.

Creating Employee Payroll Information Sheets

The practice must maintain up-to-date, accurate payroll information about each employee. You should prepare a payroll information sheet with the following information for each employee:

- The employee's name, address, Social Security number, and marital status.
- An indication that the employee has completed an Employment Eligibility Verification (**Form I-9**), verifying that the employee is a U.S. citizen, a legally admitted alien, or an alien authorized to work in the United States.
- The employer also must complete a new hire reporting form (NHR) on the employee's behalf and submit it to the applicable state agency before the employee receives her first paycheck. Usually, this form is collected along with the W-4 and I-9 forms. Each state has its own format, but the information gathered is universal. Some states allow electronic submission, while others accept the information via mail. Figure 56-11 shows an example of an NHR form.
- The employee's pay schedule, number of dependents, payroll type, and voluntary deductions.

Pay Schedule and Payroll Type On the payroll information sheet, list the employee's *pay schedule*, showing how often the employee is paid. Common pay schedules are weekly, biweekly, and monthly.

List the employee's payroll type—hourly wage, salary, or commission—on the payroll information sheet. An hourly wage is a set amount of money per hour of work. A salary is a set amount of money per pay period, regardless of the number of hours worked. A commission is a percentage of the amount an employee earns for the employer. Salespeople, for example, are often paid by commission.

TABLE 56-3	Payroll Duties
Frequency	**Duties**
Upon assuming payroll responsibilities	Apply for an employer identification number (EIN) with Form SS-4 if the physician does not already have an EIN.
When a new employee is hired	Have the employee complete an Employee's Withholding Allowance Certificate (Form W-4) and Employment Eligibility Verification (Form I-9). Record the employee's name and Social Security number from the employee's Social Security card.
Every payday	Withhold federal income tax and state and local income taxes (if any). Withhold the employee's share of FICA taxes (for Social Security and Medicare). Record matching amount for the employer's share. Calculate how much the practice must pay for each employee's federal and state unemployment tax.
Monthly or biweekly (depending on your deposit schedule)	Deposit withheld income taxes, withheld and employer Social Security taxes, and withheld and employer Medicare taxes.
Quarterly (by April 30, July 31, October 31, and January 31)	File Employer's Quarterly Federal Tax Return (Form 941). With the return, pay any taxes that were not deposited earlier. Deposit federal unemployment tax, if over $100.
At least once a year	Have all employees update their W-4 forms.
On or before January 31	Give employees their Wage and Tax Statements (Form W-2), which show total wages and various withheld taxes. File Employer's Annual Federal Unemployment (FUTA) Tax Return (Form 940) with tax amount due.
On or before February 28	File Transmittal of Wage and Tax Statements (Form W-3) along with the government's copies of the W-2 forms.

Form NHR
New Hire and Independent
Contractor Reporting Form

Rev. 01/2010
Massachusetts
Department of
Revenue

TO ENSURE ACCURACY, PRINT (OR TYPE) NEATLY IN UPPER-CASE LETTERS AND NUMBERS, USING A DARK, BALLPOINT PEN.

Employee Information

FIRST NAME*

MI

LAST NAME*

SOCIAL SECURITY NUMBER*

DATE OF HIRE OR REINSTATEMENT*

ADDRESS*

CITY/TOWN*

STATE*

ZIP*

+4(OPTIONAL)

IT'S THE LAW! - Massachusetts regulations require employers with 25 or more employees to report their new hires and independent contractors electronically.

For more information, go to **www.mass.gov/dor** and select the **For Businesses** tab located at the top of the page.

Employer Information

EMPLOYER IDENTIFICATION NUMBER*

CORPORATE NAME*

PAYROLL ADDRESS TO WHICH THE INCOME WITHHOLDING ORDER WILL BE SENT*

PAYROLL ADDRESS (Continued)

CITY/TOWN*

STATE*

ZIP*

+4(OPTIONAL)

NOTE: All fields on this form with an* are mandatory fields. Please ensure all information entered is legible and accurate prior to submitting the form to DOR.

Helpful Hint: Once you have completed your employer information, you may copy this form to save time when reporting future new hires and independent contractors.

Send Completed Form NHR to:
Massachusetts Department of Revenue, PO Box 55141, Boston, MA 02205-5141 or, you may fax the completed form to 617-376-3262.

FIGURE 56-11 New hire and independent contract reporting (NHR) form.

Number of Dependents Record the number of dependents (people who depend on the employee for financial support that will be claimed by the employee). Dependents may include a spouse, children, and other family members.

You can find the number of dependents on the Employee's Withholding Allowance Certificate (**Form W-4**), which should have been completed when the employee was hired (Figure 56-12). Remember, keep the completed W-4 forms in the physician's personnel file and update them annually.

Voluntary Deductions Voluntary deductions are those items not required by law to be deducted from the employee's paycheck. These may include additional federal withholding taxes, contributions to a 401(k) retirement plan, or payments to a company health insurance plan. Employees who want additional federal taxes taken out of their paycheck will indicate this deduction on their W-4 form.

Gross Earnings

Gross earnings refers to the total amount of income earned before deductions, and this figure must be calculated for each employee as a first step in the payroll process.

Calculating Gross Earnings For every payroll period, use data from the payroll information sheet to compute each

Form W-4 (2012)

Purpose. Complete Form W-4 so that your employer can withhold the correct federal income tax from your pay. Consider completing a new Form W-4 each year and when your personal or financial situation changes.

Exemption from withholding. If you are exempt, complete **only** lines 1, 2, 3, 4, and 7 and sign the form to validate it. Your exemption for 2012 expires February 18, 2013. See Pub. 505, Tax Withholding and Estimated Tax.

Note. If another person can claim you as a dependent on his or her tax return, you cannot claim exemption from withholding if your income exceeds $950 and includes more than $300 of unearned income (for example, interest and dividends).

Basic instructions. If you are not exempt, complete the **Personal Allowances Worksheet** below. The worksheets on page 2 further adjust your withholding allowances based on itemized deductions, certain credits, adjustments to income, or two-earners/multiple jobs situations.

Complete all worksheets that apply. However, you may claim fewer (or zero) allowances. For regular wages, withholding must be based on allowances you claimed and may not be a flat amount or percentage of wages.

Head of household. Generally, you can claim head of household filing status on your tax return only if you are unmarried and pay more than 50% of the costs of keeping up a home for yourself and your dependent(s) or other qualifying individuals. See Pub. 501, Exemptions, Standard Deduction, and Filing Information, for information.

Tax credits. You can take projected tax credits into account in figuring your allowable number of withholding allowances. Credits for child or dependent care expenses and the child tax credit may be claimed using the **Personal Allowances Worksheet** below. See Pub. 505 for information on converting your other credits into withholding allowances.

Nonwage income. If you have a large amount of nonwage income, such as interest or dividends, consider making estimated tax payments using Form 1040-ES, Estimated Tax for Individuals. Otherwise, you may owe additional tax. If you have pension or annuity income, see Pub. 505 to find out if you should adjust your withholding on Form W-4 or W-4P.

Two earners or multiple jobs. If you have a working spouse or more than one job, figure the total number of allowances you are entitled to claim on all jobs using worksheets from only one Form W-4. Your withholding usually will be most accurate when all allowances are claimed on the Form W-4 for the highest paying job and zero allowances are claimed on the others. See Pub. 505 for details.

Nonresident alien. If you are a nonresident alien, see Notice 1392, Supplemental Form W-4 Instructions for Nonresident Aliens, before completing this form.

Check your withholding. After your Form W-4 takes effect, use Pub. 505 to see how the amount you are having withheld compares to your projected total tax for 2012. See Pub. 505, especially if your earnings exceed $130,000 (Single) or $180,000 (Married).

Future developments. The IRS has created a page on IRS.gov for information about Form W-4, at *www.irs.gov/w4*. Information about any future developments affecting Form W-4 (such as legislation enacted after we release it) will be posted on that page.

Personal Allowances Worksheet (Keep for your records.)

A Enter "1" for **yourself** if no one else can claim you as a dependent . . . . **A** _____

B Enter "1" if:
- You are single and have only one job; or
- You are married, have only one job, and your spouse does not work; or
- Your wages from a second job or your spouse's wages (or the total of both) are $1,500 or less.

   B _____

C Enter "1" for your **spouse.** But, you may choose to enter "-0-" if you are married and have either a working spouse or more than one job. (Entering "-0-" may help you avoid having too little tax withheld.) . . . . . **C** _____

D Enter number of **dependents** (other than your spouse or yourself) you will claim on your tax return . . . . **D** _____

E Enter "1" if you will file as **head of household** on your tax return (see conditions under **Head of household** above) . . **E** _____

F Enter "1" if you have at least $1,900 of **child or dependent care expenses** for which you plan to claim a credit . . . **F** _____
   (**Note.** Do **not** include child support payments. See Pub. 503, Child and Dependent Care Expenses, for details.)

G **Child Tax Credit** (including additional child tax credit). See Pub. 972, Child Tax Credit, for more information.
- If your total income will be less than $61,000 ($90,000 if married), enter "2" for each eligible child; then **less** "1" if you have three to seven eligible children or **less** "2" if you have eight or more eligible children.
- If your total income will be between $61,000 and $84,000 ($90,000 and $119,000 if married), enter "1" for each eligible child . . . **G** _____

H Add lines A through G and enter total here. (**Note.** This may be different from the number of exemptions you claim on your tax return.) ▶ **H** _____

For accuracy, complete all worksheets that apply.
- If you plan to **itemize** or **claim adjustments to income** and want to reduce your withholding, see the **Deductions and Adjustments Worksheet** on page 2.
- If you are **single and have more than one job** or are **married and you and your spouse both work** and the combined earnings from all jobs exceed $40,000 ($10,000 if married), see the **Two-Earners/Multiple Jobs Worksheet** on page 2 to avoid having too little tax withheld.
- If **neither** of the above situations applies, **stop here** and enter the number from line H on line 5 of Form W-4 below.

------ **Separate here and give Form W-4 to your employer. Keep the top part for your records.** ------

Form W-4 — Employee's Withholding Allowance Certificate

Department of the Treasury, Internal Revenue Service

OMB No. 1545-0074   2012

▶ Whether you are entitled to claim a certain number of allowances or exemption from withholding is subject to review by the IRS. Your employer may be required to send a copy of this form to the IRS.

1   Your first name and middle initial   Last name   2   Your social security number

Home address (number and street or rural route)

3 ☐ Single ☐ Married ☐ Married, but withhold at higher Single rate.
Note. If married, but legally separated, or spouse is a nonresident alien, check the "Single" box.

City or town, state, and ZIP code

4   If your last name differs from that shown on your social security card, check here. You must call 1-800-772-1213 for a replacement card. ▶ ☐

5   Total number of allowances you are claiming (from line **H** above **or** from the applicable worksheet on page 2)   **5** ____

6   Additional amount, if any, you want withheld from each paycheck   **6** $ ____

7   I claim exemption from withholding for 2012, and I certify that I meet **both** of the following conditions for exemption.
- Last year I had a right to a refund of **all** federal income tax withheld because I had **no** tax liability, **and**
- This year I expect a refund of **all** federal income tax withheld because I expect to have **no** tax liability.
If you meet both conditions, write "Exempt" here . . . . ▶ **7** ____

Under penalties of perjury, I declare that I have examined this certificate and, to the best of my knowledge and belief, it is true, correct, and complete.

Employee's signature
(This form is not valid unless you sign it.) ▶   Date ▶

8   Employer's name and address (Employer: Complete lines 8 and 10 only if sending to the IRS.)   9 Office code (optional)   10 Employer identification number (EIN)

For Privacy Act and Paperwork Reduction Act Notice, see page 2.   Cat. No. 10220Q   Form **W-4** (2012)

FIGURE 56-12   Employee's Withholding Allowance Certificate (W-4) is completed upon hire and updated annually.

employee's gross earnings. For an hourly employee, use this equation:

Hourly Wage × Hours Worked = Gross Earnings

An employee who earns $12.50 per hour and works 35 hours, for example, has gross earnings of $437.50 ($12.50 × 35 hours) per week.

For a salaried employee, use the salary amount as the gross earnings for the pay period, no matter how many hours the employee worked. An employee who earns a weekly salary of $500, for example, receives that amount whether she worked 30, 40, or 50 hours during that week.

Fair Labor Standards Act The Fair Labor Standards Act primarily affects employees who earn hourly wages. It limits the number of hours they may work, sets their minimum wage, and regulates their overtime pay. It also requires the employer to record the number of hours they work, usually on a time card or in a time book.

For hourly employees, this act mandates payment of

- Time and a half (1½ times the normal hourly wage) for all hours worked beyond the normal 8 in a regular workday.
- Time and a half for all hours worked on the sixth consecutive day of the workweek.
- Twice the normal wage (double time) for all hours worked on the seventh consecutive workday.
- Double time, plus normal holiday pay, for all hours worked on a company-approved holiday.

The Fair Labor Standards Act also requires overtime payments for part-time hourly employees for every hour worked beyond the normal 8 in a day or 40 in a week.

Making Deductions

The law requires all employers to withhold money from employees' gross earnings to pay federal, state, and local (if any) income taxes and certain other taxes. In addition, employees may wish you to make certain voluntary deductions. For example, you might be asked to deduct an amount for child care, if the practice or hospital provides onsite child care. You also might deduct employee contributions to health insurance premiums.

You must deposit all employee deductions and employer payments into separate accounts, one for each deduction type. Monies from these **tax liability accounts** are used to pay taxes to appropriate government agencies.

Income Taxes Enough money must be withheld to cover the employee's federal income tax for the pay period. You can determine this amount by finding the employee's number of exemptions (from Form W-4) and referring to the tax tables in *Circular E, Employer's Tax Guide*, published by the IRS.

Consult the state and local tax tables for other income taxes.

FICA Taxes For FICA tax, withhold from the employee's check half of the tax owed for the pay period. Pay the other half from the practice's accounts. The amount of FICA tax that funds Social Security differs from the amount that funds Medicare. Report these two amounts separately. Check IRS *Circular E* for the latest FICA tax percentages and level of taxable earnings.

Unemployment Taxes Federal unemployment tax is not a deduction from the employees' paychecks but rather is based on their earnings and paid by the employer. The **Federal Unemployment Tax Act (FUTA)** requires employers to pay a percentage of each employee's income, up to a certain dollar amount. The percentage may be reduced if the employer also pays state unemployment taxes.

States calculate unemployment taxes differently. Some states tax employers and employees; others tax only employers. State unemployment tax usually varies with the employer's past employment record. Employers with few layoffs, like physicians, have lower tax rates than those with many layoffs. To compute state unemployment tax, apply the assigned tax rate to each employee's earnings, up to a maximum for the calendar year. For details, consult your state unemployment insurance department.

Workers' Compensation Some states require employers to insure their employees against possible loss of income resulting from work-related injury, disability, or disease. Although state laws vary, they typically require doctors to carry this insurance with a state insurance fund or state-authorized private insurer. Usually, a medical practice's insurance agent will audit the payroll books annually and then issue a bill for the workers' compensation premium due.

Calculating Net Earnings

Add each employee's required and voluntary deductions together to determine the total deductions. Then, subtract the total deductions from the gross earnings to get the employee's **net earnings**, or take-home pay. Use the following equation:

Gross earnings − Total deductions = Net earnings

The exception to this rule may be contributions the employee makes to the employer retirement plan, if available. When sponsored by an employer, as with a 401(k) account, these deductions are often taken before taxes are calculated, reducing the employee's taxable income, which encourages the employee to take part in these plans.

Preparing Paychecks

The way you prepare the practice's payroll will depend on the system the practice uses. In a small practice, you may write paychecks manually. In this case, write the check amount for the employee's net earnings and deduct the check amount from the office checkbook. Payroll also may be handled through electronic banking; see the Points on Practice feature.

If the practice uses a payroll service, you may supply time cards or payroll data to the service by mail or electronically. The service calculates all the deductions, prepares paychecks, and mails them to the practice for distribution.

No matter how paychecks are prepared, they should include information about how the check amount was determined. This information usually appears on the check stub. It should match the information on the employee earnings records and payroll

POINTS ON PRACTICE
Handling Payroll through Electronic Banking

An electronic funds transfer system (EFTS) enables you to handle the practice's payroll without writing payroll checks manually. The physician must sign up for EFTS with the bank and employees must supply their bank account numbers to the employer. Then, the bank electronically deposits employees' paychecks into their bank accounts, as directed.

Most employees like to have their paychecks deposited automatically. The money is available on the day of deposit and no one has to worry about losing a paycheck, getting to the bank before it closes, or carrying a paycheck around. Also, employees still receive a check stub along with a notification of deposit, so they can track their earnings and deductions. Contact your bank for more information and specific procedures for setting up EFTS and electronic payroll.

register. Procedure 56-4, at the end of the chapter, explains the process for generating payroll.

Maintaining Employee Earnings Records

You need to keep an employee earnings record for each employee (Figure 56-13). When creating the record, list the employee's name, address, phone number, Social Security number, birth date, spouse's name, number of dependents, job title, employment starting date, pay rate, and voluntary deductions.

Then, for each pay period, record the employee's gross earnings, individual deductions, net earnings, and related information. Properly completed earnings records show each employee's earning history.

Maintaining a Payroll Register

A payroll register summarizes vital information about all employees and their earnings (Figure 56-14). At the end of each pay period, record each employee's earnings to date, hourly rate, hours worked, overtime hours, overtime earnings, and total gross earnings. Also, list the gross earnings subject to unemployment taxes and FICA, all required and voluntary deductions, net earnings,

and the paycheck number. Refer to Procedure 56-4, at the end of this chapter, for an example of how to prepare and complete the payroll procedure and register.

Handling Payroll Electronically

Manual payroll preparation and related tasks may take an hour per week for each employee. To save time and to provide the convenience for employees of having their paychecks automatically deposited, some practices handle payroll tasks electronically.

If you work in a relatively small practice, you may handle all payroll tasks in the office, using accounting or payroll software. If you work in a large practice, you may prepare payroll information on the computer and transmit it by modem to an outside payroll service for processing. Depending on which system and software the practice has, you may use the computer to

- Create, update, and delete employee payroll information files.
- Prepare employee paychecks, stubs, and W-2 forms.
- Update and print employee earnings records.
- Update all appropriate bookkeeping records, such as the payroll ledger and general ledger, with payroll data.

Name _____ Soc. Sec. No. _____ Dependents _____ Year _____

Address _____ Birth Date _____ Deductions _____

Job Title _____ Pay Rate

Employed on _____

Spouse _____ Terminated on _____ Record of Changes

Phone _____ Reason _____

Date	Rate

Check Number	Period Number	Earnings			Deductions					Net Pay	Cumulative FICA
		Regular	OT	Total	FICA	Fed. Tax	State	SUI	SDI		
1st Quarter Total											
2nd Quarter Total											

FIGURE 56-13 Earnings records show the earning history of each employee at the practice.

Emp. No.	Name	Earnings to date	Hrly. Rate	Reg. Hrs.	OT Hrs.	OT Earnings	TOTAL GROSS	Earnings Subject to Unemp.	Earnings Subject to FICA	Social Security (FICA)	Medicare	Federal W/H	State W/H	Health Ins.	Net pay	Check No.
0010	Scott, B.	9,823.14	14.00	70.00			980.00	980.00	980.00	60.50	14.10	147.92	15.10	25.00	717.38	11747
0020	Wilson, J.	14,290.38	17.00	70.00	6.50	165.75	1355.75	1355.75	1355.75	83.26	19.47	160.45	15.85	67.50	1009.22	11748
0030	Diaz, J.	2,750.26	5.50	46.25			254.37	254.37	254.37	15.77	3.68	38.20	3.75		192.97	11749
0040	Ling, W.	2,240.57	6.80	30.00			204.00	204.00	204.00	12.66	2.96	26.02	3.12		159.54	11750
0050	Harris, E.	2,600.98	10.00	23.50			235.00	235.00	235.00	14.57	3.41	33.52	3.36		180.14	11751

FIGURE 56-14 The payroll register is designed to summarize information about all employees and their earnings.

To perform these payroll functions electronically, follow the specific instructions in the software manual or get instructions from the payroll service. Generally, you would follow these steps:

1. Select an option from the "Payroll" menu. Wait for the prompt and select the appropriate employee from the employee list.
2. Create a new employee file:
   a. Enter employee name, address, SSN, marital status, pay schedule, number of dependents, payroll type, and voluntary deductions.
   b. Print two copies—one for the employee and one for the personnel file.
3. Update employee payroll information after a life change such as change in marital status, birth of a child, change of address, or voluntary change in deductions:
   a. Select "Update Employee File."
   b. Make required changes.
   c. Print the form for the employee signature after he confirms information is correct.
   d. Print two signed copies—one for the employee and one for the personnel file.
   e. Payroll information must be correct and current. It should be updated yearly for each employee.
4. Delete an employee from payroll:
   a. Select "Terminate Employee."
   b. Print a copy of the file before deleting it, as the employer is required to keep employee payroll records for four years.
5. Generate paychecks and paystubs:
   a. Select the employee from the employee list.
   b. Choose the "Print Paycheck" option.
   c. Answer each prompt displayed (for example, hours worked).
   d. From the payroll information entered previously, the program calculates the employee's net earnings, generates a paycheck, and prints a pay stub with the appropriate information.
6. Create an employee earnings record.
   a. Select "Creating Employee Earnings Record."
   b. Follow the prompts to enter the required information.

c. Depending on the software program used, this information may be updated automatically with each paycheck generated.

Select an option from the "Payroll" menu. Wait for the prompt, then select the appropriate employee from a list of employees.

▶ Calculating and Filing Taxes   LO 56.7

In many practices, administrative medical assistants set up tax liability accounts for money withheld from paychecks. These accounts are used to submit this money to appropriate agencies. Visit www.irs.gov for further information.

Setting Up Tax Liability Accounts

It is important to hold the money deducted from paychecks until it can be sent to the appropriate government agencies. Deductions from employees' paychecks for federal, state, and local income taxes and FICA taxes, as well as employer payments based on payroll, like federal and state unemployment taxes, must be deposited until payment is due. For these accounts, choose a bank authorized by the IRS to accept federal tax deposits. If the practice makes other paycheck deductions, such as for workers' compensation or a 401(k) plan, maintain accurate records for this money as well.

Each time you prepare paychecks, deposit the withheld money into the proper account as dictated by your particular practice. Record the deposited amounts as debits in the practice's checking account.

Understanding Federal Tax Deposit Schedules

You will probably deposit federal income taxes and FICA taxes (which together are known as employment taxes) on a quarterly, monthly, or biweekly (every-other-week) schedule. Every November, IRS personnel decide which deposit schedule your office should use for the next year.

If the IRS does not notify you about this matter, determine your deposit schedule based on the total employment taxes your office reported on the previous year's Employer's Quarterly Federal Tax Returns (Form 941). For example, if your office reported $50,000 or less in employment taxes during the past year, you would make monthly employment tax deposits the present year. If your office reported more than $50,000 during the past year, you would make semimonthly tax deposits.

Exceptions to the monthly or semimonthly tax deposit schedules are the $500 rule and the $100,000 rule. The $500 rule applies to employers who owe less than $500 in employment taxes during a tax period (such as a quarter). These employers do not have to make a deposit for that period. The $100,000 rule applies to employers who owe $100,000 or more in employment taxes on any one day during a tax period. These employers must deposit the tax by the next banking day after the day that ceiling is reached.

Submitting Federal Income Taxes and FICA Taxes

Since January 1, 2011, businesses must submit federal income taxes and FICA taxes to the IRS by electronic funds transfer (EFT). The EFT program, known as TAXLINK, began in 1995. If for any reason, such as the office EFT process having not yet been completed, a check must be mailed, make the check payable to "Financial Agent." Put the practice EIN in the check's memo section and mail it to Financial Agent, Federal Tax Deposit Processing Center, in St. Louis, MO. If your office does not have electronic fund transfer capabilities, contact the office accountant or

FIGURE 56-15 Tax dollars filed with FUTA returns (Form 940) provide income to temporarily unemployed workers.

financial institution, who may be able to submit your tax liabilities for you (a fee is usually charged for this service).

If you work in a practice with a large payroll, you may need to make deposits every few days. In most practices, however, you will probably make deposits once a month. Then, every 3 months, a more complete accounting is required on a quarterly basis, which will be discussed in more detail a bit later.

Submitting Federal Unemployment Tax Act (FUTA) and State Unemployment Tax Act (SUTA) Taxes

FUTA taxes provide money to workers who are unemployed. If the practice owes more than $100 in federal unemployment tax at the end of the quarter, deposit the tax amount with an FTD Coupon (Form 8109). At the end of the year, file an Employer's Annual Federal Unemployment (FUTA) Tax Return (Form 940) with any final taxes owed (Figure 56-15).

Generally, an employer must pay FUTA taxes if employees' wages total more than $1500 in any quarter (3-month period) and if those employees are not seasonal or household workers. The FUTA tax, which is 6.2%, is applied to the first $7000 of income for a year.

Some states are also governed by a State Unemployment Tax Act (SUTA). These taxes are filed along with FUTA taxes. Make sure you know the laws governing unemployment taxes in your state.

Filing an Employer's Quarterly Federal Tax Return

Each quarter, file an Employer's Quarterly Federal Tax Return (Form 941) with the IRS (Figure 56-16). This tax return summarizes the federal income and FICA taxes (employment taxes) withheld from employees' paychecks.

As a general rule, you should file Form 941 at the nearest IRS office by the last day of the first month after the quarter ends.

FIGURE 56-16 Most practices make tax deposits monthly and then make a more complete accounting quarterly on the Employers' Quarterly Federal Tax Return (Form 941), the first page of which is shown here.

FIGURE 56-17 A Wage and Tax Statement (Form W-2) records the total amount of taxes withheld during the previous year for each employee.

If the practice has deposited all taxes on time, you have an additional 10 days after the due date to file.

Handling State and Local Income Taxes

Send withheld state and local income taxes to the proper agencies, using their forms, procedures, and schedules. If required, prepare quarterly or other tax forms for your state or local agency. If you are unsure of how often to submit these forms and taxes, you can visit your state website or the IRS website at www.irs.gov.

Filing Wage and Tax Statements

After the end of each year, file a Wage and Tax Statement (**Form W-2**) with the appropriate federal, state, and local government agencies for each employee who had federal income and FICA taxes withheld during the previous year (Figure 56-17). Also, supply copies of Form W-2 to each employee.

Form W-2 shows the employee's total taxable income for the previous year. It also shows the exact amount of federal income taxes and FICA taxes (for Social Security and Medicare) withheld, along with the amounts of state and local taxes withheld (if any).

Along with the W-2 forms, submit Form W-3, a Transmittal of Wage and Tax Statements (Figure 56-18). This form lists the employer's name, address, and EIN and summarizes the amount of all employees' earnings and the federal income taxes and FICA taxes withheld.

PROCEDURE 56-1 Preparing a Travel Expense Report

(Imagine that you attended the latest AAMA or AMT annual conference. Research the price of airfare from your locale to the city of the conference. Determine registration and other costs. Use these figures to perform the procedure.)

Procedure Goal: To obtain reimbursement or account for preapproved travel funds, and to provide documentation of expenses for the medical office.

OSHA Guidelines: This procedure does not involve exposure to blood, body fluids, or tissues.

Materials: Travel expense form (Figure 56-6), pen, receipts, conference web information, and a calculator.

Method: Procedure steps.

1. Ensure your travel received prior approval.
   RATIONALE: Without prior approval, your expenses may be denied.

2. Save receipts from the event.

3. Complete the personal identifying information on the form.

4. Insert the purpose of the travel, the location, dates, and number of days.

5. Place the amounts as labeled in the expense table.

6. Total the amounts.

7. Check the appropriate box to indicate if you missed work and the dates and total number of days.

8. Sign and date the form.

9. Attach receipts (generally, original receipts are submitted; keep copies for your own records).
   RATIONALE: Without receipts, the expenses will not be reimbursed.

10. Submit completed form and receipts.

DO NOT STAPLE

| 33333 | a Control number | | For Official Use Only ▶ OMB No. 1545-0008 | |

| b Kind of Payer (Check one) | 941 ☐ Military ☐ 943 ☐ 944 ☐ CT-1 ☐ Hshld. emp. ☐ Medicare govt. emp. ☐ | Kind of Employer (Check one) | None apply ☐ 501c non-govt. ☐ State/local non-501c ☐ State/local 501c ☐ Federal govt. ☐ | Third-party sick pay (Check if applicable) ☐ |

c Total number of Forms W-2	d Establishment number	1 Wages, tips, other compensation	2 Federal income tax withheld
e Employer identification number (EIN)		3 Social security wages	4 Social security tax withheld
f Employer's name		5 Medicare wages and tips	6 Medicare tax withheld
		7 Social security tips	8 Allocated tips
		9	10 Dependent care benefits
		11 Nonqualified plans	12a Deferred compensation
g Employer's address and ZIP code			
h Other EIN used this year		13 For third-party sick pay use only	12b
15 State Employer's state ID number		14 Income tax withheld by payer of third-party sick pay	
16 State wages, tips, etc.	17 State income tax	18 Local wages, tips, etc.	19 Local income tax
Contact person		Telephone number	For Official Use Only
Email address		Fax number	

Under penalties of perjury, I declare that I have examined this return and accompanying documents and, to the best of my knowledge and belief, they are true, correct, and complete.

Signature ▶   Title ▶   Date ▶

Form **W-3** Transmittal of Wage and Tax Statements   **2012**   Department of the Treasury Internal Revenue Service

Send this entire page with the entire Copy A page of Form(s) W-2 to the Social Security Administration (SSA). Photocopies are not acceptable. Do not send Form W-3 if you filed electronically with the SSA.
Do not send any payment (cash, checks, money orders, etc.) with Forms W-2 and W-3.

Reminder

Separate instructions. See the 2012 General Instructions for Forms W-2 and W-3 for information on completing this form.

Purpose of Form

A Form W-3 Transmittal is completed only when paper Copy A of Form(s) W-2, Wage and Tax Statement, is being filed. Do not file Form W-3 alone. Do not file Form W-3 for Form(s) W-2 that were submitted electronically to the SSA (see below). All paper forms **must** comply with IRS standards and be machine readable. Photocopies are **not** acceptable. Use a Form W-3 even if only one paper Form W-2 is being filed. Make sure both the Form W-3 and Form(s) W-2 show the correct tax year and Employer Identification Number (EIN). Make a copy of this form and keep it with Copy D (For Employer) of Form(s) W-2 for your records. The IRS recommends retaining copies of these forms for four years.

E-Filing

The SSA strongly suggests employers report Form W-3 and Forms W-2 Copy A electronically instead of on paper. The SSA provides two free e-filing options on its Business Services Online (BSO) website:

• **W-2 Online.** Use fill-in forms to create, save, print, and submit up to 50 Forms W-2 at a time to the SSA.

• **File Upload.** Upload wage files to the SSA you have created using payroll or tax software that formats the files according to the SSA's *Specifications for Filing Forms W-2 Electronically (EFW2).*

W-2 Online fill-in forms or file uploads will be on time if submitted by April 1, 2013. For more information, go to *www.socialsecurity.gov/employer* and select "First Time Filers" or "Returning Filers" under "BEFORE YOU FILE."

When To File

Mail Copy A of Form W-3 with Form(s) W-2 by February 28, 2013.

Where To File Paper Forms

Send this entire page with the entire Copy A page of Form(s) W-2 to:

Social Security Administration
Data Operations Center
Wilkes-Barre, PA 18769-0001

Note. If you use "Certified Mail" to file, change the ZIP code to "18769-0002." If you use an IRS-approved private delivery service, add "ATTN: W-2 Process, 1150 E. Mountain Dr." to the address and change the ZIP code to "18702-7997." See Publication 15 (Circular E), Employer's Tax Guide, for a list of IRS-approved private delivery services.

For Privacy Act and Paperwork Reduction Act Notice, see the separate instructions.
Cat. No. 10159Y

FIGURE 56-18   Submit the Transmittal of Wage and Tax Statements (Form W-3) with the W-2 forms.

PROCEDURE 56-2 Preparing an Agenda

Procedure Goal: To facilitate a meeting's organization and focus by providing a list of meeting topics, the name of the person reporting, and the order in which each topic will be addressed.

OSHA Guidelines: This procedure does not involve exposure to blood, body fluids, or tissues.

Materials: Paper and pen or computer, copy machine, and minutes from last meeting.

Method: Procedure steps.

1. Approximately one week before the meeting, e-mail or post a memo to staff offering them an opportunity to add items to the agenda. This is referred to as a *Call for Agenda Items.*
   RATIONALE: Allows an opportunity for all staff members to suggest items for discussion.

2. Place the following on top of the form used to create the agenda:
   • Name of the practice.
   • Site name, if the practice has more than one location.

- Title: *Staff Meeting Agenda.*
- Date and time the meeting is scheduled to begin and end.

3. Many offices have standing topics that go on the agenda every month; examples are
   - Introduction of new staff members.
   - Approval of minutes, if formal minutes are kept.
   - Staff news (promotions, birthdays, weddings, births, etc.).
   - Quality assurance report.
   - Policy and procedure updates.
   - Committee reports.
   - Report from individuals who may have attended a conference.

   RATIONALE: Consistency in meeting format ensures that items are not forgotten.

4. Review the minutes from the previous meeting to determine any topics that required action with the person responsible. List these on the agenda under *Old Business.*

5. Add topics obtained from the *Call for Agenda Items* and any new topics the manager wishes to discuss. List these under *New Business.*

6. Add *Other* on the agenda to allow announcements or other brief information.

7. Place the date and time of the next meeting at the end of the agenda.
   RATIONALE: Advance notice allows staff members to plan other meetings and events around previously scheduled items.

8. At least one week prior to the meeting, inform and verify persons on the agenda who will present a topic at the meeting.
   RATIONALE: Advance notice assures those presenting topics will be prepared.

9. Send agenda to staff members prior to the meeting.

10. Make copies available at the staff meeting.

PROCEDURE 56-3 Completing an Incident Report

Procedure Goal: To provide documentation of an adverse occurrence or potential risk to facilitate investigation, correction, and aid in the avoidance of future occurrences.

OSHA Guidelines: This procedure does not involve exposure to blood, body fluids, or tissues.

Materials: A paper and pen, and an incident report (Figure 56-10 may be used).

Method: Procedure steps.

1. Make sure appropriate initial first aid and appropriate assistive steps are taken to help the injured person.
   RATIONALE: The injured person must be taken care of prior to completing any paperwork.

2. Interview the person to whom the incident occurred, gathering the required facts as needed for the incident report, including contact information.
   RATIONALE: The injured person's statement should be in her own words, clarifying information as needed.

3. Interview witnesses, gathering the required facts as needed for the incident report, including contact information.
   RATIONALE: Witnesses can add information to the injured person's statement of how the incident occurred.

4. Ensure information is complete.

5. Transfer the information to the incident report form.

6. Review the form for accuracy and clarity.

7. Submit the form to the appropriate supervisor.

PROCEDURE 56-4 Generating Payroll

Procedure Goal: To handle the practice's payroll as efficiently and accurately as possible for each pay period.

OSHA Guidelines: This procedure does not involve exposure to blood, body fluids, or tissues.

Materials: Employees' time cards, employees' earnings records, payroll register, IRS tax tables, and check register.

Method: Procedure steps.

1. Calculate the total regular and overtime hours worked, based on the employee's time card. Enter those totals under the appropriate headings on the payroll register.

2. Check the pay rate on the employee earnings record. Multiply the hours worked (including any paid vacation or paid holidays, if applicable) by the rates for regular time and overtime (time and a half or double time). This yields gross earnings.

3. Enter the gross earnings under the appropriate heading on the payroll register. Subtract any nontaxable benefits, such as healthcare or retirement programs.

4. Using IRS tax tables and data on the employee earnings record, determine the amount of federal income tax to withhold based on the employee's marital status and number of exemptions. Also, compute the amount of FICA tax to withhold for Social Security (6.2%) and Medicare (1.45%).

5. Following state and local procedures, determine the amount of state and local income taxes (if any) to withhold based on the employee's marital status and number of exemptions.

6. Calculate the employer's contributions to FUTA and to the state unemployment fund, if any. Post these amounts to the employer's account.

7. Enter any other required or voluntary deductions, such as health insurance or contributions to a 401(k) fund.

8. Subtract all deductions from the gross earnings to get the employee's net earnings.

9. Enter the total amount withheld from all employees for FICA under the headings for Social Security and Medicare. Remember that the employer must match these amounts. Enter other employer contributions, such as for federal and state unemployment taxes, under the appropriate headings.

10. Fill out the check stub, including the employee's name, date, pay period, gross earnings, all deductions, and net earnings. Make out the paycheck for the net earnings.

11. Deposit each deduction in a tax liability account.

SUMMARY OF LEARNING OUTCOMES

LEARNING OUTCOMES	KEY POINTS
56.1 **Explain the basic organizational designs of the medical office and the relationship of the physician and the medical assistant with the practice manager and direct supervisors.**	In a physician-owned medical practice, the medical assistant will often report directly to the practice manager. In a company-owned practice, the medical assistant will often report to the medical director. Regardless of the practice's organizational design, the MA should always know the office chain of command and who her direct supervisor is and should consistently follow the chain of command as outlined in the organizational chart and the office policies and procedures manual.
56.2 **Describe the responsibilities of the practice manager.**	The practice manager's job description may change from practice to practice, but common responsibilities include creating, updating, and maintaining the office policies and procedures manual; making sure all licenses and certifications necessary for all healthcare providers are current and up-to-date; and ensuring all necessary contracts with payers and other providers are also current. The practice manager is also in charge of the practice's finances and budget, including overseeing the office petty cash fund. Exceptional communication and interpersonal skills are required, as on any given day, the manager may be communicating with staff, patients, healthcare providers, hospitals, insurers, vendors, contractors, government agencies, bankers, other employers, educators, attorneys, and community organizations. The manager also will evaluate and purchase equipment and systems that fit the practice's needs and budget, facilitate the installation and staff training, and then oversee the ongoing operations. Other managerial functions include ensuring availability of mailing and shipping services, inventory and supply purchases, and appropriate market and public relation strategies, which may include websites, brochures, and community event sponsorship.
56.3 **Summarize the basic human relations functions in practice management.**	The human relations role refers to how the practice manages employees and deals with elements of hiring, orienting, and training employees and terminating employees when necessary. Understanding the laws, acts, and regulations surrounding employment is also a large part of the human relations aspect of the practice manager's role.

LEARNING OUTCOMES	KEY POINTS
56.4 **Distinguish the four traits of someone with leadership skills and the importance of these skills to the healthcare team.**	Any of the following traits may be attributable to a leader: a desire to achieve both personal and organizational goals; confidence that is based on a good understanding of the situation at hand; the ability to be a team member and influence other members of the team to accomplish stated goals; excellent communication skills; the ability and willingness to accommodate change; integrity; the willingness to accept responsibility; the realization that goals are achieved best through the efforts of many; and the giving of genuine recognition to others who assist in achieving goals. All of these items and the ability to be a leader are important in a medical assistant as a healthcare team member because when the office members work together with the common goal of caring for their patients, the result is excellent patient care.
56.5 **Compare risk management and quality assurance in a medical facility.**	The term *risk management* (RM) is defined as a plan and processes that continually identify, assess, correct, and monitor functions of the medical office to prevent negative outcomes and minimize risk exposure and consequent liability. When an incident does occur, an incident report is completed to track the cause of the incident to minimize future risk. Quality assurance (QA) is procedures that ensure the services provided in the medical practice meet or exceed the requirements and standards.
56.6 **Calculate an employee's gross earnings, deductions, and net earnings for a pay period.**	To calculate an employee's gross earnings, multiply the hours worked by the hourly rate. Using state, local, and federal tax guidelines, calculate the employee's tax deductions. Add to these any voluntary deductions and subtract the total deductions to obtain the employee's net earnings. Using the employee payroll record containing the employee's name, address, SSN, and number of exemptions, record the employee's gross earnings, deductions (including mandatory and voluntary deductions), and net paycheck.
56.7 **Describe tax forms commonly used in the medical office and the purpose of the office tax liability account.**	Tax forms used in a medical practice include, but are not limited to, W-2, W-3, and W-4 forms; NHR forms; I-9s; quarterly federal tax forms; wage and tax statements; and FUTA and SUTA forms. The practice liability account is set up to hold the money deducted from employees' paychecks until the funds can be appropriately disbursed to government agencies. There may be separate accounts for federal and state taxes as well as unemployment and retirement funds. Record the tax amounts deposited in the liability account as debits in the practice's checking account.

CASE STUDY CRITICAL THINKING

Recall Cindy Chen from the beginning of the chapter. Now that you have completed the chapter, answer the following questions regarding her case.

1. What questions would be appropriate to ask Cindy when interviewing her for the position?

2. If she is hired, other staff members may also know her medical status. How should this be best handled by the practice? By Cindy?

1. (LO 56.1)In most medical practices, the medical assistant will work under the supervision of
   a. The physician
   b. The physician assistant
   c. The nurse practitioner
   d. The staff nurse
   e. Any of the above, depending on the practice structure

2. (LO 56.2)The document that is the backbone of the medical practice is its
   a. HIPAA manual
   b. Employee manual
   c. Policies and procedures manual
   d. MSDS binder
   e. OSHA guidelines

3. (LO 56.2)The practice manager is responsible for which of the following tasks?
   a. Licenses, certifications, and contract updates
   b. Budgets and financial planning
   c. Managing petty cash
   d. Schedule and travel for physicians and employees
   e. All of the above

4. (LO 56.3)Which act does NOT come under the heading of Human Resources?
   a. EEOC
   b. ADA
   c. FMLA
   d. ECOA
   e. Fair Labor Standards Act

5. (LO 56.3)Which of the following questions cannot be asked during an interview?
   a. Do you have reliable transportation?
   b. Do you have small children at home?
   c. Are you capable of performing the duties listed on the job description?
   d. We require a certification for our medical assistants; are you certified?
   e. Our hours are 8:00 a.m.–4:30 p.m. and one Saturday a month from 8:00 a.m.–1:00 p.m. on a rotating schedule; can you be available for this schedule?

6. (LO 56.4)Why are goals important in building a team?
   a. Goals keep team members busy
   b. Goals keep each person focused solely on his or her own job
   c. Creating goals keeps supervisors busy
   d. Goals increase understanding of expectations
   e. a, b, & c only

7. (LO 56.5)There are five steps to the improvement process. Which one implements the plan?
   a. Identification
   b. Assessment
   c. Correction
   d. Monitoring
   e. Reevaluation

8. (LO 56.5)When is an incident report required?
   a. Only if an employee is injured while working
   b. Only if a patient is hurt because of employee error
   c. Only if a patient is hurt through no fault of the office staff
   d. For any adverse outcome or event with risk of liability
   e. For any adverse outcome or event with no risk of liability

9. (LO 56.6)Which tax form is more commonly known as the I-9?
   a. Form NHR
   b. Employment Eligibility and Verification
   c. Employee's Withholding Allowance Certificate
   d. Transmittal of Wage and Tax Statements
   e. Employee Wage and Tax Statement

10. (LO 56.7)Which tax provides for unemployment benefits?
    a. FUTA
    b. SUTA
    c. FICA
    d. State and local taxes
    e. EFT

Emergency Preparedness

C A S E   S T U D Y

PATIENT INFORMATION

Patient Name	Gender	DOB
Mohammad Nassar	M	5/17/XX

Attending	MRN	Allergies
Elizabeth H. Williams, MD	423-90-687	NKA

Mohammad Nassar, a 15-year-old male, is a returning patient. His mother brings him to the office today with flulike symptoms including high fever and chills, muscle aches, and coughing. He has a known past medical history of asthma, which has been relatively stable on a new maintenance dose of albuterol extended-release tablets 8 mg twice a day. Mohammad states that he aches all over and feels like he is "freezing." He is the eighth person this morning who has come in with flulike symptoms. The other seven patients tested positive on a rapid test for Influenza Type A. Mohammad's rapid influenza screening test is positive. He is now the eighth positive case this morning. The office manager informs you that the local health department notified the office that there is a severe regional outbreak of a novel type of Influenza A.

Keep Mohammad (and his mother) in mind as you study this chapter. There will be questions at the end of the chapter based on the case study. The information in the chapter will help you answer these questions.

L E A R N I N G   O U T C O M E S

After completing Chapter 57, you will be able to:

57.1 Discuss the importance of first aid during a medical emergency.

57.2 Identify items found on a crash cart.

57.3 Recognize various accidental emergencies and how to deal with them.

57.4 List common illnesses that can result in medical emergencies.

57.5 Identify less common illnesses that can result in medical emergencies.

57.6 Discuss your role in caring for people with psychosocial emergencies.

57.7 Carry out the procedure for calming a patient who is under extreme stress.

57.8 Discuss ways to educate patients about how to prevent and respond to emergencies.

57.9 Illustrate your role in responding to natural disasters and pandemic illness.

57.10 Discuss your role in responding to acts of bioterrorism.

K E Y   T E R M S

automated external defibrillator (AED)
bioterrorism
cerebrovascular accident (CVA)
concussion
contusion
crash cart
dehydration
dislocation
epistaxis
hematemesis

hematoma
hyperglycemia
hypoglycemia
hypovolemic shock
palpitations
septic shock
splint
sprain
strain
ventricular fibrillation (VF)

I. A (1) Apply critical thinking skills in performing patient assessment and care

IX. C (10)(d) Explain how the following impact the medical assistant's practice and give examples: Good Samaritan Act(s)

XI. C (5) State principles and steps of professional/provider CPR

XI. C (6) Describe basic principles of first aid

XI. C (9) Discuss requirements for responding to hazardous material disposal

XI. C (11) Discuss critical elements of an emergency plan for response to a natural disaster or other emergency

XI. C (12) Identify emergency preparedness plans in your community

XI. C (13) Discuss potential role(s) of the medical assistant in emergency preparedness

XI. P (3) Develop a personal (patient and employee) safety plan

XI. P (4) Develop an environmental safety plan

XI. P (6) Participate in a mock environmental exposure event with documentation of steps taken

XI. P (9) Maintain provider/professional level CPR certification

XI. P (10) Perform first aid procedures

XI. P (12) Maintain a current list of community resources for emergency preparedness

XI. A (1) Recognize the effects of stress on all persons involved in emergency situations

XI. A (2) Demonstrate self awareness in responding to emergency situations

2. Anatomy and Physiology

Graduates:

c. Assist the physician with the regimen of diagnostic and treatment modalities as they relate to each body system

9. Medical Office Clinical Procedures

Graduates:

e. Recognize emergencies and treatments and minor office surgical procedures

o. Perform:

(5) First aid and CPR

q. Instruct patients with special needs

▶ Introduction

Emergencies of all types can occur when you are working as a medical assistant. Patients may come to your facility with an acute illness or injury. You may have to handle phone calls from patients with urgent physical or psychological problems. You could even experience a disaster—anything from a simple office fire to a bomb threat or bioterrorism. As a medical assistant, you must be prepared to determine the level of urgency and handle any emergency that arises. Remember to stay calm and think through each situation in order to respond appropriately and create the best outcome.

▶ Understanding Medical Emergencies   LO 57.1

A medical emergency is any situation in which a person suddenly becomes ill or sustains an injury that requires immediate help by a healthcare professional. Your prompt action in a medical emergency could prevent permanent disability or even death.

As a medical assistant, you may see life-threatening medical emergencies in the healthcare setting. For example, a patient in the waiting room may have chest pains that could indicate a heart attack is imminent. You also may see emergencies that are not life-threatening, such as a coworker sustaining a minor injury on the job. And you could encounter emergencies outside the office. For example, a family member might cut a finger while using a kitchen knife or a restaurant patron might choke on a piece of food. Your quick response is vital in all of these situations.

In or out of the office, a medical emergency may require you to perform first aid. First aid is the immediate care given to someone who is injured or suddenly becomes ill, before complete medical care can be obtained. Prompt and appropriate first aid can

- Save a life.
- Reduce pain.
- Prevent further injury.
- Reduce the risk of permanent disability.
- Increase the chance of early recovery.

Because most emergencies do not occur in a medical office, your role in patient education is critical. The more you teach patients about first aid and the proper way to respond to emergencies, the better equipped they will be to handle accidental injuries and illnesses. You also should make patients aware of Good Samaritan laws. These laws serve to protect people who respond, in good faith, to medical emergencies but have no medical training. Every state in the United States has Good Samaritan laws or regulations.

▶ Preparing for Medical Emergencies

LO 57.2

How prepared you are for an emergency can mean the difference between life and death for a patient. You must be able to perform procedures quickly and correctly. Keeping your skills up-to-date will enable you to handle medical emergencies effectively.

Just as important is your ability to ensure that the medical office where you work is ready to handle whatever emergencies arise. This preparedness will depend on your own organizational skills and knowledge of community resources.

Preparing the Office

First, establish with the doctor which duties are expected of you and of other office personnel in case of an emergency and determine the available resources. One of your most important allies will be the local emergency medical services (EMS) system. An EMS system is a network of qualified emergency services personnel who use community resources and equipment to provide emergency care to victims of injury or sudden illness.

Posting Emergency Telephone Numbers Although the local EMS system's telephone number is 911 in most parts of the country, some areas may not have 911 service. Post the area's EMS system telephone number at every telephone and on the **crash cart** (the rolling cart of emergency supplies and equipment) or first-aid tray. Every office employee should know this number. If the community has no EMS system, post the telephone number of the local ambulance or rescue squad. You also should post the telephone numbers of the nearest fire company, police station, poison control center, women's shelter, rape hotline, and drug and alcohol center.

When you call EMS for medical assistance and transport, speak clearly and calmly to the dispatcher and be prepared to provide the following information:

- Your name, telephone number, and location.
- Nature of the emergency.
- Number of people in need of help.
- Condition of the injured or ill patient(s).
- Summary of the first aid that has been given.
- Directions on how to reach the location of the emergency.

Do not hang up until the dispatcher gives you permission to do so.

Common Emergency and First-Aid Supplies

The crash cart or tray contains basic drugs, supplies, and equipment for medical emergencies. Most crash carts also contain a first-aid kit with supplies for managing minor injuries and ailments.

TABLE 57-1	Contents of a First-Aid Kit
Absorbent compress bandages (sterile)	
Adhesive bandages (assorted sizes)	
Adhesive tape	
Airway or breathing barrier	
Analgesics, like acetaminophen	
Antiseptic solution or spray	
Antiseptic wipes	
Aspirin (81 mg)	
Calamine lotion	
Chemical cold packs	
Diphenhydramine (Benadryl®)	
Disposable gloves	
Elastic bandages in various sizes	
Emergency blanket	
First-aid book or information card	
Gauze pads (sterile)	
Glucose tablets or sugar source	
Hand sanitizer	
Personal protective equipment (PPE): gloves, mask, and goggles or face shield, gown, shower cap, booties, pocket mask, or mouth shield	
Plastic bags	
Premoistened towelettes or hand cleaner	
Roller bandages	
Scissors	
Splints in various sizes	
Sterile gauze pads in various sizes	
Sterile rolls of gauze	
Sterile saline solution	
Sunscreen	
Thermometer (with extra batteries if digital)	
Triangular bandage	
Tweezers	
Waterproof flashlight with extra batteries	

Table 57-1 lists the usual items in a first-aid kit. The actual contents of the crash cart may vary slightly from practice to practice. Become familiar with these contents and know where they are located in the office. Procedure 57-1, at the end of this chapter, describes how to check and restock essential crash cart items.

Guidelines for Handling Emergencies

A medical emergency requires you to take certain steps. You are not responsible for diagnosing or providing medical care other than first aid. You are expected, however, to note the presence of serious conditions that threaten the patient's life and to take appropriate action, performing only those procedures you have been trained to perform.

TABLE 57-2	Personal Protective Equipment for Emergencies	
Equipment	Conditions for Use	Sample Emergencies Requiring Equipment
Gloves	Chance of contact with blood or other body secretion or excretion during emergency	Open wound, eye trauma
Goggles and mask or face shield and possible head cover	Chance of blood or other body secretion or excretion being splattered, coughed, or sprayed onto the mucus membranes of the eyes, mouth, or nose	Bleeding, vomiting, most emergency care for small children (because of squirming)
Gown and possible booties	Chance of contact with excessive bleeding or secretion and excretion	Childbirth, severe nosebleed
Pocket mask or mouth shield	Needed for CPR or rescue breathing	Heart attack (MI), respiratory arrest

Patient Emergencies Assess the situation and surroundings to determine whether it is safe for you to assist. If safe, don the appropriate PPE, such as gloves. Next, do an initial assessment to detect and immediately correct any life-threatening circulation, airway, and breathing problems. Correcting life-threatening problems is essential to survival. The initial assessment has six steps:

1. Form a general impression of the patient.
2. Determine the patient's level of responsiveness.
3. Assess the circulation (compressions or the need for them if no pulse detected), airway, and breathing status of the patient, sometimes referred to as the CABs.
4. Determine the priority or urgency of the patient's condition.
5. Conduct a focused exam.
6. Document a history.

Procedure 57-2, at the end of this chapter, provides guidelines for performing these six steps.

Telephone Emergencies Sometimes, a patient or a patient's family member calls the medical office with an emergency. If you are responsible for handling telephone calls, be prepared to triage the injuries by phone. Triaging is the classification of injuries according to severity, urgency of treatment, and place for treatment.

To handle emergency calls, follow the practice's telephone triage protocols. For example, if a parent calls to say her daughter has broken her arm and the child's bone is visible, tell her to call the local EMS system for immediate care and transport to the hospital. If, however, a parent calls to say her son swallowed half a bottle of baby bath, tell her to remain calm and give her the telephone number of the poison control center. Depending on circumstances, you may offer to make the necessary phone call yourself.

Adhere to the following general guidelines in any emergency situation:

- Stay calm.
- Reassure the patient.
- Act in a confident, organized manner.

Personal Protection Whenever you administer first aid and emergency treatment, try to reduce or eliminate the risk of exposing yourself and others to infection. Follow Standard Precautions and assume all blood and body fluids are infected with bloodborne pathogens. To protect yourself and others, take the following basic precautions. Include PPE in your first-aid kit at work and at home. Standard PPE includes gloves, goggles and mask or face shield, gown, cap, and booties. A pocket mask or mouth shield provides personal protection when you perform rescue breathing. Plan to use specific PPE based on the patient's condition. Table 57-2 provides examples of PPE to use in various emergency situations. When in doubt, wear more PPE than you may think is called for.

Wear gloves if you expect hand contact with blood, body fluids, mucous membranes, torn skin, or potentially contaminated articles or surfaces. In addition, if you have any cuts or lesions, wear PPE over the affected area.

Minimize splashing, splattering, or spraying of blood or other body fluids when performing first aid. If blood or other body fluids splash into your eyes, nose, or mouth, flush the area with water as soon as possible.

Wash your hands thoroughly with soap and water after removing the gloves. Also wash other skin surfaces that have come in contact with blood or other body fluids. Do not touch your mouth, nose, or eyes and do not eat or drink after providing emergency care until you have washed your hands thoroughly. If you have been exposed to blood or other body fluids, be sure to tell the doctor. You may need postexposure treatment.

Documentation Properly document all office emergencies in the patient's chart. Be sure to include your assessment, treatment given, and the patient's response. If the patient was transported to another facility, record the location.

Go to CONNECT to see a video about *Performing an Emergency Assessment*.

▶ Accidental Injuries

LO 57.3

No matter where you encounter an emergency, your knowledge and certifications should enable you to provide first aid for the patient until a physician or EMT arrives. To help you become familiar with how to handle various emergency situations, the following sections present accidental injuries, common illnesses, and less common illnesses.

Bites and Stings

Dog and cat bites and bee, wasp, and hornet stings are fairly common. Less common are snakebites and spider bites, which you are more likely to encounter in certain parts of the country, such as Florida or the Southwest, than in other areas.

Animal Bites An animal bite may bruise the skin, tear it, or leave a puncture wound. A wound that breaks the skin should be seen by a doctor and will need to be reported to the police, animal control officer, and local health department. If the animal can be found, it should be checked for rabies. Then, depending on the animal's rabies vaccination status, the animal may need to be quarantined. If the animal is a probable carrier of rabies and cannot be found, depending on the extent of the injury the doctor may administer rabies immunoglobulin and rabies vaccination to the patient as a precaution.

Dogs, cats, skunks, squirrels, raccoons, bats, and foxes are more likely to carry rabies than are other animals. Hamsters, gerbils, guinea pigs, and mice are rarely infected by the rabies virus.

Human bites can raise concerns about transmitting the human immunodeficiency virus (HIV) or hepatitis B virus. HIV can be transmitted only if the bite breaks the skin and if the biter has bleeding gums. Hepatitis B virus may be transmitted by a human bite that punctures the skin. In this case, a series of three injections is required to immunize against hepatitis B.

Immediate care for bites calls for washing the area thoroughly with antiseptic soap and water. If the bite caused a puncture wound, allow the wound to bleed for a few minutes to flush out bacteria. If the wound is bleeding profusely or spurting blood, apply pressure to the wound. Then wash the area with soap and water. Apply an antibiotic ointment and a dry, sterile dressing. The doctor will administer tetanus toxoid if the patient has not received it in the last 7 to 10 years.

Insect Stings Insect stings are merely a nuisance to most patients. The site of the sting can become red, swollen, itchy, and painful. If the patient was stung by a honeybee, you must first remove the stinger because it still has the ability to release venom. Remove the stinger by scraping the skin with a credit card or other flat, hard, sharp object. Be careful not to release more venom. Avoid using your fingers or tweezers because squeezing the stinger may force more venom into the wound. (If you cannot remove the stinger, call the physician.) Wash the skin with soap and water. After the stinger is removed, apply ice to the site, 10 minutes on and 10 minutes off, to reduce the pain and swelling.

A sting can be deadly to a patient who is allergic to the insect venom because anaphylaxis can develop. The symptoms of and treatment for anaphylaxis are described later in this chapter.

Snakebites Poisonous snakes in the United States include rattlesnakes, water moccasins (or cottonmouths), copperheads, and coral snakes. Because snakes are cold-blooded, they often lie on rocks to warm themselves. Most bites occur when a person steps onto, sits down on, or reaches over or between rocks where a snake is sunning itself.

The bites of most poisonous snakes produce similar symptoms: one or two puncture marks, pain, and swelling at the site; rapid pulse; nausea; vomiting; and sometimes unconsciousness and seizures. If possible, get a description of the snake so the EMS team or the hospital can procure the proper antivenin (a substance that counteracts the snake poison) ahead of time. Snakebites are dangerous, but with proper intervention, they rarely lead to death.

If a patient has been bitten by a potentially poisonous snake, call a doctor or the EMS system. If the patient must walk, have him walk slowly to prevent dispersion (spreading) of the poison through the circulation. To care for a poisonous snakebite while you await help, keep the patient calm and remove rings, watches, or tight clothing in the area. If possible, immobilize the injured part and position it below heart level. Do not apply ice or a tourniquet and do not cut or suction the wound.

Spider Bites Only two types of spiders in the United States are a serious threat to health: the black widow spider, which has a red hourglass mark on its abdomen, and the brown recluse spider, which has a violin-shaped mark on its head. The black widow bite causes swelling and pain at the site as well as nausea, vomiting, rigid abdomen, fever, rash, and difficulty breathing or swallowing. The brown recluse bite causes severe swelling and tenderness and, eventually, ulceration along the nerve closest to the location of the bite.

You are not expected to classify spiders and their bites accurately, so any patient bitten by a spider must be seen by a physician. To care for a patient with a spider bite, wash the area thoroughly with soap and water. Apply a cold compress to the area to reduce swelling and pain. If possible, elevate the area to slow the poison's spreading. Healing of the bite can sometimes take several months.

Burns

Burns involve tissue injury that occurs from heat, chemicals, electricity, or radiation. Be sure to teach patients about emergency treatment for burns and any follow-up care prescribed by the physician.

Types of Burns

Thermal Burns Thermal burns may be caused by contact with hot liquids, steam, flames, radiation, and excessive heat from fires or hot objects. Call the EMS team immediately for victims of such burns. To stop the burning process, use water to cool a burning substance or use a wet cloth or blanket to put out the fire.

Chemical Burns Chemical burns are more likely to affect workers at chemical or industrial facilities than individuals in the home. To treat this type of burn, first remove the cause of the burn. Take care not to come into contact with the chemical. Brush off any excess dry chemical and remove any clothing contaminated with the chemical. Gently flood the area with cool water for at least 15 minutes. Cover the area with a dry sterile dressing. If the burn is severe, call EMS to transport the patient to the hospital. Monitor the patient carefully for signs of shock.

Electrical Burns Electrical burns are injuries from exposure to electrical currents, including lightning. These burns occur at the site where the electricity enters the body and where the current exits the body and enters the ground. Along the current's pathway, extensive tissue damage can occur from heat followed by chemical changes to nerve, muscle, and heart tissue. Call the EMS team immediately for these types of injuries.

Classifications of Burns The severity of a burn is determined by the depth and extent of the burn area, the source of the burn, the age of the patient, body regions burned, and other patient illnesses and injuries. For more information about classifying and estimating the extent of burns, see the chapter *The Integumentary System*.

Go to CONNECT to see an animation about *Burns*.

Choking

Choking occurs when food or a foreign object blocks a person's trachea, or windpipe. The main symptom of a choking emergency is the inability to speak. A choking person who cannot talk may give the universal sign of choking—a hand up to the throat and a fearful look. If you see someone giving the universal sign, be prepared to act promptly.

Procedure 57-3, at the end of this chapter, provides guidelines for assisting an adult or a child who is responsive and choking. The American Heart Association generally considers anyone between the ages of one and eight years old a child. Procedure 57-4, at the end of this chapter, provides the guidelines for assisting an infant who is responsive and has a foreign body airway obstruction. An infant is defined by the American Heart Association as any child younger than the age of 1 year.

Ear Trauma

Treat any cut or laceration to the ear by lightly applying a bandage, with even pressure, over the injury. It may be possible to reattach a severed ear surgically. Carefully wrap the severed ear in a sterile dressing secured with a self-adherent gauze bandage. Then wrap the ear in plastic, label it, and place it in an ice chest or over an ice pack so it is kept chilled but is not in direct contact with the ice. Send it with the patient to the hospital.

Eye Trauma

Depending on its severity, eye trauma may require no more than an ice pack or cold compress, or it may require hospital care. Eye trauma may result from a fall, a blow to the eye, or a wound from a pointed object. Whatever the cause, carefully examine the eye to the best of your ability and notify the physician of the patient's condition.

Eye injuries are commonly caused by foreign objects in the eye. Tiny specks cause tearing and can be painful. To remove them, use moistened sterile gauze or a tissue. Do not use a cotton ball because it may leave behind eye-irritating cotton wisps. If an object has penetrated the eye, do not try to remove it. Seek medical attention immediately.

Falls

If a patient falls from a chair or an examining table and cannot get up, call for help. Do not move the patient until the physician or an EMT examines him. Instruct the patient not to move his head, neck, or back if injuries to those areas are suspected. If possible, have someone hold the patient's neck to stabilize it until the physician or EMT arrives. Move the patient only in a life-threatening situation, such as if the building is on fire. Arrange for transport to the hospital and document the fall and injury in the patient's chart.

If the fall results in only a bump, apply ice and observe for bruises and swelling. Give the patient time to collect himself. Be sure to notify the doctor, who should examine the patient. Then document the fall, the injury, and the treatment in the patient's chart.

Fractures, Dislocations, Sprains, and Strains

A fracture is a break in a bone. Fractures are categorized in several ways (Figure 57-1). Complete fractures go across the entire bone; incomplete fractures go through only part of the bone. Comminuted fractures are those in which the bone has broken into several fragments. In a greenstick fracture, the bone is bent, but only one side is fractured. Greenstick fractures occur most often in children because their bones are still soft and pliable. A fracture is closed if it does not cause a break in the skin. In open fractures, the bone breaks through the skin.

A **dislocation** is the displacement of a bone end from the joint. Both fractures and dislocations usually result from accidents or sports injuries. They can cause pain, tenderness, loss of function, deformity, swelling, and discoloration. The injury is usually diagnosed by X-ray.

Fracture and dislocation treatment depends on factors like the nature of the injury and the patient's age and physical condition. The basic emergency steps are

1. Keep the person calm and limit his movement.
2. Assess him for any other injuries.
3. Notify the doctor or call EMS if needed.
   - Do not try to move the person until the doctor or EMS arrives.
4. If the skin is broken, cover with a sterile dressing.
5. Immobilize the extremity with a splint or sling (Figure 57-2).
   - Use rolled-up newspaper, strips of wood, etc.
   - Immobilize the joint above and below the injury.
   - Immobilize the bone in the position it is found.
   - Do not try to put the bone back in place.
6. Place an ice pack on the affected area.
7. Monitor him for signs of shock.
8. Assess for signs of lack of circulation in the injured limb including pale or blue skin, loss of feeling, and tingling in the area.

Complete fracture Incomplete fracture Closed fracture

Open fracture Greenstick fracture Comminuted fracture

FIGURE 57-1 These illustrations show various types of fractures.

FIGURE 57-2 When using a splint, make sure you immobilize above and below the injured joint.

FIGURE 57-3 Patients should be instructed to keep the cast dry and to notify the physician if they have pain or unusual sensations.

Immobilization is sometimes provided by the application of a splint or cast. The purpose of both splints and casts is to keep an injured body part in place and protect it as it heals. A **splint** is an appliance used for conditions that do not require rigid immobilization or, as a temporary measure, for those in which swelling is anticipated. A *cast* is a rigid, external dressing, usually made of plaster or fiberglass, that is molded to the contours of the body part to which it is applied. You may assist the physician with the application of a cast (Figure 57-3). You also may educate the patient about these basic elements of cast care:

- Report any of the following to the physician immediately: pain, swelling, discoloration of exposed portions, lack of pulsation and warmth, or the inability to move exposed parts.
- Keep the casted extremity elevated for the first day.
- Avoid indenting the cast until it is completely dry.
- Check the movement and sensation of the visible extremities frequently.
- Restrict strenuous activities for the first few days.
- Avoid allowing the affected limb to hang down for any length of time.
- Do not put anything inside the cast.
- Keep the cast dry.

Follow the physician's orders regarding activity restrictions.

Sprains and strains often result from sports injuries and accidents. A **sprain** is an injury characterized by partial tearing of a ligament that supports a joint, like the ankle. A sprain also may involve injuries to tendons, muscles, and local blood vessels and contusions of the surrounding soft tissue. A **strain** is a muscle injury that results from overexertion. For example, back strain may occur when a person carries a heavy load.

Symptoms of a sprain include swelling, tenderness, pain during movement, and local discoloration. If you suspect a sprain, splint the joint, apply ice, and call the EMS system if needed. Inform the patient that an X-ray may be required to confirm there is no fracture. A strain causes pain on motion. In most cases, it should be examined by a physician, who may prescribe rest, application of heat, and a muscle relaxant.

Head Injuries

Head injuries include concussions, contusions, fractures, intracranial bleeding, and scalp hematomas and lacerations. Some head injuries can be life-threatening and require immediate medical attention.

Concussion A **concussion** is a jarring injury to the brain. It is the most common type of head injury. Someone who has a concussion may lose consciousness. Temporary loss of vision, pallor (paleness), listlessness, memory loss, or vomiting also can occur. Symptoms may disappear rapidly or last up to 24 hours. A concussion may produce slow intracranial bleeding. Teach the patient and the patient's family basic precautions after this type of injury. See the Educating the Patient section for more information on concussions.

Go to CONNECT to see an animation about *Concussion*.

Severe Head Injuries Contusions, fractures, and intracranial bleeding cause symptoms similar to, but more profound than, symptoms of concussions. Symptoms to look for are leakage of clear or bloody fluid from the ears or nose, seizures, and respiratory arrest. A patient with a severe head injury requires immediate hospitalization. Your priority is to maintain the patient's airway and to begin CPR if needed.

Scalp Hematomas and Lacerations A **hematoma** is a swelling caused by blood under the skin. A scalp hematoma causes a bump on the head. This swelling can be reduced by applying ice immediately after the injury. Because blood vessels in the scalp are close to the skin, scalp lacerations often bleed profusely and look worse than they really are. Apply direct pressure to stop bleeding from a scalp laceration, wash the area with soap and water, and apply a dry, sterile dressing over the area.

Concussion

Because a concussion can cause intracranial bleeding, handle gently a patient who is being treated for this type of injury. If bleeding is slow, it might take up to 24 hours to produce symptoms. Because intracranial bleeding may require brain surgery, use the following patient education guidelines to help ensure patient safety after a concussion:

- Inform the patient that the first 24 hours after the injury are the most critical.
- Tell the patient to refrain from strenuous activity, to rest, and to return to regular activity gradually. Instruct the patient to avoid using pain medicines other than acetaminophen, unless the drugs are approved by the physician.
- Advise the patient to eat lightly, especially if nausea and vomiting occur.
- Tell a family member to check on the patient every few hours. The family member should make sure the patient knows his own name, his location, and the name of the family member.
- Instruct the family member to call for medical assistance immediately if the patient exhibits any of these warning signs:
  - Any symptom that is getting worse, like headaches, sleepiness, or nausea, including nausea that does not go away.
  - Changes in behavior, such as irritability or confusion.
  - Dilated pupils (pupils that are bigger than normal) or pupils of different sizes.
  - Trouble walking or speaking.
  - Drainage of bloody or clear fluids from ears or nose.
  - Vomiting.
  - Seizures.
  - Weakness or numbness in the arms or legs.
  - A less serious head injury in a patient taking blood thinners or who has a bleeding disorder like hemophilia.

Hemorrhaging

Hemorrhaging (heavy or uncontrollable bleeding) is generally the result of an injury. It also may be caused by an illness. The first-aid treatment remains the same in both cases. Bleeding can be internal or external. When administering first aid to a patient who may have internal bleeding, cover the patient with a blanket for warmth, keep the patient quiet and calm, and get medical help immediately.

Control external bleeding to prevent rapid blood loss and shock. Use direct pressure, apply additional dressings as needed, elevate the bleeding body part, and put pressure over a pressure point, as described in Procedure 57-5, at the end of this chapter. Then transport the patient to an emergency care facility.

As a last resort, if medical help is more than an hour away, you may need to use a tourniquet (Figure 57-4) to save a person's life. You apply a tourniquet over the main pressure point above the wound and tighten the tourniquet until the bleeding stops. For upper limb injuries, place the tourniquet as high as possible and tighten as tight as possible. If you apply a tourniquet, make sure you write the application time on the tourniquet or the patient's forehead. New research shows that with better trauma surgery techniques, a tourniquet may be used to stop life-threatening hemorrhage without loss of the affected limb.

Go to CONNECT to see a video about *Controlling Bleeding*.

FIGURE 57-4 Apply a tourniquet as a last resort—if the bleeding cannot be stopped and medical help is more than an hour away. Record the time applied on the tourniquet or the patient's forehead.

Multiple Injuries

Sometimes, a patient sustains more than one type of injury—for example, an arm fracture, head injury, lacerations, and internal bleeding. Multiple injuries often result from a car accident or a fall. If you need to assist a patient with multiple injuries, assess the CABs, call EMS (or have someone else call), and perform CPR if needed. Once you have ensured that the patient has a pulse, an open airway, and is breathing on his own, perform first aid for the most life-threatening injuries first.

Poisoning

A poison is a substance that produces harmful effects if it enters the body. Poisoning is serious and can result in death or permanent injury if immediate medical care is not provided.

In addition to being able to handle a poisoning emergency, you need to educate patients in how to do the same. Teach them about the symptoms of and treatment for the different types of poisoning and provide them with pamphlets that describe the procedures to follow and stickers with the telephone number of the regional poison control center.

The majority of accidental poisonings happen to children younger than the age of 5. Young children are not necessarily put off by strong smells or burning sensations when they swallow something. Common causes of poisoning in children are household cleaning products, household plants, and medications. Poisons also can be caused by improperly prepared or contaminated food. These types of poisons are ingested or swallowed.

Poisoning that results from coming in contact with plants (called absorbed poisoning), like poison ivy, poison sumac, and poison oak, is common and generally fairly minor. It can be serious, however, if the poisoning occurs over a large body surface.

Poisons also can be inhaled. This situation occurs when a person inhales a poisonous gas like carbon monoxide or the fumes from burning poisonous plants.

Ingested Poisons Swallowed poison remains in the stomach only a short time. Most of it is absorbed while in the small intestine. Symptoms of poisoning include abdominal pain and cramping; nausea; vomiting; diarrhea; odor, stains, or burns around or in the mouth; drowsiness; and unconsciousness. You also should suspect poisoning if packages containing poisonous substances are near a person who has one or more of these symptoms.

It is crucial to call a poison control center (if available), hospital emergency room, doctor, or the EMS system for instructions if you think a patient has swallowed a poison. When you call, you will need to know the following:

- The patient's age.
- The name of the poison.
- The amount of poison swallowed.
- When the poison was swallowed.
- Whether or not the person has vomited.
- How much time it will take to get the patient to a medical facility.

Poisons vary in their toxicity. Some cause damage right away; others cause damage several hours later. If the patient is alert and not having convulsions, follow these steps:

1. Call the regional poison control center.
2. If directed by the poison control center, induce vomiting with syrup of ipecac.
3. Seek immediate medical attention.

Do not induce vomiting unless directed by a medical authority. The patient may have ingested a strong acid, alkali, or petroleum product, like chlorine bleach or gasoline. These products may cause further damage to the throat and esophagus during vomiting. If you do not know what the patient ingested, never induce vomiting.

Turn the patient on her left side. This position delays stomach emptying by several hours and prevents aspiration if the patient vomits. Take both poison container and vomited material to the hospital for inspection.

Food poisoning, another type of ingested poisoning, can occur when bacteria produce toxins in food. Botulism, for example, results from eating improperly canned or preserved foods contaminated with the bacterium *Clostridium botulinum*. Symptoms appear within 12 to 36 hours after eating contaminated food. Initial symptoms include dry mouth, sore throat, weakness, vomiting, and diarrhea.

Food poisoning is often difficult to detect because the signs and symptoms vary greatly. A patient with food poisoning usually has abdominal pain, nausea, vomiting, gas, frequent bowel sounds, and diarrhea. Chills, joint pain, and excessive sweating also may occur. If you suspect a patient has food poisoning, call the poison control center and arrange for immediate transport to the hospital.

Absorbed Poisons Most people have had the red, itchy rash that results from contact with poison ivy, poison sumac, or poison oak. In some people, however, the rash may be accompanied by a generalized swelling, burning eyes, headache, fever, and abnormal pulse or respirations.

To treat a patient who has come in contact with an absorbed poison, call the regional poison control center. Have the patient immediately remove all contaminated clothing. Then wash the affected skin thoroughly with soap and water, drench it with alcohol, and rinse well. To help relieve symptoms, apply wet compresses soaked with calamine lotion. Also, suggest baths in colloidal oatmeal or applications of a paste made from 3 teaspoons baking soda and 1 teaspoon water to soothe the itching. If the rash is severe, the doctor may prescribe a corticosteroid ointment. Tell the patient to seek medical assistance if a fever or swelling develops.

Inhaled Poisons A patient may inhale poisons by breathing air contaminated by chemicals in the workplace or by a malfunctioning stove or furnace in the home. The patient may not realize she has been exposed to a poisonous gas until symptoms arise. Even then, a patient may merely suspect the flu because some symptoms of inhalation poisoning mimic those of influenza. Common symptoms include headache, tinnitus (ringing in the ears), angina (chest pain), shortness of breath, muscle weakness, nausea, vomiting, confusion, and dizziness, followed by blurred or double vision, difficulty breathing, unconsciousness, and cardiac arrest. Also, a patient who has facial burns may have sustained an inhalation injury.

To treat poisoning by inhalation, first get the patient into fresh air. Have someone call the EMS system or the regional poison control center. Loosen tight-fitting clothing and wrap the patient in a blanket to prevent shock. Check the patient's CABs and begin CPR if needed.

Carbon monoxide is a major cause of inhalation poisoning in the home. It is a colorless and odorless natural gas produced by incomplete combustion of organic fuels, like coal, wood, or gasoline. Carbon monoxide is especially dangerous in closed spaces because, when inhaled, it replaces oxygen in the blood. If you suspect carbon monoxide poisoning, look for clues in the environment such as a malfunctioning furnace or a car engine left running in a closed space like a garage.

Mild carbon monoxide poisoning can cause headache and flulike symptoms without fever. Moderate poisoning may cause tinnitus, drowsiness, severe seizures, coma, and cardiopulmonary problems. Because the gas is odorless, people are often unaware they are being poisoned. They may fall asleep, lapse into unconsciousness, and die.

Weather-Related Injuries

Exposure to extreme cold, extreme heat, and the sun's damaging rays can cause weather-related injuries, which may require emergency medical attention.

Hypothermia Hypothermia, caused by exposure to cold, occurs when a person loses more body heat than he or she can produce, resulting in a body temperature below 95°F. This condition usually occurs in the very old or very young, or in chronically ill or malnourished individuals. People who are outdoors with insufficient clothing in the winter or who get wet in cold weather are more likely to suffer from hypothermia.

Hypothermia symptoms include lethargy, loss of coordination, confusion, and uncontrollable shivering. If the person's body temperature is extremely low, the person may stop shivering. If untreated, hypothermia can result in cardiac arrest and coma.

Treat hypothermia by moving the person inside if possible and covering him with blankets. If he is wet, remove his wet clothing. If he is confused or unconscious, monitor his breathing and call the EMS system. If he is awake and alert, give him warm, nonalcoholic liquids.

Frostbite When body tissues are exposed to below-freezing temperatures, frostbite can occur. Frostbite causes ice crystals to form between tissue cells, and these crystals enlarge as they extract water from the cells. Frostbite also causes obstruction to the blood supply in the form of blood clots. This aspect of frostbite prevents blood from flowing to the tissues and causes additional, severe damage to cells.

Frostbite symptoms include white, waxy, or grayish yellow skin. The affected body part feels cold, tingling, and painful. The skin surface may feel crusty and the underlying tissue soft in comparison. If the frostbite is deep, the body part may feel cold and hard and not be sensitive to pain. Blisters may appear after rewarming.

Treat frostbite by wrapping warm clothing or blankets around the affected body part or placing it in contact with a warm body part. Do not rub or massage the affected area or you may cause further damage to the frozen tissue. Call for medical assistance. If you are in a remote area, use the wet rapid rewarming method. This method involves placing the affected part in warm (100°F to 104°F) water. Hot water should be added at regular intervals to keep the temperature of the bath stable. As an alternative method, you can heat the affected area with warm compresses. Continue rewarming for 20 to 40 minutes. After the affected area becomes soft, place dry, sterile gauze between skin surfaces, such as between the toes or the fingers or between the ear and the side of the head. Do not massage the skin or break blisters.

Heatstroke Heatstroke results from prolonged exposure to high temperatures and humidity. This condition may lead to excessive loss of fluids (dehydration) and insufficient blood in the circulatory system (hypovolemic shock). High body temperature can damage tissues and organs throughout the body. If untreated, the patient will die. People most susceptible to heatstroke are children, the elderly, athletes, and patients who are obese, are diabetic, or have circulatory problems or other chronic illnesses.

Symptoms of heatstroke include hot, dry skin; high body temperature; altered mental state; rapid pulse; rapid breathing; dizziness; and weakness. If you suspect a patient has heatstroke, check the patient's CABs and call the EMS system. Move the patient to a cool place and remove outer clothing unless it is made of light cotton or other light fabric. Also, cool the patient with any means available, such as gentle spraying with a hose, movement to an air-conditioned place, vigorous fanning, or application of a wet sheet. If the humidity is above 75%, place ice packs on the patient's groin and armpits. Stop cooling when the patient's mental state improves. Keep the patient's head and shoulders slightly elevated.

Sunburn Do not dismiss a sunburn as trivial. It is a burn that can cause redness, tenderness, pain, swelling, blisters, and peeling skin and may lead to skin damage or cancer later in life.

Soak sunburned skin in cool water to help reduce the heat. Apply cold compresses, and later calamine lotion, to bring relief from the burning sensation. Have the patient elevate the legs and arms to prevent swelling. The patient also should drink plenty of water and take a pain reliever.

Educate the patient about the importance of using sunscreen and reapplying it every 2 to 3 hours when outdoors. Advise the patient to stay out of direct sunlight between 10:00 a.m. and 2:00 p.m. because the sun's rays are strongest during that period.

Wounds

A wound is an injury in which the skin or tissues under the skin are damaged. Wounds can be either open or closed. Figure 57-5 shows the various types of wounds.

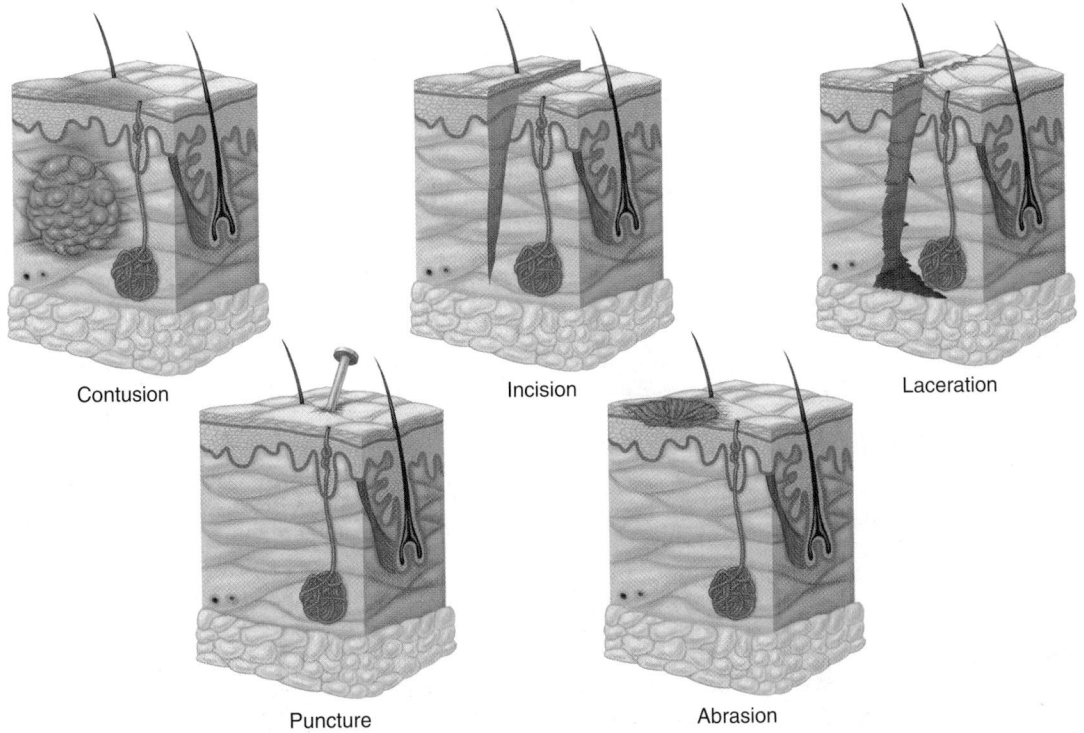

FIGURE 57-5 Different types of wounds produce different degrees of tissue damage.

Open Wounds An open wound is a break in the skin or mucous membrane. Types of open wounds include incisions, lacerations, abrasions, and punctures.

Incisions and Lacerations An incision is a clean and smooth cut, like that from a kitchen knife. A laceration has jagged edges, as may result when a child steps on a piece of broken glass in the sand at the beach. Care of minor incisions and lacerations involves controlling bleeding by covering the wound with a clean or sterile dressing and applying direct pressure. After the bleeding stops, clean and dress the wound. Procedure 57-6, at the end of this chapter, explains how to clean minor wounds. Teach the patient the importance of keeping the wound clean and checking for signs of infection, like heat, redness, pain, and swelling.

If the wound is deep and involves muscle, tendons, the face, the genitals, the mouth, or the tongue, control the bleeding with direct pressure to the wound (with a sterile dressing or clean cloth held against its surface), elevation, and use of pressure points. Contact the doctor and, if necessary, the EMS system.

Amputations If a fingertip or toe is completely or nearly severed, quick action may increase the likelihood that it can be saved. Elevate the injured extremity, cover the digit with a dry dressing, and immobilize the hand or foot. Retrieve the severed digit, wrap it in gauze, put it in a plastic bag, put the bag on ice, and send the part with the patient to the hospital.

Abrasions An abrasion is a scraping of the skin, as when someone slides across rough dirt during a softball game.

Abrasions require washing with soap and water. Be sure to remove all the dirt and debris to prevent tattooing (dark discoloration under the skin). Minor abrasions do not need a dressing or bandage, but large ones do. Various types of bandaging are shown in Figure 57-6. As with any wound, teach the patient to watch for signs of infection.

Punctures A puncture wound is a small hole created by a piercing object, like a bullet, knife, nail, or animal tooth. Puncture wounds are a potential breeding ground for tetanus bacteria because the bacteria can live and thrive in the absence of oxygen. Rinse the wound under running water for 15 minutes. Then clean the wound with soap and water and apply a dry, sterile dressing. If the patient has not had a tetanus toxoid immunization in the past 7 to 10 years, inform the physician so one can be ordered.

Closed Wounds A closed wound is an injury that occurs inside the body without breaking the skin. Closed wounds, often called **contusions** (bruises), are caused by a blunt object striking the tissue. This action produces broken blood vessels and internal, localized bleeding (hematoma) below the area that has been struck. Treat such a wound with cold compresses to reduce swelling. The affected area will turn from black and blue to green to yellow as blood pigments oxidize. Inform the patient that these color changes are part of the normal healing process.

Go to CONNECT to see a video about *Cleaning Minor Wounds.*

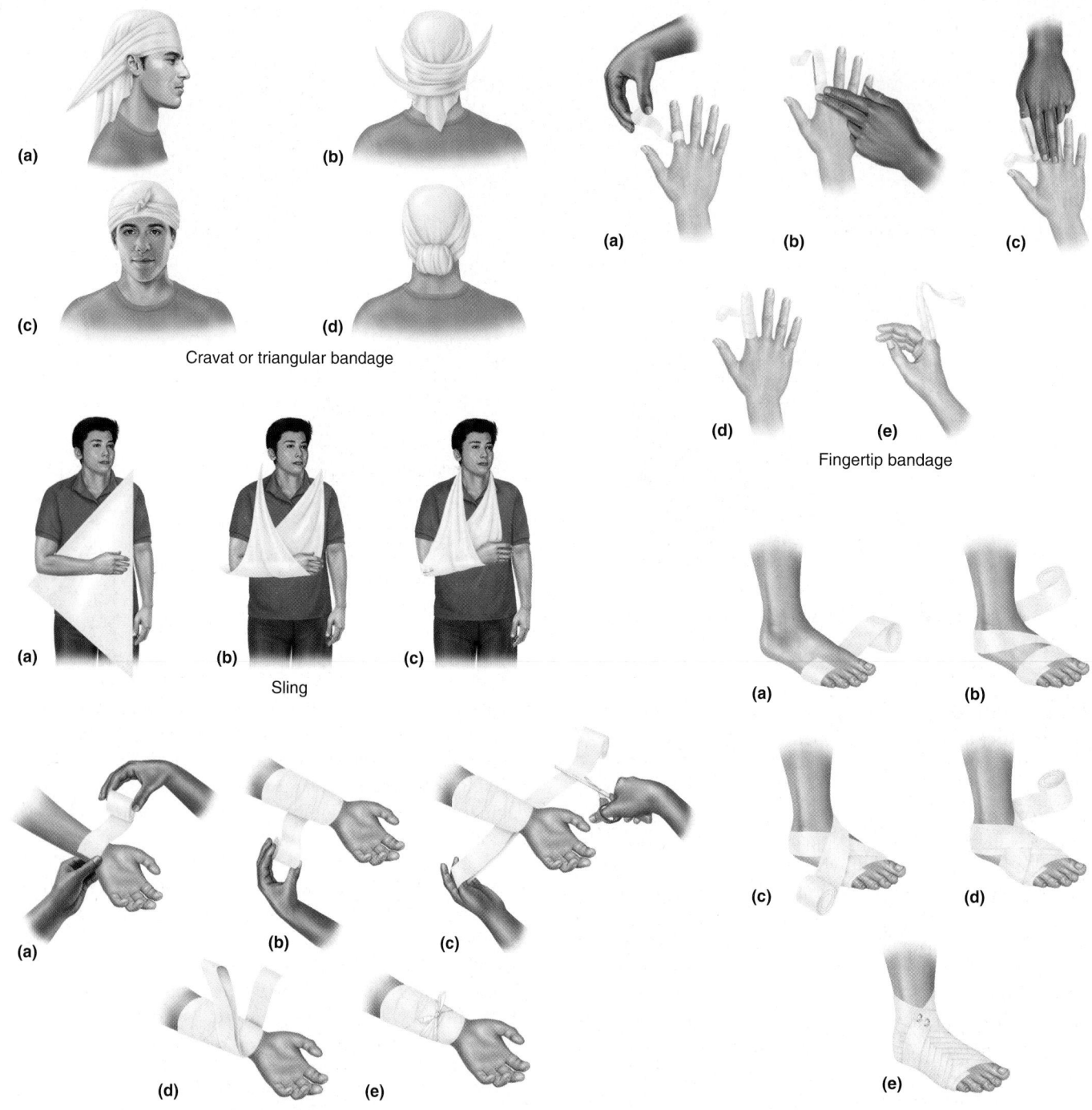

(a)

(b)

(c)

(d)

Cravat or triangular bandage

(a)

(b)

(c)

(d)

(e)

Fingertip bandage

(a)

(b)

(c)

Sling

(a)

(b)

(a)

(b)

(c)

(d)

(e)

Circular bandage

(c)

(d)

(e)

Figure eight bandage

FIGURE 57-6   Apply a bandage, as needed, to a wound.

▶ Common Disorders   LO 57.4

A variety of common disorders frequently require emergency
medical intervention. As a patient educator, you can help ensure patients recognize the symptoms of illnesses and know
when to call for medical assistance. Teaching patients the
importance of following the physician's orders for follow-up
care is also your responsibility. Common disorders include the
following:

- Abdominal pain
- Asthma
- Dehydration
- Diarrhea
- Fainting
- Fever
- Hyperventilation

- Nosebleed
- Tachycardia
- Vomiting

Abdominal Pain

Sudden, acute abdominal pain accompanied by fever may indicate an emergency that requires surgery. The pain may involve spasmodic contractions. It may feel knifelike or ache dully, and it may be localized or may radiate. The pain's location gives clues to its cause. Acute pain in the right upper quadrant, for example, may signal a gallbladder attack. Pain in the right lower quadrant may indicate appendicitis.

Other causes include internal hemorrhage, intestinal perforation or obstruction, peptic ulcer, and hernia. In women, pelvic pain can indicate a gynecologic problem. Obviously, trauma to the area, such as wounds or blows, can produce acute abdominal pain.

While waiting for patient transport, have the patient lie on his back with his knees flexed (unless there is a wound or swelling in the abdomen). This position lets the abdominal muscles relax. Keep the patient quiet and warm, and stay calm and attentive. Do not give anything by mouth, and keep an emesis (vomiting) basin handy in case the patient vomits. Do not apply heat to the abdomen as heat may exacerbate inflammation. Monitor the patient's pulse and consciousness and check for signs of shock.

Asthma

Asthma is a common disorder caused by spasmodic narrowing of the bronchi. It is often an inherited tendency and several members of one family may suffer from it. A patient who is having an acute attack wheezes, coughs, and is short of breath. She may become frightened and feel as if she cannot get enough air. If you suspect an asthma attack, check the patient's CABs and notify the doctor at once. You may assist the patient in using a respiratory inhaler if she carries one with her. If directed, administer a mininebulizer treatment with a bronchodilator (drug that opens the bronchi), like albuterol (Proventil) or epinephrine.

Dehydration

Dehydration results from a lack of adequate water in the body. The body's fluid intake is not sufficient to meet its fluid needs. Severe dehydration can result from vomiting, excessive heat and sweating, diarrhea, or lack of food or fluid intake. The following are symptoms of dehydration:

- Extreme thirst
- Tiredness
- Light-headedness
- Abdominal or muscle cramping
- Confusion (especially in elderly people)

Perform the following steps to administer first aid to a dehydrated person"

1. Move the victim into the shade or to a cool area.
2. To replace lost fluids, give the victim frequent, small amounts of decaffeinated fluids.

3. If symptoms persist or are accompanied by nausea, diarrhea, or convulsions, call for the EMS system or a physician.

Diarrhea (Acute)

Acute diarrhea can be caused by an intestinal infection, food poisoning, a bowel disorder, or medication side effects. Severe diarrhea causes dehydration and dangerous electrolyte imbalances that can lead to shock. Symptoms of shock include rapid pulse, low blood pressure, and pale, clammy skin.

Help the patient lie on his back and elevate his legs. Report the patient's condition to the doctor. As directed, prepare to assist in administering intravenous fluids to correct dehydration and restore electrolytes, and to draw blood for testing.

Fainting (Syncope)

Fainting, or syncope, is a partial or complete loss of consciousness, which usually follows a decrease in blood flow to the brain. Before fainting, patients may feel weak, dizzy, cold, or nauseated. They may perspire or look pale and anxious.

If you are with a patient who feels as if she is going to faint, tell her to lower her head between her legs and to breathe deeply. Stay with her until the feeling passes. If the patient is having difficulty breathing or faints, lay her flat on her back with her feet slightly elevated. Loosen tight clothing and apply a cold cloth to her face. Observe the patient carefully, monitoring her breathing and level of consciousness. Observe for weakness in her arms and legs. Let her rest for at least 10 minutes after she regains full consciousness. Notify the physician the patient fainted.

If your efforts do not revive a patient who has fainted, instead call the physician and the EMS system as the patient may be slipping into a coma.

Fever

Fever is a common clinical sign that often indicates infection. Mild or moderate fever can accompany a cold or an upset stomach. It can usually be managed with aspirin (in adults only), ibuprofen, or acetaminophen. A fever of 106°F or higher (hyperthermia) is dangerous, however, because irreversible brain damage can occur if the fever is not lowered immediately.

If a patient's temperature is dangerously high, you must proceed at once to check the other vital signs and the level of consciousness. Notify the doctor and be prepared to start rapid cooling measures if directed to do so. Place ice packs on the groin and axilla, or give the patient a tepid sponge bath. If the patient is a child, be prepared to manage seizures (discussed later in this chapter). Do not give a child with a fever aspirin unless directed by a physician.

Hyperventilation

Some patients who are under a great deal of stress lack the skills to deal with the stress effectively. They may seem anxious, frazzled, and more emotional than average patients. Patients under stress may begin to hyperventilate, or breathe too rapidly and too deeply. This breathing disturbs the normal balance of oxygen and carbon dioxide in the blood, and the carbon dioxide concentration falls below normal levels. Patients who are hyperventilating also may feel light-headed and as if they cannot get enough air. In addition, they may have chest pain and feel apprehensive.

Move a hyperventilating patient to a quiet area. Have the patient sit peacefully and visualize a calm and serene environment, like a beach or the mountains. With a calm and soothing voice, coach the patient to take slow, normal breaths. If the patient continues to hyperventilate after several minutes of coaching, notify the physician as this may indicate a more serious lung problem.

Nosebleed

Nosebleed, or **epistaxis,** can occur for a variety of reasons. They include blowing the nose too hard, local irritation or dryness, frequent sneezing, fragile or superficial blood vessels, high blood pressure, a blow to the nose, and a foreign body in the nose. Nosebleeds are common in children, especially at night.

Treat a nosebleed by having the patient sit up with the head tilted forward to prevent blood from running down the back of the throat. Next, have the patient gently pinch the nostrils shut at the bottom for at least 5 minutes. If that does not stop the bleeding, continue to pinch the nostrils for an additional 5 minutes. If the bleeding cannot be controlled within 10 minutes, alert the physician.

Tachycardia

Tachycardia is a rapid heart rate, generally in excess of 100 beats per minute. A patient with tachycardia may report having **palpitations,** unusually rapid, strong, or irregular pulsations of the heart. He may feel as if his heart is pounding. Help the patient lie down, take his vital signs, and, if instructed, obtain an electrocardiogram (ECG). (Electrocardiography is discussed in the *Electrocardiography and Pulmonary Function Testing* chapter.) If tachycardia is accompanied by low blood pressure and light-headedness, notify the physician immediately. These symptoms indicate the patient could faint or go into shock. Remain with the patient and keep him calm.

Vomiting

Vomiting is a symptom common to many disorders, ranging from food poisoning to various infections. When severe, it can lead to dehydration and dangerous changes in electrolyte levels, especially in patients who are very young, very old, or diabetic or who also have diarrhea. Because these problems can be severe, notify the doctor and provide appropriate care. Procedure 57-7, at the end of this chapter, describes how to provide emergency care for a patient who is vomiting.

Go to CONNECT to see a video about *Caring for a Patient Who Is Vomiting.*

▶ Less Common Disorders

LO 57.5

Even though some disorders are less common than those previously discussed, you should still be familiar enough with them to handle them effectively if a physician or EMT is not immediately available. Educate patients about symptoms they may encounter that require emergency medical intervention and about the importance of follow-up care when recovering from such illnesses or disorders. Less common disorders that may require emergency medical intervention include

- Anaphylaxis
- Bacterial meningitis
- Diabetic emergencies
- Gallbladder attack
- Heart attack (myocardial infarction)
- Hematemesis (the vomiting of blood)
- Obstetric emergencies
- Respiratory arrest
- Seizures
- Shock
- Stroke
- Toxic shock syndrome
- Viral encephalitis

Anaphylaxis

Anaphylaxis, or anaphylactic shock, is a severe, often life-threatening allergic reaction, which can be immediate or delayed up to 2 hours. It happens to people who have become sensitized to certain substances. For example, it can result from eating a type of food, being stung by an insect, or taking a particular type of medication, like penicillin.

The first sign of anaphylaxis usually comes from the patient's skin. It becomes itchy, turns red, feels hot, and develops hives. The face may also become puffy. The throat may swell so that the patient has trouble breathing and swallowing and feels as if he has a "lump in the throat." Other symptoms include pallor, perspiration, abdominal pain or nausea, and a weak, rapid, irregular pulse. If you detect these symptoms or if the patient becomes restless, has a headache, or says his throat feels as if it is closing up, take the following steps immediately.

Check the patient's CABs and then notify the doctor. As directed, administer epinephrine, oral antihistamines, and oxygen and help the patient sit up. After the patient receives epinephrine, monitor his vital signs every 2 to 3 minutes. Note skin color and monitor the airway. If he does not recover quickly, arrange for immediate transport to the hospital.

When severely allergic patients stabilize, the doctor prescribes an epinephrine autoinjector for patients to carry with them. You are responsible for teaching patients how to use this device. See the *Assisting in Other Medical Specialties* chapter for more information about using an autoinjector.

Because of the possibility of anaphylaxis, a patient who has just received any type of injection should routinely be kept in the office for 20 to 30 minutes of observation. This procedure reduces the possibility that an allergic reaction to the medication will occur while the patient is unattended.

A less severe allergic reaction to drugs or certain foods may cause sneezing, itching, slight swelling of the skin, rash, or hives. This type of reaction can usually be controlled with diphenhydramine hydrochloride (Benadryl) or another antihistamine. The patient should be monitored closely, however, to make sure the condition does not progress to anaphylaxis.

Bacterial Meningitis

Bacterial meningitis is almost always a complication of another bacterial infection, like otitis media (middle ear infection) or pneumonia. So, first find out whether the patient currently has or recently has had a bacterial infection. The signs of bacterial meningitis are fever, chills, headache, neck stiffness, and vomiting. If the patient has these signs and then develops a fever of 102°F, becomes less alert, has altered respirations, or experiences seizures, the infection has progressed to a dangerous state.

If these signs are present, assess the patient's CABs and notify the physician of the change in the patient's condition. Expect to arrange for transport to the hospital, where the patient will be treated with intravenous antibiotics.

Diabetic Emergencies

Diabetes is a fairly common disorder of carbohydrate metabolism (for more information about diabetes, see the chapters *The Endocrine System* and *Assisting in Other Medical Specialties*). The body needs insulin, a hormone secreted by the pancreas, to use blood sugar to fuel body cells. Insulin secretion is impaired in patients with diabetes.

You can teach patients who have diabetes or who are at risk for diabetes how to recognize early signs of **hypoglycemia** (low blood sugar) and **hyperglycemia** (high blood sugar) before these conditions become medical emergencies. Symptoms of hypoglycemia include dizziness; headache; confusion; hunger; weakness; full, rapid pulse; and pallor. Symptoms of hyperglycemia include dry mouth, intense thirst, muscle weakness, and blurred vision. You also should be familiar with the signs and symptoms of the two most common diabetic emergencies you will encounter: insulin shock and diabetic coma.

Insulin Shock Insulin shock is basically very severe hypoglycemia, in which a patient has too little sugar in the blood. Insulin shock occurs when insulin levels are so high that they move too much sugar from the blood into cells. Symptoms include rapid pulse; shallow respiration; hunger; profuse sweating; pale, cool, clammy skin; double vision; tremors; restlessness; confusion; and possibly fainting. Insulin shock can usually be corrected with administration of some form of sugar (candy, juice, or regular soda for a conscious patient or a sprinkle of table sugar on the tongue for an unconscious patient). If the cause of a diabetic emergency is unknown, give sugar. Patients will improve quickly if the cause is insulin shock and will not be harmed if the cause is in a diabetic coma, provided they are then transported to the hospital.

Diabetic Coma Diabetic coma is the end result of severe hyperglycemia, in which a patient has too much sugar in the blood. It occurs when insulin levels are insufficient to move blood sugar into body cells. Its symptoms include rapid, deep gulping breaths; flushed, warm, dry skin; thirst; acetone breath (a sweet or fruity odor from the mouth); and disorientation or confusion. If you suspect diabetic coma, notify the doctor at once and expect to arrange transport to the hospital.

Gallbladder Attack (Acute)

A classic acute gallbladder attack occurs after a person eats a high-fat meal rich in cholesterol. The patient may wake up in the night with acute abdominal pain (gallbladder colic) in the right upper quadrant. The pain is caused by inflammation of the gallbladder, usually related to gallstones obstructing the cystic duct, through which bile is secreted by the gallbladder. The pain may radiate to the back between the shoulder blades or be localized in the epigastric region (the upper central region of the abdomen) and the front chest area. The attack may be accompanied by nausea and vomiting. The pain is usually so severe the patient seeks medical attention; many patients think they are having a heart attack.

Gallbladder attacks caused by gallstones are more common among women who are older than age 40 and obese, and the frequency of attacks increases with age (especially after age 65). Diagnosis is usually made with the help of ultrasonography. The patient may require surgery to remove the gallbladder.

Heart Attack

A heart attack, or myocardial infarction (MI), occurs when the blood flow to the heart is reduced as a result of blockage in the coronary arteries or their branches. Chest pain is the cardinal symptom of a myocardial infarction. The patient may describe the pain as crushing, burning, heavy, aching, or like that of indigestion. The pain may radiate down the left arm or into the jaw, throat, or both shoulders. It may be accompanied by shortness of breath, sweating, nausea, and vomiting. The patient may be pale and have a feeling of doom. If you cannot easily detect pallor (paleness) because the patient has dark skin, check the patient's inner lip for paleness. Elderly patients may experience atypical symptoms of a myocardial infarction, like jaw pain, because responses to pain diminish during the aging process. The pain of a myocardial infarction is not relieved by nitroglycerin.

If you think a patient is having a myocardial infarction, follow the American Heart Association's "Chain of Survival," outlined here:

- Immediate recognition and activation of EMS.
- Early CPR.
- Rapid defibrillation.
- Advanced life support.
- Post-cardiac arrest care.

Do not let the patient walk. Loosen tight clothing and have the patient sit up to aid breathing. The physician may order you to administer oxygen at 4 to 6 liters per minute; make sure no one in the area is smoking. Stay with the patient, observe the CABs, and begin CPR if required. If directed, obtain an ECG. Take apical and radial pulses, as instructed by the physician. Be prepared to obtain medication from the crash cart or

TABLE 57-3 Key Components of Basic Life Support

Component	Recommendations		
	Adults	**Children**	**Infants**
Recognition	Unresponsive, all ages No breathing or abnormal breathing like gasping No pulse palpated within 10 seconds (healthcare professionals)		
CPR sequence	CAB	CAB	CAB
Compression rate	At least 100/min		
Compression depth	At least 2 inches	2 inches or ⅓ anteroposterior chest circumference	1½ inches or ⅓ anteroposterior chest circumference
Chest wall recoil	Complete recoil between compressions.		
Compression interruptions	Limit chest compression interruptions to less than 10 seconds if at all		
Airway	Head tilt–chin lift Healthcare professionals only—jaw thrust if indicated by trauma		
Compression to ventilation ratio	30:2 (1 or 2 rescuers)	30:2 (single rescuer) 15:2 (2 healthcare professional rescuers)	30:2 (single rescuer) 15:2 (2 healthcare professional rescuers)
Ventilations for untrained rescuer	Compressions only		
Defibrillation	Use AED as soon as possible. Minimize interruptions in chest compressions before and after shock. Resume compressions immediately after each shock.		

Adapted from *2010 American Heart Association Guidelines for Cardiopulmonary Resuscitation and Emergency Cardiovascular Care Service*, Pt. 4, tab. 1.

use a defibrillator if required. The American Heart Association Guidelines for CPR key components are found in Table 57-3.

Ventricular fibrillation (VF)—the most common cause of cardiac arrest—is an abnormal heart rhythm. During VF, the heart's rhythm becomes chaotic and the heart does not pump blood. VF treatment is defibrillation using a medical device called a defibrillator, which works by delivering an electrical shock to the heart to interrupt the chaotic rhythm. Defibrillators are effective only if used within minutes of the patient's collapse. An **automated external defibrillator (AED)** is a computerized defibrillator programmed to recognize VF and other lethal heart rhythms (Figure 57-7). These devices are found in many public places, including airports, but also may be used at the clinic where you are employed.

To use an AED, attach the adhesive electrode pads to the client's chest in a specific arrangement as determined by the manufacturer. Look at the illustration on the electrode's packing or machine. Activate the AED and it will analyze the heart's rhythm and determine if a shock is required. Pressing the "Shock" button will deliver an electrical charge to the patient's heart by way of the AED's electrode wires attached to the chest.

In order to use an AED, you must be properly trained. Training is included as part of the CPR courses of the American Red Cross and the American Heart Association. Obtaining CPR and first-aid certification will be an asset to you as a medical assistant and is necessary to receive medical assisting certification by some agencies.

Go to CONNECT to see a video about *Performing Cardiopulmonary Resuscitation (CPR)*.

FIGURE 57-7 An automated external defibrillator delivers an electric current to the heart to a stop chaotic rhythm like ventricular fibrillation.

Hematemesis

Hematemesis is the vomiting of blood. A patient who vomits bright red blood may have a gastrointestinal disorder, like a bleeding ulcer. A patient who vomits blood that looks like coffee grounds may have slow bleeding into the stomach.

Quickly check the vital signs of a patient with hematemesis. If pulse and breathing are rapid and blood pressure is low, the patient may be going into shock. Notify the doctor immediately and get the crash cart to help the doctor start an intravenous line to replace lost fluid. Then call the EMS system.

Obstetric Emergencies

If you work in an obstetric practice, you may see emergencies unique to this specialty. Although the physician handles most obstetric emergencies, you can assist by asking the patient specific questions about her problem so the physician can decide what treatment is necessary.

Set up written protocols to handle these situations. For example, if the patient calls from home and reports gushing vaginal bleeding, your protocol may be to call the EMS system for her and tell her to lie down with her feet elevated. If the patient has a miscarriage, have her bring the expelled tissue with her to the office or hospital. (See the *Assisting in Reproductive and Urinary Specialties* chapter for more information.)

Respiratory Arrest

Respiratory arrest, or lack of breathing, is usually preceded by respiratory distress symptoms, which include difficulty breathing, rapid breathing, palpitations, racing pulse, high or low blood pressure, sweating, pale or bluish skin, and decreasing level of consciousness. If a patient shows these symptoms, notify the doctor right away. If the patient develops respiratory arrest, have someone call the doctor and the EMS system while you perform CPR.

Seizures

A seizure, or convulsion, is a series of violent and involuntary muscle contractions. Seizures are usually related to brain malfunctions that can result from diseased or injured brain tissues. A seizure may be caused by high fever, epilepsy (a brain disorder that causes seizures with varying severity), meningitis, diabetic states, and many other medical problems.

Follow this emergency care for seizure patients:

1. Remove objects that may cause injury.
2. Place the patient on the floor or the ground. If possible, position him on his side with his head turned to the side to help keep the airway open and unobstructed by the tongue. This position is especially important if the patient vomits, to prevent aspiration of vomitus into the lungs.
3. Loosen restrictive clothing and never place anything in the patient's mouth.
4. Protect the patient from injury, but do not try to hold him still during convulsions.
5. After convulsions end, keep the patient at rest, positioned for drainage from the mouth.
6. Make sure the patient is breathing. If he is not, begin rescue breathing or CPR.

7. Take vital signs and monitor respirations closely.
8. Move the patient to an exam room or have him taken to a medical facility.

Shock

Generally speaking, shock is a life-threatening state associated with cardiovascular system failure. It can bring to a stop all normal metabolic functions. This condition prevents the vital organs from receiving blood.

Early symptoms of shock include restlessness; irritability; fear; rapid pulse; pale, cool skin; and increased respiratory rate. Treat a patient in shock by elevating the feet 8 to 12 inches. If you suspect a head injury, however, keep the patient flat. Monitor the patient's CABs and take steps to control bleeding. If the patient is chilly, wrap the patient in a blanket. Notify the physician and call the EMS system.

Several types of shock are possible. Anaphylactic shock, or anaphylaxis, is usually associated with an allergic reaction, as previously discussed. Hypovolemic shock and septic shock are two other types of shock.

Hypovolemic Shock **Hypovolemic shock** results from insufficient blood volume in the circulatory system. It occurs after an injury that causes major fluid loss, such as hemorrhage or burns. Patients with hypovolemic shock must be transported to an emergency facility immediately.

Septic Shock **Septic shock** results from massive, widespread infection that affects the ability of the blood vessels to circulate blood. Common causes are urinary tract infection (UTI) (especially in older adults), postpartum infection, and a variety of infections in patients with immunosuppression (as caused by chemotherapy or acquired immunodeficiency syndrome [AIDS]).

Stroke

A stroke or **cerebrovascular accident** (**CVA**) occurs when the blood supply to the brain is impaired. This impairment may cause temporary or permanent damage, depending on how long the brain cells are deprived of oxygen.

A minor stroke can cause headache, confusion, dizziness, tinnitus, minor speech difficulties, personality changes, weakness of the limbs, and memory loss. A major stroke typically produces loss of consciousness, paralysis on one side of the body, difficulty swallowing, loss of bladder and bowel control, slurred or garbled speech, and unequal pupil size. The American Stroke Association recommends using the acronym FAST to assess if someone is having a stroke.

- F—facial drooping; ask the patient to smile, do both sides of the mouth raise?
- A—arm weakness; have the patient raise both arms, do both arms stay up?
- S—speech difficulty; have the patient repeat a simple sentence, is it correct?
- T—time to call 911; don't delay, even if the patient seems to be getting better.

If a patient has a stroke in the office, notify the physician at once and call the EMS system. Maintain the patient's airway by turning the head toward the affected side to allow secretions to drain out rather than be aspirated. Loosen tight clothing. If directed by the physician, monitor vital signs and administer oxygen.

Toxic Shock Syndrome

Toxic shock syndrome (TSS) is an acute infection caused by the bacterium *Staphylococcus aureus*. The toxin produced by the bacterium can enter the body through a break in the skin or through the uterus. Although the infection is most common in menstruating women who are using tampons at the time of onset, the link between tampon use and TSS is unclear.

TSS symptoms include high fever, intense muscle aches, vomiting, diarrhea, headache, bouts of violent shivering, vaginal discharge, red eyes, and a decreased level of consciousness. A sign specific to TSS is a deep red rash on the palms of the hands and the soles of the feet. This skin then sloughs off. A menstruating patient with these symptoms should be instructed to remove the tampon immediately and replace it with a sanitary napkin.

TSS is treated with intravenous antibiotics and fluids. The patient will require hospitalization.

Viral Encephalitis

Viral encephalitis is a severe brain inflammation caused directly by a virus or secondary to a complication resulting from a viral infection. Viral encephalitis may result from an epidemic or may arise sporadically. This condition requires accurate identification and prompt treatment. Symptoms develop suddenly, beginning with fever, headache, and vomiting. They quickly progress to stiff neck and back, decreased level of consciousness (from drowsiness to coma), and paralysis and seizures.

The level of consciousness must be monitored frequently in a patient with viral encephalitis. Prepare the patient for treatment with antiviral drugs and arrange for transport to a hospital for a lumbar puncture and other diagnostic tests.

▶ Common Psychosocial Emergencies   LO 57.6

You will probably encounter psychosocial emergencies in the medical office at some point. These may result from drug or alcohol abuse, spousal abuse, child abuse, or elder abuse. Handle these situations as you were directed in the *Patient Interview and History* chapter. If you encounter patients who have overdosed on drugs, exhibit violent behavior, mention suicide, or have been raped, follow the specific clinical responsibilities described in this section.

You also may be responsible for referring patients with psychosocial emergencies to resources in the community. Some of these resources are listed in Table 57-4.

A patient who is overdosing on drugs can suffer serious medical problems and can even die. If a patient who has taken an overdose is brought to the medical office, call the EMS system immediately and arrange for transport to the hospital.

TABLE 57-4   Resources for Patient Assistance

Resource
Al-Anon Family Groups
Alcoholics Anonymous
Mothers Against Drunk Driving (MADD)
Narcotics Anonymous
National Child Abuse Hotline
National Coalition Against Domestic Violence
National Council on Child Abuse and Family Violence
National Domestic Violence Hotline
National Institute for Alcohol Abuse and Alcoholism (NIAAA)
National Institute on Drug Abuse
National Organization for Victim Assistance
Students Against Destructive Decisions

Patients on drugs may become violent during withdrawal from the substance or while under the influence. If, at any time, a patient becomes aggressive or threatening, follow office protocol for handling violent behavior. The protocol should state when to call the police, how to document the incident, and when to notify the insurance carrier.

During a psychosocial emergency, a patient may tell you he is so depressed that he has thought about killing himself. Allow the patient to talk freely. Listen carefully without interrupting. Whenever a patient mentions suicide or talks about life in ways that make you suspect suicidal tendencies, discuss your suspicions with the physician. Take comments on suicide seriously, no matter how casual they may seem.

Victims of rape may be of any age and either gender, but more than 90% are women. If a patient says she has been raped, provide privacy. Limit the number of people who ask her questions. She may feel traumatized, embarrassed, and fearful. Do not make her go through the office routine at this time.

If the physician asks you to speak to the patient, explain to her that you are legally required to contact the police so they can file a report. The patient can decide later whether she wishes to press charges.

Contact the local rape hotline and request a rape counselor come to the office to stay with the patient during the exam and police report procedures. The physician should be familiar with state laws for collecting specimens and the protocol for caring for a rape victim.

The procedure of ensuring that a specimen is obtained from the victim and is correctly identified, that the specimen is under the uninterrupted control of authorized personnel, and that the specimen has not been altered or replaced is called *establishing chain of custody*. This procedure is required for medicolegal issues like evidence of rape and for drug tests for illicit drug use. If the chain between the victim and the specimen cannot be proved to have remained unbroken, the specimen must be considered invalid. The steps for establishing a chain of custody are outlined in the *Processing and Testing Urine and Stool Specimens* chapter and are essentially the same for any specimen with a medicolegal purpose. These general steps help maintain an intact chain of custody. Always refer to your office's procedures to make sure you are meeting all relevant requirements.

▶ The Patient under Stress
LO 57.7

In emergency situations, patients and family members are under a great deal of stress. You must realize that people react differently to emergency situations. You can learn how to detect signs of extreme stress by being alert for patients whose behavior varies from that previously observed or who cannot focus or follow directions.

Your role during many emergency situations may be to keep victims and their families and friends calm. You can promote calmness by listening carefully and giving your full attention. Your first priority, at all times, is the victim's well-being. If he is very distraught, for example, hold his hand while the doctor examines him. If one of his relatives is crying and causing him to become emotional, suggest that the relative do something to help—for example, fill out paperwork in another room.

You may face special challenges when communicating with victims during emergencies. Victims may not speak your language, or they may have a visual or hearing impairment. In such instances, follow these guidelines:

- Use gestures throughout the process for non-English-speaking victims. Continue to speak, however, because they may be able to understand some English.
- Tell patients who have visual impairments what you are going to do before you do it, and maintain voice and touch contact while caring for them.
- Ask patients who have hearing impairments whether they can read lips. If they can, speak slowly to them and never turn away while you are speaking. If they cannot read lips, communicate by writing and using gestures. At all times, try to remain face to face and keep direct physical contact.

▶ Educating the Patient
LO 57.8

During minor medical emergencies, after major emergencies have been resolved, and during routine office visits, you can educate patients about ways to prevent and handle various medical emergencies. For example, you might tell them how to contact the local American Red Cross office, post notices of upcoming classes the Red Cross offers, and encourage patients and family members to learn basic first aid. You also might develop a first-aid kit checklist and make it available to patients and families.

Make sure all family members, including children, are familiar with the local EMS system and know how to contact it in an emergency. Suggest that families keep emergency numbers by the telephone. In addition, teach parents how to childproof their home for children of various ages. Remember, childproofing

differs for different children—for example, for children who can crawl as opposed to children who can walk.

Provide brief, easy-to-read handouts to reinforce the information you present to patients. Prepare handouts in multiple languages if you provide care for non-English-speaking patients. Find and use patient education resources for the types of patients seen by the practice. For example, if you work in an obstetric office, obtain educational materials for pregnant and postpartum patients from companies that provide pregnancy-related products. Ask company representatives what materials are available. Many companies provide free videos and booklets.

▶ Disasters and Pandemics
LO 57.9

Your skills in dealing with emergencies, including first-aid and CPR training, will be an enormous help to your community in the event of a disaster or pandemic illness. To be fully effective, you also must be familiar with standard protocols for responding to disasters and pandemic illness. Table 57-5 shows ways you can help in certain types of disasters. You may even want to participate in fire or other disaster drills to familiarize yourself with emergency procedures.

Evacuation and Shelter-in-Place Plans

Every office should have evacuation and shelter-in-place plans in the event of an emergency. "Shelter-in-place" refers to an interior room or rooms within your medical facility with few or no windows and is a place to take refuge. Plans should include means of communication for employees during and after the emergency. Maps of the facility with escape routes clearly marked should be posted. These plans should be in writing and there should be periodic practice drills. Employees should be trained in shelter-in-place procedures and their roles in implementing them. If a shelter-in-place option is a part of your emergency plan, be sure to implement a means of alerting your employees to shelter-in-place that is easy to distinguish from alerts used to signal an evacuation.

Pandemic Illness

A rapidly spreading influenza outbreak can overwhelm your office's resources very quickly. The influenza virus is capable of mutating, creating novel strains. Since the population has never been exposed to a novel influenza strain, no one has immunity to the new strain and the virus can spread quickly throughout the world. You must plan for pandemic illness before it occurs. Your office should have a written plan that includes

- Identification and isolation of patients with potential influenza.
- Communication and reporting.
- Occupational health.
- Education and training of patients and staff.
- Respiratory hygiene.

In the most serious scenario, a worldwide influenza outbreak may last 12 to 24 months. There may be waves of illness that

TABLE 57-5 Assisting in a Disaster

Type of Disaster	Action to Take
Weather disaster, such as a flood or hurricane	• Report to the community command post. • Have your credentials with you. • Receive an identifying tag or vest and assignment. • Accept only an assignment that is appropriate for your abilities. • Expect to be part of a team. • Document what medical care each victim receives on each person's disaster tag.
Office fire	• Activate the alarm system. • Use a fire extinguisher if the fire is confined to a small container, like a trash can. • Turn off oxygen. • Shut windows and doors. • Seal doors with wet cloths to prevent smoke from entering. • If evacuation is necessary, proceed quietly and calmly. Direct ambulatory patients and family members to the appropriate exit route. Assist patients who need help leaving the building.
Bioterrorist attack	• Be alert for rapidly increasing incidence of disease in a healthy population (clusters). • Take appropriate isolation precautions. • Use Standard Precautions when cleaning/decontaminating patient rooms and equipment. • Inform local health departments of suspected bioterrorism agent.
Chemical emergency	• Don appropriate PPE to avoid secondary contamination. • Identify the chemical if possible and report to the local authorities. • Determine if there is a protocol for the specific chemical, if known. • Assist with patient decontamination. • Monitor patient's CABs and vital signs if indicated. • Document what medical care each victim receives. • Arrange for patient transport if possible.
Radiation emergencies	• Assess for contamination (contact with radioisotope released in liquid or power form) or exposure from an external source (for example, from a nuclear power plant accident). • If victim is contaminated, use PPE appropriate for radiation protection, assess for amount of contamination, and decontaminate victim following approved decontamination procedures. • If victim is exposed, look for signs of acute radiation syndrome (ARS) and assist physician in management of multisystem ARS symptoms.
Mass casualties	• Assess the situation for safety. • If there is an explosion, do not go toward the explosion. • Report to the community command post. • Triage victims as necessary. • Render first aid as required. • Document what medical care each victim receives.

come and go every 6 to 8 weeks. Vaccines may be unavailable at first and antivirals will likely be in short supply. To reduce confusion, essential personnel and their roles should be clearly defined. The practice's plan should be flexible, as it is likely the situation will rapidly change. Having a flexible plan will more easily accommodate an evolving pandemic. For more information, see the Caution: Handle with Care feature.

▶ Bioterrorism

LO 57.10

Bioterrorism is the intentional release of a biologic agent with the intent to harm individuals. The Centers for Disease Control and Prevention (CDC) defines a biologic agent as a weapon when it is easy to disseminate, has a high potential for mortality, can cause a public panic or social disruption, and requires public health preparedness. Numerous biologic agents are

CAUTION: HANDLE WITH CARE

Planning and Implementing a Preparedness Plan for Pandemic Illness

Even a normally smooth-running medical office can quickly become a shambles during a significant influenza outbreak. The office will most likely be short staffed due to illness while the population of sick patients increases dramatically. You must be prepared for dealing with a surge of patients, decreasing numbers of staff, and dwindling supplies. The U.S. Department of Health and Human Services recommends developing a plan that includes the following information:

- Communication
  - Identify points of contact (most likely state and local health departments).
  - Assign a point person for external communications to ensure consistent communication.
  - Keep lists of healthcare facilities and their points of contact (hospitals, home healthcare agencies, social services, EMS, laboratories, Red Cross).
- Isolation and containment
  - Use phone triage of patients to determine who should be seen.
  - Cancel nonessential patient appointments.
  - Use block scheduling for flu versus nonflu patient care.
  - Implement respiratory hygiene plan, including
    - Posting cover-your-cough signs;
    - Distributing masks to ill patients; and
    - Providing tissues and hand hygiene products in convenient locations.
  - Establish a vaccine priority list for staff and patients.

- Education and training
  - Designate a person to coordinate training.
  - Impliment infection control training for staff and patients.
  - Provide patient literature regarding home care for ill family members.
- Occupational health policies
  - Develop a nonpunitive sick leave policy.
  - Determine how to handle staff who become ill at work.
  - Determine when staff may return to work after recovering from flu. When symptomatic but well enough to work, staff may return to work.
  - Determine how to deal with staff who need to care for sick family members.
  - Develop a system for evaluating symptomatic staff prior to beginning work.
  - Manage staff at increased risk for flu complications (pregnant or immunocompromised staff).
  - Provide staff's seasonal flu vaccination.
- Surge capacity plan (dealing with resource shortages)
  - Manage staffing shortages.
  - Encourage staff to establish a family care plan.
  - Establish the minimum number of staff necessary to keep the office open.
  - Anticipate consumable resource needs (masks, gloves, hand hygiene products, etc.).
  - Plan for addressing supply shortages.
  - Plan for stockpiling at least a week of supplies at first sign of pandemic illness in the United States.

identified as weapons, including anthrax, tularemia, smallpox, plague, and botulism. The CDC maintains an Internet site with current information about identified biologic agents at www.bt.cdc.gov.

Physicians' offices will be on the front lines should a biologic agent be intentionally released. It will be up to physicians and their staff to sound the alarm to public officials that something may be amiss. Physicians and medical assistants should be vigilant about cases that present themselves as well as common trends in syndromes. Be on the lookout for unusual patterns in affected patients. Indications of a bioterrorist attack might include many patients having been in the same place at the same time or an unusual distribution for common illnesses, such as an increase in chicken-pox-like illness in adults that might be smallpox.

If you suspect bioterrorism is responsible for an illness, report your suspicions to the physician. It is the responsibility of your facility to immediately contact the local public health department. The information about the patient should

be recorded and appropriate tests should be performed. The laboratory should be notified of the potential for bioterrorism. Additionally, consultations with specialists and discussions of all findings are necessary when bioterrorism is suspected. The following is a list of clues of a bioterroristic attack as defined by the American College of Physicians—American Society of Internal Medicine:

- Unusual temporal or geographic clustering of illness.
- Unusual age distribution of common disease, such as an illness that appears to be chicken pox in adults but is really smallpox.
- A large epidemic with greater caseloads than expected, especially in a discrete population.
- More severe disease than expected.
- Unusual route of exposure.
- A disease that is outside its normal transmission season or is impossible to transmit naturally in the absence of its normal vector.

- Multiple simultaneous epidemics of different diseases.
- A disease outbreak with health consequences to humans and animals.
- Unusual strains or variants of organisms or antimicrobial resistance patterns.

In any disaster, you may be asked to perform triage. When you perform triage, you give each injured victim a tag that classifies the person as emergent (needing immediate care), urgent (needing care within several hours), nonurgent (needing care when time is not critical), or dead. The triage process is outlined in Procedure 57-8, at the end of this chapter.

PROCEDURE 57-1 Stocking the Crash Cart

Procedure Goal: To ensure that the crash cart includes all appropriate drugs, supplies, and equipment needed for emergencies.

OSHA Guidelines: This procedure does not involve exposure to blood, body fluids, or tissues.

Materials: Protocol for or list of crash cart items, and crash cart.

Method: Procedure steps.

1. Review the office protocol for or list of items that should be on the crash cart.

2. Verify each drug on the crash cart and check the amount against the office protocol or list. Restock those that were used and replace those that have passed their expiration date.
   RATIONALE: Drugs on the crash cart should be available in quantities sufficient for use during an emergency. An out-of-date drug is of no use in an emergency.
   Some typical crash cart drugs are listed here:
   - Activated charcoal
   - Adenosine
   - Atropine
   - Calcium
   - Dexamethasone
   - Dextrose 50%
   - Diazepam (Valium)
   - Digoxin (Lanoxin)
   - Diphenhydramine hydrochloride (Benadryl)
   - Epinephrine, injectable
   - Furosemide (Lasix)
   - Glucagon
   - Glucose paste or tablets
   - Insulin (regular or a variety)
   - Intravenous dextrose in saline and intravenous dextrose in water
   - Isoproterenol hydrochloride (Isuprel), aerosol inhaler and injectable
   - Lactated Ringer's solution
   - Lidocaine (Xylocaine), injectable
   - Methylprednisolone tablets

   - Narcan
   - Nitroglycerin tablets
   - Phenobarbital, injectable
   - Phenytoin (Dilantin)
   - Saline solution, isotonic (0.9%)
   - Sodium bicarbonate, injectable
   - Sterile water for injection

3. Check the supplies on the crash cart against the list. Restock items that were used and make sure the packaging of supplies on the cart has not been opened.
   RATIONALE: Items on the cart must be available and ready for use at the time of an emergency.
   Some typical crash cart supplies are listed here:
   - Adhesive tape
   - Constricting band or tourniquet
   - Dressing supplies (alcohol wipes, rolls of gauze, bandage strips, bandage scissors)
   - Intravenous tubing, venipuncture devices, and butterfly needles
   - Personal protective equipment
   - Syringes and needles in various sizes

4. Check the equipment on the crash cart against the list and examine it to make sure it is in working order. Restock missing or broken equipment.
   RATIONALE: There is no time during an emergency to make sure equipment works.
   Some typical crash cart equipment is listed here:
   - Airways in assorted sizes
   - Ambu-bag, a trademark for a breathing bag used to assist respiratory ventilation
   - Automated external defibrillator (electrical device that shocks the heart to restore normal beating)
   - Endotracheal tubes in various sizes
   - Oxygen tank with oxygen mask and cannula

5. Check miscellaneous items on the crash cart against the list and restock as needed. Some typical miscellaneous crash cart items are listed here:
   - Orange juice
   - Sugar packets

PROCEDURE 57-2 Performing an Emergency Assessment

Procedure Goal: To assess a medical emergency quickly and accurately.

OSHA Guidelines:

Materials: Patient's chart, pen, gloves, and other PPE appropriate to the situation.

Method: Procedure steps.

1. Put on gloves.

2. Form a general impression of the patient, including his level of responsiveness, level of distress, facial expressions, age, ability to talk, and skin color.

3. If the patient can communicate clearly, ask what happened. If not, ask someone who observed the accident or injury.

4. Assess an unresponsive patient by tapping on his shoulder and asking, "Are you OK?" If there is no response, proceed to the next step.
   RATIONALE: You must know if a patient is unresponsive before proceeding. The patient's responsiveness will determine if you need to assess his circulation, airway, and breathing.

5. Assess the patient's circulation, airway, and breathing. Perform CPR as needed.

6. Is there any serious external bleeding? Control any significant bleeding.

7. If all life-threatening problems have been identified and treated, perform a focused exam. Start at the head and perform the following steps rapidly, taking about 90 seconds.

   a. Head: Check for deformities, bruises, open wounds, tenderness, depressions, and swelling. Check the ears, nose, and mouth for fluid, blood, or foreign bodies.

   b. Eyes: Open the eyes and compare the pupils. They should be the same size.

   c. Neck: Look and feel for deformities, bruises, depressions, open wounds, tenderness, and swelling. Check for a medical alert bracelet or necklace.

   d. Chest: Look and feel for deformities, bruises, open wounds, tenderness, depressions, and swelling.

   e. Abdomen: Look and feel for deformities, bruises, open wounds, tenderness, depressions, and swelling.

   f. Pelvis: Look and feel for deformities, bruises, open wounds, tenderness, depressions, and swelling.

   g. Arms: Look and feel for deformities, bruises, open wounds, depressions, tenderness, and swelling. Compare the arms for any differences in size, color, or temperature.

   h. Legs: Look and feel for deformities, bruises, open wounds, depressions, tenderness, and swelling. Compare the legs for any differences in size, color, or temperature.

   i. Back: Look and feel for deformities, bruises, open wounds, depressions, tenderness, and swelling. Feel under the patient for pools of blood.
   RATIONALE: Pools of blood indicate rapid hemorrhage.

8. Check vital signs and observe the patient for pallor (paleness) or cyanosis (a bluish tint). If the patient is dark-skinned, observe for pallor or cyanosis on the inside of the lips and mouth.
   RATIONALE: A patient's status may change quickly. Checking vital signs often will alert you to any changes in the patient's condition.

9. Document your findings and report them to the doctor or emergency medical technician (EMT).

10. Assist the doctor or EMT as requested.

11. Dispose of biohazardous waste according to OSHA guidelines.

12. Remove your gloves and wash your hands.

PROCEDURE 57-3 Foreign Body Airway Obstruction in a Responsive Adult or Child

Procedure Goal: To correctly relieve a foreign body from the airway of an adult or child.

OSHA Guidelines: This procedure does not involve exposure to blood, body fluids, or tissues.

Materials: Choking adult or child patient. *Caution: Never perform this procedure on someone who is not choking.*

Method: Procedure steps.

1. Ask, "Are you choking?" If the answer is "Yes," indicated by a nod of the head or some other sign, tell the patient you can help.

   A choking person cannot speak, cough, or breathe and exhibits the universal sign of choking. If the patient is coughing, observe him closely to see if he clears the object. If he is not coughing or stops coughing, use abdominal thrusts.

2. Position yourself behind the patient. Place your fist against the abdomen just above the navel and below the xiphoid process.

3. Grasp your fist with your other hand and provide quick inward and upward thrusts into the patient's abdomen.

FIGURE Procedure 57-3 Step 3 Perform abdominal thrusts on a conscious choking victim.

RATIONALE: The thrust should be sufficient to move enough air from the lungs so the object can be displaced from the airway.

Note: If a pregnant or obese person is choking, you will need to place your arms around the chest and perform thrusts over the center of the breastbone.

FIGURE Procedure 57-3 Step 3 Use a chest thrust for a choking victim who is pregnant or obese.

4. Continue the thrusts until the object is expelled or the patient becomes unresponsive.

5. If the patient becomes unresponsive, call EMS and position the patient on his back and begin chest compressions without a pulse check.
RATIONALE: A patient who becomes unresponsive is most likely not getting the necessary amount of oxygen to the brain.

6. Use the head tilt–chin lift to open the patient's airway.

7. Look into the mouth. If you see the foreign body, remove it using your index finger. **Do not perform any blind finger sweeps.**

FIGURE Procedure 57-3 Step 7 If you see the foreign body, use your index finger to remove it from the mouth. Do not perform a blind finger sweep.

8. Open the airway. If the patient is not breathing, attempt a rescue breath. Observe the chest. If it does not rise with the breath, reposition the airway and administer another rescue breath. If the chest does not rise after the second attempt, assume the airway is still blocked and continue CPR.

PROCEDURE 57-4 Foreign Body Airway Obstruction in a Responsive Infant

Procedure Goal: To correctly relieve a foreign body from the airway of an infant.

OSHA Guidelines: This procedure does not involve exposure to blood, body fluids, or tissues.

Materials: Choking infant. *Caution: Never perform this procedure on an infant who is not choking.*

Method: Procedure steps.

1. Assess the infant for signs of severe or complete airway obstruction, which include
   a. Sudden onset of difficulty in breathing.
   b. Inability to speak, make sounds, or cry.
   c. A high-pitched, noisy, wheezing sound or no sounds while inhaling.
   d. Weak, ineffective coughs.
   e. Blue lips or skin.
2. Hold the infant with his head down, supporting the body with your forearm. His legs should straddle your forearm and you should support his jaw and head with your hand and fingers. This is best done in a sitting or kneeling position.

FIGURE Procedure 57-4 Step 4   Perform five chest thrusts.

FIGURE Procedure 57-4 Step 2   Use back blows for a choking infant.

3. Give up to five back blows with the heel of your free hand, as shown in the figure above. Strike the infant's back forcefully between the shoulder blades. At any point, if the object is expelled, discontinue the back blows.
   RATIONALE: Effective back blows may successfully dislodge the object. Having the infant's head down will allow the object to fall out.
4. If the obstruction is not cleared, turn the infant over as a unit, supporting the head with your hands and the body between your forearms.

5. Keep the head lower than the chest and perform five chest thrusts.
   RATIONALE: Chest thrusts will force air out of the lungs, helping dislodge the object.
   Place two fingers over the breastbone (sternum), above the xiphoid. Give five quick chest thrusts about ½ to 1 inch deep. Stop the compressions if the object is expelled.
6. Alternate five back blows and five chest thrusts until the object is expelled or until the infant becomes unconscious. If the infant becomes unconscious, call EMS or have someone do it for you.
7. Open the infant's mouth by grasping both the tongue and the lower jaw between the thumb and fingers, and pull up the lower jawbone. *If you see the object, remove it using your smallest finger.* **Do not use blind finger sweeps on an infant.**
   RATIONALE: A blind finger sweep may push the object deeper into the airway.
8. Open the airway and attempt to provide rescue breaths. If the chest does not rise, reposition the airway (both head and chin) and try to provide another rescue breath.
9. If the rescue breaths are unsuccessful, begin CPR.
10. Open the infant's mouth and look for the foreign object. If you see an object, remove it with your smallest finger.
11. Open the airway and attempt to provide rescue breaths. If the chest does not rise, continue CPR until the doctor or EMS arrives.

PROCEDURE 57-5 Controlling Bleeding

Procedure Goal: To control bleeding and minimize blood loss.

OSHA Guidelines:

Materials: Clean or sterile dressings.

Method: Procedure steps.

1. If you have time, wash your hands and don exam gloves, face protection, and a gown.
   RATIONALE: To protect yourself from splatters, splashes, and sprays.

2. Using a clean or sterile dressing, apply direct pressure over the wound.

3. If blood soaks through the dressing, do not remove it. Apply an additional dressing over the original one.
   RATIONALE: Removing the dressing may dislodge a clot and cause more bleeding.

4. If possible, elevate the bleeding body part.

5. If direct pressure and elevation do not stop the bleeding, apply pressure over the nearest pressure point between the bleeding and the heart. For example, if the wound is on the lower arm, apply pressure on the brachial artery. For a lower-leg wound, apply pressure on the femoral artery in the groin.

6. When the doctor or EMT arrives, assist as requested.

7. After the patient has been transferred to a hospital, properly dispose of contaminated materials.

8. Remove the gloves and wash your hands.

9. Document your care in the patient's chart.

FIGURE Procedure 57-5 Step 5   Apply pressure on these pressure points to stop bleeding.

PROCEDURE 57-6 Cleaning Minor Wounds

Procedure Goal: To clean and dress minor wounds.

OSHA Guidelines:

Materials: Sterile gauze squares, basin, antiseptic soap, warm water, and sterile dressing.

Method: Procedure steps.

1. Wash your hands and don exam gloves.
2. Dip several gauze squares in a basin of warm, soapy water.
3. Wash the wound from the center outward, using a new gauze square for each cleansing motion.
   RATIONALE: To avoid bringing contaminants from the surrounding skin into the wound.
4. As you wash, remove debris that could cause infection.

FIGURE Procedure 57-6 Step 4 Using a pair of forceps, carefully remove any large debris that could cause infection.

5. Rinse the area thoroughly, preferably by placing the wound under warm, running water.
   RATIONALE: Running water will wash away debris.

FIGURE Procedure 57-6 Step 5 Rinsing the area with water or sterile saline washes debris from the wound.

6. Pat the wound dry with sterile gauze squares.
7. Cover the wound with a dry, sterile dressing. Bandage the dressing in place.
8. Properly dispose of contaminated materials and decontaminate surfaces potentially exposed to blood or body fluid.
9. Remove the gloves and wash your hands.
10. Instruct the patient on wound care.
11. Record the procedure in the patient's chart.

PROCEDURE 57-7 Caring for a Patient Who Is Vomiting

Procedure Goal: To increase comfort and minimize complications, such as aspiration, for a patient who is vomiting.

OSHA Guidelines:

Materials: Emesis basin, cool compress, cup of cool water, paper tissues or a towel, and (if ordered) intravenous fluids, electrolytes, and an antinausea drug.

Method: Procedure steps.

1. Wash your hands and don exam gloves and other PPE.
2. Ask the patient when and how the vomiting started and how frequently it occurs. Find out whether she is nauseated or in pain.
3. Give the patient an emesis basin to collect vomit. Observe and document its amount, color, odor, and consistency.

Particularly note blood, bile, undigested food, or feces in the vomit.

4. Place a cool compress on the patient's forehead to make her more comfortable. Offer water and paper tissues or a towel to clean her mouth.
5. Monitor for signs of dehydration, like confusion, irritability, and flushed, dry skin. Also monitor for signs of electrolyte imbalances, like leg cramps or an irregular pulse.
6. If requested, assist by laying out supplies and equipment for the physician to use in administering intravenous fluids and electrolytes. Administer an antinausea drug if prescribed.
   RATIONALE: To replace fluids and electrolytes if the patient becomes dehydrated.
7. Prepare the patient for diagnostic tests if instructed.
8. Remove the gloves and wash your hands.

PROCEDURE 57-8 Performing Triage in a Disaster

Procedure Goal: To prioritize disaster victims.

OSHA Guidelines:

Materials: Disaster tag and a pen.

Method: Procedure steps.

1. Wash your hands and don exam gloves and other PPE if available.
2. Quickly assess each victim.
3. Sort victims by type of injury and need for care, classifying them as emergent, urgent, nonurgent, or dead.
   RATIONALE: Sorting the victims allows for rapid treatment based on need.

4. Label the emergent patients no. 1 and send them to appropriate treatment stations immediately. Emergent patients, such as those who are in shock or who are hemorrhaging, need immediate care.
5. Label the urgent patients no. 2 and send them to basic first-aid stations. Urgent patients need care within the next several hours. Such patients may have lacerations that can be dressed quickly to stop the bleeding but can wait for suturing.
6. Label nonurgent patients no. 3 and send them to volunteers who will be empathic and provide refreshments. Nonurgent patients are those for whom timing of treatment is not critical, like patients who have no physical injuries but are emotionally upset.
7. Label patients who are dead no. 4. Ensure that the bodies are moved to an area where they will be safe until they can be identified and proper action can be taken.

SUMMARY OF LEARNING OUTCOMES

LEARNING OUTCOMES	KEY POINTS
57.1 **Discuss the importance of first aid during a medical emergency.**	Prompt and appropriate first aid can save a life, reduce pain, prevent further injury, reduce the risk of permanent disability, and increase the chance of early recovery.
57.2 **Identify items found on a crash cart.**	The crash cart should include all appropriate drugs, supplies, and equipment needed for emergencies. These include but are not limited to activated charcoal, atropine, dextrose 50%, epinephrine, lactated Ringer's solution, nitroglycerin tablets, and sodium bicarbonate.
57.3 **Recognize various accidental emergencies and how to deal with them.**	Accidental injuries you may encounter include bites and stings; burns; choking; ear trauma; eye trauma; falls; fractures, dislocations, sprains, and strains; head injuries; hemorrhaging; multiple injuries; poisoning; weather-related injuries; and wounds.
57.4 **List common illnesses that can result in medical emergencies.**	Common illnesses that may cause a medical emergency include abdominal pain, asthma, dehydration, diarrhea, fainting, fever, hyperventilation, nosebleed, tachycardia, and vomiting.
57.5 **Identify less common illnesses that can result in medical emergencies.**	Less common illnesses you may encounter in a medical office include anaphylaxis, bacterial meningitis, diabetic emergencies, gallbladder attack, myocardial infarction, hematemesis, obstetric emergencies, respiratory arrest, seizures, shock, stroke, toxic shock syndrome, and viral encephalitis.
57.6 **Discuss your role in caring for people with psychosocial emergencies.**	Psychosocial emergencies in the medical office include drug or alcohol abuse, spousal abuse, child abuse, elder abuse, and rape. As a medical assistant, you may be involved in the direct care of someone suffering a psychosocial emergency or you may arrange for his or her care at an outside agency.

LEARNING OUTCOMES	KEY POINTS
57.7 Carry out the procedure for calming a patient who is under extreme stress.	A medical assistant can help calm a patient under stress by listening carefully and giving her or his full attention.
57.8 Discuss ways to educate patients about how to prevent and respond to emergencies.	Medical assistants should educate patients about ways to prevent and handle various medical emergencies by providing brief, easy-to-read handouts containing local emergency contact numbers and a first-aid kit checklist. The handouts should be prepared in multiple languages if the practice provides care for non-English-speaking patients.
57.9 Illustrate your role in responding to natural disasters and pandemic illness.	During a disaster, a medical assistant's first-aid and CPR training will be of enormous help. A medical assistant also must be familiar with standard protocols for responding to disasters and pandemic illness.
57.10 Discuss your role in responding to acts of bioterrorism.	Physicians' offices will be on the front lines if a biologic agent is intentionally released as an act of terror. You should be aware of unusual patterns of disease in patients being seen at your office. Indications of a bioterrorist attack might include many patients having been in the same place at the same time or an unusual distribution for common illnesses, like an increase in chicken-pox-like illness in adults that might be smallpox.

CASE STUDY CRITICAL THINKING

Recall Mohammad Nassar from the beginning of the chapter. Now that you have completed the chapter, answer the following questions regarding his case.

1. What action should you take to keep Mohammad from exposing the other patients in the reception area?

2. What precautions should his mother take?

3. Mohammad tells you he feels like he is going to vomit. How should you care for Mohammad?

4. Dr. Williams tells you the office needs to implement the preparedness plan for pandemic illness. What steps should you take?

EXAM PREPARATION QUESTIONS

1. (LO 57.3) What is the first action you should take when administering first aid for an animal bite?
   a. Check to see if the animal has had a rabies vaccination
   b. Clean the wound with soap and water
   c. Call animal control
   d. Administer tetanus toxoid
   e. Put antibiotic ointment on the wound

2. (LO 57.3) A displacement of a bone end from the joint is a
   a. Fracture
   b. Sprain
   c. Dislocation
   d. Impaction
   e. Greenstick

3. (LO 57.3) Which of the following is a jarring injury to the brain?
   a. Concussion
   b. Stroke
   c. Seizure
   d. TIA
   e. Aneurysm

4. (LO 57.3) When should you apply a tourniquet to a wound?
   a. To save the limb
   b. If medical help is less than an hour away
   c. Only if the patient is alert
   d. As a last resort, if bleeding cannot be stopped
   e. Before putting pressure on a wound

5. (LO 57.5) Severe hypoglycemia is known as
   a. Insulin shock
   b. Diabetic coma
   c. High blood sugar
   d. Diabetes mellitus
   e. Diabetes insipidus

6. (LO 57.4) The medical term for fainting is
   a. Hypoglycemia
   b. Epistaxis
   c. Shock
   d. Stroke
   e. Syncope

7. (LO 57.5) A severe, often life-threatening allergic reaction is known as
   a. Anaphylaxis
   b. Bee sting
   c. Hives
   d. Toxic shock syndrome
   e. CVA

8. (LO 57.10) The intentional release of a biologic agent with the intent to harm individuals is known as
   a. Pandemic illness
   b. Natural disaster
   c. Mass casualties
   d. Bioterrorism
   e. Radiation contamination

9. (LO 57.6) Drug abuse, attempted suicide, rape, child abuse, and alcohol abuse are examples of
   a. Common illnesses
   b. Psychosocial emergencies
   c. Stress-related diseases
   d. Psychiatric diseases
   e. Medical emergencies

10. (LO 57.3) An injury characterized by partial tearing of a ligament that supports a joint is a
    a. Fracture
    b. Strain
    c. Dislocation
    d. Splint
    e. Sprain

Preparing for the World of Work

CHAPTER 58

CASE STUDY

Employee Name	Gender	DOB
Reagan Patrick	Female	09/07/XX

Position	Credentials	Supervisor
Student	In Training	Malik Katahri, CMM

EMPLOYEE INFORMATION

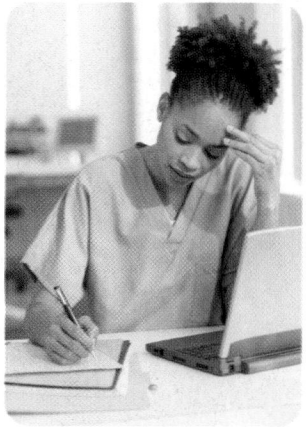

Reagan Patrick, a 25-year-old-female, is just finishing her applied training and is beginning her job search. Her applied training included venipuncture, ECG, urinalysis, assisting with exams and procedures, patient reception, insurance claim form completion, patient scheduling, and many other clinical and administrative skills. She lives in a small town but is willing to relocate. She is excited about her new career in healthcare because it is so different from working at the bank.

Keep Reagan in mind as you study this chapter. There will be questions at the end of the chapter based on the case study. The information in the chapter will help you answer these questions.

LEARNING OUTCOMES

After completing Chapter 58, you will be able to:

58.1 Carry out professionalism in all applied training scenarios.
58.2 Summarize the necessary steps for obtaining professional certification.
58.3 Describe an appropriate strategy for finding a position.
58.4 Explain key factors for a successful interview.
58.5 Describe ways of becoming a successful employee.

KEY TERMS

affiliation agreement
applied training
applied training coordinator
chronological résumé
constructive criticism
functional résumé
networking
portfolio
professional objective
reference
targeted résumé

IV. A (6) Demonstrate awareness of how an individual's personal appearance affects anticipated responses

IX. P (4) Practice within the standard of care for a medical assistant

1. General Orientation

Students will:

c. Understand medical assistant credentialing requirements and the process to obtain the credential; comprehend the importance of credentialing

d. Have knowledge of the general responsibilities of the medical assistant

e. Define scope of practice for the medical assistant, and comprehend the conditions for practice within the state that the medical assistant is employed

11. Career Development

Graduates:

a. Perform the essential requirements for employment, such as résumé writing, effective interviewing, dressing professionally, and following up appropriately

b. Demonstrate professionalism by:

(1) Exhibiting dependability, punctuality, and a positive work ethic

(2) Exhibiting a positive attitude and a sense of responsibility

(3) Maintaining confidentiality at all times

(4) Being cognizant of ethical boundaries

(5) Exhibiting initiative

(6) Adapting to change

(7) Expressing a responsible attitude

(8) Being courteous and diplomatic

(9) Conducting work within scope of education, training, and ability

▶ Introduction

After completing a medical assisting program, you may be both excited and apprehensive about beginning your new career. Such a reaction is perfectly normal. In this chapter, you will learn how to maximize your applied training experience and gain the hands-on experience you need for securing a position in medical assisting. Your applied training is an opportunity for you to explore the different responsibilities required of a medical assistant. After completing this chapter, you will understand the process for becoming a nationally certified medical assistant. You also will know how to effectively begin searching for a position in medical assisting—which includes completing a résumé, cover letter, and thank-you letter—and how to form a strategic plan to secure this position. And, as you explore this chapter, you will gain valuable interviewing techniques for successfully competing in the modern healthcare world.

▶ Training in Action   LO 58.1

An **applied training** experience is an opportunity to work within a medical facility to gain the essential on-the-job experience for beginning your new career. Some schools call this training an externship, while others call it a practicum. Whether it is called an externship or a practicum, it is an opportunity to apply—in an actual medical environment—the knowledge and skills that you have learned.

Most applied training is measured by hours attended, usually a minimum of 160 hours. Applied training is a mandatory requirement of fulfilling a medical assisting program in educational institutions that are accredited by the Accrediting Bureau of Health Education Schools (ABHES) and the Commission on Accreditation of Allied Health Education Programs (CAAHEP). Some of the applied training is completed after the didactic or academic portion of the curriculum (for example, during the last module or semester) and some is completed during the last semester. Medical assisting applied training may be performed at physician offices, laboratories, hospitals, administrative billing offices, and clinics.

The Applied Training Process

To make the applied training process possible, the educational institution where the medical assisting student is enrolled partners with local medical facilities throughout the area. Most schools have an **applied training coordinator** who is familiar with medical assisting and the medical community. The applied training coordinator procures applied training sites and qualifies or assesses them to make certain that they provide a thorough educational experience. A checklist is often designed to ensure that students are given a well-rounded, safe experience (Figure 58-1). Although student applied training experiences are unpaid, the student should be positive about the experience and appreciate the opportunity to train with the facility.

Applied Training Requirements Applied training sites are required to review and sign an **affiliation agreement.**

The affiliation agreement states the expectations of the facility and the expectations of the student. Some examples of the expectations of the applied training site include

- Providing reasonable opportunities for clinical instruction by qualified facility personnel for students participating in the program.
- Supervising students in a manner that will provide safe practice and meaningful clinical education.

In addition, the expectations of the educational institution may include

- Reinforcing patient confidentiality by having the student sign a statement of confidentiality.
- Providing professional liability insurance for the student, the educational institution, and the faculty.
- Ensuring that the student is medically able to perform the assigned duties of the applied training facility by providing proof of immunizations and health physicals.

CLINICAL SITE ASSESSMENT

Name of Site _____

Address _____

Specialty _____ Supervisor _____

Telephone # _____ Fax # _____

Number of Staff _____

Administrative/Clinical experience available to students
(check all that apply)

_____ Front office skills

_____ Word processing skills

_____ Measure/Record vital signs

_____ Blood drawing (venipuncture, fingersticks)

_____ Injections

_____ Electrocardiograms

_____ Specimen collection/diagnostic procedures
(urinalysis, blood sugar, cholesterol, etc.)

_____ Assisting with minor surgical procedures

I have determined that this site meets the need of the students in the medical assisting program.

Print name of evaluator _____

Signature of evaluator _____ Date _____

FIGURE 58-1 A form such as this clinical site assessment is often used by the applied training coordinator to help determine if a clinical site will be appropriate for medical assisting applied training.

The applied training coordinator is the liaison between the applied training site and the educational institution.

Screening The applied training coordinator places students in applied training clinical sites. It is not uncommon for the clinical site to screen students prior to their applied training. This screening can include

- Interviewing students prior to their applied training.
- Asking students to provide a urine or hair sample for drug screening prior to the applied training.
- Asking students to consent to a criminal background check prior to beginning their applied training. Some medical

facilities check only for felony convictions, and others check for misdemeanors and felonies. Honesty is the best policy for criminal background checks. Some institutions will waive some convictions as long as the student is honest and truthful about the conviction early in the process.

Time Sheets Students receive time sheets to be completed on a daily basis and faxed to the educational facility at the end of every week. The clinical preceptor and the student both sign the time sheet (Figure 58-2). Weekly telephone calls and site visits may be performed by the clinical coordinator or a medical assisting instructor for each student. Some schools

Clinical Training Time Sheet
Medical Assistant Program

Instructions:

Students are expected to attend their clinical site for a minimum of 32 hours per week, and will not receive credit for more than ten hours per day. **For shifts greater than four hours, you must include a thirty-minute meal break.**

_____ Complete the log daily and fax the log each week to the school no later than 5 p.m. Friday.

_____ For each day attended, please include a brief description of the duties performed.

_____ The time sheet must be signed and dated by both the student and the Clinical Site Supervisor.

Student Information

Name: _____

Program: _____

Home Phone: _____

Alt. Phone: _____

Clinical Site Information

Name: _____

Phone: _____

Rotation: _____

Assignment Dates: _____

Site Supervisor's Name: _____

	Date	Time In	Time Out	Total Hours	General Duties Performed*
Monday					
Tuesday					
Wednesday					
Thursday					
Friday					
Saturday					
TOTAL HOURS					

*Examples of General Duties include: Billing, Vital Signs, Lab Work, Filing, Charting, etc.

Student Signature: _____

Date: _____

Supervisor: _____

Supervisor Signature: _____

Date: _____

FIGURE 58-2 Students participating in applied training complete a weekly time sheet.

STUDENT WEEKLY PROGRESS REPORT

This form needs to be completed and signed each week. It must be faxed with the time sheet on Friday afternoon. It is designed to help you maximize your clinical training experience. Having recognizable goals is the surest way to succeed!

Name: _____ Date: _____

Class Code: _____

Clinical Site: _____

Supervisor Signature: _____

Student Signature: _____

I.   Goals for next week:
        1. _____
        2. _____
        3. _____

II.   Personal assessment of progress this week:
        _____
        _____
        _____

III.   Supervisor's assessment of progress this week:
        _____
        _____
        _____

IV.   Identify one task/item/event you are most proud of that occurred this week:
        _____
        _____

V.   Did you meet your goals for this week? Why or why not?
        _____
        _____

FIGURE 58-3 A weekly progress report is a helpful way for students to track their applied training goals and achievements.

require weekly progress reports from each student, outlining the procedures and duties the student performed during the week. Figure 58-3 provides an example of this report. When students finish their applied training, the preceptors will complete a final evaluation and the students will be graded on their applied training performance.

Expectations of Applied Training Candidates

While in an applied training program, you are expected to be and look professional, report to the applied training site as scheduled, and display initiative and a willingness to learn.

Professionalism You are expected to conduct yourself in a professional manner at all times while attending your applied training. During this experience, you may often feel that you are being criticized by the site preceptor, but this is a normal part of learning, called **constructive criticism.** Constructive criticism is aimed at giving you feedback about your performance in order to improve that performance. You are not expected to know everything during your applied training, but you are expected to be open to suggestions and ideas.

Asking questions during your applied training is expected, but you should not question why a procedure is done a certain way or why you are asked to do something. Do not argue with preceptors about their skills, and know that you may be exposed to some procedures that are not performed exactly as you were taught. After all, there is usually more than one way to get the desired result in patient care. Everything you do during your applied training is a learning experience and should be treated as such.

Your behavior at your applied training site is expected to be as professional as if you were an employee there. Foul language and inappropriate conversation are not tolerated in any workplace. You are expected to be professional with the patients under all circumstances. Medical facilities expect you to demonstrate empathy and compassion to every patient. Proper verbal skills and grammar are expected at all times. Do not use slang when communicating with office staff and patients.

Personal phone calls should not be made or accepted during working hours. Turn off your cell phone while at work and do not use the facility phone for personal calls. Park your car in the designated employee parking area, not in places reserved for patients. Many patients are older and have difficulty walking long distances. It is a professional courtesy and good customer practice to allow the patients to use the parking spots closest to the entrances.

Attendance You are expected to report to your applied training *every day* that you are assigned to a schedule. It is your responsibility to have several alternatives for babysitting and transportation. Employers are seeking dependable and punctual medical staff and do not tolerate attendance problems with their own staff, nor do they expect it from their applied training students. Chronic attendance and punctuality issues can be grounds for termination of your applied training. In the event of an emergency, you are expected to call the medical facility and the school 2 hours before the beginning of your shift, as would any other employee.

As a medical assisting student doing your applied training, also be sure to adhere to the facility's policy regarding breaks. Take breaks only when it is appropriate to do so. If you smoke, refrain from smoking during work hours, smoking only in designated areas if allowed. Many medical facilities are now considered no-smoking zones and smoking is prohibited on the grounds. Lunch breaks are permitted under facility policies. Be sure to adhere to break and lunch time frames, returning back to work on time.

Professional Appearance Medical facilities expect you to appear as a medical professional. Most facilities require a uniform that consists of a scrub top and bottom and a lab jacket. Your scrubs should be clean, pressed, and well-fitting. Shoes should be clean, white, and in good repair. Your name tag or badge should always be worn and visible to patients. Nails should be trimmed and clean. Many medical facilities will not accept students with artificial nails, like acrylics. Facial and tongue piercings are not acceptable when working with patients and visible tattoos must be covered. Your hair should be a natural color and pulled back from your face and off your collar. Makeup should be conservative and in good taste. Perfumes, colognes, scented shampoos, hair gels, and hairsprays should not be used because patients with respiratory conditions or allergies may not be able to tolerate them.

Remember that as a medical assisting student conducting your applied training, you represent several things:

- The school you attend. It is important to maintain a good reputation in the medical community. You will depend on the school's reputation to obtain a job.
- The profession of medical assisting. Participating in a medical assisting applied training program gives you an opportunity to represent the profession of medical assisting to patients and the community.
- Yourself. First impressions are lasting impressions. Make your first impression to the medical community an outstanding one. Even if you are not offered a position here, or if the site is not one where you would like a permanent position, the office will be able to give you your first professional reference and may be key to your obtaining your first position as a medical assistant.

Initiative and Willingness to Learn During your applied training, accept all assignments with enthusiasm and grace, no matter how mundane. These tasks are often a test of how well you accept assignments and work within a medical team. Ask for additional work if you are idle and look for tasks that need to be done. Keep a notebook and record the office policies and procedures. Be prepared to observe and participate in all office policies and procedures.

Make a Good Impression Often, a shy and passive medical assisting student in applied training will appear to the preceptor and facility as unmotivated or lacking initiative. It is important to be assertive and confident when working in healthcare. Remember: Every day on your applied training is "show time"! You may have to step out of your comfort zone to make a good impression.

▶ Obtaining Professional Certification

LO 58.2

Once you complete your education, you may be eligible to take a national certification exam. Some employers require—and many prefer—a medical assistant who is certified. Holding a medical assisting credential can make you more desirable in a competitive job market and enhance the possibilities of career advancement once you are hired. There are two major credentialing agencies: the American Association of Medical Assistants (AAMA) and the American Medical Technologists (AMT). The CMA (AAMA) exam is offered by the Certifying Board of the AAMA and the RMA exam is offered by the AMT. Each of these agencies has its own specific exam eligibility requirements.

Certification Qualifications

In order to sit for a national certification exam, you must meet certain criteria. Both agencies require that you be of good character, including having no felony convictions or guilty pleas to felonies. Other eligibility requirements include

- AAMA—graduation from a CAAHEP- or ABHES-accredited medical assisting program. If you are a student in a program accredited by either of these agencies, you may take the test up to 30 days prior to graduation or within 12 months after graduation.
- AMT—graduation from an ABHES- or CAAHEP-accredited medical assisting program or from a program at a college with regional accreditation and at least 720 clock hours of medical assisting skills training. If you have formal U.S. Armed Forces medical services training, you are also eligible to take the RMA exam. In addition, someone with at least 5 years of experience working as a medical assistant may take the RMA exam.

Applying for the Exam

Once you determine that you are eligible for national certification, you must apply to take the exam. There are required fees for each exam and both require completion of an application form. The steps for applying include

1. Request an application from the appropriate agency.
2. Gather required documents.
3. Review all exam policies and procedures in the examination handbooks.
4. Complete the application and mail or submit it to the appropriate agency.
5. Schedule an exam time.

Be sure to provide all the required information when completing the application. Submitting an incomplete application will delay your taking the exam, which could affect the timing of your job search.

Preparing to Take the Exam

Taking the time to prepare will increase your chances of successfully completing the exam, so never try to take the exam without knowing the following:

- Test format. The CMA (AAMA) exam is a computer-based test. The RMA is either computer-based or paper and pencil.
- Content areas. This gives you general information about the material covered on the test.

General Content Areas When you begin studying for the exam, a good starting point is to know the content covered within the exam. The areas of knowledge you should be familiar with for either exam include general medical, which includes medical terminology, anatomy and physiology, medical ethics and law, and human behavior; administrative; clinical; and laboratory. These general areas are expanded further in the content outlines available from the AAMA or AMT. Use the expanded content outlines as a study guide, making sure you review materials from each specific content area.

Study Tips At first, studying for a national exam can seem like an impossible task. You may feel overwhelmed, with no idea where to start or what to do. Do not panic. Instead, break it down. You cannot study everything at once so you must find a way to make it manageable. If you are served a 12-ounce steak, you would not put the entire steak in your mouth and try to chew it. What would you do? Cut it into pieces. That is exactly what you need to do when studying for the certification exam. Study a piece at a time.

Start by taking a practice exam that covers all the content areas of the real exam. This will give you information about your areas of weakness. Use this information to focus your studies on what you do not know. Students often make the mistake of studying what they do know because it feels good, but this will not help you in the long run. If you study what you do not know, you will ultimately spend less time studying. Once you have studied the content in your areas of weakness, take another practice test. You will most likely score higher on the second practice test. Identify the areas you are still having trouble with

and study the content in those areas. You will soon feel comfortable with the information in all areas.

During your study process, follow these general guidelines:

- Start early; do not wait until a few days before the exam. Cramming does not work.
- Study some every day.
- Create a study schedule and follow it.
- Study in a quiet place free of distractions. Turn off your phone while you are studying; most calls can wait until you are finished.
- Make flash cards with terms, definitions, and concepts.
- Use mnemonic devices to help you remember difficult material. For example, if you are learning the stages of mitosis, in order, remember the first letter of each phase; IPMAT—interphase, prophase, metaphase, anaphase, telophase.

The Day of the Test This is the time to show your knowledge. You have followed your study plan and you are ready. Now, make sure you make the best of all that studying by getting a good start on the day. To prepare for test day:

- Get a good night's sleep the night before the test. Remember, do not cram—it does not work and just tires out your brain.
- Eat a balanced breakfast. Your brain, like your car, needs fuel.
- Take a short walk if you can. Exercise helps your brain as well as your body.
- Make sure you give yourself enough time to get to the testing site and make sure you know exactly where it is. Use a map if necessary.
- Bring all necessary documents to the testing site. Do not forget your photo ID. You will have to identify yourself.
- If you are taking a pencil and paper test, bring more than one pencil with you.
- Tell yourself that you are prepared. Believing in yourself is essential.

▶ Preparing to Find a Position   LO 58.3

The next phase of beginning your new career is seeking a position as a medical assistant. Most accredited schools have a career services department. Its primary focus is job placement after graduation. The department's counselors will assist you in writing your résumé, improving your interviewing skills, and learning about positions in your field. Many employers will contact a school's career services department to recruit medical personnel.

Seeking Employment

In addition to working with a career services department, you can take advantage of a number of other resources in seeking employment within the medical assisting field. These resources include Internet sites, classified ads, employment services, and networking with classmates and others.

Internet Sites and Classified Ads Many prospective employers use employment websites and classified advertisements in area newspapers to alert potential applicants to a career opportunity within their organization. The job listing or advertisement usually describes the position's duties and responsibilities as well as the type of education and experience preferred.

When you are first beginning to seek a medical assisting position, do not become discouraged if you see advertisements asking for a specified amount of experience, such as two years. You must realize that employers place ads seeking an experienced candidate, but many will consider a new graduate because experienced candidates are not always available. Becoming credentialed will help you bridge this experience gap. A local newspaper's classified advertisements and corresponding website are often a good place to start your search. You also might check for a medical practice network website in your area. These often have lists of local medical practices along with job postings for these practices. They may even allow you to submit online job applications.

It is important to explore all the possibilities when seeking employment opportunities. A medical assistant is qualified for a number of positions. For example, new graduates can apply for the following positions:

- Unit secretary in hospitals.
- Phlebotomist in labs.
- Patient care associate or patient care technician in hospitals.
- Entry-level medical coding and billing.
- Customer service representative in medical-related companies.
- Clinical or administrative positions in physician offices and clinics.

The Internet is another useful tool when seeking employment. Internet websites for job seekers are becoming more and more popular, as they often allow job seekers to post résumés online and to respond to advertisements that are posted by employers locally or statewide. Many hospitals and larger companies will not accept paper or faxed résumés; instead, they require all applicants to fill out an electronic application and post résumés on the facility website. Newly graduated medical assistants should post their résumé and cover letter on all local hospital and physician network websites and on local employment websites during their applied training to start circulating their résumés.

Employment Services Employment and temporary agencies provide assistance in locating a specific job. Both types of agencies have a variety of job openings on file. You should call to make an appointment with an employment counselor. Agencies usually require you to fill out an application, take a basic healthcare knowledge test, and provide a résumé. If the agency has positions that match your skills, it contacts the employer. If the service has no appropriate listings, it will place your résumé on file.

Employment services are an excellent way to gain experience and select a position. You are given an opportunity to try out the office or facility with little commitment on your part. Many permanent opportunities can result from a temporary job assignment.

Networking Networking involves making contacts with relatives, friends, and acquaintances that may have information about how to find a job in your field. People in your network may be able to give you job leads or tell you about openings. Word-of-mouth referrals—finding job information by talking with other people—can be very helpful. Other people may be able to introduce you to others who work in, or know people who work in, your field. You also may find opportunities at your applied training site. Although there might not be a position available directly within your site, the practice manager may know someone who is looking for a medical assistant. Networking is a valuable tool. It can advance your career even while you are employed.

Joining a medical assisting organization and attending conferences are the easiest ways to network. Attend an organization's local chapter meetings, like the AAMA county or state chapters, and talk with as many people as possible. Always bring a pen and a notebook. Be prepared to exchange information with other attendees. Remember, networking is an exchange of information—it is not one-sided. What you learn through networking may enable you to provide others with information to help their job search or further their career.

Your classmates are often a good source of networking. It is important to build lasting friendships with your classmates and keep in touch after graduation. Oftentimes, they will know of positions as they gain employment. Networking begins in the classroom.

Creating a Résumé

Your résumé is a vital part of the employment process. It provides potential employers with information about your educational and work history and other aspects of your background.

Components of a Résumé In order to create a well-rounded, informative résumé, you need to include a wide variety of information about your background.

Personal Information Include your name, address, telephone number, cell phone number, and e-mail address. Do not include your marital status or the number of children you have. You should not include your height, weight, interests, or hobbies unless you think they are relevant to the position.

Professional Objective A **professional objective** is a brief, general statement that demonstrates a career goal. An example of an effective, professional objective is the following: "To work as a medical assistant, applying skills in patient relations and laboratory work while gaining increasing responsibility." If you want to list a specific career objective, such as applying your medical assisting skills in a pediatric medical facility, it would be best to mention it in the cover letter and not on your résumé.

Employment Experience List the title of your most recent or last job first, the dates you were employed there, and a brief description of your duties. Choose jobs that have been the most beneficial to your working career. Do not clutter your résumé with needless details or irrelevant jobs. You can elaborate on specific duties in your cover letter and in the interview. Only include jobs you have held for a longer period of time, such as 6 months to a year.

Educational Background In providing your educational history, list your highest degree first, the school attended, the dates, and the major field of study. Include educational experience that may be relevant to the job, like certification, licensing, advanced training, and intensive seminars. Do not list individual classes on your résumé. However, do list skills obtained during your training such as phlebotomy, CPT, and ICD-9 coding skills. If you have taken special classes that relate directly to the job you are seeking, list them in your cover letter.

Awards and Honors List the awards and honors related to your career or that indicate excellence. Perfect attendance, academic honors, and student-of-the-month are excellent traits that employers are seeking. Highlight this information prominently rather than writing it as an afterthought. You can make the most impact by displaying your best qualities at the beginning of this section.

Campus and Community Activities List activities that show leadership abilities and a willingness to contribute. Include any volunteer work that you may have performed.

Professional Memberships and Activities List any career-related professional memberships. Student memberships are available through the American Medical Technologists (AMT) and the American Association of Medical Assistants (AAMA). You can contact the AMT and request a copy of the student by-laws and directions on how to form a student membership in your school. The AAMA provides continuing education through their local chapters and sponsors local meetings periodically throughout the year. Employers like medical professionals who are involved in their disciplines. It demonstrates a commitment and dedication to their chosen field.

Summary of Skills As you learn clinical and administrative skills, be sure to list them on your résumé. Under headings like "Clinical Skills" or "Administrative Skills," list the skills you have acquired in school and during your applied training. Some examples of clinical skills include

- ECG
- Venipuncture
- Urinalysis
- Parenteral injections
- Aseptic technique and bloodborne pathogens
- First aid and bandaging
- CPR
- Triage and vital statistics
- Spirometry

Some examples of administrative work include

- CPT, HCPCS, and ICD-10 coding.
- Insurance claim form completion and reimbursement posting.
- Medisoft billing and reimbursement software (or any software package you have experience with).

- Medical office accounting practices.
- Keyboarding speed.
- Microsoft Office software (list the software programs you are proficient with).

Choosing a Résumé Style Three different résumé styles have been developed, each of which has specific advantages and disadvantages. You will want to choose a style or combination of styles that best describes your strengths and skills.

Functional Résumé A **functional résumé** highlights specialty areas of your accomplishments and strengths. You can organize these in an order that supports your objective. Functional résumés are useful when you change careers, re-enter the job market after an absence, or have had a variety of different, unconnected work experiences. A sample of a functional résumé is shown in Figure 58-4.

Chronological Résumé Individuals who have job experience use a **chronological résumé.** List your most recent job first and end with your first job. Chronological résumés are best when you stay in the same field as your prior jobs and when your employment history shows growth and development. Do not use a chronological résumé if you have gaps in your work history, if you have changed careers, if you have been in the same job for many years, or if you are looking for your first job. Figure 58-5 illustrates a chronological résumé.

Targeted Résumé A **targeted résumé** is best if you are focused on a specific job target. The résumé should contain a clear, concise objective about what you are looking for. This résumé should list your skills, academic achievements, student honors, and other pertinent information that correlates with your objective. This type of information adds substance to your résumé when you just graduated and do not have relevant job experience. Because the targeted résumé is an academic-type résumé, your skills, achievements, and community and volunteer work—your most significant assets—should be listed first. A sample of a targeted résumé is shown in Figure 58-6.

Writing the Résumé

One of the most daunting tasks of completing the résumé process is writing the résumé. Résumé writing is different from any other form of writing. The language you use in your résumé will affect its success, so it is important to be careful and conscientious when choosing your words.

You should use a direct, functional writing style that focuses on the use of verbs and other words that imply action on your part. Translate the facts of your academic and employment history into an active and precise résumé that will keep the reader's interest and highlight your major accomplishments in a concise, effective manner.

Writing with action words and strong verbs portrays you as an energetic, active person who is able to achieve results in his or her work. Choose words that display your strengths and demonstrate your initiative. Table 58-1 provides a list of commonly used verbs that help create a strong, active résumé.

Donna Turner-Smith
18 Kingsley Road
Olmsted Falls, OH 44138
(440) 555-4279

PUBLIC HEALTH EDUCATION:
　　Instructed community groups on HIV awareness.
　　Instructed volunteers on how to set up community programs on domestic violence
　　Facilitated workshops for parents of teenagers
　　Provided in-services for public school teachers on signs and symptoms of
　　substance abuse

COUNSELING:
　　Consulted with social workers on individual cases for suspected child abuse
　　Worked with parents from abused homes
　　Counseled individual abused children

ORGANIZATIONAL:
　　Grant writing for federal funds for HIV awareness programs
　　Served as a liaison for transitional shelters for victims of domestic violence
　　Served as a liaison between community health agencies and public schools

PROFESSIONAL WORK HISTORY:

　　2006–2011　　Project SAFE, Plymouth, Michigan
　　　　　　　　　　HIV Public Health Instructor

　　2011–2012　　Department of Child Health and Safety, Cleveland, Ohio
　　　　　　　　　　Public Health Educator

EDUCATION:
　　2006 B.S. Sociology, Eastern Michigan University, Ypsilanti, Michigan

References available upon request

FIGURE 58-4　A functional résumé is often used by people who are reentering the job market.

Below are two writing samples that differ only in their style. The first example is ineffective because it does not use action words to accent the applicant's work experiences.

Example #1
WORK EXPERIENCE

Medical Assistant
Manager of eight medical assistants from three offices. Office manager of three offices located east and west side. In charge of the daily operations of the medical office. Trainer of all new medical assistants.

Special Projects:　Coordinator and secretary for Cuyahoga County Chapter of the American Association of Medical Assistants.

Accomplishments:　Daily patient census went up 25% by implementing the "Patient First" customer service program. Patient-facility relations improved.

In the second example, below, the first paragraph has been rewritten. Notice how the tone has changed. The paragraph now sounds stronger and more active. This person accomplished goals and really did things.

Anthony Dalton
1234 West 25th Street
Park Ridge, NJ 07656
(201) 555-8311

WORK EXPERIENCE:

     September 2010–Present   NORTH BERGEN CLINIC FOUNDATION

         Lead Medical Assistant for Cardiology practice
         Patient preparation
         EKG and Holter Monitor
         Assist with Stress Testing
         Patient follow-up

     June 2002–August 2010   ST. JOSEPH HOSPITAL

         Phlebotomist–inpatient and outpatient

     March 2002–June 2002   ST. JOSEPH HOSPITAL

         Medical Assisting Externship
         Administrative and clinical responsibilities utilizing all
         medical assisting skills in the Emergency department.

- Patient triage
- Foley catheters
- EKG
- Specimen collection
- Patient intake
- Insurance verification

EDUCATION AND CERTIFICATIONS:

     Associate of Applied Science Degree, June 2008, Bergen Community College,
     Paramus, New Jersey, 07645

     Certified Medical Assistant, August 2002

References available upon request

FIGURE 58-5   A chronological résumé lists a person's job history in chronological order.

Example #2
WORK EXPERIENCE

Medical Assistant
Managed eight medical assistants from three different offices. Oversaw three offices in the Greater Cleveland area. Directed the daily operations of the medical offices. Coordinated events and served as secretary for the Cuyahoga County Chapter of the American Association of Medical Assistants. Increased daily patient census by 25% due to the success of a customer service model, "Patient First," which improved patient-facility relations during my tenure.

Résumé Writing Tips

Pay close attention to detail as you create your résumé. Here are some suggestions to help you:

- Organize your information by using a worksheet (Figure 58-7). List all the addresses, dates, phone numbers, and

Kelly Adamson
220 Terrace Avenue
Mooresburg, TN 37811
(423) 555-2657

CAREER OBJECTIVE:

To obtain a challenging position as a medical assistant in a growth oriented
ambulatory care facility

ACHIEVEMENTS:

Registered Medical Assistant
Certified Phlebotomy Technician
Registered Medical Office Specialist
Graduate of an Accredited Medical Assistant Program
OSHA Compliance Officer
American Heart BLS Instructor

SKILLS AND CAPABILITIES:

Front office and Clinical Medical Assistant Patient Triage
Specimen Collection Venipuncture
EKG and Holter Monitor Parenteral Injections
ICD-9 and CPT Coding Medical Billing

PROFESSIONAL EXPERIENCE:

September, 2011–Present   Affiliated Physician Network, Mooresburg, Tennessee
        Medical Assistant/Office Coordinator
June, 2001–September, 2006–2011,   Partners in Internal Medicine, Mooresburg,
        Tennessee Medical Assistant

EDUCATION:

Sanford Brown Institute, Diploma, Medical Assisting 2006

AFFILIATIONS:

American Medical Technologists

References available upon request

FIGURE 58-6   A targeted résumé is often used by a person who is focusing on a specific job target.

supervisors of previous positions that you have held. Write
down brief descriptions of all the responsibilities and duties
of your positions.

- List your educational institutions and their addresses, your
dates of attendance, and the type of diploma or degree, including your major.
- Choose a résumé format that best describes your experience,
education, and achievements.
- Use a computer and save your résumé on a flash drive.
- Proofread all spelling and grammar. Your completed résumé
should be perfect. Do not rely on the spell-checking feature

of your computer. Proofread your résumé line by line and
request that someone else also proofread your résumé.

- Select a high-quality, standard size (8½ by 11) résumé paper
with a weight between 20 and 25 pounds. Use an ivory or
white paper with matching envelopes.
- Use clear and concise statements and sentences. Your writing
should reflect a positive and confident tone. For example, if you
are describing your duties as a server, use sentences that focus
on customer service, cash management, and the training and
development of new servers. Avoid using the word "I" because
the reader already knows that the résumé is referring to you.

TABLE 58-1	Effective Résumé Verbs
administered	inspected
advised	introduced
analyzed	maintained
billed	managed
carried out	motivated
compiled	negotiated
completed	operated
conducted	ordered
contacted	organized
coordinated	oversaw
counseled	performed
designed	planned
developed	prepared
directed	presented
distributed	produced
established	reviewed
functioned as	supervised
implemented	taught
improved	trained

- Be truthful and honest about your strengths and abilities. Do not mislead or exaggerate any skills, talents, or experience.

Procedure 58-1, at the end of this chapter, provides information on how to write a résumé.

Writing a Cover Letter

A cover letter is an introduction to your résumé. It is a tool that markets your résumé as well as your skills and abilities. Cover letters are just as important as your résumé in your job search. An effective cover letter motivates the employer to review the résumé and interview the candidate.

Your cover letter should be direct and to the point. It should be no longer than one page and typed on paper that matches your résumé. If possible, your cover letter should be addressed to a specific person in the organization. You can call the hospital or facility and ask to whom you should address the letter. If a name is not available, it is acceptable to address the letter to "Human Resource Manager" or "Recruitment Manager." Research the facility or hospital prior to writing the letter. This information can

EMPLOYMENT WORKSHEET

Job Title _____

Dates _____

Employer _____

City, State _____

Major Duties _____

_____

_____

_____

_____

Special Projects _____

_____

_____

Accomplishments _____

_____

_____

_____

_____

FIGURE 58-7 An employment worksheet can be a useful tool in drafting a résumé.

```
                                          Your Street Address
                                          City, State, Zip Code
                                     _____


        Date

        Name of person to whom you are writing
        Title
        Company or Organization
        Street Address
        City, State, Zip Code


        Dear Dr., Mr., Mrs., Miss, or Ms. _____.

        1st Paragraph: Tell why you are writing. Name the position or general area of work that interests
        you. Mention how you learned about the job opening. State why you are interested in the job.

        2nd Paragraph: Refer to the enclosed résumé and give some background information. Indicate why
        you should be considered as a candidate, focusing on how your skills can fulfill the needs of the
        company. Relate your experiences to their needs and mention results/achievements. Do not restate
        what is said on your résumé—you want to pull together all the information and tell how your
        background fits the position.

        3rd Paragraph: Close by making a specific request for an interview. Say that you will follow up with
        a phone call to arrange a mutually convenient interview time. Offer to provide any additional
        information that may be needed. Thank the employer for his/her time and consideration.

        Sincerely,

        (your handwritten signature)

        Type your name



        Enclosure
```

FIGURE 58-8   The object of a cover letter is to convince the recipient to read your résumé.

help you tailor your letter to show how your qualifications and interests directly relate to the needs of the company or medical facility. Make sure the description of your qualifications and interests reflects the words used by the company in the advertisement. Always be truthful about the information in the cover letter; employers often verify all facts presented in your résumé and cover letter. Check each cover letter for errors in spelling, grammar, and punctuation. The format for a cover letter is shown in Figure 58-8.

Sending a Résumé

When sending a résumé, make sure you have the correct name, address, and zip code of the facility. This information should be typed on a matching envelope. Many software programs have an envelope template feature that allows you to print an envelope using the address in your cover letter. Do not handwrite envelopes; professionally appearing mail is often opened first. Make sure that you attach sufficient postage.

If you fax a résumé, verify the fax number and person or department you are faxing to. Make sure your name is on all the faxed pages. If your fax machine provides a fax completion printout, save it to verify that the fax was delivered.

Some classified ads request that you send your résumé via e-mail. In order to send your résumé in electronic form, you must first have an account with an Internet service provider (ISP). You will be asked by the ISP to select a log-in or screen name. Do not use a casual name for your log-in; prospective employers will see your log-in name in their in-box. Instead, choose a name that is conservative and professional. Most e-mail programs have an attachment feature that will allow you to send a Microsoft Word document via e-mail. Verify that your e-mail was sent by checking your sent items.

Post your résumé and cover letter on the Internet by using a career job search Internet site. Most Internet job sites have local employers posting positions daily. A job search Internet site will provide clear directions on how to post your résumé and cover letter. Some school career services departments host online job fairs and will assist you in posting your résumé.

Obtaining a Reference

Prior to the end of your applied training, meet with your preceptor and ask for a **reference**. A reference is a recommendation for employment from the facility and the preceptor. A reference can be in the form of a letter from the facility, preceptor, or physician or it can be a request to include these people on your reference list. It is professional to always ask before you list someone as a reference. References are important to career building because employers often like to inquire about a person prior to offering him or her employment. Your first references in medical assisting are your instructors and then the applied training facility.

You will want three to five references, including employment, academic, and character references. Ask instructors for a general letter before you finish your program. Fellow members of professional associations or your classmates can provide character references and your applied training facility can provide an employment reference. Make sure that you ask your references for permission to use their names and phone numbers. Do not print your references on the bottom of your résumé. List them on a separate sheet of paper so that you can provide them upon request and update the list as needed.

Preparing a Portfolio

Prior to the interviewing phase, you should organize all your employment documentation into a portfolio. A **portfolio** is a collection of documents and may include your résumé; cover letter; reference list or reference letters; awards for volunteer service in a health-related field; and student recognition certificates for student-of-the-year or month, perfect attendance, or academic honors. Include a copy of your transcript, diploma or degree, and medical assisting credentials such as your CMA (AAMA) or RMA (AMT). You also can include any other certifications you hold, like a CPR card or phlebotomy certification. Some employers request proof of immunizations, so include that in your portfolio. Give your portfolio a professional presentation by printing your documents on a high-quality printer and organizing them in a nice binder. A professional portfolio can help you obtain employment. If needed, look for a service that specializes in creating professional portfolios.

▶ Interviewing
LO 58.4

Preparation for your interview begins long before the interview itself. After you send your cover letters and résumés, you must make sure that prospective employers can reach you by telephone. You must practice how you are going to handle your interview, and you must plan what to wear and how to present yourself in the most professional way.

Before starting your job search, invest in an answering machine or voicemail to receive calls when you are not available. Be sure the outgoing message is clear, concise, and professional. Avoid cute messages or background music. An appropriate message would be, "I'm unable to take your call at the moment, but your call is important to me. Please leave your name, number, the time you called, and a brief message after the tone and I will call you back as soon as I can. Thank you." Also, make sure all household members who answer the phone (especially children) know proper phone etiquette and how to take a written message. When a prospective employer calls with an interview invitation, write down the interviewer's name, company or practice name, day, time, and location of the interview.

Interview Planning and Strategies

Just as the résumé is important for opening the door to opportunity, the job interview itself is critical for allowing you to present yourself professionally and to clearly articulate why you are the best person for the job. As you learned in the *Interpersonal Communication* chapter, being successful in a medical assisting career is centered on communication—both verbal and nonverbal. These communication skills will be assets during your job interviews. The following list provides some strategies that will help you improve your interviewing skills:

- Practice interviewing. Rehearse possible questions and be prepared to answer them directly. Have a friend or family member interview you as you sit in front of a mirror and observe your body language. Your college career center may help you prepare by offering mock interviews.

- Anticipate question types. Expect open-ended questions like "What are your strengths?", "What are your weaknesses?", "Tell me about your best work experience," and "Can you give me an example how you have worked with others to solve a problem?" Decide in advance what information and skills are pertinent to the position and reveal your strengths. For example, you could say, "While I was at school, I learned to get along with a diverse group of people."

- Learn about the company. Be prepared; research the company or medical facility. What is the type of specialty? How many physicians are there?

- Dress appropriately. Because much communication is nonverbal, dressing appropriately for the interview is important. In most situations, you will be safe if you wear clean, pressed, conservative business clothes in neutral colors. Do not wear current fashions or fad clothing to an interview. Pay special attention to grooming. Keep makeup light and wear little jewelry. Make sure that your hair and nails are clean and styled conservatively. Do not carry a large purse, backpack, books, coat, or hat. Leave extra clothing in an outside office and simply carry a pen, your portfolio with extra copies of your résumé, and a small pad for taking notes. Turn cell phones and pagers off during the interview or leave them in your vehicle.

- Be punctual. A good first impression is important and can be lasting. If you arrive late for the interview, a prospective employer may conclude that you will be late in arriving to work. Make certain you know the location and the time of the interview. Allow time for traffic, parking, and other preliminaries.

- Be professional. Being too familiar in your manner can be a barrier to a professional interview. Never call anyone by his or her first name unless you are asked to.

- Know the interviewer's title and the pronunciation of his or her name. Do not sit down until the interviewer does.

- Exhibit appropriate interview behavior. Always greet the interviewer with a smile. The interview is an opportunity to sell yourself to the employer. Offer your hand for a firm, confident handshake and be alert to the interviewer's body language. The flow of conversation during an interview should be natural. Maintain eye contact, pay attention to the interviewer, and show interest. Ask intelligent questions that you have prepared before the interview. Remember, the interview is an opportunity for both the prospective employer and the prospective employee to gather information and make a good impression. In addition to reviewing the experience listed on your résumé, the interviewer will evaluate your personality and behavior. At the same time, you will be observing the office and learning more about the position. Try to be aware of the office's atmosphere, its equipment and supplies, and the attitudes of the staff. Does it seem like a pleasant, professional place to work? Request a tour of the facility and ask yourself if you would be happy in that work environment.

- Be poised and relaxed. Avoid nervous habits like tapping your pencil, playing with your hair, or covering your mouth with your hand. Watch language such as "you know," "ah," and "stuff like that." Use proper grammar and pronunciation as you talk with the interviewer—do not use slang. Do not smoke beforehand (you will smell like smoke), chew gum, fidget, or bite your nails.

- Maintain comfortable eye contact. Look the interviewer in the eye and speak with confidence. Your eyes reveal much about you; use them to show interest, confidence, poise, and sincerity. Use other nonverbal techniques like a firm handshake to reinforce your confidence.

- Relate your experience to the job. Use every question as an opportunity to show how your skills relate to the job. Use examples taken from school, previous jobs, your applied training, volunteer work, leadership in student organizations, and personal experience to indicate that you have the personal qualities, aptitude, and skills needed for this job.

- Be honest. While it is important to be confident and stress your strengths, it is equally important to your sense of integrity to be honest. Dishonesty always catches up to you sooner or later. Someone will verify your background, so do not exaggerate your accomplishments, grade point average, or experience.

- Focus on how you can benefit the company. Do not ask about benefits, salary, or vacations until you are offered the job. During a first interview, try to show how you can contribute to the organization. Do not appear to be too eager to move up through the company or suggest that you are more interested in gaining experience than in contributing to the company.

- Close the interview on a positive note. Thank the interviewer for his or her time, shake hands, and say that you are looking forward to hearing from him or her. On the way out of the office, thank the staff members involved in the interview. Ask for a business card from anyone to whom you think you might want to send a thank-you note. After leaving the interview, write down any additional information you want to remember. Every interview provides you with information about the medical assisting profession. Even if an interview does not result in a job, you will have met new people, developed a larger network of professional contacts, and gained valuable interviewing experience.

- Follow up with a letter within two days of the interview. After an interview, it is professional to send a thank-you letter to the person or persons from the company who conducted your interview. Your letter may be brief, but it should express your appreciation for the opportunity to have met with the interviewer, reaffirm your interest in the organization, and state your desire to remain a part of the selection process. By sending a thank-you letter, you display common business courtesy, which can make a difference in the employer's hiring decision. Even if you are not interested in continuing the interview and selection process, you should thank the employer for holding the interview. Procedure 58-2, at the end of this chapter, explains how to write and send a thank-you letter.

- Complete an application. Some employers ask you to complete an employment application at an interview even when you provide a résumé. You can use your résumé to help you complete the application. Fill out the application neatly. Spell all words correctly and read and follow the instructions on the form carefully. Your application represents you; it must make a good first impression. Fill in all sections of the application—do not write "see résumé." Because an application is signed, it is a legal document and, as such, referring to your résumé, even though the information is there, is not allowed.

- Comply with other aspects of the application process. As part of the application process, employers are required by federal law to request documents that prove your identity and eligibility to work in the United States. To maintain the safety and confidentiality of the medical office, hospital, or laboratory, employers may also check your police record, credit rating, and history of chemical or alcohol abuse. A drug screen may be requested. You may be asked to provide the needed documents or to give the employer authorization to obtain them.

- Do not excessively contact the interviewer by telephone or e-mail after the interview. Prior to leaving the interview, it is acceptable to ask the interviewer when a decision will be made and if the interviewer will call to let you know whether or not an offer of employment will be made. It is acceptable to ask permission to contact the interviewer to follow up on the position.

Interview Questions

In order to prepare for your interview, you can anticipate that you may be asked any of the following questions:

- I see from your résumé that you graduated from ABC School. What did that school have to offer you that others did not?

- What is your five-year goal?
- Tell me about yourself.
- What do you consider to be your greatest strengths and weaknesses?
- How would your instructors describe you?
- What qualifications do you have that make you a good candidate for this position?
- How could you make a contribution to this facility?
- How well do you work with others?
- What is your concept of a team environment?
- How well do you work under pressure?
- Will you be able to work overtime?
- Do you have the flexibility to work various shifts?
- What has been your major accomplishment to date?
- Why did you choose medical assisting as your career?
- Do you have any questions that you would like to ask?

It is also helpful to be prepared with any questions that you may have for the interviewer about the position or the facility. Remember, however, that questions about salary and benefits are not appropriate in a first interview.

An interviewer may ask you questions that you are not obligated to answer. These questions refer to age, race, sexual orientation, marital status, or number of children. Even if the questions sound harmless or the interviewer seems nonjudgmental, these questions have nothing to do with your skills or abilities. If the interviewer asks even one of these questions, you should reconsider whether you want to work for the organization.

If you are asked an inappropriate question during an interview, be polite and remain professional in declining to answer. You may simply state that you do not believe the requested information is necessary for the employer to evaluate your qualifications for the job. Try to move the discussion onto a more relevant topic.

Reasons for Not Being Hired

Employers in business were asked to list reasons for not hiring a job candidate. Some of the biggest complaints included

1. Poor appearance, not being dressed properly, and being poorly groomed.
2. Acting like a know-it-all.
3. Not communicating clearly, as well as poor voice, diction, and grammar.
4. Lack of planning for the interview, with no purpose or goals communicated.
5. Lack of confidence or poise.
6. No interest in or enthusiasm for the job.
7. Objectionable content on personal social networking pages.
8. Being interested only in the best salary offer.
9. Inappropriate voicemail greeting.
10. Unwillingness to begin in an entry-level position.
11. Making excuses about an unfavorable record.
12. No tact.
13. No maturity.
14. No curiosity about the job.
15. Being critical of past employers.

Salary Negotiations

Medical assisting salaries are varied and differ by geographic area. When you are a new graduate, you will begin your career as an entry-level medical assistant. As you gain experience, your compensation will reflect that. Salary ranges are determined by geographic location, medical specialty, years of experience, credentialing, and the job description.

The first step in determining your compensation needs is to know how much income is required to meet your living expenses. You will need to prepare a budget. Keep track of your overall expenditures and living expenses. Itemizing your basic living expenses can help you to prepare a budget.

Establishing a budget will give you an idea of the amount of income you may need. Once your budget is established, you have a negotiating benchmark. Employers will often ask you what you are looking for with regard to salary. If you answer directly, you may risk either quoting yourself out of a job or leaving money on the table. The best response to this question is to ask the employer the range of the position. Most positions have a low-to-high range. For example, the range for a specific position could be between $23,000 and $32,000 annually. Once you know the range, quote a little higher than what your budgetary amount is, which will give the employer room to negotiate down if necessary. Allow the employer to bring up salary first.

▶ On the Job   LO 58.5

Once you have a job, you must learn how to be an effective employee. There are many ways that your initiative enables the medical team in the office, hospital, clinic, or laboratory to function effectively. You must identify the important skills in your daily duties, stay competitive and marketable through continuing education, and integrate constructive criticism from your employee evaluations into your daily work and annual goals.

Job Description

During the initial paperwork process when you begin as a new employee, you may be asked to read and sign a job description for the position for which you have been hired. The purpose of a job description is to provide the standard benchmarks of your position. It will list and describe the position's expectations and the duties to be performed. A job description includes detailed information, such as

- Essential duties and responsibilities.
- Qualifications.
- Education and experience.
- Certificates, licenses, and registrations.
- Physical demands.
- Description of the work environment.

Employee Evaluations

Employee evaluations are usually held annually. An initial employment review generally occurs after a 90-day probationary period. Evaluations describe an employee's performance and, in most situations, the employee and the employer meet to discuss this. The purpose of an annual evaluation should be to check the goals and values of both the employer and the employee to make sure they support each other.

An employee evaluation form typically outlines the most important qualities and abilities needed for the job. It evaluates the employee's strengths and weaknesses. This form also may help determine whether an employee is worthy of a merit raise, which is a raise based on performance (as opposed to a cost-of-living raise). The quantity and quality of work are assessed on this form, as are initiative, judgment, and cooperation. A completed evaluation is placed in an official record of employment.

Continuing Education

After completing a medical assisting program, you should continue your education, setting specific educational advancement goals on a yearly basis. For example, you may decide to obtain further education to learn more about the medical specialty in which you

work. Once you obtain your certification as a medical assistant, you will be required to obtain a specific number of continuing education units (CEUs) yearly to maintain your certification credential.

As medical research expands its discoveries and as new technologies emerge, the necessity for self-education increases. You must read to stay abreast of updates in medicine. The need for more highly specialized training presents you with an opportunity for growth in your education and career. Medical publications are the best source for the latest medical information. Local and state medical assisting meetings also provide information about advances in the field. And, of course, the Internet is a valuable source for staying current about today's technological advances.

Self-education is an important skill for the medical assistant. It helps you to stay up-to-date in topics about medicine, healthcare, wellness, insurance products, and pharmaceuticals. Patients may ask questions about information they have read or about the effectiveness of certain new treatments and having this knowledge will enable you to better discuss this information and to refer patients' questions to their physician for more details.

PROCEDURE 58-1 Résumé Writing

Procedure Goal: To develop a résumé that defines your career objective and highlights your skills.

OSHA Guidelines: This procedure does not involve exposure to blood, body fluids, or tissues.

Materials: Paper, pen, dictionary, thesaurus, and a computer.

Method: Procedure steps.

1. Type your full name, address (temporary and permanent, if you have both), telephone number with area code, and e-mail address (if you have one).

2. List your general career objective. You also may choose to summarize your skills. If you want to phrase your objective to fit a specific position, you should include that information in a cover letter to accompany the résumé.

3. List the highest level of education or the most recently obtained degree first. Include the school name, degree earned, and date of graduation. Be sure to list any special projects, courses, or participation in overseas study programs.

4. Summarize your work experience. List your most recent or most relevant employment first. Describe your responsibilities and list job titles, company names, and dates of employment. Summer employment, volunteer work, and student applied training also may be included.

Use short sentences with strong action words such as *directed, designed, developed,* and *organized.* For example, condense a responsibility into "Handled insurance and billing" or "Drafted correspondence as requested."
RATIONALE: Action verbs give the impression that you are an energetic and results-oriented employee.

5. List any memberships and affiliations with professional organizations alphabetically or by order of importance.

6. Do not list references on your résumé.
RATIONALE: It is easier to update your reference list if you maintain it in a separate file.

7. Do not list the salary you wish to receive in a medical assisting position. Salary requirements should not be discussed until a job offer is received. If the ad you are answering requests that you include a required salary, it is best to state a range (no broader than $5,000 from lowest to highest point in the range for an annual salary).

8. Print your résumé on an 8½- by 11-inch sheet of high-quality white or off-white bond paper. Carefully check your résumé for spelling, punctuation, and grammatical errors. Have someone else double-check your résumé whenever possible.
RATIONALE: Your résumé is a printed reflection of you, so ensuring its accuracy and completeness is essential.

PROCEDURE 58-2 Writing Thank-You Notes

Procedure Goal: To develop an appropriate, professional thank-you note after an interview or applied training.

OSHA Guidelines: This procedure does not involve exposure to blood, body fluids, or tissues.

Materials: Paper, pen, dictionary, thesaurus, computer, and a #10 business envelope.

Method: Procedure steps.

1. Complete the letter within two days of the interview or completion of the applied training. Begin by typing the date at the top of the letter.
   RATIONALE: It is considered professional behavior to follow up in a prompt manner and will help the interviewer to remember you during employment selection.

2. Type the name of the person who interviewed you (or who was your mentor in the applied training). Include credentials and title, such as Dr. or Director of Client Services. Include the complete address of the office or organization.

3. Start the letter with "Dear Dr., Mr., Mrs., Miss, or Ms. _____:"

4. In the first paragraph, thank the interviewer for his time and for granting the interview. Discuss some specific impressions; for example, "I found the interview and tour of the facilities an enjoyable experience. I would welcome the opportunity to work in such a state-of-the-art medical setting." If you are writing to thank your mentor for her time during your applied training and for allowing you to perform your applied training at her office, practice, or clinic, discuss the knowledge and experience you gained during the applied training.

5. In the second paragraph, mention the aspects of the job or applied training that you found most interesting or challenging. For a job interview thank-you note, state how your skills and qualifications will make you an asset to the staff. When preparing an applied training thank-you letter, mention interest in any future positions.

6. In the last paragraph, thank the interviewer for considering you for the position. Ask to be contacted at his earliest convenience regarding his employment decision.

7. Close the letter with "Sincerely," and type your name. Leave enough space—usually 4 spaces—above your typewritten name to sign your name.

8. Type your return address in the upper-left corner of the #10 business envelope. Then type the interviewer's name and address in the envelope's center, apply the proper postage, and mail the letter. You also can e-mail your thank-you letter. Proper letter format and professional tone and appearance still apply. Send the thank-you letter as an attachment.

SUMMARY OF LEARNING OUTCOMES

LEARNING OUTCOMES	KEY POINTS
58.1 **Carry out professionalism in all applied training scenarios.**	Students' weekly progress sheets should reveal new goals each week and progress on previous weeks' goals. Their assessment and the preceptor's assessments should be similar and show professionalism, willingness to learn, and continual progress throughout the applied training.
58.2 **Summarize the necessary steps for obtaining professional certification.**	When seeking national certification, students should determine if they are eligible to take the certification exam, gather necessary documents, apply for the exam, and study and prepare to take the exam.
58.3 **Describe an appropriate strategy for finding a position.**	Students should be able to list classified advertisements available in local papers, employment websites, networking, and employment agencies where employment assistance is available and should provide a workable, professional résumé that can be used to begin the employment search.
58.4 **Explain key factors for a successful interview.**	Students should be able to list key factors, such as portraying confidence, smiling, looking the interviewer in the eye, having questions ready for the interviewer about the position, and practicing answers to common interviewing questions. If possible, participation in a mock interview should be considered.
58.5 **Describe ways of becoming a successful employee.**	The keys to becoming a successful employee include using the job description to provide benchmarks for performance standards, using employee evaluations to improve performance, and continuing self-education throughout your career.

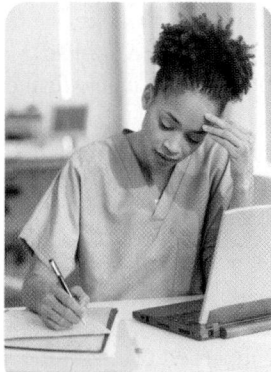

Recall Reagan from the beginning of the chapter. Now that you have completed the chapter, answer the following questions regarding her case.

1. What should be Reagan's first steps in seeking employment?
2. What style of résumé should she choose?

1. (LO 58.1) The document that states the expectations of the facility and student for the applied training site is a(n)
   a. Time sheet
   b. Affiliation agreement
   c. Progress report
   d. Applied training plan
   e. Job description

2. (LO 58.1) Feedback given in order to improve performance is
   a. Affiliation
   b. Benchmarking
   c. Training agreement
   d. Constructive criticism
   e. Negotiation

3. (LO 58.1) Which of the following personality types are generally the best for medical assisting students involved in applied training?
   a. Quiet/passive
   b. Aggressive/know-it-all
   c. Assertive/confident
   d. Shy/timid
   e. Tentative/unbending

4. (LO 58.3) Which résumé style generally works best for new medical assisting graduates seeking employment?
   a. Targeted résumé
   b. Chronological résumé
   c. Functional résumé
   d. Curriculum vitae
   e. Simple résumé

5. (LO 58.3) A reference is a recommendation for a position. Which of the following persons might you consider asking for a reference?
   a. Former supervisor
   b. Applied training supervisor/preceptor
   c. Medical assisting instructor
   d. Applied training coordinator
   e. All of the above

6. (LO 58.1) If you are unable to attend your applied training due to an emergency, you should
   a. Call your instructor and ask that he or she call the applied training site
   b. Call the applied training site and the school two hours before you are to arrive
   c. E-mail the applied training site that you will not be in
   d. E-mail your instructor that you will be absent
   e. Call the applied training site when it opens

7. (LO 58.5) Employee evaluations are usually held
   a. Each month
   b. Yearly
   c. Every 90 days
   d. At the employee's request
   e. Only if there is an issue with an employee

8. (LO 58.2) Which of the following is a certification eligibility requirement of the AAMA?
   a. Graduation from a CAAHEP- or ABHES-accredited school
   b. U.S. Armed Forces medical services training
   c. Working as a medical assistant for 5 years
   d. Teaching in a medical assisting program
   e. Attending a medical assisting program that has 720 hours of training

9. (LO 58.3) A chronological résumé is used most often when
   a. A person has gaps in his or her work history
   b. Someone has job experience
   c. A person is changing jobs
   d. A person is looking for a specific job
   e. A person has just graduated

10. (LO 58.3) A collection of documents you may take to a job interview is a/an
    a. Affiliation
    b. Application
    c. Portfolio
    d. Reference
    e. Résumé

Prefixes

a-, an- without, not
ab- from, away
ad- to, toward
ambi-, amph-, amphi- both, on both sides, around
ante- before
antero- in front of
anti- against, opposing
auto- self
bi- twice, double
brachy- short
brady- slow
cata- down, lower, under
centi- hundred
cephal- head
chol-, chole-, cholo- gall
chromo- color
circum- around
co-, com-, con- together, with
contra- against
cryo- cold
de- down, from
deca- ten
deci- tenth
demi- half
dextro- to the right
di- double, twice
dia- through, apart, between
dipla-, diplo- double, twin
dis- apart, away from
dys- difficult, painful, bad, abnormal
e-, ec-, ecto- away, from, without, outside
em-, en- in, into, inside
endo- within, inside
ento- within, inner
epi- on, above
erythro- red
eu- good
ex-, exo- outside of, beyond, without
extra- outside of, beyond, in addition
fore- before, in front of
gyn-, gyno-, gyne-, gyneco- woman, female
hemi- half
hetero- other, unlike
homeo-, homo- same, like
hyper- above, over, increased, excessive
hypo- below, under, decreased
idio- personal, self-produced
im-, in-, ir- not
in- in, into
infra- beneath

inter- between, among
intra-, intro- into, within, during
juxta- near, nearby
kata-, kath- down, lower, under
kineto- motion
leuco-, leuko- white
levo- to the left
macro- large, long
mal- bad
mega-, megalo- large, great
meio- contraction
melan-, melano- black
mes-, meso- middle
meta- beyond
micro- small
mio- smaller, less
mono- single, one
multi- many
neo- new
non-, not- no
nulli- none
ob- against
olig-, oligo- few, less than normal
ortho- straight
oxy- sharp, acid
pachy- thick
pan- all, every
par-, para- alongside of, with; woman who has given birth
per- through, excessive
peri- around
pes- foot
pluri- more, several
pneo- breathing
poly- many, much
post- after, behind
pre-, pro- before, in front of
presby-, presbyo- old age
primi- first
pseudo- false
quadri- four
re- back, again
retro- backward, behind
semi- half
steno- contracted, narrow
stereo- firm, solid, three-dimensional
sub- under
super-, supra- above, upon, excess
sym-, syn- with, together
tachy- fast
tele- distant, far
tetra- four
tomo- incision, section

trans- across
tri- three
tropho- nutrition, growth
ultra- beyond, excess
uni- one
veni- vein
xanth-, xantho- yellow

Suffixes

-ad to, toward
-aesthesia, -esthesia sensation
-al characterized by
-algia pain
-ase enzyme
-asthenia weakness
-cele swelling, tumor
-centesis puncture, tapping
-cidal killing
-cide causing death
-cise cut
-coele cavity
-cyst bladder, bag
-cyte cell, cellular
-dynia pain
-ectomy cutting out, surgical removal
-emesis vomiting
-emia blood
-esthesia sensation
-form shape
-fuge driving away
-gene, -genic, -genetic, -genesis, -genous arising from, origin, formation
-gram recorded information
-graph instrument for recording
-graphy the process of recording
-ia condition
-iasis condition of
-ic, -ical pertaining to
-ism condition, process, theory
-itis inflammation of
-ium membrane
-ize to cause to be, to become, to treat by special method
-kinesis, -kinetic motion
-lepsis, -lepsy seizure, convulsion
-lith stone
-logy science of, study of
-lysis setting free, disintegration, decomposition
-malacia abnormal softening
-mania insanity, abnormal desire
-meter measure
-metry process of measuring

-odynia pain
-oid resembling
-ole small, little
-oma tumor
-opia vision
-opsy to view
-osis disease, condition of
-ostomy to make a mouth, opening
-otomy incision, surgical cutting
-ous having
-pathy disease, suffering
-penia too few, lack, decreased
-pexy surgical fixation
-phagia, -phage eating, consuming, swallowing
-phobia fear, abnormal fear
-phylaxis protection
-plasia formation or development
-plastic molded
-plasty operation to reconstruct, surgical repair
-plegia paralysis
-pnea breathing
-rrhage, -rrhagia abnormal or excessive discharge, hemorrhage, flow
-rrhaphy suture of
-rrhea flow, discharge
-sclerosis hardening
-scope instrument used to examine
-scopy examining
-sepsis poisoning, infection
-spasm cramp or twitching
-stasis stoppage
-stomy opening
-therapy treatment
-thermy heat
-tome cutting instrument
-tomy incision, section
-tripsy surgical crushing
-trophy turning, tendency
-tropy turning, tendency
-uria urine

Word Roots

adeno- gland, glandular
adipo- fat
aero- air
andr-, andro- man, male
angio- blood vessel
ano- anus
arterio- artery
arthro- joint
bili- bile
bio- life
blasto-, blast- developing stage, bud
bracheo- arm
broncho- bronchial (windpipe)

carcino- cancer
cardio- heart
cerebr-, cerebro- brain
cephalo- head
cervico- neck
chondro- cartilage
chromo- color
colo- colon
colp-, colpo- vagina
coro- body
cost-, costo- rib
crani-, cranio- skull
cysto- bladder, bag
cyto- cell, cellular
dacry-, dacryo- tears, lacrimal apparatus
dactyl-, dactylo- finger, toe
dent-, denti-, dento- teeth
derma-, dermat-, dermato- skin
dorsi-, dorso- back
encephalo- brain
entero- intestine
esthesio- sensation
fibro- connective tissue
galact-, galacto- milk
gastr-, gastro- stomach
gingiv- gums
glosso- tongue
gluco-, glyco- sugar, sweet
gravid-, gravid- pregnant female
haemo-, hemato-, hem-, hemo- blood
hepa-, hepar-, hepato- liver
herni- rupture
hidro- sweat (perspiration)
histo- tissue
hydra-, hydro- water
hyster-, hystero- uterus
ictero- jaundice
ileo- ileum
karyo- nucleus, nut
kera-, kerato- horn, hardness, cornea
lact- milk
laparo- abdomen
latero- side
linguo- tongue
lipo- fat
lith- stone
lobo- lobe
mast-, masto- breast
med-, medi- middle
mening- meninges (covers the brain)
metro-, metra- uterus
my-, myo- muscle
myel-, myelo- marrow
narco- sleep
nas-, naso- nose
necro- dead
nephr-, nephro- kidney

neu-, neuro- nerve
niter-, nitro- nitrogen
nucleo- nucleus
oculo- eye
odont- tooth
omphalo- navel, umbilicus
onco- tumor
oo- ovum, egg
oophor- ovary
ophthalmo- eye
orchid- testicle
os- mouth, opening
oste-, osteo- bone
oto- ear
paedo-, pedo- child
palpebro- eyelid
path-, patho- disease, suffering
pepso- digestion
phag-, phago- eating, consuming, swallowing
pharyng-, pharyngo- throat, pharynx
phlebo- vein
pleuro- side, rib
pneumo- air, lungs
pod- foot
procto- rectum
psych- the mind
pulmon-, pulmono- lung
pyelo- pelvis (renal)
pyo- pus
pyro- fever, heat
reni-, reno- kidney
rhino- nose
sacchar- sugar
sacro- sacrum
salpingo- tube, fallopian tube
sarco- flesh
sclero- hard, sclera
septi-, septic-, septico- poison, infection
stomato- mouth
teno-, tenoto- tendon
thermo- heat
thio- sulfa
thoraco- chest
thrombo- blood clot
thyro- thyroid gland
tricho- hair
urino-, uro- urine, urinary organs
utero- uterus, uterine
uvulo- uvula
vagin- vagina
vaso- vessel
ventri-, ventro- abdomen
vesico- blister

Abbreviations

a   before

aa, AA   of each

ABGs   arterial blood gases

a.c.   before meals

ADD   attention deficit disorder

ADL   activities of daily living

ad lib   as desired

ADT   admission, discharge, transfer

AIDS   acquired immunodeficiency syndrome

AKA   above knee amputation

a.m.a.   against medical advice

AMA   American Medical Association

amp.   ampule

amt   amount

aq., AQ   water; aqueous

ASHD   atherosclerotic heart disease

ausc.   auscultation

ax   axis

Bib, bib   drink

b.i.d., bid, BID   twice a day

BKA   below knee amputation

BM   bowel movement

BP, B/P   blood pressure

BPC   blood pressure check

BPH   benign prostatic hypertrophy

bpm   beats per minute

BSA   body surface area

c̄   with

Ca, CA   calcium; cancer

CABG   coronary artery bypass graft

cap, caps   capsules

CBC   complete blood (cell) count

C.C., CC   chief complaint

CDC   Centers for Disease Control and Prevention

CHF   congestive heart failure

chr   chronic

cm   centimeter

CNS   central nervous system

Comp, comp   compound

COPD   chronic obstructive pulmonary disease

CP   chest pain

CPE   complete physical examination

CPR   cardiopulmonary resuscitation

CSF   cerebrospinal fluid

CT   computed tomography

CV   cardiovascular

CVA   cerebrovascular accident

CXR   chest X-ray

d   day

D&C   dilation and curettage

DEA   Drug Enforcement Administration

Dil, dil   dilute

DM   diabetes mellitus

DNR   do not resuscitate

DOB   date of birth

Dr.   doctor

DTaP   diphtheria-tetanus-acellular pertussis vaccine

DTs   delirium tremens

DVT   deep venous thrombosis

D/W   dextrose in water

Dx, dx   diagnosis

ECG, EKG   electrocardiogram

ED   emergency department

EEG   electroencephalogram

EENT   eyes, ears, nose, and throat

EP   established patient

ER   emergency room

ESR   erythrocyte sedimentation rate

FBS   fasting blood sugar

FDA   Food and Drug Administration

FH   family history

Fl, fl, fld   fluid

fl oz   fluid ounce

F/u   follow-up

FUO   fever of unknown origin

Fx   fracture

g   gram

GBS   gallbladder series

GI   gastrointestinal

Gm, gm   gram

gr   grain

gt, gtt   drop, drops

GTT   glucose tolerance test

GU   genitourinary

GYN   gynecology

HA   headache

HB, Hgb   hemoglobin

hct   hematocrit

HEENT   head, ears, eyes, nose, throat

HIV   human immunodeficiency virus

HO   history of

HPI   history of present illness

HPV   human papillomavirus

Hx   history

ICU   intensive care unit

I&D   incision and drainage

IDDM   insulin-dependent diabetes

IM   intramuscular

inf.   infusion; inferior

inj   injection

I&O   intake and output

IT   inhalation therapy

IUD   intrauterine device

IV   intravenous

KUB   kidneys, ureters, bladder

L   liter

L1, L2, etc.   lumbar vertebrae

lab   laboratory

lb   pound

liq   liquid

LLE   left lower extremity (left leg)

LLL   left lower lobe

LLQ   left lower quadrant

LMP   last menstrual period

LUE   left upper extremity (left arm)

LUQ   left upper quadrant

m   meter

M   mix (Latin *misce*)

mcg   microgram

mg   milligram

MI   myocardial infarction

mL   milliliter

mm   millimeter

MM   mucous membrane

mmHg   millimeters of mercury

MRI   magnetic resonance imaging

MS   multiple sclerosis

NB   newborn

NED   no evidence of disease

NIDDM   noninsulin-dependent diabetes mellitus

NKA   no known allergies

no, #   number

noc, noct   night

npo, NPO   nothing by mouth

NPT   new patient

NS   normal saline

NSAID   nonsteroidal anti-inflammatory drug

NTP   normal temperature and pressure

N&V, N/V   nausea and vomiting

NYD   not yet diagnosed

OB   obstetrics

OC   oral contraceptive

oint   ointment

OOB   out of bed

OPD   outpatient department

OPS   outpatient services

OR   operating room

OT   occupational therapy

OTC   over-the-counter

oz   ounce

p̄   after

PA   posteroanterior

Pap Pap smear
Path pathology
p.c., pc after meals
PE physical examination
per by, with
PH past history
PID pelvic inflammatory disease
PMFSH past medical, family, social history
PMS premenstrual syndrome
po by mouth
p/o postoperative
POMR problem-oriented medical record
P&P Pap smear (Papanicolaou smear) and pelvic examination
p.r.n., prn, PRN whenever necessary
pt pint
Pt patient
PT physical therapy
PTA prior to admission
pulv powder
PVC premature ventricular contraction
q. every
q2, q2h every 2 hours
q.a.m., qam every morning
q.h., qh every hour
qns, QNS quantity not sufficient
qs, QS quantity sufficient
qt quart
RA rheumatoid arthritis; right atrium
RBC red blood cells; red blood (cell) count
RDA recommended dietary allowance, recommended daily allowance
REM rapid eye movement
RF rheumatoid factor
RLE right lower extremity (right leg)
RLL right lower lobe
RLQ right lower quadrant
R/O rule out
ROM range of motion
ROS/SR review of systems/systems review
RUE right upper extremity (right arm)
RUQ right upper quadrant
RV right ventricle
Rx prescription, take
s̄ without
SAD seasonal affective disorder
SIDS sudden infant death syndrome
sig sigmoidoscopy
Sig directions
SL sublingual
SOAP subjective, objective, assessment, plan
SOB shortness of breath
sol solution
S/R suture removal

Staph staphylococcus
stat, STAT immediately
STI sexually transmitted infection
Strep streptococcus
subcu subcutaneous
subcut subcutaneous
subling sublingual
surg surgery
S/W saline in water
SX symptoms
T1, T2, etc. thoracic vertebrae
T&A tonsillectomy and adenoidectomy
tab tablet
TB tuberculosis
tbs., tbsp tablespoon
TIA transient ischemic attack
t.i.d., tid, TID three times a day
tinc, tinct, tr tincture
TMJ temporomandibular joint
top topically
TPR temperature, pulse, and respiration
TSH thyroid stimulating hormone
tsp teaspoon
Tx treatment
U unit
UA urinalysis
UCHD usual childhood diseases
UGI upper gastrointestinal
ung, ungt ointment
URI upper respiratory infection
US ultrasound
UTI urinary tract infection
VA visual acuity
VD venereal disease
VF visual field
VS vital signs
WBC white blood cells; white blood (cell) count
WNL within normal limits
wt weight
y/o year old

Symbols

Weights and Measures

pounds
° degrees
′ foot; minute
″ inch; second
mEq milliequivalent
mL milliliter
dL deciliter
mg% milligrams percent; milligrams per 100 mL

Mathematical Functions and Terms

number
+ plus; positive; acid reaction
− minus; negative; alkaline reaction
± plus or minus; either positive or negative; indefinite
× multiply; magnification; crossed with, hybrid
÷ , / divided by
= equal to
≈ approximately equal to
> greater than; from which is derived
< less than; derived from
≮ not less than
≯ not greater than
≤ equal to or less than
≥ equal to or greater than
≠ not equal to
√ square root
³√ cube root
∞ infinity
: ratio; "is to"
∴ therefore
% percent
π pi (3.14159)—the ratio of circumference of a circle to its diameter

Chemical Notations

Δ change; heat
⇌ reversible reaction
↑ increase
↓ decrease

Warnings

Ⓒ Schedule I controlled substance
Ⓒ Schedule II controlled substance
Ⓒ Schedule III controlled substance
Ⓒ Schedule IV controlled substance
Ⓒ Schedule V controlled substance
☠ poison
☢ radiation
☣ biohazard

Others

℞ prescription; take
□, ♂ male
○, ♀ female
† one
†† two
††† three

Infectious Diseases Caused by Bacteria

NAME	DESCRIPTION
Boil	Localized skin infection usually caused by staphylococcus bactera.
Botulism	A type of food poisoning caused by a toxin produced by the bacterium *Clostridium botulinum*.
Conjunctivitis	Commonly called pink eye, this condition is highly contagious when the cause is bacterial. Can also be caused by viruses and allergies.
Gonorrhea	Highly contagious condition transmitted by sexual intercourse and caused by gonococcus bacteria.
Impetigo	A *Staphylococcus* or *Streptococcus* infection commonly found in children that causes lesions on the face or lower leg. Impetigo is highly contagious when contact is made with the lesions. This condition is treated with antibiotics.
Legionnaire's disease	An acute type of bacterial pneumonia caused by *Legionnaire* bacillus, a gram-negative organism. It grows in standing water such as that found in commercial air conditioners, humidifiers, water heaters, and evaporative condensers.
Lyme disease	An arthropod-borne disease caused by the spirochete *Borrelia burgdorferi*. The disease is transmitted by deer ticks. The signs and symptoms include skin lesions, central nervous system and cardiac involvement, and arthritis.
Meningitis	Inflammation of the meninges. Causes include bacterial, viral, and fungal infections.
Pertussis	Also called whooping cough. Caused by bacillus bacteria.
Pneumonia	Respiratory condition in which lung tissue is inflamed, usually causing difficulty breathing and a cough. Can also be caused by fungus or chemicals.
Rheumatic fever	Febrile (characterized by fever) disease, usually occurring after a streptococcal infection.
Strep throat	Inflammation and infection of the throat caused by streptococcus bacteria.
Syphilis	Infectious venereal disease, usually transmitted by sexual contact. Caused by a spirochete bacterium.
Tetanus	Infectious disease produced by the toxins from the tetanus bacillus. The first sign is stiffness of the jaw, hence the common name "lockjaw."
Tuberculosis (TB)	A disease that primarily affects the lungs but can spread to other parts of the body. Caused by various strains of the bacterium *Mycobacterium tuberculosis*.

Infectious Disease Caused by Fungi

NAME	DESCRIPTION
Tinea (ringworm)	A fungal skin infection that gets its name because it appears serpentine like a worm. *Tinea corporis* means the location is on the trunk or body, *tinea capitis* affects the scalp, and *tinea pedis* refers to the feet, and is commonly known as athlete's foot.

Infectious Diseases Caused by Parasites

NAME	DESCRIPTION
Giardiasis	Disease transmitted by the oral-fecal route and through untreated water. Causes diarrhea.
Malaria	Disease transmitted to humans from the bite of an infected anopheles mosquito. Protozoan parasites invade the red blood cells and create symptoms such as high fever and chills.
Scabies	A highly contagious skin condition that results from a mite that burrows beneath the skin, leaving its feces behind. The feces leave red lines of inflammation on the skin.

Infectious Diseases Caused by Protozoa

NAME	DESCRIPTION
Amebic dysentery	Condition characterized by loose stools; causes inflammation of the intestines.
Trichomoniasis	Condition that affects the reproductive organs and can be transmitted through sexual intercourse.

Infectious Diseases Caused by Viruses

NAME	DESCRIPTION
Acquired immune deficiency syndrome (AIDS)	Syndrome caused by HIV (human immunodeficiency virus), resulting in decreased resistance to infections. Transmitted by blood and body fluids.
Hepatitis	Hepatitis types A, B, C, D, and E are all caused by a virus. This disease affects the liver and can cause mild to moderate symptoms or chronic illness, and possibly death. Healthcare workers are encouraged to be vaccinated for hepatitis B because they are at risk for contact with client blood and body fluids.
Herpes simplex virus types 1 and 2 (HSV-1, HSV-2)	Typically HSV-1 causes cold sores, is very contagious, and is spread through contact with infected saliva. HSV-2, known as genital herpes, is sexually transmitted. However, it should be noted that there can be crossing over, with HSV-1 infecting the genitals and HSV-2 infecting the mouth.
Human immunodeficiency virus (HIV)	Virus that destroys the immune system and can result in AIDS (acquired immune deficiency syndrome).
Human papillomavirus (HPV)	The most common sexually transmitted infection. Some strains of HPV cause harmless verrucae (warts); other strains are the greatest single risk factor for cervical cancer and may also cause other, less common cancers such as cancer of the vagina, penis, and oropharynx.
Influenza	Commonly called "the flu"; an infection of both the upper and lower respiratory tracts.
Mononucleosis	A highly contagious viral infection spread through the saliva of the infected person. Caused by either the Epstein-Barr virus or the cytomegalovirus (CMV).
Severe acute respiratory syndrome (SARS)	Highly contagious disease that causes severe flulike symptoms.
Upper respiratory (tract) infection (URI)	The term often used for the common cold, including pharyngitis (sore throat). Caused by the rhinovirus.
Varicella	Highly contagious disease caused by the varicella-zoster virus. Also called chickenpox, it is characterized by the presence of skin lesions. Shingles is also caused by varicella and is seen in patients who have previously had chickenpox.

Genetic Diseases

DISEASE	DESCRIPTION
Albinism	A genetic condition in which a person is born with little or no pigmentation in the skin, eyes, or hair.
Cystic fibrosis	A life-threatening disease that affects the lungs and pancreas. It is one of the most common inherited life-threatening disorders among Caucasians in the United States.
Down syndrome	Abnormal cell division involving chromosome 21 that results in physical abnormalities and some form of mental retardation. It is the single most common type of birth defect.
Fragile X syndrome	The most common inherited cause of learning disability, caused by a defect on one of the genes on the X chromosome. It affects boys more severely than girls.
Hemophilia	Inheritable bleeding disorder in which an essential clotting factor is low or missing, primarily affecting males.
Klinefelter's syndrome	A disorder in which males have an extra X chromosome, resulting in tall stature, pear-shaped fat distribution, small testes, sparse body hair, infertility, and slightly lower intelligence.
Muscular dystrophy	A group of genetic disorders that affect the muscular and nervous systems, most often affecting males.
Phenylketonuria (PKU)	A genetic disorder in which the body is unable to properly eliminate phenylalanine, which is an essential amino acid. Organ damage, mental retardation, and even death are possible.
Turner's syndrome	A disorder that results when females have a single X chromosome. Symptoms include a webbed neck, broad chest, short stature, and infertility. Intelligence is normal.

Common Diseases and Disorders in the United States*

DISEASE	EXAMPLES	SCREENING AND PREVENTION
Heart disease	Coronary artery disease, atherosclerosis, congestive heart failure	Monitor blood pressure and cholesterol and triglyceride levels, and have routine electrocardiograms (ECG).
Cancer	Skin, lung, breast, prostate, blood, colorectal, gynecologic, HPV-related	Have routine breast or prostate exam, Pap smear, and colonoscopy. Monitor size and shape of skin lesions. Maintain healthy eating habits and a good body weight, exercise, do not use tobacco products, and limit alcohol consumption.
Cerebrovascular diseases	Stroke, deep vein thrombosis, aneurysm, embolism	Maintain healthy eating habits and a good body weight, exercise, do not use tobacco products, and limit alcohol consumption. Have routine screening tests and physical exams.
Chronic respiratory diseases	Asthma, COPD, tuberculosis	Do not use tobacco products, avoid irritants and allergens, and monitor air quality. Have routine screening tests (TB skin test) and vaccinations.
Diabetes mellitus	Type 1, type 2, gestational	Have blood glucose tests, including fasting blood sugar, and hemoglobin A1c blood test. Maintain healthy eating habits and a good body weight, exercise, and limit alcohol and sugar consumption.
Alzheimer's disease		Maintain a healthy lifestyle and have a regular physical examination.
Influenza		Maintain a healthy lifestyle and obtain a yearly flu vaccination.
Pneumonia		Maintain a healthy lifestyle and obtain a yearly pneumonia vaccination.
Nephritis/nephrosis	Chronic renal disease (CRD), end stage renal disease (ESRD)	Have routine urinalysis. Maintain healthy eating habits and a good body weight, exercise, do not use tobacco products, and limit alcohol consumption.

*Entries ordered from most to least common.

Skin Lesions

NAME AND EXAMPLE	DESCRIPTION
Bulla	A large blister or cluster of blisters.
Cicatrix	A scar, usually inside a wound or tissue.
Crust	Dried blood or pus on the skin.
Ecchymosis	A black-and-blue mark or bruise.
Erosion	A shallow area of skin worn away by friction or pressure.
Excoriation	A scratch; may be covered with dried blood.
Fissure	A crack in the skin's surface.
Keloid	An overgrowth of scar tissue.
Macule	A flat skin discoloration, such as a freckle or a flat mole.
Nodule	A large pimple or small node (larger than 1 cm).

NAME AND EXAMPLE	DESCRIPTION
Papule	An elevated mass similar to but smaller than a nodule.
Petechiae	Pinpoint skin hemorrhages that result from bleeding disorders.
Plaque	A small, flat, scaly area of the skin.
Purpura	Purple-red bruises; usually the result of clotting abnormalities.
Pustule	An elevated (infected) lesion containing pus.
Scale	Thin plaque of epithelial tissue on the skin's surface.
Tumor	A swelling of abnormal tissue growth.
Ulcer	A wound that results from tissue loss.
Vesicle	A blister.
Wheal	Another term for hive.

Classifications of Fractures

NAME AND EXAMPLE	DESCRIPTION
Closed fracture (simple fracture)	Fracture in which the skin remains intact.
Comminuted fracture	Fracture in which the bone has broken into several fragments.
Complete fracture	Fracture that goes across the entire bone.
Greenstick fracture	Fracture commonly seen in children; occurs in bones that are not completely ossified, so there is a bending and only one side of the bone is fractured, rather than a complete breaking of bone.
Impacted fracture	Fracture in which one end of the fractured bone is driven into the interior of the other.

Classifications of Fractures (*concluded*)

NAME AND EXAMPLE	DESCRIPTION
Incomplete fracture	Fracture that goes through only part of the bone.
Open fracture (compound fracture)	Fracture in which the skin is broken.

Bone Disorders

NAME	DESCRIPTION
Arthritis	A general term meaning joint inflammation.
Bursitis	Inflammation of a bursa, which is the fluid-filled sac that cushions tendons. (Tendons attach muscles to bone.)
Carpal tunnel syndrome (CTS)	Occurs when the median nerve in the wrist is excessively compressed by an inflamed tendon (the flexor retinaculum).
Gout (gouty arthritis)	A type of arthritis associated with high uric acid levels in the blood with crystalline deposits in the joints, kidneys, and various soft tissues.
Kyphosis	An abnormal, exaggerated curvature of the spine, most often at the thoracic level. This condition is often referred to as humpback.
Lordosis	An exaggerated inward (convex) curvature of the lumbar spine. The condition is sometimes called swayback.
Osteoarthritis (OA)	Also known as degenerative joint disease (DJD) or wear-and-tear arthritis.
Osteogenesis imperfecta (brittle bone disease)	People with brittle bone disease have decreased amounts of collagen in their bones, which leads to very fragile bones.
Osteoporosis	A condition in which bones become thin (more porous) over time.
Osteosarcoma	A type of bone cancer that originates from osteoblasts, the cells that make bone tissue. It is most often seen in children, teens, and young adults, and occurs more often in males than females.
Paget's disease	Causes bones to enlarge and become deformed and weak. It usually affects people older than 40 years of age.
Rheumatoid arthritis (RA)	A chronic, systemic inflammatory disease that attacks the smaller joints such as those in the hands and feet.
Scoliosis	An abnormal, S-shaped lateral curvature of the thoracic or lumbar spine.

Classifications of Burns

NAME	DESCRIPTION
First-degree	A superficial burn that causes pain and makes the surrounding skin turn red.
Second-degree	A partial-thickness burn that extends deeper into the skin than first-degree burns; causes blistering along with pain and redness.
Third-degree	A full-thickness burn that involves all layers of the skin and requires immediate medical assistance.

Diseases and Disorders of the Integumentary System

NAME	DESCRIPTION
Acne vulgaris	An infection of the sebaceous gland(s), which causes pustules, papules, and scarring of the affected skin.
Alopecia	The absence or loss of hair, especially of the head (baldness).
Basal cell carcinoma	Skin cancer that originates from the basal layer of the epidermis and rarely metastasizes (spreads).
Cellulitis	An inflammation of the connective tissue in skin that is most often seen on the face and legs. A bacterial infection by *Staphylococcus aureus* or *Streptococcus* is the most common cause.
Comedos	Commonly known as blackheads; collections of bacteria, dead epithelial cells, and dried sebum.
Dermatitis	A general term describing any inflammation of the skin; can be caused by a wide range of disorders.

Diseases and Disorders of the Integumentary System (*concluded*)

NAME	DESCRIPTION
Eczema	A common chronic dermatitis that often has acute phases or flareups followed by periods of remission. The rash of eczema can appear anywhere on the body and appears as a red, scaly, pruritic (itchy) rash that may be painful.
Folliculitis	Inflammation of hair follicles. When it involves a single hair follicle, the condition is called a furuncle. When more than one hair follicle is involved, it is a carbuncle.
Jaundice	A yellow cast to the skin that often occurs with liver disease.
Lentigos	Commonly called liver spots or age spots; these are not caused by the liver but are the result of excessive melanin production due to overexposure to sunlight (UV rays).
Malignant melanoma	Skin cancer that arises from melanocytes and often metastasizes (spreads).
Psoriasis	A common chronic inflammatory skin condition that has an autoimmune basis.
Rosacea	A skin disorder that commonly appears as facial redness, predominantly over the cheeks and nose.
Squamous cell carcinoma	Skin cancer that arises from the upper cells of the epidermis and often metastasizes (spreads).

Diseases and Disorders of the Muscular System

NAME	DESCRIPTION
Fibromyalgia	A fairly common condition that results in chronic pain primarily in joints, muscles, and tendons. It most commonly affects women between the ages of 20 and 50.
Muscular dystrophy (MD)	A group of inherited disorders characterized by muscle weakness and a loss of muscle tissue.
Myasthenia gravis	A condition in which affected persons experience muscle weakness. In this autoimmune condition, a person produces antibodies that prevent muscles from receiving neurotransmitters from neurons.
Sprains	Injuries that excessively stretch or tear ligaments at a joint.
Strains	Caused by stretching or tearing of muscles or tendons.
Tendonitis	Painful inflammation of a tendon as well as of the tendon–muscle attachment to a bone.
Torticollis	Also known as wry neck. This condition is due to abnormally contracted neck muscles. The head typically bends toward the side of the contracted muscle and the chin rotates to the opposite side.

Diseases and Disorders of the Blood and Circulatory System

NAME	DESCRIPTION
Anemia	A symptom of an underlying disease process. Anemia occurs when the blood has less than its normal oxygen-carrying capacity. Anemia is the most common blood disorder in the United States and occurs more often in women than in men.
Aneurysm	A ballooned, weakened arterial wall. The most common locations of aneurysms are the aorta and the arteries in the brain, legs, intestines, and spleen. An aortic aneurysm is a bulge in the wall of the aorta.
Leukemia	A neoplastic condition in which the bone marrow produces a large number of WBCs that are not normal.
Thrombocythemia	A condition in which there is an increase in the platelet count. This condition is the opposite of thrombocytopenia.
Thrombocytopenia	A condition in which there are too few platelets, causing abnormal bleeding. This can be caused by a variety of situations, such as leukemia, certain medications, or idiopathic (unknown) reasons. The bleeding may be mild or life threatening.
Thrombophlebitis	A condition in which a thrombus and inflammation develop in a vein. It most commonly occurs in the deeper veins of the legs.
Varicose veins (varices or varicosities)	Tortuous or twisted, dilated veins that are usually seen in the legs. They affect women more often than men.

Diseases and Disorders of the Cardiovascular System

NAME	DESCRIPTION
Arrhythmias	Also known as dysrhythmias; abnormal heart rhythms and/or rates.
Congenital heart disease	A problem with the heart's structure and function due to abnormal heart development before birth.
Congestive heart failure (CHF)	Failure of the heart to pump effectively. The heart weakens over time and loses its ability to supply blood to the body.
Coronary artery disease (CAD)	Condition involving partial or complete blockage of major coronary arteries that supply blood to the heart.
Endocarditis	An inflammation of the innermost lining of the heart and heart valves, usually caused by bacterial infections.
Murmurs	Abnormal heart sounds. Not all murmurs indicate a heart disorder. Murmurs are graded from 1 to 6, with 6 being quite loud and the most serious.
Myocardial infarction (MI, heart attack)	Death of heart tissue due to deprivation of oxygen. The cardiac muscle sustains damage because of ischemia.
Myocarditis	An inflammation of the muscular layer of the heart caused by a viral infection. It leads to weakening of the heart wall.
Pericarditis	Inflammation of the pericardium, usually caused by complications of viral or bacterial infections, MIs, or chest injuries.

Diseases and Disorders of the Lymphatic and Immune Systems

NAME	DESCRIPTION
Allergies	Excessive immune responses to stimuli that would not ordinarily cause a reaction.
Autoimmune disease	A disease in which the immune system targets itself.
Chronic fatigue syndrome (CFS)	Causes a person to feel severe tiredness; possibly caused by the Epstein-Barr virus (EBV).
HIV/AIDS	A viral disease spread through blood and body fluids. AIDS is caused by the human immunodeficiency virus (HIV). HIV attacks T lymphocytes.
Lymphadenitis	Inflammation of lymph nodes; can be viral or bacterial.
Lymphadenopathy	Any disease involving the lymph nodes; causes can be autoimmune disease or malignancy.
Lymphedema	Blockage of lymphatic vessels; can be caused by genetics, parasitic infections, trauma to the vessels, tumors, radiation therapy, cellulitis, and surgeries.
Systemic lupus erythematosus (SLE)	Autoimmune disorder that affects women more often than men. Affects many organ systems of the body and has numerous symptoms, usually including joint pain and swelling.

Diseases and Disorders of the Respiratory System

NAME	DESCRIPTION
Allergic rhinitis	A hypersensitivity reaction to various airborne allergens.
Asthma	Hyperactivity of the bronchioles; an inflammatory response with excess mucus production.
Atelectasis	Commonly called collapsed lung; may occur after surgery or due to pleural effusion.
Bronchitis	Inflammation of the bronchi; can be acute or chronic. Often follows a cold. One common cause of chronic bronchitis is cigarette smoking.
Chronic obstructive pulmonary disease (COPD)	A group of lung disorders in which obstruction limits airflow to the lungs. COPD includes chronic bronchitis and emphysema.
Emphysema	A lung disease in which the alveolar walls are destroyed; often caused by cigarette smoking.
Laryngitis	An acute inflammation of the larynx; caused by viruses, bacteria, polyp formation, excessive use, allergies, smoking, heartburn, alcohol use, nerve damage, or stroke.
Lung cancer	The leading cancer-related cause of death in the United States. Caused by smoking or exposure to radon, asbestos, and industrial carcinogens. The three types are small cell lung cancer, squamous cell lung cancer, and adenocarcinoma.

Diseases and Disorders of the Respiratory System (*concluded*)

NAME	DESCRIPTION
Mesothelioma	A type of cancer that affects the pleura and is a result of asbestos exposure.
Pleuritis or pleurisy	A condition in which the pleura become inflamed.
Pneumonoconiosis	Lung diseases that result from years of exposure to different environmental or occupational types of dust.
Pulmonary edema	A condition in which fluids fill the alveoli of the lungs, most commonly occurring with left heart failure.
Pulmonary embolism	Blocked artery in the lungs, usually caused by a blood clot.
Respiratory distress syndrome (RDS)	Kills apparently healthy infants; the cause is unknown.
Sinusitis	Inflammation of the membranes lining the sinuses. It can be acute or chronic.
Sudden infant death syndrome (SIDS)	The sudden and unexpected death of an infant under one year of age. There is no explainable cause of death.

Diseases and Disorders of the Nervous System

NAME	DESCRIPTION
Alzheimer's disease	A progressive, degenerative disease of the gray matter of the brain that causes dementia.
Amyotrophic lateral sclerosis (ALS)	Commonly known as Lou Gehrig's disease; a fatal disorder characterized by the degeneration of neurons in the spinal cord and brain.
Bell's palsy	A disorder in which facial muscles are very weak or temporarily totally paralyzed. Results from damage to the facial nerve; causes are unknown.
Brain tumors and cancers	Abnormal growths in the brain. Malignant tumors that start in brain tissue are called primary brain cancers. Those that start elsewhere and metastasize to the brain are classified as secondary brain cancers.
Epilepsy	A condition in which the brain experiences repeated spontaneous seizures due to abnormal electrical activity of the brain.
Guillain-Barré syndrome	A disorder in which the body's immune system attacks part of the peripheral nervous system. It has a sudden and unexpected onset.
Multiple sclerosis (MS)	A chronic disease of the central nervous system in which myelin is destroyed. Some known causes are viruses, genetic factors, and immune system abnormalities.
Neuralgia	A group of disorders commonly referred to as nerve pain; most frequently occur in the nerves of the face.
Parkinson's disease	A nervous system disorder that is slowly progressive and degenerative.
Sciatica	A condition in which the sciatic nerve is damaged, commonly due to excessive pressure on the nerve from prolonged sitting.
Stroke or cerebrovascular accident (CVA)	Occurs when brain cells die because of inadequate blood perfusion of the brain.

Diseases and Disorders of the Urinary System

NAME	DESCRIPTION
Acute renal failure (ARF)	A sudden loss of kidney function due to burns, dehydration, low blood pressure, hemorrhage, allergic reactions, obstructions, poisons, alcohol abuse, or trauma.
Chronic renal failure (CRF)	A condition in which the kidneys slowly lose their ability to function due to diabetes, hypertension, kidney disease, or heart failure.
Cystitis	A urinary bladder infection caused by different types of bacteria.
Glomerulonephritis	Inflammation of the glomeruli of the kidney, caused by bacterial infections, renal diseases, and immune disorders.

Diseases and Disorders of the Urinary System (*concluded*)

NAME	DESCRIPTION
Incontinence	A condition in which an adult cannot control urination. Can be temporary or long lasting; caused by various medications, UTIs, nervous system disorders, cancers, surgery, trauma, or pregnancy.
Polycystic kidney disease (PKD)	A disorder in which the kidneys enlarge because of the presence of many cysts within them. The cause is hereditary.
Pyelonephritis	A type of complicated UTI that begins as a bladder infection and spreads up one or both ureters into the kidneys.
Renal calculi (kidney stones)	Solid masses of crystals that obstruct the ducts within the kidneys or ureters. Painful condition caused by gouty arthritis, ureter defects, overly concentrated urine, or UTIs.

Diseases and Disorders of the Male Reproductive System

NAME	DESCRIPTION
Benign prostatic hypertrophy (BPH)	The nonmalignant enlargement of the prostate gland.
Epididymitis	Inflammation of the epididymis. Most cases start as an infection of the urinary tract.
Impotence or erectile dysfunction (ED)	A disorder in which a male cannot achieve or maintain an erection to complete sexual intercourse. Can be caused by many physical or psychological conditions.
Prostate cancer	One of the most common cancers in men older than 40. A high-fat diet, increased age, and genetic predisposition all increase the risk.
Prostatitis	An inflammation of the prostate gland; can be acute or chronic. May be caused by bacterial infections, catheterization, trauma, excessive alcohol consumption, or scarring.
Testicular cancer	A malignant growth in one or both testicles. Occurs more commonly in males 15 to 30 years of age and is very aggressive.

Diseases and Disorders of the Female Reproductive System

NAME	DESCRIPTION
Breast cancer	One of the most common cancers in females. Evaluated and graded based on tumor size and how far cells have traveled from the site of origin.
Cervical cancer	This type of cancer usually develops slowly, and with early detection by a yearly Pap smear, treatment is often successful.
Cervicitis	Inflammation of the cervix, caused by an infection.
Dysmenorrhea	Condition of experiencing severe menstrual cramps that limit normal daily activities.
Endometriosis	A condition in which tissues that make up the lining of the uterus grow outside the uterus.
Fibrocystic breast change	Common condition consisting of abnormal but usually benign cysts in the breasts that vary in size related to the menstrual cycle.
Fibroids	Benign tumors that grow in the uterine wall.
Infertility	The inability to conceive a child due to scarring of the fallopian tubes, STIs, PID, endometriosis, or hormone imbalance.
Ovarian cancer	Considered more deadly than the other types of gynecological cancers because its symptoms are mild and indistinct.
Pelvic inflammatory disease (PID)	Acute or chronic infection of the reproductive tract caused by untreated STIs or bacteria.
Premenstrual syndrome (PMS)	A collection of symptoms that occur just before the menstrual period. Symptoms include anxiety, depression, irritability, bloating, and diarrhea.
Uterine (endometrial) cancer	Most common in postmenopausal women. It may be related to increased levels of estrogen.
Vaginitis	Inflammation of the vagina, associated with abnormal vaginal discharge.
Vulvovaginitis	Inflammation of the vulva and vagina.

Diseases and Disorders of the Digestive System

NAME	DESCRIPTION
Appendicitis	An inflammation of the appendix. If not treated promptly, it can be life threatening.
Cholelithiasis (gallstones)	Gallstones are hardened deposits of bile that can form in the gallbladder. Two types of calculi are cholesterol and pigment stones.
Cirrhosis	A chronic liver disease in which normal liver tissue is replaced with nonfunctional scar tissue.
Colitis	An inflammation of the large intestine. This condition can be chronic or short-lived, depending on the cause.
Colorectal cancer	Usually arises from the lining of the rectum or colon. This type of cancer is curable if diagnosed and treated early. It is the third most common cause of death due to cancer in both men and women.
Constipation	The condition of difficult defecation or elimination of feces.
Crohn's disease	A type of inflammatory bowel disease. It can affect any region of the digestive tract from the mouth to the anus, but most often affects the ileum (lower part of the small intestine).
Diarrhea	The condition of watery and frequent feces. Many cases of diarrhea do not require treatment because they are usually self-limiting and stop within a day or two.
Diverticulitis	Inflammation of diverticuli in the intestine. Diverticuli are abnormal dilations or pouches in the intestinal wall. When the diverticuli are not inflamed, the condition is known as *diverticulosis*.
Gastric or stomach ulcers	Occur when the lining of the stomach breaks down.
Gastritis	An inflammation of the stomach lining; often referred to as an upset stomach.
Gastroesophageal reflux disorder (GERD)	This occurs when stomach acids are pushed into the esophagus (also called heartburn). If not treated, GERD can cause erosion of the esophagus and even esophageal cancer.
Helicobacter pylori (H. pylori)	Organism implicated as being responsible for many diseases and disorders, including gastric ulcers.
Hemorrhoids	Varicosities (varicose veins) of the rectum or anus.
Hepatitis	Inflammation of the liver. There are many different types of hepatitis, but they all involve inflammation of the liver. Many signs and symptoms are shared, regardless of the cause of the inflammation.
Hiatal hernias	Occur when a portion of the stomach protrudes into the thoracic cavity through an opening (esophageal hiatus) in the diaphragm.
Inguinal hernias	Occur when a portion of the large intestine protrudes into the inguinal canal, which is located where the thigh and the body trunk meet. In males, the hernia can also protrude into the scrotum.
Oral cancer	Usually involves the lips or tongue but can occur anywhere in the mouth. This type of cancer tends to spread rapidly to other organs because of the high vascularity of this area.
Pancreatic cancer	The fourth leading cause of cancer death in the United States. The poor prognosis and five-year survival rate of only 5% is due to the late diagnosis in many cases.
Stomach cancer	Most commonly occurs in the uppermost (cardiac) portion of the stomach. It appears to occur more frequently in Japan, Chile, and Iceland than in the United States. This may be due to diets high in nitrates that are known to be carcinogenic.

Diseases and Disorders of Metabolism and Nutrition

NAME	DESCRIPTION
Anorexia nervosa	An eating disorder in which individuals have a perception of being overweight regardless of their actual weight.
Bulimia	An eating disorder in which the person may be of normal weight and may eat normal or even excessive amounts of food, but then vomits to rid himself or herself of the calories. Also called binge-and-purge eating.
Hypercholesterolemia	An excess of cholesterol in the blood.

Diseases and Disorders of Metabolism and Nutrition (*concluded*)

NAME	DESCRIPTION
Kwashiorkor	A type of starvation in which there is too little protein in the diet.
Malnutrition	Inadequate or excessive caloric intake.
Marasmus	A type of starvation that entails both protein and calorie insufficiency.
Metabolic syndrome	A group of symptoms such as hypertension, hyperinsulinism, excess body fat around the waist, and hypercholesterolemia. Lifestyle changes, medication, and regular appointments with a healthcare provider are essential.
Obesity	A body weight greater than 20% above the standard is considered obesity, and 50% over the standard is considered morbid obesity.
Starvation	A type of malnutrition resulting from inadequate caloric intake, inadequate resources, dietary imbalances, illness, or self-imposed starvation.

Diseases and Disorders of the Endocrine System

NAME	DESCRIPTION
Acromegaly	A condition caused by the secretion of too much growth hormone after puberty that causes the hands, feet, and face to take on unusual enlargement.
Addison's syndrome	Hyposecretion of ACTH in which patients experience anorexia, fatigue, weight loss, GI problems, and bronzing of the skin.
Diabetes insipidus	Hyposecretion of ADH. Symptoms include excessive urination, thirst, and dehydration.
Diabetes mellitus	Hyposecretion of insulin, categorized into type 1 (insulin dependent) and type 2 (non-insulin dependent).
Dwarfism (achondroplasia)	Abnormal underdevelopment of the body due to hyposecretion of growth hormone (GH). Adult height is 4 feet 10 inches or less.
Epinephrine and norepinephrine imbalances	Cause increase in blood pressure, tachycardia, and tachypnea.
Estrogen imbalances	Hyposecretion before or during menopause results in hot flashes, vaginal dryness, mood changes, depression, and loss of bone density.
Gigantism	Abnormal increase in the length of long bones due to hypersecretion of growth hormone during childhood.
Hypercalcemia	An increase in blood calcium levels, resulting in more calcium going into bone.
Hyperthyroidism	Excess secretion of thyroid hormone (TSH). Also called Grave's disease, it causes an overall increase in metabolism.
Hypocalcemia	A condition in which there is too little calcium in the blood.
Hypoglycemia	A low level of glucose in the blood.
Hypothyroidism	Too little TSH is secreted, resulting in slowing of metabolism.
Melatonin imbalances	Hyposecretion disturbs the sleep cycle and contributes to depression.
Pancreatic tumors	Malignant tumors have a poor prognosis due to difficulty in diagnosing.
Pheochromocytoma	A benign tumor of the adrenal medulla that can cause an increase in blood pressure.
Thymosin imbalances	Hyposecretion results in lack of mature T lymphocytes and a decrease in immunity.
Thyroid tumor	Abnormal growth on the thyroid gland. May be benign or malignant.

Diseases and Disorders of the Special Senses—The Eye

NAME	DESCRIPTION
Amblyopia	Commonly called lazy eye; occurs when a child does not use one eye regularly.
Astigmatism	Occurs when the cornea or lens has an abnormal shape, which causes blurred images in near or distant vision.
Blepharitis	Inflammation of the eyelid, as well as corneal abrasions (scratching of the cornea).
Cataracts	Opaque structures within the lens that prevent light from going through the lens. Over time, images begin to look fuzzy; if left untreated, cataracts may cause blindness.
Color blindness	The inability to see certain colors. May be inherited; occurs more commonly in males.
Dry eye syndrome (xerophthalmia)	One of the most common eye problems treated by physicians. This syndrome results from a decreased production of the oil within tears, which normally occurs with age.
Ectropion	Eversion of the lower eyelid.
Entropion	Inversion of the lower eyelid.
Glaucoma	Indicated by an increase in intraocular pressure, caused by a buildup of aqueous humor in the anterior chamber. If untreated, this excess pressure can lead to permanent damage of the optic nerve that can result in blindness.
Hyperopia	Farsightedness.
Macular degeneration	A progressive disease that usually affects people over the age of 50. It occurs when the retina no longer receives an adequate blood supply. It is the most common cause of vision loss in the United States.
Myopia	Nearsightedness.
Nystagmus	Rapid, involuntary eye movements. The movements may be horizontal or vertical.
Presbyopia	A common eye disorder that results in the loss of lens elasticity. It develops with age and causes a person to have difficulty seeing objects that are close up.
Retinal detachment	Occurs when the layers of the retina separate. It is considered a medical emergency and if not treated right away leads to permanent vision loss.
Strabismus	A misalignment of the eyes. Convergent strabismus is commonly referred to as crossed eyes.

Diseases and Disorders of the Special Senses—The Ear

NAME	DESCRIPTION
Cerumen impaction	Buildup of ear wax within the external auditory canal.
Meniere's disease	A disturbance in the equilibrium characterized by *vertigo* (dizziness), ringing in the ears, nausea, and progressive hearing loss.
Otitis externa	Inflammation of the outer ear.
Otitis media	Inflammation of the middle ear.
Otosclerosis	The immobilization of the stapes within the middle ear; a common cause of conductive hearing loss.
Presbycusis	Hearing loss because of the aging process.
Tinnitus	Ringing in the ears.
Vertigo	Dizziness.

Introduction

Although large electronic health record (EHR) systems were first introduced into hospital facilities in the 1960s, it wasn't until the last decade that their deployment became prolific across the broad spectrum of the healthcare community. An EHR system is a computerized, organized collection of individual patients' healthcare information in a digital format which can be stored, shared, and transmitted between healthcare facilities. Through the EHR, patients have become the beneficiary of improved medical care, greater safety, and increased control over medical records, enabling them to make important contributions to their healthcare.

Because of the changes in the way that health records are being stored, healthcare professionals must have exposure to and hands-on experience with electronic documentation. Specialization of informatics that now manage and process medical data has created the urgent need for professionals with the ability to chart using electronic clerical skills, clinical skills, and patient care in an EHR system.

The following exercises will enable you to develop the skills of inputing and retrieving healthcare data in the industry-standard SpringCharts™ EHR program.

Patient A Profile

The patient is Chris Sykes, a 12-year-old boy, born May 22, 2001. He is English-speaking. Chris lives with his parents in Sherman, Texas. He has come to the clinic with his mother because he is planning to start playing soccer and is required to obtain a pre-sports physical. His parents are concerned about the family history of hypertension and heart disease, and want to make sure it is safe for Chris to play. Chris is up to date on his immunizations.

Patient B Profile

The patient is Patti Adams, a 58-year-old married woman, born 06/25/1955. Her preferred language is English, her race is African-American, and

her ethnicity is Hispanic. Patti is an established patient who lives in Sherman, Texas. She lives with her husband and works at Flagler Technical Institute. Patti's past medical history includes left breast biopsy (2008), appendectomy (2001), occasional flu and sinus allergies, three pregnancies (G3), two live children (P2), and one miscarriage. Patti has a current diagnosis of hypertension. She arrives at the clinic today complaining of painful swelling on her left thigh.

Exercises

The 10 EHR exercises will allow you to work directly in an industry-standard EHR program that is currently used by physicians and medical staff in healthcare clinics across the country. These case studies will allow you to electronically practice the following medical assisting duties:

- Build a past medical history and family health history into a patient's fact sheet
- Record a patient's chief complaint
- Record vitals signs into an office visit note
- Order several tests
- Document the administration of patient instruction sheets

You will need to go to the Online Learning Center at www.mhhe.com/BoothMA5e. On the left side of the screen, click on the "SpringCharts EHR Activities" and then follow the instructions below.

If you have been assigned to complete the live EHR exercises, you will work in the SpringCharts EHR program. Before you

proceed, read these important tips! You need to make sure the EHR software and related files are loaded on your computer.

Step A. Is SpringCharts EHR Installed on My Computer?

SpringCharts EHR is downloaded from the *Medical Assisting* Online Learning Center (OLC), www.mhhe.com/BoothMA5e, and then installed on your individual computer or onto a flash drive.

Check to see if you have a SpringCharts icon on your desktop. See Figure IV-1. If it is not there, check with your instructor about downloading the software; you will need to follow the directions listed at www.mhhe.com/BoothMA5e. You will not be able to complete the exercises without the SpringCharts program.

Step B. How Do I Launch SpringCharts EHR?

When SpringCharts was installed on your computer or your flash drive, a shortcut icon to the SpringCharts program was placed on your desktop

- Double-click on the SpringCharts icon to open the program. You *may* receive a Windows Security Alert screen (Figure IV-2); it is designed to protect

FIGURE IV-1 SpringCharts desktop icon.

FIGURE IV-2 Windows' firewall security activation window.

your computer system. Please click the [Unblock] button to continue. You only have to do this the first time you launch the SpringCharts EHR program.

- A *Log On* window appears (Figure IV-3). On this version of SpringCharts the user name and password are hardcoded in, so you do not need to enter them. Select the [Log on] button to open the SpringCharts program.

- The program opens and automatically places two patients on the *Office Calendar* and two patients in the *Patient Tracker* (Figure IV-4). A small tutorial window displays in the center. This tutorial window appears every time you log in to this version of SpringCharts. Simply close this window by clicking on the red [X] in the upper right corner.

Congratulations! You have successfully launched SpringCharts EHR.

Check to be sure you have the correct version of SpringCharts. This may not be the first time your school has used the SpringCharts program. It is worthwhile to ensure that you have accessed the correct version of SpringCharts.

- In the opening screen of SpringCharts, click on the *Help* menu and select the *About SpringCharts* option (Figure IV-5).

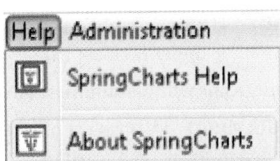

FIGURE IV-5   Accessing *AboutSpringCharts*.

- In the *Program Information* window you can find the version of SpringCharts you have launched (Figure IV-6). The correct version for this text is *2011 R 1.0.10*. If your screen displays a different version number, contact your instructor. You need the correct version to complete the exercises.

- Close the Program Information window by clicking the [Done] button. Close SpringCharts by clicking the *File* menu and selecting the *Quit* submenu. Answer *Yes* to the inquiry *Shut down SpringCharts?* Click the [No] button in the *Backup Recommended* window.

Congratulations! You are ready to begin your SpringCharts EHR adventure.

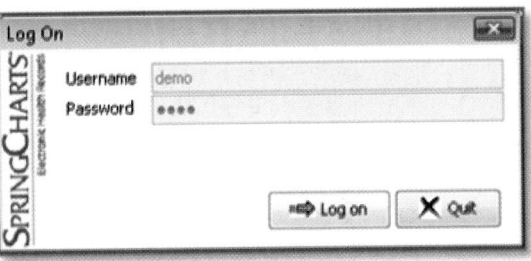

FIGURE IV-3   SpringCharts *Log On* window.

FIGURE IV-4   Opening screen of SpringCharts EHR.

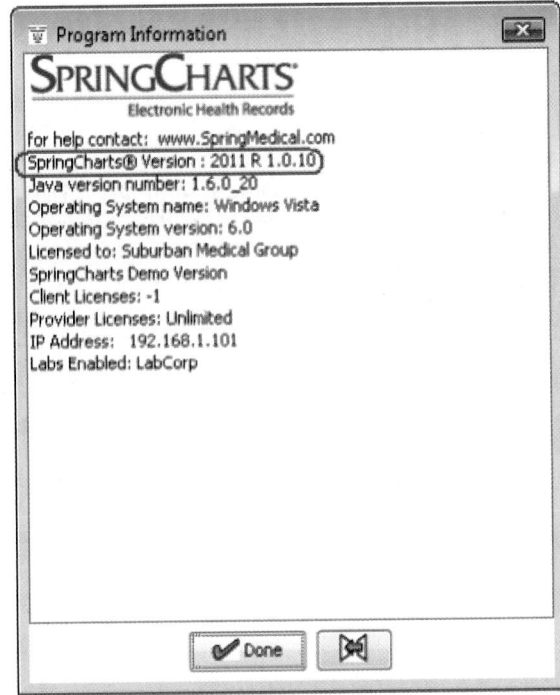

FIGURE IV-6   *Program Information* window.

Glossary

*Parenthetical numbers indicate the chapter in which the entry is a key term or is first defined in context. Entries not followed by a chapter number are important terms related to material covered but not specifically defined in the text.

10× lens (tĕn) A magnifying lens in the ocular of a microscope that magnifies an image ten times. (45*)

24-hour urine specimen (twĕn′tē fôr our yŏor′ in spĕs′ ə-mən) A urine specimen collected over a 24-hour period and used to complete a quantitative and qualitative analysis of one or more substances, such as sodium, chloride, and calcium. (47)

AAMA See **American Association of Medical Assistants.** (1)

abandonment (ə-băn′dən-mənt) A situation in which a health-care professional stops caring for a patient without arranging for care by an equally qualified substitute. (5)

ABA number (nŭm′ber) A fraction appearing in the upper-right corner of all printed checks that identifies the geographic area and specific bank on which the check is drawn. (21)

abduction (ab-dŭk′shuň) Movement away from the body. (25)

ABHES See **Accrediting Bureau of Health Education Schools.** (1)

abscess (ăb′sĕs′) A collection of pus (white blood cells, bacteria, and dead skin cells) that forms as a result of infection. (44)

absorption (əb-sôrp′shən) The process by which one substance is absorbed, or taken in and incorporated, into another, as when the body converts food or drugs into a form it can use. (51)

abuse (ə-byōōs′) A practice or behavior that is not indicative of or in line with sound medical or fiscal activity. (5)

access (ăk′sĕs) The way patients enter and exit a medical office. (7)

accessibility (ăk-sĕs′ə-bĭl′ĭ-tē) The ease with which people can move into and out of a space. (9)

accommodation (ă-kom′ə-dā-shən) The ability of the lens to change shape, allowing the eye to focus images of objects that are near or far away. (35)

accounts payable (ə-kounts′ pā′-ă-bəl) Money owed by a business; the practice's expenses. (20)

accounts receivable (ə-kounts′ rĭ-sē′ və-bəl) Income or money owed to a business. (20)

accreditation (ə-krĕd′ĭ-tā′shən) The documentation of official authorization or approval of a program. (1)

Accrediting Bureau of Health Education Schools (ABHES) (ə-′kre-dət-ing byoor-oh uhv helth edju′kei′shun sku′lz) An accrediting body that accredits private postsecondary institutions and programs that prepare individuals for entry into the medical assisting profession. (1)

acetabulum (as′ətab′yələm) The hip socket. (24)

acetylcholine (as-e-til-kō′lēn) A neurotransmitter released by the parasympathetic nerves onto organs and glands for resting and digesting. (25)

acetylcholinesterase (as′e-til-kō-lin-es′ter-ās) An enzyme within the nervous system that hydrolyzes acetylcholine to acetate and choline. (25)

acid-fast stain (ăs′ĭd făst stān) A staining procedure for identifying bacteria that have a waxy cell wall. (46)

acids (ăs′ĭds) Electrolytes that release hydrogen ions in water. (22)

acinar cells (as′i-nar sĕlz) Cells in the pancreas that produce pancreatic juice. (33)

acquired immunodeficiency syndrome (AIDS) (ə-kwīrd im′yū-nō-dē-fish′en-sē sĭn′drōm′) The most advanced stage of HIV infection; it severely weakens the body's immune system. (46)

acromegaly (ak-rō-meg′ă-lē) A disorder in which too much growth hormone is produced in adults. (34)

acrosome (ak′rō-sōm) An enzyme-filled sac covering the head of a sperm that aids in the penetration of the egg during fertilization. (32)

ACTH See **adrenocorticotropic hormone.** (34)

action potential (ăk′shən pə-tĕn′shəl) The flow of electrical current along the axon membrane. (30)

active file (ăk′tĭv fĭl) A file used on a consistent basis. (15)

active listening (ăk′tĭv lĭs′ənĭng) Part of two-way communication, such as offering feedback or asking questions; contrast with **passive listening.** (4)

active transport (ak′-tiv trans-pórt) The movement of a substance across a cell membrane from an area of low concentration to an area of high concentration. (22)

acupressure (ak-you-presh-er) Pressure applied by hands to various areas of the body to restore balance in the body's energy flow.

acupuncture (ak-you-punk-chūr) The practice of inserting needles into various areas of the body to restore balance in the body's energy flow.

acupuncturist (ăk′yŏo-pŭngk′chər-ĭst) A practitioner of acupuncture. The acupuncturist uses hollow needles inserted into the patient's skin to treat pain, discomfort, or systemic imbalances. (2)

acute (ə-kyōōt′) Having a rapid onset and progress, as acute appendicitis. (18)

ADA See **Americans with Disabilities Act.** (7)

addiction (ă-dĭk′shun) A physical or psychological dependence on a substance, usually involving a pattern of behavior that includes obsessive or compulsive preoccupation with the substance and the security of its supply, as well as a high rate of relapse after withdrawal. (36, 40)

Addison's disease (ă-dĭsuns dĭzēz) A condition in which the adrenal glands fail to produce enough corticosteroids. (34)

add-on code (ăd′on′ kōd) A code indicating procedures that are usually carried out in addition to another procedure. Add-on codes are used together with the primary code. (19)

adduction (ă-dŭk′shŭn) Movement toward the body. (25)

adenoids (ăd′n-oidz′) See **pharyngeal tonsils.** (33)

ADH See **antidiuretic hormone.** (34)

adjustment (ə-jŭst′-ment) Manual treatments given by a chiropractor that move the joints of the spine and other joints into proper alignment. (18, 44)

administer (ăd-mǐn´ǐ-stər) To give a drug directly by injection, by mouth, or by any other route that introduces the drug into the body. (51)

adrenocorticotropic hormone (ACTH) (ă-drē´nō-kōr´ti-kō-trō´pik hor´mōn) Hormone that stimulates the adrenal cortex to release its hormones. (34)

advance scheduling (ăd-văns skěj´ōōl-ǐng) Booking an appointment several weeks or even months in advance. (16)

AED See **automated external defibrillator.** (57)

aerobes (âr´ōbs´) Bacteria that grow best in the presence of oxygen. (46)

aerobic respiration (â-rō´bǐk rěs´pə-rā´shən) A process that requires large amounts of oxygen and uses glucose to make ATP. (25)

afebrile (ā-feb´ril) Having a body temperature within one's normal range. (37)

afferent arterioles (ăf´ər-ənt ar-tēr´ē-ōlz) Structures that deliver blood to the glomeruli of the kidneys. (31)

afferent nerves (ăf´ər-ənt nûrvs) A type of sensory nerves that are responsible for detecting sensory information from the environment or even from inside the body and bringing it to the CNS for interpretation. (30)

affiliation agreement (ə-fĭl´ē-ā´shənə-grē´mənt) An agreement that applied training participants must sign that states the expectations of the facility and the expectations of the student. (58)

agar (ā´gär´) A gelatin-like substance derived from seaweed that gives a culture medium its semisolid consistency. (46)

age analysis (āj ə-năl´ĭ-sĭs) The process of clarifying and reviewing past due accounts by age from the first date of billing. (20)

agenda (ə-jěn´də) The list of topics discussed or presented at a meeting, in order of presentation. (56)

agent (ā´-jənt) (legal) A person who acts on a physician's behalf while performing professional tasks; (clinical) an active principal or entity that produces a certain effect, for example, an infectious agent. (3)

agglutination (ă-glū-ti-nā´shŭn) The clumping of red blood cells following a blood transfusion. (27)

aggressive (ə-grěs´ĭv) Imposing one's position on others or trying to manipulate them. (4)

agonist (ăg´ənist) See **antagonist.** (25)

agranular leukocyte (ă-gran´-yulər lū´kō-sīt) A type of leukocyte (white blood cell) with a solid nucleus and clear cytoplasm; includes lymphocytes and monocytes. (27)

agranulocyte (ă-gran´yū-lō-sīt) See **agranular leukocyte.** (27)

AIDS See **Acquired Immune Deficiency Syndrome.** (46)

albumins (ăl-byōō´mĭns) The smallest of the plasma proteins. Albumins are important for pulling water into the bloodstream to help maintain blood pressure. (27)

alcohol-based hand disinfectants (AHD) (al´kŏ-hol bāsd hand dis-in-fek´tănts) Gels, foams, or liquids with an alcohol content of 60–95% that are used for hand disinfection. (6)

aldosterone (al-dos´ter-ōn) A hormone produced in the adrenal glands that acts on the kidney. It causes the body to retain sodium and excrete potassium. Its role is to maintain blood volume and pressure. (32)

alimentary canal (ăl´ə-měn´tə-rē kə-năl´) The organs of the digestive system that extend from the mouth to the anus. (33)

allele (ə-lēl´) Any one of a pair or series of **genes** that occupy a specific position on a specific **chromosome.** (22)

allergen (ăl´ər-jən) An antigen that induces an allergic reaction. (28)

allergic rhinitis (al´ərjik rī-nī´tis) A hypersensitivity reaction to various airborne allergens. (29)

allergist (ăl´ər-jĭst) A specialist who diagnoses and treats physical reactions to substances including mold, dust, fur, pollen, foods, drugs, and chemicals. (2)

allopathy (ə-lō-păth´-ē) The usual medical practice of physicians and other health professionals; also known as conventional medicine.

allowed charge (ə-loud´ chärj) The amount that is the most the payer will pay any provider for each procedure or service. (17)

alopecia (ăl´ə-pē´shə) The clinical term for baldness. (23)

alphabetic filing system (ăl´fə-bět´ik fī´lǐng sis´təm) A filing system in which the files are arranged in alphabetic order, with the patient's last name first, followed by the first name and middle initial. (15)

Alphabetic Index (ăl´fə-bět´ik ĭn´děks´) One of two ways diagnoses are listed in the ICD-9-CM. They appear in alphabetic order with their corresponding diagnosis codes. (18)

alternative medicine (ôl-tûr´-nə-tĭv měd´-ĭ-sĭn) The type of medicine used in place of conventional medicine to promote health and treat disease.

alveolar glands (al-vē´ō-lăr glăndz) Glands that make milk under the influence of the hormone **prolactin.** (32)

alveoli (ăl-vē´ə-lī´) Clusters of air sacs in which the exchange of gases between air and blood takes place; located in the lungs. (29)

amblyopia (am-blē-ō´pē-ă) Poor vision in one eye without a detectable cause. (35)

amenorrhea (ā-men´ŏ-rē´ă) Absence or abnormal cessation of the menses. (39)

American Association of Medical Assistants (AAMA) (ə-měr´ĭkən ə-sō´sē-ā´shən měd´ĭ-kəl ə-sĭs´tənts) The professional organization that certifies medical assistants and works to maintain professional standards in the medical assisting profession. (1)

American Medical Technologists (AMT) (ă-mer´i-kăn med´i-kăl tek-nol´ŏ-jists) The registering organization for medical assistants that provides online continuing education, certification information, and member news. (1)

Americans with Disabilities Act (ADA) (ə-měr´ĭ-kəns dĭs´ə-bĭl´ĭ-tēs ăkt) A U.S. civil rights act forbidding discrimination against people because of a physical or mental handicap. (7)

amino acids (ə-mē´nō ăs´ĭds) Natural organic compounds found in plant and animal foods and used by the body to create protein. (55)

amnion (ăm´nē-ən) The innermost membrane enveloping the embryo and containing amniotic fluid. (32)

AMT See **American Medical Technologists.** (1)

anabolism (ənab´əlĭz´əm) The stage of metabolism in which substances such as nutrients are changed into more complex substances and used to build body tissues. (55)

anaerobe (ăn´ə-rōb´) A bacterium that grows best in the absence of oxygen. (46)

anal canal (ā´nəl kə-năl´) The last few centimeters of the rectum. (33)

anaphase (an´əfāz) The period of mitosis when the centromeres divide and pull the chromosomes (formerly chromatids) toward the centrioles at opposite sides of the cell. (22)

anaphylactic shock (an´ă-fi-lak´tik shok) A severe, often fatal form of shock characterized by smooth muscle contraction and capillary dilation initiated by cytotropic (IgE class) antibodies. (2)

anaphylaxis (an´ă-fī-lak´sis)   A severe allergic reaction with symptoms that include respiratory distress, difficulty in swallowing, pallor, and a drastic drop in blood pressure that can lead to circulatory collapse. (28)

anatomical position (an´ə-tŏm´ĭ-kəl pə-zĭsh´ən)   When the body is standing upright and facing forward with the arms at the side and the palms of the hands facing forward. (22)

anatomy (ə-nătə-mē)   The scientific term for the study of body structure. (22)

anemia (ə-nē´mē-ə)   A condition characterized by low red blood cell count. This condition decreases the ability to transport oxygen throughout the body. (27)

anergic reaction (an-er´jik rē-ăk´shən)   A lack of response to skin testing that indicates the body's inability to mount a normal response to invasion by a pathogen.

anesthesia (ăn´ĭs-thē´zhə)   A loss of sensation, particularly the feeling of pain. (44)

anesthetic (ăn´ĭs-thĕt´ik)   A medication that causes anesthesia. (44)

anesthetist (ă-nes´thĕ-tist)   A specialist who uses medications to cause patients to lose sensation or feeling during surgery. (2)

aneurysm (ăn´yə-rĭz´əm)   A serious and potentially life-threatening bulge in the wall of a blood vessel. (27)

angiography (an-jē-og´ră-fē)   An x-ray examination of a blood vessel, performed after the injection of a contrast medium, that evaluates the function and structure of one or more arteries or veins. (42)

annotate (ăn´ō-tāt´)   To underline or highlight key points of a document or to write reminders, make comments, and suggest actions in the margins. (10)

anorexia nervosa (ăn´ə-rĕk´sē-ə nûr-vō´sə)   An eating disorder in which people starve themselves because they fear that if they lose control of eating they will become grossly overweight. (55)

ANS   See autonomic nervous system. (30)

antagonist (ăn-tăg´ə-nist)   A muscle that produces the oppo-site movement of the **prime mover.** (25)

antecubital space (an-te-kyū´bi-tăl spās)   The inner side or bend of the elbow; the site at which the brachial artery is felt or heard when a pulse or blood pressure is taken. (37)

anterior (ăn-tîr´ē-ər)   Anatomical term meaning toward the front of the body; also called ventral. (22)

anthracosis (an´thrə kō´sis)   Chronic lung disease caused by the inhalation of coal deposits; also known as Black Lung Disease. (29)

antibodies (ăn´tĭ-bod´ēs)   Highly specific proteins that attach themselves to foreign substances in an initial step in destroying such substances, as part of the body's defenses. (28)

antibody-mediated response (an´ti-bod-ē mē´dē-ăt-ed rĕ-spons´)   The part of our body's immune response that occurs when B cells respond to antigens by becoming plasma cells, which make antibodies that attach to antigens. (28)

anticoagulants (an´tē-kō-ag´yŭ-läntz)   Substances that prevent clotting. (48)

antidiuretic hormone (ADH) (an´tē-dī-yū-ret´ik hôr´mōn´)   A hormone that increases water reabsorption, which decreases urine production and helps to maintain blood pressure. (34)

antigen (an´tĭ-jən)   A foreign substance that stimulates white blood cells to create antibodies when it enters the body. (28)

antihistamines (ăn´tē-hĭs´tə-mēnz)   Medications used to treat allergies. (28)

antimicrobial (an´tē-mī-krō´bē-ăl)   An agent that kills microorganisms or suppresses their growth. (46)

antioxidants (ăn´tē-ŏk´sĭ-dənt)   Chemical agents that fight cell-destroying chemical substances called free radicals. (55)

antiseptic (ăn´tĭ-sĕp´tĭk)   A cleaning product used on human tissue as an anti-infection agent. (9)

antivirus software (an-tē vī´rəs so ft-wer)   Software that prevents and removes computer viruses. Such programs may also detect and remove adware and spyware. (8)

anuria (an-yū´rē-ă)   The absence of urine production. (47)

aortic semilunar valve (ā ôr´tĭk sem´ē loonər valv)   Heart valve that is a semilunar valve and that is situated between the left ventricle and the aorta. (26)

apex (ā´pěks)   The left lower corner of the heart, where the strongest heart sounds can be heard. (37)

apical (ap´i-kăl)   Located at the **apex** of the heart. (37)

apnea (ap´nēə)   The absence of respiration. (37)

apocrine gland (ap´ō-krin glănd)   A type of sweat gland. It produces a thicker type of sweat than other sweat glands and contains more proteins. (23)

aponeurosis (ap´ō-nū-rō´sis)   A tough, sheet-like structure that is made of fibrous connective tissue. It typically attaches muscles to other muscles. (25)

appendicitis (ə-pĕn´dĭ-sī´tĭs)   Inflammation of the appendix. (33)

appendicular (ap´en-dik´yū-lăr)   The division of the skeletal system that consists of the bones of the arms, legs, pectoral girdle, and pelvic girdle. (24)

applied training (ă-plīd trān´ing)   An opportunity to work within a medical facility to gain the essential on-the-job experience for beginning your new career, sometimes known as an externship or practicum. (58)

applied training coordinator (ă-plīd trān´ing kō-ōr´di-nā-tŏr)   A professional who procures applied training sites and qualifies or assesses them to make certain that they provide a thorough educational experience. May also be known as a clinical coordinator. (58)

approximate (a-prŏk´s i māt)   To bring the edges of a wound together so the tissue surfaces are close in order to protect the area from further contamination and to minimize scar and scab formation. (44)

aqueous humor (a´kwē-əs hyōō´mər)   A liquid produced by the eye's ciliary body that fills the space between the cornea and the lens. (35)

arbitration (är´bĭ-trā´shən)   A process in which opposing sides choose a person or persons outside the court system, often someone with special knowledge in the field, to hear and decide a dispute. (5)

areflexia (ā-rē-flek´sē-ă)   The absence of reflexes. (30)

areola (ă-rē´ō-lă)   The pigmented area that surrounds the nipple. (32)

aromatherapy (a-rō´-mə-thēr´-ə-pē)   The use of essential oil extracts or essences from flowers, herbs, and trees to promote health and well-being.

arrector pili (ă-rek´tōr pī´lī)   Muscles attached to most hair follicles and found in the dermis. (23)

arrhythmia (ə-rĭth´mē-ə)   Irregularity in heart rhythm. (26)

arterial blood gases (är-tîr´ē-əl blŭd găs´ses)   A test that measures the amount of gases, such as oxygen and carbon dioxide, dissolved in arterial blood.

arthritis (arth rīt´is)   A general term meaning joint inflammation. (24)

arthrography (ar-throg′ră-fē) A radiologic procedure performed by a radiologist, who uses a contrast medium and fluoroscopy to help diagnose abnormalities or injuries in the cartilage, tendons, or ligaments of the joints—usually the knee or shoulder. (50)

arthroscopy (är-thŏs′kə-pē) A procedure in which an orthopedist examines a joint, usually the knee or shoulder, with a tubular instrument called an arthroscope; also used to guide surgical procedures. (42)

articular cartilage (ar-tik′yu-lăr kär′tl-ĭj) The cartilage that covers the **epiphysis** of long bones. (24)

articulations (ärtik′yəla′shən) The area where bones are joined together; joints. (24)

artifact (är′tə-făkt′) Any irrelevant object or mark observed when examining specimens or graphic records that is not related to the object being examined; for example, a foreign object visible through a microscope or an erroneous mark on an ECG strip. (45)

asbestosis (asbestō′sis) Chronic lung disease caused by the inhalation of asbestos fibers. (29)

ascending colon (ə-sĕnd′ĭng kō′lən) The segment of the large intestine that runs up the right side of the abdominal cavity. (33)

ascending tracts (ə-sĕnd′ĭng träkts) The tracts of the spinal cord that carry sensory information to the brain. (30)

asepsis (ă-sep′sis) The condition in which pathogens are absent or controlled. (6)

assault (ə-sôlt′) The open threat of bodily harm to another. (5)

assertive (ə-sûrt′tĭv) Being firm and standing up for oneself while showing respect for others. (4)

asset (ăs′ĕt′) An item owned by the practice that has a dollar value, such as the medical practice building, office equipment, or accounts receivable. (21)

assignment of benefits (ə-sīn′mənt bĕn′ə-fĭts) An authorization for an insurance carrier to pay a physician or practice directly. (17)

asthma (az′mə) A condition in which the tubes of the bronchial tree become obstructed due to inflammation. (29)

astigmatism (ə-stĭg′mə-tĭz′əm) A condition in which the cornea has an abnormal shape, which causes blurred images during near or distant vision. (43)

astrocytes (ăs′-trō-sīts) Star-shaped cells within the nervous system that anchor blood vessels to the nerve cells. (30)

atelectasis (at′ilek′təsis) The collapse of a lung because of fluid, air, pus, or blood. (29)

atherosclerosis (ăth′ə-rō-sklə-rō′sĭs) The accumulation of fatty deposits along the inner walls of arteries. (26)

atlas (ăt′ləs) The first cervical vertebra. (24)

atoms (ăt′əmz) The simplest units of all matter. (22)

atria (ā′trē-ă) [Singular: atrium] Chambers of the heart that receive blood from the veins and circulate it to the ventricles. (26)

atrial natriuretic peptide (ā′trē-ăl nā′trēyū-ret′ik pep′tīd) A hormone secreted by the heart that regulates blood pressure. (28)

atrioventricular bundle (ā′trē-ō-ventrik′yū-lar bŭn′dl) A structure that is located between the ventricles of the heart and that sends the electrical impulse to the Purkinje fibers. (26)

atrioventricular node (ā′trē-ō-ventrik′yū-lar nōd) A node that is located between the atria of the heart. After the electrical impulse reaches the atrioventricular node, the atria contract and the impulse is sent to the ventricles. (26)

atrioventricular septum (a′treo-ventrik′yu-lar səp′təm) The wall separating the upper atrial chambers from the lower ventricular chambers of the heart. (26)

attitude (at-i-tood) A disposition to act in a certain way. (3)

audiologist (aw-dē-ol′ōjist) A healthcare specialist who focuses on evaluating and correcting hearing problems. (43)

audiometer (aw-dē-om′ĕ-ter) An electronic device that measures hearing acuity by producing sounds in specific frequencies and intensities. (43)

audit (ô′dĭt) To examine and review a group of patient records for completeness and accuracy—particularly as related to their ability to back up the charges sent to health insurance carriers for reimbursement. (11)

auricle (ôr′ĭ-kəl) The outside part of the ear, made of cartilage and covered with skin. (35)

auscultated blood pressure (ô′skəl-tāt-ĕd blŭd prĕsh′ər) Blood pressure as measured by listening with a stethoscope. (37)

auscultation (ô′skəl-tā′shən) The process of listening to body sounds. (38)

authorization (ô′thər-ĭ-zā′shən) A form that explains in detail the standards for the use and disclosure of patient information for purposes other than treatment, payment, or healthcare operations. (3)

autoclave (aw′tō-klāv) A device that uses pressurized steam to sterilize instruments and equipment. (45)

autoimmune disease (aw′tō-ĭmyoŏn di-zēz′) Any condition in which the body attacks its own antigens, causing illness to the patient. (28)

automated external defibrillator (AED) (ô′tə-mā′tĭd ĭk-stûr′nəl dē-fib′ri-lā-ter) A computerized defibrillator programmed to recognize lethal heart rhythms and deliver an electrical shock to restore a normal rhythm. (57)

automated voice response unit (aw′tō-mā′tĕd voys rĕ-spons′ yū′nit) Automated answering unit with a recorded voice that offers the caller various options for routing the call. (13)

automatic puncturing devices (aw′tō-mat′ik pungk′shŭr-ing dĕ-vīs′-iz) A type of lancet that is spring loaded, is self-contained, and has a mechanically controlled skin puncture depth. (48)

autonomic (ô′tə-nŏm′ĭk) A division of the peripheral nervous system that connects the central nervous system to viscera such as the heart, stomach, intestines, glands, blood vessels, and bladder. (30)

autonomic nervous system (ANS) (ô′tə-nŏm′ĭk nūr′vəs sĭs′təm) A system that is in charge of the body's automatic functions, such as the respiratory and gastrointestinal systems. (30)

autopsy (ô-top′-sē) The examination of a cadaver to determine or confirm the cause of death. (2)

autosome (ô′tə-sōm′) A chromosome that is not a sex chromosome. (22)

axial (ăk′sē-əl) The division of the skeletal system that consists of the skull, vertebral column, and rib cage. (24)

axilla (ăk-sĭl′ə) Armpit; one of the four locations for temperature readings. (37)

axis (ak′-səs) The second vertebra of the neck on which the head turns. (24)

axon (ăk′sŏn′) A type of nerve fiber that is typically long and branches far from the cell body. Its function is to send information away from the cell body. (30)

Ayurveda (eye-yer-vay-duh) A form of medicine, originated in India, that uses herbal preparations, dietary changes, exercises, and meditation to restore health and promote well-being.

bacillus (ba-sil′ŭs) A rod-shaped bacterium. (46)

bacterial spore (băk-tîr´ē al spôr) A primitive, thick-walled reproductive body capable of developing into a new individual; resistant to killing through disinfection. (44)

balance billing (băl´əns bĭl´ĭng) Billing a patient for the difference between a higher usual fee and a lower allowed charge. (17)

balloon angioplasty (buh-loon an´je-o-plas´tē) A procedure using a slender, hollow tube passed through a coronary artery to compress a blockage in the artery. (42)

bandwidth (bănd´wĭdth´) A measurement, calculated in bits or bytes, of how much information can be sent or processed with one single instruction. (8)

barium enema (bâr´ē-əm ĕn´ə-mə) A radiologic procedure performed by a radiologist who administers barium sulfate through the anus, into the rectum, and then into the colon to help diagnose and evaluate obstructions, ulcers, polyps, diverticuloses, tumors, or motility problems of the colon or rectum; also called a lower GI (gastrointestinal) series. (50)

barium swallow (bâr´ē-əm swŏl´ō) A radiologic procedure that involves oral administration of a barium sulfate drink to help diagnose and evaluate obstructions, ulcers, polyps, diverticuloses, tumors, or motility problems of the esophagus, stomach, duodenum, and small intestine; also called an upper GI (gastrointestinal) series. (50)

baroreceptors (bar´ō-rē-sep´ters) Structures, located in the aorta and carotid arteries, that help regulate blood pressure. (26)

Bartholin's glands (bär´ tə linz glăndz) Glands lateral to the vagina that produce mucus for lubrication of the vagina. (32)

bases (bā´sēz´) Electrolytes that release hydroxyl ions in water. (22)

basophil (bā-sō-fil) A type of granular leukocyte that produces the chemical histamine, which aids the body in controlling allergic reactions and other exaggerated immunologic responses. (27)

battery (băt´ə-rē) An action that causes bodily harm to another. (5)

behavior modification (bĭ-hāv´yər mŏd´ə-fĭ-kā-shən) The altering of personal habits to promote a healthier lifestyle. (55)

benefits (bĕn´ə-fĭts) Payments for medical services. (17)

benign (bē-nīn´) A noncancerous or nonmalignant growth or condition. (28)

benign prostatic hypertrophy (bē nīn´ prostat´ik hī pur´trə fē) A noncancerous enlargement of the prostate gland. (32)

bicarbonate ions (bī-kar´bon-āt ī´onz) Elements formed when carbon dioxide gets into the bloodstream and reacts with water. In the alimentary canal, these ions neutralize acidic chyme arriving from the stomach. (29)

bicuspids (bī-kŭs´pĭds) Teeth with two cusps. There are two in front of each set of molars. (33)

bicuspid valve (bī-kŭs´pĭd vălv) Heart valve that has two cusps and that is located between the left atrium and the left ventricle. Also known as the mitral valve. (26)

bile (bīl) A substance created in the liver and stored in the gallbladder. Bile is a bitter yellow-green fluid that is used in the digestion of fats. (33)

bilirubin (bili-rū´bin) A bile pigment formed by the breakdown of hemoglobin in the liver. (27, 40)

bilirubinuria (bil´i-rū-bi-nū´rē-ă) The presence of bilirubin in the urine; one of the first signs of liver disease or conditions that involve the liver. (47)

biliverdin (bil-i-ver´din) A pigment released when a red blood cell is destroyed. (27)

biochemistry (bĭ´ō-kĕm´ĭ-strē) The study of matter and chemical reactions in the body. (22)

bioelectromagnetic-based therapies (bī´ō-ē-lĕk´tro-mag-ne-tik basd thĕr´ə-pēs) The use of measurable energy fields in such things as magnetic therapy, millimeter wave therapy, sound energy therapy, and light therapy.

bioethics (bī-ō-ĕth´ĭks) Principles of right and wrong in issues that arise from medical advances. (5)

biofeedback (bī-ō-fēd´-băk) A type of therapy in which an individual learns how to control involuntary body responses in order to promote health and treat disease.

biofield therapies (bī-ō-field thĕr´-ə-pēs) Treatments that affect the energy fields that surround and penetrate the human body in order to promote health and well-being.

biohazardous materials (bī-ō-hăz´ərd-əs mə-tir´ē-əls) Biological agents that can spread disease to living things. (44)

biohazardous waste container (bī-ō-hăz´ərd-əs wāst kən-tā´nər) A leak-proof, puncture-resistant container, color-coded red or labeled with a special biohazard symbol, that is used to store and dispose of contaminated supplies and equipment. (44)

biohazard symbol (bī-ō-hăz´ərd sĭm´bəl) A symbol that must appear on all containers used to store waste products, blood, blood products, or other specimens that may be infectious. (45)

biopsy (bī-op´-sē) The removal and examination of a sample of tissue from a living body for diagnostic purposes. (2, 28)

biopsy specimen (bī-ŏp´sē spĕs´ə-mən) A small amount of tissue removed from the body for examination under a microscope to diagnose an illness. (44)

bioterrorism (bī-ō´tĕr´ə-rĭz´əm) The intentional release of a biologic agent with the intent to harm individuals. (57)

birthday rule (bûrth´dā´rōol) A rule that states that the insurance policy of a policyholder whose birthday comes first in the year is the primary payer for all dependents. (17)

blastocyst (blas´tō-sist) A morula that travels down the uterine tube to the uterus and is invaded with fluid. It then implants into the wall of the uterus. (32)

bloodborne pathogen (blŭd-bôrn păth´ə-jən) A disease-causing microorganism carried in a host's blood and transmitted through contact with infected blood, tissue, or body fluids.

blood-brain barrier (blŭd brān bär´ē-ər) A structure that is formed from tight capillaries to protect the tissues of the central nervous system from certain substances. (30)

B lymphocyte (bē lĭm´fə-sīt´) A type of nongranular leukocyte that produces antibodies to combat specific pathogens. (48)

board-certified physician (bōrd sĕr´ti-fĭd fĭ-zish´ŭn) A licensed practitioner who has obtained education and licensing for 9 to 12 years and taken multiple tests known as board tests. (2)

body (bod-ee) Single-spaced lines of text that are the content of a business letter. (10)

body language (bŏd´ē lăng´gwĭj) Nonverbal communication, including facial expressions, eye contact, posture, touch, and attention to personal space. (4)

body mechanics (bod´ē mĕ-kan´iks) The application of physical principles to achieve maximum efficiency and to limit risk of physical stress or injury to the practitioner of physical therapy, massage therapy, or chiropractic or osteopathic manipulation. (7)

body surface area (BSA) (bod´ē sŭr´făs är´ē-ă) The area of the external surface of the body, expressed in square meters (m²); used to calculate metabolic, electrolyte, and nutritional requirements; drug dosage; and expected pulmonary function measurements. (52)

bolus (bō´ləs) The mass created when food is combined with saliva and mucus. (33)

bone conduction (bōn kən-dŭk´shən) The process by which sound waves pass through the bones of the skull directly to the inner ear, bypassing the outer and middle ears. (35)

bookkeeping (bŏŏk´kē´pĭng) The systematic recording of business transactions. (21)

botulism (bŏch´ə-lĭz´əm) A life-threatening type of food poisoning that results from eating improperly canned or preserved foods that have been contaminated with the bacterium *Clostridium botulinum*. (25)

boundaries (baun-d(ə-)rēs) A physical or psychological space that indicates the limit of appropriate versus inappropriate behavior. (4)

Bowman's capsule (bō´mənz kap´səl) A capsule that surrounds the **glomerulus** of the kidney. (31)

brachial artery (brāk´ē-ăl är´tə-rē) An artery that provides a palpable pulse and audible vascular sounds in the antecubital space (the bend of the elbow). (37)

brachytherapy (brak-ē-thār´ă-pē´) A radiation therapy technique in which a radiologist places temporary radioactive implants close to or directly into cancerous tissue; used for treating localized cancers. (50)

bradycardia (braid uh card e uh) A slow heart rate; usually less than 60 beats per minute. (37)

brain stem (brān stēm) A structure that connects the cerebrum to the spinal cord. (30)

breach of contract (brēch kŏn´trăkt´) The violation of or failure to live up to a contract's terms. (5)

bronchi (brŏn-kī) The two branches of the trachea that enter the lungs. (29)

bronchial tree (brŏng´kē-al trē) A series of tubes that begins where the distal end of the trachea branches. (29)

bronchioles (brŏng´kē-ōlz) A part of the respiratory tract that branches from the tertiary bronchi. (29)

buccal (bŭk´ăl) Between the cheek and gum. (53)

budget (bŭj´ĕt) The total sum of money allocated for a particular purpose or period of time. (56)

buffy coat (buf´ē kōt) The layer between the packed red blood cells and plasma in a centrifuged blood sample; this layer contains the white blood cells and platelets. (48)

bulbourethral glands (bŭl´bō-yū-rē´thrăl glăndz) Glands that lie beneath the prostate and empty their fluid into the urethra. Their fluid aids in sperm movement. (32)

bulimia (bōō-lē´mē-ə) An eating disorder in which people eat a large quantity of food in a short period of time (bingeing) and then attempt to counter the effects of bingeing by self-induced vomiting, use of laxatives or diuretics, and/or excessive exercise. (55)

bundled codes (bŭn´dĕld kōds) When healthcare services that are usually separate are considered as a single entity for purposes of classification and payment. (19)

bundle of His (bŭn´ dl ov hiss) Also known as the AV bundle, this is the node located between the ventricles of the heart that carries the electrical impulse from the AV node to the bundle branches. (26)

burnout (´bər-naut) The end result of prolonged periods of stress without relief. Burnout is an energy-depleting condition that can affect one's health and career. It can be common for those who work in healthcare. (4)

bursitis (bər-sī´tĭs) Inflammation of a bursa. (24)

butterfly system (bŭt´ĕr-flī sis´tĕm) A type of needle used to draw blood from patients with small or fragile veins. Sometimes called a winged infusion set, it has flexible wings attached to the needle and a length of flexible tubing. (48)

CABG See **coronary artery bypass graft.** (42)

calcaneus (kal-kā´nē-ŭs) The largest tarsal bone; also called the heel bone. (24)

calcitonin (kal-si-tō´nin) A hormone produced by the thyroid gland that lowers blood calcium levels by activating osteoblasts. (34)

calibrate (kăl´ə-brāt) To determine the caliber of; to standardize a measuring instrument. (37)

calibration syringe (kăl´ə-brā´shən sə-rĭnj) A standardized measuring instrument used to check and adjust the volume indicator on a spirometer. (49)

calorie (kăl´ə-rē) A unit used to measure the amount of energy food produces; the amount of energy needed to raise the temperature of 1 kg of water by 1°C. (55)

calyces (kă´lĭ-sēz´) Small cavities of the renal pelvis of the kidney. (31)

CAM (kăm) The acronym for complementary and alternative medicine. Complementary medicine is used with conventional medicine. Alternative medicine is used in place of conventional medicine.

canaliculi (kan-ă-lik´yū-lī) Tiny canals that connect lacunae to each other. (24)

cancellous (kan´siləs) Bone also known as spongy bone. It contains spaces within it containing the red bone marrow. (24)

capillary (kăp´ə-lĕr´ē) Branches of arterioles and the smallest type of blood vessel. (26)

capillary puncture (kăp´ə-lĕr´ē pŭngk´chər) A blood-drawing technique that requires a superficial puncture of the skin with a sharp point. (48)

capitation (kăp´ĭ-tā´shən) A payment structure in which a health maintenance organization prepays an annual set fee per patient to a physician. (17)

carboxyhemoglobin (kärbok´sēhē´məglō´bin) The term used when the hemoglobin of red blood cells is carrying carbon dioxide. (27)

carboxypeptidase (kar-bok-sē-pep´ti-dās) A pancreatic enzyme that digests proteins.

carcinogen (kär-sĭn´ə-jən) A factor that is known to cause the formation of cancer.

cardiac catheterization (kär´dē-ăk´ kath´ĕ-ter-ĭ-zā´shun) A diagnostic method in which a catheter is inserted into a vein or artery in the arm or leg and passed through blood vessels into the heart. (42)

cardiac cycle (kär´dē-ăk´ sī´kəl) The sequence of contraction and relaxation that makes up a complete heartbeat. (49)

cardiac output (kahr´dē-ak owt´put) The product of heart rate and stroke volume, measured in liters per minute; the amount of blood that is pumped by the heart in 1 minute. (26)

cardiac rehabilitation (kahr´dē-ak rē´hă-bil´i-tā´shŭn) A systematic program of exercise and nutritional, behavioral, and vocational counseling to optimize the recovery and physiologic capacity of the patient with cardiovascular disease. (2)

cardiac sphincter (kär´dē-ăk sfingk´tər) The valve-like structure composed of a circular band of muscle at the juncture of the esophagus and stomach. Also known as the esophageal sphincter. (33)

cardiologist (kär´dē-ŏl´ə-jĭst) A specialist who diagnoses and treats diseases of the heart and blood vessels (cardiovascular diseases). (2)

carditis (kar-dī´tis) Inflammation of the heart. (26)

carpal (kär´pəl) Bones of the wrist. (24)

carpal tunnel syndrome (kär´pəl tŭn´əl sĭn´drōm´) A painful disorder caused by compression of the median nerve in the carpal tunnel of the wrist. (24)

carrier (kăr´ē-ər) A reservoir host who is unaware of the presence of a pathogen and so spreads the disease while exhibiting no symptoms of infection. (6)

cash flow statement (kăsh flō stā´tmənt) A statement that shows the cash on hand at the beginning of a period, the income and disbursements made during the period, and the new amount of cash on hand at the end of the period. (21)

cashier's check (kă-shîrz´ chĕ´k) A bank check issued by a bank on bank paper and signed by a bank representative; usually purchased by individuals who do not have checking accounts. (21)

cast (kăst) Cylinder-shaped elements with flat or rounded ends, differing in composition and size, that form when protein from the breakdown of cells accumulates and precipitates in the kidney tubules and is washed into the urine. (47)

A rigid, external dressing, usually made of plaster or fiberglass, that is molded to the contours of the body part to which it is applied; used to immobilize a fractured or dislocated bone.

catabolism (kə tab´əliz´am) The stage of metabolism in which complex substances, including nutrients and body tissues, are broken down into simpler substances and converted into energy. (55)

cataracts (kăt´ə-răkts´) Cloudy areas that form in the lens of the eye that prevent light from reaching visual receptors. (35)

categories (kat´ĕ-gōr-ez) In both ICD-9 and ICD-10, the first 3 digits of the diagnosis code. (18)

catheterization (kath´ĕ-ter-ĭ-zǎ´shun) The procedure during which a catheter is inserted into a vessel, an organ, or a body cavity. (47)

caudal (kôd´l) See **inferior**. (22)

CD-ROM (sē´dē´rŏm´) A compact disc that contains software programs; an abbreviation for "compact disc—read-only memory." (8)

cecum (sē´kəm) The first section of the large intestine. (33)

celiac disease (sē´lē-ăk´dī-zĕz´) An intolerance to gluten that causes an immune response in the body and reduces the absorption of nutrients in the small intestines. (55)

cell body (sĕl bŏd´ē) The portion of the neuron that contains the nucleus and organelles. (30)

cell-mediated response (sel mē´dē-āt-id rĕspons´) The part of our body's immune response that occurs when T cells bind to antigens on cells and attack the antigens directly. (28)

cell membrane (sĕl mĕm´brān´) The outer limit of a cell that is thin and selectively permeable. It controls the movement of substances into and out of the cell. (22)

cells (sĕlz) The smallest living units of structure and function. (22)

cellulitis (sel-yū-lī´tis) Inflammation of cellular or connective tissue. (23)

cellulose (sĕl´yə-lōs´) A type of carbohydrate that is found in vegetables and cannot be digested by humans; commonly called fiber. (33)

Celsius (centigrade) (sĕ l´sē-əs) One of two common scales for measuring temperature; measured in degrees Celsius, or °C. (37)

Centers for Medicare and Medicaid Services (CMS) (sĕn´tərs mĕd´ĭ-kâr´ mĕd´ĭ-kăd´ sûr´vĭs-əz) A congressional agency designed to handle Medicare and Medicaid insurance claims. It was formerly known as the Health Care Financing Administration. (17)

central nervous system (CNS) (sĕn´trəl nûr´vəs sĭs´təm) A system that consists of the brain and the spinal cord. (30)

central processing unit (CPU) (sĕn´trəl prŏs´es´ĭng yōō´nĭt) A microprocessor, the primary computer chip responsible for interpreting and executing programs. (8)

centrifuge (sĕn´trə-fyōoj´) A device used to spin a specimen at high speed until it separates into its component parts. (45)

centrioles (sen´trē ōlz) Two cylinder-shaped organs near the cell nucleus that are essential for cell division, by equally dividing chromosomes to the daughter cells. (22)

cerebellum (sĕr´ə-bĕl´əm) An area of the brain inferior to the cerebrum that coordinates complex skeletal muscle coordination. (30)

cerebrospinal fluid (CSF) (sĕr´ĕ-brō-spī´nəl flōō´ĭd) The fluid in the subarachnoid space of the meninges and the central canal of the spinal cord. (30)

cerebrovascular accident (ser´əbrovas´kyələr ak´sidənt) A stroke. Caused by a hemorrhage in the brain or more often by a clot lodged in a cerebral artery. (27)

cerebrum (sĕr´ə-brəm) The largest part of the brain; it mainly includes the cerebral hemispheres. (30)

Certificate of Waiver tests (sər-tĭf´ĭ-kĭt wā´vər tĕsts) Laboratory tests that pose an insignificant risk to the patient if they are performed or interpreted incorrectly, are simple and accurate to such a degree that the risk of obtaining incorrect results is minimal, and have been approved by the Food and Drug Administration for use by patients at home; laboratories performing only Certificate of Waiver tests must meet less stringent standards than laboratories that perform tests in other categories. (45)

certification (sĕr´ti-fi-kā´shŭn) The attainment of board approval and credentialing in a specialty. (1)

certified check (sûr´tə-fĭd´ chĕk) A payer's check written and signed by the payer, which is stamped "certified" by the bank. The bank has already drawn money from the payer's account to guarantee that the check will be paid. (21)

Certified Medical Assistant (CMA) (sûr´tə-fĭd´ mĕd´ĭ-kəl ə-sĭs´tənt) A medical assistant whose knowledge about the skills of medical assistants, as summarized by the 2003 AAMA Role Delineation Study areas of competence, has been certified by the Certifying Board of the American Association of Medical Assistants (AAMA). (1)

cerumen (sə-rōo´mən) A wax-like substance produced by glands in the ear canal; also called earwax. (35)

cervical enlargement (sûr´vĭ-kəl in-lär´jmənt) The thickening of the spinal cord in the neck region. (30)

cervical orifice (sûr´vĭ-kəl ôr´ə-fĭs) The opening of the uterus through the cervix into the vagina. (32)

cervicitis (ser-vi-sī´tis) Inflammation of the cervix. (32)

cervix (sûr´vĭks) The lowest portion of the uterus that extends into the vagina. (32)

cesarean section (si zer´ē ən sək´ shən) A surgical incision of the abdomen and uterus to deliver a baby transabdominally. (32)

chain of command (chān kŏ-man´d) A command hierarchy where a group of people are committed to carrying out orders from the highest authority. (56)

chain of custody (chān kŭs′tə-dē) A procedure for ensuring that a specimen is obtained from a specified individual, is correctly identified, is under the uninterrupted control of authorized personnel, and has not been altered or replaced. (57)

CHAMPVA (Civilian Health and Medical Program of the Veterans Administration) (sĭ-vĭl′yən hĕlth mĕd′ĭ-kəl prō′ğram vĕtər-enz ăd-mĭn′ĭ-strā′shən) A type of health insurance that covers the expenses of families (dependent spouses and children) of veterans with total, permanent, and service-connected disabilities. It also covers the surviving families of veterans who die in the line of duty or as a result of service-connected disabilities. (17)

chancre (shang′ker) A painless ulcer that may appear on the tongue, the lips, the genitalia, the rectum, or elsewhere. (46)

chapters (chap-tərz) The breakdown of diagnosis codes by body system or disease. There are 17 chapters in ICD-9 and 21 in ICD-10. (18)

charge slip (chärj slĭp) The original record of services performed for a patient and the charges for those services. (20)

check (chĕk) A bank draft or order written by a payer that directs the bank to pay a sum of money on demand to the payee. (21)

CHEDDAR (chĕd′er) **C:** Chief complaint. **H:** History. **E:** Examination. **D:** Details of problem and complaints. **D:** Drugs and dosage. **A:** Assessment. **R:** Return visit information or referral, if applicable. (11)

chemical digestion (kem′i-kăl di-jes′chŭn) The breaking down of food for use by the body caused by enzymes in the body such as amylase. (33)

chemistry (kĕm′ĭ-strē) The study of the composition of matter and how matter changes. (22)

chemoreceptor (kē′mo-rĭ-sĕp′tôr) Any cell that is activated by a change in chemical concentration and results in a nerve impulse. The olfactory or smell receptors in the nose are an example of a chemoreceptor. (35)

Cheyne-Stokes respirations (chain stokes RES per ra shuns) A pattern of breathing that gradually alternates between deep and shallow breaths with a period of apnea or no breathing that can last from 5 to 40 seconds. (37)

chief cells (chēf sĕlz) Cells in the lining of the stomach that secrete **pepsinogen.** (33)

chief complaint (CC) (chēf kəm-plān′t) The patient's main issue of pain or ailment. (18, 36)

chiropractor (kī′rə-prăk′tôr) A physician who uses a system of therapy, including manipulation of the spine, to treat illness or pain. This treatment is done without drugs or surgery. (2)

chlamydia (klə mid′ē ah) A common bacterial STI caused by bacterium *Chlamydia trachomatis* that can lead to PID in women. (32)

cholangiography (kō-lan-jē-og′ră-fē) A test that evaluates the function of the bile ducts by injection of a contrast medium directly into the common bile duct (during gallbladder surgery) or through a T-tube (after gallbladder surgery or during radiologic testing) and taking an x-ray. (50)

cholecystography (kō-lē-sis-tog′ră-fē) A gallbladder function test performed by x-ray after the patient ingests an oral contrast agent; used to detect gallstones and bile duct obstruction. (42)

cholesterol (kə-lĕs′tə-rôl) A fat-related substance that the body produces in the liver and obtains from dietary sources; needed in small amounts to carry out several vital functions. High levels of cholesterol in the blood increase the risk of heart and artery disease. (33, 55)

chordae tendineae (kôr′dĕ ten-din′ā) Cord-like structures that attach the cusps of the heart valves to the papillary muscles in the ventricles. (26)

choroid (kôr′oid′) The middle layer of the eye, which contains the iris, the ciliary body, and most of the eye's blood vessels. (35)

chromosome (krō′mə-sōm′) Thread-like structures composed of DNA. (22)

chronic (krŏn′ĭk) Lasting a long time or recurring frequently, as in chronic osteoarthritis. (18)

chronic obstructive pulmonary disease (COPD) (krŏn′ĭk ob-strŭk′tiv pŏŏlmə-nĕr′ē dĭ-zēz′) A disease characterized by the presence of airflow obstruction as a result of chronic bronchitis or emphysema. It is typically progressive. Cigarette smoking is the leading cause. (29)

chronological résumé (krŏn′ə-lŏj′ĭ-kəl rĕz′ŏŏ-mā′) The type of résumé used by individuals who have job experience. Jobs are listed according to date, with the most recent being listed first. (58)

chylomicron (kī-lō-mi′kron) The least dense of the lipoproteins; it functions in lipid transportation. (27)

chyme (kīm) The mixture of food and gastric juice. (33)

chymotrypsin (kī-mō-trip′sin) A pancreatic enzyme that digests proteins. (32)

cilia (sil′ēa) Hair-like projections from the outside of the cell membrane on some cell types. (22)

ciliary body (sĭl′ē-ār′ē bŏd′ē) A wedge-shaped thickening in the middle layer of the eyeball that contains the muscles that control the shape of the lens. (35)

circumduction (ser-kŭm-dŭk′shŭn) Moving a body part in a circle; for example, tracing a circle with your arm. (25)

cirrhosis (sĭ-rō′sĭs) A long-lasting liver disease in which normal liver tissue is replaced with nonfunctioning scar tissue. (33)

Civilian Health and Medical Program of the Veterans Administration See **CHAMPVA.** (17)

civil law (sĭv′əl lô) Involves crimes against persons. A person can sue another person, business, or the government. Judgments often require a payment of money. (5)

clarification (klăr′ə-fĭ′kā′shən) Asking questions that provide an increased understanding of a problem. (36)

clarity (klăr′i-tē) Clearness in writing or stating a message. (10)

class action lawsuit (klăs-ăk′shənlô′sōōt) A lawsuit in which one or more people sue a company or other legal entity that allegedly wronged all of them in the same way. (20)

clavicle (klăv′ĭ-kəl) A slender, curved long bone that connects the sternum and the scapula; also called the collar bone. (24)

clean-catch midstream urine specimen (klēn-kăch mĭd′strēm yŏŏr′ĭn spĕs′əmən) A type of urine specimen that requires special cleansing of the external genitalia to avoid contamination by organisms residing near the external opening of the urethra and is used to identify the number and types of pathogens present in urine; sometimes referred to as midvoid. (47)

clearinghouse (klĭr′ĭng-hous′) A group that takes nonstandard medical billing software formats and translates them into the standard EDI formats. (17)

cleavage (klē′vĭj) The rapid rate of mitosis of a zygote immediately following fertilization. (32)

CLIA ′88 See **Clinical Laboratory Improvement Amendments of 1988.** (1)

clinical diagnosis (klĭn′ĭ-kəldī′əg-nō′sĭs) A diagnosis based on the signs and symptoms of a disease or condition. (38)

clinical drug trial (klĭn´ĭ-kəl drŭg trī´əl) An internationally recognized research protocol designed to evaluate the efficacy or safety of drugs and to produce scientifically valid results.

Clinical Laboratory Improvement Amendments of 1988 (CLIA '88) (klē´ə) A law enacted by Congress in 1988 that placed all laboratory facilities that conduct tests for diagnosing, preventing, or treating human disease or for assessing human health under federal regulations administered by the Health Care Financing Administration (HCFA) and the Centers for Disease Control and Prevention (CDC). (1)

clitoris (klĭt´ər-ĭs) Located anterior to the urethral opening in females. It contains erectile tissue and is rich in sensory nerves. (32)

clock speed (klŏk spēd) A measurement of how many instructions per second that a CPU can process. Clock speed is measured in megahertz (MHz) or gigahertz (GHz). (8)

closed file (klōzd fīl) A file for a patient who has died, moved away, or for some other reason no longer consults the office for medical expertise. (15)

closed posture (klōzd pŏs´chər) A position that conveys the feeling of not being totally receptive to what is being said; arms are often rigid or folded across the chest. (4)

cluster scheduling (klŭs´tər skĕj´ool-ĭng) The scheduling of similar appointments together at a certain time of the day or week. (16)

CMA See **Certified Medical Assistant.** (1)

CMS See **Centers for Medicare and Medicaid Services.** (17)

CNS See **central nervous system.** (30)

coagulation (kō-ăg´yə-lā´shən) The process by which a clot forms in blood. (27)

coccus (kŏk´əs) A spherical, round, or ovoid bacterium. (46)

coccyx (kŏk´sĭks) A small, triangular-shaped bone consisting of three to five fused vertebrae. (24)

cochlea (kŏk´lē-ă) A spiral-shaped canal in the inner ear that contains the hearing receptors. (35)

cochlear implant (kok´lē-ăr im´plant) Amplification device surgically implanted with its stimulating electrodes inserted directly into the nonfunctioning cochlea. (43)

code linkage (kōd lĭng´kĭj) Analysis of the connection between diagnostic and procedural information in order to evaluate the medical necessity of the reported charges.

This analysis is performed by insurance company representatives. (19)

coinsurance (kō-ĭn-shoor´əns) A fixed percentage of covered charges paid by the insured person after a deductible has been met. (17)

colitis (kə-lī´tĭs) Inflammation of the colon.

colonoscopy (kō-lon-os´kŏ-pē) A procedure used to determine the cause of diarrhea, constipation, bleeding, or lower abdominal pain by inserting a scope through the anus to provide direct visualization of the large intestine. (42)

colony (kŏl´ə-nē) A distinct group of microorganisms, visible with the naked eye, on the surface of a culture medium. (46)

color family (kŭl´ər făm´ə-lē) A group of colors that share certain characteristics, such as warmth or coolness, allowing them to blend well together. (7)

colposcopy (kol-pos´kŏ-pē) The examination of the vagina and cervix with an instrument called a colposcope to identify abnormal tissue, such as cancerous or precancerous cells. (39)

combining vowel (kəm-bīn-ĭng vou´əl) A vowel (often an o) that is placed between a word root and suffix to ease pronunciation. (22)

Commission on Accreditation of Allied Health Education Programs (CAAHEP) (kŏ-mish´ŭn ă-kred´i-tā´shŭn al´īd helth) A voluntary organization that accredits allied health education programs. (1)

common bile duct (kŏm´ən bīl dŭkt) Duct that carries bile to the duodenum. It is formed from the merger of the cystic and hepatic ducts. (33)

compactible file (kəm-păkt´-əbəl fīl) Files kept on rolling shelves that slide along permanent tracks in the floor and are stored close together or stacked when not in use. (15)

complement (kŏm´plə-mənt) A protein present in serum that is involved in specific defenses. (28)

complementary medicine (kŏm´-plə-měn-tə-rē měd´-i-sĭn) A type of medicine that is used with conventional medicine.

complete blood (cell) count (kŏm-plēt´ blŭd kownt) A combination of the following determinations: red blood cell indices and count, white blood cell count, hematocrit, hemoglobin, platelets, and differential blood count. (48)

complete proteins (kəm-plēt´ prō´tenz´) Proteins that contain all nine essential amino acids. (55)

complex carbohydrates (kəm-plĕks´ kär´bō-hī´drāt´s) Long chains of sugar units; also known as polysaccharides. (55)

complex inheritance (kəm-plĕks´ ĭn-hĕr´ĭ-təns) The inheritance of traits determined by multiple genes. (22)

compliance plan (kəm-plī´əns plăn) A process for finding, correcting, and preventing illegal medical office practices. (19)

complimentary closing (kom-pluh-men-tuh-ree kloh-zing) The closing remark of a business letter found two spaces below the last line of the body of the letter. (10)

compound (kŏm´pound´) A substance that is formed when two or more atoms of more than one element are chemically combined. (22)

compound microscope (kŏm´pound´mī´krə-skōp´) A microscope that uses two lenses to magnify the image created by condensed light focused through the object being examined. (45)

comprehension (kom´prē-hen´shŭn) Knowledge or understanding of an object, situation, event, or verbal statement. (3)

computed tomography (kəm-pyoot´ĕd tō-mogra-fē) A radiographic examination that produces a three-dimensional, cross-sectional view of an area of the body; may be performed with or without a contrast medium. (42)

concise (kən-sīs´) Brevity; the use of no unnecessary words. (10)

concurrent care (kŏn-kŭr´ĕnt kār) Care being provided by more than one physician, such as with specialists. (19)

concussion (kən-kŭsh´ən) A jarring injury to the brain; the most common type of head injury. (57)

conductive hearing loss (kon-dŭk-tiv´hĕr´ing lôs) A type of hearing loss that occurs when sound waves cannot be conducted through the ear. Most types are temporary. (43)

condyle (kon´dīl) Rounded articular surface on a bone. (22)

cones (kōnz) Light-sensing nerve cells in the eye, at the posterior of the retina, that are sensitive to color, provide sharp images, and function only in bright light. (35)

conflict (kŏn´flĭkt´) An opposition of opinions or ideas. (4)

conjunctiva (kŏn´jŭngk-tī´və) The protective membrane that lines the eyelid and covers the anterior of the sclera, or the white of the eye. (35)

conjunctivitis (kən-jŭngk´tə-vī´tĭs)   A contagious infection of the conjunctiva caused by bacteria, viruses, and allergies. The symptoms may include discharge, red eyes, itching, and swollen eyelids; also commonly called pinkeye. (35)

connective tissue (kə-nĕk´tĭv)   A tissue type that is the framework of the body. (22)

consent (kən-´sĕnt)   A voluntary agreement that a patient gives to allow a medically trained person the permission to touch, examine, and perform a treatment. (5)

constructive criticism (kən-stre´k-tiv kr´i-tə-si-zəm)   A type of critique that is aimed at giving an individual feedback about his or her performance in order to improve that performance. (3, 58)

consultation (kon´sŭl-tā´shŭn)   Meeting of two or more physicians or surgeons to evaluate the nature and progress of disease in a particular patient and to establish diagnosis, prognosis, and/or therapy. (19)

consumable (kən-soo´mə-bəl)   Able to be emptied or used up, as with supplies. (9)

consumer education (kən-soo´mərĕj´ə-ka´shən)   The process by which the average person learns to make informed decisions about goods and services, including healthcare. (14)

contagious (kən-tā´jəs)   Having a disease that can easily be transmitted to others. (7)

contaminated (kən-tăm´ə-nāt´ĕd)   Soiled or stained, particularly through contact with potentially infectious substances; no longer clean or sterile. (6, 9)

continuing education (kŏn-tin´yū-ing ed´yū-kā´shŭn)   Systematic professional learning experiences designed to augment knowledge and skills of healthcare professionals; education completed after the initial educational program; required for relicensure in some fields. (1)

contract (kŏn´trăct´)   A voluntary agreement between two parties in which specific promises are made. (5)

contraindication (kŏn´trə-ĭn´dĭ-kā´-shən)   A symptom that renders use of a remedy or procedure inadvisable, usually because of risk. (40)

contrast medium (kŏn´trast´ mē´dē-əm)   A substance that makes internal organs denser and blocks the passage of x-rays to photographic film. Introducing a contrast medium into certain structures or areas of the body can provide a clear image of organs and tissues and highlight indications of how well they are functioning. (50)

controlled substance (kən-trōld´ sŭb´stəns)   A drug or drug product that is categorized as potentially dangerous and addictive and is strictly regulated by federal laws. (51)

control sample (kən-trōl´ săm´pəl)   A specimen that has a known value; used as a comparison for test results on a patient sample. (45)

contusion (kon-tū´shŭn)   A closed wound, or bruise. (57)

conventional medicine (kən-vĕn´-shən-əl mĕd´-ĭ-sĭn)   The usual practice of physicians and other allied health professionals, such as physical therapists, psychologists, medical assistants, and registered nurses. Also known as allopathy.

conventions (kən-vĕn´shənz)   A list of abbreviations, punctuation, symbols, typefaces, and instructional notes appearing in the beginning of the ICD-9. The items provide guidelines for using the code set. (18)

convolutions (kŏn´və-loo´shənz)   The ridges of brain matter between the sulci; also called gyri. (30)

coordination of benefits (kō-ôr´dn-ā´shən bĕn´ə-fĭts)   A legal principle that limits payment by insurance companies to 100% of the cost of covered expenses. (17)

copayment (kō´pā-mĕnt, kō´pā)   A fixed or set amount paid for each healthcare or medical service; the remainder is paid by the health insurance plan. (17)

COPD   See **chronic obstructive pulmonary disease.** (29)

cornea (kôr´nē-ə)   A transparent area on the front of the outer layer of the eye that acts as a window to let light into the eye. (35)

coronary artery bypass graft (CABG) (kor´-uh-ner-ee ahr´-tuh-ree bahy´-pas grahft)   A surgery performed to bypass a blockage within a coronary artery with a vessel taken from another area. (42)

coronary sinus (kôr´ə-nĕr´ē sī´nəs)   The large vein that receives oxygen-poor blood from the cardiac veins and empties it into the right atrium of the heart. (26)

corporation (kôr-pə-´rā-shən)   A type of business group, such as a medical practice, that is established by law and managed by a board of directors. (5)

corpus callosum (kôr´pəs ka-l´ō-səm)   A thick bundle of nerve fibers that connects the cerebral hemispheres. (30)

corpus luteum (kôr´pŭs lū-tē´ŭm)   A ruptured follicle cell in the ovary following ovulation. (32)

cortex (kôr´təks´)   The outermost layer of the cerebrum. (30)

cortisol (kôr´ti-sol)   A steroid hormone that is released when a person is stressed. It decreases protein synthesis. (34)

coryza (côrī´zə)   Another name for an upper respiratory tract infection. The common cold. (29)

costal (kos´tăl)   Cartilage that attaches true ribs to the sternum. (24)

counseling (kown´sĕl-ing)   Provision of advice and instruction by a healthcare professional to patients. (19)

counter check (koun´tər chĕk)   A special bank check that allows a depositor to draw funds from his own account only, as when he has forgotten his checkbook. (21)

courtesy title (kûr´tĭ-sē tīt´l)   A title used before a person's name, such as Dr., Mr., or Ms. (10)

covered entity (kŭv´ərd en-tə-tē)   Any organization that transmits health information in an electronic form that is related in any way with a HIPAA-covered business. (8)

cover sheet (kŭv´ər shēt)   A form sent with a fax that provides details about the transmission. (10)

Cowper's glands (kou´ pərz glăndz)   Bulbourethral glands. (32)

coxal (koks-al´)   Pertaining to the bones of the pelvic girdle. The coxa is composed of the ilium, ischium, and pubis. (24)

CPT   See *Current Procedural Terminology.* (19)

CPU   See **central processing unit.** (8)

cranial (krā´-nē-ăl)   See **superior.** (24)

cranial nerves (krā´nē-ăl nûrvs)   Peripheral nerves that originate from the brain. (30)

crash cart (krăsh kärt)   A rolling cart of emergency supplies and equipment. (57)

creatine phosphate (krē´ă-tēn fos´fāt)   A protein that stores extra phosphate groups. (25)

credentialing (krĕ-den´shăl-ing)   A formal review of the qualifications of a healthcare provider who has applied to participate in a healthcare system or plan. (5)

credit (krĕd´ĭt)   An extension of time to pay for services, which are provided on trust. (20)

credit bureau (kre´-dit byür´-ō)   A company that provides information about the creditworthiness of a person seeking credit. (20)

cricoid cartilage (krī´koyd kär´tl-ĭj)   A cartilage of the larynx that forms most of the posterior wall and a small part of the anterior wall. (29)

crime (krīm) An offense against the state committed or omitted in violation of public law. (5)

criminal law (krĭm´ə-nəl lô) Involves crimes against the state. When a state or federal law is violated, the government brings criminal charges against the alleged offender. (5)

critical care (krĭt´i-kăl kār) Care provided to unstable, critically ill patients. Constant bedside attention is needed in order to code critical care. (19)

critical thinking (krĭt´i-kăl thingk´ing) The practice of considering all aspects of a situation when deciding what to believe or what to do. (3)

cross-reference (krôs´rĕf´ər-əns) The notation within the ICD-9 of the word *see* after a main term in the index. The *see* reference means that the main term first checked is not correct. Another category must then be used. (18)

cross-referenced (krôs´rĕf´ər-ənsd) Filed in two or more places, with each place noted in each file; the exact contents of the file may be duplicated, or a cross-reference form can be created, listing all the places to find the file. (15)

cross-training (krōs-tr´ā-ning) The acquisition of training in a variety of tasks and skills. (1)

cryosurgery (krī´ō-sûr´jə-rē) The use of extreme cold to destroy unwanted tissue, such as skin lesions. (44)

cryotherapy (krī´ō-thĕr´ə-pē) The application of cold to a patient's body for therapeutic reasons. (54)

cryptorchidism (kriptôr´kidiz´əm) Congenital failure of the testes to descend into the scrotal sac. (32)

crystals (krĭs´təls) Naturally produced solids of definite form; commonly seen in urine specimens, especially those permitted to cool. (47)

cultural diversity (kŭl´chŭr-ăl di-vĕr´si-tē) The inevitable variety in customs, attitudes, practices, and behavior that exists among groups of people from different ethnic, racial, or national backgrounds who come into contact. (3)

culture (kŭl´chər) In the sociologic sense, a pattern of assumptions, beliefs, and practices that shape the way people think and act. (38)

To place a sample of a specimen in or on a substance that allows microorganisms to grow in order to identify the microorganisms present. (46)

culture and sensitivity (C&S) (kŭl´chər sĕn´sĭ-tĭv´ə-tē) A procedure that

involves culturing a specimen and then testing the isolated bacteria's susceptibility (sensitivity) to certain antibiotics to determine which antibiotics would be most effective in treating an infection. (46)

culture medium (kŭl´chər mē´de-əm) A substance containing all the nutrients a particular type of microorganism needs to grow. (46)

***Current Procedural Terminology* (CPT) (kûr´ənt prə-sē´jər-əl tûr´mə-nŏl´ə-jē)** A book with the most commonly used system of procedure codes. It is the HIPAA-required code set for physicians' procedures. (19)

cursor (kûr´sər) A blinking line or cube on a computer screen that shows where the next character that is keyed will appear. (8)

Cushing's disease (kush´ingz dĭ-zēz´) A condition in which a person produces too much **cortisol** or has used too many steroid hormones. Some of the signs and symptoms include buffalo hump, obesity, a moon face, and abdominal stretch marks; also called hypercortisolism. (34)

cuspids (kŭs´pĭdz) The sharpest teeth; they act to tear food. (33)

customized Altering something to meet individual specifications such as when creating unique settings within an EHR software program to meet the needs of a specialty physician or medical office. (12)

cyanosis (sī´ə-nō´sĭs) A bluish color of skin that results when the supply of oxygen is low in the blood. (23)

cycle billing (sī´kəl bĭl´ĭng) A system that sends invoices to groups of patients every few days, spreading the work of billing all patients over the month while billing each patient only once. (20)

cystic duct (sĭs´tĭk dŭkt) The duct from the gallbladder that merges with the hepatic duct to form the common bile duct. (33)

cystitis (sis-tī´tis) Inflammation of the urinary bladder caused by infection. (31)

cytokines (sī´tō-kīnz) A chemical secreted by T lymphocytes in response to an antigen. Cytokines increase T- and B-cell production, kill cells that have antigens, and stimulate red bone marrow to produce more white blood cells. (28)

cytokinesis (sī´tō-ki-nē´sis) Splitting of the cytoplasm during cell division. (22)

cytoplasm (sī´tə-plăz´əm) The watery intracellular substance that consists mostly of water, proteins, ions, and nutrients. (22)

damages (dăm´ijz) Money paid as compensation for violating legal rights. (20)

database (dā´tə-bās) A collection of records created and stored on a computer. (8)

dateline (dāt´līn´) The line at the top of a letter that contains the month, day, and year. (10)

debridement (dā-brēd-mont´) The removal of debris or dead tissue from a wound to expose healthy tissue. (44)

decibel (dĕs´ə-bəl) A unit for measuring the relative intensity of sounds on a scale from 0 to 130. (43)

deductible (dĭ-dŭk´tə-bəl) A fixed dollar amount that must be paid by the insured before additional expenses are covered by an insurer. (17)

deep (dēp) Anatomical term meaning closer to the inside of the body. (22)

defamation (dĕf´ə-mā´shən) Damaging a person's reputation by making public statements that are both false and malicious. (5)

defecation reflex (def-ē-kā´shŭn rē´flĕks´) The relaxation of the anal sphincters so that feces can move through the anus in the process of elimination. (33)

deflection (dĭ-flĕk´shən) A peak or valley on an electrocardiogram. (49)

dehydration (dē-hī´drā´shən) The condition that results from a lack of adequate water in the body. (55, 57)

dementia (dĭ-mĕn´shə) The deterioration of mental faculties from organic disease of the brain. (42)

demographics (dĕ-mog´ră-fiks) Statistical data relating to the population and particular groups within it. (11)

dendrite (dĕn´drīt´) A type of nerve fiber that is short and branches near the cell body. Its function is to receive information from the neuron. (30)

deoxyhemoglobin (dē-oks-ē-hē-mō-glō´bin) A type of hemoglobin that is not carrying oxygen. It is darker red in color than hemoglobin. (27)

dependent (dĭ-pĕn´dənt) A person who depends on another person for financial support. (21)

depolarization (dē-pō´lăr-i-zā-shŭn) The loss of polarity, or opposite charges inside and outside; the electrical impulse that initiates a chain reaction resulting in contraction. (49)

depolarized (dē-pō´lăr-īzd) A state in which sodium ions flow to the inside of the cell membrane, making the outside less positive. Depolarization occurs when a neuron responds to stimuli such as heat, pressure, or chemicals. (30)

depression (di´-pre-shan) The lowering of a body part. (25)

dermatitis (dûr´mə-tī´tĭs) Inflammation of the skin. (23)

dermatologist (der-mă-tol´ō-jist) A specialist who diagnoses and treats diseases of the skin, hair, and nails. (2)

dermatome (dur´mə tōm) An area of skin innervated by a spinal nerve. (30)

dermis (dûr´mĭs) The middle layer of the skin, which contains connective tissue, nerve endings, hair follicles, sweat glands, and oil glands. (23)

descending colon (dĭ-sĕnd´ĭng kō´lən) The segment of the large intestine after the transverse colon that descends the left side of the abdominal cavity. (33)

descending tracts (dĭ-sĕnd´ĭng trăkts) Tracts of the spinal cord that carry motor information from the brain to muscles and glands. (30)

detrusor muscle (dē-trŭs´or mŭs´əl) A smooth muscle that contracts to push urine from the bladder into the urethra. (31)

diabetes insipidus (dī´ə bētĭs ĭn sĭp´ĭdəs) The condition of excessive thirst and excessive urination related to hyposecretion of ADH so that water is not retained by the kidney. (34)

diabetes mellitus (dī´ə-bē´tĭs mə-lī´təs) Any of several related endocrine disorders characterized by an elevated level of glucose in the blood, caused by a deficiency of insulin or insulin resistance at the cellular level. (34)

diagnosis (Dx) (dī´əg-nō´sĭs) The primary condition for which a patient is receiving care. (18)

diagnosis code (dī´əg-nō´sĭs kōd) The way a diagnosis is communicated to the third-party payer on the healthcare claim. (18)

diagnostic radiology (dī´əg-nos´tĭk rā´dē-ŏl´ə-jē) The use of x-ray technology to determine the cause of a patient's symptoms. (50)

diapedesis (dī´ă-pĕ-dē´sĭs) The squeezing of a cell through a blood vessel wall. (27)

diaphoresis (dī´əfarē´sĭs) Excessive sweating as a result of illness or injury. (29)

diaphragm (dī´ə-frăm´) A muscle that separates the thoracic and abdominopelvic cavities. (22)

diaphysis (dī´-af´i-sis) The shaft of a long bone. (24)

diastolic pressure (dī´ə-stŏl´ĭk prĕsh´ər) The blood pressure measured when the heart relaxes. (26)

diathermy (dĭ´ə-thŭr´mē) A type of heat therapy in which a machine produces high-frequency waves that achieve deep heat penetration in muscle tissue. (54)

diencephalon (dī-en-sef´ă-lon) A structure that includes the thalamus and the hypothalamus. It is located between the cerebral hemispheres and is superior to the brain stem. (30)

dietary supplement (dī´-ĭ-tĕr-ē sŭp´-lə-mənt) Vitamins, minerals, herbals, and other substances taken by mouth without a prescription to promote health and well-being.

differential diagnosis (dĭf´ə-rĕn´shəl dī´əg-nō´sĭs) The process of determining the correct diagnosis when two or more diagnoses are possible. (38)

differently abled (dĭf´ər-ənt-lē ā´bəld) Having a condition that limits or changes a person's abilities and may require special accommodations. (7)

diffusion (di-fyū´zhŭn) The movement of a substance from an area of high concentration to an area of low concentration. (22)

digital examination (dĭj´ĭ-tl ĭg-zam´ə-nā´shən) Part of a physical examination in which the physician inserts one or two fingers of one hand into the opening of a body canal such as the vagina or the rectum; used to palpate canal and related structures. (38)

diluent (dĭl´yōō-ənt) A liquid used to dissolve and dilute another substance, such as a drug. (53)

disability insurance (dĭs´ə-bĭlĭ-tē ĭn-shōōr´əns) Insurance that provides a monthly, prearranged payment to an individual who cannot work as the result of an injury or disability. (17)

disaccharide (dī-sak´ă-rīd) A type of carbohydrate that is a simple sugar. (33)

disbursement (dĭs-bûrs´mənt) Any payment of funds made by the physician's office for goods and services. (8)

disclaimer (dĭs-klā´mər) A statement of denial of legal liability or that refutes the authenticity of a claim. (8)

disclosure (dĭ-sklō´zhər) The release of, the transfer of, the provision of access to, or the divulgence in any manner of patient information. (5)

disclosure statement (dĭ-sklō´zhər stāt´mənt) A written description of agreed terms of payment; also called a federal Truth in Lending statement. (20)

discrimination (dĭs-´skrĭm-ə-´nā-shən) Unequal and unfair treatment. (5)

disinfectant (dĭs´ĭn-fĕk´tănt) A cleaning product applied to instruments and equipment to reduce or eliminate infectious organisms; not used on human tissue. (44)

disinfection (dis-in-fek´shŭn) Destruction of pathogenic microorganisms or their toxins or vectors by direct exposure to chemical or physical agents. (9)

disk clean up (dĭsk kleen up) A computer maintenance untility designed to free up disk space on computer users' hard drive. (8)

disk defragmentation (dĭsk di-frag-men-ta-shun) A computer program designed to increase access speed by rearranging files stored on a disk to occupy contiguous storage locations, a technique commonly known as defragmenting. (8)

dislocation (dĭs´lō-kā´shən) The displacement of a bone end from a joint. (57)

dispense (dĭ-spĕns´) To distribute a drug, in a properly labeled container, to a patient who is to use it. (51)

distal (dĭs´təl) Anatomic term meaning farther away from a point of attachment or farther away from the trunk of the body. (22)

distal convoluted tubule (dĭs´təl kon´vō-lū-ted tū´byūl) The last twisted section of the renal tubule; it is located after the loop of Henle. Several of these tubules merge together to form collecting ducts. (31)

distribution (dĭs´trĭ-byōō´shən) The biochemical process of transporting a drug from its administration site in the body to its site of action. (51)

diverticula (dī´vĕr-tik´yū-lă) Pouches or sacs opening from a tubular or saccular organ, such as the gut or bladder. Plural of diverticulum. (33)

diverticulitis (dī´ver-tik-yū-lī´tis) Inflammation of the diverticuli, which are abnormal dilations in the intestine. (33)

diverticulosis (dī´ver-tik-yū-lō-sis) Abnormal outpouchings or dilations of the intestine. (29)

DNA (dē´ĕn-ā´) A nucleic acid that contains the genetic information of cells. (22)

doctor of osteopathy (dok´tər ŏs´tē-ŏp´ə-thē) A doctor who focuses special attention on the musculoskeletal system and uses hands and eyes to identify and adjust structural problems, supporting the body's natural tendency toward health and self-healing. (2)

doctrine of informed consent (dŏk-´trĭn of ĭn-fôrmd´ kən-´sēnt) The legal basis for informed consent, usually outlined in a state's medical practice act. (5)

doctrine of professional discretion (dŏk-´trĭn of prə-fĕsh´ə-nəl dĭ-skrĕsh´ən) A principle under which a physician can exercise judgment as to whether to show patients who are being treated for mental or emotional conditions their records. (5)

documentation (dŏk´yə-mən-tā´shən) The recording of information in a patient's medical record; includes detailed notes about each contact with the patient and about the treatment plan, patient progress, and treatment outcomes. (11)

dorsal (dôr´səl) See **posterior**. (22)

dorsal root (dôr´səl rōōt) A portion of a spinal nerve that contains axons of sensory neurons only. (30)

dorsiflexion (dōr-si-flek´shŭn) Pointing the toes upward. (25)

dosage (dōs´aj) The size, frequency, and number of doses. (51)

dose (dōs) The amount of a drug given or taken at one time. (51)

dot matrix printer (dŏt mā´trĭks prĭn´tər) An impact printer that creates characters by placing a series of tiny dots next to one another. (8)

double-booking system (dŭb´əl bŏŏk´ĭng sĭs´təm) A system of scheduling in which two or more patients are booked for the same appointment slot, with the assumption that both patients will be seen by the doctor within the scheduled period. (16)

douche (dōōsh) Vaginal irrigation, which can be used to administer vaginal medication in liquid form. (53)

downcoding (doun kōd-ing) Term used when the insurance carrier bases reimbursement on a code level lower than the one submitted by the provider. (19)

drainage catheter (drā´nĭj kăth´ĭ-tər) A type of catheter used to withdraw fluids. (47)

dressing (drĕs´ĭng) A sterile material used to cover a surgical or other wound. (44)

DSL (digital subscriber line) (dĭj´ĭ-tl səb-skrĭb´ərlīn) A type of modem that operates over telephone lines but uses a different frequency than a telephone, allowing a computer to access the Internet at the same time that a telephone is being used. (8)

dual coverage (dū´əl kŭv´ĕr-ăj) Term used when a patient is covered by Medicare and Medicaid. (17)

ductus arteriosus (dŭk´tŭs ar-tēr´ē-ō´sus) The connection in the fetus between the pulmonary trunk and the aorta. (32)

ductus venosus (duk´tŭs ven-ō´sus) A blood vessel that allows most of the blood to bypass the liver in the fetus. (32)

duodenum (dōō´ə-dē´nəm) The first section of the small intestine. (33)

durable item (dōŏr´ə-bəl ī´təm) A piece of equipment that is used repeatedly, such as a telephone, computer, or examination table; contrast with **expendable item.** (8)

durable power of attorney (dŏŏr´ə-bəl poúər ə-tûr´nē) A document naming the person who will make decisions regarding medical care on behalf of another person if that person becomes unable to do so. (5)

dwarfism (dwôrf´ĭzm) A condition in which too little growth hormone is produced, resulting in an abnormally small stature. (34)

dysmenorrhea (dis-men-ōr-ē´ă) Severe menstrual cramps that limit daily activity. (32, 39)

dyspnea (disp-nē´ă) Difficult or painful breathing. (29)

ear ossicles (îr os´i-klz) Three tiny bones called the malleus, the incus, and the stapes located in the middle ear cavity. They are the smallest bones of the body. (24)

eccrine gland (ek´rin glănd) The most numerous type of sweat gland. Eccrine sweat glands produce a watery type of sweat and are activated primarily by heat. (23)

ECG See **electrocardiogram.** (49)

echocardiography (ek´ō-kar-dē-og´ră-fē) A procedure that tests the structure and function of the heart through the use of reflected sound waves, or echoes. (42, 49)

E code (ē kōd) A type of code in the ICD-9. E-codes identify the external causes of injuries and poisoning. (18)

ectoderm (ek´tō-derm) The primary germ layer that gives rise to nervous tissue and some epithelial tissue. (32)

ectropion (ek-trō´pē-ŭn) Eversion of the lower eyelid. (35)

eczema (ĕk´sə-mə) Inflammatory condition of the skin. (23)

edema (ĭ-dē´mə) An excessive buildup of fluid in body tissue. (26)

EDI See **electronic data interchange.** (17)

editing (ĕd´ĭt-ĭng) The process of ensuring that a document is accurate, clear, and complete; free of grammatical errors; organized logically; and written in the appropriate style. (10)

EDTA (ethylenediaminetetraacetic acid) (eth´ĭ-lēn-dī´ă-mĕn-tet´ră-ă-sē´tik as´id) A chelating agent and anticoagulant; added to blood specimens for hematologic and other tests. (48)

effacement (i fās´mənt) Thinning of the cervix in preparation for childbirth. (32)

effectors (ĭ-fĕk´tərs) Muscles and glands that are stimulated by motor neurons in the peripheral nervous system. (30)

efferent arterioles (ĕf´ər-ənt ar-tēr´ē-ōlz) Structures that deliver blood to peritubular capillaries that are wrapped around the renal tubules of the nephron in the kidneys. (31)

efferent nerves (ĕf´ər-ənt nûrvs) Motor nerves that bring information or impulses from the central nervous system to the peripheral nervous system to allow for the movement or action of a muscle or gland. (30)

efficacy (ĕf´ĭ-kə-sē) The therapeutic value of a procedure or therapy, such as a drug. (51)

efficiency (ĭ-fĭsh´ən-sē) The ability to produce a desired result with the least effort, expense, and waste. (8)

EHR See **electronic health records.** (2, 12)

EIA See **enzyme immunoassay.** (47)

EKG See **electrocardiogram.** (49)

elderly (el´dĕr-lē) Individuals over the age of 65. (41)

elective procedure (ĭ-lĕk´tĭv prə-sē´jər) A medical procedure that is not required to sustain life but is requested for payment to the third-party payer by the patient or physician. Some elective procedures are paid for by third-party payers, whereas others are not. (17)

electrocardiogram (ECG or EKG) (ĭ-lĕk´trō-kär´dē-ə-grăm´) The tracing made by an **electrocardiograph.** (49)

electrocardiograph (ĭ-lĕk´trō-kär´dē-ə-grăf´) An instrument that measures and displays the waves of electrical impulses responsible for the cardiac cycle. (49)

electrocardiography (ĭ-lĕk´trō-kär´dē-ŏg´rə-fē) The process by which a graphic pattern is created to reflect the electrical impulses generated by the heart as it pumps. (49)

electrocauterization (ĭ-lĕk´trō-kô´tər-ī-zā´shən) The use of a needle, probe, or loop heated by electric current to remove growths such as warts, to stop bleeding, and to control nosebleeds that either will not subside or continually recur. (44)

electrodes (ĭ-lĕk′trōds′) Sensors that detect electrical activity. (49)

electroencephalography (ĭ-lĕk′trō-ĕn-sĕf′ə-lŏ′grə-fē) A procedure that records the electrical activity of the brain as a tracing called an electroencephalogram, or EEG, on a strip of graph paper. (42)

electrolytes (ĭ-lĕk′trə-līts) Substances that carry electrical current through the movement of ions. (22)

electromyography (ĭ-lĕk′trō-mī-og′rə-fē) A procedure in which needle electrodes are inserted into some of the skeletal muscles and a monitor records the nerve impulses and measures conduction time; used to detect neuromuscular disorders or nerve damage. (42)

electronic data interchange (EDI) (ĭ-lĕk-trŏn′ĭk dā′tə ĭn′tər-chānj′) Transmitting electronic medical insurance claims from providers to payers using the necessary information systems. (17)

electronic health records (EHR) (i-lek-tron-ik helth rĕ′-kôrds) Patient health record created and stored on a computer or other electronic storage device. Also known as **electronic medical records**. (2, 12)

electronic mail (ĭ-lĕk′trŏn′ĭk) A method of sending and receiving messages through a computer network; commonly known as e-mail. (8)

electronic media (i-lek-tron′-ik mee′-dee-uh) Any transmissions that are physically moved from one location to another through the use of magnetic tape, disk, compact disk media, or any other form of digital or electronic technology. (10)

electronic medical records (EMR) (i-lek-tron-ik med-i-kuhl rĕ′kôrds) Patient medical record created and stored on a computer or other electronic storage device. Also known as **electronic health records**. (12)

electronic transaction record (ĭ-lĕk′trŏn′ĭk trăn-săk′shən rĕ′-kôrd) The standardized codes and formats used for the exchange of medical data. (5)

elevation (e-lə-v′ā-shən) The raising of a body part. (25)

ELISA test See **enzyme-linked immunosorbent assay test**. (46)

embolism (ĕm′bə-lĭz′əm) An obstruction in a blood vessel. (29)

embolus (ĕm′bə-ləs) A portion of a thrombus that breaks off and moves through the bloodstream. (27)

embryonic period (em-brē-on′ik pîr′ē-əd) The second through eighth weeks of pregnancy. (32)

E/M code (ē/ĕm kōd) Evaluation and management codes that are often considered the most important of all CPT codes. The E/M section guidelines explain how to code different levels of services. (19)

empathy (ĕm′pə-thē) Identification with or sensitivity to another person's feelings and problems. (3, 4)

emphysema (em′fəsēmə) A chronic lung condition consisting of damage to the alveoli of the lungs. It is heavily associated with smoking, which causes stretching of the spaces between the alveoli and paralyzes the cilia of the respiratory system. (29)

employee handbook (em-ploy′ē handbŏk′) A synopsis of human resources policies and procedures. (56)

employment contract (ĕm-ploi′mənt kŏn′trăkt′) A written agreement of employment terms between employer and employee that describes the employee's duties and the considerations (money, benefits, and so on) to be given by the employer in exchange. (21)

empyema (em′pīē′mə) A collection of pus in the pleural cavity.(29)

EMR See **electronic medical record**. (12)

enclosures (ĕn-klō′zhərz) Materials that are included in the same envelope as the primary letter. (10)

encounter form (en-′kaun-tər form) A form that combines the charges for services rendered, an invoice for payment or insurance copayment, and all the information for submitting an insurance claim; also known as a superbill. (20)

endocardium (en-dō-kar′dē-ŭm) The innermost layer of the heart. (26)

endochondral (en-dō-kon′drăl) A type of ossification in which bones start out as cartilage models. (24)

endocrine gland (ĕn′də-kri-n glănd) A gland that secretes its products directly into tissue, fluid, or blood. (34)

endocrinologist (ĕn′də-kra-nŏl′ə-jĭst) A specialist who diagnoses and treats disorders of the endocrine system, which regulates many body functions by circulating hormones that are secreted by glands throughout the body. (2)

endoderm (ĕn′dō-derm) The primary germ layer that gives rise to epithelial tissues only. (32)

endogenous infection (ĕn′-dŏj′ə-nəs ĭn-fĕk′shən) An infection in which an abnormality or malfunction in routine body processes causes normally beneficial or harmless microorganisms to become pathogenic. (6)

endolymph (ĕn′dō-limf) A fluid in the inner ear. When this fluid moves, it activates hearing and equilibrium receptors. (35)

endometriosis (en′dō-mē-trē-ō′sis) A condition in which tissues that make up the lining of the uterus grow outside the uterus. (32)

endometrium (en′dō-mē′trē-ŭm) The innermost layer of the uterus. It undergoes significant changes during the menstrual cycle. (32)

endomysium (en′dō-miz′ē-ŭm) A connective tissue covering that surrounds individual muscle cells. (25)

endoplasmic reticulum (en′doplaz′mik ritik′yəlum) The organelles of the endoplasmic reticulum are composed of both smooth and rough types. The rough type contains ribosomes on its surface. The smooth type has no ribosomes. Both types create a network of passageways throughout the cytoplasm. (22)

endorse (ĕn-dôrs′) To sign or stamp the back of a check with the proper identification of the person or organization to whom the check is made out, to prevent the check from being cashed if it is stolen or lost. (21)

endorsement (ĕn-dôrs-mĕnt) Signature on the back of a check with the terms for accepting the check as payment. (21)

endoscopy (ĕn-dôs′kə-pē) Any procedure in which a scope is used to visually inspect a canal or cavity within the body. (42)

endosteum (en-dos′tē-ŭm) A membrane that lines the medullary cavity and the holes of spongy bone. (24)

engineered safety devices (en′ji-nēr′d sāf′tē dĕ-vīs-ez) Devices specifically designed to isolate or remove a hazard. These include needles with safety shields and self-shielding needles. (6)

entropion (en-trō′pē-ūn) Inversion of the lower eyelid. (35)

enunciation (ĭ-nŭn′sē-ā′shən) Clear and distinct speaking. (13)

enuresis Bed wetting. (40)

enzyme immunoassay (EIA) (ĕn′zīm im′yū-nō-as′ā) The detection of substances by immunologic methods. This method involves an antigen, an antibody specific for the antigen, and a second antibody conjugated to an enzyme. (47)

enzyme-linked immunosorbent assay (ELISA) test (ĕnˊzīm-lĭngkt imˊyū-nō-sōrˊbent ăsˊā tĕst)   A blood test that confirms the presence of antibodies developed by the body's immune system in response to an initial HIV infection. (46)

EOB   See **explanation of benefits.** (17)

eosinophil (ē-ō-sinˊō-fil)   A type of granular leukocyte that captures invading bacteria and antigen-antibody complexes through phagocytosis. (27)

epicardium (ep-i-karˊdē-ŭm)   The outermost layer of the wall of the heart. Also known as the **visceral pericardium.** (26)

epidermis (ĕpˊĭ-dûrˊmĭs)   The most superficial layer of the skin. (23)

epididymis (ep-i-didˊi-mis)   An elongated structure attached to the back of the testes and in which sperm cells mature. (32)

epididymitis (ep-i-did-i-mīˊtis)   Inflammation of an **epididymis.** Most cases result from infection. (32)

epiglottic cartilage (ep-i-glotˊik kärˊtl-ĭj)   A cartilage of the larynx that forms the framework of the **epiglottis.** (29)

epiglottis (ep-i-glotˊis)   The flap-like structure that closes off the larynx during swallowing. (29)

epilepsy (ĕpˊə-lĕpˊsē)   A condition that occurs when parts of the brain receive a burst of electrical signals that disrupt normal brain function; also called **seizures.** (30)

epimysium (ep-i-misˊ-ē-ŭm)   A thin covering that is just deep to the fascia of a muscle. It surrounds the entire muscle. (25)

epinephrine (ĕpˊə-nĕfˊrĭn)   An injectable medication used to treat anaphylaxis by causing vasoconstriction to increase blood pressure. (28)

A hormone secreted from the adrenal glands. It increases heart rate, breathing rate, and blood pressure. (34)

epiphyseal disk (ep-i-fizˊē-ăl dĭsk)   A plate of cartilage between the **epiphysis** and the **diaphysis.** (24)

epiphysis (e-pifˊi-sis)   The expanded end of a long bone. (24)

episiotomy (epēˊzēotˊəmē)   A surgical incision of the female perineum to enlarge the vaginal opening for delivery. (32)

epistaxis (ĕpˊi-stakˊsis)   Nosebleed. (57)

epithelial tissue (ep-i-thēˊlē-ĕl tĭshˊoo)   A tissue type that lines the tubes, hollow organs, and cavities of the body. (22)

e-prescribing (ē-prĕ-skrībˊ-ing)   Prescriptions are entered electronically and transmitted directly to the pharmacy. (51)

erectile tissue (ĭ-rĕkˊtəl tĭshˊoo)   A highly specialized tissue located in the shaft of the penis. It fills with blood to achieve an erection. (32)

ergonomics (ĕrˊgŏ-nomˊiks)   The science of workplace, tools, and equipment designed to reduce worker discomfort, strain, and fatigue and to prevent work-related injuries. (6)

erythema (er-i-thēˊmǎ)   Redness of the skin. (54)

erythroblastosis fetalis (ĕ-rithˊrō-blas-tōˊsis feˊtǎl-is)   A serious anemia that develops in a fetus with Rh-positive blood as a result of antibodies in an Rh-negative mother's body. (27)

erythrocytes (ĭ-rĭthˊrə-sītˊs)   Red blood cells. (27)

erythrocyte sedimentation rate (ESR) (ĭ-rĭthˊrə-sītˊ sĕdˊə-mən-tāˊshən rāt)   The rate at which red blood cells, the heaviest blood component, settle to the bottom of a blood sample. (48)

erythropoietin (ĕ-rith-rō-poyˊē-tin)   A hormone secreted by the kidney and responsible for regulating the production of red blood cells. (27)

esophageal hiatus (ĭ-sŏfˊə-jēˊəl hī-āˊ-ts)   Hole in the diaphragm through which the esophagus passes. (33)

ESR   See erythrocyte sedimentation rate. (48)

established patient (ĭ-stăbˊlĭsht pāˊshənt)   A patient who has seen the physician within the past 3 years. This determination is important when using E/M codes. (19)

estrogen (ĕsˊtrə-jən)   A female sex hormone; when produced during ovulation, estrogen causes a buildup of the lining of the uterus (womb) to prepare it for a possible pregnancy. (32)

ethics (ĕthˊiks)   General principles of right and wrong, as opposed to requirements of law. (5)

ethmoid (ĕthˊmoyd)   Bones located between the sphenoid and nasal bone that form part of the floor of the cranium. (24)

ethylenediaminetetraacetic acid   See **EDTA.** (48)

etiologic agent (ēˊtē-ə-lŏjˊik āˊjənt)   A living microorganism or its toxin that may cause human disease. (46)

etiology (ēˊtē-olˊŏ-jē)   The science and study of the causes of disease and their mode of operation. (18)

etiquette (ĕtˊĭ-ket)   Good manners. (13)

eustachian tube (yoo-stāˊshən toob)   An opening in the middle ear, leading to the back of the throat, that helps equalize air pressure on both sides of the eardrum. (35)

eversion (ē-verˊzhŭn)   Turning the sole of the foot laterally. (25)

exclusion (ĭk-skloozhˊən)   An expense that is not covered by a particular insurance policy, such as an eye examination or dental care. (17)

excretion (ĭk-skrēˊshən)   The elimination of waste by a discharge; in drug metabolism, the manner in which a drug is eliminated from the body. (51)

exocrine gland (ĕkˊsə-krĭn glănd)   A gland that secretes its product into a duct. (34)

exogenous infection (ĕk-sŏjˊə-nəsĭn-fĕkˊshən)   An infection that is caused by the introduction of a pathogen from outside the body. (6)

exophthalmos (ĕk-sŏf-thalˊ-məs)   Bulging of the eyeballs, often related to hyperthyroidism. (34)

expendable item (ĭk-spĕnˊdəbəl īˊtəm)   An item that is used and must then be restocked; also known collectively as supplies. Contrast with **durable item.** (8)

expiration (ĕkˊspə-rāˊshən)   The process of breathing out; also called exhalation. (29)

explanation of benefits (EOB) (ĕkˊsplə-nāˊshən ŭv bĕnˊə-fits)   Information that explains the medical claim in detail; also called **remittance advice (RA).** (17)

explanation of payment (EOP) (eksˊplə-nāˊshŭn pā-ment)   Document sent by insurance carrier when payment is made describing the terms of the payments. Also known as **explanation of benefits (EOB)** or **remittance advice (RA).** (17)

exposure control plan (eks-pōˊzhŭr kŏn-trōlˊ plan)   A written document of practices and procedures, required equipment, and facilities designed to minimize employee exposure to infectious agents or biohazardous materials. (6)

expressed contract (ĭk-sprĕstˊ kŏnˊtrăct)   A contract clearly stated in written or spoken words. (5)

extension (ĭk-stĕnˊshən)   An unbending or straightening movement of the two elements of a jointed body part. (25)

external auditory canal (ĭk-stûrˊnəl ôˊdĭ-tôrˊē kə-nălˊ)   Canal that carries sound waves to the tympanic membrane; commonly called the ear canal. (35)

extrinsic eye muscles (ĭk-strĭnˊsĭk īmŭsˊəlz)   The skeletal muscles that move the eyeball. (35)

facsimile machine (făk-sĭm´ə-lēmə-shēn´) A piece of office equipment used to send a facsimile, or fax, over telephone lines from one modem to another; more commonly called a fax machine. (8)

factual teaching (făk-chool tēch´ing) Method of teaching that provides the patient with details of the information that is being taught. (14)

facultative (fak-ŭl-tā´tiv) Able to adapt to different conditions; in microbiology, able to grow in environments either with or without oxygen. (46)

Fahrenheit (făr´ən-hīt) One of two common scales used for measuring temperature; measured in degrees Fahrenheit, or °F. (37)

fallopian tubes (fə-lō-pē-ən tūbz) Tubes that extend from the uterus on each side and that open near an ovary. (32)

family practitioner (făm´ə-lē prăk-tĭsh´ə-nər) A physician who does not specialize in a branch of medicine but treats all types and ages of patients; also called a general practitioner. (2)

fascia (fash´e-ă) A structure that covers entire skeletal muscles and separates them from each other. (25)

fascicle (făs´ĭ-kəl) Sections of a muscle divided by connective tissue called perimysium. (25)

febrile (fĕb´rəl) Having a body temperature above one's normal range. (37)

fecal occult blood test (FOBT) (fē´kăl ŏ-kŭlt´ blŭd test) A test to find hidden blood in the stool. (47)

feces (fē´sēz) Material found in the large intestine and made from leftover chyme. Feces are eventually eliminated through the anus. (33)

Federal Unemployment Tax Act (FUTA) This act requires employers to pay a percentage of each employee's income up to a certain dollar amount. (56)

feedback (fēd´băk´) Verbal and nonverbal evidence that a message was received and understood. (4)

feedback loop (fēd´băk loop) A mechanism to control hormone levels. The two types are positive and negative feedback loops. (34)

fee-for-service (fē fôr sûr´vĭs) A major type of health plan. It repays policyholders for the costs of healthcare that are due to illness and accidents. (17)

fee schedule (fē skĕj´ool) A list of the costs of common services and procedures performed by a physician. (17)

felony (fĕl´ə-nē) A serious crime, such as murder or rape, that is punishable by imprisonment. In certain crimes, a felony is punishable by death. (5)

femoral (fem´ŏ-răl) Relating to the femur or thigh. (22)

femur (fē´mər) The bone in the upper leg; commonly called the thigh bone. (24)

fenestrated drape (fĕn´ĭ-strāt´ĕd drāp) A drape that has a round or slit-like opening that provides access to the surgical site. (38)

fertilization (fĕr´til-i-zā´shŭn) The process in which an egg unites with a sperm. (32)

fetal period (fēt´l pĭr´ē-əd) A period that begins at week nine of pregnancy and continues through delivery of the offspring. (32)

fetus (fē´tŭs) The product of conception from the end of the eighth week to the moment of birth. (32)

fiber (fī´bər) The tough, stringy part of vegetables and grains, which is not absorbed by the body but aids in a variety of bodily functions. (55)

fibrinogen (fī-brin´ō-jen) A protein found in plasma that is important for blood clotting. (27)

fibroid (fī´broid) A benign tumor in the uterus composed of fibrous tissue. (32)

fibromyalgia (fī-brō-mī-al´jē-ă) A condition that exhibits chronic pain primarily in joints, muscles, and tendons. (25)

fibula (fīb´yə-lə) The lateral bone of the lower leg. (24)

file guide (fīl gīd) A heavy cardboard or plastic insert used to identify a group of file folders in a file drawer. (15)

filtration (fĭl-trā´shən) A process that separates substances into solutions by forcing them across a membrane. (22)

fimbriae (fĭm-brē-ē) Fringe-like structures that border the entrances of the **fallopian tubes.** (32)

firewall (fīr´wôl) A system that protects a computer network from unauthorized access by users on its own network or another network such as the Internet. (8)

first morning urine specimen (fûrst môr´nĭng yŏŏr´ĭn spĕs´ə-mən) A urine specimen that is collected after a night's sleep; contains greater concentrations of substances that collect over time than specimens taken during the day. (47)

fixative (fĭk´sə-tĭv) A solution sprayed on a slide immediately after the specimen is applied. It is used to preserve and hold the cells in place until a microscopic examination is performed. (9)

flaccid (flak´sid) Weak, soft; not erect. (32)

flagellum (flajel´əm) The "tail-like" structure on some cell membranes that provides cell movement. (22)

flexion (flek´shŭn) A bending movement of the two elements of a jointed body part. (25)

floater (flō´tər) A nonsterile assistant who is free to move about the room during surgery and attend to unsterile needs. (44)

fluidotherapy (floo´id-ōthĕr´ə-pē) A technique for stimulating healing, particularly in the hands and feet, by placing the affected body part in a container of glass beads that are heated and agitated with hot air. (54)

follicle (fŏl´ĭ-kəl) An accessory organ of the skin that is found in the dermis and the sites at which hairs emerge. (23)

follicle-stimulating hormone (FSH) (fŏl´ĭ-kəl stim´yū-lā-ting hôr´mōn) A hormone that in females stimulates the production of estrogen by the ovaries; in males, it stimulates sperm production. (32)

follicular cells (fə-li´-kyə-lər selz) Small cells contained in the primordial follicle along with a large cell called a primary **oocyte.** (32)

folliculitis (fŏ-lik-yū-lī´tis) Inflammation of the hair follicle. (23)

fomite (fō´mīt) An inanimate object, such as clothing, body fluids, water, or food, that may be contaminated with infectious organisms and thus serve to transmit disease. (6)

fontanel (fän-tə-n´el) The soft spot in an infant's skull that consists of tough membranes that connect to incompletely developed bone. (40)

food exchange (food ĭks-chānj´) A unit of food in a particular food category that provides the same amounts of protein, fat, and carbohydrates as all other units of food in that category. (55)

foramen magnum (fō-rā´-mən mag-nəm) The large hole in the occipital bone that allows the brain to connect to the spinal cord. (24)

foramen ovale (fō-rā´men ō-va´lē) A hole in the fetal heart between the right atrium and the left atrium. (32)

forced vital capacity (FVC) (fôrst vīt´l kə-păs´ĭ-tē) The greatest volume of air that a person is able to expel when performing rapid, forced expiration. (49)

formalin (fôr-mă-lin) A dilute solution of formaldehyde used to preserve biological specimens. (44)

formed elements (fôrmd ĕl´ə-mənts) Red blood cells, white blood cells, and platelets; compose 45% of blood volume. (48)

Form I-9 (fôrm) (Employment Eligibility Verification) A federal form for verifying the employee is a U.S. citizen, a legally admitted alien, or an alien authorized to work in the United States. (56)

formula method (fôrm´yū-lă meth´ŏd) A basic formula to calculate dosage. D/H × Q, where D: desired dose, H: dose on hand, Q: quantity of the dose. (52)

formulary (fôr´myū-lă-rē) An insurance plan's list of approved prescription medications. (17)

Form W-2 (tax form) (taks fôrm) The form that an employer must send to an employee and the IRS at the end of the year. It reports an employee's annual wages and the amount of taxes withheld from his or her paycheck. (56)

Form W-4 (tax form) (taks fôrm) A form completed by an employee to indicate his or her tax situation, such as exemptions and status, to the employer. (56)

fracture (frăk´chər) Any break in a bone. (42)

fraud (frôd) An act of deception that is used to take advantage of another person or entity. (5)

frequency (frē´kwən-sē) The number of complete fluctuations of energy per second in the form of waves. (43)

frontal (frŭn´tl) Anatomic term that refers to the plane that divides the body into anterior and posterior portions. Also called coronal. (22)

FSH See **follicle-stimulating hormone.** (32)

fulgurated (ful´gy ə rā təd) The use of heat or laser to burn or destroy tissue. (32)

full-block letter style (fool blŏk lĕt´ər stīl) A letter format in which all lines begin flush left; also called block style. (10)

functional résumé (fŭngk´shə-nəl rĕz´ōō-mā´) A résumé that highlights specialty areas of a person's accomplishments and strengths. (58)

fundus (fun´dus) The upper domed portion of an organ. (32)

fungus (fŭng´gəs) A eukaryotic organism that has a rigid cell wall at some stage in the life cycle. (46)

FUTA See **Federal Unemployment Tax Act.** (56)

FVC See **forced vital capacity.** (49)

gait (gāt) The way a person walks, consisting of two phases: stance and swing. (54)

ganglia (găng´glē-ə) Collections of neuron cell bodies outside the central nervous system. (30)

gastric juice (găs´trĭk jüs) Secretions from the stomach lining that begin the process of digesting protein. (33)

gastritis (gă-strī´tĭs) Inflammation of the stomach lining. (33)

gastroenterologist (găs´trō-ĕn-ter-ol´ō-jist) A specialist who diagnoses and treats disorders of the entire gastrointestinal tract, including the stomach, intestines, and associated digestive organs. (2)

gastroesophageal reflux disease (GERD) (gas´trō-ē-sof´ă-jē´ăl rē´flĕks dĭ-zēz´) A condition that occurs when stomach acids are pushed into the esophagus and cause heartburn. (33)

gene (jēn) A segment of DNA that determines a body trait. (22)

general duty clause (jen´ĕr-əl dū´tē klôz) An OSHA clause that requires an employer to maintain a workplace free from hazards that are recognized as likely to cause death or serious injury. (6)

general physical examination (exam) (jĕn´ər-əl fĭz´ĭ-kəl ĭg-zăm´ə-nā´shən) An examination performed by a physician to confirm a patient's health or to diagnose a medical problem. (9)

generic name (jə-nĕr´ĭk nām) A drug's official name. (51)

geriatrician (jer´ē-at´ trish´ăn) Specialists who care for elderly individuals, usually those over the age of 65. (41)

gerontologist (jĕr´ən-tŏl´ə-jĭst) A specialist who studies the aging process. (2)

GH See **growth hormone.** (34)

gigantism (jī´gan-tizm) A condition in which too much growth hormone is produced in childhood, resulting in an abnormally increased stature. (34)

glans penis (glanz pē´nĭs) A cone-shaped structure at the end of the penis. (32)

glaucoma (glou-kō´mə) A condition in which too much pressure is created in the eye by excessive aqueous humor. This excess pressure can lead to permanent damage of the optic nerves, resulting in blindness. (35)

global period (glō´bəl pîr´ē-əd) The period of time that is covered for follow-up care of a procedure or surgical service. (19)

globulins (glob´yū-linz) Plasma proteins that transport lipids and some vitamins. (27)

glomerular filtrate (glō-măr´yū-lărfĭl´trāt´) The fluid remaining in the **glomerular capsule** after **glomerular filtration.** (31)

glomerular filtration (glō-măr´yū-lăr fĭl-trā´shən) The process by which urine forms in the kidneys as blood moves through a tight ball of capillaries called the glomerulus. (31)

glomerulonephritis (glō-măr´yū-lō-nef-rī´tis) An inflammation of the glomeruli of the kidney. (31)

glomerulus (glō-măr´yū-lŭs) A group of capillaries in the renal corpuscle. (31)

glottis (glot´is) The opening between the vocal cords. (29)

glucagon (gloo´kə-gŏn´) A hormone that increases glucose concentrations in the bloodstream and slows down protein synthesis. (34)

gluten (glū´tĕn) The insoluble protein (prolamines) constituent of wheat and other grains; a mixture of gliadin, glutenin, and other proteins; believed to be an agent in celiac disease. (55)

glycogen (glī´kə-jən) An excess of glucose that is stored in the liver and in skeletal muscle. (33)

glycosuria (glī-kō-sū´rē-ă) The presence of significant levels of glucose in the urine. (47)

goiter (goi´tər) Enlargement of the thyroid gland, which causes swelling of the neck, often related to iodine insufficiency in the diet. (34)

Golgi apparatus (gôl´jē ap´ə-rat´es) The cell's Golgi apparatus synthesizes carbohydrates and also appears to prepare and store secretions for discharge from the cell. (22)

gonadotropin-releasing hormone (GnRH) (gō´na-dō-trō´pin ri-lēs´ing hôr´mōn´) Hormone that stimulates the anterior pituitary gland to release **follicle-stimulating hormone (FSH).** (32)

gonads (gō´nădz) The reproductive organs; namely, in women, the ovaries, and in men, the testes. (34)

goniometer (gō-nē-ä´-me-tər) A protractor device that measures range of motion. (54)

gout (gowt) A medical condition characterized by an elevated uric acid level and recurrent acute arthritis. (24)

G-protein (jē-prō´tēn) A substance that causes enzymes in the cell to activate following the activation of the hormone-receptor complex in the cell membrane. (34)

Gram-negative (grăm′nĕg′ə-tĭv) Referring to bacteria that lose their purple color when a decolorizer has been added during a Gram stain. (46)

Gram-positive (grăm′pŏz′ĭ-tĭv) Referring to bacteria that retain their purple color after a decolorizer has been added during a Gram stain. (46)

Gram stain (grăm stān) A method of staining that differentiates bacteria according to the chemical composition of their cell walls. (46)

granular leukocyte (grăn′yə-lər lōō′kəsīt′) A type of leukocyte (white blood cell) with a segmented nucleus and granulated cytoplasm; also known as a polymorphonuclear leukocyte. (27)

granulocyte (gran′yū-lō-sīt) See **granular leukocyte.** (27)

Grave's disease (grāvz dĭ-zēz′) A disorder in which a person develops antibodies that attack the thyroid gland. (34)

gray matter (grā măt′ər) The inner tissue of the brain and the spinal cord that is darker in color than **white matter.** It contains all the bodies and dendrites of nerve cells. (30)

grievance process (grē-văns pros′es) A mediation process through the human relations department utilized when an employee or employees feel they are treated unjustly. (56)

gross earnings (grōs ûr′nĭngz) The total amount an employee earns before deductions. (21)

group practice (grōōp prăk′tĭs) A medical management system in which a group of three or more licensed physicians share their collective income, expenses, facilities, equipment, records, and personnel. (5)

growth hormone (GH) (grōth hôr′mōn′) A hormone that stimulates an increase in the size of the muscles and bones of the body. (34)

growth plate (grōth plāt) A shaft of cartilage between the epiphysis and the diaphysis; also known as the **epiphyseal disk.** (24)

guarantor (gar′ăn-tōr) The patient, caregiver, or entity responsible for payment of the healthcare bill. (20)

gustatory receptors (gə′s-tə-tör-ēri-se′p-tərz) Taste receptors that are found on taste buds. (35)

gynecologist (gī′nĭ-kŏ′lə-jĭst) A specialist who performs routine physical care and examinations of the female reproductive system. (2)

gyri (jī′rī) The ridges of brain matter between the sulci; also called **convolutions.** (30)

hairy leukoplakia (hâr′ē lū-kō-plā′kē-ă) A white lesion on the tongue associated with AIDS. (46)

hapten (hap′tĕn) Foreign substances in the body too small to start an immune response by themselves. (28)

hard copy (härd′ kŏp′ē) A readable paper copy or printout of information. (8)

hard skills (hahrd skilz) Specific technical and operational proficiencies. (3)

hardware (härd′wâr′) The physical components of a computer system, including the monitor, keyboard, and printer. (8)

hazard label (hăz′ərd lā′bəl) A shortened version of the Material Safety Data Sheet; permanently affixed to a hazardous substance container. (6)

HCG See **human chorionic gonadotropin.** (32)

HCPCS See **Healthcare Common Procedure Coding System.** (19)

HCPCS Level II codes (hĭk-pĭks lĕv′əl tōō kōdz) Codes that cover many supplies such as sterile trays, drugs, and durable medical equipment; also referred to as national codes. They also cover services and procedures not included in the CPT. (19)

healthcare-associated infections (HAI) (helth′kār ă-sō′sē-āt-ĕd infek′shŭnz) Infections acquired by a patient in a healthcare facility. (6)

Healthcare Common Procedure Coding System (HCPCS) (hĕlth kâr kŏm′ən prə-sē′jər kōd′ĭng sĭs′təm) A coding system developed by the Centers for Medicare and Medicaid Services that is used in coding services for Medicare patients. (19)

health fraud (hĕlth frôd) A deception or trickery related to health prevention or care for profit.

Health Insurance Portability and Accountability Act See **HIPAA.** (1)

health maintenance organization (HMO) (hĕlth mān′tə-nəns ôr′gə-nĭ-zā′shən) A healthcare organization that provides specific services to individuals and their dependents who are enrolled in the plan. Doctors who enroll in an HMO agree to provide certain services in exchange for a prepaid fee. (17)

helper T-cells (hĕl′pər tē′ sĕlz) White blood cells that are a key component of the body's immune system and that work in coordination with other white blood cells to combat infection. (46)

hematemesis (hē′-mă-tem′ĕ-sis) The vomiting of blood. (57)

hematocrit (hē′mă-tō-krit) The percentage of the volume of a sample made up of red blood cells after the sample has been spun in a centrifuge. (27)

hematology (hē′mə-tŏl′ə-jē) The study of blood. (48)

hematoma (hē′mə-tō′mə) A swelling caused by blood under the skin. (48, 57)

hematopoiesis (hēmətōpōē′sis) The process of new blood cell formation in the red bone marrow of cancellous bone. (24)

hematuria (hē-mă-tu′rē-ă) The presence of blood in the urine. (47)

hemocytoblast (hē′mă-sī′tō-blast) Cells of the red bone marrow that produce most red blood cells. (27)

hemoglobin (hē′mə-glō′bĭn) A protein that contains iron and bonds with and carries oxygen to cells; the main component of erythrocytes. (23)

hemoglobinuria (hē′mō-glō-bi-nū′rē-ă) The presence of free **hemoglobin** in the urine; a rare condition caused by transfusion reactions, malaria, drug reactions, snake bites, or severe burns. (47)

hemolysis (hē-mol′ĭ-sis) The rupturing of red blood cells, which releases hemoglobin. (48)

hemolytic anemias (hē mō lit′ ik ənē′mēăz) Types of anemia that cause red blood cells to be destroyed faster than they can be made. (27)

hemoptysis (hi mop′ ti sis) The spitting up of blood from the respiratory tract. (29)

hemorrhoids (hĕm′ə-roidz′) Varicose veins of the rectum or anus. (33)

hemostasis (hē′mō-stā-sis) The stoppage of bleeding. (27)

hemothorax (hē′ mō thôr′ aks) Blood collection in the pleural cavity causing collapse of the lung. (29)

hepatic duct (hĭ-păt′ĭk dŭkt) A duct that leaves the liver carrying bile and merges with the cystic duct to form the common bile duct. (33)

hepatic lobule (he-păt′ĭk lob′yūl) Smaller divisions within the lobes of the liver. (33)

hepatic portal system (he-pat′ik pôr′tl sĭs′təm) The collection of veins carrying blood to the liver. (26)

hepatic portal vein (hĭ-păt′ĭk vān pôr′tl) A blood vessel that carries blood from the other digestive organs to the **hepatic lobules.** (33)

hepatitis (hĕp´ə-tī´tĭss) Inflammation of the liver usually caused by viruses or toxins. (33)

hepatocytes (hep´ă-tō-sītz) The cells within the lobules of the liver. Hepatocytes process nutrients in the blood and make bile. (33)

hernia (hûr´nē-ə) The protrusion of an organ through the wall that usually contains it, such as a hiatal or inguinal hernia. (33)

herpes simplex (her´pēz sĭm´plĕks) A medical condition characterized by an eruption of one or more groups of vesicles on the lips or genitalia. (23)

herpes zoster (her´pēz zos´ter) A medical condition characterized by an eruption of a group of vesicles on one side of the body following a nerve root. (23)

hierarchy (hī´ə-rär´kē) A term that pertains to Abraham Maslow's hierarchy of needs. This hierarchy states that human beings are motivated by unsatisfied needs and that certain lower needs must be satisfied before higher needs can be met. (4)

hilum (hī´lŭm) The indented side of a lymph node. (23)

The entrance of the renal sinus that contains the renal artery, renal vein, and ureter. (31)

HIPAA (Health Insurance Portability and Accountability Act) (hĭp´ə) A set of regulations whose goals include the following: (1) improving the portability and continuity of healthcare coverage in group and individual markets; (2) combating waste, fraud, and abuse in healthcare insurance and healthcare delivery; (3) promoting the use of a medical savings account; (4) improving access to long-term care services and coverage; and (5) simplifying the administration of health insurance. (1)

HIV See **human immunodeficiency virus.** (46)

HMO See **health maintenance organization.** (17)

Holter monitor (hol´tər mŏn´ĭ-tər) An electrocardiography device that includes a small portable cassette recorder worn around a patient's waist or on a shoulder strap to record the heart's electrical activity. (49)

homeopathic medicine (hō-mē-ō-păth´-ĭk mĕd´-ĭ-sĭn) A system of medicine that uses remedies in an attempt to stimulate the body to recover itself.

homeostasis (hō´mē-ō-stā´sĭs) A balanced, stable state within the body. (4)

homologous chromosome (hŏ-mŏl´ō-gŭs krō´mə-sōm´) Members in each pair of chromosomes. (22)

hormone (hôr´mōn´) A chemical secreted by a cell that affects the functions of other cells. (34)

hospice (hŏs´pĭs) Volunteers who work with terminally ill patients and their families. (4)

human chorionic gonadotropin (HCG) (hyōō´mən kō-rē-on´ik gō´nad-ō-trō´pin) A hormone secreted by cells of the embryo after implantation. It maintains the corpus luteum in the ovary so it will continue to secrete estrogen and progesterone. (32)

human immunodeficiency virus (HIV) (hyōō´mən im´yū-nō-dē-fish´en-sē vī´rəs) A retrovirus that gradually destroys the body's immune system and causes AIDS. (46)

humerus (hyü´-mə-rəs) The bone of the upper arm. (24)

humors (hyōō´mərz) Fluids of the body. (28)

hydrotherapy (hī´drə-thĕr´ə-pē) The therapeutic use of water to treat physical problems. (54)

hydrothorax (hī´drō thôr´aks) Fluid collection in the pleural cavity causing collapse of the lung. (29)

hyoid (hī´-òid) The bone that anchors the tongue. (24)

hyperextension (hī´per-eks-ten´shŭn) Extension of a body part past the normal anatomic position. (25)

hyperglycemia (hī´pər-glī-sē´mē-ə) High blood sugar. (57)

hyperopia (hī-per-ō´pē-ă) A condition that occurs when light entering the eye is focused behind the retina; commonly called farsightedness. (43)

hyperpnea (hī-per-nē´ă) Abnormally deep, rapid breathing. (37)

hyperpyrexia (hī per py rex´ ē a) An exceptionally high fever. (37)

hyperreflexia (hī´per-rē-flek´sē-ă) Reflexes that are stronger than normal reflexes.

hypertension (hī´pər-tĕn´shən) High blood pressure. (37)

hyperventilation (hī´pər-vĕn´tl-ā´shən) The condition of breathing rapidly and deeply. Hyperventilating decreases the amount of carbon dioxide in the blood. (29)

hypnosis (hĭp-nō´-sĭs) A trance-like state usually induced by another person to access the subconscious mind and promote healing.

hypodermis (hī´pə-dûr´mĭs) The subcutaneous layer of the skin that is largely made of adipose tissue. (23)

hypoglycemia (hī´pō-glī-sē´mē-ə) Low blood sugar. (57)

hyporeflexia (hī´pō-rē-flek´sē-ă) A condition of decreased reflexes. (30)

hypotension (hī´pō-tĕn´shən) Low blood pressure. (37)

hypothalamus (hī´pō-thăl´ə-məs) A region of the **diencephalon.** It maintains homeostasis by regulating many vital activities such as heart rate, blood pressure, and breathing rate. (30)

hypovolemic shock (hī´pō-vō-lē´mik shŏk) A state of shock resulting from insufficient blood volume in the circulatory system. (57)

hypoxemia (hī´pok-sē´mē-ă) Subnormal oxygenation of arterial blood, short of anoxia. (49)

hypoxia (hī pôk´ sē ə) Inadequate oxygenation of the cells of the body. (29)

hysterectomy (hĭs´tə-rĕk´tə-mē) Surgical removal of the uterus. (32)

ICD-9 See *International Classification of Diseases, Ninth Revision, Clinical Modification.* (18)

icons (ī´kŏnz´) Pictorial images; on a computer screen, graphic symbols that identify menu choices. (8)

identification line (ī-dĕn´tə-fĭ-kā´shən līn) A line at the bottom of a letter containing the letter writer's initials and the typist's initials. (10)

idiopathic (ĭd-ē-ō-path´ik) A disease or condition of unknown cause. (33)

IFFA See **immunofluorescent antibody test.** (46)

ileocecal sphincter (ĭl´ē ō sē´kəl sfĭngk´ter) A structure that controls the movement of **chime** from the ileum to the **cecum.** (33)

ileum (ĭl´ē-əm) The last portion of the small intestine. It is directly attached to the large intestine. (33)

ilium (i´-lē-əm) The most superior part of the hip bone. It is broad and flaring. (24)

immunity (ĭ-myōōn´ĭ-tē) The condition of being resistant or not susceptible to pathogens and the diseases they cause. (28)

immunization (im´yū-nī-zā-shən) The administration of a vaccine or toxoid to protect susceptible individuals from communicable diseases. (40)

immunocompromised (im´yū-nō-kom´pro-mīzd) Having an impaired or weakened immune system.

immunofluorescent antibody (IFFA) test (im´yū-nō-flūr-es´ent ăn´tī-bŏd-ē tĕst) A blood test used to confirm enzyme-linked immunosorbent assay (ELISA) test results for HIV infection. (46)

immunoglobulins (im´yū-nō-glob´yū-linz) A class of structurally related proteins that include IgG, IgA, IgM, and IgE; also called **antibodies.** (28)

impetigo (im´pĭ-tī´gō) A contagious skin infection usually caused by germs commonly called staph and strep. (23)

implied consent (im-plīd kŭn-sent) A form of consent that is not expressly granted by a person, but rather inferred from a person's actions and the facts and circumstances of a particular situation (or in some cases by a person's silence or inaction). (5)

implied contract (ĭm-plīd kŏn´trăct´) A contract that is created by the acceptance or conduct of the parties rather than the written word. (5)

impotence (ĭm´pŏ-tens) A disorder in which a male cannot maintain an erect penis to complete sexual intercourse; also called erectile dysfunction. (32)

inactive file (ĭn-ăk´tĭv fīl) A file used infrequently. (15)

incident report (in´si-dĕnt rē-pōrt´) A special form required by a facility when an adverse outcome or event with risk of liability occurs. (56)

incision (ĭn-sĭzh´ən) A surgical wound made by cutting into body tissue. (44)

incisors (ĭn-sī´zərz) The most medial teeth. They act as chisels to bite off food. (33)

incomplete proteins (ĭn´kəm-plēt´ prō´tēnz´) Proteins that lack one or more of the essential amino acids. (55)

incontinence (in-kon´ti-nens) The involuntary leakage of urine. (41)

incus (ĭng´kəs) A small bone in the middle ear, located between the malleus and the stapes; also called the anvil. (35)

indexing (in´dĕks´ing) The naming of a file. (15)

indexing rules (in´dĕks´ing rōols) Rules used as guidelines for the sequencing of files based on current business practice. (15)

indication (ĭn´dĭ-kā´shən) The purpose or reason for using a drug, as approved by the FDA. (51)

individual identifiable health information (IIHI) (in-duh-vij-oo-uhell ī-den-tuh-fī-

able hĕlth ĭn´fər-mā´shən) Any part of an individual's health information, including demographic information, collected from an individual that is received by a covered entity (e.g., a healthcare provider).

induction (in-dŭk´shŭn) The pregnant patient is admitted to the delivering healthcare facility then given medication to start uterine contractions. (39)

induration (in-də-´rā-shən) The process of hardening or of becomming hard.

infection (ĭn-fĕk´shən) The presence of a pathogen in or on the body. (28)

infectious waste (ĭn-fĕk´shəs wāst) Waste that can be dangerous to those who handle it or to the environment; includes human waste, human tissue, and body fluids as well as potentially hazardous waste, such as used needles, scalpels, and dressings, and cultures of human cells. (7)

inferior (ĭn-fĭr´ē-ər) Anatomic term meaning below or closer to the feet; also called caudal. (22)

infertility (in´fĕr-til´i-tē) Diminished ability to produce offspring; does not imply sterility. (39)

inflammation (ĭn´flə-mā´shən) The body's reaction when tissue becomes injured or infected. The four cardinal signs are redness, heat, pain, and swelling. (28)

inflammatory phase (in-flam´-a-tor-ee fāz) The initial phase of wound healing in which bleeding is reduced as blood vessels in the affected area constrict. (44)

informed consent (ĭn-fôrmd´ kən-sĕnt) The patient's right to receive all information relative to his or her condition and then make a decision regarding treatment based upon that knowledge. (5)

informed consent form (ĭn-fôrmd´ kən-sĕnt fôrm) A form that verifies that a patient understands the offered treatment and its possible outcomes or side effects. (11)

infundibulum (in-fŭn-dib´yū-lŭm) The funnel-like end of the uterine tube near an ovary. It catches the secondary oocyte as it leaves the ovary. (32)

infusion (in-fyū´zhŭn) A slow drip, as of an intravenous solution into a vein. (53)

ink-jet printer (ĭngk´jĕt´ prĭn´tər) A non-impact printer that forms characters by using a series of dots created by tiny drops of ink. (8)

innate immunity (ĭn āt ĭmyoŏn´ītē) The body's mechanisms to protect itself against pathogens in general; also called nonspecific defenses. (28)

inner cell mass (ĭn´ər sĕl măs) A group of cells in a blastocyte that gives rise to an embryo. (32)

inorganic (ĭn´ôr-găn´ĭk) Matter that generally does not contain carbon and hydrogen. (22)

insertion (ĭn-sûr´shən) An attachment site of a skeletal muscle that moves when a muscle contracts. (25)

inside address (ĭn-sīd´ ə-drĕs´) The name and address of the person to whom the letter is being sent. It appears on a business letter two to four spaces down from the date. It should be two, three, or four lines in length. (10)

inspection (ĭn-spĕk´shən) The visual examination of the patient's entire body and overall appearance. (38)

inspiration (in-spə-rā´-shən) The act of breathing in; also called inhalation. (29)

instruction set (ĭn-strŭk´shən set) Includes the groups of instructions from installed programming that a CPU can implement. (8)

insulin (ĭn´sə-lĭn) A hormone that regulates the amount of sugar in the blood by facilitating its entry into the cells. (34)

integrative medicine (ĭn´-tĭ-grāt´-tĭv mĕd´-ĭ-sĭn) The combination of components of conventional medicine with complementary and alternative medicine modalities.

integrity (in-teg´ri-tē) Adhering to the appropriate code of law and ethics and being honest and trustworthy. (3)

interactive pager (ĭn´tər-ăk´tĭv pāj´ər) A pager designed for two-way communication. The pager screen displays a printed message and allows the physician to respond by way of a mini keyboard. (13)

interatrial septum (in´tər ā´trē əl səp´təm) The wall separating the right and left atria from each other. (26)

intercalated disc (in-ter´kă-lā-ted disk) A disk that connects groups of cardiac muscles. This disc allows the fibers in that group to contract and relax together. (25)

interferon (in-ter-fĕr´on) A protein that blocks viruses from infecting cells. (28)

interim room (ĭn´tər-ĭm rōom) A room off the patient reception area and away from the examination rooms for occasions when patients require privacy. (7)

International Classification of Diseases, Ninth Revision, Clinical Modification(ICD-9) (ĭn´tər-năsh´ə-nəl klăs´ə-fīkā´shən dĭ-zēz´əz nīnth rĭ-vĭzh´ən klĭn´ĭ-kəl

mŏd´ə-fĭ-kā´shən)   Code set that is based on a system maintained by the World Health Organization of the United Nations. The use of the ICD-9 codes in the healthcare industry is mandated by **HIPAA** for reporting patients' diseases, conditions, and signs and symptoms. (18)

Internet (ĭn´tər-nĕt´)   A global network of computers. (8)

interneuron (in´ter-nū´ron)   A structure found only in the central nervous system that functions to link sensory and motor neurons together. (30)

internist (ĭn-tûr´nĭst)   A doctor who specializes in diagnosing and treating problems related to the internal organs. (2)

interpersonal skills (ĭn´tər-pûr´sə-nəl skĭlz)   Attitudes, qualities, and abilities that influence the level of success and satisfaction achieved in interacting with other people. (4)

interphalangeal (intərfələn´jēal)   Pertaining to the joints between the phalangeal bones. (24)

interphase (in´ter-fāz)   The state of a cell carrying out its normal daily functions and not dividing. (22)

interstitial cell (in-ter-stish´əl sĕl)   A cell located between the seminiferous tubules that is responsible for making testosterone. (32)

interstitial fluid (in-ter-stish´əl floōĭd)   Fluid found between tissue cells that is absorbed by lymph capillaries to become lymph. (28)

interventricular septum (in´tər ventrik´yələr səp´təm)   The wall separating the right and left ventricles from each other. (26)

intestinal lipase (ĭn-tĕs´tĭ-nəl lip´ās)   An enzyme that digests fat. (33)

intradermal (ID) (in´tră-der´măl)   Within the upper layers of the skin. (53)

intradermal test (in´tră-der´măl tĕst)   An allergy test in which dilute solutions of allergens are introduced into the skin of the inner forearm or upper back with a fine-gauge needle. (42)

intramembranous (in-trə-me´m-brə-nəs)   A type of ossification in which bones begin as tough fibrous membranes. (24)

intramuscular (IM) (in´tră-mŭs´kyū-lăr)   Within muscle; an IM injection allows administration of a larger amount of a drug than a subcutaneous injection allows. (53)

intraoperative (in´tră-ŏp´ər-ə-tĭv)   Taking place during surgery. (44)

intravenous (IV) (ĭn´trə-vē´nəs)   Injected directly into a vein. (53)

intravenous pyelography (IVP) (ĭn´trə-vē´nəs pī´ĕ-log´ră-fē)   A radiologic procedure in which the doctor injects a contrast medium into a vein and takes a series of x-rays of the kidneys, ureters, and bladder to evaluate urinary system abnormalities or trauma to the urinary system; also known as excretory urography. (50)

intrinsic factor (ĭn-trĭn´zĭk făk´tər)   A substance secreted by **parietal cells** in the lining of the stomach. It is necessary for vitamin B_{12} absorption. (33)

invasive (ĭn-vā´sĭv)   Referring to a procedure in which a catheter, wire, or other foreign object is introduced into a blood vessel or organ through the skin or a body orifice. Surgical asepsis is required during all invasive tests. (50)

inventory (ĭn´vən-tôrē)   A list of supplies used regularly and the quantities in stock. (8)

inversion (ĭn-vûr´zhən)   Turning the sole of the foot medially. (25)

invoice (ĭn´vois´)   A bill for materials or services received by or services performed by the practice. (8)

ions (ī´ənz)   Positively or negatively charged particles. (22)

iris (ī´rĭs)   The colored part of the eye, made of muscular tissue that contracts and relaxes, altering the size of the pupil. (35)

ischium (is´-kē-əm)   A structure that forms the lower part of the hip bone. (24)

islets of Langerhans (ī´lĭts lan´ger-hans)   Structures in the pancreas that secrete insulin and glucagon into the bloodstream. (34)

itinerary (ī-tĭn´ə-rĕr´ē)   A detailed travel plan listing dates and times for specific transportation arrangements and events, the location of meetings and lodgings, and phone numbers. (16)

IV   See **intravenous.** (53)

IVP   See **intravenous pyelography.** (50)

jaundice (jŏn´dĭs)   A condition characterized by yellowness of the skin, eyes, mucous membranes, and excretions; occurs during the second stage of hepatitis infection. (40)

jejunum (jə-jōō´nəm)   The mid-portion and the majority of the small intestine. (33)

journalizing (jûr´nə-līz´ĭng)   The process of logging charges and receipts in a chronological list each day; used in the single-entry system of bookkeeping. (21)

juxtaglomerular apparatus (jŭks´tă-glŏmer´yū-lăr ăp´ə-răt´əs)   A structure contained in the nephron and made up of the macula densa and **juxtaglomerular cells.**

juxtaglomerular cells (jŭks´tă-glŏmer´yū-lăr sĕlz)   Enlarged smooth muscle cells in the walls of either the afferent or efferent arterioles.

Kaposi's sarcoma (kap´ō-sēz sar-kō´mă)   Abnormal tissue occurring in the skin, and sometimes in the lymph nodes and organs, manifested by reddish-purple to dark blue patches or spots on the skin. (46)

keratin (kĕr´ə-tĭn)   A tough, hard protein contained in skin, hair, and nails. (23)

keratinocyte (kĕ-rat´i-nō-sīt)   The most common cell type in the epidermis of the skin. (23)

key (kē)   The act of inputting or entering information into a computer. (10)

KOH mount (kā´ō-āch mount)   A type of mount used when a physician suspects a patient has a fungal infection of the skin, nails, or hair and to which potassium hydroxide is added to dissolve the keratin in cell walls. (46)

Krebs cycle (krĕbz sī´kəl)   Also called the citric acid cycle. This cycle generates ATP for muscle cells. (25)

KUB radiography (kā´yōō-bē rā´dē-og´ră-fē)   The process of x-raying the abdomen to help assess the size, shape, and position of the urinary organs; evaluate urinary system diseases or disorders; or determine the presence of kidney stones. It can also be helpful in determining the position of an intrauterine device (IUD) or in locating foreign bodies in the digestive tract; also called a flat plate of the abdomen. (50)

kyphosis (kī-fō´sis)   A deformity of the spine characterized by a bent-over position; more commonly called humpback. (38, 41)

labeling (lā´bəl-ĭng)   Information provided with a drug, including FDA-approved indications and the form of the drug. (51)

labia majora (lā´bē-ă mă´jôr-ă)   The rounded folds of adipose tissue and skin that serve to protect the other female reproductive organs. (32)

labia minora (lā´bē-ă mĭ´nôr-ă)   The folds of skin between the labia majora. (32)

labor relations (lā´bŏr rĕ-lā´shŭnz)   An HR role that refers to issues that arise between employees and management. (56)

labyrinth (lăb´ə-rĭnth´)   The inner ear. (35)

laceration (lăs´ə-rā´shən)   A jagged, open wound in the skin that can extend down into the underlying tissue. (44)

lacrimal apparatus (lăk´rə-məl ăp´ə-răt´əs) A structure that consists of the lacrimal glands and nasolacrimal ducts. (35)

lacrimal gland (lăk´rə-məl glănd) A gland in the eye that produces tears. (35)

lactase (lăk´tās) An enzyme that digests sugars. (33)

lactic acid (lăk´tĭk ăs´ĭd) A waste product that must be released from the cell. It is produced when a cell is low on oxygen and converts pyruvic acid. (25)

lactiferous (lak-tif´ə rus) Pertaining to producing milk. (32)

lactogen (lak´tō-jen) Substance secreted by the placenta that stimulates the enlargement of the mammary glands. (32)

lacunae (lə-kü-na) Holes in the matrix of bone that hold osteocytes. (24)

lamella (lə-me´-lə) Layers of bone surrounding the canals of osteons. (24)

LAN (local area network) (lăn) See **local area network**. (8)

lancet (lăn´sĭt) A small, disposable instrument with a sharp point used to puncture the skin and make a shallow incision; used for capillary puncture. (48)

laryngopharynx (lă-ring´gō-far-ingks) The portion of the pharynx behind the **larynx**. (33)

larynx (lăr´ingks) The part of the respiratory tract between the pharynx and the trachea that is responsible for voice production; also called the voice box. (29)

laser printer (lā´zər prĭn´tər) A high-resolution printer that uses a technology similar to that of a photocopier. It is the fastest type of computer printer and produces the highest-quality output. (8)

last menstrual period (LMP) (lăst men´strū-ăl pēr´ē-ŏd) The date of the first day of the last menstruation; used to determine an estimated expected delivery date for a pregnant patient. (39)

lateral (lăt´ər-əl) A directional term that means farther away from the midline of the body. (22)

lateral file (lăt´ər-əl fīl) A horizontal filing cabinet that features doors that flip up and a pull-out drawer, where files are arranged with sides facing out. (15)

law (lô) A rule of conduct established and enforced by an authority or governing body, such as the federal government. (5)

law of agency (lô ā´jən-sē) A law stating that an employee is considered to be acting on the physician's behalf while performing professional duties. (5)

lead (lēd) A view of a specific area of the heart on an electrocardiogram. (49)

lease (lēs) To rent an item or piece of equipment.

legal custody (lēgəl kŭs´tə-dē) The court-decreed right to have control over a child's upbringing and to take responsibility for the child's care, including healthcare. (20)

lens (lĕnz) A clear, circular disc located in the eye, just posterior to the iris, that can change shape to help the eye focus images of objects that are near or far away. (35)

lentigo (len-tī´gō) A brown macule resembling a freckle except that the border is usually regular and microscopic proliferation of rete ridges is present; scattered melanocytes are seen in the basal cell layer. It is usually caused by sun exposure in someone of middle age or older. (41)

letterhead (lĕt´ər-hĕd´) Formal business stationery, with the doctor's (or office's) name and address printed at the top, used for correspondence with patients, colleagues, and vendors. (10)

leukemia (lōō-kē´mē-ə) A medical condition in which bone marrow produces a large number of white blood cells that are not normal. (27)

leukocyte (lōō-kə-sīt) White blood cells. (27)

leukocytosis (lū´kō-sī-tō´sis) A white blood cell count that is above normal. (27)

leukopenia (lū´kō-pē´nē-ă) A white blood cell count that is below normal. (27)

LH See **luteinizing hormone**. (32)

liability insurance (lī´ə-bĭl´ĭ-tē ĭn-shōōr´əns) A type of insurance that covers injuries caused by the insured or injuries that occurred on the insured's property. (17)

liable (lī´ə-bəl) Legally responsible. (5)

libel (lī´bəl) A false publication, as in writing, print, signs, or pictures, that damages a person's reputation. (5)

lifetime maximum benefit (līf´tīm´ măk´sə-məm bĕn´ə-fĭt) The total sum that a health plan will pay out over the patient's life. (17)

ligament (lĭg´ə-mənt) A tough, fibrous band of tissue that connects bone to bone. (24)

ligature (lĭg´ə-chōŏr´) Suture material. (44)

limbus (lĭm bŭs) The corneal-scleral junction, which is the area where the sclera (the white of the eye) gives way to the clear covering of the iris (cornea). (35)

limited check (lĭm´ĭ-tĭd chĕk) A check that is void after a certain time limit; commonly used for payroll. (21)

lingual frenulum (ling´gwăl fren´yūlŭm) A flap of mucosa that holds the body of the tongue to the floor of the oral cavity. (33)

lingual tonsils (ling´gwăl ton´silz) Two lumps of lymphatic tissue at the back of the tongue that act to destroy bacteria and viruses. (33)

linoleic acid (lin-ō-lē´ik as´id) An essential fatty acid found in corn and sunflower oils. (33)

lipid (lip´id) "Fat-soluble," an operational term describing a solubility characteristic, not a chemical substance, denoting substances extracted from animal or vegetable cells by nonpolar solvents; included in the heterogeneous collection of materials thus extractable are fatty acids, glycerides, glyceryl ethers, phospholipids, sphingolipids, long-chain alcohols, waxes, terpenes, steroids, and "fat-soluble" vitamins such as A, D, and E. (33)

lipoproteins (lip-ō-prō´tēnz) Large molecules that are fat-soluble on the inside and water-soluble on the outside and carry lipids such as cholesterol and triglycerides through the bloodstream. (27)

lithotripsy (lith´ō-trip-sē) The crushing of a stone in the renal pelvis, ureter, or bladder by mechanical force or sound waves. (31)

living will (lĭv´ĭng wĭl) A legal document addressed to a patient's family and healthcare providers stating what type of treatment the patient wishes or does not wish to receive if he becomes terminally ill, unconscious, or permanently comatose; sometimes called an advance directive. (5)

lobe (lōb) The frontal, parietal, temporal, or occipital regions of the cerebral hemisphere. (30)

local area network (LAN) (lō´kăl ār´ē-ă net´wŏrk) A network that connects computers in one building or a group of buildings. (8)

locum tenens (lō´kum tĕn´ens) A substitute physician hired to see patients while the regular physician is away from the office. (16)

loop electrosurgical excision procedure (LEEP) (lūp ĕ-lek´trō-sŭr´jik-ăl ek-sizh´ŭn prŏ-sē´jŭr) A diagnostic and therapeutic gynecologic surgical technique for removing dysplastic cells from the cervix with a small wire loop. (39)

loop of Henle (lōōp hen´lē) The portion of the renal tubule that curves back toward the renal corpuscle and twists again to become the distal convoluted tubule. (31)

lubricant (loo-bri-kə nt) A water-soluble gel used during examination of the rectum or vaginal cavity. (9)

lumbar enlargement (lŭm´bər ĕnlärj´mənt) The thickening of the spinal cord in the low back region. (30)

lunula (lū´nū-lă) The white half-moon–shaped area at the base of a nail. (23)

luteinizing hormone (LH) (lū´tē-in-izing hôr´mōn´) Hormone that in females stimulates ovulation and the production of estrogen; in males, it stimulates the production of testosterone. (32)

lymph (limf) The fluid found inside of the lymphatic vessels. (28)

lymphedema (limf´e-dē´mă) The blockage of lymphatic vessels that results in the swelling of tissue from the accumulation of lymphatic fluid. (28)

lymphocyte (lĭm´fō-sīt) An agranular leukocyte formed in lymphatic tissue. Lymphocytes are generally small. See **T lymphocyte** and **B lymphocyte.** (27, 28)

lymphokines (lĭmf´ ō kĭnz) A type of cytokine secreted by T cells that increases T-cell production and directly kills cells with antigens.(28)

lysosomes (lī´sə-sōmz) Structures that are known to perform the digestive function of the cells. (22)

lysozyme (lī´sō-zīm) An enzyme in tears that destroys pathogens on the surface of the eye. (28)

macrophage (măk´rə-făj´) A type of phagocytic cell found in the liver, spleen, lungs, bone marrow, and connective tissue. Macrophages play several roles in humoral and cell-mediated immunity, including presenting the antigens to the lymphocytes involved in these defenses; also known as monocytes while in the bloodstream. (28)

macula densa (mak´yū-lă den´sa) An area of the distal convoluted tubule that touches afferent and efferent arterioles.

macular degeneration (mak´yū-lăr dē-jen-er-ā´shŭn) A progressive disease that usually affects people older than the age of 50. It occurs when the retina no longer receives an adequate blood supply. (35)

magnetic resonance imaging (MRI) (măgnĕt´ĭk rĕz´ə-nəns ĭ-măj´ing) A viewing technique that uses a powerful magnetic field to produce an image of internal body structures. (42)

magnetic therapy (măg-nĕt´-ĭk thĕr´-ə-pē) A type of therapy in which magnets are placed on the body to penetrate and correct the body's energy fields. (51)

maintenance contract (măn´tə-nəns kŏn´trăkt´) A contract that specifies when a piece of equipment will be cleaned, checked for worn parts, and repaired. (8)

major histocompatibility complex (MHC) (mā´jər his´tō-kom-pat-ĭ-bil´i-tē kəm-plĕks) A large protein complex that plays a role in T-cell activation. (28)

malignant (mə-lĭg´nənt) A type of tumor or neoplasm that is invasive and destructive and that tends to metastasize; it is commonly known as cancerous. (28)

malleus (măl´ē-əs) A small bone in the middle ear that is attached to the eardrum; also called the hammer. (35)

malpractice claim (măl-prăk´tĭs klām) A lawsuit brought by a patient against a physician for errors in diagnosis or treatment. (5)

maltase (mawl-tās) An enzyme that digests sugars. (33)

mammary glands (mam´ă-rē glăndz) Accessory organs of the female reproductive system that secrete milk after pregnancy. (32)

mammography (mă-mŏg´rə-fē) X-ray examination of the breasts. (50)

managed care organization (MCO) (măn´ĭjd kâr ôr´gə-nĭ-zā´shən) A health-care business that, through mergers and buyouts, can deliver healthcare more cost-effectively. (2)

mandible (man´-də-bəl) A bone that forms the lower portion of the jaw. (24)

manipulation (mə-nĭp´yə-lā´shən) The systematic movement of a patient's body parts. (38)

margin (mahr-jin) The space or measurement around the edges of a form or letter that is left blank. (10)

marrow (mer´-ō) A substance that is contained in the medullary cavity. In adults, it consists primarily of fat. (24)

massage (mə-säzh) The use of pressure, kneading, stroking, and the human touch to alleviate pain and promote healing through relaxation.

massage therapist (mə-säzh´thĕr´ə-pĭst) An individual who is trained to use pressure, kneading, and stroking to promote muscle and full-body relaxation. (2)

mastoid process (mas´-toid pr´ä-ses) A large bump on each temporal bone just behind each ear. It resembles a nipple, hence the name mastoid. (24)

Material Safety Data Sheet (MSDS) (mə-tîr´ē-əl sāf´tē dā´tə shēt) A form that is required for all hazardous chemicals or other substances used in the laboratory and that contains information about the product's name, ingredients, chemical characteristics, physical and health hazards, guidelines for safe handling, and procedures to be followed in the event of exposure. (6, 8)

matrix (mā´trĭks) The basic format of an appointment book, established by blocking off times on the schedule during which the doctor is able to see patients. (16)
The material between the cells of connective tissue. (22)

matter (măt´er) Anything that takes up space and has weight. Liquids, solids, and gases are matter. (22)

maturation phase (măch´ə-rā´shən fāz) The third phase of wound healing, in which scar tissue forms. (44)

maxilla (mak-si´-lə) A bone that forms the upper portion of the jaw. (24)

Mayo stand (mā´ō stănd) A movable stainless steel instrument tray on a stand. (44)

MCO See **managed care organization.** (2)

mechanical digestion (mĕ-kan´i-kăl dī-jes´chŭn) The breaking down of food for use by the body by a physical method such as chewing. (33)

medial (mē´dē-əl) A directional term that describes areas closer to the midline of the body. (22)

mediation (mē´dē-ā-shun) Intervention in a dispute in order to resolve it. (56)

Medicaid (mĕd´ĭ-kād´) A federally funded health cost-assistance program for low-income, blind, and disabled patients; families receiving aid to dependent children; foster children; and children with birth defects. (17)

medical asepsis (mĕd´ĭ-kəl ə-sĕp´sĭs) Measures taken to reduce the number of microorganisms, such as hand washing and wearing examination gloves, that do not necessarily eliminate microorganisms; also called clean technique. (41)

medical identity theft (med´i-kăl ī-den´ti-tē theft) Using another person's name or insurance to seek healthcare. (7)

medical practice act (mĕd´i-kəl prăk´tĭs ăkt) A law that defines the exact duties that physicians and other healthcare personnel may perform. (5)

Medicare (mĕd´ĭ-kâr´) A national health insurance program for Americans aged 65 and older. (17)

Medicare + Choice Plan (mĕd´ĭ-kâr´ chois plăn) Medicare benefit in which beneficiaries can choose to enroll in one of three major types of plans instead of the **Original Medicare Plan.** (17)

Medigap (měd´ĭ-găp´) Private insurance that Medicare recipients can purchase to reduce the gap in coverage—the amount they would have to pay from their own pockets after receiving Medicare benefits. (17)

meditation (měd´-ĭ-tā-shən) A state in which the body is consciously relaxed and the mind becomes calm and focused.

medullary cavity (me´-de-ler-ē ka´-və-tē) The canal that runs through the center of the **diaphysis.** (24)

megakaryocytes (meg-ă-kar´ē-ō-sīts) Cells within red blood marrow that give rise to platelets. (27)

meiosis (mī-ō´sis) A type of cell division in which each new cell contains only one member of each chromosome pair. (22)

melanin (měl´ə-nĭn) A pigment that is deposited throughout the layers of the epidermis. (23)

melanocyte (měl´ă-nō-sīt) A cell type within the epidermis that makes the pigment **melanin.** (23)

melanocyte-stimulating hormone (MSH) (məl´ən ō sīt stim´ yū lāting hôr mōn´) A hormone released from the anterior pituitary to stimulate melanin production in the skin's epidermal cells. (34)

melatonin (měl´ə-tō´nĭn) A hormone that helps to regulate circadian rhythms. (34)

membrane potential (měm´brān´ pə-těn´shəl) The potential inside a cell relative to the fluid outside the cell. (30)

menarche (me-nar´kē) The first menstrual period. (32, 39, 40)

Meniere's disease (Mən´yerz dĭzēz) An inner-ear disease characterized by attacks of vertigo, tinnitus, and nausea. Permanent hearing loss may result.

meninges (mě-nin´jēz) Membranes that protect the brain and spinal cord. (30)

meningitis (měn´ĭn-jī´tĭs) An inflammation of the **meninges.** (30)

meniscus (mə-nĭs´kəs) The curve in the air-to-liquid surface of a liquid specimen in a container. (37)

menopause (měn´ə-pôz´) The termination of the menstrual cycle due to the normal aging of the ovaries. (32, 39)

menorrhagia (men´ŏ-rā´jē-ă) Excessively prolonged or profuse menses. (39)

menses (měn´sēz) The clinical term for menstrual flow. (32)

menstrual cycle (měn´strōō-əl sī´kəl) The female reproductive cycle. It consists of regular changes in the uterine lining that lead to monthly bleeding. (32)

menstruation (men´strū-ā´shŭn) Cyclic endometrial shedding and discharge of a bloody fluid from the uterus during the menstrual cycle. (39)

mensuration (měn´sə-rā´-shən) The process of measuring. (38)

meridian (mə-rĭd´-ē-ən) Pathways of energetic flow that are distributed symmetrically throughout the body. These pathways are used in acupuncture, traditional Chinese medicine, and Ayurveda. (2)

mesentery (me´sen´tərē) The fan-like tissue that attaches the jejunum and ileum to the posterior abdominal wall. (33)

mesoderm (mez´ō-derm) The primary germ layer that gives rise to connective tissue and some epithelial tissue. (32)

metabolism (mĭ-tăb´ə-lĭz´əm) The overall chemical functioning of the body, including all body processes that build small molecules into large ones (anabolism) and break down large molecules into small ones (catabolism). (22)

metacarpals (me-tə-k´är-pəlz) The bones that form the palms of the hand. (24)

metacarpophalangeal (met´əkar´pōfəlan´jēəl) Pertaining to the joints that join the phalanges to the metacarpals. (24)

metaphase (met´əfāz) Period of mitosis when the chromosomes line up on the spindle fibers created by the centrioles during prophase. (22)

metastasis (mǒ-tăs´tə-sĭs) The transfer of abnormal cells to body sites far removed from the original tumor; the spread of tumor cells. (24)

metatarsals (mět´ə-tär´salz) The bones that form the front of the foot. (24)

metatarsophalangeal (met´ətar´sōfəlan´jēəl) Pertaining to the joints that join the phalanges to the metatarsals. (24)

metrorrhagia (mē´trō-rā´jē-ă) Any irregular, acyclic bleeding from the uterus between periods. (39)

MHC See **major histocompatibility complex.** (28)

microbiology (mī´krō-bī-ŏl´ə-jē) The study of microorganisms. (46)

microfiche (mī´krō-fēsh´) Microfilm in rectangular sheets. (8)

microfilm (mī´krə-fĭlm´) A roll of film stored on a reel and imprinted with information on a reduced scale to minimize storage space requirements. (8)

microglia (mī-krŏg´lēa) Small cells within the nervous system that act as phagocytes, watching for and engulfing invaders. (30)

microorganism (mī´krō-ôr´gə-nĭz´əm) A simple form of life, commonly made up of a single cell and so small that it can be seen only with a microscope. (6)

micropipette (mī´krō-pī-pet´) A small pipette that holds a small, precise volume of fluid; used to collect capillary blood. (48)

microvilli (mī´krō-vil´-ī) Structures found in the lining of the small intestine. They greatly increase the surface area of the small intestine so it can absorb many nutrients. (33)

micturition (mik-chū-rish´ŭn) The process of urination. (31)

middle digit (´mi-dəl ´di-jət) A small group of two to three numbers in the middle of a patient number that is used as an identifying unit in a filing system. (15)

midlevel provider (mid-lev´ĕl prō-vī´dĕr) Refers to physician assistants and nurse practioners who provide patient care under the supervision of a physician. (56)

midsagittal (mid´saj´i-tăl) Anatomical term that refers to the plane that runs lengthwise down the midline of the body, dividing it into equal left and right halves. (22)

minerals (mĭn´ər-əlz) Natural, inorganic substances the body needs to help build and maintain body tissues and carry on life functions. (55)

minors (mī-nərs) Anyone under the age of majority—18 in most states, 21 in some jurisdictions. (5)

minutes (mi-nətz´) A report of what happened and what was discussed and decided at a meeting. (16)

mirroring (m ĭr´ər-ĭng) Restating in your own words what a person is saying. (36)

misdemeanor (mĭs´dĭ-mē´nər) A less serious crime such as theft under a certain dollar amount or disturbing the peace. A misdemeanor is punishable by fines or imprisonment. (5)

mitochondria (mīto´kon´drēə) Structures that provide energy for cells and are the respiratory centers for the cell. (22)

mitosis (mī-tō´sĭs) A type of cell division that produces ordinary body, or somatic, cells; each new cell receives a complete set of paired chromosomes. (22)

mitral valve (mī´trăl vălv) See **bicuspid valve.** (26)

mobility aid (mō´bəl-ə-tē ād) Device that improves one's ability to move from one place to another; also called mobility assistive device. (54)

modeling (mŏd´l-ĭng) The process of teaching the patient a new skill by having the patient observe and imitate it. (14)

modem (mōʹdəm) A device used to transfer information from one computer to another through telephone lines. (8)

modified-block letter style (mŏdʹə-fīd blŏk lĕtʹər stīl) A letter format similar to full-block style, except that the dateline, complimentary closing, signature block, and notations are aligned and begin at the center of the page or slightly to the right of center. (10)

modified-wave schedule (mŏdʹə-fīd wāv skĕjʹōōl) A scheduling system similar to the wave system, with patients arriving at planned intervals during the hour, allowing time to catch up before the next hour begins. (16)

modifier (mŏdʹə-fīʹər) One or more two-digit codes assigned to the five-digit main code to show that some special circumstance applied to the service or procedure that the physician performed. (19)

molars (mōʹlərz) Back teeth that are flat and are designed to grind food. (33)

mold (mōld) Fungi that grow into large, fuzzy, multicelled organisms that produce spores. (46)

molecule (mŏlʹĭ-kyōōlʹ) The smallest unit into which an element can be divided and still retain its properties; it is formed when atoms bond together. (22)

money order (mŭnʹē ôrʹdər) A certificate of guaranteed payment, which may be purchased from a bank, a post office, or some convenience stores. (21)

monocyte (monʹ-o-sīt) A type of phagocyte that is formed in bone marrow and circulates throughout the blood for a very short period of time. It then migrates to specific tissues and is called a macrophage. (27)

monokines (monʹō kīnz) A type of cytokine secreted by lymphocytes and macrophages that assists in regulating the immune response by increasing B-cell production and stimulating red bone marrow to produce more white blood cells. (28)

mononucleosis (monʹō nōō klē ōʹsis) A highly contagious viral infection caused by the Epstein-Barr virus (EBV). (28)

monosaccharide (mon-ō-sakʹă-rīd) A type of carbohydrate that is a simple sugar. (33)

mons pubis (mʹānz pyʹü-bəs) A fatty area that overlies the public bone. (32)

moral values (môrʹəl vălʹyōōz) Values or types of behavior that serve as a basis for ethical conduct and are formed through the influence of the family, culture, or society. (5)

morbidity (mōr-bidʹi-tē) The frequency of the appearance of complications following a surgical procedure or other treatment. (18)

mordant (môrʹdnt) A substance, such as iodine, that can intensify or deepen the response a specimen has to a stain. (46)

morphology (môr-fŏlʹə-jē) The study of the shape or form of objects. (48)

mortality (mōr-talʹi-tē) A fatal outcome. (18)

morula (mōrʹū-lă) A zygote that has undergone cleavage and results in a ball of cells. (32)

motherboard (mŭthʹər-bôrdʹ) The main circuit board of a computer that controls the other components in the system. (8)

motility (mōʹti li tē) To be capable of movement. (32)

motor (mōʹtər) Efferent neurons that carry information from the central nervous system to the effectors. (30)

motor nerves (mōʹtŏr nĕrvs) An efferent nerve conveying an impulse that excites muscular contraction; motor nerves in the autonomic nervous system also elicit secretions from glandular epithelia. (30)

mouse (mous) A pointing device that can be added to a computer that directs activity on the computer screen by positioning a pointer or cursor on the screen. It can be directly attached to the computer or can be wireless. (8)

moxibustion (mŏks-ĭ-bŭsʹ-chən) The application of heat at the points where the needles are inserted during acupuncture.

MRI See **magnetic resonance imaging.** (42)

MSDS See **Material Safety Data Sheet.** (6, 8)

MSH See **melanocyte-stimulating hormone.** (34)

mucocutaneous exposure (myü-kō-kyüʹ-tā-nē-əs ik-spōʹ-zhər) Exposure to a pathogen through mucous membranes. (46)

mucosa (myōō-kōʹsə) The innermost layer of the wall of the alimentary canal. (33)

mucous cells (myōōʹ-kəs sĕlz) Cells that are found in the salivary glands and the lining of the stomach and that secrete mucous. (33)

MUGA scan (mŭgʹə skăn) A radiologic procedure that evaluates the condition of the heart's myocardium; it involves injection of radioisotopes that concentrate in the myocardium, followed by the use of a gamma camera to measure ventricular contractions to evaluate the patient's heart wall. (50)

multimedia (mŭlʹtē-mēʹdē-ə) More than one medium, such as in graphics, sound, and text, used to convey information. (8)

multitasking (mŭlʹtē-tăsʹk ĭng) Running two or more computer software programs simultaneously. (8)

multi-unit smooth muscle (mŭlʹtē- yōōʹnĭt smōōth mŭsʹəl) A type of smooth muscle that is found in the iris of the eye and in the walls of blood vessels. (25)

murmur (mûrʹmər) An abnormal heart sound heard when the ventricles contract and blood leaks back into the atria. (26)

muscle fatigue (mŭsʹəl fa-tēgʹ) A condition caused by a buildup of lactic acid. (25)

muscle fiber (mŭsʹəl fīʹbər) Muscle cells that are called fibers because of their long lengths. (25)

muscle tissue (mŭsʹəl tĭshʹōō) A tissue type that is specialized to shorten and elongate. (22)

muscular dystrophy (mŭsʹkyə-lər disʹtrō-fē) A group of inherited disorders characterized by a loss of muscle tissue and by muscle weakness. (25)

mutation (myōō-taʹshən) An error that sometimes occurs when DNA is duplicated. When it occurs, it is passed to descendent cells and may or may not affect them in harmful ways. (22)

myasthenia gravis (mī-as-thēʹnē-ă gravʹis) An autoimmune disorder that is characterized by muscle weakness. (25)

myelin (mīʹə-lĭn) A fatty substance that insulates the axon and allows it to send nerve impulses quickly. (30)

myelography (mīʹĕ-logʹră-fē) An x-ray visualization of the spinal cord after the injection of a radioactive contrast medium or air into the spinal subarachnoid space (between the second and innermost of three membranes that cover the spinal cord). This test can reveal tumors, cysts, spinal stenosis, or herniated disks. (42, 50)

myocardial infarction (mīʹō-kärʹdē-ăl ĭn-farkʹshən) A heart attack that occurs when the blood flow to the heart is reduced as a result of blockage in the coronary arteries or their branches. (26)

myocardium (mīʹō-kärʹdē-əm) The middle and thickest layer of the heart. It is made primarily of cardiac muscle. (26)

myocytes (mīʹō sīts) Muscle cells; also called muscle fibers. (25)

myofibrils (mī-ō-fīʹbrils) Long structures that fill the sarcoplasm of a muscle fiber. (25)

myoglobin (mī-ō-glōʹbin) A pigment contained in muscle cells that stores extra oxygen. (25)

myoglobinuria (mī´ō-glō-bi-nū-rē-ă) The presence of myoglobin in the urine; can be caused by injured or damaged muscle tissue. (47)

myometrium (mī´ō-mē´trē-ŭm) The middle, thick muscular layer of the uterus. (32)

myopia (mī-ō´pē-ə) A condition that occurs when light entering the eye is focused in front of the retina; commonly called nearsightedness. (43)

myxedema (mik-se-dē´mă) A severe type of hypothyroidism that is most common in women older than the age of 50. (34)

nail bed (nāl běd) The layer beneath each nail. (23)

narcotic (när-kŏt´ĭk) A popular term for an opioid and term of choice in government agencies; see **opioid.** (51)

nares (ner´ēz) The openings of the nose or nostrils. (29)

nasal (nā´zəl) Relating to the nose. The nasal bones fuse to form the bridge of the nose. (24)

nasal conchae (nā´zəl kon´kē) Structures that extend from the lateral walls of the nasal cavity. (29)

nasal mucosa (nā´zəl myōō-kō´sə) The lining of the nose. (38)

nasal septum (nā´zəl sěp´təm) A structure that divides the nasal cavity into a left and right portion. (29)

nasolacrimal duct (nā-zō-lăk´rə-məl dŭkt) A structure located on the medial aspect of each eyeball. These ducts drain tears into the nose. (35)

nasopharynx (nā´zō-far´ingks) The portion of the pharynx behind the nasal cavity. (33)

National Center for Complementary and Alternative Medicine (NCCAM) (năsh´ə-nəl sěn´tər for kŏm´ -plə-měn-tə-rē and ôl-tûr´-nə-tĭv měd´-ĭ-sĭn) National organization that conducts and supports CAM research and provides CAM information to healthcare providers and the public.

natural killer (NK) cells (năch´ər-el kĭl´ər selz) Non-B and non-T lymphocytes. NK cells kill cancer cells and virus-infected cells without previous exposure to the antigen. (28)

naturopathic medicine (nă´-chə-rŏp´-ə-thĭk měd´-ĭ-sĭn) A system of medicine that relies on the healing power of the body and supports that power through various healthcare practices, such as nutritional counseling, lifestyle counseling, and exercise.

needle biopsy (nēd´l bī´ŏp´sē) A procedure in which a needle and syringe are used to aspirate (withdraw by suction) fluid or tissue cells. (44)

negligence (něg´lĭ-jəns) A medical professional's failure to perform an essential action or performance of an improper action that directly results in the harm of a patient. (5)

negotiable (nĭ-gō´shē-ə-bəl) Legally transferable from one person to another. (21)

neonatal period (nē-ō-nā´təl pĭr´ē-əd) The first 4 weeks of the postnatal period of an offspring. (32)

neonate (nē´ə-nāt´) An infant during the first 4 weeks of life. (32)

nephrologist (ne-frol´ō-jĭst) A specialist who studies, diagnoses, and manages diseases of the kidney. (2)

nephrons (nef´ronz) Microscopic structures in the kidneys that filter blood and form urine. (31)

nerve fiber (nûrv fī´bər) A structure that extends from the cell body. It consists of two types: axons and dendrites. (30)

nerve impulse (nûrv ĭm´pŭls´) Electrochemical messages transmitted from neurons to other neurons and effectors. (30)

nervous tissue (nûr´vəs tĭsh´ōō) A tissue type located in the brain, spinal cord, and peripheral nerves. (22)

netbook (´net bŭk) A small portable laptop computer designed for wireless communication and access to the Internet. (8)

net earnings (nět ûr´n ĭngz) Take-home pay, calculated by subtracting total deductions from gross earnings. (56)

network (nět´wûrk´) A system that links several computers together. (8)

networking (nět´wûrk´ĭng) Making contacts with relatives, friends, and acquaintances that may have information about how to find a job in your field. (58)

neuralgia (nōō-răl´jə) A medical condition characterized by severe pain along the distribution of a nerve. (30)

neuroglia (nûr-ŏg´lēə) Structures that function as support cells for other neurons, including astrocytes, microglia, and oligodendrocytes. See also **neuroglial cells.** (30)

neuroglial cell (nū-rog´lē-ăl sěl) Non-neuronal type of nervous tissue that is smaller and more abundant than neurons. Neuroglial cells support neurons. (30)

neurologist (nōō-rəl´ə-jist) A specialist who diagnoses and treats disorders and diseases of the nervous system, including the brain, spinal cord, and nerves. (2)

neuron (nōōr´ŏn´) A nerve cell; it carries nerve impulses between the brain or spinal cord and other parts of the body. (30)

neurotransmitter (nōōr´ō-trăns´mĭt-ər) A chemical within the vesicles of the synaptic knob that is released into the postsynaptic structures when a nerve impulse reaches the synaptic knob. (30)

neutrophil (nū´trō-fil) A type of granular leukocyte that aids in phagocytosis by attacking bacterial invaders; also responsible for the release of pyrogens. (27)

new patient (nōō pā´shənt) Patient that, for CPT reporting purposes, has not received professional services from the physician within the past 3 years. (19)

NK cells See **natural killer cells.** (28)

nocturia (nok-tū´rē-ă) Excessive nighttime urination. (41)

nomogram (nō´mō-gram) A form of line chart showing scales for the variables involved in a particular formula in such a way that corresponding values for each variable lie in a straight line intersecting all the scales. (52)

noncompliant (nŏn´kəm-plī´ent) The term used to describe a patient who does not follow the medical advice given. (11)

noninvasive (non-in-vā´siv) Referring to procedures that do not require inserting devices, breaking the skin, or monitoring to the degree needed with invasive procedures. (50)

nonsteroidal hormone (non-stěr´oyd-al hôr´mōn´) A type of hormone made of amino acids and proteins. (34)

norepinephrine (nōr´ep-i-nef´rin) A neurotransmitter released by sympathetic neurons onto organs and glands for fight-or-flight (stressful) situations. (25)

no-show (nō shō) A patient who does not call to cancel and does not come to an appointment. (16)

nosocomial infection (nos-ō-kō´mē-ăl ĭn-fěk-shən) An infection contracted in a hospital.

notations (nō-tā´shənz) Information found at the end of a business letter indicating enclosures included with the letter and the names of other people who will be receiving copies of the letter. (10)

Notice of Privacy Practices (NPP) (nō´tĭs prī´və-sē prăk´tis-əs) A document that informs patients of their rights as outlined under **HIPAA.** (5)

NPP See **Notice of Privacy Practices.** (5)

nuclear medicine (noo´klē-ər měd´ĭ-sĭn) The use of radionuclides, or radioisotopes (radioactive elements or their compounds), to evaluate the bone, brain, lungs, kidneys, liver, pancreas, thyroid, and spleen; also known as radionuclide imaging. (50)

nucleases (nū´klē-ās-ez) Pancreatic enzymes that digest nucleic acids. (33)

nucleus (noo´klē-əs) The control center of a cell; contains the chromosomes that direct cellular processes. (22)

numeric filing system (noo-měr´ĭkfīl´ĭng sĭs´təm) A filing system that organizes files by numbers instead of names. Each patient is assigned a number in the order in which she joins the practice. (15)

nutrient (nū´trē-ěnt) A constituent of food necessary for normal physiologic function. (33)

nystagmus (nis-tag´mŭs) Rapid involuntary eye movements that may be the result of drug or alcohol use, brain injury or lesion, or cerebrovascular accident (CVA). (35)

O&P specimen (ō ənd pē spěs´ə-mən) An ova and parasites specimen, or a stool sample, that is examined for the presence of certain forms of protozoans or parasites, including their eggs (ova). (47)

objective (əb-jěk´tĭv) Pertaining to data that are readily apparent and measurable, such as vital signs, test results, or physical examination findings. (11)

objective data (əb-jěk´tĭv dā´tə) Information about the patient's condition that is readily apparent or measureable. (36)

objectives (ob-jek´tĭvs) The set of magnifying lenses contained in the nosepiece of a compound microscope. (45)

occipital (ŏk-sĭp´ĭ-tl) Relating to the back of the head. The occipital bone forms the back of the skull. (24)

occult blood (ə-kŭlt blŭd) Blood contained in some other substance, not visible to the naked eye. (9)

Occupational Safety and Health Act See **OSHA.** (1, 6)

OCR See **optical character recognition.** (8)

ocular (ŏk´yə-lər) An eyepiece of a microscope. (45)

oil-immersion objective (oil ĭ-mûr´zhən əb-jěk´tĭv) A microscope objective that is designed to be lowered into a drop of immersion oil placed directly above the prepared specimen under examination, eliminating the air space between the microscope slide and the objective and producing a much sharper, brighter image. (45)

ointment (oint´mənt) A form of topical drug; also known as a salve. (53)

Older Americans Act of 1965 (ōl´dər ə-měr´ĭ-kəns ăkt) A U.S. law that guarantees certain benefits to elderly citizens, including healthcare, retirement income, and protection against abuse. (7)

olfactory (ŏl-făk´tə-rē) Relating to the sense of smell. (35)

oligodendrocytes (ŏl´ĭgōden´drəsīts) Specialized neuroglial cells that assist in the production of the myelin sheath. (30)

oliguria (ol´i-gu´re-ah) Insufficient production (or volume) of urine. (47)

OMM See **osteopathic manipulative medicine.** (2)

oncologist (ŏn-kŏl´ə-jĭst) A specialist who identifies tumors and treats patients who have cancer. (2)

onychectomy (ŏn-i-kek´tō-mē) The removal of a fingernail or toenail. (44)

oocyte (ō´ō-sīt) The immature egg. (32)

oogenesis (ō-ō-jen´ě-sis) The process of egg cell formation. (32)

open-book account (ō´pən boŏkə-kount´) An account that is open to charges made occasionally as needed. (20)

open-hours scheduling (ō´pən ourz skěj´ool-ĭng) A system of scheduling in which patients arrive at the doctor's office at their convenience and are seen on a first-come, first-served basis. (16)

open posture (ōpən pŏs´chər) A position that conveys a feeling of receptiveness and friendliness; facing another person with arms comfortably at the sides or in the lap. (4)

ophthalmologist (ŏf-thəl-mŏl´ə-jĭst) A medical doctor who is an eye specialist. (35)

ophthalmoscope (of-thal´mō-skōp) A hand-held instrument with a light; used to view inner eye structures. (43)

opioid (ō´-pē-óid) A natural or synthetic drug that produces opium-like effects. (51)

opportunistic infection (ŏp´ər-toon ĭs´tĭk ĭn-fěk-shən) Infection by microorganisms that can cause disease only when a host's resistance is low. (6)

optical character reader (OCR) (ŏp´tĭ-kəl kär´ək-tər rēd ər) An electronic scanner that can "read" typed letters. (10)

optical character recognition (OCR) (ŏp´tĭ-kəl kär´ək-tər rek-uhg-nish-uhn) The process or technology of reading data in printed form by a device that scans and identifies characters. (8)

optical microscope (op´ti-kəl mī´krə-skōp´) A microscope that uses light, concentrated through a condenser and focused through the object being examined, to project an image. (45)

optic chiasm (ŏp´tĭk kī´azm) A structure located at the base of the brain where parts of the optic nerves cross. It carries visual information to the brain. (35)

optician (ŏp-tĭ´shən) An eye professional who fills prescriptions for eyeglasses and contact lenses. (35)

optometrist (ŏp-tŏm´ĭ-trĭst) A trained and licensed vision specialist who is not a physician. (35)

orbicularis oculi (ōr-bik´yū-lā´ris ok´yū-lī) The muscle in the eyelid responsible for blinking. (35)

orbit (ôr´bĭt) The eye socket, which forms a protective shell around the eye. (35)

organ (ôr´gan) Structure formed by the organization of two or more different tissue types that carries out specific functions. (22)

organ of Corti (ôr´gən əv kôr´tē) The organ of hearing, located within the cochlea of the inner ear. (35)

organelle (ôr´gə-nəl´) A structure within a cell that performs a specific function. (22)

organic (ôr-găn´ĭk) Pertaining to matter that contains carbon and hydrogen. (22)

organism (ôr´gə-nĭz´əm) A whole living being that is formed from organ systems. (22)

organization (ōr´găn-ī-zā´shŭn) A facility or set of coordinated facilities that provide health care. (3)

organizational chart (ōr´găn-ī-zā´shŭn-əl chart) A formal drawing of the supervisory structure and reporting relationships of an organization such as a medical facility. (56)

organ system (ôr´gən sĭs´təm) A system that consists of organs that join together to carry out vital functions. (22)

orifice (ôr´i fis) An opening. (32)

origin (ôr´ə-jĭn) An attachment site of a skeletal muscle that does not move when a muscle contracts. (25)

Original Medicare Plan (ə-rĭj´ə-nəl měd´ĭ-kâr´ plăn) The Medicare fee-for-service plan that allows the beneficiary to choose any licensed physician certified by Medicare. (17)

oropharynx (ōr´ō-far´ingks) The portion of the pharynx behind the oral cavity. (33)

orthopedist (ôr´thə-pēd´ĭst) A specialist who diagnoses and treats diseases and disorders of the muscles and bones. (2)

orthopnea (ôr thop´nē a) Condition of difficulty breathing except while in an upright position. (29)

orthostatic hypotension (ôr´-thə-stăt´-ĭk hi´pō-těn´ shən) A situation in which blood pressure becomes low and the pulse increases when a patient is moved from a lying to standing position; also known as postural hypotension. (37)

OSHA (Occupational Safety and Health Act) (ō´shə) A set of regulations designed to save lives, prevent injuries, and protect the health of workers in the United States. (1, 6)

osmosis (ŏz-mō´s ĭs) The diffusion of water across a semipermeable membrane such as a cell membrane. (22)

ossicles (os´i-kĕls) Small bones; specifically, one of the bones of the tympanic cavity or middle ear. (35)

ossification (ä-sə-fə-kā´-shən) The process of bone growth. (24)

osteoarthritis (os´tē-ō-ahr-thrī´tis) Arthritis characterized by erosion of articular cartilage, which becomes soft, frayed, and thinned with eburnation of subchondral bone and outgrowths of marginal osteophytes; pain and loss of function result; mainly affects weight-bearing joints and is more common in women, the overweight, and older people. (41)

osteoblast (os´tē-ō-blast) Bone-forming cells that turn membrane into bone. They use excess blood calcium to build new bone. (24)

osteoclast (os´tē-ō-klast) Bone-dissolving cells. When bone is dissolved, calcium is released into the bloodstream. (24)

osteocyte (äs´-tē-ə-sīt) A cell of osseous tissue; also called a bone cell. (24)

osteon (äs´-tē-ən) Elongated cylinders that run up and down the long axis of bone. (24)

osteopathic manipulative medicine (OMM) (ŏs´tē-ō-păth´ĭk mə-nĭp´ū-lă´tĭv měd´ĭ-sĭn) A system of hands-on techniques that help relieve pain, restore motion, support the body's natural functions, and influence the body's structure. Osteopathic physicians study OMM in addition to medical courses. (2)

osteoporosis (ôs´tē-ō-pə-rō´sĭs) An endocrine and metabolic disorder of the musculoskeletal system, more common in women than in men, characterized by hunched-over posture. (41)

osteosarcoma (os´tē-ō-sar-kō´mă) A type of bone cancer that originates from osteoblasts, the cells that make bony tissue. (24)

OT See **oxytocin**. (32)

otologist (ō-tol´ŏ-jist) A medical doctor who specializes in the health of the ear. (43)

otorhinolaryngologist (ō-tō-rī´nō-lar-ing-gol´ŏ-jist) A specialist who diagnoses and treats diseases of the ear, nose, and throat. (2)

otosclerosis (ō-tō-sklŭ rō-sis) Hardening or immobilization of the stapes within the inner ear. (35)

out guide (out gīd) A marker made of stiff material and used as a placeholder when a file is taken out of a filing system. (15)

ova (ō va) Eggs. (32)

oval window (ō´vəl wĭn´dō) The beginning of the inner ear. (35)

overbooking (ō´vər-bŏŏk´ĭng) Scheduling appointments for more patients than can reasonably be seen in the time allowed. (16)

oviduct (ō´ və´duct) A Fallopian tube. (32)

ovulation (ŏ´vyə-lā´shən) The process by which the ovaries release one ovum (egg) approximately every 28 days. (32)

ovum (ō vəm) One egg. The female "egg" that unites with the male sperm to begin reproduction. (22)

oxygenated (ok´səjənātəd) Oxygenated blood refers to blood that has been to the lungs and is carrying oxygen in the hemoglobin. (23)

oxygen debt (ok´s ĭ-jən det) A condition that develops when skeletal muscles are used strenuously for a minute or two. (29)

oxyhemoglobin (oks-ē-hē-mō-glō´bin) Hemoglobin that is bound to oxygen. It is bright red in color. (29)

oxytocin (OT) (ok-sē-tō´sin) A hormone that causes contraction of the uterus during childbirth and the ejection of milk from mammary glands during breast-feeding. (32)

package insert (pak´ăj in´sərt) A manufacturer's printed guideline for the use and dosing of a drug; includes the pharmacokinetics, dosage forms, and other relevant information about a drug. (51)

packed red blood cells (păkt rĕd blud sĕlz) Red blood cells that collect at the bottom of a centrifuged blood sample. (48)

palate (pal´ăt) The roof of the mouth. (33)

palatine (pa´-lə-tīn) Bones that form the anterior portion of the roof of the mouth and the **palate**. (24)

palatine tonsils (pal´ă-tīn tŏn´sils) Two masses of lymphatic tissue located at the back of the throat. (33)

palpation (păl-pā´shən) A type of touch used by healthcare providers to determine characteristics such as texture, temperature, shape, and the presence of movement. (38)

palpatory method (pal-pa´tôr´ē měth´əd) Systolic blood pressure measured by using the sense of touch. This measurement provides a necessary preliminary approximation of the systolic blood pressure to ensure an adequate level of inflation when the actual auscultatory measurement is made. (37)

palpitations (păl´pĭ-tā´shənz) Unusually rapid, strong, or irregular pulsations of the heart. (57)

pancreatic amylase (pan-krē-at´ik am´il-ās) An enzyme that digests carbohydrates. (33)

pancreatic lipase (pan-krē-at´ik lip´ās) An enzyme that digests lipids. (33)

panel (păn´əl) Tests frequently ordered together that are organ or disease oriented. (19)

papillae (pə-pĭl´ē) The "bumps" of the tongue in which the taste buds are found. (35)

paranasal sinuses (par-ă-nā´zəl sī´nŭs-ĕz) Air-filled spaces within skull bones that open into the nasal cavity. (29)

parasite (păr´ə-sīt´) An organism that lives on or in another organism and relies on it for nourishment or some other advantage to the detriment of the host organism. (46)

parasympathetic division (păr´ə-sĭm´pə-thĕt´ĭk) A division of the autonomic nervous system that prepares the body for rest and digestion. (30)

parathyroid glands (para-ă-thī royd glăndz) Four small glands embedded in the posterior thyroid gland that secrete parathyroid hormone (PTH); also known as parathormone. (34)

parathyroid hormone (PH) (par-ă-thī´royd hôr´mōn´) A hormone that helps regulate calcium levels in the bloodstream. It increases blood calcium by decreasing bone calcium. (32)

parenteral nutrition (pă-ren´ter-əl nōō-trĭsh´ən) Nutrition obtained when specially prepared nutrients are injected directly into patients' veins rather than taken by mouth. (55)

paresthesias (par-es-thē´zē-ăs) Abnormal sensations ranging from burning to tingling. (30)

parietal (pă-rī´ĕ-tăl) Bones that form most of the top and sides of the skull. (24)

parietal cells (pă-rī′ĕ-tăl sĕlz) Stomach cells that secrete hydrochloric acid, which is necessary to convert **pepsinogen** to **pepsin.** Parietal cells also secrete **intrinsic factor,** which is necessary for vitamin B$_{12}$ absorption. (33)

parietal pericardium (pă-rī′ĕ-tăl per-i-kar′dē-ŭm) The layer on top of the visceral pericardium. (26)

parietal peritoneum (pă-rī′ĕ-tăl per-ə-tŏ-nē′əm) The lining of the abdominal cavity. (33)

parotid glands (pă-rot′id glăndz) The largest of the salivary glands. The parotid glands are located beneath the skin just in front of the ears. (33)

participating physicians (pär-tĭs′ə-pāt′ĭng fĭ-zĭsh′ənz) Physicians who enroll in managed care plans. They have contracts with MCOs that stipulate their fees. (17)

participatory teaching (pahr-tis′i-pă-to′rē tēch′ing) Method of teaching that includes demonstrations of techniques that may be necessary to show that something has been learned. (14)

partnership (pärt′nər shĭp) A form of medical practice management in which two or more parties practice together under a written agreement, specifying the rights, obligations, and responsibilities of each partner. (5)

parturition (pär′tur ish′ən) The act of giving birth. (32)

passive listening (păs′ĭv lĭs′ən-ing) Hearing what a person has to say without responding in any way; contrast with **active listening.** (4)

patch test (păch tĕst) An allergy test in which a gauze patch soaked with a suspected allergen is taped onto the skin with nonallergenic tape; used to discover the cause of contact dermatitis. (42)

patella (pə-té-lə) The bone commonly referred to as the kneecap. (24)

pathogen (păth′ə-jən) A microorganism capable of causing disease. (6)

pathologist (pă-thŏl′ə-jĭst) A medical doctor who studies the changes a disease produces in the cells, fluids, and processes of the entire body. (2)

patient advocacy (pā′shĕnt ad′vŏ-kă-sē) The act of speaking and acting on behalf of the patient's needs and well-being. (3)

patient compliance (pā′shənt kəm-plī′əns) Obedience in terms of following a physician's orders. (41)

patient ledger card (pā′shənt lĕj′ər kärd) A card containing information

needed for insurance purposes, including the patient's name, address, telephone number, Social Security number, insurance information, employer's name, and any special billing instructions. It also includes the name of the person who is responsible for charges if this is anyone other than the patient. (21)

patient record/chart (pā′shənt rĕk′ərd/chärt) A compilation of important information about a patient's medical history and present condition. (11)

payee (pā-ē′) A person who receives a payment. (21)

payer (pā′ər) A person who pays a bill or writes a check. (21)

pay schedule (pā skĭej′ool) A list showing how often an employee is paid, such as weekly, biweekly, or monthly. (21)

pectoral girdle (pĕk′tər-əl gr-dl) The structure that attaches the arms to the axial skeleton. (24)

pediatrician (pē′dē-ə-trĭ-shən) A specialist who diagnoses and treats childhood diseases and teaches parents skills for keeping their children healthy. (2)

pediculosis (pədik′yoolō′sis) The medical term for lice. (23)

pegboard system (pĕg′bôrd sĭs′təm) A bookkeeping system that uses a lightweight board with pegs on which forms can be stacked, allowing each transaction to be entered and recorded on four different bookkeeping forms at once; also called the one-write system. (21)

pelvic girdle (pĕl′vik gr-dl) The structure that attaches the legs to the axial skeleton. (24)

pepsin (pep′sin) An enzyme that allows the body to digest proteins. (33)

pepsinogen (pep-sin′ō-jen) Substance that is secreted by the chief cells in the lining of the stomach and becomes **pepsin** in the presence of acid. (33)

peptidases (pep′ti-dās-ez) Enzymes that digest proteins. (33)

percussion (pər-kŭsh′ən) Tapping or striking the body to hear sounds or feel vibration. (38)

percutaneous exposure (per-kyū-tā′nē-ŭs ĭk-spō′zhər) Exposure to a pathogen through a puncture wound or needlestick. (46)

pericardium (per-i-kar′dē-ŭm) A membrane that covers the heart and large blood vessels attached to it. (26)

perilymph (per′i-limf) A fluid in the inner ear. When this fluid moves, it activates hearing and equilibrium receptors. (35)

perimetrium (peri-mē′trēŭm) The thin layer that covers the myometrium of the uterus. (32)

perimysium (per-i-mis′ē-ŭm) The connective tissue that divides a muscle into sections called fascicles. (25)

perineum (per i nē′üm) In the male, the area between the scrotum and anus; in the female, the area between the vagina and rectum. (32)

periosteum (pĕr′ē ŏs′tē əm) The membrane that surrounds the **diaphysis** of a bone. (24)

peripheral nervous system (PNS) (pə-rĭf′ər-əl nûr′vəs sĭs′təm) A system that consists of nerves that branch off the central nervous system. (30)

peristalsis (pĕr′ĭ-stôl′sĭs) The rhythmic muscular contractions that move a substance through a tract, such as food through the digestive tract and the ovum through the fallopian tube. (32, 34)

persistence (pĕr-sis′tĕns) Survival despite opposition or adverse environmental conditions. (3)

personal health record (PHR) (pĕr′sŏn-ăl helth rek′ŏrd) A health record that provides a summary of medical information, maintained in electronic or other format by an individual, that can be shared with anyone of the patient's choosing. (12)

personal protective equipment (PPE) (pur-sə-nəl prə-tek-tiv i-kwip-mənt) Any type of protective gear worn to guard against physical hazards. (6)

personal space (pûr′sə-nəl spās) A certain area that surrounds an individual and within which another person's physical presence is felt as an intrusion. (4)

PET See **positron emission tomography.** (42, 50)

petty cash fund (pĕt′ē kăsh fŭnd) Cash kept on hand in the office for small purchases. (21)

PH See **parathyroid hormone.** (32)

phagocyte (făg′ə-sīt′) A specialized white blood cell that engulfs and digests pathogens. (28)

phagocytosis (fag′ō-sī-tō′sis) The process by which white blood cells defend the body against infection by engulfing invading pathogens. (28)

phalanges (fə-lan′-jēz) The bones of the fingers. (24)

pharmaceutical (fär′mə-soo′tĭ-kəl) Pertaining to medicinal drugs. (51)

pharmacodynamics (far′mă-kō-dī-nam′iks) The study of what drugs do to the body: the mechanism of action, or how they work to produce a therapeutic effect. (51)

pharmacognosy (far-mă-kog′nō-sē) The study of characteristics of natural drugs and their sources. (51)

pharmacokinetics (far′mă-kō-kinet′iks) The study of what the body does to drugs: how the body absorbs, metabolizes, distributes, and excretes the drugs. (51)

pharmacology (făr′ma-kŏl′ə-jē) The study of drugs. (51)

pharmacotherapeutics (far′mă-kō-thĕr′ə-pyōō′tĭks) The study of how drugs are used to treat disease; also called clinical **pharmacology.** (51)

pharyngeal tonsils (fă-rin′jē-ăl tŏn′səls) Two masses of lymphatic tissue located above the palatine tonsils; also called adenoids. (33)

pharynx (făr′ĭngks) Structure below the mouth and nasal cavities that is an organ of the respiratory system as well as the digestive system. (29)

phenylketonuria (PKU) (fen′il-kē′tō-nū′rē-ă) A genetically inherited disorder in which the body cannot properly metabolize the nutrient phenylalanine, resulting in the buildup of phenylketones in the blood and their presence in the urine. The accumulation of phenylketones results in mental retardation. (22, 47)

PHI See **protected health information.** (5)

philosophy (fĭ-lŏs′ə-fē) The system of values and principles an office has adopted in its everyday practice. (14)

phlebotomy (flĭ-bŏt′ə-mē) The insertion of a needle or cannula (small tube) into a vein for the purpose of withdrawing blood. (48)

photometer (fō-tŏm′ĭ-tər) An instrument that measures light intensity. (45)

PHR See **personal health record.** (12)

physiatrist (fiz-ī′ă-trist) A physical medicine specialist, who diagnoses and treats diseases and disorders with physical therapy. (2)

physical therapy (fĭz′ĭ-kəl thĕr′ə-pē) A medical specialty that uses cold, heat, water, exercise, massage, traction, and other physical means to treat musculoskeletal, nervous, and cardiopulmonary disorders. (54)

physician assistant (PA) (fĭ-zĭsh′ən ə-sĭs′tənt) A healthcare provider who practices medicine under the supervision of a physician. (2)

physician's office laboratory (POL) (fĭ-zĭsh′ənz ô′fĭs lăb′rə-tôr′ē) A laboratory contained in a physician's office; processing tests in the POL produces quick turnaround and eliminates the need for patients to travel to other test locations. (45)

physiology (fĭz′ē-ŏl′ə-jē) The science of the study of the body's functions. (22)

pineal body (pin′ē-ăl bŏd′ē) A small gland located between the cerebral hemispheres that secretes melatonin. (34)

pitch (pĭch) The high or low quality in the sound of a person's speaking voice. (13)

PKU See **phenylketonuria.** (22, 47)

placebo effect (plə′-sē-bō ĭ-fĕkt′) The belief that a medication or treatment works even though it is not scientifically substantiated. In research, a placebo is an inactive substance or preparation used as a control to determine the effectiveness of a medicinal drug.

placenta (plə-sĕn′tə) An organ located between the mother and the fetus. It permits the absorption of nutrients and oxygen. In some cases, harmful substances such as viruses are absorbed through the placenta. (32)

plantar flexion (plan′tăr flek′shŭn) Pointing the toes downward. (25)

plasma (plăz′mə) The fluid component of blood, in which formed elements are suspended; makes up 55% of blood volume. (48)

plastic surgeon (plăs′tĭk sûr′jən) A specialist who reconstructs, corrects, or improves body structures. (2)

platelets (plāt′lĭts) Fragments of cytoplasm in the blood that are crucial to clot formation; also called thrombocytes. (27)

pleura (plūr′ă) The membranes that surround the lungs. (29)

pleural effusion (plŏŏr′ əl if yōō′zhən) A buildup of fluid within the pleural cavity. (29)

pleurisy (ploor′əsē) Also known as pleuritis; this is an inflammation of the parietal pleura of the lungs. (29)

pleuritis (ploor-ī′-tis) A condition in which the **pleura** become inflamed, which causes them to stick together. It can also cause an excess amount of fluid to form between the membranes. (29)

plexus (plĕk′səs) A structure that is formed when spinal nerves fuse together. It includes the cervical, brachial, and lumbosacral nerves. (30)

PMS See **premenstrual syndrome.** (32)

pneumoconiosis (nŭmŏ kō′nēō′sĭs) This is the name given to lung diseases that result

from years of exposure to different environmental or occupational types of dust. (29)

pneumothorax (nū-mō-thŏr′aks) The presence of air or gas in the pleural cavity. The lung typically collapses with pneumothorax. (29)

PNS See **peripheral nervous system.** (30)

podiatrist (pə-dī′-ə-trist) Physician who specializes in the study and treatment of the foot and ankle. (2)

POL See **physician's office laboratory.** (45)

polar body (pō′lər bŏd′ē) A nonfunctional cell that is one of two small cells formed during the division of an oocyte. (32)

polarity (pō-lăr′ĭ-tē) The condition of having two separate poles, one of which is positive and the other, negative. (49)

polarized (pō′lə-rīzd′) The state in which the outside of a cell membrane is positively charged and the inside is negatively charged. Polarization occurs when a neuron is at rest. (30)

policies and procedures (P&P) (pol′i-sēz prŏ-sē′jŭrz) A key written communication tool in the medical office that covers all office policies for administrative and clinical procedures. (56)

polypharmacy (pol′ē-fahr′mă-sē) The administration of many drugs at the same time. (41)

polysaccharide (pol-ē-sak′ă-rīd) A type of carbohydrate that is a starch. (33)

POMR (pē′ō-ĕm-är) The problem-oriented medical record system for keeping patients' charts. Information in a POMR includes the database of information about the patient and the patient's condition, the problem list, the diagnostic and treatment plan, and progress notes. (11)

portfolio (pôrt-fō′lē-ō′) A collection of an applicant's résumé, reference letters, and other documents of interest to a potential employer. (58)

positive tilt test (pŏz′-ĭ-tĭv tĭlt tĕst) When the pulse rate increases more than 10 beats per minute (bpm) and the blood pressure drops more than 20 points while taking vital signs in the lying, sitting, and standing positions. (37)

positron emission tomography (PET) (pah′-zih-tron ee-mih′-shun toh-mah′-gruh-fee) A radiologic procedure that entails injecting isotopes combined with other substances involved in metabolic activity, such as glucose. These special isotopes emit positrons, which a computer processes and displays on a screen. (42, 50)

postcoital (pōst-kō´i-tăl) After sexual union. (39)

posterior (pŏ-stîr´ē-ar) Anatomic term meaning toward the back of the body. Also called dorsal. (22)

postnatal period (pōst-nā´tăl pîr´ē-əd) The period following childbirth. (32)

postoperative (pōst-ŏp´ər-ə-tĭv) Taking place after a surgical procedure. (44)

postural hypotension (pŏs-chĕr-ăl hī-pō-tĕn-shŭn) A situation in which blood pressure becomes low and the pulse increases when a patient is moved from a lying to a standing position; also known as orthostatic hypotension. (37)

posture (pŏs´chər) Body position and alignment. (54)

power of attorney (pou´ər ə-tûr´nē) The legal right to act as the attorney or agent of another person, including handling that person's financial matters. (21)

PPE See **personal protective equipment.** (6)

PPO See **preferred provider organization.** (17)

practitioner (prăk-tĭsh´ə-nər) One who practices a profession. (1)

preauthorization (prē ô´thər-ĭ-zā´shən) Authorization or approval for payment from a third-party payer requested in advance of a specific procedure. (17)

pre-certification (prē sûr´tə-fĭ-kā´shən) A determination of the amount of money that will be paid by a third-party payer for a specific procedure before the procedure is conducted. (17)

preferred provider organization (PPO) (pr ĭ-fûrd´ prə-vīd´ər or gə-nĭ-zā´shən) A managed care plan that establishes a network of providers to perform services for plan members. (17)

prefix (prē-fĭks) A word part that comes at the beginning of a medical term that alters the meaning of the term. (22)

premenstrual syndrome (PMS) (prē-me´n-strŭ-al sin´-drōm) A syndrome that is a collection of symptoms that occur just before the menstrual period. (32)

premium (prē´mē-əm) The basic annual cost of healthcare insurance. (17)

prenatal period (prē-nā´tăl pîr´ē-əd) The period that includes the embryonic and fetal periods until the delivery of the offspring. (32)

preoperative (prē-ŏp´ər-ə-tĭv) Taking place prior to surgery. (44)

prepuce (prē´pūs) A piece of skin in the uncircumcised male that covers the glans penis. (32)

presbyopia (prez-bē-ō´pē-ă) A common eye disorder that results in the loss of lens elasticity. Presbyopia develops with age and causes a person to have difficulty seeing objects close up. (43)

prescribe (pr ĭ-skr īb´) To give a patient a prescription to be filled by a pharmacy. (51)

prescription (pr ĭ-skr ĭp´shən) A physician's written order for medication. (51)

prescription drug (pr ĭ-skr ĭp´shən drŭg) A drug that can be legally used only by order of a physician and must be administered or dispensed by a licensed healthcare professional. (51)

preventive medicine (prĕ-ven´tiv med´i-sin) The branch of medical science concerned with the prevention of disease and with promotion of physical and mental health, through study of the etiology and epidemiology of disease processes. (2, 41)

primary care physician (PCP) (pr ī´mĕr´ē kâr fĭ-zĭsh´ən) A physician who provides routine medical care and referrals to specialists. (2)

primary diagnosis (prī´mar-ē dī-ăg-nō´sis) The diagnosis given as the primary reason for the patient seeking care. (18)

primary germ layer (pr ī´mĕr´ē jûrm lā´ər) An inner cell mass that organizes into layers: the ectoderm, mesoderm, and endoderm. (32)

prime mover (pr īm moo´vər) The muscle responsible for most of the movement when a body movement is produced by a group of muscles. (25)

primordial follicle (pr ī-mōr´dē-ălfŏl´ĭ-kəl) A structure that develops in the ovarian cortex of a female infant before she is born. (32)

principal diagnosis (prin´si-păl dī´ăg-nō´sis) The diagnosis that is found, after testing and study, to be the main reason for the patient's need for healthcare services. (18)

prioritizing (prī-ôr-ĭ-tīz´-ing) Sorting and dealing with matters in the order of urgency and importance. (3)

Privacy Rule (pr ī´və-sē rool) Common name for the **HIPAA** Standard for Privacy of Individually Identifiable Health Information, which provides the first comprehensive federal protection for the privacy of health information. The Privacy Rule creates national standards to protect individuals' medical records and other personal health information. (5)

PRL See **prolactin.** (34)

probationary period (prō-bā-shŭn-ār-ē pĕr´ē-ŏd) A trial period where the employer may terminate the new employee without cause. (56)

problem solving (prob´lĕm sŏlv-ing) A step-by-step approach that uses critical thinking and good judgment to deal with situations or occurrences that need resolution. (3)

procedure code (prə-sē´jər kōd) Codes that represent medical procedures, such as surgery and diagnostic tests, and medical services, such as an examination to evaluate a patient's condition. (19)

proctologist (prok-tŏl´ə-jĭst) Physician who diagnoses and treats disorders of the anus, rectum, and intestines. (2)

proctoscopy (prok-tos´kō-pē) An examination of the lower rectum and anal canal with a 3-inch instrument called a proctoscope to detect hemorrhoids, polyps, fissures, fistulas, and abscesses. (42)

professional development (prŏ-fesh´ŭn-ăl dĕ-vel´ŏp-mĕnt) The skills and knowledge attained for both personal development and career advancement. (1)

professional objective (prŏ-fesh´un-ăl ŏb-jek´tiv) A brief, general statement that demonstrates a career goal. (58)

proficiency testing program (prə-fī´shən-cē tĕst´ing prō´grăm´) A required set of tests for clinical laboratories; the tests measure the accuracy of the laboratory's test results and adherence to standard operating procedures. (45)

progesterone (prō-jĕs´tə-rōn´) A female steroid hormone primarily produced by the ovary. (32)

prognosis (prŏg-nō´sĭs) A prediction of the probable course of a disease in an individual and the chances of recovery. (38)

prolactin (PRL) (prō-lak´tin) A hormone that stimulates milk production in the mammary glands. (34)

prolapse (prō´laps) A sinking of an organ or other part, especially its appearance at a natural or artificial orifice. (41)

proliferation phase (prə-lif´ər-ā´shən fāz) The second phase of wound healing, in which new tissue forms, closing off the wound. (44)

pronation (prō-nā´shŭn) Turning the palms of the hand downward. (25)

pronunciation (prə-nun´cē-ā´shən) The sounding out of words. (13)

proofreading (proof´rēd´ĭng) Checking a document for formatting, data, and mechanical errors. (10)

prophase (prōfaz) Movement of the replicated centrioles to the opposite ends of the cell, creating spindle-like fibers during mitosis. (22)

proportion method (prō-pōr′shŭn meth′ŏd) A fraction formula based on ratios and proportions that is used to calculate dosage. (52)

prostaglandin (pros-tă-glan′din) A local hormone derived from lipid molecules. Prostaglandins typically do not travel in the bloodstream to find their target cells because their targets are close by. This hormone has numerous effects, including uterine stimulation during childbirth. (34)

prostate gland (prŏs′tāt′ glănd) A chestnut-shaped gland that surrounds the beginning of the urethra in the male. (32)

prostatitis (pros-tă-tī′tis) Inflammation of the prostate gland, which can be acute or chronic. (32)

protected health information (PHI) (prə-těkt-əd hělth ĭn′fər-mā′shən) Individually identifiable health information that is transmitted or maintained by electronic or other media, such as computer storage devices. The core of the **HIPAA Privacy Rule** is the protection, use, and disclosure of protected health information. (5)

protein (prō′tēn) Macromolecules consisting of long sequences of α-amino acids [$H_2N-CHR-COOH$] in peptide (amide) linkage (elimination of H_2O between the α-NH_2 and α-COOH of successive residues). Protein is three-fourths of the dry weight of most cell matter and is involved in structures, hormones, enzymes, muscle contraction, immunologic response, and essential life functions. The amino acids involved are generally the 20 α-amino acids (glycine, l-alanine) recognized by the genetic code. Cross-links yielding globular forms of protein are often effected through the –SH groups of two sulfur-containing l-cysteinyl residues, as well as by noncovalent forces (e.g., hydrogen bonds, lipophilic attractions). (55)

proteinuria (prō-tē-nū′rē-ă) An excess of protein in the urine. (47)

protozoan (prō′-tə-zō′ən) A single-celled eukaryotic organism much larger than a bacterium; some protozoans can cause disease in humans. (46)

protraction (prō-trăk′shən) Moving a body part anteriorly. (25)

proximal (prok′si-măl) Anatomic term meaning closer to a point of attachment or closer to the trunk of the body. (22)

proximal convoluted tubule (prok′simăl kon′vō-lū-ted tū′byūl) The portion of the renal tubule that is directly attached to the glomerular capsule and becomes the loop of Henle. (31)

psoriasis (sə-rī′ə-sĭs) A common skin condition characterized by reddish-silver scaly lesions most often found on the elbows, knees, scalp, and trunk. (23)

puberty (pyoo′bər-tē) The period of adolescence when a person begins to develop secondary sexual traits and reproductive functions. (40)

pubis (pyü′-bəs) The area that forms the front of a hip bone. (24)

pulmonary circuit (pool′mə-nĕr′ē sûr′kĭt) The route that blood takes from the heart to the lungs and back to the heart again. (26)

pulmonary circulation (pul′mŏ-nar-ē sĭr′kyū-lā′shŭn) The passage of blood from the right ventricle through the pulmonary artery to the lungs and back through the pulmonary veins to the left atrium. (26)

pulmonary function test (pool′mə-nĕr′ē fŭngk′shən tĕst) A test that evaluates a patient's lung volume and capacity; used to detect and diagnose pulmonary problems or to monitor certain respiratory disorders and evaluate the effectiveness of treatment. (49)

pulmonary semilunar valve (pool′mə-nĕr′ēsem′ē loonər valv) A heart valve that is a semilunar valve. It is situated between the right ventricle and the pulmonary trunk. (26)

pulmonary trunk (pool′mə-nĕr′ē trŭngk) A large artery that branches into the pulmonary arteries and carries blood to the lungs. (26)

punctuality (pŭngk-choo-al-i-tē) Showing up on appointed dates and at appointed times. (3)

puncture wound (pŭngk′chər wound) A deep wound caused by a sharp, pointed object. (44)

punitive damages (pyoo′nĭ-tĭv dăm′ĭjez) Money paid as punishment for intentionally breaking the law. (20)

pupil (pyoo′pəl) The opening at the center of the iris, which grows smaller or larger as the iris contracts or relaxes, respectively; it regulates the amount of light that enters the eye. (35)

purchase order (pûr′chĭs ôr′dər) A form that authorizes a purchase for the practice. (8)

purchasing groups (pur′chĭs-ĭng groops) Groups of medical offices associated with a nearby hospital that order supplies through the hospital to obtain a quantity discount. (8)

Purkinje fibers (per′kin-jē fi′bərz) Cardiac fibers that are located in the lateral walls of the ventricles. (26)

pyelonephritis (pī′ĕ-lō-ne-frī′tis) A urinary tract infection that involves one or both of the kidneys. (31)

pyloric sphincter (pī-lôrĭk sfingk′tər) The valve-like structure composed of a circular band of muscle at the juncture of the stomach and small intestine. (33)

pyothorax (pī ō thôr′ aks) Pus or infected fluid in the pleural cavity causing collapse of the lung. (29)

pyrogens (pī′rō-jenz) Fever-producing substances released by neutrophils. (48)

QC See **quality control.** (45)

qi (chē) According to traditional Chinese medicine, a vital energy that flows throughout the body.

quadrants (kwŏd′rəntz) Four equal sections, such as those into which the abdomen is figuratively divided during an examination. (38)

qualitative analysis (kwŏl′ĭ-tā′tĭv-ənăl′ĭ-sĭs) In microbiology, identification of bacteria present in a specimen by the appearance of colonies grown on a culture plate. (46)

qualitative test response (kwŏl′ĭ-tā′tĭv tĕst rĭ-spŏns′) A test result that indicates the substance tested for is either present or absent. (45)

quality assurance program (kwŏl′ĭ-tē ə-shoor′əns prō′gram′) A required program for clinical laboratories designed to monitor the quality of patient care, including quality control, instrument and equipment maintenance, proficiency testing, training and continuing education, and standard operating procedures documentation. (45)

quality control (QC) (kwŏl′ĭ-tē kən-trōl′) An ongoing system, required in every physician's office, to evaluate the quality of medical care provided. (46)

quality control program (kwŏl′ĭ-tē kəntrōl′ prō′grăm′) A component of a quality assurance program that focuses on ensuring accuracy in laboratory test results through careful monitoring of test procedures. (45)

quantitative analysis (kwŏn´tĭ-tā´tĭv ə-năl´ĭ-sĭs) In microbiology, a determination of the number of bacteria present in a specimen by direct count of colonies grown on a culture plate. (46)

quantitative test results (kwŏn´tĭ-tā´tĭv tĕst rĭ-zŭlt´) The concentration of a test substance in a specimen. (45)

quarterly return (kwŏr´tar-lē rĭ-tûrn´) The Employer's Quarterly Federal Tax Return, a form submitted to the IRS every 3 months that summarizes the federal income and employment taxes withheld from employees' paychecks. (21)

qui tam (kwē - ´tăm) Latin, meaning "to bring action for the king and for one's self." (5)

RA See **explanation of benefits, remittance advice.** (17)

radial artery (rā´dē-əl är´tə-rē) An artery located in the groove on the thumb side of the inner wrist, where the pulse is taken on adults. (37)

radiation therapy (rā´dē-ā´shən thĕr´ə-pē) The use of x-rays and radioactive substances to treat cancer. (50)

radiography (rā´dē-og´rə-fē) Examination of any part of the body for diagnostic purposes by means of x-rays with the record of the findings usually impressed on a photographic film. (50)

radiologist (rā´dē-ŏl´ə-jĭst) A physician who specializes in taking and reading x-rays. (2)

radius (rā-dē-əs) The lateral bone of the forearm. (24)

rales (ralz) Noisy respirations usually due to blockage of the bronchial tubes. (37)

RAM See **random access memory.** (8)

random access memory (RAM) (răn´dəm ăk´sĕs mĕm´ə-rē) The temporary, or programmable, memory in a computer. (8)

random urine specimen (răn´dəm yŏŏr´ĭn spĕs´ə-mən) A single urine specimen taken at any time of the day; the most common type of sample collected. (47)

range of motion (ROM) (rānj mō´shən) The degree to which a joint is able to move. (54)

rapport (ră-pôr´) A harmonious, positive relationship. (4)

RBRVS See **resource-based relative value scale.** (17)

read only memory (ROM) (rĕd ōn´lē mĕm´ə-rē) A computer's permanent memory, which can be read by the computer but not changed. It provides the

computer with the basic operating instructions it needs to function. (8)

reagent (rē-ā´jənt) A chemical or chemically treated substance used in test procedures and formulated to react in specific ways when exposed under specific conditions. (45)

reconciliation (rĕk´ən-sĭl´ē-ā´shən) A comparison of the office's financial records with bank records to ensure that they are consistent and accurate; usually done when the monthly checking account statement is received from the bank. (21)

records management system (rĕ-kôrdz măn´ĭj-mənt sĭs´təm) How patient records are created, filed, and maintained. (15)

recovery position (rĭ-kŭv´ər-ē pə-zĭsh´ən) The position a person is placed in after receiving first aid for choking or cardiopulmonary resuscitation. (57)

rectum (rĕk´təm) The last section of the sigmoid colon that straightens out and becomes the anal canal. (33)

Red Flags Rule (rĕd flăgz rūl) A law requiring certain businesses, including most medical offices and other healthcare facilities, to develop written programs to detect the warning signs, or red flags, of identity theft. (7)

reference (rĕf´ər-əns) A recommendation for employment from a facility or a preceptor. (5)

reference laboratory (rĕf´ər-əns lăb´rə-tôr´ē) A laboratory owned and operated by an organization outside the physician's practice. (45)

referral (rĭ-fûr´əl) An authorization from a medical practice for a patient to have specialized services performed by another practice; often required for insurance purposes. (17)

reflection (rĭ-flĕk´shən) When a thought, idea or opinion is formed as a result of deeper thought. (36)

reflex (rē´flĕks´) A predictable automatic response to stimuli. (30)

reflexology (rē -flĕk-sŏl´-ə-jē) Manual therapy to the foot and/or hand in which pressure is applied to "reflex" points mapped out on the feet or hands.

refraction (rĭ-frăk´shən) The bending of light by the cornea, lens, and eye fluids to focus light onto the retina. (35)

refraction examination (rĭ-frăk´shən ĭg-zăm´ə-nā´shən) An eye examination in which the patient looks through a succession of different lenses to find out which ones create the clearest image. (43)

refractometer (rē-frak-tom´ĕ-ter) An optical instrument that measures the refraction, or bending, of light as it passes through a liquid. (47)

Registered Medical Assistant (RMA) (rĕj´ĭ-stərd mĕd´ĭ-kəl ə-sĭs´tənt) A medical assistant who has met the educational requirements and taken and passed the certification examination for medical assisting given by the American Medical Technologists (AMT). (1)

registration (rĕj´ĭs-trā´shŭn) The recording of information (e.g., licensure, birth or death date). (1)

Reiki (ray-key) The use of visualization and touch to balance energy flow and bring healthy energy to affected body parts.

relaxin (rē-lak´sin) A hormone that comes from the corpus luteum. It inhibits uterine contractions and relaxes the ligaments of the pelvis in preparation for childbirth. (32)

remedy (rĕm´-ĭ-dē) A treatment prescribed by a homeopath in small amounts that in large doses would produce the same symptoms seen in the patient.

remittance advice (RA) (rĭ-mĭt´nsăd-vīs´) A form that the patient and the practice receive for each encounter that outlines the amount billed by the practice, the amount allowed, the amount of subscriber liability, the amount paid, and notations of any service not covered, including an explanation of why that service is not covered; also called an **explanation of benefits.** (17)

renal calculi (rē´nəl kăl´kyə-lī´) Kidney stones. (31)

renal column (rē´nəl kŏl´əm) The portion of the **renal cortex** between the **renal pyramids.** (31)

renal corpuscle (rē´nəl kôr´pə-səl) Corpuscle that is composed of the glomerulus and the glomerular capsule. The filtration of blood occurs here. (31)

renal cortex (rē´nəl kôr´tĕks´) The outermost layer of the kidney. (31)

renal medulla (rē´nəl mĭ-dŭl´ə) The middle portion of the kidney. (31)

renal pelvis (rē´nəl pĕl´vĭs) The internal structure of the kidney. Urine flows from the renal pelvis down the ureter. (31)

renal pyramids (rē´nəl pĭr´ə-mĭdz) Triangular-shaped areas in the medulla of the kidney. (31)

renal sinus (rē´nəl sī´nəs) The medial depression of a kidney. (31)

renal tubule (rē´nəl tū´byūl) Structure that extends from the glomerular capsule of a nephron and is composed of the proximal convoluted tubule, the loop of Henle, and the distal convoluted tubule. (31)

renin (rĕn´in) A hormone secreted by the kidney that helps to regulate blood pressure. (31)

repolarization (rē´pō-lăr-i-zā´shŭn) The process of returning to the original polar (resting) state. (30, 49)

reputable (rĕp-yə-tə-bəl) Having a good reputation. (8)

requisition (rĕk´wĭ-zĭsh´ən) A formal request from a staff member or doctor for the purchase of equipment or supplies. (8)

reservoir host (rĕz´ər-vwär´ hōst) An animal, insect, or human whose body is susceptible to growth of a pathogen. (6)

resident normal flora (´re-zə-dənt, ´nôr-məl, ´flōr-ə) Bacteria, fungi, and protozoa that have taken up residence either in or on the human body. Some of these organisms neither help nor harm the host and some are beneficial, creating a barrier against pathogens.

res ipsa loquitur (rees ip-suh loh-kwi-ter) Latin, meaning "the thing speaks for itself," which is also known as the doctrine of common knowledge. (5)

resource-based relative value scale (RBRVS) (rē´sôrs´ băst rĕl´ə-tĭv văl´yōō skāl) The payment system used by Medicare. It establishes the relative value units for services, replacing the providers' consensus on usual fees. (17)

respiratory distress syndrome (res´pə-rə-tôr´ē distres sin´drəm) Condition found usually in premature babies, who lack the substance surfactant in their lungs, causing the lungs to collapse on expiration. (29)

respiratory hygiene/cough etiquette (rĕs´pər-ə-tôr´ē hī´jēn´kôf ĕt´ĭ-kĭt) Infection control guideline that includes teaching the patient to cover his or her mouth/nose when coughing and dispose of tissues in the proper receptacle. (38)

respiratory volume (rĕs´pər-ə-tôr´ē vŏl´yōōm) The different volumes of air that move in and out of the lungs during different intensities of breathing. These volumes can be measured to assess the healthiness of the respiratory system. (29)

respondeat superior (rehs-pond-dee-at soo-peer-ee-or) Latin, meaning "let the master answer," a doctrine under which an employer is legally liable for the acts of his or her employees, if such acts were performed within the scope of the employee's duties. (5)

restatement (rē-stāt´ment) Repeating what a patient says in your own words back to the patient. (36)

résumé (rĕz´ŏŏ-mā´) A typewritten document summarizing one's employment and educational history. (1)

retention schedule (rĭ-tĕn´shənskĕj´ōōl) A schedule that details how long to keep different types of patient records in the office after they have become inactive or closed and how long the records should be stored. (15)

retina (rĕt´n-ə) The inner layer of the eye; contains light-sensing nerve cells. (35)

retraction (rĭ-trăk´shən) Moving a body part posteriorly. (25)

retrograde pyelography (rĕt´rə-grād´pī´ĕ-log´ră-fē) A radiologic procedure in which the doctor injects a contrast medium through a urethral catheter and takes a series of x-rays to evaluate function of the ureters, bladder, and urethra. (50)

retroperitoneal (re-trō-per-ə-tə-nē´-əl) An anatomic term that means behind the peritoneal cavity. It is where the kidneys lie. (31)

return demonstation (rĭ-tûrn´dĕm´ən-strā´shən) Participatory teaching method in which the technique is first described to the patient and then demonstrated to the patient; the patient is then asked to repeat the demonstration. (14)

review of systems (rē-vū´ sis´tĕmz) A process of gathering information about a patient's health history regardless of apparent relevance to the chief complaint. (11)

rhabdomyolysis (rab´dō-mī-ol´i-sis) A condition in which the kidneys have been damaged due to toxins released from muscle cells. (25)

Rh antigen (är´ āch an´tĭ-jən) A protein first discovered on the red blood cells of rhesus monkeys, hence the name Rh. (27)

RhoGAM (rō´găm) A medication that prevents an Rh-negative mother from making antibodies against the Rh antigen. (27)

ribosomes (rībəsōmz) The organelle within the cytoplasm responsible for protein synthesis. (22)

RMA See **Registered Medical Assistant.** (1)

RNA (är´ĕn-ā´) A nucleic acid used to make protein. (22)

rods (rŏdz) Light-sensing nerve cells in the eye, at the posterior of the retina, that function in dim light but do not provide sharp images or detect color. (35)

ROM See **read only memory.** (8)

rosacea (rō-zā´shē-ă) A condition characterized by chronic redness and acne over the nose and cheeks. (23)

rotation (rō-tā´shən) Twisting a body part. (25)

route (rōōt) The way a drug is introduced into the body. (51)

rugae (rōō´gā) The expandable folds of an organ. (32) The folds of the stomach lining. (33)

sacrum (sa´-krəm) A triangular-shaped bone that consists of five fused vertebra. (24)

sagittal (saj´i-tăl) An anatomic term that refers to the plane that divides the body into left and right portions. (22)

salutation (săl´yə-tā´shən) A written greeting, such as "Dear," used at the beginning of a letter. (10)

sanitization (săn´ĭ-tĭ-zā´shən) A reduction of the number of microorganisms on an object or a surface to a fairly safe level. (9)

sarcolemma (sar´kō-lem´ă) The cell membrane of a muscle fiber. (25)

sarcoplasm (sar´-kō-pla-zim) The cytoplasm of a muscle fiber. (25)

sarcoplasmic reticulum (sar-kō-plaz´mik re-tik´yū-lŭm) The endoplasmic reticulum of a muscle fiber. (25)

SARS (severe acute respiratory syndrome) (särz; sivĕr əkyōōt res´pərətôr´ē sin´drəm) A severe and acute respiratory illness characterized by fever and a nonproductive cough that progresses to the point at which insufficient oxygen is present in the blood. (29)

saturated fat (săch´ə-rā´tĭd făt) Fats, derived primarily from animal sources, that are usually solid at room temperature and that tend to raise blood cholesterol levels. (55)

scabies (skā´bēz) Skin lesions that are very itchy and caused by a burrowing mite. Scabies is most commonly found between the fingers and on the genitalia. (23)

scanner (skăn´ər) An optical device that converts printed matter into a format that can be read by the computer and inputs the converted information. (8)

scapula (sk´a-pyə-la) Thin, triangular-shaped, flat bones located on the dorsal surface of the rib cage; also called shoulder blades. (24)

Schwann cell (shwahn sĕl) A neuroglial cell whose cell membrane coats the axons. (27)

sciatica (sī-ăt´ĭ-kə) Pain in the low back and hip radiating down the back of the leg along the sciatic nerve. (30)

sclera (sklĭr´ə) The tough, outermost layer, or "white," of the eye, through which light cannot pass; covers all except the front of the eye. (35)

scoliosis (skō´lē-ō´sĭs) A lateral curvature of the spine, which is normally straight when viewed from behind. (24, 38)

scored (skōrd) An indented line on a tablet where the medication can be broken into pieces. (53)

scratch test (skrăch tĕst) An allergy test in which extracts of suspected allergens are applied to the patient's skin and the skin is then scratched to allow the extracts to penetrate. (42)

screening (skrēn´ĭng) Performing a diagnostic test on a person who is typically free of symptoms. (14)

screen saver (skrēn sāv´ər) A program that automatically changes the monitor display at short intervals or constantly shows moving images to prevent burn-in of images on the computer screen. (8)

scrotum (skrō´təm) In a male, the sac of skin below the pelvic cavity that contains the testes. (32)

sebaceous (sĭ-bā´shəs) A type of oil gland found in the dermis. (23)

sebum (sē´bŭm) An oily substance produced by sebaceous glands. (23)

secondary diagnosis (sek´ŏn-dār-ē dī-ăg-nō´sis) Diagnosis other than the primary diagnosis for other conditions that are also affecting the patient at the time of the visit. (18)

Security Rule (sĭ-kyŏŏr´ĭ-tē rōōl) The technical safeguards that protect the confidentiality, integrity, and availability of health information covered by **HIPAA.** The Security Rule specifies how patient information is protected on computer networks, the Internet, disks, and other storage media. (5)

seizure (sē´zhər) A series of violent and involuntary contractions of the muscles; also called a convulsion. (30)

self-confidence (self-kŏn-fĭ-dĕns) Believing in oneself; assured. (3)

sella turcica (sel´ă tŭr´sē-kă) A deep depression in the sphenoid bone where the pituitary gland sits. (24)

semen (sē´mən) Sperm and the various substances that nourish and transport them. (32)

semicircular canals (sĕm´ē-sŭr´kyə-lər kə-nălz´) Structures in the inner ear that help a person maintain balance; each of the three canals is positioned at right angles to the other two. (35)

seminal vesicles (sem´-ə-năl ves´i-klz) A pair of convoluted tubes that lie behind the bladder. These tubes secrete a fluid that provides nutrition for the sperm. (32)

seminiferous tubules (sem´i-nif´er-ŭs tū´byūlz) These tubes contain spermatogenic cells and are located in the lobules of the testes. (32)

sensorineural hearing loss (sen´sŏr-i-nūr´ăl hîr´ĭng lôs) This type of hearing loss occurs when neural structures associated with the ear are damaged. Neural structures include hearing receptors and the auditory nerve. (43)

sensory (sĕn´sə-rē) Afferent neurons that carry sensory information from the periphery to the central nervous system. (30)

sensory adaptation (sĕn´sə-rē ăd´ăp-tā´shən) A process in which the same chemical can stimulate receptors only for a limited amount of time until the receptors eventually no longer respond to the chemical. (35)

sensory teaching (sen´sŏr-ē tēch´ing) Method of teaching that provides patient with a description of the physical sensations he or she may have as part of the learning or the procedure involved. (14)

septic shock (sĕp´tĭk shŏk) A state of shock resulting from massive, widespread infection that affects the blood vessels' ability to circulate blood. (57)

sequential order (sĭ´kwĕn´shəl ôr´dər) One after another in a predictable pattern or sequence. (15)

serosa (se-rō´să) The outermost layer of the alimentary canal; also known as the visceral peritoneum. (35)

serous cells (sēr´ŭs sĕlz) One of two types of cells that make up the salivary glands. These cells secrete a watery fluid that contains amylase. (33)

serum (sēr´ŭm) The liquid portion of blood (plasma) when all of the clotting factors have been removed. (27)

serum separators (sēr´ŭm sep´ăr-ā´tŏrz) A type of blood collection tube with an additive that, when spun, forms a gel-like barrier between serum and the clot in a coagulated blood sample. (48)

service contract (sûr´vĭs kŏn´trăkt´) A contract that covers services for equipment that are not included in a standard maintenance contract. (8)

severe acute respiratory syndrome See **SARS.** (29)

sex chromosome (sĕks krō´mə-sōm´) Chromosome of the 23rd pair. (22)

sex-linked trait (sĕks lĭngk trāt) Traits that are carried on the sex chromosomes, or X and Y chromosomes. (22)

sexual harassment (sek´shū-ăl hăr´ăs-ment) Unwelcome verbal, visual, or physical conduct of a sexual nature that is severe or pervasive and affects working conditions or creates a hostile work environment. (56)

sigmoid colon (sig-mòid kō-lən) An S-shaped tube that lies between the **descending colon** and the **rectum.** (33)

sigmoidoscopy (sig´moy-dos´kŏ-pē) A procedure in which the interior of the sigmoid area of the large intestine, between the descending colon and the rectum, is examined with a sigmoidoscope, a lighted instrument with a magnifying lens. (42)

sign (sīn) An objective or external factor, such as blood pressure, rash, or swelling, that can be seen or felt by the physician or measured by an instrument. (11, 38)

signature block (sig´-nuh-cher blok´) The writer's name and business title found four lines below the complimentary closing in a business letter. (10)

silicosis (sil´i kō´sis) Chronic lung disease caused by the inhalation of silica dust. (29)

simplified letter style (sĭm´plə-fīd´ lĕt´ər stīl) A modification of the full-block style in which the salutation and complimentary closing are omitted and a subject line typed in all capital letters is placed between the address and the body of the letter. (10)

single-entry account (sĭng´gəl-ĕn´trē ə-kount´) An account that has only one charge, usually for a small amount, for a patient who does not come in regularly. (20)

sinoatrial node (sī´nō-ā´trē-ăl nōd) A small bundle of heart muscle tissue in the superior wall of the right atrium that sets the rhythm (or pattern) of the heart's contractions; also called sinus node or pacemaker. (26)

sinusitis (sī´nə-sī´tĭs) Inflammation of the lining of a sinus. (29)

skinfold test (skĭn´fōld tĕst) A method of measuring fat as a percentage of body weight by measuring the thickness of a fold of skin with a caliper. (55)

skip (skĭp) A patient who has moved without leaving a forwarding address and his bill is unpaid. (20)

slander (slăn´dər) The speaking of defamatory words intended to prejudice others against an individual in a manner that jeopardizes his or her reputation or means of livelihood. (5)

SLE See **systemic lupus erythematosus.** (28)

sleep apnea (slēp ap-nē´ah) A condition characterized by pauses in breathing during sleep. (49)

slit lamp (slĭt lămp) An instrument composed of a magnifying lens combined with a light source; used to provide a minute examination of the eye's anatomy. (43)

smear (smîr) A specimen spread thinly and unevenly across a slide. (46)

SNS See **somatic nervous system.** (30)

SOAP (sōp) An approach to medical records documentation that documents information in the following order: S (**subjective** data), O (**objective** data), A (assessment), P (plan of action). (11)

soft skills (sawft skilz) Personal attributes that enhance an individual's interactions, job performance, and career prospects. (3)

software (sôft´wâr´) A program, or set of instructions, that tells a computer what to do. (8)

sole proprietorship (sōl prə -prī´-ə-tər shĭp) A form of medical practice management in which a physician practices alone, assuming all benefits and liabilities for the business. (5)

solution (sə-loō´shən) A homogeneous mixture of a solid, liquid, or gaseous substance in a liquid, such as a dissolved drug in liquid form. (53)

somatic (sō-măt´ĭk) A division of the peripheral nervous system that connects the central nervous system to skin and skeletal muscle. (30)

somatic nervous system (SNS) (sō-măt´ĭk nûr´vəs sĭs´təm) A system that governs the body's skeletal or voluntary muscles. (30)

SOMR Source-oriented medical record. (11)

SPECT (spĕkt) Single photon emission computed tomography; a radiologic procedure in which a gamma camera detects signals induced by gamma radiation and a computer converts these signals into two- or three-dimensional images that are displayed on a screen. (50)

speculum (spĕk´yə-ləm) An instrument that expands the vaginal opening to permit viewing of the vagina and cervix. (39)

spermatids (sper´mă-tidz) Immature sperm before they develop their flagella (tails). (32)

spermatocytes (sper´mă-tō-sīts) The cells that result when spermatogonia undergo mitosis. (32)

spermatogenesis (sper´mă-tō-jen´ĕ-sis) The process of sperm cell formation. (32)

spermatogenic cells (sper´mă-tō-jen´ik sĕlz) The cells that give rise to sperm cells. (32)

spermatogonia (sper´mă-tō-gō´nē-ă) The earliest cell in the process of **spermatogenesis.** (32)

sphenoid A bone that forms part of the floor of the cranium. (24)

sphincter (sfĭngk´tər) A valve-like structure formed from circular bands of muscle. Sphincters are located around various body openings and passages. (25, 33)

sphygmomanometer (sfig´mō-mă-nom´ĕter) An instrument for measuring blood pressure; consists of an inflatable cuff, a pressure bulb used to inflate the cuff, and a device to read the pressure. (37)

spinal nerves (spī´năl nûrvs) Peripheral nerves that originate from the spinal cord. (30)

spirillum (spī-ril´ŭm) A spiral-shaped bacterium. (46)

spirometer (spī-rom´ĕ-ter) An instrument that measures the air taken in and expelled from the lungs. (49)

spirometry (spī-rom´ĕ-trē) A test used to measure breathing capacity. (49)

splenectomy (splən ek´ tō me) Surgical removal of the spleen. (28)

splint (splĭnt) A device used to immobilize and protect a body part. (57)

splinting catheter (splĭnt´ĭng kăth´ĭ-tər) A type of catheter inserted after plastic repair of the ureter; it must remain in place for at least a week after surgery. (47)

spores (spōrz) A resistant form of certain species of bacteria. (9)

sprain (sprān) An injury characterized by partial tearing of a ligament that supports a joint, such as the ankle. A sprain may also involve injuries to tendons, muscles, and local blood vessels and contusions of the surrounding soft tissue. (57)

stain (stān) In microbiology, a solution of a dye or group of dyes that imparts a color to microorganisms. (46)

standard (stăn´dərd) A specimen for which test values are already known; used to calibrate test equipment. (45)

standardization (stăn-dər-dĭ-zā´-shən) The consistency of the active ingredient(s) in a supplement from batch to batch and from manufacturer to manufacturer.

Standard Precautions (stăn´dərd prĭ-kô´shənz) A combination of Universal Precautions and Body Substance Isolation guidelines; used in hospitals for the care of all patients. (6)

stapes (stā´pēz) A small bone in the middle ear that is attached to the inner ear; also called the stirrup. (35)

statement (stāt´mənt) A form similar to an invoice; contains a courteous reminder to the patient that payment is due. (20)

State Unemployment Tax Act (SUTA) Some states are also governed by this act; these taxes are filed along with FUTA taxes. (56)

statute of limitations (stăch´ootl ĭm´ĭ-tā´shənz) A state law that sets a time limit on when a collection suit on a past-due account can legally be filed. (20)

stent (stĕnt) A metal mesh tube used to hold a vessel open. (42)

stereoscopy (ster-ē-os´kŏ-pē) An x-ray procedure that uses a specially designed microscope (stereoscopic, or Greenough, microscope) with double eyepieces and objectives to take films at different angles and produce three-dimensional images; used primarily to study the skull. (50)

sterile field (stĕr´əl fēld) An area free of microorganisms used as a work area during a surgical procedure. (44)

sterile scrub assistant (stĕr´əl skrŭb ə-sĭs´tənt) An assistant who handles sterile equipment during a surgical procedure. (44)

sterilization (stĕr´ə-lĭ-zā´shən) The destruction of all microorganisms, including bacterial spores, by specific means. (9)

sterilization indicator (stĕr´ə-lĭ-zā´shən ĭn´dĭ-kā´tor) A tag, insert, tape, tube, or strip that confirms that the items in an autoclave have been exposed to the correct volume of steam at the correct temperature for the correct amount of time. (9)

sternum (st´ər-nəm) A bone that forms the front and middle portion of the rib cage; also called the breastbone or breast plate. (24)

steroidal hormone (stĭr´oid´əlhôr´mōn´) A hormone derived from steroids that are soluble in lipids and can cross cell membranes very easily. (34)

stethoscope (stĕth´ə-skōp´) An instrument that amplifies body sounds. (37)

strabismus (strə-bĭz´məs) A condition that results in a lack of parallel visual axes of the eyes; commonly called crossed eyes. (35)

strain (strān) A muscle injury that results from overexertion or overstretching. (57)

stratum basale (strat´ŭm bā-sā´lē) The deepest layer of the epidermis of the skin. (23)

stratum corneum (strat´ŭm kōr´nē ŭm) The most superficial layer of the epidermis of the skin. (23)

stratum germinativum (strat´ŭm jur´minə tē´vŭm) The deepest layer of the epidermis; also known as stratum basale. (23)

stressor (stres´or) Any stimulus that produces stress. (34)

stress test (strĕs tĕst) A procedure that involves recording an electrocardiogram while the patient is exercising on a stationary bicycle, treadmill, or stair-stepping ergometer, which measures work performed. (44)

striations (strī-ā´shŭns) Bands produced from the arrangement of filaments in myofibrils in skeletal and cardiac muscle cells. (25)

stroke (strōk) A condition that occurs when the blood supply to the brain is impaired. It may cause temporary or permanent damage. (57)

stylus (stī´ləs) A pen-like instrument that records electrical impulses on ECG paper. (49)

subarachnoid space (sŭb-ă-rak´noyd spās) An area between the arachnoid mater and the pia mater. (30)

subcategories (sŭb-kăt-ĭ-gôr´ēz) The 4th digits added to many ICD-9 codes giving further specificity to the diagnosis. (18)

subclinical case (sŭb-klin´i-kăl kās) An infection in which the host experiences only some of the symptoms of the infection or milder symptoms than in a full case. (6)

subcutaneous (subcut) (sŭb´kyoo-tā´nē-əs) Under the skin. (53)

subjective (səb-jĕk´tĭv) Pertaining to data that are obtained from conversation with a person or patient. (11)

subjective data (səb-jĕk´tĭv dā´tə) Information about the patient's condition that includes thoughts, feelings, and perceptions. (36)

subject line (sŭb´jĭkt līn) Optional line of two to three words that appears three lines below the inside address of a business letter. (10)

sublingual (sŭb-ling´gwăl) Under the tongue. (53)

sublingual gland (sŭb-ling´gwăl glănd) The smallest of the salivary glands. (50)

submandibular gland (sŭb-man-dib´yu-lăr glănd) The gland that is located in the floor of the mouth. (33)

submucosa (sŭb-mū-kō´să) The layer of the alimentary canal located between the mucosa and the muscular layer. (33)

subpoena (sə-pē´nə) A written court order that is addressed to a specific person and requires that person's presence in court on a specific date at a specific time. (5)

subpoena duces tecum (sə-pee-nə doo-seez tee-kəm) Latin; a legal document that requires the recipient to bring certain written records to court to be used as evidence in a lawsuit. (5)

substance abuse (sŭb´stəns ə-byoos´) The use of a substance in a way that is not medically approved, such as using diet pills to stay awake or consuming large quantities of cough syrup that contains codeine. Substance abusers are not necessarily addicts. (36, 40)

sucrase (sū´krās) An enzyme that digests sugars. (33)

sudoriferous (soo´dərif´ərəs) The sweat glands. (23)

suffix (sŭ-fĭks) A word part that comes at the end of a medical term that alters the meaning of the term. (22)

sulci (sŭl´si) The grooves on the surface of the cerebrum. (30)

superbill (soo´pər-bĭl´) A form that combines the charges for services rendered, an invoice for payment or insurance copayment, and all the information for submitting an insurance claim; also known as an encounter form. (20)

superficial (soo´pər-fĭsh´əl) Anatomic term meaning closer to the surface of the body. (22)

superior (soo´-pîr´-ē-ər) Anatomic term meaning above or closer to the head; also called cranial. (22)

supernatant (sū-per-nā´tănt) The liquid portion of a substance from which solids have settled to the bottom, as with a urine specimen after centrifugation. (47)

supination (sū´pi-nā´shŭn) Turning the palm of the hand upward. (25)

surfactant (sər fak´ tənt) Fatty substance secreted by some alveolar cells that helps maintain the inflation of the alveoli so that they do not collapse in on themselves between inspirations. (29)

surgeon (sûr´jən) A physician who uses hands and medical instruments to diagnose and correct deformities and treat external and internal injuries or disease. (2)

surgical asepsis (sûr´jə-kəl ă-sep´sis) The elimination of all microorganisms from objects or working areas; also called sterile technique. (44)

susceptible host (sə-sĕp´təbal hōst) An individual who has little or no immunity to infection by a particular organism. (6)

SUTA See **State Unemployment Tax Act**. (56)

suture (soo´chər) Fibrous joints in the skull. (30)

A surgical stitch made to close a wound. (24, 44)

symmetry (sĭm´ĭ-trē) The degree to which one side of the body is the same as the other. (38)

sympathetic division (sĭm´pə-thĕt´ĭk) A division of the autonomic nervous system that prepares organs for fight-or-flight (stressful) situations. (30)

symptom (sĭm´təm) A subjective, or internal, condition felt by a patient, such as pain, headache, or nausea, or another indication that generally cannot be seen or felt by the doctor or measured by instruments. (11, 38)

synaptic knob (si-nap´tik nŏb) The end of the axon branch. (30)

synaptic space (si-nap-tik spās) The space between the axon of one neuron and the dendrite of the next. (30)

synergist (sĭn´ər-jist´) Muscles that help the **prime mover** by stabilizing joints. (25)

synovial (sin-ō-vē-əl) A type of joint, such as the elbow or knee, that is freely moveable. (24)

systemic circuit (sĭ-stĕm´ĭk sûr´kĭt) The route that blood takes from the heart through the body and back to the heart. (26)

systemic circulation (sĭ-stĕm´ĭk sir´kyū-lā´shŭn) The circulation of blood through the arteries, capillaries, and veins of the general system, from the left ventricle to the right atrium. (26)

systemic lupus erythematosus (SLE) (si-stĕm´ĭk loo´pəs ĕr´ə- thē´mə-tō´sĭs) An autoimmune disorder in which a person produces antibodies that target the person's own cells and tissues. (28)

systolic pressure (sĭ-stŏl´ĭk prĕsh´ər) The blood pressure measured when the left ventricle of the heart contracts. (26)

tab (tăb) A tapered rectangular or rounded extension at the top of a file folder. (15)

tablet PC (´ta-blət pē sē) A laptop or slate-shaped mobile computer, equipped with a touchscreen or graphics tablet to operate the computer with a digital pen, or a fingertip instead of a keyboard or mouse. (8)

Tabular List (tăb´yə-lər lĭst) One of two ways that diagnoses are listed in the **ICD-9**. In the Tabular List, the diagnosis codes are listed in numerical order with additional instructions. (18)

tachycardia (tak´i-kar´dē-ă) Rapid heart rate, generally in excess of 100 beats per minute. (37)

tachypnea (tăk´ĭp-nē´ə)   Abnormally rapid breathing. (37)

targeted résumé (tär´gĭt-əd rĕz´ōō-mā´)   A résumé that is focused on a specific job target. (58)

tarsals (tär´-səlz)   Bones of the ankle. (24)

taste bud (tāst bŭd)   A structure that is made of taste cells (a type of chemoreceptor) and supporting cells. (35)

tax liability account (tăks lī´ə-bĭl´ĭ-tē ă-kownt)   Money withheld from employees' paychecks and held in a separate account that must be used to pay taxes to appropriate government agencies. (56)

teamwork (tēm-wûrk´)   Working with others in the best interest of completing the job. (3)

telecommunication device for the deaf (TDD) (tel´ĕ-kŏ-myū´ni-kā´shŭn dĕ-vīs´ def)   Telephone accessory that transmits and receives text over standard telephone lines. Also referred to as teletypewriter (TTY) and text telephone (TT). (13)

telephone triage (tĕl´ə-fōn´ trē-äzh´)   A process of determining the level of urgency of each incoming telephone call and how it should be handled. (13)

teletherapy (tel-ĕ-thăr´ăpē)   A radiation therapy technique that allows deeper penetration than brachytherapy; used primarily for deep tumors. (50)

teletype (TTY) device (tĕl´ə-tīp)   A specially designed telephone that looks very much like a laptop computer with a cradle for the receiver of a traditional telephone. It is used by the hearing impaired to type communications onto a keyboard. (7)

telophase (tel´əfāz)   The final stage of mitosis; chromosomes reach the centrioles and the division creating two cells, each with a complete set of chromosomes, is completed. (22)

template (tĕm´plĭt)   A guide that ensures consistency and accuracy. (10)

temporal (temp´-or-al)   Bones that form the lower sides of the skull. (24)

temporal mandibular joint (TMJ) (tĕmp or al man dĭb yū lər joints)   The location where the mandible attaches to the temporal bone. (24)

temporal scanner (temp´-or-al skăn-ĕr)   An instrument used to measure the body temperature by scanning the temporal artery in the forehead. (37)

tendon (tĕn´dən)   A cord-like fibrous tissue that connects muscle to bone. (25)

tendonitis (ten dŭn ī tis)   Inflammation of a tendon. (25)

terminal (tûr´mə-nəl)   Fatal.

terminal digit (tûr´mə-nəl dĭj ĭt)   A small group of two to three numbers at the end of a patient number that is used as an identifying unit in a filing system. (15)

testes (tĕs´tēz)   The primary organs of the male reproductive system. Testes produce the hormone **testosterone**. (32)

testosterone (tĕs-tŏs´tə-rōn´)   A hormone produced by the testes that maintains the male reproductive structures and male characteristics such as deep voice, body hair, and muscle mass. (32)

tetanus (tĕt´n-əs)   A disease caused by *Clostridium tetani* living in the soil and water; more commonly called lockjaw. (25)

thalamus (thăl´ə-məs)   Structure that acts as a relay station for sensory information heading to the cerebral cortex for interpretation; a subdivision of the **diencephalon**. (30)

thalassemia (thal´ə sē´mēə)   An inherited form of anemia with a defective hemoglobin chain causing micocytic (small), hypochromic (pale), and short-lived red blood cells. (27)

therapeutic team (thĕr´ə-pyōō´tĭk tēm)   A group of physicians, nurses, medical assistants, and other specialists who work with patients dealing with chronic illness or recovery from major injuries. (54)

therapeutic touch (thĕr´-ə-pyōō-tĭk tŭch)   The use of touch to detect and correct a person's energy fields, thus promoting healing and health.

thermography (ther-mog´ră-fē)   A radiologic procedure in which an infrared camera is used to take photographs that record variations in skin temperature as dark (cool areas), light (warm areas), or shades of gray (areas with temperatures between cool and warm); used to diagnose breast tumors, breast abscesses, and fibrocystic breast disease. (50)

thermometer (ther-mom´ə-ter)   An instrument, either electronic or disposable, that is used to measure body temperature. (37)

thermotherapy (ther´mō-thăr´ă-pē)   The application of heat to the body to treat a disorder or injury. (54)

third-party check (thûrd pär´tē chĕk)   A check made out to one recipient and given in payment to another, as with one made out to a patient rather than the medical practice. (21)

third-party payer (thûrd pär´tē pā´ər)   A health plan that agrees to carry the risk of paying for patient services. (17)

thoracocentesis (thôr´ə kō´sen tē´ sis)   Medical procedure where a sterile needle is introduced into the chest to remove fluid and pus. (29)

thoracostomy (thor´ə kos´ tə mē)   The surgical insertion of a chest tube to provide continuous drainage of the thoracic (chest) cavity. (29)

thorax (thôr´aks)   The chest cavity. (29)

thrombocytes (throm´bō-sīts)   See **platelets.** (27)

thrombophlebitis (thrŏm´bō-flĕ-bī´tis)   A medical condition that most commonly occurs in leg veins when a blood clot and inflammation develop. (27)

thrombus (thrŏm´bəs)   A blood clot that forms on the inside of an injured blood vessel wall. (27)

thymosin (thī´mō-sin)   A hormone that promotes the production of certain lymphocytes. (34)

thymus gland (thī´məs glănd)   A gland that lies between the lungs. It secretes a hormone called **thymosin.** (34)

thyroid cartilage (thī´roid´ kär´tl-ĭj)   The largest cartilage in the larynx. It forms the anterior wall of the larynx. (29)

thyroid gland (thī´roid gland)   An endocrine gland, consisting of irregularly spheroid follicles, lying in front and to the sides of the upper part of the trachea, in a horseshoe shape, with two lateral lobes connected by a narrow central portion, the isthmus; occasionally an elongated offshoot, the pyramidal lobe, passes upward from the isthmus in front of the trachea. It is supplied by branches from the external carotid and subclavian arteries, and its nerves are derived from the middle cervical and cervicothoracic ganglia of the sympathetic system. It secretes thyroid hormone and calcitonin. (34)

thyroid hormone (thī´roid´ hôr´mōn´)   A hormone produced by the thyroid gland that increases energy production, stimulates protein synthesis, and speeds up the repair of damaged tissue. (34)

thyroid-stimulating hormone (TSH) (thī´roid´stim´yū-lā-ting hôr´mōn´)   A hormone that stimulates the thyroid gland to release its hormone. (34)

tibia (ti-bē-ə)   The medial bone of the lower leg; commonly called the shin bone. (24)

tickler file (tĭk´lər fīl)   A reminder file for keeping track of time-sensitive obligations. (15)

timed urine specimen (tīmd yōor´ĭn spĕs´ə-mən)   A specimen of a patient's urine collected over a specific time period. (47)

time management (tīm man´ăj-mĕnt)
Utilizing time in an effective manner to accomplish the desired results. (3)

time-specified scheduling (tīm spĕs´ə-fīd skĕj´ool-ĭng) A system of scheduling where patients arrive at regular, specified intervals, assuring the practice a steady stream of patients throughout the day. (16)

tinea (tin ē´ă) A fungal infection. (23)

tinnitus (ti-nī´tus) An abnormal ringing in the ear. (43)

tissue (tĭsh´oo) A structure that is formed when cells of the same type organize together. (22)

T lymphocyte (tē lĭm´fə-sīt) A type of nongranular leukocyte that regulates immunologic response; includes helper T cells and suppressor T cells. (48)

tonometer (tō-nom´ĕ-tĕr) An instrument for determining pressure or tension, especially determining ocular tension. (43)

topical (tŏp´ĭ-kəl) Applied to the skin. (44)

tort (tôrt) In civil law, a breach of some obligation that causes harm or injury to someone. (5)

torticollis (tôr´tikol´is) A muscular disease causing a cervical deformity in which the head bends toward the affected side while the chin rotates to the opposite side. (25)

touchpad (tŭch păd) A type of pointing device common to laptop and notebook computers that directs activity on the computer screen by positioning a pointer or cursor on the screen. It is a small, flat device or surface that is highly sensitive to touch. (8)

touch screen (tŭch skrēn) A type of computer monitor that acts as an intake device, receiving information through the touch of a pen, wand, or hand directly to the screen. (8)

tourniquet (tŭr´ni-kĕt) An instrument for temporarily arresting the flow of blood to or from a distal part by pressure applied with an encircling device. (48)

tower case (tou´ər kās) A vertical housing for the system unit of a personal computer. (8)

toxicology (tŏk´sĭ-kŏl´ə-jē) The study of poisons or poisonous effects of drugs. (51)

TPO See **treatment, payments, and operations.** (5)

trachea (trā´kē-ə) The part of the respiratory tract between the larynx and the bronchial tree that is tubular and made of rings of cartilage and smooth muscle; also called the windpipe. (29)

trackball (trăk bôl) A pointing device with a ball that is rolled to position a pointer

or cursor on a computer screen. It can be directly attached to the computer or can be wireless. (8)

tracking (trăk´ĭng) (financial) Watching for changes in spending so as to help control expenses. (21)

traction (trăk´shən) The pulling or stretching of the musculoskeletal system to treat dislocated joints, joints afflicted by arthritis or other diseases, and fractured bones. (54)

trade name (trād nām) A drug's brand or proprietary name. (51)

traditional Chinese medicine (TCM) (trə -dĭsh´-ə -nəl chī-nēz mĕd´-ĭ-sĭn) An ancient system of medicine originating in China that involves herbal and animal source preparations to treat illness. TCM includes various treatments such as acupuncture and acupressure.

transcription (trăn-skrĭp´shən) The transforming of spoken notes into accurate written form. (11)

transcutaneous absorption (trans-kyū-tā´nē-ŭs əb-sorp´shən) Entry (as of a pathogen) through a cut or crack in the skin. (9)

transdermal (trans-der´mel) A type of topical drug administration that slowly and evenly releases a systemic drug through the skin directly into the bloodstream; a transdermal unit is also called a patch. (53)

transfer (trăns-fûr´) To give something, such as information, to another party outside the doctor's office. (11)

transurethral resection of prostate (trans´yoŏ rĕ thrəl rĕ-sək´ shən) Removal of the prostate through the urethra.

transverse (trăns-vûrs´) Anatomic term that refers to the plane that divides the body into superior and inferior portions. (22)

transverse colon (trăns-vûrs´ kō´lən) The segment of the large intestine that crosses the upper abdominal cavity between the ascending and descending colon. (32)

traveler's check (trăv´əl-rz chĕk) A check purchased and signed at a bank and later signed over to a payee. (21)

treatment, payments, and operations (TPO) (trēt´mənt pā´mənts ŏp´ə-rā´shəns) The portion of **HIPAA** that allows the provider to use and share patient health-care information for treatment, payment, and operations (such as quality improvement). (5)

triage (trē-äzh´) To assess the urgency and types of conditions patients present as well as their immediate medical needs. (2)

TRICARE (trī´kâr) A program that provides healthcare benefits for families of military personnel and military retirees. (17)

trichinosis (trik-i-nō´sis) A disease caused by a worm that is usually ingested from undercooked meat. (25)

tricuspid valve (trī-kŭs´pid vălv) A heart valve that has three cusps and is situated between the right atrium and the right ventricle. (26)

triglycerides (trī-glĭs´ə-rīd´z) Simple lipids consisting of glycerol (an alcohol) and three fatty acids. (33)

trigone (trī´gōn) The triangle formed by the openings of the two ureters and the urethra in the internal floor of the bladder. (31)

troubleshooting (trŭb´əl-shoo´tĭng) Trying to determine and correct a problem without having to call a service supplier. (8)

Truth in Lending Statement (trūth lending stāt´mĕnt) A written description of the agreed terms of payment between the patient and medical practice when payment will be made in more than four installments. (20)

trypsin (trip´sin) A pancreatic enzyme that digests proteins. (33)

TSH See **thyroid-stimulating hormone.** (34)

TTY device See **teletype device.** (7)

tubular reabsorption (tū´byū-lăr re-ab-sôrp´shən) The second process of urine formation in which the glomerular filtrate flows into the proximal convoluted tubule. (31)

tubular secretion (tū´byū-lăr sĭ-krē´shən) The third process of urine formation in which substances move out of the blood in the peritubular capillaries into renal tubules. (31)

tutorial (too-tôr´ē-əl) A small program included in a software package designed to give users an overall picture of the product and its functions. (8)

tympanic membrane (tĭm-păn´ĭk mĕm´brān´) A fibrous partition located at the inner end of the ear canal and separating the outer ear from the middle ear; also called the eardrum. (35)

tympanic thermometer (tim-pan´ik thermom´ĕ-ter) A type of electronic thermometer that measures infrared energy emitted from the tympanic membrane. (37)

ulna (əl´-nə) The medial bone of the lower arm. (24)

ultrasonic cleaning (ŭl´trə-sŏn´ĭk klēn´ĭng) A method of sanitization that involves placing instruments in a cleaning solution in a special receptacle that generates sound waves through the cleaning solution, loosening contaminants. Ultrasonic cleaning is safe for even very fragile instruments. (9)

ultrasound (ŭl´trə-sound) The noninvasive therapeutic or diagnostic use of very high frequency sound waves for examination of internal body structures. (50)

umami (oo-mom´ē) Savory taste produced by glutamic acid (monosodium glutamate), recognized as the fifth taste sensation. (35)

umbilical cord (ŭm-bĭl´ĭ-kəl kôrd) The rope-like connection between the fetus and the placenta. It contains the umbilical blood vessels. (32)

unbundling (ŭn-bŭnd´ling) Use of several *Current Procedural Terminology* codes for a service when one inclusive code is available. (19)

underbooking (ŭn´dər-bŏŏkĭng) Leaving large, unused gaps in the doctor's schedule; this approach does not make the best use of the doctor's time. (16)

uniform donor card (yōō´nə-fôrm´ dō´nər kärd) A legal document that states a person's wish to make a gift upon death of one or more organs for medical research, organ transplants, or placement in a tissue bank. (5)

unit (yōō´nĭt) A part of an individual's name or title, described in indexing rules. (15)

unit price (yōō´nĭt prīs) The total price of a package divided by the number of items that comprise the package. (8)

Universal Precautions (yōō´nə-vur´səl prĭ-kô´shənz) Specific precautions required by the Department of Health and Human Services' Centers for Disease Control and Prevention (CDC) to prevent healthcare workers from exposing themselves and others to infection by bloodborne pathogens. (6)

unsaturated fats (ŭn-săch´ə-rā´tĭd făts) Fats, including most vegetable oils, that are usually liquid at room temperature and tend to lower blood cholesterol. (55)

upcoding (ŭp kōd-ing) Coding to a higher level of service than that provided to obtain higher reimbursements. (19)

upper respiratory (tract) infection (upper res´pərətôr´ē tract infek´shən) The common cold. (29)

urea (yōō-rē´ə) Waste product formed by the breakdown of proteins and nucleic acids. (31)

ureters (yōō-rē´tərz) Long, slender, muscular tubes that carry urine from the kidneys to the urinary bladder. (31)

urethra (yōō-rē´thrə) The tube that conveys urine from the bladder during urination. (31)

uric acid (yōōr´ĭk as´id) Waste product formed by the breakdown of proteins and nucleic acids. (31)

urinalysis (yōōr´ə-năl´ĭ-sĭs) The physical, chemical, and microscopic evaluation of urine to obtain information about body health and disease. (47)

urinary catheter (yōōr´ə-nĕr´ē kăth´ĭ-tər) A sterile plastic tube inserted to provide urinary drainage. (47)

urinary pH (yōōr´ə-nĕr´ē pē´äch) A measure of the degree of acidity or alkalinity of urine. (47)

urine specific gravity (yōōr´ĭn spĭ-sĭf´ĭk grăv´ĭ-tē) A measure of the concentration or amount (total weight) of substances dissolved in urine. (47)

urobilinogen (yūr-ō-bī-lin´ō-jen) A colorless compound formed by the breakdown of hemoglobin in the intestines. Elevated levels in urine may indicate increased red blood cell destruction or liver disease, whereas lack of urobilinogen in the urine may suggest total bile duct obstruction. (47)

urologist (yōō-rŏl´ə-jĭst) A specialist who diagnoses and treats diseases of the kidney, bladder, and urinary system. (2)

use (yōōs) The sharing, employing, applying, utilizing, examining, or analyzing of individually identifiable health information by employees or other members of an organization's workforce. (5)

uterus (yōō´tər-əs) A hollow, muscular organ that functions to receive an embryo and sustain its development; also called the womb. (32)

uvula (yōō´vyə-lə) The part of the soft palate that hangs down in the back of the throat. (33)

uvulotomy (yōō´vyəlot´əmē) Surgical procedure removing all or part of the uvula of the soft palate. (29)

vaccine (văk-sēn´) A special preparation made from microorganisms and administered to a person to produce reduced sensitivity to, or increased immunity to, an infectious disease. (6)

vagina (və-jī´nə) A tubular organ that extends from the uterus to the labia. (32)

vaginal introitus (vaj´ i-nəl in trō´itəs) The vaginal os or orifice. The opening of the vagina to the outside of the body. (32)

vaginitis (vaj-i-nī´tis) Inflammation of the vagina characterized by an abnormal vaginal discharge. (32)

varicose veins (văr´i-kōs vānz) Distended veins that result when vein valves are destroyed and blood pools in the veins, causing these veins to dilate. (26)

vas deferens (văs´ dĕf´ər-ənz) A tube that connects the epididymis with the urethra and that carries sperm. (32)

vasectomy (və-sĕk´tə-mē) A male sterilization procedure in which a section of each vas deferens is removed. (39)

vasoconstriction (vā´sō-kon-strik´shŭn) The constriction of the muscular wall of an artery to increase blood pressure. (26)

vasodilation (vā-sō-dī-lā´shŭn) The widening of the muscular wall of an artery to decrease blood pressure. (26)

V code (vē kōd) A code used to identify encounters for reasons other than illness or injury, such as annual checkups, immunizations, and normal childbirth. (18)

vector (vĕk´tər) A living organism, such as an insect, that carries microorganisms from an infected person to another person. (6)

venipuncture (ven´i-pŭnk-chŭr) The puncture of a vein, usually with a needle, for the purpose of drawing blood. (48)

ventilation (vĕn´tə-lā´shən) Moving air in and out of the lungs; also called breathing. (29)

ventral (vĕn´trəl) See **anterior.** (22)

ventral root (vĕn´trəl rōōt) A portion of the spinal nerve that contains axons of motor neurons only. (30)

ventricle (vĕn´trĭ-kəl) Interconnected cavities in the brain filled with cerebrospinal fluid. (30)

ventricular fibrillation (VF) (ven-trik´yū-lăr fĭ-bri-lā´shŭn) An abnormal heart rhythm that is the most common cause of cardiac arrest. (57)

verbalizing (vûr´bə-līz´-ĭng) Stating what you believe the patient is suggesting or implying. (36)

vermiform appendix (ver´mi-fôrm ə-pĕn´dĭks) A structure made mostly of lymphoid tissue and projecting off the cecum. It is commonly referred to as simply the appendix. (33)

vertical file (vûr´tĭ-kəl fīl) A filing cabinet featuring pull-out drawers that usually contain a metal frame or bar equipped to handle letter- or legal-sized documents in hanging file folders. (15)

vertigo (vûr´tĭ gō) Dizziness. (35)

vesicles (vĕs´ĭ-kəlz) Small sacs within the synaptic knobs that contain chemicals called neurotransmitters. (30)

vestibule (ves ti b´yōol) The space enclosed by the labia minora. (32)

The area in the inner ear between the semicircular canals and the cochlea. (35)

VF See **ventricular fibrillation.** (57)

vial (vī´əl) A small glass bottle with a self-sealing rubber stopper. (44)

vibrio (vib´rē-ō) A comma-shaped bacterium. (46)

virtual private network (VPN) (vur - choo-ul prī-vit net-wurk) These are used to connect two or more computer systems. (8)

virulence (vĭr´yə-ləns) A microorganism's disease-producing power. (6)

virus (vī´rəs) One of the smallest known infectious agents, consisting only of nucleic acid surrounded by a protein coat; can live and grow only within the living cells of other organisms. (46)

visceral pericardium (vis´er-ăl per-i-kar´dē-ŭm) The innermost layer of the pericardium that lies directly on top of the heart; also known as the epicardium. (26)

visceral peritoneum (vĭs´er-ăl per-ə-tōnē´əm) Also known as the serosa, the outermost layer of the abdominal organs that secretes serous fluid to keep the organs from sticking to each other. (33)

visceral smooth muscle (vĭs´ər-əl smōoth mŭs´əl) A type of smooth muscle containing sheets of muscle that closely contact each other. It is found in the walls of hollow organs such as the stomach, intestines, bladder, and uterus. (25)

vitamins (vī´tə-mĭnz) Organic substances that are essential for normal body growth and maintenance and resistance to infection. (55)

vitreous humor (vĭt´rē-əs hyōo´mər) A jelly-like substance that fills the part of the eye behind the lens and helps the eye keep its shape. (35)

voice mail (vois māl) An advanced form of answering machine that allows a caller to leave a message when the phone line is busy.

void (void) (legal) A term used to describe something that is not legally enforceable. (5)

volume (vŏl´yōom) The amount of space an object, such as a drug, occupies. (52)

vomer (vō´mər) A thin bone that divides the nasal cavity. (24)

voucher check (vou´chər chĕk) A business check with an attached stub, which is kept as a receipt. (21)

VPN See **virtual private network.** (8)

vulva (vul´vah) External female genitalia. (32)

vulvovaginitis (vul vō vaj´i-nī´tis) Inflammation of the external female genitalia and vagina. (32)

walk-in (wôk´ĭn) A patient who arrives without an appointment. (16)

WAN (wŏn) See **wide area network.** (8)

warranty (wôr´ən-tē) A contract that specifies free service and replacement of parts for a piece of equipment during a certain period, usually a year.

warts (wôrts) Flesh-colored skin lesions with distinct round borders that are raised and often have small finger-like projections; also called verruca. (23)

wave scheduling (wāv skĕj´ōol-ĭng) A system of scheduling in which the number of patients seen each hour is determined by dividing the hour by the length of the average visit and then giving that number of patients appointments with the doctor at the beginning of each hour. (16)

weight (wāt) The product of the force of gravity, defined internationally as 9.81 (m/sec)/sec, × the mass of the body. (52)

wellness (wĕl´nĕs) A philosophy of life and personal hygiene that views health as not merely the absence of illness but the fullest realization of one's physical and mental potential, as achieved through positive attitudes, fitness training, a diet low in fat and high in fiber, and the avoidance of unhealthful practices. (2)

Western blot test (wĕs´tərn blŏt tĕst) A blood test used to confirm enzyme-linked immunosorbent assay (ELISA) test results for HIV infection. (46)

wet mount (wĕt mount) A preparation of a specimen in a liquid that allows the organisms to remain alive and mobile while they are being identified. (46)

white matter (hwīt măt´ər) The outer tissue of the spinal cord that is lighter in color than **gray matter.** It contains myelinated axons. (30)

whole blood (hōl blŭd) The total volume of plasma and formed elements, or blood in which the elements have not been separated by coagulation or centrifugation. (48)

whole-body skin examination (hōl bŏd´ē skĭn ĭg-zăm´ə-nā´shən) An examination of the visible top layer of the entire surface of the skin, including the scalp, genital area, and areas between the toes, to look for lesions, especially suspicious moles or precancerous growths. (42)

whole foods (hōl fūdz) Foods that have little or no processing before they are eaten. (2)

wide area network (WAN) (wīd ār´ē-ă net´wŏrk) A computer network in which the computers connected may be far apart, generally having a radius of half a mile or more. (8)

Wood's light examination (wŏodz līt ĭg-zăm´ə-nā´shən) A type of dermatologic examination in which a physician inspects the patient's skin under an ultraviolet lamp in a darkened room. (42)

word root (wûrd rōot) The base meaning of a medical term.

work ethic (wŏrk eth´ik) A set of values of hard work held by employees. (3)

work practice controls (wŏrk prak´tis kŏn-trōl´z) Controlling workplace injuries by altering the way a task is performed. (6)

work quality (work kwahl´i-tē) Striving for excellence in doing the job; pride in one's performance. (3)

World Health Organization (WHO) (wŏrld helth ŏr´găn-ĭ-zā´shŭn) A unit of the United Nations devoted to international health problems. (18)

write-it-once (pegboard) system (rīt it wŭns pĕg-bôrd´ sis´tĕm) A manual bookkeeping system where the daily log has prepunched holes on the right or left side of the log. Prepunched charge sheets (of NCR paper) are placed in designated areas on top of the day sheet, which has been placed on the pegboard. The patient ledger card is placed between the day sheet and the charge sheet and an entry is made; it appears on all three documents at the same time. (21)

written-contract account (rīt´n kŏn´trăkt´ə-kount´) An agreement between the physician and patient stating that the patient will pay a bill in more than four installments. (20)

X12 837 Health Care Claim (hĕlth kâr klām) An electronic claim transaction that is the **HIPAA** Health Care Claim or Equivalent Encounter Information ("HIPAA claim"). (17)

xeroradiography (zē´rō-rā´dē-og´ră-fē) A radiologic procedure in which x-rays are developed with a powder toner, similar to the toner in photocopiers, and the x-ray image is processed on specially treated xerographic paper; used to diagnose breast cancer, abscesses, lesions, or calcifications.

xiphoid process (zif´oyd pros´es) The lower extension of the breast-bone; the cartilaginous tip of the sternum. (24)

yeast (yēst) A fungus that grows mainly as a single-celled organism and reproduces by budding. (46)

yoga (yō´-gə) A series of poses and breathing exercises that provide awareness of the unity of the whole being. The practice of yoga also increases flexibility and strength.

yolk sac (yōk săk) The sac that holds the materials for the nutrition of the embryo. (32)

Zip drive (zĭp drīv) A Zip drive is a high-capacity floppy disk drive developed by Iomega®. Zip disks are slightly larger and about twice as thick as a conventional floppy disk. Zip drives can hold 100 to 750 MB of data. They are durable and relatively inexpensive. They may be used for backing up hard disks and transporting large files. (8)

zona pellucida (zō´nă pe-lū´sid-ă) A layer that surrounds the cell membrane of an egg. (32)

Z-track method (zē´trăk mĕth´əd) A technique used when injecting an intramuscular (IM) drug that can irritate subcutaneous tissue; involves pulling the skin and subcutaneous tissue to the side before inserting the needle at the site, creating a zigzag path in the tissue layers that prevents the drug from leaking into the subcutaneous tissue and causing irritation. (53)

zygomatic (zī-gə-m´a-tik) The bones that form the prominence of the cheeks. (24)

zygote (zī´gōt) The cell that is formed from the union of the egg and sperm. (32)

Credits

Photo Credits

permission from Spring Medical Systems, Inc. All rights reserved. Figure 16.5: From Helen Houser and Terri Wyman, ADMINISTRATIVE MEDICAL ASSISTING: A WORKFORCE READINESS APPROACH, 1/e. © 2012 McGraw Hill Companies, Inc. Reprinted with permission. Figure 16.6: From Helen Houser and Terri Wyman, ADMINISTRATIVE MEDICAL ASSISTING: A WORKFORCE READINESS APPROACH, 1/e. © 2012 McGraw Hill Companies, Inc. Reprinted with permission. Figure 16.7: From Helen Houser and Terri Wyman, ADMINISTRATIVE MEDICAL ASSISTING: A WORKFORCE READINESS APPROACH, 1/e. © 2012 McGraw Hill Companies, Inc. Reprinted with permission. Figure 16.10: From Helen Houser and Terri Wyman, ADMINISTRATIVE MEDICAL ASSISTING: A WORKFORCE READINESS APPROACH, 1/e. © 2012 McGraw Hill Companies, Inc. Reprinted with permission.

CHAPTER 17
Figure 17.1: The Kaiser Family Foundation, Kaiser Fast Facts. Data Source: Kaiser/HRET Survey of Employer-Sponsored Health Benefits, 1999–2011; KPMG Survey of Employer-Sponsored Health Benefits, 1993, 1996; The Health Insurance Association of America (HIAA), 1988. Available at http://facts.kff.org/chart.aspx?ch=2285. Figure 17.4: From Helen Houser and Terri Wyman, ADMINISTRATIVE MEDICAL ASSISTING: A WORKFORCE READINESS APPROACH, 1/e. © 2012 McGraw Hill Companies, Inc. Reprinted with permission. Figure 17.7: From Helen Houser and Terri Wyman, ADMINISTRATIVE MEDICAL ASSISTING: A WORKFORCE READINESS APPROACH, 1/e. © 2012 McGraw Hill Companies, Inc. Reprinted with permission. Figure 17.8: From Helen Houser and Terri Wyman, ADMINISTRATIVE MEDICAL ASSISTING: A WORKFORCE READINESS APPROACH, 1/e. © 2012 McGraw Hill Companies, Inc. Reprinted with permission. Figure 17.9: From Helen Houser and Terri Wyman, ADMINISTRATIVE MEDICAL ASSISTING: A WORKFORCE READINESS APPROACH, 1/e. © 2012 McGraw Hill Companies, Inc. Reprinted with permission. Figure 17.10: From Helen Houser and Terri Wyman, ADMINISTRATIVE MEDICAL ASSISTING: A WORKFORCE READINESS APPROACH, 1/e. © 2012 McGraw Hill Companies, Inc. Reprinted with permission. Figure 17.11: From Helen Houser and Terri Wyman, ADMINISTRATIVE MEDICAL ASSISTING: A WORKFORCE READINESS APPROACH, 1/e. © 2012 McGraw Hill Companies, Inc. Reprinted with permission. Figure 17.12: From Helen Houser and Terri Wyman, ADMINISTRATIVE MEDICAL ASSISTING: A WORKFORCE READINESS APPROACH, 1/e. © 2012 McGraw Hill Companies, Inc. Reprinted with permission.

CHAPTER 18
Figure 18.3: From Helen Houser and Terri Wyman, ADMINISTRATIVE MEDICAL ASSISTING: A WORKFORCE READINESS APPROACH, 1/e. © 2012 McGraw Hill Companies, Inc. Reprinted with permission. Figure 18.4: From Helen Houser and Terri Wyman, ADMINISTRATIVE MEDICAL ASSISTING: A WORKFORCE READINESS APPROACH, 1/e. © 2012 McGraw Hill Companies, Inc. Reprinted with permission. Figure 18.5: From Helen Houser and Terri Wyman, ADMINISTRATIVE MEDICAL ASSISTING: A WORKFORCE READINESS APPROACH, 1/e. © 2012 McGraw Hill Companies, Inc. Reprinted with permission. Figure 18.6: From Helen Houser and Terri Wyman, ADMINISTRATIVE MEDICAL ASSISTING: A WORKFORCE READINESS APPROACH, 1/e. © 2012 McGraw Hill Companies, Inc. Reprinted with permission. Figure 18.7: From Helen Houser and Terri Wyman, ADMINISTRATIVE MEDICAL ASSISTING: A WORKFORCE READINESS APPROACH, 1/e. © 2012 McGraw Hill Companies, Inc. Reprinted with permission. Figure 18.8: From Helen Houser and Terri Wyman, ADMINISTRATIVE MEDICAL ASSISTING: A WORKFORCE READINESS APPROACH, 1/e. © 2012 McGraw Hill Companies, Inc. Reprinted with permission. Figure 18.9: From Helen Houser and Terri Wyman, ADMINISTRATIVE MEDICAL ASSISTING: A WORKFORCE READINESS APPROACH, 1/e. © 2012 McGraw Hill Companies, Inc. Reprinted with permission. Figure 18.10: From Helen Houser and Terri Wyman, ADMINISTRATIVE MEDICAL ASSISTING: A WORKFORCE READINESS APPROACH, 1/e. © 2012 McGraw Hill Companies, Inc. Reprinted with permission.

CHAPTER 19
Figure 19.1: Reprinted with permission from the American Medical Association. Figure 19.2: Reprinted with permission from the American Medical Association. Page 414: Example boxes: From Helen Houser and Terri Wyman, ADMINISTRATIVE MEDICAL ASSISTING: A WORKFORCE READINESS APPROACH, 1/e. © 2012 McGraw Hill Companies, Inc. Reprinted with permission. Figure 19.3: Reprinted with permission from the American Medical Association. Page 415, Example boxes: From Helen Houser and Terri Wyman, ADMINISTRATIVE MEDICAL ASSISTING: A WORKFORCE READINESS APPROACH, 1/e. © 2012 McGraw Hill Companies, Inc. Reprinted with permission. Table 19.1: From Helen Houser and Terri Wyman, ADMINISTRATIVE MEDICAL ASSISTING: A WORKFORCE READINESS APPROACH, 1/e. © 2012 McGraw Hill Companies, Inc. Reprinted with permission. Page 416, Example box (top): Reprinted with permission from the American Medical Association. Page 416, Example box (bottom): From Helen Houser and Terri Wyman, ADMINISTRATIVE MEDICAL ASSISTING: A WORKFORCE READINESS APPROACH, 1/e. © 2012 McGraw Hill Companies, Inc. Reprinted with permission. Table 19.2: Reprinted with permission from the American Medical Association. Table 19.3: Reprinted with permission from the American Medical Association. Figure 19.4: From Helen Houser and Terri Wyman, ADMINISTRATIVE MEDICAL ASSISTING: A WORKFORCE READINESS APPROACH, 1/e. © 2012 McGraw Hill Companies, Inc. Reprinted with permission. Figure 19.5: From Helen Houser and Terri Wyman, ADMINISTRATIVE MEDICAL ASSISTING: A WORKFORCE READINESS APPROACH, 1/e. © 2012 McGraw Hill Companies, Inc. Reprinted with permission. Figure 19.6: Screen captures of SpringCharts™ Electronic Health Records software are reprinted with permission from Spring Medical Systems, Inc. All rights reserved.

CHAPTER 20
Figure 20.1: From Helen Houser and Terri Wyman, ADMINISTRATIVE MEDICAL ASSISTING: A WORKFORCE READINESS APPROACH, 1/e. © 2012 McGraw Hill Companies, Inc. Reprinted with permission. Figure 20.3: From Helen Houser and Terri Wyman, ADMINISTRATIVE MEDICAL ASSISTING: A WORKFORCE READINESS APPROACH, 1/e. © 2012 McGraw Hill Companies, Inc. Reprinted with permission. Figure 20.4: From Helen Houser and Terri Wyman, ADMINISTRATIVE MEDICAL ASSISTING: A WORKFORCE READINESS APPROACH, 1/e. © 2012 McGraw Hill Companies, Inc. Reprinted with permission. Figure 20.5: From Helen Houser and Terri Wyman, ADMINISTRATIVE MEDICAL ASSISTING: A WORKFORCE READINESS APPROACH, 1/e. © 2012 McGraw Hill Companies, Inc. Reprinted with permission. Figure 20.6: From Helen Houser and Terri Wyman, ADMINISTRATIVE MEDICAL ASSISTING: A WORKFORCE READINESS APPROACH, 1/e. © 2012 McGraw Hill Companies, Inc. Reprinted with permission. Figure 20.7: From Helen Houser and Terri Wyman, ADMINISTRATIVE MEDICAL ASSISTING: A WORKFORCE READINESS APPROACH, 1/e. © 2012 McGraw Hill Companies, Inc. Reprinted with permission. Figure 20.8: From Helen Houser and Terri Wyman, ADMINISTRATIVE MEDICAL ASSISTING: A WORKFORCE READINESS APPROACH, 1/e. © 2012 McGraw Hill Companies, Inc. Reprinted with permission.

CHAPTER 21
Figure 21.2: From Helen Houser and Terri Wyman, ADMINISTRATIVE MEDICAL ASSISTING: A WORKFORCE READINESS APPROACH, 1/e. © 2012 McGraw Hill Companies, Inc. Reprinted with permission. Figure 21.3: From Helen Houser and Terri Wyman, ADMINISTRATIVE MEDICAL ASSISTING: A WORKFORCE READINESS APPROACH, 1/e. © 2012 McGraw Hill Companies, Inc. Reprinted with permission. Figure 21.4: From Helen Houser and Terri Wyman, ADMINISTRATIVE MEDICAL ASSISTING: A WORKFORCE READINESS APPROACH, 1/e. © 2012 McGraw Hill Companies, Inc. Reprinted with permission. Figure 21.6: From Helen Houser and Terri Wyman, ADMINISTRATIVE MEDICAL ASSISTING: A WORKFORCE READINESS APPROACH, 1/e. © 2012 McGraw Hill Companies, Inc. Reprinted with permission. Figure 21.7: From Helen Houser and Terri Wyman,

ADMINISTRATIVE MEDICAL ASSISTING: A WORKFORCE READINESS APPROACH, 1/e.
© 2012 McGraw Hill Companies, Inc. Reprinted with permission. Figure 21.8: From Helen Houser and Terri Wyman, ADMINISTRATIVE MEDICAL ASSISTING: A WORKFORCE READINESS APPROACH, 1/e. © 2012 McGraw Hill Companies, Inc. Reprinted with permission. Figure 21.9: From Helen Houser and Terri Wyman, ADMINISTRATIVE MEDICAL ASSISTING: A WORKFORCE READINESS APPROACH, 1/e. © 2012 McGraw Hill Companies, Inc. Reprinted with permission.

CHAPTER 22
Figure 22.8: From David Shier et al., HOLE'S HUMAN ANATOMY & PHYSIOLOGY, 12/e. © 2010 McGraw Hill Companies, Inc. Reprinted with permission. Figure 22.9: From David Shier et al., HOLE'S HUMAN ANATOMY & PHYSIOLOGY, 12/e. © 2010 McGraw Hill Companies, Inc. Reprinted with permission.

CHAPTER 23
Figure 23.1: From David Shier et al., HOLE'S HUMAN ANATOMY & PHYSIOLOGY, 12/e. © 2010 McGraw Hill Companies, Inc. Reprinted with permission. Figure 23.3: From David Shier et al., HOLE'S HUMAN ANATOMY & PHYSIOLOGY, 12/e. © 2010 McGraw Hill Companies, Inc. Reprinted with permission.

CHAPTER 24
Figure 24.1: From David Shier et al., HOLE'S HUMAN ANATOMY & PHYSIOLOGY, 12/e. © 2010 McGraw Hill Companies, Inc. Reprinted with permission. Figure 24.4: From David Shier et al., HOLE'S HUMAN ANATOMY & PHYSIOLOGY, 12/e. © 2010 McGraw Hill Companies, Inc. Reprinted with permission. Figure 24.5: From David Shier et al., HOLE'S HUMAN ANATOMY & PHYSIOLOGY, 9/e. © 2010 McGraw Hill Companies, Inc. Reprinted with permission. Figure 24.6: From David Shier et al., HOLE'S HUMAN ANATOMY & PHYSIOLOGY, 12/e. © 2010 McGraw Hill Companies, Inc. Reprinted with permission. Figure 24.7: From David Shier et al., HOLE'S HUMAN ANATOMY & PHYSIOLOGY, 12/e. © 2010 McGraw Hill Companies, Inc. Reprinted with permission. Figure 24.8: From David Shier et al., HOLE'S HUMAN ANATOMY & PHYSIOLOGY, 12/e. © 2010 McGraw Hill Companies, Inc. Reprinted with permission. Figure 24.9: From Rod Seeley et al., SEELEY'S ANATOMY & PHYSIOLOGY, 9/e. © 2011 McGraw Hill Companies, Inc. Reprinted with permission. Figure 24.10(a, b): From David Shier et al., HOLE'S HUMAN ANATOMY & PHYSIOLOGY, 12/e. © 2010 McGraw Hill Companies, Inc. Reprinted with permission. Figure 24.12: From David Shier et al., HOLE'S HUMAN ANATOMY & PHYSIOLOGY, 12/e. © 2010 McGraw Hill Companies, Inc. Reprinted with permission. Figure 24.13: From David Shier et al., HOLE'S HUMAN ANATOMY & PHYSIOLOGY, 12/e. © 2010 McGraw Hill Companies, Inc. Reprinted with permission.

CHAPTER 25
Figure 25.1: From David Shier et al., HOLE'S HUMAN ANATOMY & PHYSIOLOGY, 12/e. © 2010 McGraw Hill Companies, Inc. Reprinted with permission. Figure 25.2: From David Shier et al., HOLE'S HUMAN ANATOMY & PHYSIOLOGY, 12/e. © 2010 McGraw Hill Companies, Inc. Reprinted with permission. Figure 25.6: From David Shier et al., HOLE'S HUMAN ANATOMY & PHYSIOLOGY, 12/e. © 2010 McGraw Hill Companies, Inc. Reprinted with permission. Figure 25.7: From David Shier et al., HOLE'S HUMAN ANATOMY & PHYSIOLOGY, 12/e. © 2010 McGraw Hill Companies, Inc. Reprinted with permission. Figure 25.9: From David Shier et al., HOLE'S HUMAN ANATOMY & PHYSIOLOGY, 12/e. © 2010 McGraw Hill Companies, Inc. Reprinted with permission.

CHAPTER 26
Figure 26.1: From David Shier et al., HOLE'S HUMAN ANATOMY & PHYSIOLOGY, 12/e. © 2010 McGraw Hill Companies, Inc. Reprinted with permission. Figure 26.2: From David Shier et al., HOLE'S HUMAN ANATOMY & PHYSIOLOGY, 12/e. © 2010 McGraw Hill Companies, Inc. Reprinted with permission. Figure 26.3: From David Shier et al., HOLE'S HUMAN ANATOMY & PHYSIOLOGY, 12/e. © 2010 McGraw Hill Companies, Inc. Reprinted with permission. Figure 26.4: From David Shier et al., HOLE'S HUMAN ANATOMY & PHYSIOLOGY, 12/e. © 2010 McGraw Hill Companies,

PROFESSIONALS, 4/e. © 2012 McGraw Hill Companies, Inc. Reprinted with permission. Medication label copyright Pfizer Inc. Reproduced with permission. Figure 52.4: Kathryn A. Booth et al., MATH & DOSAGE CALCULATIONS FOR HEALTHCARE PROFESSIONALS, 4/e. © 2012 McGraw Hill Companies, Inc. Reprinted with permission. Medication label copyright © Abbott Pharmaceuticals Division. Reproduced with permission. Figure 52.5: Label reproduced with permission from Teva Pharmaceuticals. This label is a representation only and should not be used for any official purposes. Figure 52.6: Kathryn A. Booth et al., MATH & DOSAGE CALCULATIONS FOR HEALTHCARE PROFESSIONALS, 4/e. © 2012 McGraw Hill Companies, Inc. Reprinted with permission. Medication label copyright © Abbott Pharmaceuticals Division. Reproduced with permission. Figure 52.7: Kathryn A. Booth and James Whaley, MATH AND DOSAGE CALCULATIONS FOR MEDICAL CAREERS, 2/e. © 2007 McGraw Hill Companies, Inc. Reprinted with permission. Page 1073, Label for Cyanocobalamin: Reprinted with permission of APP Pharmaceuticals, LLC.

CHAPTER 53

Figure 53.1(a): Screen captures of SpringCharts™ Electronic Health Records software are reprinted with permission from Spring Medical Systems, Inc. All rights reserved. Figure 53.1(b): Screen captures of SpringCharts™ Electronic Health Records software are reprinted with permission from Spring Medical Systems, Inc. All rights reserved. Figure 53.2: Reprinted with permission of APP Pharmaceuticals, LLC. Figure 53.8: Kathryn A. Booth et al., MATH & DOSAGE CALCULATIONS FOR HEALTHCARE PROFESSIONALS, 4/e. © 2012 McGraw Hill Companies,

Inc. Reprinted with permission. Figure 53.9: Kathryn A. Booth et al., MATH & DOSAGE CALCULATIONS FOR HEALTHCARE PROFESSIONALS, 4/e. © 2012 McGraw Hill Companies, Inc. Reprinted with permission. Figure 53.14(a): Kathryn A. Booth et al., MATH & DOSAGE CALCULATIONS FOR HEALTHCARE PROFESSIONALS, 4/e. © 2012 McGraw Hill Companies, Inc. Reprinted with permission.

CHAPTER 54

Figure 54.6: Kathryn A. Booth, HEALTH CARE SCIENCE TECHNOLOGY: CAREER FOUNDATIONS, 1/e. © 2003 McGraw Hill Companies, Inc. Reprinted with permission. Figure 54.10: Kathryn A. Booth, HEALTH CARE SCIENCE TECHNOLOGY: CAREER FOUNDATIONS, 1/e. © 2003 McGraw Hill Companies, Inc. Reprinted with permission.

CHAPTER 56

Figure 56.2: From Helen Houser and Terri Wyman, ADMINISTRATIVE MEDICAL ASSISTING: A WORKFORCE READINESS APPROACH, 1/e. © 2012 McGraw Hill Companies, Inc. Reprinted with permission. Figure 56.3: From Helen Houser and Terri Wyman, ADMINISTRATIVE MEDICAL ASSISTING: A WORKFORCE READINESS APPROACH, 1/e. © 2012 McGraw Hill Companies, Inc. Reprinted with permission. Figure 56.6: From Helen Houser and Terri Wyman, ADMINISTRATIVE MEDICAL ASSISTING: A WORKFORCE READINESS APPROACH, 1/e. © 2012 McGraw Hill Companies, Inc. Reprinted with permission. Figure 56.8: From Helen Houser and Terri Wyman, ADMINISTRATIVE MEDICAL ASSISTING: A WORKFORCE READINESS APPROACH, 1/e. © 2012 McGraw Hill Companies, Inc. Reprinted with permission. Figure 56.9: From Helen Houser and Terri

Wyman, ADMINISTRATIVE MEDICAL ASSISTING: A WORKFORCE READINESS APPROACH, 1/e. © 2012 McGraw Hill Companies, Inc. Reprinted with permission. Figure 56.10: From Helen Houser and Terri Wyman, ADMINISTRATIVE MEDICAL ASSISTING: A WORKFORCE READINESS APPROACH, 1/e. © 2012 McGraw Hill Companies, Inc. Reprinted with permission. Figure 56.11: From Helen Houser and Terri Wyman, ADMINISTRATIVE MEDICAL ASSISTING: A WORKFORCE READINESS APPROACH, 1/e. © 2012 McGraw Hill Companies, Inc. Reprinted with permission. Figure 56.13: From Helen Houser and Terri Wyman, ADMINISTRATIVE MEDICAL ASSISTING: A WORKFORCE READINESS APPROACH, 1/e. © 2012 McGraw Hill Companies, Inc. Reprinted with permission. Figure 56.14: From Helen Houser and Terri Wyman, ADMINISTRATIVE MEDICAL ASSISTING: A WORKFORCE READINESS APPROACH, 1/e. © 2012 McGraw Hill Companies, Inc. Reprinted with permission.

CHAPTER 57

Page 1195, Chain of Survival: Reprinted with permission 2010 American Heart Association Guidelines for CPR and ECC, Part 4: CPR Overview, circulation. 2010;122[suppl 3]:S676-S684 © 2010, American Heart Association, Inc. Table 57.3: Adapted from: 2010 American Heart Association Guidelines for Cardiopulmonary Resuscitation and Emergency Cardiovascular Care Service, Part 4 Table 1. Page 1201, List of clues of a bioterroristic attack: Epidemiological Clues of a Bioterroristic Attack: Clinical Information, Bioterrorism and Disaster Preparedness. Pocket Guide. Used with permission from the American College of Physicians.

Index

Page numbers in **boldface** indicate figures. Page numbers followed by b indicate box features, p procedures, and t tables, respectively.

Employer identification number (EIN), applying for, 1166
Employer's Quarterly Federal Tax Return, 1171–1172, **1174**, 1174–1175, **1175**
Employment, seeking
    applied training, 1212–1216
    employment services, 1218
    interviewing, 1225–1227
    networking, 1218
    obtaining professional certification, 1216–1217
    preparing portfolio, 1225
    reasons for not being hired, 1227
    resume writing, 1218–1223, 1228p
    salary negotiations, 1227
    sending resume, 1224–1225
    writing cover letter, 1223–1224, **1224**
    writing thank-you notes, 1228p–1229p
Employment contract, 64–65
Employment Eligibility Verification (Form I-9), 1166
Employment laws, 93
Employment services, 1218
Employment taxes, 1171–1172
Employment verification, 442–443
EMS system, calling, 1182
Enamelware, 191
Encephalitis, 815t
    viral, 1198
Encephalopathy, 815–816
Enclosure notation, in business letter, **209,** 210
Encounter form, 337, **338,** 368, **369,** 437, 454
Endocarditis, 552b, 812t
Endocardium, 541, **542**
Endochondral ossification, 512
Endocrine gland, 475, 658
Endocrine system, 658–667
    aging and, 796
    diseases and disorders, 663b–667b, 812, 814, 815t
    hormones, 658–660, 660t
    ICD-10 coding guidelines, 402
    major organs of, **659,** 660–663, 660t
    negative and positive feedback loops, 658–660, **661**
    stress response, 663
    structure and function of, **479**
    surgical coding, 424
Endocrinologist, 16
Endocrinology, 16
    disease and disorder, 812, 814, 815t
    examination for, 819
    as specialty, 810
Endoderm, 633, **633**
Endogenous infection, 106
Endolymph, 679
Endometrial cancer, 811t
Endometriosis, 631b, 757t
Endometrium, 628, **628**
    polyps, 757t
Endomysium, **527,** 528

Endoplasmic reticulum, 485–486, **486**
Endorsement of checks, **460,** 461–462
Endoscope, chemical sterilization, 866
Endoscopy, 548b, 819–820, **820**
Endosteum, 512
Endotracheal tube, 191
Enema
    barium, 1026t, 1027–1028
    retention, 1100p
Engineered safety devices, 113
Entrances, medical office, 135
Entropion, 678b
Enunciation, telephone calls, 276
Enuresis, 781
Envelopes
    address format, 221–222, **222**
    address placement, 221, **221**
    for overnight delivery, 222
    preparing envelopes, **221,** 221–222, 222t
    types of, 205
Environmental Protection Agency (EPA), disposal of needles and sharps, 1081, **1081**
Enzyme immunoassay (EIA), 948, 957p
Enzyme-linked immunosorbent assay (ELISA) test, 907, 983
Enzymes, 572
    from pancreas, 649
EOB. *See* Explanation of benefits
Eosinophils, 560, **561,** 884t, 976t, 979
Epicardium, 541, **542**
Epicondyle, 515t
Epidermis, 496–497, **497**
Epididymis, 621, 622, **622**
Epididymitis, 626b, 758t
Epidural space, 597
Epiglottic cartilage, 581, **582**
Epiglottis, 581, **582**
Epilepsy, 606b, 815t
Epimysium, **527,** 528
Epinephrine, 576b, **659,** 660t, 662, 1193
    use in minor surgery, 869
Epinephrine autoinjector, 809b
Epiphyseal disk, 512
Epiphysis, 511
Episodic tension headaches, 607b
Epistaxis, 1194
Epithelial cells
    casts, 950, **950**
    in urine specimens, **949,** 949–950
Epithelial tissue, 475–476, **476**
Epocrates, 1051
E-prescibing, 1055, 1055b
    EHR and, 259, 264
    renewing by telephone, 287p–288p
Epstein-Barr virus (EBV), 577b, 906t, 977t
Equal Credit Opportunity Act (ECOA), 440t, 442
Equal Employment Opportunity Commission (EEOC), 1160
Equal Pay Act, 1160
Equestrian therapy, 1106b

Equifax Inc., 443
Equilibrium, 679
Equipment
    filing, 312–313
    for laboratory, 896
    laboratory, using, 884–887
    for mail, 222
    for measurement, 886–887
    sanitizing, disinfecting and sterilizing equipment, 862
Erectile dysfunction, 626b
Erectile tissue, 625
Erection, 625, 629
Ergonomics, 104–105
Erikson, Erik, 45
Erosion, **498,** 499t
Errors
    in documents, 217
    in office supply orders, 180
Erythema, 1084, 1110
Erythroblastosis fetalis, 564, **565**
Erythrocyte count (RBC), 975t
Erythrocytes, 475, 559
Erythrocyte sedimentation rate (ESR), 975t, 976t, 980
Erythropoietin, 560, 612, 663
ESBLs, 913
E-scheduling, 330
Escherichia coli, 106, 912t, 914t
Esophageal hiatus, 646
Esophageal sphincter, 647
Esophagus, **644, 646,** 646–647
    cancer of, 811t
ESR. *See* Erythrocyte sedimentation rate (ESR)
Essential amino acids, 651, 1129
Established patient, procedure coding and, 420
Esteem needs, 45, **47**
Estrogen, 627, 629, 635, 658, **659,** 660t, 663
Ethics. *See also* Legal issues
    code of, 90–91
    confidentiality and mandatory disclosure, 88–90
    defined, 63
Ethmoid bone, 515, **515**
Ethnic groups, patients of diverse.
    See Cultural differences and considerations
Etiologic agent, 923
Etiologic Agent label, 923, **923**
Etiology, 403
Etiquette, for telephone calls, 275–277
Eukaryotic cells, 904, 905t
Eustachian tube, 678, **679**
Evacuation systems, 967, 984p–986p
Evaluation and management codes (E/M codes), **419,** 419–420
Evaluations, filing systems, 321b
Eversion, 529, **530, 1108**
Ewing's family of tumors (EFT), 521b
Examination, CHEDDAR format, 244

Muscle relaxant, 1048t
Muscle strength testing, 1106–1107
Muscle tissue, 476–477, **477**
   cardiac, 476–477
   chest pain from sore, 548b
   electrical stimulation of, in physical
      therapy, 1113–1114
   microbial diseases of, 916t
   skeletal, 476–477, **477**
   smooth, 476–477
Muscular dystrophy, 535b–536b
Muscular system, 526–537. *See also*
      Orthopedics
   abdominal muscles, **531, 533, 534**
   aging and, 535, 795
   ankle, foot and toes, **531,** 533, 535
   of arm, **531, 532,** 533
   attachment and action of muscles, 528–529,
      529, 530
   diseases and disorders of, 535b–537b
   examination of, in general physical
      examination, 735
   function of muscles, 526
   of head, 531, **531**
   leg muscles, **531,** 533
   muscle fatigue, 528
   muscle strains and sprains, 534b
   oxygen debt, 528
   pectoral girdle, **531,** 533, **534**
   production of energy for muscles, 528
   respiratory muscles, 533, **534**
   structure and function of, **478**
   types of muscles, 526–528, **527,** 527t
   of wrist, hand and fingers, **531, 532,** 533
Musculoskeletal system
   diseases and disorders, 816, 816t
   ICD-10 coding guidelines, 404
   surgical coding, 422–423
Music, in reception area, 130
Music therapy, 1106b
Mutations, 487
Mutual agreement, extending credit,
      443–444
Myasthenia gravis, 536b
Mycobacteria, 913
Mycobacterium avium complex (MAC)
      infection, 908
Mycobacterium leprae, 913, 914t
Mycobacterium tuberculosis, 912t, 913, 914t
Mycoplasma, 913
Mycoplasma pneumoniae, 912t, 914t
Mydriatic, 1048t
Myelin, 596
Myelography, 822, 823, 1026t, 1032–1033
Myocardial infarction, 546, 548b, 554b,
      812, 812t
Myocardial infarction (MI), 1195–1196
Myocarditis, 552b, 812t
Myocardium, 541, **542**
Myocytes, 528
Myofibrils, 526, **527**
Myoglobin, 528

Myoglobinuria, 948
Myometrium, 628, **628**
Myopia, 832, **832**
MyPlate, 1136, **1136**
Myxedema, **667,** 667b, 814

N

Nägele's rule, 748
Nail bed, 501, **501**
Nail polish, infection control and, 115
Nails, 501, **501**
   general appearance of, 733
Names
   of drugs, 1046
   generic, 1046
   microorganisms, 905
   rules for alphabetic filing of personal
      names, 315, 316t, 317b
   trade, 1046
Narcotics, 1053
   storage of, 173
Narcotics Anonymous, 1198t
Nares, 581
Nasal cavity, 581, **582,** 645, **646**
   sense of smell, **671,** 671–672
Nasal conchae, 581
Nasal inhaler, 1085, 1097p–1098p
Nasal mucosa, 733
Nasal septum, 581
Nasal smears, 884t
Nasal specula, 191, 196, **196,** 197t
Nasolacrimal duct, 674, **674**
Nasopharynx, 644, 645, **646**
National AIDS Hotline, 299t
National Alliance for Health Information
      Technology (NAHIT), 258
National Association of Claims Assistance
      Professionals (NACAP), 22t
National Association of Emergency Medical
      Technicians, 23t
National Association for Health Professionals
      (NAHP), 5
National Board of Medical Examiners
      (NBME), 6
National Board of Surgical Technology and
      Surgical Assisting, 23t
National Cancer Institute, 299t
National Center for Competency Testing
      (NCCT), 5
National Certified Medical Assistant
      (NCMA), 5
National Certified Medical Office Assistant
      (NCMOA), 5
National Childhood Vaccine Injury Act, 778
National Clearinghouse for Alcohol and Drug
      Information, 299t
National Coalition Against Domestic Abuse,
      1198t
National Committee for Clinical Laboratory
      Standards (NCCLS), 968
National Committee on Quality Assurance
      (NCQA), 1164

National Council on Radiation Protection and
      Measurements (NCRP), 1035
National Domestic Violence Hotline, 1198t
National Healthcare Association (NHA), 5
National Health Information Center, 299t
National Institute for Alcohol Abuse and
      Alcoholism (NIAAA), 1198t
National Institute for Occupational Safety and
      Health (NIOSH), 104–105, 968–969
National Institute on Drug Abuse, 1198t
National Institutes of Health, 156t, 802b
National Kidney Foundation, 299t
National Library of Medicine, 156t
National Notifiable Disease Surveillance
      System, 116
National Organization for Rare Disorders
      (NORD), 299t
National Organization for Victim
      Assistance, 1198t
National Organization of Competency
      Assurance (NOCA), 5
National Patient Safety Goals, 25, 25t
National Pharmacy Technician
      Association, 23t
National Phlebotomy Association (NPA), 23t
National Practitioner Data Bank, 79–80
National Provider Identifier (NPI), 354
Natural killer (NK) cells, 573
Naturally acquired active immunity, 574
Naturally acquired passive immunity, 575
NBME. *See* National Board of Medical
      Examiners (NBME)
NCCLS. *See* National Committee for Clinical
      Laboratory Standards (NCCLS)
Nearsightedness, 832
Near vision, 834, 843p
Neatness, of patient records, 247
Neck, examination of, 733
Needle biopsy, 825p, 854
Needle holders, 859
Needles
   for blood specimens, 968
   choosing, 1081–1082, 1082t
   disposable, 198
   disposal of, 1081, **1081**
   engineered safety devices, 113
   engineered safety devices for blood
      specimens, **969,** 969–970
   parts of, 1082, **1082**
   sharing and AIDS/HIV infection, 907
   sterilization, 197t
   suture, 859, **859**
   work practice controls, 113
Needlestick Safety and Prevention Act, 113
   engineered safety devices, 113
   work practice controls, 113
Needs, hierarchy of, 45–46, **47**
Negative feedback loop, 658–660, **661**
Negative verbal communication, 47–48
Neglect
   child, 785
   elderly patient, 802–803